TEXTBOOK OF SMALL ANIMAL MEDICINE

TEXTBOOK OF SMALL ANIMAL MEDICINE

Edited by

John K. Dunn MA, MVetSc, BVM&S, DSAM, DipECVIM, MRCVS

Department of Clinical Veterinary Medicine
University of Cambridge, UK

W. B. Saunders

London Edinburgh New York Philadelphia Sydney Toronto

W.B. SAUNDERS
An imprint of Harcourt Publishers Limited

© Harcourt Brace and Company 1999. All rights reserved.
© Harcourt Publishers Limited 2000. All rights reserved.

No part of this publication may be reproduced, stored in a retrieval system, or transmitted in any form or by any means, electronic, mechanical, photocopying or otherwise, without the prior permission of the publishers (Harcourt Publishers Limited, Robert Stevenson House, 1–3 Baxter's Place, Leith Walk, Edinburgh EH1 3AF), or a licence permitting restricted copying in the United Kingdom issued by the Copyright Licensing Agency, 90 Tottenham Court Road, London W1P 0LP.

ISBN 0-7020-1582-2

British Library Cataloguing in Publication Data
A catalogue record for this book is available from the British Library

Library of Congress Cataloging in Publication Data
A catalog record for this book is available from the Library of Congress

Medical knowledge is constantly changing. As new information becomes available, changes in treatment, procedures, equipment and the use of drugs become necessary. The authors and Publishers have, as far as it is possible, taken care to ensure that the information given in the text is accurate and up to date. However, readers are strongly advised to confirm that the information, especially with regard to drug usage, complies with latest legislation and standards of practice.

The Publishers and authors have made every effort to trace the copyright holders for borrowed material. If they have inadvertently overlooked any, they will be pleased to rectify the matter at the first opportunity.

Commissioning Editor: Catriona Byers
Development Editor: Tim Kimber
Project Supervisor: Mark Sanderson
Senior Project Editor: Carol Parr

Typeset by Phoenix Photosetting, Chatham, Kent
Printed in China

The Publisher's policy is to use **paper manufactured from sustainable forests**

Contents

List of Contributors   vii

Preface   xi

SECTION I: Problem-oriented medicine

1. Introduction to medical problem solving   3
   J. K. Dunn
2. Anorexia and polyphagia   13
   J. K. Dunn
3. Weight loss and weight gain   18
   P. J. Watson and J. K. Dunn
4. Fever and hypothermia   28
   J. K. Dunn
5. Vomiting   39
   J. K. Dunn
6. Dysphagia, regurgitation and ptyalism   51
   C. M. Elwood
7. Diarrhoea   58
   C. M. Elwood
8. Defecatory tenesmus   66
   C. M. Elwood
9. Polydipsia and polyuria   70
   J. K. Dunn
10. Persistent nasal discharge   82
    J. P. Bray
11. Dyspnoea   87
    L. G. King
12. Chronic cough   93
    L. G. King
13. Cardiac murmurs   99
    J. K. Dunn
14. Pallor   107
    J. K. Dunn
15. Cyanosis   118
    J. K. Dunn
16. Hyperaemia and congestion   123
    J. K. Dunn
17. Jaundice   126
    J. K. Dunn
18. Peripheral oedema and ascites   136
    K. J. Dunn
19. Abdominal pain   146
    K. J. Dunn
20. Lymphadenopathy   151
    J. K. Dunn
21. Abnormal haemostasis   160
    J. K. Dunn
22. Urinary incontinence and abnormal micturition   168
    S. P. Gregory
23. Haematuria   176
    J. K. Dunn
24. Alopecia   186
    R. Bond
25. Pruritus   194
    R. Bond
26. Scaling and crusting disorders   201
    R. Bond
27. Joint, bone and muscle pain   207
    R. Whitelock
28. Episodic weakness and collapse   218
    A. Boswood
29. Disturbances of cardiac rhythm   225
    A. Boswood
30. Ataxia   232
    J. K. Dunn
31. Paresis and paralysis   236
    J. K. Dunn
32. Seizures   242
    M. P. Targett
33. Depression, disorientation, stupor and coma   249
    M. P. Targett

SECTION II: Systems medicine

34 **Diseases of the cardiovascular system** 255
J. K. Dunn, J. Elliott and M. E. Herrtage

35 **Diseases of the respiratory system** 345
W. T. Clark

36 **Diseases of the alimentary tract** 371
C. P. Sturgess

37 **Diseases of the liver and biliary tract** 448
J. Rothuizen

38 **Diseases of the exocrine pancreas** 498
D. A. Williams

39 **Diseases of the endocrine system** 526
M. E. Herrtage

40 **Diseases of the reproductive system** 574
G. C. W. England

41 **Diseases of the urinary system** 612
D. F. Senior

42 **Diseases of the nervous system** 662
R. S. Bagley and S. J. Wheeler

43 **Muscle diseases of the dog and cat** 695
R. E. McKerrell

44 **Diseases of bones and joints** 719
C. May

45 **Diseases of blood and blood-forming organs** 765
J. D. Littlewood

46 **Diseases of the eye** 820
S. M. Petersen-Jones

47 **Skin diseases of the dog and cat** 871
S. E. Shaw and S. E. Kelly

48 **Specific infections of the dog** 921
I. A. P. McCandlish

49 **Infectious diseases of the cat** 959
R. M. Gaskell and M. Bennett

50 **Principles of cancer therapy** 985
J. M. Dobson

51 **Behaviour problems** 1029
V. O'Farrell

Index 1043

Colour plate 556–557

Contributors

Rodney S. Bagley
Washington State University
Department of Veterinary Clinical
Medicine and Surgery
College of Veterinary Medicine
Pullman, WA
USA

Malcolm Bennett
Department of Veterinary Pathology
University of Liverpool
Leahurst
Neston
South Wirral
UK

Ross Bond
Department of Small Animal
Medicine and Surgery
Royal Veterinary College
Hawkshead Lane
North Mymms, Hatfield
Herts
UK

Adrian Boswood
Department of Small Animal
Medicine and Surgery
Royal Veterinary College
Hawkshead Lane
North Mymms, Hatfield
Herts
UK

Jonathan P. Bray
The Queen's Veterinary School Hospital
University of Cambridge
Madingley Road
Cambridge
UK

William T. Clark
Department of Applied Veterinary Medicine
Murdoch University
Murdoch
Western Australia
Australia

Jane M. Dobson
Department of Clinical Veterinary Medicine
University of Cambridge
Madingley Road
Cambridge
UK

John K. Dunn
Department of Clinical Veterinary Medicine
University of Cambridge
Madingley Road
Cambridge
UK

Katie J. Dunn
Vetstream
Langford Arch
Sawston
Cambridge
UK

Jonathan Elliott
Department of Veterinary Basic Sciences
Royal Veterinary College
Royal College Street
Camden
London
UK

Clive M. Elwood
Davies White
Manor Farm Business Park
Higham Gobion
Hitchin
Herts
UK

Gary C. W. England
Royal Veterinary College
University of London
Hawkshead Lane
North Mymms
Hatfield
Herts
UK

Rosalind M. Gaskell
Department of Veterinary Pathology
University of Liverpool
Leahurst, Neston
South Wirral
UK

Sue P. Gregory
Department of Small Animal
Medicine and Surgery
Royal Veterinary College
Hawkshead Lane
North Mymms
Hatfield
Herts
UK

Michael E. Herrtage
Department of Clinical Veterinary Medicine
University of Cambridge
Madingley Road
Cambridge
UK

Susan E. Kelly
Department of Applied Veterinary Medicine
Murdoch University
Murdoch
Western Australia
Australia

Lesley G. King
Section of Critical Care
School of Veterinary Medicine
University of Pennsylvania
3900 Delancey Street
Philadelphia, PA
USA

Janet D. Littlewood
Animal Health Trust
Lanwades Park
Kentford
Newmarket
Suffolk
UK

Chris May
Willows Referral Service
78 Tanworth Lane
Shirley
Solihull
West Midlands
UK

Irene A. P. McCandlish
IDEXX Laboratories
Grange House
Sandbeck Way
Wetherby
W Yorkshire
UK
(Previously at University of Glasgow Veterinary
School, Department of Veterinary Pathology)

Rosemary E. McKerrell
Ongars
Dunmow Road
Hatfield Heath
Bishop's Stortford
Herts
UK

Valerie O'Farrell
Royal (Dick) School of Veterinary Studies
University of Edinburgh
Department of Veterinary Clinical Studies
Summerhall
Edinburgh
UK

Simon M. Petersen-Jones
Department of Small Animal Clinical Sciences
College of Veterinary Medicine
Michigan State University
East Lansing, MI
USA

Jan Rothuizen
Department of Clinical Sciences
of Companion Animals
Faculty of Veterinary Medicine
University of Utrecht
Utrecht
The Netherlands

David F. Senior
Department of Veterinary Clinical Sciences
School of Veterinary Medicine
Louisiana State University
Baton Rouge, LA
USA

Susan E. Shaw
Department of Veterinary Clinical Science
University of Bristol
Langford House
Langford
Bristol
UK

Christopher P. Sturgess
Department of Clinical Veterinary Science
University of Bristol
Langford House
Langford
Bristol
UK

Michael P. Targett
Department of Clinical Veterinary Medicine
University of Cambridge
Madingley Road
Cambridge
UK

Penny J. Watson
Department of Clinical Veterinary Medicine
University of Cambridge
Madingley Road
Cambridge
UK

Simon J. Wheeler
Royal Veterinary College
Hawkshead Lane
North Mymms
Hatfield
Herts
UK

Richard Whitelock
Davies White
Unit 5
Manor Farm Business Park
Higham Gobion
Hitchin
Herts
UK

David A. Williams
Department of Small Animal
Medicine and Surgery
College of Veterinary Medicine
Texas A & M University
College Station, TX
USA

Preface

The last two decades have seen major advances in the field of small animal medicine. Indeed, this progress continues at a pace which at times must seem overwhelming both to undergraduate veterinary students trying to come to terms with this wealth of knowledge for the first time, and busy small animal practitioners who are simply trying to stay abreast of current developments. During this period many new conditions have been identified and our understanding of the pathophysiological mechanisms of disease has improved considerably. Furthermore the advent of more sophisticated diagnostic techniques, particularly ultrasonography, and the introduction of many new forms of therapy has greatly enhanced our ability to effectively treat and more objectively assess the progress of animals placed under our care.

My main aim has been to provide an easy-to-read reference source for undergraduate veterinary students and small animal practitioners, including those who have opted for periods of postgraduate training or who are studying for the RCVS Certificate or Diploma in Small Animal Medicine, or the Diploma of the European College of Veterinary Internal Medicine (Small Animals). With this in mind, every attempt has been made to make the text accessible and to present information in a way that is concise and clinically relevant.

This textbook covers diseases of the dog and cat in one volume. I have been fortunate to recruit the services of 31 authors from the United Kingdom, mainland Europe, United States of America and Australasia. All are authorities in their own clinical disciplines and are respected internationally for their individual contributions to both teaching and research. There is no shortage of illustrations; many, including those depicting diseases of the skin, eyes and blood, are repeated in colour in the plate section.

The book is divided into two sections. The first consists of 33 chapters devoted to specific clinical problems all of which are commonly encountered in day-to-day practice. An attempt has been made to retain a uniform format throughout. The emphasis is very much focused on clinical problem solving. A unique feature of this textbook is the production of checklists for history and physical examination. These checklists, which have been used in preference to algorithms, take the form of questions or a series of prompts designed to ensure that essential historical and clinical details are not omitted.

Each chapter starts with a brief introduction (including relevent anatomy and underlying pathophysiology). This is followed by sections on the use and interpretation of relevant diagnostic techniques and, finally, management of the problem under investigation. References in this section have been kept to a minimum; those that have been cited relate to points of contention. Information concerning specific diseases is cross referenced to the appropriate systems chapters in Section II.

Section II comprises 18 chapters, each describing the diseases of a specific organ or body system. In order to provide rapid retrieval of information, each chapter is preceded by a table of contents. This is followed by a review of the clinical examination of each body system and an in-depth discussion of specific conditions. Diseases of the dog and cat are dealt with separately where appropriate and each chapter is extensively referenced.

Textbooks of this nature rely heavily on the goodwill and cooperation of many people. I extend my sincere thanks to all the contributing authors, without whose enduring patience this project would never have been completed. My thanks also go out to my colleagues and staff at the University of Cambridge Vet School who provided enthusiastic support throughout. A particular debt is due to John Fuller for his artwork. His magnificent illustrations and line drawings have added a degree of continuity and enhanced the overall appearance of this textbook. The editorial staff at W.B. Saunders, in particular Catriona Byres, Tim Kimber, Carol Parr and latterly Deborah Russell, have been instrumental in guiding me through the lows and highs during preparation of the manuscripts. Thank you for your hard work and for keeping me on track. Finally, very special thanks are due to my family and friends who must have wondered whether this textbook would ever see the light of day.

Regardless of how long we have practised the art of veterinary medicine, we all strive to improve our clinical expertise and practical skills in the knowledge that it is far easier to become complacent and stagnate than to expand our base of acquired knowledge. I hope this textbook contributes in some small way to this upward learning curve that we refer to as continued professional development.

John K. Dunn

SECTION I

PROBLEM-ORIENTED MEDICINE

1	Introduction to medical problem solving	3	
2	Anorexia and polyphagia	13	
3	Weight loss and weight gain	18	
4	Fever and hypothermia	28	
5	Vomiting	39	
6	Dysphagia, regurgitation and ptyalism	51	
7	Diarrhoea	58	
8	Defecatory tenesmus	66	
9	Polydipsia and polyuria	70	
10	Persistent nasal discharge	82	
11	Dyspnoea	87	
12	Chronic cough	93	
13	Cardiac murmurs	99	
14	Pallor	107	
15	Cyanosis	118	
16	Hyperaemia and congestion	123	
17	Jaundice	126	
18	Peripheral oedema and ascites	136	
19	Abdominal pain	146	
20	Lymphadenopathy	151	
21	Abnormal haemostasis	160	
22	Urinary incontinence and abnormal micturition	168	
23	Haematuria	176	
24	Alopecia	186	
25	Pruritus	194	
26	Scaling and crusting disorders	201	
27	Joint, bone and muscle pain	207	
28	Episodic weakness and collapse	218	
29	Disturbances of cardiac rhythm	225	
30	Ataxia	232	
31	Paresis and paralysis	236	
32	Seizures	242	
33	Depression, disorientation, stupor and coma	249	

1

Introduction to Medical Problem Solving

J. K. Dunn

WHY USE A PROBLEM-ORIENTED APPROACH?

The field of small animal medicine is one of the most rapidly expanding areas of veterinary science, and veterinary students are now required to assimilate and absorb more factual information than ever before. More importantly, each student must learn how to apply this vast wealth of information to clinical situations which are geared to providing the best possible quality of patient care in terms of diagnosis and management. In this respect the problem-oriented approach, in addition to being an integral part of the diagnostic process, is an invaluable educational tool. Whereas older diagnostic systems to a large extent relied on ruling out differential diagnoses based simply on clinical impressions of the case in question, problem-oriented medicine places more emphasis on critical identification of the patient's problems and an understanding of the pathophysiological mechanisms responsible for each problem, thereby providing the framework for a more logical and structured approach to diagnosis and management, which in turn promotes a higher quality of patient care. By concentrating more on scientific logic rather than 'gut feelings', the problem-oriented approach eliminates much of the guesswork and discourages hasty and misguided presumptive diagnoses. It ensures that the clinician, having accurately identified specific problems, then places them in proper perspective and investigates them accordingly. By recording all the problems identified from the history and physical examination, plus any laboratory and/or radiographic findings, a more complete and ultimately more reliable, clinical picture is obtained. Insignificant problems, or problems which at first may appear irrelevant if taken in the context of the primary presenting complaint, are therefore less likely to be forgotten and can be recalled if necessary at a later stage of the investigative process.

THE PROBLEM-ORIENTED VETERINARY MEDICAL RECORD

The problem-oriented approach emphasizes the need for accurate and complete medical records, and a well-prepared medical record is fundamental to the concept of quality patient care. It should record details of the animal's history, clinical findings and results of ancillary tests. For hospitalized patients, it should chart a daily assessment of the animal's progress together with plans for further investigations, and should include a discharge summary. In this respect the medical record serves as an important form of communication between technical and professional staff as well as a source of material for retrospective studies. Finally it should be remembered that a medical record is also a legal document which may be called upon in cases of litigation.

The components of the problem-oriented veterinary medical record (POVMR) can be conveniently divided into four groups:

1. Collection of baseline information (usually referred to as the database);
2. Formulation of a master problem list (problem definition);
3. Initial assessment and diagnostic plan;
4. Progress notes (to include daily assessment, follow-up plans, and discharge summary).

COLLECTION OF BASELINE INFORMATION (DATABASE)

The database consists of problems identified from the history and physical examination. At the outset the clinician should record each problem separately, regardless of whether or not it appears relevant to the primary presenting complaint. Remember most problems identified from either the history or physical examination which warrant further medical investigation are not diagnoses. Depending on the extent of the previous investigations and nature of the illness the database may also include the results of preliminary laboratory screening tests (urinalysis, routine haematology and the results of a limited biochemical screen) and/or radiographic findings. As the case progresses the database expands as the results of further diagnostic tests become available (e.g. electrocardiographic/echocardiographic findings, biopsy reports etc.). As the database expands, problems which were identified at the outset become progressively more defined until a specific diagnosis is reached.

History

The history begins with a description of the animal (age, sex, breed). Special care should be taken when interpreting problems described by the owner. Although their observations may be accurate, owners often tend to exaggerate the importance of some problems whilst underestimating the significance of others. A complete and detailed history is therefore absolutely essential in developing the minimum database. Question design is extremely important when taking a history.

Questions should be phrased in such a way so as to obtain a factual rather than an inferential answer, i.e. care should be taken not to ask a question in such a way that only one answer is implied; by providing several possible answers the clinician is less able to bias the owner's response. Responses which are equivocal, i.e. answers such as 'I don't know' or 'I'm not sure' or 'Perhaps—well yes I think so' should be listed as questionable on the master problem list so that they may be recalled as such at a later date. For the owner's peace of mind it is best to focus attention, at least initially, on the primary presenting complaint. The clinician should ask questions in a systematic manner so that the problems which are identified can be arranged in chronological order. The open-ended technique where an owner is asked to 'describe his/her pet's problem(s)' is probably the least satisfactory from a chronological viewpoint.

The following general items of information should be obtained from the owner (readers are requested to consult Section II of this book for more detailed points relating to the history-taking for a specific body system or organ):

- Past medical/surgical history, including vaccination status, parasite control and previous therapy
- Time in owner's possession and details of present environment (rural/urban)
- The nature of the primary complaint; if necessary ask the owner to describe the course of events
- Contact with other pets in the household
- General activity/demeanour
- Diet
- Appetite
- Water consumption
- Vomiting or diarrhoea
- Coughing or sneezing
- Weight loss/gain
- Lameness
- Reproductive history (particularly intact bitches)

It is important to communicate with clients at a level that they are familiar with and are able to understand. For clarification, the main problems identified during the history taking can be summarized on completion of a full physical examination.

Physical examination

Detailed accounts of the clinical examination of each body system are included in Section II. In order to obtain consistent and meaningful information the general physical examination should be performed in a systematic manner. Haste is probably the most common reason for errors and omissions during a physical examination. For this reason the clinician should not be tempted to take short cuts or be distracted by the nature of the primary complaint, and the same routine should be used for each examination.

The physical examination serves two useful functions: (1) to detect congenital abnormalities in the young animal and (2) to establish the seriousness of a problem in a sick animal. A full physical examination should be performed on every animal preferably when it is presented for its first vaccination to identify any congenital abnormalities which may be present (cardiac murmurs, umbilical hernias and cryptorchidism).

Regardless of how localized the primary complaint may appear, a *full* physical examination should be performed on *every* patient. Once the general examination has been completed, particular attention may then be given to the body system(s) in which dysfunction is suspected from the history. To a certain extent, the emphasis of the general physical examination may be influenced by the age of the patient. Congenital defects, particularly those involving the heart, are more common in animals less than six months of age, whereas geriatric patients may show clinical signs of multiple organ dysfunction associated with age-related degenerative changes in the heart, lungs, liver, kidneys, joints and eyes.

The history and general physical examination are best recorded separately (Fig. 1.1). A written check-off list is invaluable, and if possible should be incorporated into the medical records to ensure that each body system is examined in sequence. A series of tick boxes are provided on the form and these are filled as each system examination is completed and any abnormalities are recorded in writing below the boxes (Fig. 1.1). On completion, the sheet should be signed or initialled by the person performing the examination.

GENERAL PHYSICAL EXAMINATION OF THE DOG AND CAT

A step by step check list for performing a full general physical examination is given below.

■ Inspection

The first part of the examination involves inspecting the animal from a distance, e.g. as it enters the examination room, and certainly before lifting it onto the examination table. Observations should be made regarding the following:

- The animal's general body condition (note whether thin or obese, hair coat quality and cleanliness)
- Demeanour (bright, disinterested or depressed)
- Attitude (friendly, wary or aggressive)
- Conformation and symmetry
- Locomotion/gait
- Neurological deficits, e.g. loss of vision, head tilt, ataxia, circling or knuckling of a limb

■ Physical examination

Before progressing with the second part of the examination the clinician should familiarize himself with the patient. The examination then proceeds by recording the animal's body weight, temperature, pulse and respiratory rate.

As a rough guide the normal resting temperature, pulse and respiratory rate (TPR) for the dog and cat are given below (considerable overlap exists between these ranges of normal values):

Temperature (°C)	37.5–39.0
Pulse rate (beats per minute)	
small dogs/cats (<10 kg)	110–115
medium-sized dogs (10–25 kg)	80–120
large dogs (>25 kg)	70–90
Respiratory rate (respirations per minute)	20–40

Rectal temperature

Remember the animal's temperature will increase with physical activity, excitement and high environmental temperatures. A dog's temperature may rise after a long car journey on a hot day. A brief examination of the anus, anal sacs, perineal region and external genitalia may be performed while taking the temperature, and the consistency and colour of the faeces on the end of the thermometer should be noted (hard, soft, diarrhoeic, pale, bloody etc.).

Pulse

The pulse should be counted for at least 15, and preferably 30 seconds. Both femoral arteries should be palpated, placing the fingers on the artery from the front of the leg. Note and record rate, character, rhythm, tension and type of wave.

Respiratory rate

Note the rate and character of respiration by watching the movement of the thoracic wall at the thoracic arch. Count for at least 30 seconds and note the type of movement, depth and rhythm of respiration. This is especially important in cats where changes in respiratory pattern may be subtle.

Head

Nares: check for symmetry, patency, altered pigmentation and discharges.

Lips: check for symmetry, presence of lesions and pigmentation.

a

Case No: _____ Date: _____

Owner's name: _____ Reason for appointment: _____

Patient's name: _____

Age: _____ /

Sex: ☐ M ☐ F

☐ Entire ☐ Neuter

Amount (if known) _____ _____ _____

Immunisation

☐ Distemper   ☐ Panleucopenia   ☐ Tetanus
☐ Hepatitis   ☐ FVR/Calici   ☐ Influenza
☐ Leptospirosis ☐ Other ( )
☐ Parvovirus   ☐ Boosters
☐ Other ( )
☐ Boosters

BIOP _____

Previous problems: 1. _____

2. _____

3. _____

4. _____

Other animals:
(where relevant) _____

Environment: ☐ Urban   ☐ Suburban   ☐ Rural

Details if relevant
e.g. bedding,
type of management: _____

_____

_____

_____

_____

_____

HISTORY

CASE NO: _____
OWNER'S NAME: _____
PATIENT'S NAME: _____   DATE: _____
_____ T: _____ P: _____ R: _____ WEIGHT: _____ KG.

	Normal	Abnormal	No exam		Normal	Abnormal	No exam
1. General appearance	☐	☐	☐	8. Musculoskeletal Joints	☐	☐	☐
				Bones	☐	☐	☐
2. Attitude	☐	☐	☐	Muscles	☐	☐	☐
3. Locomotion	☐	☐	☐	9. Perineum Anus	☐	☐	☐
4. Head & Face Eyes	☐	☐	☐				
Ears	☐	☐	☐	Vulva/ Testicles	☐	☐	☐
Nose	☐	☐	☐	Mamm. gland/ Penis	☐	☐	☐
5. Oral cavity Mucous membrane	☐	☐	☐	Prostate	☐	☐	☐
Gingiva	☐	☐	☐	10. Abdominal cavity	☐	☐	☐
Teeth	☐	☐	☐	11. Respiratory	☐	☐	☐
Tonsils	☐	☐	☐	12. Cardiovascular	☐	☐	☐
6. Lymph nodes	☐	☐	☐	13. Nervous system	☐	☐	☐
7. Integument	☐	☐	☐				

DETAILED EXAMINATION
(Auscultation, Percussion, Rectal, etc)

_____
_____
_____
_____
_____
_____
_____
_____
_____
_____
_____

Signed _____

PHYSICAL EXAMINATION

Figure 1.1 History and physical examination forms used to compile the problem-oriented medical record at the Queen's Veterinary School Hospital, University of Cambridge. BIOP, been in owner's possession; FVR, feline viral rhinotracheitis.

Oral cavity: check colour and moistness of oral mucous membranes. Normal capillary refill time is less than 2 seconds. Inspect gingivae for signs of inflammation or masses, and teeth for evidence of calculus formation. Open the mouth gently to examine the oral and occlusal surfaces of the teeth, tongue, hard/soft palate, pharynx and tonsils. To visualize the latter it is usually necessary to depress the tongue with a spatula or finger; cat's tonsils are particularly difficult, and sometimes almost impossible, to examine without some form of sedation. The underside of the tongue should be examined for evidence of a linear foreign body, such as a thread or piece of string in any animal that is vomiting.

Eyes: a superficial examination of each eye should include an examination of the conjunctival mucous membranes, eyelids, cornea, iris and lens. Pupillary light reflexes should be evaluated with a pen torch and the conjunctival mucous membranes for changes in colour (pallor, erythema, jaundice). The ocular sclera is particularly useful for detecting early jaundice.

Ears: examine the pinnae for skin lesions, swellings etc. and check each external auditory meatus for the presence of abnormal odours, discharges or other signs of inflammation.

Superficial lymph nodes and salivary glands

- Palpate the submandibular, prescapular (superficial cervical) and popliteal lymph nodes. Generalized lymphadenopathy such as that which occurs with multicentric lymphoma may also result in palpable enlargement of the axillary and inguinal lymph nodes.
- Palpate the submandibular and parotid salivary glands.

Neck

- Palpate the larynx and thyroid region particularly in older cats.
- Gently pinch the trachea to see if this elicits a cough.
- Assess hydration status by 'tenting' the skin over the dorsal aspect of the neck or top of the head.

The trunk and legs

- Palpate and observe for symmetry, size and shape.
- Examine skin and hair coat.
- Palpate the mammary glands for swellings, lumps, discharges and ulceration.
- Palpate the ribs for old fractures etc.
- Palpate the muscles and flex the joints; note any pain, swelling or crepitation.
- Examine the external genitalia, i.e. penis, prepuce and scrotum/testes in the male, and vulva in the female. When examining the vulva check the colour of the mucosal surface and note the presence of any discharge.

Thorax

Physical examination of the thorax involves palpation, auscultation and percussion. Auscultation should be carried out in a quiet room and if the dog is panting it will be necessary to ask the owner to gently close the animal's mouth. This is particularly important when attempting to classify or categorize a cardiac murmur. Purring in a contented cat is not easily overcome; blowing gently into each nostril may sometimes help. Both components of the endpiece of the stethoscope should be utilized when auscultating the heart and lungs (the bell detects low pitched sounds and the diaphragm the higher pitched sounds). With experience the clinician will learn to differentiate artefactual sounds such as hair rubbing on the stethoscope diaphragm, fine muscle fasciculations, gastrointestinal sounds, sniffing or purring, which may interfere with, or be superimposed on normal respiratory and cardiovascular sounds. Always auscultate both sides of the thorax.

Heart

- Palpate the chest wall to locate the apex beat (the area where the palpable shock, produced when the apex of the heart beats against the chest wall during each systole, is strongest). This point coincides roughly with the region of the mitral valve.
- Assess the heart sounds for loudness and clarity. The first heart sound (S1) corresponds to the vibration which occurs during closure of the atrioventricular (mitral and tricuspid) valves followed by the rapid ejection of blood from the ventricles. The second heart sound (S2) is associated with the closure of the pulmonic and aortic valves. Other 'normal' heart sounds (e.g. S3 and S4 sounds) and murmurs may be auscultated particularly in disease states (see Chapters 13 and 14). The pulmonic, aortic and mitral valves are most readily auscultated on the left side of the chest, the tricuspid valve on the right side. While listening to the heart the femoral pulse should be simultaneously

palpated. A pulse deficit is the term used to describe a set of heart sounds without a corresponding pulse and indicates a dysrhythmia.

Respiratory system

- Auscultate the larynx, trachea and thorax. Upper airway noises, particularly harsh crackles or wheezes, may be transmitted downwards and heard over the lungs (referred lung sounds).
- Respiratory sounds may be referred to as normal or adventitious.

Normal respiratory sounds

These may be classified as bronchial or vesicular, or a combination of the two (bronchovesicular). *Bronchial* (or tracheal) sounds are the result of air passing through larger airways. These harsh sounds may be heard if the stethoscope is placed over the larynx or trachea; similar sounds may be heard over the middle third of the thorax as air in the intrathoracic trachea passes caudally towards the coryna. They occur with equal duration during the inspiratory and expiratory phases of respiration, and decrease in intensity caudal to the hilar region. Increased bronchial sounds with or without increased vesicular sounds occur with excitement and panting, and also in young or thin-chested dogs. *Vesicular sounds* are the softer low pitched rustling sounds which can be heard during normal respiration. They are slightly louder on inspiration. Vesicular sounds have been attributed to the vortices of air which form as the terminal bronchioles open into the alveoli. *Bronchovesicular sounds*, as the term implies, are intermediate in quality between bronchial and vesicular sounds. Feline respiratory sounds are generally less audible than those of the dog and bronchial sounds tend to predominate.

Adventitious respiratory sounds

Adventitious sounds indicate the presence of a pathological process. They may originate from the bronchi, lungs and pleura. *Crackles* (rales) are discontinuous or intermittent sounds which are superimposed on the normal bronchovesicular respiratory noises. They are usually classified as fine or course (synonymous with the sounds previously referred to as dry and moist crackles respectively). Fine crackles occur with interstitial oedema, interstitial pneumonia and pulmonary fibrosis, and are most commonly heard during late inspiration. Course crackles generally indicate fluid accumulation in the bronchi, bronchioles or alveoli (e.g. bronchopneumonia or advanced pulmonary oedema). They have a more gurgling or bubbling quality and tend to be more pronounced during early inspiration. *Wheezes* (previously referred to as rhonchi), in contrast to crackles, are continuous sounds which are generated by air passing through a narrowed airway which results in vibration of the airway wall. They possess a musical, often whistling, quality and can be described as high pitched (sibilant) or low pitched (sonorous). Wheezes are a feature of chronic obstructive pulmonary disease, usually occurring during expiration. Lower pitched wheezes may be associated with secretions in the airway and therefore may be heard with course crackles. Inspiratory stridor is the more specific term used to describe the wheezes which are frequently associated with stenosis or partial obstruction of the upper respiratory tract (larynx, trachea or mainstem bronchi). *Pleural frictional sounds* are fine crackling noises caused by the rubbing together of roughened parietal and visceral pleural surfaces. These relatively rare sounds tend to be higher pitched and more focal in distribution than pulmonary crackles. Although not continuous, they are consistent in that they occur during the same phase of respiration (usually late inspiration).

Absence of lung sounds

A reduction in the intensity or complete absence of lung sounds is likely to occur if free fluid or air accumulates in the thoracic cavity. Other causes of reduced lung sounds include obesity, large space-occupying intrathoracic masses, diaphragmatic hernia and severe, diffuse terminal airway disease resulting in consolidation of one or more lung lobes.

Percussion

Percussion is a less useful diagnostic technique in small animals than it is for large animal species. The middle finger of one hand is placed over an intercostal space and struck with the middle finger of the other hand between the distal interphalangeal joint and the finger nail. Increased resonance occurs with pneumothorax or possibly severe pulmonary emphysema; decreased resonance may be expected with pleural effusions or large intrathoracic masses. The anterior thorax should be palpated in any dyspnoeic cat. Normally this area can be compressed easily between the thumb and fingers of one hand; failure to do so is highly suggestive of an anterior thoracic mass. *Dyspnoeic cats are serious risks for any type of examination and sedation may be necessary to avoid struggling and further respiratory embarrassment.*

Abdomen

The abdomen should be palpated gently between the fingers of both hands. Altering the position of the animal, for example by raising the forelimbs or placing in lateral recumbency, may occasionally aid palpation of an organ or mass that would otherwise not be palpable. The following structures may be palpated in the abdomen:

1. *Anterior abdomen*
- small intestine
- liver (if enlarged)
- stomach (if distended)

2. *Mid-abdomen*
- small intestine
- mesenteric lymph nodes (if enlarged)
- kidneys; in the cat especially, the left kidney is extremely mobile and easy to palpate and it is usually possible also to palpate the posterior pole of the right kidney, partially hidden under the right costal arch.
- ± spleen

3. *Caudal abdomen*
- small intestine
- faeces in the descending colon or rectum
- uterus (if distended)
- bladder (if moderately distended with urine)
- prostate gland (only if grossly enlarged)

Rectal examination

A rectal examination should, if possible, be performed on every sick animal and certainly in every middle-aged male dog as part of a full physical examination. It should be combined with a simultaneous single-handed palpation of the caudal abdomen to include the following:

- Direct digital examination of the rectal mucosa and anal sacs (check for perineal hernias, rectal diverticulae, rectal polyps or tumours, anal sac impaction, abscessation or tumours)
- Palpation per rectum of the prostate gland, bladder neck, pelvic urethra, uterus, cervix and dorsal wall of the vagina
- Note the consistency of faeces and presence of any blood

THE INITIAL PROBLEM LIST

The initial problem list consists of problems which have been identified from the history, clinical examination and results of preliminary laboratory screening tests. To begin with, it is best if each problem is listed separately in chronological order. This ensures that problems which at first sight appear to be unrelated to the main presenting complaint are not forgotten and can be recalled if the need arises at a later stage of the investigative process. It may also be helpful, particularly with the more complex cases, to establish a priority list of high and low priority problems At this stage it is often a good idea to review the problem list with the owner. This ensures that the owner has an insight into the complexity of the case and is aware of the high priority problems which warrant the most urgent attention.

When listing the problems, each problem should be stated at its highest level of refinement, i.e. its current level of understanding. Care should be taken not to overstate a problem or group of problems. A problem may be defined in one of four different forms:

1. A problem identified from the history or a clinical sign (e.g. pica, polydipsia, anorexia, altered behaviour, etc.)
2. An abnormal laboratory finding (e.g. increased blood urea, leucocytosis, persistent proteinuria, etc.)
3. A pathophysiological process or syndrome (e.g. anaemia, uraemia, nephrotic syndrome, etc.)
4. A specific diagnosis (e.g. keratoconjunctivitis sicca, perineal hernia, valvular endocardiosis)

Having identified the problem(s), an attempt should be made to localize each problem to a specific organ or body system. To this end, it is usually possible to refine and condense the list of problems under investigation. For example, problems which lack specificity and which cannot be localized to one system (anorexia, weight loss, lethargy, etc.) can often be grouped with problems such as vomiting or diarrhoea which are more likely to reflect specific organ dysfunction. Since polyuria and polydipsia generally occur simultaneously (in most cases polyuria is secondary to primary polydipsia) it is logical to consider the two problems as one. It may also be possible to group together problems which relate to the same body system or which arise from a common underlying pathophysiological mechanism. For example, erythema, exudation and crusting may be grouped together as one problem (moist exudative dermatitis). Grouping problems in this way is helpful in that it allows a clinician to be more selective in formulating his/her initial diagnostic plan.

As a case progresses, additional problems may be added to the problem list and it may be possible to condense and refine problems which have already been identified. For example, an initial problem list in a middle-aged male Dobermann may consist of five separate problems (exercise intolerance, weight loss, non-productive cough, 4/6 systolic heart murmur and tachycardia). If thoracic radiography subsequently reveals generalized cardiomegaly and evidence of pulmonary oedema, the problems may be refined and grouped as one, in this case, the syndrome of congestive heart failure. The problem list therefore, is constantly re-defined and amended as the results of further diagnostic procedures become available, until a specific diagnosis is reached.

A *master problem list* should be placed at the front of the patient's record. This consists of a numbered list of every problem, active or resolved, preferably in chronological order. The date of onset and resolution of each problem should be recorded on this sheet. In most cases the master problem list is a condensed version of the initial problem list since it may list diagnoses rather than separate problems. One advantage of such a list is that it helps colleagues who are not familiar with the case to gain an immediate picture of the patient's past and present medical history.

FORMULATING A PLAN

This is one of the most critical steps in the investigative process. A plan of action may be divided into three components: (1) a diagnostic plan, (2) a therapeutic plan and (3) client education.

Diagnostic plan

Initially it may be necessary to draw up a plan for each problem identified, concentrating on the most serious problem(s) first. The differential diagnoses or rule-outs for each problem (or group of problems) are listed in decreasing order of probability. The aim of the initial diagnostic plan should be to confirm or rule out conditions which appear either at the top of the list or as differentials for more than one problem. Having considered the potential pathophysiological mechanisms responsible for each of the problems under investigation, the clinician must then decide which laboratory tests or diagnostic procedures are the most appropriate. Furthermore, from an owner's point of view, it is important that the tests selected are cost-effective.

Therefore tests which specifically rule in or out the differential diagnosis in question should be chosen in preference to those which are more likely to yield equivocal results. With life-threatening problems, it may be necessary to investigate several possible diagnoses simultaneously, e.g. acute renal failure, diabetic ketoacidosis, liver failure, hypoadrenocorticism and pyometra are possible differential diagnoses for a severely dehydrated, semi-comatose middle-aged bitch which is presented with a history of vomiting, polydipsia, polyuria and depression, and each differential must be investigated accordingly. Each test or procedure to be performed should be accompanied by a tick-off box in the medical record.

Therapeutic plan

The therapeutic plan should state the goal of therapy and whether the therapy is specific, symptomatic, supportive, or simply palliative. Details of treatment received should be recorded in the medical record, i.e. medication, dose, frequency and route of administration. Details relating to intravenous fluid therapy and urine output, e.g. type and volume of fluid to be administered, rate of administration, cumulative totals for fluid received and volume of urine produced, are best recorded on a separate form. Ideally, treatment should be withheld until the cause of the problem has been accurately identified since some drugs, most notably glucocorticoids, significantly influence the results of biochemical tests, thereby making the interpretation of results considerably more difficult. Where this is not possible, for example in an animal which presents with life-threatening signs, an attempt should be made to obtain all the necessary diagnostic specimens (e.g. urine, blood, samples for bacteriological culture etc.) *before* treatment commences since this may provide useful baseline data to compare with post-treatment laboratory results.

Client education

The final part of the plan involves keeping the owner fully informed on the animal's progress (response to therapy, results of tests, diagnosis, prognosis), and/or any new problems which may have arisen. Not least of all an owner of a hospitalized patient should be provided with a written estimate of the costs likely to be incurred at each step of the investigative process.

ASSESSMENT AND PROGRESS NOTES

Each problem should be evaluated separately at appropriate intervals (usually once daily for hospitalized patients but the frequency will depend on the severity and nature of the problem, and also the rate at which haematological, biochemical and other physiological parameters change). The progress notes should be organized using either the SOAP or DAP formats outlined below.

The SOAP format consists of four sections:

1. *Subjective data*: Record history obtained from the owner and subjective observations such as changes in mental attitude, activity, appetite, etc. Is the animal's condition improving, remaining stable or deteriorating?
2. *Objective data*: Record objective clinical information, i.e. clinical findings (include normal findings if necessary) and the results of laboratory tests and special examinations.
3. *Assessment*: Interpret the significance of the subjective and objective data paying particular attention to new abnormalities or complications which may have arisen. If appropriate re-evaluate the prognosis.
4. *Plan*: Update and/or revise the diagnostic and therapeutic plans on the basis of the above. Update the owner with regard to the animal's progress.

The DAP (Data, Assessment and Plan) system is essentially a condensed version of the SOAP format. The sections containing the subjective and objective observations are combined into one section (D for Data). By repeating the SOAP (or DAP) system on a daily basis, the clinician is forced to assess each active problem in a logical and organized manner until the problem is either resolved or no further progress can be made.

DISCHARGE SUMMARY

A discharge summary should be prepared for the owner and, if appropriate, the referring veterinary surgeon. This should include the diagnosis (or tentative diagnosis), details of therapy (and response to therapy), prognosis and advice concerning the short-term and long-term management of the patient.

2

Anorexia and Polyphagia

J. K. Dunn

REGULATION OF FOOD INTAKE

In veterinary medicine the terms appetite and hunger are often used synonymously. *Appetite*, defined as a desire for food, is essentially a psychological process which is stimulated by the sight, smell and thought of food and accompanied by the flow of saliva in the mouth and gastric juice in the stomach. In contrast, *hunger* can be defined as an excessive desire for food and is a normal physiological response to meet the body's demand for more food. *Satiety* is the opposite of hunger and represents the sensation that occurs after eating a meal which fulfils the energy and nutritional requirements of the animal.

Food intake is regulated by internal (central) and peripheral control mechanisms. These include: (1) mechanical stimulation of the gastrointestinal tract; (2) hormonal responses to the sight, smell and ingestion of food; (3) body stores of fat and glycogen, and (4) ovarian and testicular hormones. In addition food intake is modified by several external factors including environmental temperature.

Food intake can be divided into two phases. First, initiation of feeding is due to physiological stimulation of the *appetite centre* located in the ventrolateral hypothalamus. The feeding centre is activated by alpha-adrenergic mechanisms and inhibited by beta-adrenergic and dopaminergic input. The satiety centre directly inhibits activity of the feeding centre. The onset of feeding is brought about by a reduction in negative signals from the satiety centre to the appetite centre. Lesions which destroy the feeding centre lead to progressive anorexia and weight loss.

Second, termination of feeding is due to increased activity of the satiety centre represented by a group of nuclei in the ventromedial hypothalamus. Lesions which destroy the ventromedial nuclei result in a voracious appetite. The satiety centre receives input from preabsorptive and postabsorptive receptors. Preabsorptive receptors are located in the oropharynx, stomach and intestines. Mechanoreceptors respond to gastric filling and generate afferent vagal impulses to the satiety centre. Postabsorptive signals to the satiety centre are thought to arise primarily as a result of alterations in glucose metabolism in the liver, meal-induced increases in insulin concentrations and insulin:glucagon ratio, and possibly also postprandial changes in amino acid balance.

Factors regulating food intake

Both the appetite and satiety centres are influenced by higher centres in the cerebral cortex which explains why feeding behaviour may be modified by pain, or the stress or anxiety related to alterations in an animal's daily routine or immediate surroundings. Factors which influence calorific balance may be expected to influence food intake. In the short term, a caloric deficit promotes hunger and caloric excess activates the satiety centre (see Chapter 3 on weight loss/gain). Other factors which are known to influence food intake include alterations in taste and smell sensation, basal metabolic rate, body temperature, plasma concentrations of glucose and amino acids, and the central nervous system concentrations of neurotransmitters, such as serotonin and its precursor tryptophan. Several hormones (e.g. insulin, glucagon, growth hormone, thyroid hormones and oestrogen) and gut peptides, released during feeding, have also been implicated in appetite control, for example cholecystokinin is known to promote satiety.

ANOREXIA

Anorexia refers to a complete loss of appetite and/or disinterest in food. Inappetence infers a partial loss of appetite or depressed food intake (the term partial anorexia is also sometimes used in this context). Anorexia may be psychological, physiological or pathological in origin. Many diseases cause anorexia by interfering with the normal neural, humoral and mechanical control mechanisms which regulate food intake.

Classification

Primary anorexia

Primary anorexia implies either some disease process acting directly on the hypothalamic appetite centre, e.g. an expanding hypothalamic or pituitary tumour, or the presence of some psychological factor which interferes with the neural control of feeding. In contrast to humans where anorexia nervosa is a relatively common disorder, primary anorexia in small animals is uncommon or at least rarely diagnosed. For example a hypothalamic tumour is probably unlikely to be diagnosed as a cause of anorexia until it expands to a point that it results in other signs of neurological dysfunction. Psychological factors resulting in 'stress' such as a change of home or new environment (especially cats), a sudden change in diet to one which is less palatable, alterations in daily routine, fear, anxiety, excitement or severe pain may influence food intake and should be considered as possible causes of anorexia particularly in the absence of more specific clinical signs.

Secondary anorexia

Most cases of anorexia in small animals occur secondary to some other disease process which affects the neural and endocrine regulation of food intake. The net result is decreased stimulation of the appetite centre or increased activity of the satiety centre despite the fact that the animal may already be in a state of negative caloric or protein balance. Cases of secondary anorexia are often associated with other clinical signs in particular vomiting and diarrhoea. Most disorders which result in nausea or vomiting also cause anorexia or inappetance implying that the feeding control centres and the vomiting centre, which is also located in the hypothalamus, may be interconnected. Cancer is an important differential diagnosis which should be ruled out in any animal presenting with chronic anorexia and weight loss (see Chapter 50). Most patients with cancer become anorectic (cancer cachexia). Sometimes anorexia may develop only during the terminal stage of the disease whereas in others it may be the primary complaint before other signs of cancer become apparent. It has been shown that some tumour-bearing experimental animals have high CNS levels of the neurotransmitter tryptophan which together with other peptides are thought to inhibit the feeding centre.

Primary or secondary anorexia should be differentiated from causes of *pseudoanorexia* where an animal shows an interest in food but is either unable to eat due to a problem affecting prehension, mastication or swallowing, or is reluctant to eat because it elicits pain. Causes of pseudoanorexia should be readily identified on the basis of the history and clinical examination. They include oropharyngeal disease (tooth root abscess, severe periodontal disease and gingivitis, buccal ulceration, foreign bodies), maxillary/mandibular fractures or temperomandibular joint luxation, hypoglossal or mandibular paralysis, temporal myositis, tetanus and oesophagitis.

Common causes of primary and secondary anorexia are listed in Table 2.1. In most cases of secondary anorexia the exact pathophysiogical mechanism is uncertain.

INVESTIGATION OF ANOREXIA

The main objective of the investigations should be to identify the underlying cause using an approach that is both logical and cost effective. Since anorexia is a non-specific finding, emphasis should be placed on attempting to identify additional significant historical, clinical or laboratory findings towards which more specific investigations may be directed.

HISTORY CHECKLIST

❏ **Duration?**

❏ **Accompanied by weight loss?**
If the answer is yes, may reflect degree of chronicity.

❏ **Change to less palatable (low calorie) diet?**

❏ **Amount fed and frequency of feeding?**

❏ **Breed and nervous disposition?**
Some oriental breeds of cat are fussy eaters; highly strung dogs may have variable appetites.

❏ **Can animal prehend, chew and swallow food normally?**

❏ **Other clinical signs of systemic disease?**
Evidence of systemic disease such as lethargy,

Table 2.1 Causes of primary and secondary anorexia

Primary anorexia

Neurological dysfunction
Destruction of the appetite centre, e.g. by an expanding pituitary or hypothalamic tumour
Increased intracranial pressure (hydrocephalus or cerebral oedema)
Altered smell or taste sensation

Psychological factors
Sudden change of diet (less palatable food)
Change in environment
Altered daily routine
Excitement, fear, anxiety, stress

Secondary anorexia

Fever (anorexia possibly mediated by endogenous pyrogens such as tumour necrosis factor, interferons and interleukin-1)

Pain (especially severe abdominal pain)

Toxins/drugs
Bacterial endotoxins, e.g. pyometra
Endogenous toxins released in association with uraemia, hepatic failure, ketosis (ketoacidotic diabetic)
Exogenous toxins (cardiac glycosides, chemotherapy with cytotoxic agents; anorexia may be associated with vomiting and nausea via a direct action of the drug on the chemoreceptor trigger zone in the medulla oblongata)

Infectious disease (may be associated with fever, endotoxaemia etc.)

Inflammation/neoplasia of abdominal viscera, e.g. stomach, small and large intestine, kidneys, pancreas or liver (may be associated with pain and vomiting)

Distension of stomach or small intestine, e.g. foreign body obstruction (probably associated with pain and vomiting)

Uterine enlargement/distension, e.g. late pregnancy or pyometra (with the latter, release of toxins may contribute to anorexia and vomiting)

Endocrine and metabolic disorders, e.g. hypoadrenocorticism, hypercalcaemia, hepatic lipidosis in cats

Neoplasia (cancer cachexia)

High environmental temperatures

Miscellaneous disorders
Cardiac failure (cardiac cachexia)
Motion sickness/inner ear disease

fever, vomiting/diarrhoea, pain, polydipsia/polyuria, oculonasal discharge, cough or respiratory distress, CNS signs or altered behaviour may help to localize the cause of the anorexia.

- Change in animal's environment or daily routine?
- Record details of previous treatment or current medication, e.g. digitalis or cytotoxic agents.

PHYSICAL EXAMINATION

Since anorexia is a non-specific sign of so many different disorders a full physical examination is absolutely essential in attempting to establish the cause, particularly in cases where anorexia may be the sole presenting complaint. The presence of additional signs of localized or systemic disease may provide vital clues and almost certainly will be helpful in determining the direction which further investigations should take. The animal should be weighed on a regular basis. Anorexia accompanied by progressive weight loss and/or fever often indicates the presence of systemic disease.

It is important to rule out immediately those conditions which interfere with the mechanical processes of prehending, chewing or swallowing food. If necessary food may be offered to confirm that there is no desire to eat. A full physical examination should include detailed examination of the following:

- Check the oral cavity for pain on opening mouth, tooth root abscesses, fractured teeth, periodontal disease, stomatitis, gingivitis, buccal or lingual ulceration and foreign bodies.
- Check the bones of the face, mandibles and the muscles of mastication (for fractures/dislocations and pain/swelling over temporal muscles).

An initial diagnostic plan for the patient with persistent anorexia should include the following:

- Full routine haematological examination
- Complete biochemistry screen
- Urinalysis
- Lateral radiographs of the thorax and abdomen
- Feline leukaemia virus and feline immunodeficiency virus assays in cats

Additional tests are based on the history, clinical findings and results of the initial database

Symptomatic therapy of anorexia

Symptomatic therapy of anorexia or inappetence is only indicated if the cause cannot be ascertained, i.e. animals which are not showing clinical or laboratory evidence of systemic disease.

Appetite may be stimulated in the following ways:

1. Improve the odour of the diet for example the addition of tuna, sardines, gravy etc. may stimulate the appetite of the fussy eater.
2. B complex vitamins either per os or by injection.
3. Diazepam (0.25 mg kg^{-1} body weight once daily).

Dehydration and any underlying electrolyte or acid–base disturbances should be corrected beforehand. Nasogastric or pharyngostomy tube feeding should be considered when anorexia is persistent and the metabolic consequences of not eating become life-threatening, for example the cat with hepatic lipidosis.

POLYPHAGIA

Polyphagia can be defined as a ravenous or voracious appetite which results in the ingestion of food in quantities in excess of the calculated normal intake. It should be differentiated from pica which is the craving for abnormal substances such as soil or paper. Polyphagia may be psychological, physiological or pathological in origin and can be classified as either primary or secondary.

Primary polyphagia

Polyphagia is the result of increased activity of the feeding centre and inhibition of the satiety centre. Lesions which destroy the ventromedial hypothalamic nuclei, for example hypothalamic tumours, are rare causes of polyphagia. Overfeeding can be regarded as a psychological form of polyphagia and is the most common cause of obesity in small animals. Under normal circumstances a positive caloric balance would activate the satiety centre. In obese dogs the normal control mechanisms fail and affected animals continue to eat excessively even in the face of increased body fat deposits. The reason for this failure of negative feedback on the appetite centre is not known but the fact that certain breeds of dog have a tendency to become obese suggests a genetic predisposition (see Chapter 3).

Secondary polyphagia

Diseases that either induce a negative caloric balance (e.g. maldigestion/malabsorption syndromes) or increase basal metabolic rate (e.g. hyperthyroidism) result in secondary polyphagia. In these cases polyphagia is pathological and represents a compensatory response to sustain increased nutritional requirements and maintain body weight (Table 2.2). This compensatory mechanism is generally inadequate and the polyphagia is usually accompanied by a variable degree of weight loss and muscle wasting. An appropriate physiological increase in appetite may occur in response to gestation, lactation, strenuous exercise and exposure to cold environmental temperatures. Certain drugs such as glucocorticoids, progestagens (e.g. megoestrol acetate), diazepam and the anticonvulsive agents phenobarbitone, primidone and phenytoin are also potent appetite stimulants.

INVESTIGATION OF POLYPHAGIA

Overfeeding, often associated with insufficient exercise, is the most common cause of weight gain and obesity in small animals. In most cases where polyphagia is associated with progressive weight loss the history and physical examination will usually provide evidence of additional problems. The next part of the investigation can then be directed towards ruling out diseases which create negative caloric and/or nitrogen balance or which result in an increased metabolic rate (see Table 2.2).

HISTORY CHECKLIST

❏ **Duration?**

❏ **Accompanied by weight loss or weight gain?**
If weight loss or muscle wasting, rule out disorders which increase metabolic rate or which create a negative energy balance (maldigestion/malabsorption syndromes, diabetes mellitus, hyperthyroidism, hyperadrenocorticism). If animal has gained weight rule out overfeeding.

❏ **Has there been a change to a more palatable (calorie dense) diet?**

❏ **Amount fed and frequency of feeding. Table scraps and tit-bits?**

Table 2.2 Classification and causes of polyphagia

Primary polyphagia
Destruction of the satiety centre, e.g. by a hypothalamic tumour (rare)
Overfeeding (may be psychological in origin and the tendency to become obese may involve a genetic predisposition)

Secondary polyphagia
Physiological causes
Gestation
Lactation
Strenuous exercise
Exposure to cold environmental temperatures

Pathological causes
Disorders inducing negative caloric balance
    Maldigestion (e.g. exocrine pancreatic insufficiency)
    Malabsorption syndromes (e.g. infiltrative diseases of the small intestine)
    Diabetes mellitus
    Hyperadrenocorticism
    ±Hypoglycaemia, e.g. insulinoma

Disorders resulting in increased basal metabolic rate
    Hyperthyroidism
    Phaeochromocytoma

Drug-induced
Glucocorticoids
Progestagens (e.g. megoestrol acetate)
Anticonvulsants (phenobarbitone, primidone and phenytoin)
Diazepam

❏ **Other clinical signs of systemic disease?**
Other clinical signs such as lethargy, exercise intolerance, tachycardia, vomiting/diarrhoea, polydipsia/polyuria, alopecia, central nervous system signs or altered behaviour (e.g. irritability, restlessness) may help establish the cause of the polyphagia.

❏ **Record details of previous treatment or current medication**
e.g. glucocorticoids, progestagens or anticonvulsants.

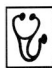

PHYSICAL EXAMINATION

The animal's weight should be recorded on a regular basis. Polyphagic animals which lose weight may be expected to show additional clinical signs consistent with the underlying disorder.

- Diarrhoea? Consider maldigestion or malabsorption.
- Polydipsia/polyuria? Consider diabetes mellitus, hyperadrenocorticism, hyperthyroidism.
- Alopecia? Consider hyperadrenocorticism.
- CNS signs or altered behaviour? Consider hypoglycaemia or hyperthyroidism.
- Palpably enlarged liver? Consider diabetes mellitus, hyperadrenocorticism or hyperthyroidism.

The initial diagnostic plan should consist of the following:

- Full routine haematological examination
- Complete biochemical screen
- Urinalysis
- Lateral radiographs of the thorax and abdomen

When polyphagia is accompanied by a history of diarrhoea or steatorrhoea the following additional tests should be performed:

- Faecal worm egg count
- Faecal culture and sensitivity
- Faecal smears for undigested starch, fat and muscle fibres
- Serum trypsin-like immunoreactivity (TLI), folate and vitamin B_{12} assays
- ± oral fat, xylose or differential sugar absorption tests.

Additional tests may be necessary to investigate thyroid function (T_4 assay may help to rule out hyperthyroidism) and the pituitary–adrenal axis (adrenocorticotropic hormone response test or low-dose dexamethasone suppression test to screen for hyperadrenocorticism).

■ Management

Symptomatic therapy for secondary polyphagia is not appropriate and the main objective should be to remove or treat the underlying cause. Dietary restriction and/or the feeding of a low calorie/high fibre diet is indicated only when polyphagia is associated with overfeeding and results in obesity. Management of obesity is covered in greater detail in Chapter 3.

3

Weight Loss and Weight Gain

P. J. Watson and J. K. Dunn

INTRODUCTION

Weight loss or obesity occur if the intake of calories does not match expenditure, particularly if the imbalance is prolonged or the body's normal homeostatic adaptation to changes in calorie intake fails. Rapid changes in weight may be due to changes in total body water, such as weight gain in ascites or pericardial effusion or weight loss due to dehydration or diuretic therapy. Repeated weight measurements, although important, must therefore be interpreted with caution along with other clinical findings and a general assessment of body condition. Weight loss or gain is usually considered significant if there is a 10% increase or decrease in body weight not associated with fluid changes. It should be noted that fluid retention, such as ascites, may mask concurrent weight loss and owners may confuse fluid retention with obesity.

Two commonly quoted measures of energy requirement are basal energy requirement (BER) and maintenance energy requirement (MER). MER is about twice BER in dogs and 1.4 times BER in cats. BER is the amount of energy used in thermoneutral conditions following sleep and 12–18 hours after food consumption, whereas MER is the amount of energy used in thermoneutral conditions by a moderately active animal including the energy needed to obtain and use food in the amounts necessary to maintain body weight. It does not include the energy needed for additional physical activity or production.

To calculate average BER, the following linear approximations may be used (where W = weight in kg):

$$\text{BER (kcal day}^{-1}) = 70 + 30\,W \text{ for dogs}$$
$$\text{BER (kcal day}^{-1}) = 50\,W \text{ for cats}$$

Alternatively, the following equations for MER may be used:

$$\text{MER (kcal day}^{-1}) = 110\,W^{0.75} \text{ for dogs}$$
$$\text{MER (kcal day}^{-1}) = 70\,W \text{ for cats or } 80\,W$$
for active outdoor cats

It should be stressed that any formula is only an average for the species and individual animals may vary as much as 30% above or below this even in health. In disease, the variation is even more marked.

WEIGHT LOSS

Weight loss results from negative caloric balance and is usually associated with depletion of total body reserves of nitrogen (lean body mass) as well as fat. Even in controlled weight loss programmes in obese humans 15–40% of weight loss is said to be lean body mass. In conditions causing hypermetabolism (trauma, many systemic diseases, stress, burns, neoplasia) loss of lean body mass is even more significant. Weight loss is therefore of concern even in an obese dog or cat, especially if it has concurrent disease.

Emaciation is the term used to describe a state of severe weight loss induced by prolonged malnutrition or undernutrition.

Cachexia describes the general physical wasting and malnutrition associated particularly with malignancy (cancer cachexia) and chronic congestive cardiac failure (cardiac cachexia). The precise pathophysiological mechanisms causing it are not understood although humoral factors and anorexia, intestinal malabsorption, uncoupling of metabolism by tumours, hypoproteinaemia and poor tissue perfusion causing tissue hypoxia have all been implicated. The presence of cachexia is a poor prognostic indicator in both neoplasia and heart failure.

Causes of weight loss

Many conditions may result in weight loss and it is most appropriate to divide the causes into the following categories (Table 3.1):

Table 3.1 Causes of weight loss

Inadequate intake of nutrients
Primary causes
Poor quality diet, i.e. low calorie, low protein or poor digestibility
Nutritionally acceptable diet in inadequate amounts for normal animal
Nutritionally acceptable diet in inadequate amounts for stage of life or lifestyle

Note: MER and thus daily calorie requirements are increased by approximate amounts shown in brackets
  Pregnancy (1.1–1.3 MER during last trimester in dog; up to 1.25 MER cat)
  Lactation (2.0–4.0 MER during peak lactation)
  Growth (1.2–2.0 MER depending on stage and breed)
  Strenuous exercise (up to 4.0 MER for sled dog)
  Cold (1.25–1.75 MER)
  Heat (up to 2.5 MER in tropical climates)

Secondary causes
Inability to prehend, chew or swallow food (oropharyngeal disease, e.g. glossopharyngeal or mandibular paralysis; mandibular/maxillary fractures; temporomandibular luxation; severe periodontal or tooth disease, gingivitis or stomatitis; oropharyngeal foreign body or neoplasia; temporal myositis; cricopharyngeal achalasia)
Nausea and vomiting (see Chapter 5)
Regurgitation (megaoesophagus, oesophagitis, oesophageal obstruction)
Anorexia or inappetence associated with drug therapy or localized or systemic disease (see Chapter 2)

Increased nutrient requirements due to pathology
Reduced nutrient assimilation
Maldigestion (exocrine pancreatic insufficiency, bile salt deficiency or degradation of bile salts by small intestinal bacterial overgrowth)
Malabsorption (inflammatory or neoplastic infiltration of the small intestine, vascular congestion, may occur as a component of cardiac and cancer cachexia)
'Short bowel syndrome' (malabsorption and maldigestion following extensive resection of small intestine)

Increased nutrient metabolism and/or impaired synthesis of body protein
Hyperthyroidism
Diabetes mellitus
Hypermetabolism due to trauma, stress or systemic disease
Pyrexia (13% rise in BER for every 1°C temperature increase)
Neoplasia (cancer cachexia)
Congestive heart failure (cardiac cachexia)
Chronic liver disease (decreased synthesis of albumin and globulins except γ-globulins)
Phaeochromocytoma

Increased nutrient loss
Protein-losing enteropathy (lymphangiectasia, lymphosarcoma and severe inflammatory bowel disease: both albumin and globulin fractions lost)
Protein-losing nephropathy (glomerular disease: mainly albumin lost)
Chronic blood loss (serum proteins lost)
Severe burns (serum proteins lost)
Severe pyoderma (serum proteins lost)
Draining purulent conditions, e.g. pyothorax (serum proteins lost)

1. Feeding a diet insufficient for normal physiological needs
   (a) Feeding poor quality, low calorie, low protein or poorly digestible diet to normal animal
   (b) Feeding insufficient amounts of nutritionally acceptable diet to a normal dog (a and b amount to neglect or ignorance and are uncommon)
   (c) Failing to provide the necessary increase in calories and protein for a demanding stage of life (pregnancy, lactation, growth, hard work, extremes of cold or heat).
2. Impaired desire or ability to eat (see Chapter 2)
3. Increased nutrient requirements due to a disease process
   (a) Reduced nutrient assimilation
   (b) Increased nutrient metabolism and/or impaired synthesis of body protein
   (c) Increased nutrient loss

Consequences of weight loss

In a normal fasting animal, the reduction in blood glucose caused by negative caloric balance leads to a reduction in insulin secretion which causes reduced conversion of thyroxine (T4) into the more active tri-iodothyronine (T3). This results in a lowering of basal metabolic rate so reducing the caloric requirement. The concurrent increase in circulating glucagon caused by hypoglycaemia stimulates hepatic glycogenolysis and glucose release, hepatic gluconeogensis from amino acids, lactic acid and glycerol, and the release of glycerol and fatty acids from fat stores (lipolysis). Lipolysis is facilitated by the reduction in insulin secretion and fatty acids are converted in the liver into ketone bodies which can be used as fuel.

If fasting continues, glycogen reserves are depleted rapidly (within a few days in humans but faster in dogs and cats). Body protein is then initially used as the main source of energy. Over about a week, there is a gradual change to using stored fat as the predominant fuel because increased blood ketone levels induce enzyme changes in peripheral tissues, including brain and heart, to increase ketone body use and reduce glucose use. There is a continued, moderate protein loss mainly to provide glucose for obligate glucose users (red blood cells, renal medullary cells, nervous tissue and fibroblasts in wound repair) but protein does not become the predominant source of energy again until late in the course of fasting when all fat reserves have been used. The animal is suffering severe malnutrition by this stage.

Unfortunately in many animals with weight loss, not only is there negative calorie balance but also concurrent stress, injury or disease which accelerates loss of lean body mass as a result of 'hypermetabolism'. The reduced intake or increased loss of calories in these animals starts the same metabolic changes described above but the neuroendocrine responses to stress counteract the down-regulation of basal metabolic rate. Sympathetic nervous system stimulation and release of catecholamines, adrenocorticoids, glucagon and growth hormone act to stop the reduction in conversion of T4 into T3 and cause increased glucose production from glycogen and protein, increased lipolysis and increased protein synthesis for tissue repair. Hypermetabolic animals are often hyperglycaemic and peripherally insulin resistant in spite of negative calorie balance. There is an increase in the rate and depth of respiration and oxygen consumption (due to increased fat oxidation) and increased heart rate. Blood is shunted from the spleen and splanchnic areas to the brain and muscles and cardiac output may be increased 2 to 3 times. In addition, if the animal is pyrexic, its energy requirements are increased by an estimated 13% per degree centigrade temperature rise. Fibroblasts in healing wounds and many neoplasms have increased glucose requirements, which they metabolize anaerobically to produce lactic acid.

Therefore, animals in negative energy balance with concurrent disease have increased protein and fat requirements compared with normal animals. They cannot supply all their calorie needs with carbohydrate due to metabolic changes including peripheral insulin resistance.

In animals with weight loss, muscle protein breakdown occurs more slowly than changes in other body proteins, so by the time muscle loss is obvious clinically many other important physiological changes have occurred. There is no 'stored protein' in the body so any protein loss involves the use of structural or functional proteins. About half of body protein is in a state of dynamic flux and is relatively metabolically labile. This is used first and includes plasma, visceral and muscle protein. The other half is relatively metabolically stable and is found in bones, ligaments, tendons and cartilage. This protein is not used until weight loss is marked. In the first few days of negative calorie balance, liver and plasma proteins are lost and there is a marked reduction in hepatic protein synthesis. Then, protein is taken from the gastrointestinal tract resulting in a reduction in mass and enzyme activity and an increase in intestinal transit time. The immune system is also affected relatively early in the course of weight loss. There is depression of humoral immunity with a reduced ability to synthesize antibodies, particularly IgA and reduced interferon synthesis. There is a reduction in cell-mediated immunity with fewer T lymphocytes. The barrier functions of the skin and mucosal surfaces are disrupted and inflammatory responses are reduced. There is a reduction in the levels of most complement proteins except C4 and reduced leucocyte mobility and bactericidal activity. Skeletal muscle is only affected after these other changes are underway with reduced synthesis and increased degradation of muscle protein.

Weight loss may therefore lead to serious changes in the immune system and viscera which may significantly impair recovery from surgery and disease and lead to further complications. Hypermetabolism was said to have contributed to more than 85% of deaths in a human surgical intensive care unit (Donoghue, 1989) and patients with tumours and concurrent cachexia suffer more complications associated with chemotherapy, radiotherapy and surgery than those without cachexia (Hammer, 1994). If an animal has significant weight loss, it is obviously important to find and treat the cause and provide sufficient calorie and protein intake as soon as possible.

INVESTIGATION OF WEIGHT LOSS

A detailed history and physical examination should provide important clues to the pathogenesis and body system involved.

HISTORY CHECKLIST

❑ **Age, breed, sex**
Growing, pregnant, lactating?

❑ **Temperament and general demeanour**
Hyperexcitable, nervous, lethargic, depressed?

❑ **Quality of diet, amount fed, frequency of feeding**
Is amount fed sufficient for age, degree of physical activity and ambient temperature?

❑ **Severity and progression of weight loss?**
Remember to note the effects of fluid imbalance

❑ **Appetite**
Depressed, normal or increased?

❑ **Polydipsia/polyuria?**

❑ **Vomiting and/or diarrhoea?**

❑ **Exercise intolerance?**

❑ **Coughing?**

❑ **Current medication?**

PHYSICAL EXAMINATION

Most chronic infectious, inflammatory or neoplastic disorders and some metabolic and endocrine problems are characterized by non-specific signs such as weight loss, anorexia and lethargy. In malignancy, weight loss may be apparent in the early stages before more specific clinical signs develop. This is particularly the case with neoplasms involving the gastrointestinal tract, pancreas, liver, spleen, lymph nodes or bone marrow. Physical examination should therefore include careful and systematic palpation of the abdomen and peripheral lymph nodes.

The initial diagnostic plan for an animal with unexplained weight loss should include:

- Full routine haematological examination
- Complete biochemical profile including total plasma protein concentration and albumin:globulin ratio
- Urine analysis
- Lateral radiographs of chest and abdomen
- Faecal worm egg count
- Cats: feline leukaemia virus and feline immunodeficiency virus ± feline coronavirus assays

Additional tests are based on the history, clinical findings and results of the initial database listed above. The reader should consult other Chapters for more detailed discussion of common clinical problems that may be associated with weight loss.

Symptomatic treatment

Management of weight loss is directed primarily at correcting the underlying cause. In many chronic diseases, weight loss is associated with anorexia and it is essential to ensure these animals are obtaining sufficient protein and calories to prevent catabolism and loss of lean body mass with the consequences outlined above. This might be achieved by feeding a highly palatable, high quality food, but it will be necessary to tube feed some patients to ensure sufficient intake. In most animals, some form of enteral feeding is possible with nasogastric tubes being indicated in the short term and gastrostomy tubes for more prolonged support. If a diet designed for use in cats or dogs is used, vitamins and minerals will be correctly balanced to energy intake, although extra B vitamin supplementation may be considered in cats, particularly if they have concurrent polyuria as urinary loss can be marked in this species. Total parenteral nutrition is difficult and potentially dangerous and is only indicated in animals with severe, intractable vomiting or extensive gastrointestinal disease. The reader is referred to texts on critical care nutrition for more detailed coverage of tube feeding.

WEIGHT GAIN

Obesity, resulting from the intake of calories exceeding expenditure, is the commonest cause of weight gain in small animals and the most frequent form of 'malnutrition' seen in practice. It has been estimated that if a dog or cat regularly consumes 1% more calories than is necessary it will be almost 25% overweight by middle age. The incidence varies in different studies and countries but 25–44% of dogs and 6–40% of cats seen in veterinary practices are obese (Markwell and Butterwick, 1994). This may overestimate the incidence in the general population as obesity predisposes animals to a number of diseases, but it is clearly a significant problem. Other causes of weight gain include increases in total body water, large masses such as splenic tumours and unsuspected pregnancy.

Humans are defined as obese if they are 10–20% above ideal weight with reference to optimal height–weight standards. There are extensive data on this in humans but much less in dogs (pure-breds only and not cross-breds) and none in cats. It may, therefore, be more appropriate to define obesity physiologically in small animals as a pathological accumulation of fat much in excess of that necessary for optimal body function (Markwell and Butterwick, 1994).

Causes of obesity

Obesity may be defined as uncomplicated, resulting primarily from excessive calorie intake, or complicated, arising from other causes. In humans, only 5% of cases of obesity are 'complicated' and the fraction is probably similar in dogs and cats. In other words, most animals are obese because they are fed too much relative to the amount of exercise or other work they perform. Other factors described below, such as breed and neutering, may predispose to obesity but the primary cause remains owner-induced overfeeding and/or under-exercising and therefore the primary cure is to reduce calorie intake and increase exercise. Some of the owner-related factors predisposing to obesity are listed in Table 3.2. It is important to feed each individual according to its energy needs and adjust intake as necessary to maintain a constant weight. Owners often fail to do this and also do not take into account extra energy obtained from snacks and tit-bits. Exercise may be inadequate due to lack of time or owner or animal illness or unwillingness, and food may be provided as a palliative to exercise. It has been shown that indoor cats are more likely to become obese than those allowed outside probably due to reduced exercise. In addition, owners often encourage feeding behaviour, such as begging in dogs, which increases calorie intake. Obesity in owners has been associated with an increased incidence of obesity in dogs. The reasons for this are unclear but may include lack of exercise, consumption of high calorie tit-bits or failure to recognize obesity in the animal as a problem.

Table 3.2 Owner-related factors predisposing to obesity in dogs and cats

Failure to adjust food intake to individual calorie needs Failure to recognize some dogs require less food than average (normal variation) Failure to recognize reduced needs with age, neutering, orthopaedic and other diseases reducing exercise
Failure to take into account additional energy obtained from snacks or supplements
Encouraging appetite/feeding behaviour as a sign of health Encouraging begging behaviour Standing over animal while it eats (aggressive attitude which may 'force' dog to eat when not hungry)
Failure to exercise sufficiently Inadequate exercise due to lack of time or owner or animal illness Providing food as a palliative instead of exercise Keeping a cat indoors
Obesity in owners (often related to obesity in dogs)

Factors other than owner behaviour predisposing to obesity in dogs and cats are summarized in Table 3.3. In humans, obesity is recognized as a complex phenomenon involving genetic, cultural and social factors. *Genetic factors* also appear to be involved in dogs, with some breeds being more prone to obesity than others. For example, Labrador retrievers, cairn terriers, cocker spaniels, long-haired dachshunds, Shetland sheepdogs, Basset hounds, beagles and cavalier King Charles spaniels appear to be prone to obesity whereas German shepherd dogs, greyhounds, Yorkshire terriers, dobermanns, Staffordshire bull terriers, lurchers and whippets are relatively resistant to weight gain (Edney and Smith, 1986). Breed incidence of obesity seems to relate to poor regulation

Table 3.3 Factors other than owner behaviour predisposing to obesity in dogs and cats

---
Diet fed
Home-made diet – tends to be high fat, lacks consistency in calorie content and lack feeding guides
High sugar diet – fructose is used more efficiently than glucose
High fat diet – increases palatability and caloric density: fat stored and used more efficiently than carbohydrate or protein

Genetic factors – some breeds of dog are predisposed to obesity (see text)

Social interactions with other animals – competition for food

Neutering – approximately doubles the incidence of obesity in cats and dogs of both sexes

Age
Hyperplasia of adipose cells if obese while growing
Reduced metabolic rate and exercise with increasing age encourages obesity

---

of food intake when presented with a highly palatable diet, which is similar to the behaviour often observed in obese humans. It is presently unclear whether similar breed predispositions occur in pedigree cats.

Social interactions with other animals in a household may also predispose to obesity with animals eating large amounts quickly to avoid competition or dominant animals consuming another's food.

Neutering approximately doubles the incidence of obesity in dogs and cats of both sexes. This appears to be due to a number of factors including reduced exercise due to less 'roaming' behaviour, loss of the inhibitory effect of oestrogen on appetite in spayed bitches and queens, and lowering of testosterone levels postcastration allowing increased efficiency of food utilization.

Age has an effect on the incidence and consequences of obesity. It is important to ensure growing puppies and kittens do not become obese as overfeeding in the first 4–6 months of life may cause an increase in the number (hyperplasia) of adipose cells as opposed to simply an increase in cell size (hypertrophy) which occurs in the mature adult. The hyperplasia is irreversible and permanently predisposes the animal to obesity in later life. Animals require less calories as they get older because their basal metabolic rate decreases due to a reduction in lean body mass and there is also a tendency towards reduced physical activity with age.

Finally, the *type of food* fed influences the incidence of obesity, particularly if the food is given ad lib and the animal is expected to regulate its own intake. High fat diets predispose to obesity as fat increases both the palatability and caloric density of the food. Fat is also utilized as an energy source and stored as fat more efficiently than carbohydrate or protein. Increasing dietary sugar also predisposes to obesity. Sugar (sucrose) consists of fructose and glucose whereas starch is composed of glucose only. Fructose is used more efficiently than glucose so high sugar foods are more likely to cause obesity than high starch foods. Animals on home-made diets are more prone to obesity as the constituents tend to be high in fat and the ingredients, and thus calorie content, lack consistency from day to day. In addition, manufactured foods are sold with feeding guides for average dogs whereas homemade diets have no guides making it difficult to estimate daily requirements.

The factors described above all increase the risk of 'uncomplicated' weight gain. 'Complicated' obesity, secondary to systemic disease or drug-induced, is uncommon but must be ruled out before contemplating a weight reduction programme. The latter is unlikely to be successful in these cases unless the primary cause is treated. The commonest causes of complicated obesity are listed in Table 3.4. Endocrine causes include hypothyroidism in dogs which causes weight gain by reducing the basal metabolic rate, hyperadrenocorticism in dogs and

Table 3.4 Causes of complicated obesity

Endocrine disorders
Hypothyroidism (dogs; cats only following bilateral thyroidectomy and rare congenital cases)
Hyperadrenocorticism (dogs and cats)
Insulinoma (dogs and very rare cases in cats)
Acromegaly (dogs and cats)
Hypogonadism (dogs and cats)

Drug-induced
Progestagens
Glucocorticoids
Diazepam
Anticonvulsants, e.g. primidone

Primary hyperlipidaemia

Bilateral destruction of hypothalamic satiety centre (very rare)

cats which results in polyphagia and increased fat deposition, and insulinomas in dogs and very rarely in cats which also stimulate polyphagia and fat deposition. Animals with hypogonadism, acromegaly and primary hyperlipidaemias may also show weight gain. Some drugs induce polyphagia and/or increased fat deposition. These include progestagens such as megoestrol acetate, glucocorticoids, diazepam and primidone. Bilateral destruction of the satiety centre (for example by a tumour) results in polyphagia and obesity but this is very rare.

Consequences of obesity

It is important to treat obesity in small animals as it will certainly reduce the quality of life and also probably reduce the lifespan. Much work has been done in humans on the links between obesity and disease and particularly the associated increases in cardiovascular and gall-bladder disease and diabetes mellitus. There is much less information on dogs and even less in cats but the following associations have been found or proposed in small animals.

Respiratory embarrassment is frequent in obese dogs and is thought to be largely due to narrowing of the laryngeal and pharyngeal areas by fatty deposits which interfere with the airway. This contrasts with humans where the respiratory difficulties associated with weight gain are due to increased weight on the chest wall (Markwell and Butterwick, 1994). An increased risk of *circulatory problems* has been proposed due to the increase in cardiac output required to perfuse excess adipose tissue and weakening of cardiac muscle by fatty infiltrate. However, this has only been shown in dogs which are grossly obese and not those which are only moderately so (Edney and Smith, 1986; Markwell and Butterwick, 1994). There is a strong association in humans between *hypertension* and obesity and an increased incidence of hypertension has also been shown in obese dogs (Hand *et al.*, 1989).

It is commonly proposed in both humans and dogs that there is an increased incidence of *osteoarthritis* in obese individuals. However, no conclusive links between obesity and increased joint damage have been shown in either species except with gross obesity. Dogs with osteoarthritis tend to exercise less and be relatively old. Older dogs are also at increased risk of obesity so any association between osteoarthritis and obesity may not be causative. However, it would seem sensible to control the weight of dogs already affected with osteoarthritis both to reduce the stress imposed on joints and to counteract the tendency to become obese with the reduction in exercise caused by joint pain.

Obesity appears to be associated in dogs with an *increased risk from infectious diseases*.

Obesity appears to be associated with some cases of *diabetes mellitus* in dogs and cats in a similar way to humans. In obese dogs, the degree of hyperinsulinaemia and insulin resistance seen are directly related to the degree of obesity, as in humans. The insulin resistance is due to a reduction in the number of insulin receptors with an additional postreceptor defect in some cases. Recent work in cats has shown that obesity is also a risk factor in the development of diabetes mellitus in this species and that the effect of obesity on insulin kinetics may contribute to the transient diabetes mellitus seen in some cats.

Obesity also causes *fatty infiltration in the liver* of dogs which may result in a subclinical decrease in hepatic function. More importantly, obesity is a major predisposing factor for the development of *idiopathic hepatic lipidosis* in cats which is potentially life-threatening, although the exact mechanisms behind its development are unclear.

Obesity increases *surgical* and *anaesthetic risk*. There are technical difficulties associated with operating on a fat individual leading to prolonged surgery time; healing is slowed and there is an increased risk of wound breakdown and fat necrosis following surgical trauma. Obesity alters the kinetics of anaesthetic drugs and anaesthesia is further complicated by the possibility of obesity-induced respiratory, cardiovascular and hepatic compromise.

Obesity also *complicates clinical examination* and *diagnosis* with muffling of heart and lung sounds on auscultation and difficulty in palpating the abdomen.

Feline lower urinary tract disease is linked epidemiologically with obesity although the reason is unclear. One theory suggested is that, as a result of consuming a general excess of food, the overweight cat also consumes excess minerals including magnesium which are excreted in the urine and contribute to urolithiasis.

Obesity has also been implicated as one of the factors predisposing to *pancreatitis* in dogs and cats.

A number of other associations between obesity and disease in dogs and cats have been suggested. However, a survey of a large number of overweight dogs showed no clear relationships between obesity and skin or reproductive problems or neoplasia (Edney and Smith, 1986).

INVESTIGATION OF OBESITY

It is important to examine every animal before embarking on a weight control programme to rule out other reasons for weight gain and check for any primary or predisposing causes of obesity or any of the secondary consequences outlined above. Management factors relating to diet and exercise should be discussed with the owners to identify any areas which need addressing.

 ## HISTORY CHECKLIST

❏ **Age, breed, sex**
Young or old? neutered? breed predisposed to obesity?

❏ **Lifestyle**
Exercise? indoor cat?

❏ **Type of diet and quantity fed**
Homemade? tit-bits? begging behaviour?

❏ **Any other pets**
Competition at feeding time?

❏ **Appetite?**

❏ **Polydipsia/polyuria?**

❏ **Exercise intolerance or collapse?**

❏ **Lameness?**

❏ **Current medication**
Diazepam; glucocorticoids; progestagens; anticonvulsants?

It should be noted that, if the owner of an obese animal insists the daily food intake is small but the animal is not losing weight, they may be right. Obesity, at least in humans, appears to be divided into two phases: dynamic and static. During the dynamic phase, an increase in calorie intake results in an increase in weight. As this occurs, there is also an increase in lean body mass which increases basal energy requirements. When this offsets the excessive calorie intake there is no further weight gain and the individual is in the static phase of obesity. During the static phase, calorie intake may even be reduced but the same body weight maintained. This is thought to be due to a reduction in meal-induced heat production in obese individuals.

 ## PHYSICAL EXAMINATION

Full physical examination is important to assess the degree of obesity, rule out other causes of weight gain and look for evidence of predisposing or secondary disease. Examination should include careful abdominal palpation to rule out unsuspected pregnancy, splenic or other masses, or hepatomegaly suggestive of hyperadrenocorticism. Changes in the skin and/or hair coat may indicate endocrine disease and the animal should be assessed for evidence of ascites, pericardial effusion or other fluid accumulation which may account for the weight gain.

The degree of obesity should be assessed to allow estimation of a target weight after dieting. This may be achieved by weighing the animal and comparing its weight with standards for the breed but there are several disadvantages to this approach in dogs: there may be a wide variation in size even within one breed; cross-breds do not have a 'standard' weight and assessing weight alone fails to take account of body composition so a dog may seem overweight if it has substantial muscle development. It is also difficult to assess puppies in this way as ideal weights are usually quoted for adults. Absolute weight is a more helpful indication of obesity in cats where there is much less variation in adult body size than dogs. Generally, a healthy non-obese adult domestic shorthaired cat weighs 3.5–4.5 kg, although some individuals with larger frames may be heavier. In dogs, measurement of weight should be combined with a 'condition score' to assess the degree of obesity. Probably the easiest method is to palpate the layer of tissue overlying the ribs. If this is 0.5 cm or more in thickness but the ribs are still palpable then the dog is moderately overweight whereas if the tissue layer is so thick the ribs cannot be palpated then the animal is frankly obese. The tissue over the loins may also be palpated for obesity. Cats are more difficult to assess manually and visually. They tend to store excess fat intra-abdominally and in the inguinal region and although obesity is relatively easy to recognize in cats, assessment of the degree of obesity can be more difficult. Other methods of assessing obesity have been used in dogs but most of them, such as densitometry, X-ray absorptiometry, ultrasonography or magnetic resonance imaging are not practical in clinical situations. In humans, obesity can be quantified by measuring the subcutaneous fat layer with calipers on a skinfold but this method cannot be used in dogs because the skin lifts from the underlying fat in this species.

The **initial diagnostic plan** for an obese animal should ideally include:

- Full routine haematological and biochemical profiles including plasma cholesterol to rule out endocrine disease;
- Urinalysis to rule out secondary diabetes mellitus;
- Additional tests as necessary if endocrine disease is suspected: adrenocorticotropic hormone (ACTH) stimulation test or low dose dexamethasone suppression test for hyperadrenocorticism; thyroid stimulating hormone (TSH) or thyrotropin releasing hormone (TRH) stimulation test for hypothryroidism; insulin/glucose ratios or intravenous glucose tolerance test for insulinoma.

These tests are not necessary in all obese animals examined but are important if the physical examination shows evidence of complicating disease or if the animal fails to respond as expected to the weight loss programme.

Management of obesity

The stages in the management of uncomplicated obesity are outlined in Table 3.5. It is possible to manage obesity in dogs by hospitalization and starvation for a number of weeks but this is generally unacceptable for humane reasons unless the obesity is life-threatening. It is also unsatisfactory as the owner is not involved so management faults remain uncorrected and obesity is likely to recur. In addition, studies in humans show that during short-term starvation more protein and water is lost relative to fat than on calorie-controlled diets.

Table 3.5 Stages in controlled weight reduction (after Markwell and Butterwick, 1994)

1. Identification of obese animal and assessment of degree of obesity (weight, condition score)
2. Clinical examination for other causes of weight gain, primary causes of obesity or secondary consequences
3. Client counselling to identify any management problems and convince them of the benefits of weight reduction
4. Assessment of target weight: 12–15% less than present in dogs, 13% less than present in cats
5. Selection of type and quantity of diet: 40–60% of MER at target weight in dogs, 60% of MER at target weight in cats
6. Regular re-evaluation: reduce food intake by 10% if no weight lost in target period. Set new target weights as necessary
7. Selection of type and quantity of maintenance diet when target weight achieved
8. Regular follow-up to prevent recurrence of obesity

For this reason, it has been suggested in humans that weight loss in excess of 1% per week requires special justification. Starvation is contraindicated in cats due to the risk of hepatic lipidosis in this species. Weight loss in cats should be controlled and it is particularly important to ensure obese cats continue to eat after diet changes to prevent this potentially fatal problem from developing.

Owner compliance is essential. Management problems will have been identified while taking the history and should be addressed and the benefits of weight loss and possible consequences of obesity should be explained. Diplomacy and care are necessary at this stage as the owner should be happy and convinced of the benefits of weight loss in their animal if the programme is to be successful.

Obesity management should ideally start with prevention in the puppy and kitten. Feeding and the long-term consequences of juvenile obesity should be discussed at the first vaccination and the animal weighed and condition scored on every visit to the surgery. Particular attention should be paid to dietary advice in susceptible breeds and at times when weight gain is likely such as after neutering or orthopaedic surgery.

Dieting of the obese adult animal begins with setting a target weight. In very obese animals, it is advisable to diet in steps by setting several targets rather than aiming to lose all the necessary weight at once. This provides a psychological stimulus for the owner and allows reassessment by the veterinarian to give a more accurate final target weight. The target generally aimed for in dogs is 12–15% weight loss over 12 weeks. In cats, it is important to control the rate of weight loss carefully but a mean loss of 13.5% over 18 weeks has been found to be safe (Butterwick et al., 1994).

When the target has been set, the type and quantity of diet fed should be considered. The animal may be fed a reduced amount of its normal diet but this has several disadvantages. The nutrient content of pet food is balanced to the energy content so feeding significantly less than maintenance may result in nutrient deficiencies. In addition, owner compliance may be improved by a change in diet particularly if feeding inappropriate food contributed to the problem in the first place. Commercial low calorie diets are formulated to minimize the risk of nutrient deficiencies. They rely on either an increased fibre content or a formulation without a high fibre content but with low energy density. Fibre has traditionally been used because it is thought to reduce the feeling of hunger, but recent work suggests it has little effect on long-term satiety and the regulation of energy intake, hence the introduction of non-fibre based diets. The type of fibre may be important, with soluble fibre inducing satiety more effectively than insoluble, but soluble fibre may also cause bloating and loose faeces which are generally unacceptable (Markwell and Butterwick, 1994). High-fibre diets have been used successfully in cats as well as dogs although it is presently unclear how well normal cats cope metabolically with increased dietary fibre (Maskell and Graham, 1994).

The amount of food to be fed is calculated from the target weight and MER of the animal. In dogs, the MER for the target weight should be calculated and the animal given a calorie intake of 40–60% of this. If sufficient loss is not achieved after 12 weeks then calorie intake may be reduced by a further 10%. It is obviously important to avoid tit-bits and high energy supplements. In cats, it is recommended that 60% of the MER at target weight is fed, using the equation for active cats of MER = 80 kcal kg^{-1} bodyweight day^{-1}. Again, if satisfactory weight loss is not achieved over 18 weeks then the calorie intake may be reduced by 10%.

It is advisable to offer food in two or three meals a day rather than one to increase the energy lost via meal-induced thermogenesis. On average, 10% of the body's energy expenditure is in the form of meal-induced heat, some as a result of energy expended on food utilization and the rest produced by brown adipose tissue and sustained for several hours following a meal. The amount of thermogenesis by brown adipose tissue varies with environmental temperature and calorie intake. It is stimulated by the sympathetic nervous system and increases when energy intake exceeds requirement. There appears to be a genetic element to this response, at least in humans and mice, where obesity is associated with a reduction in heat production after a meal which appears to be part of the cause, rather than the effect, of weight gain. Unfortunately, meal-induced thermogenesis tends to reduce in weight loss programmes. This to some extent counteracts the efforts to lose weight.

Increasing exercise can help energy expenditure and weight loss but its contribution to reducing obesity should not be overexaggerated and it should be used as an alternative to reducing calorie intake. The benefits of exercise have not been properly quantified in obese cats and dogs but it has been calculated that energy requirements are increased to 11.3% above resting levels in a 25 kg dog undergoing typical levels of activity. The effect of exercise on energy expenditure is therefore limited but it is wise to increase exercise as well as reduce calorie intake, provided both owner and pet are physically capable of this.

Increasing exercise is relatively easy in dogs but more difficult in cats where it may involve allowing them outdoors or encouraging play.

During the weight loss programme, the animal should be frequently reassessed and weighed and new targets set or changes in food intake implemented as necessary. Once the target weight has been achieved, the animal should be maintained on an appropriate maintenance diet which may involve either continuing with the low calorie diet or changing to another commercial food. Feeding home-made diets should be strongly discouraged due to the increased incidence of obesity on these. The animal should be fed sufficient to maintain a stable body weight and it has been suggested that this is equivalent to no greater than 10% more than the final calorie intake during treatment. It is important to re-examine the animal frequently, at least initially, to ensure that the weight is maintained with no recurrence of obesity.

Finally, various pharmacological means of managing uncomplicated obesity have been tried in humans and dogs. These include thyroid hormone, growth hormone, ketosteroids, β-adrenergic agonists, α-adrenergic antagonists and anorectic drugs such as fenfluramine. Work on these is limited and their long-term use is unproven so drug therapy is not presently applicable for the obese dog, except specifically to treat a complicating cause.

REFERENCES

Butterwick, R.F., Wills, J.M., Sloth, C and Markwell, P.J. (1994) A Study of obese cats on a calorie-controlled weight reduction programme. *Veterinary Record* **134**, 372–377.

Donoghue, S. (1989) Nutritional support of hospitalised patients. *Veterinary Clinics of North America: Small Animal Practice* **19**, 475–495.

Edney, A.T.B. and Smith, P.M. (1986) Study of obesity in dogs visiting veterinary practices in the United Kingdom. *Veterinary Record* **118**, 391–396.

Hammer, A.S. (1994) Nutrition and cancer. In: *The Waltham Book of Clinical Nutrition of the Dog and Cat* (Eds. Wills, J.M. and Simpson, K.W.) Pergamon, pp. 75–85.

Hand, M.S., Armstrong, P.J. and Allen, T.A. (1989) Obesity: occurrence, treatment and prevention. *Veterinary Clinics of North America: Small Animal Practice* **19**, 447–474.

Markwell, P.J. and Butterwick, R.F. (1994) Obesity. In: *The Waltham Book of Clinical Nutrition of the Dog and Cat* (Eds. Wills, J.M. and Simpson, K.W.) Pergamon, pp. 131–148.

Maskell, I.E. and Graham, P.A. (1994) Endocrine disorders. In: *The Waltham Book of Clinical Nutrition of the Dog and Cat* (Eds. Wills, J.M. and Simpson, K.W.) Pergamon, pp. 373–389.

4

Fever and Hypothermia

J. K. Dunn

FEVER

Fever (pyrexia), defined as an increase in body temperature, is a common manifestation of numerous clinical disorders. To understand the significance of fever in a clinical setting it is necessary to have a basic understanding of normal thermoregulation and the pathophysiological mechanisms which may give rise to a febrile state.

Thermoregulation

In humans and experimental animals it has been shown that body temperature is subject to daily variation, being lowest in the morning and highest in the evening. Body temperature is controlled by the thermoregulatory centre located in the preoptic region of the anterior hypothalamus. The thermal 'set-point' is maintained by a delicate equilibrium between heat production and heat loss mechanisms (Fig. 4.1). Normal body temperature is maintained within a relatively narrow range (37.8–39.3°C in dogs; 38.0–39.2°C in cats) despite exposure to a wide range of environmental temperatures. Alterations in ambient and core body temperatures are sensed by peripheral and central thermoreceptors; the effector arm of the reflex arc consists of those organs or systems which are capable of either conserving or dissipating body heat, i.e. skin, muscle and respiratory system. Specific mediators such as noradrenaline and 5-hydroxytryptamine, act on the thermoregulatory centre to alter (raise) the thermal set-point in the febrile state. True fever should be differentiated from other hyperthermic states where the thermal set-point is not increased (see below).

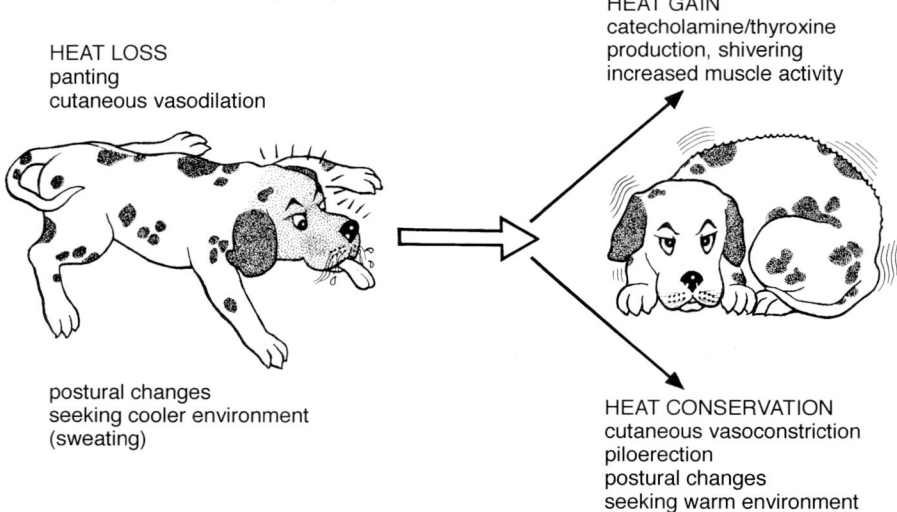

Fig. 4.1 Normal thermoregulation. The mechanisms for increasing body temperature are generally mediated by the sympathetic nervous system whereas those which lower body temperature are regulated by the parasympathetic nervous system. Dogs and cats possess few sweat glands and lose excess body heat by panting.

PATHOPHYSIOLOGY

Exogenous pyrogens

Numerous agents, termed exogenous pyrogens, may induce a febrile response. These include Gram-negative and Gram-positive bacteria, bacterial endotoxin, viruses, fungi, parasites, toxins, tumours, bile acids, drugs (including certain steroids and tetracyclines) and substances released from necrotic tissue. Strictly speaking the term exogenous pyrogen is misleading since most exogenous pyrogens are not themselves directly pyrogenic, i.e. they do not act directly on the thermoregulatory centre. They do so via the release of a group of common cell-derived chemical mediators referred to collectively as endogenous pyrogens.

Endogenous pyrogens

Most endogenous pyrogens are thought to be low-molecular-weight polypeptides which can cross the blood–brain barrier. They act directly on the thermoregulatory centre and increase the thermal set-point by induction of prostaglandin E synthesis. There are a number of sources of endogenous pyrogen: bone marrow-derived polymorphonuclear leucocytes (neutrophils, eosinophils) and mononuclear macrophages, either circulating (monocytes) or fixed in organs (Kupffer cells of the liver, splenic and alveolar macrophages). Several immunological mediators released by endotoxin-activated macrophages can be classified as endogenous pyrogens. These mediators include interleukin-1 (IL-1), tumour necrosis factor (TNF), interferons and prostaglandins. Some of these mediators, for example TNF, in turn elicit the production and release of other cytokines (eicosanoids) which are also capable of inducing a febrile response. Although structurally distinct, IL-1 and TNF share many of the same biological properties; for example both are involved in the generation of the acute phase response and both are thought to be responsible for the systemic effects (e.g. anorexia and depression) which are usually associated with fever. Sensitized lymphocytes release soluble cytokines which stimulate the production of endogenous pyrogens from leucocytes and macrophages. Some tumour cells release endogenous pyrogen without prior stimulation by an exogenous agent. In addition to prostaglandin E, other chemical mediators such as prostaglandin precursors, cyclic AMP and the monoamines, noradrenaline and 5-hydroxytryptamine, released in inflammatory and non-inflammatory conditions, may also contribute to the production of fever.

ADVERSE VERSUS BENEFICIAL EFFECTS OF FEVER

The beneficial effects of fever are often overlooked. The decision to suppress a febrile response should be made after weighing up the adverse effects of fever against those for allowing it to run its course. Interleukin-1 is one of the major mediators of the acute phase response which is characterized by fever, decreased serum concentrations of iron and zinc, and the synthesis and release by the liver of acute phase proteins, including haptoglobin, ceruloplasmin, C-reactive protein and fibrinogen. The decrease in serum iron in particular is thought to play an important role in inhibiting the replication of bacteria and certain viruses for which iron is an essential element. In addition to promoting a period of rest, fever is known to alter the immune response in several ways. Endogenous pyrogens can increase granulocyte mobility and enhance the bactericidal and phagocytic activities of granulocytes and macrophages. IL-1 and TNF enhance lymphocyte transformation, T cell activation and T cell responses during antigen presentation. It has also been shown that animals with experimentally induced sepsis have a higher mortality rate if they do not develop a febrile response (Hardie *et al.*, 1986). In most cases, therefore, there is an argument for allowing moderate fevers to run their course. Whenever possible, treatment should be specifically directed at the primary disease process responsible for the fever and symptomatic treatment using antipyretic agents should only be considered if the fever and the non-specific clinical signs which accompany it (weight loss, anorexia, lethargy etc.) become particularly severe or prolonged, or the cause of the fever cannot be ascertained.

TYPES OF FEVER

Fever can be classified on the basis of duration and periodicity as follows.

- *Intermittent (undulating) fever* is characterized by febrile episodes lasting one or more days

with intervening periods of normal temperature.
- *Sustained (persistent) fever* typically lasts for several days or even weeks with minimal variation between successive meaurements.
- *Remittent (septic) fevers* are usually caused by acute bacterial infections and are characterized by daily increases in body temperature (fever 'spikes') with intervening periods of normal or subnormal temperature.

True fever should be differentiated from non-pyrogenic causes of hyperthermia in which the thermal set-point is not raised. Causes of non-pyrogenic hyperthermia include heat stroke, malignant hyperthermia, over-exertion, primary hypothalamic lesions, drug reactions, grand mal seizure activity (increased muscle activity) and hypermetabolic states such as hyperthyroidism and phaeochromocytoma. Temperatures greater than 41°C (105.8°F) generally are usually not true fevers. They are nevertheless potentially life-threatening and require emergency treatment to prevent irreversible damage to the brain (cerebral oedema), liver and kidneys.

FEVER OF UNKNOWN ORIGIN

The term fever of unknown origin (FUO) describes a syndrome characterized by prolonged or intermittent febrile episodes where there are no other specific clinical signs that would define a separate syndrome. In humans the criteria for defining FUO are as follows:

- Fever of more than three weeks duration associated with non-specific signs of illness such as lethargy, anorexia and weight loss;
- Temperature at least 0.8°C (1.5°F) above normal on several occasions;
- Diagnosis uncertain after one week of hospitalization and routine laboratory tests.

Fulfilment of these criteria can be helpful in eliminating short-lived pyrexias of infectious origin, postoperative fevers and hyperthermia due to heat stroke and over-exertion. It is doubtful, however, whether these same criteria can be used to define FUO in dogs and cats since, in a practical setting at least, the definition of 'fever of unknown origin' will be influenced by the extent and nature of the initial laboratory investigations employed. For this reason it could be argued that a true FUO case is one where the diagnosis is still obscure after performing a series of preliminary screening tests such as those described below.

Pathophysiological basis of fever of unknown origin

The major causes of FUO can be discussed under four major headings:

1. Localized and systemic infections
2. Immune-mediated disorders
3. Neoplasia
4. Miscellaneous disorders

In one survey, infections (40%), immune-mediated disorders (20%) and neoplasia (20%) accounted for the majority of FUO cases (Feldman, 1980). Approximately 10% of cases can be attributed to miscellaneous causes; the remaining 10% represent those cases which remain undiagnosed and are truly FUO. A retrospective survey undertaken at the Department of Clinical Veterinary Medicine, University of Cambridge showed that approximately 32% of FUO cases had primary bone marrow problems (leukaemias, myeloma or true aplastic anaemia) or solid tumours (mostly lymphomas) and 22% had immune-mediated disorders (mostly inflammatory polyarthropathies). Infection was confirmed in only 16%; miscellaneous causes (portosystemic shunts, sterile, steroid-responsive meningitis and metaphyseal osteopathy) accounted for 12%, and 18% remained undiagnosed (Dunn and Dunn, 1998).

Infection

Bacterial endocarditis resulting in intermittent thromboembolic episodes is reported to be the most common systemic infection causing FUO in the dog (Feldman, 1980). Systemic mycoses are often characterized by persistent or intermittent fever associated with chronic wasting, skin lesions, ophthalmic lesions, osteomyelitis, and granulomatous lesions in many viscera including the lungs. Early cases of pyothorax or inhaled bronchial foreign bodies may present without obvious respiratory signs. Other localized infections such as uterine stump pyometra, pyelonephritis and prostatic abscesses should also be considered as potential causes of unexplained fever. Viral infections are generally self-limiting. In the cat the feline leukaemia virus (FeLV) and its associated diseases, and feline immunodeficiency virus (FIV) are important causes of FUO since the immunosuppressive and, in the case of FeLV, myelodysplastic effects of these viruses predispose the host to recurrent bacterial infections.

The conditions most commonly associated with bacteraemia in one study were malignant neoplasms, discospondylitis and infections of the cardiovascular and urogenital systems. Bacteraemia, in the absence of an obvious source of infection, appears to be rare but may occur with aplastic anaemia and certain myeloproliferative disorders which result in persistent neutropenia (Gorman and Evans, 1987).

Immune-mediated disorders

Antigen–antibody complexes activate complement which leads to the release of several potent inflammatory-inducing agents, most notably $C3_a$ and $C5_a$ which attract neutrophils and macrophages to the site(s) of immune complex deposition. The ensuing removal of immune complexes is associated with the release of endogenous pyrogen by phagocytic cells. Immune-mediated polyarthritis, either the primary or idiopathic form or less frequently as a manifestation of systemic lupus erythematosus (SLE), is probably the most common cause of FUO in the dog. Feline infectious peritonitis is the most common multisystemic immune complex disease in cats.

A number of primary (congenital) and secondary (acquired) immunodeficiency syndromes have been recognized in the dog. Many of these occur in certain breeds (Table 4.1).

Neoplasia

Fever may be a manifestation of malignancy long before the underlying tumour becomes apparent (Feldman, 1980). Some tumour cells produce and release endogenous pyrogen without prior stimulation by exogenous pyrogen. Lymphoproliferative and myeloproliferative disorders often present with a history of intermittent fever spikes which may reflect altered humoral or cellular immune function or defective neutrophil function and a predisposition to transient bacteraemic episodes. Neutropenia, occurring either as part of a preleukaemic syndrome or as a result of bone marrow infiltration with neoplastic haemopoietic cells, also predisposes to secondary infection.

Table 4.1 Causes of primary and secondary immunodeficiency

Primary defects in non-specific immunity
- Immotile cilia syndrome resulting in recurrent respiratory infections (springer spaniel, old English sheepdog, English setter, West Highland white terrier, pointers and other breeds)
- Canine cyclical haemopoiesis (grey collies)
- Canine granulocytopathy in Irish setters (deficiency of leucocyte adhesion proteins)
- Bone marrow dyscrasia in miniature and toy poodles
- Defective neutrophil bactericidal activity in Dobermanns
- Complement (C3) deficiency in Brittany spaniels
- Pelger–Huet anomaly (foxhounds)
- Neutrophil function defect in collie breeds?

Defects in specific immunity
- Combined immunodeficiency syndrome in dachshunds, corgis and basset hounds
- Thymosin-responsive wasting syndrome in growth hormone deficient weimeraners
- Chronic rhinitis and pneumonia in Irish wolfhounds with low serum IgA levels
- Immunodeficiency syndrome characterized by low serum IgA and IgG concentrations in weimeraners
- Transient hypogammaglobulinaemia (samoyeds)
- Selective IgA deficiency (beagles, Chinese shar pei, German shepherd dog)
- Selective IgM deficiency (Dobermanns)
- T cell immunodeficiency in weimeraners
- Lethal acrodermatitis (bull terriers)

Secondary immunodeficiency syndromes
Immunodeficiency may occur secondary to a number of infections (e.g. generalized demodicosis, canine distemper and parvovirus infections, ehrlichiosis, aspergillosis and protracted bacterial infections) and haemopoietic neoplasia. Nutritional problems (e.g. zinc deficiency), drugs (e.g. prolonged glucocorticoid therapy, cytotoxic agents), and endocrinopathies (hyperadrenocorticism and diabetes mellitus) may also predispose to recurrent infection.

Miscellaneous disorders

Miscellaneous causes of FUO include metaphyseal osteopathy, panosteitis, liver disease (portosystemic shunts or hepatic necrosis, which may result in intermittent endotoxaemia), inflammatory or granulomatous bowel disease, pulmonary thromboembolism and drug reactions.

Table 4.2 Conditions which can present with fever of unknown origin

Dogs	Cats
Systemic infections	*Systemic infections*
Bacterial endocarditis	Feline immunodeficiency virus (FIV) infection
Bacteraemias from an inapparent focus	Feline leukaemia virus (FeLV) infection
Protozoal infections (disseminated toxoplasmosis, neosporosis, leishmaniasis, babesiosis)	Feline infectious anaemia (*Haemobartonella felis*)
Lyme disease (acute)	Feline infectious peritonitis (FIP)
Leptospirosis	Bacteraemias from an inapparent focus
Mycobacterium sp.	Sytemic mycoses (e.g. histoplasmosis, cryptococcosis)
Rickettsial disease (e.g. ehrlichiosis, haemobartonellosis)	
Disseminated mycotic infections (e.g. histoplasmosis, blastomycosis, cryptococcosis, coccidioidomycosis)	
Psittacosis	
Localized infections	*Localized infections*
Bacterial endocarditis	Pyothorax and lung infections (e.g. pulmonary abscess, bronchopneumonia)
Urogenital infections (e.g. pyelonephritis, chronic prostatitis/prostatic abscess, stump pyometra)	Occult hepatitis abscess or cholangiohepatitis
Pyothorax and lung infections (e.g. inhaled pulmonary foreign bodies/pulmonary abscess, bronchopneumonia)	Urogenital infections (e.g. pyelonephritis)
Occult hepatic abscess or cholangitis	Localized peritonitis
Localized peritonitis	Osteomyelitis
Discospondylitis	Cat bite abscess/cellulitis
Osteomyelitis (especially disseminated haematogenous osteomyelitis in young dogs)	
Neoplasia	*Neoplasia*
Lymphoproliferative or myeloproliferative disease	FeLV-related lymphoproliferative and myeloproliferative disorders
Large neoplasms (especially hepatic tumours) with necrotic centres	
Immune-mediated disease	*Immune-mediated disease*
Systemic lupus erythematosus (SLE)	Feline infectious peritonitis
Immune-mediated polyarthropathy:	Systemic lupus erythematosus (rare in cats)
rheumatoid arthritis (erosive)	Chronic progressive polyarthropathy:
idiopathic polyarthritis (non-erosive)	ankylosing (periosteal proliferative) form
Autoimmune haemolytic anaemia	luxating (erosive) form
Immune-mediated thrombocytopenia	Autoimmune haemolytic anaemia
Sterile steroid-responsive meningitis (immune-mediated?)	Immune-mediated thrombocytopenia
Miscellaneous disorders	*Miscellaneous disorders*
Drug reactions: tetracycline, sulphonamides, penicillin, amphotericin B, quinidine	Drug reactions: tetracycline, levamisole
Metaphyseal osteopathy	
Panosteitis	
Inflammatory/granulomatous bowel disease	
Hepatic necrosis	
Pulmonary emboli	
Nodular panniculitis	
Pansteatitis	
Hypervitaminosis A	

INVESTIGATION OF FUO

The list of differential diagnoses for FUO is extensive (Table 4.2). Infection is responsible for many cases of unexplained fever and should be ruled out first. Since the initial presenting signs are often non-specific and tend to vary in intensity, repeated physical examinations and laboratory tests are usually necessary to detect new clinical signs as soon as they develop so that further investigations may be directed towards a specific body system. The main aim of the diagnostic investigations is to define a syndrome other than FUO.

HISTORY CHECKLIST

❏ **Age, sex, breed?**

❏ **Vaccination status?**

❏ **Diet?**
An exclusively fish diet may lead to pansteatitis.

❏ **Geographical location and travel outside the United Kingdom?**

❏ **Lifestyle?**
Free-roaming cats are more susceptible to FeLV and FIV infections.

❏ **Duration of illness?**

❏ **Recurring or persistent clinical signs?**

❏ **Previous illness or recent surgery?**

❏ **Trauma?**

❏ **Localized or shifting lameness?**

❏ **Recent drug administration?**
A favourable response to antibiotics implies an infectious aetiology. Prior injudicious treatment with glucocorticoids may not only mask clinical signs but can significantly influence the results of laboratory tests.

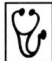

PHYSICAL EXAMINATION

❏ **Pyrexic?**
When taking an animal's temperature the degree of stress or excitement, the environmental temperature, and the distance travelled to the surgery should be considered. An increase in body temperature up to 39.5°C (103°F) is less likely to be significant than a temperature greater than 40°C (104°F) which in most cases can be regarded as a significant clinical finding. Having established the animal is febrile the type of fever (sustained, intermittent or remittent) should be ascertained early in the course of the investigation by recording the temperature three or four times daily over at least a 24 h period (preferably over a 72 h period).

❏ **Lymphadenopathy?**

❏ **Enlargement of liver, spleen or kidneys?**

❏ **Petechial or ecchymotic haemorrhages on the skin, mucosae or retinae?**

❏ **Cardiac murmurs (systolic or diastolic)?**
A murmur which develops during the course of the disease is suggestive of bacterial endocarditis although the absence of a murmur does not preclude this diagnosis.

❏ **Localized pain (neck, back or abdomen)?**

❏ **Ulcerative skin lesions or oral ulcers?**

❏ **Joint pain, joint effusion or periarticular soft tissue swelling?**
Immune-mediated polyarthropathies frequently involve the carpal and tarsal joints first whereas infective arthritides tend to involve the larger more proximal joints.

❏ **Rectal examination (prostatomegaly)?**

❏ **Ophthalmic examination (chorioretinitis, retinal detachment and/or haemorrhage, anterior uveitis)?**
Many disseminated infections (FeLV, toxoplasmosis, feline infectious peritonitis and systemic mycoses) can present with ocular lesions.

INITIAL DIAGNOSTIC PLAN

In the absence of localizing clinical signs the diagnostic plan may be divided conveniently into two phases. The first phase consists of a series of simple screening tests to establish the presence of a septic, inflammatory or neoplastic focus. The more elaborate diagnostic procedures which comprise the second phase of the investigation are based on the results of the preliminary screening tests and/or the presence of new clinical signs or laboratory findings.

■ Preliminary screening tests

- Routine haematology (including a platelet count)
- Complete biochemical profile
- Routine urinalysis including microscopic examination of urine sediment
- Total plasma protein and plasma fibrinogen concentrations. (In small animals hyperfibrinogenaemia is a non-specific indicator of an inflammatory process)
- FeLV and FIV assays in cats
- Lateral thoracic and abdominal radiographs to localize a septic, inflammatory or neoplastic focus. Long bones and joints should also be radiographed in cases with a history of shifting leg lameness.
- ±Urine culture and sensitivity
- ±Faecal examination (worm egg count, culture, occult blood) especially if there is a history of diarrhoea.

■ Additional diagnostic procedures

The index of suspicion for a particular disease, based on the results of the preliminary screening tests, dictates the most appropriate test(s) for any one situation. The indications for the procedures listed below are summarized in Table 4.3.

Blood cultures

Blood cultures are indicated in most FUO cases (more specific indications are given in Table 4.3). In order to maximize the chances of a positive result, three or four blood samples should be collected aseptically over a 24 h period and submitted for aerobic and anaerobic culture. Each blood sample should, if possible, be collected from a different vein using standard aseptic technique. In order to minimize the risk of contamination a fresh needle should be attached to the syringe before transferring the blood to the appropriate culture media. The most frequently isolated bacteria in one study were *Staphylococcus* spp. and *Enterobacter* spp. (Hirsch *et al.*, 1984). Traditionally blood is taken either during a febrile episode or as the temperature is rising (although there is some evidence to suggest that culture during a febrile episode does not increase the frequency of positive results; Dow and Jones, 1989). Since bacteraemia in dogs with endocarditis is continuous the timing of the blood cultures is less important. Bacterial isolation rates in dogs with bacterial endocarditis vary between 50% and 80% (Calvert, 1982; Elwood *et al.*, 1993); a negative culture result does not rule out bacteraemia (repeated negative results can occur in confirmed cases of bacterial endocarditis). Antibiotics should be discontinued for at least two to seven days before sampling since they may delay or inhibit bacterial growth. Culture media which contain the anticoagulant polyanetholsulphate or antibiotic inhibitors in the form of drug-destroying enzymes or antibiotic resins, may improve detection rates. A result can be considered positive if at least two culture bottles, each taken at a different time, contain the same bacterial species.

Bone marrow aspiration

Bone marrow aspiration is indicated when fever is associated with an unexplained cytopenia (anaemia, neutropenia or thrombocytopenia), leucocytosis (neutrophilia, lymphocytosis or large numbers of atypical blood cells in the circulation) and hypergammaglobulinaemia. Bone marrow aspiration and biopsy techniques are described in Chapter 45.

Synovial fluid aspirates

Aspiration of joint fluid is indicated when fever is accompanied by a history of intermittent or shifting leg lamenes, joint pain or periarticular soft tissue swelling.

Electrocardiography and echocardiography

Electrocardiography is indicated in patients showing clinical signs of heart failure or which have cardiac arrhythmias (bacterial endocarditis involving the mitral or aortic valves may progress to congestive heart failure or occasionally result in thromboembolic myocarditis associated with premature ventricular contractions). Echocardiography is the most useful diagnostic aid for confirming the presence of vegetative thrombi on the heart valves or mural endocardium.

Immunodiagnostic screening tests

Most immunodiagnostic screening tests employ species-specific reagents, often antiglobulins. The results of such tests should always be interpreted in association with appropriate clinical signs and

Table 4.3 Fever of unknown origin: indications for diagnostic procedures

Diagnostic procedure	Indications based on problems identified from the history, physical examination and initial laboratory and radiographic procedures
Blood culture	Systolic or diastolic cardiac murmur Neutropenia or neutrophilia (± left shift) Shifting leg lameness Back, bone or joint pain
Bone marrow aspiration	Anaemia, thrombocytopenia and/or neutropenia Leucocytosis/suspected leukaemia (e.g. unexplained neutrophilia, lymphocytosis or large numbers of atypical white blood cells in peripheral blood)
Synovial fluid aspiration (joint tap)	History of shifting leg lameness with back or joint pain and periarticular swelling Neutrophilia ±hyperfibrinogenaemia
Electrocardiography	Congestive heart failure especially if dysrhythmia (e.g. myocarditis)
Echocardiography	Cardiac murmur±dysrhythmia suggestive of bacterial endocarditis
Immunodiagnostic screening tests	
Rheumatoid factor	As for joint aspirates and blood culture
Antinuclear antibodies	As for joint aspirates and blood culture Ulcerative/vesicular cutaneous or oral lesions Persistent proteinuria
Direct antiglobulin test (Coombs' test)	Haemolytic anaemia Thrombocytopenia (especially if positive for antiplatelet antibodies)
Antiplatelet antibodies	Thrombocytopenia Coombs' positive anaemia
Serum protein electrophoresis ±immunoelectrophoresis	Abnormal total serum/plasma proteins Hypergammaglobulinaemia
Serology (toxoplasmosis, borreliosis, feline infectious peritonitis, ehrlichiosis, aspergillosis and other systemic mycoses)	Fundic lesions e.g. chorioretinitis, retinal detachment (toxoplasmosis, FIP, systemic mycoses) Anterior uveitis (FIP, toxoplasmosis, systemic mycoses) Discospondylitis (*Brucella canis*) Polyarthropathy (Lyme disease) Increased total serum/plasma proteins, especially if increased globulin fraction (FIP, ehrlichiosis)
Immune function tests, e.g. immunoelectrophoresis, neutrophil function tests, complement assays, lymphocyte blastogenesis	Cause of FUO cannot be established; congenital or acquired immunodeficiency syndrome suspected
Specialized radiographic techniques	
Double contrast cystography (with abdominal ultrasound examination)	Prostatomegaly
Barium meal	Persistent melaena
Technetium-^{99m}-labelled leucocyte scan	Unable to establish cause of FUO
Exploratory laparotomy	Abdominal mass Enlarged spleen or liver Unexplained abdominal pain
Biopsy	Abnormal renal or hepatic function tests Ulcerative/vesicular cutaneous or oral lesions (additional immunofluorescent studies may be indicated)
Therapeutic trial	Diagnosis cannot be established after extensive investigation

other laboratory test results. Consideration should be given to the diagnostic significance of positive results since all of the tests described below can produce false negative and false positive results and the significance of a given titre is influenced by the type of test and the methodology used.

Rheumatoid factor (RF)

Rheumatoid factor is an IgM autoantibody that is directed against the animal's native IgG (IgG and IgA rheumatoid factors have also been detected). RF titres of 1:16 or greater are generally considered positive and consistent with a diagnosis of rheumatoid arthritis in cases where there are appropriate clinical and radiographic signs. Like most immunodiagnostic screening tests false negative and false positive results may occur. Not every dog with rheumatoid arthritis for example has a RF titre, and low titres may be recorded in healthy dogs and in dogs with SLE and bacterial endocarditis.

Antinuclear antibody (ANA)

Antinuclear antibodies are directed against constituents of the cell nucleus and nuclear membrane (double stranded DNA and other soluble nuclear proteins). Low ANA titres have been reported in normal dogs but titres greater than 1:20 (or 1:80 depending on the substrate) are usually considered significant. Some cases of canine SLE remain ANA-negative throughout the course of the disease and conversely, some dogs with non-immunological diseases such as lymphoma, bacterial endocarditis and myelogenous leukaemia may have positive ANA tests.

Direct antiglobulin test (Coombs' test)

The direct antiglobulin (Coombs') test detects autoantibodies or complement components (usually C3) bound to the patient's red cells. The test should be performed at 4°C and 37°C to detect both warm and cold agglutinating antibodies. It has been shown that some healthy dogs and cats have a low agglutinating titre at 4°C and positive Coombs' tests have been documented in animals with numerous infectious, inflammatory and neoplastic disorders including malignant lymphoma, myeloproliferative disease and bacterial endocarditis. Positive titres therefore require cautious interpretation especially when there is no clinical or laboratory evidence of haemolysis. Causes of false positive and false negative tests are given in Chapter 45.

Antiplatelet antibodies

Direct and indirect fluorescent antibody tests and an Elisa test for detecting the presence of antiplatelet antibodies are described in Chapter 45 (see immune-mediated thrombocytopenia).

Serum protein electrophoresis and immunoelectrophoresis

Protein electrophoresis is indicated when a chronic inflammatory process is suspected or when the total plasma protein concentration is abnormal. A polyclonal increase in the gamma-globulin fraction is most commonly associated with viral infections, especially feline infectious peritonitis, chronic bacterial infections, parasitic infections such as ehrlichiosis and leishmaniasis, and immune-mediated disorders such as SLE, autoimmune haemolytic anaemia or thrombocytopenia and idiopathic polyarthritis. A monoclonal gamma globulin peak is more consistent with plasma cell myeloma and, less frequently, functional B cell lymphomas; a monoclonal gammopathy may also occasionally occur with cases of ehrlichiosis.

Decreased gammaglobulin concentrations usually occur with concomitant decreases in other serum protein fractions and are associated with numerous debilitating disorders such as lymphoma and other malignant neoplasms. Low concentrations of specific immunoglobulin subclasses may occur with various primary immunodeficiency syndromes, for example, a syndrome characterized by chronic rhinitis and pneumonia occurs in association with low serum IgA levels in Irish wolfhounds (see Table 4.1).

Serology

Serological tests are available for toxoplasmosis, feline infectious peritonitis, borreliosis (Lyme disease), brucellosis and numerous mycotic infections, including aspergillosis.

The first of paired serum samples should be collected in the evaluation of the patient with FUO, especially if ocular lesions are present, and stored at −20°C. A rising titre, based on a second sample taken 2–3 weeks later, is usually regarded as being diagnostically significant.

Immune function tests

Certain primary immunodeficiency syndromes are associated with a decrease in the serum concentration of a specific immunoglobulin subclass (see above under immunoelectrophoresis). *Tests to evaluate neutrophil function* require specialized equipment and must be performed on fresh cells within two hours of collection. Diagnosis of neutrophil dysfunction involves in vitro assessment of their chemotactic, adhesion and bactericidal properties. One of the more commonly used neutrophil function tests is the nitroblue tetrazolium dye reduction test. This test assays the respiratory burst of the neutrophil following phagocytosis and provides a measurement of the cell's metabolic activity.

Complement activity can be measured using a 50% haemolytic complement (CH_{50}) assay. Specific components of the complement cascade, for example C3, can be assayed by radial immunodiffusion. Immune complex disease may result in a decrease in CH_{50} activity. The concentration of complement may also decrease with many infectious and non-infectious diseases as well as neoplasia. Complement assays must be performed the same day otherwise the serum should be frozen at –90°C.

The cell-mediated arm of the immune system can be evaluated in vitro by measuring *lymphocyte blastogenesis* and the uptake of tritiated thymidine in response to various mitogens.

Specialized radiographic techniques

The indications for contrast radiographic techniques are given in Table 4.3.

^{99m}Technetium-labelled leucocyte scan

Leucocytes can be labelled with ^{99m}technetium hexamethyl-propylene amine oxime (^{99m}Tc HMPAO). Technetium scans are widely used in human medicine for localizing various forms of inflammatory disease and infections. They are used as an aid to the diagnosis of inflammatory bowel disease, postoperative sepsis and acute and chronic osteomyelitis. Their use with regard to the investigation of fever of unknown origin has not been fully established. The essential requirement for their success is that the disease to be localized is associated with a neutrophilic (purulent or pyogenic) inflammatory response.

In dogs 20–30 ml of blood are collected into citrate phosphate dextrose (CPD) anticoagulant to provide approximately 3–4 ml of labelled leucocytes depending on the total white blood cell count. Leucocytes are separated following exposure to the technetium complex to provide a mixed leucocyte suspension. The labelled cells are re-injected in a bolus via an intravenous catheter. A major advantage of the scanning procedure is that no anaesthesia is required. Although this technique has yet to be fully evaluated in the diagnosis of FUO in dogs and cats and controlled studies have not been performed, preliminary results, using doses of technetium of 300–500 MBq per dog, at the Department of Clinical Veterinary Medicine, University of Cambridge have proved encouraging.

Exploratory laparotomy and surgical biopsy

Exploratory laparotomy and/or surgical biopsies are only indicated if the clinical signs or laboratory data indicate specific organ or system dysfunction.

Therapeutic trial

A therapeutic trial should only be undertaken when the cause of the fever cannot be ascertained. Corticosteroids, with appropriate antibiotic cover, should be administered with extreme caution and only after an animal fails to respond to broad spectrum antibiotics alone or to symptomatic treatment with non-steroidal antipyretic analgesic drugs.

MANAGEMENT OF FEVER

The symptomatic treatment of fever should be considered only when attempts to identify the underlying cause have proved unsuccessful and when patient discomfort is particularly severe. Fluid support and antibiotic cover should be given if necessary, for example, where fever is associated with life-threatening endotoxaemia. The doses for some of the common antipyretic drugs are given in Table 4.4. The antipyretic action of the non-steroidal anti-inflammatory group of drugs, which includes acetylsalicylic acid (aspirin), indomethacin and flunixin meglumine, is due to their antiprostaglandin action. In addition to its antipyretic properties the specific cyclo-oxygenase blocking action of flunixin meglumine may be of use in treating dogs with endotoxaemia since prostaglandins are important lipid mediators of endotoxic shock. Glucocorticoids block the synthesis of tumour necrosis factor, a cytokine mediator of endotoxic shock produced by activated macrophages. One practical disadvantage, however, is that these drugs are most effective if given before the onset of endotoxaemia, a point that is difficult if not impossible to predict. Prolonged use of non-steroidal anti-inflammatory drugs (NSAID) is not advised since side effects such as vomiting associated with gastric ulceration and haemorrhage are not uncommon. The dose of aspirin for cats is considerably less than that for dogs because of the marked reduction in hepatic clearance in this

Table 4.4 Doses of antipyretic agents used in dogs and cats

Drug	Dogs	Cats
Acetylsalicylic acid (aspirin)	10–25 mg kg^{-1} p.o. every 8–24 h	10 mg kg^{-1} p.o. every 48–72 h
Acetaminaphen	10–20 mg kg^{-1} p.o. every 12–24 h	Contraindicated
Dipyrone	25 mg kg^{-1} i.v., i.m. or s.c. every 8 h	As for dogs
Flunixin meglumine	0.5–1.0 mg kg^{-1} i.v., i.m. or p.o. once daily; maximum 3 days dosage	Not recommended

i.v., intravenously; i.m., intramuscularly; s.c., subcutaneously; p.o., per os.

species. The repeated use of dipyrone has been associated with bone marrow suppression and relatively small doses of paracetamol (1/4 of a 250 mg tablet) can result in Heinz body haemolytic anaemia in cats.

Management of non-pyrogenic causes of hyperthermia

Probably the most common example of non-pyrogenic hyperthermia is heat stroke. The animal's temperature may rise to 41–41.5°C and prompt and aggressive action is necessary to prevent irreversible damage to vital organs. Cold intravenous fluids (normal saline) should be administered and if possible the animal placed in a cold-water bath. Glucocorticoids (e.g. intravenous dexamethasone or betamethasone) are usually indicated to combat shock. Close patient monitoring is advised after the body temperature has returned to normal since some cases progress to disseminated intravascular coagulation 48–72 h after making an apparent recovery.

HYPOTHERMIA

Hypothermia occurs when the normal thermoregulatory mechanisms are no longer able to maintain core body temperature. Most frequently, hypothermia occurs in neonatal, geriatric or severely debilitated patients. Possible causes include acute decompensated congestive heart failure (cardiogenic shock associated with myocardial failure), severe hypothyroidism, prolonged immobilization either during surgical intervention or during anaesthetic recovery, and prolonged exposure to extreme cold. Clinical signs associated with hypothermia are shivering, decreased level of consciousness, bradycardia, weak pulse, depressed respiration and muscle stiffness. Treatment consists of actively rewarming the animal and minimizing further heat loss. Any underlying disease or acid–base disturbance should be treated appropriately. The animal should be placed on a heating pad or wrapped in blankets. 'Bubble wrap' also provides adequate insulation for the hypothermic patient. Warm intravenous fluids should be administered and if necessary peritoneal dialysis undertaken using warm normal saline. The patient should be rewarmed at a rate not exceeding 0.5–1.0°C h^{-1} and close monitoring is required to ensure ventricular fibrillation does not occur during the rewarming period.

REFERENCES

Calvert, C.A. (1982) Valvular bacterial endocarditis in the dog. *Journal of the American Veterinary Medical Association* **180**, 1080–1084.

Dow, S.W. and Jones, R.L. (1989) Bacteraemia: Pathogenesis and diagnosis, *Compendium of Continuing Education* **11**, 432–443.

Dunn, K.J. and Dunn, J.K. (1998) Diagnostic investigations in one hundred and one dogs with pyrexia of unknown origin. *Journal of Small Animal Practice* (in press).

Elwood, C.M., Cobb, M.A. and Stepien, R.L. (1993) Clinical and echocardiographic findings in 10 dogs with vegetative bacterial endocarditis. *Journal of Small Animal Practice* **34**, 420–427.

Feldman, B.F. (1980) Fever of undetermined origin. *Compendium of Continuing Education* **2**, 970–977.

Gorman, N.T. and Evans, R.J. (1987) Myeloproliferative disease in the dog and cat: Clinical presentations, diagnosis and treatment. *Veterinary Record* **121**, 490–496.

Hardie, E.M., Rawlings, C.A. and Calvert, C.A. (1986) Severe sepsis in selected small animal surgical patients. *Journal of the American Animal Hospital Association* **22**, 33–41.

Hirsch, C.C., Jang, S.S. and Biberstein, E.L. (1984) Blood culture of the canine patient. *Journal of the Veterinary Medicine Association* **84**, 175–178.

5

Vomiting

J. K. Dunn

Vomiting is an active process involving the coordinated, vigorous contraction of the abdominal, thoracic and diaphragmatic muscles and resulting in the forceful ejection of vomitus from the mouth. The act of vomiting may be preceded by a period of nausea characterized by depression, salivation, licking of the lips and repeated attempts to swallow. Regurgitation (see Chapter 6) is a passive process associated with minimal movement of the thoracic and abdominal muscles.

PATHOPHYSIOLOGY

The reflex act of vomiting involves the vomiting centre situated in the lateral reticular formation of the medulla oblongata. Neurones of the vomiting centre can be stimulated directly or indirectly via afferent impulses received from the chemoreceptor trigger zone, vestibular apparatus, higher centres in the cerebrocortex and peripheral receptors in the pharynx and abdominal viscera.

Direct stimulation of the vomiting centre

An increase in cerebrospinal fluid (CSF) pressure (e.g. hydrocephalus), cerebral oedema (e.g. following trauma), or central nervous system inflammation, infection or neoplasia may result in direct stimulation of the neurones of the vomiting centre.

Indirect stimulation of the vomiting centre

Indirect stimulation of the vomiting centre may occur via:
1. The chemoreceptor trigger zone (CTZ) located on the floor of the fourth ventricle. The CTZ may be stimulated by
   (a) drugs such as apomorphine, cardiac glycosides and certain antineoplastic agents (some drugs/toxins may directly stimulate the vomiting centre)
   (b) metabolic toxins associated with uraemia, hepatic failure and diabetic ketoacidosis (ketones)
   (c) bacterial endotoxins associated with Gram-negative sepsis (e.g. pyometra).
2. Vestibular afferent input via the vestibular branch of the eighth cranial nerve either as a result of inflammatory vestibular disease or motion sickness.
3. Stimulation of higher centres in the cerebrocortex e.g. severe pain, 'stress' or excitement (psychogenic vomiting).
4. Visceral afferent impulses from peripheral receptors located in the pharynx (via the glossopharyngeal nerve) or abdominal viscera, visceral peritoneum and urogenital tract (via the vagus and sympathetic nerves) which respond to distension, inflammation, rapid changes in osmolality and noxious chemicals or irritants.

Vomiting can be classified as acute or chronic, and gastric or non-gastric in origin (Tables 5.1 and 5.2). Acute gastritis is probably the single most common cause of transient vomiting in small animals although often a specific cause is not identified (transient vomiting in most young animals is often attributed to some form of dietary indiscretion). The normal gastric mucosal barrier with its layer of mucus is resistant to gastric acid and the proteolytic enzyme pepsin. Damage to the gastric mucosa results in back diffusion of acid into the submucosa, the release of histamine from mast cells and initiation of an inflammatory response. The proximal small intestine is frequently involved in the inflammatory process resulting in gastroenteritis with vomiting and diarrhoea.

Table 5.1 Gastric and non-gastric causes of acute vomiting

	Aetiology
Gastric causes	
Acute gastritis/gastroenteritis	
Dietary indiscretion	Ingestion of grass, foreign bodies, contaminated or decomposing food or rubbish; sudden change in diet or overeating; dietary intolerance
Toxins	Plant toxins, bacterial enterotoxins, uraemic toxins
Poisons	Ethylene gycol, heavy metals, cleaning agents, certain herbicides
Drugs	Non-steroidal anti-inflammatory drugs, e.g. aspirin, phenylbutazone, indomethacin, ibuprufen and flunixin; prolonged high doses of dexamethasone following intervertebral disc surgery
Infectious disease	
Viral	Canine distemper virus; canine parvovirus; infectious canine hepatitis virus (canine adenovirus 1); canine coronavirus
Bacterial	Leptospirosis (*Leptospira canicola*, *L. icterohaemorrhagiae*); salmonellosis; campylobacteriosis
Parasitic	Toxocariasis (vomiting occasionally associated with a heavy *Toxocara canis* burden)
Haemorrhagic gastroenteritis	Possibly represents an anaphylactic response to bacterial (?clostridial) toxins
Gastric dilatation	
Simple acute gastric dilatation	Usually seen in young pups and is associated with overeating
Gastric dilatation with volvulus	Seen most frequently in large deep-chested dogs (e.g. setters, boxers, Irish wolfhounds); possibly associated with the feeding of a large meal followed by a period of exercise
Non-gastric causes	
Acute complete obstruction of the proximal small intestine	Foreign body; intussusception; volvulus; strangulated hernia
Acute pancreatitis	May be associated with adbominal trauma, pancreatic surgery, feeding of high fat diets to obese dogs, prolonged administration of high doses of dexamethasone following intervertebral disc surgery
Acute hepatitis	Infectious causes, e.g. leptospirosis, infectious canine hepatitis; toxins
Acute renal failure	Acute interstitial nephritis, e.g. leptospirosis (*L. canicola*); acute glomerulonephritis; acute tubular necrosis (e.g. ethylene glycol toxicity, aminoglycoside toxicity, prolonged hypercalcaemia), renal ischaemia (e.g. associated with severe hypovolaemia)
Peritonitis	Intestinal perforation; bladder rupture; pancreatitis, ruptured pyometra
Pyometra	Vomiting due to endotoxaemia
Diabetic ketoacidosis	Direct action of ketone bodies on chemoreceptor trigger zone
Acute urethral obstruction	Urethral calculi or occasionally neoplasia (e.g. transitional cell carcinoma)
Hypoadrenocorticism	Acute Addisonian crisis; chronic form of the disease may cause intermittent vomiting
Acute vestibular disease	Motion sickness; vestibulitis; hydrocephalus; CNS neoplasia
Increased intracranial pressure	Cerebral oedema (head trauma); hydrocephalus; CNS neoplasia
Colitis	Vomiting associated with visceral pain (increased sympathetic activity?)

Table 5.2 Gastric and non-gastric causes of chronic vomiting

	Aetiology
Gastric causes	
Gastric retention	Vomiting occurs at a variable interval after feeding and occasionally may be described as projectile.
Pyloric stenosis	
Congenital	Most commonly recognized in brachycephalic breeds, e.g. boxers. Animal starts to vomit after weaning; condition caused by intrinsic hypertrophy of the circular smooth muscle of the pylorus.
Acquired	Occurs in association with antral polyps, gastric foreign bodies, gastric ulceration or neoplasia, and hyperplastic gastropathy.
Pylorospasm	Has been attributed as a primary cause of gastric outflow obstruction in toy or miniature breeds especially in young, very nervous or excitable animals; others suggest that the delayed gastric emptying represents an abnormality in gastric motility, i.e. gastric stasis. Gastric stasis may be associated with hypokalaemia, anticholinergic therapy, or as sequel to acute parvoviral enteritis or chronic gastric distension
Gastrointestinal obstruction	Vomiting may be a feature of (1) a gastric foreign body which intermittently either partially or completely obstructs the pylorus or (2) a partial intestinal obstruction associated with a foreign body, stricture, intussusception or neoplasia, e.g. adenocarcinoma of the small intestine.
Chronic gastritis	
Non-erosive	
Chronic superficial gastritis	Infiltration of the gastric mucosa with plasma cells and lymphocytes suggests an immune-mediated pathogenesis. Diagnosis: full thickness gastric biopsy
Chronic atrophic gastritis	Parietal cells replaced by mucus-producing cells which may result in secondary bacterial overgrowth and diarrhoea. Diagnosis: full thickness gastric biopsy
Chronic hyperplastic gastropathy	Macroscopic thickening of the gastric mucosa and rugal folds may result in gastric outflow obstruction. Aetiology uncertain; two known causes of gastric mucosal hypertrophy and ulceration are systemic mastocytosis (with resultant release of histamine) and hypergastrinaemia. Diagnosis: barium study, e.g. double contrast gastrogram, to show thickened rugal folds and a full thickness gastric biopsy
Eosinophilic gastritis	Diffuse infiltration of the stomach wall with eosinophils (occasionally discrete granulomatous nodules).
Erosive (see causes of gastric ulceration below)	
Gastric ulceration	Common sites for peptic ulcers are pyloric antrum, lesser curvature of the stomach and the proximal duodenum; may be associated with gastric neoplasia (see below), foreign bodies, pyloric stenosis and chronic gastritis; may occur as superficial erosions or deep indurated ulcer. Other causes include drugs (non-steroidal anti-inflammatory drugs and corticosteroids), chronic renal failure (uraemic gastropathy), hepatic failure, 'stress', systemic mastocytosis or mastocytomas (with release of histamine) and the Zollinger–Ellison syndrome associated with gastrin-producing tumours of the pancreas (gastrinomas). Diagnosis: contrast studies of the stomach, gastroscopy, laparotomy and gastric biopsy.
Gastric neoplasia	Adenocarcinomas in older dogs (>8 years old) and may involve pyloric antrum and cause gastric outflow obstruction. Diagnosis as for gastric ulceration.
Non-gastric causes	
Chronic renal failure	Associated with hypergastrinaemia which results in the increased secretion of gastric acid.
Chronic hypoadrenocorticism (see Table 5.1)	
Chronic liver disease/hepatic failure	Chronic active hepatitis, cholangiohepatitis, cirrhosis, hepatic neoplasia and portosystemic shunts
Chronic relapsing pancreatitis or pancreatic neoplasia	

COMPLICATIONS OF VOMITING

Dehydration

The loss of water with sodium via gastrointestinal tract secretions exacerbated by decreased fluid intake results in *dehydration* which, if severe enough, may lead to prerenal azotaemia especially in an animal which already has compromised renal function e.g. chronic renal insufficiency.

Electrolyte and acid–base disturbances

Persistent vomiting may result in *hyponatraemia*. The loss of sodium in excess of water causes the extracellular fluid to become hypotonic and water is taken into the cells by osmosis (hypotonic dehydration). This transfer of fluid to the cells further reduces the volume of the already depleted extracellular fluid compartment and may lead to vascular collapse (shock).

Persistent and profuse vomiting may lead to a deficit of total body potassium and *hypokalaemia*, signs of which include gastrointestinal ileus and muscle weakness. Hypokalaemia may also impair the ability of the renal tubules to concentrate urine which may worsen the dehydration.

Pyloric outflow obstruction or high duodenal obstruction resulting in the loss of hydrochloric acid may lead to *hypochloraemia* and the development of metabolic alkalosis. The latter may be accompanied by a paradoxical aciduria as the kidneys attempt to conserve bicarbonate ions to protect against the anion (chloride) deficit.

INVESTIGATION OF VOMITING

The severity and frequency of the vomiting (acute versus chronic), the nature (appearance) of the vomitus, the degree of weakness and depression, and the presence of serious, potentially life-threatening clinical signs such as dehydration, shock, collapse, fever or abdominal pain dictate the extent of the initial diagnostic investigations. Most cases of acute, uncomplicated gastritis or gastroenteritis caused by simple dietary indiscretion may be expected to resolve within 24–48 h and require only conservative management and supportive care, hence extensive laboratory and radiographic examinations are not justified.

HISTORY CHECKLIST

❑ Vomiting, regurgitating or retching?

True vomiting, as described above, must be differentiated from pharyngeal retching and regurgitation. Pharyngeal retching occurs immediately after the prehension of food. The animal becomes visibly distressed and has difficulty in swallowing (see Chapter 6 on dysphagia). Food and saliva may be expelled from the mouth and fluids may pass down the nose producing a bilateral nasal discharge. Inhalation of food particles results in paroxysms of non-productive coughing and ultimately aspiration pneumonia. It is also worth noting that paroxysmal bouts of coughing, regardless of the cause, frequently end with the animal gagging or retching and bringing up small amounts of clear mucus, phlegm or saliva, hence some owners may even confuse coughing with vomiting.

Regurgitation is indicative of an oesophageal lesion. The animal passively ejects food and saliva sometimes in the shape of a semi-formed tubular 'cast' with the head lowered and minimal contraction of the thoracic and abdominal muscles.

Causes of pharyngeal retching and regurgitation are listed in Table 5.3.

❑ Breed, age, sex and vaccination status?

Consider infectious causes of vomiting, e.g. canine distemper virus, canine parvovirus or feline panleukopenia virus infections in young animals which are not vaccinated. Gastric dilatation and volvulus is more common in large deep-chested breeds (setters, boxers, Irish wolfhounds). Pyloric stenosis is more common in brachycephalic breeds especially boxers.

❑ Age of animal when first started to vomit?

If the onset of vomiting is associated with weaning consider a vascular ring anomaly, pyloric stenosis or abnormality in gastric motility resulting in poor gastric emptying. If gastric outflow obstruction, vomiting may be projectile.

❑ Onset (acute or chronic), frequency and duration of vomiting?

An animal which has been vomiting only once or twice per day for 2–3 days and remains relatively bright and alert is less likely to require an extensive diagnostic work-up than an animal which has been vomiting intermittently for weeks/months and is showing signs of systemic disease (see below).

Table 5.3 Causes of pharyngeal retching and regurgitation

Pharyngeal retching	Comments
Pharyngitis/tonsillitis	
Cricopharyngeal achalasia	Possibly inherited in cocker spaniels
Retropharyngeal foreign body	
Animals may retch and bring up clear phlegm following a paroxysmal bout of coughing	
Regurgitation	
Megaoesophagus	
Congenital	Highest incidence in German shepherds, great Danes and Irish setters
Acquired	Idiopathic or associated with myasthenia gravis, polymyopathy, hypothyroidism, hypoadrenocorticism and lead poisoning; may also occur in association with a vascular ring anomaly, oesophageal stricture or oesophagitis (see below).
Oesophageal foreign body	Higher incidence in terrier breeds
Oesophageal diverticulum (congenital or acquired)	May be associated with broncho-oesophageal fistula
Oesophageal stricture (congenital or acquired)	*Intraluminal* Congenital: fibrous band constricts oesophageal lumen Acquired: scar tissue following ingestion of an oesophageal foreign body or primary oesophageal neoplasia (rare) *Extraluminal* Congenital: associated with a congenital vascular ring anomaly (oesophageal stricture occurs over base of heart) Acquired: compression of the oesophagus by a large neoplastic intrathoracic mass, e.g. lymphoma involving the thymus or bronchial lymph nodes, or other large mediastinal masses; iatrogenic form occasionally occurs 2–14 days after the administration of gaseous anaesthesia via an endotracheal tube (more common in cats).
Oesophagitis	Rare; usually a sequel to an oesophageal foreign body or associated with gastro-oesophageal reflux
Oesophageal neoplasia	Rare; sarcomas with *Spirocerca lupi* infection
Vascular ring anomaly	German shepherds and Irish setters predisposed
Hiatal hernia	Rare
Gastro-oesophageal intussusception	Rare

❑ **Amount, colour and consistency of vomitus?**

The presence of bile rules out a complete pyloric obstruction. Under normal circumstances all food should have left the stomach 6–8 h after a meal. The vomitus of animals with gastric outflow obstruction contains partially digested food and saliva with little or no bile. Haematemesis (the presence of blood in the vomitus) warrants a more aggressive diagnostic approach. Flecks or clots of fresh blood indicate recent mucosal damage whereas digested blood which has been in the stomach for some time has a typical 'coffee grounds' appearance.

❑ **Colour and consistency of faeces?**

Is the vomiting accompanied by diarrhoea and if so which came first? Many animals with simple gastritis initially vomit before developing diarrhoea and signs more consistent with gastroenteritis. Has there been evidence of either fresh blood in the stool (e.g. canine parvoviral gastroenteritis, haemorrhagic gastroenteritis) or melaena (bleeding lesion higher up the gastrointestinal tract e.g. intestinal or gastric tumour)?

❑ Diet and appetite?
Consider frequency of feeding, amount fed, recent dietary changes and relationship of vomiting to feeding or drinking. Is dog a scavenger or showing signs of pica? Consider the possibility of ingestion of foreign bodies, contaminated food or toxins.

❑ Signs of systemic disease or other clinical signs?
Many clinical signs associated with vomiting such as depression, lethargy, weakness and inappetence are non-specific and of limited diagnostic value. They may simply reflect a state of nausea or a mild degree of dehydration. Other more specific historical data such as polydipsia and polyuria, halitosis, jaundice and abdominal pain are suggestive of specific organ dysfunction.

❑ Is vomiting associated with travel?

❑ Previous medical or surgical problems and recent or current medication?
Non-steroidal anti-inflammatory drugs such as aspirin, phenylbutazone, ibuprofen and flunixin may cause vomiting as a side effect.

PHYSICAL EXAMINATION

❑ Temperature, pulse and respiration?
Fever may indicate an infectious process or possibly severe abdominal pain. Signs of hypovolaemic shock may be apparent with severe dehydration, i.e. a 10–15% fluid deficit or dogs with acute hypoadrenocorticism (Addisonian crisis).

❑ Clinical evidence of dehydration?
'Tenting' of the skin provides a rough indicator of hydration status but is unreliable in very thin or obese animals. The first clinical signs of water loss and extracellular fluid (ECF) volume contraction become evident when body weight is reduced by 5–8%. The signs become more obvious by 10% and with 15% loss of body weight signs of hypovolaemic shock become evident. Signs of ECF volume depletion include a weak, rapid pulse, dry mucous membranes with prolonged capillary refill time, decreased skin elasticity, sunken eyes, decreased urine output and microcardia on thoracic radiographs.

❑ Icteric mucous membranes?
Icteric mucous membranes may occur with primary liver disease (e.g. acute or chronic hepatitis), or as a result of occlusion or compression of the bile duct in association with acute pancreatitis or pancreatic neoplasia.

❑ Enlarged peripheral lymph nodes?
Dogs with lymphoma may vomit as a result of organ dysfunction or the hypercalcaemia which frequently accompanies the malignancy.

❑ Halitosis and/or oral or lingual ulceration?
Consider chronic renal failure or possibly the ingestion of caustic substances.

❑ Abdominal palpation
A thorough physical examination should include a careful systematic examination of the abdomen. Elevating the animal's forelimbs may permit palpation of organs in the cranial abdomen and occasionally gastric foreign bodies. The presence of any abnormal abdominal masses should be recorded. Particular attention should be paid to the size, shape and consistency of the kidneys and liver (palpation of the latter usually indicates hepatomegaly). The uterus may be palpable if it is distended (pyometra or pregnancy). Abdominal pain may be associated with acute gastritis or gastroenteritis, pancreatitis, hepatitis, pyelonephritis, peritonitis, closed pyometritis, and acute intestinal obstruction associated with the ingestion of foreign bodies or intussusception. Abdominal pain is an inconsistent finding in dogs with hypoadrenocorticism.

❑ Rectal examination
Where appropriate, a rectal examination may confirm an owner's suspicion of melaena.

Based on the history and clinical findings a more extensive laboratory and radiographic investigation is indicated if:

1. the vomiting is frequent and accompanied by systemic signs such as fever, dehydration, shock, collapse or acute abdominal pain;
2. the vomitus contains a significant amount of blood;
3. the vomiting is an intermittent or recurrent problem;
4. the initial episode of vomiting fails to respond to conventional symptomatic treatment for acute non-specific gastritis or gastroenteritis.

FURTHER INVESTIGATION

Routine haematological examination

Many vomiting animals may show a 'stress leucogram' characterized by a mild mature neutrophilia, lymphopenia and eosinopenia. A more pronounced neutrophilia, often accompanied by a left shift, is indicative of an inflammatory disease process or sepsis, e.g. pyometra. Leucopenia (usually the result of a neutropenia with or without a *degenerative* left shift) may be associated with acute Gram-negative sepsis (e.g. acute salmonellosis) or the acute phase of most viral infections including parvoviral gastroenteritis. If the animal survives the initial 24–48 h period the neutropenia gives way to a neutrophilia and *regenerative* left shift. Eosinophilia is an inconsistent feature of eosinophilic gastroenteritis; eosinophilia with an accompanying lymphocytosis occasionally occurs with hypoadrenocorticism. The packed cell volume (PCV) and total plasma protein (TPP) concentration provide only a very rough assessment of an animal's hydration status. An increase in PCV and TPP concentration may indicate dehydration. Anaemia may be associated with bleeding gastrointestinal lesions, chronic renal failure, acute or chronic hepatitis and hypoadrenocorticism. Chronic haemorrhage from a gastrointestinal lesion may result in the typical non-regenerative microcytic, hypochromic anaemia associated with iron deficiency.

Complete biochemical screen

A complete biochemical screen provides early diagnosis of many of the potentially life-threatening metabolic causes of acute or chronic vomiting such as diabetic ketoacidosis, hypoadrenocorticism, chronic renal failure and hepatic failure. Electrolyte concentrations are particularly important since they may not only indicate the cause of the vomiting but should be taken into consideration when planning fluid therapy. For example hyperkalaemia when accompanied by hyponatraemia is highly suggestive of hypoadrenocorticism and the administration of additional potassium in intravenous fluids is contraindicated. Similarly an animal which is vomiting because it is hypercalcaemic should be diuresed with isotonic (0.9%) sodium chloride. Lipase and amylase assays should be performed to rule out pancreatitis especially if acute vomiting is associated with abdominal pain and plain abdominal radiographs are inconclusive.

Urinalysis

Increased plasma urea and creatinine concentrations should always be interpreted in association with urine specific gravity to differentiate prerenal azotaemia associated with severe dehydration or hypovolaemia from primary renal disease. Hence it is important to obtain a urine sample before intravenous fluids are administered. Calculation of the urinary fractional excretion of sodium may also assist in differentiating prerenal azotaemia from acute renal failure (normal less than 1%).

Examination of faeces

A faecal sample should be submitted for a worm egg count and bacteriological examination especially when vomiting is accompanied by diarrhoea.

pH of the vomitus

The pH of the vomitus may help differentiate true vomiting from regurgitation associated with oesophageal disease. Regurgitated fluid and/or food containing salivary secretions is alkaline whereas vomitus of gastric origin has a pH of 4 or less.

Arterial blood gas analysis and pH

When appropriate facilities are available the acid–base status should be assessed by measuring the pH and total concentration of carbon dioxide of arterial blood (or failing this the plasma concentration of bicarbonate).

Electrocardiography

An ECG should be performed if hypoadrenocorticism is suspected, i.e. vomiting is associated with bradycardia and signs of hypovolaemic shock. Hyperkalaemia may result in an absence of P waves (atrial standstill), peaked T waves and, if the bradycardia is pronounced, a sinoventricular escape rhythm.

Radiography

Plain lateral and ventrodorsal views of the abdomen frequently provide useful diagnostic information. With acute pancreatitis an ill-defined area of opacity due to localized peritonitis may be seen in the cranial abdomen with 'fixation' and dilation of the duodenal loop. The size of the liver can be assessed by examining the position of the gastric axis. Hepatomegaly may be seen with primary (e.g. cholangiohepatitis or hepatic neoplasia) or secondary liver disease (e.g. diabetes mellitus). Hepatic disorders leading to hepatic insufficiency or hepatic failure (e.g. hepatic fibrosis or cirrhosis, or portosystemic shunts) may cause a reduction in the size of the liver. In cases where regurgitation cannot be differentiated from vomiting on a historical basis a lateral radiograph of the thorax may help rule out megaoesophagus. A small heart (microcardia) especially if accompanied by hyperlucency (underperfusion) of the lung fields suggests hypovolaemia and is suggestive of hypoadrenocorticism.

Contrast studies of the gastrointestinal tract are generally reserved for cases of chronic or recurrent vomiting when a diagnosis cannot be made from the history, clinical signs, initial laboratory tests or plain radiographs. For routine use, commercially prepared barium preparations are the safest and best since they are well tolerated even in dehydrated animals. When perforation of the gastrointestinal tract is suspected, preference is given to a water-soluble organic iodine preparation (e.g. Conray, Mallinckrodt Medical UK Ltd or Gastrografin, Schering Health Care) since leakage of barium into the mediastinum or peritoneal cavity can elicit a granulomatous inflammatory response. For the same reason care should be exercised if performing gastrointestinal surgery on an animal to which barium has recently been administered. Organic iodine preparations should be used cautiously in hypovolaemic or dehydrated animals since they are hypertonic and draw fluid into the intestinal lumen.

Contrast examination of the oesophagus

Contrast examination of the oesophagus may be necessary when regurgitation cannot be differentiated from true vomiting. Lateral views of the neck and thorax are taken immediately after swallowing a thick viscous barium paste (E-Z Paste; E-Z-EM Inc.) or after feeding tinned dog food mixed with a quarter of its volume of 100% w/v barium sulphate suspension (Polibar Rapid; E-Z-EM Inc.). The latter may demonstrate more fully the severity of the megaoesophagus and provide a more accurate assessment of its functional capacity.

Contrast examination of the stomach and small intestine

A full barium study evaluates gastric emptying and follows the passage of contrast material through the small and large intestines. It also permits a subjective assessment of the size, shape and position of the stomach and intestines in relation to other viscera. Adequate patient preparation is essential in order to obtain an optimal study. The animal should be fasted for 12–24 h and given a soapy water enema 1–2 h before the study is due to start (usually best if scheduled for early morning). If necessary the patient may be sedated with acepromazine since this drug has a minimal effect on gastrointestinal motility. For reference, plain radiographs of the abdomen should always be taken before the administration of the contrast agent, usually a fine 100% w/v suspension of barium sulphate (Polibar Rapid; E-Z-EM Inc.). The barium can be given either via a large syringe attached to a flexible rubber tube or via a stomach tube (8–12 ml kg^{-1} bodyweight for small and medium sized dogs and cats; 5–7 ml kg^{-1} bodyweight for large dogs). Lateral and ventrodorsal views of the abdomen are taken immediately and approximately 15 min, 30 min, 1, 2 and 4 h thereafter. The intervals at which the later films are taken will vary slightly depending on the rate at which barium passes through the gastrointestinal tract (GIT) as well as the segment of the GIT which is of particular interest. In most animals the duodenum is filled within 15–30 min and the jejunum after 1 h. Barium usually reaches the caecum between 1.5 and 2 h and is present in the colon after 3–4 h. The study should be continued until barium has left the small bowel. In most cases all barium should have left the stomach after 4–6 h although occasionally a small quantity of barium is still visible in the stomach after this period. Gastric emptying may be delayed in very nervous or excited dogs. A final radiograph should be taken the following morning, i.e. approximately 24 h after the administration of the barium to define lesions in the small intestine or colon which retain barium. Significant lesions should be visible as consistent filling defects on successive films.

Contrast examination of the stomach

If a gastric foreign body is suspected but is not visible on plain survey radiographs, a small quantity (10–20 ml) of 100% w/v barium suspension may be given to coat the surface of the foreign body without obscuring it. Four views of the stomach should be taken immediately and at 15 min intervals thereafter (see following section on double contrast gastrography). If no foreign body is detected a full barium study with follow through as described above can be performed.

Double contrast gastrogram

A double contrast gastrogram (DCG) provides a more detailed evaluation of gastric mucosal integrity. A DCG is indicated in any animal with a history of chronic vomiting and/or haematemesis when an ulcerative inflammatory or neoplastic lesion involving the gastric wall is suspected. The dog is first sedated with acepromazine; the intravenous administration of hypotonic agents such as glucagon delays gastric emptying and allows adequate distension of the stomach with air (see Table 5.4 for dose). A high density 170–200 w/v barium sulphate suspension (Baritop Plus; Bioglan Laboratories Ltd) is administered via stomach tube (2 ml kg^{-1} bodyweight) followed by approximately 20 ml kg^{-1} bodyweight of air. The stomach tube is removed and the animal is rotated through 360° to ensure barium coats the entire mucosal surface. Four views of the abdomen are taken immediately (Fig. 5.1a, b, c, d) and at 15 min intervals thereafter. The right lateral (RL) (Fig. 5.1b) and dorsoventral (DV) (Fig. 5.1c) views concentrate barium in the dependent portions of the stomach (pyloric antrum and body of the stomach, respectively) with gas in the upper portions; on the left lateral (LL) (Fig. 5.1a) and ventrodorsal (VD) (Fig. 5.1d) views barium is concentrated in the fundus with gas in the pyloric region.

Table 5.4 Intravenous dose of glucagon for a double contrast gastrogram

Bodyweight (kg)	Dose of glucagon (mg)
1–8	0.1
9–20	0.2
21–40	0.3
>40	0.35

Endoscopy

Gastroscopy, using a long flexible fibreoptic endoscope is a useful non-invasive technique for identifying the presence of gastric mucosal lesions such as ulcers, tumours and polyps when radiographic findings are either negative or equivocal. It may also be possible to remove small gastric foreign bodies or to obtain 'grab' biopsies of mucosal lesions using grasping forceps introduced via the biopsy channel of the endoscope. The major disadvantages of gastroscopy are that, although providing an excellent view of the gastric mucosa, it is not possible to assess gastric wall thickness and, in the hands of an inexperienced operator, some lesions may not be detected. In some cases a superficial 'grab' biopsy may be less informative or even misleading when compared to a full thickness biopsy of the gastric wall obtained at surgery.

Exploratory laparotomy

Blind surgical exploration of the abdomen in the absence of extensive laboratory and radiographic examinations is rarely productive. How many dogs with megaoesophagus have been subjected to unnecessary abdominal surgery because their chests were not radiographed beforehand? Exploratory laparotomy is only indicated when:

1. Radiographic or endoscopic findings are inconclusive;
2. Confirmation of a tentative diagnosis requires histological examination of a full thickness gastric or intestinal biopsy, or complete resection of the lesion;
3. A more accurate assessment of the severity and extent of the lesion is required prior to possible resection. Some gastric tumours for example do not penetrate the mucosal surface and yet nevertheless cause a significant degree of pyloric outflow obstruction because of the extensive submucosal/serosal infiltration.

GENERAL MANAGEMENT AND TREATMENT OF THE VOMITING ANIMAL

The immediate aims of treatment are (1) to correct or remove the primary cause of the vomiting, (2) to control the vomiting episodes thereby alleviating the further loss of fluid and electrolytes,

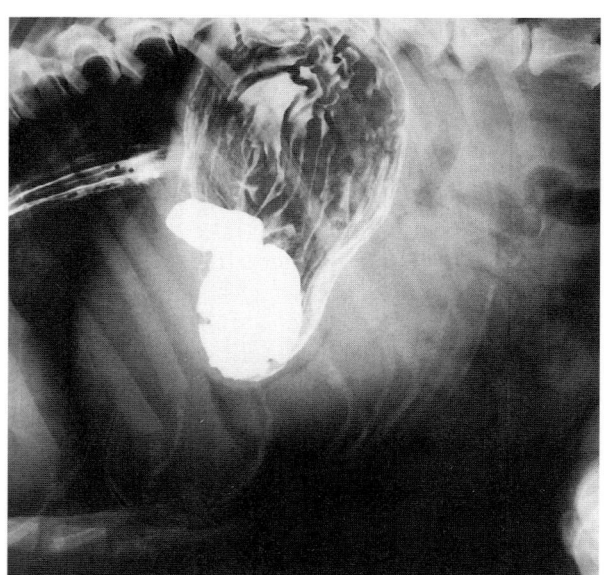

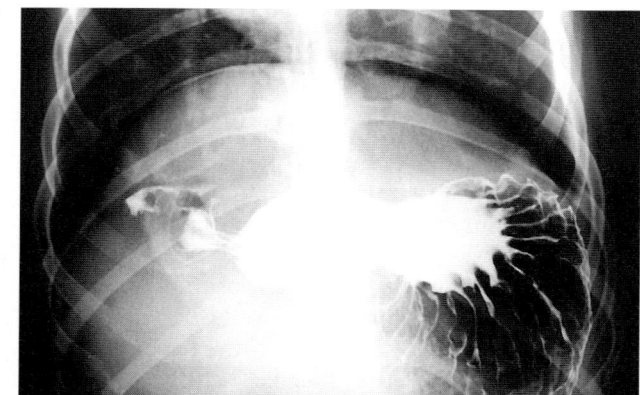

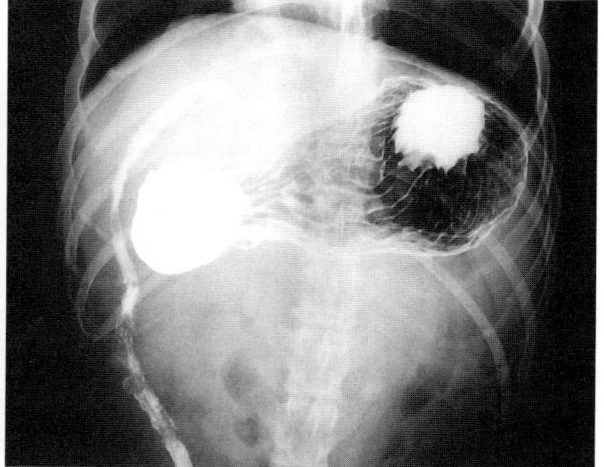

Figure 5.1 Four views of a double contrast gastrogram from a normal 6-year-old Bernese mountain dog. (a) (left lateral projection) Barium is filling the fundus and air is present in the pyloric antrum. (b) (right lateral projection) Barium is filling the pyloric antrum and air is outlining the rugal folds within the fundus. (c) (dorsoventral projection) Barium is filling the ventral parts of the stomach body and pyloric antrum. Gas is outlining the rugal folds in the dorsal parts of the fundus. (d) (ventrodorsal projection) Barium is filling the fundus and pyloric antrum. Air is outlining the rugal folds in the body of the stomach. Barium is starting to leave the stomach. Photographs courtesy of Michael Herrtage.

and (3) to correct any fluid, electrolyte or acid–base disturbances which may be present. The treatment of specific diseases which cause vomiting is discussed in Section II.

Most cases of acute, non-specific gastritis or gastroenteritis are self-limiting or respond within 24–48 h to symptomatic therapy consisting of the following.

1. Withhold all food for 24 h (water for 12 h).
2. After 12 h offer a small amount of water or icecubes

3. After 24 h, if water is tolerated, introduce a bland carbohydrate consisting of cooked rice, lean minced beef, chicken, cottage cheese, baby food or a commercial prescription diet (e.g. Waltham Low Fat Diet). Avoid diets high in fat or protein. Initially split total daily requirement into three or even four small meals. Consider an exclusion or hypoallergenic diet containing mutton and rice, or a prescription diet (e.g. Waltham Hypoallergenic Diet) if allergic gastritis is diagnosed or suspected.

Persistent vomiting results in dehydration and electrolyte and acid–base abnormalities, the severity of which depend on the frequency and cause of the vomiting and the volume of fluid lost from the gastrointestinal tract.

Fluid therapy

Fluids are best administered via the intravenous route since subcutaneous fluids are poorly absorbed in dehydrated animals. Intravenous fluids must supply maintenance requirements (40–60 ml kg^{-1} bodyweight 24 h^{-1}), must correct any existing fluid deficit, and replace continued losses as they occur. The fluid deficit may be calculated as follows:

Fluid required (deficit in ml) = BW (kg) × % dehydration × 1000 + maintenance (40–60 ml kg^{-1} 24 h^{-1}) + extraordinary losses (estimated fluid losses due to vomiting and diarrhoea)

About 75% of the total fluid deficit may be replaced over the first 24 h and the remainder over the next 12 h. If facilities for measuring electrolytes and acid–base status are not available an isotonic balanced electrolyte solution such as Hartmann's solution is generally satisfactory. Vomiting results in the loss of sodium, potassium and chloride. The most common abnormality is hypokalaemia accompanied by a metabolic acidosis which may be at least partially compensated by a respiratory alkalosis. Hence, it may be necessary in many cases to supplement with additional potassium; 20 mmol of potassium chloride may safely be added to each litre of fluids and, if renal function is normal, infused at a rate not exceeding 0.5 mmol of potassium per kg bodyweight per hour. When vomiting is severe and associated with gastric outflow obstruction, a hypokalaemic, hypochloraemic metabolic alkalosis with paradoxical aciduria may develop. If a metabolic alkalosis is suspected 0.9% saline is the fluid of choice; correction of the chloride deficit results in the renal excretion of bicarbonate with conservation of potassium. The use of an alkali buffering solution such as lactated Hartmann's solution is only indicated in cases of confirmed metabolic acidosis.

Antiemetics

Antiemetics are indicated only when vomiting is so severe and profuse that fluid, electrolyte and acid–base abnormalities are difficult to control. They should be administered only after the possibility of pyloric obstruction or a gastrointestinal foreign body has been ruled out. Antiemetic drugs act by blocking the chemoreceptor zone (CTZ), the vomiting centre or the vestibular apparatus. Common antiemetic drugs used in veterinary practice include the following.

1. *Antihistamines* (e.g. promethazine, diphenhydramine) block the CTZ and depress input from the vestibular apparatus. Indications: control of motion sickness or vomiting associated with vestibular disease.
2. *Phenothiazines* (acetylpromazine, chlorpromazine, prochlorperazine) block the CTZ but also possess weak anticholinergic properties. They are effective in blocking viscerally stimulated vomiting of acute gastritis but will not block vomiting induced by severe visceral pain or spasm. Chlorpromazine is an effective antiemetic and has minimal tranquillizing action. Phenothiazines have an alpha-adrenergic action which causes arteriolar vasodilation and hypotension. The use of these drugs is therefore contraindicated in dehydrated or hypovolaemic animals.
3. *Parasympatholytic drugs* (atropine sulphate, propantheline bromide) decrease visceral motility, spasm and gastrointestinal secretions by inhibiting visceral afferent vagal impulses. They are the least effective of the antiemetics and their prolonged use (i.e. greater than three days) may induce gastric atony and intestinal stasis. The main indications for their use are for the treatment of suspected cases of congenital pyloric stenosis (contraindicated if gastric outflow obstruction is due to an organic lesion).
4. *Metoclopramide* increases the tone and amplitude of oesophageal and gastric contractions, relaxes the pyloric sphincter thereby promoting gastric emptying, and increases duodenal peristalsis. The actions of metoclopramide are mediated by its antidopaminergic effects on the

CTZ. Indications: (a) early morning bilious vomiting, (b) vomiting associated with cancer chemotherapy, (c) acute non-specific gastritis, (d) acute viral gastroenteritis, and (e) treatment of delayed gastric emptying associated with gastric ulceration or neoplasia (except when the outflow obstruction is associated with an organic lesion, e.g. neoplasia involving the pyloric antrum or gastric foreign body).

Histamine blocking drugs

Histamine blocking drugs such as cimetidine or ranitidine block the H_2 receptors on gastric parietal cells resulting in a marked decrease in gastric acid secretion. Indications: gastric or duodenal ulceration, reflux oesophagitis, uraemic gastropathy and chronic gastritis.

Antacids

Antacids such as aluminium hydroxide, magnesium hydroxide or magnesium trisilicate must be given every 2–4 hours to effectively buffer gastric acid. Indications: gastric or duodenal ulceration, oesophagitis associated with gastro-oesophageal reflux of acid), and management of dogs with chronic renal failure (aluminium hydroxide binds dietary phosphate). Both aluminium hydroxide and magnesium hydroxide may inhibit the absorption of orally administered cimetidine.

Antibiotics

Antibiotics are indicated only for the treatment of specific bacterial infections. The use of corticosteroids should be restricted to cases of immune-mediated gastritis or gastroenteritis, e.g. chronic eosinophilic gastritis.

Oral protectants

Oral protectants such as kaolin, kaopectate and bismuth preparations are rarely indicated since they do not effectively coat the damaged gastric mucosa.

6

Dysphagia, Regurgitation and Ptyalism

C. M. Elwood

Dysphagia is difficulty swallowing, regurgitation (in relation to alimentary function) is the flowing back of undigested food, and ptyalism is excessive salivation. These clinical signs are often associated with disorders of swallowing function.

NORMAL ANATOMY AND PHYSIOLOGY OF SWALLOWING

The process of swallowing passes food from the mouth through the oropharynx, the laryngopharynx, the oesophagus and the gastro-oesophageal junction to the stomach. There are three phases of normal swallowing, *oropharyngeal*, *pharyngeal* and *gastro-oesophageal*. All of these phases require sequential, coordinated reflex actvity of a number of nerves and muscles.

The normal pharynx consists of three regions; the oropharynx ventrally and the nasopharynx dorsally, divided by the soft palate, and the caudal common chamber, the laryngopharynx. The pharynx has four openings: to the nasal cavity, the oral cavity, the larynx and the oesophagus. It receives innervation from cranial nerves V, IX and X. The activity of pharyngeal and palatine muscles is under reflex control.

Following prehension and chewing of food or drinking of fluid, a bolus is formed at the base of the tongue and is passed voluntarily into the oropharynx. This initiates a series of reflex events. Afferent impulses pass from receptors in and around the pharynx, via the trigeminal and glossopharyngeal nerves, to the tractus solitarius, thence to the nucleus tractus solitarius and reticular formation and on to the swallowing centre. The swallowing centre sends inhibitory impulses to cease respirations and excitatory signals to the cranial nerve nuclei V, VII, IX, X and XII. As a result of these signals, there is contraction of palatine muscles to raise the soft palate and close off the opening to the nasal cavity, there is closure of the glottis, the larynx is pulled rostrally, elevating the epiglottis, and there is a sequential contraction of pharyngeal muscles from a rostral to a caudal direction which propels the bolus caudally. Relaxation of the thyropharyngeus and cricopharyngeus muscles allows passage of the bolus into the cranial oesophagus, via the upper oesophageal sphincter. This initiates the oesophageal phase of swallowing.

The oesophagus is a long muscular tube consisting of four layers, the mucosa, the submucosa, the muscularis and the adventitia. In the dog there are two layers of oblique striated muscle throughout the length of the oesophagus, whereas in the cat there is a gradual transition such that the distal one third is predominantly smooth muscle. The oesophagus receives and sends nervous impulses via the vagus nerve. When a food bolus reaches the oesophagus a peristaltic wave of contraction of oesophageal muscle is required to push the bolus aborally into the stomach, through the lower oesophageal sphincter. This is a reflex event under central control, coordinated via the swallowing centre and the nucleus ambiguus of the vagus nerve. Primary peristaltic waves are initiated as part of the swallowing reflex, and may be sufficient to propel liquids distally, but often a bolus of food will not pass to the stomach following primary peristalsis; in this case a 'secondary peristaltic wave' is initiated. Secondary peristalsis requires sensory input from receptors in the oesophagus, which recognize distension of the lumen, and travel to the tractus solitarius of the spinal cord to the nucleus tractus solitarius and thence to the swallowing centre. The motor characteristics of secondary peristalsis appear to be indistinguishable from primary peristalsis.

The lower oesophageal sphincter consists of a

number of functional portions: (a) interdigitating rugal folds, (b) the right diaphragmatic crus, (c) the oblique implantation of the oesophagus into the stomach, (d) a muscular sling from gastric smooth muscle and (e) a short intra-abdominal segment which allows compression of the terminal oesophagus by positive intra-abdominal pressure. Lower oesophageal sphincter tone is partially under the control of the vagus nerve, but also has receptors for histamine (H_1 type), gastrin and acetylcholine. Relaxation of the lower oesophageal sphincter allows passage of a food bolus from the oesophagus to the stomach.

Normal swallowing is accompanied by the production of lubricating saliva which occurs following a number of stimuli, including (a) anticipation of eating, (b) sight, smell and taste of food, (c) mechanical stimulation of the upper mouth and oesophagus, (d) stimulation of the vomiting reflex, (e) intense tastes (e.g. bitters), and (f) direct stimulation of muscarinic acetylcholine receptors in the salivary gland. Saliva is normally swallowed and passes into the stomach.

PATHOPHYSIOLOGY

Dysphagia

Interference with the normal swallowing process causes dysphagia. Thus, obstruction, sensory abnormalities, pain or neuromuscular dysfunction in the mouth, pharynx, oesophagus or lower oesophageal sphincter can all elicit signs of dysphagia (Table 6.1).

Regurgitation

Regurgitation usually manifests when food boluses cannot pass through the upper oesophageal sphincter, the oesophagus or the lower oesophageal sphincter. This may be the result of obstruction, immotility, or pain (Table 6.1).

Ptyalism

This occurs either as a result of an excessive production of saliva or an inability to swallow saliva (Table 6.1).

INVESTIGATION OF DYSPHAGIA, REGURGITATION AND PTYALISM

HISTORY CHECKLIST

❑ **Age, breed and sex?**
Congenital disorders are most likely to manifest in younger animals, often at weaning. Conditions to consider in young animals include congenital megaoesophagus, vascular ring anomalies and congenital cricopharyngeal stricture or achalasia.

❑ **Is the animal regurgitating, vomiting or retching?**
Distinguishing between these three presentations is extremely important: the distinction will usually not be made by the owner.
Vomiting is a reflex activity, in which the animal may show initial salivation, followed by lowering of the head, active contraction of the abdominal muscles and return of gastric contents (which may sometimes be tinged yellow by bile).
Regurgitation is a passive return of food or fluid, there are usually no preceding signs of nausea and no warning of its occurrence; ingesta returns with minimal effort from the animal. Food is undigested, but may remain in the oesophagus for some time after ingestion, thus time between eating and return of food does not distinguish between vomiting and regurgitation.
Retching is the act of clearing the upper airway, often following a bout of coughing. It may be productive or non-productive and is usually accompanied by a 'gagging' noise.

❑ **Is there a combination of vomiting and regurgitation?**
Signs of both vomiting and regurgitation may be seen with conditions of the lower oesophageal sphincter region (e.g. hiatal hernia) or with reflux oesophagitis subsequent to vomition of irritant gastric juices.

❑ **Appetite?**
A decrease in appetite suggests pain, nausea or systemic illness. Non-painful diseases such as idiopathic megaoesophagus are not associated with decreased appetite unless there are complications (e.g. aspiration pneumonia).

❑ **Is there a difference in the ability to swallow fluids compared with solids?**
Partial obstruction or painful conditions (e.g. oesophagitis, vascular ring anomalies) may allow an animal to swallow fluids better that solids.

Table 6.1 Conditions associated with clinical signs of dysphagia, and/or regurgitation, and/or ptyalism

	Dysphagia	Regurgitation	Ptyalism
Systemic disease			
Hepatic encephalopathy			√
Nausea from other disease			√
Tongue disorders			
Neoplasia	√		(√)
Necrosis	√		(√)
Glossitis	√		(√)
Paralysis (CN XII)	√		(√)
Oral cavity disease			
Dental disease	√		√
Gingivitis	√		√
Neoplasia	√		√
Cleft palate	√		
Foreign body/trauma	√		√
Pharyngeal disorders			
Foreign bodies	√		√
Neoplasia	√		√
Retropharyngeal lymphadenopathy	√	√	√
Salivary gland enlargement	√	√	(√)
Rabies	√		√
Botulism	√		√
CNS disease (CN IX, X)	√	√	√
Tonsillar enlargement	√		√
Cricopharyngeal stenosis	√	√	
Cricopharyngeal achalasia	√		
Laryngeal disease			
Paralysis	√		
Neoplasia	√		
Chondritis	√		
Retropharyngeal disease			
Foreign bodies	√		√
Neoplasia	√		√
Lymphadenopathy	√		(√)
Sialadenitis	√		√
Salivary gland necrosis	√		(√)
Megaoesophagus			
Idiopathic	(√)	√	(√)
Myasthenia gravis	(√)	√	(√)
Myopathy	(√)	√	(√)
Myositis	(√)	√	(√)
Toxins	(√)	√	(√)
Hypothyroidism	√	√	(√)
Neuropathy/neuritis	(√)	√	(√)
Oesophageal diverticulum	√	√	(√)
Dysautonomia	√	√	(√)
Gastro-oesophageal junction			
Hiatal hernia	√	√	√
Gastro-oesophageal intussusception	√	√	√
Neoplasia	√	√	√
Intraoesophageal narrowing			
Stricture	√	√	√
Neoplasia	√	√	√
Granulomata	√	√	√
Foreign body	√	√	√
Abcess	√	√	√
Oesophagitis			
Infectious	√	√	√
Toxic/irritant	√	√	√
Reflux	√	√	√
Extraoesophageal compression			
Vascular ring anomaly	√	√	√
Thoracic neoplasia	√	√	√
Granulomas	√	√	√
Cervical neoplasia	√	√	√

√ common; (√) occasional.

> **Table 6.2** A diagnostic approach to regurgitation, dysphagia and ptyalism
>
> 1. **Identify likely site of disease (oral, pharyngeal, oesophageal, systemic)**
>   History and physical examination
>   Observation of eating behaviour
>
> 2. **Rule out systemic disease**
>   Haematology, biochemistry and urinalysis
>
> 3. **Rule out infectious disease if suspected**
>   Serology
>
> 4. **Rule out mass lesions, radiolucent foreign objects, megaoesophagus, thoracic disease**
>   Plain radiographs of pharynx/larynx, neck and thorax
>   Ultrasonography
>
> 5. **Examine pharynx, larynx and oesophagus**
>   Laryngoscopy
>   Endoscopy
>
> 6. **Rule out functional disorders**
>   Contrast examinations
>   Fluoroscopy
>
> 7. **Rule out neuromuscular diseases**
>   Exercise testing
>   Neurological examination
>   'Tensilon' testing

Conditions that are associated with defects in the sensory pathways or with prehension abnormalities (e.g. dental pain) may allow better swallowing of solids than liquids.

❏ **Is there blood in the saliva or regurgitated matter?**
The presence of blood suggests erosion or ulceration of the mucosa which can occur with neoplasia, trauma, foreign bodies or mucosal irritation (e.g. oesophagitis).

❏ **Signs of nasal disease?**
Sneezing, snorting, epistaxis and nasal discharge may all be seen as a result of reflux into the nasal chamber when there is regurgitation, but can also be an indication of disorders of the caudal nares and nasopharynx.

❏ **Signs of upper and lower airway disease?**
It is important to recognize signs of upper and lower airway disease (coughing, tachypnoea) because they may indicate aspiration pneumonia and influence diagnostic and therapeutic decisions. In rare cases of broncho-oesophageal fistulation, pneumonia may occur as a direct result of passage of ingesta through the fistula. Respiratory difficulty may also be reported when space-occupying thoracic lesions impinge on lung tissue as well as the oesophagus. Intermittent dyspnoea may accompany a sliding hiatal hernia.

❏ **Voice change?**
Alteration in character of voice may indicate concurrent laryngeal disease, for example due to idiopathic laryngeal paralysis, laryngeal neoplasia, or extralaryngeal compressive lesions. Laryngeal paralysis may be seen as a result of intrathoracic masses that impinge upon the recurrent laryngeal nerve as well as the oesophagus.

❏ **Is exercise tolerance normal?**
Poor exercise tolerance, in the absence of other causes, could indicate generalized neuromuscular disease. Myasthenia gravis is associated with normal muscle function that rapidly deteriorates with exercise and may be restored by the administration of an acetylcholine esterase inhibitor (the 'Tensilon test' q.v.), whereas with myopathy and myositis weakness may manifest from the start of exercise.

❏ **Other neuromuscular signs?**
Generalized weakness or stiffness may suggest myopathy; myositis may be accompanied by muscular pain. Signs of brain disease such as stupor, poor mentation, abnormal behaviour (e.g. head pressing, aimless circling) or cranial nerve function deficits may suggest central nervous system disease and involvement of cranial nerve nuclei of the swallowing reflex. Dysfunction of the mandibular branch of the trigeminal nerve causes an inability to close the mouth.

❏ **Has there been a history of recent trauma or recent foreign body ingestion?**
Trauma to soft tissue, teeth or bones can all cause dysphagia. Trauma to the pharynx can occur from a recent stick injury, and retropharyngeal abcessation can occur as a consequence of entrapment of foreign matter following such an injury. Oesophageal obstruction can occur following ingestion of foreign bodies such as toys, bones and chews. Acute onset of signs is typical of foreign body ingestion or trauma.

❏ **Recent general anaesthetic?**
Reflux of gastrointestinal contents during general anaesthesia can cause oesophagitis and oesophageal stricture formation. Signs typically occur a few days after the reflux event.

- ❏ **Other history or signs of systemic or infectious disease?**

Signs of hepatic encephalopathy (e.g. apparent blindness, head pressing, mania, depression) may accompany ptyalism in cats with portosystemic shunts. Other metabolic, gastrointestinal or abdominal or neurologic diseases (e.g. vestibular syndrome) that are associated with nausea may show ptyalism as a component of the clinical presentation. Dysphagia and ptyalism are early signs of rabies encephalitis. Owners should therefore be questioned regarding vaccination status, possible exposure, travel abroad etc.

- ❏ **Exposure to toxins or irritants?**

Access to decomposing matter contaminated with *Clostridium botulinum* can cause botulism, with dysphagia occurring in association with generalized muscle weakness. Botulism may be more common in kennelled dogs (e.g. hounds). Ingestion of caustics or locally irritating plants, or even stinging insects can cause superficial irritation and/or swelling of the mouth, pharynx and oesophagus with consequent dysphagia, ptyalism or regurgitation. Recent therapy with insecticides containing pyrethrin/pyrethroid or organophosphate can be a cause of ptyalism.

 ## PHYSICAL EXAMINATION

The main aim of the general physical examination is to identify systemic, complicating or intercurrent disease. Particular emphasis should be placed on the following aspects.

- ❏ **Oral examination**

A thorough oral examination should be performed to identify oropharyngeal or dental disease. In most dogs, digital palpation of the dental arcade, oropharynx and laryngopharynx may be performed, and will help identify painful foci, swellings and foreign bodies.

- ❏ **Examination of head and neck**

The head, neck, retropharyngeal region and salivary glands should be carefully examined visually and aurally and palpated to identify pain, swelling and assymetry. A distended, fluid-filled oesophagus may be palpable in the ventral cervical region in some cases of megaoesophagus. Discharging sinuses or a fluctuating subcutaneous swelling may be seen consequent to a retained foreign body (e.g. a stick) in the retropharyngeal or cervical region.

- ❏ **Thoracic examination and auscultation**

This should identify signs of aspiration pneumonia (localized crackles and whistles, pleural rubs or decreasing sounds). Other findings, for example, tachypnoea, decreased audibility of heart or lung sounds, displacement of the apex beat of the heart, and fluid lines upon thoracic percussion are more suggestive of intrathoracic masses.

- ❏ **Chest compressibility**

Masses in the anterior thorax of cats particularly (e.g. thymic lymphosarcoma) may reduce the compressibility of the thoracic cage anterior to the heart.

- ❏ **Examination of the neuromuscular system**

This should identify signs of myopathy/myositis, cranial nerve deficits, generalized neurological disease and dysautonomia (xerostomia, hypolacrimation, mydriasis, constipation, bladder distension).

- ❏ **Watching the animal eat and drink**

This is a critical part of the examination. Observing the formation and swallowing of a bolus will help the clinician localize signs of dysphagia to the oral cavity, the pharynx and cranial to the upper oesophageal sphincter, or the oesophagus. The absence of dysphagia in cases of ptyalism or regurgitation reduces the number of possible differential diagnoses.

FURTHER INVESTIGATION

Haematology, biochemistry and urinalysis screens

Neutrophilia with or without a left shift may be seen with inflammatory diseases, such as retropharyngeal abscessation, aspiration pneumonia or retained foreign bodies. Increased serum bile acids, low urea, red cell microcytosis and urate crystalluria may all be seen in cases of portosystemic shunting. Laboratory findings of hepatic or renal dysfunction may indicate reasons for ptyalism as a consequence of nausea. Lymphoid leukaemia may sometimes accompany retropharyngeal lymphadenopathy in severe lymphosarcoma. Hypochloraemia and hypokalaemia can occur as a result of loss of acidic gastric contents and metabolic alkalosis, and suggest that vomition is occurring. Increased creatine kinase (CK) can be seen with myopathy and myositis, and in hypothyroidism. Increased serum cholesterol may also be increased with hypothyroidism.

Serology

Serology may be used to detect infectious diseases such as toxoplasmosis, feline leukaemia virus (FeLV) and feline immunodeficiency virus (FIV) which can cause neurologic disease, focal infection or neoplasia (FeLV). Thyroid function testing (TSH or TRH stimulation tests and TSH/T4 assays) may be useful in cases of myopathy, neuropathy and undiagnosed megaoesophagus. Increased concentrations of anti-acetylcholine receptor antibodies in serum are diagnostic of myasthenia gravis; this may cause generalized muscle weakness or megaoesophagus alone.

Radiography and ultrasonography

Plain radiographs of the thorax will identify megaoesophagus, intrathoracic masses, oesophageal foreign bodies, some cases of hiatal herniation, gastro-oesophageal intussusception, oesophageal diverticula and oesophageal fistula. Plain cervical radiographs may identify and help to localize cervical mass lesions and radio-opaque foreign bodies. Plain radiographs of the pharynx and larynx can identify mass lesions and foreign bodies.

The pharynx and oesophagus may be further evaluated by performing a barium swallow with barium paste (70% w/v), suspension (30% w/v) or barium mixed with food. Barium paste will outline the pharynx and upper oesophagus, barium suspension is useful for evaluating the oesophagus, and barium with food will outline both pharynx and oesophagus. Where oesophageal tears or ruptures are suspected, or where a risk of aspiration exists, iodine-based contrast media should be used. A contrast examination may identify megaoesophagus, sites of luminal narrowing in the oesophagus, oesophageal diverticula, broncho-oesophageal fistulae, gastro-oesophageal intussusception, some cases of hiatal hernia, radiolucent foreign bodies and mucosal mass lesions of the oesophagus.

Fluoroscopy

Fluoroscopy is a useful technique for evaluating swallowing function in the pharynx and oesophagus, particularly if used in association with contrast media (see above). The animal should be unsedated and offered both liquid barium and barium with food. To completely evaluate swallowing function, it may be necessary to record the passage of boluses along the complete length of pharynx to stomach. The most critical phases of the study are evaluation of bolus formation in the oropharynx and passage into the cranial oesophagus; this process relies upon normal pharyngeal sensation, normal pharyngeal anatomy and muscle function, and normal relaxation of the upper oesophageal sphincter. Repeated swallowing attempts in which a bolus fails to pass into the oesophagus suggest dysfunction in the upper oesophageal sphincter (e.g. pain, foreign bodies, cricopharyngeal stenosis). During fluoroscopy the larynx and trachea should also be evaluated for evidence of aspiration of contrast material.

Ultrasonography

Ultrasonography may be used to evaluate structures in and around the head and neck. It may allow identification of mass lesions and foreign bodies. Intrathoracic masses may be further evaluated using ultrasonography and biopsies may also be obtained under ultrasonographic guidance. Ultrasonography has been used in the identification and characterization of liver disease and portosystemic shunts.

Laryngoscopy

This facilitates full and careful visual examination of the larynx and pharynx, and is best performed under light general anaesthesia. During the procedure, digital palpation of the pharynx, larynx and upper oesophageal sphincter may also be performed. Visual examination of the vocal cords should be performed with the animal in dorsal recumbency as it is regaining conciousness. Lack of movement of one or both vocal cords suggests laryngeal paralysis, but an extremely light plane of anaesthesia is required to avoid false diagnosis.

Endoscopic examination

Endoscopy is extremely useful for the evaluation of the pharynx, larynx, oesophagus and lower oesophageal sphincter. Although endoscopy does not often provide functional information, it can identify foreign bodies, megaoesophagus, strictures, extra-oesophageal compression, oesophagitis and neoplasia. Both rigid endoscopes and flexible fibreoptic endoscopes can be used, although only the latter allows full insufflation of the oesophagus and effective examination of the lower oesophageal sphincter. Using either a retroflexed flexible endoscope or a dental mirror, the nasopharynx may be examined for the presence of disease. The wide diameter of rigid endoscopes makes them extremely useful in the management of oesophageal foreign bodies because they allow passage of rigid instruments. The wide diameter is a disadvantage, however, in the evaluation of felines and in cases of oesophageal narrowing. Flexible endoscopy also has therapeutic applications; it can be used, for example, for removal of foreign bodies, perendoscopic balloon dilatation of strictures and placement of tubes for provision of nutritional support.

Tissue biopsy and fine needle aspiration

Masses identified by palpation, radiography, ultrasonography, laryngoscopy or endoscopy should be further characterized by either biopsy or fine needle aspiration. In addition to histopathology/cytology, tissue may also be submitted for bacterial culture and antibiotic sensitivity testing.

Computed tomography/magnetic resonance imaging

These imaging techniques may be applicable when further evaluation of suspected central nervous system disease is required. They also have potential for identification of mass lesions in the head, neck and thorax where other techniques have proved unrewarding.

The 'Tensilon' test

Clinical signs of myasthenia gravis may be either exercise intolerance, determined by exercise testing, or megaoesophagus. A diagnosis of myasthenia gravis may be pursued by performing a 'Tensilon' test. In myasthenia gravis the clinical signs may be abrogated by the administration of the short-acting acetylcholine esterase inhibitor, edrophonium chloride (0.11–0.22 mg kg^{-1} i.v. (dog); 2.5 mg per cat i.v.). When performing a 'Tensilon' test a syringe containing atropine (0.04 mg kg^{-1}) and an appropriate endotracheal tube should be readily available, in case of severe muscarinic effects of the edrophonium. The response of megaoesophagus to edrophonium must be monitored by fluoroscopy and responses appear to be less predictable.

Anti-acetylcholine receptor antibodies (Anti-AChR)

Anti-AChR may now be measured in a serum sample for both dogs and cats. In cases of acquired myasthenia gravis increased titres of anti-AChR are considered diagnostic. This test is particularly useful when 'Tensilon' testing is equivocal and also to monitor subsequent immunosuppressive therapy.

Toxicology

Toxicological investigations might include whole blood acetylcholine esterase (organophosphate toxicity), blood lead, or urinary δ-aminolaevulenic acid levels.

Exploratory surgery

Where foreign bodies are suspected (e.g. appropriate history and/or presence of discharging sinuses) or where mass lesions have been identified, exploratory surgery may be useful to either remove or resect the offending object or obtain biopsy material.

Dietary trial

When diagnostic efforts have failed to produce a treatable diagnosis, or where further investigation is not possible, a dietary trial may be useful. It is difficult to predict in a given individual which dietary option is most likely to succeed, so choice of feeding is usually by trial and error. Feeding regimes that may be successful include feeding little and often, feeding from a height, feeding liquidized food paste, feeding a liquid food, and feeding a dry diet as opposed to a wet diet (or vice versa). In exceptional circumstances, animals may be maintained by placement of permanent feeding tubes (e.g. percutaneous gastrostomy).

7

Diarrhoea

C. M. Elwood

Diarrhoea is defined as increased volume or fluidity of faeces or increased frequency of defecation. Dysfunction or diseases of the small and large intestines, the pancreas and the liver may all cause diarrhoea; these may be primary or secondary to systemic disease.

NORMAL INTESTINAL FUNCTION

Ingested food enters the stomach where the combination of an acid environment, pepsin proteolytic activity and active gastric motility leads to the production of semi-fluid chyme, which is then passed into the duodenum in controlled quantities. The duodenum also receives intestinal and pancreatic secretions and bile, which are mixed with chyme to continue the digestive process. Pancreatic secretions contain sodium bicarbonate which neutralizes gastric acid, as well as various enzymes including lipase, amylase and trypsin. Bile contains bile salts and bile pigments; bile salts are important for the emulsification of undigested fats into micelles, which greatly increases exposure to the fat digesting enzyme lipase.

Carbohydrate digestion is initiated by salivary amylase and continued by pancreatic amylase. These processes produce disaccharides and oligosaccharides, which are further digested by disaccharidase (lactase and sucrase) and oligosaccharidase enzymes in the small intestinal brush border. Monosaccharides are absorbed into the mucosal cell by co-transport with sodium (glucose, galactose) or by facilitated diffusion (fructose).

Protein digestion is initiated by pepsin in the stomach and continued by pancreatic proteolytic enzymes (including trypsin and chymotrypsin) and by peptidases of the intestinal brush border. Amino acids are absorbed into the mucosal cell by various carriers and enter the blood stream by both simple and facilitated diffusion.

Emulsified fat micelles are digested by pancreatic lipase to produce free fatty acids and monoglycerides; these passively diffuse into the mucosal epithelial cell where they are re-esterified to triglyceride (fatty acids with less than 10–12 carbon atoms pass directly into the portal blood), thus maintaining the diffusion gradient. Triglycerides, cholesterol and cholesterol esters are synthesized, with protein and phospholipid, into chylomicrons which pass into the lacteal ducts and thence to the thoracic duct and systemic circulation.

Mixing of ingesta and secreted digestive components in the small intestine is facilitated by segmental contraction of the bowel wall; this activity also promotes digestion and absorption at the brush border by maximizing contact with luminal contents. Ingesta is passed distally along the intestine by peristaltic waves, which also promote intestinal health in the interdigestive period by sweeping undigested contents and luminal bacteria aborally. Eventually this material enters the colon via the ileocolic valve.

The large intestine performs a number of functions, including storage and co-ordinated elimination of faecal material and dehydration of faeces (by absorbing approximately 90% of the water entering). This latter function is extremely efficient, but it should be recognized that the colon only accounts for approximately 10–15% of total water absorption in the gastrointestinal tract; most occurs in the jejunum and ileum. The net flux of water through the gastrointestinal tract is at least $0.15 \, l \, kg^{-1}$ bodyweight day^{-1} and this means that small intestinal disease can cause significantly greater fluid losses from the body than large intestinal disease.

PATHOPHYSIOLOGY

Osmotic diarrhoea occurs when there is an increased luminal osmotic load, often as a result of maldigestion or malabsorption, which retains moisture within the lumen and increases the fluidity and bulk of faeces.

Abnormal intestinal motility causes diarrhoea either because of increased delivery of faeces to the colon and/or rectum, or consequent to poor absorptive function when there is intestinal stasis. It may occur for a number of reasons, e.g. drug therapy or intestinal inflammation.

Increased intestinal secretion overloads the normal absorptive capacity of the intestine and typically leads to voluminous watery stools. It can occur in response to a number of luminal or systemic factors such as increased concentrations of intraluminal hydroxy fatty acids produced by bacterial hydrolysis of ingested fat, intestinal inflammation or bacterial enterotoxins.

Increased permeability means that absorbed electrolytes (normally absorbed against a concentration gradient by active or facilitated diffusion) cannot be retained, and that fluid is not absorbed. Further increases in permeability lead to loss of macromolecules and tissue fluid, with consequent osmotic effects adding to the faecal fluid loss. The normal intestinal mucosa is relatively impermeable to electrolytes and macromolecules and this permeability barrier is maintained, in part, by tight junctions between epithelial cells. Maintenance of this permeability barrier is critical for normal absorptive capacity. Increased intestinal permeability occurs when there is damage to the normal mucosa, such as occurs with viral or bacterial enteritides, intestinal lymphosarcoma, intestinal ischaemia or intestinal inflammation.

Many diseases that cause diarrhoea do so by a combination of these mechanisms. In inflammatory bowel diseases, for example, there may be damage or immaturity of the normal villous mucosa leading to maldigestion, malabsorption and consequent osmotic effects, there may be increased intestinal permeability, and inflammatory mediators may influence epithelial cell secretion and cause aberrant motility.

INVESTIGATION OF DIARRHOEA

 ### HISTORY CHECKLIST

❏ **Age and breed?**
Certain breeds are more commonly seen with certain conditions; German shepherd dogs, for example, appear to be over represented among dogs with small intestinal bacterial overgrowth (SIBO) and exocrine pancreatic insufficiency (EPI); histiocytic ulcerative colitis is most often seen in boxer dogs. Young animals appear to be at greater risk of clinically significant intestinal helminthiasis, infectious diarrhoea or foreign body ingestion. Intestinal neoplasia is more common in older animals.

❏ **Signs of small intestinal disease or large intestinal disease?**
A number of presenting features will often enable the clinician to localize signs to the small or large intestine (Table 7.1). This is an extremely important step because the differential diagnoses, diagnostic approaches and management differs between the two (Tables 7.2–7.5).

❏ **Are the signs acute or chronic?**
The differential diagnoses of acute and chronic diarrhoea are different, and require different approaches to diagnosis and management. Chronic diarrhoea is generally considered to be present when signs have been apparent for longer than 4 weeks, and is an indication for diagnostic investigation and specific

Table 7.1 Clinical parameters used to distinguish between large and small bowel diarrhoea

Clinical sign	Small intestinal diarrhoea	Large intestinal diarrhoea
Defecatory frequency	3–4/day	Up to 10/day
Stool volume	Increased	Small amounts, total volume normal or increased
Faecal consistency	Soft to fluid	Soft
Defecatory tenesmus	Rare	Usual
Vomiting	Occasional	Rare
Weight loss	Often	Occasional
Inappetence	Variable	Occasional
Blood on stool	Rare	Common
Mucus on stool	Occasional	Common

Table 7.2 The differential diagnosis of small bowel diarrhoea

Extraintestinal disease
  Exocrine pancreatic insufficiency
  Acute pancreatitis
  Hepatic disease
  Renal failure
  Hypoadrenocorticism
Dietary intolerance
  Lactase deficiency
  Abrupt diet change
  Dietary indiscretion
Dietary allergy
  Immediate-type hypersensitivity
  Gluten sensitive enteropathy
Bacterial infection
  Salmonella spp.
  Campylobacter jejuni
  Bacillus piliformis
  Enteropathogenic *E. coli*
Viral infection
  Canine parvovirus
  Feline parvovirus
  Feline leukaemia virus
  Feline infectious peritonitis
  Feline immunodeficiency virus
  Canine distemper virus
  Canine corona virus
  Rotavirus
  Astrovirus
Parasitic infection
  Helminths
    Strongyloides spp.
    Trichuris volpis (dog only)
    Ancylostoma spp. (dog only)
    Uncinaria stenocephala (dog only)
    Toxocara spp.
    Toxascaris leonina (cat only)

Fungal/protozoal infection
  Giardia spp.
  Cryptosporidia spp.
Small intestinal bacterial overgrowth
  Idiopathic
  Secondary to intestinal anomalies, increased intake (e.g. coprophagia), chronic obstruction, deranged intestinal motility, mucosal immune defects, EPI, maldigestion/malabsorption, achlorhydria.
Foreign bodies
  Complete obstruction
  Partial obstruction
  Linear
Anomalies and malformations
  Lymphangiectasia
  Intestinal stricture
  Intussusception
  Intestinal volvulus
  Congenital malformation e.g. short bowel
Toxicities
  Heavy metals
  Drugs
  Insecticides
Idiopathic inflammatory bowel diseases
  Lymphoplasmacytic enteritis
  Eosinophilic enteritis
  Immunoproliferative enteropathy of Basenjis
Neoplasia
  Lymphosarcoma
  Other (e.g. plasmacytoma, carcinoma, adenocarcinoma, leiomyoma, leiomyosarcoma)

Table 7.3 The differential diagnosis of large bowel diarrhoea

Dietary intolerance
Dietary indiscretion
Dietary allergy
Bacterial infection
  Salmonella spp.
  Campylobacter jejuni
  Enteropathogenic *E. coli*
  Clostridium perfringens
  Yersinia enterocolitica
Parasitic infestation
  Trichuris vulpis
  Giardia spp.

Inflammatory bowel diseases
  Eosinophilic colitis
  Lymphoplasmacytic colitis
  Histiocytic ulcerative colitis
  Granulomatous colitis
  Fibrinopurulent colitis
Foreign bodies
Intestinal malformations and anomalies
  Caecal inversion
  Ileocolic inversion
Neoplasia
  Lymphosarcoma
  Other neoplasia

Table 7.4 A diagnostic approach to small bowel diarrhoea

1. **Determine duration, extent and severity of disease**
   History
2. **Initiate non-specific therapy, if appropriate (diet, antibiotics and anthelmintics), and/or pursue diagnosis**
3. **Rule out infectious disease**
   Faecal culture and parasitology
   Serological testing
   Virus antigen detection
4. **Rule out systemic involvement**
   Haematology
   Biochemistry
   Urinalysis
5. **Rule out exocrine pancreatic insufficiency**
   Trypsin-like immunoreactivity
   Faecal proteolytic activity
6. **Rule out intestinal obstruction, foreign bodies, mass lesions, mucosal thickening, anomalies**
   Plain and contrast radiography
   Ultrasonography
7. **Perform non-invasive tests of small intestinal function**
   Serum folate and cobalamin concentrations
   Sugar permeability and function tests
   Breath hydrogen testing
8. **Rule out dietary intolerance**
   Appropriate dietary trial
9. **Consider repeating faecal culture and parasitology**
10. **Rule out intraluminal or mucosal disease**
    Endoscopic examination or exploratory laparotomy
    Mucosal biopsy and duodenal juice sampling

Table 7.5 A diagnostic approach to large bowel diarrhoea

1. **Determine duration, extent and severity of disease**
   History
2. **Initiate non-specific therapy if appropriate (diet, antibiotics and anthelmintics), and/or pursue diagnosis**
3. **Rule out infectious disease**
   Faecal culture and parasitology
4. **Rule out *Clostridium perfringens* infection and examine for mucosal inflammation**
   Faecal cytology
5. **Rule out systemic disease**
   Haematology
   Biochemistry
   Urinalysis
6. **Rule out intestinal obstruction, foreign bodies, mass lesions, mucosal thickening, anomalies**
   Plain and contrast radiography
   Ultrasonography
7. **Rule out dietary intolerance**
   Appropriate dietary trial
8. **Consider non-specific therapy**
   Non-steroidal anti-inflammatory drugs (e.g. olsalazine, mesalazine)
   High fibre diet
   Motility modifiers
9. **Rule out intraluminal or mucosal disease**
   Endoscopy/proctoscopy
   Mucosal biopsy

therapy. Acute diarrhoea is often self-limiting and/or is easily managed by symptomatic and supportive therapy, and may not require definitive diagnosis. Profuse, acute diarrhoea, however, accompanied by systemic signs (such as fever, leucocytosis, leucopenia or dehydration) is consistent with more severe disease (e.g. infectious enteritis), and more vigorous investigation and aggressive therapy are warranted in such cases.

❑ Is the animal vaccinated and wormed?
Unvaccinated animals are at increased risk of viral enteritides. Lack of appropriate prophylaxis may increase the risk of parasitic infestation; anthelmintics may be indicated in such cases without further investigation if clinical signs are consistent.

❑ What is the animal's normal environment?
Kennelled animals are at greater risk of infectious bacterial enteritis and intestinal parasitism if appropriate husbandry is not applied.

❑ Appetite?
Increased appetite may be seen with maldigestion/malabsorption syndromes where the animal is systemically well (e.g. EPI, intestinal lymphangiectasia, inflammatory bowel disease (IBD)). Normal appetite is often a feature of large intestinal disease. Decreased appetite may be seen with infectious enteritides, SIBO, IBD, foreign bodies, neoplasia, intestinal obstruction and primary systemic disease.

❑ Dietary history?
Signs triggered by a particular foodstuff suggest dietary intolerance. Ingestion of milk can cause osmotic diarrhoea in lactase-deficient animals. Previously administered diets/foodstuffs should be avoided when formulating therapeutic dietary regimes.

❑ Weight loss/poor growth?
Weight loss/poor weight gain suggests negative protein-calorie balance, either as a result of inadequate ingestion due to poor appetite,

maldigestion/malabsorption, or the catabolic effects of systemically released mediators (e.g. inflammatory cytokines).

❏ **In contacts?**
Disease in in-contact animals suggests either a common environmental factor such as diet, toxins or infectious disease.

❏ **Signs of involvement of other body systems or systemic illness?**
Certain systemic diseases (e.g. renal failure, hypoadrenocorticism) can cause diarrhoea. Similarly, diarrhoeic diseases can cause systemic illness (e.g. viral or bacterial enteritides, protein-losing enteropathies).

❏ **Exposure to potential toxins (e.g. lead, iron, detergents or drugs (e.g. cathartics, laxatives)**

❏ **Abdominal pain?**
Signs of abdominal pain (e.g. guarding of abdomen, relief postures, vocalization) can be associated with foreign body ingestion, acute infectious enteritides, excessive intestinal gas, intestinal anomalies, intestinal obstruction, intestinal spasm, focal neoplasia, lead poisoning and metabolic diseases. Pain is uncommon in EPI, IBD, lymphosarcoma and lymphangiectasia.

❏ **Is foreign body ingestion a possibility?**
Has the animal had access to foreign objects (e.g. toys, string, bones)? Are any household objects missing?

❏ **What is the character of the stool?**
Voluminous, pale, extremely malodorous stools with a soft to semi-solid consistency are characteristic of maldigestion, especially EPI. Blood in the stool suggests loss of mucosal integrity. Partially digested blood and tissue may be seen when there is necrosis and sloughing of small intestinal mucosa (e.g. in parvoviral enteritis).

❏ **Does the diarrhoea respond to withholding food?**
Diarrhoea that is predominantly the result of osmotic effects will stop when food is withheld and recur upon reintroduction. Primary secretory diarrhoea will show no response to withholding of food.

PHYSICAL EXAMINATION

The main aim of the general physical examination is to identify disease in other body systems.

❏ **Signs of malnutrition**
Poor hair coat, muscle wasting, pot-bellied appearance and poor skin condition can all be indicators of poor nutritional status, suggestive of chronic maldigestive or malabsorptive diseases.

❏ **Abdominal palpation**
Thorough abdominal palpation should be performed to identify organomegaly, intestinal thickening or enlargement, aggregated bowel loops, mesenteric lymphadenopathy, excess intestinal fluid or gas, focal pain or intestinal tympany. The opportunity should be taken to repeat this examination if the animal is relaxed (e.g. following sedation or general anaesthesia).

❏ **Rectal examination**
A rectal examination should be performed in every case of chronic diarrhoea. This allows identification of rectal disease and visual examination of faecal character, as well as facilitating collection of faeces for laboratory testing.

FURTHER INVESTIGATION OR SYMPTOMATIC TREATMENT?

Following a complete history and physical examination the clinician must decide upon an appropriate course of action. Non-specific therapy may be appropriate for acute diarrhoea or when mild, chronic signs are present. When there is pronounced chronic diarrhoea or systemic illness is apparent, then aggressive supportive therapy and further diagnostic endeavours are appropriate. These decisions must be made by the clinician on a case-by-case basis.

CLINICAL AND LABORATORY INVESTIGATION OF DIARRHOEA

Faecal culture

Routine faecal culture should be performed to identify and obtain sensitivity spectra for *Salmonella* spp. and *Campylobacter* spp. In some centres it is possible to detect virulence genes and factors in enteropathogenic strains of *Escherichia coli* using molecular techniques, and assays can be employed that identify bacterial toxins in faeces (e.g. *Clostridium perfringens* enterotoxin).

Faecal virology

Canine parvoviral infection may be confirmed by use of ELISA to detect viral antigen in faecal material. In exceptional circumstances electron microscopy can be used to identify viral particles in faeces.

Faecal parasitology

Faecal examinations for parasites should be performed to rule out intestinal helminth infections (e.g. *Trichuris*, *Ancylostoma*) and intestinal protozoal infections (*Giardia*, *Cryptosporidia*). Faecal ELISA tests have been evaluated for the diagnosis of giardiasis in dogs but appear to offer little benefit over multiple (three or four) zinc sulphate flotation tests to identify cysts.

Faecal examinations

Faecal microscopy may be used to identify fats and fatty acids (Sudan III staining), undigested muscle fibres and undigested starch (iodine staining); positive findings suggest maldigestion (fats, muscle, starch) and malabsorption (fatty acids). Positive faecal occult blood (following 3 days on a white meat diet), suggests loss of mucosal integrity (inflammation, infection, neoplasia).

Faecal and rectal cytology

Smears of faecal mucus or superficial rectal mucosal cells (collected via digital rectal examination) may be examined following rapid cytological staining for the presence of inflammatory cells (neutrophils, eosinophils etc.), organisms (e.g. *Histoplasma*) and bacteria or bacterial spores. *C. perfringens* spores may be identified as oval bodies with pale central regions; more than two or three spores per high power field is usually considered to be significant.

Haematology

Routine haematology can identify systemic disease and inflammatory responses and may show mild anaemia with chronic disease or blood loss. Panleucopenia is seen in canine and feline parvoviral infection. Red cell microcytosis is seen with iron deficiency following chronic intestinal blood loss. Eosinophilia may be seen with parasitism, idiopathic eosinophilic conditions, mast cell neoplasia and hypoadrenocorticism.

Biochemistry

Serum/plasma biochemistry screening should identify systemic involvement in the disease process. Hyponatraemia and hyperkalaemia are typical of hypoadrenocorticism, but similar abnormalities have also been seen in cases of intestinal salmonellosis, trichuriasis and ulceration (so called 'pseudo-Addisonian' syndrome); an ACTH stimulation test provides a definitive diagnosis of hypoadrenocorticism. In the absence of indicators of hepatic failure or an increased urine protein:creatinine ratio, hypoalbuminaemia is most likely due to protein-losing enteropathy, the most common causes of which are IBD, lymphangiectasia and lymphosarcoma. In PLE, hypoalbuminaemia is often accompanied by hypoglobulinaemia.

Urinalysis

Urinalysis should be performed as part of the screen for systemic disease.

Serology and toxicology

Where appropriate, specific infection or intoxication may be confirmed by appropriate tests (e.g. feline leukaemia virus, feline immunodeficiency virus, lead poisoning).

Tests for EPI

Trypsin-like immunoreactivity (TLI) is measured by immunoassay in serum or plasma, and is therefore species specific. A canine TLI assay is routinely available and a feline TLI assay is available through selected centres. TLI measures circulating trypsinogen (or trypsin) and the concentration is reduced in EPI. Because of its ease and availability, this test should be performed early in the investigation of chronic small bowel diarrhoea.

Where feline TLI is unavailable, faecal proteolytic activity may be measured by casein or azocasein digestion, which is performed on a radial enzyme diffusion plate.

The bentiromide-para-aminobenzoic acid (BT-PABA) test has been superseded by measurement of serum TLI.

Tests of small intestinal function

Serum folate and cobalamin concentrations can be used as intestinal function tests in the investigation of canine small bowel disease. Folate is absorbed in the jejunum and decreased blood levels are consistent with diseases of the upper small intestine (e.g. dietary hypersensitivity). Because bacteria synthesize folate, increased serum folate has been associated with SIBO, but this is not a specific finding. Cobalamin is bound to intrinsic factor (produced by the stomach and pancreas in dogs) and the complex is absorbed in the ileum after binding to a specific carrier protein. Low serum cobalamin levels suggest either defective intrinsic factor production (not reported in the dog), bacterial binding of cobalamin (e.g. SIBO) or defective uptake in the ileum, either as a result of ileal disease or a receptor defect (which has been reported in giant Schnauzers and Border collies). The combination of low serum cobalamin and high serum folate has a high specificity but low sensitivity for SIBO.

Other tests that have been used to evaluate small intestinal function and permeability include plasma turbidity testing following fat administration (to test for lipid malassimilation) and xylose absorption and PABA absorption tests (to test for carbohydrate malassimilation). These tests have fallen out of favour recently because of cost, lack of specificity, variability (especially in relation to intestinal motility and blood flow) and their time-consuming nature. In contrast, some centres are now using tests of intestinal permeability that involve administration of pairs of sugars (e.g. mannitol/cellobiose, lactulose/rhamnose), one of which is well absorbed by the normal mucosa (e.g. rhamnose) and one of which is absorbed poorly (most likely via paracellular channels, e.g. lactulose). The ratio of the large sugar to the small (e.g. lactulose/rhamnose), either in urine or blood, is considered a measure of the 'leakiness' of the gut. Increased ratios may be associated with intestinal damage, and the tests can be used to demonstrate improvement following therapy. The use of two sugars and expression of the results as a ratio eliminates variables such as dose, gastric emptying, intestinal transit time and mucosal blood flow. In addition, a further sugar pair (e.g. xylose and 3-*O*-methyl-glucose (3MG)) may be added to the preparation. Xylose absorption appears to be rate limited according to the functional capacity of carriers in the intestinal brush border, whereas 3MG is completely absorbed. Reductions in the ratio xylose/3MG may be attributed to reduced function in the intestinal brush border. Although these sugar absorption tests are not without pitfalls, and require continued evaluation in a clinical setting, they can prove a useful part of the armoury in the investigation and management of canine and feline small intestinal disease.

Sequential measurement of breath hydrogen concentrations following sugar administration has also been used as a clinical tool; hydrogen is produced by enteric bacterial metabolism of carbohydrate. An early peak of hydrogen concentration following administration suggests either high proximal small intestinal bacterial numbers (i.e. SIBO) or rapid intestinal transit.

Radiographic examination

Plain abdominal radiographs can identify radio-opaque intestinal foreign objects, intestinal obstruction and large masses. Positive contrast radiographic examinations of the upper gastrointestinal tract (using barium liquid or barium impregnated plastic spheres) allow evaluation of gastric emptying and intestinal transit times, and can identify intestinal obstruction and anatomic anomalies. In addition, liquid barium can identify radiolucent foreign objects, focal and diffuse intestinal thickening, and mucosal abnormalities. A barium enema may be used to demonstrate similar changes in the large intestine. Negative contrast examination of the upper gastrointestinal tract (enteroclysis) has also been described but is not in common clinical use.

Ultrasonographic examinations

Ultrasonographic examinations can be complementary to, and in some cases alternative to, contrast examinations of the small and large bowel. In experienced hands, ultrasonography can identify mucosal thickening (focal or diffuse), intestinal mass lesions, intestinal obstruction, foreign bodies and anomalies (e.g. intussusceptions). In addition, focal mass lesions of a sufficient size to avoid luminal perforation can be biopsied using automated, spring-loaded biopsy instruments. This procedure should not be attempted by the inexperienced operator.

Dietary trial

Suspected dietary intolerance may be ruled out by performing a careful dietary trial. This should consist of feeding either a proprietary or homemade diet which contains a limited range of protein and carbohydrate sources (ideally one of each), none of which the animal has encountered before, and should therefore be based upon a thorough and careful dietary history. For homemade diets, possible carbohydrate sources include maize, rice or potatoes and possible protein sources include rabbit, chicken, turkey, fish or low-fat cottage cheese. These diets should be fed for a minimum of 4 weeks (authorities vary on this point) and the owners should be instructed to ensure that the animal is exposed to no other foodstuffs throughout this period (including treats or sweets).

High fibre diets may be useful for the management of chronic large intestinal diarrhoea, and may be fed early in the course of investigation if infectious disease is ruled out and clinical signs are mild.

Endoscopic examination

Endoscopy allows minimally invasive visualization and mucosal biopsy of the stomach, duodenum, colon and, occasionally, the ileum. It also facilitates collection of samples such as duodenal juice for microscopic and microbiological investigation. Abnormal visual findings during endoscopy include mucosal thickening/corrugation, mucosal erythema, excessive mucus, increased mucosal friability (all consistent with inflammation or neoplasia), luminal stricture, mucosal bleeding, mass lesions, and ulcers or erosions. The absence of visual abnormalities does not rule out significant microscopic disease.

Biopsy

Whenever performing an endoscopic examination, or when exploratory surgery is non-diagnostic (or unremarkable), multiple mucosal biopsies should be obtained. These may be either mucosal pinch biopsies during endoscopy or full thickness biopsies during surgery (dermatological biopsy punches are useful for this). Biopsies should be placed in fixative for subsequent histopathological examination. Histopathology will help identify and characterize mucosal inflammatory infiltration, mucosal neoplasia, lymphangiectasia, and some cases of infection or parasitic infestation.

Exploratory laparotomy and biopsy

Indications for exploratory laparotomy include discrete lesions identified by palpation, endoscopy, radiography or ultrasonography, and the need to obtain full thickness biopsy specimens from the length of the small bowel. Exploratory laparotomy should be performed only after ruling out systemic/metabolic disease and infectious disease. Duodenal juice may also be aspirated during exploratory laparotomy, using a syringe and needle passed obliquely through the bowel wall.

Duodenal juice examination and culture

Duodenal juice may be examined under phase contrast microscopy for the presence of parasites (e.g. *Giardia* trophozoites) and may be submitted for quantitative bacterial culture which is the only means of definitively diagnosing SIBO.

8

Defecatory Tenesmus

C. M. Elwood

Tenesmus is excessive straining to defecate or urinate. The investigation of abnormal urination and urinary incontinence is dealt with in Chapter 22. This chapter therefore concentrates on the investigation of defecatory tenesmus.

NORMAL DEFECATION

Normal defecation is achieved by a combination of voluntary control and reflex activity, coordinated in the lumbosacral spinal cord. The urge to defecate occurs in response to stimulation of the rectum, and is transferred in afferent fibres of the parasympathetic nervous system to the spinal cord, via the pelvic nerves. Sensations associated with stimulation of the anus and stretch of the muscles of the pelvic diaphragm also travel to the lumbosacral spinal cord and play a role in both maintaining continence and initiating defecation. Continence mechanisms allow an animal to reach a site appropriate for defecation, at which point conscious inhibition of the defecatory reflex is removed and the animal adopts a squatting posture. There is relaxation of the external anal sphincter (striated muscle innervated by the pudendal nerve), contraction of the levator ani muscle (first coccygeal nerve) and coccygeus muscle (third sacral nerve), inhibition of tone in the internal anal sphincter and contraction of rectal smooth muscle (parasympathetic fibres in the pelvic nerve). By closing the glottis, contracting the diaphragm and contracting the abdominal musculature, intra-abdominal pressure increases and the faecal bolus is extruded.

PATHOPHYSIOLOGY OF DEFECATORY TENESMUS

The clinical sign of defecatory tenesmus results from continued stimulation of the defecatory reflexes. These stimuli may be appropriate, when there is actual or functional obstruction to normal passage of faeces, or inappropriate, arising from either continued stimulation of stretch receptors and/or mucosal irritation. Functional obstruction to the passage of faeces may result from weakness/paralysis of the smooth muscle of the bowel, spasm of the muscles (due to pain or neuromuscular disease), an inability to increase intra-abdominal pressure (pain, muscle weakness, breach of the abdominal cavity wall) or an inability to maintain the normal posture for defecation (pain, weakness). Differential diagnoses for defecatory tenesmus are listed in Table 8.1.

INVESTIGATION OF DEFECATORY TENESMUS

HISTORY CHECKLIST

❏ **Age, breed, sex?**
Very young animals with defecatory tenesmus should be examined for imperforate anus or intestinal atresia; congenital megacolon is also a possibility. Entire male dogs are at greater risk of prostatic enlargement and perineal herniation, which may cause both urinary and defecatory tenesmus.

❏ **Is it urinary or defecatory tenesmus?**
These may be distinguished by establishing that there is normal function in the other system, and by determining the nature of the abnormal function. Occasionally, there may be disease affecting both systems (e.g. prostatomegaly causing urinary obstruction and defecatory tenesmus).

❏ **Obstruction or irritation?**
Persistent straining following the passage of faeces suggests mucosal irritation whereas straining before passage is more consistent with obstruction.

Table 8.1 The differential diagnosis of defecatory tenesmus

Defecatory tenesmus with empty colon
Large intestinal diarrhoea
Caecal inversions
Colonic neoplasia
Extracolonic compression
Intussusception
Acute pancreatitis
Proctitis
Defecatory tenesmus with full colon and abnormal rectal examination
Anal sac abscessation
Anal sac neoplasia
Faecal impaction
Foreign body
Imperforate anus
Intestinal atresia
Intrapelvic mass
Pararectal neoplasia
Pelvic narrowing
Perianal abscess
Perianal fistula
Perineal hernia
Prostatic enlargement (neoplasia, hyperplasia, abscess, cyst)
Rectal neoplasia
Rectal stricture
Trauma
Defecatory tenesmus with full colon and normal rectal examination
Benign colonic stricture
Dysautonomia
Dehydration
Drugs (opiates and opioids, anticholinergics, sucralfate, kaolin)
Foreign body
Megacolon
Colonic neoplasia
Extraluminal compression of the colon
Musculoskeletal pain or weakness
Inability to raise intra-abdominal pressure (e.g. inguinal hernia, diaphragmatic rupture)

❏ **Diarrhoea?**
Diarrhoea is increased frequency of effective defecation, increased faecal volume or increased faecal fluidity. Tenesmus due to causes of large bowel diarrhoea is often associated with the production of small volumes of semi-liquid faeces, often very mucoid with surface haemorrhage. If large volumes of watery diarrhoea are produced, small bowel involvement should be suspected.

❏ **Constipation?**
Defecatory tenesmus with infrequent passage of a stool, suggests either a functional disorder of the normal defecatory apparatus (e.g. megacolon, perineal hernia) or partial/incomplete obstruction to the passage of faeces (e.g. intrapelvic mass, faecal impaction).

❏ **Haematochezia?**
Blood on the stool, without diarrhoea, suggests focal lesions of the colon, rectum or anus (e.g. colonic neoplasia, early colitis, rectal trauma, anal sac abscess).

❏ **Dyschezia?**
Painful defecation may be manifested as constipation, crying out upon defecation or reluctance to defecate. Dyschezia with tenesmus may be seen with painful conditions such as anal sac abscessation, rectal or colonic neoplasia, proctitis, rectal trauma or foreign body, prostatic disease and intrapelvic neoplasia.

❏ **Stool character?**
Stools with a ribbon-like shape imply luminal stricture in the rectum.

❏ **Trauma/foreign body?**
Recent foreign body ingestion may suggest tenesmus is due to colorectal irritation/obstruction. A history consistent with trauma to the anus, rectum, perineum or pelvis may indicate a possible functional or actual obstruction.

❏ **Abdominal pain?**
Signs of abdominal pain include crying upon handling or abdominal palpation, boarding of the abdominal musculature, 'colicky' behaviour and performance of relief postures. Pain may be seen with traumatic diseases of the defecatory apparatus and with neoplasia. Other causes of pain must also be considered, because they can prevent adoption of normal voiding posture or manoeuvres to increase intra-abdominal pressure.

❏ **Signs of neuromuscular disease?**
Possible weakness and/or paresis, ataxia, hind limb muscle wasting, muscle pain or back pain should all be questioned to evaluate possible generalized spinal or neuromuscular disease as a cause of defecatory tenesmus.

❏ **Weight loss?**
Weight loss suggests either systemic involvement

in a disease process (e.g. neoplasia, infection) or gastrointestinal disease.

❏ Recent medication?
A history of recent drug administration should be obtained, because certain drugs can cause constipation (Table 8.1).

❏ Dysautonomia
Regurgitation, dry mouth, dry eye, mydriasis and protrusion of the nictitating membranes may accompany defecatory (and urinary) tenesmus in cases of dysautonomia.

PHYSICAL EXAMINATION

❏ General physical examination
This should identify complicating or intercurrent disease. The perineum should be examined for asymmetry, swelling, discoloration and pain. The inguinal and umbilical regions should be examined for herniation. Dyspnoea following a road-traffic accident may be associated with diaphragmatic herniation, and may be accompanied by reduced heart or lung sounds on thoracic auscultation. Herniations and ruptures can prevent the normal increase in intra-abdominal pressure during defecation.

❏ Abdominal palpation
Abdominal palpation should particularly attempt to identify the colon and prostate (which may move into the abdomen when enlarged). A large colon full of hard faecal boluses may be detected when there is constipation or obstipation. Mass lesions of the colon, bladder or caudal abdomen may be detectable. Abdominal palpation should be repeated at every opportunity, particularly when the animal is relaxed (e.g. during sedation or general anaesthesia for other diagnostic procedures).

❏ Rectal examination
Rectal palpation should be performed in every dog but may not be feasible in cats. Features to note on rectal palpation include anal tone, the character of faeces, the presence or absence of blood on the glove, the diameter of the pelvic canal, the size, firmness and sensitivity of the intrapelvic urethra, breakdown of the pelvic diaphragm consistent with perineal herniation, the size, shape, surface regularity, consistency and sensitivity of the prostate gland (male dogs) and the presence of rectal mass lesions, foreign bodies or rectal strictures.

❏ Neuromuscular examination
When the general history or physical examination suggests possible neuromuscular or musculoskeletal disease, neurological and musculoskeletal examinations are appropriate.

FURTHER INVESTIGATION

■ Observation

The clinician should observe the actions of the animal when showing tenesmus. This may allow confirmation of the nature of the tenesmus (urinary versus defecatory). The normal postures for defecation and urination differ in both the canine and the feline and may help to localize signs. If a normal posture is adopted, neuromuscular or orthopaedic conditions become less likely. If straining produces signs of pain or discomfort, then musculoskeletal disease should be considered. Observation also allows further confirmation of historical points already covered.

■ Investigation of large intestinal disease

Where history and physical examination suggest that large intestinal diarrhoea is present, investigations should be pursued based upon the appropriate differential diagnosis (see Chapter 7).

■ Haematology/biochemistry

Haematology and biochemistry screens should be obtained to rule out metabolic or infectious disease. Complications of conditions causing tenesmus include hypercalcaemia secondary to anal sac adenocarcinoma or peritonitis.

■ Microbiology

Microbiological examination of faeces is indicated where large bowel diarrhoea is a feature, or where there is a proctitis.

■ Parasitology

These examinations may be necessary to rule out parasitic causes of defecatory tenesmus (e.g. *Trichuris vulpis*).

Plain radiographic examinations

Radiographic examinations play a major role in the investigation of defecatory tenesmus. Plain lateral abdominal radiographs should always image the anus and rectum; it is easy to collimate out structures such as the terminal rectum and fail to detect perineal herniation. Plain abdominal radiographs allow identification of enlarged organs, megacolon, intra-abdominal masses, radio-opaque foreign bodies, some intussusceptions, prostatic or paraprostatic enlargements, perineal herniation and skeletal disease.

Barium enema

Following thorough bowel cleansing, a barium enema may be administered to provide contrast examination of the lower bowel. This may outline foreign bodies, intussusceptions, mucosal irregularities, mucosal thickenings or mass lesions, strictures, and extraluminal compression.

Ultrasonography

Ultrasonography may be extremely useful to evaluate the gastrointestinal tract and prostate. Ultrasonography can detect masses of the intestinal wall, intraluminal foreign bodies, intra-abdominal masses, intussusception, intrapelvic masses and prostatic enlargement. Ultrasound may also be used to guide aspiration or biopsy of focal abnormalities.

Needle biopsy

This may be appropriate for the further assessment of masses identified by observation, palpation or imaging.

Prostatic wash or ejaculate analysis

These investigations may be appropriate where prostatic disease is a suspected cause of defecatory tenesmus (see Chapter 41).

Faecal cytology

Following the passage of faeces or rectal examination, surface mucus on the stool or glove may be smeared for cytological examination. This may reveal inflammatory cells, infectious organisms (e.g. *Histoplasma* spp. in North America), or spores of toxin-producing *Clostridium perfringens*.

Proctoscopy/colonoscopy

To evaluate the large bowel and rectum visually, and to obtain mucosal biopsies of any identified lesions, proctoscopy or colonoscopy may be performed. These techniques may be achieved with rigid instruments (which only evaluate the rectum and descending colon) or flexible fibreoptic instruments (which can evaluate the whole length of the large intestine). Thorough patient preparation and cleansing of the colon is indicated to allow adequate visualization of the mucosa. These techniques will detect mucosal inflammation, parasitic infestation, neoplasia, stricture, foreign bodies, extraluminal compression, intussusceptions and caecal inversion.

The diagnostic approach to defecatory tenesmus is summarized in Table 8.2.

Table 8.2 A diagnostic approach to defecatory tenesmus

1. Determine general health and nature of defecation History
2. Evaluate anus, rectum, colon and abdominal cavity Physical examination Abdominal palpation Rectal examination
3. Signs of large bowel diarrhoea/colitis/proctitis See Chapters 7 and 36
4. Rule out systemic disease or complications Haematology Biochemistry Urinalysis
4. If obstruction suspected, attempt to localize/ characterize Plain abdominal radiographs Ultrasonography Contrast radiography Proctoscopy/colonoscopy Tissue sampling procedures

9
Polydipsia and Polyuria

J. K. Dunn

Polyuria signifies the formation and excretion of large volumes of urine (50 ml kg^{-1} 24 h^{-1}) usually of low specific gravity. *Polydipsia* can be defined as increased thirst resulting in the consumption of increased volumes of fluid (>100 ml kg^{-1} 24 h^{-1}). Depending on the water content of the diet a healthy dog drinks on average 50–60 ml kg^{-1} 24 h^{-1}; normal urine output varies between 20 and 40 ml kg^{-1} 24 h^{-1}.

NORMAL WATER BALANCE

The balance between water input and output is so precise that daily fluctuations in body weight rarely exceed 1%. Water may be taken into the body by drinking or in food (hence the moisture content of the diet may influence the volume of water drunk); it is also produced in the body from the oxidation of carbohydrate, fat and protein. Water is lost from the body in urine, faeces and by evaporation from the skin and respiratory tract. Under normal circumstances the amount of water lost in faeces is minimal compared to the volumes lost in urine and by evaporation. Adjustments to the rate of release of antidiuretic hormone (ADH) from the neurohypophysis ensure that the urine is maximally concentrated and that the volume is the minimum required for the obligatory excretion of the end-products of protein metabolism (urea, sulphate and phosphate ions). Water contained in the diet plus the volume of water drunk after a meal are sufficient to meet this obligatory urine loss. Similarly the increased volumes of water drunk by animals in hot weather or during periods of activity are sufficient to immediately match the increased evaporative losses and prevent dehydration.

The two main mechanisms responsible for normal water balance are: (1) the thirst mechanism and (2) the renal concentration mechanisms. In most cases polydipsia compensates for obligatory polyuria, i.e. polyuria is the primary problem and results in a secondary or compensatory polydipsia. This is true for all the disorders which are commonly associated with polydipsia with the exception of primary or psychogenic polydipsia (compulsive water drinking) where polyuria is secondary and occurs in response to the excess water load.

Providing the thirst and renal concentrating mechanisms are intact polyuria is accompanied by compensatory polydipsia so that the volume of total body fluids is maintained within normal limits. Simultaneous defects in the thirst and renal concentration mechanisms may result in two possible outcomes.

1. Polyuria which occurs without compensatory polydipsia results in volume depletion of both the extracellular and intracellular compartments leading to hypernatraemia, hypovolaemia and cellular dehydration.
2. If polydipsia occurs without compensatory polyuria the cells become overhydrated which may have consequences on cerebral and pulmonary function. The same problem may occur with iatrogenic volume overload following the overzealous administration of intravenous fluids especially to patients with impaired renal tubular function or renal 'shutdown'.

Water balance is partly regulated by the osmolality of the extracellular fluid (ECF) and is therefore closely related to sodium homeostasis since the osmolality of ECF is almost entirely determined by the concentration of sodium ions (Fig. 9.1).

THIRST

The 'thirst' centres are located in the hypothalamus. The neurones of the thirst centre respond to increases in ECF osmolality and decreases in

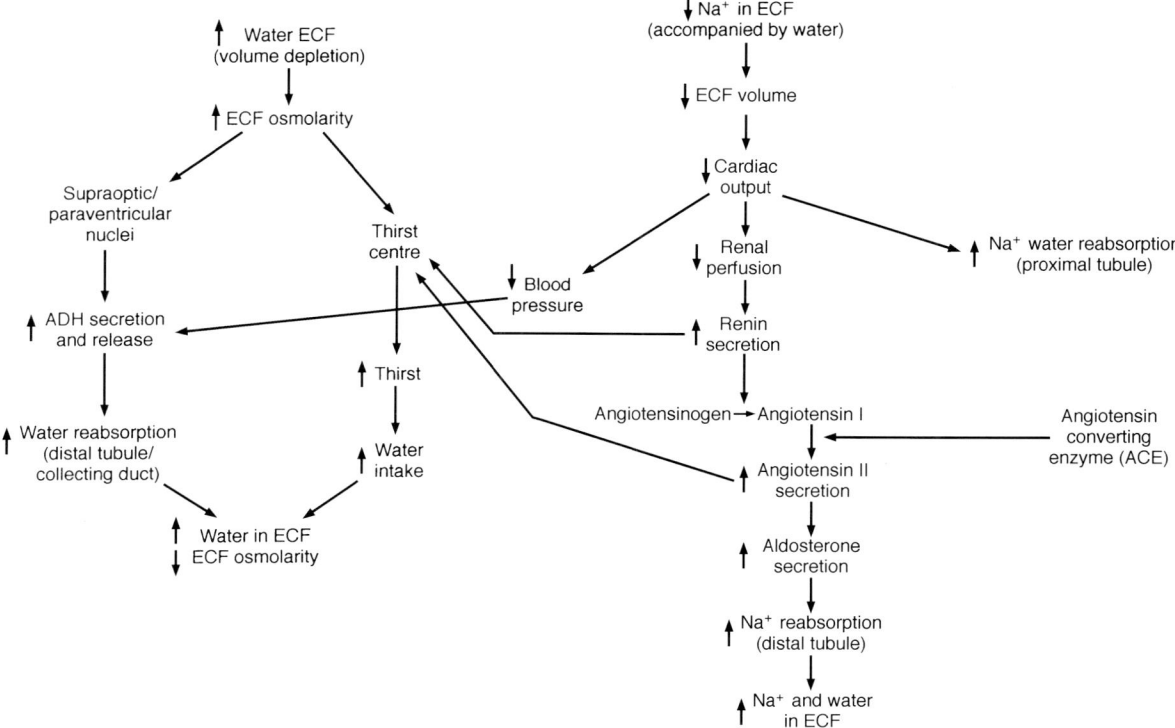

Figure 9.1 Water and sodium balance. ECF, extracellular fluid.

effective blood (ECF) volume. The normal day to day control of water balance involves interaction between osmoreceptors in the hypothalamus and pressure receptors located in the left atrium and major vessels (carotid sinus and aortic arch).

RENAL CONCENTRATING MECHANISMS

Secretion of antidiuretic hormone

ADH (or vasopressin) is synthesized by the supraoptic and paraventricular nuclei of the hypothalamus and stored in nerve endings in the posterior pituitary (neurohypophysis). The osmoreceptors of the hypothalamus are located in close proximity to the ADH synthesizing cells. The stimuli for ADH release are plasma hypertonicity and hypovolaemia. Sodium and its anions contribute more than 95% to the total osmotic pressure and are the most potent stimulators of ADH secretion. A 1% increase in osmolality is sufficient to evoke a significant change in ADH secretion via osmoreceptors in the hypothalamus whereas an 8–10% reduction in blood volume is required to stimulate ADH release.

ADH increases the permeability of the cells of the distal renal tubules and collecting ducts to water via a specific receptor mechanism. In response to ADH, water is reabsorbed along concentration gradients established in the renal medulla by the countercurrent multiplier system involving the loop of Henle and vasa recta. High concentrations of sodium and urea in the medullary interstitium preserve this concentration gradient which is necessary for ADH to exert its maximal antidiuretic effect. A loss of renal medullary hypertonicity ('medullary washout') reduces the ability of the kidney to concentrate urine in response to ADH.

The ability of the kidney to concentrate urine therefore depends on the following factors:

1. The amount of circulating ADH.
2. The responsiveness of the distal tubules and collecting ducts to ADH.
3. The degree of hypertonicity of the renal medulla and the presence of a normal concentration gradient.
4. The concentration of solute in the glomerular filtrate.

Renal tubular function

Glomerular filtrate is isosthenuric, i.e. has a specific gravity similar to that of plasma (1.008–1.012). Approximately 70% of the filtered sodium load is actively reabsorbed in the proximal tubule by a process which is dependent on the activity of a cellular sodium-potassium ATPase pump. The continuous reabsorption of sodium and other solutes including glucose sets up osmotic gradients so that water is reabsorbed passively with the sodium. Approximately 25% of the sodium load is reabsorbed with chloride from the thick ascending limb of the loop of Henle, a process which can be blocked by loop diuretics such as frusemide. Reabsorption of sodium from the loop of Henle contributes significantly to the maintenance of medullary hypertonicity. Since this part of the nephron is relatively impermeable to water the glomerular filtrate is actively diluted and is therefore hypotonic as it enters the distal tubule. In the distal tubule sodium (less than 10% of the filtered load) and water are reabsorbed under the action of aldosterone, while potassium is actively secreted into the tubular lumen. Finally, in the presence of ADH, water is reabsorbed with urea from some distal tubule segments and the collecting ducts resulting in the formation of concentrated urine.

Aldosterone

Aldosterone is produced by the zona glomerulosa of the adrenal cortex and acts on the cells of the distal tubule to promote the reabsorption of sodium and excretion of potassium and hydrogen ions. Increased plasma potassium concentrations increase aldosterone secretion via a direct effect of potassium on the adrenal cortex. Alterations in plasma sodium concentration affect aldosterone release via the renin–angiotensin system (Fig. 9.1).

Sodium depletion causes a reduction in circulating blood volume which decreases renal perfusion. In response to this decrease in renal perfusion specialized myoepithelial cells in the juxtaglomerular apparatus secrete the proteolytic enzyme renin. Conditions such as dehydration, shock, haemorrhage or congestive heart failure which decrease ECF volume and/or arterial blood pressure therefore activate the renin–angiotensin system.

Renin cleaves angiotensin I from angiotensinogen, a plasma alpha-2 globulin produced in the liver. Angiotensin converting enzyme (ACE) converts angiotensin I into angiotensin II. Angiotensin II is a powerful vasoconstrictor which increases peripheral vascular resistance. It also has a direct negative feedback effect on the secretion of renin and stimulates the release of aldosterone from the adrenal cortex thereby restoring the ECF volume deficit and increasing arterial blood pressure.

Activation of the renin–angiotensin system and the increased circulating levels of aldosterone may partly explain why dogs with congestive heart failure, particularly those in the early stages of decompensation, tend to be mildly polydipsic. In addition to providing a stimulus for ADH release angiotensin has a direct stimulatory effect on the thirst centre.

Natriuretic factors

Natriuretic factors are peptides that influence sodium balance in the short term by promoting the urinary excretion of sodium. One such factor, atrial natriuretic peptide, is released in response to left atrial volume overload.

PATHOPHYSIOLOGY OF POLYURIA

In many cases the cause of polyuria is multifactorial, for example the polyuria associated with chronic liver disease may be partly due to renal medullary washout (decreased urea production), and partly to decreased renin catabolism or possibly the reduced metabolism of glucocorticoids resulting in interference with the action of ADH. The proposed pathophysiological mechanisms for the numerous non-endocrine and endocrine disorders which cause polyuria/polydipsia are described in Tables 9.1 and 9.2. The mechanisms responsible for the polyuria/polydipsia associated with many of the non-endocrine disorders frequently involve an endocrine component, for example interference with the action of ADH.

Solute diuresis

Osmotic diuresis occurs when the glomerular filtrate contains a large amount of solute (e.g. glucose, urea or sodium) which exceeds the

Table 9.1 Non-endocrine causes of polyuria and polydipsia

Condition	Mechanism for polyuria/polydipsia
Chronic renal failure	Decrease in number of functional nephrons; osmotic diuresis
Chronic liver disease	Decreased medullary hypertonicity; hypercortisolaemia; impaired action and release of ADH and aldosterone
Pyometra and other toxaemic states	Renal tubular insensitivity to ADH induced by *E. coli* endotoxins; immune-complex glumerulonephritis
Primary (psychogenic) polydipsia	Failure of collecting ducts to respond to ADH; medullary washout
Primary renal glycosuria	Osmotic diuresis
Fanconi syndrome	Osmotic diuresis
Hypercalcaemia, e.g. hypercalcaemia associated with malignancy, metastatic bone tumours, renal dysplasia	Nephrocalcinosis may result in chronic renal insufficiency; impaired action of ADH on renal tubular/collecting duct receptors
Hypokalaemia, e.g. excessive loss of potassium via the gastrointestinal tract or urinary tract (diabetes mellitus, diuretics)	Intracellular dehydration results in stimulation of thirst centre; medullary washout; failure of collecting duct to respond to ADH
Congestive heart failure	Activation of the renin–angiotensin–aldosterone system (angiotensin has a direct stimulatory action on the thirst centre)
Hyperviscosity syndromes, e.g. polycythaemia, hypergammaglobulinaemia	Uncertain

Table 9.2 Endocrine causes of polyuria and polydipsia

Condition	Mechanism for polyuria/polydipsia
Diabetes insipidus (central or nephrogenic forms)	Decreased secretion of ADH (central) or distal tubules/collecting ducts unresponsive to ADH (nephrogenic)
Diabetes mellitus (may be associated with hyperadrenocorticism)	Osmotic diuresis
Hyperadrenocorticism (may be associated with diabetes mellitus)	Excessive production of cortisol interferes with action of ADH on renal tubules/collecting ducts; ?inhibition of ADH release
Hypoadrenocorticism (approximately 15% of chronic cases are polyuric/polydipsic)	Medullary washout (increased urinary excretion of sodium); hypovolaemia stimulates ADH release
Hyperthyroidism	Uncertain; probably multifactorial (may interfere with action of ADH; increased renal blood flow may result in medullary washout)
Acromegaly (either iatrogenic due to prolonged progestagen administration or arises spontaneously during dioestrus phase of oestrus cycle)	Excessive production of growth hormone results in insulin-resistant diabetes mellitus
Hypercalcaemia, e.g. primary hyperparathyroidism (usually parathyroid adenomas); hypervitaminosis D	As for non-endocrine causes of hypercalcaemia (Table 9.1)
Hypocalcaemia, e.g. idiopathic hypoparathyroidism; thyroid carcinoma resulting in hypercalcitonism (rare)	Uncertain

reabsorptive capacity of the proximal tubular epithelial cells. The osmotic gradient set up means that water is retained in the glomerular filtrate so that, even if adequate amounts of ADH are present, the volume of fluid presented to the collecting duct overwhelms its capacity to reabsorb water resulting in the obligatory excretion of water. Diabetes mellitus, chronic renal failure and the diuresis that occurs after successful relief of a urethral obstruction are examples of osmotic diuresis.

■ Water diuresis

ADH alters the permeability of the cells of the distal tubules and collecting ducts to water by attaching to receptors on the peritubular side of the cell. This results in activation of adenyl cyclase and an increase in the intracellular concentration of cyclic AMP. The ingestion of a large volume of water for example in dogs with primary polydipsia expands the extracellular space and plasma volume, i.e. the animal becomes overhydrated and as a result ADH secretion is inhibited (in this case a *relative* deficiency of ADH). Water diuresis may be the result of an *absolute* (total or partial) deficiency of ADH (central diabetes insipidus). Several drugs, hormones and disease conditions alter the renal tubular responsiveness to ADH by altering the interaction of ADH with its receptor, the activation of adenyl cyclase or the catabolism of cAMP (nephrogenic diabetes insipidus). The result is the excretion of large volumes of solute-free urine.

■ Renal medullary washout

The corticomedullary gradient is maintained by the efflux of high levels of urea and sodium chloride from the loop of Henle and collecting ducts. Conditions which deplete the concentration of urea or sodium in the renal medullary interstitium or diseases which cause pronounced polydipsia over a prolonged period may result in a loss of medullary hypertonicity and an inability to concentrate urine maximally even in the presence of adequate amounts of ADH. In addition to causing polyuria, medullary washout may create problems when interpreting the various diagnostic tests used to differentiate between primary (psychogenic) polydipsia and both the central and nephrogenic forms of diabetes insipidus.

INVESTIGATION OF POLYDIPSIA AND POLYURIA

Endocrine and non-endocrine causes of polyuria/polydipsia and the pathophysiological mechanisms are summarized in Tables 9.1 and 9.2.

An accurate history and thorough physical examination are prerequisite if unnecessary and expensive laboratory tests are to be avoided. Consideration should be given to the general health of the patient, diet, environmental factors, reproductive history, and recent or current drug administration.

HISTORY CHECKLIST

❏ **How much water is the animal drinking?**
Verify and quantitate the polydipsia. The volume of water drunk should be quantitated on a daily (24 hour) basis at an early stage of the investigations. For animals from multi-pet households this may require a short period of hospitalization. In most cases, including animals with diabetes insipidus, the polydipsia is secondary to an obligatory polyuria. Tables 9.1 and 9.2 list the major causes of polyuria and polydipsia; mild transient increases in water intake may occur in response to dehydration or hypovolaemia caused by or associated with high environmental temperatures, strenuous exercise, dyspnoea or prolonged hyperventilation, acute haemorrhage, lactation, vomiting and diarrhoea and severe burns.

Animals with diabetes insipidus or primary polydipsia are usually severely polydipsic with a four- to sixfold increase in water consumption. Some animals with diabetes insipidus may drink from puddles or toilets; some even drink their own urine making it difficult to obtain an accurate estimate of the volume drunk. Primary polydipsia is a rare condition where water consumption exceeds the body's demand and results in a compensatory polyuria. Specific causes include central nervous system (e.g. hypothalamic) lesions and psychogenic polydipsia (compulsive water drinking). With the latter, hospitalization alone may significantly reduce the volume of water drunk presumably by removing any precipitating emotional or stress factor that may be present.

❏ **Urinary incontinence or nocturia?**
An owner may seek veterinary attention either because the animal is drinking more water or suddenly is unable to retain large volumes of urine at night. Nocturia refers to the conscious

(voluntary) act of urinating at night which may simply be a consequence of the amount of water drunk. Sphincter mechanism incompetence (or oestrogen-responsive incontinence) typically occurs in obese, middle-aged, medium to large breed speyed bitches and is characterized by the passive dribbling of urine when the dog is either lying down resting or sleeping. Polyuria may initiate or exacerbate both nocturia and urinary incontinence.

❑ Breed, age and sex (sexually intact or neutered)?
Pyometra should be ruled out in middle-aged intact bitches. Poodles are predisposed to diabetes mellitus and hyperadrenocorticism; lhasa apsos and shih tzus to familial renal dysplasia; Basenjis and elkhounds to primary renal glycosuria; Bedlington terriers to copper storage hepatopathy. Psychogenic polydipsia, although a relatively rare condition, tends to occur in larger breeds of dog. The three major differential diagnoses for polydipsia in an elderly cat are chronic renal insufficiency, diabetes mellitus and hyperthyroidism.

❑ Appetite and diet?
Composition of the diet influences the volume of fluid drunk. This is especially true in cats which derive a higher percentage of their total daily fluid requirements from food. Animals fed an all-in-one dry diet invariably drink more water than do those fed a moist or semi-moist diet. Many of the non-endocrine causes of polyuria/polydipsia cause inappetence or anorexia; in contrast, animals with psychogenic polydipsia and some of the endocrine causes such as hyperadrenocorticism, hyperthyroidism (unless the apathetic form) and diabetes mellitus (unless ketoacidotic) may have normal or increased appetites.

❑ General health?
Has the animal been showing signs of systemic or metabolic disease such as weight loss, lethargy, depression, anorexia, vomiting or diarrhoea? If the answer is yes, consider toxaemia (pyometra), uraemia, ketoacidosis, hypoadrenocorticism and hypercalcaemia.

❑ Exercise intolerance or generalized weakness?
Muscle atrophy, especially pronounced over the temporal region, and progressive muscle weakness occur in dogs with hyperadrenocorticism hence their typical pot-bellied appearance.

❑ CNS signs or behavioural changes?
CNS signs or behavioural changes (ataxia, apparent blindness, aimless wandering, stupor and seizures) may be seen with hepatic encephalopathy and in some dogs with hyperadrenocorticism (especially those with a large expanding pituitary adenoma).

❑ Reproductive history?
Recent oestrus or recent oestrogen administration? Pyometra typically occurs in middle-aged bitches and is characterized by a purulent and/or sanguineous vaginal discharge (usually first noticed 4–8 weeks after oestrus, i.e. during or immediately after the dioestrus phase of the cycle). Pyometra may occur in younger animals following the administration of oestrogens for misalliance. Hyperadrenocorticism may be associated with prolonged anoestrus or a history of reduced libido in the stud dog.

❑ Environmental changes?
Occasionally a precipitating stress factor (moving house, new baby etc.) may be identified in dogs with primary psychogenic polydipsia.

❑ Trauma?
Acquired diabetes insipidus has been reported in dogs and cats following trauma to the head resulting in disruption of the pituitary stalk.

❑ Recent/current drug administration?
Many drugs can induce polyuria/polydipsia and can modify urine specific gravity. Hence for diagnostic purposes it is important to obtain a urine sample before the animal is given intravenous fluids or diuretics. The administration of frusemide, dextrose, mannitol or intravenous crystalloid solutions results in an obligatory solute diuresis. Glucocorticoids and anticonvulsant drugs such as phenytoin, primidone and phenobarbitol interfere either with the release of ADH from the pituitary or the action of ADH on the renal tubules.

PHYSICAL EXAMINATION

❑ General demeanour?
Dogs with the central form of diabetes insipidus or psychogenic polydipsia may be excitable and nervous but otherwise appear healthy.

❑ Weigh and assess hydration status
Skin 'tenting' provides only a very rough assessment of an animal's hydration status and is unreliable in the very obese or emaciated patient or in animals with hyperadrenocorticism.

❏ Peripheral lymphadenopathy?
Multicentric lymphadenopathy should be considered and the plasma calcium concentration checked. The most common cause of hypercalcaemia in small animals is that associated with lymphoma.

❏ Palpable thyroid mass?
Hyperthyroidism in the cat is usually caused by a benign thyroid adenoma (less frequently a thyroid carcinoma).

❏ Bradycardia?
Consider electrolyte imbalances e.g. hyperkalaemia (hypoadrenocorticism) or hypercalcaemia.

❏ Abdomen
Are the kidneys enlarged (glomerulonephritis, amyloidosis, pyelonephritis) or small and misshapen (chronic interstitial nephritis, congenital renal hypoplasia)?

Is the liver enlarged (diabetes mellitus, hyperadrenocorticism, chronic active hepatitis, feline lymphocytic cholangiohepatitis, hepatic neoplasia) or small (hepatic fibrosis or cirrhosis, portosystemic shunt)?

Is the uterus distended (closed-cervix pyometra)?

Is the abdomen pendulous with or without the skin changes described below (hyperadrenocorticism)?

❏ External genitalia
Is there a vaginal discharge (open-cervix pyometra) or testicular atrophy (hyperadrenocorticism)?

❏ Skin
Endocrine alopecia, thin, non-elastic skin, comedone formation if associated with a pendulous abdomen are characteristic of hyperadrenocorticism.

❏ Cataract formation?
This may suggest diabetes mellitus.

LABORATORY INVESTIGATION OF POLYDIPSIA/POLYURIA

■ Urinalysis

Urine protein
Low molecular weight proteins up to the size of albumin are filtered by the glomeruli and pass into the renal tubular lumen. Normal urine has a trace of protein; healthy dogs and cats excrete small amounts of protein (usually <30 mg kg^{-1} day^{-1}). Dipstick reagent strips are sensitive for albumin but do not detect globulins or Bence-Jones proteins; a trace protein measurement equates to only 5–20 mg dl^{-1} of protein. Most animals with chronic interstitial nephritis do not pass large quantities of protein in urine (there may be trace or 1+ reading on a dipstick). If 3+ or 4+ proteinuria persists, calculation of the urinary protein:creatinine ratio may help to rule out protein-losing nephropathy (see below). The urinary protein content may be increased by the presence of red blood cells, white blood cells and bacteria and this should be taken into consideration when interpreting the results. False positive readings may occur if urine contaminated with quaternary ammonium antiseptics or chlorhexidine or if urine is highly alkaline; damp strips may also give a false positive result. False negative readings may occur if the predominant protein is not albumin or if urine is very dilute.

Turbimetric tests induce precipitation of protein by the addition of chemical reagents, e.g. nitric acid, hot acetic acid and sulphosalicylic acid (SSA). The density of the precipitate is quantified by optical densitometry. Turbimetric tests detect albumin, globulins, Bence-Jones proteins and glycoproteins. False positives occur if sulphonamide metabolites, penicillin, cephalosporin or iodinated radiographic contrast agents are present in urine.

Mechanisms of proteinuria

- *Prerenal (preglomerular) or glomerular overload*: Intravascular haemolysis (haemoglobinaemia); rhabdomyolysis (free myoglobin); immunoglobulin light chain monomers or dimers (Bence-Jones proteins) with plasma cell myeloma
- *Glomerular*: Damage to glomerular filtration barrier e.g. glomerulonephritis, renal amyloidosis
- *Postglomerular*
  (a) Defective proximal tubular cell function resulting in failure to reabsorb low molecular weight proteins, e.g. Fanconi syndrome, acute tubular necrosis (heavy metal or aminoglycoside toxicity)
  (b) Urogenital inflammation resulting in exudation of protein into urine, e.g. pyelonephritis, cystitis, prostatitis, urolithiasis and transitional cell carcinoma

- *Functional proteinuria?* In humans functional proteinuria is associated with strenuous exercise, fever, exposure to extremes of temperature, stress, congestive heart failure and systemic arterial hypertension

Assessing the significance of proteinuria

Consider the magnitude of proteinuria in relation to urine specific gravity, for example 2+ proteinuria in a very dilute urine could be significant. Examine urinary sediment to rule out contamination with blood or inflammatory exudate.

If proteinuria is not associated with haematuria or an inflammatory exudate (i.e. an active urinary sediment), check *urine protein:urine creatinine ratio (UP:UC ratio)* to quantify the extent of the protein loss (centrifuge the urine first).

$$\text{UP:UC} = \frac{\text{Urine protein concentration (mg dl}^{-1})^*}{\text{Urine creatinine concentration (mg dl}^{-1})^*}$$

Conversion factors:
Protein g l^{-1} to mg dl^{-1} (multiply × 100)
Urine creatinine μmol l^{-1} to mg dl^{-1} (divide by 88.4)

The UP:UC ratio on a single sample correlates well with the measured 24 hour urinary protein excretion.

Interpretation of UP:UC ratios

- A UP:UC ratio of <1.0 is normal for dogs and cats; most dogs have a UP:UC ratio <0.5
- If the UP:UC ratio is between 1.0 and 5.0 consider preglomerular, mild glomerular or postglomerular lesions (the latter should be associated with an active sediment)
- A UP:UC ratio between 5 and 13 usually indicates severe postglomerular proteinuria or glomerulonephropathy
- A UP:UC ratio >13 indicates severe glomerulonephropathy

Urine glucose

The presence of a 3+ or 4+ reading for glucose on a dipstick when accompanied by an increased plasma glucose concentration (see below) is consistent with a diagnosis of diabetes mellitus. Affected animals may also test positive for the presence of ketones. Transient glycosuria (1+ or occasionally 2+ readings) and hyperglycaemia may be seen in the urine of cats which are severely stressed, for example during the blood sampling procedure. Primary renal glycosuria and Fanconi syndrome should be ruled out in an animal that has significant glycosuria but a normal plasma glucose concentration.

Urinary tract infection

Evidence of urinary tract infection may be expected with pyelonephritis and in most dogs with hyperadrenocorticism and diabetes mellitus. Even if bacteria are not seen on microscopic examination a urine sample, preferably collected by cystocentesis, should be submitted for bacteriology if either of the last two disorders is suspected.

The interpretation of other abnormalities on urinalysis, for example the presence of bilirubin, and a more detailed discussion on the microscopic examination of urine sediment are included in Chapters 17 and 23, respectively.

Urine specific gravity

The specific gravity (SG) of urine depends on the molecular size and weight as well as the total number of solute molecules. An approximate relationship exists between the SG and the total concentration of urinary solute. Typical values for urine SG in the dog and cat are shown in Table 9.3. On the basis of urine SG a patient may be classified into one of four categories as follows:

Hyposthenuric range:	SG 1.001–1.007; urine more dilute than plasma
Isosthenuric range:	SG 1.008–1.012; urine concentration equals that of plasma i.e. 'fixed range' urine typical of end-stage renal failure
Range of minimal concentration	SG 1.013–1.029; urine concentration is submaximal
Hypersthenuric	SG >1.030; evidence of adequate concentrating ability

The production of large volumes of persistently dilute solute-free urine with a SG less than 1.007 is suggestive of a deficiency of, or lack of responsiveness to ADH. It does not, however, indicate abnormal tubular function or lack of functional nephrons since urine is *actively* diluted in the ascending limb of the loop of Henle.

Urine osmolality

Osmolality represents the concentration of osmotically active particles in solution and is expressed in mOsm kg^{-1}. Osmolality is directly related to osmotic pressure and is not influenced by molecular weight or particle size. Normal

Table 9.3 Urine specific gravity (SG), urine and plasma osmolality: normal values

	Urine SG (typical values)	Urine SG (extreme values)	Urine osmolality (mOsm kg^{-1})	Plasma osmolality (mOsm kg^{-1})
Dog	1.015–1.045	1.001–1.065	500–1400	275–305
Cat	1.035–1.060	1.001–1.080	1250–2100	275–305

values for plasma and urine osmolality are given in Table 9.3. The measurement of urine and plasma osmolalities is a more accurate method of assessing an animal's ability to concentrate urine in response to water deprivation (see below for investigation of persistent hyposthenuria).

Routine haematological examination

The following haematological findings may be of significance when investigating an animal with polydipsia and polyuria.

Non-regenerative anaemia
- Chronic renal failure
- Chronic liver disease
- Hypoadrenocorticism; occasionally regenerative if acute gastrointestinal haemorrhage.

Increased PCV
- Consider dehydration especially if plasma concentrations of total plasma proteins urea, creatinine, sodium and chloride are also increased; dogs with central diabetes insipidus are often slightly dehydrated.

Neutrophilic leucocytosis
- Closed-cervix pyometra; total and differential white blood cell counts may be normal if cervix is open
- Pyelonephritis
- A neutrophilia, often accompanied by lymphopenia and/or eosinopenia (stress haemogram), may be associated with hyperadrenocorticism or other severe metabolic disorders such as diabetes mellitus

Eosinophilia and lymphocytosis
- Occasionally seen with hypoadrenocorticism

Complete biochemical screen

A complete biochemical screen should include glucose, urea, creatinine, sodium, potassium, chloride, calcium, phosphate, alanine aminotransferase (ALT), alkaline phosphatase (ALP), gammaglutamyl transferase (gamma-GT) and total plasma protein determinations. It provides a cost-effective means of identifying or ruling out many of the conditions associated with polyuria/polydipsia, especially some of the more obscure electrolyte abnormalities such as the hyponatraemia and hyperkalaemia typical of hypoadrenocorticism, or the hypercalcaemia which may be associated with malignancy. Hypoproteinaemia (hypoalbuminaemia) may occur with chronic liver disease and glomerulonephropathy. A blood sample for glucose determination should be collected in a tube containing fluoride/oxalate; storage in heparin may artificially lower the plasma glucose concentration. Biochemical abnormalities which may be of relevance in the investigation of polydipsia and polyuria are summarized in Table 9.4.

Radiography

Lateral thoracic and abdominal radiographs should be examined for the following:

- Evidence of hyperadrenocorticism (bronchial/tracheal calcification, hepatomegaly, calcification along fascial planes or calcinosis cutis, osteoporosis, occasionally mineralization of adrenal gland if neoplastic);
- Microcardia and hyperlucent lungfields (hypoadrenocorticism);
- Cardiomegaly ± signs of CHF (hyperthyroidism);
- Hepatomegaly (diabetes mellitus, hyperadrenocorticism, hyperthyroidism and primary liver disease) or small liver (cirrhosis/fibrosis and portosystemic shunts);
- Kidneys which are small (chronic interstitial nephritis) or large (glomerulonephropathy);
- Enlarged, distended uterus (pyometra);
- Skeletal osteoporosis (primary hyperparathyroidism or hyperadrenocorticism);
- Hyperostosis of the skull with soft tissue swelling of the head, neck, limbs and oropharyngeal region (acromegaly).

Table 9.4 Biochemical abnormalities and their possible causes in the investigation of polydipsia and polyuria

Biochemical abnormality	Possible causes
Increased urea, creatinine ±phosphate	Renal insufficiency or renal failure Prerenal azotaemia due to hypovolaemia (e.g. hypoadrenocorticism) or severe dehydration; if the latter, sodium and chloride levels may also be increased. *Low* urea levels may occur with chronic liver disease especially portosystemic shunts.
Increased liver enzymes (ALT, ALP and gamma-GT)	Primary liver disease (NB liver enzymes may be normal with chronic liver disorders such as cirrhosis) Hyperadrenocorticism Diabetes mellitus Hyperthyroidism Acromegaly
Hyperglycaemia	Diabetes mellitus Hyperadrenocorticism Acromegaly Stress/excitement in the cat
Hypoglycaemia	Mild hypoglycaemia occurs occasionally with liver disease, especially hepatic neoplasia, and hypoadrenocorticism
Electrolyte abnormalities *Hypercalcaemia*	Primary hyperparathyroidism Malignancy (especially lymphoma) Vitamin D toxicity Hypoadrenocorticism (usually mild hypercalcaemia)
Hypocalcaemia	Idiopathic hypoparathyroidism Occasionally thyroid carcinomas
Hyperkalaemia and hyponatraemia (with a sodium/potassium ratio often less than 25:1)	Hypoadrenocorticism
Hypernatraemia/hyperchloraemia	Severe dehydration
Hypokalaemia	Excessive loss via the gastrointestinal or urinary tracts
Hyperphosphataemia	Chronic renal insufficiency or renal failure Hypoparathyroidism (increased phosphate may be associated with hypocalcaemia) Occasionally acromegaly
Hypoproteinaemia (hypoalbuminaemia)	Chronic liver disease Glomerulonephropathy

■ Ultrasonography

Ultrasonography may be used to visualize the structure of the liver, kidneys, adrenal glands and uterus.

■ Additional diagnostic tests

- The ACTH response test, low dose dexamethasone suppression (LDDS) test and urinary cortisol:creatinine ratio are screening tests for hyperadrenocorticism. The ACTH and LDDS tests are dynamic tests which evaluate the pituitary–adrenal axis.
- An oral T3 suppression test or intravenous thyroid stimulating hormone response may be used to evaluate thyroid function in cats with suspected hyperthyroidism but which have equivocal T4 results.
- Water deprivation and ADH response tests are indicated for the investigation of persistent hyposthenuria (see below).

Investigation of the polyuric/polydipsic animal with persistent hyposthenuria

Persistent hyposthenuria may be caused by:

- A complete or partial deficiency of ADH (central diabetes insipidus). A partial deficiency of ADH may result in the production of urine within the isosthenuric range.
- Disorders affecting the distal tubules and collecting ducts which interfere with the action of ADH (nephrogenic diabetes insipidus).
- Excessive water intake, e.g. primary polydipsia. Dogs with psychogenic polydipsia tend to be overhydrated and have a relative deficiency of ADH.

The aims of the diagnostic tests are twofold. First, an attempt must be made to differentiate primary polydipsia from diabetes insipidus, and secondly if diabetes insipidus is diagnosed the central form should be differentiated from the nephrogenic form since the prognosis and management for each is quite different.

The investigation of persistent hyposthenuria involves an assessment of an animal's ability to concentrate urine in response to water deprivation and after the administration of exogenous vasopressin (ADH).

Water deprivation test

The protocol for the standard water deprivation test is as follows:

1. Fast animal for 12 h
2. Catheterize and empty bladder
3. Check urine specific gravity
4. Record body weight
5. If possible record urine and plasma osmolality, packed cell volume, total plasma proteins and plasma urea
6. Withhold all water
7. Catheterize bladder and record parameters 3, 4 and 5 every one or two hours.

The test is discontinued when the animal has lost 5% of its body weight or if the urine SG exceeds 1.030. Values between 1.020 and 1.030 are equivocal and indicate submaximal concentration. Equivocal results may be obtained in animals with a partial deficiency of ADH or when polydipsia results in renal medullary washout. A urine:plasma osmolality ratio less than 1 and failure to concentrate above 1.010 is highly suggestive of diabetes insipidus.

Modified or partial water deprivation test

The modified water deprivation test is indicated when the results of the standard water deprivation test or ADH response test are equivocal and renal medullary washout is suspected. The modified water deprivation test restores medullary hypertonicity and may therefore help differentiate primary polydipsia associated with renal medullary washout from diabetes insipidus but will not differentiate between the central and nephrogenic forms of diabetes insipidus. Water intake is reduced gradually (5–10% daily) over a period of three days. Daily water intake should not exceed 100 ml kg^{-1}. Hydration status and urine SG are monitored daily. Failure to concentrate urine above the SG values previously obtained suggests that renal medullary washout is not a factor in the animal's ability to concentrate urine.

Both forms of water deprivation test are contraindicated in animals which are azotaemic, hypercalcaemic or dehydrated.

Response to exogenous ADH

An ADH response test is indicated if an animal fails to concentrate its urine in response to water deprivation. Used on its own a positive response to exogenously administered ADH does not confirm a diagnosis of central diabetes insipidus since normal dogs and dogs with other polyuric conditions (e.g. dogs with hyperadrenocorticism) with appropriate levels of ADH will respond to ADH. A positive response to ADH is not significant unless it has been demonstrated that the animal cannot concentrate its urine in response to water deprivation. ADH may be administered immediately after a water deprivation test. The animal may be fed beforehand and offered *small* amounts of water before starting the test. Large amounts of water given either during or immediately after the test may result in signs of water intoxication. The protocol for the ADH response test is as follows:

1. Catheterize and empty the bladder; check urine SG
2. Inject vasopressin (DDAVP, Ferring) intramuscularly. Dose: 2.0 µg for small dogs <15 kg (and cats); 4.0 µg for dogs >15 kg.
3. Catheterize and check urine SG at 30 min intervals for 2 hours.

A positive response to ADH (urine SG >1.025 or in most cases 1.030) is consistent with a diagnosis of central diabetes insipidus. Failure to concentrate urine above SG 1.010 and a urine:plasma osmolality ratio <1 suggests the nephrogenic form of diabetes insidipus. Equivocal results, i.e. SG values <1.025, may be due to the effects of renal medullary washout and such cases may show a more convincing response if ADH is administered on two or three consecutive days.

Hickey–Hare test

The development of CNS signs due to sodium overload is a potential hazard which has restricted extensive use of this test which involves the administration of an intravenous bolus of hypertonic saline. The protocol is as follows:

1. Give 20 ml kg^{-1} of water by stomach tube
2. Catheterize and empty bladder
3. Infuse 2.5% sodium chloride intravenously at a rate of 2.5 ml kg^{-1} min^{-1} over 45 min
4. Measure urine volume, SG and osmolality every 15 min after the start of the infusion. In normal dogs' urine volume progressively decreases as the SG and osmolality increase. Failure to do so is suggestive of central or nephrogenic diabetes insipidus.

10

Persistent Nasal Discharge

J. P. Bray

INTRODUCTION

A nasal discharge and sneezing are the two classical signs of upper respiratory tract disease. However, with more chronic disease, the intensity or frequency of sneezing may become reduced, as this reflex becomes obtunded. It is therefore more typical for animals to present for investigation of a persistent nasal discharge.

Many nasal diseases present with an identical clinical picture, and the presence of a discharge may provide little immediate clue to the underlying disease process. Careful history taking, physical examination and diagnostic evaluation are necessary to elucidate the aetiology. Some diseases have recognizable 'foot-prints' and a methodical clinician will usually be rewarded for his or her investigation.

NASAL ANATOMY AND PHYSIOLOGY

The nose of the dog and cat is a bi-chambered cavity that functions to (1) warm and humidify the inspired air, and (2) entrap and eliminate small airborne particles. The nose functions so efficiently as a heat-exchanger that dogs can exhale air 16.5°C below body temperature, saving 75% of the water and 80% of the heat in dry air at 0°C. The nose also contains an extensive olfactory mucous membrane which is located in the caudodorsal area of each fossa.

The nose of the dog and cat is evenly divided by a central wall, the nasal septum. Each half, or fossa, provides a separate passageway for air between the nostrils and the openings into the nasopharynx. The fossae are almost filled with conchae, scrolls of bone and cartilage that project medially from the sides and roof. The conchae are richly vascular and are lined with glandular mucosal epithelium. There are three separate conchae in the dog and cat – dorsal, middle and ventral. Their size and formation is more varied in the dog, but remarkably uniform in the cat. The ventral concha is the most complex and occupies the rostral and ventral quarter of the nasal fossa. The dorsal surface of the ventral concha is thrown into numerous (>30) folds of varying complexity. The remaining conchae are ethmoturbinates and have a more simplistic arrangement. The conchae fill the nasal fossa so tightly that air-flow is restricted to three narrow channels between the chonchal folds – the dorsal, middle and ventral meatus. Even slight inflammation of the turbinates or accumulation of discharge within the airway can obstruct air-flow.

The nose is the first line of defence for the respiratory system against airborne particles and inspired antigens. Nasal secretions from mucus-producing cells in the epithelium, submucosal and nasal glands entrap small particles as air moves over the conchal folds. Immunoglobulins (IgA), complement, opsonin proteins and other immunological factors in the secretions recognize and deactivate antigens and, following stimulation, can initiate an inflammatory response. The conchae are lined with pseudostratified ciliated columnar epithelium which creates a mucociliary blanket that sweeps the secretions in a caudal direction at a rate of about 6 mm min^{-1}. Once in the nasopharynx, the secretions can be swallowed. The development of a *discharge* from the nostrils of a dog or cat implies that the capacity of this mucociliary apparatus has been exceeded either due to obstruction of the clearance pathway (e.g. neoplasia, inflammation) or increased production of mucus or inflammatory exudate.

Sneezing is also an important component of the respiratory defence mechanism, producing an explosive rush of air through the nose to dislodge and expel foreign material, mucus and debris. Sneezing is a reflex which is initiated following stimulation of subepithelial receptors. These receptors can be activated by a number of mechanical, inflammatory, chemical or infectious causes. *Reverse sneezing* is an important condition to recognize because its occurrence can promote anxious calls from owners who consider their animal to be either suffocating or having a fit. Reverse sneezing is caused by spasms of the nasopharynx and is typified by violent, paroxysmal inspiratory efforts. Reverse sneezing accurately localizes the site of irritation to the nasopharynx and diagnostic investigation should therefore focus more specifically on this region.

The role of the frontal and the maxillary paranasal sinuses of dog and cat is obscure. The frontal sinus is the biggest and is separated in two by a median septum. In the dog, each half is further divided into three separate cavities (rostral, medial and lateral) which open individually into the nasal fossa. The sinuses are lined with ciliated epithelium and mucus secreting cells, and may be primarily or secondarily involved in a disease process of the upper respiratory tract.

INVESTIGATION OF PERSISTENT NASAL DISCHARGE

HISTORY CHECKLIST

❏ **Age, sex, breed?**
Congenital conditions (e.g. cleft palate, nasopharyngeal polyps) are more likely to contribute to nasal disease in the young (< 1 year old) animal. Conversely, nasal tumours occur more commonly in the older animal (mean age 9–10 years). Geriatric animals are also more likely to suffer from dental conditions which can be the cause of significant nasal disease. Nasal aspergillosis is seen more commonly in the young adult with 77% of cases occurring in animals less than eight years of age.

Few breed-specific nasal diseases are recognized. However, the conformational disruption of the upper airway in brachycephalic dogs can contribute to noisy, stertorous breathing. Nasal aspergillosis is limited almost exclusively to the long-nosed (doliocephalic, mesaticephalic) breeds.

An increased incidence of disease in male animals has been recognized in certain conditions (e.g. nasal aspergillosis, feline nasal tumours).

❏ **Onset of signs?**
The time of onset of nasal signs may provide some clues to the underlying aetiology. Nasal foreign bodies are often associated with an acute onset of violent and persistent sneezing which eventually acquiesces to be replaced by a thick, purulent discharge. In contrast, nasal aspergillosis, neoplasia and dental disease may have a more insidious onset of signs, and are associated with infrequent sneezing. Intermittent nasal signs associated with allergic conditions may occur after exposure to the appropriate environmental conditions, plants or chemical agents.

❏ **Nature of discharge?**
Certain historical features of the discharge are important to identify. The type of discharge (serous, mucoid, purulent, bloody, containing plant or food material) and previous response to treatment should be determined. Did the discharge begin unilaterally or bilaterally? Animals may clear small quantities of discharge from their noses by constant licking or frequent swallowing, and the owner may not appreciate an overt nasal discharge. Occasionally, however, hyperaemia or moist pyoderma of the upper lip may provide evidence of this cleaning behaviour. In cats, soiling of the dorsum of the paws and antebrachium may indicate increased grooming of the face.

❏ **Nasal obstruction?**
Owners may be aware of nasal obstruction either due to an increase in mouth breathing by their animal or the development of unusual sounds during respiration. Physical airway obstruction caused by turbinate swelling, discharge, neoplasia, foreign body or polyp can produce a high-pitched wheeze as air flows through a narrowed passage. Affected animals may also have reduced exercise tolerance. If nasal obstruction is severe, animals may be reluctant to eat as they are unable to breathe simultaneously through their nose. Anorexia may also occur due to reduced olfaction or severe dental disease.

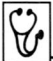

PHYSICAL EXAMINATION

A complete physical examination should be completed in all animals before focusing specific attention on the skull, oral cavity and upper respiratory tract. Although there are few systemic manifestations of nasal disease, attention should be made of the general body condition and mental status of the animal, presence of other neoplastic processes which may have metastasized to the nose, and evidence of other allergic reactions (e.g. interdigital hyperaemia, otitis externa). Dogs with nasal aspergillosis are often dull, withdrawn or depressed and may hold their head low when sitting.

❏ Facial symmetry?

Palpation and visual evaluation of the skull should be performed to identify the presence of any facial swelling, pain or distortion. Facial distortion is more commonly associated with neoplasia and soft fluctuant masses may be palpable if a tumour has eroded through the nasal or frontal bones. Retrobulbar extension of a nasal tumour may cause exophthalmus which may be appreciable on direct observation or with light digital pressure on the globe. Blepharospasm may be seen in association with paranasal extension of aspergillosis. Aspergillosis can also cause pain over the face, particularly on palpation of the frontal sinuses. Atrophy of the temporal muscles is also a feature of this disease. The nostrils should also be assessed for symmetry, obstruction or distortion. Neoplastic erosion of the nares (e.g. by a squamous cell carcinoma) may cause epistaxis and sneezing, but may be difficult to detect without careful inspection. Feline cryptococcus infection may cause a fungal granuloma of the nares with significant distortion of the nasal cartilages. Depigmentation or ulceration of one or both nostrils is almost pathognomonic for aspergillosis.

❏ Nasal obstruction?

Air-flow through both nostrils can be assessed by placing a few strands of cotton-wool in front of each nostril. Movement of the cotton should be observed during both inspiration and expiration from both nostrils. The author prefers to assess air-flow by gently obstructing each nostril with a thumb. Both nostrils are assessed independently with the mouth closed. The normal animal should be able to breath without distress through the other, patent, nostril. Any increase in noise or respiratory embarrassment during occlusion localizes disease to that side of the nose.

❏ Oral examination

Dental pathology is commonly overlooked during the investigation of nasal disease but can be a significant cause of chronic irritation. Attention should be given to both the hard and soft palates for signs of congenital lesions or tumour extension/invasion. The dental arcade should be examined closely for evidence of dental or periodontal disease.

❏ Regional lymph nodes

Chronic disease of the nasal chamber may cause a regional lymphadenopathy due to antigenic stimulation. Although few nasal tumours have distant metastases, fine needle aspiration and cytological investigation of enlarged nodes should be performed.

■ FURTHER INVESTIGATION

■ Clinical pathology

Systemic manifestations of nasal disease are infrequent and evaluation of haematological and biochemical parameters rarely contributes to identification of the underlying aetiology. However, for the investigation of epistaxis, a complete haematological profile (for assessment of anaemia and evaluation of platelet numbers) and coagulation panel (including von Willebrand's factor) is essential. In the cat, serological testing for feline leukaemia and feline immunodeficiency virus infections should be performed. Serological testing for aspergillosis can be performed using agar gel double diffusion, counter-immunoelectrophoresis and enzyme-linked immunosorbent assay techniques. Although all techniques are useful, test sensitivity varies and both false-positive and false-negative results can occur. Complete reliance on a serological result for diagnosis of nasal aspergillosis should therefore be resisted.

■ Diagnostic imaging

Radiography is one of the more common techniques for assessing the upper airway. However, due to the fine features of some of the anatomical structures, and the potential for obscured detail by numerous overlying structures, careful positioning and quality processing is essential. General anaesthesia is required for optimal patient positioning. At least three views are recommended – lateral skull, dorsoventral intra-oral and a rostrocaudal horizontal view for evaluation of the frontal sinuses. If dental disease is suspected, oblique views of the maxilla will highlight the apices of the tooth roots. The intra-oral view is the best for evaluating the nasal cavity and the use of non-screen film will increase resolution of fine turbinate detail in this area. The natural symmetry of the nose can be utilized to assess changes in turbinate detail and density between each nasal cavity. Destructive changes of the turbinates and nasal septum are more typically associated with either aspergillosis or neoplasia. Although neoplasia is more likely to cause erosion of the nasal or facial bones, aspergillosis infection may also cause an osteomyelitis and periosteal reaction of the facial bones. An increase in soft tissue density within the nasal chambers may be associated with neoplasia, a polypoid growth or accumulation of discharge. Aspergillosis typically causes a reduction in density and, in severe cases, the nasal chamber can appear almost empty. However, the profuse discharge which occurs with fungal infection will increase radiodensity in focal areas of the nose and careful interpretation is necessary.

Computed tomography has particular value in the investigation of nasal disease as it provides high resolution, cross-sectional slices through the nose. Turbinate detail, frontal sinus involvement, and the degree of extranasal extension of tumour can all be accurately assessed, which greatly improves diagnostic success rate. These facilities are increasingly available to the general practitioner at regional centres.

Rhinoscopy

Visual evaluation of each nasal chamber is one of the most valuable aspects of nasal investigation and should be performed in every case. Both anterior and posterior (retrograde) rhinoscopy should be completed. Although the use of a simple otoscope has been described for anterior rhinoscopy, this equipment only permits examination of the rostral few centimetres beyond the nares. Rarely is this investigation rewarding and, as a consequence, reliance on this technique may frustrate the clinician into considering rhinoscopy a 'worthless' procedure. Examination with a rigid 2.7 or 3.0 mm arthroscope permits a thorough inspection of all structures within each nasal fossa. With experience, the operator should be able to navigate the scope along the dorsal, middle and ventral meati and thereby examine completely all regions of the nose. The middle meatus is of greatest interest and navigation into the caudal aspect permits evaluation of the ventral conchae and ethmoturbinates.

One of the more frustrating elements of rhinoscopy is obstruction of the visual field by blood or discharge. This complication can be resolved simply by constantly flushing the nose with a saline drip during the examination. Saline can be administered either via a purpose-built arthroscopic cannula which surrounds the rigid arthroscope, or by placing a Foley catheter around the back of the soft palate and flushing towards the scope. The pharynx must be carefully packed and a cuffed endotracheal tube must be in place to prevent aspiration during a flushed rhinoscopic examination.

Retrograde rhinoscopy permits evaluation of the nasopharynx and choanal region. Although examination of this area should ideally be performed in every case of nasal discharge, it is absolutely essential if the animal is reported to have 'reverse sneezing' as a clinical feature of its disease. Although a dental mirror can provide some visualization of this area (particularly if the soft palate is retracted with a spay hook), the best inspection is afforded by retroflexing a small flexible endoscope over the soft palate.

Culture

The increased financial cost involved in identifying the type and antibiotic sensitivity of a suspected pathogen is usually unrewarding in terms of providing curative treatment for most nasal discharges. True primary bacterial rhinitis and sinusitis are rare in the dog and cat. Secondary bacterial infection will, however, develop with any nasal disease regardless of the underlying aetiology (e.g. neoplasia, aspergillosis, foreign body, allergy). Bacteriological results from swabs obtained from the upper airway should therefore be interpreted with care, regardless of collection technique. Positive fungal cultures can be obtained from normal noses and this finding is therefore of little value in the diagnosis of aspergillosis.

Nasal flush

Cytological examination of fluid collected during vigorous flushing of the nasal cavity with saline may occasionally provide additional clues to the underlying aetiology, particularly if neoplasia is suspected. Unfortunately, the diagnostic yield with this technique is low. Occasionally, larger pieces of tissue may be dislodged during the flushing procedure which can be investigated histologically. In recent years, attention has focused on immunoglobulin assay of the nasal wash solution to provide a definitive diagnosis for allergic rhinitis. This work is mirroring advances in the human field and may hold some promise for investigation of this troublesome condition.

Histopathology

Histological inspection of biopsies from turbinate tissue or suspected tumour is often essential in order to establish a definitive diagnosis. Unfortunately, one of the remaining frustrations of nasal investigations is the inability to obtain biopsy samples accurately and consistently from a specific area of interest. Although samples of nasal tissue can be obtained by alligator forceps, clamshell biopsy forceps or plastic catheters, these techniques must be performed blindly and sample collection is therefore random. Retrieval of non-diagnostic specimens is therefore a frustration, particularly if the pathology is focal. In addition, these techniques are very traumatic and may be associated with significant haemorrhage. Newer arthroscopes enable biopsy forceps to be attached to their front, which offers the potential for visually guided biopsies. In some cases, however, this addition makes the unit more bulky and therefore more difficult to navigate through the nose.

Exploratory rhinotomy

Very few diseases are considered to benefit from complete turbinectomy and the indications for rhinotomy are now limited. Occasionally, however, less invasive diagnostic investigations may be thwarted by the enclosed and tightly packed arrangement of the nose. Exploratory surgery is then indicated to obtain definitive biopsy samples or to retrieve foreign material. The nasal cavity may be approached from either the dorsal or ventral route. The ventral route is considered to provide satisfactory access to all regions of the nasal cavity and nasopharynx, with superior cosmetic results. Rhinotomy is invasive and can be associated with considerable haemorrhage. Complications are minimized by swiftness, and by packing off areas of the nose during exploration to control blood loss. The nose can be packed prior to closure, with packing material removed via the nostril after surgery. Postoperative complications include haemorrhage, subcutaneous emphysema and dyspnoea. Confining the exploration to one side of the nasal cavity will reduce the incidence of complications associated with postoperative nasal obstruction.

11

Dyspnoea

L. G. King

The term 'dyspnoea' refers to a sensation of breathlessness and is clinically recognizable as respiratory distress. Dyspnoea is a challenging emergency situation that requires a careful and logical approach.

PATHOPHYSIOLOGY

Ventilation

Respiration is controlled by chemoreceptors near the respiratory centres of the medulla oblongata. Impulses from the brainstem are transmitted through the spinal cord to the phrenic and intercostal nerves. Contraction of the diaphragm causes it to flatten and displace the abdominal contents caudally, whereas contraction of the intercostals lifts and spreads the ribs. The negative pressure exerted by the potential space between the pleura is transmitted to the lungs, resulting in their expansion during inspiration. Movement of air into the chest (ventilation) may be impeded by a variety of disorders (Table 11.1).

Minute ventilation is defined as the product of the number of breaths per minute and the tidal volume. There is an inverse linear relationship between the partial pressure of plasma carbon dioxide ($Pa\text{CO}_2$), and the minute ventilation. In other words, the more air moved in and out of the lungs each minute, the lower the $Pa\text{CO}_2$. Because CO_2 is such a highly diffusible gas, clinical changes in $Pa\text{CO}_2$ are almost always related to the minute ventilation rather than to the presence of pulmonary abnormalities that might affect gas exchange.

Brainstem control usually results in the maintenance of normal $Pa\text{CO}_2$; any increase in $Pa\text{CO}_2$ results in increased respiratory drive. Hypoventilation results in hypoxia due to decreased delivery of air to the alveoli. Animals with a disease that is causing hypoventilation have clinical signs of respiratory distress because the combination of high $Pa\text{CO}_2$ and hypoxia causes dramatically increased respiratory drive.

Gas exchange

Once air has been moved into the lungs, gas exchange occurs by diffusion. In the normal

Table 11.1 Common causes of respiratory distress due to hypoventilation and increased $Pa\text{CO}_2$ in dogs and cats

- Anaesthesia
- Brainstem disease
- Spinal cord compression or disease above the level of C3
- Lower motor neurone paralysis of the phrenic or intercostal nerves
- Neuromuscular junction disorders such as myasthenia gravis
- Myopathies affecting the diaphragm or other respiratory muscles
- Orthopaedic injury to the ribcage or sternum including flail chest
- Tension pneumothorax
- Pleural effusion
- Diaphragmatic hernia or other space-occupying extrapulmonary lesion
- Upper airway obstruction such as laryngeal paralysis or brachycephalic airway syndrome
- Metabolic alkalosis (mild compensatory hypoventilation)
- End-stage lung disease

animal, the large surface area for contact between the alveoli and capillary blood results in a minimal barrier for diffusion of oxygen. In the presence of serious lung disease, diffusion of oxygen across the alveolar walls may be limited by thickening of the alveolar membrane, oedema or inflammation.

For normal gas exchange to occur, ventilation (delivery of oxygen) and perfusion (flow of blood through capillaries) must be matched at each alveolus. Ventilation/perfusion mismatch is the most common cause of hypoxia in the clinical patient. If bronchi are obstructed or if alveoli are atelectatic or filled with fluid, air cannot enter that part of the lung. The deoxygenated blood that perfuses the underventilated area mixes with oxygenated blood from the normal areas of the lung, resulting in a decrease in arterial oxygen (PaO_2). The most extreme form of ventilation/perfusion mismatch, called 'shunting', occurs when large volumes of blood completely bypass the lungs and deoxygenated haemoglobin is returned to the systemic circulation. Common causes of hypoxia are listed in Table 11.2.

If lung disease is so severe that profound arterial hypoxia results, stimulation of cells in the carotid and aortic bodies may trigger an increased respiratory effort. In the presence of severe lung disease, therefore, control by $PaCO_2$ may be over-ridden by the presence of profound hypoxia. Thus, hyperventilation and decreased $PaCO_2$ are common in dogs and cats with severe pulmonary disease.

Oxygen transport

Once oxygen has diffused into the plasma, it binds to haemoglobin for delivery to the tissues. The relationship between the amount of oxygen dissolved in plasma (PaO_2) and the saturation of the haemoglobin with oxygen (SaO_2) is defined by a sigmoid curve (Fig. 11.1). The plateau of the curve allows a considerable margin for decrease in PaO_2 before desaturation occurs. Mild to moderate lung disease, which results in minor decreases in PaO_2, may not be associated with desaturation as long as PaO_2 remains greater than 60 mmHg. Thus, oxygen delivery to the tissues remains adequate at rest and the mucous membranes still appear pink. Once the lung disease has progressed to a PaO_2 lower than 60 mmHg, minor worsening of lung disease or manipulation of the animal may result in significant decreases in haemoglobin saturation.

CLINICAL RECOGNITION OF DYSPNOEA

Progressive respiratory dysfunction results in defective gas exchange and increased work of breathing. Normal respiration is characterized by almost imperceptible concurrent excursion of the chest and abdominal walls. As respiratory drive increases, there is increased recruitment of the secondary muscles of respiration. Clinically, this results in an increased rate and depth of respiration, the use of abdominal wall muscles and postural adaptations that minimize resistance to air flow (Table 11.3).

Increased work of breathing may eventually result in fatigue of respiratory muscles and the development of paradoxical respiration, which signals imminent respiratory failure. Paradoxical respiration is recognized by loss of the synchronous movement of the thoracic and abdominal walls; observation of the animal reveals that during inspiration the thoracic wall expands but the caudal ribcage and the abdominal walls collapse inwards. This paradoxical movement opposes the normal expansion of the lungs and signifies severe respiratory dysfunction.

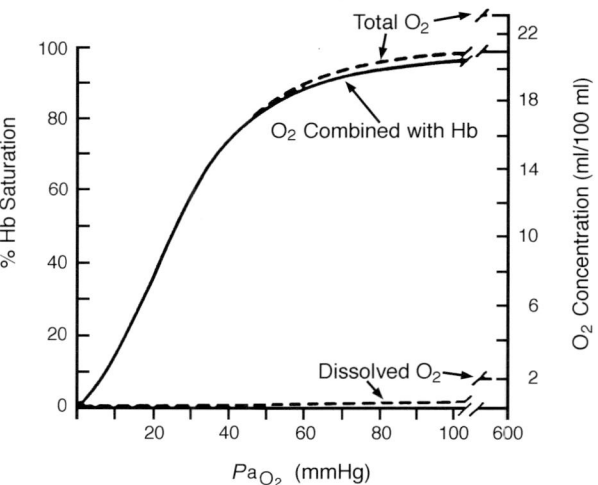

Figure 11.1 Oxygen haemoglobin dissociation curve (solid line). Once the PaO_2 is greater than 60 mmHg, haemoglobin is saturated with oxygen and the mucous membranes of the animal appear pink. Due to the sigmoid shape of the curve, rapid desaturation occurs at PaO_2 values less than 60 mmHg. (Reproduced with permission from West JB (1985) Respiratory Physiology – The Essentials, 3rd edn. Williams and Wilkins, Baltimore).

Table 11.2 Common causes of respiratory distress due to gas exchange abnormalities and hypoxia in dogs and cats

Pneumonia: bacterial, viral, fungal, protozoal
Neoplasia: primary or metastatic
Cardiogenic pulmonary oedema
Haemorrhage due to trauma or coagulopathy
Vasculitis: non-cardiogenic pulmonary oedema and acute respiratory distress syndrome
Atelectasis
Inflammatory lung disease such as pulmonary infiltrate with eosinophils or lymphomatoid granulomatosis
Thromboembolic disease
Airway obstruction and absorption atelectasis
Chronic bronchitis and bronchiectasis
Bronchial smooth muscle spasm (cats only)
Emphysema
Right to left shunt, for example reverse patent ductus arteriosus
Hypoventilation
Lung lobe torsion

Table 11.3 Postural adaptations that minimize resistance to air flow in dyspnoeic animals

Nasal flare
Open-mouthed breathing
Lifting and extending head and neck
Standing, sitting or lying in sternal recumbency
Abduction of elbows

INVESTIGATION OF DYSPNOEA

Once dyspnoea is recognized clinically, the clinician must make rapid decisions regarding clinical management. In animals who may not tolerate manipulation, these decisions are often based solely on a truncated physical examination and brief history.

 HISTORY CHECKLIST

❏ **Age, breed, sex?**
Young animals may suffer from congenital anomalies such as pectus excavatum or broncho-oesophageal fistula, whereas older animals are more prone to neoplastic lung disease or heart failure.

❏ **Previous preventative medicine?**
Vaccination status may be important to rule out distemper virus infection. Heartworm status (previous testing or use of heartworm prophylaxis) should be determined in areas where dirofilariasis is endemic.

❏ **Duration of signs?**
Chronic respiratory signs such as snoring in English bulldogs with brachycephalic airway disease, or coughing in a Yorkshire terrier with a collapsing trachea, may provide supportive evidence that the current episode of dyspnoea is an escalation of a chronic disorder. Caution should be exercised in interpretation of apparently acute disorders. Many pet owners do not recognize the early clinical signs of respiratory distress, or interpret them as 'normal' for that particular animal. Some animals, such as cats, may lead a sedentary lifestyle and may not manifest problems until their disease becomes so severe that they decompensate.

❏ **Inciting incidents, toxic exposures, or previous illness?**
Diagnosis of the cause of respiratory distress may be easy when the owner rushes in an animal who has just been hit by a car. In contrast, careful questioning may be necessary to elicit a history of exposure to toxins such as anticoagulant rodenticides or paraquat. A history of recent illness may provide clues that the animal has developed aspiration pneumonia or pulmonary manifestations of a systemic disorder.

❏ **Respiratory signs in other animals?**

❏ **Previous therapy and response?**
In particular, knowledge of any response to previous antibiotic, diuretic or corticosteroid therapy may provide helpful information.

PHYSICAL EXAMINATION

❏ Observation of respiratory pattern

Animals with pulmonary or pleural disease tend to have a *restrictive* breathing pattern: rapid shallow respirations which may involve a considerable abdominal component. Those with upper airway obstruction tend to have prolonged, deep inspiration and respiratory *stridor* if the obstruction is located at the larynx. Dogs with paradoxical respiration may show signs of respiratory muscle fatigue.

❏ Mucous membrane colour

Mucous membrane colour depends on SaO_2, the amount of blood flow through the tissues, and the haemoglobin concentration of the blood. Cyanosis (bluish/purple mucous membranes) is a serious sign of desaturation that warrants immediate action. Pink mucous membranes merely indicate a PaO_2 greater than 60 mmHg, and therefore do not rule out clinically significant hypoxia. Pale mucous membranes are difficult to interpret. If there is limited flow of haemoglobin through the tissues, such as might occur in animals with decreased peripheral perfusion or severe anaemia, the clinician cannot make any estimate of haemoglobin oxygenation status.

❏ Palpation

The whole airway from the nares to the thoracic inlet should be palpated and observed for evidence of discharge, swelling, asymmetry or traumatic injury. If possible, without stressing the animal, the mouth should be opened to observe the pharynx and tonsils. Evidence of oral mucosal ulceration may suggest non-cardiogenic pulmonary oedema in a puppy that bit an electrical cord. The presence of nasal discharge may be an important indicator of infectious processes such as distemper virus infection or bacterial pneumonia. Dogs with traumatic injuries to the trachea or mainstem bronchi may have subcutaneous emphysema. Animals with neoplasia may have palpable mass lesions obstructing air flow in the cervical area. The cranial thoracic cavity may appear solid and difficult to compress in cats with cranial mediastinal masses. Percussion may demonstrate increased resonance in animals with pneumothorax, or increased dullness in animals with fluid or mass lesions.

❏ Auscultation

Ideally, the patient should be auscultated while standing. Since panting and open-mouthed breathing may be associated with shallow respiration and increased extraneous upper airway noise, the mouth should be briefly held closed during auscultation. If possible, without inducing undue stress, animals with shallow respiration should be encouraged to breathe deeply once or twice by holding off the nares. Referred sounds from the upper airway can be distinguished from lower airway sounds by auscultation of the cervical trachea. Harsh lung sounds indicate turbulent air flow through airways narrowed by inflammation, oedema or mucus. Dullness or lack of air movement may signal pleural effusion or pneumothorax. Crackles usually indicate the presence of fluid in the airways or alveoli, which could be due to oedema, haemorrhage, mucus or purulent material. Since congestive heart failure is a common cause of dyspnoea in dogs and cats, the heart should be carefully auscultated. Careful attention should be paid to the presence of murmurs, a gallop rhythm or other arrhythmia.

❏ Rectal temperature

Fever, an elevation of the hypothalamic set-point for thermoregulation, signals inflammation or infection. Hyperthermia is common in animals with upper respiratory obstruction, as the limited flow of air over the tongue prevents heat exchange and the increased work of respiration generates an increased heat load.

FURTHER INVESTIGATION

Diagnostic testing may initially be limited in dyspnoeic animals. The most distressed animals can decompensate with relatively minimal manipulation, such as might be required for venepuncture or thoracic radiography. If faced with such a situation, the clinician must treat empirically to stabilize the animal, and forego diagnostics until the animal is more stable. Immediate management should include oxygen therapy and establishment of venous access. Diagnostic thoracocentesis may be considered prior to radiography if historical information and/or physical examination suggest the presence of pleural air or fluid. Rational drug therapy may be initiated based on a reasonable assessment of the most common causes of respiratory distress. Assuming that the animal is stable enough for diagnostic testing, the following may be considered.

❑ Radiography

Thoracic radiographs should be evaluated for the presence of pleural effusion (scalloping of lung lobes, pleural fissures or a fluid line) or elevation of the heart and collapsed lung lobes that might indicate pneumothorax. The cardiac silhouette should be examined to detect chamber enlargement that might indicate congestive heart failure or pericardial effusion, and the pulmonary vasculature should be evaluated to detect venous distension. The lung fields should be carefully evaluated for the presence of air bronchograms which indicate an alveolar pattern. A peribronchial pattern, especially if accompanied by lung hyperinflation, is suggestive of feline asthma. Normal or near normal thoracic radiographs should prompt consideration of airway disease, and a lateral radiograph of the neck should be obtained to evaluate the oropharyngeal region and trachea. Masses or foreign bodies can occasionally be seen outlined by the negative contrast of air in the trachea and larynx.

❑ Fluoroscopy

Fluoroscopy allows real-time, dynamic determination of airway motion for diagnosis of tracheal and mainstem bronchial collapse. In rare instances of diaphragmatic paralysis, fluoroscopy may be required to assess diaphragmatic function.

❑ Thoracocentesis

Thoracocentesis represents both a diagnostic and a therapeutic aid for stabilization of animals in respiratory distress. A needle connected to a short piece of tubing and a three-way stopcock is carefully introduced into the pleural cavity via the seventh or eighth intercostal space. Suction by a syringe allows withdrawal of fluid or air until negative pressure is obtained. Samples of fluid should be submitted for cytological analysis and for aerobic and anaerobic culture.

❑ Tests of pulmonary function

Tests of pulmonary function provide quantitative information about the severity of respiratory dysfunction but they provide limited qualitative information regarding the cause of the problem. The gold standard for estimation of pulmonary function is arterial blood gas analysis which is expensive and relatively invasive. Two non-invasive, indirect instruments are available.

Pulse oximetry provides continuous estimation of SaO_2, allowing quantitation of hypoxia and monitoring response to therapy or tolerance of diagnostic procedures. The instrument is a dual wavelength spectrophotometer which determines the absorption of light shone through tissue using a probe which is placed on the tongue, lip, ear pinna or toe of the animal. Poor tissue perfusion and excessive movement of the animal result in difficulty obtaining accurate readings with this instrument.

End-tidal capnography provides an estimation of pulmonary venous carbon dioxide by analysis of CO_2 in exhaled air. Most veterinary instruments are 'side-stream' samplers that are introduced into an anaesthetic circuit by means of a T junction or sample exhaled air directly from the nares in the awake animal. The CO_2 concentrations in the air obtained at the end of exhalation are related to those of the pulmonary venous blood and thereby reflect the ventilation status of the animal. High respiration rate and panting result in erroneous measurements using these instruments.

❑ Blood tests

A complete blood count may provide evidence of infection if there is an elevated white blood cell count. Some cats with feline asthma and dogs with eosinophilic pneumonia may present with an eosinophilia. Many animals with pneumonia, however, have perfectly normal white blood cell counts. An increased haematocrit (i.e. secondary polycythaemia) may indicate dehydration or chronic hypoxia resulting in increased erythropoietin production. Although a chemistry panel does not provide direct information about the respiratory tract, important information about concurrent systemic disease may provide clues to the aetiology of respiratory distress. Other specific blood tests may be indicated depending on the type of respiratory disease. Cats, for example, may require testing for feline leukaemia virus, and dogs with possible pulmonary thromboembolism may require evaluation for the presence of hyperadrenocorticism.

❑ Laryngoscopy and bronchoscopy

Direct visualization of the respiratory tract in the dyspnoeic dog or cat is limited to those crises that are thought to be caused by airway obstruction. Since general anaesthesia is required there is considerable risk to the unstable animal. Additionally, if airway obstruction is present, recovery from anaesthesia can be fraught with difficulty unless the airway obstruction has been resolved. The animal should be lightly anaesthetized with a short-acting drug that does not affect laryngeal function (typically thiopental or propofol). The larynx is then carefully observed to determine whether vocal cord motion is present and symmetrical, and whether the motion is occurring at the appropriate phase of respiration. Bronchoscopy may be required if a tracheobronchial mass or foreign body is suspected.

❑ Cytological and bacteriological examination of the respiratory tract

Samples for bacteriological and cytological examination may be obtained from the respiratory tract by transtracheal wash, bronchoalveolar lavage (BAL), or fine needle lung aspirates. Pharyngeal swabs provide little useful information since they are easily contaminated with oral microorganisms. Fine needle aspirates may be obtained with relatively little stress in animals with consolidated lung or focal mass lesions. Some dyspnoeic animals may tolerate a transtracheal wash (a catheter is inserted percutaneously through a needle into the trachea, and sterile saline is instilled and withdrawn to provide a sample for bacteriological culture and cytology), but the animal should be carefully observed for deterioration during this procedure.

❑ Other diagnostic procedures

Some animals may benefit from sophisticated imaging techniques such as scintigraphy, computed tomography or magnetic resonance imaging. Assessment of lung compliance and airway resistance may be considered. Finally, exploratory surgery may be required to effect diagnosis and resolution of some respiratory disorders such as pulmonary masses or lung lobe torsions.

12

Chronic Cough

L. G. King

A chronic cough may be defined as a cough that has been present for more than two months. Since coughing is a sign of airway disease, but not a diagnosis in itself, dogs and cats with chronic coughing often present the clinician with both a diagnostic and a therapeutic dilemma.

PATHOPHYSIOLOGY

Chronic coughing is a non-specific response to inflammation or physical stimulation of the airways. Inflammation may be a sequel of a variety of insults, including viral, bacterial or other infections, allergic or hypersensitivity responses, foreign material, external compression, structural abnormalities or neoplasia. Common causes of chronic coughing in dogs and cats are listed in Tables 12.1 and 12.2.

When the airways become inflamed, the pathological manifestations include erythema and hyperaemia, mucosal oedema, increased mucus production with proliferation of goblet and Clara cells, and infiltration of inflammatory cells. The types of inflammatory cell vary depending on the aetiology of the inflammation. For example, a cat with feline asthma may have an eosinophilic infiltrate, whereas a puppy with *Bordetella bronchiseptica* tracheobronchitis may have predominantly neutrophilic and lymphocytic infiltrates. Normally, the mucociliary escalator, backed up by alveolar macrophages and bronchus-associated lymphoid tissue, are the most important protective mechanisms of the lower airways. The cough reflex comes into play as a vital defence mechanism when these mechanisms have been overwhelmed by an increased volume of exudate or mucus, or by the presence of foreign material. The cough reflex may also be triggered by repeated local mechanical stimulation, such as might occur in dogs with structural abnormalities such as collapsing trachea or compression of the left mainstem bronchus.

The cough reflex is a cholinergic vagal reflex that is triggered by local inflammation or physical stimuli in the airways. A cough begins as a maximal inspiration, followed by initial forced exhalation against a closed glottis (Valsalva manoeuvre). Sudden opening of the glottis results in rapid expulsion of air under considerable pressure, which assists in removal of debris, foreign material and mucus from the respiratory tract. This is

Table 12.1 Some causes of chronic coughing in dogs

- Collapsing trachea
- Chronic bronchitis
- Compression of the left mainstem bronchus
- Left-sided congestive heart failure, often mitral regurgitation or dilated cardiomyopathy
- Chronic bronchopneumonia
- Bronchiectasis
- Tracheal or bronchial foreign bodies
- Tracheal or bronchial masses or neoplasms (intraluminal or extraluminal)
- Pulmonary neoplasia such as bronchogenic carcinoma
- Parasitic infestations (lungworms such as *Capillaria aerophila, Filaroides* spp., *Crenosoma vulpis*, migration of ascarids)
- Heartworms (*Dirofilaria immitis, Angiostrongylus vasorum*)
- Fungal infections such as blastomycosis or aspergillosis
- Inflammatory pulmonary disorders such as pulmonary infiltrate with eosinophils or lymphomatoid granulomatosis

Table 12.2 Some causes of chronic coughing in cats

- Feline asthma (bronchospasm mediated by hypersensitivity response)
- Chronic bronchitis
- Bronchiectasis
- Emphysema
- Parasitic infestation (lungworms such as *Aelurostrongylus abstrusus*, migration of Ascarids, other)
- Aspirated tracheobronchial foreign bodies
- Chronic bronchopneumonia
- Pulmonary fungal infections (cryptococcosis)
- Cranial mediastinal masses
- Heartworms (*Dirofilaria immitis*)

assisted by simultaneous contraction of the bronchial smooth muscle which narrows the airways, further increasing the force at which material is expelled.

Coughing may be defined as productive or non-productive. A productive cough occurs when material is expectorated from the trachea into the pharynx. In dogs and cats this material is usually swallowed, but it can occasionally be expectorated to the exterior. Clinically, a productive cough sounds moist and low-pitched, and the animal often swallows immediately afterwards. In contrast, the more common non-productive chronic cough is usually harsh, high-pitched or even honking. Expectoration of mucus may occur occasionally, but is usually not a feature. Dogs with chronic non-productive coughing frequently suffer from paroxysms of coughing which are of great concern to their owners.

INVESTIGATION OF CHRONIC COUGH

A cough that has been present for more than two months is usually a marker for significant disease in the animal. The disease may be confined to the airways, or may represent more extensive pulmonary or even systemic disease such as neoplasia. Many of these disorders are slowly progressive and most do not resolve spontaneously. Early treatment is often the most important tool to delay progression. Every animal that has suffered from a cough for more than two months, therefore, deserves at least a basic work-up to determine the best course of management required to prevent progression of the disease.

HISTORY CHECKLIST

❏ **Age, breed, sex?**
Chronic coughing is most common in older animals, resulting from lesions such as chronic bronchitis or collapsing trachea, congestive heart failure and neoplasia. Younger animals may be more likely to suffer from infectious or parasitic infections, especially if they are in a high-stress environment. Breed predispositions exist for certain disorders, for example collapsing trachea is common in Yorkshire terriers and miniature poodles. Feline asthma is most commonly a problem of middle-aged cats.

❏ **Previous preventative medicine?**
Worming history may be important in evaluation of animals with suspected lungworms. Heartworm status (previous testing or use of prophylaxis) should be determined in areas where dirofilariasis is endemic.

❏ **Duration of signs?**
By definition, dogs and cats with chronic coughing have had problems for more than two months. Many will have suffered mild symptoms for years, with recent exacerbation of signs that may prompt consultation with a veterinarian. Particular attention should be paid to the presence and duration of other systemic signs such as weight loss or vomiting, which could indicate a more serious systemic disorder such as neoplasia.

❏ **Inciting incidents or illness?**
Many animals with chronic coughing have no history of any predisposing cause. Occasionally, however, historical information can be

extremely helpful. A previous history of vomiting or regurgitation can indicate the presence of chronic aspiration pneumonia or systemic neoplasia. Chronic bronchitis may occur as a sequel of infectious tracheobronchitis or necrotizing tracheitis due to smoke inhalation. Recent travel to areas endemic for lungworms, heartworms or fungal infections may be of diagnostic significance.

❏ **Respiratory signs in other animals?**
Most animals with a chronic cough are the only affected animal in the household. The presence of multiple affected animals suggests an environmental, infectious or parasitic aetiology.

❏ **Previous therapy and response?**

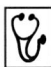 **PHYSICAL EXAMINATION**

❏ **Observation**
Observation of the animal at rest can provide vital information about the extent of disease within the respiratory system. Most animals with mild to moderate chronic bronchitis, collapsing trachea, or even partial airway obstruction are normal at rest between paroxysms of coughing. These dogs typically have no signs of increased effort, paradoxical respiration or cyanosis. Unfortunately, many of these animals may be anxious or panting which can make it difficult to assess respiratory function. Every effort should be made to observe them in a relaxed and calm environment. In contrast, animals with severe airway, heart or lung disease often have increased respiratory rate and effort at rest. They may have a considerable abdominal component to their respiration, with nasal flare and postural adaptation. The most severely affected animals have paradoxical respiration and signs of respiratory muscle fatigue.

❏ **Examination of the pharynx**
Assuming that the animal tolerates the manipulation while awake, the pharynx should be observed by opening the mouth and briefly depressing the tongue. If the larynx is visible, this suggests a defective gag reflex, which might be accompanied by aspiration pneumonia. If the tonsils are enlarged and protruding from the tonsillar crypts, or the pharynx appears erythematous, local inflammation may be present. Unilateral enlargement of one tonsil should prompt suspicion of tonsillar neoplasia.

❏ **Palpation**
The whole airway, particularly the cervical trachea, should be carefully palpated. Attention should be paid to the presence of any kind of compressive mass lesion in the neck or thoracic inlet. The trachea itself should be palpated and compressed to induce coughing. In normal dogs and cats, the trachea is cylindrical and the dorsal membrane can only be palpated with difficulty. Dogs with collapsing trachea may have obvious softening of the tracheal cartilage and airway deformity (tracheal rings become C-shaped). A brief, dry cough can be induced in most normal dogs and cats when the trachea is compressed. In contrast, paroxysms of coughing and wheezing may be elicited in animals with pre-existing inflammation caused by tracheal collapse, chronic bronchitis or feline asthma. Induction of a moist or productive cough should prompt suspicion of bronchopneumonia, bronchiectasis or other serious lung disease.

❏ **Auscultation**
Auscultation is a vital part of the evaluation of any animal with a chronic cough. The first important question, particularly in dogs, is whether or not there is evidence of heart disease. Coughing can be an early sign of left-sided congestive heart failure in dogs with mitral regurgitation or dilated cardiomyopathy. Interestingly, cats with heart failure rarely cough, but instead become dyspnoeic. It is important to recognize that the mere presence of a murmur is not enough to prompt a diagnosis of congestive heart failure (see Chapter 13). Many animals that are actually suffering from chronic bronchitis or collapsing trachea also have some degree of mild mitral endocardiosis but are not actually in heart failure. Therapy for heart disease in such animals will not result in resolution of the cough, which instead should be treated with antitussives and bronchodilators. Some animals with mitral regurgitation may have significant enlargement of the left atrium due to regurgitant flow. In this instance, compression of the left mainstem bronchus may result in coughing that is unrelated to heart failure.

Next, all lung fields and the cervical trachea should be carefully auscultated for the presence of abnormal sounds. The most common finding is increased upper airway sounds, particularly in animals with chronic bronchitis, collapsing trachea or airway obstruction. In animals with tracheal obstruction, the sounds are loudest when the bell of the stethoscope is placed over the cervical trachea. Wheezes (musical sounds produced by movement of air through narrowed airways) are often auscultated in cats with feline asthma. Dull areas may indicate the presence of collapsed or consolidated lung lobes, or masses. Crackles are a serious finding, suggesting the presence of fluid within the airways or alveoli, for example cardiogenic oedema or pneumonia. Dogs with chronic end-stage bronchial or lung disease may also have generalized coarse crackles which are probably caused by early closure and opening of small bronchi rather than the presence of fluid.

❏ **Rectal temperature**

Most animals with chronic coughing do not have a fever, but fever may accompany chronic fungal or bacterial infections or neoplasms. Hyperthermia may occur in animals with upper airway obstruction due to poor air movement over the surface of the tongue, and diminished capacity for evaporative cooling.

❏ **Other**

A complete physical examination, including abdominal palpation, should be performed in every animal with chronic coughing. Abdominal distension attributable to hepatomegaly and hyperadrenocorticism can contribute to coughing due to craniad pressure on the diaphragm by abdominal contents. The presence of a fluid wave may indicate ascites and right-sided heart failure. Palpable abdominal masses could represent neoplasia which may have metastasized to the lungs.

FURTHER INVESTIGATION

As previously mentioned, every animal with a chronic cough should be carefully evaluated before definitive therapy is initiated. Many of these animals require life-long therapy and most have slowly progressive disease. In particular, management of disorders such as collapsing trachea, chronic bronchitis and congestive heart failure can be extremely frustrating for both owner and veterinarian. Before committing an animal to life-long therapy for these chronic illnesses it is vital that a correct diagnosis is made and that reversible or curable disorders are ruled out.

Blood tests

Most of these animals deserve a basic clinical work-up including full routine haematology, a biochemistry panel, urinalysis and if applicable, heartworm testing. The intent is to determine the presence of organic or systemic disease which may be contributing to the chronic cough. For example, animals with fungal pneumonia may have an eosinophilia or increased white blood cell count, and those with hyperadrenocorticism may have increased liver enzymes. If therapy with drugs such as corticosteroids, angiotensin-converting enzyme inhibitors or digoxin is to be considered, then knowledge of liver and kidney function and electrolyte status is vital. In animals in which fungal or protozoal disease is a possible diagnosis, serological titres for agents such as *Cryptococcus* spp., *Aspergillus* spp. or *Toxoplasma gondii* may be helpful. In cats, testing for feline leukaemia virus, feline immunodeficiency virus, or feline infectious peritonitis may be indicated.

Radiography

Thoracic (and sometimes cervical) radiographs are vital in evaluation of animals with chronic coughing. Dogs with chronic bronchitis or collapsing trachea usually have normal radiographs or a peribronchial pattern, suggesting the presence of peribronchial infiltrates. Sometimes a collapsing trachea can be demonstrated by radiographs obtained during inspiration and during exhalation, or by using flexed and extended neck views. Caution should be exercised in interpretation of these views, however. Animals with chronic tracheal collapse or bronchitis usually do not have evidence of pulmonary alveolar disease. If there are any signs of alveolar disease, other disorders such as bronchopneumonia, neoplasia or congestive heart failure should be considered. Bronchiectasis can be evident as a cylindrical dilation of bronchi as they extend to the periphery of the lung lobes, rather than their usual tapering appearance. Masses may be evident in lung lobes or compressing the airways and radio-opaque foreign bodies may be seen. Lastly, intraluminal masses, abscesses, parasitic nodules or foreign bodies may be outlined by the negative contrast of air in the major airways.

Fluoroscopy

Fluoroscopy is a very useful additional tool to confirm a diagnosis of collapsing trachea or compression or collapse of a mainstem bronchus. Plain radiographs of the airways, even when carefully taken at different phases of respiration and in different neck positions, can be deceptive or in some cases non-diagnostic. Fluoroscopy provides a non-invasive, dynamic, real-time representation of the motion of the airways.

Faecal flotation for parasites

Pulmonary migration of ascarids can cause chronic cough especially in heavily infested puppies or kittens. In areas where lungworms are endemic, a Baermann flotation technique should be performed to detect the presence of lungworm larvae in the stool. It must be remembered that lungworm larvae may not always be present in the stool, as their numbers may be low or they may be intermittently shed. Usually, faecal samples are evaluated three days in a row. If the index of suspicion for lungworms is high, anthelminthic therapy should be initiated even if the results are negative.

Bronchoscopy

Bronchoscopy is a very useful tool for evaluation of the chronically coughing dog. Dynamic collapse of the airways can be easily seen, and bronchoscopy is the 'gold standard' for diagnosis of collapsing trachea. Foreign bodies may be visualized and even removed. The airways can be evaluated for the presence of inflammation and exudate, and samples for bacteriological and cytological examination can be obtained directly from affected areas. Bronchoalveolar lavage can provide diagnostic information in cases of fungal or neoplastic lung disease. Bronchoscopy can only be carried out under general anaesthesia, which limits its use to the stable animal.

Cytological and bacteriological examination of the respiratory tract

Bronchoscopy and bronchoalveolar lavage (BAL) is the most specific method by which samples can be obtained from the respiratory tract. To perform a BAL, the tip of the bronchoscope is wedged in an affected bronchus. Several aliquots of saline are instilled into the bronchus through a narrow-bore tube which has been inserted into the bronchus through the biopsy channel of the bronchoscope, and then as much as possible is aspirated from the lung lobe. This technique provides samples from deep within the parenchyma of the lung. When a bronchoscope is not available, however, diagnostic samples may still be obtained by use of techniques such as transtracheal or endotracheal washing. A catheter is inserted into the trachea either percutaneously or through a sterile endotracheal tube and sterile saline is instilled and withdrawn to provide a sample from the upper airways (rather than from the parenchyma as is obtained using BAL). Because of the inherent risks associated with anaesthesia and exacerbation of tracheal inflammation, these techniques should be used cautiously in dogs with collapsing trachea.

Bacterial and fungal cultures of samples obtained from the airways may be diagnostic if bronchopneumonia is present, but the results should not be over-interpreted in the presence of chronic bronchitis or collapsing trachea. Although positive bacterial cultures are obtained in some animals with chronic airway disease they are usually opportunistic pathogens colonizing the inflamed airway, and should not be regarded as primary pathogenic agents. Treatment with antibiotics may cause temporary improvement but does not usually result in long-term resolution of signs. Cytological examination of BAL or transtracheal wash samples may show evidence of toxoplasma tachyzoites, fungal yeast forms, lungworm larvae and occasionally neoplasia. The type of inflammatory cell can also provide useful information, for example a predominant population of eosinophils in tracheal wash fluid may suggest parasitic or fungal infection, a hypersensitivity response, or pulmonary infiltrate with eosinophils.

Tests of pulmonary function

Arterial blood gas analysis, pulse oximetry and end-tidal capnography are usually normal in animals with mild to moderate airway disease. Oxygenation may decrease with severe airway disease due to progressive ventilation–perfusion mismatch. Ventilation and $PaCO_2$ are usually normal unless there is an airway obstruction preventing air flow.

Measurement of airway resistance, lung compliance and the generation of tidal breathing flow volume loops also provide very useful information in animals with airway disease. These techniques are currently being evaluated in cats with bronchitis and feline asthma, and in dogs with chronic bronchitis. They require the use of sophisticated computerized instruments and are only available to a limited number of veterinarians.

■ Other diagnostic procedures

Left-sided congestive heart failure is a common cause of chronic coughing in dogs, which may require evaluation by echocardiography and electrocardiography. Some dogs or cats with chronic coughing may have mass lesions in the lung which may require surgical exploration and resection. Some of these animals may also benefit from additional imaging modalities such as computed tomography or magnetic resonance imaging of the thorax.

13

Cardiac Murmurs

J. K. Dunn

The audible characteristics of a cardiac murmur are determined by many cardiac and non-cardiac factors. Not all murmurs indicate cardiac pathology; some are benign and may disappear spontaneously. Likewise, the presence of a heart murmur, even if it is considered to be pathological, should not be taken as evidence that the animal has congestive heart failure. Indeed, most cases of mitral valve endocardiosis during the early stages at least have normal myocardial contractility and although there may be a significant regurgitant fraction of blood entering the left atrium the animal may show no signs of cardiac decompensation. It is therefore important when performing a clinical examination to record the particular characteristics of a murmur to allow comparisons with later observations which may or may not correlate with an altered clinical presentation.

CARDIAC AUSCULTATION

Auscultation of the thorax should be performed in a quiet room. All of the cardiac valve areas should be auscultated systematically, using both the bell and diaphragm of the stethoscope, and the point of maximal intensity in relation to a specific valve and the presence/absence of a precordial thrill should be noted. Certain murmurs, e.g. the murmur associated with patent ductus arteriosus can be localized to a small area of the chest wall. If a murmur is audible, other areas of the thorax including the thoracic inlet should be auscultated since murmurs often radiate across the chest wall. Fig. 13.1 illustrates the approximate sites on the chest wall for placement of the stethoscope head to auscultate each of the four cardiac valves.

Left side
- Mitral valve region: fifth intercostal space at the level of the costochondral junction approximately one quarter of the distance from the

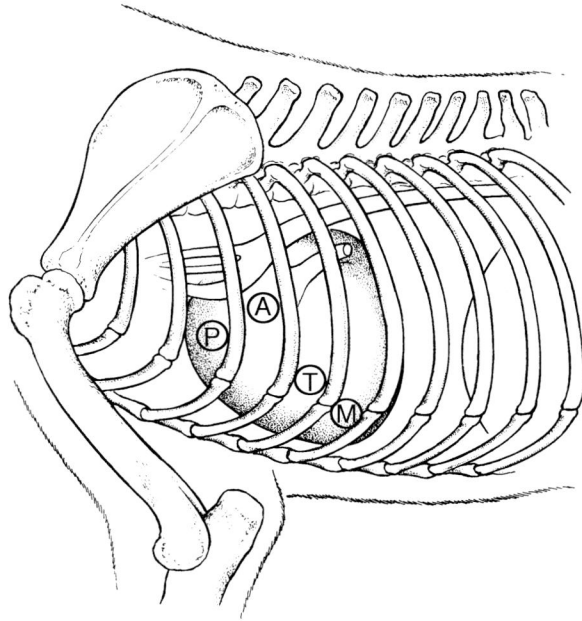

Figure 13.1 Points of auscultation for the mitral (M), tricuspid (T), pulmonic (P) and aortic (A) valves.

sternum to the vertebrae. In the cat this position may be slightly further back i.e. fifth or sixth intercostal space.
- Aortic valve region: third–fourth intercostal space level with the point of the shoulder (second–third intercostal space in the cat just dorsal to pulmonic valve region).
- Pulmonic valve region: second–third intercostal space just above the costochondral junction i.e. just ventral to the aortic valve region (second–third intercostal space in the cat).

Right side
- Tricuspid valve region: fourth intercostal space at the level of the costochondral junction (fourth–fifth intercostal space in the cat).

Table 13.1 Acquired and congenital causes of cardiac murmurs in dogs and cats

Systolic murmurs		Breed, sex and age predisposition	Character of murmur
Mitral insufficiency			
Acquired	Endocardiosis	Small, toy or miniature breeds of dogs; increased incidence in dogs >7 years of age.	Harsh low to medium frequency holosystolic murmur with PMI over the AV valve (occasional musical 'squeaky' quality); loud murmurs over the mitral valve may be heard on the right side; first heart sound may be accentuated whereas second may be difficult to detect
	Dilated cardiomyopathy	Giant breeds (Irish wolfhound, great Dane), Dobermanns, old English sheepdogs, cocker spaniels and cats	
	Hypertrophic cardiomyopathy	Boxers and cats	
	Bacterial endocarditis	Large breed dogs, often male, 2–7 years of age	
Congenital	Mitral dysplasia	German shepherds and great Danes especially males; one of the most common congenital defects in cats	
Tricuspid insufficiency			
Acquired	Endocardiosis (may involve the tricuspid and mitral valves; rarely the tricuspid valve on its own)	As for mitral insufficiency	As for mitral insufficiency
Congenital	Tricuspid dysplasia (rare)	Less common than mitral dysplasia; large breed dogs especially males, e.g. Dobermanns, setters and retrievers; one of the most common defects in cats	
Aortic stenosis		Newfoundlands (inherited), boxers, German shepherds, golden retrievers, German short-haired pointers; in cats may be associated with hypertrophic cardiomyopathy	High frequency crescendo–decrescendo murmur with PMI over the aortic valve region; radiates to thoracic inlet and up carotid arteries; occasionally severe murmurs may be auscultated on top of the cranium; may be associated with a precordial thrill; weak femoral pulse; may be an early diastolic component to the murmur if aortic regurgitation
Pulmonic stenosis		Bulldogs, beagles, chihuahuas, miniature schnauzers, cocker spaniels, samoyeds, fox terriers and brachycephalic breeds; rare in cats	High frequency crescendo–decrescendo murmur with PMI over the pulmonic valve region; intensity often correlates with degree of stenosis; ±precordial thrill; ±split second heart sound (S2)
Ventricular septal defect		Keeshounds (inherited), ?increased incidence in bulldogs, cats	Harsh holosystolic 'diagonal' murmur with PMI over right 2nd–4th intercostal space at costochondral junction; also audible over left mitral valve area; ±split S2; ±precordial thrill at PMI; murmur may disappear if pulmonary hypertension develops and shunt reverses direction i.e. if blood flows right to left
Atrial septal defect		–	Soft systolic murmur over pulmonic region (relative aortic stenosis if large flow rate across the valve); split S2
Tetralogy of Fallot		Keeshounds (inherited), bulldogs	Holosystolic murmur right side (VSD); systolic over pulmonic valve region left side (pulmonic stenosis); ±precordial thrill over pulmonic valve region if murmur severe
Diastolic murmurs			
Aortic or pulmonic regurgitation		Aortic insufficiency may be associated with congenital subaortic stenosis or bacterial endocarditis involving the aortic valve; pulmonic insufficiency may be associated with dirofilariasis	High-pitched low-grade decrescendo murmur during early diastole; may be systolic murmur of aortic stenosis
Mitral or tricuspid stenosis		–	Low-grade systolic murmur
Continuous murmurs			
Patent ductus arteriosus		Miniature poodles (inherited), cocker spaniels, German shepherds, Irish setters, pomeranians, collies, Shetland sheepdogs and keeshounds	'Machinery-type' murmur localized to the aortic/pulmonic valve region; may be accompanied by a systolic murmur of mitral regurgitation; occasionally radiates to thoracic inlet; strong femoral pulse with rapid diastolic fall off (waterhammer pulse)

AV, atrioventricular; PMI, point of maximal intensity; IVS, interventricular septum.

Radiographic features	Echocardiographic features	Electrocardiographic features
Presence of murmur does not indicate animal has CHF and intensity of murmur does not necessarily correlate with the degree of valvular incompetence; radiographic findings are therefore variable and relate to the degree of regurgitation, e.g. left atrial enlargement (marked with mitral dysplasia); ±left ventricular enlargement, ±pulmonary venous congestion, ±pulmonary oedema; severe left-sided failure may progress to signs of right-sided failure, e.g. right heart enlargement, enlarged posterior vena cava, hepatomegaly, ascites and pleural effusion. Generalized cardiomegaly with dilated cardiomyopathy; radiographs may be unremarkable with hypertrophic cardiomyopathy	*Endocardiosis:* thickened AV valve leaflets; left atrial ±left ventricular enlargement; increased fractional shortening unless myocardial failure; prolapse of mitral valve into left atrium; chaotic fluttering of mitral valve if chordae tendinae rupture. *Dilated cardiomyopathy:* severe enlargement of all four chambers; increased left ventricular systolic and diastolic internal dimensions; increased E-point to septum separation; left ventricular hypokinesis and reduced fractional shortening. *Hypertrophic cardiomyopathy:* decreased left ventricular systolic and diastolic dimensions; increased thickness of interventricular septum and left ventricular free wall during systole and diastole; hypertrophy of left ventricular papillary muscles; increased fractional shortening; may be associated with subaortic stenosis	Wide P waves (left atrial enlargement); ±tall/wide QRS complexes (left ventricular enlargement); supraventricular arrhythmias (e.g. atrial fibrillation) common with dilated cardiomyopathy; ventricular arrhythmias or bundle branch block especially with hypertrophic cardiomyopathy in cats
Right atrial ±right ventricular enlargement	As for mitral insufficiency	Deep Q waves ±right axis shift consistent with right atrial and right ventricular enlargement
Radiographs often unremarkable; ±post-stenotic dilatation on lateral and DV views; left ventricular enlargement ±signs of left-sided CHF	Subaortic fibrous ring; post-stenotic dilatation; premature aortic closure; systolic fluttering of the aortic valve; systolic anterior motion of the mitral valve; diastolic fluttering of the mitral valve; left ventricular hypertrophy with normal or increased fractional shortening	ECG often normal; ±signs of left atrial/ventricular enlargement; arrhythmias common
May be normal; if clinically significant, right atrial/right ventricular enlargement; post-stenotic dilatation of main pulmonary artery produces 2 o'clock 'bulge' on DV view; may be decreased pulmonary vascularity	Abnormal thickening or doming of pulmonic valve; post-stenotic dilatation of main pulmonary artery; ±right ventricular hypertrophy; flattened or paradoxical motion of the interventricular septum	Deep S and Q waves (leads I, II, III and aVF) and right axis shift consistent with right ventricular enlargement; arrhythmias common
May be normal if defect is small; left-sided cardiomegaly with pulmonary overcirculation ±oedema; right ventricular enlargement; enlarged main pulmonary artery segment	Defect high in interventricular septum; left atrial and left ventricular dilation; hyperkinetic left ventricle if defect is large (right ventricle usually normal)	Changes consistent with biventricular enlargement; ±right bundle branch block
Pulmonary overcirculation; ±right ventricular enlargement	–	–
Right ventricular enlargement; hypoperfused lung fields and small pulmonary arteries; ±post-stenotic dilatation of pulmonary artery; ±displaced aortic arch	High ventricular septal defect; right ventricular hypertrophy, pulmonic stenosis; over-riding aorta; hypertrophy of interventricular septum and flattened or paradoxical IVS motion	Deep S and Q waves (leads I, II, III and aVF) and a right axis shift consistent with right ventricular enlargement
If associated with endocarditis often signs of left-sided CHF	–	–
Left or right atrial enlargement but ventricles normal; pulmonary venous engorgement ±oedema	–	–
Left-sided cardiomegaly ± right ventricular enlargement if pulmonary hypertension; pulmonary overcirculation ±pulmonary oedema; three 'bulges' on DV view: enlargement of descending aortic arch (1 o'clock), main pulmonary artery (2 o'clock) and left auricular appendage (3 o'clock)	Difficult to image; confirm left atrial and left ventricular enlargement; exaggerated septal motion; in advanced cases may be decreased contractility; with Doppler may appreciate continuous flow disturbance and high-grade retrograde flow toward the pulmonic valve	Left atrial and left ventricular enlargement (in severe cases pronounced P mitrale ±P pulmonale), wide tall QRS complexes with ST slurring

PATHOPHYSIOLOGY

Cardiac murmurs are caused by a disruption to the normal laminar flow of blood either within the heart or as blood exits the heart and enters the major vessels. Murmurs may be classified as pathological, functional or benign. A pathological murmur is the result of a congenital or acquired structural defect involving either the heart or great vessels (ventricular outflow tracts). A murmur may be generated as blood flows through a narrowed outflow tract (e.g. aortic stenosis), an abnormal vascular or chamber communication (e.g. patent ductus arteriosus or ventricular septal defect), or an abnormal valve orifice (e.g. mitral valve incompetence). Valvular incompetence of the atrioventricular (AV) valves may occur if the valve cusps become thickened (endocardiosis) or if the atrioventricular annulus dilates to a point that the valve cusps are unable to close properly (dilated cardiomyopathy). In both these situations the retrograde flow of blood through the valve orifice may be expected to produce a cardiac murmur.

Functional (physiological) murmurs are associated with extra-cardiac factors, i.e. high output states such as fever, pregnancy, chronic anaemia and hyperthyroidism which result in tachycardia and an increase in blood flow velocity. The haemic murmurs associated with severe chronic anaemia (packed cell volume usually less than 0.15 l/l) can be attributed to a decrease in blood viscosity and a compensatory increase in cardiac output in response to chronic hypoxia. They are generally soft, low grade (no greater than 3/6), early–mid systolic, ejection-type murmurs with a point of maximal intensity over the mitral or aortic valves.

Innocent or benign murmurs are functional murmurs which are typically heard in young puppies and kittens and occasionally in some narrow-chested breeds of dog. They are associated with alterations in the flow velocity through the

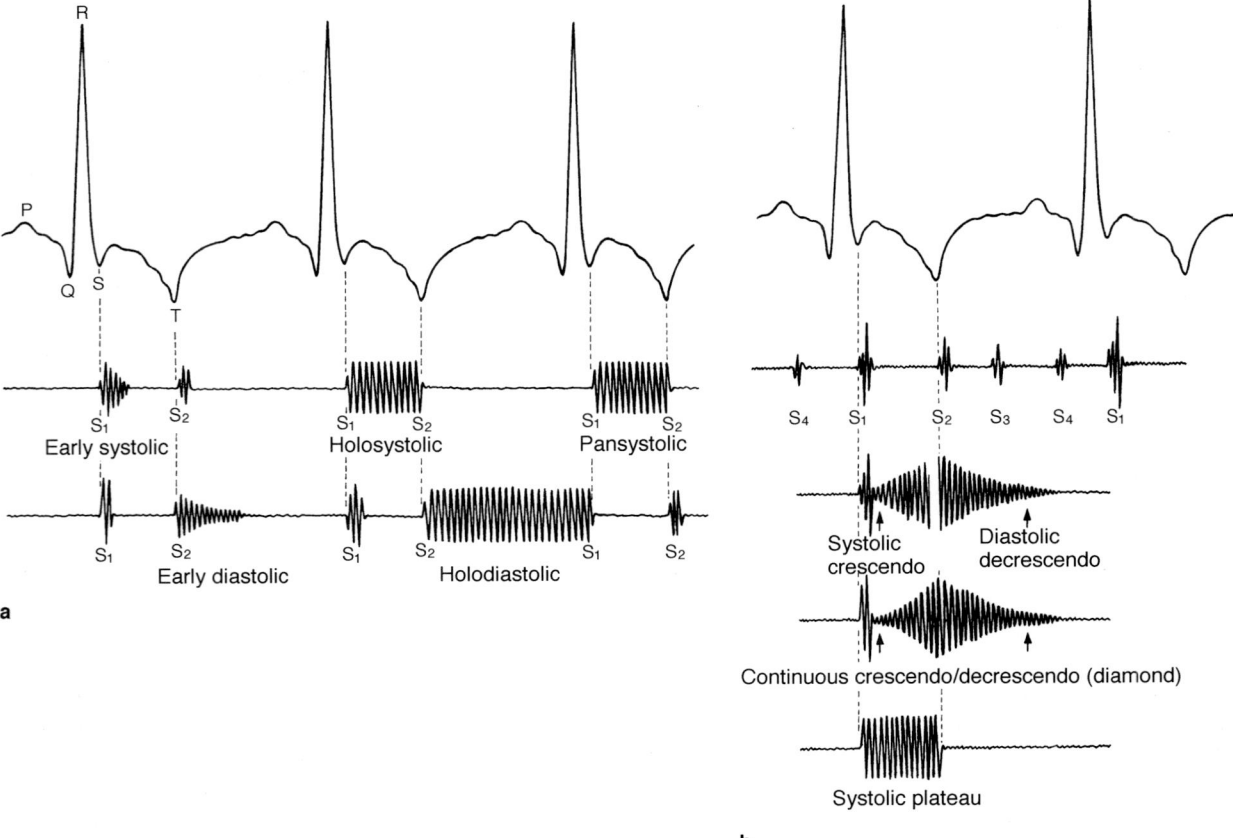

Fig. 13.2 (a and b) Diagrams showing the timing of cardiac murmurs in relation to the four heart sounds and phase of the cardiac cycle. The phonocardiographic characteristic (shape) of each type of murmur is also shown. After Gompf (1988).

ventricular outflow tracts. The intensity of such murmurs is therefore influenced by heart rate (being more pronounced if the animal is tachycardic), stroke volume and ejection velocity. Innocent murmurs are generally soft, low grade (no greater than 2/6), early systolic, ejection type murmurs. On auscultation they tend to be loudest over the mitral or aortic valve regions or at the thoracic inlet and they radiate poorly. In many young animals the murmur may be expected to disappear by 4–5 months of age. The conditions which may give rise to different types of cardiac murmur are summarized in Table 13.1.

CLASSIFICATION OF CARDIAC MURMURS

A murmur may be characterized on the basis of the following features: timing, duration, intensity, pitch, quality (shape), location and radiation.

Timing and duration

A murmur can be classified according to its timing in the cardiac cycle and relationship to the normal S1 and S2 heart sounds (see Fig. 13.2). A systolic murmur describes a murmur occurring between S1 and S2. An early systolic murmur stops before mid-systole; a holosystolic murmur extends throughout systole but ends before S2 and a pansystolic murmur extends throughout systole and obscures the S2 sound. Systolic murmurs may be caused by AV insufficiency (commonly involving the mitral valve), aortic or pulmonic stenosis, and atrial or ventricular septal defects. Functional and innocent murmurs are also systolic.

A diastolic murmur is one occurring after S2 and before the next S1 of the cardiac cycle. Diastolic murmurs are relatively rare; they may be heard with aortic insufficiency (e.g. bacterial endocarditis of the aortic valve or in association with aortic stenosis), dirofilariasis, and stenosis of an AV valve.

A continuous murmur is one which starts after S1, continues through S2 and stops before the next S1. The most common cause of a continuous murmur is a left to right shunting patent ductus arteriosus (if the direction of the shunt reverses the murmur may disappear). Occasionally aortic stenosis is complicated by a degree of aortic regurgitation resulting in a murmur with both systolic and an early diastolic components.

Intensity

The intensity of a murmur does not reflect flow volume and therefore, in some cases, bears no correlation to the severity of the underlying defect, i.e. small defects may produce loud murmurs and vice versa. Intensity is generally graded on a scale of I–VI as follows:

- Grade I   Murmur barely audible; careful auscultation required, i.e. this is the softest audible murmur.
- Grade II   A very soft murmur but it is heard as soon as the stethoscope is applied to the chest wall.
- Grade III Approximately the same intensity as normal heart sounds.
- Grade IV   Louder than normal heart sounds but no precordial thrill is present.
- Grade V   Can be heard with the stethoscope barely touching the thorax and a palpable precordial thrill present.
- Grade VI   Can be heard with the stethoscope away from the animal's chest.

Pitch (quality or frequency)

A murmur may be classified as having a low, medium, high or mixed frequency. Sharp ejection-type murmurs caused by blood flowing at an increased velocity through a stenosed ventricular outflow tract tend to be of higher frequency than the harsher regurgitant murmurs typical of valvular insufficiency (although some of the latter possess a distinctive 'squeaky' quality). A harsh continuous 'machinery' type murmur is a feature of patent ductus arteriosus.

Shape (modulation)

The shape of a murmur refers to its phonocardiographic characteristics (Fig. 13.2). A crescendo murmur starts softly and gets louder before it stops; a decrescendo murmur does exactly the opposite. A crescendo–decrescendo (diamond-shaped) murmur starts softly then becomes louder before dying away softly. The shape of a murmur may indicate a certain valvular abnormality. The systolic regurgitant murmurs associated with AV insufficiency or ventricular septal defect (VSD) are usually plateau-shaped murmurs; the systolic ejection type murmurs typical of aortic or pulmonic stenosis are usually described as being crescendo–decrescendo murmurs. Diastolic murmurs, associated with aortic insufficiency or AV valve stenosis, are rare and are usually decrescendo in shape.

Location and radiation

The location of a murmur is represented by the point of maximal intensity (PMI). When a murmur is the result of a valvular lesion the PMI may help identify the valve involved. Even if the murmur is caused by a non-valvular lesion, e.g. patent ductus arteriosus or ventricular septal defect the PMI of the murmur (and also its pitch and quality) may provide clues as to the possible cause. Having identified the PMI, continued auscultation is necessary to determine whether the murmur radiates to other parts of the thorax, including the thoracic inlet. Severe regurgitant murmurs associated with AV valve incompetence typically radiate cranially and dorsally; the ejection murmur associated with aortic stenosis often radiates to the thoracic inlet and up the carotid vessels in the neck (severe murmurs may even be auscultated on top of the head).

Miscellaneous 'murmurs'

Systolic clicks

Systolic clicks are mid to late high frequency systolic sounds which in humans are associated with mitral valve prolapse. In the dog the cause and clinical significance of systolic clicks are unknown but they are thought to indicate early mitral valve disease.

'Respiratory' murmurs

'Respiratory' murmurs may be heard in deep-chested breeds of dog especially if they are panting. These sounds, which mimic low-grade systolic murmurs, are of no clinical significance. The fact that 'respiratory' murmurs tend to wax and wane in intensity and may disappear if the animal is sedated for radiography suggests that they are probably benign functional flow murmurs.

INVESTIGATION OF A CARDIAC MURMUR

The investigation of any cardiac murmur is similar for any animal although the urgency for specific diagnostic tests will be determined by the animal's age and whether it is showing clinical signs of cardiac decompensation. The presence of a murmur in a twelve-week old animal presented for routine vaccination which appears otherwise healthy should be investigated at the earliest opportunity. The majority of such murmurs are the result of congenital cardiac defects and accurate diagnosis is essential if the owner is to be provided with an accurate, long-term prognosis. In contrast, a murmur detected in an older animal is more likely to be associated with clinical signs of congestive heart failure (CHF). A detailed history may therefore not only confirm the absence or presence of signs consistent with CHF but may also provide an approximate assessment of the degree of cardiac decompensation.

HISTORY CHECKLIST

☐ **Breed, age and sex?**

A young (<6 months old) animal which presents with a loud (>3/6) murmur will almost certainly have a congenital cardiac defect. Certain congenital defects have a much higher incidence in some breeds than others (Table 13.1). The majority of middle-aged or old dogs (>4 years old) will either have mitral insufficiency or dilated cardiomyopathy. Murmurs associated with mitral insufficiency due to endocardiosis are more common in smaller (toy) breeds of dog particularly in animals greater than 7 years of age although certain breeds, for example cavalier King Charles spaniels, can develop murmurs when 3 years old or less. Not infrequently these animals may present with no clinical signs. Dogs with dilated cardiomyopathy tend to present slightly earlier, often between 4 and 7 years of age, and the murmur is often associated with signs suggestive of CHF or low output failure (although this may be influenced by the breed of animal).

The presence of a murmur in a cat nearly always indicates cardiac pathology unless there is evidence to suggest the animal is severely anaemic. The most common feline congenital cardiac defects are listed in Table 13.2. The most common cause of a murmur (often accompanied by a gallop rhythm and/or tachycardia) in an older cat is hypertrophic or, less frequently, dilated cardiomyopathy.

☐ **Is the animal showing signs of cardiac decompensation i.e. backward (congestive) and/or forward (low output) heart failure?**

- Exercise intolerance?
- Systemic signs such as weakness, anorexia,

Table 13.2 Some of the more common causes of congenital heart disease in the cat

- Mitral valve dysplasia
- Tricuspid valve dysplasia
- Ventricular septal defect
- Aortic stenosis
- Persistent common atrioventricular canal
- Endocardial fibroelastosis
- Patent ductus arteriosus
- Tetralogy of Fallot

weight loss (cardiac cachexia)?; if systemic signs are associated with a history of intermittent febrile episodes and/or lameness in a young to middle-aged large breed dog then consider bacteraemia due to bacterial endocarditis as a possible cause.
- If animal is young, is it growing normally or does it appear stunted?
- Cough or altered respiratory pattern?
- Abdominal distension (ascites)?
- Syncope?

PHYSICAL EXAMINATION

❏ **Characterize the murmur**
The type of murmur may provide important diagnostic clues especially with congenital heart disorders. When auscultating the heart always simultaneously palpate the femoral pulse and note pulse pressure and the presence of a pulse deficit. The femoral pulse may be weak with aortic stenosis; PDA is characterized by a strong pulse with a rapid diastolic fall-off ('waterhammer' pulse).

❏ **Normal mucous membranes?**
Pale with anaemia or hypoxia; cyanotic with right to left shunts in a young animal with left-sided heart failure resulting in severe pulmonary oedema.

❏ **Prolonged capillary refill time?**
Indicates poor peripheral perfusion.

❏ **Dyspnoeic?**
Can a cough be elicited on tracheal palpation?

❏ **Adventitious lung sounds?**
Crackles and wheezes may indicate pulmonary oedema.

❏ **Hepatomegaly?**

❏ **Evidence of ascites, peripheral oedema or a jugular pulse?**

❏ **Always palpate the cervical region of cats for the presence of a thyroid mass.**

FURTHER INVESTIGATION

Radiography

Lateral and dorsoventral thoracic radiographs
Check for:
- Enlargement of the cardiac silhouette
- Evidence of pulmonary venous congestion, oedema or pulmonary overcirculation (left-sided failure) or accumulation of fluid in the pleural space (right-sided failure)

Lateral ± ventrodorsal abdominal radiographs
Check for:
- Hepatomegaly (passive venous congestion of the liver)
- Increased diameter of posterior vena cava
- Ascites

Electrocardiography

Electrocardiographic evidence of chamber enlargement should always be interpreted in association with the radiographic findings. Signs of left atrial and/or left ventricular enlargement tend to be non-specific; signs of right atrial/ventricular enlargement are usually more significant (seen most frequently with tetralogy of Fallot or pulmonic stenosis). The presence of ectopic supraventricular or ventricular complexes in an animal with a heart murmur generally indicates severe myocardial dilatation or hypertrophy and resultant myocardial hypoxia.

Echocardiography

With echocardiography it is usually possible to:
- Ascertain the nature of the cardiac defect responsible for the murmur (with the exception of the small PDA);
- Assess chamber dimensions and thickness of

the left ventricular free wall and interventricular septum, i.e. it is possible to differentiate the dilated and hypertrophic forms of cardiomyopathy;
- Assess myocardial contractility which is important for both prognostic and therapeutic purposes;
- Detect abnormal valve formation and/or function, and the presence of valvular or mural thrombi;
- Detect the presence of pericardial fluid.

Angiography

With the increased use of ultrasonography angiography is less frequently performed. Occasionally it may be required to investigate a congenital cardiac defect when the results of echocardiography are equivocal.

Routine haematology and biochemistry screening

If the animal which has a murmur appears quite fit and healthy there is probably no initial justification for submitting haematological specimens to the laboratory. Animals with cardiac disorders are more likely to show haematological and/or biochemical abnormalities if there is evidence of the following:

- Right to left (reverse) shunting of blood. Young animals with tetralogy of Fallot are usually hypoxaemic and as a result may develop secondary polycythaemia.
- Animals with congestive heart failure may have increased numbers of circulating normoblasts despite the fact they are not anaemic (presumably this also may be attributed to mild hypoxia resulting in erythropoietin-mediated stimulation of the bone marrow). Animals with significant pleural or abdominal effusions are often mildly hypoproteinaemic (hypoalbuminaemic).
- Renal function (urea, creatinine and urine protein:creatinine ratio) should be checked in animals with dilated cardiomyopathy since reduced renal perfusion may result in prerenal azotaemia. Liver enzymes (ALP and ALT) may also be slightly increased due to passive venous congestion of the liver.
- Dogs with subacute bacterial endocarditis may have a neutrophilia with or without a left shift, a monocytosis and increased plasma fibrinogen concentration.

Serum or plasma T3 and T4 assays

T3 and T4 assays should be performed in all cats with cardiac murmurs.

REFERENCE

Gompf, R.E. (1988) The clinical approach to heart disease: History and physical examination. In *Canine and Feline Cardiology* (Ed. P.R. Fox). Churchill Livingstone, New York, pp. 29–42.

14

Pallor

J. K. Dunn

Pallor of the mucous membranes may reflect either decreased red cell mass, i.e. anaemia, or decreased peripheral perfusion as occurs with cardiogenic, hypovolaemic or vasculogenic shock. Cardiogenic shock implies a marked reduction in cardiac output due to acute myocardial failure (pump failure) or as a result of a tachydysrhythmia associated with myocardial dysfunction. Hypovolaemic shock occurs after acute blood loss (loss of 30–40% of total blood volume), severe thermal burns or crush injuries (loss of plasma), or severe dehydration (resulting from either water deprivation or mixed water and electrolyte loss). In vasculogenic shock blood volume is normal but there is relative hypovolaemia as the volume of blood stored in the venous capacitance vessels increases. This type of shock may be mediated by neurogenic reflexes (e.g. trauma) or may occur when there is loss of sympathetic tone (sympathetic blockade). Other causes include endotoxaemia, which results in the release of vasodilator substances such as histamine and vasoactive kinins, and adrenal insufficiency (an acute Addisonian crisis).

INVESTIGATION OF PALE MUCOUS MEMBRANES

In most cases, the history and clinical examination will provide sufficient clues for the clinician to be able to decide whether pallor is the result of anaemia or decreased peripheral perfusion (shock) so the diagnostic approach to each situation will be discussed separately.

ANAEMIA

Anaemia is characterized by a decrease in the number of circulating erythrocytes, haemoglobin concentration and packed cell volume (PCV).

Pathophysiology and clinical manifestations

An absolute decrease in the number of circulating red cells may occur in three ways:

1. Haemorrhage;
2. Increased red cell destruction usually associated with a decrease in red cell lifespan;
3. Inadequate production of red cells by the bone marrow either as a result of reduced proliferation of red cell precursors (hypoproliferative anaemias) or the defective synthesis of haemoglobin or nuclear chromatin (maturation defect anaemias).

Anaemias due to haemorrhage or haemolysis are typically regenerative; hypoproliferative and maturation defect anaemias are non-regenerative (see section on classification of anaemias).

The clinical signs associated with anaemia reflect the reduced oxygen-carrying capacity of the blood (hypoxaemia) and also the various physiological mechanisms which come into play. The severity of signs depends on four factors:

1. Rate of onset and severity of the anaemia, i.e. acute or chronic.
2. The degree of physiological compensation. Older animals are generally less able to compensate for severe reductions in blood volume and the effects of tissue hypoxia because the reserve capacity of their cardiovascular and respiratory systems is reduced.
3. The degree of exertional stress to which the animal is subjected.
4. The associated effects of any underlying disease which may be present.

Tissue hypoxia and decreased blood viscosity result in a reflex tachycardia. On auscultation, heart sounds may be accentuated and with most severe anaemias (packed cell volume (PCV) usually <0.15 l l^{-1}) a cardiac 'haemic' murmur develops. These low grade (usually no more than 2/6 or

3/6 in intensity), mid-systolic murmurs can be attributed to decreased blood viscosity and increased flow velocity and are audible over the left cardiac apex. Such murmurs usually disappear when the anaemia is corrected; failure to do so indicates concurrent cardiac pathology.

With acute blood loss, left ventricular function is suppressed and signs of hypovolaemic shock predominate. The arterial (femoral) pulse becomes weak and rapid, and capillary refill time is prolonged (greater than 2 s). In an attempt to maintain tissue oxygenation the heart rate increases in order to increase cardiac output (cardiac output=heart rate × stroke volume). In addition, oxygen more readily dissociates from haemoglobin and is taken up by tissues. In contrast, with severe chronic anaemias or anaemias where blood is lost more slowly, fluid moves from the tissues into the circulation thereby maintaining circulatory volume. The heart rate in these cases may be normal or only slightly elevated and the pulse pressure may be increased. The increase in cardiac output is the result of an increase in stroke volume brought about by ventricular dilatation and hypertrophy. In older animals with pre-existing heart disease this increase in cardiac workload may ultimately lead to myocardial decompensation and signs of congestive heart failure.

INVESTIGATION OF ANAEMIA

The main objective of the initial investigations is to classify the anaemia as either regenerative or non-regenerative on the basis of the reticulocyte count and red cell indices. The next step involves accurately identifying the pathophysiological mechanism or underlying disease process responsible for the anaemia. Having done this, the clinician should be able to provide the owner with a more accurate prognosis and initiate an appropriate treatment programme.

HISTORY CHECKLIST

❑ **Age, breed and sex?**
Certain congenital bleeding disorders have a higher incidence in certain breeds, e.g. von Willebrand's disease in Doberman pinschers and German shepherd dogs. Some bleeding disorders such as haemophilia A are sex-linked and occur only in males. Affected animals may be expected to show a bleeding tendency at a relatively early age.

❑ **Rate of onset?**
A rapid onset of anaemia is highly suggestive of either haemorrhage or haemolysis, whereas anaemia which is more insidious in onset and follows a chronic course, especially if it is associated with fever or signs of recurrent infection, is more indicative of a primary bone marrow disorder, for example a myeloproliferative or lymphoproliferative disorder.

❑ **Trauma?**
Consider the possibility of internal haemorrhage especially if there is a history of trauma.

❑ **Evidence of sepsis?**
See comments above concerning rate of onset.

❑ **Exposure to toxins**
Consider the possibility of exposure to toxic drugs or chemicals, e.g. anticoagulant rodenticides (e.g. warfarin), oestrogenic compounds, non-steroidal analgesics or cytotoxic agents (e.g. cyclophosphamide).

❑ **Evidence of external haemorrhage?**
Signs such as epistaxis, haemoptysis, haematemesis, haematuria or haemoglobinuria and melaena may indicate a more generalized bleeding tendency.

❑ **Lethargy, anorexia, depression, weight loss, fever?**
These non-specific signs occur in most anaemic patients and are of little help in establishing a diagnosis. The severity of these signs depends on the severity and rate of onset of the anaemia.

❑ **Exercise intolerance, respiratory distress and/or syncope?**
The absence or presence of exercise intolerance and syncope reflects the severity of the anaemia and, more significantly, the rate of onset. Similar signs may be observed in animals with acute cardiogenic shock.

❑ **Evidence of other systemic signs?**
The presence of systemic signs such as vomiting, diarrhoea, polydipsia and polyuria suggests that an underlying systemic or metabolic disorder is responsible for the anaemia (e.g. chronic renal insufficiency or hypoadrenocorticism).

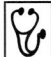 PHYSICAL EXAMINATION

The comments above regarding pathophysiology and clinical manifestations of anaemia should be considered.

❏ **Generalized weakness, exercise intolerance or signs of respiratory distress?**

An animal with a slowly progressive anaemia may appear quite bright and alert at rest and may show respiratory signs only when excited or exercised whereas an animal which becomes acutely anaemic may be expected to show signs of respiratory distress (tachypnoea or dyspnoea) at rest.

❏ **Quality and rate of arterial pulse?**

Assess pulse rate (increased or normal?) and strength (weak or bounding?).

❏ **Tachycardia?**

❏ **Cardiac murmur?**

❏ **Pyrexic?**

Fever indicates an underlying infectious, inflammatory or neoplastic disease process. Acute intravascular haemolysis may be associated with a febrile response due to release of red cell pyrogens.

❏ **Jaundiced?**

The increased destruction of red cells may result in jaundice (consider acute intravascular haemolysis if jaundice is severe).

❏ **Evidence of ecchymotic or petechial haemorrhages?**

Check gingivae, conjunctivae, sclerae, external genitalia and skin, especially areas where the skin is thin and more susceptible to trauma, e.g. inguinal region for signs of haemorrhage. The most common cause of petechial and ecchymotic haemorrhages is thrombocytopenia. Retinal haemorrhages may occasionally be detected by ophthalmoscopic examination in severely thrombocytopenic animals.

❏ **Hepatomegaly or splenomegaly?**

Enlargement of the spleen and/or liver in an anaemic animal may be caused by extramedullary erythropoiesis, increased extravascular destruction of opsonized red cells or platelets, or neoplastic infiltration (e.g. lymphoproliferative or myeloproliferative disease).

❏ **Lymphadenopathy?**

Rule out lymphoma or systemic immune-mediated disorders such as polyarthritis or systemic lupus erythematosus.

❏ **Abdominal pain/abdominal masses?**

Rule out acute intra-abdominal haemorrhage. Splenic neoplasms, particularly haemangiosarcoma or lymphoma, occasionally rupture and the resultant haemorrhage into the abdominal cavity may be potentially life threatening.

INITIAL DIAGNOSTIC PLAN

A minimal diagnostic plan for the investigation of anaemia should include the following:

- Full routine haematological examination including reticulocyte and platelet counts
- Examination of a blood film for the presence of red cell parasites (*Haemobartonella* sp., *Babesia* sp.)
- A complete biochemical profile. (A complete biochemical screen at the Department of Clinical Veterinary Medicine, University of Cambridge, includes urea, creatinine, glucose, alanine aminotransferase (ALT), aspartate aminotransferase (AST), alkaline phosphatase (ALP), gamma-glutamyl transferase (GGT), creatine kinase (CK), calcium, phosphate, sodium, potassium and chloride.)
- Urinalysis
- Lateral radiographs of the thorax and abdomen
- Cats should be screened for the feline leukaemia (FeLV) and feline immunodeficiency (FIV) viruses.

Based on the results of the above more specific tests to detect abnormalities in iron metabolism (see below), abnormalities in blood clotting, red cell antibodies (direct Coombs' test) and faecal occult blood may be indicated. Bone marrow aspiration or biopsy may help to define more accurately the cause of the anaemia.

Interpretation of haematological results

Physiological alterations

When interpreting the red cell parameters, consideration should be given to the age and breed of animal. The total red cell count, haemoglobin concentration, packed cell volume (PCV) and total plasma protein content are generally lower in young animals less than 6 months of age, for example a PCV of $0.30-0.35\,l\,l^{-1}$ is not unusual for a 3-month-old pup or kitten, although for the first three weeks after birth the PCV may be normal due to the increased size of the red cells. During pregnancy the red cell count, haemoglobin concentration and PCV decrease before returning to normal during lactation. The same three parameters are increased in most greyhounds (PCV 0.55–0.60 l l^{-1}); some poodles also have a high PCV due to the presence of macrocytic erythrocytes.

Artefactual results

Poor sample collection and handling may also influence haematological results. For example, a delay in transit or exposure to high environmental temperatures may result in significant haemolysis which can lower the total red cell count, PCV and mean cell volume (MCV), and increase the total plasma protein concentration and mean cell haemoglobin concentration (MCHC). Excessive anticoagulant (e.g. EDTA) in the collection tube caused by the addition of an inadequate volume of blood can decrease the PCV and affect the validity of the MCV and MCHC calculations. Gross lipaemia may increase the haemoglobin concentration.

Total plasma protein concentration

Most laboratories include the total plasma protein (TPP) concentration as part of a routine haematological examination. The TPP concentration should always be interpreted in association with the PCV. A low TPP concentration accompanied by a low PCV is indicative of ongoing or recent haemorrhage (taking into account the age-related changes described above). Severe dehydration may increase both the PCV and TPP concentration and therefore may mask the true degree of anaemia.

Reticulocyte counts

Reticulocytes on a blood film are best demonstrated using a supravital stain such as new methylene blue. On routine Romanowsky-stained films, reticulocytes appear as large (macrocytic) cells with bluish/pink (polychromatophilic) cytoplasm. Small numbers of reticulocytes, usually less than 1%, are present in the blood of healthy dogs and cats. The presence of large numbers of circulating reticulocytes in response to haemorrhage or haemolysis increases the mean cell volume (MCV) and indicates increased erythropoietic activity. Thus regenerative anaemias generally show marked anisocytosis and a variable degree of poikilocytosis. The magnitude of the reticulocyte response generally correlates with the degree of erythropoietic activity. After an acute haemorrhagic or haemolytic episode reticulocytes do not appear in the circulation for up to 48–72 h, reaching maximal production by 7 days. Reticulocytosis may be classified as mild (1–4%), moderate (5–20%) or marked (>20%). An increase in the number of reticulocytes is usually accompanied by a concomitant increase in the numbers of circulating nucleated red blood cells (normoblasts).

Inappropriate red cell response

An inappropriate red cell response is one in which the numbers of normoblasts exceeds the numbers of reticulocytes present. Such a response may be an indicator of damage to the marrow stroma (e.g. myeloproliferative disease or myelodysplasia). A similar type of response may occur in dogs with congestive heart failure, presumably in response to chronic hypoxia, or with lead poisoning.

Reticulocyte correction factors

Prolonged stimulation of the erythroid marrow results in the release of younger, larger 'shift' reticulocytes which have a longer maturation time and circulating half-life. The observed percentage of reticulocytes may therefore overestimate the degree of marrow responsiveness at any one time since it does not take into account variations in circulating red cell numbers and changes in reticulocyte maturation time.

- Absolute reticulocyte count corrects for variation in red cell number i.e. the degree of anaemia

$$\text{Absolute reticulocyte count } (\times 10^9 \text{ l}^{-1}) = \text{observed \% reticulocytes} \times \text{RBC count } (\times 10^{12} \text{ l}^{-1}) \times 10$$

An absolute reticulocyte count >60×10^9 l^{-1} in the dog (>50×10^9 l^{-1} in the cat) is evidence of a responsive anaemia.

- Corrected reticulocyte count also corrects for variation in red cell number

$$\text{Corrected reticulocyte count (\%)} = \frac{\text{observed reticulocyte count (\%)} \times \text{measured PCV (l l}^{-1})}{\text{average PCV for species (0.45 l l}^{-1}\text{ dog; 0.40 l l}^{-1}\text{ cat)}}$$

A corrected reticulocyte count greater than 1% is indicative of active erythropoiesis

- Reticulocyte production index (RPI) applies a further factor to take into account the prolonged maturation time of younger reticulocytes.

$$\text{RPI} = \frac{\text{corrected reticulocyte count (\%)}}{\text{maturation factor}}$$

Maturation factor (days)	PCV (l l^{-1})
1.0	0.45
1.5	0.35
2.0	0.25
2.5	0.15

RPI <1 indicates anaemia is non-regenerative
RPI between 1 and 2 indicates erythropoietically active marrow, e.g blood loss
RPI >2 indicates accelerated erythropoiesis; RPI >3 more consistent with haemolysis

Tests to detect abnormalities in iron metabolism

Different causes of anaemia can lead to abnormalities in the transport, utilization, storage and distribution of iron reserves within the body. These alterations in iron metabolism may therefore be helpful in differentiating between the various causes of anaemia (particularly non-regenerative anaemia).

Serum iron

Iron measured in serum is bound to the transport protein transferrin. Since haemoglobin synthesis takes precedence over the demands for other iron compounds, the haemoglobin pool of iron may be the last pool to show the effects of iron deficiency. For this reason serum iron levels begin to fall only when iron stores are virtually depleted and usually before anaemia develops. Causes of low serum iron levels include chronic haemorrhage (true iron deficiency), portosystemic shunts and anaemia associated with chronic inflammatory or neoplastic disease processes (anaemia of chronic disease). With true iron deficiency the stores of non-haem iron in the liver and bone marrow are depleted; with anaemia of chronic disease the stores of non-haem iron are typically increased. The concentration of serum iron, therefore, does not on its own provide an accurate estimate of total body iron reserves.

Increases in serum iron concentration occur with chronic haemolysis and in some cases of aplastic or hypoplastic anaemia. The administration of glucocorticoids can increase serum iron concentration in dogs. Normal values for serum iron in the dog are 101±23 µg dl^{-1} (approx. 18.1±4.1 µmol l^{-1}).

Total iron binding capacity (TIBC)

In normal animals transferrin is only one-third saturated with iron. Transferrin can be assayed by its ability to bind additional iron (unbound iron binding capacity; UIBC) and is measured in terms of iron content of serum after it has been saturated with iron (total iron binding capacity; TIBC). Hence serum iron+UIBC=TIBC. In most species the TIBC usually increases during the early stages of iron depletion and precedes the fall in serum iron. In dogs the normal TIBC is 334±26 µg dl^{-1} (approx. 59.8±4.7 µmol l^{-1}) (Smith, 1989) and the TIBC does not change significantly with true iron deficiency. Anaemia of chronic disease is associated with low or low normal TIBC.

Percentage saturation of transferrin

The percentage saturation of transferrin is the ratio of serum iron to TIBC (serum iron/TIBC) and may provide a more accurate indicator of an animal's iron status than either serum iron or TIBC alone. Alterations in the ratio are summarized in Table 14.1.

Serum ferritin

Serum ferritin assays have been developed and validated for use in the dog although they are not yet routinely available (Weeks et al., 1989; Andrews et al., 1992). The concentration of ferritin correlates well with the concentration of non-haem iron in the liver and spleen and provides a reliable means of estimating iron stores in dogs (Weeks et al., 1989). Ferritin concentrations have been reported in normal dogs using an ELISA assay (Weeks et al., 1989). Serum ferritin concentrations in 61 normal healthy dogs, determined by using a double monoclonal antibody assay, ranged from 80 to 800 ng ml^{-1} (conventional units) with a mean of 252 ng ml^{-1} (Andrews et al., 1992). Ferritin is an acute phase protein and

Table 14.1 Interpretation of serum iron, total iron binding capacity, percentage saturation of transferrin and ferritin assays in the dog

Parameter	Chronic haemorrhage	Anaemia of chronic disease	Chronic haemolysis
Serum iron	Decreased	Decreased	Increased
Total iron binding capacity	Usually no significant change	Decreased or low normal	Decreased?
% Transferrin saturation	Decreased	Decreased	Increased
Ferritin	Decreased	Increased	Increased

any increase should be measured relative to the concentration of other acute phase proteins such as ceruloplasmin or haptoglobin.

Bone marrow iron stores

Bone marrow iron (haemosiderin) stores can be stained with Prussian blue and provide a reasonable estimate of storage iron.

A semi-quantitative assessment of bone marrow iron can be helpful in differentiating true iron deficiency anaemia from the anaemia of chronic disease in which there is impaired release of iron from bone marrow reticuloendothelial stores.

LABORATORY CLASSIFICATION OF ANAEMIA

Anaemia may be classified morphologically on the basis of the red cell indices, i.e. mean corpuscular volume (MCV), mean corpuscular haemo-

Table 14.2 Classification of anaemia based on red cell morphology

Morphological classification	Possible aetiology
Macrocytic, hypochromic (increased MCV, decreased MCHC)	Haemorrhage or haemolysis, i.e. regenerative anaemias
Normocytic, normochromic (normal MCV, normal MCHC)	Following acute blood loss before erythroid regeneration occurs
	Most non-regenerative anaemias caused by primary or secondary failure of erythropoiesis, i.e. hypoproliferative anaemias
Macrocytic, normochromic (increased MCV, normal MCHC)	Myeloproliferative disease (e.g. erythraemic myelosis); FeLV infection; ?vitamin B_{12}/folate deficiency (nuclear maturation defect anaemia)
Microcytic, hypochromic (decreased MCV, decreased MCHC)	Iron deficiency anaemia due to chronic blood loss (cytoplasmic maturation defect anaemia); portosystemic shunts; anaemia of chronic disease

Table 14.3 Normal haematological parameters in the dog[a]

Parameter	Units	Normal range
Total red blood cells (RBC)	$\times 10^{12}$ l^{-1}	5.5–8.5
Packed cell volume (PCV)	$l\, l^{-1}$	0.37–0.55
Haemoglobin (Hb)	g dl^{-1}	12–18
Mean corpuscular volume (MCV)	fl	60–77
Mean corpuscular haemoglobin (MCH)	pg	19.5–24.5
Mean corpuscular haemoglobin concentration (MCHC)	g dl^{-1}	32–37
Reticulocytes	%	0–1.5
Nucleated RBCS	number/100 WBCS	
Total white blood cell (WBC)	$\times 10^9$ l^{-1}	6–17
Band neutrophils		0–0.3
Neutrophils		3–11.5
Lymphocytes		1–4.8
Monocytes		0.2–1.5
Eosinophils		0.1–1.3
Basophils		0
Platelets	$\times 10^9$ l^{-1}	175–500
Plasma protein	g l^{-1}	55–80

[a] Reference ranges vary with different laboratories. The above values are those of the Department of Clinical Veterinary Medicine (Central Diagnostic Services), University of Cambridge.

globin (MCH) and mean corpuscular haemoglobin concentration (MCHC) as follows:
- Macrocytic and hypochromic
- Normocytic and normochromic
- Macrocytic and normochromic
- Microcytic and hypochromic

Some of the more common causes of each of these types of anaemia are given in Table 14.2. Normal haematological values for the dog and cat are given in Table 14.3.

Alternatively, anaemia can be classified on a pathophysiological and aetiological basis taking into account the degree of bone marrow responsiveness (regenerative or non-regenerative).

The major differentiating features of regenerative and non-regenerative anaemias are summarized in Table 14.4.

REGENERATIVE ANAEMIAS

Regenerative anaemias are caused by either haemorrhage or haemolysis. They are characterized by increased numbers of large immature reticulocytes and nucleated red blood cells (normoblasts) in the circulation. As a result, examination of a blood film shows marked anisocytosis and the anaemia is typically macrocytic and hypochromic. It may be possible to differentiate between haemorrhage and haemolysis by the extent of the regenerative features and total

Table 14.4 Features of regenerative and non-regenerative anaemias

Feature	Regenerative	Non-regenerative
Reticulocytosis i.e. > 5% reticulocytes or evidence of polychromasia	Yes	No
Anisocytosis	Yes	No
Poikilocytosis	Yes	No
Normoblastosis	Yes	Possible in myeloproliferative disease or if damage to marrow stroma
Increased numbers of Howell–Jolly bodies	± (especially cats)	No
Increased numbers of Heinz bodies	± (especially cats)	No
Reactive leukocytosis	Yes	No

Table 14.5 Differentiating features of haemorrhagic and haemolytic anaemias

Haemorrhage	Haemolysis
Normocytic during first 48–72 h then macrocytic (MCV increased)	As for haemorrhage
Normochromic during first 48–72 h then hypochromic (MCHC decreased)	As for haemorrhage
Moderate anisocytosis ± poikilocytosis	Marked anisocytosis ± poikilocytosis (e.g. spherocytes or schistocytes)
Moderate polychromasia and reticulocytosis	Marked polychromasia and reticulocytosis
Decreased plasma proteins	Normal plasma proteins
Thrombocytosis (large shift platelets)	± RBC parasites e.g. *Haemobartonella* sp., *Babesia* sp.
Microcytic/hypochromic if iron stores depleted and progressing to state of true iron deficiency (chronic haemorrhage)	±Increased numbers of Heinz bodies (paracetamol poisoning)

plasma protein concentration (see Table 14.5). Regardless of the cause, most regenerative anaemias are accompanied by a reactive neutrophilia with a variable left shift.

Haemorrhage

Acute haemorrhage

For the first 24 hours after an acute haemorrhagic episode the PCV does not reflect the degree of blood loss. Indeed most if not all the red cell parameters may initially be within normal limits since red cells and plasma are lost in proportions similar to whole blood. In addition, splenic contraction may help offset any fall in PCV. Only when compensatory mechanisms have expanded the blood volume (movement of interstitial fluid into the vascular space) will the typical laboratory signs of anaemia become apparent, the decrease in PCV usually being accompanied by a decrease in total plasma protein concentration. Since there is also a lag phase of 24–48 h in the production and release of reticulocytes into the circulation following blood loss, the anaemia initially appears normocytic, normochromic and non-regenerative. Following a severe acute haemorrhagic episode it may take as long as 2 weeks for the PCV to return to normal. The reticulocyte response is frequently accompanied by a neutrophilic leucocytosis and left shift especially after haemorrhage into a body cavity. Platelet numbers also increase and large granular 'shift' platelets are released into the circulation.

Chronic haemorrhage

Chronic blood loss gradually results in depletion of bone marrow iron stores and ultimately an iron-deficient state. As iron stores become depleted the reticulocyte response diminishes. The anaemia progresses through a normocytic phase as reticulocyte numbers decrease becoming microcytic, hypochromic and non-regenerative once iron stores have been exhausted completely. Thrombocytosis is a relatively consistent feature of chronic haemorrhage, for example, platelet numbers in dogs with bleeding gastrointestinal tumours may exceed $1000 \times 10^9 \, l^{-1}$. The most common causes of acute and chronic haemorrhage are listed in Table 14.6.

Haemolysis

Haemolytic anaemias can be classified on a pathophysiological basis as intrinsic or extrinsic. *Intrinsic haemolytic anaemias* are exceedingly rare

Table 14.6 Causes of acute and chronic haemorrhage

Acute haemorrhage
- Following trauma or surgery
- Bleeding gastrointestinal ulcers or tumours
- Renal/bladder neoplasia
- Rupture of large vascular splenic tumours, e.g. haemangiosarcoma or lymphoma
- Congenital defects in haemostasis, e.g. von Willebrand's disease, haemophilia A
- Acquired defects in haemostasis, e.g. warfarin poisoning, severe liver disease, DIC, immune-mediated thrombocytopenia
- Parasites, e.g. hookworms, *Haemonchus* sp., *Coccidia* sp.

Chronic haemorrhage
- Ongoing blood loss from any of the above causes
- Heavy lice and flea infestations; hookworms

and are associated with an inherent metabolic defect in the red cell, e.g. red cell pyruvate kinase deficiency in Basenjis and red cell phosphofructokinase deficiency of springer spaniels. *Extrinsic haemolytic anaemias* involve external factors that render the red cell or red cell membrane abnormal, e.g. drugs or red cell parasites, or antibodies directed against the red cell membrane, the net result being a reduction in red cell lifespan. Red cells are destroyed extravascularly in the liver, spleen or bone marrow, or intravascularly (or by a combination of both mechanisms).

Autoagglutination of red cells or a positive direct Coombs' test are indicative of immune-mediated haemolysis. The major causes of extrinsic haemolytic anaemia are summarized in Table 14.7. The pathophysiology, diagnosis and management of immune-mediated haemolytic anaemia and other causes of haemolysis are discussed at length in Chapter 45.

Fragmentation or micro-angiopathic haemolytic anaemias are characterized by the presence of schistocytes (fragmented erythrocytes). Red cells are cleaved and fragmented as they pass through a meshwork of fibrin in the microvasculature (e.g. disseminated intravascular coagulation) or the abnormal vasculature channels comprising large parenchymatous neoplasms such as splenic haemangiosarcoma.

NON-REGENERATIVE ANAEMIAS

A non-regenerative anaemia is defined as an anaemia of greater than five days duration with an

Table 14.7 Causes of extrinsic haemolytic anaemia

Immune-mediated
- Intravascular haemolysis; often via activation of complement attached to IgM antibody
- Extravascular haemolysis; frequently IgG antibodies directed against red cell membrane ± complement (C3) activation

Primary
- Idiopathic autoimmune haemolytic anaemia

Secondary
- Associated with myeloproliferative or lymphoproliferative disease red cell parasites
- Red cell parasites, e.g. *Haemobartonella* sp., *Babesia* sp.
- Drug-induced
- Neonatal isoerythrolysis

Oxidant damage to red cells
- Paracetamol toxicity resulting in Heinz body haemolytic anaemia

Infectious agents
- Leptospirosis (*Leptospira icterohaemorrhagiae*)

Poisonous plants
- Onion toxicity (dogs)

Miscellaneous
- Lead poisoning (dogs)

---

inappropriately low reticulocyte count. Non-regenerative anaemias can be classified as either hypoproliferative anaemias or maturation defect anaemias.

HYPOPROLIFERATIVE ANAEMIAS

Most non-responsive anaemias in small animals are normocytic, normochromic hypoproliferative anaemias and are insidious in onset. Failure of erythropoiesis may be the result of a primary bone marrow disorder or more commonly it is a secondary manifestation of some other disease process (Table 14.8).

Primary failure of erythropoiesis

Hypoproliferative anaemias due to primary failure of erythropoiesis occasionally are the result of a selective depletion of erythroid precursors only. More commonly, however, the anaemia is accompanied by a concurrent cytopenia (neutropenia or thrombocytopenia) or in some cases a deficiency of all marrow-derived blood cells in the circulation (true pancytopenia). Such anaemias are generally severe (PCV <0.10–0.15 l l^{-1}) although clinical signs relating to the anaemia may only be noted by the owner at a late stage in the progression of the disease. Serum iron concentrations may be increased and a bone marrow aspirate and/or trephine biopsy is usually necessary in order to obtain a definitive diagnosis (see Chapter 45 for a discussion of specific causes).

Secondary failure of erythropoiesis

The anaemia which occurs in association with numerous inflammatory, metabolic and neoplastic disorders is caused by a mild, selective depletion of erythroid precursors (Table 14.7). The *anaemia of inflammatory disease* is usually mild to moderate in severity (PCV often 0.20–0.35 l l^{-1}) and may be accompanied by an inflammatory blood picture (e.g. neutrophilic leucocytosis). Increased numbers of leptocytes (target cells) may be present. The pathogenesis involves a defect in iron metabolism which results in the relative unavailability of iron for red cell precursors. Serum iron concentration may be normal or decreased although bone marrow examination frequently shows abundant haemosiderin deposits in marrow macrophages. Thus, evaluation of a bone marrow aspirate for iron may help differentiate the anaemia associated with inflammatory disease from that associated with true iron deficiency; although both are associated with low serum iron concentrations, marrow iron

Table 14.8 Causes of non-regenerative anaemia

Primary causes	Secondary causes
• Pure red cell aplasia/erythroid hypoplasia, i.e. *selective* depletion of red cell precursors in the bone marrow. • Aplastic anaemia, i.e. *generalized* bone marrow suppression reflected in blood as a pancytopenia. Pancytopenia may also be caused by diffuse infiltration of the bone marrow with neoplastic cells (myelophthisis) resulting in suppression of normal haemopoiesis. • Myeloproliferative disease (MPD), e.g. acute myelogenous or chronic granulocytic leukaemia. • Lymphoproliferative disease, e.g. multicentric lymphoma (with bone marrow involvement), acute lymphoblastic or chronic lymphocytic leukaemia and plasma cell myeloma. • Myelofibrosis (infiltration of bone marrow with fibrous tissue) • Myelodysplasia (preleukaemia or atypical MPD); in the cat myelodysplasia is often associated with FeLV infection	• Chronic inflammatory disease or neoplasia (anaemia of chronic disease) • Renal disease • Chronic liver disease • Endocrine disorders, e.g. hypoadrenocorticism (Addison's disease), hypothyroidism

(haemosiderin) stores will be severely depleted or even absent with the latter. The anaemia associated with inflammatory and neoplastic conditions is often referred to collectively as the *anaemia of chronic disease* and is the single most common cause of anaemia in small animals. Other mechanisms of anaemia associated with malignancy include haemorrhage, myelophthisis, disseminated intravascular coagulation and haemolysis.

Maturation defect anaemias

Maturation defect anaemias are relatively rare. In contrast to hypoproliferative anaemias the bone marrow is usually hypercellular with increased numbers of red cell precursors. However, because either nuclear or cytoplasmic maturation is abnormal, erythropoiesis is ineffective and the red cells are not readily released into the circulation. Examples of *cytoplasmic maturation defect anaemias* include (1) the microcytic, hypochromic anaemia associated with iron deficiency (chronic blood loss) and lead poisoning. With *nuclear maturation defect anaemias* the production of large megaloblastic red cell precursors in the bone marrow is reflected by the appearance of macrocytic, normochromic erythrocytes in the peripheral blood. Megaloblastic anaemia may occur in cats in association with FeLV infection; in dogs megaloblastosis has been associated with prolonged therapy with anticonvulsive agents (phenytoin, phenobarbitol and primidone) and folate antagonists (methotrexate and trimethoprim), and a folate-responsive macrocytic anaemia occasionally is associated with small intestinal malabsorption, neoplasia, liver disease and prolonged anorexia.

THERAPY OF ABNORMAL ERYTHROPOIESIS

The prime aim of treating any anaemic patient is to identify and treat any underlying disorder that may be present. The treatment of hypoproliferative anaemias due to primary bone marrow disorders is to a large extent supportive and consists of whole blood transfusion or transfusion of packed red cells and anabolic steroids, although some of the myeloproliferative disorders require more specific therapy. Where an immune-mediated pathogenesis is suspected, immunosuppressive agents are indicated. Iron supplementation is indicated only for cases of confirmed iron deficiency (more specific details are given in Chapter 45).

CARDIOVASCULAR CAUSES OF PALLOR

Pallor of the mucous membranes may be associated with poor peripheral perfusion and/or a marked reduction in cardiac output. Since cardiac output is a function of stroke volume and heart rate, disorders that decrease stroke volume or cause a marked decrease in heart rate may lead to a clinically significant reduction in cardiac output. Causes of decreased stroke volume include myocardial failure (decreased myocardial contractility), pericardial effusion, peripheral vasodilation (e.g. overzealous administration of vasodilating agents) and shock (e.g. hypovolaemic shock associated with acute haemorrhage or hypoadrenocorticism). Severe disturbances in cardiac rhythm such as atrial fibrillation or ventricular tachycardia may also result in a marked decrease in cardiac output.

Investigation of cardiovascular causes of pallor

Where poor peripheral perfusion is the result of primary myocardial failure (dilated cardiomyopathy) or a severe tachydysrhythmia animals may be expected to show signs attributable to low output ('forward') cardiac failure and congestive ('backward') cardiac failure. Signs of low output failure associated with myocardial failure include exercise intolerance, syncope, tachycardia and a weak, rapid arterial pulse. A cardiac murmur is frequently present. Anaemic or hypovolaemic animals may exhibit similar clinical signs, however such animals usually have no preceding history or signs of 'backward' failure such as a cough, pulmonary oedema or pleural effusion. Dogs with pericardial effusion frequently have a history of a rapid onset of ascites and laboured respiration. Heart sounds may be muffled on auscultation. Having established, on the basis of routine haematology, that the animal is not anaemic, thoracic and abdominal radiography, electrocardiography and, if available, echocardiography should be performed to ascertain the nature and severity of cardiac dysfunction. The plasma concentrations of sodium and potassium should be determined and if necessary an ACTH response test performed to rule out hypoadrenocorticism (Addison's disease).

The management of myocardial failure, pericardial effusion, hypoadrenocorticism and shock is dealt with in Chapters 34 and 39.

REFERENCES

Andrews, G.A., et al. (1992) An improved canine ferritin assay for canine sera. *Veterinary Clinical Pathology* 21, 57–60.

Smith, J.E. (1989) Iron metabolism and its diseases. In: *Clinical Biochemistry of Domestic Animals 4th Edition* (Ed. J.J. Kaneko) Academic Press, San Diego pp. 256–273.

Weeks, B.R., et al. (1989) Relationship of serum ferritin and iron concentrations and serum total iron-binding capacity to non-heme iron stores in dogs *American Journal of Veterinary Research* 50, 198–200.

15

Cyanosis

J. K. Dunn

Cyanosis refers to the bluish discoloration of the skin and mucous membranes caused by excessive levels of reduced (deoxygenated) haemoglobin in the blood. Cyanosis therefore implies that an animal is hypoxaemic, i.e. has a reduced partial pressure of oxygen in arterial blood (PaO_2) and that, as a result, less oxygen is available for the body tissues (hypoxia). Conversely, the absence of visible cyanosis does not mean that a degree of cellular hypoxia is not present since cyanosis only becomes apparent when the mean capillary concentration of reduced haemoglobin exceeds 5%. Furthermore, cyanosis may be masked in severely anaemic patients since, although the proportion of reduced haemoglobin relative to the total haemoglobin concentration may be quite large, the *absolute* amount of reduced haemoglobin will be small and insufficient to cause cyanosis. For the same reason, cyanosis may be more apparent in animals with severe polycythaemia. Despite having higher than normal arterial oxygen saturation, localized passive venous congestion in these cases results in increased levels of reduced haemoglobin in the vessels supplying a given area.

Pathophysiological mechanisms for cyanosis

- Arterial hypoxaemia. Normal arterial oxygen saturation (95–97%) is maintained at sea level by a PaO_2 of 85–100 mmHg; a decrease in arterial PaO_2 leads to decreased PO_2 in capillary blood.
- Increased extraction of oxygen from capillary blood.
- Increased concentration of poorly oxygenated blood in cutaneous vessels due to passive venous congestion (see Chapter 16 on hyperaemia and congestion).
- Increase in the concentration of circulating abnormal haemoglobin pigments, e.g. methaemoglobin or sulphhaemoglobin.

CENTRAL CYANOSIS

Central cyanosis involving the skin and mucous membranes is caused by arterial hypoxaemia or less frequently by circulating abnormal haemoglobin pigments. For cyanosis to become clinically apparent PaO_2 must be less than 50% which corresponds to an arterial oxygen saturation of approximately 80%.

Arterial hypoxaemia

There are a number of causes of arterial hypoxaemia including the following.

The oxygen concentration in inspired air may be reduced, for example at high altitudes or due to anaesthetic error.

Alveolar hypoventilation is always associated with an increase in PaO_2 which results in respiratory acidosis if severe. Possible causes of hypoventilation include drug-induced central nervous system depression (barbiturates, morphine, muscle relaxants), damage to the respiratory control centre in the brainstem (trauma, haemorrhage, inflammation) or severe trauma to the cervical spinal cord, trauma to the chest wall, neuromuscular disease (e.g. myasthenia gravis) resulting in paralysis of the respiratory muscles, severe upper airway obstruction (laryngeal oedema or paralysis, tracheal collapse, tracheal foreign body) or bronchoconstriction (feline allergic bronchitis).

The impaired diffusion of oxygen between alveoli and haemoglobin in capillary blood is probably a less important cause of cyanosis because the diffusion reserves of normal lung tissue are enormous. Under resting conditions the PO_2 of capillary blood equilibrates with PO_2 of the alveolar gas very rapidly. This occurs when the red cell is only about one third of its way along the capillary and any difference between alveolar gas and end-capillary blood PO_2 is unmeasurably small. A large part of this diffusion reserve is utilized during strenuous exercise when increased pulmonary blood flow reduces the time for oxygen transfer. However, $P\text{a}O_2$ usually only falls under such circumstances if additional factors come into play, e.g. at high altitudes where the PO_2 of the inspired air is lower or if the alveolar–capillary membrane is thickened by a disease process, for example alveolar destruction, severe pulmonary fibrosis, or inflammatory or neoplastic pulmonary infiltrates. With diffusion impairment $P\text{a}O_2$ is usually not increased and may be decreased if the hypoxaemic state stimulates hyperventilation.

Ventilation–perfusion mismatch or inequality occurs when a poorly ventilated area of lung is perfused. The result is inefficient gas exchange and arterial hypoxaemia. This common cause of hypoxaemia occurs with most severe pulmonary parenchymal diseases involving the interstitial tissue and/or alveoli, e.g. pulmonary oedema, bronchopneumonia, aspiration pneumonia, pulmonary thromboembolism, atelectasis, pulmonary contusion and shock lung (adult respiratory distress syndrome).

Right to left cardiovascular shunts occur in some congenital cardiac defects in which non-oxygenated venous blood from the right heart mixes with oxygenated blood returning to the left side of the heart without entering the pulmonary circulation. Examples include tetralogy of Fallot, Eisenmenger's syndrome and reverse shunting ventricular septal defects (VSD). A dog with a reverse shunting patent ductus arteriosus (PDA) may show differential cyanosis of the posterior extremities only because the shunted non-oxygenated blood enters the aorta after the bifurcation of the subclavian vessels. Other congenital heart disorders which result in cyanosis are associated with a degree of pulmonary artery outflow obstruction (pulmonary stenosis) or pulmonary hypertension, or both. The cyanosis is invariably exacerbated by exercise or excitement. Cyanosis due to a right to left cardiac shunt may be differentiated from that associated with severe primary lung disease by administering 100% oxygen; the cyanosis due to cardiac shunts is usually unaffected whereas cyanosis due to lung disease may be expected to decrease.

Intrapulmonary arteriovenous shunts or fistulae develop with severe lobar consolidation where a lung lobe is still perfused but underventilated (see ventilation–perfusion mismatch above).

Circulating abnormal haemoglobin pigments

Central cyanosis may be associated with circulating abnormal pigments. Congenital haemoglobinopathies are extremely rare in small animals. One case of exercise intolerance associated with an abnormal haemoglobin has been reported in a dog (Jones et al., 1978) and congenital methaemoglobinaemia has been reported in dogs with a hereditary deficiency of the enzyme methaemoglobin reductase (Harvey et al., 1991). Methaemoglobin is produced when haem iron is oxidized to the ferric state and is unable to bind to oxygen. Acquired methaemoglobinaemia occurs if haemoglobin is exposed to oxidant chemicals such as paracetamol, nitrates, nitrites, benzocaine, phenacetin, anilidine dyes, phenazopyridine and certain sulphonamides (sulphanilamide, sulphathiazole and sulphapyridine). Cats are especially sensitive to the effects of oxidant chemicals since they are deficient in the enzyme glucuronyl transferase and are unable to conjugate these drugs with glucuronic acid in the liver. Both phenacetin and acetanilid can cause methaemoglobinaemia and sulphhaemoglobinaemia in cats, and in the dog onion toxicity can produce methaemoglobinaemia.

PERIPHERAL CYANOSIS

Peripheral cyanosis is the result of a circulatory disturbance in peripheral vascular beds; cyanosis is therefore restricted to the extremities. Although the $P\text{a}O_2$ is usually normal, the PO_2 at the venous end of the capillary bed is reduced.

Causes of peripheral cyanosis include:

- Peripheral vasoconstriction in response to cold or as a compensatory mechanism in congestive heart failure;
- Hypovolaemic shock;
- Localized arterial obstruction by thromboemboli, e.g. feline cardiomyopathy, bacterial endocarditis and other hypercoagulable states such as glomerulonephropathy, hyperadrenocorticism, dirofilariasis and cold agglutinin disease.
- Localized venous obstruction (e.g. due to thrombophlebitis) or venous stasis where sluggish capillary blood flow results in increased oxygen extraction (e.g. polcythaemia or acute myocardial failure resulting in cardiogenic shock).

Cinical signs associated with cyanosis

The clinical signs which accompany cyanosis reflect the underlying cause for the cyanosis. In most cases cyanosis is associated with severe respiratory distress which may be due to acute upper airway obstruction, decompensated congestive heart failure or severe pulmonary disease (see other sections of this book for a more detailed description of the clinical signs associated with each of these conditions).

INVESTIGATION OF CYANOSIS

HISTORY CHECKLIST

❏ Age?
If the animal is young, cyanosis is probably the result of a congenital cardiac defect associated with a right to left cardiovascular shunt. In older animals congestive heart failure or severe pulmonary disease are more likely causes of cyanosis.

❏ Breed?
Tracheal collapse, congestive heart failure due to mitral insufficiency and chronic bronchitis are conditions which have a higher incidence in small or toy breeds.

❏ Trauma?
Severe damage to chest wall and/or pulmonary parenchyma resulting in pulmonary contusion or severe pneumothorax.

❏ Drug administration?
For example paracetamol or other oxidant drugs.

❏ Syncope or abnormal gait?
True syncopal episodes are suggestive of heart disease or acute respiratory obstruction. Episodic weakness associated with collapse can be caused by generalized neuromuscular problems such as myasthenia gravis.

PHYSICAL EXAMINATION

❏ Severe respiratory distress?
Inspiratory stridor is indicative of upper airway obstructive disease whereas expiratory dyspnoea is more suggestive of lower airway disease (see causes of arterial hypoxaemia).

❏ Pale mucous membranes?
Pale mucous membranes may indicate poor peripheral perfusion (e.g. due to myocardial failure) or anaemia (e.g. Heinz body haemolytic anaemia due to paracetamol poisoning).

❏ Cardiac murmur?
Cardiac murmurs may be caused by primary heart disease or severe anaemia. A murmur may not be audible with a reverse (right to left) shunting patent ductus arteriosus or ventricular septal defect.

❏ Hindlimb paralysis (unilateral or bilateral)?
Cats with cardiomyopathy are susceptible to thromboembolic disease. Formation of a 'saddle' thrombus at the bifurcation of the two iliac arteries results in severe hindlimb weakness and the pads of the affected limbs become cyanotic, pale and cold.

❏ Adventitial lung sounds such as crackles or wheezes?
See pulmonary causes of arterial hypoxaemia.

INITIAL DIAGNOSTIC PLAN

A minimum database should include the following.

Haematology

Methaemoglobinaemia?

Check a drop of blood on filter paper (methaemoglobin stains filter paper brown). Oxygen bubbled into a test tube containing blood from a patient with suspected methaemoglobinaemia will not produce oxyhaemoglobin and its associated red colour.

Polcythaemia?

Right to left cardiovascular shunts result in chronic hypoxia and increased erythropoietin secretion by kidneys.

Increased numbers of Heinz bodies and anaemic

The presence of increased numbers of circulating Heinz bodies is highly suggestive of paracetamol poisoning. Note that normal healthy cats can have up to 10% Heinz bodies.

Thoracic radiography

- Abnormal cardiac size/shape, e.g. cardiomegaly (left-sided, right-sided or generalized)?
- Evidence of pulmonary overcirculation or oedema?
- Changes involving pulmonary parenchyma?
- Evidence of a tracheal foreign body?

Bronchoscopy

Bronchoscopy is indicated if signs of upper airway obstruction are present to evaluate the upper airways and if necessary remove a tracheal foreign body.

Electrocardiography

Most congenital heart disorders resulting in cyanosis are associated either with right to left shunts or a degree of pulmonary outflow obstruction and/or pulmonary hypertension which results in changes on an ECG consistent with right ventricular enlargement, e.g. deep S waves in leads I, II and III, or deep Q waves in leads I, II, III and aVF. Severe chronic pulmonary disease can also result in secondary pulmonary hypertension and right ventricular hypertrophy (cor pulmonale).

Echocardiography

Echocardiography is indicated to establish the nature of the congenital cardiac defect and to provide an assessment of myocardial contractility. A 'bubble' study or Doppler echocardiography can be used to confirm the presence of a right to left shunt.

Arterial blood gas analysis

- Normal or decreased PaO_2?
- Normal or increased $PaCO_2$?

Angiocardiography

A non-selective angiogram performed via a cephalic or jugular vein injection may help confirm the presence of a right to left shunt if echocardiography is not available or the results are inconclusive.

THERAPY

Initial treatment of cyanosis is symptomatic with the main aim being to improve short-term survival. Symptomatic treatment may include relieving the upper airway obstruction (tracheostomy if necessary), administration of oxygen via an intranasal tube or face mask, and the use of bronchodilators. Specific treatment should be directed at the underlying cause; for example, diuretics, positive inotropic drugs, vasodilators and possibly anti-arrhythmic agents may be used to treat congestive heart failure due to dilated cardiomyopathy.

Paracetamol poisoning requires prompt and specific treatment in the form of *acetylcysteine* (140 mg kg^{-1} body weight orally or intravenously as a 5% solution, then 70 mg kg^{-1} body weight every 4 hours for three to five treatments). Other drugs have proved useful in the treatment of methaemoglobinaemia namely:

- *Sodium sulphate:* 50 mg kg^{-1} body weight given as a 1.6% solution every 4 hours for a total of six treatments.
- *Methylene blue:* 1–2 mg kg^{-1} body weight given as a 1% solution intravenously over a 5 min period and repeated as necessary or orally at a dose of 100–300 mg kg^{-1} body weight daily. In toxic doses methylene blue may induce Heinz body formation and intravascular haemolysis.
- *Cimetidine:* initially 10 mg kg^{-1} body weight orally then 5 mg kg^{-1} body weight every 6 h for 48 h.
- *Ascorbic acid:* 30 mg kg^{-1} body weight orally every 6 h for seven treatments.

REFERENCES

Harvey, J.W., *et al.* (1991). Methaemoglobin reductase deficiency in dogs. *Comparative Haematology International* **1**, 55–59.

Jones, D.R.E., *et al.* (1978). Reduced exercise tolerance in a dog associated with abnormal haemoglobin. *Veterinary Record* **102**, 105.

16

Hyperaemia and Congestion

J. K. Dunn

The terms hyperaemia and congestion refer to an increased volume of blood in an affected tissue. In the context of a physical examination hyperaemia or congestion causes the affected tissues (mucous membranes, skin or sclerae) to appear redder than normal.

Active hyperaemia occurs when arterial or arteriolar dilation produces an increased flow of blood through capillary beds. Hyperaemia may be localized and involve the opening of capillaries which are normally inactive. The redness which occurs as a component of the acute inflammatory response is the result of sympathetic stimulation and/or vasoactive substances which are released locally. More generalized hyperaemia and flushing of the skin and mucosae occurs when body heat must be dissipated for example in febrile states or strenuous exercise, or it may reflect a systemic disorder such as *polycythaemia* (see Chapter 45). The accompanying clinical signs reflect the underlying cause. A febrile animal, almost certainly will show non-specific signs of lethargy, depression, anorexia and possibly also weight loss if the pyrexia is sustained for a few days. In addition the animal may shiver in an attempt to conserve heat and raise the core body temperature to the new, raised thermoregulatory set-point, or may pant in order to dissipate excess body heat as the fever subsides.

Dogs with absolute polycythaemia (primary or secondary) have an increased red cell mass and as a result there is sludging of red cells in the small capillaries. The hyperaemia which develops is therefore active but also has an inactive component (see congestion below). A rare cause of generalized hyperaemia is phaeochromocytoma, a catecholamine-secreting tumour of the adrenal medulla, which has been reported to cause intermittent blanching and flushing of the skin.

The term *injected* is sometimes used to refer to the congested scleral blood vessels which occur with episcleritis, glaucoma, keratoconjunctivitis and anterior uveitis.

Passive hyperaemia or *congestion* occurs as a result of obstruction of blood flow from a given area, i.e. impaired venous drainage. Congestion imparts a bluish-red discoloration to the affected area, the bluish tinge being due to an increase in deoxygenated haemoglobin in the blood (cyanosis). The most common cause of systemic congestion is heart failure (congestive heart failure) which results in damming back of blood through the left or right side of the heart (or both) into the venous capacitance vessels. Congestion may occasionally be localized, for example if the return of venous blood from an extremity is obstructed by a large neoplastic mass. The increased hydrostatic pressure which develops in the affected area of tissue with both localized and systemic congestion contributes to the development of oedema, hence congestion and oedema often exist together. For example, left-sided congestive heart failure leads to pulmonary congestion and oedema; right-sided congestive heart failure is associated with passive venous congestion of the liver, ascites, oedema of the extremities and pleural and pericardial effusion.

INVESTIGATION OF HYPERAEMIA AND CONGESTION

Localized hyperaemia of the skin (erythema) associated with inflammation is usually accompanied by other changes which characterize the acute inflammatory response such as heat, pain and soft tissue swelling. Investigation of localized congestion and oedema may involve biopsying the affected area or the space-occupying lesion responsible for obstructing venous and lymphatic drainage.

If the problem appears generalized, an initial diagnostic plan should include a full routine haematological examination (to rule out polycythaemia), thoracic and abdominal radiographs and, if possible, arterial blood gas measurements.

Management of disorders causing localized or generalized hyperaemia should be directed at treating the underlying cause.

POLYCYTHAEMIA

Polycythaemia is defined as an increase in haemoglobin concentration, total red cell count and packed cell volume (PCV). Polycythaemia can be classified as relative or absolute.

Relative polycythaemia

Relative polycythaemia is characterized by an increase in PCV and total plasma protein concentration. The total red cell mass is normal. Relative polycythaemia is usually caused by a disturbance in body fluid balance, for example, decreased plasma volume due to severe dehydration.

Absolute polycythaemia

With absolute polycythaemia the total red cell mass and PCV are increased but the total plasma protein concentration is normal. Absolute polycythaemia may be primary or secondary. Plasma volume is usually normal or, in some cases of primary absolute polycythaemia, it may be slightly decreased.

Primary absolute polycythaemia, also known as polycythaemia vera or primary proliferative polycythaemia, is regarded as a chronic myeloproliferative disorder (see Chapter 45). The total red cell count, haemoglobin concentration and PCV are usually markedly increased (PCV often in the range 0.65–$0.80\, l\, l^{-1}$). Serum erythropoietin levels are low or non-detectable.

Secondary absolute polycythaemia is associated with increased erythropoietin secretion. The polycythaemia which develops with certain congenital cardiac disorders (resulting in the right to left shunting of blood), chronic pulmonary disease and high altitude acclimatization represents an appropriate response to chronic hypoxia (low arterial oxygen saturation). In some cases of secondary polycythaemia the erythropoietin response occurs in the absence of tissue hypoxia, i.e. there is an inappropriate erythropoietin response. This is seen most commonly with renal tumours.

Clinical manifestations of absolute polycythaemia

Clinical signs of absolute polycythaemia relate to the increased red cell mass and resultant hyperviscosity, and include lethargy, weight loss, exercise intolerance, polydipsia and polyuria. The mucosae appear intensely congested and on ophthalmoscopic examination the retinal vessels appear distended and tortuous. Affected animals may also show a variety of central nervous system signs, most frequently hind limb ataxia or collapse, and have a tendency towards haemorrhagic diatheses.

Initial diagnostic plan

Relative polycythaemia, for example due to severe dehydration, can be confirmed and treated with little difficulty, depending of course on the underlying cause. The differentiation of primary and secondary absolute polycythaemia is difficult in the dog and cat; unlike humans, primary polycythaemia is rarely associated with concurrent leucocytosis, thrombocytosis and splenomegaly. The initial investigations should therefore be directed towards ruling out possible causes of secondary polycythaemia.

Arterial blood oxygen saturation

Arterial blood oxygen saturation is usually within normal limits (greater than 90%; PaO_2 greater than 60 mmHg) in dogs with primary polycythaemia and cases where polycythaemia is secondary and associated with an inappropriate release of erythropoietin.

Determination of serum or urinary erythropoietin concentration

As mentioned above, primary polycythaemia is associated with low or undetectable erythopoietin concentrations whereas with secondary polycythaemia, erythropoietin levels are usually increased (although there is an area of overlap which means that in some cases it is difficult to differentiate between the primary and secondary forms of the disease). The concentration of serum erythropoietin should be measured *before* phlebotomy.

Radiography

Plain radiographs of the thorax should be taken to rule out primary cardiac or respiratory disease. Radiographs of the abdomen and, if necessary, intravenous urography should be performed to rule out renal neoplasia as a cause of secondary polycythaemia. Renal angiography is occasionally indicated to detect abnormalities in renal vasculature.

Bone marrow aspiration and core biopsy

Bone marrow aspiration and biopsy is rarely helpful in confirming a diagnosis of primary polycythaemia. The ratio of myeloid cells to erythroid cells may be decreased or normal. Erythroid hyperplasia is a consistent finding but the maturation and distribution of erythroid cells is often normal. Megakaryocyte numbers may be increased. Stores of haemosiderin in cases of primary polycythaemia may be reduced. Progression to myelofibrosis or acute myeloid leukaemia has not been documented in the dog.

Total red cell mass and plasma volume

Direct measurement of the total red cell mass can be performed using radioactive chromium (^{51}Cr)-labelled red cells and plasma volume can be determined using radioactive iodine (^{125}I)-labelled serum albumen to differentiate relative from absolute polycythaemia.

Management of polycythaemia

Relative polycythaemia due to dehydration is treated by the administration of intravenous fluids. The management of primary and secondary absolute polycythaemia may require repeated phlebotomy or chemotherapy and is discussed more fully in Chapter 45.

17

Jaundice

J. K. Dunn

The terms jaundice and icterus describe the yellow discoloration of the skin, sclerae and mucous membranes caused by excessive levels of bilirubin in the circulation (hyperbilirubinaemia) and tissues. Hyperbilirubinaemia indicates either severe (usually acute) haemolysis or hepatobiliary disease.

PATHOPHYSIOLOGY OF HYPERBILIRUBINAEMIA

Between 70 and 80% of the total plasma concentration of bilirubin is derived from haemoglobin released from senescent red blood cells phagocytosed by macrophages in the liver and spleen. A smaller proportion is derived from haem-containing enzymes in the liver (cytochromes, catalase, peroxidase), myoglobin and the destruction of immature red cells in the bone marrow. Haemoglobin is broken down into its haem and globin components. Haem is metabolized to free iron and stored as ferritin or haemosiderin primarily in the reticuloendothelial cells of the liver and bone marrow. Like the protein (globin) component of the haemoglobin molecule iron is re-used to produce more haemoglobin. Bilirubin is the only major breakdown product from haemoglobin which requires excretion. The protoporphyrin ring of the haemoglobin molecule is opened by the enzyme haem oxygenase and is converted into biliverdin which in turn is reduced to bilirubin in the liver under the action of another enzyme biliverdin reductase.

Unconjugated (free or indirect) bilirubin is insoluble in water and is bound to albumin for transport to the liver. The albumin–bilirubin complex is too large to diffuse out of the vascular space so that unbound bilirubin passes across cell membranes to enter tissues only if the binding capacity is exceeded. The following factors are known to decrease the amount of bilirubin which binds to albumin:

- Decrease in plasma albumin concentration;
- Decreased number or availability of binding sites on the albumin molecule, e.g. drugs such as salicylates, thyroxin, digoxin, diazepam and sulphonamides compete for and decrease the number of available binding sites;
- Acidosis (which decreases the affinity of albumin for bilirubin).

Before entering the hepatocyte, bilirubin dissociates from albumin. The movement of bilirubin from plasma to hepatocyte is bidirectional and is thought to involve an active carrier transport mechanism. A small amount of bilirubin entering the hepatocyte remains unconjugated and returns to plasma.

Inside the hepatocyte bilirubin binds Y and Z proteins. These proteins 'trap' the bilirubin which is then conjugated with glucuronic acid to form bilirubin monoglucuronide and diglucuronide under the action of the enzyme glucuronyl transferase. Conjugated or direct bilirubin is water soluble and is therefore excreted in the urine (its lipid insolubility limits back diffusion into hepatocytes and also reabsorption from the intestines so that most is excreted in faeces). Conjugated bilirubin is excreted from the hepatocytes into the bile canaliculi probably via a specific carrier mechanism and then via the bile duct (common bile duct in the dog) into the gut lumen.

Conjugated bilirubin is then deconjugated and reduced to urobilinogen by microflora in the large intestine. Most urobilinogen is oxidized to stercobilin (urobilin) and is excreted in the faeces. Approximately 5–10% is returned via the portal blood (enterohepatic circulation) to the liver where it is removed by hepatocytes and re-excreted into bile although a small amount enters the systemic circulation and is excreted in the urine (see Fig. 17.1).

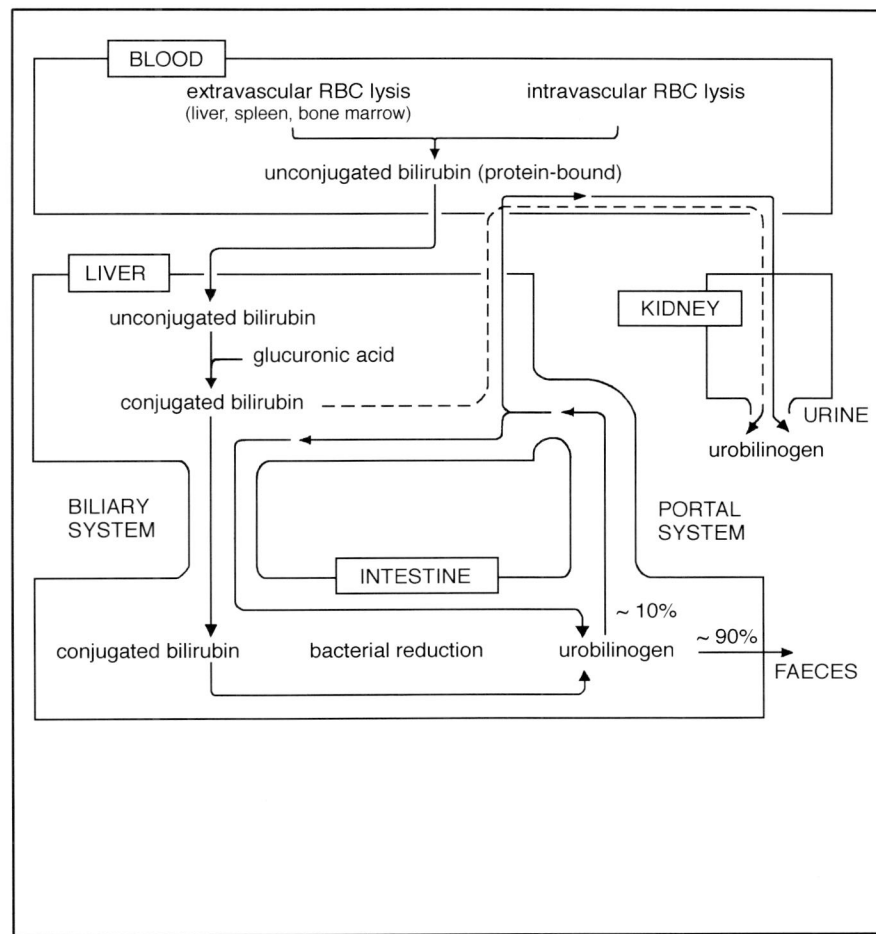

Fig. 17.1 Bilirubin excretion. The broken line indicates the small amount of conjugated bilirubin which is excreted by the kidneys in healthy dogs. In dogs the renal threshold for bilirubin is extremely low and 1+ bilirubinuria is common especially if the urine sample is concentrated (specific gravity >1.035). Bilirubinuria is not a normal finding in the cat. RBC, red blood cells. From Dunn (1992), courtesy of *In Practice*.

■ Hyperbilirubinaemia

Increased plasma concentrations of bilirubin may occur via three mechanisms.

1. *Increased production of bilirubin as a result of increased red blood cell destruction.* Most cases of immune-mediated or autoimmune haemolytic anaemia do *not* present with jaundice. This is because most of the opsonized red cells are destroyed extravascularly in the liver and spleen, and the haemoglobin which is released binds to plasma haptoglobin and is metabolized via normal pathways into its haem and globin components. Jaundice is therefore more likely to occur as a result of an acute intravascular haemolytic episode when a marked increase in red cell destruction not only saturates the plasma haptoglobin system but overwhelms the ability of the liver to take up and conjugate the bilirubin presented to it. Moreover, it is possible that liver function may be slightly impaired during an acute haemolytic episode as a result of hepatocellular hypoxia, and that this may contribute to the decreased capacity of the liver to conjugate and excrete bilirubin. This may partly explain why, at 48–72 hours after an acute haemolytic episode, the concentrations of unconjugated and conjugated bilirubin in the plasma equilibrate. Haemoglobin which is not bound to plasma haptoglobin will be filtered by the glomeruli and imparts a characteristic port wine discoloration to the urine (haemoglobinuria).

2. *Decreased hepatic uptake and conjugation of bilirubin.* Interference to the normal uptake and/or conjugation of bilirubin is often associated with altered excretion of conjugated bilirubin due to intrahepatic cholestasis (see below). Hepatocellular injury primarily damages the sensitive excretory transport mechanism within the hepatocyte whereas the ability of the cell to take up and conjugate bilirubin is preserved. The net result of hepatocellular damage is therefore a build-up of conjugated bilirubin in plasma.

3. *Decreased excretion of conjugated bilirubin in bile due to intrahepatic or posthepatic cholestasis (or both).* Invariably, diffuse hepatocellular damage leads to a degree of intrahepatic cholestasis as the hepatocytes swell and the bile canaliculi may become partially occluded by inflammatory debris. The converse is also true, i.e. intra- or posthepatic cholestasis, regardless of cause, causes a variable degree of hepatocellular damage. Posthepatic cholestasis is caused by partial or complete obstruction of the bile duct, e.g. by a primary bile duct tumour (rare) or tumour of the pancreas.

Common causes of hyperbilirubinaemia and jaundice in the dog and cat are listed in Table 17.1.

INVESTIGATION OF JAUNDICE

The objectives of diagnostic investigations are twofold. The clinician should first attempt to classify the type of jaundice before proceeding with the more specific diagnostic tests required to reach a definitive diagnosis.

The preliminary database

The preliminary database for the jaundiced patient should consist of the following.

- History and clinical findings
- Full haematological examination. A blood film should be screened for the presence of large numbers of Heinz bodies, intracellular red cell parasites (e.g. *Haemobartonella felis*), and checked for evidence of autoagglutination. If haemolysis is suspected and autoagglutination is not evident blood should be submitted for direct antiglobulin (Coombs') and antinuclear antibody tests (see Chapters 14 and 45 for causes of intra- and extravascular haemolysis).
- Complete biochemical screen (to include total/conjugated bilirubin, liver enzymes, amylase and lipase determinations)
- Urinalysis
- Abdominal radiography to subjectively assess the size of the liver and spleen. A check should also be made for any radiographic evidence of pancreatic disease.
- In cats feline leukaemia virus and feline immunodeficiency virus status should be ascertained and a thorough ophthalmoscopic examination should be performed.
- A T_4 assay should be performed in older cats (with or without palpable thyroid masses) since hyperthyroidism can be associated with clinical signs (including occasionally jaundice) and biochemical findings suggestive of liver disease.

Although a complete biochemical screen may be extremely helpful, especially in the acutely ill patient, particular attention should be paid to the plasma concentrations of bilirubin (total/conjugated), tests for hepatocellular damage and cholestasis, and liver function tests. Most tests which detect hepatocellular damage or dysfunction unfortunately lack specificity and fail to provide information regarding the type or distribution of lesion(s) within the liver, i.e. they cannot differentiate diffuse, albeit relatively mild hepatobiliary damage, from a more severe but localized inflammatory or neoplastic lesion.

INTERPRETATION OF LABORATORY TESTS IN THE JAUNDICED ANIMAL

Bilirubin and other bile pigments

Plasma bilirubin

Bilirubin can be assayed colorimetrically using the van den Bergh reaction. The blood sample should be as fresh as possible since direct exposure to sunlight or some fluorescent lighting can reduce the bilirubin content by as much as 50% per hour.

Measurement of total bilirubin concentration (conjugated plus unconjugated bilirubin) in plasma quantitates the degree of jaundice, and the percentage of unconjugated and conjugated fractions is sometimes helpful in differentiating between the different types of jaundice. The total, conjugated and unconjugated bilirubin concentrations should always be interpreted in association with liver enzymes and/or results of liver function tests.

Bilirubinuria

A trace of bilirubin (conjugated form) is common in concentrated urine samples (specific gravity greater than 1.035) from healthy dogs. This is partly due to the much lower renal threshold for bilirubin in this species and also the fact that canine renal tubular epithelial cells contain glucuronyl transferase and are therefore capable of conjugating a small amount of bilirubin. Mild bilirubinuria is occasionally associated with fever

Table 17.1 Common causes of jaundice in dogs and cats

	Dogs	Cats
Haemolytic jaundice	Autoimmune haemolytic anaemia Neonatal isoerythrolysis Incompatible blood transfusion Bacteraemia/septicaemia (± hepatocellular component to the jaundice) Dirofilariasis	Haemobartonellosis Heinz body haemolytic anaemia, e.g. paracetamol poisoning (± hepatocellular component) Autoimmune haemolytic anaemia (may be associated with FeLV infection) Bacteraemia/septicaemia (± hepatocellular component)
Hepatocellular jaundice (in many cases intrahepatic cholestasis contributes significantly to the jaundice)	Hepatic fibrosis/cirrhosis Cholangitis/cholangiohepatitis Chronic active hepatitis Copper toxicosis of Bedlington terriers (also reported in West Highland white terriers and Doberman pinschers) Drug-induced or 'toxic' hepatitis (prolonged anticonvulsant therapy, mebendazole, levamisole, aflatoxins, thiacetarsamide) Hepatic neoplasia (primary or secondary) Infectious canine hepatitis Leptospirosis (*L. icterohaemorrhagiae*)	Ascending cholangiohepatitis Progressive lymphocytic cholangitis Hepatic lipidosis (may be associated with diabetes mellitus) Hyperthyroidism Hepatic neoplasia (especially lymphoma) Feline infectious peritonitis
Obstructive (post-hepatic) jaundice	Neoplasia compressing the bile duct (e.g. pancreatic carcinoma or primary bile duct carcinoma) Acute pancreatitis (with concurrent duodenitis and occlusion of the bile duct) Cholelithiasis Traumatic rupture of the bile duct or gall bladder	Neoplasia compressing the bile duct Cholelithiasis Traumatic rupture of the bile duct or gall bladder

or starvation in dogs. An increased amount of bilirubin in a canine urine sample (e.g. 3+ or 4+ on a stick test) frequently precedes hyperbilirubinaemia and is therefore a reliable indicator of impending jaundice. The presence of bilirubin, even in trace amounts in the urine of a cat, is unusual and usually indicates either hepatocellular damage or cholestasis.

Urine urobilinogen

The amount of urobilinogen present in the urine is extremely variable and is dependent on many factors. Although the presence of urobilinogen infers that the bile duct is at least partially patent, an absence of urobilinogen does not necessarily mean that the bile duct is completely obstructed since many apparently healthy dogs produce urine with no measurable urobilinogen. One explanation for this may be that, like bilirubin, urobilinogen is sensitive to fluorescent lighting so that any delay in testing a sample exposed to such lighting may lead to a false negative result. The amount of urobilinogen excreted in the urine also depends on the amount excreted in the faeces, the activity of the gastrointestinal microflora and intestinal transit time. Severe haemolysis, constipation and gastrointestinal haemorrhage all may increase the amount of urobilinogen present.

Tests for detecting liver damage

Liver damage may be hepatocellular or biliary in origin, and the activities of various liver enzymes in the plasma or serum can be used to assess such injury. It is important to note, however, that liver enzymes which either leak from damaged hepatocytes or are secreted in response to hepatocellular injury provide little or no information about the functional capacity of the liver. For example, in dogs with advanced cirrhosis or young animals with congenital portosystemic shunts there may be very little active hepatocellular damage despite a significant reduction in hepatic function. Not infrequently, therefore, liver enzymes in such animals may fall within normal limits. Haemolysis interferes with many of the liver enzyme assays, in particular alanine aminotransferase and aspartate aminotransferase. For this reason separated plasma or serum should be submitted to a laboratory rather than whole blood.

Hepatocellular injury

Hepatocellular injury results in a change in cell membrane permeability which allows leakage of cytosolic enzymes into the extracellular fluid (plasma). The magnitude of the increase in any particular enzyme generally reflects the number of hepatocytes affected. Invariably, hepatocellular damage regardless of the underlying cause, is usually associated with a degree of intrahepatic cholestasis presumably because swelling of hepatocytes partially occludes the bile canaliculi.

Alanine aminotransferase (ALT)

ALT is found in high concentrations in canine and feline hepatocytes and is considered to be liver specific in these species. Hepatocellular necrosis or degeneration results in altered membrane permeability and increased levels of the enzyme in the circulation. Since the half-life of the enzyme in plasma is relatively short, high levels may be expected only during the phase of acute cell damage; thereafter, circulating levels of the enzyme decline rapidly. The magnitude of the increase in ALT does not distinguish irreversible 'toxic' or neoplastic hepatocellular damage from reversible degenerative changes commonly associated with a number of extrahepatic problems such as severe anaemia, cardiac insufficiency, and certain metabolic and inflammatory disorders. A reduction in the ALT concentration in plasma by approximately 50% over a 24–48 h period generally indicates a more favourable prognosis, whereas persistently high values indicate continued hepatocellular damage. Certain drugs, most notably glucocorticoids and barbiturates, also cause ALT to increase.

Aspartate aminotransferase (AST)

AST is found in the cytoplasm and mitochondria of several cell types (hepatocytes, cardiac and skeletal muscle, and intestinal mucosa) and therefore cannot be regarded as liver specific. As with ALT the serum half-life of AST is extremely short (approximately 5 h in the dog and less than 80 min in the cat). When ALT and AST assays are performed simultaneously, the increase in ALT usually exceeds the increase in AST. Like ALT, changes in cell membrane permeability result in the release of AST from the cytoplasm. Because ALT is released in significant amounts more readily than AST an increase in AST if accompanied by a concomitant increase in ALT and alkaline phosphatase (ALP) is indicative of severe hepatocellular damage. AST may be a more sensitive indicator of hepatobiliary disease in the cat.

Glutamate dehydrogenase (GLDH)

In dogs an increase in the mitochondrial enzyme GLDH is considered to be a reliable indicator of acute hepatic necrosis.

Lactate dehydrogenase (LDH)

Numerous isoenzymes of LDH are widely distributed in animal tissues (liver, skeletal and cardiac muscle, kidney, lung and lymphoreticular tissue). As red cells also contain a significant amount of LDH, a haemolysed blood sample is unsuitable for LDH determination. Total LDH activity is therefore an unreliable and non-specific indicator of liver damage in most species. Because there is considerable species variation in the distribution of the various isoenzymes interpretation of LDH isoenzyme patterns must be undertaken with great care.

Cholestasis

Cholestasis implies an interference with bile flow. The occlusion of bile canaliculi (intrahepatic cholestasis) may be caused by swelling of hepatocytes, hepatic fibrosis or cirrhosis. In the cat, cholestasis may be associated with ascending cholangiohepatitis and progressive lymphocytic cholangitis. The most common cause of extrahepatic cholestasis in older dogs is obstruction of the bile duct by pancreatic adenocarcinoma. Jaundice is a common presenting feature of all these diseases.

Alkaline phosphatase (ALP)

A number of membrane-bound isoenzymes of ALP may be found in several tissues (liver, bone, intestine, kidney, placenta and granulocytes). Most liver ALP is located in the canalicular membranes of the hepatocytes. In response to cholestasis, increased amounts of ALP are synthesized and released into the circulation. The half-life of the hepatic enzyme is approximately 3 days in the dog and 6 h in the cat. The isoenzymes derived from placenta and intestines are rapidly cleared from blood, and renal ALP is excreted directly into urine so these sources are not important causes of increased concentrations of ALP in the plasma. Active osteoblasts secrete ALP and this explains the increased levels seen in young growing animals less than 6–8 months of age. Levels of ALP in this age group rarely exceed the normal range of values by more than two- or threefold. Less commonly, ALP may be increased in other conditions where there is extensive osteolysis and bone remodelling.

Glucocorticoids (either endogenous or exogenous) induce the synthesis and release of a specific isoenzyme which partly explains the marked increase in ALP seen in dogs with Cushing's disease (affected animals also have diffuse hepatic lipidosis). Anticonvulsants such as primidone and phenobarbital also induce the release of hepatic enzymes including ALP. In some dogs, certain non-hepatic malignant tumours, e.g. mammary carcinoma, may be associated with high ALP levels. Cats do not have a corticosteroid isoenzyme and there is no evidence to suggest that other drug-induced increases in ALP occur.

For the reasons mentioned above an increase in ALP alone should not be regarded as evidence of liver damage (a marked increase in ALP with only a very slight increase in ALT occasionally occurs in cases of complete bile duct obstruction). Since most cases of intrahepatic cholestasis occur secondary to hepatocellular damage or hepatocyte swelling, increases in ALP are usually accompanied by an increase in ALT, and probably also AST. An increase in the hepatic isoenzyme of ALP is also often parallelled by an increase in GGT (see below). In the dog, persistently high ALP *and* ALT are indicative of ongoing hepatic damage. In the cat, because the half-life of the enzyme is extremely short, ALP levels are generally much lower than those of the dog both in health and disease. A relatively mild increase therefore may be significant and ALP values, if taken with ALT, may still be useful indicators of liver disease in this species.

Gamma-glutamyltransferase (GGT)

GGT is an enzyme which is found in the cell surface membranes of several organs (liver, kidney, pancreas, intestine and lung). Most of the GGT in the plasma is derived from the liver where it is located in the canalicular membranes of hepatocytes. Like ALP, GGT appears in plasma as a result of increased synthesis rather than as a result of leakage from the cell. In most cases, changes in GGT mimic those of ALP in the dog although the biliary response of GGT is generally less sensitive than ALP. In the dog, increased levels of GGT occur in response to cholestasis, hepatocellular disease and glucocorticoids. Therefore, unless an animal has received glucocorticoids, a simultaneous increase in both enzymes suggests (1) that the liver is the source of the ALP, and (2) a more serious degree of cholestasis is present. The current feeling is that GGT in small animals offers no real advantages over ALP in the diagnosis of hepatobiliary disease except that it is more liver specific. In cats, GGT concentrations tend to be negligible in all but the most severe forms of liver disease.

Tests for assessing liver function

A decrease in functional hepatic mass and/or a reduction in hepatic blood flow leads to hepatic insufficiency and ultimately liver failure. The laboratory tests for detecting liver dysfunction in a jaundiced animal are described below. These include:

1. Concentration of endogenous substances normally excreted by the hepatobiliary system, e.g. bilirubin (see above) or bile salts (bile acids);
2. Plasma urea, plasma ammonia or the ammonia tolerance test;
3. Total plasma protein concentration;
4. Ratio of plasma branched chain to aromatic amino acids (to assess amino acid metabolism).

Plasma bile salts (bile acids)

Bile acids (cholic and chenodeoxycholic acids) are synthesized by hepatocytes, conjugated primarily with glycine and taurine, and secreted as bile salts into bile. Most (95%) of bile salts are recirculated, i.e. they are taken up from the gut (terminal ileum) and transported via the portal circulation to the liver where they are cleared by hepatocytes and resecreted into the bile (enterohepatic circulation). Fasting animals, in which the concentration of bile salts is equivocal, should be fed and the assays repeated two hours postprandially. Increases in pre- and/or postprandial circulating bile salt concentrations, occur with most (but not all) congenital or acquired portosystemic shunts and most hepatobiliary disorders in the dog and cat, especially those associated with cholestasis due to posthepatic biliary obstruction. Glucocorticoid-induced hepatopathy rarely causes a significant increase in bile salts. As tests of hepatic function, bile salt assays provide a simpler and more convenient alternative to the bromosulphophthalein (BSP) and indocyanine green (ICG) tests. In comparison to these dye retention tests, bile salt assays also have greater sensitivity for detecting a variety of hepatobiliary disorders. Moreover, unlike the BSP clearance test, bile salt assays can be performed in jaundiced animals. Both the hepatocellular uptake and excretion of bilirubin are competitively inhibited by BSP hence the results of a BSP clearance test are rendered meaningless in an animal which is jaundiced (retention values are falsely increased).

Ammonia

Microbial deamination of amino acids in the intestinal tract is the major source of ammonia. Ammonia, absorbed from the intestine into portal venous blood, is removed and converted into urea in the liver. Blood ammonia concentration is a useful test of functional hepatic mass. One major disadvantage of a blood ammonia determination is the instability of ammonia in the blood sample. Handling of samples is therefore extremely important. The blood sample should be placed on ice immediately after collection, the plasma separated within 30 min, and the assay performed on the separated plasma within 60 min.

Reference values for ammonia vary considerably in different laboratories. In most cases of portocaval shunting, an increased plasma ammonia concentration is accompanied by a decrease in plasma urea (additional evidence for a portosystemic shunt may be obtained by the presence of ammonium biurate crystals in the urine). False increases in plasma ammonia concentrations may occur with increased ammonia production in the gut due to haemorrhage or feeding a high protein diet.

An *ammonia tolerance test* has been described which involves the oral administration of ammonium chloride (20%w/v solution is given via stomach tube at a dose of 0.5ml kg^{-1} body weight) after a 12 h fast. Blood samples are obtained before and 30 min after administering the ammonium chloride; normal postprandial values are usually no more than 2–2.5 times the baseline values. Increased postprandial ammonia levels may precipitate signs of encephalopathy in animals with portosystemic shunts.

Plasma proteins

The liver is the sole site for albumin synthesis. Hypoalbuminaemia is a common terminal feature of *chronic* liver disease, occurring when functional hepatic mass has been reduced to 20% or less. Non-hepatic causes of hypoalbuminaemia include glomerulonephropathy, protein-losing enteropathy, maldigestion and malabsorption, protein malnutrition, and cardiogenic ascites.

Although some globulins are synthesized in the liver, immunoglobulins are synthesized exclusively in lymphoid tissue. Polyclonal increases in the gammaglobulin fraction may occur with liver disease in many species. In the cat, two diseases, feline infectious peritonitis and progressive lymphocytic cholangitis, are frequently associated with marked hypergammaglobulinaemia.

Clotting factors and clotting tests

The liver is the major site for the production of numerous clotting factors (fibrinogen, prothrombin and factors V, VII, IX, X, XII, and possibly also XIII). Although few dogs with liver disease present with a clinical bleeding problem, laboratory abnormalities of coagulation (increased one-stage prothrombin and activated partial thromboplastin times) frequently occur. Bleeding is only likely to occur in cases of acute severe liver failure associated with diffuse inflammatory changes (e.g. infectious canine hepatitis or hepatic necrosis) or severe neoplastic infiltration. Such patients are more likely to develop disseminated intravascular coagulation which may further increase the bleeding tendency.

CLASSIFICATION OF JAUNDICE

Jaundice is usually classified on a pathophysiological basis as haemolytic (prehepatic), hepatocellular (intrahepatic) or obstructive (posthepatic) jaundice. The differentiating historical, clinical and laboratory features of each type of jaundice are summarized below. The reader is referred to Chapters 37, 38, 45 and 48 for a more detailed discussion of the causes of jaundice listed in Table 17.1.

The history and clinical signs associated with each type of jaundice will depend on the pathogenesis and the duration of the underlying disorder. Jaundice becomes clinically detectable when the plasma (serum) concentration of bilirubin exceeds 26 µmol l^{-1} (1.5 mg dl^{-1}). At this concentration of bilirubin plasma will appear icteric to the naked eye (plasma usually develops a yellowish tinge before there is clinical evidence of jaundice). Early jaundice is best detected on the sclerae, the thinner, non-pigmented, hairless areas of skin, and the inner surfaces of the pinnae. The intensity of the jaundice reflects the plasma concentration of bilirubin. The onset of jaundice usually does not coincide with the onset of associated clinical signs (e.g. with liver disease, jaundice may occur several days or possibly even weeks after the more acute signs of hepatic disease such as vomiting or diarrhoea have become apparent). Similarly, jaundice usually takes longer to resolve than the causative disease.

HISTORY CHECKLIST

Haemolytic jaundice

- Sudden onset of anorexia, weakness and collapse?
- Are mucous membranes visibly pale?
- Febrile?
- Splenomegaly and/or hepatomegaly suggestive of increased red blood cell destruction?
- Urine discoloured (haemoglobinuria)?
- Recent drug administration, e.g. paracetamol?

Hepatocellular jaundice

- Have signs of systemic disease such as anorexia, lethargy, weight loss, vomiting and diarrhoea preceded onset of jaundice (may be a few days, or in some cases, weeks)?
- Evidence of abdominal pain?
- Polyuria/polydipsia?
- Abdominal distension?
- CNS signs or behavioural changes (seizures, circling, stupor, blindness, disorientation, etc.)?
- Evidence of external haemorrhage (increased bleeding tendency)?

Obstructive jaundice

- Vomiting/diarrhoea (may precede onset of jaundice)?
- Abdominal pain?
- Evidence of haemorrhage?
- Pale, fatty faeces?

CLINICAL AND LABORATORY FEATURES OF JAUNDICE

Haemolytic jaundice

- **Jaundice may be relatively mild**
Initially, the production of bilirubin exceeds the capacity of the liver to conjugate it so that a higher proportion (80–90%) of bilirubin is unconjugated (unconjugated bilirubin is insoluble in water and is less likely to stain tissues). After 48–72 h, however, the concentrations of unconjugated and conjugated bilirubin equilibrate so that 50% or more may be conjugated. This is partly because liver function is impaired and as a result the liver's ability to excrete conjugated bilirubin is diminished.

- **ALT and ALP may be slightly increased**
Although the jaundice is not of hepatocellular origin liver enzymes may be increased as a result of hepatocellular hypoxia.

- **Haemoglobinaemia/haemoglobinuria**
Excess haemoglobin which is not bound to plasma haptoglobin is excreted in the urine and is potentially toxic for renal tubular epithelial cells.

- **Increase in urine bilirubin**
Initially this may be minimal since unconjugated bilirubin is not filtered by the glomeruli.

- **Regenerative anaemia**
Typically this is a macrocytic hypochromic anaemia, providing sufficient time (at least 48–72 h) has elapsed following the haemolytic crisis to allow the bone marrow to respond; also marked anisocytosis, poikilocytosis, polychromasia and increased numbers of circulating nucleated red blood cells and reticulocytes. Spherocytes, if present, are highly suggestive of autoimmune haemolytic anaemia (AIHA) although their absence does not preclude such a diagnosis. The presence of autoagglutination confirms an immune-mediated mechanism for the haemolysis. If there is no evidence of autoagglutination, blood should be submitted for a direct antiglobulin (Coombs') test. Anaemia is usually accompanied by a reactive leucocytosis (neutrophilia ± left shift).

Hepatocellular jaundice

- **Jaundice tends to be more severe**
Total bilirubin levels are usually higher with

greater than 50% conjugated. Total bilirubin levels rarely exceed 85 µmol l^{-1} in small animals.

- **Mild to moderate increases in ALT and ALP.**

- **Significant bilirubinuria**

- **Plasma proteins**
With chronic liver disease, i.e. hepatic failure, total plasma proteins may be low (hypoalbuminaemia) although the globulin fraction may be increased; blood urea may be low (<2.5 mmol l^{-1}) and clotting times (OSPT and APTT) may be prolonged.

- **Packed cell volume decreased or normal**
Animals with liver disease may be mildly anaemic (anaemia of chronic disease). Increased numbers of acanthocytes are sometimes seen with diffuse liver disease. Variable total WBC count (the total WBC count will reflect the pathogenesis).

- **Liver size variable**
Liver may be small with cirrhosis or enlarged with cholangiohepatitis.

Obstructive jaundice

- **Obstructive jaundice**
This is usually associated with the highest bilirubin levels and at least 50% (in many cases greater than 75%) of the bilirubin is conjugated.

- **Marked increase in ALP ± GGT with a more moderate increase in ALT**

- **Significant bilirubinuria**

- **Absorption of vitamin K**
Complete biliary obstruction may lead to the decreased absorption of vitamin K and hence decreased synthesis of vitamin K-dependent clotting factors (II, VII, IX and X) with a resultant increase in clotting times (especially OSPT). The clotting defect may be at least partially corrected by the parenteral administration of vitamin K$_1$. In contrast the increased bleeding tendency which occurs with diffuse hepatocellular injury and/or hepatic failure is multifactorial and does not respond to vitamin K$_1$ therapy. Complete obstruction of the bile duct may result in steatorrhoea and the passage of pale acholic faeces.

FURTHER INVESTIGATION

If haemolysis is suspected and the cause cannot be ascertained using any of the tests described above *blood cultures* should be performed to rule out possible infectious (bacteraemic or septicaemic) causes (see Table 17.1).

In cases where the jaundice is considered to be of hepatocellular origin the following procedures are indicated.

Ultrasonographic examination of the liver

Ultrasonography is useful for evaluating the size and consistency of the liver, the hepatic vasculature and the biliary system.

Liver biopsy

Liver biopsy is frequently necessary in cases showing biochemical evidence of hepatobiliary damage or liver dysfunction. In particular, a liver biopsy may be helpful in (1) establishing the nature of the pathology and/or aetiology, (2) the potential for reversibility, and (3) the degree of hepatocellular regeneration. If the liver is uniformly enlarged, liver biopsy may be performed safely via percutaneous needle biopsy (preferably using ultrasound guidance). If the liver is small then the technique is best performed via a laparotomy incision or via laparoscopy. *Clotting tests should always be performed before surgical intervention in any animal with liver disease.*

MANAGEMENT OF JAUNDICE

The specific management of jaundice depends on the aetiology and, in the absence of a definitive diagnosis, treatment is primarily supportive. The reader is referred to Chapter 37 for a more detailed discussion of therapy for specific diseases which can cause jaundice. The following points are worthy of consideration when treating any jaundiced animal.

- Adequate caloric and fluid supplementation should be provided (Ringers solution ± additional glucose and potassium if necessary).
- Supplement with B complex and fat-soluble vitamins.

- Some antibiotics are concentrated in bile and are more effective against enteric Gram-negative and/or anaerobic organisms which are likely to be involved. These include ampicillin, amoxycillin, cephalosporins, chloramphenicol and metronidazole (the latter is particularly effective against anaerobic organisms and may be used in combination with ampicillin). The use of tetracyclines, neomycin, streptomycin and sulphonamides should be avoided.
- Immunosuppressive agents such as prednisolone are only indicated when the jaundice has an immune-mediated pathogenesis, e.g. immune-mediated haemolytic disease, lymphocytic cholangiohepatitis, chronic active hepatitis and possibly feline infectious peritonitis.
- Hydrochloretic agents, e.g. bile acids such as dehydrocholic acid may stimulate the flow of watery bile in animals with cholestasis (recommended dose 10–15 mg kg^{-1} body weight per os three times daily for 7–10 days).

REFERENCES

Dunn, J. K. (1992) Assessment of liver damage and dysfunction. *In Practice* **14**, 193–200.

18

Peripheral Oedema and Ascites

K. J. Dunn

ASCITES

The peritoneum is a serous membrane lining the abdominal cavity. Its main functions are protection (by walling off areas of inflammation), lubrication and absorption of transudates/exudates. True ascites refers to the accumulation of serous or serosanguinous fluid in the peritoneal space. A more generalized description would include distension of the abdomen with other fluids, e.g. chyle, blood and inflammatory exudates. Ascites is always a sign of disease therefore investigation should be aimed at identifying the primary underlying problem.

Ascites may be caused by a number of inflammatory, infectious, metabolic, degenerative and neoplastic disease processes. The biochemical and cytological characteristics of the ascitic fluid may help to differentiate the cause of the abdominal effusion (Table 18.1).

Pathophysiology

There are four primary pathophysiological mechanisms for the development of ascites:

- Transudation
- Exudation
- Neoplastic cell exfoliation
- Vessel or viscus rupture

Transudates are morbid accumulations of fluid which build up due to a hydrostatic imbalance despite normal vascular permeability. In hepatic failure, ascites develops as a result of portal hypertension and sodium retention; hypoalbuminaemia may contribute to the tendency to accumulate fluid but is rarely the primary problem. Portal hypertension must be sustained for ascites to develop. A transient increase in portal venous pressure is compensated for by increased lymph flow from the bowel.

Modified transudates arise as a result of the leakage of fluid from lymphatic or blood vessels increasing the protein content of the transudate. Accumulation of fluid irritates the mesothelium and results in exfoliation of mesothelial cells and secondary inflammatory changes. Most neoplastic effusions are modified transudates.

Exudates arise due to increased vascular permeability. Exudates may be septic or non-septic. The release of inflammatory mediators increases vascular permeability and induces a chemotactic response of inflammatory and phagocytic cells. In acute inflammation, arteriolar dilatation occurs and the increased blood flow and pressure in the small vessels means that capillary hydrostatic pressure may exceed the colloid oncotic pressure of plasma. Low molecular weight solutes and fluid pass into the intracellular space in larger volumes. In inflamed tissue separation of adjacent endothelial cells in the vessel walls produces holes through which larger molecules such as proteins can escape. Lymphatic flow rate is initially increased to take up the proteins but once this capacity is exceeded the interstitial oncotic pressure increases and more fluid is drawn out of the circulation. In addition, the large proteins present in the interstitial tissues are broken down to smaller molecules which further increases the oncotic pressure.

INVESTIGATION OF ASCITES

Investigation of ascites is aimed at identifying the underlying cause.

HISTORY CHECKLIST

❏ Rate of fluid accumulation?
The rate of abdominal distension may be important in establishing the aetiology of the condition and can influence the severity of clinical signs. Ascites often develops relatively slowly in right-sided congestive heart failure, e.g. dilated

Table 18.1 Differential diagnosis of ascites

Transudate
- Hypoproteinaemia
    Protein-losing enteropathy (e.g. lymphangiectasia)
    Glomerulonephropathy
    Hepatic failure
- Portal hypertension (sustained)

Modified transudate
- Cardiac disease (usually right-sided congestive heart failure, e.g. pericardial effusion, dilated cardiomyopathy)
- Portal venous obstruction (thrombosis, stricture, vascular anomaly)
- Abdominal neoplasm obstructing lymphatic or venous drainage

Exudate
- Septic
    Intestinal perforation
    Ruptured pyometra
    Ruptured abscess
    Extension of infection from abdominal organs
- Non-septic
    Acute pancreatitis
    Feline infectious peritonitis
    Ruptured urinary bladder
    Ruptured gall bladder

Miscellaneous
- Chyle (referred to as chylous ascites or chyloperitoneum); rare in small animals
    Ruptured lymphatics, e.g. trauma
    Lymphangiectasia
    Portal obstruction
    Increased hydrostatic pressure
- Haemorrhage
    Trauma resulting in rupture of spleen/liver
    Neoplasia (especially splenic haemangiosarcoma or lymphoma)
    Bleeding disorder (e.g. warfarin poisoning)
    Thrombosis
    Torsion of the stomach or spleen
    Phaeochromocytoma eroding blood vessel

cardiomyopathy, whereas more rapid fluid accumulation occurs with pericardial effusions as cardiac tamponade develops. If fluid accumulates slowly the animal has time to accommodate to the changes associated with the ascites.

❑ **Presence of other signs of systemic illness?**
Dyspnoea may be associated with increased abdominal pressure resulting in displacement of the diaphragm cranially. Cardiac disease may cause dyspnoea due to pulmonary oedema and/or pleural effusion. The presence of other signs such as wasting, polydipsia/polyuria, diarrhoea, vomiting and appetite changes may indicate a systemic disease process, e.g. chronic liver disease. Coughing or exercise intolerance are more indicative of cardiac disease.

 ## PHYSICAL EXAMINATION

❑ **Palpation of the abdomen**
To identify distension, increased abdominal pressure or pain if peritonitis is present.

❑ **Ballotment for detection of a fluid thrill**
Tapping on one side of the abdomen whilst placing the palm of the other hand flat on the opposite abdominal wall may allow detection of a fluid wave moving across the abdomen (fluid thrill). False positive fluid thrills are rare but it is difficult to detect the presence of small amounts of fluid by this method.

❑ **Subcutaneous oedema?**
Although a rare finding in small animals, oedema may be present particularly in the dependent areas of limbs, ventral abdomen and prepuce.

❑ **Femoral pulses**
These should be palpated and will often be thready if abdominal pressure is increased or in cases where ascites is due to cardiac decompensation. Weak pulses in multiple sites suggests cardiac insufficiency rather than a local lesion.

❑ **Full cardiological examination**
Check particularly for signs of right-sided failure, e.g. distension of jugular veins, jugular pulses or oedema. The presence of murmurs, pulse deficits or other signs of cardiac dysfunction should also be noted.

FURTHER INVESTIGATION

Measurement of central venous pressure

Central venous pressure (CVP) is controlled by interaction of circulating blood volume, cardiac function and alterations in the vascular bed. To measure CVP a long catheter is placed in the external jugular vein. A three-way stopcock is attached to the catheter and connected to two intravenous lines. Normal saline is run through one of the lines while the other is taped vertically and then filled with fluid from the first line. When the vertical fluid line is connected to the jugular vein the CVP is measured from the midpoint of the trachea at the thoracic inlet to the height of the liquid column. Normal CVP in the dog is −1 to 5 cm of water. Values greater than 10 cm water are abnormal and a CVP above 15 cm is most commonly seen with congestive heart failure.

Radiography

Abdominal radiographs will show a typical 'groundglass' appearance to the abdomen. This makes identification of abdominal organs and/or masses difficult (Fig. 18.1).

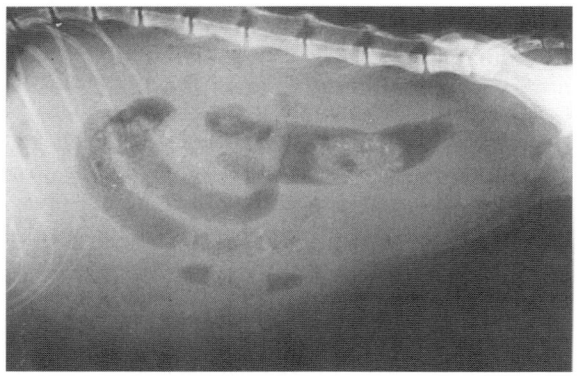

Figure 18.1 Lateral radiograph of a cat with feline infectious peritonitis (effusive form). Note the 'groundglass' appearance of the abdomen. Photograph courtesy of Michael Herrtage.

Thoracic radiography should be performed to investigate potential cardiac pathology as a cause of the ascites.

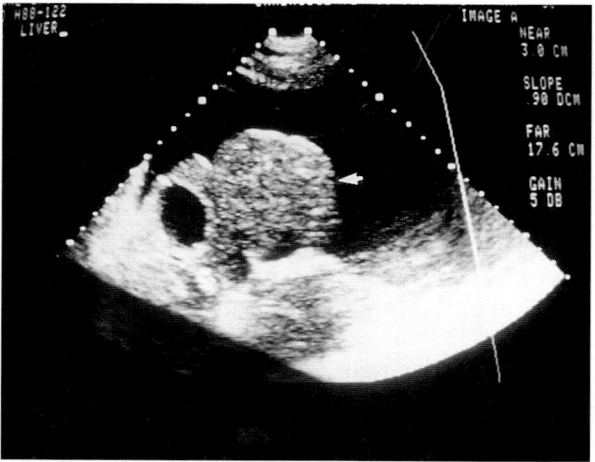

Figure 18.2 Ultrasound picture of the ascitic abdomen of a 6-year-old German shepherd dog. Note the fluid outlining a liver lobe (arrow). Photograph courtesy of Michael Herrtage.

Ultrasonography

Abdominal ultrasonography is ideally suited to imaging in the presence of fluid (Fig. 18.2). Examination should be made of all parenchymatous organs to assess their size and structure. Echocardiography is indicated to rule out pericardial effusion, endocardiosis, dysplasia of the tricuspid valve and dilated cardiomyopathy.

Electrocardiography

Electrocardiographic signs of right-sided enlargement or conduction disturbances may be present in cardiac conditions such as pulmonic stenosis, tricuspid dysplasia, tetralogy of Fallot, reverse patent ductus arteriosus and severe heartworm disease (see Chapter 34).

Laboratory data

Initially, full haematological and biochemical screens, including bile salts, should be performed as part of the minimum database. Peritonitis may present with a peracute (neutropenia with degenerative left shift) or an acute (neutrophilia with regenerative left shift) inflammatory response.

Total plasma protein concentration

The total plasma protein concentration and albumin:globulin ratio must be determined in all cases. Hypoalbuminaemia must be very severe ($<10\,g\,l^{-1}$) to cause ascites in its own right. Ascites may occur with albumin concentration of $20\,g\,l^{-1}$ and concurrent portal hypertension. Feline infectious peritonitis and cholangiohepatitis may present with markedly increased total plasma protein concentrations (hypergammaglobulinaemia).

Renal function

Urea and creatinine concentrations should be assessed in conjunction with urine specific gravity since the presence of ascites can also cause venous stasis and reduced renal blood flow (pre-renal failure).

Hepatic enzymes and bile salts

The concentrations of alkaline phosphatase (ALP), alanine aminotransferase (ALT), aspartate aminotransferase (AST), gamma glutamyl transferase (GGT) and serum bile salts should be measured.

Pancreatic enzymes

Plasma concentrations of amylase, lipase and possibly trypsin-like immunoreactivity (TLI) should be measured especially if there are signs consistent with pancreatitis and cytological examination of fluid is consistent with inflammatory exudate. The concentrations of these enzymes in the abdominal effusion may also be useful in assessing damage to the pancreas.

Urinalysis

Urinary protein detected on a dipstick must be assessed in relation to urine specific gravity (2+ protein in dilute urine may be significant). Normal dogs and cats excrete some protein in the urine (usually <30 mg kg^{-1} day^{-1}). A protein:creatinine ratio should be calculated and values >1 are significant. Urinary protein:creatinine ratios are usually >3 in primary protein-losing nephropathy, e.g. glomerulonephropathy. Single urine protein:creatinine ratios correlate well with 24 hour protein excretion values.

Technique for abdominocentesis

In most cases abdominocentesis can be performed without sedation and carries minimal risk to the patient. The ventral mid-abdomen should be clipped at the level of the umbilicus and prepared in a sterile fashion. Local anaesthesia can be infiltrated into the skin and subcutis if required. The animal is restrained in lateral recumbency. Performing the procedure with the animal standing may allow a sample of fluid to be collected when the volume of ascites is small. A 25 mm, 20 gauge needle or 'over the needle' catheter is inserted through the midline, 1–2 cm caudal to the umbilicus and a sample of fluid can be collected for analysis. If blood is aspirated, then one sample should be collected into anticoagulant and a second allowed to stand to see if it clots. A sample of fluid should be collected into EDTA for cytological analysis, total protein estimation and specific gravity measurement. Samples collected into plain tubes can be submitted for bacteriological examination and triglyceride/cholesterol concentrations.

Abdominal fluid analysis

The type of effusion is classified according to its protein content and cell count but the categories are not mutually exclusive and there is wide overlap, for example, between modified transudates and exudates with respect to protein content

Table 18.2 Classification of abdominal effusions

	Normal	Transudate	Modified transudate	Exudate
Gross appearance	Clear, straw colour	Clear, straw colour	Yellow or blood-tinged, turbid	Turbid
Protein concentration (g l^{-1})	<25	<25; often <15	Variable; usually >25	>25; usually >30
Specific gravity (serum scale)	<1.015	<1.015	1.015–1.025	>1.025
Nucleated cell count ($\times 10^9$ l^{-1})	<3.0	<0.5–1.0	1.0–7.0	>7.0
Predominant cell type	Mesothelial cells/macrophages	Mesothelial cells/macrophages	Mesothelial cells/macrophages ± increasing numbers of non-degenerate neutrophils ± small lymphocytes	Neutrophils/macrophages; neutrophils degenerate if bacterial infection
Typical causes	–	Hypoproteinaemia; congestive heart failure (CHF)	Result of chronic transudation (e.g. associated with CHF, neoplasia etc.)	Feline infectious peritonitis; bacterial, e.g. *Actinomyces* sp., *Nocardia* sp.

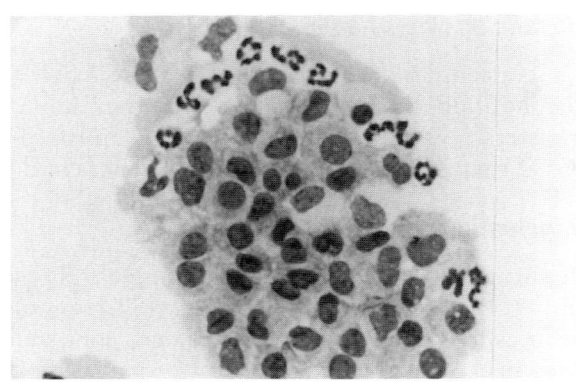

Figure 18.3 (a) Modified transudates are frequently either straw coloured or, as in this case, serosanguinous. (b) Peritoneal fluid from a dog with congestive heart failure. This shows a cluster of reactive mesothelial cells surrounded by non-degenerate neutrophils. As mesothelial cells become more reactive their cytoplasm becomes vacuolated and less intensively basophilic, the nuclei become more pleomorphic, and the cells have the appearance of peritoneal macrophages (Giemsa; original magnification ×125; photographs J.K. Dunn reproduced courtesy of *In Practice*).

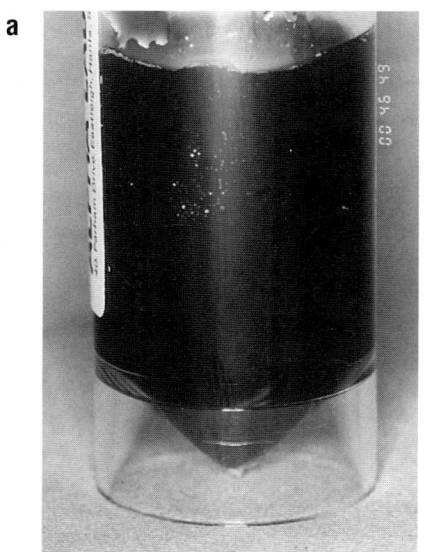

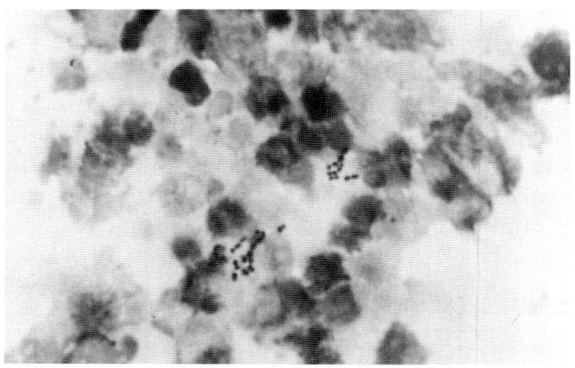

Figure 18.4 (a) Gross appearance of abdominal fluid from a dog with peritonitis following perforation of the small intestine (photograph courtesy of Michael Herrtage). (b) Peritonitis. Neutrophils are showing severe karyolytic changes. Two neutrophils contain ingested bacteria (Giemsa ×250; photograph J.K. Dunn reproduced courtesy of *In Practice*).

(Table 18.2). Transudates contain few, non-phagocytic cells (mesothelial cells and macrophages), as they become modified, cell counts rise and an increasing number of neutrophils are seen (Fig. 18.3a,b). Septic exudates contain bacteria, degenerate neutrophils and macrophages and/or neutrophils with intracellular bacteria (Fig. 18.4a,b). In non-septic exudates neutrophils with age-related changes predominate and no bacteria are present (Fig. 18.5a,b). Chylous effusions are white or pinkish opaque fluids, containing small numbers of mature lymphocytes and fat droplets. Increasing numbers of neutrophils and macrophages appear with time. Chyle has a

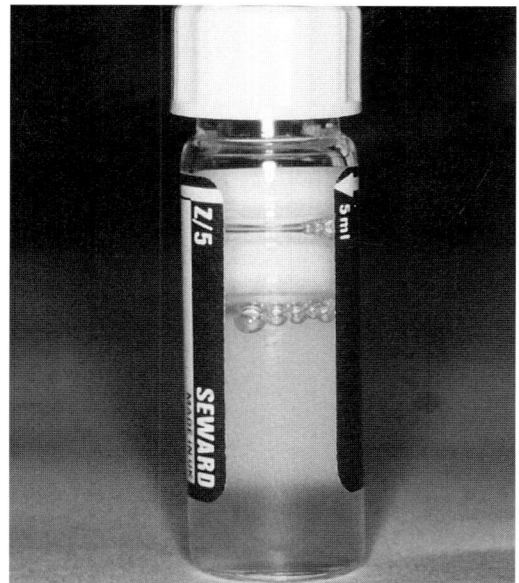

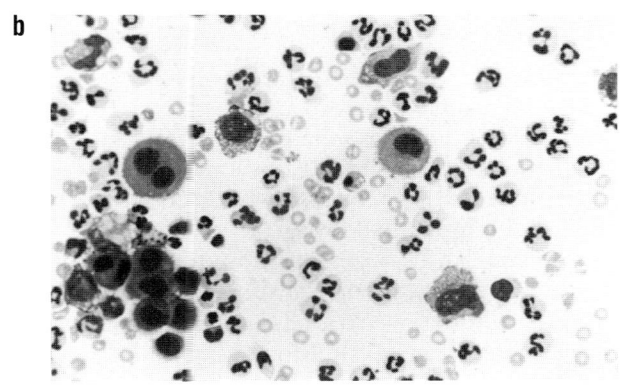

Figure 18.5 (a) Gross appearance of abdominal fluid from a cat with effusive feline infectious peritonitis (FIP). The fluid is typically straw coloured and may contain fibrin flecks. Due to the high protein (primarily globulin) concentration effusions from cats with FIP often froth when shaken. (b) Peritoneal fluid from a dog with acute pancreatitis and associated peritonitis. Numerous red blood cells, non-degenerate neutrophils and reactive mesothelial cells are present. Note the binucleate mesothelial cells. This is an example of a non-septic exudate (Giemsa; original magnification ×125; photographs J.K. Dunn reproduced courtesy of *In Practice*).

high triglyceride content with a cholesterol: triglyceride ratio <1.0. The triglyceride content of chyle is greater than that of serum and cholesterol concentration is lower (the reverse is true for non- or pseudochylous effusions).

True chylous effusions should clear on addition of ethanol but not on centrifugation.

SYMPTOMATIC THERAPY

Treatment should be aimed at addressing the underlying problem whenever possible. However, in many cases therapy is not available and symptomatic treatment must be employed. In human patients with chronic hepatic failure ascites is known to be deleterious to health. There is no evidence to suggest that this is the case in dogs.

Ascitic fluid should not be drained unless the volume of fluid present is compromising the animal's respiration or ambulation. If large volumes are to be removed it is safer to insert an indwelling polyethylene intravenous catheter as described above. This minimizes the risk of organ laceration. The urinary bladder should be drained before abdominocentesis to prevent damage to this organ. Unless plasma transfusions are given, abdominocentesis should be performed as infrequently as possible to reduce further loss of albumin. Diuretics, such as frusemide, can be administered though response is often disappointing, especially in animals with right-sided congestive heart failure. Complications of therapy such as potassium depletion, dehydration and reduced glomerular filtration rate can be minimized by using pulse–dose intermittent therapy. When cardiac ascites is present, spironolactone in combination with frusemide and/or angiotensin-converting enzyme inhibitors (ACE inhibitors), may be more effective and may help to minimize the risk of hypokalaemia.

Shunt devices can be placed to transport ascitic fluid to the central venous system. Complications are common with these devices and in view of the poor long-term prognosis of the underlying condition in most cases their use in animals, certainly in practice situations, is not feasible. Open drainage and/or indwelling drains can be considered if the fluid is accumulating at a rapid rate.

PERIPHERAL OEDEMA

Oedema is defined as an excessive accumulation of fluid within the intercellular space. The interstitial fluid is trapped in pockets among a network of proteoglycan filaments, the result of which is the production of a fluid with gel-like properties. Fluid diffuses rather than flows through this gel. In the normal state this gel matrix prevents fluid flow to lower areas of the body as a result of gravity and prevents spread of bacteria and other agents from one tissue area to another.

The presence of a predetermined amount of fluid in the interstitium depends on a finely balanced system of filtration and absorption. In normal tissue the vascular walls are freely permeable to water and electrolytes but not proteins. Water and solutes which are filtered into the interstitium are returned to the circulation via the lymphatics. The extensive lymphatic network present in most tissues is also able to take up any protein which inadvertently leaks into the interstitium. Oedema is relatively rare in small animals; right-sided heart failure is more likely to cause ascites than oedema.

PATHOPHYSIOLOGY

The forces driving fluid out of blood vessels are as follows.

1. *Hydrostatic pressure in the vessel*: the vascular hydrostatic pressure is the pressure gradient between fluid leaving the arteriolar end of the capillary bed and that resorbed at the venous end.
2. *Colloid osmotic pressure (oncotic pressure) of interstitial fluid*: usually there is little protein present in the interstitial fluid and excess protein is removed via the lymphatics so this is not a significant factor.

The forces drawing fluid into the vessels are as follows.

1. *Tissue tension*: this factor is important in relation to the distribution of the oedema, i.e. increased tissue tension in the pads reduces the likelihood of oedema occurring there. As tissue tension rises less fluid escapes from the blood vessels and so the volume of oedema fluid is controlled.
2. *Colloid osmotic pressure (oncotic pressure) of plasma*: this is generated by the proteins in plasma and, of these, albumin is the most important as it is present in a high concentration and has a low molecular weight.

The mechanisms which control the balance of fluid entering and leaving the vessels have a reserve capacity. For example, capillary hydrostatic pressure must double or plasma colloid oncotic pressure drop from 28 mmHg to less than 10 mmHg before oedema forms.

Oedema arises by a variety of mechanisms:

- Increased capillary hydrostatic pressure;
- Reduced capillary oncotic pressure;
- An increase in the inherent permeability of capillaries to water or increased surface area of capillaries or capillary bed (the filtration coefficient);
- Reduced lymphatic drainage;
- Iatrogenic, i.e. overzealous administration of intravenous fluids particularly if the animal is already volume overloaded, i.e. has congestive heart failure or renal shutdown.

Oedema can be classified as generalized or localized.

Generalized oedema

The oedema involves both the hind and fore limbs and its presence suggests a systemic disease. Furthermore, if ascites is present in association with oedema a diagnosis of cardiac dysfunction is more likely. If no ascites is present hypoproteinaemia is the more likely cause.

Localized oedema

This is more usually associated with an inflammatory, infectious or traumatic lesion.

Localized oedema can be divided into four types:

1. *Bilateral forelimb involvement* usually indicates cranial vena cava obstruction, e.g. lymphatic or heart base tumour.

2. *Bilateral hindlimb involvement*: if ascites is present the lesion is cranial to the renal vein; if no ascites present then the lesion is probably within the pelvic canal, e.g. obstruction to the common iliac veins.
3. *Head and neck*: angioneurotic oedema (of allergic origin) is most likely but check the retropharyngeal and submandibular lymph nodes for evidence of enlargement which may be the result of neoplasia (lymphoma) or inflammation.
4. *Extremity of one limb*: localized disease most likely so examine the affected limb thoroughly.

Occasionally an animal with systemic disease may develop local oedema. This is most frequently seen in 'pre-oedematous states' where there is increased interstitial fluid pressure but no overt oedema. Oedema may then develop in the limb beneath the animal when it is recumbent, due to reduction in venous drainage (hypostatic congestion). Localized oedema may occur in multiple sites, particularly in primary lymphoedema, giving the impression of generalized oedema.

Oedema may result in tissue damage as it increases the distance between the blood vessels and tissue cells and hence interferes with the diffusion of oxygen, glucose, amino acids and other cellular nutrients.

INVESTIGATION OF PERIPHERAL OEDEMA

Causes of oedema are summarized in Table 18.3.

In order to shorten the list of possible differential diagnoses a thorough history should be taken and physical examination performed prior to laboratory investigation.

HISTORY CHECKLIST

❏ **Has the animal shown any other signs of systemic illness?**

Polydipsia/polyuria may indicate renal disease. Polydipsia may also be seen in cardiac disease but more common findings would be exercise intolerance or lethargy. Concurrent vomiting and diarrhoea may be seen with protein-losing enteropathy and with toxaemia due to hepatic or renal disease.

❏ **Has the animal had any similar problems previously?**

This may be important with respect to the possibility of compressive lesions or allergic reactions.

Table 18.3 Differential diagnosis of oedema

Increased capillary hydrostatic pressure caused by functional/structural obstruction to blood flow
- Congestive cardiac failure (right-sided)
- Venous obstruction, e.g. intraluminal thrombus
- Compression of vessel by extraluminal mass
- Arteriovenous fistula
- Hypostasis

Reduced capillary oncotic pressure (hypoalbuminaemia)
- Protein-losing enteropathy or glomerulonephropathy (nephrotic syndrome)
- Chronic liver disease, i.e. reduced hepatic synthesis of protein
- Protein malnutrition
- Exudative lesions, e.g. severe burns/peritonitis

Increased vascular permeability
- Type 1 immediate hypersensitivity response (local release of vasodilators)
- Chronic inflammatory disease
- Vasculitis (infectious/immune-mediated) or vascular trauma
- Toxins

Reduced lymphatic drainage (lymphoedema)
- Congenital
- Acquired
  Neoplastic
  Traumatic
  Compression of lymphatics (recumbency)

Increased interstitial gel matrix
- Myxoedema (hypothyroidism)

❏ **Distribution of lesions (localized vs generalized)?**
Has the distribution changed with time? Is the distribution variable?

❏ **Has the oedema progressed or is it resolving?**

❏ **Is the animal ascitic?**

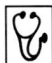

PHYSICAL EXAMINATION

- The swelling should be palpated for evidence of pitting to confirm that true oedema is present. Heat, pain and redness may indicate inflammation whereas cool, non-painful swellings are seen with vascular occlusion and decreased lymphatic drainage.
- The size and consistency of local lymph nodes should be evaluated.
- With localized oedema the affected limb, its blood supply and drainage lymph node must

be examined. The swollen limb should be palpated for the presence of masses and auscultated (a continuous murmur can often be heard over an AV fistula).
- If oedema is present in one or more limbs the animal should be examined for lameness and gait abnormalities.
- Rectal examination should be performed to check for the presence of pelvic masses in the case of hindlimb oedema.
- If hindlimb oedema is present femoral pulse quality should be assessed.
- Observe the animal eating and drinking to see if there are any problems with swallowing (may indicate submandibular or laryngeal/pharyngeal swelling).
- Animals with submandibular oedema may become dyspnoeic.
- If the oedema is generalized the aim of the physical examination is to rule out primary systemic disease and detailed examinations of the cardiac, renal, hepatic and gastrointestinal systems should be performed.
- Check for evidence of chronic inflammatory disease, cardiac disease, allergy, evidence of trauma.

Laboratory data

Initially, full routine haematological and biochemical profiles should be performed and must include the following.

- *Total plasma protein concentration* as well as an albumin:globulin ratio should be measured. If albumin and globulin levels are both low then the possibility of gastrointestinal loss, e.g. protein-losing enteropathy, should be investigated by examination of faecal samples for parasites and occult blood. Further investigations such as gut biopsy may be required for definitive diagnosis of enteropathies such as lymphangiectasia.
- *Liver enzymes* should be measured although these may be within normal limits in chronic liver disease, e.g. cirrhosis or fibrosis. Hepatic function should be assessed by the use of specific hepatic function tests, e.g. serum bile salts or plasma ammonia concentrations.

Urinalysis

Urine should be checked for the presence of an excessive amount of protein if the animal is hypoalbuminaemic (see section on ascites).

FURTHER INVESTIGATION

Radiography

This should include thoracic radiography to assess cardiac size and shape, the size of the caudal vena cava, and to screen for the presence of intrathoracic masses and pericardial or pleural effusions.

Abdominal radiographs should be assessed for alterations in hepatic size or the presence of ascites. Hepatomegaly may indicate passive venous congestion associated with right-sided congestive heart failure and microhepatica will be seen in cirrhosis and in many cases of portosystemic shunting. The visualization of enlarged kidneys may suggest a diagnosis of glomerulonephritis.

Ultrasonography

Examination should include echocardiography in cases of suspected cardiac dysfunction. Examination of the larger vessels may detect the presence of venous obstruction such as thrombosis. Hepatic ultrasonography may show hepatic venous stasis and cirrhosis. Doppler ultrasonographic examination may be very useful for identifying arteriovenous fistulae. If the kidneys are enlarged, renal ultrasonography is indicated to identify any abnormalities in renal architecture.

Venous pressure measurements

If possible, central venous pressure should be measured and postcapillary venous pressure measurements can also be performed (normal –1 to 5 cm of water).

Angiography

Identification of arteriovenous fistulae requires arterial injection of contrast agent which is probably beyond the scope of most small animal practitioners. Venous angiograms can be performed in cases of suspected venous obstruction. These are simple to perform and require the injection of a water-soluble, iodine-based contrast agent into a vein distal to the suspected occlusion.

Lymphangiography

This is also a technically skilled procedure whereby the lymphatic vessels in the affected area are identified and surgically exposed. An oily contrast agent (Lipiodol Ultra-fluid) is introduced into the vessel and radiographs taken immediately. Water-based agents are not suitable for this procedure as they extravasate too quickly. However, intradermal injection of 10 ml of a water-soluble, iodine-based contrast agent will be taken up into the lymphatics. The disadvantage of this technique is that if oedema is affecting one limb the procedure must be repeated on the unaffected leg to provide a normal lymphangiogram. The intradermal injection of this volume of contrast can cause severe skin sloughs.

Radiolabelled albumin excretion studies

This is a specialized technique not readily available. The presence of intravenously injected ^{51}Cr-labelled albumin in the faeces is quantitated in 24 h faecal collections on three consecutive days postinjection. The amount of labelled albumin in the faeces is compared to the amount injected to determine the percentage loss. Normal dogs lose 5.5% of injected ^{51}Cr in the first 72 h. Dogs and cats with protein-losing enteropathies can lose 10–84% of the injected material within three days.

Cytological and/or histological examination of biopsy material

Cytological or histological examination of affected tissue or enlarged lymph nodes may provide evidence of inflammation or neoplasia.

THERAPY

Treatment is largely directed at the underlying cause. Oedema often develops as a result of a combination of predisposing factors. Identification and correction of these may reverse the oedematous state. Symptomatic therapy may also help, e.g. a plasma transfusion will temporarily correct a hypoproteinaemic state and orthostatic oedema may be reduced by the use of support bandages or physiotherapy to promote venous return.

19

Abdominal Pain

K. J. Dunn

Pain results from the physical or chemical stimulation of nociceptive nerve endings or nerve fibres. Abdominal pain can be classified as visceral, deep somatic or referred. Like the skin, the parietal surfaces of the abdominal organs are richly innervated with many fibre types including fast (delta) fibres. This allows appreciation of a wide variety of pain sensations such as pricking, aching and burning, and since there is abundant innervation, the sensation is localized over the painful area. The gastrointestinal mucosa has a similar distribution of pain receptors to the skin and thus is quite sensitive to irritation and painful stimuli. Stimuli causing diffuse stimulation of pain nerve endings throughout a viscus cause more pain than localized damage, e.g. surgical incision through a bowel loop is relatively painless but ischaemia of a bowel loop is very painful.

Visceral pain is usually due to excessive tension on nerve endings in smooth muscle activating the mechanoreceptors of C fibres. Most visceral pain is transmitted through type C fibres which can only transmit burning or aching pain. The parenchyma of the liver is almost insensitive to painful stimuli but the bile ducts, ureters, fallopian tubes and peritoneum are extremely sensitive.

Pain is primarily localized by the brain to the spinal segment corresponding to the nerves which are stimulated. The accuracy of localization therefore depends on the size of the area of innervation synapsing at a given spinal segment. Referred pain is pain which occurs in addition to (or in the absence of) true visceral or deep pain. Referred pain is felt at a site other than that of stimulation, in deep or superficial structures supplied by the same or adjacent neural segments. Pain is usually referred to other parts of the same nerve segment but may spread to adjacent segments, or occasionally corresponding segments on the opposite side of the body. Pain is referred more commonly to the ventral rather than dorsal parts of the body.

PATHOPHYSIOLOGY

Abdominal pain results from one of five distinct mechanisms.

1. Distension of a hollow viscus, e.g. bowel obstruction (caused by tumour or foreign body), or a urinary calculus lodged in the ureter or urethra.
2. Traction on peritoneum or mesentery, e.g. torsion of bowel or some other organ.
3. Ischaemia caused by severe stretching of an organ (e.g. gastric dilation) or compromised blood supply (e.g. splenic torsion).
4. Inflammation of or chemical damage to viscera.
5. Spasm of smooth muscle of a hollow viscus.

MANIFESTATIONS OF ABDOMINAL PAIN

Physiological response

- Tachycardia
- Tachypnoea
- Pupillary dilation
- Hyperthermia ± sweating

Behavioural response

- Abnormal posture and gait, e.g. arching of the back, unwillingness to move, praying stance (elevation of hindquarters whilst crouching at the front (Fig. 19.1)).
- Vocalization.
- Failure to take in adequate food and water.
- Pacing/restlessness (displacement activity).
- Disinclination to be examined, e.g. palpation of the abdomen provokes a withdrawal or defence response (abdominal guarding).

The numerous causes of abdominal pain are listed in Table 19.1.

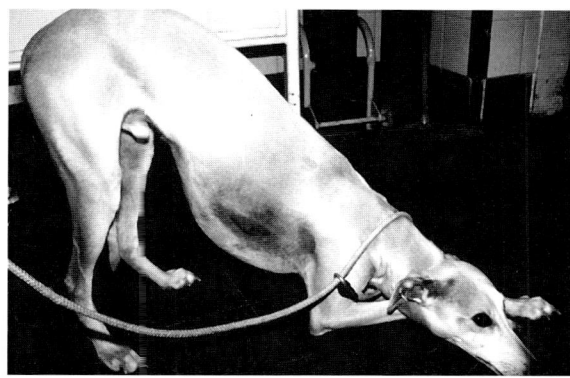

Figure 19.1 A 6-year-old whippet adopting the 'praying stance' due to cranial abdominal pain. Photograph courtesy of Michael Herrtage.

INVESTIGATION OF ABDOMINAL PAIN

 HISTORY CHECKLIST

❏ **Does the animal show signs of abdominal discomfort?**

Owners may recognize abdominal pain because the animal is obviously uncomfortable (it may pace, lick its abdomen, growl when picked up or it may adopt an abnormal posture, e.g. a 'praying stance' (see Fig. 19.1) with cranial abdominal pain associated with acute pancreatitis.

❏ **Are the signs continuous or intermittent?**

Cramping abdominal pains are usually the result of rhythmic spastic contractions of smooth muscle, e.g. gastroenteritis, constipation, ureteral obstruction.

❏ **If signs are intermittent, do they occur at specific times of the day or are they associated with feeding?**

Periodicity and duration of signs and association with other events may help to indicate the underlying cause. With gastric ulceration, pain is caused by acid or irritants in contact with the hypersensitive submucosa. Pain is reduced by eating but increases again after an interval, and vomiting relieves pain.

❏ **Is the animal eating and drinking normally?**

Inappetance and reduced water intake are often associated with pain. The presence of polydipsia may indicate more specific organ disease, e.g. glomerulonephropathy or hepatitis.

Table 19.1 Differential diagnoses of abdominal pain

Gastrointestinal
- Gastritis/gastroenteritis, e.g. campylobacteriosis, salmonellosis.
- Ulceration
- Dilation/volvulus of stomach or intestine (ischaemia)
- Perforation (peritonitis)
- Obstruction (intestinal foreign body, neoplasia or intussusception)

Hepatobiliary tract
- Acute hepatitis (rapid enlargement of the liver results in capsular stretching)
- Cholelithiasis (bile ducts and gall bladder very sensitive to stretch)

Pancreas
- Pancreatitis
- Neoplasia

Spleen
- Torsion
- Neoplasia (large splenic tumours may be painful, probably due to stretching of capsule and ligaments)
- Infection (rare)

Peritoneum
- Peritonitis (associated with pancreatitis, ruptured pyometra, perforation of gastrointestinal tract, or leakage of urine or bile)

Urogenital
- Pyelonephritis or lower urinary tract infection
- Bladder muscle spasm, e.g. inflammatory disease (cystitis)
- Ureteral spasm, e.g. renal calculus lodged in ureter
- Obstruction ± rupture
- Metritis (endometritis/pyometra)
- Acute prostatitis
- Neoplasia (prostate, bladder, ovary, retained testicle)
- Testicular/uterine torsion (rare occurrences in small animals)

Miscellaneous
- Abdominal haemorrhage, e.g. ruptured splenic haemangiosarcoma or lymphoma
- Hypoadrenocorticism (Addisons' disease)
- Lead poisoning
- Vasculitis
- Referred pain (disc disease, fractures, abscesses)
- Steatitis (cats)

❏ **Any lameness or stiffness, locomotor or gait abnormalities?**

These signs may be the result of primary orthopaedic or spinal problems which may result in referred abdominal pain, although any animal in pain may be reluctant to move.

❏ **Any other signs of systemic illness noted?**

Depression is commonly associated with pain. Vomiting and diarrhoea are also non-specific signs which may be associated with pain or they may be attributable to specific organ involvement, e.g. pancreatitis or hepatitis.

❏ **Any weight change?**
Ascites may be mistaken for obesity by owners. If pain is caused by neoplasia there may be associated weight loss.

PHYSICAL EXAMINATION

Initial observation may suggest the presence of abdominal pain, e.g. abnormal movement of the abdominal walls during respiration, adoption of an abnormal posture or crying when lifted.

The initial objective of the physical examination is to localize the site of pain. It is important to ensure that the pain is arising from the abdomen itself. Pain may be referred to the abdomen from extra-abdominal sites; for example spinal pain (disc disease), polyarthritis, myositis and pleurisy may be manifested as apparent abdominal pain. Once pain has been localized to the abdomen detailed abdominal palpation may help to localize the pain more specifically. Further investigation therefore is directed towards determining the nature of the lesion.

❏ **Palpation of the abdomen**
The abdomen should be palpated gently at first and then in more detail, examining each organ in turn. In dogs the small intestine, large intestine and urinary bladder can be readily palpated and in cats and non-obese dogs the kidneys should be easily located. Where possible, pain should be localized to a particular organ or abdominal quadrant. The cranial left abdominal quadrant contains the liver, stomach, head of spleen, pancreas, left adrenal gland and kidney. The cranial right abdominal quadrant includes the pancreas, liver, pylorus, proximal small intestine, right adrenal gland and kidney. The caudal quadrants contain intestine, kidneys, ovaries, uterus (female), ureters, bladder, prostate (male) and the left also has the spleen and colon. Abdominal organomegaly and abnormal masses in the caudal abdomen can usually be palpated unless there is a significant amount of free abdominal fluid or the animal is obese. If pain is diffuse, such as in peritonitis, the abdomen may be acutely tender with boarding of the abdominal muscles, or it may be tympanitic if gas-producing organisms are present. In some cases further palpation may be impossible without analgesia or sedation/anaesthesia.

Abdominal pain may be obvious during physical examination but it is important not to miss subtle clues like abdominal tenseness or a tendency for the animal to move away during palpation of certain areas. If possible pain should be classified as diffuse or localized.

❏ **Rectal examination**
Rectal examination of the prostate gland is an important part of the clinical examination in male dogs. In both sexes the pelvic canal, distal urogenital tract and both anal sacs can be palpated per rectum.

FURTHER INVESTIGATION

Radiography

In cases where abdominal palpation is difficult, abdominal imaging is essential. In the absence of ascites, plain radiography will demonstrate organ size and shape, or the presence of dilated segments of bowel and radio-opaque foreign bodies. Localized areas of peritonitis, characterized by reduced abdominal detail, may also be identified (Fig. 19.2). If abnormalities are detected or if pain has been localized to a specific organ then more detailed contrast radiography may be performed, for example, a double contrast gastrogram, barium meal, intravenous urogram, double contrast cystogram or retrograde urethrogram.

Laboratory data

The choice of laboratory tests will depend on the acuteness, severity and area in which the pain is localized. Observation may be the only necessary action in the first instance but, in cases of severe or chronic

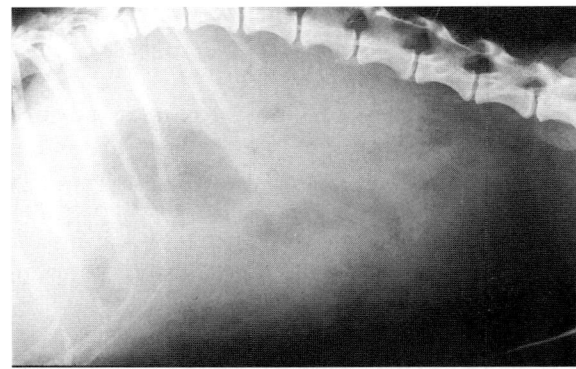

Figure 19.2 Lateral abdominal radiograph of an 8-year-old Yorkshire terrier with acute pancreatitis showing poor abdominal detail particularly in the cranioventral abdomen. Photograph courtesy of Michael Herrtage.

pain, additional laboratory investigation may be required. In many cases radiography may be the most valuable additional investigation but full haematological and biochemical screens are indicated if radiography fails to identify an obvious lesion.

Haematological examination

The presence of a neutrophilia with a regenerative left shift may indicate acute inflammation or infection. In conditions resulting in endotoxaemia (e.g. acute sepsis) and certain viral conditions (e.g. canine parvovirus infection), neutropenia may be noted. Haemograms should be evaluated for the presence of anaemia. An intensely regenerative anaemia may indicate the presence of acute haemorrhage into the abdominal cavity (e.g. splenic haemorrhage from haemangiosarcoma or lymphoma should be considered). Chronic haemorrhage into the gastrointestinal tract resulting from gastrointestinal neoplasia or ulceration may result in iron deficiency anaemia.

In all bleeding animals where a cause cannot be established, a platelet count should be performed, and a coagulation profile, including one-stage prothrombin time, activated partial thromboplastin time and fibrin degradation products, is indicated to detect coagulopathies and congenital or acquired defects in haemostasis.

Biochemical screen

A complete biochemical profile should include urea, creatinine, total plasma proteins, albumin, liver enzymes, electrolytes, glucose, lipase, amylase and trypsin-like immunoreactivity (TLI) (especially cats). Urea and creatinine may be increased in acute renal disease or urinary tract obstruction. Globulin levels are often increased in chronic inflammatory conditions and hypoproteinaemia may be due to protein loss from the gastrointestinal or urinary tract, chronic haemorrhage or chronic hepatic disease. Pancreatitis often results in marked elevations of amylase, lipase levels or TLI, and albumin and calcium levels are often low. A decreased sodium:potassium ratio (often in association with mild hypercalcaemia) may indicate hypoadrenocorticism. Marked hypercalcaemia should be investigated further. In addition bile salts and bilirubin should be measured if there is any suggestion of hepatic disease.

Urinalysis

Urinalysis, particularly specific gravity in conjunction with plasma urea and creatinine concentrations, provides an indication of renal tubular function. The presence of significant proteinuria (see Chapters 9 and 41) suggests glomerulonephropathy. Urine sediment should be examined cytologically for evidence of urinary tract neoplasia, infection or crystalluria.

Faecal analysis

In all cases of suspected gastrointestinal haemorrhage, faeces should be examined for the presence of melaena. This may be intermittent in nature so faecal samples should be observed over a number of days. Analysis for occult blood may be performed by feeding a meat-free diet for 3–4 days and then collecting a number of faecal samples for examination. In dogs and cats this test is notoriously unreliable. False positives are common due to meat proteins present in the diet or as a result of cimetidine or iron therapy. False negatives may also occur due to poor mixing of blood in the faeces or intermittent bleeding.

Faecal culture for *Salmonella* and *Campylobacter* species should be performed in all cases where diarrhoea is associated with abdominal pain.

Abdominal ultrasonography

This is indicated in almost all causes of abdominal pain. However, in many cases ultrasonography is difficult without heavy sedation/analgesia because the pressure of the probe over painful areas causes extreme discomfort. Ultrasonographic examination of the abdomen is extremely important when the presence of free abdominal fluid makes radiographic imaging techniques less sensitive (Fig. 19.3). Examination of liver, spleen, kidneys, bladder and prostate should be possible in virtually all animals. Pancreatic, adrenal, gastric and intestinal ultrasonography is possible in the hands of an experienced operator and ultrasonographic examination of the genital tract may be useful where abnormalities are present, e.g. uterine enlargement or a retained testicle.

Endoscopy

This may be indicated where primary gastric or upper gastrointestinal pathology is suspected, e.g. gastric or small intestinal (jejunal) ulceration.

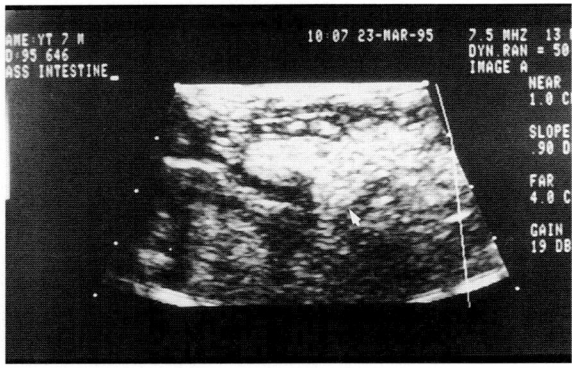

Figure 19.3 Abdominal ultrasonograph of the same animal as in Fig. 19.2 demonstrating a mass-like structure around the proximal small intestine in the region of the pancreas (arrow). Note the presence of a small amount of free abdominal fluid. Photograph courtesy of Michael Herrtage.

Abdominocentesis

If free abdominal fluid is present, a sample of fluid may be collected by abdominocentesis for cytological and biochemical analysis (see Chapter 18 for technique).

MANAGEMENT OF ABDOMINAL PAIN

The aim is to remove the cause if possible, or to provide supportive therapy whilst treating pain symptomatically if necessary.

Symptomatic therapy

The use of analgesia can be very dangerous in cases of abdominal pain where a diagnosis has not been reached. Potent analgesics (particularly opiates) may mask pain and allow a potentially life-threatening condition to develop unnoticed. Non-steroidal anti-inflammatory drugs should be used with caution due to their tendency to predispose to gastrointestinal ulceration and haemorrhage which may exacerbate a pre-existing condition. Antispasmodics such as atropine or hyoscine are also probably best avoided until a definitive diagnosis has been reached.

20

Lymphadenopathy

J. K. Dunn

During routine physical examination the submandibular, superficial cervical (prescapular), popliteal and inguinal lymph nodes may be palpated in a normal animal; other lymph nodes such as the retropharyngeal, cervical and axillary are usually palpable only in very thin animals or if they are enlarged. A loss of surrounding fat in geriatric or cachectic animals may make normal lymph nodes appear more prominent.

The strict definition of lymphadenopathy is disease of the lymph nodes but since most inflammatory, infectious or neoplastic diseases involving lymph nodes result in their enlargement the term is often used synonymously to describe the enlargement of one or more lymph nodes.

A lymph node represents an accumulation of lymphoid tissue located along the course of lymphatic vessels. They are sites of lymphocyte production and form part of the reticuloendothelial system, now referred to as the monocyte phagocyte system (MPS). As such, they play a critical role in the body's defence against noxious stimuli such as bacteria and toxins. The lymphatic system also functions to return interstitial fluid to the bloodstream. Lymph flow is unidirectional and each set of lymph nodes is responsible for draining a specific area of the body.

Lymph nodes are composed of T and B lymphocytes. B lymphocytes are located primarily in the cortex of the lymph node and are arranged in small follicles each with a germinal centre. The paracortical regions of lymph nodes are composed of dense accumulations of lymphocytes (primarily T lymphocytes) in close apposition to macrophages and dendritic cells. The dendritic and interdigitating cells of lymph nodes function as macrophages. These cells possess surface receptors for C_3 and the F_c fragment of immunoglobulin, and can be stimulated to express major histocompatability complex (MHC) class II antigens. Their main function is the phagocytosis of particulate material and the presentation of antigen to lymphocytes.

Lymphocytes originate in the bone marrow, the largest lymphopoietic tissue, from committed lymphoid stem cells and mature in bone marrow and thymus (primary lymphoid organs). In mammals, B cells mature in the bone marrow; some stem cells seed the thymus where they are processed to become T lymphocytes. The production of pre-B cells in the bone marrow and T cells in the thymus occurs independently of antigenic stimulation. Lymphocytes migrate from the primary lymphoid organs to secondary lymphoid organs where subsets of B and T cells develop in response to antigenic stimulation. B cells migrate to the lymphoid follicles of lymph nodes, spleen and gut-associated lymphoid tissue; T cells migrate to the paracortical regions of lymph nodes, periarterial sheaths and parafollicular areas of the gut-associated lymphoid tissue.

Most B cells are to be found in the bone marrow and spleen whereas the thymus, lymph nodes and thoracic duct lymph are composed primarily of T cells. B cells are generally short-lived in contrast to most T cells which are long-lived and recirculate from blood to lymph nodes via the lymphatic vessels and then back to blood again.

FUNCTIONS OF B AND T LYMPHOCYTES

B lymphocytes

Antigenic stimulation of B cells results in their blastic transformation to plasma cells which then synthesize and store immunoglobulin. Antibody production occurs mainly in the lymph nodes. Some B cells, like macrophages, can present antigen to T cells. B cells recognize antigen via their surface membrane-bound immunoglobulin.

T lymphocytes

T cells play an important role in cell-mediated immunity and also modulate the humoral immune response. T suppressor cell dysfunction is often implicated in the pathogenesis of autoimmunity. Both stimulated B and T lymphocytes (T helper cells especially) produce soluble substances known as lymphokines which are important in the pathogenesis of inflammatory and immunological responses. These substances include interferons, interleukin-2 and macrophage activating factor.

T helper (T_h) cells

The T_h cell receptor interacts with specific antigen presented with class II MHC antigen expressed on the surface of an antigen presenting cell such as a macrophage. Activated, T_h cells stimulate the transformation of B cells into plasma cells, and they also activate cytotoxic T cells.

T suppressor (T_s) cells

T suppressor cells are regulatory lymphocytes which specifically suppress the immune response to a specific antigen by releasing suppressor factors that inhibit T_h and B cells.

Null cells

Null cells possess receptors for the F_c component of immunoglobulin and T and B cell markers. This population of cells, which have the morphology of large granular lymphocytes, includes lymphocytes with killer (K) and natural killer (NK) activity.

CAUSES OF LYMPH NODE ENLARGEMENT

Lymph node enlargement may be generalized or may involve a single node (Table 20.1). The cause of the lymphadenopathy can often be established on the basis of cytological examination of a fine needle aspirate of the enlarged node. Possible causes include neoplasia (primary, e.g. lymphoma, or metastatic tumour deposits) and inflammation (either infection or antigenic stimulation associated with immune-mediated disease). Extramedullary haemopoiesis or myeloid metaplasia are rare causes of lymph node enlargement.

Isolated lymph node enlargement

Acute inflammation of a lymph node usually results in heat, tendernesss and reddening of the overlying skin. Inflammation is often associated with staphylococcal or streptococcal infections and abscess formation (suppurative lymphadenitis). If infection becomes chronic the lymph node may either abscess and eventually rupture or it may progress to a chronic granulomatous or pyogranulomatous response. This is especially true of deep-seated fungal infections or with infections associated with *Nocardia* spp., *Actinomyces* spp. and mycobacteriaceae. Many dogs and cats with periodontal disease have mild to moderately enlarged submandibular lymph nodes.

If, on cytological examination, signs of localized inflammation are absent, neoplasia for example, isolated lymphoma should be suspected. It is worth noting that large lymphomatous lymph nodes may develop necrotic centres. Consequently a fine needle aspirate taken from the centre of such a node may not be representative of the primary disease process responsible for the lymphadenopathy. Foci of metastatic tumour deposits within a lymph node cause it to enlarge because they stimulate lymphoid hyperplasia and a concurrent inflammatory response (occasionally tumour metastasis can occur without obvious lymph node enlargement). The affected lymph node not infrequently becomes 'fixed' to surrounding tissues. Carcinomas are the most common solid tumours to metastasize via lymphatic channels (sarcomas do so much less frequently); other tumours which spread preferentially via lymphatics include malignant melanomas, mast cell tumours and transmissable venereal tumours.

Generalized lymph node enlargement

Mild generalized lymph node enlargement may be associated with septicaemia/bacteraemia, the early phase of many viral infections (e.g. feline leukaemia virus infection), generalized demodicosis, ehrlichiosis, leishmaniasis, and immune-mediated disorders such as autoimmune haemolytic anaemia and the immune-mediated polyarthropathies. Mild transient generalized lymph node enlargement may occur after vaccination. Neoplastic causes include multicentric lymphoma which occasionally may involve just one lymph node (see above) or more frequently either a group of nodes (e.g. submandibular lymph nodes)

Table 20.1 Causes of isolated or generalized lymph node enlargement

Cause	Comment
Infection in adjacent tissues, e.g. abscess formation, cellulitis, deep pyoderma	Often isolated enlargement of drainage lymph node associated with suppurative lymphadenitis, pyogranulomatous lymphadenitis or lymphoid hyperplasia
Periodontal disease	Mild/moderate enlargement of submandibular lymph nodes
Septicaemia/bacteraemia or the acute phase of most viral infections, e.g. FeLV or FIV	Mild generalized lymphadenopathy
Generalized skin disease (e.g. demodicosis, sarcoptic mange, flea bite allergic dermatitis) hypereosinophilic syndrome (cats), leishmaniasis, ehrlichiosis	Mild/moderate generalized lymphadenopathy
Immune-mediated disease, e.g. autoimmune haemolytic anaemia, immune-mediated polyarthropathy	Mild generalized lymphoid hyperplasia
Lymphoma	May involve one lymph node or one group of nodes, e.g. submandibular lymph nodes; more often generalized lymphadenopathy; lymph nodes often extremely large, firm but non-painful; lymph node size may fluctuate spontaneously especially with low-grade forms
Primary haemopoietic neoplasms, e.g. lymphoma (see above), leukaemias, plasma cell myeloma and systemic or malignant histiocytosis	These primary bone marrow disorders may result in secondary infiltration of lymph nodes with neoplastic cells and mild generalized peripheral lymphadenopathy
Metastatic neoplasia	Often one lymph node involved which may become 'fixed' to surrounding tissues
Vaccination	Mild transient generalized lymphadenopathy may occur after vaccination

or all peripheral and internal lymph nodes. With lymphoma, the lymph nodes are often extremely large, firm but non-painful. Lymph node size may fluctuate spontaneously especially with the rarer low-grade forms of the disease.

INVESTIGATION OF LYMPHADENOPATHY

HISTORY CHECKLIST

❏ **Age?**
Lymphoma is a more likely cause of generalized lymph node enlargement in animals more than 5–6 years of age.

❏ **History of recent travel or vaccination?**

❏ **Size of node and rate of growth?**
With lymphoma, lymph nodes tend to be much larger and increase in size quite rapidly.

❏ **With cats, has there been a history of fighting resulting in bite wounds/abscesses, recurrent lameness, episodes of pyrexia, etc?**
Localized abscessation is more likely to give rise to enlargement of a single node.

❏ **Is node painful and hot?**
If so, probably associated with infection.

❏ **Have any masses been removed previously from the skin or adjacent soft tissues?**
If so suspect tumour metastasis in the node.

❏ **Has animal shown signs of systemic illness, e.g. anorexia, weight loss, lethargy, pyrexia, vomiting, diarrhoea, polydipsia, polyuria?**
In this context it is worth noting that many dogs with multicentric lymphoma appear quite bright on initial presentation.

PHYSICAL EXAMINATION

When examining a young cat or dog the lymph nodes may appear more prominent than they do in older animals because they are not obscured by large amounts of body fat. Having established a lymph node is increased in size an attempt should be made to record the size of the node(s) as accurately as possible with a pair of calipers. If an isolated lymph node is involved repeated examinations are essential to ensure that other nodes in the lymphatic chain do not become involved. The consistency of the node should be recorded together with the presence of any pain. When one or more lymph nodes are enlarged, the overlying skin and adjacent soft tissues and/or bony structures which drain to the affected node should be examined for the presence of an inflammatory or neoplastic lesion. With infection there may be heat, tenderness and erythema of the overlying skin or possibly even abscess formation involving the soft tissues adjacent to the node. Lymph nodes which contain metastatic tumour deposits are also often firm, warm and painful and may be 'fixed' to underlying tissues. Palpation of the node may reveal 'cording' or thickening of efferent lymphatic vessels suggesting lymphatic spread of a tumour. In contrast, with lymphoma, although the nodes may be extremely large and firm they are usually mobile and non-painful. Occasionally a large lymphomatous lymph node is associated with lymphoedema of the surrounding soft tissues resulting from partial obstruction of lymphatic drainage. Massively enlarged submandibular or tracheobronchial lymph nodes may result in stertorous respiration or dyspnoea. A full physical examination of an animal with generalized lymphadenopathy should include careful palpation of the abdomen for evidence of splenic and/or hepatic enlargement. A rectal examination should be performed to check for the presence of enlarged sublumbar lymph nodes.

INITIAL DIAGNOSTIC PLAN

Fine needle lymph node aspirate

Fine needle aspiration (FNA) is simple, inexpensive and easy to perform and is a technique which may be used to obtain cells for cytological examination from any soft tissue mass. Fine needle aspiration of an enlarged lymph node in most cases will differentiate lymphoid hyperplasia, i.e. a reactive node from one which is lymphomatous or contains metastatic tumour deposits. Lymph node cytology may detect a specific infection such as leishmaniasis, toxoplasmosis or infection with *Mycobacteria* spp.

An aspirate should always be taken before treatment commences since corticosteroids and cytotoxic therapy may considerably alter cellular morphology. During microscopic examination of the smear, the slide should always be scanned under low power magnification first in order to detect small focal clusters of metastatic tumour cells with different morphology and staining characteristics.

Technique for fine needle aspiration of a lymph node (see Chapter 50)

1. Clip and surgically prepare the skin over the lymph node.
2. Immobilize the mass between thumb and forefinger (if the node can be immobilized by an assistant, both hands are freed to aspirate).
3. Introduce the needle (usually one inch × 21 guage) with the syringe attached and direct it towards the centre of the lymph node. Alternatively, the needle can be inserted separately and the syringe attached afterwards
4. Apply strong negative pressure by withdrawing the plunger one half to threequarters the volume of the syringe. Then redirect the needle and repeat the aspiration procedure taking care not to withdraw the needle from the mass when redirecting.
5. Maintain slight negative pressure and withdraw the needle quickly from the mass.
6. Remove the needle and draw air into the syringe.
7. Replace the needle and forcefully expel the aspirated contents onto a clean glass slide; always prepare several smears in case special stains are required. A suitable technique for preparing a smear is illustrated in Fig. 20.1. The smearing technique requires practice since lymphoid cells are easily smudged or distorted by excessive pressure during spreading (Fig. 20.2).

Lymph node cytology

A fine needle aspirate taken from a normal lymph node consists primarily of small and medium-sized lymphocytes, a smaller number of lymphoblasts (usually less than 15%), a few plasma cells and the occasional macrophage. The cytological appearance varies depending on the patho-

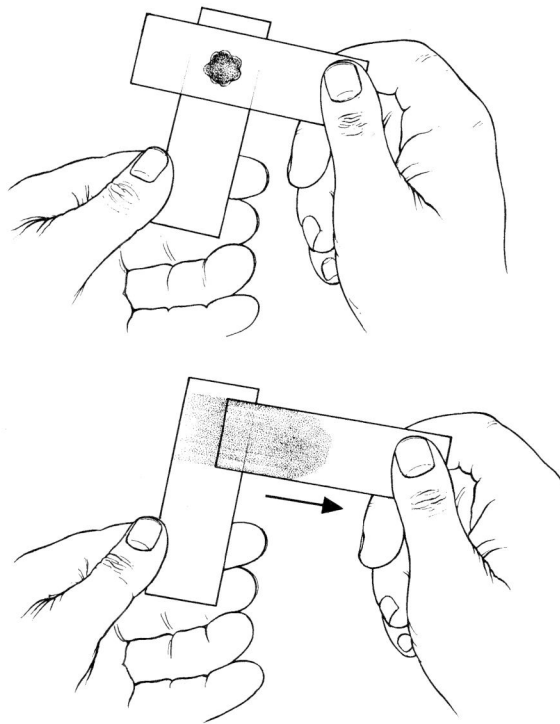

Figure 20.1 Lymph node aspiration: preparing a smear for cytological examination.

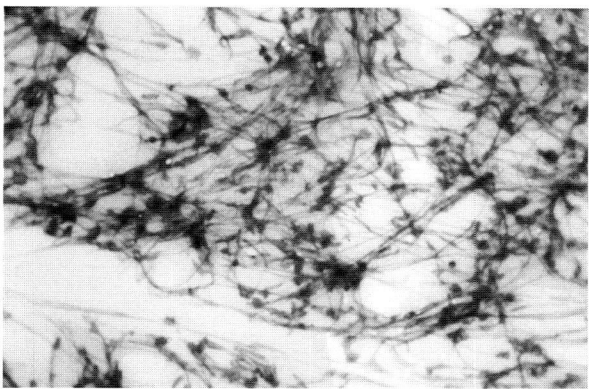

Figure 20.2 A non-diagnostic lymph node aspirate. Poor technique during smear preparation has resulted in severe cellular and nuclear disruption. (May–Grünwald Giemsa; original magnification ×125.) See colour plate.

logical process responsible for the lymph node enlargement.

Acute suppurative lymphadenitis is characterized by increased numbers of neutrophils showing moderate to severe degenerative changes. Large neoplastic lymph nodes may undergo similar central inflammatory or necrotic changes which may obscure the underlying neoplastic process (Fig. 20.3). There may also be increased numbers of reactive macrophages, lymphocytes and plasma cells. Increased numbers of macrophages are a feature of *granulomatous* or *pyogranulomatous responses* associated with fungal agents and intracellular bacteria (e.g. *Mycobacterium* spp., *Nocardia* spp.). Occasionally bacteria are present in neutrophils or macrophages.

Lymphoid hyperplasia indicates a more chronic response to non-infectious antigenic stimuli (e.g. inflammatory mediators or antigen–antibody complexes). Lymphoid hyperplasia is characterized by a predominance of small and medium-sized lymphocytes with a variable number of lymphoblasts and plasma cells (the number reflecting the degree of antigenic stimulation).

The larger more reactive lymphocytes typically show marked chromatin clumping (Fig. 20.4a). There may also be increased numbers of neutrophils, macrophages, mast cells and eosinophils in reactive lymph nodes (Fig. 20.4b). Submandibular lymph node aspirates taken from animals with dental disease/gingivitis frequently contain significant numbers of neutrophils and macrophages. Aspirates taken from the lymph nodes of cats with flea bite allergic dermatitis or hypereosinophilic syndrome contain increased numbers of eosinophils.

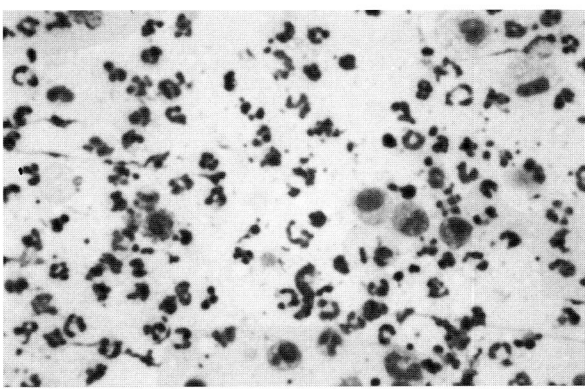

Figure 20.3 Fine-needle aspirate taken from the necrotic centre of an enlarged submandibular lymph node. This aspirate consisted of a large number of degenerate neutrophils and fewer macrophages. There was no clear indication that this node was neoplastic although subsequent histopathological examination showed that this was the case (lymphoma). (May–Grünwald Giemsa; ×50.) See colour plate.

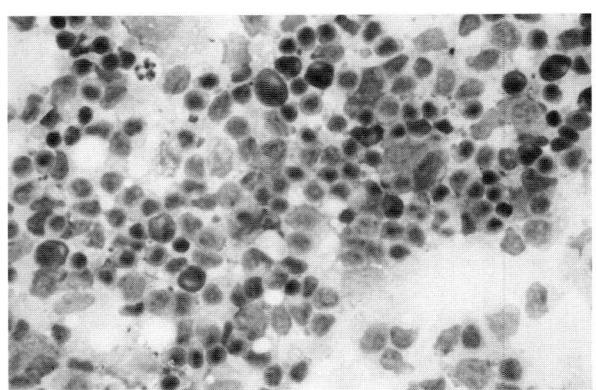

Figure 20.4 (a) Fine needle aspirate of a reactive lymph node showing lymphoid hyperplasia. The aspirate is moderately haemodiluted. The nucleated cells, present with the exception of the single neutrophil, are small or medium-sized lymphocytes showing clumping of nuclear chromatin. (b) Fine needle aspirate of a lymph node from a dog with immune-mediated polyarthritis. This consists of a mixed population of small and medium-sized lymphocytes, plasma cells, neutrophils and macrophages. The number of lymphoblasts comprised less than 10% of the nucleated cells counted. The increased number of plasma cells present suggests a degree of antigenic stimulation. (May–Grünwald Giemsa, (a) ×250; (b) ×50.) See colour plate.

With *lymphoma* the normal cell population is replaced by a monomorphic population of lymphoblasts showing varying degrees of cellular, nuclear and nucleolar pleomorphism (Fig. 20.5). Lymphomas may be classified on a cytological basis as low, intermediate or high grade tumours. Classification of cell type requires careful attention to nuclear size and shape, nucleolar size, shape and number, chromatin pattern and mitotic rate. The size of the lymphocyte nuclei compared to the size of a red blood cell acts as a useful guide in determining cell size. The nucleus of a mature small lymphocyte is approximately equal in diameter to a red blood cell (RBC). The criteria used in the National Cancer Institute Working Formulation classification system are given in Table 20.2.

Tumour metastases may be focal or, in some cases, so extensive that the normal population of cells is replaced by sheets or large clusters of neoplastic cells. Focal tumour deposits are often associated with a concurrent inflammatory response and/or lymphoid hyperplasia (Fig. 20.6).

Full haematological examination

This should include a reticulocyte count (if anaemic) and a platelet count. The blood film should be checked for the presence of neoplastic lymphoid cells or lymphocytes with atypical morphology. Many cases of lymphoma, including some in which bone marrow aspiration cytology confirms marrow involvement, may have normal haematology. Animals with a more severe, diffuse infiltrate may present with one or more cytopenias. Infectious or inflammatory/immune-mediated disease may result in a neutrophilic leucocytosis and a high plasma fibrinogen concentration. Septicaemia and bacteraemia may cause neutropenia and a degenerative left shift; lymphopenia is a common feature of the acute phase of most viral infections. Animals with lym-

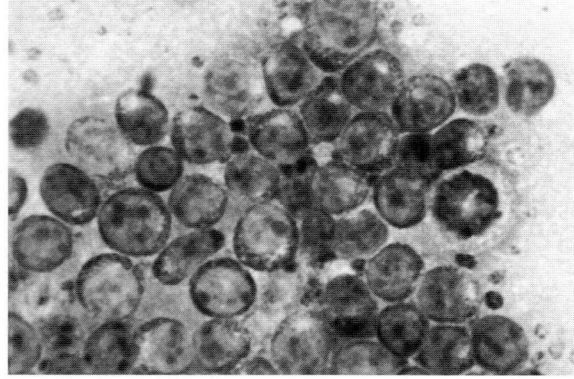

Figure 20.5 Fine needle aspirate of the submandibular lymph node of a dog showing unequivocal evidence of lymphoid malignancy (lymphoma). A monomorphic population of pleomorphic lymphoblasts is present. Note the extreme variation in nucleolar size, shape and number. The cytology in this case is consistent with a diagnosis of lymphoblastic lymphoma. (May–Grünwald Giemsa ×250.) See colour plate.

Table 20.2 Cytological classification of lymphoma

Grade of tumour	Comments
Low grade	
Diffuse small lymphocytic	Cells indistinguishable from benign small lymphocytes; mitotic rate is low; nuclei approximately one RBC in diameter; uniform chromatin pattern with one small nucleolus; most are B cell tumours; respond poorly to chemotherapy but overall survival is better than average.
Follicular (small cleaved or mixed)	Follicular forms are rare in the dog
Intermediate grade	
Follicular large	Difficult to diagnose on a cytological basis; cells similar in appearance to those of the diffuse large non-cleaved form, i.e. large nuclei at least $2 \times$ RBC in diameter with multiple nucleoli; high mitotic rate.
Diffuse small cleaved	Low mitotic rate; nuclei less than one RBC in diameter; dense staining nuclei (may obscure linear clefts); coarse, condensed chromatin pattern with one small nucleolus; B and T cell phenotypes; prognosis not established.
Diffuse mixed	Occasional mitotic figure; population of small cleaved cells with a minority of large cells; difficult to differentiate from benign hyperplasia but with diffuse mixed lymphoma usually only two cell types
Diffuse large non-cleaved	High mitotic rate; nuclei 1.5–2.0 times larger than an RBC in diameter; nuclei round/ovoid with uniform to cribriform chromatin pattern and multiple large, pale nucleoli; cytoplasm pale staining and easily ruptured; prognosis average to good; most are B cell tumours.
High grade	
Immunoblastic	High mitotic rate; nuclei vary in size (usually about $1.5 \times$ RBC in diameter); nuclei round/ovoid with cribriform chromatin pattern; single or occasionally two very large prominent central nucleoli; moderate to abundant basophilic cytoplasm with clear Golgi zone; almost all are B cell tumours; prognosis average (approximately 20% survive one year with standard chemotherapy).
Lymphoblastic	Mitotic rate may be extremely high; convoluted (common) or non-convoluted (rare) forms; nuclei about $1.0–1.5 \times$ RBC in diameter; homogenous chromatin pattern may obscure several small nucleoli; irregular undulating nuclear outline; 'cap' of cytoplasm; associated with mediastinal masses and hypercalcaemia; almost all are T cell tumours; prognosis poor (only 5% survive one year).
Diffuse small cleaved	High mitotic rate; round/ovoid nuclei approximately $1.5 \times$ RBC in diameter and slightly irregular in outline; cribriform chromatin pattern with multiple prominent small to large nucleoli; variable amount of basophilic cytoplasm; most are B cell tumours; prognosis average.

RBC, red blood cell.

phoma or any neoplastic or chronic debilitating disease process, be it infectious or inflammatory, frequently have a mild non-regenerative anaemia.

■ Full biochemistry screen

Pronounced generalized lymphadenopathy warrants a full biochemistry screen, to include urea, creatinine, liver enzymes (alanine aminotransferase, alkaline phosphatase and gamma-glutamyl transferase), calcium, albumin and albumin:globulin ratio. Animals with multicentric lymphoma not infrequently are hypercalcaemic which may affect renal function. Liver enzymes may be increased in cases where the liver is infiltrated (in these cases, bile salts should be assayed to assess liver function).

■ Urinalysis

Urinalysis should be performed to assess renal function in all animals with lymphoma especially those which are hypercalcaemic. Urine should also be checked before commencing chemotherapy since many cytotoxic drugs are eliminated via the kidneys.

■ Radiography

Lateral screening radiographs of the thorax and abdomen are indicated unless the enlarged lymph node is unequivocally the result of a localized acute inflammatory process. In cases of lymphoma, particularly if there is evidence of multicentric involvement, thoracic radiographs may confirm involvement of the intrathoracic (sternal, mediastinal and tracheobronchial) lymph nodes or evidence of pulmonary metastases (thoracic radiographs should be taken in any animal with documented evidence of malignancy to rule out the possibility of pulmonary metastases). Abdominal radiographs may be helpful in confirming the presence of enlarged intra-abdominal (sublumbar/iliac and possibly mesenteric) lymph nodes and hepatosplenomegaly. Fine needle aspirates may be obtained from large masses or organs (e.g.

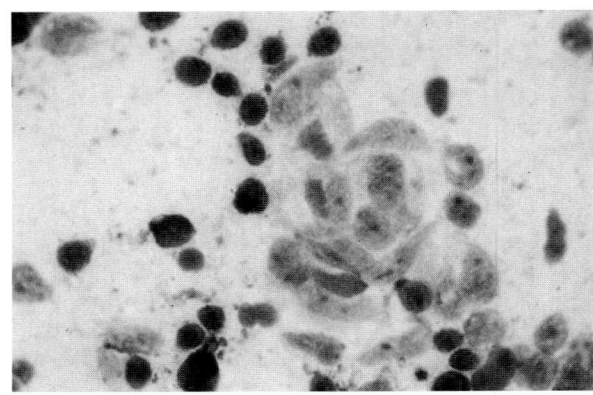

Figure 20.6 Fine needle aspirate of a submandibular lymph node showing a central cluster of non-lymphoid, spindle-shaped cells. These cells represented a metastatic tumour deposit from a fibrosarcoma. (May–Grünwald Giemsa ×250.) See colour plate.

lymph nodes, spleen or liver) under ultrasound guidance for cytological examination.

■ Feline leukaemia virus and feline immunodeficiency virus assays

■ Lymph node biopsy

If the results of the fine needle aspirate are equivocal a lymph node biopsy or preferably an excised intact lymph node should be submitted for histopathological examination. Having excised the node an impression smear for cytological examination can be made from the cut surface. Excision of the lymph node is also justified in cases of solitary lymphoma.

■ Bone marrow aspiration and/or biopsy

Since multicentric lymphoma may involve the bone marrow, a bone marrow aspirate is indicated particularly if leukaemic cells, atypical lymphocytes or other haematological abnormalities are present. Animals with lymphoma which have normal haematological results may nevertheless have marrow involvement. It is also worth noting that *primary* bone marrow disorders, e.g. the acute and chronic leukaemias, may result in secondary infiltration of peripheral lymph nodes with neoplastic cells.

Lymphangiography

This contrast technique involves cannulation of a peripheral lymphatic vessel in an anaesthetized animal. It is used to evaluate the presence or absence of lymphatic vessels, lymph flow and lymph node function.

Lymphoscintigraphy

This non-invasive technique is limited to a few referral centres and involves the use of radionuclides to image regional lymph node drainage patterns. General anaesthesia is not required. The procedure is useful for demonstrating obstructive lymphatic disease.

MANAGEMENT OF LYMPHADENOPATHY

The management of the various causes of lymph node enlargement depends on the cause. The treatment of lymphoma and leukaemias is covered in Chapter 50. When an infectious cause is suspected appropriate antibiotic therapy should be instituted. The management of an enlarged node containing metastatic tumour deposits will depend on the extent of spread of the primary tumour and the degree of malignancy. Treatment options include chemotherapy, radiotherapy and surgery.

21

Abnormal Haemostasis

J. K. Dunn

Normal haemostasis involves the interaction of vessel wall, platelets and coagulation factors. Vessel wall defects, decreased platelet numbers or abnormal platelet function, or a deficiency of one or more extrinsic or intrinsic coagulation factors may result in prolonged bleeding.

NORMAL HAEMOSTASIS

Primary haemostasis

Trauma to the vessel wall causes reflex vasoconstriction and platelets adhere to the exposed collagen. During this adhesion process the platelets change shape and release several substances which are potent platelet aggregators such as adenosine diphosphate (ADP), serotonin, prostaglandin (thomboxane A_2), and platelet factors 3 and 4. Platelet aggregation then leads to formation of the primary platelet or haemostatic plug. Von Willebrand factor is required for normal platelet adherence and primary haemostasis.

Thromboxane A_2, synthesized in platelets via the arachidonic acid pathway, promotes platelet aggregation and is a potent vasoconstrictor. A similar prostaglandin (PGI_2) is synthesized in the vascular endothelium. PGI_2 is an inhibitor of platelet aggregation and relaxes vascular smooth muscle. The production of thromboxane A_2 and PGI_2 is finely balanced; vascular injury upsets the

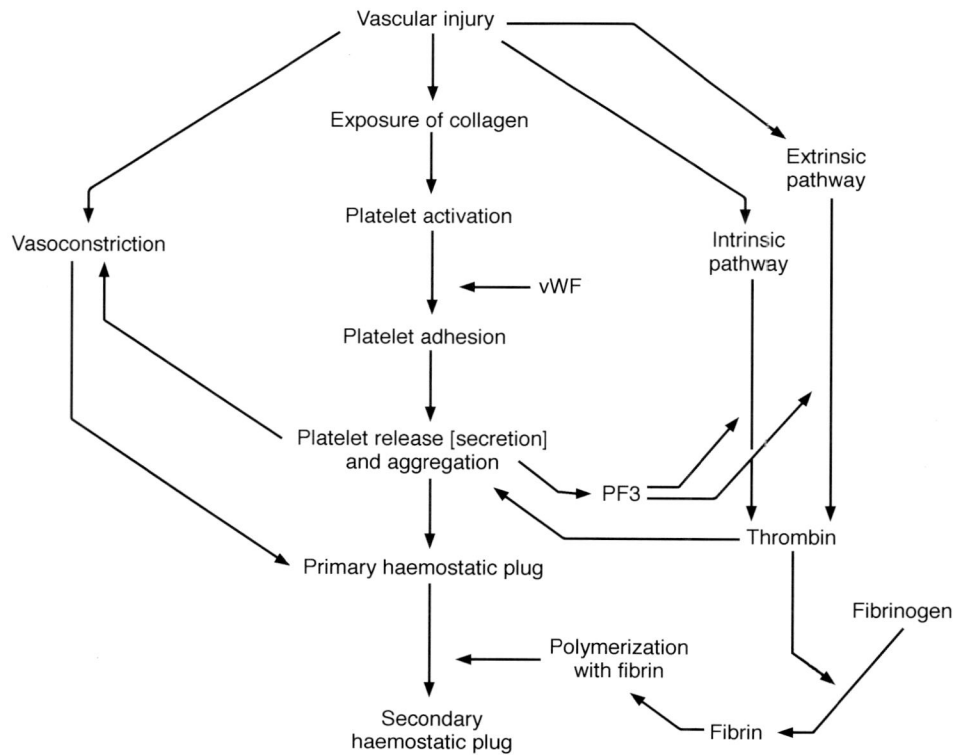

Figure 21.1 Simplified diagram of normal haemostasis. vWF, von Willebrand factor; PF3, platelet factor 3.

balance in favour of thromboxane leading to formation of the primary haemostatic plug. Certain non-steroidal analgesic drugs such as aspirin and phenylbutazone interfere with platelet secretion and aggregation by inhibiting the production of platelet thromboxane A_2.

Secondary haemostasis

Thrombin converts fibrinogen into fibrin monomer, and fibrin strands are incorporated into the primary platelet plug. Platelets become emeshed in a fibrin network resulting in stabilization of the platelet plug.

The series of events leading to formation of a stabilized platelet plug are outlined in Fig. 21.1.

Coagulation cascade

Platelet adherence and aggregation create favourable conditions for activation of the coagulation cascade. Coagulation factors are activated sequentially so that inactive precursors are converted into active enzymes or cofactors which activate the next factor in the sequence.

A simplified diagram of the coagulation pathways is shown in Fig. 21.2. The coagulation cascade classically is divided into intrinsic and extrinsic pathways which share a terminal common pathway. Most clotting factors (II, V, VII, IX and X) are synthesized in the liver.

The *extrinsic system* is activated by the release of tissue thromboplastin (factor III), a lipoprotein

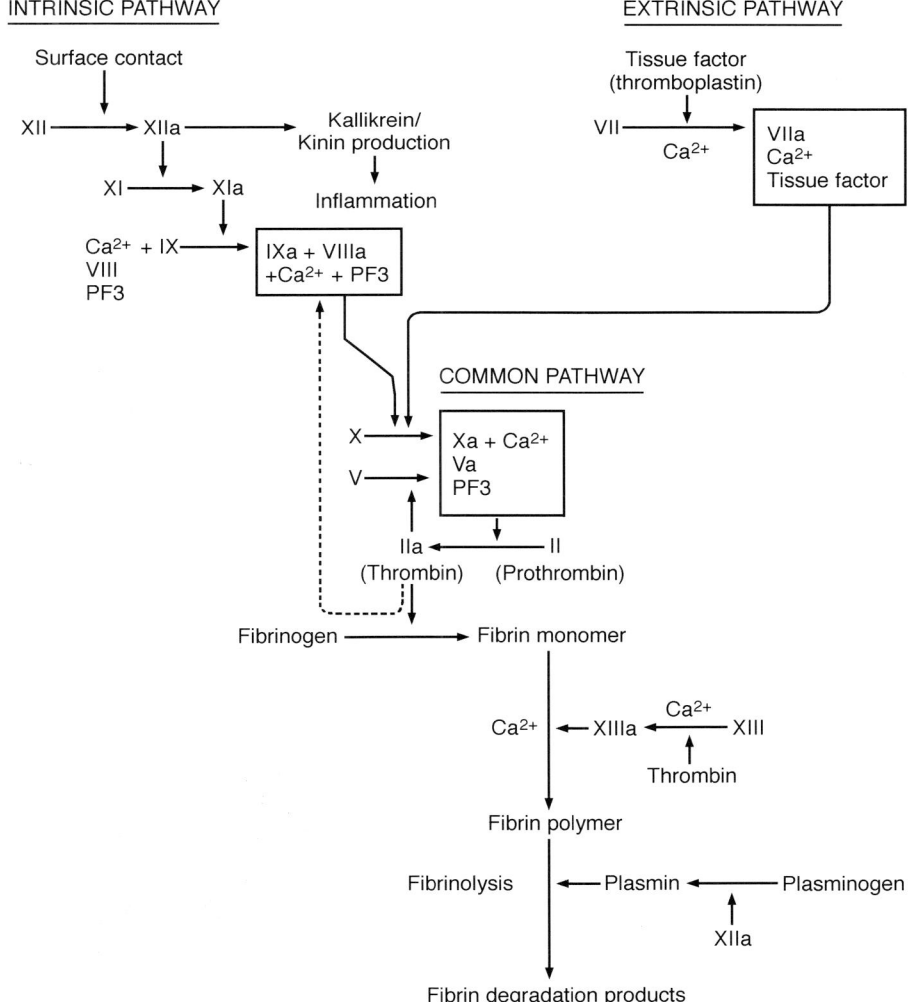

Figure 21.2 The intrinsic and extrinsic pathways of the coagulation cascade.

complex present on most cell membranes. The *intrinsic system* is activated by surface contact and involves the interaction of activated factor XII and high molecular weight kininogen which results in the production of kallikrein and kinin, two important mediators of inflammation. The *common pathway* involves the conversion of prothrombin (factor II) into thrombin (factor IIa). Thrombin converts fibrinogen into fibrin which stabilizes the primary platelet plug, and is also involved in the activation of factor XIII. The conversion of thrombin is controlled by naturally occurring inhibitors in plasma such as antithrombin III and protein C.

Fibrinolysis

Plasminogen is converted into plasmin under the action of factor XIIa, a process controlled by plasminogen activator inhibitors. The activation of plasmin results in degradation of the stabilized platelet plug and the production of fibrin degradation products. Activated factors and fibrin degradation products are cleared from the circulation by the liver. Excessive fibrinolytic activity leads to impaired secondary haemostasis and rebleeding from the site of injury.

Both the extrinsic and intrinsic systems interact *in vivo*. Many reactions take place on the surface of platelets and platelet factor 3 (PF3) is required for the conversion of factor X and prothrombin into factor Xa and thrombin, respectively. Calcium ions are essential for several reactions including the activation of prothrombin.

Production and release of platelets

Megakaryocytes are derived from pluripotent stem cells in the bone marrow. The earliest recognizable megakaryocyte precursor cell is the *megakaryoblast*. The differentiation of colony forming units – megakaryoblast (CFU-Meg) to *promegakaryocytes* and finally to *megakaryocytes* is regulated initially by a specific megakaryocyte colony stimulating factor (Meg-CSF) and then by thrombopoietin. Platelets are produced by cytoplasmic fragmentation of mature megakaryocytes. The entire process of megakaryocyte differentiation and maturation takes approximately three days in the dog. The number of bone marrow megakaryocytes is regulated by the circulating platelet mass (the number of platelets × platelet volume). Hence thrombocytopenia caused by increased destruction or consumption of platelets is usually followed by megakaryocytic hyperplasia and a rebound thrombocytosis although there is a lag phase of approximately three days before increased platelet production is evident in the blood. The circulating lifespan of a platelet is approximately six days. Up to 20–30% of the circulating platelet mass can be sequestered in the normal spleen; with splenomegaly this figure may be as high as 90%. Senescent platelets are removed from the circulation by macrophages in the spleen, liver, bone marrow and lungs.

An adequate number of functional platelets is essential for normal haemostasis and clot retraction. Platelets interact with endothelial cells to help maintain vascular integrity. They provide platelet phospholipid (platelet factor 3) which plays an important role in the coagulation pathways. Platelets also release vasoactive amines and activate chemotactic substances which contribute to the inflammatory response. They also possess limited phagocytic and bactericidal properties.

INVESTIGATION OF ABNORMAL HAEMOSTASIS

Differences in clinical presentation may help differentiate hereditary (congenital) from acquired bleeding disorders. Haemostatic abnormalities may also be classified on a pathophysiological basis as (1) defects in vascular integrity, (2) platelet disorders (either thrombocytopenia or abnormal platelet function), and (3) deficiencies in one or more extrinsic or intrinsic clotting factors (Table 21.1).

HISTORY CHECKLIST

❑ Age, breed and sex?

Some inherited coagulopathies have a higher incidence in certain breeds, e.g. von Willebrand's disease is most common in Doberman pinschers, Scottish terriers, German shepherds, corgis and golden retrievers. A particularly severe form of haemophilia A occurs in German shepherds; the condition is sex-linked and affects males only, although females may be asymptomatic carriers. With severe inherited coagulation defects bleeding may occur at an early age; mild inherited defects may not be detected until early adulthood when an animal is subjected to elective surgery. Idiopathic

Table 21.1 Hereditary and acquired causes of abnormal haemostasis

Vascular abnormalities	
Congenital	Ehlers–Danlos syndrome
Acquired	Immune-complex vasculitis (systemic lupus erythematosus, rheumatoid arthritis, drug-induced); hyperadrenocorticism (prolonged bleeding and bruising after venepuncture)
Platelet disorders	
Thrombocytopenia	*Failure of platelet production* Primary bone marrow disease (e.g. lymphoproliferative disease, myeloproliferative disease, myelofibrosis); aplastic anaemia (e.g. oestrogen toxicity or hyperoestrogenism associated with a functional Sertoli cell tumour) Chemotherapy (cyclophosphamide, doxyrubicin) Thrombocytopenia associated with the production of macroplatelets in cavalier King Charles spaniel (affected animals rarely have bleeding episodes). *Premature platelet destruction* Immune-mediated thrombocytopenia: primary (idiopathic) or secondary, e.g. may occur in association with lymphoproliferative or myeloproliferative disease (occasionally solid tumours), immune-mediated haemolytic anaemia, systemic lupus erythematosus (SLE) and ehrlichiosis, or as a sequel to viral infection or live virus vaccination; occasionally drug-induced, e.g. an SLE-like syndrome has been reported following the administration of potentiated sulphonamides (sulphadiazine/trimethoprim combination) particularly in Dobermanns. *Excessive consumption of platelets* Disseminated intravascular coagulation Acute, severe haemorrhage (usually transient thrombocytopenia followed by a rebound thrombocytosis) Splenomegaly (sequestration of large numbers of platelets in an enlarged spleen)
Platelet dysfunction	
Congenital	Chediak–Higashi syndrome in cats Inherited thrombocytopathy in Otterhounds and Bassett hounds (North America)
Acquired	Drug-induced, e.g. non-steroidal anti-inflammatory drugs (may cause bleeding especially if given to an animal with a pre-existing bleeding disorder), plasma expanders, heparin Von Willebrand's disease Acute pancreatitis Severe uraemia Hypergammaglobulinaemia (e.g. plasma cell myeloma) Disseminated intravascular coagulation Ehrlichia canis infection Megakaryocytic leukaemia
Coagulation factor abnormalities	
Congenital	Von Willebrand's disease Haemophilia A (classic haemophilia due to factor VIII deficiency) Haemophilia B (Christmas disease or factor IX deficiency) Haemophilia C (factor XI deficiency) in dogs Hypoprothrombinaemia (boxers) Factor VII deficiency Factor X deficiency (cocker spaniels) Factor XII deficiency (cats) Multifactorial coagulopathy in Devon rex cats
Acquired	Vitamin K antagonism (poisoning with anticoagulant rodenticides such as warfarin and related hydroxycoumarin derivatives) Severe diffuse liver disease Disseminated intravascular coagulation (may be triggered by endotoxaemia, disseminated neoplasia, liver disease, heat stroke, acute pancreatitis, acute viral infections, dirofilariasis, severe trauma)

immune-mediated thrombocytopenia is more common in young to middle-aged females, and toy poodles, cocker spaniels and Doberman pinschers appear to be over-represented.

❏ **Previous episodes of haemorrhage and if so at what age did they occur?**
Acquired bleeding disorders tend to manifest in older animals with no previous history of recurrent bleeding episodes.

❏ **Haemorrhage?**
Haemorrhage may be spontaneous or precipitated by trauma, surgery (e.g. ovariohysterectomy, castration or dew claw removal), loss of deciduous teeth or onset of pro-oestrus. The severity and extent of haemorrhage is dependent on the nature of the bleeding defect (vascular abnormality, platelet disorder or coagulation factor deficiency) and reflects the severity of the abnormality present. For example haemophilia A may affect dogs with varying degrees of severity. Severely affected animals with less than 1% normal factor VIII levels bleed spontaneously at an early age and many fail to reach adulthood.

❏ **Bleeding in related animals or littermates?**

❏ **Drug administration (e.g. non-steroidal anti-inflammatory drugs, oestrogens) or exposure to toxins (e.g. anticoagulant rodenticides such as warfarin and related derivatives)?**

❏ **Signs of concurrent systemic disease?**
Presence of systemic signs may reflect an underlying disease and suggests that the bleeding tendency is acquired.

❏ **Type of haemorrhage (see physical examination below)?**

 PHYSICAL EXAMINATION

❏ **Type of haemorrhage?**
Platelet and vascular abnormalities result in capillary bleeding due to impaired formation of the primary platelet plug at the site of vascular injury. Capillary bleeding is characterized by multifocal pinpoint (petechial) or larger ecchymotic haemorrhages most commonly on the skin, mucosal surfaces and sclerae. An examination of the mucosal surfaces should include the gums, conjunctivae and external genitalia. The ventral abdomen and inguinal region should be examined closely for evidence of petechial or ecchymotic haemorrhages since the skin in these areas is thinner and more susceptible to trauma. Melaena, epistaxis, haematuria, haematemesis and intraocular or retinal haemorrhage are common manifestations of severe thrombocytopenia or functional platelet defects. Coagulation factor abnormalities more commonly give rise to subcutaneous or intramuscular haematomata, intra-articular haemorrhage or haemorrhage into a body cavity.

❏ **Pale mucous membranes and/or signs of hypovolaemic shock?**

❏ **Lameness (haemarthrosis), abdominal pain (intra-abdominal haemorrhage) or dyspnoea (pulmonary or intrathoracic haemorrhage)?**

Laboratory investigation of haemostasis

The laboratory investigation of haemostasis should be preceded by a full routine haematological examination and biochemical screen. The tests which follow can be divided into two categories: (1) a series of preliminary screening tests designed to evaluate the extrinsic, intrinsic and common pathways of the coagulation cascade and (2) specific factor assays and tests to evaluate platelet function. Common causes of abnormal haemostatic screening tests are given in Table 21.2.

Sample collection

Blood should be collected using plastic syringes and specimen tubes. Samples for routine haematological examination (including a platelet count) should be collected into EDTA; sodium citrate (nine volumes of blood mixed with one volume of 3.8% sodium citrate) is the preferred anticoagulant for measuring one stage prothrombin and activated partial thromboplastin times and specific factor assays.

Screening tests

❏ **Bleeding time**
The bleeding time is a screening test for vascular and platelet disorders since it measures the time to formation of the primary haemostatic plug. Common causes of prolonged bleeding time (vascular abnormalities, thrombocytopenia and platelet function disorders) are listed in Table

Table 21.2 Screening tests for haemostasis: common causes of abnormal results

Abnormal screening test	Possible causes
Increased bleeding time	Vascular abnormalities Platelet disorders, e.g. thrombocytopenia and functional platelet defects (see Table 21.1 for specific causes) Von Willebrand's disease
Increased whole blood clotting time (or activated whole blood clotting time)	Intrinsic factor deficiency, e.g haemophilia A or haemophilia B Warfarin toxicity Severe liver disease Disseminated intravascular coagulation Severe thrombocytopenia
Increased one-stage prothrombin time (OSPT)	Warfarin toxicity resulting in vitamin K antagonism (increase in OSPT precedes increase in APTT due to short half-life of factor VII) Dietary deficiency or inadequate absorption of vitamin K (rare; latter may occur with post-hepatic obstruction leading to biliary stasis) Severe liver disease Disseminated intravascular coagulation Prothrombin deficiency
Increased activated partial thromboplastin time (APTT)	Deficiency of one or more of the intrinsic factors, e.g factor VIII (haemophilia A), IX (haemophilia B), XI (haemophilia C) and XII Deficiency of a common pathway factor, e.g. factor II (prothrombin) or factor X (Stuart factor deficiency) will cause increase in OSPT and APTT Warfarin poisoning Severe liver disease Disseminated intravascular coagulation
Increased thrombin time	Hypofibrinogenaemia (chronic liver disease or disseminated intravascular coagulation) Circulating heparin

OSPT, one-stage prothrombin time; APTT, activated partial thromboplastin time.

21.1. Disposable spring-loaded devices are available which make two standardized incisions on the inside of the upper lip (see Chapter 45). Blood oozing from the edges of the incisions is gently blotted with a piece of filter paper taking care not to touch the incision itself. A normal bleeding time should be less than 4 minutes (prolonged by aspirin, phenylbutazone and other non-steroidal anti-inflammatory drugs). A modification of the procedure described above is the *cuticle bleeding time*. This technique, which involves clipping the cuticle of a toe nail under light anaesthesia, has been advocated as a presurgical screening test for von Willebrands disease.

❏ Whole blood clotting time and activated clotting time

The whole blood clotting time (WBCT) (Lee–White method) measures the time taken for 1 ml of whole blood to clot in a prewarmed glass tube at 37°C. After 2–3 min the tube should be gently tilted every 30 s until a clot forms. The test should be performed in triplicate taking the mean of the three values. A normal value for the dog is 6.1±0.2 min (Osbaldiston *et al.*, 1970). The WBCT is a simple albeit insensitive test which detects severe deficiencies of one or more of the intrinsic coagulation factors (Table 21.2). Prolongation of the WBCT occurs with warfarin poisoning or haemophilia A. WBCT may also increase with severe thrombocytopenia. The *activated clotting time* (ACT) is a modification of the WBCT. The ACT is the time required for fibrin clot formation when blood is added to a commercially prepared tube containing a substance that potentiates surface activation. The ACT is more sensitive than the WBCT and detects defects in the intrinsic and common pathways. A factor must be less than 5% of normal to prolong the ACT thus making this a less sensitive test than the activated partial thromboplastin time (see below). Like the WBCT the ACT is prolonged with severe thrombocytopenia. Normal ACT in the dog and cat varies between 60 and 90 s.

❑ **Clot retraction**

A fibrin clot should normally retract 50% in 1–2 h. Poor clot retraction, when the serum fails to separate from the clot, is indicative of thrombocytopenia or abnormal platelet function.

❑ **Platelet count**

Platelet counts should be performed within 4 h; when this is not possible a quick semiquantitative assessment of platelet numbers can be made by examination of a Romanowsky-stained air-dried blood film. Under high-power (×100) magnification platelet numbers can be estimated as shown in Table 21.3.

Normal platelet numbers in the dog and cat are approximately $175–400 \times 10^9$ l^{-1}. Spontaneous haemorrhage rarely occurs with platelet counts greater than 50×10^9 l^{-1}. The presence of large platelets, for example following acute haemorrhage, may be associated with a rebound thrombocytosis and generally indicates active thrombopoiesis. A decrease in mean platelet volume has been noted during the early stages of immune-mediated thrombocytopenia; the presence of larger platelets during the later stages of the disease correlates with increased platelet production. Thrombocytopenia has been documented in otherwise healthy cavalier King Charles spaniels. Affected animals rarely bleed spontaneously even with platelet counts less than 50×10^9 l^{-1}. Electronic platelet counts are artificially low because the platelets are extremely large and are counted as small red cells. Platelet counts from cavalier King Charles spaniels should therefore always be checked manually.

Blood (collected in EDTA) from thrombocytopenic patients may be checked for the presence of *antiplatelet antibodies* using a direct fluorescent antibody technique on a peripheral blood smear (a similar technique has been described using a bone marrow smear to check for the presence of antimegakaryocyte antibodies; Joshi and Jain, 1976). An ELISA test has also been developed to detect circulating antiplatelet antibodies (Campbell et al., 1984) and an indirect fluorescent antibody test to detect antiplatelet antibodies in plasma has been described (Kristensen et al., 1994). A *bone marrow aspirate* should be considered if a primary bone marrow disorder is suspected, if the results of immunological screening tests are equivocal or if immune-mediated thrombocytopenia fails to respond to conventional immunosuppresssive therapy. Causes of thrombocytopenia are listed in Table 21.1.

❑ **The one-stage prothrombin and activated partial thromboplastin times**

Both the one-stage prothrombin time (OSPT) and activated partial thromboplastin time (APTT) should be performed using citrated plasma. Plasma should be separated immediately and frozen in several aliquots at –20°C. Failure to do so may result in depletion of coagulation factors and erroneous results. Both tests should be performed in duplicate using plasma from a healthy dog as a control sample.

The OSPT is the principal test for evaluating the extrinsic and common pathways. Plasma is incubated with tissue thromboplastin and clotting is initiated by the addition of calcium. The OSPT is prolonged by deficiencies of factors V, VII, X, prothrombin and fibrinogen. Prolongation of more than 3 s over the control value (normal approximately 7–10 s) is suggestive of an extrinsic defect. The OSPT is consistently prolonged with warfarin toxicity (OSPT increases before APTT due to the early depletion of factor VII; Table 21.2).

The APTT, sometimes referred to as the kaolin–cephalin clotting time, evaluates the intrinsic and common pathways. Plasma is activated under controlled conditions in the presence of phospholipid and then clotting is initiated by the addition of calcium. An increase of more than 5–7 s over the control time (normal approximately 15–25 s) is generally considered abnormal. Prolongation of APTT occurs only with a severe deficiency of a single factor (factor at least 30% of normal values). The APTT is not affected by severe thrombocytopenia (Table 21.2).

❑ **Thrombin time**

The thrombin time (TT) is the time taken for the fibrin clot to form following the addition of bovine thrombin to citrated plasma, i.e. it measures the speed of conversion of fibrinogen into fibrin and therefore evaluates the common pathway. Prolongation of the TT occurs with hypofibrinogenaemia, increased circulating fibrin

Table 21.3 Estimation of platelet numbers from a blood film

Platelets per high power field	Platelet count ($\times 10^9$ l^{-1})
>20	450
5–7	150
3–4	100
0–2	50
Occasional	15

degradation products (e.g. with disseminated intravascular coagulation), or if circulating heparin is present (Table 21.2).

❏ Russell's viper venom time

The Russell's viper venom time (RVVT) is a rarely used test which measures the activity of the common pathway clotting factors (factors V, X, prothrombin and fibrinogen). The Russell's viper venom acts as an intrinsic thromboplastin and the test is useful for defining deficiencies of factor X. The RVVT is dependent on the release of phospholipid from platelets in test plasma and is therefore also prolonged with thrombocytopenia. It is also a crude test of platelet function. Normal RVVT is 10–14 s.

❏ Fibrinogen

Fibrinogen can be assayed directly by spinning two haematocrit tubes filled with blood (collected in EDTA) for 5 min. The total protein content of the plasma from one of the tubes is measured with a hand refractometer. The second tube is placed in a water bath at 56°C to precipitate the fibrinogen and the total protein content is measured after recentrifugation. The difference in total protein values equals the fibrinogen concentration. Hypofibrinogenaemia occurs with severe chronic liver disease and disseminated intravascular coagulation.

❏ Fibrinogen (fibrin) degadation products

Commercial test kits are available to evaluate the fibrinolytic system. These use latex particles coated with antibodies against human fibrin degradation products (FDPs). Blood is collected into a special tube which contains thrombin, to clot the sample, and an inhibitor of fibrinolysis to prevent further fibrin breakdown. The most common cause of increased FDPs is disseminated intravascular coagulation (DIC). In severe cases of DIC with extremely low plasma fibrinogen concentrations blood may fail to clot in the collection tube and this may be regarded as a poor prognostic indicator. An FDP concentration >40 µg ml^{-1} is the maximum value that can be measured using a 1:20 dilution of serum (normal FDP concentration <4 µg ml^{-1}).

Specific factor assays

Specific factor assays are generally performed using citrated plasma. Assays are available for factor VIII and the concentration of von Willebrand factor antigen can be measured by immunoelectrophoresis. Dogs with haemophilia A have low levels of factor VIII. The concentration of factor VIII varies in affected males (<1% of normal if severe). Carrier females have factor VIII levels between 50 and 60% and normal or increased von Willebrand factor levels. Dogs with von Willebrand's disease have low (<50% of normal) levels of von Willebrand antigen and factor VIII concentrations are usually also decreased.

Platelet function tests

Platelet aggregometry assesses the *in vitro* ability of platelets to aggregate in response to various chemical stimuli (ADP, serotonin, collagen and arachidonic acid). Certain drugs, most notably non-steroidal drugs such as aspirin and phenylbutazone, significantly impair platelet aggregation and prolong bleeding time.

MANAGEMENT

Management of specific bleeding disorders is covered in Chapter 45.

REFERENCES

Campbell, K.C. et al. (1984). Application of the enzyme-linked immunosorbent assay for the detection of platelet antibodies in dogs. *American Journal of Veterinary Research* 45, 2561–2564.

Joshi, B.C. and Jain, N.C. (1976). Detection of antiplatelet antibody in serum and on megakaryocytes of dogs with autoimmune thrombocytopenia. *American Journal of Veterinary Research* 37, 681–685.

Kristensen, A.T. et al. (1994). Detection of antiplatelet antibody with a platelet immunofluorescence assay. *Journal of Veterinary Internal Medicine* 8, 36–39.

Osbaldiston, G.D. et al. (1970). Blood coagulation: Comparative studies in dogs, cats, horses and cattle. *British Veterinary Journal* 126, 512-521.

22

Urinary Incontinence and Abnormal Micturition

S. P. Gregory

Micturition (urination) is the process whereby the bladder is emptied of urine via the urethra. This process is usually a conscious act which, in the normal adult animal, is under voluntary control. Abnormalities of micturition include: difficulty passing urine, painful urination, passing an abnormal stream, urinary frequency and urgency. Terms which are commonly used to describe abnormal micturition are:

- *Dysuria* – difficult or painful passage of urine;
- *Stranguria* – straining or hesitancy prior to or after urination;
- *Pollakiuria* – increased frequency of urination;
- *Nocturia* – the urge or need to urinate at night.

Urinary incontinence is the involuntary passage of urine and may occur with or without abnormal micturition. *Enuresis* is the unconscious leakage of urine from a sleeping animal and should not be confused with nocturia.

It is common for stranguria and pollakiuria to accompany dysuria. In general dysuria indicates primary disease affecting the lower urinary tract, i.e. the bladder and urethra, although the upper urinary tract may be secondarily involved. Urinary incontinence usually also occurs as a result of abnormalities affecting the lower urinary tract although in some cases, e.g. ectopic ureter, an abnormality affecting the upper urinary tract may be present. Urinary incontinence may also be associated with some neurological diseases.

It is important when presented with an owner complaining that their animal has abnormal micturition and/or urinary incontinence to differentiate these problems from poor house training or behavioural abnormalities.

PATHOPHYSIOLOGY

In the normal animal urine produced by the kidneys is collected in the urinary bladder and stored until an appropriate time and place is found for urination. The bladder is composed of smooth muscle which is lined by urothelium. It is a hollow organ with good compliance, that is, it can store large volumes of urine with very little change in pressure. Bladder filling and emptying is regulated by the autonomic nervous system with the somatic and central nervous systems contributing to the overall control of micturition in the normal animal.

The urethra is confluent with the bladder and is also composed predominantly of smooth muscle with a urothelial lining. There is no discrete urethral sphincter and urethral closure is maintained by a combination of factors which include: resting smooth muscle tone, peri-urethral striated muscle tone and reflex activity, interlocking folds of urethral mucosa and the effect of intra-abdominal pressure acting concomitantly on the bladder neck and proximal urethra.

Normal urination is dependent on urethral patency and good co-ordination between sensory and motor components of the autonomic, somatic and central nervous systems. In the normal animal anatomical factors which are of particular importance in maintaining urinary continence are normal ureterovesical junctions, a urethra of 'normal length' for the size of the animal and an intra-abdominal bladder neck.

Bladder filling and urine storage are primarily controlled by the *sympathetic nervous system*. This is mediated by spinal segments (L1–L4 in the dog, L2–L5 in the cat) and the *hypogastric nerve*. Release of noradrenaline from postganglionic nerve fibres acts on β-adrenergic receptors within the detrusor muscle causing smooth muscle relaxation. Noradrenaline also acts on α-adrenergic receptors in the bladder neck and urethra resulting in smooth muscle contraction and increased outflow resistance.

The *parasympathetic nervous system* primarily controls bladder emptying, which is mediated via sacral segments (S1–S3) of the spinal cord and the *pelvic nerve*. Stretch receptors within the bladder wall detect bladder filling and impulses are sent via the pelvic nerve to the spinal cord. Local reflexes, which are modulated by the brain and spinal cord, cause acetylcholine release from postganglionic parasympathetic nerve endings. Muscarinic receptors in the detrusor muscle are stimulated resulting in bladder contraction.

The *somatic nervous system* is important in controlling peri-urethral striated muscle. It is mediated via sacral segments (S1–S3) of the spinal cord and the *pudendal nerve*. Striated muscle contraction raises urethral pressure and contributes to continence. The integrity of the central nervous system is very important as it allows the animal voluntarily to control urine storage and elimination and also provides fine tuning and co-ordination of the whole process.

In very general terms, abnormal micturition may occur as a result of abnormal anatomy causing abnormal function or abnormal function with no gross anatomical change. Possible causes of abnormal micturition are listed in Table 22.1. In practice, urinary tract infection, urolithiasis, prostatic disease, trauma and neoplasia are the commonest causes of abnormal micturition in dogs. In cats the commonest causes of abnormal

Table 22.1 Causes of abnormal micturition in dogs and cats

Abnormal function associated with anatomical abnormalities visible on radiographic and ultrasonographic investigations	Bladder	• neoplasia – benign, e.g. leiomyoma, or malignant, e.g. transitional call carcinoma • inflammatory lesions, e.g. polypoid cystitis or chronic cystitis → bladder wall thickening • calculi • foreign bodies, e.g. catheters • developmental lesions, e.g. urachal diverticulum, ureterocoele • trauma, e.g. bladder rupture, blood clot, sloughed tissue • bladder entrapment/displacement
	Urethra	• calculi/urethral plugs • neoplasia, benign or malignant, focal or diffuse • strictures • granulomatous urethritis • urethral tear/trauma • diverticula • compression by external structure, e.g. vaginal neoplasm or other pelvic masses
	Prostate	• benign prostatic hypertrophy • prostatitis (acute/chronic) • prostatic abscess • prostatic cysts (para/intraprostatic) • prostatic neoplasia • squamous metaplasia • prostatic calculi
Abnormal function with no evidence of anatomical abnormalities on radiographic and ultrasonographic investigations	Bladder	• urinary tract infection usually bacterial, rarely secondary to yeast, mycoplasma or parasitic infection • toxic cystitis, e.g. cyclophosphamide • idiopathic cystitis, e.g. FLUTD • bladder atony, e.g. following excessive stretch during urethral obstruction • detrusor instability • neurological disease
	Urethra	• reflex dysynergia • urethritis • neurological disease

FLUTD = feline lower urinary tract disease (previously FUS)

micturition are the spectrum of conditions seen in feline lower urinary tract disease (FLUTD) including idiopathic cystitis and urethritis with an unclear aetiology, and urinary tract/spinal trauma. Some potential causes listed in Table 22.1 are extremely rare, e.g. parasitic and fungal infections.

Urinary incontinence may also be the result of abnormal anatomy causing abnormal function, e.g. ectopic ureter, or abnormal function with no anatomical change, e.g. urethral sphincter mechanism incompetence. However, neurological disease is also a significant cause of incontinence in animals and so urinary incontinence is usually classified as being *neurogenic* or *non-neurogenic*. Potential causes of urinary incontinence are listed in Table 22.2.

In some animals abnormal micturition and urinary incontinence may co-exist. The commonest examples are conditions which cause partial obstruction to urine outflow, resulting in unconscious urine leakage when bladder pressure rises. This form of incontinence is termed *paradoxical* or *obstructive incontinence*. Another example of abnormal urination and urinary incontinence is *overflow incontinence* frequently seen in animals with neurological disease. These animals typically have large, easily expressible bladders but are unable to void unaided.

INVESTIGATION OF ABNORMAL URINATION AND URINARY INCONTINENCE

When presented with an animal with abnormal micturition/urinary incontinence a core investigation based on history, physical examination, routine laboratory tests, radiographic and ultrasonographic examinations can be followed in

Table 22.2 Causes of urinary incontinence in dogs and cats

Non-neurogenic urinary incontinence	Urinary incontinence associated with anatomical abnormalities visible on radiographic and ultrasonographic investigations	• ectopic ureter • pelvic bladder and short urethra associated with SMI (+/–vaginal abnormality in cats) • bladder hypoplasia • prostatic disease • intersexuality • bladder neoplasia • urethral obstructions • ureterovaginal fistula • vesicovaginal fistula • vaginal neoplasia • pelvic masses • perineal rupture • pervious urachus
	Urinary incontinence with no evidence of anatomical abnormalities on radiographic and ultrasonographic investigations	• SMI • cystitis • detrusor instability • bladder atony
Neurogenic urinary incontinence		Lesions may affect the brain, spinal cord, autonomic or peripheral nervous systems. Underlying causes of neurological disease are variable but important categories include: • trauma • tumour • degeneration • infection • congenital/developmental • other

SMI = urethral sphincter mechanism incompetence.

most cases with a good diagnostic return. In some cases, however, extra or more specialized investigations may also be required.

HISTORY CHECKLIST

❏ Age, breed and sex?
Abnormal micturition as a result of urinary tract neoplasia is uncommon in young animals. Prostatic disease and vaginal neoplasia which may interfere with urethral function are more common in entire animals, Urolithiasis may be associated with metabolic abnormalities in certain breeds of dog, e.g. urate calculi in the Dalmatian. The commonest cause of urinary incontinence in juvenile dogs is ureteral ectopia, whereas urethral sphincter mechanism incompetence is most common in neutered female, medium to large breed dogs.

❏ What is the owner's complaint?
During the consultation it is important to establish the owner's complaint as well as the animal's problem and confirm that they are the same. In cases of suspected abnormal micturition and urinary incontinence it is always important to consider that tenesmus, abnormal posturing, genital bleeding and apparent urine leakage may be caused by disease affecting the genital or lower gastrointestinal tracts.

❏ What is the duration of their complaint?
It is important to establish if the problem is acute or chronic. Acute urinary tract obstructions are commonly caused by calculi whereas gradually progressive dysuria is more commonly associated with neoplasia. It should be remembered, however, that owners may not always notice minor changes to micturition and a chronic problem may present as an acute emergency. In cases of urinary incontinence, establishing whether the animal has been incontinent since puppy/kittenhood or whether the incontinence is of recent onset can provide very useful information when considering potential differential diagnoses.

❏ Is the animal urinating or not?
This is an essential question in the animal presented with abnormal micturition. A negative answer may imply acute urinary tract obstruction which requires emergency treatment; alternatively the owner may admit to not observing their animal and so may not know the answer. This is common in cats that have free access to outside the house. In incontinent animals lack of urination may be associated with a bladder that doesn't contain urine, e.g. animals with bilateral ureteral ectopia and bladder hypoplasia, or it may be seen in animals with neurological disease and overflow incontinence.

❏ If urinating, what is the animal doing, how is it passing urine, what is the appearance and smell of the urine passed and where is it coming from?
Is the animal's stream of urine normal or weak/interrupted? Is there frequency/urgency? Is the animal straining and does it appear uncomfortable? Does the urine contain blood or have an abnormal smell? Where is the urine coming from, e.g. from the penis/vulva, from a urethrostomy or from another orifice?

❏ If it is not urinating, how long has it been since anybody saw the animal urinate?
In cases of acute urinary tract obstruction the duration of obstruction will affect the degree of azotaemia and hyperkalaemia which in turn will influence the immediate care the animal requires.

❏ Do the owners usually observe urination and, if so, are they familiar with their pet's normal urinary habits and urine appearance?
Unless owners know what their animal was doing before investigation and treatment, the response to treatment the animal receives may be difficult to assess. This is particularly important with signs which may be intermittent in nature, e.g. incontinence associated with urethral sphincter mechanism incompetence.

❏ Is the animal incontinent? If so, when does it leak, where does the leakage come from and is the leakage continual or intermittent?
Dogs with urethral sphincter mechanism incompetence tend to leak urine when recumbent and the leakage is often intermittent with the animal having good/bad days whereas animals with ectopic ureters tend to leak continually. Rarely, an animal may leak urine from its anus if a urethrorectal fistula is present or from another abnormal orifice, e.g. previous urachus.

❏ Has the owner noticed any abnormal discharge?
This may be pus or blood from the animal's penis or vulva and the animal may have been licking its external genitalia excessively. Blood dripping from the penis in male dogs is commonly associated with prostatic disease, whereas vulval bleeding in a bitch may originate from the urethra rather than the vagina and be an indicator of urethral malignancy.

❑ **Has the animal received any recent medical treatment?**

If so what was it, when did it finish and what was the outcome? Recent courses of antibiotics may interfere with urine bacteriology; diuretics and corticosteroids may cause polydipsia and polyuria resulting in frequency and urgency, nocturia and incontinence. Cyclophosphamide can cause sterile cystitis. Response to treatment, e.g. sympathomimetic drugs for urethral sphincter mechanism incompetence (SMI), may provide additional support for a presumptive diagnosis, particularly where there is no single diagnostic finding which can definitively confirm the diagnosis.

❑ **Have their been any recent traumatic episodes, surgery or apparently unrelated illness?**

Urethral strictures/ruptures may occur following bites to the perineum in cats. Recent catheterization can cause iatrogenic trauma to the urethra or introduce a urinary tract infection. Poor tissue handling during surgery to the caudal abdomen may result in a ureteral or bladder injury. SMI may occur following ovariohysterectomy. Hyperadrenocortism and diabetes mellitus predispose to urinary tract infection.

❑ **Are the signs getting better, worse or staying static since they were first noticed and does the problem occur daily or intermittently?**

This information is important for determining the progression of the problem, e.g. dysuria of gradually increasing severity is more likely to be associated with anatomical obstructions such as neoplasia. It is important to establish the pattern of signs before any treatment is started. If the signs are intermittent a longer follow-up may be required before the success of any treatment can be established.

❑ **Are the animal's signs confined to the urinary tract or is it systemically ill?**

An animal with a portosystemic shunt can present with primary urinary tract signs but on closer questioning, the owner may also have noticed signs of hepatic encephalopathy; an animal with a urinary tract infection, particularly if it involves the upper urinary tract, may be systemically ill.

❑ **When did the animal last urinate?**

It is essential to know this before examining the animal. If the animal has just passed urine or is incontinent, a full bladder is likely to be significant, compared to an animal which has a full bladder but has not had an opportunity to urinate. Similarly an empty bladder may reflect incontinence or it may be that the animal has voided urine normally.

❑ **Where and how does the animal prefer to urinate?**

It can be very useful before hospitalizing an animal, to know where and how the animal normally chooses to urinate. In many hospitals, for hygienic reasons, animals may not have access to grass or soil and some may try to 'hold on' until a suitable environment becomes available. Knowledge of the animal's dislikes/preferences can make assessment of urination during hospitalization much easier as can the use of specific commands, e.g. 'spend' is the toileting command often used by the Guide Dog for the Blind Association.

❑ **When was the animal last in season?**

In female animals a recent season or treatment with exogenous oestrogens result in vaginal enlargement. This may interfere with vaginourethrography, particularly urethral filling. If the investigation is elective it may be preferable to postpone it until the effect of the oestrogen has subsided.

PHYSICAL EXAMINATION

❑ **General physical examination**

This should include the animal's body condition, demeanour, hydration status as well as a risk assessment for general anaesthesia.

❑ **Abdominal and bladder palpation**

Is the bladder empty or full? If empty can any masses/thickening of the bladder wall be palpated? Can it be expressed and if so what is the subjective degree of resistance? Is the abdomen distended, painful or does it contain fluid?

❑ **Examination of external genitalia**

Urethral bleeding may be the first indicator of a urethral neoplasm or prostatic disease. Pus dripping from the penis may indicate a prostatic abscess. Male cats with feline lower urinary tract disease may have a gelatinous plug visible at the external urethral orifice. The external genitalia may appear ambiguous in intersex animals. Unconscious leakage of urine confirms urinary incontinence.

❑ **Examination of perineum and inguinal regions**

Bladder entrapment in a perineal or inguinal hernia may cause dysuria or acute urinary tract obstruction.

❏ Urethral examination
In the dog the urethra should be examined along its length by rectal (and vaginal) palpation of the intrapelvic urethra and external palpation of the perineum and penis. In the male dog or cat the penis should be exposed and the external urethral orifice examined. Calculi and focal/diffuse neoplasms may be palpable on urethral examination.

❏ Examination of the prostate
The prostate should be palpated per rectum or using a combination of rectal and abdominal palpation. Its size, position, consistency and symmetry should be assessed. The normal prostate is not painful on palpation and is firm and bilobed on rectal palpation.

❏ Observe urination
Urination should be observed to corroborate the owner's description. Check whether the stream is continuous or intermittent and assess if urination is initiated normally.

❏ Passage of a urethral catheter
In the male dog a catheter can be passed to help establish urethral patency. In the bitch or cat it is advisable to wait until the animal is sedated or anaesthetized before attempting to pass a catheter. Passage of a catheter, although useful, does not exclude a physical obstruction since a catheter may be advanced beyond small calculi and soft tissue masses may allow passage of a catheter, but act as a valve to the antegrade passage of urine. Passage of a catheter is also a useful means of emptying the bladder and assessing the residual volume of urine. Following urination the normal residual volume is between 0.2 and 0.4 ml kg^{-1}.

❏ Neurological examination
Animals with abnormal micturition secondary to neurological disease usually have neurological deficits and a history of other abnormalities, e.g. spinal disease, faecal incontinence. The examination of all animals with abnormal micturition and urinary incontinence should include examination of the sacral reflexes. If the perineal and bulbospongiosus reflexes are intact, there is normal anal tone, and sensation over the caudal back, perineum and tail is present; the sacral reflexes and pudendal nerve function can be considered normal. In cases of suspected neurological disease, a full neurological examination should be performed remembering that apparently unrelated deficits may indicate a multifocal disease, e.g. anisocoria or bilateral mydriasis with dysautonomia.

Laboratory investigations

Urine examination
Urine from all animals with abnormal micturition and urinary incontinence should routinely be collected and submitted for urinalysis and bacterial culture. Ideally the best method of collection, as it is least likely to be contaminated by normal flora residing in the external genitalia, is cystocentesis. However in some animals, particularly those which are fat, large and incontinent, this may be difficult to achieve without the aid of ultrasound guidance. Catheterization is a practical alternative although attention to technique is required and a quantitative culture should be requested. Samples should be collected in suitable containers and transported to the laboratory without delay.

Urinalysis should include determination of the urine pH, specific gravity, protein content, as well as routine biochemical tests. The sediment should be examined and the presence, appearance and number of red and white blood cells recorded. The presence of casts, bacteria, epithelial cells and type of crystals should also be noted. Although urinalysis may suggest a bacterial infection, bacteriology should be performed to definitively diagnose urinary tract infections and provide *in vitro* antibiotic sensitivities.

Haematology and biochemistry
Routine haematology and biochemistry should be considered in all animals with abnormal micturition and/or urinary incontinence and not just reserved for elderly animals and those with systemic disease. Useful information can often be gained from routine screening and may reveal or suggest an underlying cause for the urinary tract disease, e.g. diabetes mellitus and hyperadrenocorticism frequently predispose to urinary tract infection, hypercalcaemia may frequently predispose to calcium oxalate uroliths and urate calculi are frequently associated with hepatic encephalopathy.

Serology
Urinary incontinence in cats has been associated with feline leukaemia virus infection (FeLV) and, therefore, it is prudent to test incontinent cats for FeLV prior to investigation.

Radiographic and ultrasonographic investigations
Radiographic investigation, plain and contrast studies, and ultrasonography are the most

important techniques used in the investigation of abnormal micturition and urinary incontinence. Plain films can reveal renal enlargement or irregularity which may be secondary to abnormalities affecting the lower urinary tract. The size of the bladder can be assessed and the presence of radio-opaque calculi determined both within the bladder and at other sites along the urinary tract. Secondary changes suggestive of malignancy may be seen, in particular enlarged sublumbar lymph nodes and bony changes affecting the pelvis and vertebrae in advanced cases of prostatic neoplasia. In the male dog prostatic enlargement may be apparent, as may lesions affecting the os penis or penile soft tissues. Absence of a bladder shadow or evidence of abdominal fluid may indicate urinary tract rupture particularly following trauma.

The most useful radiographic investigations involve the use of contrast media and these studies demonstrate urinary tract anatomy. Physical obstructions, such as strictures, radiolucent calculi and soft tissue masses or bladder/urethral tears, are most usefully demonstrated with these techniques but a negative study may also provide very useful information by ruling out an anatomical lesion thereby suggesting a functional abnormality. The most useful contrast studies include positive contrast urethrocystography (vagino-urethrography in the female), double contrast cystography and intravenous urography. Pneumocystography, although commonly used, in practice provides no additional information to the above studies and is more likely to be associated with a missed diagnosis.

Ultrasonographic examination of the urinary tract is complementary to radiography. Ultrasound is particularly good for examining the urinary bladder as well as the kidneys and prostate. There may be limited access and sensitivity when examining the urethra and normal ureters, respectively. Therefore, contrast radiography is in general a better method of examining these structures, although dynamic ultrasound imaging of ureteral emptying is an excellent way of confirming that the ureters empty into the bladder in incontinent animals.

In order to make the best use of these techniques and in particular contrast radiography, good radiographic technique should be used. When the investigation is elective animals should be properly prepared for the examination with enemas, so as to avoid faeces in the rectum obscuring intrapelvic detail. If malignancy is suspected, thoracic films and ultrasound examination of the liver and sublumbar lymph nodes should also be performed.

FURTHER INVESTIGATION

The above diagnostic investigations tend to form the core investigation for the majority of animals presented with abnormal micturition and urinary incontinence. Specific extra investigations based on the animal's history and outcome of the tests detailed above include the following.

Specific investigation of the prostate

Prostatic disease is a common cause of abnormal micturition and urinary incontinence in entire male dogs and as such warrants a slightly more in depth investigation. Common prostatic diseases are detailed in Table 22.1. The above approach applies to the investigation of dogs with prostatic disease but additional specific tests may also include:

- prostatic aspiration/fine needle aspiration
- core biopsy/incisional biopsy
- prostatic washes pre- and postprostatic massage
- semen evaluation

Calculus analysis

Calculi obtained as the result of voluntary voiding, surgical removal, catheter or endoscopic retrieval or voiding hydropropulsion should be quantitatively analysed using physical techniques such as X-ray diffraction crystallography since chemical analysis can be inaccurate. All calculi should be sectioned before analysis to establish if they are composite in nature and if so what each layer is composed of. In cases of recurrent urinary tract infection culture of a calculus is also useful.

Biopsy

Biopsy of masses involving the urinary tract is important in the differentiation of malignant from benign lesions. Biopsies may be achieved in a number of ways, many obviating the need for surgery. As the bladder and urethra are hollow organs the more commonly used methods of non-invasive tissue collection such as fine needle aspirates and core needle biopsies may be inappropriate. A useful technique for obtaining tissue from the urethra and bladder is by catheter suction biopsy, guided by digital palpation and/or ultrasound. In larger female dogs biopsies may be made using direct visualization via a cystoscope. However, for some lesions there will be no alternative to collecting a biopsy surgically.

Cystoscopy

Endoscopy of the lower urinary tract can be used to directly visualize and biopsy lesions within the bladder and urethra in dogs and cats. Rigid paediatric cystoscopes are most commonly used and may provide useful information about congenital (e.g. openings of ectopic ureters) as well as acquired lesions (e.g. neoplasms, calculi). Examination of the bladder and urethra is limited by penile anatomy in male dogs unless a long flexible scope is used, although prepubic percutaneous cystoscopy is possible with a rigid scope. In some small cats and dogs the use of biopsy forceps may be restricted and overall the availability of suitable equipment and expertise in veterinary practice is limited. However, cystoscopy is a useful procedure and is currently considered to be the optimum method of discriminating idiopathic cystitis from other causes of feline lower urinary tract disease.

Urodynamic investigation and other electrophysiological tests

Much has been written on the use of urodynamics in the investigation of abnormal micturition and urinary incontinence in the veterinary literature. The techniques most appropriate to the investigation of abnormal urination and incontinence are *cystometry, uroflowmetry* and *urethral pressure profilometry*. These investigative techniques play a large role in the investigation of urinary tract disease in humans but unfortunately have been applied rarely to the investigation of clinical cases in the veterinary field. This is mainly due to the lack of co-operation received from veterinary patients compared to humans. Cystometry measures the relationship between bladder pressure and volume during bladder filling. Uroflowmetry measures urine flow against time and urethral pressure profilometry measures urethral tone over urethral length. The use and interpretation of the results obtained from these investigations is specialized and they are only available at a few referral centres. Electromyography is also useful in the investigation of suspected neurological causes of abnormal micturition and urinary incontinence.

Advanced imaging techniques

These techniques include myelography, computed tomography and magnetic resonance imaging. They have a role to play in certain cases of abnormal micturition and urinary incontinence but are perhaps most useful in the investigation of neurological causes of lower urinary tract disease.

Drug trial

In some dogs with abnormal micturition and urinary incontinence no obvious anatomical, infectious or neurological cause for the dysuria can be found. In these animals a functional abnormality is assumed to be present. The cause of the functional abnormality can be difficult to diagnose definitively but the animal may respond to symptomatic treatment with a variety of drugs which may support the presumptive diagnosis. Possible causes of such functional abnormalities include detrusor instability and reflex dyssynergia.

Detrusor instability is a functional abnormality whereby the bladder is hyperactive and poorly compliant. In humans it is a common cause of urinary incontinence. It is thought to exist as a primary entity in dogs, but is probably most commonly seen secondary to urinary tract infections. Definitive diagnosis is made by cystometry but response to 'bladder calming drugs' such as the antimuscarinics oxybutynin and propantheline supports the presumptive diagnosis.

Reflex dyssynergia is another functional abnormality which is most commonly seen in animals with neurological disease, however it may also occur in animals without obvious neurological deficits. The affected animal starts micturition but the striated muscle round the urethra contracts causing a functional urethral obstruction with passage of no or only small spurts of urine. Treatment with a smooth and skeletal muscle relaxant frequently helps, e.g. diazepam and phenoxybenzamine.

When investigating animals with abnormal micturition and urinary incontinence it should be remembered that it is common for two or more conditions to co-exist. Some abnormalities may predispose to other conditions, e.g. urinary tract infection predisposes to struvite calculi, ectopic ureter predisposes to infection and many of these conditions can cause abnormal micturition and urinary incontinence in their own right. It is important therefore that the investigation is thorough and additional disease is not overlooked. The management of specific conditions affecting the bladder, urethra and prostate is detailed in Chapter 41.

23

Haematuria

J. K. Dunn

Haematuria is the presence of blood in the urine. Haematuria which is visible to the naked eye (gross haematuria) warrants further investigation. Microscopic haematuria (haematuria detected only on examination of urine sediment) may be of little clinical significance. Small numbers of erythrocytes are lost via the urinary tract in healthy dogs and cats (usually less than five to seven red cells per high power field). Moreover, the technique (catheterization or cystocentesis) used to collect the sample may also result in contamination of urine with red blood cells. Microscopic haematuria is more likely to be significant if (1) it is a persistent finding and (2) on examination of urine sediment there are more than five to seven red blood cells per high power field.

DIFFERENTIATION OF HAEMATURIA FROM HAEMOGLOBINURIA AND MYOGLOBINURIA

It is important to differentiate haematuria from *haemoglobinuria*. The latter also imparts a reddish colour to urine and may be accompanied by haemoglobinaemia resulting in red discoloration of separated plasma. Haemoglobinuria occurs when a large amount of haemoglobin, released from red cells during a haemolytic crisis, exceeds the liver's capacity to convert it into bilirubin and is filtered by the renal glomeruli. Filtered haemoglobin is toxic to renal tubules and may result in tubular necrosis. In acidic urine haemoglobin appears more brown than red so that haemoglobinuria is often characterized by a brownish red or 'port wine' discoloration of urine (Fig. 45.7; Chapter 45). Haemoglobin is also released from lysed red cells in 'aged' urine samples. If a urine sample is allowed to stand for 15–20 min or is centrifuged, intact red cells settle out in the sediment and the supernatant becomes clear whereas with haemoglobinuria the supernatant retains its original colour. Others have advocated the use of an occult blood test on urine sediment; a negative occult reaction on the sediment and an absence of red cells, with a positive occult blood response on the supernatant suggests either haemoglobin or myoglobin is present.

Severe muscle necrosis, trauma (severe crushing injuries) or the exertional rhabdomyolysis seen in greyhounds may result in myoglobinuria and a reddish brown discoloration of urine. Like haemoglobin, myoglobin is toxic to renal tubules. Animals with myoglobinuria are likely to present with generalized muscle pain, muscle swelling, weakness and raised muscle enzymes (alanine aminotransferase, creatine kinase and lactate dehydrogenase).

Other pigments such as porphyrins, certain drugs (phenytoin, sulphonamides) and some dyes in foodstuffs are rare causes of red or pink discolored urine.

CAUSES OF HAEMATURIA

Haematuria may arise from lesions in the kidneys or lower urinary tract. Lesions involving internal and external genitalia may also result in significant haematuria. Hence haematuria may be classified according to the anatomical site of origin (Table 23.1).

INVESTIGATION OF HAEMATURIA

The objectives of the initial investigations are firstly to localize the haematuria to an anatomical site and then to identify the cause. The presence of free intact red cells and red cell casts indicates haemorrhage into renal tubules or severe glomerular disease allowing red cells to enter the tubules. Systemic disorders, most commonly abnormalities in haemostasis such as thrombocytopenia or coagulation factor deficiencies, may cause diffuse bleeding throughout the entire

Table 23.1 Causes of haematuria based on site of origin

Kidney	Diffuse bleeding
• Pyelonephritis • Glomerulonephropathy • Acute tubular necrosis (e.g. gentamycin toxicity) • Leptospirosis (rare) • Neoplasia (usually primary) • Renal calculi • Renal cysts • Infarction, e.g. subacute bacterial endocarditis, cardiomyopathy • Trauma • Idiopathic renal haematuria • Recurring haematuria of Welsh corgis • *Dirofilaria immitis* (microfilaria) • *Dioctophyma renale*	• Bleeding disorders, e.g. thrombocytopenia, coagulation factor deficiencies • Heat stroke (probably due to DIC) • Violent exercise **Accessory sex organs, internal and external genitalia** • Prostatic disease (prostatitis, prostatic abscess, prostatic cyst, benign prostatic hyperplasia, neoplasia) • Uterus (oestrus, infection, subinvolution of the placenta, neoplasia) • Vagina (oestrus, benign polyps, trauma, neoplasia, e.g. transitional cell carcinoma or transmissible venereal tumour) • Penis (trauma, neoplasia, e.g. transmissible venereal tumour)
Lower urinary tract (ureter, bladder and urethra)	**Iatrogenic haematuria caused by technique used for collecting urine sample**
• Infection • Calculi • Inflammation, e.g. feline lower urinary tract disease or obstructive uropathy (usually occurs in the absence of infection) • Neoplasia (e.g. transitional cell carcinoma) • Trauma (resulting in bladder or urethral rupture) • Retention cystitis, e.g. spinal cord damage resulting in upper motor neurone lesion • Cyclophosphamide (sterile haemorrhagic cystitis) • *Capillaria plica*	• Catheterization or cystocentesis; manual expression of the bladder

length of the urinary tract which may be associated with other clinical signs such as petechiation of the skin and mucosae.

HISTORY CHECKLIST

❏ Age, sex and breed?
Females in general have a higher incidence of urinary tract infections and some breeds of dog are predisposed to the formation of certain types of urinary calculi (see Chapter 41).

❏ Is this the first episode of haematuria?
If not, note frequency, severity and outcome of previous episodes.

❏ Does blood appear throughout urination?
Blood which is present throughout urination indicates disease of the kidneys, ureters or bladder. Haematuria at the beginning of micturition is more consistent with disease of the lower urinary tract, i.e. prostate, urethra, penis, uterus or vagina. Haematuria confined to the end of micturition is characteristic of bladder or prostatic disease although dogs with prostatic disease often may pass drops of blood independent of urination.

❏ Are other signs of urinary tract disease present?
These may be dysuria (painful or difficult urination), stranguria (painful, often non-productive attempts to urinate) or pollakiuria (increased frequency of urination). Haematuria caused by inflammation and/or infection of the lower urinary tract, prostate or genitalia, or disorders which result in obstruction of the urinary tract (e.g. cystitis, calculi or neoplasia) is often associated with abnormal micturition. In this context it is worth noting that owners of cats with lower urinary tract disease, especially those with obstructive uropathy, often confuse stranguria with constipation. Occasionally animals that are severely dysuric may also become incontinent (urge-type of urinary incontinence associated with persistent mechanical stimulation of the lower urinary tract by calculi).

❏ **Is animal showing systemic signs of disease, e.g. weight loss, anorexia, lethargy?**

The presence of such signs suggests that either renal or prostatic disease may be responsible for the haematuria. Vomiting, diarrhoea, polydipsia and polyuria may be evident in dogs with end-stage pyelonephritis and bitches with pyometra.

❏ **Is there evidence of abdominal pain, i.e. does the animal appear restless, uncomfortable and stand with its back arched?**

Pyelonephritis, ureteral calculi and acute prostatitis may cause abdominal pain which may be difficult to localize.

❏ **Has there been other evidence of external haemorrhage such as epistaxis, melaena, cutaneous or mucosal haemorrhage?**

❏ **History of previous surgery?**

❏ **Trauma?**

❏ **Exposure to drugs (e.g. cyclophosphamide) or toxins (e.g. anticoagulant rodenticides)?**

❏ **If an intact female, is she or has she recently been in oestrus?**

PHYSICAL EXAMINATION

❏ **Is there evidence of dysuria or stranguria and can the animal pass a good continuous flow of urine?**

In many cases it may be necessary to hospitalize the animal in order to confirm the owner's observations or suspicions. The presence or absence of dysuria for example is important in establishing the origin and cause of the haematuria and in some cases the owner may not be able to provide this information. This is especially true in cats which do not use an indoor litter tray.

❏ **Is there evidence of cutaneous or mucosal haemorrhages?**

❏ **Is the animal's gait normal?**

Dogs with acute prostatitis may appear ataxic.

❏ **Examination of the abdomen should include careful palpation of the kidneys and bladder; the uterus may be palpated if it is distended with fluid.**

Large prostatic masses for example paraprostatic cysts may be identified on abdominal palpation.

The kidneys may be enlarged and painful (glomerulonephritis, pyelonephritis) or enlarged and non-painful (hydronephrosis or polycystic kidneys, amyloidosis or neoplasia, e.g. lymphoma). Tumours and vesicular calculi if large enough can sometimes be detected on palpation; multiple calculus formation may result in crepitation within the bladder lumen. The bladder of a cat with obstructive uropathy is firm, distended and extremely painful.

❏ **The prostate, pelvic urethra and cervix should be palpated per rectum**

The causes of prostatic enlargement are listed in Table 23.1. A large painful prostate suggests acute prostatitis; a large asymmetrical and painless prostate with irregular surface contours is more consistent with neoplasia.

❏ **The external genitalia should be examined**

The external genitalia should be examined for evidence of trauma, inflammation and/or infection, ulceration, petechiation and neoplasia.

INITIAL DIAGNOSTIC PLAN

Many isolated episodes of haematuria are the result of infection which resolve with appropriate antibiotic therapy (see later). In these uncomplicated cases a minimum database at the very least should include urinalysis. A more aggressive diagnostic approach is warranted for animals which either fail to respond to antibiosis or which have persistent or recurrent haematuria. In these cases it is important to rule out factors which may predispose to recurrent infection, and also systemic disorders and bleeding defects as possible causes for the haematuria. If the patient is in shock or is suspected to be severely anaemic, thoracic and abdominal radiographs should be taken to check for evidence of trauma and appropriate laboratory tests should be performed to evaluate haemostasis (see Chapter 21).

Urinalysis

When interpreting the results of urinalysis it is important to remember that the method used to collect the urine sample and the way in which it is subsequently handled can influence the results. For example a midstream voided sample which is usually used for initial routine urine analysis may be contaminated by blood, bacteria and exudate present in the prepuce or vagina. Traumatization of the urethra during catheterization may result in microscopic or occasionally gross haematuria and at the same time may introduce infection into the bladder. Cystocentesis is the preferred method of obtaining a representative sample of urine from the bladder.

Urinalysis should be performed on a freshly collected uncontaminated urine sample within 30 min. If urinalysis cannot be performed within 2 h the sample should be refrigerated at 4°C and brought back to room temperature before it is analysed. Routine urinalysis consists of (1) checking the colour, turbidity, smell and specific gravity; (2) performing a series of biochemical tests using multitest dipsticks and (3) microscopic examination of centrifuged urine sediment (5 min at 2000 rpm).

Confirming gross or microscopic haematuria

Although contamination with red cells may still occur in a sample collected by cystocentesis this is usually minimal if a fine 22 gauge needle is used. If blood is absent from a sample collected by cystocentesis and present in a voided specimen then it must originate in the lower urinary tract distal to the bladder. As a general rule of thumb the sediment of urine collected by cystocentesis should have no more than 0–3 red cells per high power field (hpf), catheterized samples 0–5 red cells/hpf and midstream voided samples 0–7 red cells/hpf on microscopic examination.

Urine dipsticks give a false positive reading for blood if haemoglobin or myoglobin is present in the sample. Haemolysis occurs in hypotonic urine (sp. gr. < 1.008) or if the urine is very acidic or alkaline. Similar false positive results may occur if a urine sample or the test pad on the dipstick is contaminated with an oxidizing agent such as povidone iodine or hypochlorite.

Urine pH

Most dogs and cats have a urine pH between 5.5 and 7.0. A sample of urine which is allowed to stand open at room temperature will become alkaline. In small animals the presence of haematuria in association with an increase in urine pH (often greater than 7.5) is suggestive of a urinary tract infection caused by urease-producing bacteria (e.g. *Staphylococcus* spp., *Proteus* spp. and *Klebsiella* spp.).

Glycosuria

Glucose is most easily detected using the test pad on urine dipsticks. The presence of glucose in the urine of cats in most cases is the result of fear or the stress associated with obtaining the urine or blood sample. Glycosuria is accompanied by hyperglycaemia and often a marked lymphocytosis. If glucose is detected in a canine urine sample further investigations are warranted to rule out diabetes mellitus and hyperadrenocorticism both of which may be associated with recurrent urinary tract infections.

Proteinuria (see Chapter 9 for a more detailed account of investigation and significance of proteinuria)

Dipstick reagent strips detect albumin; they do not test for globulins or Bence-Jones proteins. Turbimetric tests such as the sulphosalicylic acid test detect albumin, globulins, Bence-Jones proteins and glycoproteins. The protein concentration should be interpreted in light of the urine specific gravity (sp. gr.). A 1+ reaction in an isosthenuric sample is probably more significant than a similar reading in a sample which has a sp. gr. of 1.045. Urine with a sp. gr. >1.020 may be expected to contain a trace or 1+ protein; rarely does normal urine contain more than 2+ protein. Any loss of red cells into the urinary tract will contribute towards the protein content although it generally requires massive bleeding to cause 3+ or 4+ proteinuria. The urine protein content may also be influenced (increased) by the presence of urinary tract inflammation and/or infection; proteinuria which occurs without significant numbers of white or red blood cells is suggestive of glomerular damage. The significance of persistent 3+ or 4+ proteinuria can be more accurately assessed by determining the urine protein:creatinine ratio which has a close correlation with the quantitative 24 h urine protein determination (see Chapter 9).

■ Microscopic examination of urine sediment

Pyuria (increased numbers of white blood cells)

Normal voided urine should contain less than eight leucocytes per hpf (for samples obtained by catheterization and cystocentesis the figures are less than five and less than three, respectively). Contamination of the urine sample with a purulent preputial or vaginal discharge may result in an increased number of white blood cells (pyuria). Persistent pyuria in a urine sample collected by cystocentesis is indicative of urinary tract inflammation. In most cases the inflammatory changes are the result of infection, either uncomplicated bacterial cystitis or urethritis, or infection associated with neoplasia or urolithiasis. Certain types of cystic or urethral calculi in the dog, for example urates or oxalates, can cause pronounced inflammation in the absence of infection, and in the cat naturally occurring cases of lower urinary tract disease are rarely associated with an infectious agent although recent studies have implicated the involvement of viruses (feline calici virus and a cell-associated herpes virus). Conversely it is not unusual for an animal which is producing exceptionally dilute urine or which has deficient granulocyte function (e.g. one with diabetes mellitus or hyperadrenocorticism) to have a concurrent urinary tract infection but no microscopic evidence of pyuria. Urine which contains increased numbers of leucocytes should be routinely submitted for bacteriological examination (culture and sensitivity) regardless of whether bacteria are seen on microscopic examination of the sediment (see below). Similarly urine from diabetic and cushingoid animals should be cultured even if there is no clinical or laboratory evidence of urinary tract disease.

Leucocyte esterase activity is detected on a dipstick only when more than 15×10^3 organisms ml^{-1} of urine are present. It is therefore an insensitive screen for pyuria in small animals. Oxidants such as cephalosporins and gentamycin may produce false positive results.

Bacteriuria

The presence of bacteria, often with increased numbers of red and white blood cells, in a urine sample collected by cystocentesis usually indicates a urinary tract infection (UTI) originating in the bladder or less frequently ureters or kidneys, although the reflux of urine from the proximal urethra into the bladder in dogs with prostatic disease can result in similar laboratory findings. In contrast, the presence of bacteria in association with pyuria in voided or catheterized samples may indicate infection at any point in the urinary tract or contamination of the sample by a preputial or vaginal discharge. The presence of bacteria in a sample containing few leucocytes suggests contamination by cutaneous or faecal organisms. Greater than 10^4 bacilli ml^{-1} and 10^5 cocci ml^{-1} must be present in urine before the organisms are readily seen on microscopic examination of urine sediment. Yeast infections (e.g. *Candida* spp.) are not easily detected on routine urinalysis since typically few organisms are seen. For these reasons urine samples showing evidence of haematuria, pyuria or both should be cultured even if organisms are not seen during routine microscopic examination.

The nitrite test band on urine dipsticks is generally considered to be an unreliable indicator of infection since the diet of small animals usually contains insufficient nitrate and not all bacteria reduce nitrate to nitrite. A positive test result is an indication for urine sediment examination and urine culture.

Epithelial cells

A few small and large epithelial cells may be seen in the urine sediment of most normal animals. Infection and inflammation of the lower urinary tract results in exfoliation of increased numbers of urothelial cells. Large numbers of epithelial cells and particularly the presence of irregularly arranged cell clusters should be regarded with suspicion. Clusters of epithelial cells showing variation in nuclear to cytoplasmic ratio are highly suggestive of neoplasia, in particular transitional cell carcinoma (Fig. 23.1). When large numbers of epithelial cells are seen on routine examination of a wet unstained preparation of urine sediment an air-dried slide of freshly centrifuged sediment (preferably using a cytospin technique) should be stained with a Romanowsky-type stain (e.g. Giemsa or new methylene blue) to provide more detailed morphological assessment of the cells. The administration of cytotoxic agents such as cyclophosphamide and high concentrations of radiographic contrast agents may result in increased numbers of degenerate and morphologically atypical epithelial cells.

Cylindruria (increased numbers of casts in the urine)

Most urine samples from healthy animals contain no casts; certainly there should be no more than 0–1 granular casts/hpf and 0–2 hyaline casts/hpf. A cast represents a cylindrical mould of aggregated protein or cells, or both, which is formed within the renal tubular lumen. Excessive numbers of casts indicate renal disease although in some cases the renal pathology is secondary and is completely reversible. Nephrons that are

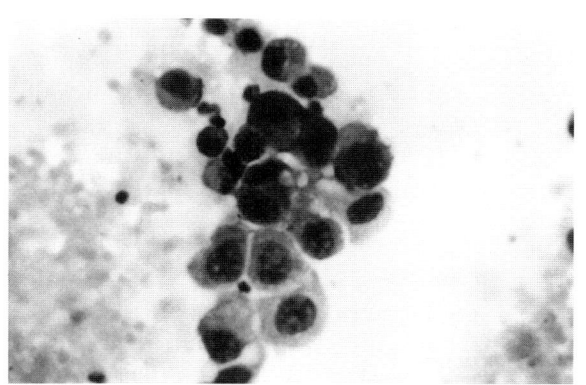

Figure 23.1 A cluster of neoplastic urothelial cells in a Giemsa-stained preparation of urine sediment from a dog with a transitional cell carcinoma of the bladder wall. Note the irregular way in which the cells are arranged and the variable nuclear:cytoplasmic ratio. May–Grünwald Giemsa ×125. See colour plate.

ischaemic or become obstructed excrete mucoprotein resulting in an increased tendency towards cast formation. The presence of cellular casts is usually abnormal and is indicative of renal disease. Increased numbers of casts can be shed although renal tests may be normal, for example during early aminoglycoside toxicity; conversely an absence of casts does not preclude renal disease. The causes and significance of each type of cast are summarized in Table 23.2.

Crystalluria

Crystals occur commonly in urine but are often of little diagnostic significance. The presence of crystals in urinary sediment implies the urine is supersaturated and does not indicate urolithiasis. The solubility and concentration of the crystalloid determine whether crystals form in urine. The solubility of crystals is pH dependent, for example struvite crystals are common in alkaline urine. In some cases the urine is rendered alkaline by the presence of urease-splitting bacteria and if the infection is not treated appropriately or recurs after treatment, persistent alkalinity may result in formation of struvite uroliths. Urine specific gravity and the temperature at which the urine sample is stored also influence the number of crystals present (cooling urine after collection increases the number of crystals present). The increase in pH which occurs in stale urine favours struvite crystallization. The urine of many normal dogs and cats contains struvite and occasionally calcium oxalate crystals. Uric acid or urate crystals are frequently noted in the urine of Dalmations. The presence of

Table 23.2 Causes and clinical significance of different types of urinary cast

Type of cast	Composition	Causes and significance of increased numbers
Hyaline casts	Pure aggregates of mucoprotein (Tamm–Horsfall mucoprotein) and small amounts of serum albumin	Dehydration (increased numbers during rehydration and diuresis); severe proteinuria; urine with acid pH; least significant of all the casts
Granular casts (coarse or fine)	Granules represent particles from degenerate tubular epithelial cells in a mucoprotein matrix	Severe dehydration (seen during rehydration); aminoglycoside toxicity.
WBC casts	Composition similar to granular casts plus white blood cells	Usually pyelonephritis, i.e. WBC casts indicate renal inflammation (usually infection); acute tubular necrosis.
RBC casts	As for granular casts plus red blood cells	Glomerulonephritis, vasculitis, renal infarction, renal tumour; presence indicates haemorrhage into renal tubules or severe glomerular disease (e.g. glomerulonephritis or neoplasia).
Renal tubular cell casts		Heavy metal intoxication, tubular hypoxia, acute oliguric renal failure; indicative of severe tubular damage.
Waxy casts	Represent old degenerate granular casts	Numerous renal diseases (see granular casts).
Fatty casts	Type of granular cast in which fat droplets accumulate in tubular cells as they degenerate	Numerous renal diseases especially in cats; may be seen in dogs with nephrotic syndrome

Table 23.3 Types of crystal found in the urine of dogs and cats

Type of crystal	Clinical significance
Struvite (magnesium ammonium phosphate)	Common in neutral or alkaline urine; may be associated with urinary tract infections (especially infections with urease splitting bacteria which increase urinary pH).
Calcium oxalate	Normal or may indicate ethylene glycol toxicity
Ammonium urate/uric acid	Normal in Dalmations but also found in other breeds. The presence of biurate crystals is virtually pathognomonic for a congenital portosystemic shunt.
Cystine	Cystinuria is due to an inherited renal tubular transport defect involving cystine and other amino acids. Cystine crystals may be observed in acid urine. Increased incidence in dachshunds, Yorkshire terriers and basset hounds.
Calcium phosphate	Normal or associated with struvite calculi.
Calcium carbonate	Rare in small animals.
Bilirubin	May be present in normal dogs especially if urine is concentrated or has a high bilirubin concentration.
Cholesterol	May be present in normal dogs and cats.
Leucine and tyrosine	Possibly associated with hepatic disease.
Hippurate	Significance uncertain.
Sulphonamide	May occur following the administration of sulphonamides especially if urine is concentrated or urine output is inadequate.

ammonium biurate, leucine or tyrosine crystals is almost pathognomonic for hepatic dysfunction (portosystemic shunts). Large numbers of oxalate crystals if associated with clinical signs and laboratory findings suggesting renal failure support a diagnosis of ethylene glycol (antifreeze) toxicity. Bilirubin crystals may be seen in normal dog urine, and some drugs, for example trimethoprim, can crystallize when excreted into the urine. The different types of crystals found in urine are summarized in Table 23.3. A more detailed description of the different types of urolith and their significance is included in Chapter 41.

Urine culture and sensitivity

Culture and sensitivity may not be justified in patients which present for the first time with haematuria especially if other clinical signs consistent with urinary tract infection (UTI) are present since many cases respond to appropriate antibiotic therapy. However if an upper UTI or prostatic disease is suspected or if the UTI recurs after antibiotic therapy, urine culture is an essential part of the diagnostic investigations. Quantitative culture may help to determine the significance of any organism isolated. The presence of greater than 10^5 bacteria ml^{-1} represents significant bacteriuria.

Radiography

Plain lateral and ventrodorsal views of the abdomen should be taken to check for the presence of uroliths, prostatic enlargement or enlarged kidneys. Some calculi are radiodense (e.g. struvite and oxalates); others (e.g. urates) are radiolucent. Cystine calculi have an intermediate density.

Full haematological examination

Haematology should include a platelet count if blood loss is persistent or severe. Check for evidence of inflammation and/or infection (neutrophilia with pyelonephritis, pyometra, prostatitis or prostatic abscess) and anaemia (bladder tumours, coagulopathies).

Limited biochemical screen

- Increased urea, creatinine and phosphate concentrations increase with renal disease, post-

renal obstruction (occlusion of the urethra by calculi, bladder neck tumours or extensive prostatic carcinomas) and bladder rupture.
- ± Hyperkalaemia with prolonged obstruction to urine outflow
- ± Mild hypocalcaemia (as a result of hyperphosphataemia).
- Hyponatraemia sometimes associated with bladder rupture.
- Check liver enzymes and bile salts. Occasionally urethral obstruction occurs in dogs with portosystemic shunts due to the formation of multiple small urate calculi.

FURTHER INVESTIGATION

The following procedures are indicated if the results from the above tests are uninformative or if the source of haematuria cannot be localized.

Clotting profile

One-stage prothrombin and activated partial thromboplastin tests are indicated if a coagulopathy is suspected, for example if large numbers of red cell casts are present in the urine suggesting haematuria of renal origin.

Urine protein:creatinine ratio

Urine protein to creatinine ratio should be calculated in cases with persistent 3+ or 4+ proteinuria to assess the significance of the protein loss. Check serum albumin concentration and submit serum and urine for protein electrophoresis. Glomerulonephropathy is usually characterized by significant proteinuria and hypoalbuminaemia.

Radiographic contrast studies

Pneumocystography and *double contrast cystography* are useful techniques for demonstrating irregularities or thickening of the bladder mucosal surface (bladder neoplasia, chronic cystitis) and the presence of intraluminal masses (cystic calculi). *Retrograde urethrography* is more helpful for diagnosing urethral calculi, urethral tumours (rare), urethral rupture and prostatic disease (especially prostatic neoplasia).

Intravenous urography detects irregularities in renal size and shape as well as abnormalities and filling defects involving the renal pelvis and renal calyces (e.g. pyelonephritis, renal or ureteral calculi, renal neoplasia, renal cysts, renal infarcts, ureteral rupture (rare) and idiopathic haematuria.

Ultrasonography of bladder, prostate and kidneys

Ultrasonography may help to differentiate renal or prostatic cysts from neoplastic lesions. Fine needle aspiration of an enlarged kidney or prostate may be performed under ultrasound guidance (see below).

Arteriography

Arteriography can be used to detect vascular abnormalities but is rarely performed since ultrasonography may detect similar abnormalities.

Prostatic wash/ejaculation

Cytological examination of a prostatic wash or ejaculated fluid may help to differentiate infection (e.g. bacterial prostatitis or a prostatic abscess; Fig. 23.2) from benign hyperplasia (Fig. 23.3), squamous metaplasia (Fig. 23.4) and neoplasia of the prostate gland (Fig. 23.5).

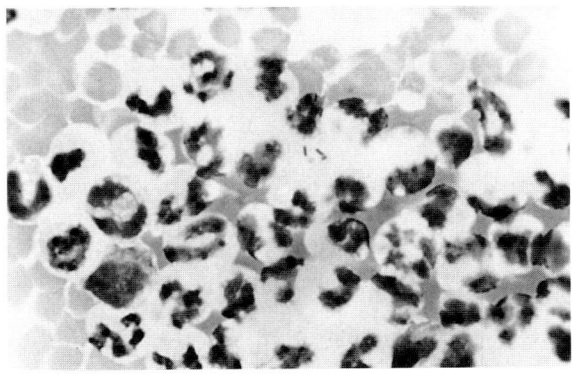

Figure 23.2 Prostatic wash from a dog with acute prostatitis. Note the degenerate appearance of the neutrophils, a few of which contained intracellular bacteria. May–Grünwald Giemsa ×250. See colour plate.

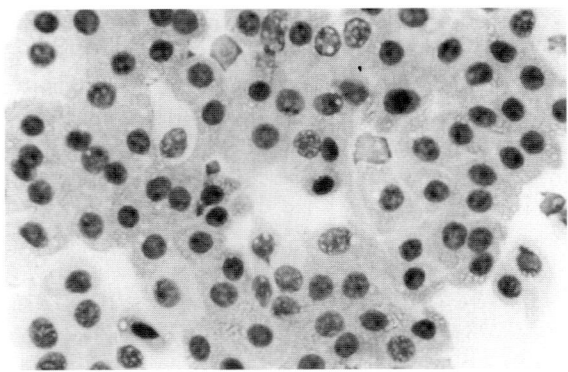

Figure 23.3 Prostatic wash from a dog with benign hyperplasia of the prostate gland. Large sheets of epithelial cells are present. The cells appear uniform with respect to size and shape. May–Grünwald Giemsa ×125. See colour plate.

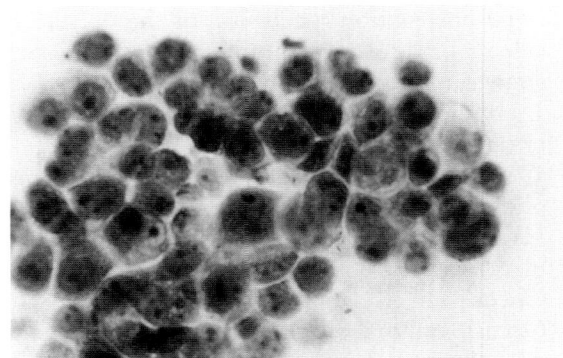

Figure 23.5 This fine needle aspirate of the prostate gland from a dog with a large prostatic carcinoma was taken under ultrasound guidance. An irregular cluster of urothelial cells is present. The cells are showing marked variation in cell size, nuclear:cytoplasmic ratio, and nucleolar number, size and shape. May–Grünwald Giemsa ×125. See colour plate.

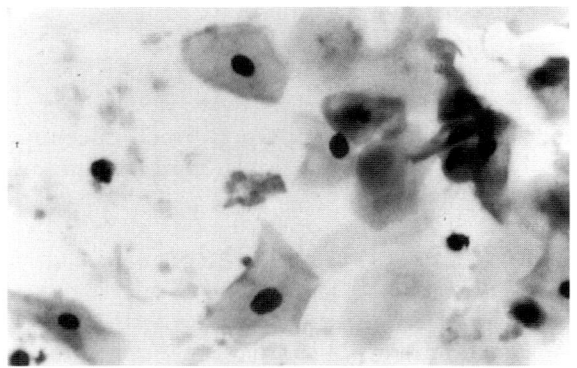

Figure 23.4 This prostatic wash contains large numbers of keratinized or partially keratinized urothelial cells consistent with squamous metaplasia of the prostate gland. Squamous metaplasia may be seen with functional Sertoli cell tumours in response to high circulating oestrogen levels. May–Grünwald Giemsa ×125. See colour plate.

Fine needle aspiration or biopsy

Fine needle aspiration of an enlarged kidney or prostate gland is best performed under ultrasound guidance. Vaginal, penile or preputial masses can either be surgically biopsied or fine needle aspirates or impression smears may be submitted for cytological examination.

Cystoscopy

Cystoscopy is a rarely used technique with limited applications in veterinary practice. It involves passing a narrow gauge flexible fibre-optic endoscope via the urethra into the bladder (bitches only). Using this technique it may be possible non-invasively to identify and biopsy neoplastic masses, thereby allowing the early differentiation of malignant tumours from benign polyps involving the bladder or urethral mucosa.

Exploratory laparotomy

Exploratory laparotomy is indicated only in cases when the source of haematuria cannot be identified or if the blood loss into the urinary tract is particularly severe and suspected to be of renal origin. After administration of a diuretic the ureters are catheterized separately via the bladder and the urine collected from each is checked for the presence of blood.

MANAGEMENT OF HAEMATURIA

Most cases of haematuria are the result of a urinary tract infection or infection of the accessory sex organs, e.g. the prostate gland. In some cases the infection is associated with urolithiasis or neoplasia. Animals which present with haematuria for the first time and which are not severely dysuric or showing systemic signs are therefore often treated empirically with a 10–14 day course of an appropriate antibiotic. Ampicillin or trimethoprim sulphadiazine have been shown to be good first choice antibiotics for most urinary tract infections. Ampicillin is almost 100% effective against streptococci and staphylococci; 80% of infections involving *Escherischia coli* or *Enterobacter* spp. are susceptible to trimethoprim sulphadiazine. A case which fails to respond to antibiotics, or which recurs, warrants further investigation to identify the cause. Failure to respond to antibiotic therapy indicates either a non-infectious cause of haematuria or that the wrong antibiotic has been chosen. Recurrence of haematuria following an initial response to antibiotics may be due to recurrence of the infection so that the urine becomes infected with the same organism or in some cases the urine may become reinfected with different microbes. Patients which present with recurrent urinary tract infections, even if each episode may be antibiotic responsive, should be investigated further to rule out the possibility of urolithiasis, neoplasia, renal or prostatic involvement, or the presence of concurrent disease (e.g. hyperadrenocorticism or diabetes mellitus).

A patient showing signs of severe dysuria should first be catheterized to ensure the urethra is not obstructed by calculi. If the catheter cannot be passed, for example in a dog with a urethral calculus or a cat with obstructive uropathy associated with the formation of a urethral plug, the animal should be managed as follows.

- First stabilize the animal with intravenous fluids (normal saline) to correct any fluid and electrolyte imbalances which may be present and to supply maintenance fluid requirements. The animal's general demeanour will often reflect the degree of dehydration associated with the postrenal azotaemia.
- Relieve the obstruction and re-establish urine flow. This can be achieved by catheterizing the animal and back flushing the sabulous plug or calculus with sterile saline (retropulsion). Cystocentesis, if performed beforehand, may relieve the urethral spasm and allow easier passage of the catheter. The plasma concentrations of urea, creatinine and potassium and urine output should be monitored closely after the obstruction is relieved. Postobstructive diuresis may result in the further urinary loss of potassium.
- Remove the calculus surgically (cystotomy) or attempt to dissolve struvite stones by dietary management (see Chapter 41).
- Following surgery, medical management consists of eradicating the infection if one is present and stimulating polyuria by adding salt to the diet.

The long-term management and prevention of canine urolithiasis and feline lower urinary tract disease, including obstructive uropathy due to urolith or urethral plug formation, are discussed in Chapter 41.

24

Alopecia

R. Bond

INTRODUCTION

Abnormalities of the hair coat of dogs and cats are usually obvious to owners early in the course of a disease. Alopecia, absence of hair in an area where it is normally present, or hypotrichosis, partial hair loss, is a common consequence of skin infections or ectoparasitic infestations. Alopecia may also be a manifestation of internal diseases such as endocrinopathies. In other cases, the alopecia may represent no risk to the patient and may be nothing more than a cosmetic problem, albeit one which may cause the owner considerable distress. A methodical approach and accurate diagnosis are prerequisites for successful management of these cases. This chapter describes the mechanisms by which alopecia may develop and suggests an approach to the diagnosis of alopecia in these species.

PATHOPHYSIOLOGY

In mammals, a cyclical pattern of hair shedding followed by new growth and replacement has evolved. The growing or 'anagen' phase is characterized by the production of a hair shaft. Anagen usually accounts for 80–90% of the duration of the hair growth cycle. The cessation of active hair grow heralds the onset of 'catagen', a short transitional phase during which the inferior portion of the hair follicle undergoes regression. The 'telogen' or resting phase is characterized by a period of apparent inactivity during which the fully grown hair remains anchored in the follicle by an expanded and keratinized base known as a 'club'. Shedding of the hair occurs only after the next anagen phase has progressed such that a new hair shaft enters the follicular canal. The intrinsic rhythmical follicular activity is modified by systemic factors such as thyroidal, adrenal and gonadal hormones. In the dog and cat, the hair growth cycle in each body region is asynchronous and hairs are replaced in a mosaic pattern.

Diseases of hair follicles have been classified based on pathophysiological processes which might lead to alopecia (Dunstan, 1995). Diseases characterized by alopecia can be divided into *scarring* (or potentially scarring) and *non-scarring* disorders. In scarring alopecia, the follicle is damaged such that hair growth is not possible. This usually results from a severe inflammatory process targeting the hair follicle, such as furunculosis secondary to bacterial infections and demodicosis. Less commonly, scarring alopecia may occur because of dermal inflammation which involves the adnexal structures secondarily. Non-scarring alopecias are caused by either structural or growth cycle abnormalities of the hair without follicular inflammation; they can be classified into four types (Table 24.1).

Atrophic follicular diseases associated with endocrinopathies are the most common cause of bilaterally symmetrical, non-pruritic alopecia in the dog. In contrast, traumatic alopecia accounts for most cases of symmetrical alopecia in cats. Follicular dysplasias or dystrophies, diseases characterized by incompletely or abnormally formed hair follicles and hair shafts, are uncommon causes of non-pruritic alopecia in dogs which often closely resemble endocrine diseases. Follicular dystrophies are very rare in cats. Scarring disorders associated with follicular inflammation, which often present with patchy, multifocal areas of alopecia, are common in dogs but less frequent in cats.

INVESTIGATION OF ALOPECIA

A general medical and dermatological history is required in all cases of skin disease. Points of particular relevance in cases of alopecia are discussed below.

Table 24.1 Types of non-scarring alopecia according to the classification of Dunstan (1995)

Subtypes	Mechanism	Examples
Traumatic alopecias	Hair removed in pruritic or psychogenic disease	Alopecia in allergic skin diseases
Atrophic alopecias	Abnormal hair cycle leading to shortened anagen – prolonged telogen (follicles are 'asleep').	Hypothyroidism, hyperadrenocorticism
Follicular dystrophies	Disorder of morphogens or structural proteins causing malformation of shaft or follicle such that hair growth is impossible.	Congenital alopecia in Chinese crested dogs
Matrix cell – melanocyte abnormalities	Abnormal dispersal of melanosomes and/or disruption of matrix cells	Colour dilution alopecia

HISTORY CHECKLIST

❏ **Breed predilections?**
Follicular dysplasias have been recognized in curly coated retrievers, Irish water spaniels, Portuguese water dogs, Siberian huskies, Doberman pinschers and other breeds. Breed predilections have also been described for some canine endocrinopathies (Table 24.2). Acquired pattern alopecia is most often seen in dachshunds (Table 24.3).

❏ **Age of onset?**
Congenital ectodermal defects causing alopecia from birth are occasionally encountered.

Table 24.2 Atrophic hair follicle diseases of dogs associated with endocrinopathies which commonly present with symmetrical alopecia

Disease	Underlying pathology	Breed predilection	Age of onset	Clinical signs (other than skin)	Special dermatological features
Hypothyroidism	Lymphocytic thyroiditis or idiopathic atrophy	Various. Large breeds	6–10 years	Lethargy, weight gain, exercise intolerance, corneal lipid deposits, bradycardia	Cool, puffy, thickened skin (uncommon)
Hyperadrenocorticism (spontaneous)	Pituitary or adrenal neoplasia	Various. Boxers, poodles, dachshunds, terriers	6–12 years	Abdominal enlargement, hepatomegaly, muscle wasting, testicular atrophy	Calcinosis cutis, thin skin, prominent superficial vessels
Adrenal sex hormone imbalance/'Growth hormone-responsive dermatosis'	Abnormal adrenocortical steroidogenesis due to adrenal enzyme deficiency?	Pomeranians, keeshund, poodle, chow chow	1–3 years	Nil	Hair regrowth at sites of biopsy or other trauma to the skin
Sertoli cell tumour (male)	Functional testicular neoplasia	Not reported	Adult	Testicular mass, retained testis, prostatomegaly, attractiveness to male dogs, gynaecomastia, pendulous prepuce	Linear preputial erythema?
Hyperoestrogenism (female)	Ovarian 'cysts' or functional neoplasia	Not reported	Adult	Enlarged nipples and vulva, irregular or prolonged oestrus, or prior oestrogen therapy?	Nil

Intended only as a guide. In some cases, the listed features may be absent. Reproduced with permission of the British Small Animal Veterinary Association.

Table 24.3 Atrophic hair follicle diseases of dogs of unknown or non-hormonal aetiology which may present as symmetrical alopecia

Disease	Underlying pathology	Breed predilection	Age of onset	Clinical signs (other than skin)	Main diagnostic features
Telogen effluvium	Synchronous cessation of anagen, followed by shedding and regrowth	Nil	Variable	Often nil. Previous systemic disease or physiological stress	Rapid spontaneous resolution. Stressful event 1–3 months previously
Seasonal flank alopecia	Unknown. Related to photoperiod? Mediated via pineal gland – melatonin?	Boxers, Dobermanns, Airedale terriers, schnauzers	1–12 years (usually 2–6 years)	Nil	Cyclical or seasonal course. Exclude other diseases
Oestrogen-responsive dermatosis	Unknown	Not reported	Adult	Infantile vulva? Urinary incontinence?	Exclude other diseases. Response to therapy
Testosterone-responsive dermatosis	Unknown	Not reported	Adult	Nil	Exclude other diseases. Response to therapy
Acquired pattern alopecia (pattern baldness)	Unknown	Dachshund, Manchester terrier, Boston terrier, whippet	6–12 months	Nil	Histopathology: miniaturization of hair follicles

Intended only as a guide. In some cases, the listed features may be absent.
Reproduced with permission of BSAVA.

Symmetrical, grossly non-inflammatory alopecia acquired during the first year of life is suggestive of some follicular dystrophies, matrix cell/melanocyte abnormalities, or congenital endocrine diseases such as congenital hypothyroidism or pituitary dwarfism. Hypothyroidism and hyperadrenocorticism are usually seen in middle-aged or elderly dogs. Generalized demodicosis and dermatophytosis are most common in young animals.

❑ **Presence and degree of pruritus?**
A history of moderate or severe pruritus in a dog with alopecia may indicate a traumatic aetiology or a scarring (inflammatory) disease. Non-scarring alopecia is typically non-pruritic. However, secondary microbial infections, most often caused by staphylococci, may lead to pruritus in these diseases. If the distribution and severity of the pyoderma lesions do not correlate with the degree of alopecia, then the clinician should suspect an atrophic or dystrophic follicular disease underlying the skin infection. Re-evaluation after antimicrobial therapy may be helpful in such cases.

❑ **Evidence of transmission or contagion?**
Ectoparasitic infestations and dermatophytosis should be suspected when in-contact animals or humans are affected.

❑ **Signs of internal disease?**
Clinical signs associated with abnormalities in other organ systems are seen with endocrine diseases such as hypothyroidism and hyperadrenocorticism; these are described in detail in Chapter 39. Telogen defluxion (telogen effluvium) is a transient disorder of excessive hair shedding which results from synchronous cessation of anagen induced by a stressful event such as pregnancy, lactation, or a severe illness which occurred 1–3 months previously. Anagen defluxion, a rare disease reported in cats, is characterized by a transient abnormality of cellular proliferation within the hair matrix which leads to malformation and breakage of the hair shaft (Table 24.4). Cytotoxic drugs or systemic diseases are usually implicated as causal factors.

❑ **Seasonal or cyclical episodes of alopecia?**
Seasonal or cyclical episodes of non-inflammatory symmetrical truncal alopecia followed by spontaneous hair regrowth is a typical feature of seasonal flank alopecia (Table 24.3). Cyclical episodes of alopecia are seen occasionally in cases of follicular dystrophies, such as that of the Portuguese water dog.

❑ **Reproductive history?**
Male dogs with oestrogen-producing testicular tumours may be attractive to male dogs. Anoestrus and infertility may be reported in hypothyroid bitches, and prolonged oestrus has been reported in bitches with ovarian disorders and hyperoestrogenism.

❑ **Previous drug administration?**
The response, or lack of response, to previous therapy may also be helpful; for example, failure of hair regrowth after 3–5 months of supplementation with thyroxine at an appropriate dose suggests that hypothyroidism is unlikely. Long-term glucocorticoid therapy may cause iatrogenic Cushing's disease, and oestrogens and cytotoxic drugs such as cyclophosphamide may also interfere with hair growth. A previous response to antibacterial therapy might suggest relapsing pyoderma as a cause of multifocal, inflammatory alopecia.

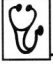 **PHYSICAL EXAMINATION**

A general physical examination may reveal clinical signs in other systems which may be related to the skin disease, particularly in dogs with hypothyroidism, hyperadrenocorticism and disorders associated with reproductive hormones (Tables 24.2 and 24.3). Although it is important to appreciate that clinical signs may be confined to the skin in some dogs with these diseases, additional physical findings can be very helpful in listing differential diagnoses in order of priority, enabling further tests to be performed in a rational order.

Clinical examination of the skin, in association with the history, should allow the clinician to determine whether the alopecia reflects traumatic alopecia associated with pruritus, follicular inflammation leading to scarring alopecia, or growth disturbances associated with either atrophic disorders or dystrophic diseases. Scarring alopecias may be associated with erythema, papules, pustules, furuncles and crusts, and the alopecia is more likely to be patchy rather than symmetrical (Table 24.5). Traumatic alopecia in the dog is usually accompanied by a complaint of pruritus. Alopecia without cutaneous inflammation in dogs suggests either an atrophic disease, a follicular dystrophy, or matrix cell/melanocyte abnormalities. Colour dilution alopecia should be strongly suspected if the dog has a dilute coat colour (for example, blue Dobermanns) and only dilute coloured areas are affected. Black hair follicular dysplasia should be considered if the alopecia is confined to black (or dark) haired areas. Both these diseases usually develop during the first year of life.

Dogs with symmetrical alopecia should be carefully evaluated for additional skin lesions. Comedones (blackheads), which are dilated hair follicles plugged with keratin and sebaceous debris, commonly develop in endocrine disease but may also be seen with demodicosis and with primary defects of keratinization. Thinning of the skin with prominent subcutaneous vessels occurs with hyperadrenocorticism, whereas dogs with hypothyroidism may have thickened skin due to increased deposition of dermal mucin (myxoedema). Calcinosis cutis, the deposition of calcium salts along dermal collagen fibres, is characterized by yellow or white papules, nodules and plaques which feel firm and gritty when palpated. Calcinosis cutis should be considered indicative of hyperadrenocorticism until proven otherwise.

Intense hyperpigmentation of the alopecic areas is most commonly seen in dogs with seasonal flank alopecia and adrenal sex hormone imbalances/growth hormone-responsive dermatosis (Table 24.2). A lightening of the coat colour (leucotrichia) is not uncommon in dogs with hyperadrenocorticism. Changes in coat colour and coat quality are also seen in many of the follicular dysplasias. The presence of miniaturized ('vellus') hairs is a key feature in acquired pattern alopecia (pattern baldness, Table 24.3), a rare disease usually seen in dachshunds, which presents with symmetrical, non-inflammatory alopecia of the pinnae and/or the ventrum.

Symmetrical alopecia or hypotrichosis is a common presentation in cats (Table 24.4). Areas commonly affected include the ventral abdomen, medial thighs, dorsolateral thorax or medial aspect of both forelegs. Owners frequently report excessive grooming to a degree sufficient to cause the alopecia. However, some cats groom secretly and the history might,

Table 24.4 Diseases of cats which may present with symmetrical alopecia

Disease	Pathophysiology	Additional signs	Diagnostic methods
Flea allergy dermatitis	Traumatic. Hypersensitivity response to flea saliva	Nil other than alopecia and pruritus (not always reported by owner) *or* papules, crusts *or* eosinophilic plaques	Evidence of fleas, response to therapy, intradermal test
Dietary sensitivity	Traumatic. Hypersensitivity response or intolerance to food or food additive	As above	Response to dietary restriction plus relapse on rechallenge
Atopy	Traumatic. Hypersensitivity response to environmental allergens	As above	Clinical signs, exclude other differentials, intradermal tests
Telogen defluxion (telogen effluvium)	Synchronous cessation of anagen, followed by shedding and regrowth	Often nil. Previous systemic disease or physiological stress	Rapid spontaneous resolution. Stressful event 1–3 months before
Anagen defluxion	Sudden transient interruption of cell proliferation in hair matrix	Severe systemic disease or cytotoxic drug therapy?	Plucked hairs show irregularities and dysplastic changes
Demodicosis	Inflammation targeting follicles infested by demodicid mites	Comedones, scales, follicular casts, pyoderma	Skin scrapings, biopsy (rare in cats)
Dermatophytosis	Inflammation targeting follicles infected by dermatophytes	Papules, scales, crusts, epidermal collarettes	Microscopy, Wood's lamp, culture, biopsy
Hyperadrenocorticism	Atrophic alopecia	Fragile skin, polyuria, polyphagia, enlarged abdomen	Blood and urine analyses. ACTH stimulation test
Hyperthyroidism	Traumatic. Excessive grooming	Variable. Weight loss, hyperactivity, polyphagia, polyuria, tachycardia	Basal thyroxine concentration
Diabetes mellitus	Unclear. Protein catabolism and hair growth cycle arrest?	Variable. Polyuria, polyphagia, weight loss	Persistent fasting hyperglycaemia and glycosuria
Hereditary hypotrichosis	Not well-defined	Otherwise healthy	Siamese and Devon rex. Exclude other causes
Psychogenic alopecia	Traumatic. Psychosis?	Otherwise healthy	Exclude *all* other possible causes

Intended only as a guide; not comprehensive.

incorrectly, suggest a failure of hair growth. Examination of the distal end of the hair shafts for evidence of self-trauma is most helpful in determining the true mechanism in such cases (see under hair plucks). Pruritus associated with hypersensitivity disorders, especially flea allergy, is the commonest cause of symmetrical alopecia in cats. Remarkably, there may be no additional gross signs of inflammatory skin disease. Psychogenic alopecia may present in a similar manner but such cases should have exhaustive investigations to exclude pruritic diseases. Hair regrowth following glucocorticoid therapy suggests that an inflammatory disease is more likely than a psychogenic disorder.

INITIAL DIAGNOSTIC PLAN

The historical and clinical features should enable the clinician to propose a list of differential diagnoses in order of priority. A diagnostic plan can then be discussed with the client and pursued in accordance with their wishes. Laboratory tests are required for the definitive diagnosis of most cases of alopecia.

LABORATORY INVESTIGATION

Skin scrapings

The microscopic examination of skin scrapings for evidence of ectoparasitism is warranted in all cases of alopecia in the dog and cat. Fungal spores and hyphae may be found in skin scrapings from dogs and cats with dermatophytosis.

Hair plucks

In dogs, dystrophic diseases and melanocytic disorders are often characterized by the production of hairs with structural abnormalities which can be detected on microscopy; for example, large melanin clumps with hair shaft distortion and fracture may be seen in colour dilution alopecia and black hair follicular dysplasia. Alternatively, the presence of large numbers of easily epilated, 'club' hairs suggests arrest of the hair growth cycle in the telogen phase, as seen in endocrine diseases.

In cats, the microscopic examination of the distal ends of plucked hairs aids in the differentiation of traumatic alopecia and alopecia associated with disturbances of hair growth. In traumatic alopecia, the end of the hair has a ragged or chewed appearance, whereas pointed ends are observed in disturbances of hair growth. Fungal spores and hyphae may be observed in hairs plucked from dogs and cats with dermatophytosis.

Skin biopsies

Skin biopsy is required for the diagnosis of follicular dystrophies and matrix cell/melanocyte

Table 24.5 Examples of diseases of the dog and cat which may present with focal alopecia

Disease	Pathophysiology	Additional signs	Diagnostic methods
Pyoderma	Inflammation targeting follicles infected by bacteria (rare in cats)	Papules, pustules, crusts, epidermal collarettes	Cytology, cultures, biopsy, response to treatment
Dermatophytosis	Inflammation targeting follicles infected by dermatophytes	Papules, scales, crusts, epidermal collarettes	Microscopy, Wood's lamp, culture, biopsy
Demodicosis	Inflammation targeting follicles infested by demodicid mites (rare in cats)	Comedones, scales, follicular casts, pyoderma	Skin scrapings, biopsy
Pelodera dermatitis	Inflammation targeting follicles infested by nematodes (rare)	Erythema, papules, scales, crusts	Recovery of nematodes on skin scrapings and biopsies
Scabies	Traumatic. Hypersensitivity response to mite allergens	Scales, crusts, erythematous papules, marked pruritus	Skin scrapings, response to therapy
Flea allergy dermatitis	Traumatic. Hypersensitivity response to flea saliva	Papules, erythema, crusts or alopecia alone	Evidence of fleas, response to therapy, intradermal skin test
Atopy	Traumatic. Hypersensitivity response to environmental allergens	Erythema, hyperpigmentation, lichenification, pyoderma or yeast infection	Clinical signs, exclude other differentials, intradermal or serological tests
Dietary sensitivity	Traumatic. Hypersensitivity response or intolerance to food or food additive	Erythema, hyperpigmentation, lichenification, pyoderma or yeast infection	Response to dietary restriction *plus* relapse on rechallenge
Alopecia areata	Immune assault on inferior portion of hair follicle (rare)	Well-demarcated alopecia without other signs	Biopsy
Pemphigus foliaceus	Autoimmune disease directed against desmosomes in epidermis. Reduced keratinocyte cohesion (rare)	Pustules, focal crusts	Biopsy

abnormalities. They are also helpful in many of the scarring disorders associated with follicular inflammation although the diagnosis can often be confirmed by other means in such cases (Table 24.5). As a general rule in cases of diffuse, non-inflammatory alopecia, multiple biopsy specimens should be obtained from the most alopecic areas; samples from marginal areas may be confusing because growing hairs may still be present. Primary lesions such as pustules and papules should be biopsied if inflammatory diseases are suspected. Few of the atrophic diseases can be diagnosed definitively by histopathological examination of skin alone; other clinical or laboratory data are usually required. The histopathological changes in hair follicle diseases can be subtle and it is preferable to submit biopsy specimens to a veterinary pathologist with a special interest in skin disease.

Haematology, blood biochemistry and urinalysis

Blood for haematology and biochemistry, and urine samples should be obtained for routine analyses in dogs and cats suspected of having endocrine or systemic diseases. The laboratory findings may support a diagnosis of a particular endocrine disease, and specific hormone assays can then be performed as indicated. For example, hypothyroid dogs may have a normocytic, normochromic, non-regenerative anaemia and hypercholesterolaemia, whereas dogs with hyperadrenocorticism often show lymphopenia, eosinopenia, and increased plasma concentrations of alkaline phosphatase and cholesterol. In general, dynamic tests of endocrine function are preferred because basal hormone concentrations may fluctuate widely in response to both physiological and pathological factors.

Tests designed to assess thyroid and pituitary/adrenal function are described in Chapter 39. Thyroid and pituitary/adrenal function should also be routinely assessed in dogs that have atrophic follicular diseases without other historical, clinical and laboratory features of endocrine diseases because the more typical features of hypothyroidism and hyperadrenocorticism do not occur in all cases. Basal oestradiol concentrations are elevated in some dogs with hyperoestrogenism associated with testicular neoplasia.

A protocol for the assessment of adrenal hormones before and after adrenocorticotrophin hormone (ACTH) stimulation has been described for use in dogs suspected of having adrenal sex hormone imbalances (Table 24.2) once hypothyroidism and hyperadrenocorticism have been excluded by specific tests (Schmeitzel et al., 1995). The pathogenesis of this disorder is poorly understood. It has been hypothesized that an abnormality of adrenal steroid synthesis related to a partial deficiency of an enzyme, 21-hydroxylase, might explain the elevated progesterone and androgen concentrations observed before and/or after ACTH stimulation in these dogs. Normal values for 17-hydroxyprogesterone before and after ACTH stimulation have been established by a UK based laboratory. In the USA, a wider array of hormones can be evaluated but this is expensive.

THERAPEUTIC PLAN

Specific therapy is available for many of the endocrine diseases of dogs and cats. In general, the treatment of dogs and cats with symmetrical alopecia by hormonal supplementation, without a specific indication based on laboratory testing, is to be discouraged. The therapy for hypothyroidism and hyperadrenocorticism is described elsewhere (Chapter 39). Only palliative therapy is available for dogs with follicular dystrophies and matrix cell/melanocyte abnormalities.

Dogs with adrenal sex hormone imbalances may respond to castration, methyltestosterone, lysodren or growth hormone. Castration of the intact male dog may be the first treatment of choice. Lysodren may also be effective; an initial dose of 15–25 mg kg^{-1} daily for 5 days is followed by maintenance doses of 15–25 mg kg^{-1} every 7–14 days. These dogs should be carefully monitored for signs of hypocortisolaemia, hyperkalaemia and hyponatraemia, particularly during initial therapy. Hair regrowth is often evident within 4–12 weeks. Although some dogs respond favourably to growth hormone supplementation, this hormone is potentially diabetogenic and is difficult to obtain. Therapy is not currently available for seasonal flank alopecia; however, it has been reported that the predicted episodes of alopecia may be prevented by melatonin supplementation. There is no rationale for supplementation with thyroid, reproductive and growth hormones in seasonal flank alopecia.

Inflammatory diseases associated with follicular infections and ectoparasitic infestations should be treated with appropriate antimicrobial and antiparasitic agents. *Staphylococcus inter-*

medius, the most common cause of canine pyoderma, is often susceptible to antibiotics such as potentiated sulphonamides, lincomycin or cephalexin. Systemic antifungal therapy with griseofulvin is generally indicated in dogs and cats with dermatophytosis. Adjunctive topical therapy is useful in reducing environmental contamination and the risk of transmission. Traumatic alopecia is best treated by identification and correction of the underlying cause; the reader is referred to Chapter 25 for an account of the approach to such cases.

REFERENCES

Dunstan, R.W. (1995) A pathomechanistic approach to diseases of the hair follicle. *Veterinary Dermatology Newsletter* **17**, 37–41.

Schmeitzel, L.P., Lothrop, C.D. and Rosenkrantz, W.S. (1995) Congenital adrenal hyperplasia-like syndrome. In: *Kirk's Current Veterinary Therapy XII*. (Ed. J.D. Bonagura). W.B. Saunders, Philadelphia, pp. 600–604.

25

Pruritus

R. Bond

INTRODUCTION

Pruritus, an unpleasant itching sensation which provokes the desire to scratch, lick or chew, is a common complaint in small animal medicine. The pathophysiology of pruritus is poorly understood but is thought to reflect stimulation of unmyelinated nerve endings by chemical mediators such as histamine, endopeptidases, substance P and leukotrienes. Pruritic skin diseases are a common source of client frustration and dissatisfaction, and uncontrolled pruritus also presents a significant welfare problem. Most pruritic skin diseases can be succesfully treated and controlled or cured, provided a structured approach is adopted. Although there is often a temptation to provide symptomatic relief of pruritus with glucocorticoids, this approach is seldom satisfactory in the longer term, and it is contraindicated in some diseases. The clinician should always attempt to establish a definitive diagnosis, so that subsequent management and treatment can be optimized. If a diagnosis cannot be obtained, then symptomatic therapy should be carefully adjusted to maximize benfits for the patient while minimizing the potential for adverse side effects.

The purpose of this chapter is to provide a framework for the investigation and management of pruritic skin diseases in dogs and cats. Obtaining a detailed history and performing a careful clinical examination are pivotal to the approach. Laboratory examinations for ectoparasites should be performed in the majority of cases, and additional investigative procedures are often required to achieve a definitive diagnosis.

INVESTIGATION OF PRURITUS

 ### HISTORY CHECKLIST

A general medical history should be obtained in all animals with skin disease. Signs of ill-health relating to other organ systems may be present in some systemic diseases with cutaneous manifestations, or there may be an unrelated disorder which requires investigation and therapy. Breed predilections for pruritic diseases can assist the clinician in prioritizing differential diagnoses but they should not prevent a consideration of other differential diagnoses. Breeds predisposed to atopic disease include small terriers, retrievers, Shar peis, boxers, German shepherd dogs and English setters. Basset hounds, Cocker spaniels and West Highland white terriers are predisposed to *Malassezia* dermatitis. The following historical points should be addressed.

❏ Age of onset?

The age predilections for pruritic diseases can be helpful. For example, pruritus in young puppies or kittens is most likely to be associated with ectoparasitic infestation with fleas, *Sarcoptes scabiei*, *Cheyletiella* spp. or *Otodectes cynotis*. Hypersensitivity disorders usually develop in young to middle-aged animals; the typical age of onset of canine atopy is 6 months to 3 years, with a range of up to 7 years. Thus, pruritus in an aged animal, previously free of skin disease, is more likely to reflect an infection or ectoparasitic infestation rather than atopic disease. Cutaneous lymphoma is a rare cause of pruritus in older animals.

❏ Development and progression of the disease?

Pruritus may manifest as scratching, licking, chewing, rubbing or rolling. Therefore, simply asking owners whether their animal scratches is not sufficient; some dogs and cats with extreme pruritus may chew constantly without scratching. It is useful to determine the owner's impression of the severity of the pruritus. Canine scabies is among the most pruritic diseases encountered, whereas pruritus associated with demodicosis may be mild. The comments of observant owners or an examination of detailed case records should allow the clinician to evaluate any progression of the disease. The sudden development of intense pruritus in an animal previously free of skin disease suggests an acquired infestation or infection; in contrast, allergic diseases may have a more gradual onset.

With hypersensitivity disorders such as atopic disease, the first sign noted by the owner is often pruritus with no or few skin lesions. In contrast, pruritus associated with canine pyoderma often develops after the appearance of primary lesions such as papules and pustules. Thus, enquiring whether the patient has a 'rash that itches' or an 'itch that rashes' can assist in determining whether any eruptive lesions represent a primary or secondary problem.

Some diseases have characteristic regional distributions, particularly during the early stages. For example, flea allergy dermatitis in dogs primarily affects the caudal regions of the trunk, especially the dorsolumbar area. In contrast, canine atopic disease is often characterized by pruritus of the face, ears, distal limbs and/or ventrum. With scabies, the lesions often initially involve the ears, elbows, hocks or ventral thorax. Canine superficial pyoderma most often affects the ventral abdomen, medial thighs or dorsal trunk.

Pruritus in cats may manifest as excessive grooming which results in symmetrical traumatic alopecia. In some cases, the cats do this secretly and the owners are not aware that the cat is removing the hair; microscopical examination of the hair shafts can help determine whether the hair is falling out or being removed (see later under hair plucks).

❏ **Lifestyle?**

Animals with free or regular access to outdoor environments are at greater risk from infections, ectoparasitic infestations, and hypersensitivity associated with pollen allergens than animals confined to the home. Recent visits to shows, grooming parlours and training classes may be of significance if a transmissible disease is suspected. There may be a history of contact with foxes in cases of canine scabies, and wild rodents are a potential source of dermatophytes for hunting dogs such as Jack Russell terriers.

❏ **Seasonality?**

Seasonal pruritus is most often associated with flea allergy dermatitis, atopy caused by pollen allergens, harvest mite (*Neotrombicula autumnalis*) infestations or, less commonly, contact dermatitis associated with outdoor plants. In the UK, harvest mites are usually a problem from July to September, whereas clinical signs associated with tree and grass pollens may be observed during the spring or early summer. A history of previously seasonal pruritus which has become perennial is suggestive of progressive atopic disease; some dogs with pollen allergies eventually develop sensitivity to indoor allergens such as housedust mites.

❏ **Evidence of transmission or contagion?**

A history of contagion to other animals strongly suggests ectoparasitism (with the exception of demodicosis) or dermatophytosis. Zoonotic skin disease is commonly seen with fleas, cheyletiellosis, scabies and dermatophytosis, and rarely with *Otodectes cynotis*, feline poxvirus and sporotrichosis.

❏ **Treatments used and response?**

A list of all treatments given in each case should be made. Recent treatments may influence clinical signs and laboratory test results, and in some cases, pruritus may reflect an adverse reaction to a treatment. The response to treatment with certain agents with specific effects can be helpful. For example, response to antibacterial therapy suggests that pyoderma is involved. Response, or lack of response, to properly administered antiparasitic therapy may suggest, or refute, a diagnosis of ectoparasitism. Response to glucocorticoid therapy is less helpful because many different types of inflammatory skin disease will improve. The pruritus associated with hypersensitivity disorders such as atopic disease, when uncomplicated by concurrent microbial infection, is usually readily controlled with glucocorticoids whereas the response in cases of dietary sensitivity is more variable. Glucocorticoid treatment is less often helpful in treating pruritus associated with scabies, demodicosis or dermatophytosis, and it may exacerbate clinical signs in the latter two diseases.

PHYSICAL EXAMINATION

A general physical examination should be accompanied by a close inspection of the entire skin surface. The nature and distribution of any skin lesions are of vital importance in determining the aetiology of the disease. When considered together with the historical features, the clinical signs in each case should allow the clinician to propose either a tentative diagnosis or a list of differential diagnoses. Laboratory tests or treatments can then be selected. It is beyond the scope of this chapter to provide a detailed description of the clinical signs associated with each inflammatory skin disease of dogs and cats; the reader is referred to other chapters in this text for further details. Tables 25.1–25.3 summarize the types of lesions and their distribution in common pruritic diseases of dogs and cats.

It is not uncommon for pruritic animals, especially dogs, to have more than one factor contributing to the pruritus. The concepts of allergic threshold and summation are important in the management of pruritus. Microbial infections such as pyoderma or *Malassezia* dermatitis frequently occur in association with parasitic, allergic, endocrine or keratinization disorders in dogs. Some dogs and cats with hypersensitivity disorders have multiple allergies; for example, atopic patients may have concurrent flea allergy or dietary sensitivity. Sequential treatment and removal of the contributing factors are required for diagnosis and management. In some animals with multiple contributing factors, successful treatment of one factor may reduce the level of pruritus below a threshold level such that the other disorders become asymptomatic.

Pruritic cats may present with one or more types of cutaneous reaction pattern. 'Miliary dermatitis' is characterized by a red–brown papulocrustuous eruption. Although most cases reflect flea allergy, other ectoparasitic and hypersensitivity disorders may be responsible. Eosinophilic plaques are highly pruritic, moist, glistening, well-demarcated lesions which usually occur on the abdomen or medial thighs. They are usually a manifestation of hypersensitivity and sometimes occur in association with miliary dermatitis. Symmetrical, traumatic alopecia on either the dorsum, ventrum or limbs is another common manifestation of allergic skin disease in the cat. For some years these cats were supected of having endocrine disease because pruritus was not always observed and the alopecic skin did not look inflamed.

INITIAL DIAGNOSTIC PLAN

The historical and clinical features should enable the clinician to propose either a tentative diagnosis or a list of differential diagnoses, and to select appropriate laboratory procedures and treatments. It is important to discuss with the owner the options for therapy and investigation, and the likely course of the disease. For example, hypersensitivity disorders are seldom cured but may be

Table 25.1 Types of skin lesions and their significance in dogs with pruritic skin disease

Lesion type	Pathophysiology	Principal differential diagnoses
Erythema ± traumatic alopecia	Vasodilatation/inflammation	Hypersensitivity diseases Irritant contact dermatitis Ectoparasitism
Erythema + greasy exudation	Inflammation + increased activity of skin glands	Pyoderma *Malassezia* dermatitis
Erythema + marked scale formation ± alopecia	Inflammation plus accelerated epidermopoiesis *or* infiltration with neoplastic lymphocytes	Ectoparasitism Dermatophytosis Pyoderma, *Malassezia* dermatitis Cutaneous lymphoma
Papules	Accumulation of inflammatory cells in dermis/epidermis	Hypersensitivity diseases Pyoderma Irritant contact dermatitis
Pustules	Accumulation of inflammatory cells (esp. neutrophils) in epidermis–dermis	Pyoderma Pemphigus foliaceus Drug eruptions, sterile pustular diseases
Comedones ± follicular casts	Accumulation of keratinous debris in follicular infundibulum ± hair growth cycle arrest	Demodicosis Keratinization defects Endocrinopathies
Focal crusts	Dried exudate on skin surface; cellular exocytosis	Scabies and other parasites Pyoderma, dermatophytosis Pemphigus foliaceus Drug eruptions, sterile pustular diseases

Table 25.2 Types of skin lesions and their significance in cats with pruritic skin disease

Lesion type	Pathophysiology	Principal differential diagnoses
Traumatic alopecia	Pruritus *or* psychogenic	Hypersensitivity diseases Ectoparasitism Psychogenic disorder
Crusted papules ('miliary dermatitis')	Accumulation of inflammatory cells in dermis/epidermis; cellular exocytosis	Hypersensitivity diseases Ectoparasitism Dermatophytosis (uncommon) Bacterial folliculitis (rare)
Erythema + marked scale formation ± alopecia	Inflammation plus accelerated epidermopoiesis *or* infiltration with neoplastic lymphocytes	Ectoparasitism Dermatophytosis Hypersensitivity diseases Cutaneous lymphoma
Focal yellow/white crust (cf. reddish crusted papules in miliary dermatitis)	Dried exudate on skin surface; cellular exocytosis	Dermatophytosis Pemphigus foliaceus Ectoparasitism Bacterial folliculitis (rare)
Eosinophilic plaque	Self-trauma, underlying hypersensitivity	Hypersensitivity diseases Idiopathic, neoplasia

Table 25.3 Distribution patterns for pruritic skin diseases

Region affected	Principal differential diagnoses
Feet	Atopy, dietary sensitivity, contact dermatitis demodicosis, tromiculidiasis, hookworm dermatitis, deep pyoderma, *Malassezia* dermatitis
Ears	Atopy, dietary sensitivity, contact dermatitis, scabies, tromiculidiasis, *Otodectes* infestation
Muzzle	Atopy, dietary sensitivity, contact dermatitis, *Malassezia* dermatitis
Ventral abdomen	Atopy, dietary sensitivity, contact dermatitis, superficial pyoderma, *Malassezia* dermatitis, flea allergy dermatitis
Dorsal trunk	Flea allergy dermatitis, cheyletiellosis, pediculosis, superficial pyoderma

controlled. Microbial infections may be treated successfully but often relapse if an underlying cause cannot be identified and corrected. Securing the client's cooperation and understanding is critical to the successful management of pruritic skin disease in dogs and cats.

LABORATORY AND OTHER DIAGNOSTIC TESTS

Laboratory tests are often required in the investigation of pruritic skin diseases. Simple, inexpensive and potentially very rewarding tests such as skin scrapings, coat brushings and cytological examinations should be routinely performed. Failure to perform these basic procedures at an early stage during the investigation of dermatological disease can lead to an incorrect diagnosis and inappropriate therapy, sometimes with serious consequences for the welfare of the patient. Additional tests, listed below, may also be warranted depending on the clinical presentation.

Skin scrapings, hair plucks and coat brushings

Skin scrapings should be obtained from every dermatology case unless the clinician is certain that the lesions could not be caused by a parasite (which is not very often in this author's experience). Skin scraping is primarily utilized in the diagnosis of ectoparasitism but can also be useful in the diagnosis of dermatophytosis. All dogs and cats with inflammatory skin disease, scaling and/or alopecia should be scraped. Identification of a single parasite or egg allows a diagnosis of infestations such as cheyletiellosis or scabies. However, failure to demonstrate *Sarcoptes scabiei* mites or eggs does not exclude a diagnosis of canine scabies, and trial therapy is always indicated whenever scabies is suspected. In most cases of demodicosis, numerous mites in all stages of development will be readily identified. However, skin biopsy is sometimes required to demonstrate mites, especially in pedal lesions and areas of thickened skin.

The observation of arthrospores on, or hyphae within, hair shafts and corneocytes provides convincing evidence of dermatophytosis. Abnormal hairs should be examined using the × 40 objective for evidence of invasion by hyphae. Fungal elements can be difficult to visualize and may not be found even when examined by experienced mycologists, and other investigative techniques including culture and Wood's lamp examination should be routinely employed when dermatophytosis is suspected but fungi are not found in scrapings.

Scales and debris collected by brushing the coat over a table can be mounted in liquid paraffin for microscopic examination; this method is useful for the diagnosis of cheyletiellosis. Brushings can also be spread on moistened white tissue paper for evidence of flea faeces; a red–brown stain on the tissue paper differentiates flea faeces from other particulate debris.

Examination of hair plucks may demonstrate the eggs of lice or *Cheyletiella* spp. attached to hair shafts, and *Demodex* spp. lying around the proximal portions of the hair. In cats with alopecia, examination of the distal ends of hairs can aid in the differentiation of traumatic alopecia from disorders of hair growth. With traumatic alopecia, the hair has a ragged, chewed end whereas with disorders of hair growth, a normal, pointed end to the hair shaft is observed.

Cytological examination

Cytological examinations are principally used to demonstrate superficial microbes such as bacteria and *Malassezia pachydermatis*. Pustule contents can be smeared onto a glass slide, stained using a rapid stain such as Diff-Quik, and examined using the oil immersion (× 100) microscope objective. With pyoderma, neutrophils (often degenerate) are the dominant cell type, and intracellular and extracellular bacteria (usually cocci) may be observed. In pemphigus foliaceus, large numbers of acantholytic (rounded, nucleated) epithelial cells can often be seen among 'healthy' neutrophils. The presence of numerous bacteria in pustule contents should prompt antibacterial therapy, whereas biopsies should be performed in dogs and cats suspected of having pemphigus foliaceus or other sterile pustular diseases.

Populations of the yeast, *M. pachydermatis*, can be rapidly assessed by clipping the hair and applying a strip of clear adhesive tape onto the affected skin. This is removed, stained using Diff-Quik and examined using the oil immersion (× 100) microscope objective. Numerous squames should be readily identified. *M. pachydermatis* is a monopolar-budding yeast with a characteristic 'peanut' or 'bottle-shaped' morphology. The distinction between normal and abnormal populations is rather arbitrary but it is difficult to find more than just an occasional yeast cell in specimens from healthy skin. Populations should be considered increased when the yeast is readily found in several fields. If the clinical signs are consistent with '*Malassezia* dermatitis', then trial therapy is indicated to determine the significance of the yeast. In some cases, large numbers of bacteria are found, either alone or in association with the yeast, and antibacterial therapy should be given in these circumstances.

Microbial cultures

The principal bacterial pathogen of canine skin, *Staphylococcus intermedius*, is often isolated from healthy dogs. Profuse growth from a swab specimen implies that it is present in large numbers and antibacterial therapy may be warranted. Empirical selection of anti-staphylococcal antibacterial agents is acceptable in superficial pyoderma but culture and sensitivity is justified in relapsing cases or in deep pyoderma.

Cultures should be performed in dogs and cats suspected of having dermatophytosis. Although dermatophytes can be cultured in practice laboratories, dermatophyte isolation and identification is a skilled process best performed in specialist mycology laboratories. Quantitative cultures of *M. pachydermatis* using contact plates, small agar dishes which can be applied directly onto lesional skin, are a useful adjunct to cytology in determining whether trial antifungal therapy is indicated.

Intradermal and serological tests for hypersensitivity disorders

These tests are used in dogs and cats suspected of having atopic disease or flea allergy dermatitis. Intradermal tests, wherein a panel of pollen and indoor allergens are injected into the skin on the flank, detect reaginic (mainly IgE) antibodies bound to dermal mast cells. Serological tests are designed to detect increased levels of allergen-specific IgE or IgG_d in the serum. In Europe, most dogs diagnosed as atopic have 'positive' reactions to housedust mites when tested with either method. Pollen reactions occur less frequently. However, it is important to note that healthy dogs also frequently show positive reactions with both of these tests, most commonly to housedust mites; this is especially a problem with the serological tests. Therefore, intradermal and serological tests are of very limited value in diagnosis. The diagnosis of atopy should be based primarily on historical and clinical features, and a positive serological or intradermal test is merely supportive. The principal role of these tests is in the selection of allergens for subsequent immunotherapy (hyposensitization); therefore, these tests are arguably not justified unless the owner wishes to pursue this form of therapy.

Elimination diets

The currently available intradermal and serological tests are of no value in the diagnosis of dietary sensitivity ('food allergy') in dogs and cats. Currently, feeding an elimination diet followed by provocative exposure is the only reliable way to establish this diagnosis. Unfortunately, this is a difficult procedure which requires a dedicated owner. A home-cooked diet comprising a novel single protein source, such as turkey, rabbit or fish, should be fed to the absolute exclusion of all else for a period of at least 4–6 weeks, or possibly longer. A carbohydrate source such as potato or rice should also be given. If a response is seen, the original diet should be fed again to confirm that the dietary change is responsible for the improvement. Home-cooked diets are considered to be nutritionally incomplete, especially with regard to calcium, thiamin, iron and in cats, taurine, and are therefore not suitable for long-term management.

Commercially prepared 'hypoallergenic' diets can also be used for diagnosis but it is preferable to reserve these for the management of proven cases because they contain a wider range of nutrients and additives than home-prepared diets.

Skin biopsy

Skin biopsies are indicated whenever an autoimmune or immune-mediated disease, cutaneous neoplasia or a keratinization defect is suspected; recognition of characteristic histopathological features is usually required to confirm these diagnoses. This technique may aid the diagnosis of pyoderma and cutaneous fungal infections, although these disorders can often be recognized by clinical signs, cytology and culture results. Biopsies are often much less helpful for diagnosing parasitic and hypersensitivity disorders, with the exception of demodicosis where the parasites are often readily observed within hair follicles. In other types of ectoparasitism, it is unusual to observe the mites within biopsy specimens. Unfortunately, pathognomonic histopathological features of each of the various types of hypersensitivity disorder (atopy, food, contact, flea) have not been recognized. Although a skilled pathologist may be able to suggest which type of hypersensitivity is most likely, it is ultimately the clinician's responsibility to differentiate these. Thus, skin biopsies are often of limited value in the investigation of suspect allergic cases, although they may enable the clinician to exclude other differential diagnoses.

FORMULATING A THERAPEUTIC PLAN

Parasitic disorders are among the commonest pruritic skin diseases and exclusion by laboratory tests and response to trial parasiticidal therapy early in the course of the investigation is desirable. It is important to treat the environment and in-contact animals when adopting the trial therapy approach. Trial antimicrobial therapy is indicated whenever the clinical signs and cytological or cultural investigations suggest that bacterial infection or *Malassezia* dermatitis is likely. Many clinicians routinely give antibacterial therapy in conjunction with glucocorticoids but, in general, this is to be discouraged. Antimicrobial therapy alone often has tremendous antipruritic effects, and more information is gained when only the antimicrobial agent is given. Examining a pruritic dog with a pyoderma after 14–21 days of antibacterial therapy allows the clinician to determine whether the pyoderma and pruritus has resolved. If the infection has resolved but the pruritus persists, then the dog should be evaluated for ectoparasitic and hypersensitivity disorders. Pyoderma may occur in association with non- or mildly pruritic diseases such as endocrinopathies or primary keratinization defects. A similar approach is required to determine the importance of *M. pachydermatis*; response to topical or systemic antiyeast therapy coupled with a reduction in yeast numbers would imply a pathogenic role.

Dogs and cats with hypersensitivity disorders such as atopy, dietary sensitivity or contact dermatitis usually remain pruritic despite parasiticidal, antibacterial and antiyeast treatment. Elimination diets, contact restriction studies, and intradermal and serological tests can then be performed as indicated. The author routinely investigates dietary sensitivity in such cases because allergen avoidance is often practicable whenever this disease is diagnosed. In contrast, allergen avoidance is seldom a practical solution for atopic disease and some cases of contact dermatitis, and lifelong glucocorticoid or other anti-inflammatory therapy is then often required.

The sequential performance of these trial procedures can lead to a lengthy investigation and it is often useful to combine some of the initial steps. For example, in a suspect atopic dog, concurrent dietary and parasite trials could be given initially to exclude dietary sensitivity and flea allergy. No response would support a diagnosis of atopic disease but if a marked response was seen, rechallenge with the original diet would differentiate dietary sensitivity from flea allergy. Symptomatic therapy with antibacterial or glucocorticoid agents may be required in severely pruritic animals while awaiting the results of laboratory tests, dietary manipulations and parasiticidal therapy. However, care must be taken to ensure that such treatments do not interfere with subsequent investigations such as intradermal tests.

26

Scaling and Crusting Disorders

R. Bond

INTRODUCTION

Scaling and crusting disorders represent a significant proportion of the dermatological case load in small animal practice. Scaling refers to the accumulation of fragments of the cornified layer of the epidermis. Crusting is indicative of an accumulation of dried exudate which is usually composed of serum, inflammatory cells or blood. In common with other dermatological signs, scaling or crusting can be seen in a wide array of skin diseases. Scaling disorders are common in dogs but are less often seen in cats. The purpose of this chapter is to describe briefly the pathophysiological processes which lead to scaling or crusting, and to describe an approach to diagnosis in such cases. Achieving a definitive diagnosis gives the clinician the best chance of instituting successful therapy. Detailed descriptions of individual diseases can be found in Chapter 47.

PATHOPHYSIOLOGY

The skin is covered by a continuous stratified keratinizing epithelium, the epidermis, which terminates at the mucocutaneous junctions. The epidermis is composed of layers occupied by viable keratinocytes (stratum basale, stratum spinosum, stratum granulosum) and non-viable, fully differentiated corneocytes (stratum corneum). The three principal processes of the self-renewal system which operate within the epidermis are proliferation, differentiation and desquamation. Cellular proliferation in the canine epidermis is confined to the basal cell layer. Cells migrate upwards from the basal layer and commit to terminal differentiation. During this process, termed keratinization, the living cell is ultimately transformed into a dead corneocyte or squame which is composed of aggregates of keratin filaments invested by a chemically resistant proteinaceous cell envelope. The canine stratum corneum is composed of approximately 40 layers of tightly-packed corneocytes.

The continual renewal of the epidermal cell population allows the skin to react to different physiological and pathological stimuli. During the normal process of desquamation, fully cornified cells are lost individually or in small groups not visible to the naked eye.

Clinical signs may result from alterations of

Table 26.1 Primary defects of keratinization and associated breed predilections

Disease	Breed predilections
Idiopathic seborrhoea	Cocker and springer spaniel, West Highland white terrier, Irish setter, Dobermann, shar pei, Labrador
Vitamin A-responsive dermatosis	Cocker spaniel, miniature schnauzer, Labrador
Zinc-responsive dermatosis	Alaskan malamute, Siberian husky, samoyed
Sebaceous adenitis	Standard poodle, akita, vizsla, samoyed
Ichthyosis	West Highland white terrier
Lethal acrodermatitis	Bull terrier
Epidermal dysplasia	West Highland white terrier
Idiopathic nasodigital hyperkeratosis	Cocker and springer spaniel
Ear margin dermatosis	Dachshund

either proliferation, differentiation or desquamation, in any combination. Enhanced proliferation and desquamation is a common reaction of the skin to inflammation; this process may be beneficial to the host when surface pathogens such as dermatophytes are present. Scaling may also occur in non-inflammatory diseases such as endocrine and nutritional disturbances reflecting the important role of hormones, proteins, trace elements and essential fatty acids in epidermal maturation. The term *primary defect of keratinization* is used to describe skin diseases characterized clinically by excessive scaling and histologically by epidermal abnormalities which result from unknown causes or as a direct consequence of abnormal keratinization (Table 26.1) Keratinization defects secondary to ectoparasites, microbial infections, inflammatory diseases and endocrinopathies are much more common.

Crusting indicates a previous episode of exudation. Histologically, the crust can be classified according to the nature of its components. Serous crust is composed primarily of plasma, cellular crust consists of degenerate polymorphonuclear cells, most commonly neutrophils, and palisading crusts develop as a consequence of episodic bursts of neutrophilic exocytosis. Palisading crusts are seen most commonly in dermatophytosis and dermatophilosis.

INVESTIGATION OF SCALING AND CRUSTING DISORDERS

 HISTORY CHECKLIST

A general medical history should be obtained in every case because scaling and crusting disorders sometimes reflect internal diseases. Alternatively, a general history may reveal evidence of other, unrelated diseases which require attention. Points of particular relevance in animals with scaling and crusting disease are discussed below.

❏ **Breed?**
Important breed predilections of value in prioritizing differential diagnoses are recognized in many defects of keratinization of dogs (Table 26.1). Primary defects of keratinization are very rare in cats, although primary idiopathic seborrhoea has been reported in Persian kittens. Lethal acrodermatitis is a symmetrical erythematous and crusting disorder of young bull terriers associated with an autosomal recessive defect in zinc metabolism.

❏ **Age of onset?**
Ichthyosis, a rare congenital disorder of keratinization characterized by scaling and/or retention of the stratum corneum, has been identified in cats and in dogs of various breeds including West Highland white terriers, Yorkshire terriers, Jack Russell terriers and Cavalier King Charles spaniels. Many of the primary defects of keratinization, such as idiopathic seborrhoea, develop during the first year of life. Ectoparasitic disorders and dermatophytosis occur in all age groups but are most common in young animals. Endocrine, metabolic and neoplastic causes of scaling are most frequent in middle-aged or elderly dogs. Nutritional disorders can occur at any age.

❏ **Development and progression of the disorder?**
The distribution and progression of skin lesions can be helpful. Pruritus is an early feature in canine scabies. Lesions most commonly develop on the pinnal margins, elbows or hocks but then may advance to involve wider areas of the limbs and ventral trunk. Dermatophytosis in dogs is often characterized by peripheral spreading from an area of scale or alopecia. Generalized skin involvement early in the course of the disease is usually a feature of ichthyosis and primary idiopathic seborrhoea.

❏ **Degree of pruritus?**
Pruritus is usually a major feature of ectoparasitic infestations and is also commonly observed with bacterial folliculitis, *Malassezia* dermatitis and dermatophytosis. Epidermal dysplasia is a controversial 'disease' of West Highland white terriers which is characterized clinically by severe pruritus (see later under clinical signs). Endocrine, nutritional and metabolic disorders, and primary defects of keratinization are usually non- or only mildly pruritic. However, secondary infection with bacteria or *Malassezia pachydermatis* commonly results in moderate or severe pruritus in such cases.

❏ **Signs of systemic disease?**
In general, dogs and cats with ectoparasitic disorders and primary defects of keratinization are otherwise healthy. Signs of systemic disease may be observed in animals with endocrine and metabolic diseases. Hypothyroid dogs may be lethargic, intolerant of exercise, and may gain weight without increased food intake. Dogs with hyperadrenocorticism may show polyuria/polydipsia, polyphagia, exercise intolerance and muscle

weakness. Weight loss, reduced appetite and polyuria/polydipsia may be observed in dogs with metabolic epidermal necrosis (superficial necrolytic dermatitis, 'hepatocutaneous syndrome'). Dogs living in or imported from southern Europe with skin disease caused by protozoan parasites of the genus *Leishmania* may present with haematological, renal, hepatic, musculoskeletal or ocular signs. Generalized scaling may be seen in cats with diabetes mellitus or hyperthyroidism.

❏ **Diet?**

Nutritional deficiencies and imbalances sufficient to cause skin disease are unlikely in dogs and cats fed on good quality commercial diets. Nutritional diseases can be observed when owners feed unbalanced home-prepared diets, and in animals with gastrointestinal disease or genetic disorders of metabolism. Zinc-responsive dermatosis may be seen in Arctic breeds such as the Alaskan malamutes; a genetic defect causing decreased zinc absorption is suspected in these dogs. Zinc-responsive dermatosis can occur in other breeds fed on diets high in phytates or minerals which inhibit zinc absorption, but this is now less often seen because manufacturers have increased the zinc content of their diets.

❏ **Evidence of transmission or contagion?**

A history of contagion to other animals strongly suggests ectoparasitism (with the exception of demodicosis) or dermatophytosis. Zoonotic skin disease is commonly seen with fleas, cheyletiellosis, scabies and dermatophytosis. Rarely, multiple animals in the household may be affected if all are fed on a nutritionally incomplete diet.

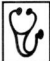 **PHYSICAL EXAMINATION**

A consideration of the nature and distribution of skin lesions in association with the historical findings should allow the clinician to prioritize the differential diagnoses in each case. Recognition of the type of skin lesions is helpful in differentiating possible causes.

Scaling may occur on its own or in association with other skin lesions. Scaling alone may result from parasitic infestations such as cheyletiellosis or leishmaniasis, and environmental factors such as dry heat. Rarely, dermatophytosis may present as localized or generalized scaling without alopecia, especially in canine infections caused by *Microsporum persicolor*. Scaling accompanied by symmetrical, non-inflammatory alopecia is suggestive of endocrine disease. Cutaneous lymphoma may present as an exfoliative erythroderma and/or nodules, plaques and ulceration of the skin, or mucous membrane ulceration.

Widespread scaling accompanied by pruritus, erythema, traumatic alopecia and varying degrees of hyperpigmentation and lichenification occur with hypersensitivity disorders, especially those which are complicated by bacterial or *M. pachydermatis* infections. Similar signs have been reported in West Highland white terriers with a primary keratinization defect termed epidermal dysplasia; high skin populations of *M. pachydermatis* are usually present in such cases.

Comedones (blackheads), dilated hair follicles plugged with keratinous debris occur with demodicosis, endocrine disease and primary defects of keratinization. Follicular casts result from the accumulation and adherence of keratinous material to the hair shaft extending beyond the follicular ostia. They indicate abnormal keratinization within the follicular infundibulum and are often a prominent feature, in addition to scaling, of sebaceous adenitis, idiopathic seborrhoea and vitamin A-responsive dermatosis. Follicular casts may also be seen in demodicosis and dermatophytosis.

Multifocal circular crusts suggest an eruptive process and often evolve from papules or pustules. These lesions are most commonly seen in canine pyoderma but also occur in sterile pustular diseases such as pemphigus foliaceus. Pyoderma lesions usually involve the ventral abdomen and trunk whereas pemphigus foliaceus often affects the face and ears. With pemphigus foliaceus, a combination of individual focal lesions and areas of coalescing crusts is often seen.

Circular, crusting lesions with alopecia occur in dermatophytosis. A gradual outward progression of the lesion may be observed with central healing and more active inflammation at the periphery. Multifocal lesions are more common in feline dermatophytosis but individual lesions are often less numerous in dogs; pyoderma is the most common cause of expanding, ring-like lesions in the latter species. Superficial pyoderma in short-coated dogs occasionally presents as diffuse truncal scaling accompanied by a subtle papular eruption and patchy alopecia. Erythematous, crusting papules are frequently observed in dogs with scabies.

The presence of symmetrical skin lesions often suggests a systemic disease (Table 26.2). Symmetrical per-orificial crusting occurs in metabolic epidermal necrosis and in zinc-responsive

Table 26.2 Scaling or crusting disorders which commonly present with symmetrical skin lesions

Disease	Pathophysiology	Clinical features	Diagnostic procedures
Idiopathic seborrhoea	Hyperproliferative basal keratinocytes	Scaling, comedones, follicular casts, hyperkeratotic plaques	History, exclude other differential diagnoses, skin biopsies
Vitamin A-responsive dermatosis	Idiopathic keratinization defect. Systemic deficiency unlikely	Scaling, comedones, follicular casts, hyperkeratotic plaques	History, exclude other differential diagnoses, skin biopsies, response to therapy
Zinc-responsive dermatosis	Abnormal keratinization leading to diffuse parakeratosis	Symmetrical tightly adherent scale. Footpad hyperkeratosis is occasionally seen	Skin biopsies, response to trial zinc supplementation
Ear margin dermatosis	Idiopathic keratinization defect	Follicular casts along pinnal margins. Non-pruritic	History, clinical signs, skin biopsies. Rule out scabies and vasculopathy
Metabolic epidermal necrosis	Unclear. Hypoaminoacidaemia secondary to hepatic disease or glucagonoma?	Footpad hyperkeratosis and fissures. Peri-orificial erosions, crusting and fissures. Weight loss, polyuria, poor appetite	Skin biopsies, biochemical tests, abdominal ultrasonography
Pemphigus foliaceus	Autoimmune disease. Damage to desmosomal proteins causing loss of keratinocyte cohesion	Pustules (transient) and crusts, often on face, ears. May involve footpads and trunk	Skin biopsies
Canine scabies	Hypersensitivity response to presence of mites in the epidermis	Crusted papules, especially ear margins, elbows, hocks. Pruritus is often severe. Contagion?	Skin scrapes. Response to trial acaricidal therapy
Leishmaniasis	Proliferation of protozoan parasite within macrophages and other cells	Exfoliative dermatitis, or nodules, or ulcers/crusts. Variable systemic signs	Demonstration of parasite in lymph node or bone marrow aspirates or skin biopsies

and other nutritional dermatoses. Metabolic epidermal necrosis is an uncommon disease of dogs characterized by symmetrical erosions, fissures, crusting and footpad hyperkeratosis. Most cases reflect a vacuolar hepatopathy or hepatic cirrhosis although rare cases are associated with pancreatic glucagonomas. In some cases, skin lesions precede clinical signs of internal disease. Erosions and fissures are less often seen with nutritional disturbances.

INITIAL DIAGNOSTIC PLAN

The historical and clinical findings should enable the clinician to propose a list of differential diagnoses. Diagnostic and therapeutic plans should then be formulated based on these features and the wishes and expectations of the client. If the cause of the problem is not immediately obvious, then initial investigations should centre on the exclusion of ectoparasitic infestations and microbial infections by skin scrapings, coat brushings, cytology and cultures.

LABORATORY AND OTHER DIAGNOSTIC TESTS

Laboratory tests should be selected on the basis of the historical and clinical findings.

Skin scrapings, hair plucks and coat brushings

These should be collected and examined in all cases presenting with scaling or crusting; techniques are described in Chapter 25.

Microbial cultures

Culture of skin scrapings and hair plucks is indicated whenever dermatophytosis is suspected. Cultures may also be used to demonstrate the presence of *Staphylococcus intermedius* and *Malassezia pachydermatis*; however, merely isolating these commensal organisms does not prove they are pathogenic. Profuse growth of the organism should increase the index of suspicion of a pathogenic role but response to trial therapy may ultimately be required to establish their significance.

Haematological and biochemical investigations

Blood samples for haematological and biochemical profiles should be obtained from animals suspected of having endocrine or metabolic disorders. Hypothyroid dogs may have a normocytic, normochromic, non-regenerative anaemia and elevated plasma cholesterol concentrations. A mature neutrophilia, lymphopenia and eosinopenia, accompanied by elevations of plasma cholesterol and alkaline phosphatase may be observed in dogs with hyperadrenocorticism. Dogs with metabolic epidermal necrosis often have non-regenerative anaemia, hypoalbuminaemia and increased plasma concentrations of liver enzymes. Fasting and postprandial bile acid concentrations are usually increased when metabolic epidermal necrosis is associated with hepatic disease. Concurrent diabetes mellitus characterized by hyperglycaemia and glycosuria is recognized in some cases. Dogs with leishmaniasis may have anaemia, thrombocytopenia, hyperglobulinaemia, azotaemia or increased hepatic enzymes. Hormone assays and dynamic function tests are indicated whenever endocrine diseases are suspected. Detailed descriptions of these procedures are given in Chapters 39 and 47.

Skin biopsies

The examination of skin biopsy specimens is often of considerable diagnostic value because many scaling and crusting disorders have relatively distinctive histopathological features (Table 26.3). Punch biopsy specimens can often be obtained

Table 26.3 Scaling and crusting diseases with diagnostic or suggestive histopathological features

Disease	Principal lesion type	Main histopathological features
Pyoderma	Papules, pustules or crusts	Neutrophilic folliculitis or furunculosis. Absence of fungal elements and *Demodex* spp.
Dermatophytosis	Alopecia, crusts	Pyogranulomas centred on hair follicles *or* hyperplastic superficial perivascular dermatitis. Fungal hyphae or spores in hair shafts or stratum corneum
Demodicosis	Alopecia, comedones, scale, crust	Lymphoplasmacytic mural folliculitis and perifolliculitis *or* suppurative folliculitis and pyogranuloma formation. Intrafollicular mites
Leishmaniasis	Scaling, nodules, ulcers or crusts	Variable. Nodular or diffuse granulomatous dermatitis or plasmacytic perivascular dermatitis. Amastigote form of parasite within macrophages
Sebaceous adenitis	Scaling, follicular casts, alopecia	Follicular hyperkeratosis and inflammatory cell infiltrate targeting sebaceous glands *or* absence of sebaceous glands in multiple biopsy specimens
Primary idiopathic seborrhoea	Scaling, comedones, follicular casts, hyperkeratotic plaques	Marked surface and follicular hyperkeratosis. Non-inflammatory in absence of infection
Pemphigus foliaceus	Pustules, crusts	Subcorneal pustules with acantholysis. Rafts of acantholytic epithelial cells in crusts
Cutaneous lymphoma	Scaling, erythroderma, alopecia, nodules, plaques	Infiltration of superficial dermis and/or epithelium with neoplastic lymphocytes
Metabolic epidermal necrosis	Symmetrical crusts, erosions, fissures	Parakeratosis, intracellular oedema of upper epidermis, superficial dermal infiltrate of mononuclear cells

from the trunk using local anaesthesia and sedation. It is important that the site is not surgically prepared prior to sampling because removal of the scale and crust may eliminate important histopathological features. Primary lesions such as papules and pustules should be biopsied where identified.

Response to trial therapy

Trial acaricidal therapy is indicated whenever scabies is suspected. Three applications of phosmet or amitraz at intervals of 2 weeks are normally effective. All in-contact dogs must be treated. Cocker spaniels and other breeds with vitamin-A responsive dermatosis should improve within 4 weeks of commencing therapy with 10 000 IU of retinol per day, and a complete response should occur within 10 weeks. Zinc sulphate at an oral dose of 10 mg kg^{-1} daily resolves lesions of zinc-responsive dermatosis within 2–6 weeks in most dogs.

FORMULATING A THERAPEUTIC PLAN

Trial parasiticidal or antimicrobial therapy should be considered when ectoparasitism or skin infection are suspected. If clinical signs persist and pruritus is present, then evaluation for allergic disorders might be indicated (see Chapter 25). In animals with minimal pruritus, endocrine, nutritional and metabolic diseases should be considered. Skin biopsies are indicated whenever primary keratinization defects, autoimmune disorders and cutaneous neoplasia are suspected, and when routine tests and initial treatments are nonproductive. A consideration of the historical, clinical and histopathological features, in association with exclusion of other differential diagnoses, should suggest a diagnosis in the majority of cases.

SYMPTOMATIC TOPICAL THERAPY OF SCALING DISORDERS

A wide array of different shampoos is available for the treatment of scaling disorders. A knowledge of the indications and actions of the different products is essential if optimal results are to be obtained. Table 26.4 serves as a guide to the selection of shampoos in different clinical presentations. Frequent applications with adequate contact time are prerequisites for good results; many products should be used twice weekly, allowing 10 minutes of contact time before thorough rinsing.

Table 26.4 Guide to the selection of shampoos for the symptomatic therapy of scaling disorders in dogs

Presentation	Treatments	Comments
Dry scaling	Sulphur–salicylic acid Fatty acid–emollient products	Use of a humectant rinse may be helpful
Greasy scaling	Tar–sulphur–salicylic acid Benzoyl peroxide Selenium sulphide	Occasionally irritating; contraindicated in cats Drying and occasionally irritating Some additional anti-*Malassezia* and antiparasitic activity
Scaling plus bacterial infection	Chlorhexidine	Adjunctive treatment only; 3% products more useful than 0.5%, where available
	Benzoyl peroxide	Adjunctive treatment only; drying; antibacterial efficacy limited
	Ethyl lactate	Adjunctive treatment only. Antibacterial efficacy limited
Scaling or greasy exudation associated with *M. pachydermatis*	2% chlorhexidine–2% miconazole combination Selenium sulphide	Good antibacterial and antiyeast activity, also degreasing Less effective than chlorhexidine–miconazole. More effective if combined with enilconazole rinse

27

Joint, Bone and Muscle Pain

R. Whitelock

Painful stimuli from the joints, bones or muscles of the appendicular skeleton almost invariably cause lameness. Multiple limb involvement or axial skeletal pain is frequently not so readily apparent, and the owner's complaint and presenting signs may be more diverse. It is imperative that the owner's complaint is identified and an accurate history is obtained before examining the animal.

INITIAL INVESTIGATION

HISTORY CHECKLIST

- ❏ **Lameness or gait abnormality?**
- ❏ **Lethargy or exercise intolerance?**
- ❏ **Stiffness?**
- ❏ **Overt signs of pain e.g. vocalization, licking, panting, tachycardia, restlessness?**
- ❏ **Behavioural change e.g. aggression?**
- ❏ **Reluctance to be groomed?**
- ❏ **Hunched appearance?**
- ❏ **Breed, age, sex?**

Certain diseases have typical breed, age and sex predispositions (for example, osteochondrosis has a predisposition for large breed dogs and clinical signs are normally first noticed between 4 and 9 months)

- ❏ **Any change in temperament?**
- ❏ **Diet?**
- ❏ **Any presence of similar signs in littermates?**

- ❏ **Response to medication?**

For example has there been an improvement on non-steroidal anti-inflammatory drugs?

Where lameness is evident, it is helpful to know the onset and duration of the signs, as well as its pattern. The following should be noted about the pattern of lameness:

- Intermittent or consistent?
- Progressive, static or improving?
- Severity over a 24 hour period?
- Cyclical?
- Effect of exercise/rest?
- Effect of weather?

 ### PHYSICAL EXAMINATION

A general physical examination should always be performed, regardless of the presenting signs, and in some cases thorough orthopaedic and neurological examinations are also indicated. Lameness does not always arise from limb pain, and both physical or mechanical deformities (for example joint ankylosis, limb deformity, muscle contracture) and neurological abnormalities need to be identified.

The physical examination should be based on observation, palpation and manipulation. In those joints, bones and muscles that are palpable the site of pain may be localized by careful examination. The shoulder and hip joints are exceptions, as they are well covered by muscle and it may be extremely difficult to accurately localize the site of pain by palpation alone. Similarly, it may be difficult to accurately localize pain of spinal origin to a particular bone, muscle or joint due to the intimate anatomical relationships of the individual structures. In these cases, appropriate use of further tests is indicated to facilitate the diagnosis. In order to enable a complete examination of the animal, the painful area should be examined last.

JOINT PAIN

When examining joints, the following features should be noted:

- range of movement
- joint stability
- swelling
- deformity
- pain
- number of joints affected

Careful palpation may enable localization of pain to specific structures, such as collateral ligaments or sesamoid bones. Many conditions, however, are more diffuse, such as inflammatory (infective or immune-mediated) synovitis or degenerative joint disease, and further diagnostic tests are necessary to establish the diagnosis.

Animals with polyarthritis are generally lame or stiff and may be pyrexic. Occasionally they are so badly affected that they are barely able to stand. The clinical signs nevertheless are often episodic.

Temporomandibular joint pain (Table 27.1)

Opening of the jaw is resented by animals with temporomandibular joint pain, which must be distinguished from masticatory eosinophilic myositis and mandibular fractures.

Shoulder joint pain (Table 27.2)

Shoulder joint pain may be intrinsic (involving the joint itself) or extrinsic (involving the soft tissues immediately adjacent to the joint). It is not always possible to distinguish the two by palpation alone. Conditions which must be distinguished from joint pain include bicipital tenosynovitis, luxation of the biceps tendon, brachial plexus tumours, nerve root pain (referred pain), cervical spinal pain and muscle pain. Care should be taken in the assessment of joint stability as normal joints have a degree of inherent instability.

Elbow pain (Table 27.3)

It may be difficult to distinguish shoulder and elbow pain in some animals due to the reciprocal arrangement of the two joints, and careful repeated examination is required. Extrinsic conditions which may resemble joint pain include panosteitis, interosseous (radius/ulna) pain and pain in adjacent muscles. The integrity of the collateral ligaments is best examined with the joint in flexion.

Carpal joint pain (Table 27.4)

The carpus is readily palpated due to minimal soft tissue coverage. Intrinsic carpal pain should be distinguishable from extrinsic pain. Accurate localization of focal pain (e.g. collateral ligament injury) is possible, as is a diagnosis of instability.

Metacarpo(tarso)-phalangeal and interphalangeal joint pain (Table 27.5)

The joints of the digits are readily palpated individually, and minimal soft tissue coverage facilitates accurate localization of pain. Collateral ligament support should be tested with the joints in extension. Causes of 'foot pain' such as laceration of the pads, penetrating foreign bodies and paronychia should not be overlooked.

Table 27.1 Causes of temporomandibular joint pain

Joint stability	Aetiology	Further diagnostic tests
Stable	Neoplasia	Diagnostic imaging
	Dysplasia[a]	Diagnostic imaging
	Degenerative joint disease	Diagnostic imaging, arthrotomy
	Meniscal injury	Diagnostic imaging, arthrotomy
Unstable	Luxation (congenital[a] or acquired)	Diagnostic imaging
	Fracture (condyle, glenoid)	Diagnostic imaging

[a] Predominantly seen in skeletally immature animals.

Table 27.2 Causes of shoulder joint pain

Joint stability	Aetiology	Further diagnostic tests
Stable	Osteochondrosis[a]	Diagnostic imaging, arthroscopy, arthrotomy
	Dysplasia[a]	Diagnostic imaging, arthroscopy, arthrotomy
	Trauma (sprain, haemarthrosis)	Diagnostic imaging, arthrocentesis, arthroscopy, arthrotomy
	Fracture (scapula, proximal humerus)	Diagnostic imaging, arthrotomy
	Degenerative joint disease	Diagnostic imaging, arthroscopy, arthrotomy
	Neoplasia	Diagnostic imaging, arthroscopy, arthrotomy
	Infective arthritis	Diagnostic imaging, arthrocentesis (synovial biopsy)
	Immune-mediated arthritis	Diagnostic imaging, arthrocentesis, synovial biopsy, serology
Unstable	Subluxation	Diagnostic imaging
	Luxation (congenital[a] or acquired)	Diagnostic imaging
	Fracture (scapula, proximal humerus)	Diagnostic imaging

[a] Predominantly seen in skeletally immature animals.

Table 27.3 Causes of elbow joint pain

Joint stability	Aetiology	Further diagnostic tests
Stable	Osteochondrosis[a] (fragmented coronoid process, osteochondritis dissecans, ununited anconeal process)	Diagnostic imaging arthroscopy, arthrotomy
	Dysplasia[a]	Diagnostic imaging, arthroscopy, arthrotomy
	Subluxation[a] (short radius/ulna syndrome)	Diagnostic imaging
	Congenital luxation[a]	Diagnostic imaging
	Trauma (sprain, haemarthrosis)	Diagnostic imaging, arthrocentesis, arthroscopy, arthrotomy
	Fracture (distal humerus, proximal radius/ulna)	Diagnostic imaging, arthrotomy
	Degenerative joint disease	Diagnostic imaging, arthroscopy, arthrotomy
	Neoplasia	Diagnostic imaging, arthroscopy, arthrotomy
	Infective arthritis	Diagnostic imaging, arthrocentesis, (synovial biopsy)
	Immune-mediated arthritis	Diagnostic imaging, arthrocentesis, synovial biopsy, serology
	Hypervitaminosis A (cat)	Diagnostic imaging
Unstable	Collateral ligament disruption	Diagnostic imaging, arthrotomy
	Luxation	Diagnostic imaging
	Fracture (distal humerus, proximal radius/ulna)	Diagnostic imaging, arthrotomy

[a] Predominantly seen in skeletally immature animals.

Table 27.4 Causes of carpal joint pain

Joint stability	Aetiology	Further diagnostic tests
Stable	Dysplasia[a]	Diagnostic imaging, arthroscopy, arthrotomy
	Subluxation[a] (short radius/ulna syndrome)	Diagnostic imaging
	Trauma (sprain, haemarthrosis)	Diagnostic imaging, arthrocentesis, arthroscopy arthrotomy
	Fracture (distal radius, carpal bone)	Diagnostic imaging, arthrotomy
	Degenerative joint disease	Diagnostic imaging, arthroscopy, arthrotomy
	Neoplasia	Diagnostic imaging, arthroscopy, arthrotomy
	Infective arthritis	Diagnostic imaging, arthrocentesis, (synovial biopsy)
	Immune-mediated arthritis	Diagnostic imaging, arthrocentesis, synovial biopsy, serology
Unstable	Hyperextension	Diagnostic imaging
	Collateral ligament disruption	Diagnostic imaging, arthrotomy
	Shear injury	Diagnostic imaging
	Subluxation (chronic erosive arthritis)	Diagnostic imaging, arthrocentesis, synovial biopsy, serology
	Luxation (of individual bones/joints)	Diagnostic imaging
	Fracture (distal radius/ulna, carpal or metacarpal bones)	Diagnostic imaging

[a] Predominantly seen in skeletally immature animals.

Table 27.5 Causes of metacarpo(tarso)-phalangeal and interphalangeal joint pain

Joint stability	Aetiology	Further diagnostic tests
Stable	Palmar sesamoid disease	Diagnostic imaging, local anaesthesia
	Trauma (sprain, haemarthrosis)	Diagnostic imaging, arthrocentesis, arthroscopy arthrotomy
	Fracture (sesamoid)	Diagnostic imaging, arthrotomy
	Degenerative joint disease	Diagnostic imaging, arthroscopy, arthrotomy
	Neoplasia	Diagnostic imaging, arthroscopy, arthrotomy
	Infective arthritis	Diagnostic imaging, arthrocentesis, (synovial biopsy)
	Immune-mediated arthritis	Diagnostic imaging, arthrocentesis, synovial biopsy, serology
Unstable	Collateral ligament disruption	Diagnostic imaging, arthrotomy
	Subluxation (chronic erosive arthritis)	Diagnostic imaging, arthrocentisis, synovial biopsy, serology
	Luxation	Diagnostic imaging
	Fracture (distal metacarpal/tarsal or phalangeal bones)	Diagnostic imaging

Coxofemoral joint pain (Table 27.6)

Localization of pain to the hip joint is not always easy and accurate identification of the source is hampered by the mass of periarticular muscle. Hip joint pain must be distinguished from spinal pain (particularly lumbosacral pain), pelvic fracture, proximal femoral bone pain, peripheral (sciatic) nerve and muscle pain.

Tarsal joint pain (Table 27.8)

As for the carpus, this joint has little soft tissue coverage and accurate localization of tarsal joint pain is possible. The collateral ligament support should be examined with the tarsocrural joint in flexion and extension. The stability of the dorsal and plantar ligamentous support should also be tested.

Table 27.6 Causes of coxofemoral joint pain

Joint stability	Aetiology	Further diagnostic tests
Stable	Ischaemic necrosis of the femoral head[a]	Diagnostic imaging
	Trauma (sprain, haemarthrosis)	Diagnostic imaging, arthrocentesis, arthroscopy, arthrotomy
	Fracture (acetabulum, femoral head/neck)	Diagnostic imaging, arthrotomy
	Degenerative joint disease (including remodelled hip dysplasia)	Diagnostic imaging, arthrocentesis, arthroscopy, arthrotomy
	Neoplasia	Diagnostic imaging, arthroscopy, arthrotomy
	Infective arthritis	Diagnostic imaging, arthrocentesis, (synovial biopsy)
	Immune-mediated arthritis	Diagnostic imaging, arthrocentesis, synovial biopsy, serology
Unstable	Subluxation (hip dysplasia[a])	Diagnostic imaging
	Luxation (developmental[a] or acquired)	Diagnostic imaging
	Fracture (femoral head/neck, acetabulum)	Diagnostic imaging

[a] Predominantly seen in skeletally immature animals.

Stifle joint pain (Table 27.7)

In contrast to the coxofemoral joint, extrinsic causes of stifle pain may be more readily separated from true joint pain. Collateral stability as well as cranial drawer stability should be tested; this may require sedation or general anaesthesia when the condition is painful or the animal is nervous.

Multiple joint pain (polyarthritis) (Table 27.9)

The presence of pain in more than one joint should raise the suspicion of immune-mediated disease, but the history and presenting signs must be taken into consideration before launching into exhaustive investigations. Animals with chronic erosive inflammatory disease frequently have

Table 27.7 Causes of stifle joint pain

Joint stability	Aetiology	Further diagnostic tests
Stable	Osteochondrosis[a]	Diagnostic imaging, arthroscopy, arthrotomy
	Avulsion of long digital extensor tendon[a]	Diagnostic imaging, arthrotomy
	Permanent patella luxation[a]	Diagnostic imaging
	Trauma (sprain, haemarthrosis)	Diagnostic imaging, arthrocentesis, arthroscopy, arthrotomy
	Fracture (distal femur, proximal tibia/fibula, fabella, patella)	Diagnostic imaging, arthrotomy
	Degenerative joint disease	Diagnostic imaging, arthroscopy, arthrotomy
	Neoplasia	Diagnostic imaging, arthroscopy, arthrotomy
	Infective arthritis	Diagnostic imaging, arthrocentesis, (synovial biopsy)
	Immune-mediated arthritis	Diagnostic imaging, arthrocentesis, synovial biopsy, serology
Unstable	Cranial cruciate rupture	Diagnostic imaging
	Collateral ligament disruption	Diagnostic imaging, arthrotomy
	Luxation (congenital[a] or acquired)	Diagnostic imaging
	Intermittent patella luxation	Diagnostic imaging
	Fracture (distal femur, proximal tibia/fibula, patella)	Diagnostic imaging

[a] Predominantly seen in skeletally immature animals.

deformed, thickened, unstable and painful joints. More acute cases may only present with peri-articular soft tissue swelling.

Intervertebral joint pain (Table 27.10)

Spinal pain can rarely be localized to an individual joint, bone or muscle on the basis of clinical examination. The division of spinal pain in this chapter is purely for convenience and it is more likely that the diagnosis of intervertebral joint disease will be made only after diagnostic imaging. Great care should be taken in attempting to demonstrate spinal instability.

Further diagnostic tests

Diagnostic imaging

Conventional radiology is adequate in the vast majority of cases and two standard projections at right angles to each other should be taken. Stressed views are invaluable in the examination of joint stability, for example to identify collateral ligament injuries or to identify the level of disruption following carpal hyperextension. Contrast studies are occasionally useful, for example shoulder arthrography in the investigation of bicipital tenosynovitis.

Computed tomography is an excellent but relatively expensive method of imaging structures which are obscured by superimposed tissues (e.g. the medial coronoid process of the elbow, the lumbosacral joint and the temporomandibular joint). Magnetic resonance imaging enables the soft tissues and the bones of a joint to be individually distinguished from one another, and can for example, accurately image meniscal injuries, ligament injuries, cartilage lesions, and spinal cord or nerve root compression.

Scintigraphy is useful for identifying areas of

Table 27.8 Causes of tarsal joint pain

Joint stability	Aetiology	Further diagnostic tests
Stable	Osteochondrosis[a]	Diagnostic imaging, arthroscopy, arthrotomy
	Trauma (sprain, haemarthrosis)	Diagnostic imaging, arthrocentesis, arthroscopy, arthrotomy
	Fracture (distal tibia, tarsal bone)	Diagnostic imaging, arthrotomy
	Degenerative joint disease	Diagnostic imaging, arthroscopy, arthrotomy
	Neoplasia	Diagnostic imaging, arthroscopy, arthrotomy
	Infective arthritis	Diagnostic imaging, arthrocentesis, (synovial biopsy)
	Immune-mediated arthritis	Diagnostic imaging, arthrocentesis, synovial biopsy, serology
Unstable	Subluxation (bone or joint)	Diagnostic imaging
	Collateral ligament disruption	Diagnostic imaging, arthrotomy
	Shear injury	Diagnostic imaging
	Luxation (bone or joint)	Diagnostic imaging
	Fracture (distal tibia/fibula, tarsal or metatarsal bones)	Diagnostic imaging, arthrotomy

[a] Predominantly seen in skeletally immature animals.

Table 27.9 Causes of multiple joint pain

Aetiology	Further diagnostic tests
Degenerative joint disease	Diagnostic imaging, arthrocentesis, (arthroscopy, arthrotomy)
Infective arthritis	Diagnostic imaging, arthrocentesis, (synovial biopsy)
Immune-mediated polyarthritis	Diagnostic imaging, arthrocentesis, synovial biopsy, serology

Table 27.10 Causes of intervertebral joint pain

Aetiology	Diagnostic test
Degenerative disc disease	Diagnostic imaging
Facet degenerative joint disease	Diagnostic imaging
Spondylosis (usually clinically insignificant)	Diagnostic imaging
Discospondylitis	Diagnostic imaging
Atlanto-axial subluxation	Diagnostic imaging
Intervertebral instability	Diagnostic imaging

abnormal blood flow, radiopharmaceutical uptake, or bone turnover, and may be of use where localization of the source of pain is difficult. Image resolution is poor compared to other imaging modalities, and having identified an area of increased activity, detailed radiographs should be taken. Scintigraphy is not often used in small animal orthopaedics.

Ultrasonography of periarticular soft tissue structures is possible, but examination of the joint itself is limited by differences in acoustic impedances between soft tissue and bone.

Arthrocentesis

Synovial fluid analysis is an extremely useful technique in the investigation of joint pain. Samples of synovial fluid are relatively easy to obtain from the joints of the appendicular skeleton in the sedated or anaesthetized animal, and do not require expensive equipment for basic analysis. Cytological examination alone will often provide a diagnosis of acute or chronic haemarthrosis, degenerative joint disease, immune-mediated joint disease and infective synovitis. In most cases additional useful information may be gained by submitting synovial fluid for further analysis.

Synovial fluid analysis should include the following:

- Volume
- Gross appearance (viscosity, turbidity, colour)
- Microscopic appearance (cytology, crystals)
- Biochemical analysis (protein, glucose, enzymes)
- Immunological examination (rheumatoid factor, antinuclear antibody, immunoglobulins or immunocomplexes, complement)
- Mucin clot test
- Bacterial culture (aerobic and anaerobic)

Arthroscopy/arthrotomy

Direct examination of the structures of the joint may be necessary to accurately identify the cause of joint pain (e.g. a partial tear of the cranial cruciate ligament). Arthroscopy has the advantage over arthrotomy in being minimally traumatic, and rapid return to activity following the surgery can be expected. It is, however, time-consuming, requires specialist equipment and training, and may require subsequent arthrotomy for treatment.

Synovial membrane biopsy

Full thickness biopsies of the synovium may be collected by either arthroscopy or arthrotomy. Immune-mediated joint disease and low-grade infective synovitis may require synovial biopsy for confirmation if synovial fluid analysis is inconclusive. Neoplasia involving the joint (e.g synovial cell sarcoma) requires biopsy for confirmation. Synovial fluid analysis is extremely unreliable as the majority of soft tissue tumours involving the joint capsule do not exfoliate and, in addition, structural information on the tumour is required for histological diagnosis.

Serology

Lyme disease is an uncommon cause of mono- or pauciarthritis in dogs that have been exposed to ticks, and the diagnosis is supported by demonstration of elevated circulating antibodies to *Borrelia burgdorferi*.

Joint anaesthesia

If the presence of joint pain is equivocal, long-acting local anaesthetic agents (e.g. bupivacaine) may be injected into the joint space under short-acting sedation or general anaesthesia. An improvement in lameness confirms the presence of joint pain.

BONE PAIN

When examining the bones, the following features should be noted:

- integrity of the overlying skin
- swelling
- deformity
- asymmetry
- instability
- pain

Digital pressure may be painful in some diseases. Apparent bone pain may be induced by palpation of soft tissue superimposed on bone. This is most marked if a peripheral nerve is palpated as it courses over bone (e.g. radial nerve running over the distolateral humerus, or peroneal nerve caudolateral to the stifle joint). If a fracture is suspected, careful palpation is necessary to avoid causing penetration of skin by sharp bony fragments, and unnecessary soft tissue trauma. Causes of bone pain are listed in Tables 27.11 and 27.12.

Further tests

Diagnostic imaging

Having established the presence of bone pain, radiological examination is almost invariably the most appropriate diagnostic test. Two standard views at right angles to each other should be taken and the painful nature of the condition may require general anaesthesia in order to obtain radiographs of adequate quality.

In the presence of multiple sites of bone pain or if the location of disease is not certain scintigraphic examination using technetium 99m may

Table 27.11 Causes of monostotic bone pain

	Aetiology	Further diagnostic tests
History of trauma	Fracture	Diagnostic imaging
	Periostitis	Diagnostic imaging
No history of trauma	Panosteitis[a]	Diagnostic imaging
	Primary bone tumour	Diagnostic imaging, bone biopsy
	Osteomyelitis	Diagnostic imaging, bone biopsy, haematology
	Stress fracture	Diagnostic imaging
	Vascular bone infarct	Diagnostic imaging

[a] Predominantly seen in skeletally immature animals.

Table 27.12 Causes of polyostotic bone pain

	Aetiology	Further diagnostic tests
History of trauma	Fracture	Diagnostic imaging
No history of trauma	Panosteitis[a]	Diagnostic imaging
	Metaphyseal osteopathy[a]	Diagnostic imaging
	Hypertrophic osteopathy[a]	Diagnostic imaging
	Craniomandibular osteopathy[a]	Diagnostic imaging
	Osteomyelitis (haematogenous)	Diagnostic imaging, bone biopsy, haematology
	Metastatic bone disease (rare)	Diagnostic imaging, bone biopsy
	Metabolic bone disease	Diagnostic imaging, bone biopsy, haematology

[a] Predominantly seen in skeletally immature animals.

be invaluable. Accurate radiological examination should then follow localization of the lesion(s).

Computed tomography provides three-dimensional imaging, enhancing structures normally masked by superimposition. It is particularly useful for imaging the skull and vertebrae.

Bone biopsy

The most common indications for bone biopsy include the diagnosis of neoplasia, bacterial infection and less commonly metabolic bone disease. Histopathological examination and anaerobic/aerobic bacterial culture of bone may, therefore, be required to establish the diagnosis. Having localized a lesion both clinically and radiographically, core biopsies may be taken using a Jamshidi needle or a trephine (e.g. Michele trephine) through a stab incision ('closed' technique). If the exact location for biopsy is unclear or if exact positioning of the biopsy instrument is difficult, the lesion may be identified using a surgical approach before biopsy ('open' technique). It may be useful to re-radiograph the animal post-biopsy to confirm the site of biopsy. Generalized bone disease may also require biopsy for diagnosis, in which case, superficial biopsy sites should be chosen to facilitate the 'closed' technique.

Haematology

Haematological changes may accompany bone disease (e.g. eosinophilia in panosteitis, neutrophilia in osteomyelitis). Serum biochemical analysis is also useful, for example in the investigation of osteopenia where renal secondary hyperparathyroidism or hyperadrenocorticism need to be ruled out. Serum calcium or phosphorus levels are of limited use in the investigation of nutritional hyperparathyroidism as compensatory mechanisms usually correct any abnormalities in the plasma concentrations of these two electrolytes.

Blood culture is advised in cases of osteomyelitis/discospondylitis. Samples for culture should be taken before administration of antimicrobial therapy.

MUSCLE PAIN

Muscle pain may be focal (e.g. muscle tear) or generalized (polymyositis), and palpation of the muscles/tendons themselves is required to differentiate it from pain of bone or joint origin. Manipulation of a joint may result in a painful response due to compression or stretching of painful muscles.

When examining the muscles, the following features should be noted:

- symmetry – most muscles are paired
- atrophy (disuse, neurogenic)
- hypertrophy
- swelling
- disruption/defects
- muscle tone/myotatic reflexes
- weakness
- contracture
- pain on palpation

Most myopathies are in fact not painful, resulting more often in weakness, stiffness and gait abnormalities. Focal muscle pain may accompany a traumatic tear or contusion, or possibly bacterial myositis. In a complete muscle tear (grade 3), a palpable defect may be present, and surgical intervention may be warranted. More generalized muscle pain may indicate polymyositis or exertional myopathy ('cramp'). Causes of muscle pain are listed in Table 27.13.

Further tests

Diagnostic imaging

Conventional radiology is of little use in the investigation of muscle disease, except to identify radiopaque foreign bodies or gas-producing bacterial infection (e.g. *Clostridium* spp.). Similarly, ultrasonography is rarely required for the diagnosis of muscle pain but its use has been reported. Magnetic resonance imaging is an excellent technique for assessing muscle integrity and the presence of neoplasia, but is likely to be normal in metabolic/inflammatory muscle diseases.

Table 27.13 Causes of muscle pain

	Aetiology	Further diagnostic tests
History of trauma	Sprain, contusion	Diagnostic imaging, haematology/serum biochemistry
	Muscle tear	Diagnostic imaging
No history of trauma	Muscle tumour (e.g. rhabdomyosarcoma)	Diagnostic imaging, muscle biopsy
	Bacterial myositis	Diagnostic imaging, haematology/serum biochemistry, muscle biopsy
	Polymyositis	Diagnostic imaging, electromyography, haematology/serum biochemistry, muscle biopsy
	Eosinophilic myositis	Diagnostic imaging, electromyography, haematology/serum biochemistry, muscle biopsy
	Exertional myopathy	Haematology/serum biochemistry, muscle biopsy
	Myositis ossificans	Diagnostic imaging, haematology/serum biochemistry, muscle biopsy
	Dermatomyositis of collies and Shetland sheepdogs	Electromyography, haematology/serum biochemistry, muscle biopsy

Electromyography

This technique provides information on the electrical activity of the muscle. Thus abnormalities may be present in diseases which involve either muscle or motor nerve control. Some myopathies will have electromyographic abnormalities as well as pain.

Serum biochemistry

Elevated levels of serum creatine kinase are relatively specific for muscle disease whereas increases in aspartate aminotransferase and lactate dehydrogenase are less so. These may be elevated in some muscle diseases but interpretation of the results observed must be done in the light of the clinical signs.

Muscle biopsy

Muscle biopsy is not a difficult technique to perform, but interpretation should be performed by an experienced pathologist. Surgical biopsy is preferable to needle biopsy as a larger sample of tissue is retrieved and muscle fibre orientation is retained. Tissue may be cryopreserved or formalin fixed, depending on the requirements of the laboratory. Indications for biopsy include neoplasia, inflammatory/immune-mediated and metabolic disease.

28

Episodic Weakness and Collapse

A. Boswood

Signs of weakness and collapse can occur with almost any severe disease. This chapter considers possible aetiologies and the diagnostic investigation of those patients which are presented primarily for their signs of weakness or collapse. It is difficult to provide a definition which adequately covers all the types of clinical signs that are described as collapse. A useful working definition would be intermittent non-fatal episodes of recumbency with or without loss of consciousness.

AETIOLOGY OF COLLAPSE

There are numerous body systems which must function normally in an individual in order for weakness and collapse not to occur. Consideration of those processes which prevent a normal dog or cat from collapsing can provide some idea of the vast number of potential causes.

In order for an animal to remain standing:

- Postural muscles must be functioning normally;
- The skeleton on which the postural muscles are working must be intact;
- Sensory and motor innervation must be intact;
- Neural information regarding position must be integrated and appropriate stimuli provided to maintain tone of the postural muscles;
- The centre of neural regulation (primarily the brain and spinal cord) and the effector organs (the muscles) must receive an adequate blood supply;
- The blood reaching the tissues must be carrying sufficient oxygen and substrates (glucose, fatty acids etc.) for cellular metabolism;
- Cellular metabolic processes must be functioning normally;
- Adequate venous drainage must be present to allow removal of by-products of metabolism from the musculature and nervous system.

In the light of this, what is remarkable is not the frequency with which animals collapse, but rather the frequency with which they do not.

From the above considerations one can construct a list of categories of disease which may give rise to collapse:

1. Cardiovascular
2. Respiratory
3. Neurological
4. Neuromuscular
5. Musculoskeletal
6. Metabolic/endocrine
7. Haematological

Examples of diseases in each category which may give rise to collapse are shown in Table 28.1. It is not intended that the table should provide a comprehensive list of all diseases that can lead to collapse but rather to illustrate a few of the more frequently encountered conditions. The reader is referred to the systems based sections for a more detailed discussion of diseases of each body system.

DEFINITIONS

Syncope

Syncope is a sudden transient loss of consciousness caused by a temporary interruption of cerebral oxygen supply. Cerebral oxygen supply is compromised sufficiently and for a long enough period to lead to a cessation of normal cerebral metabolism which results in temporary loss of consciousness. Interruption of cerebral oxygen supply can come about due to inadequate cerebral perfusion, inadequate oxygenation of haemoglobin in the blood perfusing the brain, or inadequate haemoglobin within the blood perfusing the brain.

Table 28.1 Diseases which may give rise to collapse

Type of disease	Examples
Cardiovascular	Aortic stenosis
	Bradydysrhythmias
	Tachydysrhythmias
	Cyanotic congenital heart disease
	Thromboembolism
	Vasovagal syncope
	Congestive heart failure
	Pericardial tamponade
Respiratory	Laryngeal paralysis
	Brachycephalic obstructive airway syndrome
	Collapsing trachea
Neurological	Idiopathic epilepsy
	Wobbler syndrome
	Intervertebral disc disease
	Lumbosacral disease
Neuromuscular	Myasthenia gravis
	Type II myopathy
	Myotonia
Musculoskeletal	Luxating patellae
	Hip dysplasia
Metabolic/endocrine	Hypoglycaemia, e.g. insulinoma
	Hypocalcaemia, e.g. hypoparathyroidism
	Hepatic encephalopathy
	Addison's disease
	Hypothyroidism
Haematological	Anaemia
	Coagulopathy
	Polycythaemia
Miscellaneous	Splenic neoplasia
	Exercise-induced hyperthermia

■ Seizure

A seizure is an involuntary, paroxysmal disturbance of brain function usually manifested as uncontrolled muscular activity and a loss of consiousness.

■ INVESTIGATION OF EPISODIC WEAKNESS AND COLLAPSE

 HISTORY CHECKLIST

The investigation of episodic weakness and collapse can prove frustrating because, by virtue of the episodic nature of the problem, patients frequently do not demonstrate clinical signs when presented for evaluation. This means that it is essential to obtain a detailed and thorough description of the episodes from the owner who has usually observed the signs on at least one occasion. A number of features of the history are of particular importance.

❏ **Breed?**
Many conditions associated with intermittent weakness and collapse have breed associations, e.g. aortic stenosis in boxers and golden retrievers; brachycephalic obstructive airway disease in bulldogs; type II myopathy in Labrador retrievers.

❏ **Age at onset of clinical signs?**
Congenital diseases are more likely to result in clinical signs in a young individual. Patients with conditions such as idiopathic epilepsy usually first present as young adults.

❏ **Sex?**
Some congenital and acquired diseases which can result in collapse are sex-associated, e.g. dilated cardiomyopathy occurs more commonly in male Dobermanns; sick sinus syndrome in female schnauzers.

❏ **Family history?**
Some problems leading to intermittent collapse may be hereditary or familial in nature and a history of affected relatives can be relevant.

A general history should be taken but it is most important to establish the answers to the following

❏ **When do the episodes occur?**
- When was the first episode observed?
- How many episodes in total have been observed?
- Are episodes more likely to occur during exercise or at rest? Seizures tend to occur in patients at rest and/or soon after waking, whereas exercise-induced weakness is more likely to be due to cardiovascular, respiratory or musculoskeletal causes.
- Are the episodes in any way related to feeding? If they are, do they more frequently occur before or after feeding? Hypoglycaemia is more likely to occur after fasting. Hepatic encephalopathy is more likely to occur following feeding. Narcolepsy can result in collapse at meal times.
- Is the frequency of episodes affected by environmental conditions such as temperature and humidity?

❑ **What happens at the time of episodes?**
- Is there any premonitory behaviour? Patients who have idiopathic epilepsy may give the impression that they know a seizure is about to occur.
- Is there a complete loss of consciousness? If there is a complete loss of consciousness the patient is likely to be experiencing either syncope or seizures.
- Are there signs of respiratory distress? Respiratory distress is most likely to be associated with diseases of cardiovascular or respiratory systems.
- Does the animal become recumbent? If so, does the animal choose to lie down or is the animal unable to stand? Voluntary recumbency is more likely to be associated with muscular weakness or musculoskeletal pain whereas involuntary recumbency is more likely to be associated with syncope or neurological abnormalities.
- Is there evidence of involuntary muscular activity? True syncope can be flaccid (although sometimes muscular activity is observed due to cerebral hypoxia) whereas seizures are usually associated with tonic clonic muscular activity.
- Is the pattern of collapse consistent in timing and behaviour?
- Are any changes in mucous membrane colour observed? Pallor can be caused by hypotension or anaemia whereas cyanosis suggests compromised peripheral oxygen delivery.
- How long does it take before the animal is normal again? Is there any 'postictal' behaviour? Animals may recover rapidly from syncopal episodes whereas there are often postictal behavioural changes or neurological deficits following seizures.

❑ **Other information**
- Is the animal completely normal between episodes? If not, in what way does it differ from normal?
- Is there any relevant history of previous diseases or trauma?
- Is the patient on any medication for any other condition? Many medications have the capacity to induce periods of weakness e.g. beta-blockers, vasodilators.
- Is there any access to toxins?

Having taken an accurate history the clinician should be in a position to be able to distinguish seizures from syncope and possibly to narrow down the body systems likely to be implicated in the aetiology of the episodes.

PHYSICAL EXAMINATION

A thorough and complete physical examination should be performed on any animal with a history of episodic weakness or collapse.

In this discussion particular emphasis will be placed on those systems most likely to be responsible for collapse but this is not meant to imply that other systems should be less carefully evaluated.

Before a hands on examination, the animal should be observed at rest to note the character, depth and rate of respiration as this is likely to change while the patient is undergoing examination. Inappropriate behaviour may also be noted at this time such as circling, restlessness, depression and obvious lameness or neurological deficits.

Oral, ocular and genital mucous membranes should be examined. Colour of membranes and capillary refill time (CRT) should be evaluated. Pallor is likely to indicate poor peripheral perfusion or anaemia; brick red mucous membranes may occur with polycythaemia; cyanotic mucous membranes imply poor peripheral delivery of haemoglobin (see Chapter 15). Prolonged CRT is consistent with poor peripheral perfusion, however individuals with significant cardiovascular disease can often have a normal CRT.

The pulse rate, rhythm and quality should be assessed. Bradycardia or tachycardia may indicate a cardiac rhythm disturbance. Cardiac rhythm disturbances, when irregular, can result in pulse deficits, where the peripheral pulse rate is less than the audible heart rate. When pulse deficits are present the pulse also frequently varies considerably in intensity from beat to beat. Pulse quality is a subjective but valuable assessment of the character of the pulse. A bounding pulse may be present for a number of reasons including anaemia, patent ductus arteriosus or aortic insufficiency. A weak pulse may suggest abnormalities including hypovolaemia, cardiac disease, e.g. aortic stenosis and rhythm disturbances.

The precordium should be palpated before auscultation to evaluate the site, rate and intensity of the apex beat. The presence of precordial thrills associated with high-grade murmurs may be detected.

Careful auscultation of the heart should be undertaken to evaluate the intensity of the normal heart sounds and the presence of any additional heart sounds such as murmurs, gallop sounds or splitting of the normal sounds (see Chapter 34). Where additional heart sounds are present they should be carefully characterized. The rate and rhythm of the heart should be noted and the heart rate compared to the pulse rate (see above).

The respiratory rate, depth and effort should be noted. If there is more effort associated with one phase of respiration this may be significant. Inspiratory dyspnoea is frequently associated with upper respiratory tract obstructive lesions such as laryngeal paralysis and brachycephalic obstructive airway syndrome. Expiratory dyspnoea can be associated with alveolar and small airway disease (see Chapter 35). Auscultation of the lung fields should be carried out to determine the intensity of the normal respiratory sounds and the presence of any abnormal sounds such as wheezes and crackles.

In addition careful examination of the musculoskeletal system should be carried out (see Chapters 43 and 44). A full neurological examination should also be performed to determine if a neurological abnormality is present which may account for the collapse (see Chapters 30–33).

INITIAL DIAGNOSTIC PLAN

Where a specific problem, for example a heart murmur or cardiac rhythm disturbance, has been identified during clinical examination an appropriate series of tests should be undertaken to evaluate the problem more specifically, especially where it is felt that the identified problem may account for the collapsing episodes. For description of the appropriate diagnostic evaluation the reader is referred to other chapters of this textbook.

It is frequently the case that no specific problem is identified during the clinical examination of the patient since animals are often completely normal between collapsing episodes. In these cases a rational series of diagnostic tests must be carried out in order to screen the animal for the greatest number of differential diagnoses with the least number of diagnostic tests. There is no point at this stage carrying out diagnostic tests that will only rule in or out a single disease process, unless the suspicion of that disease process is very high on the basis of the history and clinical examination.

The following questions should be considered:

- Is it necessary to investigate the problem further in this patient? If a patient has had a single collapsing episode and physical examination is unremarkable it is debatable whether further investigation is necessary (consider how few people undergo diagnostic investigation following a single fainting episode). Diagnostic evaluation is much more likely to identify an abnormality if an animal is collapsing regularly and/or where a pattern of collapse has been established.
- If further investigation is necessary which diagnostic tests will be most likely to identify or rule out diseases potentially responsible for the collapsing episodes? At this point it is wise to try to decide whether the animal appears to be having seizures or syncopal episodes or whether generalized weakness is responsible for the collapse. For diagnostic investigation of seizures the reader is referred to Chapter 32.

For patients suffering from syncope or generalized weakness the following diagnostic tests are likely to be of the greatest value.

Biochemistry profile

A biochemistry profile should include the following.

- Sodium and potassium may help to rule out Addison's disease, hypokalaemic polymyopathy of cats and various other metabolic and neurological diseases.
- Calcium: hypocalcaemia may result in seizures and muscular weakness; hypercalcaemia can also be accompanied by signs of weakness.
- Glucose: hypoglycaemia may result in collapse and seizures; hyperglycaemia is often a result of diabetes mellitus and this can result in signs of ketoacidosis and collapse.
- Ammonia: hyperammoniaemia is present in hepatic encephalopathy and can result in seizures and collapse.
- Bile acids may indicate compromised hepatic function.
- Creatine kinase (CK) and aspartate aminotransferase (AST) may be increased in conditions such as myositis or hypokalaemic myopathy.

Haematology profile

Examples of abnormalities which may predispose to collapsing episodes and which may result in abnormalities on a haematology profile include anaemia, some neoplastic diseases and chronic inflammatory diseases.

Electrocardiogram

An electrocardiogram should be recorded to determine whether there is evidence of a cardiac rhythm disturbance. A wide variety of rhythm disturbances may be associated with episodic weakness. The electrocardiogram (ECG) may also suggest the existence of ventricular hypertrophy, electrolyte disturbances or myocardial hypoxia.

Thoracic and abdominal radiography

Thoracic radiographs allow assessment of the size and shape of the cardiac silhouette, the great vessels, the pulmonary parenchyma, airways and vasculature. When thoracic radiographs are normal a large number of cardiac and respiratory causes of episodic weakness and collapse can be ruled out. Abdominal radiographs may assist in the detection of intra-abdominal disease that could be contributing to collapsing episodes, e.g. splenic neoplasia, which may lead to collapse either through intermittent haemorrhage or cardiac rhythm disturbances.

Echocardiography

If there is evidence of cardiac disease on clinical examination, radiography or ECG, echocardiography is indicated. When performed in a patient where there are no indicators of cardiac disease it is much less likely to be valuable.

Arterial blood gas measurement

Many respiratory causes of collapse and also some cardiac causes are accompanied by arterial hypoxia (inadequate arterial partial pressure of oxygen). Hypoxia can be present without obvious cyanosis. Pulse oximetry is a less sensitive way of determining whether or not an animal is hypoxic.

Blood pressure measurement

Hypotension or hypertension may predispose to collapse. Possible causes of hypotension include hypovolaemia and cardiac or vascular disease. Hypertension is usually a secondary problem in small animals and may accompany various endocrine and metabolic disorders.

Stress testing

When the clinical signs for which the patient has presented are consistently associated with exercise it is often worth exercising the patient, and if it is considered safe, attempting to precipitate the clinical signs of weakness/collapse. It may be worth carrying out some diagnostic tests before and after exercise in order to compare results. The demonstration of a change in one or more of the parameters following exercise may be highly significant. Following exercise repeat:

- Clinical examination, especially temperature, pulse and respiration;
- Biochemistry profile, especially glucose, CK, electrolytes and lactate;
- ECG.

In the author's experience animals that collapse infrequently and unpredictably which are normal on clinical examination often show no abnormality even after the series of tests described above. These are perhaps the most problematic cases. One should not dismiss the animal's problem as it is obviously of concern to the owner, however one could continue to investigate extensively and still find no evidence of an abnormality. One should view a normal series of diagnostic tests as a favourable indicator of health rather than a disappointing outcome of the investigation. Often, reassuring the owner that no significant problem has been identified and stressing the diseases that have been ruled out will be sufficient to put their mind at rest. The collapsing episodes may spontaneously resolve or continue infrequently without detriment to the animal. After initial evaluation, if the animal continues to experience episodes of weakness/collapse the owners can be asked to specifically observe mucous membrane colour and palpate the femoral pulse or apex beat. This will provide useful additional information for the clinician who is unlikely to observe the episodes. If the problem increases in frequency or the clinical signs change this may represent progression of an underlying disease and investigation at this stage is more likely to result in an abnormality being identified and the correct diagnosis being reached. Cases where the episodes progress and eventually result in the death of the patient are very rare in the absence of detectable underlying disease. In a survey of human patients undergoing diagnostic evaluation for syncope, the long-term survival of those where a problem had been identified was compared to the long-term survival of those in whom no problem was identified. The group in which no problem was identified had the better long-term survival. The implication here is that if a series of screening tests shows no abnormality that person is less likely to be suffering from a potentially life-threatening disease and therefore a negative test result is the most favourable outcome for the patient who is collapsing.

■ Specific diagnostic tests

More specific diagnostic testing should be carried out where a particular disease process is suspected on the basis of the investigative procedures already undertaken. It is not necessary to carry out these tests in all collapsing individuals. Examples of these tests and their indications are given below.

Tensilon (edrophonium chloride) test

Edrophonium chloride is a short-acting cholinesterase inhibitor which prevents the breakdown of acetylcholine and hence increases its local concentration at the neuromuscular junctions. This has the effect of improving muscle function in individuals with myasthenia gravis. To carry out the test the patient is typically exercised to the point where muscular weakness becomes apparent. Edrophonium chloride is then administered intravenously. An improvement in muscle strength indicates a positive response (suggesting the presence of myasthenia). The administration of an anticholinergic drug can result in a cholinergic crisis so the attending clinician should be prepared to administer atropine and ventilate the patient if necessary.

Acetylcholine receptor antibody test

Animals with acquired myasthenia gravis may have detectable antibody against acetylcholine receptors in their plasma (currently a validated canine assay is not available in the UK).

Adrenocorticotrophic hormone (ACTH) stimulation test

The ACTH stimulation test is useful for investigating the capacity of the adrenal glands to produce cortisol in response to a supraphysiological dose of ACTH. This can be used to diagnose Addison's disease or Cushing's disease both of which can result in episodic weakness.

Evaluation of thyroid status

Hypothyroidism in dogs and hyperthyroidism in cats may both predispose to episodes of weakness or collapse. Thus in cats, the assessment of serum total T_4 levels may be indicated. In dogs the assessment of serum total T_4 levels may not be adequate to reach a diagnosis of hypothyroidism and dynamic testing such as a thyroid-stimulating hormone (TSH) or thyrotropin releasing hormone (TRH) response tests may be indicated. Simultaneous assessment of serum total T_4 and thyroid-stimulating hormone levels may also assist in the diagnosis of hypothyroidism (see Chapter 39).

Plasma insulin concentration

The demonstration of an elevated plasma insulin level in the face of hypoglycaemia, or an inappropriate insulin to glucose ratio may confirm the presence of an insulinoma. Other tests which may assist in the diagnosis of an insulinoma include intravenous glucose tolerance testing, abdominal ultrasonography and ultimately exploratory laparotomy and biopsy.

Ambulatory ECG monitoring (Holter monitoring)

Indications for Holter monitoring include a high index of suspicion that a dysrhythmia is contributing to the collapsing episodes and the identification of a dysrhythmia on a routine ECG.

The Holter monitor recording can demonstrate the frequency and severity of the dysrhythmia over a longer period and may help establish whether the dysrhythmia is significant, or requires treatment. The wide range of normal, the inherent variability of rate and the 'normal' occurrence of occasional premature depolarizations in dogs make interpretation of the ambulatory ECG difficult. Unless the animal collapses while wearing the device and the collapse is observed and recorded one can never be certain of the significance of the observed disturbances of rhythm. Ambulatory ECG recording is not practical in cats because of the size and weight of the equipment used and the lack of cooperation of most feline patients.

Electromyography (EMG) and nerve conduction velocities

Where a myopathy, neuropathy or myasthenia is suspected a recording of the electrical activity of the muscles, measurement of nerve conduction velocities, and response of muscles to repetitive stimulation may help to demonstrate and localize the abnormality.

Muscle biopsy

Histological examination of a muscle biopsy may help demonstrate the presence of a myopathy or myositis.

CONCLUSIONS

Episodic weakness and collapse are common presenting signs in small animal practice and a vast number of underlying diseases may be responsible for the collapsing episodes. Careful consideration of the history and clinical signs will often help to determine the underlying cause of the collapse and indicate which diagnostic tests are likely to prove the most informative. In a proportion of patients who experience intermittent collapse the cause is not apparent even after detailed evaluation.

29
Disturbances of Cardiac Rhythm

A. Boswood

Disturbances of cardiac rhythm occur in a variety of disease states. Animals with cardiac rhythm disturbances (dysrhythmias) essentially fall into three categories:

1. Animals with a dysrhythmia but no clinical signs;
2. Animals with a dysrhythmia and clinical signs as a consequence of the rhythm disturbance;
3. Animals with a dysrhythmia and clinical signs associated with an underlying disease which is also responsible for the development of the dysrhythmia.

In order to rationally investigate a patient where a dysrhythmia has been detected it is necessary to understand the factors which give rise to the development of rhythm disturbances.

AETIOLOGY OF DYSRHYTHMIAS

Any disturbance of the normal rhythm of the heart can be described as a dysrhythmia. Although it is beyond the scope of this chapter to enter into a detailed discussion of the genesis of dysrhythmias it is germane to consider factors associated with their development.

Normal cardiac rhythm depends on the regular generation and normal conduction of the cardiac depolarization. The normal pattern of cardiac depolarization is for the sinoatrial node to depolarize spontaneously. The atrial myocardium, the atrioventricular (AV) node and the ventricular myocardium subsequently depolarize as the wave of depolarization, initiated in the sinoatrial node, is conducted throughout the heart. Any factor which leads to an abnormality of generation or conduction of the depolarization can predispose to the development of a rhythm disturbance. Mechanisms of cardiac rhythm disturbances and examples of the resulting abnormal rhythms are provided in Table 29.1.

Table 29.1 Mechanisms and examples of cardiac dysrhythmias

Mechanism	Example of rhythm disturbance
Abnormalities of generation of cardiac depolarization	
Increased automaticity	Ventricular tachycardia Accelerated idioventricular rhythm Atrial tachycardia Junctional tachycardia
Failure of automaticity	Sinus arrest
Abnormalities of conduction of the cardiac depolarization	
Conduction failure (block)	Atrioventricular block Sinoatrial block Bundle branch blocks (not strictly a disturbance of rhythm)
Re-entry	
Organized re-entry	Supraventricular tachycardias (Wolf–Parkinson–White syndrome) Ventricular tachycardia
Disorganized re-entry	Atrial fibrillation Ventricular fibrillation
Abnormalities of signal generation and conduction	Parasystole

In order for the cardiac depolarization to be conducted normally the heart must be structurally normal, both microscopically and macroscopically. The heart must also have normal metabolism both regionally and globally. Normal cardiac depolarization depends on the maintenance of normal intracellular and extracellular ion concentrations. This is an energy-consuming process. As an illustration of how energy consuming this can be, it has been estimated that 25–28%

of the energy expended by a dog's heart, beating at a normal rate, is used to maintain normal ionic gradients within the heart. The remainder of the energy utilized is predominantly expended during contraction and relaxation. Any disease process that compromises cardiac metabolism, or the provision and utilization of metabolic substrates and oxygen to areas of the heart, will predispose to the development of dysrhythmias.

As a rough guide the factors which are likely to lead to the development of rhythm disturbances can be considered under the following headings. Examples are given in Table 29.2.

1. Intrinsic cardiac disease
2. Hypoxia
3. Disturbances of autonomic tone
4. Metabolic or endocrine diseases
5. Mechanical disturbance to myocardial function
6. Electrolyte and acid–base disturbances
7. Drug therapy.

To some extent these categories overlap, however it is useful to consider them when faced with a patient with an unexplained dysrhythmia as it will assist in the investigation of the problem.

Table 29.2 Potential causes of cardiac dysrhythmias

Potential cause of dysrhythmia	Example
1. Intrinsic cardiac disease	Dilated cardiomyopathy Hypertrophic cardiomyopathy Mitral insufficiency
2. Hypoxia/Ischaemia	Pneumonia Pulmonary fibrosis Laryngeal paralysis Vascular disease leading to myocardial infarction
3. Disturbances of autonomic tone	Stress/anxiety Increased intracranial pressure
4. Metabolic or endocrine diseases	Hyperthyroidism Hypoadrenocorticism (Addison's disease) Phaeochromocytoma
5. Mechanical disturbance to myocardial function	Thoracic trauma Myocarditis
6. Electrolyte disturbances	Hyperkalaemia Hypokalaemia Hypocalcaemia
7. Drug therapy	Digoxin Dobutamine

PATHOGENESIS OF DYSRHYTHMIAS

Cardiac dysrhythmias usually result in clinical signs as a consequence of their ability to compromise cardiac output. Consider the simple physiological equation relating the cardiac output (CO), stroke volume (SV) and heart rate (HR):

$$CO = SV \times HR$$

Cardiac dysrhythmias decrease cardiac output either by decreasing heart rate, or decreasing stroke volume. Heart rate will be low when the patient has a bradydysrhythmia (cardiac rhythm disturbance leading to an abnormally low heart rate). The stroke volume is often compromised when a tachydysrhythmia (cardiac rhythm disturbance leading to an abnormally high heart rate) is present. At sufficiently high heart rates the length of diastole is shortened to the extent that stroke volume can fall. Despite the increase in heart rate, if diastole is compromised to a greater extent a drop in cardiac output will result. Where cardiac output is reduced over a prolonged period the efforts of the patient's cardiovascular system to compensate may result in clinical signs of congestive heart failure.

The main concerns associated with a cardiac rhythm disturbance are:

- Why is this rhythm disturbance present?
- Is this dysrhythmia resulting in compromised cardiac output?
- Is this rhythm disturbance likely to progress to one more likely to adversely affect cardiac output or to one which may be potentially fatal (i.e. ventricular asystole or fibrillation)?

INVESTIGATION OF DYSRHYTHMIAS

The diagnostic investigation of a patient with a dysrhythmia should involve confirmation of the existence of the dysrhythmia and then evaluation of the patient for evidence of cardiac or extra-cardiac disease.

HISTORY CHECKLIST

A complete and detailed history should be taken from every animal in which a cardiac rhythm disturbance is detected or suspected.

❏ Age, breed, sex?

Dysrhythmias may be a consequence of diseases likely to present in individuals of particular ages. Congenital heart disease is more likely to give rise to clinical signs in young animals. Acquired valvular disease is likely to occur in older animals.

Some breeds appear prone to particular rhythm disturbances, e.g. West Highland white terriers, sinus node dysfunction; German shepherd dogs, hereditary ventricular arrhythmias (in the US); springer spaniels, persistent atrial standstill.

Some diseases predisposing to arrhythmias occur with a greater frequency in a particular sex, e.g. dilated cardiomyopathy in male Dobermanns.

❏ Are clinical signs of cardiac disease present?

It should be ascertained whether the owners have observed signs which could be attributed either to the presence of a dysrhythmia or an underlying cardiac disease. These would include signs of inadequate cardiac output such as exercise intolerance, weakness and collapse, or signs of congestive heart failure such as dyspnoea, ascites or peripheral oedema.

❏ Has the animal shown signs of concurrent systemic disease?

A wide variety of systemic diseases can predispose to the development of cardiac rhythm disturbances and therefore any abnormalities observed by the owners may provide an insight to the underlying aetiology.

❏ Drug therapy?

Some drugs used for the treatment of cardiac and non-cardiac disease and anaesthetic agents have the potential to cause dysrhythmias and therefore any medication which the patient has received could be relevant.

❏ History of previous diseases?

Dysrhythmias may be a consequence of a previous disease process, e.g. parvoviral myocarditis in young dogs doxorubicin toxicity following chemotherapy. Therefore a history of recent illness, even when the clinical signs are no longer present, may be relevant.

PHYSICAL EXAMINATION

A complete physical examination should be carried out on any animal where a cardiac rhythm disturbance is suspected or known to be present. Although emphasis is placed on the cardiovascular examination it is not intended to suggest that this should be concentrated on to the exclusion of other systems.

The aims of the physical examination are to confirm the presence of a cardiac rhythm disturbance (although an intermittent dysrhythmia need not be present all the time) and to detect the existence of any cardiac or extracardiac disease which may have led to the development of the dysrhythmia.

❏ Cardiovascular system

Careful examination of the cardiovascular system should be undertaken. Particular emphasis should be placed on auscultation, palpation of the femoral pulse and assessment of peripheral perfusion. Often with intermittent rhythm disturbances prolonged auscultation is necessary to detect the dysrhythmia and determine the frequency with which it is occurring. Simultaneous palpation of the femoral pulse will enable the presence of a pulse deficit to be determined. Often when a rhythm disturbance is present there is marked variability in the quality of the femoral pulse with weak or undetectable pulses associated with very short interbeat intervals and potentiation of the pulse strength occurring after long diastolic pauses. Such pauses often follow premature depolarizations (post-extrasystolic potentiation).

When a rhythm disturbance is present the clinician should attempt to decide if the rhythm disturbance is regular or irregular. Some rhythm disturbances are irregularly irregular, for example the chaotic heart sounds of atrial fibrillation; some rhythm disturbances are regularly irregular, for example ventricular bigeminy where the audible beats arise consistently in pairs. Some cardiac dysrhythmias are very regular, for example the ventricular escape rhythm in third degree heart block. An attempt should be made to describe the audible rhythm disturbance.

Methodical auscultation over all areas where the heart is audible should enable the clinician to detect if there is any evidence of concurrent structural cardiac disease which may be suggested by the presence of a murmur or a gallop rhythm. A gallop rhythm may only be detectable during periods of regular cardiac rhythm; marked dysrhythmia may preclude their detection.

❏ Other systems

The remaining body systems should be carefully examined in an effort to detect the presence of a systemic disease that may be initiating or exacerbating the detected dysrhythmia.

FURTHER INVESTIGATION

Further investigation of a dysrhythmia should proceed in two stages. Firstly, every effort should be made to document and diagnose the dysrhythmia; secondly, where necessary, an attempt should be made to determine the underlying cause of the rhythm disturbance.

The electrocardiogram

An electrocardiogram (ECG) is an essential part of the investigation and treatment of cardiac rhythm disturbances. Every effort should be made to obtain a good quality ECG which should include a period of the rhythm disturbance. This should enable an accurate diagnosis of the dysrhythmia to be made. A short guide to interpretation of the ECG will be provided but for more detail the reader is referred to Chapter 34.

The following questions should be asked when interpreting an ECG:

1. Is the ECG free from artefact, within the confines of the ECG paper and calibrated for both paper speed and centimetres per millivolt vertically?
2. What is the heart rate?
3. Is there a P wave for every QRS complex? If QRS complexes arise without a preceding P wave this implies that there was no organized atrial depolarization prior to ventricular depolarization. This will imply the presence of:
   (a) atrial fibrillation
   (b) atrial standstill
   (c) ventricular depolarization.
   Where an ectopic complex arises it should be determined whether the complex occurs earlier than the next anticipated complex (i.e. is it premature?) or later than the next anticipated complex where it may represent an escape complex.
4. Is there a QRS complex for every P wave? If a P wave is not followed by a QRS complex it implies that there has been failure of conduction of atrial depolarization through the AV node. This is described as AV block:
   (a) First degree (1°) AV block. There is prolonged conduction through the AV node but every P wave is conducted. This results in a long P-Q (or P-R) interval on the ECG.
   (b) Second degree (2°) AV block. There is occasional failure of AV nodal conduction but most of the QRS complexes appear normal and supraventricular in origin (unless accompanied by aberrant conduction). A variety of types of 2° block occur.
   (c) Third degree (3°) AV block is characterized by complete failure of AV conduction. No P waves are conducted to the ventricles and a lower pacemaker develops an escape rhythm. This is often a ventricular escape rhythm and is described as an idioventricular rhythm. Although the rhythm is usually regular it is often very slow at a rate of about 30–40 beats per minute.
5. Are the P waves all of the same configuration and are the QRS complexes all of the same configuration? Variation in configuration of P waves may be normal and is described as a wandering pacemaker. Negative P waves in leads I, II or III are usually abnormal and imply atrial ectopy. QRS complexes may show variation due to occasional aberrant conduction or ectopy. Where abnormal complexes exist it should be determined if they are premature, or late relative to the next anticipated normal depolarization.
6. Are the P waves and QRS complexes consistently and reasonably related? If there are regular P waves and regular QRS complexes but they are not consistently related this may imply the presence of AV dissociation. If they are reasonably related then the rhythm is likely to be atrial and probably sinus in origin.
7. Is the heart rhythm regular or irregular? Some irregularity can be normal, and some abnormal rhythms can be very regular. Therefore regularity need not mean a normal rhythm and an irregular rhythm need not be abnormal.
8. Are the QRS complexes narrow, or wide and bizarre? Supraventricular depolarizations usually lead to normal narrow QRS complexes. Depolarizations that arise within the ventricles typically lead to wide and bizarre QRS complexes. Occasionally supraventricular complexes can appear wide and bizarre if they are conducted aberrantly through the ventricle but in this situation the QRS complex may be preceded by a P wave and there is often a characteristic pattern to the QRS complex.
9. What is the mean electrical axis?

10. What is the amplitude and duration of the P waves and QRS complexes?

Recording an ECG over a greater period of time will increase the likelihood of capturing a period of the dysrhythmia. The other advantage of prolonged ECG recording is that it allows the patient to relax during the period of recording thereby reducing stress and anxiety. Stress and anxiety are associated with sympathetic stimulation and catecholamine release which can have a considerable influence on cardiac rhythm and possibly provide an erroneous impression of the frequency and severity of the detected rhythm disturbance.

Methods of recording a prolonged ECG include the following:

- Prolonged recording with a normal 'paper-trace' ECG. Instead of recording a short rhythm strip a more prolonged recording for 5 or 10 min may be useful. This generates a lot of paper but this problem can be minimized by slowing the paper recording speed.
- Monitoring an oscilloscope trace. The patient can be hospitalized and kennelled for this and may therefore be more relaxed than when manually restrained for a traditional ECG. The disadvantage is that the oscilloscope has to be watched continuously and some animals will not tolerate prolonged connection to ECG leads. Not all monitors enable a 'hard copy' of the ECG to be obtained. Some monitors record a period of the most recently elapsed ECG and therefore if a period of dysrhythmia is observed during this time it may be possible to review this and print it out.
- Holter monitoring, a technique by which the ECG is recorded over a 24 h period onto a tape which is then 'de-coded' by a dedicated computer (some hospitals offer a commercial decoding service). This is the ideal method of recording an ECG over a prolonged period and, as the patient is in its normal environment, provides the most accurate impression of the patient's cardiac rhythm without the influence of sympathetic stimulation. The disadvantages of the technique are that it requires specialized and expensive equipment and is not practical in small dogs and cats because of the size of the recording equipment.

Attempts to document dysrhythmias can prove frustrating in animals where they are intermittent and infrequent. Further evaluation of the patient without knowledge of the underlying rhythm disturbance is rarely helpful and treatment of a patient with a dysrhythmia without an accurate rhythm diagnosis may be harmful.

When a rhythm diagnosis has been reached the significance of the dysrhythmia and the nature of the underlying diseases should be considered. Some cardiac rhythm disturbances are more frequently associated with systemic disease (e.g. ventricular tachycardia) whereas others are almost always indicative of intrinsic cardiac disease (e.g. atrial fibrillation in dogs and cats).

Some benign cardiac dysrhythmias may require no further investigation. Examples of this include sinus bradycardia, second degree AV block, sinoatrial block and sinus arrest in individuals who are showing no other clinical signs. These represent 'physiological' dysrhythmias reflecting increased vagal tone and are therefore often of no clinical significance.

For a more detailed account of which dysrhythmias are associated with which diseases the reader is referred to Chatper 34.

Further investigation is recommended if:

- there are clinical signs present which may be a direct consequence of the dysrhythmia;
- it is possible that the dysrhythmia represents a manifestation of a significant underlying disease;
- the patient has abnormalities on clinical examination other than those directly associated with the dysrhythmia.

When the dysrhythmia is the primary abnormality detected, further investigation should consist of a series of tests to evaluate the patient for evidence of diseases listed in Table 29.2). Where problems suggesting involvement of other organ systems have been identified then specific investigation of those problems is recommended. The reader is referred to the appropriate chapters of this textbook.

When intrinsic cardiac disease is suspected this can be investigated further with the use of the following diagnostic aids.

Thoracic radiography

This should enable assessment of the cardiac silhouette, pulmonary vasculature and pulmonary parenchyma to detect the presence of cardiac or respiratory disease.

Echocardiography

When a patient presents with a cardiac dysrhythmia of unknown aetiology, whether or not there is other evidence of cardiac disease on physical examination, echocardiography may help to demonstrate a structural or functional abnormality indicative of the underlying cause.

▪ Tests for extracardiac disease

To investigate for the presence of extracardiac disease which may be influencing the cardiac rhythm the following tests may be indicated.

- Haematology and biochemistry profiles and urinalysis are helpful for ruling out concurrent systemic disease. Of particular importance is the assessment of electrolytes, especially potassium, calcium and magnesium.
- Abdominal radiography and ultrasonography are used to determine if there is any significant intra-abdominal disease present. Examples of intra-abdominal diseases that can result in dysrhythmias include splenic neoplasia, gastric dilatation volvulus and acute pancreatitis.
- Arterial blood gas analysis and/or pulse oximetry are used to determine the presence of hypoxia or acid/base disturbances.
- Serology to detect evidence of infectious disease that may affect the heart, e.g. *Borrelia burgdorferi* (Lyme disease), *Toxoplasma gondii*, *Neospora caninum* and, in imported dogs, *Trypanosoma* spp. and *Dirofilaria immitis*.

▪ Specialized tests

Where a dysrhythmia appears to be a primary problem, i.e. it is not associated with detectable systemic or structural cardiac disease, the aetiology and mechanism of the dysrhythmia can be investigated further with more specialized testing.

Atropine response test

This can be used to determine the influence of the parasympathetic nervous system in the aetiology of some dysrhythmias. Various protocols are described. The author recommends 0.03 mg kg^{-1} of atropine administered intramuscularly with an ECG recorded before and 45 min after administration. The normal response to atropine is the development of sinus tachycardia. If a bradydysrhythmia resolves after administration of atropine this suggests that a physiological or pathological increase in vagal tone is responsible for the observed dysrhythmia. The atropine response test is only indicated for the investigation of bradydysrhythmias.

Response to vagal manoeuvre and antidysrhythmic therapy

The determination of the mechanism of certain supraventricular tachycardias can be assisted by temporarily inhibiting AV nodal conduction whilst recording an ECG. This can result in unconducted P waves in cases of atrial tachycardias and can result in termination of the dysrhythmia in individuals with re-entrant dysrhythmias involving the AV node in their pathway. Atrioventricular nodal conduction can be inhibited by increasing parasympathetic tone by carrying out a vagal manoeuvre such as massaging the carotid sinus or applying pressure to the eyes (with the eyelids closed). Drugs such as esmolol can be used to temporarily inhibit AV nodal conduction.

Manoeuvres affecting AV nodal conduction and parasympathetic tone are unlikely to result in any alteration in ventricular rhythm disturbances.

Electrophysiology

Recording electrical potentials and providing programmed stimuli at various endocardial sites within the cardiac chambers is used extensively in people, and has been used occasionally in animals, to determine the origin and mechanism of supraventricular and ventricular rhythm disturbances.

▪ MANAGEMENT

The management of patients with dysrhythmias depends on a number of considerations.

- Where the dysrhythmia is associated with clinical signs of compromised cardiac output or congestion, or it is felt that the dysrhythmia may progress to a life-threatening rhythm disturbance, the dysrhythmia requires appropriate treatment as a primary problem.
- Where the dysrhythmia is associated with an underlying disease the most appropriate course of action is to treat the underlying disease and monitor the dysrhythmia. If the underlying disease is successfully managed the dysrhythmia may well resolve.

- Where a dysrhythmia is present but
  (a) is not associated with clinical signs of compromised cardiac output or congestion, or
  (b) is considered unlikely to progress to a life-threatening rhythm disturbance, or
  (c) there is no detectable underlying disease, or the underlying disease is either untreatable or does not require treatment,

the dysrhythmia can be left untreated and re-evaluated at regular intervals for evidence of progression or spontaneous resolution.

CONCLUSIONS

The presence of a dysrhythmia is often an indicator of the presence of an underlying disease. As such, the investigation of a patient with a dysrhythmia involves an accurate diagnosis of cardiac rhythm followed by a thorough evaluation for evidence of underlying cardiac and non-cardiac diseases. Treatment of dysrhythmias should only be considered after accurate ECG diagnosis of the dysrhythmia and in the light of the primary disease process responsible for the rhythm disturbance.

30

Ataxia

J. K. Dunn

Ataxia represents a failure of muscular coordination resulting from disruption of sensory pathways. This lack of coordinated movement may or may not be accompanied by other neurological or neuromuscular signs such as paresis, spasticity or other involuntary movements depending on the nature and location of the neurological lesion. With truncal ataxia there is an uncontrollable swaying of the body and uncoordinated limb movement. Animals will frequently adopt a wide-based stance when standing or will cross their legs when attempting to walk.

PATHOPHYSIOLOGY AND CLASSIFICATION OF ATAXIA

Ataxia may be caused by lesions involving the cerebellum, vestibular system or proprioceptive pathways and is a sign of specific sensory dysfunction. The differentiating features and major causes of cerebellar and vestibular ataxia are discussed below. Sensory ataxia (loss of proprioception) is usually associated with motor deficits and is therefore discussed separately in Chapter 31. The reader is referred to Chapter 42 for a more detailed discussion of specific diseases which can cause ataxia.

CEREBELLAR ATAXIA

The main function of the cerebellum is to coordinate activity of muscle groups thereby ensuring that movements are smooth and accurate. The cerebellum, with the vestibular system, is also responsible for the maintenance of normal balanced posture.

A diagnosis of cerebellar disease is usually based on the clinical signs. Similarly, it is usually possible to differentiate cerebellar ataxia from the vestibular and sensory forms. The signalment and history may help determine the aetiology (see Table 30.1 for causes of cerebellar ataxia).

Table 30.1 Causes of cerebellar disease

- Congenital cerebellar hypoplasia (Irish setters, wire-haired fox terriers, samoyeds, beagles and Labradors)
- Feline panleukopenia virus infection
- Herpes virus infection (puppies)
- Cerebellar neuronal abiotrophy
- Lysosomal storage diseases
- Infection (viral, bacterial, protozoal, fungal)
- Trauma
- Neoplasia

INVESTIGATION OF CEREBELLAR ATAXIA

HISTORY CHECKLIST

Consider the breed and age of animal; an animal with a congenital cerebellar defect may be expected to show signs as soon as it becomes ambulatory and certainly before six months of age. An infectious or neoplastic cause is more likely in an older animal.

PHYSICAL EXAMINATION

A full physical examination should be followed by a detailed neurological examination. Cerebellar disease is characterized by incoordinated movement of the head, neck and all four limbs. The ataxia in most cases will be symmetrical. The animal appears dysmetric (usually hypermetric) and tends to adopt a wide-based stance. A fine head tremor or more obvious bobbing of the head will be apparent which becomes noticeably worse when the animal attempts to initiate a specific task such as eating or drinking (hence the term intention tremor). In addition, animals with cerebellar disease have difficulty in judging distances which makes simple tasks such as drinking and eating difficult if not impossible. Involvement of the anterior lobe of the cerebellum may result in increased extensor tone or even opisthotonus. The lack of coordination may cause the animal to fall over especially when performing a manoeuvre requiring any degree of precision. Paresis is not a feature of cerebellar disease (i.e. limb strength is preserved) and conscious proprioception, sensation and spinal reflexes are normal. A fine tremor of the eyeballs may also be evident; this should not be confused with true nystagmus since there are no discrete slow and fast components (see vestibular ataxia). With severe cerebellar disease the menace response may be decreased or absent.

INITIAL DIAGNOSTIC PLAN

Routine haematological and biochemical screens are rarely helpful in establishing the cause. Cerebrospinal fluid (CSF) analysis may confirm active infection or occasionally neoplasia. A magnetic resonance imaging (MRI) scan provides the most reliable means of confirming the presence of a space occupying lesion. The thickness of the bone surrounding the caudal fossa makes interpretation of computerized axial tomography (CAT) scans of the cerebellum difficult, especially in cats. *In vivo* assessment of cerebellar degeneration generally relies on clinical signs and ruling out other causes.

VESTIBULAR ATAXIA

The asymmetrical ataxia which is a feature of vestibular disease is associated with clinical signs which constitute a vestibular syndrome, i.e. head tilt, circling, rolling or loss of balance and nystagmus. How many of these signs develop depends on the severity of the vestibular deficit.

Vestibular dysfunction may be peripheral or central in origin. The peripheral vestibular system consists of the inner ear receptors and the vestibular nerve (the vestibular branch of the eighth cranial nerve) which leaves the internal accoustic meatus to enter the brainstem at the junction of pons and medulla. The central vestibular structures include the brainstem vestibular nuclei and the flocculonodular lobe of the cerebellum. The vestibular nuclei are arranged in four groups (rostral, medial, lateral and caudal groups). Axons from the vestibular nuclei extend rostrally in the medial longitudinal fasciculus and synapse in the nuclei of the cranial nerves which ennervate the muscles controlling eyeball position and movement, i.e. III (oculomotor), IV (trochlear) and VI (abducens). Other axons project to the cerebellum (via cerebellar peduncles). The vestibular system, with the cerebellum, is responsible for maintaining balance and coordination of movement.

Pathophysiology and clinical signs of vestibular dysfunction

Head tilt and circling

The head tilt and direction of circling are generally towards the same side as the lesion with the exception of paradoxical vestibular syndrome (see below). Middle ear lesions on their own may cause a head tilt; affected animals show no other signs of vestibular imbalance unless there is extension to the inner ear. Some focal forebrain lesions may produce lateral deviation of the head and circling.

Nystagmus

Vestibular nystagmus occurs in normal animals in response to movement of the head and must be differentiated from the spontaneous nystagmus which is indicative of vestibular disease. Lateral movement of the head in a normal animal results in horizontal nystagmus. The eyes first deviate slowly away from the direction in which the head is turning (slow phase) and then quickly flick back in the direction the head is moving (fast phase). Similarly if the head is moved upwards vertical nystagmus occurs with the fast phase upwards.

Vestibular disease results in spontaneous nystagmus and the fast phase is generally directed away from the side with the lesion i.e. the less active side. With peripheral vestibular lesions involving either the semicircular canals or the vestibular nerve the nystagmus is often horizontal or rotatory; spontaneous vertical nystagmus or nystagmus which changes direction with different head positions usually indicates a central vestibular lesion involving the vestibular nuclei or the flocculonodular lobe of the cerebellum.

Positional strabismus may also be seen with vestibular disease and reflects the influence of a vestibular imbalance on the function of cranial nerves III, IV and VI. If the head is straightened and the nose is elevated there is downward deviation (ventral strabismus) of the eyeball on the affected side.

Paresis (hemiparesis)

With peripheral vestibular disease, superficial and deep sensation and spinal reflexes in the limbs are intact. Evidence of sensory deficits or motor dysfunction indicates the presence of a central vestibular lesion. Axons from the vestibular nuclei extend to the spinal cord via the vestibulospinal tract and descending medial longitudinal fasciculus. The vestibulospinal tract axons synapse on the internuncial neurones in the ventral grey matter which are excitatory for the ipsilateral extensor muscles and inhibitory for the contralateral extensors. A left-sided vestibular lesion may therefore result in an ipsilateral increase and a contralateral decrease in extensor muscle tone. Hence the animal will tend to fall or lean towards the same side as the head tilt and the direction of circling. Occasionally with central vestibular lesions (especially with lesions involving the caudal cerebellar peduncle) signs such as the head tilt and the direction of circling are directed away from the side with the lesion (paradoxical vestibular syndrome).

Vomiting

Some of the axons from the vestibular nuclei extend to the reticular formation and the vomiting centre. Animals with acute severe signs of vestibular imbalance may therefore vomit or show other signs of motion sickness (nausea, salivation etc.).

Cranial nerve deficits

The facial nerve (VII) and sympathetic nerve fibres pass through the middle ear hence it is not uncommon for animals with peripheral vestibular signs associated with middle or inner ear disease to have unilateral facial nerve paralysis or Horner's syndrome. The latter is characterized by miosis, ptosis and enophthalmos. Facial nerve paralysis results in an inability to move the eyelid or lip on the affected side. The lip therefore droops and the nose tends to deviate away from the affected side. If the branches of the nerve which supply the salivary glands are involved the oral mucous membranes may appear dry. The involvement of cranial nerves in addition to the facial and vestibular nerves indicates the presence of a central lesion, e.g. a tumour at the cerebellomedullary angle may result in trigeminal nerve deficits (masseter and temporal muscle atrophy and a loss of facial sensation). The presence of medial strabismus and inability to retract the eyeball indicates involvement of the abducens nerve (VI).

Investigation of vestibular disease

A diagnosis of vestibular disease may be based on the clinical signs. A good history may help differentiate peripheral vestibular from central vestibular disease. Clearly this is important since peripheral vestibular disease generally carries a more favourable prognosis. The differentiating features are summarized in Table 30.2 and are also discussed in Chapter 42. The numerous causes of central and peripheral vestibular disease are given in Table 30.3.

Table 30.2 Differentiating features of peripheral and central vestibular dysfunction

Clinical abnormality	Peripheral vestibular syndrome	Suspect central vestibular lesion
Nystagmus	Usually horizontal; occasionally rotatory	May be vertical or changes direction with different head positions
Extensor tone	Normal	Decreased on side with lesion; increased on contralateral side
Hemiparesis and/or proprioceptive or postural deficits	Absent	Present (usually ipsilateral hemiparesis ± postural or proprioceptive deficits); occasionally signs of cerebellar involvement
Cranial nerve deficits	Facial nerve (VII) paralysis or Horner's syndrome (disruption of sympathetic fibres); ± deafness with congenital vestibular disease	Involvement of any other cranial nerve, e.g. trigeminal (V) or abducens (VI) in addition to VII
Other CNS signs, e.g. behavioural changes, seizures	Absent	Occasionally present

Note: An animal with bilateral vestibular disease may present with symmetrical ataxia and no nystagmus.

Table 30.3 Causes of peripheral and central vestibular disease

Peripheral
Congenital vestibular disease (German shepherds, Doberman pinschers, beagles, Siamese and Burmese cats)
Otitis media/interna; extension of middle ear disease to the inner ear
Ototoxic drugs (streptomycin, neomycin, gentamycin, kanamycin)
Trauma
Neoplasia
Central
Granulomatous meningoencephalitis
Encephalitis (viral, bacterial or fungal)
Trauma
Neoplasia
Thiamine deficiency (cats fed an all-fish diet)
Cerebrovascular disease (rare)
Miscellaneous (aetiology uncertain)
Idiopathic vestibular syndrome (cats)
Canine geriatric vestibular syndrome (probably peripheral vestibular disease)

HISTORY CHECKLIST

❑ **Breed and age?**

Congenital vestibular disorders occur in German shepherds, Doberman pinschers, beagles, Siamese and Burmese cats; affected animals may also be deaf. Check if similar problems in any of the litter mates.

❑ **Vaccination status?**

❑ **History of previous ear infections, chronic tonsillitis or pharyngitis?**

❑ **Trauma?**

❑ **Administration of ototoxic drugs (streptomycin, neomycin, gentamycin, kanamycin)?**

❑ **Other CNS signs present?**

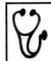

PHYSICAL EXAMINATION

A full physical examination should include an otoscopic examination of both ears and palpation of the osseous bullae. This should be followed by a detailed neurological examination to determine whether the vestibular signs are peripheral or central in origin (see Table 30.2). The answers to the following questions will help identify the location of the lesion.

❑ **Direction of head tilt and circling?**

A left-sided lesion should cause a head tilt to the left and the animal should circle in the same direction (see paradoxical vestibular syndrome for the exception to this rule). With acute severe vestibular deficits the animal may continuously roll over towards side of lesion.

❑ **Nystagmus?**

If spontaneous nystagmus is present, ascertain whether it is horizontal, vertical or rotatory; the fast component is directed away from the lesion. Positional strabismus may be seen with both vestibular and peripheral vestibular lesions.

❑ **Evidence of motor dysfunction or sensory ataxia?**

Check postural reflexes (hopping and placing reflexes) and proprioception. Suspect a central lesion if conscious proprioceptive deficit or hemiparesis is evident.

Serial neurological examinations may be required to accurately assess the prognosis. Although acute vestibular syndromes (e.g. geriatric vestibular syndrome) may present with particularly severe deficits initially, animals may be expected to improve rapidly.

INITIAL DIAGNOSTIC PLAN

- Routine haematological and biochemical screens rarely provide much diagnostic information.
- Radiograph the tympanic bullae (ventrodorsal, left and right lateral oblique, and open mouth projections). Tympanic bulla radiography has been largely superseded by MRI and CAT scans which provide greater information. In cases where advanced imaging is being considered then bulla radiography is unnecessary.
- CSF analysis; submit for cytological examination and protein content; one or both parameters may be increased with infectious or neoplastic central vestibular lesions.
- CAT scan or MRI.
- Caloric testing. The external ear canal is irrigated with ice cold or hot water. With cold water, horizontal nystagmus should develop with the fast component directed away from the ear being tested; with hot water, the fast component is towards the ear being tested. A lack of response to caloric testing indicates a lesion on that side.

31

Paresis and Paralysis

J. K. Dunn

Before discussing the diagnostic approach for animals with signs of sensory and motor dysfunction it is pertinent to define several terms:

- *Paresis* describes the deficit(s) of voluntary movement associated with partial motor paralysis which may occur in one or more limbs. Paresis presents as muscular weakness which must be differentiated from ataxia.
- *Plegia* is the term used to describe complete voluntary motor paralysis in one or more limbs.

Paresis and paralysis may be accompanied by sensory deficits within the affected limb depending upon the causative pathology. The distribution of the functional deficits forms the basis for further classification:

- *Monoplegia/paresis* is used to describe paralysis or paresis affecting a single limb.
- *Paraplegia/paresis* is used to describe paralysis or paresis affecting the hindlimbs.
- *Hemiplegia/paresis* is used to describe paralysis or paresis affecting both limbs on one side of the body.
- *Quadriplegia/paresis* is used to describe paralysis or paresis affecting all four limbs.
- *Proprioception* is position sense, i.e. the ability of an animal to recognize the position and movement of the limbs in relation to the rest of the body.
- *Ataxia* is a disruption in co-ordinated muscular activity produced by a disturbance in proprioceptive information.

LOCALIZATION OF LESIONS RESPONSIBLE FOR PARESIS AND PARALYSIS

The nature and distribution of the motor deficits usually allow the location of the causative lesion to be identified. The nature of the deficits and

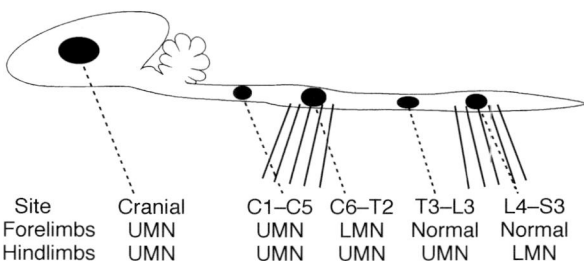

Figure 31.1 Segmental localization of lesions in the central nervous system.

associated clinical signs allow the lesions to be differentiated into signs of upper motor neurone (UMN) or lower motor neurone (LMN) damage (see Chapter 42). LMN paresis/paralysis is suggestive of a lesion within the peripheral nerves supplying the affected limb(s) or the central grey matter in which those nerves originate. UMN paresis/paralysis is suggestive of a lesion within the CNS cranial to the grey matter in which the peripheral nerve outflow to the affected limb(s) is located (Figure 31.1). It is important to remember that the spinal level refers to the spinal cord grey matter segment which does not always coincide with the vertebra with the same notation.

PATHOLOGICAL LESIONS CAUSING PARESIS AND PARALYSIS

A wide range of pathological processes within the nervous system can be associated with paresis/paralysis (see Chapter 42):

- Transection
- Static compression
- Dynamic compression
- Concussion
- Degeneration

- Vascular disease
- Infection
- Inflammation
- Neoplasia (primary or secondary).

In many instances more than one of these pathological processes will be occurring concurrently, i.e. intervertebral disc prolapse will result in both concussive and static compressive insult to the overlying spinal cord.

INVESTIGATION OF PARESIS AND PARALYSIS

The investigation of all cases of paralysis or paresis is similar. The initial examination should aim to define the lesion to a single region of the neuromuscular system, either a single spinal segment, the peripheral nervous system, or to multifocal sites. This allows the appropriate advanced diagnostic tests to be performed.

HISTORY CHECKLIST

❏ Age and breed?
Specific congenital spinal cord or vertebral abnormalities occur in certain breeds, e.g. spinal dysraphism in weimeraners and hemivertebrae in English bulldogs. Distemper myelitis is more likely in a young animal; degenerative or neoplastic processes are more common in older animals. Larger breeds are more susceptible to fibrocartilaginous emboli. Intervertebral disc disease occurs more commonly in dachshunds, cocker spaniels, beagles and Jack Russell terriers. Degenerative myelopathy (DM) occurs particularly in German shepherds older than 5 years of age. Atlantoaxial subluxation occurs most frequently in toy breed dogs and, in such breeds of dog, a history of signs attributable to an upper cervical lesion should alert the clinician to the degree of care needed in handling these dogs during examination until this diagnosis has been ruled out.

❏ Acute onset or insidious and slowly progressive?
An acute onset is more consistent with trauma, acute (Hansen Type I) intervertebral disc protrusion or fibrocartilaginous emboli. A chronic course is more typical of inflammatory lesions, Hansen Type II intervertebral disc protrusion, DM or neoplastic lesions.

❏ Difficulty jumping or climbing stairs?
This may indicate spinal pain associated with intervertebral disc protrusion, discospondylitis, spinal cord tumour or trauma, e.g. a fractured vertebra.

❏ Difficulty moving neck?
Cervical spinal pain is often associated with 'guarding' of the neck, a low head carriage and reluctance to lower the head for eating or drinking. Cervical spinal pain can be associated with cervical intervertebral disc protrusion, discospondylitis, atlantoaxial subluxation, cervical spinal cord tumour, polymyositis or meningitis.

❏ Evidence of forelimb involvement?
Confirm with neurological examination (see below).

❏ Evidence of systemic disease or other CNS signs?
Consider distemper myelitis, toxicities, infectious or metabolic disease.

❏ Abdominal discomfort/spinal pain?
Spinal pain will often present with signs of abdominal guarding which should be differentiated from abdominal pain by careful palpation and observation. Pain on rising on the hindlimbs or jumping is often associated with a lesion affecting the lumbosacral spinal cord.

❏ Continent?
Bladder and bowel function are controlled by nerves originating within the sacral spinal nerve roots. Differentiation between UMN and LMN bladder dysfunction will help in lesion localization (See Chapter 22).

❏ Tail function?
Tail carriage and function can provide a useful indication of lesion localization.

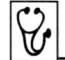 PHYSICAL AND NEUROLOGICAL EXAMINATIONS

The main aim of a detailed neurological examination is firstly to localize the lesion to a specific level of the spinal cord, and secondly to assess the severity of spinal cord or nerve root involvement in order to provide the owner with as accurate a prognosis as possible.

Quadriparesis/plegia

Single focal lesions producing symptoms in all four limbs must be located cranial to or within the cervical outflow of the spinal cord. Lesions producing these signs are summarized in Table 31.1.

Hemiparesis/plegia

Lesions affecting only one side of the body are relatively rare. Whilst traumatic lesions can produce hemiparesis, this is more usually seen with neoplastic, vascular and intracranial lesions.

Paraparesis/plegia

True paraparesis is produced by lesions caudal to the cervical outflow tracts. Due to the peripheral location of spinal tracts to the pelvic limbs, however, the clinical signs attributable to cervical spinal lesions may be more severe in the forelimbs, i.e. 'wobbler' syndrome. In such

Table 31.1 Disorders which cause quadriparesis/plegia

Degenerative/developmental
  'Wobbler' syndrome (Dobermann, rottweiler, great Dane)
  Intervertebral disc disease
  Atlantoaxial subluxation/occipitoatlantoaxial malformation
  Ascending or descending myelomalacia
  Dural ossification
  Dermoid sinus (Rhodesian ridgeback)
  Demyelinating diseases
  Storage diseases
  Multiple cartilagenous exostoses
  Subarachnoid cyst
  Hereditary myelopathy of Afghans

Inflammatory or infectious
  Meningitis
  Discospondylitis
  Distemper myelitis
  Rabies
  Toxoplasmosis
  Neosporosis
  Systemic mycoses
  Abscessation
  Feline infectious peritonitis (non-effusive form)
  Granulomatous meningoencephalomyelitis

Trauma
  Fractured vertebra
  Vertebral subluxation

Neoplasia
  Primary spinal cord tumours may be intramedullary (astrocytoma, ependymoma, glioma) or extramedullary (neurofibroma or neurofibrosarcoma, meningioma)
  Nerve root tumours (schwannoma)
  Metastatic tumours can involve a vertebral body (e.g. mammary adenocarcinoma, prostatic carcinoma, haemangiosarcoma, multiple myeloma) or epidural space (lymphoma, especially in cats)

Vascular
  Fibrocartilaginous embolus
  Spontaneous spinal cord haemorrhage (rare)

Nutritional
  Hypervitaminosis A (cats)

Table 31.2 Disorders which cause paraparesis/plegia

Degenerative
  Acute   Type I intervertebral disc protrusion
          Ascending or descending myelomalacia
  Chronic Type 2 intervertebral disc protrusion
          Degenerative myelopathy
          Dural ossification
          Demyelinating diseases
          Spondylosis deformans (rarely causes ataxia)
          Storage diseases
          Congenital spinal or vertebral malformations, e.g. spinal dysraphism and hemivertebra
          Hereditary myelopathy of Afghans

Inflammatory or infectious
  Discospondylitis
  Distemper myelitis
  Rabies
  Toxoplasmosis
  Neosporosis
  Systemic mycoses
  Abscessation
  Feline infectious peritonitis (non-effusive form)
  Granulomatous meningoencephalomyelitis

Trauma
  Fractured vertebra
  Vertebral subluxation

Neoplasia
  Primary spinal cord tumours may be intramedullary (astrocytoma, ependymoma, glioma) or extramedullary (neurofibroma or neurofibrosarcoma, meningioma)
  Nerve root tumours (schwannoma)
  Metastatic tumours can involve a vertebral body (e.g. mammary adenocarcinoma, prostatic carcinoma, haemangiosarcoma, multiple myeloma) or epidural space (lymphoma, especially in cats)

Vascular
  Fibrocartilaginous embolus
  Aortic embolism (cats)
  Spontaneous spinal cord haemorrhage (rare)

Nutritional
  Hypervitaminosis A (cats)

Table 31.3 Muscular, neurological and neuromuscular conditions presenting with generalized lower motor neurone signs

Degenerative/developmental
  Myotonia (Chow Chows, Labradors, Irish terriers)
  Muscular dystrophy ('floppy Labradors')
  Peripheral neuropathy of Boxers
  Giant axonal neuropathy (German shepherds)
  Myasthenia gravis (Jack Russell terriers, Springer spaniels, Fox terriers); also an acquired (immune-mediated) form of the disease
  Distal denervating disease

Inflammatory or infectious
  Distemper myelitis
  Toxoplasmosis
  Neosporosis

Immune-mediated
  Acute or chronic (relapsing) polyradiculoneuritis
  Idiopathic polymyositis (?immune-mediated)
  Acquired myasthenia gravis

Metabolic
  Polyneuropathy occasionally associated with diabetes mellitus, insulinoma, hypothyroidism, hypoadrenocorticism, vincristine therapy)

Trauma
  Brachial plexus avulsion
  Facial paralysis

Toxic
  Botulism
  Tick paralysis

Neoplasia
  Peripheral nerve neoplasia (schwannoma)

Vascular
  Fibrocartilaginous embolus/myelomalacia (affecting central grey matter)

---

cases a thorough neurological examination should indicate tetraparesis. In Schiff–Sherrington syndrome a severe thoracolumbar spinal cord injury may result in extensor rigidity of the forelimbs with paraplegia. Disorders producing paraparesis/plegia are summarized in Table 31.2.

LMN lesions

Muscular, neurological and neuromuscular causes of quadriparesis, quadriplegia or ataxia of all four limbs presenting with generalized lower motor neurone signs are summarized in Table 31.3.

INITIAL DIAGNOSTIC PLAN

Blood tests

Routine haematological and biochemical screens may be justified if a metabolic disorder or toxicity is suspected. Serological tests to rule out protozoal diseases, e.g. toxoplasmosis, neosporosis may be indicated.

Plain radiography

Radiological evaluation of suspected spinal lesions should include both plain lateral and ventrodorsal projections of the whole of the relevant spinal levels. Good radiographic technique is needed to allow interpretation of spinal radiographs since accurate positioning is essential. Accurate positioning can only be achieved in most instances under general anaesthesia. In the case of toy breed dogs with suspicion of a cranial cervical lesion, however, conscious radiography should be performed. Evidence of dynamic lesions may require flexed and extended radiographic views; however, these should be performed with caution since general anaesthesia will remove protective muscle spasm and manipulation of the cervical region may result in increased trauma to the spinal cord. Care should be exercised with traumatically induced lesions when a spinal fracture is suspected; whenever possible the initial diagnosis is best made from radiographs of the conscious patient.

Radiography should also be performed as appropriate for investigation of any other concurrent systemic disease, eg metastatic neoplasia.

Myelography

Myelography is an extremely useful diagnostic test for evaluation of the spinal cord. Myelography involves the introduction of a radiodense contrast medium into the cerebrospinal fluid within the subarachnoid space. Subsequent radiography allows identification of regions of spinal cord compression or swelling. It allows lesions to be assigned into the intramedullary, intradural–extramedullary or extradural compartments. As with plain radiography, both lateral and ventrodorsal views should be performed; oblique views are occasionally necessary to fully outline the lesion(s).

In most instances a CSF sample can also be collected prior to injection of the contrast material into the subarachnoid space. The introduction of contrast material can be performed by the cisternal or lumbar route (see Chapter 42). Choice of location depends on the suspected site of the lesion. For thoracic, thoracolumbar or mid- to cranial lumbar lesions, the lumbar site of injection is most likely to prove to be diagnostic, whilst for mid- to caudal cervical and caudal lumbar lesions the cisternal site is indicated. Cranial cervical lesions are sometimes difficult to fully outline. The caudal lumbar and lumbosacral region is often not outlined by myelography and epidurography or other advanced imaging techniques may be more appropriate.

The whole of the implicated spinal region should be examined since multiple lesions are not uncommon. In some cases, especially neoplasia, it may be necessary to perform myelography by both the cisternal and lumbar routes concurrently to full elucidate the lesion.

CSF analysis

CSF is routinely collected from the subarachnoid space via the foramen magnum (see Chapter 42). If a single thoracolumbar lesion is suspected, a more diagnostic CSF sample may be collected by subarachnoid puncture in the lumbar region. For cytological examination the sample should be collected into EDTA (plain tube for bacteriology). The sample should be centrifuged, preferably using a cytospin technique, and a slide suitable for cytological examination prepared within 30 min of collection because cells in CSF degenerate rapidly.

Normal CSF is water clear, colourless and does not coagulate. A red or pinkish discoloration in most cases represents faulty collection technique (contamination with red blood cells). A yellow (xanthochromic) supernatant is indicative of previous haemorrhage. Normal CSF of dogs and cats is free of red cells and contains less than $0.008 \times 10^9 \, l^{-1}$ nucleated cells. CSF becomes visibly turbid when the cell count exceeds $0.3–0.5 \times 10^9 \, l^{-1}$. In normal dogs the nucleated cell count of cisternal CSF is slightly higher than that of lumbar CSF.

Normal CSF contains low numbers of mononuclear cells (lymphocytes and a few monocytes). Neutrophils should not be present unless the sample is haemodiluted. Pleocytosis is the term used to describe an increase in the CSF nucleated cell count. CNS lesions may result in an increase in the number of normal cells or, with certain disorders, an increase in the number of a specific cell type (see below). Unfortunately, many CNS and spinal lesions do not consistently cause changes in the composition of CSF. They are more likely to do so if the affected area is in direct contact with CSF. Discrete tumours involving either the brain or spinal cord frequently either do not alter the CSF or at best cause a mild non-specific pleocytosis, i.e. increased numbers of normal mononuclear cells. Neoplastic cells are rarely seen unless the meninges are infiltrated. Acute spinal cord compression with myelomalacia may result in increased numbers of neutrophils whereas chronic compression more often results in a mild increase in the number of mononuclear cells. CSF findings with fibrocartilaginous emboli are variable and non-specific; a mixed pleocytosis may be evident. Other types of cellular response are described in Chapter 42.

In most cases an increased nucleated cell count is accompanied by an increase in the CSF protein content. CSF is an ultrafiltrate of plasma so low-molecular-weight proteins such as albumin predominate. Increases in CSF protein may be seen with haemorrhage, increased blood–CSF barrier permeability or increased intrathecal protein (globulin) synthesis. Increased permeability of the blood–CSF barrier may occur as a result of space occupying lesions as well as vascular, degenerative and inflammatory conditions. Normal CSF protein content is approximately $25–30 \, mg \, dl^{-1}$. The protein content of lumbar CSF is slightly higher than that of cisternal CSF. Occasionally CSF protein increases without an increase in cell numbers.

FURTHER INVESTIGATION

Magnetic resonance imaging

Magnetic resonance imaging (MRI) of the spinal cord requires advanced technology which is at present limited to specialist referral centres but is becoming more widely available. Resolution of detail within the spinal cord is often limited and, at present, greater information may often be obtained by myelography. Investigation of the lumbosacral region by MRI is however much superior to myelography which is frequently non-diagnostic. For the investigation of intracranial lesions MRI is invaluable.

MRI produces two-dimensional cross-sectional images dependent upon the quantity and nature of protons within the tissue of interest. A series of different imaging protocols can be used to produce different contrast patterns within the images. The most widely used protocols produce T1- and T2-weighted images. T1 imaging can be combined with the use of a gadolinium-based contrast agent. The contrast agent indicates regions of disruption of blood–brain barrier function within the CNS. T2-weighted images produce information about the relative water content of tissue and tend to highlight areas of oedema within the tissue. Due to the good architectural information produced by such images it is possible to differentiate between lesions with a mass effect and those occurring within normal tissue boundaries.

Computerized axial tomography (CAT)

CAT uses digital computer analysis to produce two-dimensional cross-sectional images through tissue using X-ray technology. It is an extremely useful technique for the investigation of bony lesions, and may be preferable to MRI for some lesions, i.e. degenerative joint disease of the articular joint facets. The information provided about soft tissue structures is however limited and for investigation of the spinal cord per se, the technique may be less useful than MRI. It can be combined with myelography and produces greater spatial information about lesion localization than is achievable by normal myelography.

Electrophysiology

A range of electrophysiological techniques are available for the investigation of the nervous system.

Electromyography measures the spontaneous electrical activity produced within muscles fibres. LMN pathology results in spontaneous abnormal electrical activity in affected muscle bellies consisting of fibrillation potentials and positive sharp waves. It takes at least seven days for these changes to develop and so cannot be used to investigate acute lesions. Spontaneous electrical activity is produced in response to damage to all parts of the affector pathway including the spinal cord grey matter, the motor axon and the affector muscle. The nature of the electrical activity is not specific in most cases for any given pathological lesion.

Nerve conduction studies are useful for the investigation of LMN lesions. Disruption of the integrity of myelin sheaths will result in a reduction in the speed and integrity of the passage of impulses along the motor axon.

Peripheral nerve/muscle biopsy

Peripheral nerve/muscle biopsy may be indicated for the investigation of certain LMN disorders.

32

Seizures

M. P. Targett

Seizure activity (a fit or convulsion) represents a paroxysmal disturbance of brain function that is sudden in onset, ceases spontaneously and has a tendency to recur. The sudden uncontrolled discharge of neurones may be the result of a primary brain lesion or may be secondary to a metabolic abnormality, e.g. hypoglycaemia. True idiopathic epilepsy describes recurrent seizures of unknown cause (see Chapter 42).

A seizure has several components.

- *Preictal phase* characterized by altered behaviour (aura). During this phase the animal may become restless, apprehensive or seek the attention of its owner.
- *Ictus* or seizure episode.
- *Postictal phase* during which the animal returns to normal. Typically, during the postictal phase which may last only a few minutes or several hours, the animal becomes confused, restless, ataxic or possibly even blind.
- *Status epilepticus* refers to the condition of continual seizure activity with incomplete recovery between seizures.

PATHOGENESIS

The initial seizure focus may involve only a small unstable group of neurones which intermittently spontaneously depolarize. This focus may then spread to involve adjacent neurones so that the seizure becomes more generalized. Certain populations of neurones in the brain such as those in the hippocampus are more likely to develop seizure activity. The membrane potential of a neurone is influenced by synapses with inhibitory (gamma-aminobutyric acid, taurine and noradrenaline) and facilitatory (acetylcholine, glutamate and serotonin) neurotransmitter activity and it is the summation of this activity which determines the activity of the neurone. The seizure threshold of a neurone or group of neurones is determined by events that regulate neuronal excitability. Thus the activity of a neurone is influenced by factors which alter the neuronal cell membrane, the number and location of inhibitory and excitatory synapses, the synthesis and degradation of neurotransmitter substances, and the glial environment. It has also been suggested that seizure threshold may be genetically predetermined since it varies between individual animals. Any structural or biochemical alterations in the environment of the neurone may trigger its spontaneous discharge. In this context a structural alteration refers to a primary brain lesion whereas biochemical alterations are generally the result of extracranial disorders, e.g. toxaemia or some other metabolic abnormality.

Idiopathic epilepsy refers to the recurrent seizure activity which occurs in animals with no detectable intra- or extracranial disease. Idiopathic epileptics may have a particularly low seizure threshold and it is possible that affected animals may have some genetically determined alteration in neuronal morphology and/or physiology which allows the neurones to depolarize spontaneously in the absence of a detectable stimulus.

CLASSIFICATION OF SEIZURES

The type of seizure may be classified on a clinical basis as partial or generalized (although partial seizures may become generalized). The clinical signs may indicate the location of the seizure focus. Seizures which originate from a focus in the motor region of the cerebrum are characterized by contralateral turning of the head, tonus/clonus of one or more limbs, and flexion of the trunk. Seizure foci located in the limbic system (e.g. hippocampus, amygdala and temporal cortex) initiate psychomotor seizure activity characterized by altered behaviour and complex motor activity. A psychomotor seizure may be manifested as somnolence, confusion, apparent blindness, failure to recognize objects, viciousness, screaming or hysterical barking, chewing, licking, jaw snapping or excessive salivation.

Generalized seizures

Generalized seizures are the most common type of seizure in the dog and represent an extended spread of seizure activity. Most can be described as grand mal, tonic/clonic seizures characterized by visceral and somatic motor activity. The seizure (ictus) is preceded by a variable preictal phase characterized by abnormal behaviour, restlessness and attention seeking. The ictal period is characterized by a combination of visceral and somatic motor activity. The animal loses contact with its environment, falls on its side and becomes transiently apnoeic. The first phase of the seizure consists of tonic, rigid extension of the limbs and opisthotonus which may persist for approximately 10–30 s. This is followed by a period of clonic limb activity characterized by continuous paddling and running movements. During the seizure the pupils appear dilated and the animal may champ its jaws and salivate profusely. Some animals void urine or faeces either during or after the seizure. Most seizures typically last only 1–2 min. Generalized tetanic-type seizures characterized by tonic extension of the limbs, opisthotonus and apnoea are a feature of strychnine poisoning. The seizures are easily triggered by noise or sudden movement and vigourous running/paddling movements are absent. In status epilepticus, coma or death may ensue as a result of hyperthermia, circulatory collapse, acidosis, hypoxia and respiratory failure.

Petit mal seizures consist of extremely brief (a few seconds) loss of consciousness and a generalized loss of muscle tone but no motor activity. It is doubtful if petit mal seizures occur in dogs or cats.

Partial seizures

Partial seizures have a seizure focus which does not spread. Motor activity may be restricted to one group of muscles of one limb if the initial seizure focus is confined to the *contralateral* motor cortex. For example seizure activity in the left thoracic limb indicates pathology in the right cerebral cortex and vice versa. A focal motor or Jacksonian seizure is a partial seizure which begins in one group of muscles and spreads to adjacent muscle groups in the same limb and then to the ipsilateral limb. A partial seizure may become generalized if electrical activity spreads to the diencephalon to discharge both cerebral hemispheres. 'Fly catching' in cavalier King Charles spaniels may represent some form of partial seizure activity, possibly focal sensory seizures originating in the visual cortex.

PATHOPHYSIOLOGY

Extracranial causes of seizure activity

Seizures which are the result of extracranial causes often occur in the absence of central nervous system (CNS) signs during the interictal period. This group includes a large number of metabolic disorders which alter neuronal function and metabolism.

Hypoglycaemia

In older dogs the most common cause of persistent hypoglycaemia is an insulin-secreting tumour of the beta cells of the pancreatic islets (insulinoma). A dog with an insulinoma may show a variety of behavioural and CNS signs including generalized seizures (which may be precipitated by exercise, excitement or feeding a large meal), ataxia, paresis, stupor and apparent blindness. Such signs may be expected to respond rapidly to the intravenous or oral administration of glucose. A fasting plasma glucose concentration <3 mmol l^{-1} with a concomitant insulin concentration >20 U l^{-1} is highly suggestive of an insulin-secreting tumour.

Other causes of hypoglycaemia such as hypoadrenocorticism, liver disease (especially hepatocellular carcinoma), hypoglycaemia in toy breeds and exercise-induced hypoglycaemia in hunting dogs are less likely to cause seizure activity.

Chronic hepatic insufficiency

Portosystemic shunts are a common cause of hepatic encephalopathy. Affected animals may show a variety of CNS and behavioural signs in addition to seizure activity, e.g. stupor, aimless bidirectional circling, head pressing or 'star gazing', ataxia and blindness. Clinical signs often become apparent after feeding and can be attributed in part to the effects of the increased blood ammonia concentration on the brain.

Hypocalcaemia

Hypocalcaemia associated with postpartum eclampsia or primary idiopathic hypoparathyroidism is often associated with tetanic seizures and behavioural changes. Hypocalcaemic seizures may also be expected to occur postoperatively in hyperthyroid cats if, during surgery to remove both thyroid glands, at least one set of parathyroid glands is not preserved. Other disorders such as acute or chronic renal failure and acute pancreatitis may result in a milder degree of hypocalcaemia which is usually insufficient to elicit CNS signs. Hypocalcaemic seizures require prompt attention and may be alleviated in the short term by the administration of calcium gluconate (4 ml 10% solution per kg bodyweight).

Renal disease

Seizures occasionally occur as a terminal feature of prolonged uraemia (uraemic encephalopathy). The CNS manifestations of uraemia are more likely to be apparent in younger dogs with congenital renal disease, e.g. congenital renal hypoplasia or renal dysplasia.

Hypoxia

Hypoxia associated with cardiovascular or pulmonary disease usually results in collapse rather than seizures. However, repeated episodes of cerebral hypoxia may lead to irreversible brain damage and the formation of scar tissue which may act as a seizure focus.

Intestinal parasitism

Young pups with severe toxascariasis may have seizures via a mechanism that has not been established.

Other extracranial causes

Other less common extracranial causes of seizures include hyperlipoproteinaemia (a familial form has been reported in miniature Schnauzers), hyperkalaemia, absolute polycythaemia and hyperthermia.

Intracranial causes of seizure activity

The presence of behavioural and/or CNS signs between seizures, especially if the signs are progressive, generally indicates structural brain disease. Intracranial causes of seizure activity are listed below. Chapter 42 gives a more detailed discussion of specific diseases.

Idiopathic epilepsy

Idiopathic epilepsy is undoubtedly the most common cause of seizures in small animals. Although epilepsy almost certainly falls into the intracranial category the cause of the seizures is unknown. Idiopathic epilepsy is known to be hereditary in certain breeds, e.g. German shepherds, keeshounds, beagles and dachshunds and it has been suggested that the seizure threshold in affected individuals is influenced and determined by genetic factors so that groups of neurones spontaneously depolarize at a lower threshold potential.

Diagnosis of idiopathic epilepsy in most instances is made on the basis of history (in particular a description of the seizures and the absence of CNS signs during the interictal period) and by ruling out extracranial and other intracranial causes of seizure activity. The onset of seizures generally occurs between one and three years of age. The frequency and intensity of the seizure may be quite variable. There may be clusters of seizure activity interspersed with periods during which the animal appears quite normal. A characteristic preictal phase (aura) may precede the seizure. In most cases the seizures are generalized and tonic/clonic in nature lasting from 30 s to several minutes. During the immediate postictal period the animal may appear depressed, ataxic or blind.

Encephalitis

- Canine distemper virus
- Toxoplasmosis
- Rabies
- Cryptococcosis
- Feline infectious peritonitis
- Non-suppurative polioencephalomyelitis (cats)
- Granulomatous meningoencephalitis
- Neosporosis

Neoplasia

- Primary tumours, e.g. meningiomas, gliomas
- Metastatic tumours, e.g. malignant mammary tumours

Clinical signs associated with brain tumours are extremely variable and depend on the location and the rate of growth of the lesion which determine whether there is a significant increase in intracranial pressure.

Developmental defects

- Hydrocephalus (abnormal accumulation of cerebrospinal fluid (CSF) results in dilatation of the ventricular system)
- Lissencephaly (congenital absence of the convolutions of the cerebral cortex; seen in lhasa apsos)
- Porencephaly (cystic malformation of the cerebrum)

Head trauma

Although CNS signs may have been apparent at the time of the original injury seizures may not occur until weeks or months afterwards.

Neuronal degeneration

- Nutritional: Thiamine deficiency
- Toxicity: Lead poisoning
  Chlorinated hydrocarbons (especially cats)
  Ethylene glycol
  Organophosphates
  Metaldehyde
  Mercury
  Strychnine
- Storage diseases (see Chapter 42)

INVESTIGATION OF SEIZURES

The complexity of the investigations will depend on the frequency and severity of the seizures as well as the age of the animal.

HISTORY CHECKLIST

An informative history is, to a large extent, dependent on an accurate description of events by the owner since few dogs have seizures while in the consulting room. The followings points of information may prove helpful in attempting to ascertain the cause of the seizures.

❏ Age?

If less than one year of age consider hydrocephalus, distemper, idiopathic epilepsy, lead poisoning, gastrointestinal parasitism, portocaval shunts and storage diseases. The animal with hydrocephalus not infrequently has visual deficits and unusual behavioural changes, e.g. alternating periods of stupor and hyperexcitability. Neoplastic causes (insulinomas or primary brain tumours) are more common in animals greater than five years of age.

❏ Breed?

Idiopathic epilepsy is particularly common in the German shepherd breed; hypoglycaemia occurs occasionally in toy breeds.

❏ Vaccination status?

Consider distemper virus infection if (1) the animal is either not fully vaccinated or has been vaccinated during the preceding fortnight; (2) seizures and/or other CNS signs are preceded by oculonasal discharge, coughing, sneezing, vomiting, diarrhoea etc.; (3) seizures are associated with multifocal CNS signs including trismus of masticatory muscles and chorea.

❏ Description of the seizure

- Is the seizure preceded by behavioural changes?
- Are CNS signs or behavioural abnormalities evident during the interictal periods? If so, assess progression of signs. CNS signs or behavioural changes associated with primary or metastatic brain tumours, although often quite variable, are usually slowly progressive and depend on the location and rate of growth of the lesion. In this context check that there has been no recent history of neoplasia or tumour removal. Mammary tumours occasionally metastasize to the brain.
- What signs, if any, are present during the immediate postictal period?
- Is the seizure partial or generalized?
- Duration and severity (intensity)?
- Involuntary paddling and/or running movements, defecation, urination?
- Loss of consciousness?
- Are seizures precipitated by or associated with exercise or excitement or did seizure occur after sleep? Seizures associated with strychnine poisoning are easily triggered by movement and noise.
- Any relationship with feeding?
- Frequency/length of time between successive seizures?
- Clusters, i.e. several in one day?

Description of the seizure can often be aided by observing a video of the episodic behaviour.

❏ Environment?

- If applicable, are littermates showing similar signs (rule out distemper)?

- Source of lead, e.g. paint or linoleum? With lead poisoning CNS signs may be accompanied by gastrointestinal signs.
- Exposure to toxins, e.g. metaldehyde, chlorinated hydrocarbons, organophosphate insecticides or phenols?

❏ **Diet?**

Cats fed an exclusively fish diet containing thiaminase may show signs of thiamine deficiency.

❏ **History of previous trauma?**

❏ **Other signs of systemic or endocrine diseases such as polyuria, polydipsia, polyphagia, alopecia etc.?**

Occasionally dogs with large pituitary adenomas show CNS signs including seizures.

PHYSICAL EXAMINATION

A full physical examination followed by detailed neurological and ophthalmoscopic examinations should be performed. The reader is referred to Chapter 42 for a more comprehensive account of the neurological examination and its use in the localization of CNS lesions (unifocal versus multifocal lesions). Neurological or behavioural signs which persist during the interictal phase suggest structural brain disease although the converse need not necessarily apply since a small focal lesion may cause intermittent seizure activity with no interictal signs.

INITIAL DIAGNOSTIC PLAN

Haematology and biochemistry

A full routine haematological examination, a complete biochemical screen and urinalysis are indicated to rule out lead poisoning, renal disease, hepatic encephalopathy and polycythaemia as well as most of the inflammatory and metabolic causes of seizures. The biochemical screen should include plasma calcium and fasting glucose concentrations. The plasma should be checked for the presence of gross lipaemia. Liver enzymes should be checked before anticonvulsive therapy commences since the commonly used barbiturate anticonvulsants induce an increase in the synthesis of microsomal liver enzymes.

Cerebrospinal fluid analysis

The analysis of CSF should include total nucleated cell and red blood cell counts, specific gravity, protein content and cytological examination. Unfortunately, CSF analysis is rarely helpful in establishing the specific cause of the seizures since CSF in most dogs with idiopathic epilepsy and metabolic disorders is normal. Similarly, with most space occupying lesions CSF is either completely unremarkable or shows a mild non-specific increase in the number of normal cells (mixed pleocytosis) and an increased protein content. Neoplastic cells are rarely seen.

The following types of cellular response may be observed in CSF:

Neutrophilic pleocytosis

Increased numbers of neutrophils in CSF occurs with bacterial infection, e.g. bacterial encephalitis or meningitis, although a similar response may occur with non-infectious inflammatory conditions, e.g. sterile meningitis. The increased cell count is usually associated with a marked increase in CSF protein content. Eosinophilic meningoencephalitis (a condition occasionally reported in dogs) is associated with an *eosinophilic pleocytosis*.

Pleocytosis of mixed cell types

- Mycotic encephalitis; neutrophils, eosinophils and mononuclear cells
- Viral encephalitis; although total cell count may be low, up to 80% of the cells present may be lymphocytes.
- Granulomatous meningoencephalitis; primarily mononuclear cells with lymphocytes predominating.
- Neoplasia; neoplastic cells rarely seen unless meningeal involvement, CNS lymphoma or metastatic carcinoma; often a mild to moderate increase in the number of mononuclear cells present.
- Fibrocartilaginous emboli; a mixed and variable population of mononuclear cells, macrophages, lymphocytes and a few neutrophils.
- Toxoplasmosis; lymphocytes predominate.

A CSF tap is contraindicated in animals where an increase in intracranial pressure is suspected, e.g. hydrocephalus, cerebral oedema or intracranial haemorrhage, since the sudden release of CSF pressure may result in herniation of the brain stem through the foramen magnum.

Radiography

Lateral and dorsoventral radiographs of the skull may help rule out previous trauma resulting in proliferation of new bone. Neoplasms are only likely to be visible if they are adjacent to the wall of the cranium and/or result in the erosion of bone (e.g. meningiomas).

FURTHER INVESTIGATION

Ultrasonography

Ultrasonography can be used, in cases where the fontanelles are still open, to investigate ventriculomegaly.

Blood lead concentration (if appropriate)

Electroencephalography (EEG)

EEG facilities are not routinely available to most practitioners therefore the use of this technique almost certainly necessitates referral to a specialist centre. Interpretation of results is difficult and in many cases similar information can be obtained from advanced imaging techniques.

Magnetic resonance imaging and computerized axial tomography

The advent and increasing availability of these techniques has revolutionized the diagnosis and treatment of intracranial space occupying lesions. They have superseded available contrast radiographic techniques such as angular venography and ventriculography. These techniques allow the identification and characterization of intracranial space occupying lesions. Advanced imaging studies should be considered as a first line diagnostic procedure in the investigation of seizure activity in animals older than five years of age.

TREATMENT OF SEIZURES

The first line treatment of seizures consists of treatment of the underlying cause where identified. The symptomatic treatment of seizures generally involves the use of anticonvulsant drugs either singly or in combination. Phenothiazine tranquillizers are generally contraindicated.

Anticonvulsant drugs in common use are listed in Table 32.1.

Complications

With most anticonvulsive drugs hepatotoxicity is a problem especially when the drugs are used in combination. Phenobarbital, primidone and phenytoin all cause an increase in serum alkaline phosphatase (ALP) via microsomal enzyme induction. The increase in ALP is usually accompanied by a smaller increase in alanine aminotransferase (ALT) and bile salt concentrations. Liver enzymes and liver function should therefore be checked periodically in animals receiving anticonvulsant medication over a prolonged period.

Aims of anticonvulsant therapy

Owner compliance is extremely important in order to maintain steady state concentrations of

Table 32.1 Anticonvulsant drugs commonly used in small animal practice

Drug	Dose	Therapeutic Range
Phenobarbital	Dog: 5–10 mg kg^{-1} bodyweight per os daily in divided doses; cat: 3–5 mg kg^{-1}	Dog: 20–40 µg ml^{-1}; cat: 10–30 µg ml^{-1}
Primidone	Dog: 10–15 mg kg^{-1} bodyweight per os daily (in divided doses up to a maximum daily dose of 35 mg kg day^{-1})	20–40 µg ml^{-1} (phenobarbital)
Potassium bromide	Dog: 30–40 mg kg^{-1} as an add-on in cases refractory to other drugs	0.7–2.0 mg ml^{-1}
Phenytoin	Dog: 10 mg kg^{-1} bodyweight per os TID up to a maximum of 20–35 mg kg^{-1} TID	10–20 µg ml^{-1}
Diazepam	Dog and cat: 0.5–1.0 mg kg^{-1} intravenously. Can be given to dogs in 5–10 mg boluses during a fit. Rarely effective on its own in controlling grand mal type seizures; best used in combination with phenobarbital or primidone	

Note: phenobarbital and diazepam are the only anticonvulsant drugs recommended for use in cats.

the drug in plasma. With most drugs it is usually necessary to increase the dose to achieve satisfactory seizure control. Therapy should be directed at decreasing the frequency and severity of the seizures. Treatment is unlikely to abolish the seizures completely in severe epileptics and many dogs will require treatment for life. Combinations of anticonvulsant drugs are best avoided unless absolutely necessary, i.e. only when seizures cannot be controlled by the use of one drug alone. It is important to monitor the blood level of the therapeutic agent to ensure that it is within the therapeutic range, remembering that the long half life of these compounds means that it takes several days to reach a steady state after any change in dose.

Therapy of status epilepticus consists initially of diazepam in an attempt to arrest the seizure activity (5–10 mg boluses every 10–20 min). If this proves ineffective phenobarbital should be administered intravenously to effect (3–15 mg kg^{-1} bodyweight). Oxygen should be given as necessary, via an endotracheal tube if the animal remains unconscious. Blood samples for diagnostic purposes (calcium and glucose determinations in the first instance) should be taken before initiating therapy and an indwelling intravenous catheter inserted to facilitate treatment of the patient. Animals which are hypoglycaemic should be given 50% dextrose solution intravenously (hypoglycaemia may occur as a result of the severe muscle exertion associated with generalized prolonged seizure activity). If hypocalcaemia is suspected calcium gluconate (5–10 ml of 10–20% solution) can be given intravenously taking care to monitor the heart rate while doing so. Bicarbonate may be administered with intravenous fluids to overcome lactic acidosis. Body temperature should be checked regularly. If the body temperature exceeds 42°C the animal should be cooled with ice baths.

33

Depression, Disorientation, Stupor and Coma

M. P. Targett

Behavioural changes such as depression, disorientation or confusion, stupor and coma reflect an altered level of consciousness and indicate abnormal function of the limbic system or frontal lobe of the cerebral cortex. The level of consciousness is maintained by sensory stimuli which act through the ascending reticular activating system (ARAS) which extends from the midbrain to the thalamus and subthalamus with diffuse projections to the cortex. The ARAS is stimulated by all major sensory pathways including those associated with touch, pain, temperature, hearing and vision. Stimulation of the ARAS results in stimulation of the cerebral cortex and vice versa. The ARAS interacts with an adrenergic system that projects from nuclei in the midbrain and caudal diencephalon. The latter, together with reticular formation structures of the pons and rostral medulla, influence sleep patterns and any alteration in the balance between the two systems can produce signs ranging from hyperexcitability to coma.

An alteration in mental status may be manifested as:

- *Depression:* the animal appears lethargic and is less responsive to its environment although still retains the capacity to respond to external stimuli in a normal manner. Most sick animals appear depressed.
- *Confusion or disorientation (impaired mentation):* the animal responds but in an inappropriate manner, e.g. there may be an apparent loss of learned behaviour.
- *Stupor:* this represents a partial loss of consciousness characterized by lethargy, immobility and diminished response to external stimuli. The animal may appear almost asleep although may still respond to strong painful stimuli.
- *Coma:* the animal is unconscious and does not respond to any stimulus except by reflex activity.

An animal showing signs of stupor or confusion may show additional behavioural or central nervous system (CNS) signs, e.g. seizure activity, especially if lesions involve other parts of the cortex. Diffuse lesions involving the frontal lobe of the cortex may produce other behavioural abnormalities such as continual pacing or head pressing. Animals with lesions involving the occipital lobes of the cerebral cortex may show a loss of learned behaviour and may appear blind (this can be described as a central blindness since direct and consensual pupillary light reflexes remain intact). The sensorimotor cortex is important for voluntary motor activity and lesions in this area may result in mild hemiparesis and postural deficits although the animal may be able to stand and walk with relatively little difficulty. Localizing signs if present are usually contralateral to the side of the lesion.

PATHOPHYSIOLOGY

Stupor and coma may be caused by diffuse bilateral cerebral disease, metabolic or toxic encephalopathies, and compressive or destructive lesions involving the rostral brainstem and midbrain.

Diffuse bilateral cerebral disease

Voluntary activity and postural reactions are depressed or absent. Central blindness may be evident. Meningeal irritation due to subarachnoid haemorrhage or infection results in head and/or neck pain, rigid neck muscles and reluctance to flex the neck. Normal vestibular eye movement is usually intact.

Metabolic or toxic encephalopathies

The signs are similar to those described for diffuse cerebral disease since cortical function is suppressed before brainstem function is affected. Depending on the cause an animal may show additional signs, for example many toxins can produce seizures (organophosphate insecticides can cause muscle fasciculations etc).

Compression or destruction of the rostral brainstem

Space-occupying lesions (tumours, abscesses) may either compress or destroy the pons and midbrain. Increased intracranial pressure (e.g. hydrocephalus or cerebral oedema) can cause caudal displacement of the cerebral hemispheres under the tentorium cerebelli or the cerebellum may herniate through the foramen magnum resulting in compression of the brainstem and profound respiratory depression.

Table 33.1 Disorders which may present with signs of decreased consciousness and/or altered mentation

Congenital/familial disorders
Lysosomal storage diseases
Hydrocephalus (most common in Chihuahuas and brachycephalic breeds)
Narcolepsy
Inflammation/infection
Encephalitis
Meningitis
Neoplasia (cerebral cortex or brainstem)
Metabolic disorders
Hypoglycaemia
Hepatic encephalopathy
Uraemic encephalopathy
Diabetic (ketoacidotic) coma
Hypoadrenocorticism
Heat stroke
Hypoxia
Increased intracranial pressure
Trauma resulting in cerebral oedema or intracranial haemorrhage
Acquired hydrocephalus
Toxins
Barbiturates
Heavy metals
Carbon monoxide
Ethylene glycol
Nutritional disorders
Thiamine deficiency (cats)
Miscellaneous
Postictal phase of idiopathic epilepsy

Disorders which can be associated with varying degrees of altered consciousness and other behavioural abnormalities are listed in Table 33.1.

INITIAL INVESTIGATION

HISTORY CHECKLIST

☐ **Breed and age?**
Hydrocephalus is common in toy breeds; with affected animals often presenting at a very early age (often less than 3 months of age). Periods of stupor and depression may be interspersed with periods of hyperexcitability or seizures. Portosystemic shunts should also be considered in the young animal which shows signs of stupor and depression punctuated by periods of hyperexcitability, aggressiveness, irritability or restlessness characterized by compulsive circling or pacing. The latter signs reflect involvement of the limbic system and the frontal and temporal lobes of the cortex.

☐ **Head trauma?**

☐ **Access to CNS depressant drugs or other toxins?**

☐ **Rate of onset and progression of clinical signs?**
Are other behavioural changes or CNS signs such as seizures, head pressing, aimless pacing present?

☐ **Are there other signs of systemic disease?**

PHYSICAL AND NEUROLOGICAL EXAMINATIONS

- If the animal is comatose check for evidence of trauma and signs of shock (temperature, pulse, respiratory rate and colour of mucous membranes should be monitored continually until level of consciousness improves).
- Check the pupillary light reflexes (fixed dilated pupils with severe brainstem compression).

Neurological examination should pay particular attention to vision and postural reactions. Often there are no localizing signs with cerebral oedema or encephalopathies whereas neoplasia and some cases of hydrocephalus may present with unilateral neurological signs (deficits contralateral to side of lesion).

- Is there head or neck pain (meningeal irritation)?
- Is there evidence of central blindness and/or postural deficits?

The following signs indicate severe midbrain/hindbrain disease and should be regarded as poor prognostic indicators in a comatose animal:

- Fixed dilated pupils
- Loss of normal vestibular nystagmus or negative caloric test
- Ventrolateral strabismus
- Extensor rigidity of the limbs or opisthotonus.

INITIAL DIAGNOSTIC PLAN

Routine haematological and biochemical screens

Routine haematological and biochemical screens should be performed to rule out metabolic disease. A complete biochemical screen for a young animal should include a bile salt assay to evaluate liver function even if liver enzymes are within normal limits.

Radiography

Lateral and dorsoventral projections of the skull should be taken to rule out fractures of the cranial vault. Radiographic assessment of hydrocephalus is unreliable, however ultrasonography may be helpful in determining the size of the lateral ventricles if the cranial fontanelles are open. Contrast radiographic techniques for investigating the size of the lateral ventricles are reported, however magnetic resonance imaging (MRI) has superseded these techniques. The differentiation between asymptomatic ventriculomegaly and symptomatic hydrocephalus can be difficult in certain breeds such as the Cavalier King Charles spaniel.

CSF analysis

CSF analysis should be undertaken if the above parameters are normal. A CSF tap is contraindicated if increased intracranial pressure is suspected and should be performed after MRI/CAT if these are to be performed. Assess CSF pressure during collection; submit for cytology, protein concentration and bacteriology if sample appears even faintly turbid on visual inspection.

FURTHER INVESTIGATION

Magnetic resonance imaging/computerized axial tomography

Advanced imaging techniques, where available, are useful for investigating altered behaviour, allowing the identification of neoplasia, cerebral oedema, haemorrhage and focal inflammatory lesions.

Electroencephalography (EEG)

EEG is a measure of the bulk electrical activity within the brain. Facilities for this technique are not widely available and test results are difficult to interpret. Lesion localization and identification can often be more accurately obtained by MRI/CAT (see Chapter 32).

SECTION II

SYSTEMS MEDICINE

34	Diseases of the cardiovascular system	255
35	Diseases of the respiratory system	345
36	Diseases of the alimentary tract	371
37	Diseases of the liver and biliary tract	448
38	Diseases of the exocrine pancreas	498
39	Diseases of the endocrine system	526
40	Diseases of the reproductive system	574
41	Diseases of the urinary system	612
42	Diseases of the nervous system	662
43	Muscle diseases of the dog and cat	695
44	Diseases of bones and joints	719
45	Diseases of blood and blood-forming organs	765
46	Diseases of the eye	820
47	Skin diseases of the dog and cat	871
48	Specific infections of the dog	921
49	Infectious diseases of the cat	959
50	Principles of cancer therapy	985
51	Behaviour problems	1029

34

Diseases of the Cardiovascular System

J. K. Dunn, J. Elliot and M. E. Herrtage

Introduction	255	Primary myocardial disease in the cat	291
Normal cardiac physiology	255	Secondary myocardial disease in the cat	298
Investigation of the cardiovascular system	256	Congenital pericardial disease	299
Heart failure	271	Acquired pericardial disease	299
Acquired heart disease	278	Congenital heart disease	309
Myocardial disease	284	Management of heart failure	321
Primary myocardial disease in the dog	284	Management of cardiac arrhythmias	328
Secondary myocardial disease in the dog	289		

INTRODUCTION

Recent advances in veterinary cardiology, most notably in the areas of diagnostic imaging and cardiovascular therapeutics, have considerably added to our understanding of cardiac disease in small animals. Some disorders, for example pulmonic stenosis, which previously would have been considered untreatable are now managed with a reasonable degree of success. In particular, the increased awareness of the pathophysiological mechanisms of heart failure has led to a more rational and ultimately more effective approach to cardiovascular therapy.

NORMAL CARDIAC PHYSIOLOGY

Muscle cells in the atria and ventricles contract almost simultaneously. The electrical impulse is generated in the sinoatrial (SA) node which is situated at the junction of the right atrium and the cranial vena cava. This sinoatrial impulse spreads across the atria to the atrioventricular (AV) node resulting in atrial depolarization. The AV node lies in the septal wall of the right atrium dorsal to the septal cusp of the right atrioventricular (tricuspid) valve. The impulse slows down as it passes through the AV node which results in a delay before ventricular depolarization. From the AV node the impulse is conducted through the common bundle of His which divides into left and right bundle branches. The right bundle branch travels down the right side of the ventricular septum to the right ventricle; the left bundle branch travels down the left side of the ventricular septum and divides into two branches (anterior and posterior fascicles). Purkinje fibres are the subendocardial terminations of the bundle branches in the walls of the ventricles.

Innervation of the heart

Parasympathetic nerves are distributed mainly to the SA node, atrial myocardium, AV node and proximal part of the ventricular conduction system. Sympathetic nerves are distributed mainly to the AV node and ventricular myocardium although some fibres also terminate in the SA node and atrial myocardium (Allert, 1990). The heart rate is dependent on the rate of discharge of the SA node. Parasympathetic activity slows SA nodal discharge and prolongs AV nodal conduction time. Sympathetic stimulation increases the rate of SA nodal discharge and shortens AV nodal conduction time. During rest or sleep the vagal inhibitory effects on the SA and AV nodes predominate over the sympathetic excitatory effects.

Variation in vagal tone occurs during inspiration and expiration. Clinically and electrocardiographically this may be manifested as sinus arrhythmia. Sinus arrhythmia is the term used to describe the regular alterations in heart rate caused by the variation in vagal tone which occur during inspiration and expiration. The heart rate increases during inspiration and slows down during expiration. In dogs sinus arrhythmia, even when pronounced and associated with sinoatrial block or sinoatrial arrest, is rarely of clinical significance. In the cat, however, sinus arrhythmia is abnormal and should be investigated further.

Increased sympathetic activity, for example during exercise or excitement, increases the rate and force of the cardiac contractions, that is, it causes positive inotropic and positive chronotropic effects.

INVESTIGATION OF THE CARDIOVASCULAR SYSTEM

History

As always, the animal's vaccination status, past medical history, diet and details of any previous or present treatment (including the response to any treatment given) should be recorded.

Dogs, and to a lesser extent, cats in heart failure often present with a history of coughing. In most cases this is due to pulmonary venous congestion and oedema, or is caused by an enlarged left atrium impinging on the bronchi at or slightly below the level of the carina. The frequency and time of day when the cough appears most pronounced should be noted. A cough of cardiac origin may become worse with exercise or excitement, or at night when the animal has been lying on one side (a nocturnal cough is highly suggestive of cardiac disease). Frequently the cough is paroxysmal terminating with an episode of pharyngeal retching and the production of clear phlegm (a productive cough).

Depending on the severity, pulmonary oedema or pleural effusion may result in orthopnoea, tachypnoea or dyspnoea (unlike pulmonary oedema a pleural effusion generally does not cause coughing). Young animals with congenital heart defects may fail to thrive and will appear stunted; this failure to gain weight should be differentiated from weight loss which may occur during the later stages of heart failure. Cardiac decompensation often results in a mild degree of polydipsia. Cardiac disorders resulting in a significant decrease in cardiac output (low output heart failure) may result in exercise intolerance, syncope and/or cyanosis of the mucous membranes. The inappetence and weight loss which is often associated with the more advanced stages of cardiac decompensation is usually attributed to cardiac cachexia.

Physical examination

Examination of the cardiovascular system can be broken down into five phases: (1) inspection; (2) temperature, pulse and respiration; (3) auscultation; (4) palpation; (5) percussion.

Inspection

Does the animal appear thin or cachexic? Is there evidence of tachypnoea or dyspnoea? Animals (particularly cats) with pleural effusion become dyspnoeic and develop a characteristic posture with elbow abduction. Jugular distension or the presence of a jugular pulse indicates an increase in central venous pressure and possible right-sided congestive heart failure. Other signs of right-sided heart failure include ascites and oedema of the ventral abdomen or limbs.

Temperature, pulse and respiration

The mucous membranes should be examined for signs of pallor or cyanosis. Pallor of the mucous membranes may be due to anaemia or poor peripheral perfusion. Cyanosis implies inadequate oxygenation of blood and may occur with congenital right to left cardiovascular shunts, severe pulmonary oedema (due to impaired diffusion of oxygen across the alveolar membrane) and acute airway obstruction. The normal capillary refill time is less than 2 s.

Palpation

The position of the apex beat over the 5th intercostal space on the left side at the level of the costochondral junction should be ascertained. Displacement of the apex beat may occur with large intrathoracic masses. The presence of a precordial thrill generally indicates a severe murmur. Both femoral pulses should be assessed noting rate, rhythm, quality and presence of a pulse deficit. Finally, the abdomen should be palpated for evidence of hepatomegaly and ascites (presence of a fluid thrill) indicative of right-sided congestive heart failure.

Percussion

Percussion of the thoracic wall is a more useful technique in cattle and horses when it can be used to outline the cardiac silhouette and detect the presence of a fluid line.

Auscultation

Auscultation of the thorax is discussed in Chapters 1 and 13. Auscultation should be performed in a quiet room, preferably when the animal is not panting, using both the bell and diaphragm of the stethoscope to detect low and high frequency tones, respectively. The heart rate, rhythm and intensity of the heart sounds and the presence of a heart murmur or abnormal respiratory sounds should be recorded. The regions of the thorax over which the mitral, tricuspid, aortic and pulmonic valves can be auscultated are described in detail in Chapter 13. The approximate location of each valve is shown in Fig. 34.1.

Obesity, pericardial or pleural effusion, diaphragmatic hernia or a large intrathoracic (for example mediastinal) mass may result in muffled heart sounds; conversely heart sounds may be accentuated with tachycardia, anaemia, excitement and in deep-chested animals.

Normal heart sounds and their association with the cardiac cycle

The four heart sounds are referred to as S1, S2, S3 and S4. In dogs and cats the presence of a third (S3) or fourth (S4) heart sound is considered abnormal and usually indicates cardiac pathology. The relationship of the normal heart sounds to the cardiac cycle is shown diagrammatically in Fig. 34.2.

The first (S1) heart sound is associated with the closure of the atrioventricular valves and is preceded by a rapid increase in intraventricular pressure. The S1 sound therefore indicates the onset of systole (ventricular depolarization) and correlates with the onset of the QRS complex on the ECG. Splitting of the first heart sound occasionally occurs in large breeds and is best heard over the cardiac apex and mitral valve region of the heart. S1 splitting is due to asynchronous closure of the AV valves. In some cases, for example in large breeds of dog, it may be regarded as a normal finding; in others it may be associated with bundle

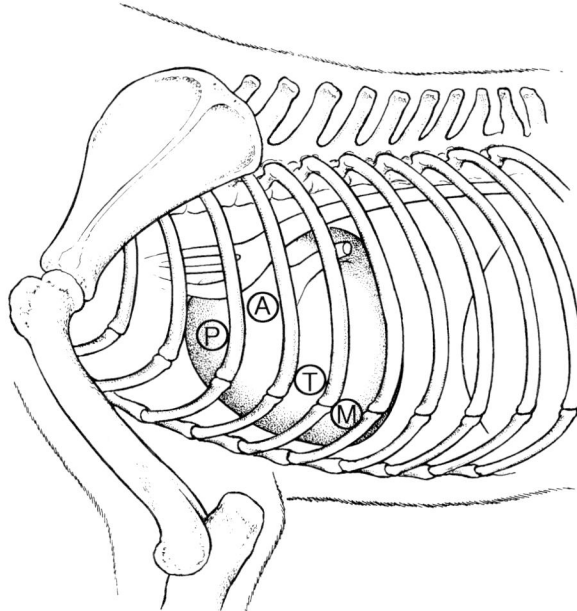

Figure 34.1 Schematic representation of the canine thorax showing the points of maximal intensity for auscultation of murmurs associated with the heart valves. M, mitral valve: 5th intercostal space on the left side at the level of the costochondral junction. T, tricuspid valve: 4th intercostal space on the right side at the level of the costochondral junction. A, aortic valve: 3rd–4th intercostal space on the left side level with the point of the shoulder. P, pulmonic valve: 2nd–3rd intercostal space on the left side just above the costochondral junction.

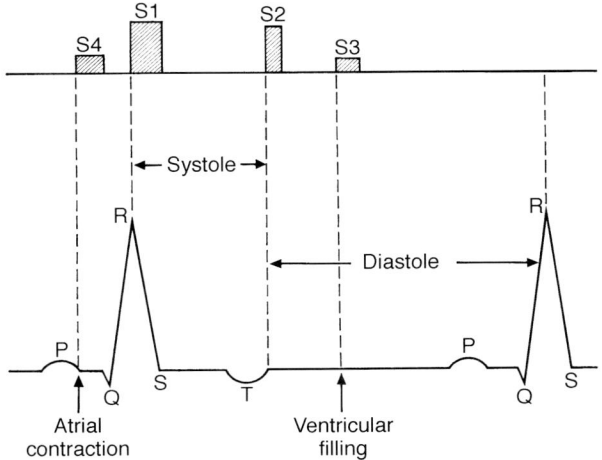

Figure 34.2 Diagram showing the relationship of the heart sounds and components of the normal electrocardiogram to the different phases of the cardiac cycle.

branch block or ventricular premature contractions.

The second (S2) heart sound is associated with the closure of the pulmonary and aortic valves which occurs once the pressure in the ventricles drops below that in the aorta and pulmonary artery. The S2 sound signifies the onset of the diastolic phase of the cardiac cycle. Splitting of the second heart sound is, in most cases, pathological and may occur with pulmonary hypertension, pulmonic stenosis, bundle branch block and ventricular premature contractions. Occasionally S2 splitting can be heard in normal dogs during inspiration.

The third (S3) heart sound is caused by rapid ventricular filling which occurs early in diastole. During diastole the pressure in the ventricles approximately equals atmospheric pressure and is slightly less than the atrial pressures therefore blood flows passively through the atrioventricular valves. Rapid ventricular filling allows the ventricles to fill to approximately 70% of their diastolic volume before the sinoatrial node discharges and the atria contract. The S3 sound is not normally heard in dogs and cats and its presence indicates ventricular dilation. It is a low frequency sound best heard over the cardiac apex or mitral valve region. It occurs towards the end of the T wave on an ECG.

The fourth (S4) heart sound is not normally heard in dogs and cats. It immediately precedes S1 and like the S3 sound its presence is usually associated with atrial and/or ventricular dilation. The S4 sound represents blood flowing rapidly into the ventricles as a result of atrial contraction (which accounts for the remaining 30% of the diastolic volume). It is a low pitched sound best heard over the pulmonic and aortic valve regions.

Systolic clicks are audible between the first and second heart sounds and may or may not be associated with a murmur. Their clinical significance is uncertain. The presence of a systolic click may indicate an abnormality in the formation and therefore the closure of the atrioventricular valves. Many animals with systolic clicks develop a mitral insufficiency murmur within 6–12 months (Gompf, 1983).

Gallop rhythms

A gallop rhythm consists of three beats. The most common type of gallop rhythm in dogs is a protodiastolic gallop which represents an accentuation of the third (S3) heart sound (Ettinger and Suter, 1970). This may occur in cases of mitral or tricuspid insufficiency when rapid ventricular filling results in diastolic overloading of the ventricles. A summation gallop is caused by fusion of the third (S3) and fourth (S4) heart sounds. The third heart sound produced is audible during diastole and its presence always indicates cardiac pathology (for example ventricular dilation). A presystolic gallop represents accentuation of the fourth (S4) heart sound and is occasionally heard in dogs with mitral insufficiency.

Cardiac murmurs

Cardiac murmurs are caused by alterations in blood flow through the heart or its major outflow tracts which produce turbulence. It is important to record details of a murmur for comparison with later observations (possibly by a different clinician) which may in turn correlate with an altered clinical presentation. The criteria used to characterize a cardiac murmur are discussed in greater detail in Chapter 13. It is important to realize that the intensity of a murmur does not necessarily correlate with the severity of the cardiac pathology responsible for its production or presence of congestive heart failure.

Timing (systolic, diastolic or continuous)

A pansystolic or holosystolic murmur extends throughout systole, that is between the first and second heart sounds; a diastolic murmur occurs after the second heart sound. A continuous murmur has both systolic and diastolic components.

Intensity

The intensity of a murmur can be graded subjectively on a scale of 1–6 as follows:

Grade 1: Careful auscultation required; murmur barely audible.
Grade 2: Very soft murmur but heard immediately when the stethoscope is applied to the chest wall.
Grade 3: Murmur approximately the same intensity as normal heart sounds.
Grade 4: Louder than normal heart sounds but no precordial thrill.
Grade 5: Murmur can be heard with stethoscope barely touching chest wall; palpable precordial thrill present.
Grade 6: Murmur heard with stethoscope away from the animal's chest.

Pitch (frequency)

High frequency ejection-type murmurs associated with aortic or pulmonic stenosis have a sharp, blowing quality compared to the low frequency, harsh regurgitant murmurs more typical of atrioventricular insufficiency. Other murmurs may be described as squeaky or musical.

Shape

The shape of a murmur refers to its modulation or quality. Does the murmur vary in intensity? A crescendo murmur is one which increases in intensity; a decrescendo murmur decreases in intensity. A crescendo–decrescendo murmur (diamond-shaped) murmur builds up to peak intensity and then falls away.

Radiation

The capacity of a murmur to radiate to different areas of the thoracic cavity reflects its origin and pathogenesis. The murmurs of aortic or pulmonic stenosis often radiate to the thoracic inlet (in the case of aortic stenosis the murmur may radiate up the carotid arteries). Murmurs associated with severe mitral insufficiency radiate cranially and dorsally.

Laboratory investigation of cardiac disease

Routine haematology and a full biochemistry screen may help to exclude the presence of an underlying disease process as a cause for a cardiac abnormality, for example anaemia may be ruled out as a cause of a systolic murmur. Arrhythmias may be the result of electrolyte or acid–base disturbances, or endotoxaemia. Feline hyperthyroidism is frequently associated with myocardial disease therefore, where appropriate, thyroid hormones should be assayed.

There are presently no specific laboratory tests for assessing myocardial damage. Lactate dehydrogenase may be released from damaged myocardium but other tissues, most notably kidney, skeletal muscle and liver also contain high concentrations of the enzyme. Low output cardiac failure may result in a significant increase in the plasma concentrations of urea and creatinine due to prerenal azotaemia; passive venous congestion of the liver associated with right-sided congestive heart failure usually results in a moderately increased level of plasma alkaline phosphatase (ALP) and alanine aminotransferase (ALT).

Haematological examination of animals with congestive or low output cardiac failure is often unremarkable. Hypoxia may result in increased numbers of circulating normoblasts and animals with severe ascites and/or pleural effusion may have low or low normal concentrations of total plasma proteins due to hypoalbuminaemia.

Electrocardiography

An electrocardiogram provides a graphic record of the voltage produced by cardiac muscle cells during atrial and ventricular depolarization and repolarization plotted against time. The electrical forces produced possess both direction and magnitude and can therefore be regarded as true cardiac vectors. The cardiac or mean electrical axis (MEA) represents the summation of many different forces. The MEA is the cardiac vector representing the average direction of spread of the depolarization wave through the ventricles as viewed from the frontal plane, that is the heart is viewed from the front with the animal standing up on its hind limbs (Fig. 34.3).

Each lead on an ECG represents a hypothetical line drawn between two sites on the body surface to which electrodes are attached. Each lead has a positive and negative pole and views the heart and the cardiac vector from a slightly different position. In most cases a hexaxial lead system (Bailey's hexaxial lead system) will provide an ECG of diagnostic quality. This combines three bipolar limb leads (leads I, II and III) with three unipolar limb leads (aVR, aVL and aVF).

The main uses of an ECG are as follows:

- Evaluation of chamber enlargement due to hypertrophy or dilation. ECG changes which suggest chamber enlargement should always be interpreted in association with radiographic abnormalities.
- Detection of cardiac arrhythmias. An ECG may be helpful in determining the type, origin and severity of an arrhythmia.
- Evaluation of cardiac therapy, for example with cardiac glycosides or anti-arrhythmic drugs.
- Detection of electrolyte or metabolic disturbances.

260 DISEASES OF THE CARDIOVASCULAR SYSTEM

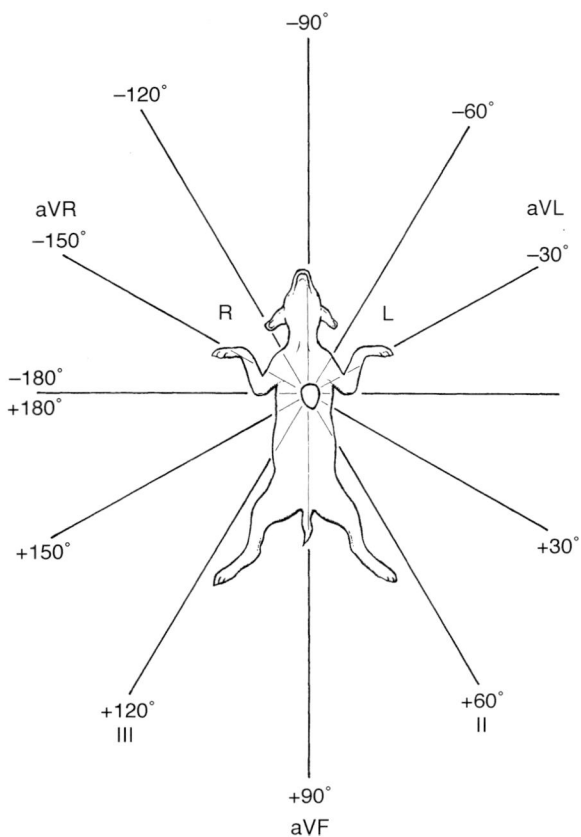

Figure 34.3 Mean electrical axis (MEA) viewed from the frontal plane.

- Evaluation of the prognosis and progression of a disease process.
- Anaesthetic monitoring during surgery.

An ECG is normally performed with the animal placed in right lateral recumbency on a rubber topped table or a blanket to prevent 50 cycles interference. With cats or any critically ill animal, especially those which are severely dyspnoeic, the ECG is best performed with the animal placed in sternal recumbency or in any position which the animal finds comfortable. The position of the animal should be taken into consideration when interpreting the ECG; sternal recumbency increases the amplitude of the P and R waves and may shift the mean electrical axis by as much as 10° to the left (Gompf and Tilley, 1979).

Continuous 24 hour ambulatory electrocardiography

A routine ECG records only a brief period of heart rhythm yielding information relevant only to the time of assessment. Certain types of arrhythmia such as paroxysmal ventricular tachycardia may only be precipitated by exercise or excitement and, therefore, may not be detected on a routine ECG. As a result, episodes of collapse, even if truly cardiogenic in origin, may remain undiagnosed because many cases appear clinically normal when examined. Continuous 24 hour ambulatory ECG monitoring circumvents this problem and provides a reliable and simple means of correlating clinical signs with disturbances of cardiac rhythm in the animal's home environment.

In one study, continuous ECGs performed on a series of healthy dogs showed marked sinus arrhythmia with associated long sinus pauses (5–7 s in some dogs) in both brachycephalic and non-brachycephalic breeds during sleep. Intermittent ventricular premature complexes were also noted (Hall *et al.*, 1991). Twenty-four hour ECG monitoring has proved useful for monitoring the progress and response to therapy in German shepherds with an inherited form of ventricular ectopy which may result in sudden death between 4 and 8 months of age (Moise and Gilmour, 1992).

The ECG and the cardiac cycle

The phases of the cardiac action potential are the result of sequential changes in cell membrane ion permeability and movement of ions into and out of the myocardial cells. Each phase of the cardiac cycle corresponds to a specific segment on the ECG trace (Fig. 34.2). The P wave represents atrial depolarization; the right atrium contracts fractionally before the left atrium. Enlargement of the atria, particularly the left atrium, accentuates this asynchrony and results in widening and notching of the P wave. The QRS complex represents ventricular depolarization and the T wave ventricular repolarization. The first negative deflection on lead II is the Q wave which is produced by discharge of the middle and apical portions of the ventricular system. Depolarization of the left and right ventricular free walls produces the R wave (under normal circumstances, the R wave represents depolarization of the left ventricle which is thicker; the deflection produced by the thinner right ventricle is essentially cancelled out). The R wave is the first positive deflection of the QRS complex on lead II. The S wave is the negative deflection which terminates the R wave; it is often difficult to define accurately and does not consistently appear on every ECG. The P–R interval represents the delay in conduction of the sinoatrial impulse through the atrioventricular node.

Basic principles of ECG interpretation

Normal ECG parameters, the criteria used for documenting chamber enlargement, and the electrocardiographic features of the more common arrhythmias are given in Tables 34.1–34.3 (see also Chapter 29). ECG abnormalities should always be interpreted in conjunction with the radiographic findings. An ECG does not differentiate between dilatation and hypertrophy.

The following questions should be answered before the ECG is analysed in detail.

- Is there a P wave for every QRS complex?
- Is the relationship of the P waves to QRS complexes constant? Slight differences in the duration of the P–R interval due to variation in vagal tone are acceptable, but should not exceed 0.01–0.02 s.
- Are all the P waves and QRS complexes similar? Altered configuration may indicate an ectopic focus or an abnormal (blocked) conduction pathway.

Ectopic impulses caused by foci of abnormal electrical discharge may originate outside the sinoatrial (SA) node in the atria, atrioventricular junctional tissue (AV node) or ventricles. Supraventricular ectopic impulses result in normal or near normal QRS complexes and altered or absent P waves. Ventricular ectopic impulses result in distorted, often biphasic QRS complexes which are wider than normal and are not associated with a P wave.

Radiological examination

Thoracic radiographs are essential in the evaluation of animals with suspected heart disease. Changes in the cardiac silhouette and lung fields provide direct information about the heart size, the condition of the lungs and volume load in the circulation. Thoracic radiography may facilitate or confirm a diagnosis suspected on the basis of physical examination, help in assessing the severity of known heart disease, or aid in the evaluation of the efficacy of treatment.

Good quality radiographs are required for accurate diagnosis and assessment. Attention to detail during the making of the radiograph is important. Accurate positioning is essential. The use of rare earth intensifying screens and a high kilovoltage (kV) technique will help to minimize movement artefact. Exposure should be made at full inspiration so that the lung fields are fully expanded and aerated. Both right lateral and dorsoventral (DV) rather than ventrodorsal projections should be made. These projections are preferred since the heart lies in a more consistent position.

Radiographs should be examined carefully and systematically for the following criteria.

Size of the cardiac silhouette

Wide variations in shape and size of the heart occur in different breeds of dogs, for example in

Table 34.1 Normal ECG parameters for the dog and cat[a]

Parameter	Normal values (dog)	Normal values (cat)
Heart rate	70–160 bpm[b]	160–200 bpm[c]
P wave duration	0.04 s (maximum)	0.04 s (maximum)
P wave amplitude	0.4 mV (maximum)	0.2 mV (maximum)
P–R interval	0.06–0.13 s	0.05–0.09 s
QRS duration	0.06 s (maximum)	0.04 s (maximum)
R wave amplitude	2.5–3.0 mV	0.9 mV (maximum)
Q–T interval	0.15–0.25 s	0.12–0.18 s
T wave	Usually less than 1/4 the height of the R wave (0.3 mV maximum in cats); may be positive, negative or biphasic but should not change polarity within any one lead	
Mean electrical axis	+40° to +100°	0 to +160°

[a] Measured on lead II.
[b] May be greater than 180 bpm in toy breeds and puppies.
[c] May be greater than 180 bpm in nervous cats and kittens.

Table 34.2 Abnormal ECG parameters and their significance in dogs and cats

Abnormal ECG parameter	Significance
Wide P wave (P mitrale); P wave may also be notched	Left atrial enlargement
Tall, peaked P waves; occasionally atrial T waves (T_a waves) may be seen as a negative deflection within the P–R segment. T_a waves represent repolarization of the atria	Right atrial enlargement
P waves tall, wide and often notched	Bilateral atrial enlargement
Wide QRS complexes; tall R waves; S–T slurring (coving); very occasionally there is deviation of the MEA to the left (see below)	Left ventricular enlargement; wide, usually biphasic QRS complexes, each preceded by a P wave are also seen with left and right bundle branch block and right ventricular hypertrophy (see below)
Deep S waves in leads I, II and III (usually also aVF); deep Q waves in leads I, II, III and aVF; S and Q waves must be greater than 0.5 mV to be classified as deep	Right ventricular enlargement (usually hypertrophy); deep Q waves are probably less reliable an indicator of right ventricular enlargement since they may occur in smaller dogs with biventricular enlargement and in deep chested breeds
Left axis deviation (MEA usually between −30° and −90°)	Left anterior fascicular branch block (MEA usually normal with complete left bundle branch block); a left axis shift is rarely seen with left ventricular enlargement
Right axis shift (MEA >100° for dogs and >160° for cats)	Right ventricular enlargement or right bundle branch block
Prolongation of P–R interval (first degree atrioventricular block)	Excessive vagal tone, e.g. in brachycephalic breeds (may be associated with marked sinus arrhythmia, a 'wandering pacemaker' and second degree AV block); drug therapy (early sign of digitalis toxicity but may also occur with beta blockers, calcium channel blockers and certain antidysrhythmic drugs); disease of the atrial myocardium or AV node; hyperkalaemia; endotoxaemia
S–T segment depression (S–T segment more than 0.2 mV below the baseline)	Myocardial ischaemia or hypoxia; often associated with signs of left atrial and left ventricular enlargement (e.g. is a common finding in dogs with dilated cardiomyopathy showing signs of severe IV congestive heart failure); occasionally S–T segment is elevated above the baseline
Tall, peaked T waves	Hyperkalaemia
Small, biphasic T waves	Hypokalaemia
T waves reverse polarity or increase in height in any one lead	Myocardial hypoxia
Prolongation of Q–T interval	Hypocalcaemia; hypokalaemia; hyperkalaemia
Shortening of Q–T interval	Hypercalcaemia; digitalis administration

deep chested breeds the heart is tall, narrow and upright whereas in barrel-chested breeds it is almost globular. On the lateral radiograph, the craniocaudal width of the normal heart is between 2.5 and 3.5 intercostal spaces and its height is approximately two-thirds the height of the thoracic cavity. The trachea normally diverges from the thoracic spine except in the case of barrel-chested breeds in which it may run parallel to the spine. On the dorsoventral projection, the normal heart should occupy no more than two-thirds the width of the thoracic cavity with the apex to the left of the midline.

The cat shows far less variation in size, although the angle of the long axis does vary. The width of the normal feline heart taken perpendicular to the long axis on the lateral projections should be less than 2.25 intercostal spaces.

The size of the cardiac silhouette is increased in congestive heart failure, pericardial effusion and peritoneopericardial diaphragmatic hernia. The cardiac silhouette may be decreased in size (microcardia) due to hypovolaemia.

Enlargement of individual cardiac chambers

The normal position of the cardiac chambers is indicated on Figs 34.4 and 34.5. Radiographic changes that occur with left-sided, right-sided and

Table 34.3 Electrocardiographic features and possible causes of commonly encountered arrhythmias

	Electrocardiographic features	Possible causes
Sinoatrial node arrhythmias		
Sinus arrhythmia	Variation in the intervals between successive P waves with alternating periods of slower and more rapid heart rates which are related to respiration	Variation in vagal tone during inspiration (heart rate increases) and expiration (heart rate decreases); more pronounced in brachycephalic breeds; physiological in dogs but pathological in cats
Wandering pacemaker	Variation in amplitude and/or polarity of P wave; relationship to QRS complex remains constant	Occurs with pronounced sinus arrhythmia and reflects variation in vagal tone (more common in brachycephalic breeds); digitalis toxicity
Sinus arrest or sinoatrial block	Delay between two successive P waves equal to or greater than two times the normal R–R interval	Increased vagal tone (more common in brachycephalic breeds); occurs in association with sinus arrhythmia and wandering pacemaker; usually asymptomatic and should be abolished with atropine or exercise; may occur with digitalis toxicity and occasionally mediastinal masses
Sinus bradycardia	Heart rate less than 70 bpm (dog) or 160 bpm (cat); rhythm is regular; may be associated with junctional or ventricular escape complexes	Hypothyroidism; hypoadrenocorticism; hypothermia; digitalis toxicity; physiological in a fit dog; may be asymptomatic or associated with weakness, lethargy and collapse
Sinus tachycardia	Heart rate greater than 160 bpm (dog) or 220–240 bpm (cat); P waves may be 'lost' in preceding T waves	Nervousness, fear or pain; fever; hyperthyroidism; shock/hypotension; anaemia; congestive heart failure; infection; phaeochromocytoma; drugs (vasodilators, atropine)
Sick sinus syndrome	Severe sinus bradycardia or sinoatrial block; heart rate often less than 40 bpm; intermittent bouts of supraventricular tachycardia or supraventricular premature complexes; concurrent AV nodal disease may result in AV block	Disease of the atria and/or AV node, e.g. fibrosis; small breeds of dog affected, e.g. miniature schnauzers and pugs; if associated with weakness or syncope give atropine (0.04 mg kg^{-1} i.m.) and repeat ECG
Atrial arrhythmias		
Atrial premature complex (APC)	A premature QRS complex is usually followed by a pause; the P wave, although still related to the QRS complex, is abnormal and precedes the QRS complex or is sometimes hidden in the preceding T wave; P–R interval may be normal, shorter or longer. Atrial bigeminy occurs when every other complex is an APC	Atrial enlargement (dilatation) associated with volume overload associated with AV insufficiency, cardiomyopathy or congenital heart disease; tumour infiltration of the myocardium; toxaemia; uraemia; digitalis toxicity; severe heartworm disease; excessive vagal tone; anaesthesia
Atrial tachycardia	Four or more APCs in a row; may be paroxysmal or sustained (usually intermittent); regular tachycardia with constant R–R intervals; P waves positive in lead II but a different shape and a P wave present for every QRS complex; QRS complexes appear normal	Severe mitral insufficiency: same diseases that cause APCs

Table 34.3 (contd.)

	Electrocardiographic features	Possible causes
Atrial fibrillation (AF)	Heart rate usually greater than 180 bpm in the dog; rhythm is typically irregular (R–R intervals variable); P waves absent and replaced by fibrillatory 'f' waves (occasionally saw-tooth pattern of atrial flutter); normal QRS complexes (or changes consistent with left ventricular enlargement); aberrant conduction at heart rates greater than 200 bpm occasionally results in abnormal QRS complexes; also S–T segment and T wave changes.	Severe distension of atria due to AV insufficiency, cardiomyopathy or congenital heart disease. Clinically, AF is characterized by pronounced exercise intolerance, syncope and signs of congestive heart failure. The heart rhythm is typically chaotic with pronounced pulse deficits. The femoral pulse varies in intensity. AF with a slow ventricular response rate occurs in some clinically 'normal' large giant breeds
Atrial standstill	Bradycardia (heart rate usually less than 60 bpm) associated with a slow sinoventricular rhythm; rhythm may be regular or irregular; P waves absent; QRS complexes normal or wide if concurrent bundle branch block; T wave often tall with hyperkalaemia; S–T segment elevated or depressed	Transient atrial standstill occurs with hyperkalaemia and digitalis toxicity; persistent atrial standstill has been reported in dogs, especially springer spaniels, with a form of muscular dystrophy resembling Emery–Dreifuss muscular dystrophy in humans (Miller and Tilley, 1995). Electrolytes are normal in these cases.
Arrhythmias involving the AV node or junctional tissue		
Junctional premature complex (JPC)	P wave usually negative in lead II and may be hidden within the QRS complex or may precede or follow it (P–R interval therefore variable); QRS complex of premature contraction appears normal or near normal and JPC may be followed by a pause	Atrial enlargement due to AV insufficiency, cardiomyopathy or congenital heart disease; digitalis toxicity
Junctional tachycardia	Heart rate usually within normal limits and rhythm regular (ectopic focus at AV junction acts as primary pacemaker); run of JPCs, i.e. P waves negative and P wave for every QRS but they may be hidden in preceding T waves or seen following QRS complexes	As for junctional premature complexes
Ventricular arrhythmias		
Ventricular premature complex (VPC)	Normal heart rate but rhythm broken by premature beat followed by a pause; wide, bizarre QRS complex which is not associated with a P wave; P wave may be lost in the VPC; ectopic complexes may be of identical shape (unifocal) or of variable shape (multiform) depending on whether they originate from one or more foci; VPCs which are superimposed on the preceding T waves (R on T phenomenon) are usually multifocal and may precede transition to ventricular tachycardia	*Cardiac causes*: congestive heart failure; cardiomyopathy; myocarditis; pericarditis; myocardial ischaemia and infarction; neoplastic infiltration of myocardium; congenital heart disease; inherited ventricular ectopy has been reported in German shepherds (Moise and Gilmour, 1992) *Non-cardiac causes*: endotoxaemia; uraemia; hyperthyroidism; gastric dilatation–volvulus; pancreatitis; electrolyte imbalance; hypoxia (e.g. due to severe anaemia); drugs (digitalis, anaesthetic agents)

	Electrocardiographic features	Possible causes
Ventricular tachycardia	May be paroxysmal or continuous; ventricular rate greater than 100 bpm; runs of VPCs followed by a pause before normal sinus rhythm resumes; P waves unrelated to the abnormal QRS complexes; fusion and capture beats present; may progress to ventricular flutter or ventricular fibrillation	Same cardiac and non-cardiac causes as for ventricular premature contractions
Ventricular flutter	Usually terminal event; smooth rhythmical undulations of the baseline; no P waves, QRS complexes or T waves seen	As for ventricular tachycardia
Ventricular fibrillation	Terminal event which progresses to cardiac arrest; fibrillation described as coarse or fine; jagged, irregular undulations of the baseline	As for ventricular tachycardia
Fusion beat	A ventricular premature contraction occurs simultaneously with the arrival of a normal sinus impulse; fusion complexes have a configuration midway between a normal QRS complex and a VPC; usually preceded by a P wave; seen with ventricular tachycardia	See ventricular tachycardia
Capture beat	The occasional P wave occurs at the right time and 'captures' the ventricles for one beat to produce a normal QRS complex; seen with ventricular tachycardia	See ventricular tachycardia
Escape rhythms	May be junctional or ventricular in origin; a single spontaneous impulse from a lower pacemaker constitutes an escape complex; a run of three or more such complexes is an escape rhythm. The heart rate is usually slow (usually less than 60 bpm); with junctional escape complexes QRS configuration is usually normal and P wave is negative and may precede, be superimposed on or follow the QRS complex; with ventricular escape complexes QRS configuration is similar to that of a VPC and P waves are absent unless complete third degree AV block is present in which case P waves are unrelated to the QRS complexes	Escape rhythms occur when the activity of the pacemaker with highest automaticity (usually the SA node) slows or when the SA nodal impulses are blocked completely. Heart rhythm is maintained at a slower rate by spontaneous discharge of a lower pacemaker located either in the AV junctional tissue or ventricles. May be associated with hyperkalaemia, digitalis toxicity, increased vagal tone or sick sinus syndrome

Table 34.3 (contd.)

	Electrocardiographic features	Possible causes
Atrioventricular heart block		
First degree AV block	Normal rhythm; P waves and QRS complexes normal and P wave for every QRS complex; P–R interval prolonged (>0.13 s in the dog and >0.09 s in the cat)	Digitalis toxicity; quinidine toxicity; hyperkalaemia; increased vagal tone; other drugs which slow heart rate (beta blockers, calcium channel blockers); may be seen in older dogs with mitral insufficiency
Second degree AV block	*Mobitz type I*: slow or normal heart rate; intermittent P waves with no associated QRS complexes; P waves and QRS complexes normal; gradual prolongation of successive P–R intervals until a P wave is blocked. *Mobitz type II*: as for type I but a fixed ratio of non-conducted P waves to QRS complexes, i.e. two or three P waves for every QRS complex; P–R interval constant although may be longer than normal; may progress to third degree AV block	Hereditary in pugs; Mobitz type I with digitalis toxicity and increased vagal tone; Mobitz type II usually associated with cardiac disease (prognosis tends to be less favourable)
Third degree (complete) AV block	No relationship between P waves and QRS complexes (P waves may be 'lost' in QRS complexes); heart rate usually <60 bpm (dog) or <100 bpm (cat); P waves normal; QRS complexes often abnormal due to bundle branch block or presence of ventricular escape complexes (idioventricular escape rhythm); occasionally complexes may be normal if block high in AV node	Congenital heart defects; severe digitalis toxicity with concurrent underlying cardiac pathology; neoplastic infiltration of the myocardium; idiopathic myocardial fibrosis involving the myocardium and/or conduction pathways; hypertrophic cardiomyopathy; bacterial endocarditis; myocardial infarction, hyperkalaemia and Lyme disease (Tilley, 1992)
Bundle branch block		
Left bundle branch block (LBBB)	QRS complexes wider than normal (>0.8 s in the dog and >0.06 s in the cat); QRS complexes positive in leads I, II, III and aVF and negative in leads aVR and aVL; QRS complex preceded by a normal P wave	Myocardial disease (dilated cardiomyopathy or myocardial ischaemia); congenital subvalvular aortic stenosis
Right bundle branch block (RBBB)	QRS complexes wider than normal (criteria for LBBB); right axis deviation with deep wide S waves in leads I, II, III and aVF; QRS complexes positive in leads aVR and aVL	May occur in normal dogs and rarely causes haemodynamic problems; seen with myocardial disease, valvular fibrosis (endocardiosis), congenital heart disease and cardiac neoplasia
Left anterior fascicular block	QRS complexes of normal duration; marked left axis deviation with deep S waves in leads II, III and aVF; small Q waves and tall R waves in leads I and aVL	Hypertrophic cardiomyopathy especially in cats; myocardial ischaemia and infarction
Electrical alternans	P waves, QRS complexes or T waves alternate in height within the same lead (usually recognized in the R wave); heart rate and rhythm normal or increased (may be supraventricular tachycardia); R waves may be small; P waves always related to QRS complexes	Pericardial effusion; pleural effusion

generalized cardiomegaly are shown diagrammatically in Figs 34.6–34.8.

Assessment of the pulmonary vasculature

The pulmonary arteries and veins should be of similar size and run on either side of the bronchi. The arteries are dorsal and the veins ventral on the lateral projection and the diameter of the cranial lobe vessels should be smaller than the proximal third of the fourth rib. On the dorsoventral projection the right and left caudal lobe vessels can be identified. The arteries are lateral to the veins. They should be of equal size and should not exceed the diameter of the ninth rib where they cross. The pulmonary vessels should be assessed for signs of tortuosity, pruning and loss of margination. Conditions which increase the size of the pulmonary vessels include left-to-right shunting (for example patent ductus arteriosus, ventricular septal defect), congestive heart failure, heartworm disease and iatrogenic fluid overload. The pulmonary vessels may be reduced in right-to-left shunting (for example tetralogy of Fallot), severe pulmonic stenosis, hypovolaemia and pulmonary thromboembolism.

Assessment of the pulmonary patterns

Pulmonary congestion and oedema may be seen predominantly in the dorsocaudal lung fields in chronic left-sided cardiac failure. In acute left-sided failure, alveolar oedema is seen more diffusely throughout the lung fields. In cats, pulmonary oedema often appears as an interstitial rather than alveolar pattern.

Assessment of the caudal vena cava

The normal caudal vena cava is usually parallel sided and of similar size to the aorta. On the lateral projection, it slopes slightly cranioventrally before merging with the caudal outline of the heart. Enlargement of the caudal vena cava and liver is evidence of right-sided heart failure. Pleural effusion and ascites can also be seen in some cases.

Assessment of the great vessels

Post-stenotic dilatation of the great vessels can be seen in some cases of congenital subaortic or pulmonic stenosis and results in filling of the cranial cardiac waist.

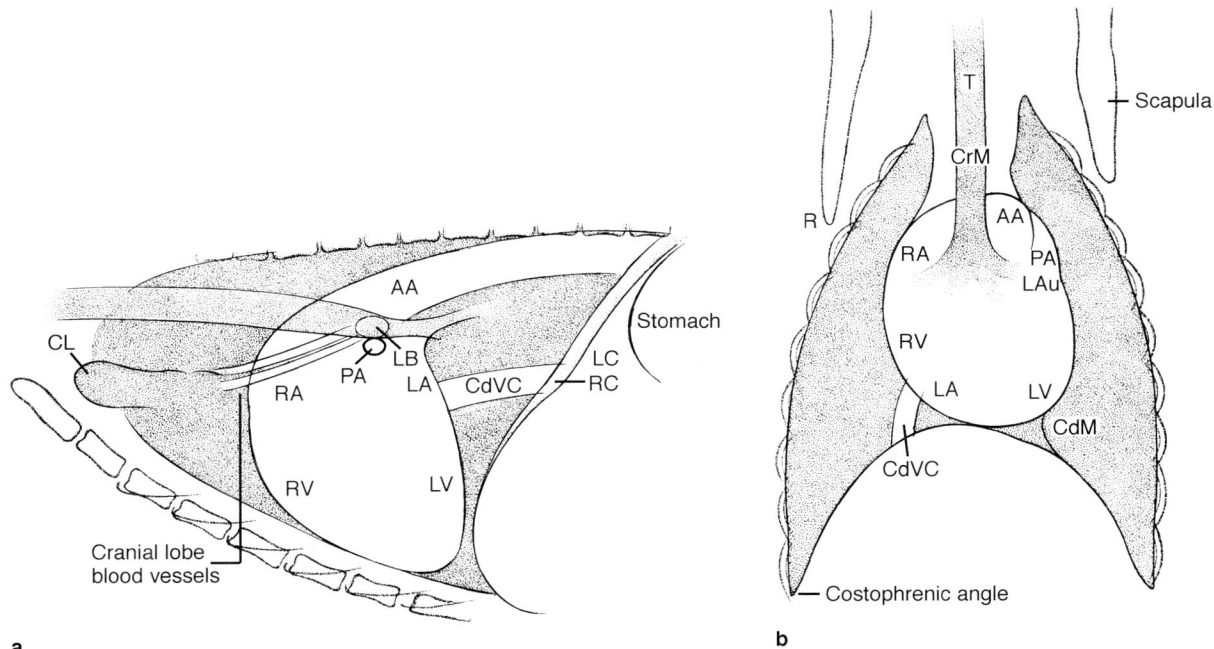

Figure 34.4 (a) Drawing from a right lateral thoracic radiograph of a normal dog showing the position of the major anatomical structures. (b) Drawing from a dorsoventral thoracic radiograph of a normal dog showing the position of the major anatomical structures. AA, aortic arch; RA, right atrium; RV, right ventricle; LA, left atrium; LAu, left auricular appendage; LV, left ventricle; PA, pulmonary artery; CdVC, caudal vena cava; T, trachea; CL, cranial extremity of left cranial lobe; LB, common opening to the left cranial and middle lobe bronchi; CrM, cranial mediastinum; CdM, ventral caudal mediastinum; RC, right crus; LC, left crus.

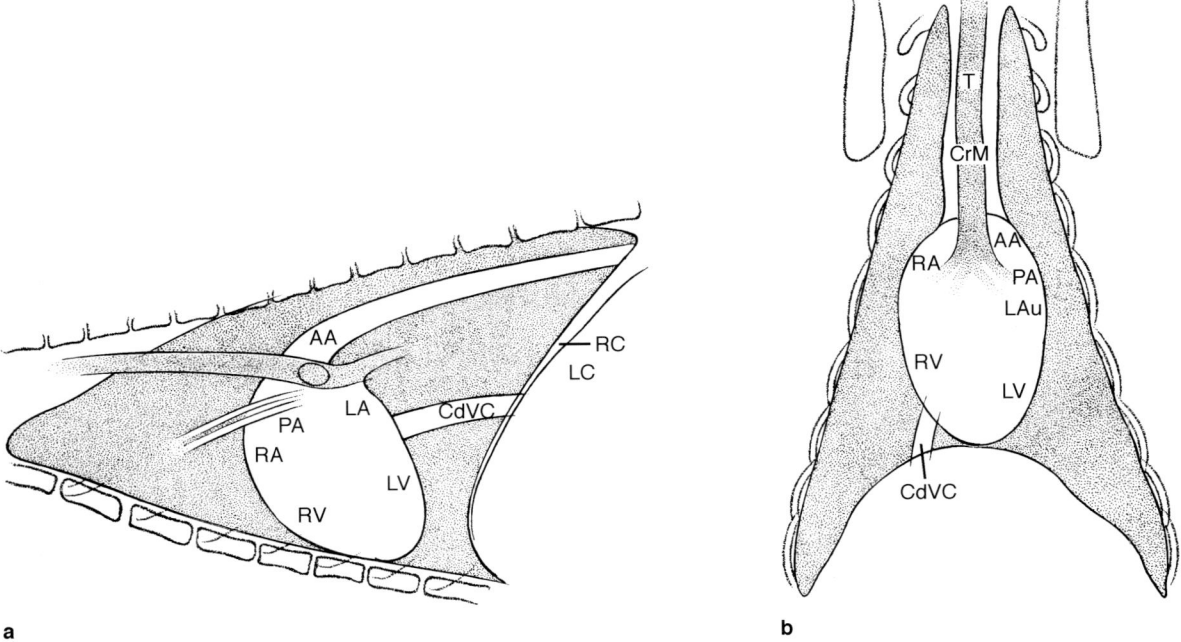

Figure 34.5 (a) Drawing from a right lateral thoracic radiograph of a normal cat showing the position of the major anatomical structures. (b) Drawing from a dorsoventral thoracic radiograph of a normal cat showing the position of the major anatomical structures. Abbreviations are the same as for Figure 34.4.

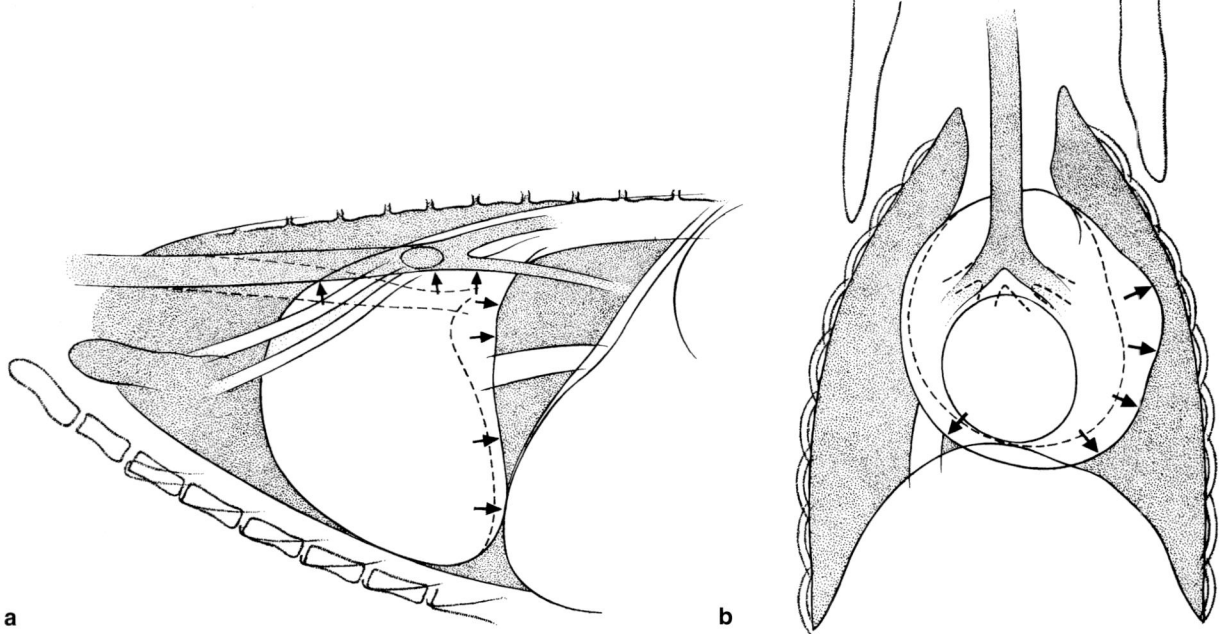

Figure 34.6 (a) Drawing from a right lateral thoracic radiograph of a dog with left-sided heart enlargement showing elevation of the trachea, straightening of the caudal border of the heart, tenting of the left atrium with loss of the caudal heart waist and splitting of the caudal lobe bronchi. The normal heart outline is represented by the dotted line. (b) Drawing from a dorsoventral thoracic radiograph of a dog with left-sided heart enlargement showing widening of the cardiac silhouette, enlargement of the left auricular appendage, double opacity of the enlarged left atrium superimposed over the heart base, displacement of the caudal lobe bronchi around the left atrium, rounding of the left ventricular border and displacement of the apex to the right. The normal heart outline is represented by the dotted line.

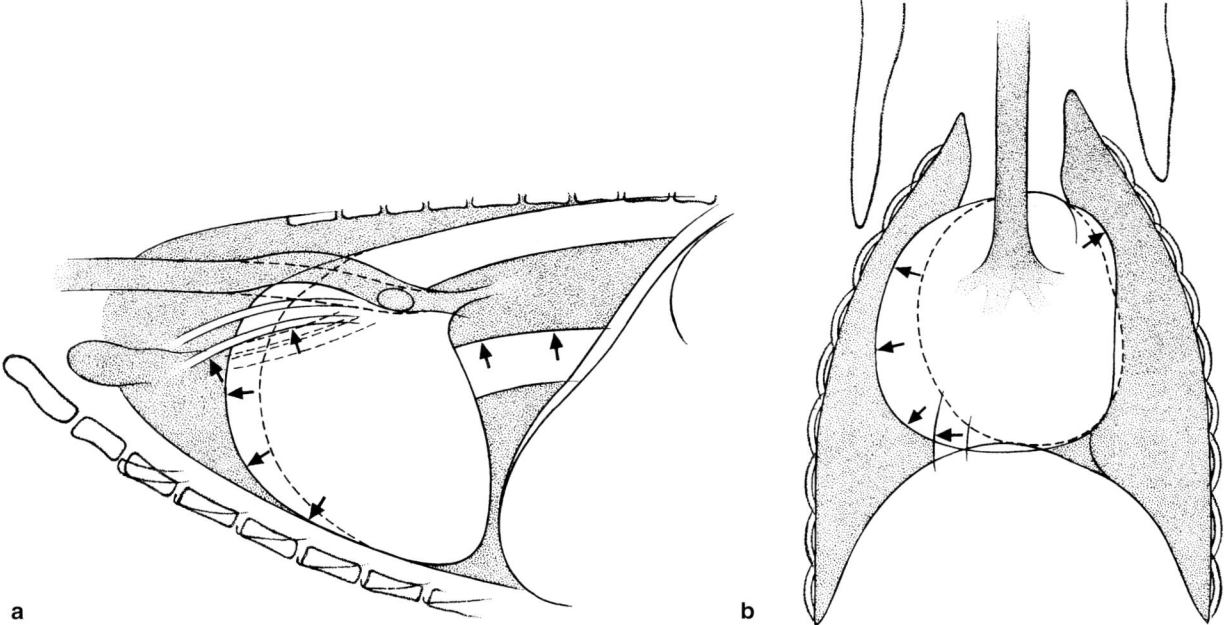

Figure 34.7 (a) Drawing from a right lateral thoracic radiograph of a dog with right-sided heart enlargement showing elevation of the trachea cranial to the heart base, increased sternal contact, rounding of the cranial heart border with loss of the cranial waist, dorsal displacement of the right cranial lobe vessels over the enlarged right atrium, enlargement and dorsal elevation of the caudal vena cava. The normal heart outline is represented by the dotted line. (b) Drawing from a dorsoventral thoracic radiograph of a dog with right-sided heart enlargement showing rounding of the right heart border which may cause the cardiac silhouette to assume an inverted 'D' shape, displacement of the apex to the left, enlargement of the caudal vena cava and possibly enlargement of the pulmonary artery segment. The normal heart outline is represented by the dotted line.

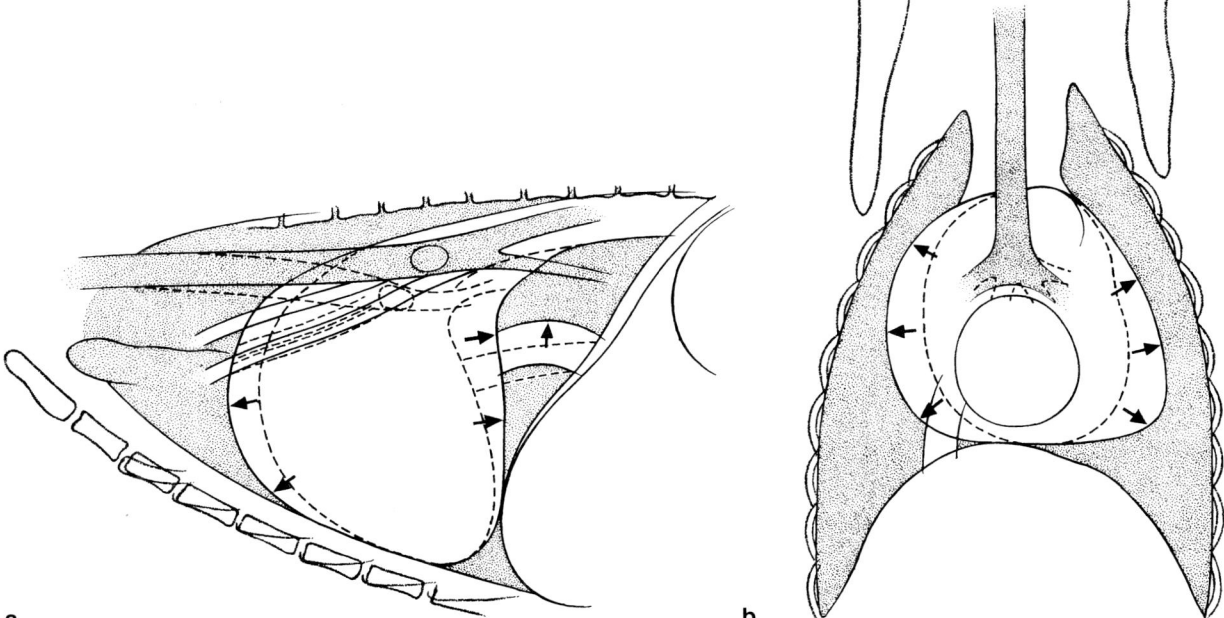

Figure 34.8 (a) Drawing from a right lateral thoracic radiograph of a dog with generalized heart enlargement showing radiological signs of left- and right-sided enlargement often with pulmonary oedema and ascites. The normal heart outline is represented by the dotted line. (b) Drawing from a dorsoventral thoracic radiograph of a dog with generalized heart enlargement showing radiological signs of left- and right-sided enlargement often with pulmonary oedema and ascites. The normal heart outline is represented by the dotted line.

Echocardiography

Diagnostic ultrasound provides a safe, non-invasive technique of obtaining qualitative and quantitative data about cardiac anatomy and function. The information gained is complementary to that obtained from thoracic radiography. Real time, two-dimensional (2D) imaging provides the most easily recognizable and understandable images of the heart. Complete examination of the heart requires a systematic approach using both the right and left parasternal acoustic windows (Fig. 34.9).

M-mode echocardiography allows measurement of chamber size and wall thickness and provides characterization and timing of motion relative to the ECG during the cardiac cycle. M-mode has a high sampling rate which facilitates accurate resolution and definition of rapidly moving structures. M-mode can be used to measure left ventricular indices, mitral valve measurements and systolic time intervals.

Doppler echocardiography provides information about the flow of blood within the heart chambers, across the valves and in the great vessels. It is complementary to 2D and M-mode echocardiography and provides a more complete, non-invasive evaluation of cardiac function.

There are two basic Doppler techniques: **continuous wave** and **pulsed wave** Doppler. A con-

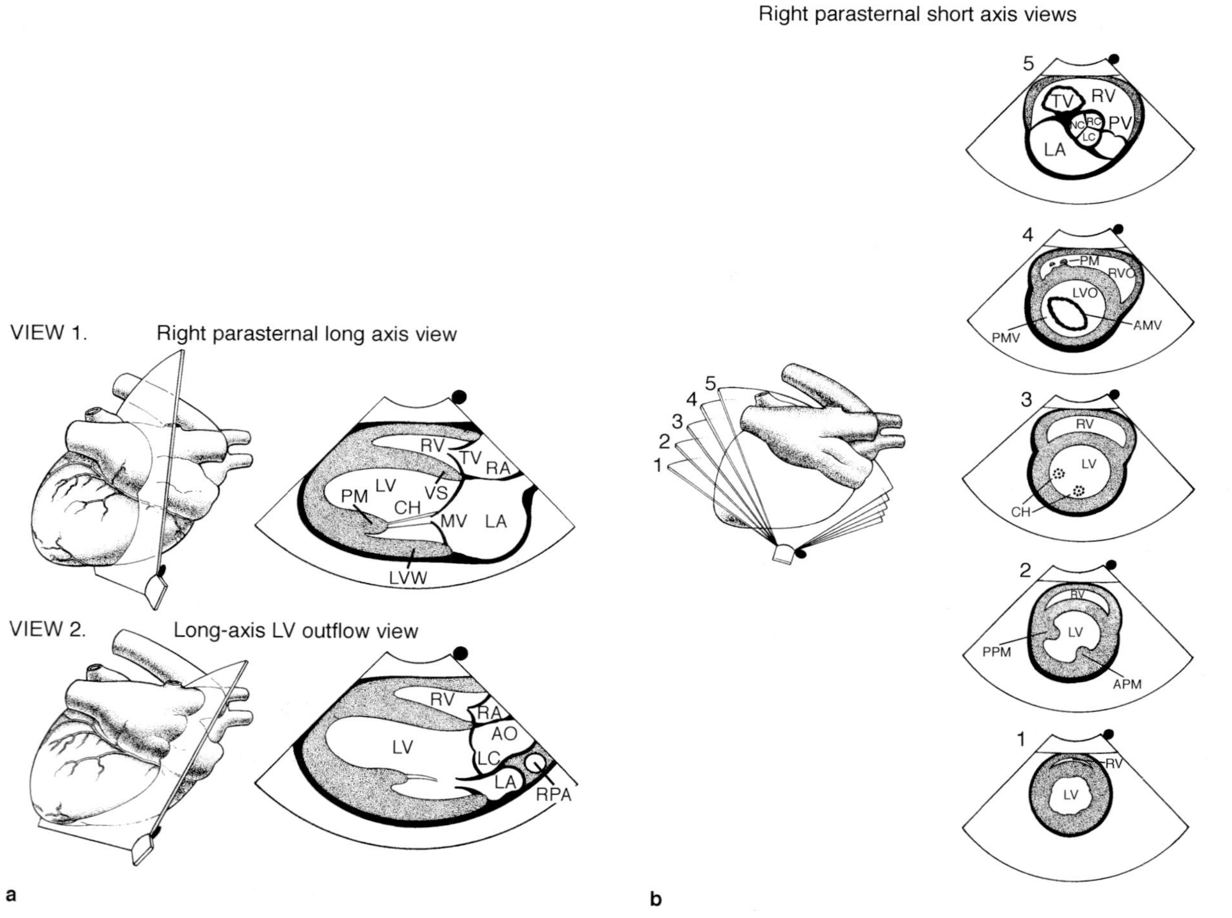

Figure 34.9 Drawings taken from ultrasound scans of a normal dog's heart. (a) Ultrasound scans taken from the right parasternal position to show the long axis views of the heart. View 1 is optimized for the left atrium and mitral valve, View 2 is optimized for the left ventricular outflow tract and aorta. (b) Ultrasound scans taken from the right parasternal position to show the short axis views of the heart. Views 1–5 are scans taken from ventral to dorsal. RA, right atrium; TV, tricuspid valve; RV, right ventricle; LA, left atrium; MV, mitral valve; AMV, anterior mitral valve leaflet; PMV, posterior mitral valve leaflet; CH, chordae tendineae; LV, left ventricle; L(R)C, left (right) coronary cusp of aortic valve; Ao, aorta; RPA, right pulmonary artery; VS, ventricular septum; LVW, left ventricular wall; PM, papillary muscle; APM, anterior papillary muscle; PPM, posterior papillary muscle. (Adapted from Thomas et al., 1993.)

tinuous wave Doppler transducer has two piezoelectric crystals, one to transmit a continuous wave of ultrasound and the other to receive backscattered echoes. This system is very sensitive and allows the measurement of high maximum velocities. The pressure gradient across a valve can be calculated using the modified Bernoulli equation:

$$\text{Pressure gradient} = 4 \times (\text{maximum velocity})^2$$

An important drawback of continuous wave Doppler, however, is that all velocities along the length and width of the ultrasound beam are recorded and as no structural information is gained, the region of abnormal flow cannot be localized accurately.

This problem is circumvented by using pulsed wave Doppler, which uses a single crystal to transmit ultrasound in pulses and is then set up to receive echoes after a time delay. In this way reflected signals are recorded only from a particular depth and localization within an echocardiographic image is then possible. However, the pulsed wave system is unable to detect high frequency Doppler shifts (that is high velocities) due to a phenomenon known as aliasing. This disadvantage is greatly reduced by **colour flow mapping**, a two-dimensional version of pulsed wave Doppler.

Cardiac catheterization and angiocardiography

The use of cardiac catheterization and angiocardiography has declined with the advent of echocardiography. However, the technique is still indicated in some cases when the diagnosis proves difficult to make or during interventional procedures for the management of heart disease, for example balloon valvuloplasty.

It is essential to obtain a good concentration of contrast medium within the heart. This is best achieved by injecting the contrast medium through a catheter positioned in the jugular vein close to the heart (*non-selective angiocardiography*) or directly into a specific cardiac chamber or great vessel (*selective angiocardiography*). Low osmolar water-soluble contrast media should be used in patients with compromised cardiac function. A pressure injector is necessary in large dogs to deliver the required amount of contrast rapidly. The flow of contrast through the heart can be recorded using a rapid film changer or on video from image intensified fluoroscopy.

Selective angiocardiography is the most versatile and reliable method of angiocardiography and provides optimal information when supplemented with pressure measurements and blood gas analyses from the cardiac chambers and great vessels. Various types of catheter are available and are designed to assist the positioning of the catheter tip in selected chambers or vessels. The placing of the catheter must be monitored by image intensification or spot films. Careful planning before the investigation and continuous monitoring of the patient during the examination are essential to increase the quality and safety of the procedure.

HEART FAILURE

The cardiovascular system has enormous compensatory reserves and heart failure only occurs when the reserve capacity is overwhelmed.

Cardiovascular reserves

- *Venous oxygen reserves*. The normal end-capillary or venous oxygen tension is 30–50 mm Hg. Providing this figure remains greater than 30 mm Hg increased oxygen can be extracted by the tissues as the demand for oxygen increases. Anaerobic metabolism occurs below a critical level of 21–22 mm Hg and results in lactic acid production in skeletal muscle tissue and signs of exercise intolerance.
- *Maximum effective heart rate*. In dogs this is approximately 180 beats per minute. Above this figure there is inadequate filling of the ventricles during diastole with a resultant decrease in cardiac output.
- *Stroke volume*. Normally only 50–65% of the diastolic volume is ejected during each cardiac cycle (Detweiler *et al.*, 1993). This figure increases as the demand for oxygen increases.
- *Coronary reserve*. Coronary blood flow can be increased to meet the increased oxygen demand of the myocardium.
- *Cardiac enlargement*. In response to an increased work load the heart either hypertrophies or dilates to maintain cardiac output and tissue perfusion.

Preload and afterload

Preload is defined as the stretching force that determines the precontraction length of each cardiac muscle fibre. A moderate increase in preload results in a greater contractile force (Frank–Starling relationship). Hence preload is related to left ventricular end-diastolic pressure. Afterload represents the tension which develops in a muscle fibre before contraction occurs, that is, the tension in the myocardium which is necessary to overcome the forces opposing ventricular ejection. As the ventricles increase in size, more tension must be generated to produce a given pressure (Laplace's law).

■ Pathophysiology of heart failure

Heart failure, by definition, occurs when cardiac output is insufficient to provide the tissues with adequate blood flow and/or when the venous return to the heart is greater than the amount of blood that the heart can expel at normal filling pressure. Most animals with heart failure show signs of both forward and backward failure. *Forward failure* refers to the inability of the heart to pump sufficient blood forward and the inadequate tissue perfusion which ensues. *Backward failure* occurs when the left and/or right ventricular end-diastolic pressure (preload) increases. This leads to increased venous pressure behind the affected chambers and the development of passive venous congestion of the lungs, liver and other tissues.

Numerous compensatory neurohumoral mechanisms become operative when cardiac output starts to fall. These compensatory changes are entirely appropriate for low output failure caused by circulatory shock, for example hypovolaemic shock, and are designed to maintain cardiac output at a level which is at least sufficient to ensure adequate tissue perfusion when the animal is at rest. If, however, a cardiac abnormality is responsible for the low output then, in the longer term, these compensatory responses become inappropriately regulated to a point that they are detrimental to the animal, further increasing the workload on the heart and setting up a self-perpetuating cycle of ventricular dysfunction (Fig. 34.10). Sustained compensatory mechanisms trigger adaptive changes in the heart and blood vessels leading to further compromise in cardiac function and signs of passive venous congestion (Packer, 1992a). Thus, clinically, signs of low output failure are usually associated with varying degrees of circulatory congestion. The cardiac function curves shown in Fig. 34.11 demonstrate these two situations of low output failure and congestive failure. Clinical cases can occur anywhere between these extremes and therefore may show a combination of low output and congestive signs depending on the level of activity attempted and the cardiac output required to maintain adequate tissue perfusion.

On a pathophysiological basis heart failure may be divided into four components: myocardial

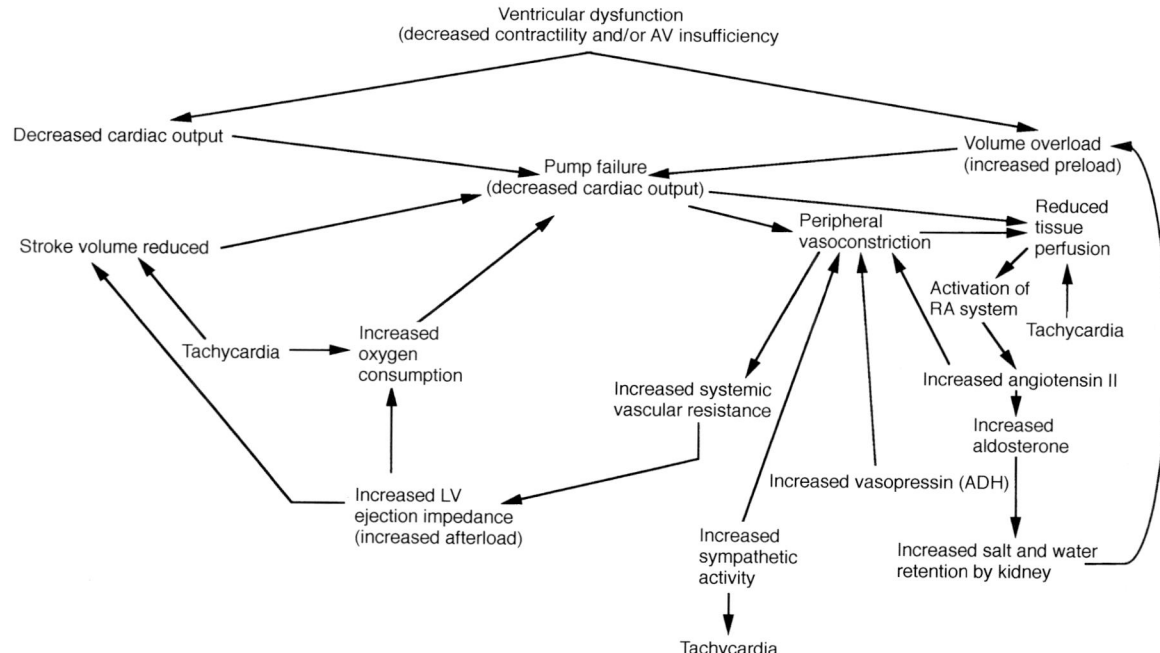

Figure 34.10 Flow diagram of the pathophysiology of heart failure. RA system = renin–angiotensin system.

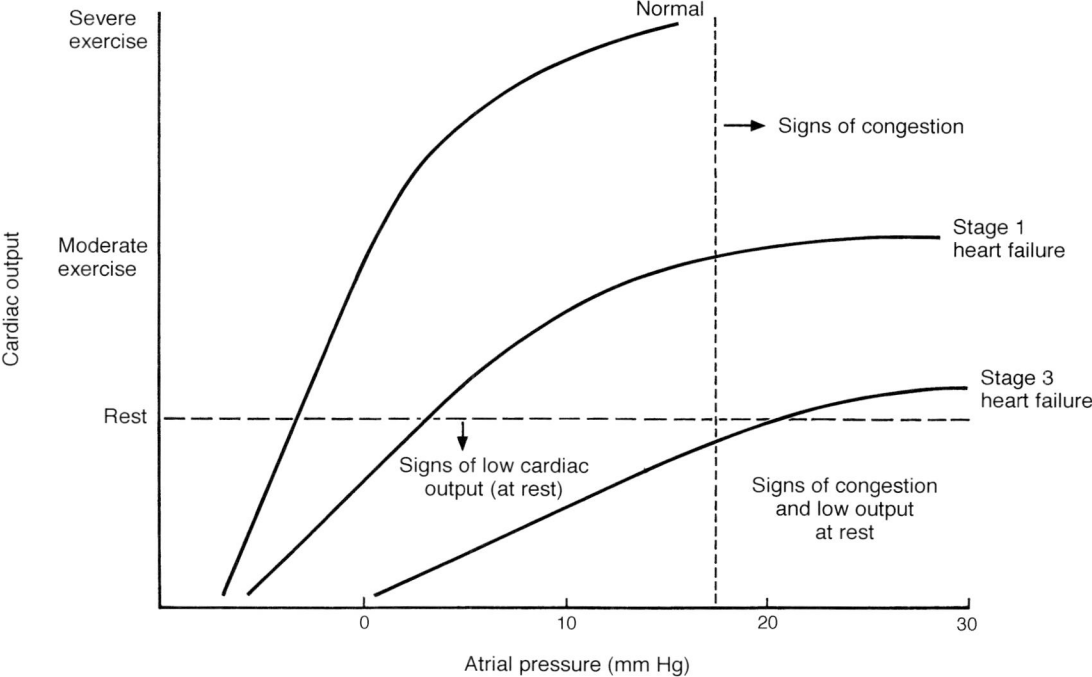

Figure 34.11 Cardiac function curves. This diagram shows the steep relationship which normally exists between cardiac filling pressure and cardiac output (normal). Early in a disease state leading to cardiac insufficiency, compensatory mechanisms will allow the heart to function at higher filling pressures to achieve sufficient cardiac output to meet the tissue requirements for moderate exercise without signs of low output or congestion developing (Stage 1 heart failure), but no cardiac reserve exists. With chronic heart disease, compensatory mechanisms become less effective and may even lead to a deterioration in cardiac function. Clinical signs of congestion occur even at rest (Stage 3 heart failure) and the heart is heavily dependent on the maintenance of extremely high filling pressures to achieve adequate cardiac output and prevent signs of low output failure at rest.

failure, volume overload, pressure overload and compliance failure.

Myocardial failure

Impaired myocardial contractility leads to systolic dysfunction which is characterized by a reduction in stroke volume and signs of low output (forward) failure. Myocardial failure may be primary (for example cardiomyopathy) or may occur secondary to prolonged volume overload. The myocardial failure which is a feature of dilated cardiomyopathy usually follows a more chronic course and numerous compensatory mechanisms come into operation to counteract the impaired myocardial function and decrease in cardiac output (see section on compensatory mechanisms).

Volume overload (increased preload)

Volume overload results in ventricular dilatation to a point where the ventricle decompensates, that is, myocardial contractility decreases and signs of both congestive heart failure and low output failure occur. Signs of congestive heart failure associated with the regurgitation of blood into the atria and volume overload may occur before myocardial decompensation and it has been shown that myocardial contractility is often normal or only mildly abnormal in dogs with congestive heart failure due to chronic mitral endocardiosis (Kittleson et al., 1984).

Causes of volume overload include the following.

- Atrioventricular insufficiency. Incompetence of the atrioventricular valves leads to regurgitation of blood from the ventricles to the atria. This may be due to endocardiosis, endocarditis, dilation of the atrioventricular annuli as

occurs with dilated cardiomyopathy, and ruptured chordae tendineae.
- Left to right cardiovascular shunts which overload the left side of the heart via the lungs. Examples include patent ductus arteriosus, ventricular septal defect and atrial septal defect.
- Sodium and water retention (see section on compensatory mechanisms).

Pressure overload (increased afterload)
Conditions which cause increased vascular resistance and which impede the ejection of blood through the ventricular outflow tracts result in ventricular hypertrophy.

Causes of pressure overload include:

- Aortic or pulmonic stenosis
- Hypertrophic cardiomyopathy
- Pulmonary hypertension (for example chronic obstructive pulmonary disease, dirofilariasis or pulmonary thrombosis).
- Increase in systemic vascular resistance (for example systemic hypertension associated with chronic renal insufficiency).

Compliance failure
Compliance failure implies a loss of myocardial elasticity so that the ventricle is unable to relax and distend properly during diastolic filling. The haemodynamic abnormalities therefore reflect diastolic dysfunction rather than systolic dysfunction which occurs with myocardial failure. Compliance failure may be associated with ventricular hypertrophy, myocardial fibrosis and pericardial effusion (cardiac tamponade).

Extracardiac factors such as excitement, heat stress, overexertion, infection, trauma, anaemia, shock, obesity, pregnancy or any severe systemic or metabolic disease process can also contribute to cardiac decompensation in an animal with pre-existing cardiac disease.

Circulatory disturbances can cause similar cardiac dysfunction either by reducing cardiac output or by creating high output states which overload the heart.

Low output states may be caused by:

1. Decreased preload, for example,
   - Overzealous use of diuretics and/or vasodilators to treat congestive heart failure
   - Hypovolaemia due to haemorrhage or hypoadrenocorticism
   - Reduced venous return (for example compression of the posterior vena cava by a large abdominal mass, ascites, gastric torsion)
2. Dysrhythmias (either tachy- or bradydysrhythmias)

High output states which overload the heart may be associated with:

1. Chronic anaemia, arteriovenous fistulae (for example cardiovascular shunts) and hyperthyroidism
2. Overzealous administration of intravenous fluids

Compensatory mechanisms in heart failure

The normal physiological mechanisms regulating the cardiovascular system are primarily concerned with the maintenance of arterial blood pressure which is adequate for cerebral perfusion. A fall in cardiac output and therefore arterial blood pressure will activate the following neurohormonal systems:

1. The sympathetic nervous system
2. The renin–angiotensin–aldosterone system
3. The renal body fluid system

The resultant effects of these neurohormonal systems are as follows.

- Blood vessels constrict, reducing the capacitance of the circulation and mobilizing blood from the venous side thereby increasing cardiac chamber filling pressures and, via the Frank–Starling mechanism, the force with which the heart muscle contracts. In addition, constriction of the arterioles diverts blood away from so called non-essential tissues towards the heart and the brain.
- The heart beats more forcefully and at a faster rate.
- The extracellular fluid volume increases which increases cardiac filling pressure.

The neuroendocrine systems listed above all interact to produce the compensatory effects which maintain cardiac output at a reasonable level to match tissue requirements. Central to this interaction is the renin–angiotensin–aldosterone system (RAAS) as shown in Fig. 34.10.

The sympathetic nervous system stimulates contraction of arterial and venous smooth muscle, an effect mediated by alpha adrenoceptors (primarily of the alpha$_1$ subtype). The cardiac effects of sympathetic stimulation are an increase in heart rate and force of cardiac muscle contraction, effects which are mediated primarily by beta$_1$-adrenoceptors. The increase in noradrenaline levels in dogs with congestive heart failure (CHF) correlates with the clinical severity, and dogs with dilated cardiomyopathy tend to have higher noradrenaline levels than those with chronic mitral valve disease (endocardiosis). There appears to be no correlation, however, between noradrenaline concentrations and myocardial function as measured by the end-systolic volume index (Ware et al., 1990).

In addition to the above, an increase in sympathetic tone via renal sympathetic nerves increases renin secretion by the juxtaglomerular apparatus of the kidney resulting in activation of the RAAS. Renin metabolizes angiotensinogen to produce angiotensin I which in turn is converted by angiotensin converting enzyme (present in many tissues) to produce the active hormone, angiotensin II. Angiotensin II also causes vasoconstriction, particularly of arterial smooth muscle and has a negative feedback effect on the production of renin. In addition, it increases release of noradrenaline from sympathetic nerve endings, thus potentiating the vascular and cardiac effects of the sympathetic system. Angiotensin II itself also has direct effects on cardiac muscle which result in increases in the rate and force of contraction and in cardiac muscle hypertrophy. Indeed, there is now good evidence for local production of renin and angiotensin II in a number of tissues, including the myocardium (Baker et al., 1992) where up-regulation of the system is thought to occur with increased ventricular wall stress (Dzau, 1992). There are also direct renal effects of angiotensin II. In the proximal convoluted tubule, angiotensin II increases the absorption of salt and water. Angiotensin II stimulates the adrenal cortex to secrete aldosterone which acts on the distal convoluted tubule of the kidney to enhance sodium retention. Salt and water homeostasis is also affected by the effects of angiotensin II in the brain where it is thought to increase thirst (possibly via a direct action on the hypothalamic thirst centres), salt appetite and the secretion of antidiuretic hormone (ADH), another potent vasoconstrictor (Hamlin, 1988).

The RAAS is also activated by decreased renal perfusion. The kidney senses poor perfusion both by a decrease in flow of tubular fluid, detected by the macula densa of the juxtaglomerular apparatus, and by reduced pressure in the afferent arterioles. Both are signals for increased renin secretion and therefore activation of the RAAS. Reduced renal blood flow therefore results in increased aldosterone secretion and enhanced salt and water retention by the kidney. Glomerular filtration rate is sustained at a normal level by angiotensin II constricting the efferent arteriole more than the afferent arteriole. The fractional amount of renal plasma flow which is filtered therefore rises, leaving peritubular capillary hydrostatic pressure low and oncotic pressure high. Both these factors favour enhanced aldosterone-induced reabsorption of tubular fluid, that is, salt and water retention (Hamlin, 1988).

It has been shown that the progressive increase in plasma aldosterone concentration which occurs in dogs with heart failure correlates with the clinical status of the animal (Knowlen et al., 1983).

As stated above, all these compensatory factors increase the work load for the heart by raising circulating volume, increasing venous return and thereby increasing the filling pressure of the heart. The effect of this increase in preload is to stretch the heart muscle and increase the end-diastolic length of the muscle which, by Starling's law, results in a greater contractile force. Stretching of the heart muscle, by Laplace's law, means that the amount of energy required to raise the pressure within the ventricle during the isovolumetric phase of contraction increases since the radius of the ventricle has increased and the wall thickness has decreased. In addition, the increase in arteriolar tone (i.e. peripheral vasoconstriction mediated by catecholamines, angiotensin II, ADH and other vasoactive peptides) also increases the isometric wall tension which must be attained before the aortic valve opens and the ejection phase of systole can commence (i.e. the resistance to cardiac output has increased). Both of these factors contribute to the increased cardiac afterload and a reduction in stroke volume.

Mechanisms which moderate these compensatory effects

If the compensatory mechanisms go unchecked their effects on cardiac function would be detrimental. A number of other mechanisms moderate their effects.

- Increased atrial stretch by raised atrial filling pressures stimulates the release of atrial natriuretic peptide (ANP) and atrial stretch receptors elicit reflex responses (Goetz, 1988). Both these hormonal and neural reflex responses to stretch tend to limit salt and water retention by the kidney and limit the high vascular resistance against which the heart has to pump. ANP itself inhibits release of noradrenaline from sympathetic nerve endings, reduces secretion of aldosterone and has direct vasodilatory and natriuretic effects. Atrial natriuretic peptide (ANP) concentrations in dogs with CHF increase as much as sixfold (Vollmar et al., 1991). Neural reflexes also reduce traffic in sympathetic nerve fibres and stimulate the release of a non-peptide natriuretic factor from the hypothalamus.

- Cardiac muscle hypertrophy occurs, increasing the thickness of the muscular ventricular wall. This tends to reduce wall stress (distributing it among an increased number of sarcomeres) and therefore the work required to raise the tension within the ventricular wall during the isovolumetric phase of systole.

These factors tend to create a delicate balance allowing the compensatory mechanisms to restore cardiac function back towards normal while, at the same time, ensuring that the cost in terms of myocardial energy consumption is minimal.

Adaptive consequences of sustained neurohormonal activation

If the neurohormonal compensatory mechanisms are activated for sustained periods of time, adaptive changes in the heart and circulation ensue which tip the balance away from compensation towards uncontrolled salt and water retention, vasoconstriction, and the detrimental consequences which lead to clinical congestive heart failure (Packer, 1992a).

The myocardium

Prolonged ventricular distension leads to a loss of the ability of the heart to increase its output in response to increases in ventricular volume. The sarcomeres are stretched to their limits and further increases in venous return have no more benefit in terms of force of subsequent contraction. In short, the Starling curve becomes depressed and flattened. Further stretch can compromise the function of the atrioventricular valves, further reducing cardiac output. In humans it has been shown that prolonged stretch of the atria leads to depletion of ANP and reduced release in response to stretch (Moe et al., 1991). Neural reflexes in response to atrial stretch also become blunted such that atrial baroreceptors are no longer able to moderate sympathetic outflow from the vasomotor centre (Zucker et al., 1977). Chronic stimulation of heart muscle by the sympathetic nervous system leads to a reduction in density of $beta_1$-adrenoceptors and a decrease in the efficiency of coupling between the remaining receptors and adenylate cyclase (so-called 'down regulation' of $beta_1$-adrenoceptors). Thus, one of the main neurohormonal mechanisms increasing the force of contraction of the heart becomes less effective.

As the work load on the heart increases so too does myocardial oxygen consumption. Although cardiac muscle hypertrophy, initially at least, can be regarded as a beneficial compensatory mechanism, with time, the hypertrophied muscle becomes deprived of oxygen as the blood supply fails to keep pace with muscle growth. The development of pulmonary venous congestion and oedema may result in hypoxia and further embarrassment of left ventricular function. An ischaemic myocardium is more susceptible to arrhythmias which may also adversely affect cardiac output.

Peripheral vasculature

Vascular adaptation to sustained neurohormonal activation in heart failure includes an increase in the responsiveness of systemic blood vessels to $alpha_1$-adrenoceptor stimulation (Forster and Armstrong, 1990). Structural changes in the walls of the blood vessels (due to sodium and water retention) occur in chronic heart failure and lead to a non-specific lack of response to vasodilator agents. More specifically, ANP production is reduced as described above and once released, it loses its ability to vasodilate peripheral vessels and reduce aldosterone release. In addition, release of endothelium-derived relaxing factor is reduced in human heart failure patients (Kubo et al., 1991). Thus, the mutual amplification which occurs between neurohormonal mechanisms of RAAS and the sympathetic nervous system can occur virtually unopposed resulting in vasoconstriction. In humans, heart failure results in increased circulating levels of endothelin, a locally active peptide mediator. If produced in excess it is thought that endothelin may have widespread vasoconstrictor effects (Margulies et al., 1990). Similar increases have been documented in dogs with heart failure, the highest levels occurring in dogs with atrial fibrillation (Elliott et al., unpublished data).

Sodium retention

With the decrease in ANP production and the loss of sensitivity of the kidney to its effects, the salt-retaining activities of the RAAS proceed unopposed.

Pathophysiology of heart failure related to the underlying cause

The above pathophysiological scenario is applicable to heart failure in patients regardless of the underlying cause. For example, in myocardial diseases such as dilated cardiomyopathy, the underlying problem is one of poor systolic function. During the chronic stages of this disease, the compensatory mechanisms and adaptive changes referred to above lead to volume overload and congestive signs which may hasten the deterioration of myocardial function.

Regurgitant valvular heart disease and congenital abnormalities causing left to right shunts also cause cardiac volume overload with the same mechanisms attempting to compensate for a reduction in cardiac output. Although cardiac muscle function may be normal in these diseases, prolonged activation of the compensatory mechanisms described above may eventually lead to detrimental effects on cardiac muscle function (cardiomyopathy of overload; Katz, 1990).

Diseases which affect diastolic function to reduce cardiac output will also activate the same neurohormonal mechanisms. Examples include hypertrophic cardiomyopathy and pericardial disease. In the former case, the problem is one of lack of ability of the cardiac muscle to relax and fill properly during diastole and it is characterized by concentric ventricular muscle hypertrophy. Here, expansion of the circulating volume and increased venous return fail to stretch the diseased muscle and circulatory congestion results. With pericardial disease, raised pericardial pressure opposes ventricular filling (particularly of the more compliant right ventricle). Compensatory changes raising venous return and filling pressure are essential if cardiac output is to be maintained. Fortunately, congestion of the systemic circulation is less life-threatening in its effects than congestion and oedema of the lungs.

Valvular diseases which cause stenosis (aortic and pulmonic stenosis) lead to pressure overload of the respective ventricles. Concentric muscle hypertrophy results from the increased work load encountered in overcoming the obstruction to cardiac output. Such animals usually show signs of syncope on exercise and develop fatal arrhythmias before compensatory mechanisms for poor cardiac output lead to circulatory congestion.

In conclusion, the compensatory and adaptive changes which occur in cardiac failure are the same regardless of the underlying cause. Inappropriate regulation of these mechanisms in chronic heart failure contributes to the self-perpetuating cycle of events leading to cardiac decompensation and signs of both forward and backward failure. For this reason, medical management strategies are aimed at counteracting some of these compensatory and adaptive changes and knowledge of the underlying cause will assist in determining the most appropriate treatment regime.

Causes and clinical signs of congestive heart failure

The clinical signs of congestive heart failure (CHF) are a direct consequence of volume overload. A large regurgitant fraction is required before signs of CHF become apparent. With mitral incompetence, the rate at which progression occurs depends on the size of the regurgitant fraction and also the compliance (distensibility) of the left atrium. In many cases signs of CHF will be accompanied by signs of low output failure, for example, cases of dilated cardiomyopathy where the signs of CHF are secondary to primary myocardial failure.

Left-sided CHF

The principal causes of left-sided CHF in the dog are acquired mitral valve incompetence (for example valvular endocardiosis or endocarditis), dilated cardiomyopathy (less frequently the hypertrophic form), congenital mitral valve dysplasia, aortic stenosis, ventricular septal defect and patent ductus arteriosus.

Interstitial or alveolar pulmonary oedema compounded by the presence of an enlarged left atrium impinging on the mainstem bronchi causes coughing, one of the early signs of left-sided failure. The cough may be more noticeable at night or first thing in the morning. Frequently the cough is paroxysmal with each bout terminating with the animal retching up phlegm or, in severe cases, flecks of blood. The animal may show exercise intolerance or may be overtly dyspnoeic. Severe pulmonary oedema may interfere with gaseous exchange and result in cyanosis of the mucous membranes especially with exertion. Some animals may become restless and have difficulty in breathing when lying down (orthopnoea).

Right-sided CHF

Disorders which may be associated with signs of right-sided CHF include pericardial effusion (cardiac tamponade), dilated cardiomyopathy, endocardiosis or endocarditis involving the tricuspid valve, dirofilariasis, cor pulmonale, congenital tricuspid valve dysplasia, pulmonic stenosis and tetralogy of Fallot. Increased right ventricular end-diastolic pressure and increased central venous pressure may produce jugular distension. Hepatomegaly and less frequently splenomegaly may be evident; the former may be associated with portal hypertension, ascites and moderate increases in plasma alkaline phosphatase (ALP) and alanine aminotransferase (ALT) concentrations. The ascites always precedes subcutaneous oedema which may develop later during the course of the disease. Fluid, usually a modified transudate, may accumulate in the thoracic cavity (hydrothorax) and/or pericardial sac (hydropericardium).

Right-sided failure may occur secondary to left-sided failure. Pulmonary venous hypertension leads to an increase in pulmonary arterial and right ventricular end-diastolic pressures. The right ventricle hypertrophies in response to right ventricular pressure overload. Central venous and capillary hydrostatic pressures increase as the right ventricle becomes overloaded and signs of right-sided failure become apparent.

Not infrequently dogs with dilated cardiomyopathy (especially those in atrial fibrillation), pericardial effusion or ruptured chordae tendineae undergo acute decompensation and may present with signs of both left and right-sided CHF as well as signs of acute low output failure.

Causes and clinical signs of low output failure

Causes of low output failure include primary myocardial failure (for example dilated cardiomyopathy), decreased myocardial compliance (for example hypertrophic cardiomyopathy, myocardial fibrosis, pericardial effusion), hypovolaemia (for example acute haemorrhage), congenital cardiovascular shunts, severe valvular incompetence and tachy- or bradydysrhythmias. A marked reduction in preload, for example, obstruction to venous return by a large abdominal mass, ascitic fluid or the overzealous administration of diuretics to an animal with impaired myocardial function (particularly if the animal is already receiving a vasodilating drug) may significantly reduce cardiac output.

Low output failure may be classified as acute or chronic depending on the severity and rate of onset of clinical signs. Acute low output failure is characterized by signs of tissue hypoperfusion and cardiogenic shock with collapse or syncope, weakness, recumbency or possibly even coma, pale mucous membranes (venous $PO_2 < 30$ mm Hg in dogs) and a weak femoral pulse. Plasma urea and creatinine concentrations may be increased (prerenal azotaemia). The clinical signs of chronic low output failure may only become apparent with excitement or exercise. Typically the animal may experience episodes of exercise intolerance, weakness or collapse, the differential diagnoses for which include numerous metabolic, neuromuscular and central nervous system disorders.

Cardiac cachexia

Cardiac cachexia refers to the severe wasting that occurs in association with chronic congestive heart failure. The weight loss which can be rapidly progressive is usually accompanied by lethargy, generalized weakness, inappetence and poor hair coat. Affected animals generally show severe signs of CHF and are moderately hypoproteinaemic. Cardiac cachexia has been attributed to a combination of factors including poor tissue perfusion, cellular hypoxia, malabsorption and anorexia

Functional classification of heart failure

The functional classification of heart failure has recently been reviewed by the International Small Animal Cardiac Health Council (1994). The new classification scheme consists of three stages, the criteria for each being based on the anatomic diagnosis and severity of clinical signs at rest (Table 34.4).

ACQUIRED HEART DISEASE

The incidence of acquired heart disease increases with age, for example endocardiosis is more common in dogs greater than 5 years of age. Numerous breed dispositions exist for certain diseases.

Endocardiosis (chronic valvular disease)

Endocardiosis is the most common cause of cardiac disease in dogs. An overall incidence of 17–40% has been reported (Keene, 1988); in one survey 58% of dogs over 9 years of age which were presented for necropsy were affected (Whitney, 1974). The condition is characterized

Table 34.4 Functional classification of heart failure (International Small Animal Cardiac Health Council System)

The asymptomatic patient	No clinical signs of heart failure apparent but heart disease present. Cardiac murmur usually detectable; may be radiographic and/or echocardiographic evidence of chamber enlargement. ECG usually unremarkable; occasionally an arrhythmia is present. This stage can be subdivided as follows: (a) Signs of heart disease present but no signs of compensation evident; (b) Signs of heart disease present in conjunction with radiographic or echocardiographic evidence of compensation in response to volume or pressure overload. Medical treatment at this stage may or may not be justifiable.
Mild to moderate heart failure	Clinical signs of heart failure evident at rest or with mild exercise which adversely affect quality of life. Typical signs include exercise intolerance, cough, tachypnoea, mild respiratory distress, and mild to moderate ascites. Usually no evidence of hypoperfusion. Medical treatment at home is indicated at this stage.
Advanced heart failure	Clinical signs of advanced heart failure are immediately obvious. These signs include severe exercise intolerance, dyspnoea and marked ascites. Evidence of hypoperfusion at rest and in the most severe cases the animal is moribund due to cardiogenic shock. Death is likely without prompt and aggressive medical therapy. This stage can be subdivided as follows: (a) Home care is possible; (b) Hospitalization essential because of cardiogenic shock, life-threatening pulmonary oedema, refractory ascites or pleural effusion present.

by chronic nodular fibrous thickenings of the free edges of the atrioventricular valve cusps which interfere with normal closure of the valves. Valvular incompetence results in regurgitation of blood from the ventricles into the atria during ventricular systole. The specific cause of the condition is not known. The lesions appear degenerative rather than inflammatory and primarily affect the mitral valve. Most cases of endocardiosis involve the mitral valve only; approximately one third of cases involve both the mitral and tricuspid valves. Isolated tricuspid valve disease is rare as are lesions involving the aortic and pulmonary valves. There is a higher incidence in older male dogs of small breeds such as chihuahuas, miniature poodles, miniature pinschers and whippets (Thrushfield et al., 1985). Endocardiosis is particularly common in cavalier King Charles spaniels in which a multifactorial polygenic threshold trait has been demonstrated (Swensen et al., 1996). The disease in this breed is unusual in that a significant percentage of animals develop murmurs at five years or younger (Darke, 1987; Beardow and Buchanan, 1993; Haggstrom et al., 1995). Endocardiosis is rare in cats.

Clinical signs

With mitral insufficiency regurgitation of blood into the left atrium during systole causes the left atrium to dilate which causes displacement of the mitral valve leaflets and dilation of the atrioventricular annuli thereby increasing the degree of mitral regurgitation. Pulmonary venous hypertension develops secondary to the increased left atrial pressure until eventually pulmonary oedema occurs. The clinical signs of mitral insufficiency are those of left-sided congestive heart failure; involvement of both atrioventricular valves may be expected to produce signs of left- and right-sided failure (see previous sections on the pathophysiology and clinical signs of congestive heart failure). Rupture of the chordae tendineae occasionally occurs resulting in acute and ultimately fatal cardiac decompensation.

The first sign of endocardiosis is usually the production of a holosystolic systolic murmur with a point of maximal intensity over the affected atrioventricular valve although high-grade murmurs tend to radiate dorsally and cranially throughout the thoracic cavity. Echocardiographic studies in cavalier King Charles spaniels have shown a good correlation between the intensity of the murmur and the severity of chronic valvular disease and heart failure class (Haggstrom et al., 1995). The intensity of the murmur does not, however, correlate with either the severity of clinical signs or the degree of regurgitation. With severe mitral regurgitation an S3 sound may occasionally be detected.

Table 34.5 Clinical features and therapy of heart failure due to chronic acquired degenerative valvular disease (endocardiosis) using the International Small Animal Cardiac Health Council System

Stage of heart failure	Clinical signs	Radiographic, echocardiographic and electrocardiographic findings	Therapy
Asymptomatic (Stage 1)	No visible clinical signs of heart disease present. Systolic murmur over mitral and/or tricuspid valve; the murmur typically becomes louder and pansystolic as valvular regurgitation increases.	*Radiography:* May be normal or mild to moderate left atrial/left ventricular enlargement. *Echocardiography:* Normal or mild to moderate left atrial/left ventricular enlargement depending on severity; mitral valve leaflets may appear thickened; may be evidence of mitral valve prolapse. *ECG:* Often normal at this stage; occasionally P wave abnormalities or evidence of left ventricular enlargement.	Treatment at this stage probably not indicated although there is some evidence to suggest that treatment of the more severe cases with angiotensin converting enzyme (ACE) inhibitors may be beneficial
Advanced heart failure (Stage 3)	Systolic murmur as above. Marked exercise intolerance, coughing, dyspnoea at rest, nocturnal restlessness and rapid progressive weight loss (cachexia). Pallor of mucous membranes and/or syncope due to low cardiac output. Pulmonary oedema may result in pulmonary crackles. Distended jugular veins, hepatomegaly and severe ascites if advanced right-sided failure. Arterial pulse weak or normal. Arrhythmias common.	*Radiography:* As above but evidence of pulmonary oedema (hilar or diffuse). Marked cardiomegaly especially left atrium and left auricular appendage. May be hepatomegaly and evidence of ascites in cases of advanced right-sided failure. *Echocardiography:* Mitral valve leaflets markedly thickened; evidence of mitral valve prolapse (or flail if chordae tendineae rupture). Severe left atrial and left ventricular enlargement. Decreased myocardial function (increased end-diastolic diameter) during later stages of mitral regurgitation; shortening fraction may be normal or slightly decreased. *ECG:* Arrhythmias common (usually atrial fibrillation but occasionally ventricular tachydysrhythmias also observed.	*Home care possible* Frusemide with or without another diuretic, ACE inhibitor, cardiac glycoside, e.g. digoxin. Consider hydralazine titration (best done in hospital) in combination with ACE inhibitor if refractory to the above but beware of hypotension. In addition exercise restriction, sodium restricted diet, antiarrhythmic therapy if indicated, nitrates, theophylline and codeine or other cough suppressants. *If hospitalized* Oxygen therapy, intravenous frusemide, reduce preload with topical nitroglycerine, reduce afterload with hydralazine or sodium nitroprusside, intravenous dobutamine, morphine theophylline, antiarrhythmic therapy if indicated, theophylline. Thoracocentesis may be required to alleviate life-threatening pleural effusion. Consider other diuretics, for example hydrochlorothiazide and spironolactone in combination with frusemide for refractory right-sided failure.

Radiographic findings

The radiographic findings vary according to the severity of the mitral incompetence and the size of the regurgitant fraction (see Table 34.5). The first chamber to enlarge is the left atrium; marked enlargement of the left atrium may result in compression of the left mainstem bronchus. Left ventricular or in severe cases biventricular enlargement may also be evident. Volume overload of the left atrium and left ventricle leads to pulmonary venous engorgement and eventually pulmonary oedema develops. The latter initially may be confined to the perihilar region or, in more severe cases, may manifest as a diffuse interstitial and/or alveolar lung pattern (Fig. 34.12). Right ventricular failure is characterized by hepatomegaly with distension of the caudal vena cava, ascites and the presence of pleural effusion.

Electrocardiography

The ECG may be normal or may show evidence of left atrial, left ventricular or biventricular enlargement (see Tables 34.1 and 34.2). Mean electrical axis is usually normal. With severe atrial dilatation a supraventricular arrhythmia may be present (for example premature atrial complexes or atrial fibrillation).

Echocardiography

Echocardiography is useful for confirming thickened AV valve leaflets and defective valve function as well as left atrial and left ventricular enlargement. Several echocardiographic studies have shown that myocardial contractility during the early stages of mitral regurgitation is either normal or in some cases there may even be a compensatory increase in contractility (Kittleson *et al.*, 1984). Echocardiography may also demonstrate thickened chordae tendineae and prolapse of the mitral valve into the left atrium. In cavalier King Charles spaniels it has been shown that mitral valve prolapse occurs as early as one to two years of age and predisposes to endocardiosis and mitral regurgitaion (Pedersen, 1996). Doppler studies show increased diastolic mitral inflow velocities (Bonagura, 1994). Rupture of the chordae tendineae results in a chaotic fluttering of the mitral valve.

Diagnosis

A diagnosis of mitral insufficiency is based on the clinical, radiographic, electrocardiographic and echocardiographic findings. The differential diagnosis of mitral (or tricuspid) endocardiosis includes the following:

a
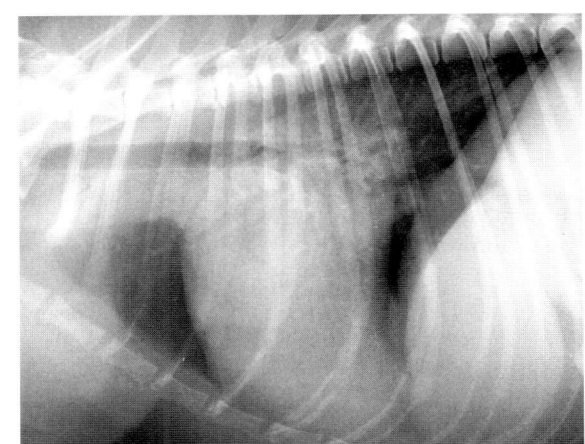

b
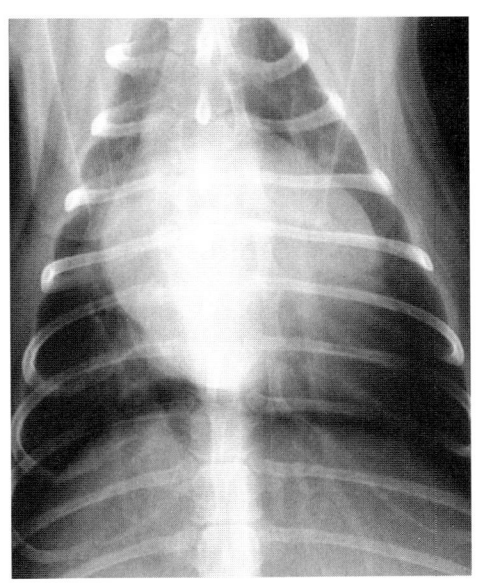

Figure 34.12 Lateral (a) and dorsoventral (b) thoracic radiographs of a 12-year-old miniature poodle with mitral valve endocardiosis. Note the prominent left atrium in both views.

- Other causes of AV valvular insufficiency, for example that associated with dilated cardiomyopathy, congenital heart disease, bacterial endocarditis, ruptured chordae tendineae and atrial and ventricular dysrhythmias.
- Other congenital and acquired causes of cardiac murmurs (see Chapter 13)
- Chronic pulmonary disease and other causes of chronic coughing (see Chapter 12) for example chronic bronchitis, bronchopneumonia, pulmonary foreign body, pulmonary neoplasia, *Filaroides osleri* infection, eosinophilic pneumonia (pulmonary infiltrate with eosinophils), collapsing trachea, dirofilariasis and systemic mycoses.
- Cor pulmonale where primary disease of the lung and/or pulmonary vasculature can lead to right ventricular hypertrophy and ultimately signs of right-sided congestive heart failure.

Treatment of congestive heart failure associated with mitral insufficiency

The treatment and general management of mitral and/or tricuspid endocardiosis essentially involves treating the signs of congestive heart failure (CHF) as they arise on a stage by stage basis. The staging scheme drawn up by International Small Animal Cardiac Health Council (see Tables 34.4 and 34.5) is useful for establishing a therapeutic protocol although a certain amount of controversy exists concerning the time at which many of the cardiovascular drugs should be administered (see below and section on cardiovascular therapeutics). Client education is extremely important especially since most of the conditions associated with mitral insufficiency are slowly progressive and their management requires a great deal of owner compliance.

Bacterial endocarditis

Bacterial endocarditis is an acute or, more commonly, a subacute condition characterized by the formation of septic vegetative thrombi on the valves and/or mural endocardium. Thrombus formation most frequently involves the mitral or aortic valves and the highest incidence occurs in large breed, male dogs older than four years of age (Calvert, 1982; Lombard and Buergelt, 1983; Sisson and Thomas, 1984). The German shepherd breed appears predisposed (Calvert, 1982; Sisson and Thomas, 1984). The pathogens most frequently isolated include *Streptococcus* sp., *Staphylococcus aureus*, *Escherichia coli*, *Pseudomonas aeruginosa*, *Corynebacterium* sp. *Aerobacter aerogenes* and *Erysipelothrix rhusiopathiae*.

Pathogenesis

Numerous predisposing factors have been implicated in the pathogenesis of valvular bacterial endocarditis. First, the valve must be damaged, for example by the turbulent blood flow associated with a congenital cardiac defect. Bacterial endocarditis involving the aortic valve has been reported in association with subaortic stenosis (Muna *et al.*, 1978; Roth, 1994). The stenosis leads to 'jetting' of blood through the aortic valve which damages the valve leaflets and may eventually result in a degree of aortic regurgitation. Secondly, transient bacteraemic episodes are presumably necessary to infect the sterile thrombi which form initially. The source of infection in many cases is speculative; infections involving the gastrointestinal tract, skin, lung, urogenital tract, oral cavity, bone and subcutaneous abscesses have been implicated in the pathogenesis as have other factors such as indwelling intravenous catheters, previous surgery and immunosuppressive drug therapy (Calvert, 1982; Bonagura, 1983; Anderson and Dubielzig, 1984; Dunn *et al.*, 1987). The vegetations which form on the valves are friable and tend to form emboli. The lesions also alter valve structure and function and may result in mitral and/or aortic regurgitation which may lead ultimately to signs of congestive heart failure.

Clinical signs

The clinical manifestations of bacterial endocarditis reflect (1) altered valve function, (2) bacteraemia, (3) the dissemination of septic emboli with subsequent infarction and localization of infection in joints, kidneys, muscle, myocardium, lungs and central nervous system (CNS) tissue, and (4) the host immune response which may result in immune complex deposition in synovial membranes and glomeruli.

The clinical signs vary depending on which organs are involved. Typically the animal may present with rather non-specific signs (for example anorexia, lethargy, weight loss) in association with a fever. The pyrexic episodes are often intermittent and may last for several days before appearing to resolve spontaneously. Bacterial endocarditis should be considered as a differential diagnosis in an animal which presents with a history of recurrent pyrexia in the absence of more specific localizing signs (see Chapter 4).

Cardiac signs

A heart murmur may be present although this may develop late in the course of the disease. The murmur may be systolic if the mitral valve is involved or diastolic if due to aortic insufficiency. Embolization of the coronary blood supply leading to myocardial infarction or myocarditis may result in dysrhythmias (particularly ventricular dysrhythmias) or atrioventricular block (Fregin *et al.*, 1972; Berry *et al.*, 1984). Some cases may develop cardiomegaly and signs of left-sided congestive heart failure.

Extracardiac signs

Extracardiac signs include lethargy, anorexia, pyrexia due to transient, bacteraemic thromboembolic episodes, lameness, muscle stiffness, petechial or ecchymotic haemorrhages due to thrombocytopenia, dyspnoea and seizures. Direct extension of the infection to one or more joints may result in a septic polyarthritis or prolonged antigenic stimulation may lead to immune complex deposition in the synovial membranes and the development of a non-septic (non-erosive) immune-mediated polyarthropathy.

Many of the clinical signs associated with bacterial endocarditis mimic those of systemic lupus erythematosus or the immune-mediated polyarthropathies since not only may the joints be involved but some animals test positive for anti-red cell, antiplatelet or antinuclear antibodies (Bennett *et al.*, 1978; Calvert, 1982; Calvert *et al.*, 1985).

Diagnosis

Ante-mortem diagnosis is often difficult particularly if a cardiac murmur is not present.

Full haematological examination and complete biochemical screen
A mild to moderate non-regenerative anaemia, neutrophilia with or without a left shift, and monocytosis may be evident. The anaemia may be attributed to the chronic inflammatory response; in a few cases there may be an immune-mediated component. Systemic thromboembolism may result in impaired renal function and/or liver damage or dysfunction. Increased alkaline phosphatase (ALP) activity, hypoglycaemia and hypoalbuminaemia are common findings in bacteraemic dogs (Calvert and Greene, 1986).

Urine analysis and bacteriology
Urinary tract infections, including those originating in the prostate gland, are a potential source of blood-borne infection. Bacteraemia is often associated with bacteriuria hence a urine sample, preferably one obtained by cystocentesis, should be submitted for routine analysis and bacteriological culture/sensitivity (Calvert *et al.*, 1985; Calvert and Greene, 1986).

Radiographic findings
Thoracic radiographs are often uninformative. Signs of congestive heart failure with left atrial and left ventricular enlargement and possibly pulmonary oedema may be evident in some dogs during the terminal stages of the disease.

Echocardiography
Echocardiography is the most useful and reliable technique for confirming a diagnosis of bacterial endocarditis ante-mortem (Pipers *et al.*, 1981; Lombard and Buergelt, 1983; Elwood *et al.*, 1993). Moderate-sized vegetations can be visualized on the heart valves or mural endocardium.

Blood cultures
Bacteraemia in dogs with endocarditis is usually continuous. The timing of the blood cultures is less important and culturing blood during febrile episodes does not increase the frequency of positive results in dogs with endocarditis (Dow and Jones, 1989). Bacterial isolation rates between 50 and 80% have been reported (Calvert, 1982; Elwood *et al.*, 1993). A negative blood culture does not preclude a diagnosis of bacterial endocarditis and repeated negative results have been reported in confirmed cases. In order to maximize the chances of obtaining a positive culture 2–3 blood samples should be collected, preferably at least one hour apart, over a 24 h period. Each blood sample should be collected from a different vein (jugular or cephalic) using standard aseptic technique. To minimize the risk of contamination a fresh needle should be attached to the syringe before the blood is transferred to the appropriate culture medium. Each sample should be submitted for aerobic and anaerobic culture. If possible, antibiotics should be discontinued at least 2 days beforehand since they may delay bacterial growth.

Synovial aspirates
Multiple joint taps should be obtained from animals with suspected joint involvement, that is

those showing signs of shifting lameness. Synovial fluid should be submitted in EDTA for protein concentration and cytology, and in a sterile plain glass tube bacteriology.

Immunological screening tests

Some cases of bacterial endocarditis test positive for anti-red cell, antiplatelet and antinuclear antibodies making differentiation from SLE difficult (Bennett *et al.*, 1978; Calvert, 1982).

Treatment

The prognosis for subacute bacterial endocarditis is guarded. Bactericidal antibiotics should be administered for a minimum of 4–6 weeks (parenterally for the first two weeks and thereafter by the oral route) at doses well above the minimum inhibitory concentration. The choice of antibiotic ideally should be based on the blood culture results. Pending these results or in cases where the results are negative but bacterial endocarditis is either suspected or has been diagnosed, a combination of broad spectrum antibiotics should be given. A standard protocol is as follows.

- Ampicillin (20–40 mg kg^{-1} body weight TID) and gentamycin (2 mg kg^{-1} bodyweight TID) in combination should be given intravenously for at least the first 5–10 days.
- Thereafter, ampillin or cephalexin (20 mg kg^{-1} bodyweight) can be given orally for a further 2–4 weeks. Additional treatment for congestive heart failure should be given as appropriate.

MYOCARDIAL DISEASE

Causes of myocardial damage include infection, inflammation, degeneration, trauma, neoplasia, toxins, drugs and ischaemia. Myocardial dysfunction results in a loss of myocardial contractility and a gradual reduction in cardiac reserve capacity. Clinical signs reflect the reduction in cardiac output with most cases progressing to congestive heart failure. The reduction in cardiac output may be exacerbated by the development of a cardiac conduction disturbance or abnormality in cardiac rhythm. Groups of damaged myocardial cells become electrically unstable and may act as ectopic pacemakers. Spontaneous discharge of these foci of electrical activity can give rise to supraventricular or ventricular arrhythmias; lesions which damage the normal conducting tissue may result in atrioventricular heart block and severe bradycardia.

Myocardial disease in dogs and cats is usually classified as primary or secondary depending on whether the lesions can be attributed to an underlying disease process.

PRIMARY MYOCARDIAL DISEASE IN THE DOG

Idiopathic dilated cardiomyopathy

Dilated cardiomyopathy (DCM), next to valvular endocardiosis, is the most commonly diagnosed cardiac disorder in dogs. In most cases the cause is not apparent; the most popular concept is that the aetiology for DCM in dogs is multifactorial (Cobb, 1992). Cases of DCM in association with a deficiency of myocardial L-carnitine have been reported in one family of boxers suggesting that nutritional factors may be involved in the pathogenesis (Keene *et al.*, 1991). L-Carnitine is necessary for the transport of long chain fatty acids into the mitochondria of cardiac muscle cells and a deficiency results in impaired mitochondrial energy production. More recently, it has been shown that some dogs with DCM have reduced plasma taurine levels (Kramer *et al.*, 1995). In humans, cardiomyopathy is associated with depression of the cellular Na$^+$, K$^+$-ATPase pump (Norgaard *et al.*, 1988) and a reduction ('down regulation') of myocardial beta-adrenergic receptors (Denniss *et al.*, 1989). Whether a similar situation exists in dogs with DCM is not clear. A recent study reported no significant difference in the beta receptor density in four dogs with DCM compared to normal dogs (Hoey *et al.*, 1991). Immune-mediated disease with the production of antibodies against altered myocardial proteins, for example following viral infection, is a known cause of cardiomyopathy in humans but has not been recognized in dogs (Bouvagnet *et al.*, 1985).

The high incidence in certain breeds of dog suggests that genetic influences may also be important. Dilated cardiomyopathy is more common in medium-sized and large, giant breeds of dog with the highest incidence occurring in English cocker spaniels, old English sheepdogs, boxers, Dobermanns, Irish wolfhounds, great Danes and Saint Bernards. There is an increased incidence in males and the average age of onset is 4–6 years of age (occasionally earlier especially in certain breeds, for example, cocker spaniels).

Pathophysiology

Dilated cardiomyopathy results in impairment of systolic function. Progressive dilatation of the atria and ventricles causes reduced myocardial contractility and increased end-diastolic pressures. As the chambers of the heart dilate so too does the fibrous atrioventricular annulus supporting the atrioventricular valve cusps. Affected animals may, therefore, be expected to show signs of low output failure due to myocardial dysfunction and also signs of congestive heart failure associated with regurgitation of blood into the atria.

History

Dilated cardiomyopathy is characterized by lethargy, inappetence or anorexia, generalized weakness, exercise intolerance and weight loss; the latter may be rapidly progressive once cardiac function becomes severely compromised. Animals which develop cardiac dysrhythmias, the most common of which is atrial fibrillation, may experience acute syncopal episodes.

Clinical signs

The clinical signs of dilated cardiomyopathy are those of left and/or right-sided congestive heart failure. In most animals there are signs consistent with both low output failure and congestive heart failure.

Severely affected animals may present with acute dyspnoea due to pulmonary oedema, pleural effusion or both. Increased bronchovesicular lung sounds with pulmonary crackles and pallor of the mucous membranes with prolongation of the capillary refill time may be evident. In some cases right-sided signs may predominate with evidence of jugular distension, hepatosplenomegaly and ascites. The heart sounds may be muffled due to the presence of pleural fluid. A systolic murmur associated with atrioventricular regurgitation and/or a gallop rhythm due to accentuation of the third (S3) heart sound may be present.

Electrocardiography

The electrocardiographic findings are variable. Changes consistent with severe left atrial and left ventricular enlargement (wide, sometimes notched P waves, wide QRS complexes, tall R waves and ST slurring) are often present. The most common arrhythmia associated with DCM is atrial fibrillation which is characterized by an irregular tachycardia with variable R–R intervals and an absence of P waves (see Figs 34.34c and 34.34d). In certain breeds (see below) ventricular arrhythmias are more common and occasionally atrial fibrillation may co-exist with ventricular premature complexes.

Radiographic findings

Dilated cardiomyopathy is usually characterized by generalized cardiomegaly although in some breeds (for example Dobermanns and boxers) thoracic radiographs often appear remarkably normal or show signs only of left atrial and mild left ventricular enlargement (Fig. 34.13). There may be evidence of pulmonary venous congestion with an interstitial or mixed interstitial/alveolar lung pattern typical of pulmonary oedema involving the perihilar and dorsocaudal regions of the lungs (Fig. 34.14).

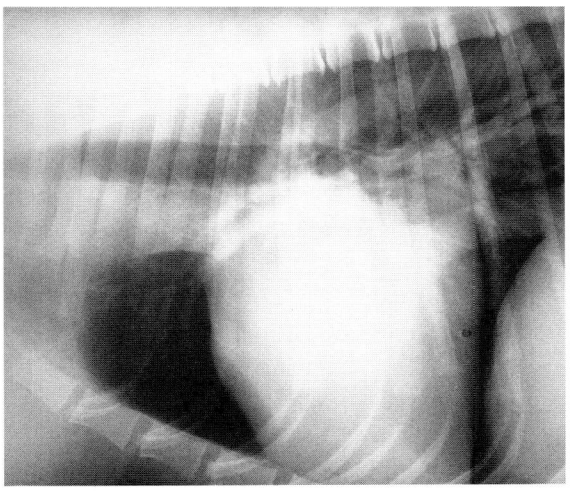

Figure 34.13 Lateral thoracic radiograph of a 3-year-old Irish wolfhound with dilated cardiomyopathy showing a large left atrium and increased size of pulmonary veins.

Echocardiography

The echocardiographic features of dilated cardiomyopathy include (Fig. 34.15):

- An increased left ventricular internal dimension (LVID) during systole and diastole;
- Reduced fractional shortening (FS) of the left ventricle during systole indicating decreased myocardial contractility;
- Increased mitral valve E-point septal separation (EPSS);

286 | DISEASES OF THE CARDIOVASCULAR SYSTEM

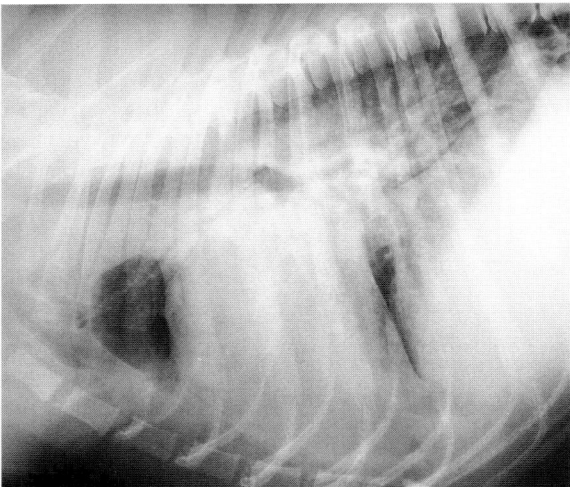

Figure 34.14 Lateral thoracic radiograph of an 8-year-old Dobermann with dilated cardiomyopathy and pulmonary oedema.

- Decreased thickness of the interventricular septum during systole and diastole;
- Evidence of pericardial fluid indicative of right-sided failure (usually the volume of fluid is minimal).

Clinicopathological findings

Dogs with reduced renal perfusion may become azotaemic. Passive venous congestion of the liver causes mild increases in liver enzymes. The total plasma protein concentration is frequently reduced especially in dogs which are ascitic.

A few cases of DCM, particularly in Dobermanns and great Danes, have been associated with hypothyroidism (Panciera, 1994). Total and free T4 levels should be checked in breeds which are susceptible to hypothyroidism although it should be noted that T4 levels may be depressed in dogs with DCM because of a 'sick' euthyroid syndrome.

Prognosis

The prognosis for DCM is invariably extremely guarded since many dogs fail to survive 6 months. Dogs which survive longer than seven months have a good probability of being long-term survivors (up to 40 months after diagnosis in some cases). The presence of pleural effusion or pulmonary oedema appear to be the poorest independent prognostic indicators in dogs with DCM (Monnet *et al.*, 1995).

Breed variations in clinical presentation

Boxer cardiomyopathy

There is a higher incidence of dilated cardiomyopathy in male boxers, the average age of onset being approximately 8.0–8.2 years (Harpster, 1983). During the early stages of the disease animals may show no clinical signs or may present with signs of weakness or syncope.

The clinical features may be divided into three categories (Harpster, 1983; Fox, 1988a):

1. asymptomatic with arrhythmias;
2. syncope or episodic weakness with signs of congestive heart failure;

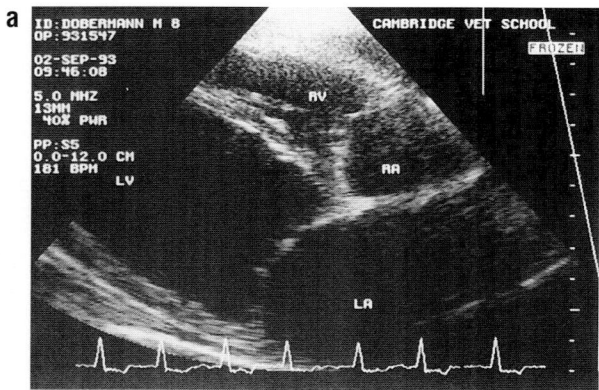
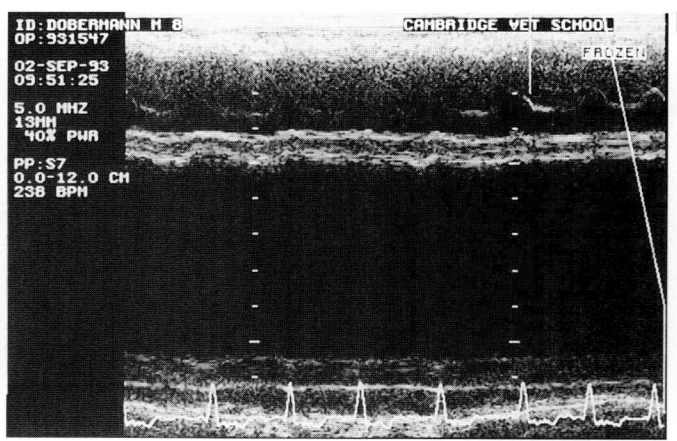

Figure 34.15 (a) 2-D right parasternal long axis view of the Dobermann illustrated in Fig. 34.14 (b) showing a massively dilated left atrium (LA) and left ventricle (LV); (b) M-mode echocardiogram of the same dog showing reduced contractility of the left ventricle.

3. signs of left sided or biventricular congestive heart failure with arrhythmias.

Approximately 50% of cases may have a murmur due to mitral insufficiency. Ventricular arrhythmias (ventricular premature contractions or paroxysmal ventricular tachycardia) are common. The ventricular extrasystoles are typically of a left bundle branch block type.

Asymptomatic cases and dogs which have syncopal episodes but which are not showing signs of congestive heart failure may show few significant radiographic abnormalities. Cardiomegaly and pulmonary oedema occur only with advanced cardiac failure; pleural effusions are uncommon. The prognosis for long-term survival is poor especially in dogs with congestive heart failure and/or arrhythmias. Many dogs fail to survive 6 months and sudden death is common (Harpster, 1983).

Cardiomyopathy of Dobermann pinschers
Dilated cardiomyopathy in Dobermanns may resemble classic DCM seen in large giant breeds of dog (generalized cardiomegaly with signs of biventricular congestive heart failure). Affected Dobermanns often present with severe dyspnoea and acute signs of low output failure. Usually there is a marked reduction in left ventricular contractility and increased left ventricular end-systolic dimensions (fractional shortening of the left ventricle during systole may be less than 10%). There is a subset of dogs, however, which present with radiographic signs of left atrial enlargement (rather than generalized cardiomegaly) and engorgement of the cranial lobar pulmonary veins. Pulmonary oedema if present tends to be diffuse rather than perihilar in distribution (Calvert, 1986). Ventricular arrhythmias are common and tend to persist throughout the course of therapy.

The prognosis is usually extremely poor with many dogs dying within 3–6 weeks of diagnosis. A few dogs may appear clinically normal but nevertheless have radiographic evidence of mild left atrial enlargement and, echocardiographically, a reduction in left ventricular contractility. Most of these dogs may be expected to develop signs of acute left-sided congestive heart failure within 12–15 months. Sudden death is common (Calvert, 1986).

English cocker spaniel cardiomyopathy
Dilated cardiomyopathy has been reported in young to middle-aged cocker spaniels. Affected animals vary in age from 2 to 9 years and an increased incidence in males has been reported (Staaden, 1981; Gooding et al., 1982; Thomas, 1987; Fox, 1988a). A familial predisposition has been suggested (Thomas, 1987). Clinical signs include a cough, exercise intolerance and dyspnoea; sudden death may occur. Unlike other breeds the clinical signs may be preceded by a long asymptomatic period. During this time ECG abnormalities consistent with left ventricular enlargement (tall R waves, ST slurring) may be noted. Deep Q waves and supraventricular arrhythmias (atrial premature contractions) are relatively common. Radiographs may show biventricular enlargement and evidence of pulmonary oedema. Echocardiographic findings are more variable; left ventricular end-systolic dimensions may be increased but myocardial function may be less suppressed than in other breeds with dilated cardiomyopathy. Progressive systolic dysfunction usually results in congestive heart failure (Gooding et al., 1986).

Treatment of dilated cardiomyopathy

- Dogs which show signs of acute decompensation should be given oxygen and confined to a kennel. Intravenous frusemide (2–4 mg kg^{-1} body weight) and nitroglycerine, a venodilator, can be administered to alleviate the pulmonary oedema and reduce cardiac preload (approximately 1 cm of nitroglycerine ointment 2% can be applied cutaneously, usually on the medial surface of the pinna, every 6–8 h). Morphine (0.2–0.3 mg kg^{-1} body weight) can be given subcutaneosly or intramuscularly.
- The use of cardiac glycosides such as digoxin as positive inotropic agents is controversial. The myocardium of dogs with dilated cardiomyopathy generally has little or no contractile reserve capacity and any improvement in myocardial contractility is minimal especially in dogs which are still in sinus rhythm (Bright, 1983; Kittleson et al., 1985a). A more significant clinical response may be observed in dogs which are in atrial fibrillation but this is not due to improved myocardial contractility but to the negative chronotropic effect of cardiac glycosides. This results in a reduction in the ventricular response rate which in turn leads to improved diastolic filling and increased cardiac output.

Large dogs may develop signs of digitalis toxicity at relatively low doses, thus it is important to calculate the dose of digoxin on a body surface area basis (see section on cardiovascular therapeutics). Renal function should be evaluated beforehand; digoxin is excreted intact by the kidneys and compromised renal function may result in digitalis toxicity. Slow oral 'digitalization' is preferred to fast intravenous 'digitalization'. Digoxin is contraindicated if multiple ventricular premature complexes are present on the ECG since even therapeutic levels of digoxin may aggravate ventricular arrhythmias during the first week of therapy (Calvert, 1986).

- Sympathomimetic drugs such as dopamine and dobutamine have yet to be fully evaluated in the treatment of dilated cardiomyopathy. Although both drugs have to be administered by slow intravenous infusion they may have a role to play in the treatment of animals which are showing signs of acute cardiogenic shock.
- Angiotensin converting enzyme (ACE) inhibitors such as captopril, enalapril and benazapril have been shown to significantly improve exercise intolerance and short-term survival times in dogs with dilated cardiomyopathy (COVE Study Group, 1995). The reduction in ejection impedance leads to increased cardiac output, a reduction in left ventricular end-diastolic pressure, increased myocardial perfusion and a decrease in myocardial oxygen demand. Enalapril (0.5 mg kg^{-1} body weight once or twice daily) has been shown to significantly reduce heart rate, blood pressure and mean capillary wedge pressure (PCWP). The reduction in PCWP is reflected clinically by decreased oedema formation in dogs with DCM (IMPROVE Study Group, 1995).

Atrial fibrillation

If digoxin fails to significantly reduce the ventricular response rate the use of beta adrenergic blocking drugs such as propranolol, or calcium blockers such as verapamil or diltiazem, should be considered. Both types of drug are negative inotropes and should be given in combination with digoxin. In humans, beta blockers have been shown to increase myocardial responsiveness to inotropic stimulation by up-regulating beta-adrenergic receptor function (Heilbrunn et al., 1989). Calcium blockers may potentiate digitalis toxicity and the dose of digitalis should be adjusted accordingly.

■ Hypertrophic cardiomyopathy

The incidence of primary (idiopathic) hypertrophic cardiomyopathy (HCM) is much lower in dogs than it is in cats. Males appear to be predominantly affected and there may be a higher incidence in boxers and German shepherd dogs (Fox, 1988a; Marks, 1993). The disease is characterized by hypertrophy of the left ventricular free wall and interventricular septum. The aetiology of primary HCM has not been determined.

Pathophysiology

Myocardial hypertrophy results in decreased left ventricular compliance (increased myocardial 'stiffness') and diastolic dysfunction. Systolic function is usually adequate. Myocardial hypertrophy results in increased myocardial tension and afterload. This in turn leads to progressive myocardial ischaemia and the development of cardiac arrhythmias which are usually ventricular in origin. In most cases the hypertrophy is asymmetric with disproportionate thickening of the interventricular septum compared to the left ventricular free wall (at necropsy, septal to left ventricular free wall ratio in affected cases is greater than 1.1:1). Asymmetric hypertrophy may cause functional left ventricular outflow obstruction (Liu et al., 1979; Thomas et al., 1984a). Ventricular hypertrophy may also be associated with focal or diffuse endocardial fibrosis which further reduces ventricular compliance.

Clinical signs

Dogs with HCM may be asymptomatic or present with a history of weakness, exercise intolerance and syncope; a few cases may show more obvious signs of congestive heart failure such as coughing, dyspnoea, pleural effusion, hepatomegaly and ascites (Liu et al., 1979). A low-grade ejection-type systolic heart murmur is occasionally detected over the region of the aortic valve.

Electrocardiographic findings

The ECG may be unremarkable. Conduction disturbances such as atrioventricular block and bundle branch block have been reported (Liu et al., 1979).

Radiographic abnormalities

In many cases thoracic radiographs may be normal. Occasionally there is evidence of mild left atrial and left ventricular enlargement but signs of left-sided congestive heart failure rarely occur.

Echocardiography

Echocardiography typically shows hypertrophy of the left ventricular free wall and interventricular septum and a reduction in the internal dimension of the left ventricle during systole and diastole. The left ventricular papillary muscles appear hypertrophied. Indices of left ventricular function may be normal or increased. Evidence of mitral regurgitation may be present. Echocardiography can be used to rule out subaortic stenosis as a cause of myocardial hypertrophy in the younger dog.

Differential diagnoses

The major differential diagnosis in a young dog is congenital subaortic stenosis which usually results in concentric symmetrical hypertrophy of the left ventricle and interventricular septum. Left ventricular hypertrophy may occur in athletic or working dogs; echocardiographic evidence of left ventricular hypertrophy has been reported in healthy fit greyhounds (Page *et al.*, 1993). It may also occur secondary to arterial hypertension in dogs with chronic renal disease (Cowgill and Kallet, 1986).

Prognosis

The prognosis for hypertrophic cardiomyopathy is extremely guarded. The condition is progressive and although medical management may be palliative, sudden unexplained death is common even in animals which have previously been asymptomatic.

Treatment

Medical management should be directed towards the signs of congestive heart failure or controlling any arrhythmia which may be present. Beta blocking agents may increase ventricular compliance and thereby improve diastolic filling although there have been no controlled studies to confirm that this is the case. The use of calcium blocking drugs such as diltiazem has not been fully evaluated.

SECONDARY MYOCARDIAL DISEASE IN THE DOG

Infective myocarditis

Viral (see also Chapter 48)
Parvoviral myocarditis occasionally occurs in young dogs which are infected *in utero* or as neonates (Atwell and Kelly, 1980; Ware and Bonagura, 1986; Van Fleet and Ferrans, 1986). Peracute disease may result in sudden death from heart failure in pups aged 3–8 weeks (Lenghaus *et al.*, 1980; Lenghaus and Studdert, 1982). Milder lesions may result in dilated cardiomyopathy and signs of congestive heart failure or arrhythmias in older pups up to the age of 6 months. There is also experimental evidence to suggest that canine distemper virus can cause severe myocardial damage in very young pups (Higgens *et al.*, 1981).

Bacterial
Focal suppurative myocarditis may occur as a sequel to bacteraemia associated with bacterial endocarditis or pericarditis (Van Fleet and Ferrans, 1986). Affected animals may show systemic signs (fever, weight loss and depression) and an arrhythmia is often evident on an ECG. Serial blood cultures should be performed in an animal showing appropriate clinical signs. Myocarditis has been reported in a dog which was seropositive for *Borrelia burgdorferi* (Lyme disease; Levy and Duray, 1988).

Protozoal
Infection of the myocardium with *Toxoplasma gondii* occasionally occurs in immunosuppressed animals. *Neospora caninum* infection has been reported as a cause of myocarditis and sudden death in a dog (Odin and Dubey, 1993). *Trypanosoma cruzi* infection (Chagas' disease) is associated with granulomatous myocarditis in young dogs in the southeastern United States (Williams *et al.*, 1977).

Fungal
Myocardial involvement has been reported with systemic mycotic infections, for example cryptococcosis, coccidioidosis and aspergillosis (Maddy, 1958; Wood *et al.*, 1978; Edwards and Rebhun, 1979; Mullaney *et al.*, 1983).

Traumatic myocarditis

Traumatic myocarditis may be caused by penetrating wounds or blunt trauma for example after a road traffic accident. Myocardial ischaemia, haemorrhage or contusion may result in severe ventricular arrhythmias which may not be apparent until 12–48 h after the traumatic episode (Macintire and Snider, 1984). Serious life-threatening arrhythmias require prompt and aggressive therapy; less severe arrhythmias associated with minimal haemodynamic changes may resolve spontaneously after a few days.

Diagnosis of myocarditis

The diagnosis of myocarditis is often presumptive and based on the history and clinical and electrocardiographic findings. Infectious myocarditis should be suspected when persistent or intermittent pyrexia is accompanied by an arrhythmia and/or signs of congestive heart failure (CHF). In the absence of signs of CHF thoracic radiographs are often unremarkable. Serial blood cultures should be taken if possible during a pyrexic episode, and serological tests for specific diseases, for example canine parvovirus or toxoplasmosis, may also be indicated.

Treatment of myocarditis

Therapy should be directed toward the underlying disease process as well as management of congestive heart failure and any arrhythmia which may be present. A broad spectrum antibiotic should be used if an infectious cause is suspected; the administration of corticosteroids for their anti-inflammatory properties may also be justified.

Myocardial neoplasia

Primary myocardial tumours are rare. Haemangiosarcoma involving the right atrium is the most common primary cardiac tumour with most cases occurring in older German shepherd dogs (Kleine et al., 1970; Pearson and Head, 1976; Aronsohn, 1985; Brown et al., 1985). Chemodectomas or heart base tumours (most are aortic body tumours rather than carotid body tumours) arise from the base of the aorta and/or pulmonary artery. They tend to be locally invasive and have a predilection for brachycephalic breeds such as boxers and Boston terriers (Patnaik et al., 1975). Metastatic tumours (for example lymphoma or haemangiosarcoma) also may infiltrate the myocardium. The clinical signs of myocardial neoplasia vary depending on the location of the mass and degree of myocardial infiltration. Arrhythmias and atrioventricular conduction blocks are common; animals with pericardial involvement may develop a pericardial effusion resulting in cardiac tamponade and signs of right-sided congestive heart failure.

Confirmation of myocardial and pericardial neoplasia is best achieved by the use of echocardiography which may reveal echodense foci or masses within the myocardium.

Toxins

The ventricular arrhythmias which are often associated with gastric dilatation–volvulus and acute pancreatitis may be the result of myocardial ischaemia and necrosis. The pathogenesis of these lesions is uncertain; myocardial depressant factors have been implicated (Muir and Weisbrode, 1982; Ware and Bonagura, 1986).

Chronic administration of the anthracycline drug, doxorubicin, results in progressive myocardial degeneration with clinical signs which are similar to those of dilated cardiomyopathy. The acute effects of cardiotoxicity (reduced left ventricular filling and decreased cardiac output) may occasionally occur after initial therapy and are thought to be mediated by histamine and catecholamine release. Signs of chronic toxicity (left ventricular enlargement and congestive heart failure) may occur with median cumulative doses greater than 150 mg m^{-2} BSA (Mauldin et al., 1992). Left ventricular dilatation is associated with a marked decrease in myocardial contractility and arrhythmias (supraventricular and ventricular arrhythmias as well as conduction abnormalities) are common. ECG changes may occur at cumulative doses less than 90 mg m^{-2} and may precede signs of congestive heart failure (Mauldin et al., 1992). Regular ECG and echocardiographic monitoring of patients receiving doxorubicin is essential therefore and therapy should be discontinued if abnormalities are noted.

Myocardial ischaemia

Myocardial ischaemia, necrosis and infarction is not a major cause of death in dogs as it is in humans. Microscopic focal myocardial infarction has been associated with thrombotic diseases, for example bacterial endocarditis, following thromboembolic occlusion of the coronary artery (Nielson and Nielson, 1954; Ware and Bonagura, 1986). Similar microscopic infarcts and focal areas of myocardial necrosis and fibrosis may occur in older dogs with valvular endocardiosis although the significance of these lesions is uncertain (Johnsson, 1972). The pathogenesis of these lesions is not known; one possibility is that they are caused by coronary vasoconstriction in response to increased levels of circulating catecholamines. Myocardial ischaemia may also occur as an important and sometimes life-threatening complication in dogs with acute gastric dilatation–volvulus and acute pancreatitis. Less frequently it has been reported with atherosclerosis in hypothyroid dogs which are hypercholesterolaemic (Liu et al., 1986).

PRIMARY MYOCARDIAL DISEASE IN THE CAT

The cardiomyopathies and thromboembolic complications which often result represent the most common cardiovascular disorders in the cat. If secondary cardiomyopathies are taken into consideration (that is cases where the cardiomyopathy is associated with an underlying systemic or metabolic disease) the incidence has been estimated at 12–15% (Bond and Fox, 1984).

Dilated cardiomyopathy

The aetiology of primary dilated cardiomyopathy in the cat is unknown. Recent work has indicated a close association between dietary taurine deficiency and dilated cardiomyopathy (Pion et al., 1987; Pion, 1989; Novotny et al., 1994). In the cat, taurine is an essential amino acid which is required for the conjugation of bile acids. The premise that taurine deficiency is one of the causative factors in the pathogenesis of DCM is based on the fact that many cats on taurine-deficient diets develop myocardial failure which can be reversed with taurine supplementation (Pion et al., 1992b; Novotny et al., 1994).

However, not all cats on taurine-depleted diets develop DCM and some which do develop cardiomyopathy fail to respond to taurine supplementation. About 38% of cats with DCM in one study failed to respond to taurine supplementation and died within the first 30 days of treatment. Hypothermia and thromboembolism were found to increase the risk of early death (Pion et al., 1992b).

It is also known that cats on apparently adequate diets can nevertheless become taurine deficient. The minimal concentration of taurine in the diet required to prevent signs of deficiency varies with the type of diet. For example, it has been shown that much higher concentrations (2000–2500 mg taurine/kg dry matter) of taurine are required in canned diets compared to dry cat foods since heating during the canning process produces products which increase the enterohepatic loss of taurine (Morris et al., 1990). Low plasma taurine levels have been reported in cats fed a taurine replete but potassium depleted diet containing 0.8% ammonium chloride as a urinary acidifier (Dow et al., 1992) suggesting a possible association between taurine and potassium balance in cats. Dietary acidification exacerbates potassium depletion in cats by decreasing gastrointestinal absorption of potassium (Dow et al., 1990).

It has been suggested therefore that the aetiology of feline DCM, like that of DCM in dogs, is multifactorial (Pion et al., 1992b). There is some evidence to show that genetic factors may play a role in feline DCM (Lawler et al., 1993). Burmese, Siamese and Abyssinian cats appear predisposed (Fox, 1988b; Bonagura, 1989). The incidence of DCM is higher in young to middle-aged cats; the evidence for a sex predilection is equivocal (Harpster, 1986).

Pathophysiology

Impairment in myocardial contractility leads to systolic dysfunction and increased end-diastolic pressures. Progressive dilatation of the ventricles results in distortion of the atrioventricular valve apparatus and mitral regurgitation which, together with the reduction in myocardial contractility, contributes to the reduction in stroke volume and decreased cardiac output.

Clinical signs

The clinical signs may be gradual in onset and are often rather vague (lethargy, reduced activity and decreased appetite). Many of the presenting signs are similar to those of hypertrophic cardiomyopathy (see below) making differentiation between the two diseases on a clinical basis difficult. Cats which are dyspnoeic may be dehydrated and hypothermic with weak femoral pulses. There may be obvious pallor or cyanosis of the mucosae with a prolonged capillary refill time. Increased respiratory crackles in association with a gallop rhythm and systolic murmur are common findings; the presence of a large volume of pleural fluid may result in muffled heart sounds. Less frequently there is also evidence of right-sided failure (jugular distension, and hepatomegaly); ascites is a rare finding.

Electrocardiography

The electrocardiographic changes do not help differentiate DCM from the hypertrophic form of the disease. Some cats remain in a relatively slow sinus rhythm. Tall R waves and wide P waves and QRS complexes may be apparent in Lead II.

Arrhythmias, especially ventricular premature complexes, have been recorded in more than 50% of cases (Harpster, 1986). The mean electrical axis is often within normal limits.

Radiographic findings

Thoracic radiographs typically show evidence of generalized cardiomegaly; enlargement of the left atrium may be particularly marked (Fig. 34.16). The cardiac silhouette is often obscured by the presence of a bilateral pleural effusion. Pulmonary venous congestion and oedema may be present but these changes are usually mild and are often masked by the presence of fluid in the pleural space. The caudal vena cava is often dilated and there may be evidence of hepatomegaly.

Echocardiography

Echocardiography offers the most reliable means of differentiating DCM from hypertrophic cardiomyopathy. The interventricular septum and left ventricular free wall appear thin and poorly contractile with a marked reduction in fractional shortening. Both ventricles and the left atrium appear dilated and left ventricular end-diastolic and end-systolic internal dimensions are increased.

Laboratory findings

Normal plasma taurine levels are greater than 60 nmol l^{-1} (Anantharaman and Ballevre, 1993); most cats with DCM have plasma taurine concentrations less than 20 nmol l^{-1} and often less than 10 nmol l^{-1} (Pion et al., 1987, 1992a; Novotny et al., 1994). Taurine-deficient cats with thromboembolism may have slightly higher plasma taurine concentrations due to reperfusion hyperkalaemia (Pion et al., 1992a). Whole blood taurine has been reported to be less sensitive to acute changes in taurine intake and provides a better indication of long-term taurine intake. Whole blood taurine concentrations greater than 280 nmol l^{-1} are considered adequate (Anantharaman and Ballevre, 1993).

Prerenal azotaemia is a common finding in cats with DCM because of reduced renal perfusion. The pleural effusion which develops with feline DCM is typically a serosanguineous modified transudate; true chylous effusions have been reported in association with right heart failure (Fossum et al., 1994).

Angiocardiography

Non-selective angiocardiography can be used to demonstrate dilatation of all cardiac chambers. The slow circulation time in cats with DCM increases the risk of thromboembolus formation

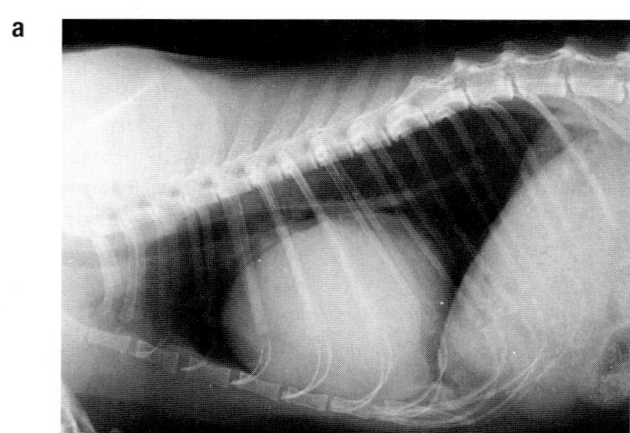
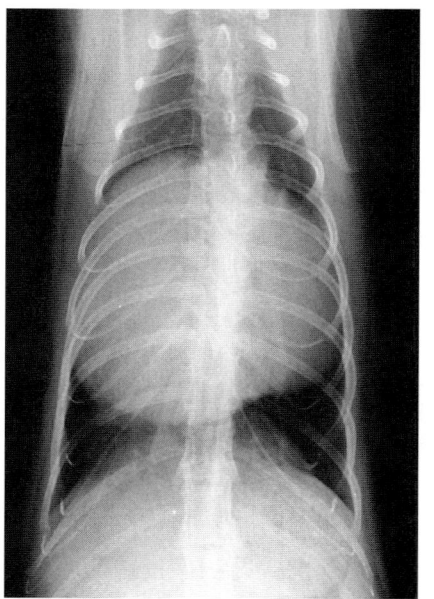

Figure 34.16 Lateral (a) and dorsoventral (b) thoracic radiographs of a 5-year-old domestic shorthaired cat with dilated cardiomyopathy showing generalized cardiomegaly.

during this procedure and decompensated cases should be stabilized beforehand (Fox and Bond, 1983).

Treatment

Cats which are severely dyspnoeic should be given oxygen, kept warm and placed in a cage. Dyspnoeic animals, particularly those with suspected pleural effusion, should be handled with care and should not be placed in dorsal or lateral recumbency for radiography. A dorsoventral radiograph taken with the animal resting in sternal recumbency is usually sufficient to confirm the presence of pleural fluid. Thoracocentesis should be attempted before a more detailed radiographic examination is performed. Other therapeutic strategies are summarized below.

- Digoxin improves myocardial contractility in some but not all cats with DCM and it has been suggested that the drug may act synergistically with taurine in this respect (Atkins et al., 1990). The liquid form of the drug is unpalatable and is generally not well tolerated. There is considerable individual variation in the way in which cats respond to digoxin (Atkins et al., 1989). The maintenance oral dose is 0.01 mg kg^{-1} every 48 h for an average 3–4 kg cat which is less than one quarter of a 62.5 µg tablet every other day (Snyder and Atkins, 1992). Cats with DCM are more susceptible to digoxin toxicity and tend to show toxic signs when the plasma concentration of digoxin is approximately 50% of the level which would be considered toxic in a normal healthy cat (Fox, 1988b). Approximately 50% of cats given 0.01 mg kg^{-1} body weight every 48 h show signs of toxicity (Atkins et al., 1989).
- Other positive inotropic agents such as dopamine and dobutamine must be given by constant slow intravenous infusion and are, therefore, not used as extensively. Both drugs can be given at a rate of 1–5 µg kg^{-1} body weight min^{-1} (Bonagura, 1989); with dobutamine, seizures have been reported with infusion rates as low as 5 µg kg^{-1} min^{-1} in cats (Fox, 1988b).
- Frusemide (initially 1.0 mg kg^{-1} body weight intravenously twice daily; for maintenance 1–2 mg kg^{-1} body weight per os once or twice daily)
- Mixed arteriovenous vasodilators such as captopril (3.12–6.25 mg kg^{-1} body weight per os twice or three times daily; this dose equates to approximately one-eighth to one quarter of a 25 mg tablet; Fox, 1988b) or venodilators such as 2% nitroglycerine ointment (⅛–¼ inch applied three times daily to the inside of the pinna; Luis Fuentes, 1992) can be given although the beneficial effects of these drugs have yet to be evaluated fully in cats with DCM. They should not be given to cats with cardiogenic shock since they may potentiate the fall in cardiac output especially if used in conjunction with diuretic agents.
- Animals which are severely hydrated may require intravenous or subcutaneous fluid therapy, for example 0.45% saline with 2.5% dextrose solution may help combat the effects of circulatory failure. The recommended rate of infusion is 25–35 ml kg^{-1} body weight day^{-1} given in two or three divided doses (Fox, 1988b). Care should be taken so that the rate of infusion optimizes cardiac output but minimizes the risk of exacerbating pulmonary oedema or a pleural effusion.
- Aspirin (25 mg kg^{-1} body weight every 72 h)
- Taurine supplementation (250–500 mg per os twice daily) may result in a dramatic clinical improvement within 1–2 weeks when DCM is associated with taurine deficiency although echocardiographic evidence of improved cardiac performance is usually not evident until after at least three weeks of treatment (Pion et al., 1992b).
- Sodium restricted diet

Prognosis

The prognosis for cats which fail to resond to taurine therapy is poor. About 93% of early deaths occur within the first two weeks; few survive longer than one month (Pion et al., 1992b). Taurine supplementation can eventually be discontinued if adequate taurine intake is provided for in the food.

Hypertrophic cardiomyopathy

The incidence of hypertrophic cardiomyopathy (HCM) is higher in the cat than it is in the dog. HCM can be classified as primary or secondary. The aetiology of the primary or idiopathic form is unknown. A recent survey of 74 cases of HCM showed no apparent breed predilection (Atkins et al., 1992); others have suggested that the Persian breed may be predisposed (Fox, 1988b). The disease rarely occurs in the Siamese, Burmese and Abyssinian breeds in which there is a much higher incidence of dilated cardiomyopathy (Fox, 1988b). Secondary HCM most commonly occurs in association with hyperthyroidism.

Idiopathic HCM typically occurs in young to middle-aged cats (mean age 6.5 years) and males are more commonly affected (Liu *et al.*, 1981; Bond and Fox, 1984; Harpster, 1986).

Pathophysiology

- HCM is characterized by symmetrical hypertrophy of the interventricular septum and left ventricular free wall. Occasionally there may be evidence of left ventricular outflow obstruction especially if there is disproportionate hypertrophy of the septum (Tilley *et al.*, 1977; Liu *et al.*, 1981). Partial aortic outflow obstruction may also be caused by anterior motion of the mitral valve during early systole but this appears to be a rare occurrence in feline HCM. Indeed, echocardiographic studies have shown that most cats with HCM do not have left ventricular outflow gradients and it appears therefore that obstructive HCM, as occurs in dogs, is rare in cats (Bright *et al.*, 1992).
- Left ventricular hypertrophy results in decreased myocardial compliance, interference with normal diastolic filling due to impaired myocardial relaxation, and an increase in left ventricular end-diastolic pressure (despite a normal or often reduced end-diastolic volume). Decreased myocardial compliance may be aggravated by focal or diffuse endocardial fibrous tissue deposition. Pressure overload within the left ventricle may also be associated with mitral valve dysfunction and regurgitation leading to left atrial enlargement (Bright *et al.*, 1992).
- The decrease in stroke volume ultimately leads to a reduction in cardiac output and decreased coronary perfusion resulting in myocardial ischaemia. Abnormal myocardial handling of calcium may be a factor in the pathogenesis of HCM (an increase in intracellular calcium inhibits complete myocardial relaxation which may explain why calcium blocking drugs have been shown to improve diastolic function significantly in affected cats (Bright *et al.*, 1991).
- More recently, excessive circulating levels of growth hormone has been implicated in the pathogenesis of HCM. Cats with acromegaly due to functional pituitary tumours have HCM (Peterson *et al.*, 1990). It has also been shown that non-acromegalic cats with HCM have significantly increased levels of growth hormone compared to normal cats and cats with other forms of cardiac disease but whether this is cause or effect is not clear (Kittleson *et al.*, 1992).

Clinical signs

Recent studies have demonstrated the heterogeneity of feline HCM with regard to the wide spectrum of clinical, electrocardiographic, radiographic and echocardiographic features of the disease (Bright *et al.*, 1992; Peterson *et al.*, 1993). Some cases of HCM remain asymptomatic until the cat is stressed. The clinical signs of HCM are typically those of left-sided congestive heart failure. Bright and others showed that 61% of cats with HCM had a history of respiratory distress characterized by the acute onset of dyspnoea progressing to mouth breathing (Bright *et al.*, 1992). Affected cats become lethargic, anorexic and may cough. Occasionally heart sounds may be muffled due to the presence of pleural or pericardial fluid. Clinical examination may reveal diffuse pulmonary crackles and the presence of a gallop rhythm and/or systolic murmur. Other more variable signs include prolonged capillary refill time and pallor or cyanosis of the tongue and mucous membranes. Animals showing severe signs of cardiac failure are often hypothermic with weak femoral pulses. The increased tendency towards thrombus formation may result in acute onset of hindlimb (less frequently forelimb) paralysis or lameness with cold limb extremities (see section on arterial thromboembolism).

Electrocardiography

Almost 70% of cases may be expected to have an abnormal ECG. Abnormalities reported include increased amplitude and width of P and R waves (P waves >0.04 s and >0.2 mV; QRS complexes >0.04 s and R waves >0.9 mV in lead II), arrhythmias (atrial or ventricular premature contractions) and conduction disturbances. Left anterior fascicular bundle branch block, with deep S waves in leads I, II and III and left axis deviation, is particularly common (Bright *et al.*, 1992).

Radiographic findings

Radiographic abnormalities consisting of mild to moderate left atrial and left ventricular enlargement or biventricular enlargement with evidence of pulmonary venous congestion and/or oedema are present in more than 80% of cases (Bright *et al.*, 1992). Biventricular enlargement may lead to elevation of the trachea and increased sternal contact and, on the dorsoventral view, the enlarged atria may result in a 'valentine-shaped' heart (Fig. 34.17). Occasionally there may also be radiographic signs of right heart failure (right

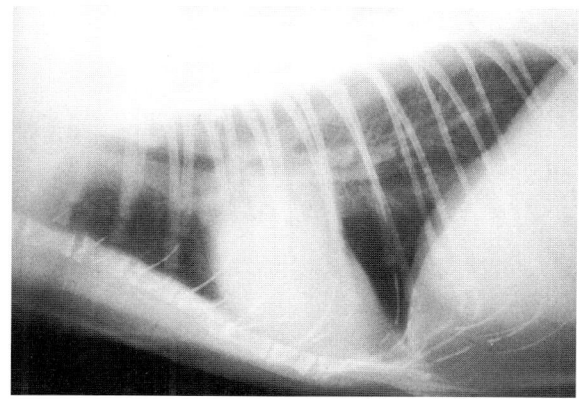
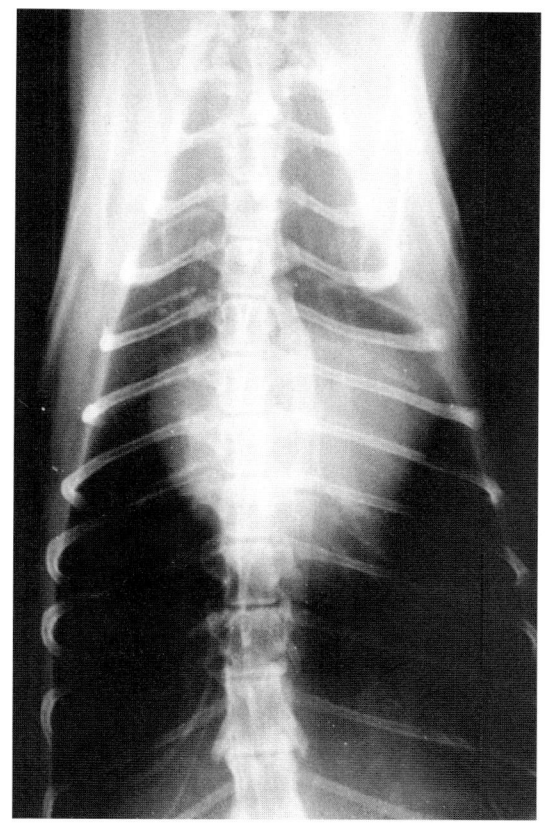
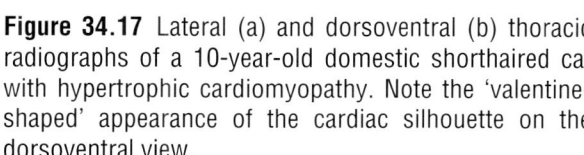

Figure 34.17 Lateral (a) and dorsoventral (b) thoracic radiographs of a 10-year-old domestic shorthaired cat with hypertrophic cardiomyopathy. Note the 'valentine-shaped' appearance of the cardiac silhouette on the dorsoventral view.

ventricular enlargement, hepatomegaly and ascites (Bright et al., 1992).

Echocardiography

HCM is characterized by symmetric or less frequently asymmetric hypertrophy of the interventricular septum and left ventricular free wall, and enlarged hypertrophied papillary muscles which contribute to a marked reduction in left ventricular internal dimensions (Fig. 34.18). Most cases show evidence of a moderate degree of left atrial dilation and fractional shortening is usually normal or increased. Occasionally there is systolic anterior motion of the septal mitral valve leaflet and Doppler studies may show mitral regurgitation (Bonagura, 1994). Mild pericardial effusion may be evident.

Angiocardiography

With the increased use of ultrasound angiocardiography is rarely required. In the absence of ultrasound facilities, non-selective angiocardiography (injection of the contrast agent via the jugular vein) can be used to demonstrate the hypertrophied left ventricle and papillary muscles and regurgitation of contrast into the dilated left atrium. Circulation time is usually normal (Bright et al., 1992).

Prognosis

The prognosis for HCM is guarded and other causes of left ventricular hypertrophy such as systemic hypertension, hyperthyroidism, acromegaly, chronic anaemia and congenital subaortic stenosis (rare in the cat) should be excluded. Plasma T3 and T4 concentrations should always be determined even when no thyroid nodules can be palpated in the neck.

Treatment

- Cats presented with severe respiratory distress should be given oxygen and confined to a cage in the first instance. Initially frusemide may be given intravenously or intramuscularly (1–2 mg kg^{-1} body weight); thereafter it may be given orally at a dose rate of 1 mg kg^{-1} body weight two or three times daily. One of the main aims of therapy should be to reduce the

296 DISEASES OF THE CARDIOVASCULAR SYSTEM

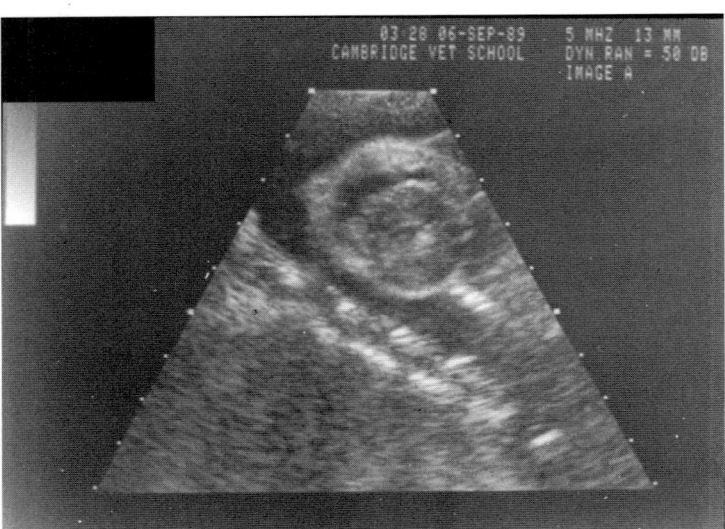

Figure 34.18 Ultrasound HCM cat (T/F).

heart rate to less than 180 beats per minute in order to improve cardiac filling.
- Diltiazem not only decreases the heart rate in cats with HCM but increases myocardial relaxation, decreases myocardial oxygen demand and dilates the coronary vasculature. It has minimal negative inotropic and peripheral vasodilating properties compared to other calcium blocking agents such as verapamil. A dose of 1.75–2.4 mg kg^{-1} body weight per os three times daily (mean effective dose 1.78 mg kg^{-1}) has been shown to effectively reduce pulmonary congestion and improve left ventricular filling with no apparent side effects (Bright et al., 1991).

Recent work has shown that the survival times of cats with HCM may be prolonged with the use of calcium blocking agents such as diltiazem. About 94% of cats in one study receiving diltiazem survived longer than 6 months (Bright et al., 1992). Cats which show no clinical signs on initial presentation and those with heart rates less than 200 beats per minute survive significantly longer than do cats with emboli or congestive heart failure, 60% of which fail to survive 6 months (Atkins et al., 1992).
- Beta-blocking drugs such as propranolol (2.5–5.0 mg per os twice or three times daily) slow the heart rate and improve diastolic filling. Propranolol is the antidysrhythmic drug of choice for cats but its effects on myocardial compliance in cases of feline HCM have not been documented (Luis Fuentes, 1992).
- Although vasodilators are generally contraindicated in cats with HCM, captopril (3.12–6.20 mg twice or three times daily) may be useful in cases with severe mitral regurgitation and signs of refractory congestive heart failure (Luis Fuentes, 1992).
- The administration of digoxin is contraindicated in cats with HCM since myocardial contractility is often normal or increased.
- Aspirin (25 mg kg^{-1} body weight every 72 h) should be given to minimize the risk of thromboembolic disease although there is no evidence to date to suggest that aspirin, if given prophylactically, decreases the incidence of arterial thrombosis in cats with HCM.

Intermediate (intergrade) cardiomyopathies

Certain forms of cardiomyopathy cannot be classified as either hypertrophic or dilated on the basis of the clinical, radiographic, echocardiographic and angiographic features. A cat with an intermediate cardiomyopathy may show signs of both systolic and dystolic dysfunction.

Restrictive cardiomyopathy

Restrictive cardiomyopathy (RCM) occurs in older cats and no convincing sex predilection has been reported (Fox, 1988b). It is the least common form of primary myocardial disease in the cat. The aetiology is not known.

The haemodynamic effects are similar to those of restrictive pericarditis. Focal or diffuse endocardial and subendocardial fibrosis impairs diastolic filling and leads to an increased left ventricular end-diastolic pressure.

The clinical signs of RCM are similar to those of the hypertrophic and dilated forms of the disease. Signs of both left- and right-sided failure may be apparent and the disease is associated with a high incidence of thromboembolic disease.

Electrocardiographic abnormalities have been recorded in up to 70% of affected cats. Changes consistent with left atrial enlargement and left ventricular enlargement may be evident and ventricular and supraventricular arrhythmias are common (Fox, 1988b).

Radiographic abnormalities include generalized cardiomegaly (left atrial enlargement is often pronounced), pulmonary congestion and oedema, and pleural effusion. Hepatomegaly and ascites may also be present. Echocardiography may show thickening of the interventricular septum and left ventricular free wall and left atrial dilation. Paradoxically, both ventricles may appear dilated (Fox, 1988b; Bonagura, 1994). Myocardial contractility is often normal or slightly reduced. A mild degree of pericardial effusion may be evident. Non-selective angiocardiography may show filling defects within the left ventricle and a grossly dilated left atrium.

Treatment is similar to the other forms of cardiomyopathy. Other causes of ventricular hypertrophy such as systemic hypertension and hyperthyroidism should be considered as possible differentials.

The prognosis as with the other forms of cardiomyopathy in the cat is guarded.

Excessive left ventricular moderator bands

This is a rare form of myocardial failure associated with abnormal moderator band networks bridging the interventricular septum, left ventricular free wall and papillary muscles. There are few clinical differentiating features and diagnosis is largely based on echocardiographic detection of the abnormal moderator bands using two-dimensional echocardiography. Conduction abnormalities (bundle branch blocks and atrioventricular blocks) appear to be common. Post-mortem examination of affected animals has shown that left ventricular hypertrophy is more common in younger cats (mean age 4 years) whereas older cats tend to show ventricular dilatation (Liu et al., 1982).

■ Arterial thromboembolism

Cats with any form of cardiomyopathy have a predilection to form intracardiac thrombi in the left atrium; the incidence is highest in cats with hypertrophic cardiomyopathy (Liu et al., 1975). These thrombi often become lodged at the bifurcation of the iliac arteries; less frequently they may occlude the brachial, coeliac or renal arteries.

Pathophysiology

Altered blood flow and vascular stasis predispose to thrombus formation. Localized release of vasoactive substances such as serotonin and thromboxane at the site of vascular occlusion result in vasoconstriction of the collateral blood supply adjacent to the occluded vessel (Schaub et al., 1982). Moreover, the release of serotonin induces platelets to aggregate which further potentiates clot formation. Occlusion at the iliac bifurcation (a so called 'saddle' thrombus) results in ischaemic damage to the muscles and nerves of both hind limbs (ischaemic neuromyopathy).

Clinical signs

Iliac thrombosis is characterized by the sudden onset of crying and hindlimb paresis which results in dragging of one or both hind limbs (occlusion of a brachial artery may cause similar signs in a forelimb). The cat may present with acute dyspnoea and mouth breathing and the mucous membranes may appear cyanotic (particularly if a pulmonary artery is thrombosed). The affected muscles become firm and painful to touch after 24 hours. One or both femoral pulses may be absent and the paws and distal limbs are hypothermic (pink pads may appear pale).

Diagnosis

Diagnosis is usually based on the history and clinical signs. Since most cases of iliac thrombosis are associated with cardiomyopathy echocardiography should be performed as soon as the cat is stabilized. Non-selective angiocardiography may be helpful to determine the extent of the thrombosis and also the integrity of the collateral blood supply. Acute muscle damage results in increased plasma concentrations of aspartate aminotransferase (AST) and creatine kinase (CK). Urea and creatinine concentrations may increase after embolization of a renal artery.

Since the clinical signs of iliac thrombosis resemble those of lower motor neurone paralysis, spinal cord lesions, for example, acute spinal cord trauma, intervertebral disc protrusion (rare in the cat) or haemorrhage, and intravertebral tumours (lymphosarcoma) should be considered as differential diagnoses.

Treatment

Treatment should be directed at alleviating signs associated with the thrombus as well as the underlying cardiac disorder responsible for its formation. Aspirin (25 mg kg^{-1} body weight per os every 72 h) should be given to inhibit platelet function. One study showed that the administration of aspirin resulted in significant preservation of collateral blood supply in cats after experimental induction of iliac thrombosis and a shortening of the recovery period (Schaub et al., 1982). However, there is evidence to suggest that aspirin is not effective in preventing further embolic episodes (Pion and Kittleson, 1989). The use of acepromazine (0.2–0.4 mg kg^{-1} bodyweight subcutaneously three times daily) has been advocated for its vasodilator properties. Heparin may be given to prevent further activation of the coagulation process (an initial intravenous dose of 1000 USP followed 3 h later by 50 USP units kg^{-1} body weight subcutaneously and thereafter 50 USP units kg^{-1} bodyweight every 6–8 h). Regular daily monitoring of activated partial thromboplastin time (APTT) is advised so that the APTT is not prolonged by more than 1.5–2.0 times the preheparin baseline values (Pion and Kittleson, 1989). Morphine (0.1 mg kg^{-1} bodyweight) can be given as an analgesic for the first 24–48 h (Flanders, 1986).

The use of the serotonin antagonist, cyproheptadine, and thrombolytic agents such as streptokinase, urokinase and tissue plasminogen activator (t-PA) have yet to be fully evaluated and to date the results have been equivocal.

Prognosis

The prognosis is at best guarded. Many animals fail to respond to medical management or succumb to the underlying cardiomyopathy. Recurrence is common. Spontaneous recanalization of the clot may occur with or without drug therapy after 2–4 days. Many cats are left with signs of residual peripheral nerve damage. Full recovery may take up to 4–6 weeks.

SECONDARY MYOCARDIAL DISEASE IN THE CAT

Infective myocarditis

Myocarditis is rare in the cat and diagnosis, as in the dog, is extremely difficult. A tentative diagnosis of myocarditis may be based on the history and clinical signs but confirmation in many cases is possible only after post-mortem examination.

Toxoplasmosis

Infection with *Toxoplasma gondii* may cause myocarditis in immunosuppressed cats, for example in association with feline leukaemia virus infection, however infection is often asymptomatic and may only be discovered as an incidental finding during post-mortem examination (Dubey and Carpenter, 1993).

Bacterial myocarditis

Bacterial myocarditis occurs occasionally in cats as a sequel to bacterial endocarditis involving the mitral valve (Harpster, 1986). The early signs of myocarditis are often non-specific and may go unrecognized. Myocarditis should be considered as a differential diagnosis if fever and other signs of systemic disease are accompanied by an arrhythmia. A neutrophilic leucocytosis with a left shift may be evident on haematological examination.

Cardiomyopathy due to thyrotoxicosis

Hyperthyroidism in the cat is usually the result of benign functional adenomas (occasionally adenocarcinomas). One or both thyroid glands may be involved and the condition typically occurs in cats older than 10 years of age. The increased levels of circulating thyroxine (T4) and triiodothyronine (T3) have a direct stimulary effect on the sinoatrial node. In addition concurrent sympathetic stimulation results in increased catecholamine release which increases cardiac workload. This leads to myocardial hypertrophy and hypercontractility. A high output state ensues until ultimately the heart decompensates and signs of congestive heart failure develop. The cardiac manifestations of hyperthyroidism include tachycardia (heart rates in excess of 200 beats per minute are common), a prominent apex beat, gallop rhythm and systolic murmur. Electrocardiographic, radiographic and echocardiographic findings are similar to those associated with hypertrophic cardiomyopathy. The non-cardiac signs of hyperthyroidism include weight loss, polyphagia, polydipsia and polyuria, hyperactivity, vomiting, diarrhoea and increased faecal volume. The diagnosis and management of feline hyperthyroidism is discussed more fully in Chapter 39.

Cardiac neoplasia

Primary heart tumours are rare in the cat and tumours such as lymphoma and haemangiosarcoma which infiltrate the myocardium usually represent secondary metastases (Tilley *et al.*, 1981).

Toxins

The cardiotoxic effects of doxorubicin are similar to those reported in the dog although it appears that cats can tolerate higher cumulative doses of the drug compared to dogs (Mauldin *et al.*, 1992).

CONGENITAL PERICARDIAL DISEASE

Congenital peritoneopericardial diaphragmatic hernia

Congenital peritoneopericardial diaphragmatic hernia (CPDH) is a complete or partial absence of the pericardial membrane which allows protrusion of liver, bowel and/or omentum into the pericardial sac. A small hernia may be asymptomatic. Large hernias may result in reduced cardiac output but rarely cause congestive heart failure or cardiac tamponade. Occasionally the contents become strangulated resulting in signs of gastrointestinal obstruction. A high incidence of CPDH has been reported in weimaraners (Evans and Biery, 1980).

Diagnosis

Gastrointestinal sounds may be auscultated over the heart. Thoracic radiographs may show generalized cardiomegaly with different densities superimposed over the cardiac silhouette (Fig. 34.19). An upper gastrointestinal contrast study may help to confirm the presence of loops of intestine in the pericardial sac. Alternatively, echocardiography can be used to obtain a definitive diagnosis. The differential diagnosis for peritoneopericardial diaphragmatic hernia includes other causes of cardiomegaly in a young dog, for example other congenital cardiac defects, rarely dilated cardiomyopathy, benign (idiopathic) pericardial effusion and possibly diaphragmatic hernia.

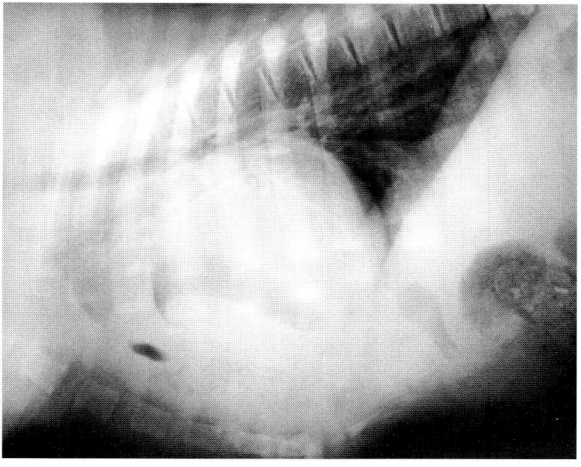

Figure 34.19 Lateral thoracic radiograph of a 3-month-old Rhodesian ridgeback with a congenital peritoneopericardial diaphragmatic hernia. Tubular gas shadows are superimposed on a large cardiac silhouette and there is merging of the caudal border of the heart and ventral border of the diaphragm. The colon is displaced cranially towards the diaphragm.

ACQUIRED PERICARDIAL DISEASE

Pericardial effusion

A build up of fluid in the pericardial sac results in compression of the heart and progressive diastolic dysfunction. A large volume of pericardial fluid reduces ventricular compliance and therefore limits diastolic filling. Central venous pressure increases and stroke volume and cardiac output decrease. This sequence of events is commonly known as cardiac tamponade. The major causes of different types of pericardial effusion in the dog and cat are summarized in Table 34.6.

Disorders causing pericardial effusion in the dog

Benign idiopathic pericardial effusion
Benign pericardial effusion is typically a disease of young to middle aged large or giant breed dogs. The aetiology is unknown. Saint Bernards, golden retrievers and great Danes are most commonly affected. Pericardiocentesis usually yields a dark, haemorrhagic, port wine-coloured effusion which fails to clot (Gibbs *et al.*, 1982; Berg *et al.*, 1984).

Cardiac and intrapericardial neoplasia
Cardiac neoplasia is often associated with pericardial effusion in older dogs. Primary cardiac

Table 34.6 Classification and causes of pericardial effusion in the dog and cat

Transudate	Congestive heart failure
	Hypoalbuminaemia
	Peritoneopericardial diaphragmatic hernia
Exudate	Septic; bacterial or fungal infections
	Sterile; feline infectious peritonitis, toxoplasmosis, occasionally seen with canine distemper, leptospirosis, feline panleucopenia and uraemia
Haemorrhage	Idiopathic (most common)
	Coagulopathies
	Cardiac rupture (e.g. rupture of the right atrial appendage with haemangiosarcoma)
	Trauma
Neoplasia	Haemangiosarcoma (especially German shepherds), metastatic lymphosarcoma, heart base tumours (especially boxers), pericardial mesothelioma (rare)

tumours are more common in the dog than they are in the cat (Tilley et al., 1981). The German shepherd is predisposed to right atrial haemangiosarcoma although the tumour may also occur in other breeds. This tumour is extremely malignant and pulmonary metastases are common. Occasionally rupture of the right auricular appendage occurs resulting in acute haemorrhage into the pericardial sac. Heart base tumours (chemodectomas) have a predilection in brachycephalic breeds such as the boxer. Chemodectomas tend to be locally invasive and rarely metastasize; they may exist concurrently with testicular tumours in some brachycephalic animals (Patnaik et al., 1975). Lymphosarcoma occasionally metastasizes to the heart and results in pericardial effusion. Primary pericardial mesothelioma is an extremely rare malignancy of the pericardial sac.

Right-sided congestive heart failure

A variable volume of pericardial fluid (modified transudate) may be present in some dogs with dilated cardiomyopathy especially those which have pleural effusion and other signs of right-sided failure. Therapeutic drainage of the pericardial effusion is rarely necessary.

Pericarditis and pericardial fibrosis (constrictive pericarditis)

Pericarditis is rare in both dogs and cats. Infection within the pericardial sac results in the development of fibrous adhesions between the epicardium and pericardium which further impair diastolic function. Penetration of the pericardial sac by a foreign body (for example gunshot pellet) may result in septic pericarditis (Thomas et al., 1984b). Sterile inflammatory effusions have been associated with canine distemper, leptospirosis and chronic uraemia.

Intrapericardial cysts

Pericardial cysts have been reported in young dogs and are rare causes of pericardial effusion (Sisson et al., 1993). Pericardial granulomas may be associated with *Actinomyces* infection.

Disorders causing pericardial effusion in the cat

In cats with hypertrophic cardiomyopathy pleural effusion and ascites is frequently accompanied by pericardial effusion (Rush et al., 1990). Sterile pericardial effusions may occur with systemic infections such as feline infectious peritonitis, toxoplasmosis and occasionally feline panleucopenia. Other less frequent causes include coagulopathies and end-stage renal failure. Cats with end-stage renal failure and pericardial effusion often have evidence of left ventricular hypertrophy, probably due to systemic hypertension (Rush et al., 1990). The most common tumour associated with pericardial disease is disseminated lymphosarcoma. Idiopathic pericardial effusions have not been documented.

Clinical signs of pericardial effusion

Pericardial effusion causes signs of low output failure which may progress to cardiogenic shock (weakness, lethargy, exercise intolerance and syncope). Signs of right-sided congestive heart failure tend to predominate with cardiac tamponade because the right ventricular wall, being thinner than the left, is more susceptible to the compressive effects of the pericardial fluid. Ascites may develop rapidly, often within 48 h. The heart sounds are muffled and the femoral pulses weak. Occasionally a rapid fall in pulse pressure may be noted during inspiration (pulsus paradoxicus).

In addition, signs of systemic disease (fever, anorexia and depression) may be apparent with infectious causes of pericardial effusion. Infection results in the formation of fibrous adhesions and a more gradual limitation in diastolic filling. The pericardial sac becomes thickened and the volume of pericardial fluid which forms is usually much smaller than with benign idiopathic effusions. Affected animals therefore tend to show signs of mild chronic cardiac tamponade and signs of right-sided failure may be more apparent than signs of low output failure. Friction-type murmurs are rare except during the early stages of pericarditis.

Electrocardiography

Classically, pericardial effusion causes a reduction in R wave amplitude (often less than 1 mv) and electrical alternans (Table 34.3). However, it should be noted that these ECG abnormalities occur infrequently and that some giant breed dogs, without any evidence of pericardial disease, may also have low amplitude complexes. Neoplastic infiltration of the myocardium may result in arrhythmias or conduction disturbances (Cobb and Brownlie, 1992).

Radiographic findings

Pericardial effusion results in generalized cardiomegaly and a loss of the normal contours of the cardiac chambers (Fig. 34.20). The heart assumes a globular appearance with a sharp outline, although not infrequently pleural and/or mediastinal fluid may obscure the cardiac silhouette. Additional signs of right-sided failure (hepatomegaly and ascites) may be evident on abdominal radiographs.

Pneumopericardiography

Pneumopericardiography is a useful technique for detecting the presence of intrapericardial masses, although its use as a diagnostic aid has now been superseded by echocardiography. To obtain reliable results the pericardial effusion should be completely drained and a volume of room air or CO_2 equivalent to between 50% and 75% of the volume of fluid aspirated injected by syringe. Radiographs are obtained immediately using multiple projections to highlight different areas of the heart (Thomas *et al.*, 1984c).

Echocardiography

Two-dimensional echocardiography is the most sensitive and specific method for detecting pericardial fluid, which appears as an echolucent space between the epicardium and pericardium. The technique is also useful for confirming the presence of pericardial mass lesions/adhesions and assessing the volume of pericardial fluid (Fig. 34.21). The heart should be examined from multiple transducer locations. Serial echocardiographic assessments may be helpful especially for

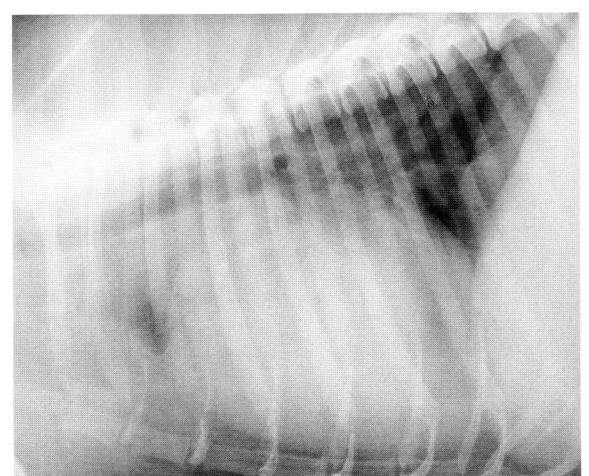
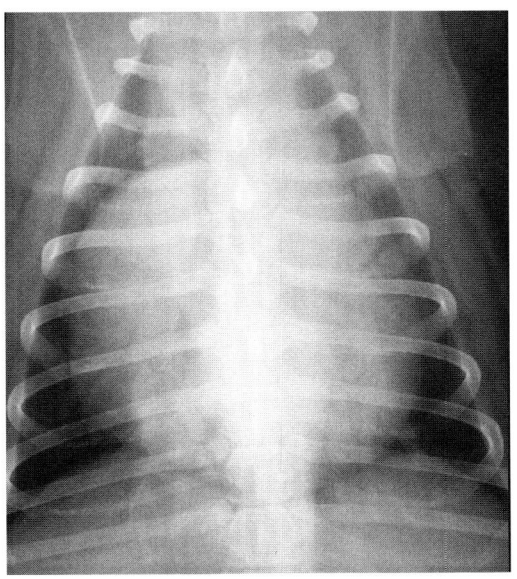

Figure 34.20 Lateral (a) and dorsoventral (b) thoracic radiographs of a 7-year-old golden retriever with pericardial effusion. The heart has a globular appearance. The outline to the cardiac silhouette is sharp and there is no enlargement of any specific cardiac chamber.

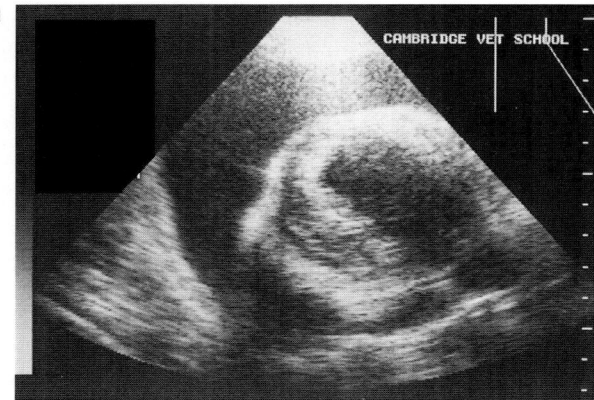 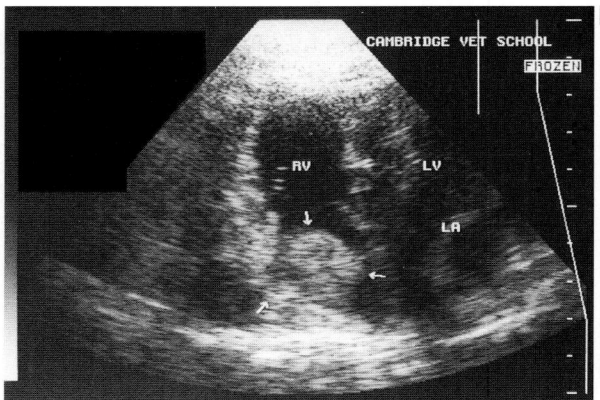

Figure 34.21 2-D left parasternal echocardiogram from the same dog as in Fig. 34.20. (a) Shows massive pericardial effusion with collapse of the right ventricle; (b) taken post-drainage shows improved diastolic function and a mass lesion in the right atrium (arrows). Subsequent post-mortem examination confirmed right atrial haemangiosarcoma.

detecting diffuse tumours such as mesotheliomas (Cobb and Brownlie, 1992).

Pericardiocentesis

Pericardiocentesis is often performed on the right side to minimize the risk of puncturing the lungs and the large coronary arteries. In the authors' experience, however, the procedure may also be performed safely on the left side. An 8 cm long 16 gauge over-the-needle intravenous catheter ensures the pericardial sac is adequately penetrated for maximal drainage of fluid. The site of entry is usually between the fourth and sixth ribs at a point approximately one quarter the way up the chest wall from the sternum. Having penetrated the pericardium, the fluid is removed using a 50 ml syringe with a three-way valve attached to the catheter. The volume of fluid varies; volumes in excess of one litre are frequently aspirated from large dogs with the idiopathic effusions whereas the volume of fluid in a cat is usually less than 50 ml.

Clinicopathological findings

Pericardial fluid should be submitted for cytological, biochemical and bacteriological examination. Cytological examination of pericardial fluid rarely differentiates neoplastic from non-neoplastic effusions although it may help to rule out infection (Sisson et al., 1984; Cobb and Brownlie, 1992). Idiopathic effusions are typically dark, port wine-coloured effusions; they do not clot and are sterile. They contain abundant red blood cells and clusters of reactive mesothelial cells which, because of the degree of blastic transformation, are difficult to differentiate from neoplastic cells. Occasionally increased numbers of plasma cells and lymphocytes may be seen. The protein content is extremely variable ranging from 9 to 57 g l^{-1} (Sisson et al., 1984).

Neoplastic effusions and those resulting from acute haemorrhage (for example due to a coagulopathy or a ruptured right atrium) often have a similar appearance although the presence of platelets and macrophages demonstrating erythrophagocytosis may provide a clue that the haemorrhage is more recent. Centrifugation of the effusion and examination of a buffy coat preparation has been advocated as a method to improve the rate of detection of malignant cells. Chemodectomas may yield an effusion which more closely resembles a modified transudate.

True inflammatory exudates are characterized by the presence of increased numbers of nucleated cells and a much higher protein content. They may be classified as septic or sterile (see Table 34.6). Haematology may show a neutrophilic leucocytosis.

Management of pericardial effusion

Pericardiocentesis should be performed to remove as much of the pericardial effusion as possible. After pericardiocentesis signs of right-sided failure (ascites and pleural effusion) usually resolve within 48 hours and during this period there is often a dramatic reduction in the animal's body weight. Partial or complete pericardectomy should be considered as an alternative to repeated pericardiocentesis especially if there is rapid recurrence of the effusion. Surgical intervention not only expedites drainage of the fluid but permits biopsy of the pericardial sac or any other mass lesion which may be present. Antibiotics should be administered if the effusion is a septic exudate. The use of corticosteroids is more controversial and is based on the possibility that idiopathic pericardial effusions may have an immune-mediated pathogenesis. The prognosis for most cases of intrapericardial neoplasia is poor.

Cor pulmonale

Cor pulmonale is the term used to describe the alterations in the structure or function of the right ventricle which may be induced by pulmonary hypertension secondary to primary lung disease.

Pathophysiology of cor pulmonale

Cor pulmonale may be acute or chronic. Alveolar hypoxia and hypoxaemia, respiratory acidosis and hypercapnoea combine to increase pulmonary vascular resistance. Pulmonary hypertension results in acute or chronic right ventricular pressure overload, right ventricular hypertrophy and eventually signs of right-sided failure.

Acute cor pulmonale caused by pulmonary thromboembolism or heartworm disease is often fatal and in most cases may not be diagnosed. Pulmonary thromboembolism can occur as a complication of chronic renal disease (especially glomerulonephropathy), hyperadrenocorticism, immune-mediated haemolytic anaemia and pancreatitis.

Chronic cor pulmonale may occur as a sequel to chronic obstructive pulmonary disease. It has been associated with chronic bronchitis, bronchiectasis, pulmonary fibrosis, infiltrative lung disease (for example neoplasia), chronic partial upper airway obstruction due to collapsing trachea, laryngeal paralysis or elongation of the soft palate, and heartworm disease.

Clinical signs of cor pulmonale

Animals with acute cor pulmonale due to pulmonary thrombosis present with severe dyspnoea and are often cyanotic. The mortality rate is high. The clinical signs of chronic cor pulmonale depend on the nature and severity of the underlying respiratory disorder. A chronic cough and/or wheezing is common in dogs with chronic bronchitis, bronchiectasis and collapsing trachea; dogs with chronic partial upper airway obstruction due to an elongated soft palate or laryngeal dysfunction may become progressively dyspnoeic with signs of inspiratory stridor/stertor. Failure to treat the underlying problem may lead to signs of right-sided congestive heart failure.

Electrocardiography

Pulmonary hypertension and resultant right ventricular hypertrophy may result in tall P waves (right atrial enlargement) and deep Q or S waves in leads I, II, III and aVF (right ventricular enlargement). The mean electrical axis may shift to the right and myocardial hypoxia may result in ST segment depression.

Radiographic findings

Acute pulmonary thromboembolism results in pulmonary hypoperfusion and lobar hyperlucency. Pulmonary vessels may appear truncated especially towards the periphery. A minimal amount of pleural fluid may be present. Right ventricular enlargement is a feature of chronic cor pulmonale and many animals will show concurrent radiographic changes consistent with chronic lung disease, for example a diffuse bronchial and/or interstitial pattern or bronchiectasis.

Clinicopathological findings

Blood gas analysis

Hypoxia (PaO_2 <80 mm Hg), hypercapnoea ($PaCO_2$ >40 mm Hg) and acidosis (pH <7.4) reflect the severity of the underlying pulmonary pathology (Spaulding and Owens, 1985). Chronic hypoxia occasionally results in secondary polycythaemia. Animals with acute pulmonary thromboembolism may become thrombocytopenic and show other laboratory evidence of disseminated intravascular coagulation (see Chapters 21 and 45). Pulmonary hypertension and right ventricular pressure overload result in an increase in central venous pressure.

In addition to the above, diagnostic investigations such as bronchoscopy and tracheal or bronchoalveolar lavage should be performed where appropriate to establish the nature of the underlying respiratory disorder responsible for the cardiac changes.

Treatment

Treatment of the underlying pulmonary condition should be instituted as quickly as possible. Acute pulmonary thromboembolism should be treated with cage rest, oxygen and antithrombotic drugs such as heparin and aspirin. The prognosis is generally poor if signs of right-sided heart failure are present.

Dirofilariasis

Canine heartworm disease caused by *Dirofilaria immitis* is endemic in most temperate and tropical coastal zones of the world (United States, Japan and Australia especially). Heartworm disease is occasionally diagnosed in imported dogs in the United Kingdom (Thomas, 1985; Matic and Herrtage, 1987). Affected animals are often between 4 and 7 years of age although the condition has been diagnosed in animals less than one year of age.

Life cycle of Dirofilaria immitis

When a mosquito bites an infected dog circulating microfilaria (first stage larvae) are ingested and develop into third stage (L3) larvae which migrate to the mouth parts of the mosquito. The third larval stage of the heartworm (*Dirofilaria immitis*) stage enters the subcutaneous tissues of the host via a bite from an infected mosquito. Young adult worms (L5 stage) reach the right side of the heart by 90–100 days postinfection. There is a prepatent time of approximately 6 months before microfilaria appear in the circulation. Occult infections occur where there is an absence of circulating microfilaria (Rawlings *et al.*, 1982).

Pathophysiology of heartworm disease

Adult worms live most commonly in the right ventricle, main pulmonary artery and parenchymal pulmonary arteries. As the number of heartworms increases they enter the right atrium and eventually migrate into the caudal vena cava. Large numbers of worms may obstruct the caudal vena cava and flow of blood to the right atrium (vena caval syndrome).

Adult worms initiate a parasite–host reaction which damages the pulmonary artery endothelium. Histologically this reaction is characterized by the proliferation of smooth muscle cells on the endothelial surface of the vessels. Circulating antibodies trap the microfilaria within the pulmonary arteries which results in pulmonary infarction and areas of consolidation around the affected vessels. Alveolar hypoxia increases pulmonary vascular resistance and leads to pulmonary hypertension. Pulmonary hypertension results in increased right ventricular afterload, right ventricular hypertrophy and eventually signs of right-sided heart failure (cor pulmonale).

Clinical signs

The clinical signs of heartworm disease, once apparent, are usually severe and progress rapidly. Damage to the pulmonary arteries results in coughing, haemoptysis, dyspnoea and decreased exercise tolerance. There is a rapid loss of body condition and pulmonary hypertension leads to right-sided heart failure. Tricuspid valve murmurs may be heard due to mechanical interference with valvular function by the adult worms (Hoskins *et al.*, 1984).

Some infected dogs show few if any clinical signs. Those with occult heartworm disease develop an allergic pneumonitis characterized by severe coughing and dyspnoea. Two conditions which may have an immune-mediated pathogenesis, eosinophilic granulomatosis and pulmonary infiltrates with eosinophilia (eosinophilic pneumonia), may also occur in association with heartworm disease (Calvert and Rawlings, 1988). Severe pulmonary artery disease may result in thromboembolic complications and thrombocytopenia especially after adulticide therapy.

Haemolysis and haemoglobinuria may occur when a large number of worms obstruct the caudal vena cava and result in fragmentation of red cells. Dogs with the caval syndrome become severely dyspnoeic and show signs of acute hypotension (tachycardia, pale mucous membranes and prolonged capillary refill time).

Electrocardiography

Electrocardiographic signs of right ventricular enlargement may be evident especially in dogs showing signs of right-sided heart failure.

Radiographic findings

Radiographic changes develop early during the course of heartworm infection. Typical abnormalities include right ventricular enlargement and a bulging pulmonary artery segment with enlarged lobar pulmonary arteries (Fig. 34.22). As the disease progresses the peripheral pulmonary

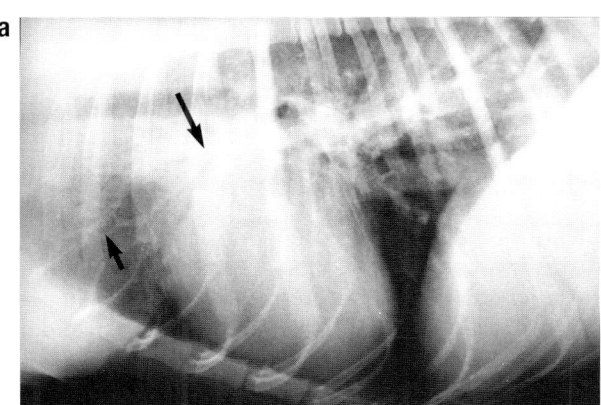
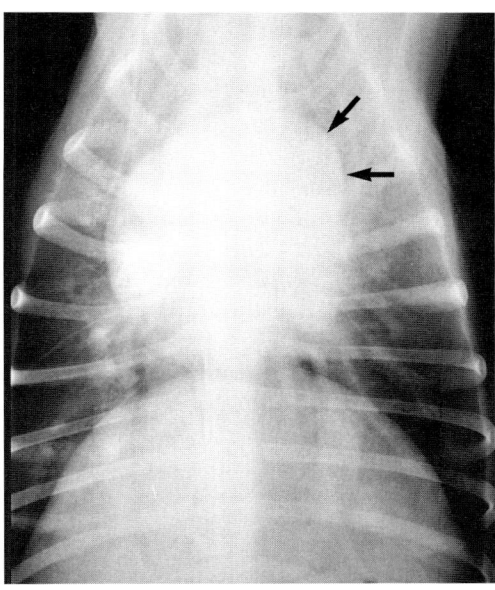

Figure 34.22 Lateral (a) and dorsoventral (b) thoracic radiographs of a 4-year-old Labrador with dirofilariasis. The lateral view shows moderate right-sided cardiac enlargement and dilation of the cranial lobe pulmonary arteries (large arrow) which appear truncated and pruned towards the periphery (small arrow). An alveolar lung pattern can be seen in the caudal lung fields with a predominantly interstitial pattern elsewhere. A pleural line can be seen over the caudal border of the heart. The dorsoventral view shows an enlarged main pulmonary artery segment (arrowed) in addition to the features noted on the lateral radiograph. Fine fissures due to a small amount of pleural fluid can be seen between the lung lobes on both sides of the chest.

arteries become truncated and tortuous especially in the caudal lung lobes. Patchy alveolar densities may be apparent especially after adulticide therapy.

Clinicopathological findings

Eosinophilia often accompanied by basophilia are the most consistent haematological abnormalities, occurring once the young adult worms enter the circulation. A mild regenerative anaemia may be present and neutrophilia may occur following adulticide treatment. Platelet numbers are often reduced as a result of increased consumption in response to endothelial damage. Liver enzymes may be increased especially if signs of right-sided cardiac failure are present; total plasma proteins may also be increased due to an increase in the globulin fraction. Proteinuria occurs in 20–30% of cases; some animals develop a glomerulonephropathy and nephrotic syndrome, and become hypoalbuminaemic (Calvert and Rawlings, 1988).

Diagnosis

The presence of microfilaria on a peripheral blood film implies the presence of adult worms. *Dirofilaria immitis* microfilaria should be differentiated from those of *Dipetalonema reconditum* and other *Dipetalonema* species which cause asymptomatic infections in dogs. This can be done by examining the acid phosphatase staining pattern of filter-treated microfilariae (Acevedo et al., 1981; Ortega-Mora et al., 1989). The blood of young dogs from endemic areas should be screened annually for the presence of microfilaria using a Knott's test. With occult infections, no circulating microfilaria are present and diagnosis is dependent on the detection of appropriate radiographic abnormalities and the results of other serodiagnostic tests.

An indirect fluorescent antibody test detecting antibodies to microfilarial antigens is useful in the diagnosis of occult heartworm disease. An ELISA test for detecting antibodies against adult worms has proved to be less satisfactory because of the high incidence of false positive results, although a negative ELISA result can be regarded as reliable evidence that occult heartworm disease is not present. More recently, ELISA tests using monoclonal antibodies against circulating adult antigens have been developed which appear to be more sensitive and specific than tests which detect adult antibodies (Calvert and Rawlings, 1988).

Treatment

Adulticide therapy

Thiacetarsamide (2.2 mg kg^{-1} body weight intravenously twice daily for two days) eliminates a high percentage of the adult heartworms (young female heartworms are often resistant). The second dose should be given not more than 10 hours after the first (Henry and Dillon, 1994). Treatment with thiacetarsamide should be delayed in dogs with radiographic signs of severe pulmonary artery disease since such animals are at risk from developing thromboembolic complications and thrombocytopenia post-treatment. Toxic reactions to thiacetarsamide occasionally occur; these include anorexia, vomiting, depression, fever, diarrhoea and the presence of tubular casts in the urine. Adulticide treatment is usually followed 4–6 weeks later by the administration of a microfilaricide (see below). The benefits of giving a microfilaricide three weeks before treatment with thiacetarsamide are questionable.

Levamisole has been used as an alternative adulticide drug but is less effective than thiacetarsamide. It is more effective as a microfilaricidal drug but toxic side effects (vomiting and CNS signs) are common.

The prophylactic use of aspirin to combat the potential thromboembolic complications has been questioned. Recent studies have shown that even doses of aspirin greater than 50 mg kg^{-1} in some dogs will not prevent thromboembolism or intimal hyperplasia associated with heartworm emboli (Boudreaux et al., 1991).

Corticosteroids are indicated if there is evidence of an eosinophilic pulmonary infiltrate. Heparin has been recommended for dogs showing signs of chronic or low-grade disseminated intravascular coagulation (DIC).

Microfilaricide treatment

Levamisole, milbemycin and ivermectin are available for use as microfilaricides (the last two can also be used prophylactically). The American Heartworm Society currently recommends that either ivermectin (50 µg kg^{-1}) or milbemycin (500 µg kg^{-1}) be given 3–4 weeks after treatment with adulticide (Soll, 1992). Treatment of dogs with large numbers of microfilaria may lead to circulatory collapse due to rapid death of the microfilaria. Dogs should therefore be observed for 6–8 h after treatment. The use of ivermectin and milbemycin in collies and collie cross breeds has been associated with anaphylactic reactions and, in some cases, death; although both the microfilaricidal and the preventative doses of these drugs are reportedly safe in susceptible collies other drugs, for example levamisole (10 mg kg^{-1} day^{-1} for 7 days) have been recommended for this breed (Dillon, 1989).

Prevention of heartworm disease

Chemoprophylaxis should be initiated 2–3 weeks after administration of a microfilaricide providing no microfilariae are detected in the blood; if microfilariae are still present microfilaricidal treatment should be repeated (Soll, 1992). In endemic areas, either ivermectin (6–12 µg kg^{-1}) or milbemycin (500–999 µg kg^{-1}) can be administered once a month. Young pups can be treated prophylactically from 6–8 weeks of age onwards. Although both drugs can be safely given to dogs which may already have circulating microfilariae, they only kill *D. immitis* larvae during the first six weeks of their development. Both drugs are also known to induce sterility in adult worms therefore dogs greater than 6 months of age on monthly preventative treatment should be tested for antigen to detect occult infections which may develop within 6 months of starting monthly macrolide administration (Henry and Dillon, 1994).

Angiostrongylosis

Angiostrongylus vasorum is a metastrongyloid parasite of dogs and foxes which primarily parasitizes the pulmonary artery and its branches; it may also inhabit the right ventricle. Natural *A. vasorum* infection has been reported in a number of European countries including Ireland, Denmark, southwest France, Spain, Italy and parts of the UK. In the UK the majority of reported cases have been confined to southwest England and south Wales (Martin and Neal, 1992; Patteson et al., 1993). The parasite was first encountered in the UK in racing greyhounds imported from Ireland (Jacobs and Prole, 1975).

Life cycle of *Angistrongylus vasorum*

Adult worms lay eggs in the terminal pulmonary arteries after a pre-patent period of 38–60 days. The first stage larvae hatch into the alveoli, pass up the bronchial tree and are swallowed and shed in the faeces. Several species of slugs and snails act as intermediate hosts. Transmission of the infective L3 larvae is thought to occur if the snails are ingested or if the dog's food becomes contaminated with faeces or slime. When ingested the third stage larvae migrate via the mesenteric lymph nodes and portal system to the liver before passing to the right ventricle and pulmonary arteries.

Clinical signs

Clinical signs include tachypnoea, coughing, haemoptysis, anaemia and haematoma formation. Some dogs with natural or experimental infections either have no clinical signs referrable to the disease or show only mild exercise intolerance; others may develop signs of acute right-sided heart failure and die within a few days of the onset of clinical signs (Patteson et al., 1993).

Radiographic findings

A diffuse interstitial/bronchial pattern with patchy coalescing alveolar densities especially in the caudal lung lobes may be visible. The latter are thought to represent focal areas of pneumonitis and haemorrhage. The right atrium and right ventricle may become enlarged and the pulmonary arteries may appear truncated. Occasionally there is evidence of pulmonary emphysema or pneumothorax.

Clinicopathological findings

Identification of A. vasorum larvae in faecal samples is the best method of diagnosing patent infections. Occult infections occur and the absence of faecal larvae does not preclude A. vasorum infection, since adult worms shed eggs intermittently. Haematological findings are inconsistent; an eosinophilia associated with larval migration may be present and some cases may be anaemic. Serum protein electrophoresis may reveal beta 2 and/or gamma globulin peaks (Patteson et al., 1993).

The increased bleeding tendency has been attributed to a consumptive coagulopathy resembling chronic compensated disseminated intravascular coagulation which results in low platelet numbers and prolongation of the activated partial thromboplastin time (Ramsey et al., 1996). Decreased factor V concentrations have been reported in experimental infections (Schelling et al., 1986).

Treatment

A. vasorum infections have been treated effectively with fenbendazole (20 mg kg^{-1} once daily for 10 days), levamisole (10 mg kg^{-1} daily for three days) and ivermectin (200 µg kg^{-1} given subcutaneously as a single dose) (Patteson et al., 1993). The ability of these drugs to completely eliminate adult worms and/or larvae has yet to be determined.

■ Hypertension

The methods for measuring blood pressure and reported normal blood pressure measurements in small animals are extremely variable. Blood pressure should be measured with the animal unsedated, relaxed and minimally restrained. Heart rate should be within normal resting limits (an increased heart rate tends to increase the diastolic blood pressure measurement). Direct measurements can be performed by percutaneous puncture of the femoral artery connected to pressure sensing and recording equipment. Non-invasive indirect measurements can be obtained using Doppler ultrasound or, in dogs, oscillometric techniques. Normal direct and indirect measurements for dogs and cats are given in Table 34.7.

In dogs, hypertension should be suspected if systolic and diastolic measurements greater than

Table 34.7 Normal blood pressure measurements in dogs and cats

Method of measurement (reference)	Dogs (systolic)	Dogs (diastolic)
Direct (Cowgill and Kallet, 1986)	148 ± 16 mm Hg	87 ± 8 mm Hg
Doppler (Remillard et al., 1991)	147 mm Hg (mean)	80 mm Hg (mean)
Oscillometric (Coulter and Keith, 1984)	144 ± 27 mm Hg	91 ± 20 mm Hg
	Cats (systolic)	Cats (diastolic)
Direct (Gordon and Goldblatt, 1967)	171 ± 22 mm Hg	123 ± 17 mm Hg
Doppler (Kobayashi et al., 1990)	118.4 ± 10.6 mm Hg	83.8 ± 12.2 mm Hg

180 mm Hg and 100 mm Hg respectively, are obtained using an indirect Doppler ultrasound technique (Remillard et al., 1991). In cats, hypertension is defined as sustained systolic and diastolic pressures greater than 170 mm Hg and 100 mm Hg, respectively, using a Doppler technique (Morgan, 1986); systolic/diastolic pressures greater than 200/145 should certainly be regarded as abnormal (Cowgill and Kallet, 1986).

Hypertension can be classified as primary (essential) or secondary. Most cases of hypertension in small animals are secondary to other diseases (Cowgill and Kallet, 1986). Regulation of arterial blood pressure depends on the interaction of a number of neural, cardiac, renal and humoral factors which affect cardiac output, plasma volume and vascular tone. Deregulation of these pressor and volume homeostatic mechanisms may initiate a hypertensive state. Activation of the renin–angiotensin–aldosterone system, altered adrenergic activity, and the release of vasopressor substances by the kidney and antidiuretic hormone from the neurohypophysis (the latter in response to increased angiotensin II levels) act together to increase peripheral vascular resistance and retain sodium and water. Increased vascular 'stiffness' associated with atherosclerosis and arteriosclerosis may also play a role in creating a hypertensive state (Cowgill and Kallet, 1983).

Primary (essential) hypertension

Spontaneous hypertension has been reported in dogs, including a colony of primary hypertensive dogs bred from two naturally occurring cases (Bovee et al., 1986; Littman et al., 1988). Diagnosis of primary hypertension essentially involves ruling out secondary causes. Since spontaneous hypertension can result in secondary renal changes (glomerulosclerosis) and renal insufficiency, identification of the primary disease process is often extremely difficult (Littman et al., 1988). High sodium diets have been implicated in the pathogenesis of primary hypertension (Turner et al., 1990). A high sodium diet may be expected to accelerate the disease process if fed to an animal with pre-existing hypertension; it is not clear, however, if a high sodium load alone can result in hypertension.

Secondary hypertension

In the cat, renal disease and hyperthyroidism are both common causes of hypertension (Kobayashi et al., 1990; Littman, 1994). Primary renal disease is the most common cause of hypertension in dogs (Cowgill and Kallet, 1986). Hypertension may also be associated with hypothyroidism, hyperadrenocorticism, diabetes mellitus, phaeochromocytoma, primary hyperaldosteronism, hyperparathyroidism (resulting in hypercalcaemia), acromegaly and hyperoestrogenism. Other potential, but less well documented, causes include polycythaemia, anaemia, renin-producing tumours, coarctation of the aorta, obesity and ageing (Dukes, 1992).

Clinical signs

Hypertension leads to glomerulosclerosis and a loss of functional nephrons. If renal function is already compromised hypertension may accelerate progression towards end-stage renal failure (Littman et al., 1988). Hypertension also results in concentric hypertrophy of the left ventricle which predisposes the myocardium to ischaemia and the development of arrhythmias. Hypertensive retinopathy is characterized by choroidal haemorrhage and focal retinal detachments. Some animals present with sudden onset blindness due to complete retinal detachment, papilloedema, intraocular haemorrhage or glaucoma (Paulsen et al., 1989). Neurological signs are usually attributed to cerebral haemorrhage; cerebral infarction associated with atherosclerosis of the cerebral arteries is occasionally seen in dogs with hypothyroidism (Liu et al., 1986).

Treatment

The main objective is to identify and treat appropriately the underlying disease (for example renal failure). When a specific disease cannot be identified and primary hypertension is suspected, therapy should be directed against the mechanism responsible for the hypertension, that is an attempt should be made to reduce the circulating blood volume, decrease sympathetic tone and/or inhibit the renin–angiotensin–aldosterone pathway. Suitable therapeutic strategies are summarized below (Cowgill and Kallet, 1986; Dukes, 1992).

- Reduce sodium intake to 0.1–0.3% of the diet (10–40 mg kg^{-1} dry matter). Sodium restriction potentiates the action of antihypertensive drug therapy (see below). Prescription diets are available which fulfil these requirements.
- Diuretics. Frusemide has a natriuretic action and can be used in the face of renal failure. Spironolactone is a more appropriate drug for treating hyperaldosteronism.

- Beta-adrenergic blocking drugs decrease cardiac output and decrease renin release by blocking the beta receptors on the juxtaglomerular apparatus. Their use is indicated in feline hyperthyroidism where hypertension is due to excessive adrenergic stimulation.
- Alpha-adrenergic blocking drugs such as prazosin can be used as balanced vasodilators and can be used safely in animals with renal dysfunction.
- Hydralazine is an arterial vasodilator. It lowers blood pressure but does not protect the kidney against glomerulosclerosis. Hydralazine may result in reflex sympathetic stimulation and renin release and therefore may have to be given with beta blockers.
- Calcium channel blockers such as verapamil and diltiazem cause vasodilation. Verapamil is a renal vasodilator and may transiently increase glomerular filtration rate.
- Angiotensin converting enzyme inhibitors are balanced vasodilators. The decreased production of aldosterone results in increased salt and water excretion. These drugs are nephrotoxic so care should be taken if there is evidence of renal dysfunction.

CONGENITAL HEART DISEASE

The prevalence of canine congenital heart defects in veterinary clinic populations is approximately 0.5–1.0% (Darke, 1986; Patterson, 1989); the prevalence in cats is slightly higher at 2% (Liu, 1977). Congenital heart defects are more common in pure bred dogs with certain breeds predisposed to specific cardiac anomalies (Table 34.8). Most of the common defects are inherited in a complex manner consistent with a polygenic basis and it is likely that the genes involved act additively to increase susceptibility to a specific defect during embryological development of the heart (Patterson, 1989).

Control measures

A reduction in the frequency of any genetic defect can only be accomplished by selection to reduce the frequency of genes involved. Pups should be screened for congenital heart disease (most significant congenital defects produce heart murmurs) at the time of their first immunization, that is 8–10 weeks of age. The primary role of a veterinarian in dealing with a suspected congenital heart defect is to:

- Provide accurate diagnosis, prognosis and appropriate treatment;
- Provide genetic counselling for cases in which a genetic cause is known or suspected.

All affected animals should be identified and eliminated from the breeding programme. Breeders should be dissuaded from breeding from the offspring of affected animals, even if clinically normal, since they may be potential carriers of the genes involved.

Most congenital heart defects cause stunted growth and clinical signs relating to cardiac dys-

Table 34.8 Breed specific predispositions to the more common congenital cardiac defects in dogs

Defect	Breed
Patent ductus arteriosus	Miniature poodle; collie, pomeranian; Shetland sheepdog; German shepherd
Pulmonic stenosis	Bulldog; fox terrier; chihuahua; beagle; samoyed; miniature schnauzer
Subaortic stenosis	German shepherd; boxer; Newfoundland; German short-haired pointer; golden retriever; rottweiler
Persistent right aortic arch	German shepherd; Irish setter
Tetralogy of Fallot	Keeshound[a]
Ventricular septal defect	Bulldog; keeshound[a]
Atrial septal defect	Samoyed
Tricuspid dysplasia	Great Dane; weimeraner; Labrador retriever
Mitral dysplasia	Great Dane; bulldog; chihuahua; bull terrier

[a] Part of a spectrum of conotruncal malformations produced by the same underlying genetic defect.

function are usually apparent before one year of age. Most are associated with a murmur; however, not all murmurs in this age-group are pathological. It is necessary, therefore, to differentiate pathological murmurs from those that can be classified as innocent or benign. Moreover, as some murmurs, particularly left ventricular outflow (ejection-type) murmurs can be delayed in onset, all normal pups should be re-examined once they have attained adult body size.

Patent ductus arteriosus is the most common defect in dogs (approximately 25–30% of all congenital defects in most studies) followed by, in decreasing order of frequency, aortic stenosis, pulmonic stenosis, ventricular septal defects, persistent right aortic arch and tetralogy of Fallot (Patterson, 1968; Mulvihill and Priester, 1973; Buchanan, 1992). The most common congenital cardiac defects in the cat are, in descending order of frequency, mitral valve dysplasia, tricuspid valve dysplasia, ventricular septal defect and aortic stenosis, especially the supravalvular form (Liu, 1977).

Patent ductus arteriosus

In the fetus, the ductus arteriosus functions to bypass the pulmonary circulation. It is a short arterial connection arising from the sixth aortic arch which carries blood from the pulmonary artery to the aorta and systemic circulation. The ductus normally closes in the first few weeks after birth to form the ligamentum arteriosum. Closure is regulated by prostaglandin synthetase inhibition and also by the changes which occur in blood oxygen saturation.

Patent ductus arteriosus (PDA) occurs as a graded defect varying in severity according to the diameter of the ductal lumen. In some cases a ductus diverticulum forms when the ductal lumen closes at its pulmonary artery end but remains open over the rest of its length (Patterson, 1989).

Pathophysiology

A ductus which remains patent after birth allows the shunting of blood during systole and diastole from the high pressure in the aorta to the pulmonary artery. PDA therefore represents an arteriovenous fistula since oxygenated blood from the aorta mixes with venous blood of the pulmonary artery. Shunting of blood through the right side of the heart leads to pulmonary overcirculation, left ventricular volume overload, pulmonary venous and arterial hypertension and ultimately signs of left-sided congestive heart failure. Left ventricular and left atrial enlargement leads to mitral regurgitation which contributes to the volume overload and pulmonary venous engorgement. Pulmonary hypertension leads to pressure overload in the right ventricle and the direction of the shunt can reverse. The incidence of left heart failure and pulmonary hypertension, and the rapidity of onset of clinical signs, is associated with the size of the ductal lumen (Patterson, 1989). Occasionally PDA occurs in association with other congenital cardiac defects, for example ventricular septal defect and pulmonic stenosis.

The incidence is highest in miniature poodles, German shepherds, Border collies, Shetland sheepdogs, pomeranians and Irish setters and a predisposition for females has been reported. A polygenic mode of inheritance is suspected in most of these breeds (Patterson, 1989).

Clinical signs

Most dogs with PDA show clinical signs before one year of age and only a few cases reach adulthood undiagnosed. The clinical signs are those of left-sided heart failure. A few animals may experience syncopal episodes. Advanced cases may show signs of biventricular failure. The characteristic feature of PDA is the presence of a continuous 'machinery-type' murmur over the aortic/pulmonic valve region which may radiate to the thoracic inlet. Most 'machinery-type' murmurs are confined to a very narrow region and are associated with a palpable precordial thrill over the cranial thorax; in many cases an additional systolic murmur associated with mitral regurgitation can be located over the mitral valve region. The femoral pulse becomes jerky ('waterhammer' pulse) because of the sharp fall off in arterial pulse pressure.

Once pulmonary hypertension develops the direction of the shunt reverses. Initially the diastolic component of the murmur disappears but as the shunt reverses the murmur may disappear completely. Shunt reversal is associated with differential cyanosis. Since the patent ductus joins the aorta distal to the aortic arch the blood supply to the head and neck is preserved and only the caudal extremities become cyanotic giving rise to hindlimb weakness.

Electrocardiography

Wide P waves, tall R waves and prolonged QRS complexes reflect left atrial and left ventricular enlargement. The presence of deep Q waves and S waves in leads I, II, III and aVF is indicative of right ventricular enlargement. T waves are often deep and negative in leads II, III and aVF. Arrhythmias (atrial fibrillation and ventricular premature complexes) may be noted especially in older dogs showing severe signs of decompensation (Goodwin and Lombard, 1992). The mean electrical axis, in most cases, is within normal limits.

Radiographic findings

Left atrial and left ventricular enlargement is usually associated with signs of pulmonary over-circulation (enlargement of both the pulmonary arteries and veins) and pulmonary oedema. Classically, three knuckles or bulges may be present on the dorsoventral projection (Fig. 34.23); these represent (1) the dilated aortic arch at the one o'clock position, (2) the enlarged pulmonary artery segment at the two o'clock position and (3) the enlarged left auricular appendage at the three o'clock position. Pulmonary hypertension may result in right ventricular enlargement.

Echocardiography

Echocardiography will confirm left atrial and left ventricular enlargement. In advanced cases there may be evidence of right ventricular enlargement and chronic volume overload may result in decreased left ventricular contractility. Septal motion may be exaggerated. The patent ductus is often difficult to image. Continuous flow disturbance or turbulence and high velocity retrograde flow toward the pulmonic valve can be detected if a pulsed Doppler sample gate is placed in the main pulmonary artery.

Angiocardiography and intracardiac pressure studies

A selective injection of contrast material into the ascending aorta or aortic root should result in simultaneous opacification of the pulmonary artery and aorta. A non-selective study, using a large diameter intravenous catheter placed into the jugular vein will demonstrate a left to right shunting PDA only after contrast has reached the aorta; for this reason serial radiographs should be taken 1, 5 and 10 s after the injection of the contrast agent.

Pressure studies can be performed beforehand. Pressures in the right ventricle and pulmonary artery are increased with the pulmonary artery pressure being greater than that in the right ventricle. The pressures in the left heart may be normal. Pulmonary artery Po_2 is usually increased and is greater than the Po_2 in the right ventricle.

Prognosis

The prognosis for a young animal showing no clinical or radiographic signs of heart failure is good and surgical correction of the PDA may result in near normal life expectancy. The prognosis becomes less favourable for dogs showing signs of cardiac decompensation, especially

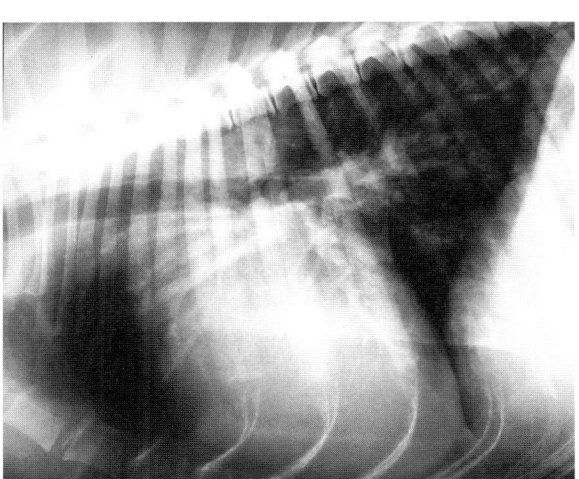
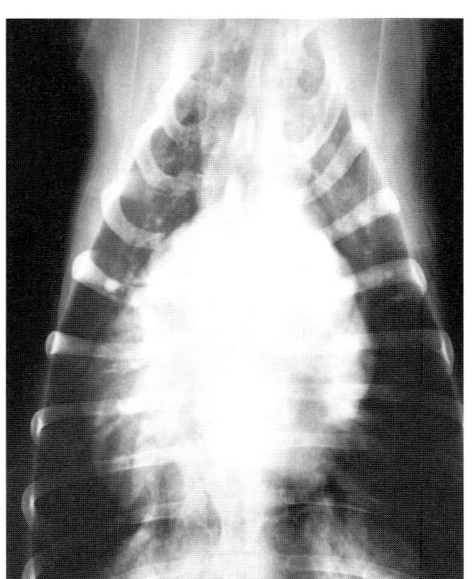

Figure 34.23 Lateral (a) and dorsoventral (b) thoracic radiographs of a 2.5-year-old female German shepherd dog with patent ductus arteriosus. Three 'knuckles' are present on the dorsoventral view representing the aorta, pulmonic artery and left auricular appendage.

where echocardiography demonstrates decreased myocardial contractility.

Treatment

Treatment of PDA usually involves double ligation of the patent vessel. A large diameter PDA may occasionally recanalize after ligation. Surgery is generally contraindicated if there is evidence of a right to left shunt. Congestive heart failure should be managed appropriately and the animal stabilized before surgery.

Aortic stenosis

Aortic stenosis can occur at three levels: (1) subvalvular; (2) valvular; and (3) supravalvular. Subvalvular aortic stenosis is the most common form in dogs; in severe cases a distinct fibrous band forms below the valve. Valvular lesions are relatively rare in the dog. Supravalvular stenosis is more common in the cat and is always associated with malformation of the aortic valve (Liu, 1977).

Pathophysiology

Aortic stenosis results in left ventricular outflow obstruction and pressure overload. The clinical presentation of aortic stenosis, as with pulmonic stenosis, relates to the severity of the outflow obstruction, the pressure gradient which develops across the aortic valve and the degree of compensatory left ventricular hypertrophy. A progressive increase in left ventricular workload leads to myocardial ischaemia which predisposes to arrhythmias and left ventricular failure. In severe cases, symmetrical concentric hypertrophy of the left ventricle and outflow tract contributes to the outflow obstruction and results in impaired diastolic filling (decreased myocardial compliance). Turbulence of blood through the stenotic region results in post-stenotic dilatation of the ascending aorta. Damage to the aortic valve leaflets and left ventricular pressure overload may result in the concurrent regurgitation of blood through aortic and mitral valves, respectively.

The highest incidence of aortic stenosis occurs in boxers, golden retrievers, German short-haired pointers and German shepherds (Patterson, 1968; Mulvihill and Priester, 1973). A genetic trait has been identified in the Newfoundland breed (Pyle et al., 1976). The high incidence in golden retrievers suggests a mode of inheritance similar to that of Newfoundlands (O'Grady et al., 1989).

Clinical signs

Dogs with mild defects often show no clinical signs and may have normal life expectancy (O'Grady et al., 1989). More severe stenosis is associated with exercise intolerance, muscular weakness and syncopal episodes. The onset of clinical signs often occurs between 6 and 10 months of age. Left-sided heart failure is uncommon in dogs with aortic stenosis; most animals die suddenly and unexpectedly probably as a result of severe ventricular arrhythmias.

Aortic stenosis is characterized by the presence of a low-grade systolic ejection-type crescendo–decrescendo murmur with a point of maximal intensity over the aortic valve region; occasionally there is a diastolic component due to aortic insufficiency. The intensity of the murmur tends to correlate with the magnitude of the outflow obstruction. The murmur may radiate up the carotid arteries and severe murmurs can occasionally be auscultated over the cranium and may be associated with a palpable precordial thrill. The murmur may also be audible over the right third or fourth intercostal spaces. The femoral pulse becomes attenuated as cardiac output falls.

Electrocardiography

Mild aortic stenosis is unlikely to cause significant electrocardiographic abnormalities. More severe lesions may result in increases in R wave amplitude and QRS duration (left ventricular enlargement), depression of the ST segment (myocardial hypoxia) and ventricular or supraventricular arrhythmias.

Radiography

Radiographs are often unremarkable. Post-stenotic dilatation of the ascending aorta may result in an enlarged aortic arch on the dorsoventral view, although this 'knuckle' may be hidden within the mediastinum, and filling of the cardiac waist on the lateral projection (Fig. 34.24). Signs of left atrial and left ventricular enlargement and left-sided failure may be present with more severe lesions or if the aortic stenosis is complicated by mitral regurgitation (O'Grady et al., 1989).

Echocardiography

Echocardiography may reveal a ring of fibrous tissue below the level of the aortic valve and is useful for confirming the presence of post-stenotic dilatation and left ventricular hypertro-

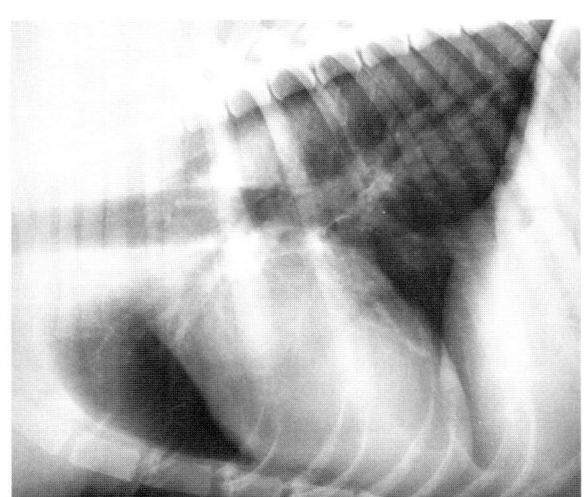
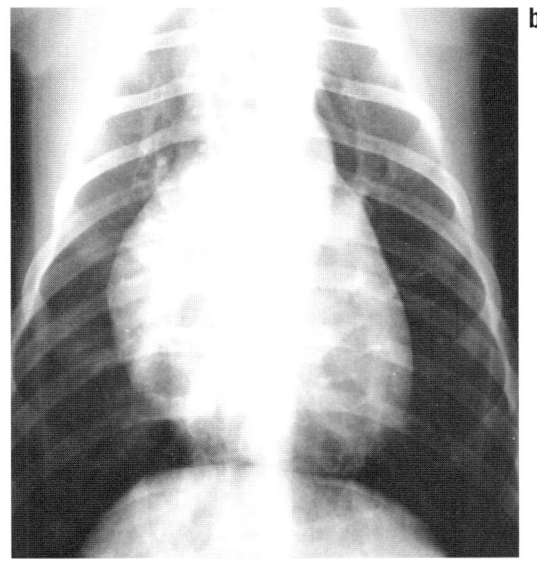

Figure 34.24 Lateral (a) and dorsoventral (b) thoracic radiographs of a 4-year-old Labrador with aortic stenosis. The cardiac silhouette is within normal dimensions for the breed but a prominent aortic knuckle is visible.

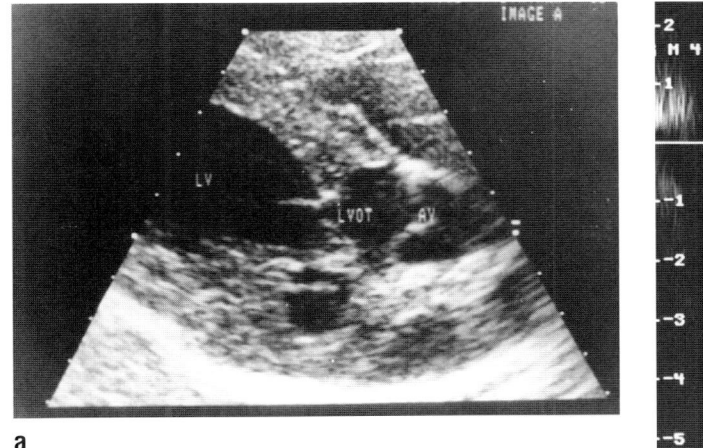
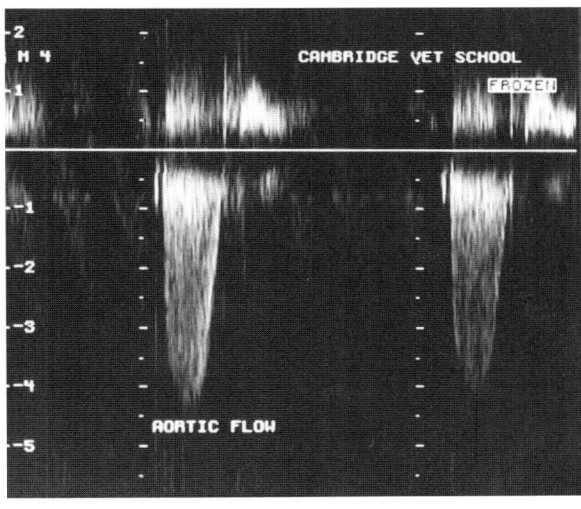

Figure 34.25 (a) Right parasternal long axis echocardiogram from a 2-year-old male Boxer with aortic stenosis showing a fibrous ring just below the aortic valve (AV) causing stenosis of the left ventricular outflow tract (LVOT). The severity can be assessed by Doppler interrogation of blood flow. (b) Continuous wave Doppler through the aortic outflow tract from a substernal approach showing peak velocity across the aortic valve of 4.25 m s^{-1} which equates to a pressure gradient of 72 mm Hg.

phy (Fig. 34.25a). Premature closure of the aortic valve during mid-systole may be evident in severe cases. Other echocardiographic features include systolic fluttering of the aortic valve, and systolic anterior motion and diastolic fluttering of the mitral valve. Left ventricular fractional shortening may be normal or increased. The severity of the lesion can be assessed by Doppler echocardiography (Fig. 34.25b). The flow velocity and pressure gradient across the aortic valve can be measured non-invasively using the Bernoulli equation (pressure = 4 × flow velocity^2) and the results correlate well with those obtained via intracardiac catheterization. Flow velocities less than 5 m s^{-1} by the time the dog reaches maturity may not significantly reduce longevity or quality of life; normal maximum aortic flow velocity is 1.5 m s^{-1} (O'Grady et al., 1989). Doppler echocardiography may also demonstrate retrograde flow of blood through the aortic valve due to aortic regurgitation. An unusual form of subaortic stenosis in combination with mitral valve dysplasia has been reported in golden retrievers (Buoscio et al., 1994).

Angiocardiography and pressure studies

Maximum pressure gradient across the aortic valve should not exceed 9 mm Hg. Moderately severe lesions have pressure gradients greater than 40 mm Hg; a pressure gradient greater than 80 mm Hg is consistent with severe stenosis and surgery is indicated.

A selective injection of contrast material into the left ventricle can be used to demonstrate left ventricular hypertrophy, subvalvular stenosis and post-stenotic dilatation (Fig. 34.26).

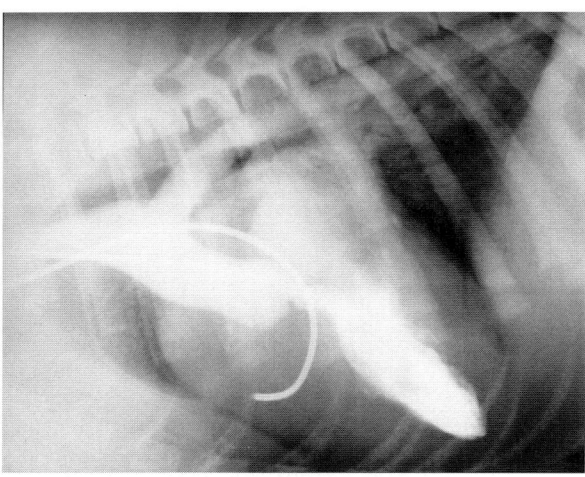

Figure 34.26 Right lateral thoracic radiograph of a 6-month-old rottweiler with aortic stenosis. Left ventricular injection of contrast demonstrates severe stenosis below the aortic valve. The curled catheter is in the right ventricle.

Prognosis

Whereas the long-term survival of dogs with untreated mild to moderate subaortic stenosis is favourable (30–50 months) most dogs with pressure gradients greater than 80 mm Hg die before three years of age (median survival 19 months; Kienle et al., 1994).

Treatment

The administration of beta-adrenergic blockers as prophylactic antiarrhythmic agents and their effect on myocardial compliance has not been fully investigated in dogs with aortic stenosis. It has been suggested, on the basis of favourable clinical reports, that beta blockers may improve diastolic filling and, by decreasing heart rate, decrease myocardial oxygen demand.

Pulmonic stenosis

Pulmonic stenosis can occur at three levels: (1) infundibular or subvalvular pulmonic stenosis may occur secondary to the valvular form and is caused by a ring of fibrous tissue surrounding the right ventricular outflow tract; (2) the valvular form which is the most common form in dogs; and (3) the supravalvular form is rare. Pulmonic stenosis is one of the components of tetralogy of Fallot. Isolated pulmonic stenosis is rare in cats.

Pathophysiology

Valvular pulmonic stenosis represents a form of pulmonic valve dysplasia. The valve leaflets are often fused or thickened and in most cases there is secondary hypertrophy of the infundibular portion of the right ventricular outflow tract (Fingland et al., 1986). The clinical signs are related to the degree of right ventricular outflow obstruction. Pulmonic stenosis causes an increased systolic pressure in the right ventricle with a systolic pressure gradient across the valve. Many dogs have mild lesions and show no clinical signs. More severe lesions lead to a pressure gradient across the pulmonic valve and pressure overload in the right ventricle. Concentric hypertrophy of the right ventricle may contribute to the outflow obstruction and a further increase in myocardial oxygen consumption. The jetting of blood through the stenotic valve may damage the valve leaflets resulting in pulmonic regurgitation and right ventricular overload. Some cases of pulmonic stenosis may be complicated by tricuspid valvular insufficiency.

The incidence of pulmonic stenosis is highest in English bulldogs, fox terriers, miniature schnauzers, chihuahuas and samoyeds (Patterson, 1989). A hereditary basis has been postulated in the beagle breed (Patterson, 1984). No sex predisposition has been reported.

Clinical signs

Clinical signs associated with pulmonic stenosis often do not become apparent until 6 months of age or older although before this the animal may appear stunted and ill thriven. The most common presenting sign is reduced exercise tolerance; more severe lesions may result in syncopal episodes and occasionally dyspnoea, cyanosis and signs of right-sided cardiac decompensation. A prominent jugular pulse due to increased right atrial pressure may be present (Fingland *et al.*, 1986). A crescendo–decrescendo systolic murmur can be heard over the pulmonic valve region; the murmur may also be audible at the thoracic inlet. Pulmonary hypertension may lead to delayed closure of the semilunar valves and a split S_2 sound. Severe murmurs may be associated with a precordial thrill.

Electrocardiography

Moderate to severe lesions consistently cause a right axis shift (>120°) and signs consistent with right ventricular enlargement (deep S and Q waves in leads I, II, III and aVF). Ventricular arrhythmias are relatively common.

Radiography

Post-stenotic dilatation of the main pulmonary artery segment may lead to an absence of the cranial waist on the lateral view and a bulge at the two o'clock position on the dorsoventral view. Right ventricular hypertrophy is manifested as a typical reverse D shape with shifting of the cardiac apex towards the left on the dorsoventral view (Fig. 34.27). Pulmonary vascularity may appear decreased.

Echocardiography

Echocardiographic findings include right ventricular hypertrophy, post-stenotic dilatation of the main pulmonary artery, abormal thickening of the pulmonic valve leaflets and flattening of the interventricular septum with paradoxical motion due to right ventricular pressure overload. The severity of the outflow obstruction can be assessed by Doppler echocardiography. A systolic pressure gradient of more than 15 mm Hg between the right ventricle and the pulmonic artery is suggestive of pulmonic stenosis.

Angiocardiography and intracardiac pressure studies

Angiocardiography and catheterization pressure studies are rarely required since both the diagnosis

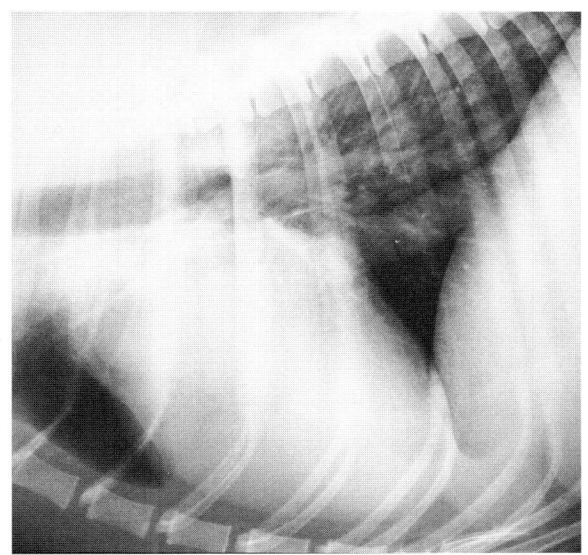
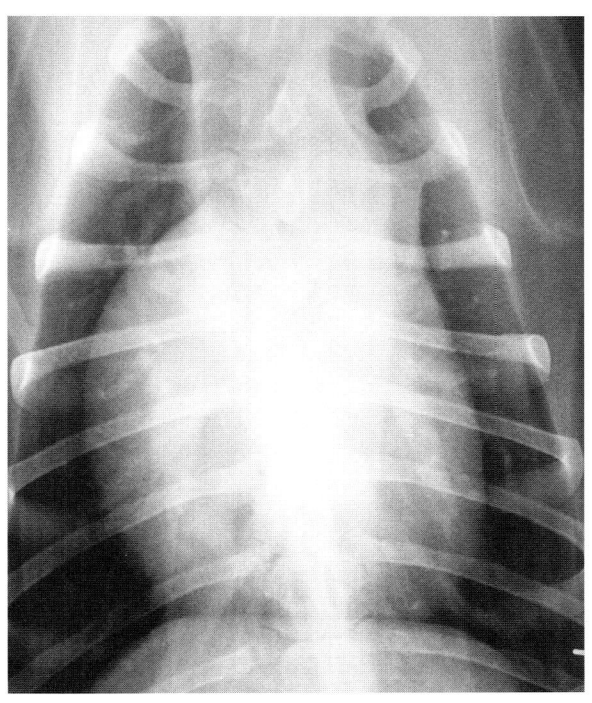

Figure 34.27 Lateral (a) and dorsoventral (b) thoracic radiographs of a 15-month-old Labrador with pulmonic stenosis. Note the increased sternal contact and filling of the cranial waist of the heart on the lateral view. A prominent pulmonic 'bulge' is evident on the dorsoventral view.

and the pressure gradient across the pulmonic valve can be assessed non-invasively by echocardiography. Non-selective or selective angiocardiographic techniques may be performed.

Treatment

The pressure gradient across the pulmonic valve should be determined before contemplating surgery. Surgery is generally indicated if the pressure gradient across the valve exceeds 70 mm Hg with evidence of severe right ventricular hypertrophy in a dog showing clinical signs. Surgical management consists of balloon dilatation of the pulmonic valve (Brownlie et al., 1991). Dogs with right ventricular systolic pressures greater than 120 mm Hg have higher 5 year mortality than dogs with right ventricular pressures less than 120 mm Hg (Fingland et al., 1986).

■ Ventricular septal defect

Ventricular septal defects (VSD) occur most frequently in keeshounds and English bulldogs and are one of the more common cardiac defects in cats (Mulvihill and Priester, 1973; Liu, 1977).

Pathophysiology

Most VSD involve the upper membranous portion of the interventricular septum and can be classified as high VSDs. The haemodynamic abnormalities, the clinical signs and progression are determined by the size of the defect. Blood normally flows from the left to the right ventricle only during systole; if pulmonary hypertension develops the direction of blood flow may reverse. An animal with a small defect may show no clinical signs. A large VSD will initially produce pulmonary overcirculation and left ventricular volume overload. Increased vascular resistance may lead to pulmonary hypertension, right ventricular pressure overload, and hypertrophy of the right ventricle and right ventricular outflow tract. Hypertrophy of the right ventricular outflow tract results in infundibular pulmonic stenosis which contributes to the right ventricular pressure overload and eventual reversal of the shunt (Eisenmenger syndrome). As with most congenital cardiac defects a VSD can occur as an isolated defect or in conjunction with other defects such as atrial septal defect, patent ductus arteriosus, aortic or pulmonic stenosis. Ventricular septal defect is also one of the components of tetralogy of Fallot. In cats most ventricular septal defects are associated with tricuspid valve dysplasia (Liu, 1977).

Clinical signs

A 'diagonal' systolic murmur with a point of maximal intensity between the 2nd and 4th right intercostal spaces and the 5th and 6th left intercostal spaces is highly suggestive of a VSD. A precordial thrill may be present. Pulmonary hypertension may be associated with splitting of the second heart sound. Shunt reversal results in attenuation of the murmur, cyanosis and ultimately signs of right-sided congestive heart failure.

Electrocardiography

Changes indicative of left ventricular, right ventricular or biventricular enlargement may be noted with a severe VSD. Arrhythmias and conduction disturbances, for example bundle branch block, have also been reported (Olivier, 1988).

Radiographic findings

Small defects are unlikely to be associated with radiographic abnormalities. The radiographic changes seen with a larger VSD are similar to those associated with a patent ductus arteriosus except that the aortic knuckle is absent and the left ventricular enlargement tends to be less pronounced. There may be evidence of generalized cardiomegaly and pulmonary overcirculation; the left atrium may appear particularly prominent. Right ventricular or biventricular enlargement is more likely to occur if the shunt reverses.

Echocardiography

A VSD high in the interventricular septum should be demonstrated in several planes. Pulsed Doppler signals from the right ventricle show high systolic blood velocities across the defect with varying degrees of turbulence and can confirm the direction of the shunt. In some dogs there may be evidence of aortic regurgitation (Sisson et al., 1991a). The left ventricle may appear hyperkinetic if the shunt is large and both the left atrium and left ventricle appear dilated. The right ventricle usually appears normal unless the shunt reverses.

Angiocardiography

Selective angiocardiography with injection of contrast material into the left ventricle can be used to confirm the presence of a left to right shunting VSD and results in simultaneous opacification of the left and right ventricles as well as the aorta and pulmonary artery.

Treatment

Small defects often require no treatment. Pulmonary banding may be considered in mature dogs with normal or only mildly increased vascular resistence to reduce flow of blood through the shunt. Anatomic repair of the defect is the only treatment likely to be effective in dogs with left to right shunts and high vascular resistance (pulmonary banding could reverse shunt flow in such cases). Dogs with bidirectional or reverse shunting VSDs are not surgical candidates.

Atrial septal defect

Atrial septal defects (ASD) are rarely diagnosed in dogs. Three types of defect have been identified: (1) a high sinus venosus ASD involves the atrial septum near the junction of the pulmonary vein and left atrium; (2) an ostium secundum ASD involves the middle portion of the atrial septum; (3) an ostium primum ASD involves the ventral atrial septum, with the ventral border of the ASD being formed by the ventricular septum or atrioventricular valves (Olivier, 1988).

Pathophysiology

An ASD usually creates a left to right shunt resulting in volume overload of the right atrium, right ventricle and pulmonary vessels. Severe dilation of the right ventricle occasionally leads to dysfunction of the tricuspid valve and tricuspid regurgitation. Occasionally an ASD occurs in combination with pulmonic stenosis.

The highest incidence of atrial septal defects occurs in Old English sheepdogs, boxers and samoyeds (Olivier, 1988).

Clinical signs

Dogs with small defects often show no clinical signs and have normal life expectancy. A more severe defect may be associated with signs of congestive heart failure (primarily respiratory signs because of the pulmonary overcirculation) and syncope. With large shunts a soft systolic murmur may be audible over the pulmonic valve region, with increased blood resulting in relative pulmonic stenosis and splitting of the second heart sound.

Electrocardiography

Electrocardiographic changes with ASD are non-specific; signs of right ventricular enlargement are occasionally present with large shunts.

Radiography

Radiographic evidence of right ventricular enlargement and pulmonary overcirculation occurs only with large shunts.

Echocardiography

A suspect ASD should be imaged in several planes and Doppler echocardiography can be used to confirm the direction of blood flow through the shunt. A non-selective injection of contrast (for example an echocardiographic bubble study) may be used in cases when reversal of the shunt is suspected.

Angiocardiography and intracardiac catheterization

The selective injection of a contrast agent into the pulmonary artery provides the most reliable method of confirming an ASD. Oxygen saturation (Sat) levels can be measured beforehand and the pulmonary to systemic flow ratio ($Q_p:Q_s$) calculated using the following equation:

$$Q_p:Q_s = (Sat_{ao} - Sat_{cvc})/(Sat_{ao} - Sat_{pa})$$

where ao=aorta, cvc=cranial vena cava and pa=pulmonary artery. Ratios greater than 2.0 are usually considered to be haemodynamically significant (Olivier, 1988).

Treatment

Most dogs with ASD do not require surgery. Surgical closure of an ASD is indicated if (1) there is progression of signs of congestive heart failure, (2) the defect is large and the $Q_p:Q_s$ is greater than 2.5, or (3) there is evidence of increased pulmonary vascular resistance and/or a right to left shunt.

Persistent common atrioventricular canal in cats

Persistent common atrioventricular canal is a common cardiac anomaly in the cat. A large ostium primum defect occurs in association with a high ventricular septal defect at the level of the coronary sinus, forming a common atrioventricular canal which is shared by all four chambers of the heart. Generalized cardiomegaly develops due to volume overload and signs of heart failure usually occur between 6 and 10 months of age. The condition is usually associated with malformation of the atrioventricular valves (Liu, 1977).

Tetralogy of Fallot

The four components of tetralogy of Fallot are (1) pulmonic stenosis (valvular, infundibular or both), (2) high ventricular septal defect, (3) compensatory right ventricular hypertrophy (secondary to pulmonic stenosis) and (4) an overriding or dextraposed aorta which means the aorta may arise from both ventricles or from the right ventricle alone.

Pathophysiology

The haemodynamic abnormalities associated with tetralogy of Fallot depend largely on the size of the VSD and degree of pulmonic stenosis. Right ventricular systolic pressure increases resulting in a variable degree of right ventricular hypertrophy. A large VSD accompanied by a minimal degree of pulmonic stenosis results in a left to right or bi-directional shunt, pulmonary overcirculation and volume overload of the left side of the heart. A minimal amount of venous, non-oxygenated blood enters the systemic circulation via the overriding aorta and therefore cyanosis is not apparent. In comparison, severe pulmonic stenosis and a large VSD leads to an increase in pulmonary vascular resistance and the development of a right to left vascular shunt. Hypertrophy of the right ventricular outflow tract and/or hypoplasia of the pulmonary artery may contribute to the pulmonic stenosis. Dogs with severe pulmonary hypertension may develop signs of right-sided heart failure.

Tetralogy of Fallot is more common in smaller breeds of dog (for example English bulldogs, poodles, and terrier breeds); in the keeshond breed tetralogy has a polygenic mode of inheritance (Patterson et al., 1974; Patterson, 1989).

Clinical signs

Most dogs with tetralogy show clinical signs during the first 6–12 months of life. Clinical signs associated with severe right to left shunts include syncope, cyanosis, and dyspnoea which may be apparent even at rest. Affected dogs often appear severely stunted and show marked exercise intolerance. Chronic hypoxia, due to shunting of unsaturated blood across the VSD, may lead to secondary polycythaemia. A systolic murmur, and occasionally a precordial thrill, typical of pulmonic stenosis can often be heard over the left 3rd intercostal space although this may become attenuated as the pressure within the right ventricle equilibrates with that in the left ventricle and blood is shunted preferentially through the aorta. A harsher holosystolic 'diagonal-type' murmur more suggestive of a VSD may be detected in cases where the pulmonic stenosis is less severe.

Electrocardiography

Most cases of tetralogy showing clinical signs have ECG changes consistent with right ventricular enlargement and a right axis shift. Signs of left-sided enlargement may be present in cases with a left to right shunting VSD.

Radiography

The classical features of tetralogy of Fallot are right ventricular enlargement and an enlarged pulmonary artery segment. Displacement of the aorta may result in a loss of the cranial waist. A right to left shunting VSD may result in hyperlucency of the lung fields due to pulmonary hypoperfusion (Fig. 34.28).

Echocardiography

Echocardiography can be used to image the high VSD, pulmonic stenosis and dextraposition of the aorta, and to confirm right ventricular hypertrophy. Other findings include reduced left atrial and left ventricular internal dimensions; hypertrophy with flattening or paradoxical motion of the interventricular septum may also be apparent. A non-selective contrast (bubble) study may help to confirm the presence of a right to left shunting VSD.

Angiocardiography and intracardiac catheterization

The non-selective injection of contrast via the jugular vein or a selective injection into the right ventricle results in simultaneous opacification of the pulmonary artery and aorta with no apparent left ventricular filling. Post-stenotic dilatation of the main pulmonary artery is usually evident (Fig. 34.29).

Right ventricular pressure increases (normal less than 35 mm Hg) and a systolic pressure gradient develops across the pulmonic valve.

CONGENITAL HEART DISEASE | 319

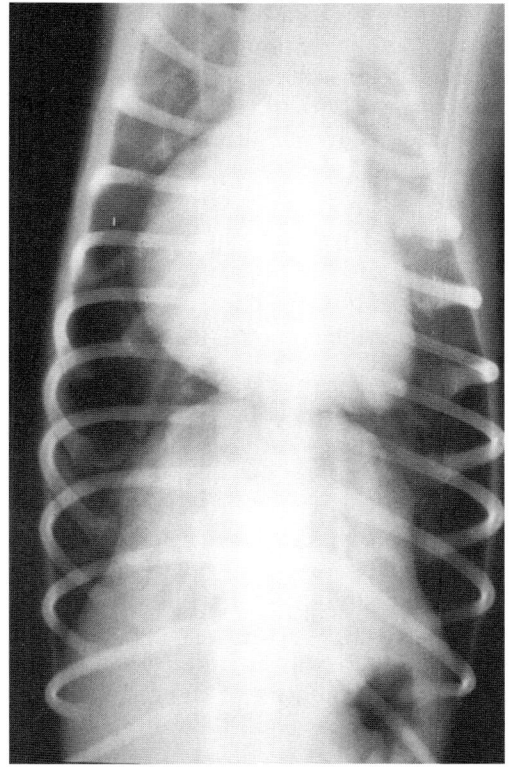

Figure 34.28 Lateral (a) and dorsoventral (b) thoracic radiographs of a month old whippet with tetralogy of Fallot. Note the hyperlucent lung fields on the lateral view and the pulmonic knuckle and prominent right ventricle on the dorsoventral view.

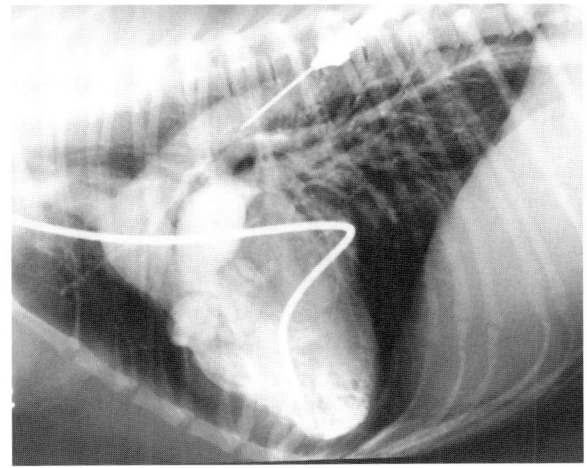

Figure 34.29 Lateral thoracic radiograph of a 14-month-old miniature poodle with tetralogy of Fallot following injection of contrast into the right ventricle. Note the simultaneous opacification of the aorta and pulmonic vasculature and the post-stenotic dilatation of the pulmonic artery. The needle is one of the ECG electrodes.

Treatment

Dogs with low pressure gradients across the pulmonic valve (less than 30 mm Hg) and a left to right shunt can be managed conservatively. The prognosis for more severe right to left shunting cases which are cyanotic is generally poor and few animals survive beyond 12–18 months of age. Although definitive surgical correction is only possible with cardiopulmonary bypass (Herrtage et al., 1983), creation of a systemic–pulmonary artery shunt, for example between the aorta and pulmonary artery (Potts anastomosis) or subclavian artery and pulmonary artery (Blalock–Taussig procedure), may increase pulmonary blood flow and systemic oxygenation (Ringwald and Bonagura, 1988). Animals which are significantly polycythaemic (PCV greater than $0.60 \, l^{-1}$) may be given aspirin to minimize the risk of thromboembolic complications. The administration of beta-adrenergic blocking drugs has been advocated although their value has not been determined.

Eisenmenger syndrome

Eisenmenger syndrome is the clinical syndrome or disease caused by the Eisenmenger complex (ventricular septal defect and pulmonary vascular disease or pulmonary hypertension resulting in the secondary right to left shunting of blood). Less precisely, Eisenmenger syndrome refers to any abnormal atrial, ventricular or vascular connection between the pulmonary and systemic circulations which results in pulmonary hypertension and the creation of a right to left shunt. The clinical signs of Eisenmenger syndrome are therefore similar to those of a reverse shunting VSD and tetralogy of Fallot.

Malformations of the atrioventricular valves

Mitral valve dysplasia

Congenital malformation of the mitral valve leaflets or associated chordae tendineae and papillary muscles is a relatively rare disorder in the dog but is probably the most common congenital cardiac defect reported in the cat (Liu, 1977). The affected valve cusps are often thickened and incomplete closure of the valve during systole results in regurgitation of blood into the left atrium. Clinical signs of left-sided congestive heart failure develop at an early age (in most cases before 6 months of age). German shepherds, great Danes, bulldogs, bull terriers and chihuahuas appear predisposed with a higher incidence in males (Mulvihill and Priester, 1973).

The pathophysiology and clinical signs of mitral dysplasia are similar to those of severe decompensated acquired mitral insufficiency. A harsh holosystolic murmur is present over the left atrioventricular valve. Electrocardiography shows changes consistent with left atrial and left ventricular enlargement and arrhythmias are common. Radiographic abnormalities include generalized or left-sided cardiomegaly (the left atrium in particular is often markedly enlarged) and pulmonary venous congestion or oedema. Echocardiography may demonstrate thickened or fused mitral valve leaflets and wide excursions of the valve leaflets during systole and diastole (Bonagura, 1994). Initially, fractional shortening may increase as the preload increases but eventually chronic volume overload leads to dilation of the left ventricle and a progressive decrease in myocardial contractility.

The prognosis for mitral dysplasia is poor. Medical management of the congestive heart failure in the form of a low salt diet, cardiac glycosides (if myocardial contractility is impaired), diuretics and vasodilators may reduce the volume of the regurgitant fraction and temporarily alleviate the clinical signs. Mitral valve replacement with a biprosthetic valve is possible with cardiopulmonary bypass (White *et al.*, 1995).

Mitral stenosis

Congenital mitral stenosis occurs infrequently in dogs often in association with subaortic stenosis; Newfoundlands and bull terriers appeared predisposed (Lehmkuhl *et al.*, 1994). A genetic basis may exist in bull terriers (Lehmkuhl *et al.*, 1994).

Mitral stenosis is usually caused by thickening and fusion of the mitral valve leaflets resulting in obstruction to the transmitral flow of blood. A diastolic pressure gradient is created across the mitral valve. Mean left atrial pressure increases resulting in left atrial enlargement and pulmonary venous congestion. Clinical signs include coughing, dyspnoea, exercise intolerance and syncope. Unlike humans where mitral stenosis is usually associated with a low-grade diastolic murmur, dogs with mitral stenosis often have a murmur typical of mitral regurgitation since most dogs develop concurrent mitral insufficiency. Radiographs show pronounced left atrial enlargement. Supraventricular arrhythmias are relatively common and echocardiography reveals abnormal diastolic motion of the mitral valve and thickened valve cusps with poor leaflet separation. Echocardiography may also detect diastolic doming of the septal mitral valve leaflet into the left ventricle in some dogs.

Dogs showing signs of congestive heart failure should be managed medically. Vasodilators and diuretics should be used cautiously since they may lead to hypotension (Lehmkuhl *et al.*, 1994).

Tricuspid valve dysplasia

Tricuspid dysplasia is less common than mitral dysplasia, the highest incidence occurring in male large breed dogs (great Danes, German shepherds, Labrador retrievers and weimaraners appear to be predisposed). In cats, tricuspid dysplasia is the second most common congenital defect next to mitral dysplasia (Liu, 1977). A harsh, regurgitant holosystolic murmur is present over the trucuspid valve region radiating across to the left side. Tricuspid regurgitation eventually leads to right ventricular volume overload and signs of right-sided congestive heart failure. A jugular pulse may be present in severe cases. An ECG may show changes consistent with right atrial and right ventricular enlargement. Radiographic evidence of tricuspid regurgitation (right-sided cardiomegaly and an enlarged caudal vena cava) is usually present. Echocardiography may show flattened or paradoxical septal motion and can be used to confirm right atrial and right ventricular dilation.

Cor triatriatum dexter

Cor triatriatum dexter is a rare congenital malformation resulting from abnormal embryonic development of the heart. Persistence of the valve of the sinus venosus results in the partitioning of the right atrium by the membranous valvular remnant into two chambers. The cranial chamber normally receives blood from the cranial vena cava and communicates with the right ventricle via a normal tricuspid valve; the caudal chamber receives blood from the caudal vena cava and communicates with the cranial chamber only via a small orifice. Affected dogs therefore tend to present with a type of right heart failure characterized by ascites and portal hypertension. The occasional dog may remain asymptomatic (Brayley et al., 1994). Definitive diagnosis of cor triatriatum is based on the results of echocardiography and non-selective angiocardiography. Selective cardiac catheterization and pressure studies may demonstrate a pressure gradient between the caudal vena cava and right atrium. Surgical removal of the anomalous septal remnant may result in resolution of clinical signs.

Persistent right aortic arch

A persistent right aortic arch is the most common vascular ring anomaly reported in dogs. The oesophagus becomes entrapped within a ring formed by the persistent right aortic arch, the left ligamentum arteriosus, the main pulmonary artery and the base of the heart. The highest incidence of vascular ring anomalies occurs in German shepherds and Irish setters and the condition may be hereditary in these breeds. Affected animals are usually stunted and thin when first presented. Food is regurgitated shortly after weaning and aspiration pneumonia may result in fever and respiratory signs.

A plain lateral thoracic radiograph may show a dilated oesophagus and ventral deviation of the trachea cranial to the heart. On the dorsoventral projection the mediastinum may appear widened with the descending aorta displaced to the right. A barium swallow can be performed to confirm constriction of the oesophagus over the heart base and dilation of the oesophagus cranial to the stricture. The condition is managed surgically by separation of the vascular ring.

MANAGEMENT OF HEART FAILURE

Understanding the pathophysiology of heart failure is the key to a logical approach to medical management. Many of the compensatory neurohormonal mechanisms which are activated in heart failure, with time, become detrimental to the animal with compromised cardiac function. This is particularly true when adaptive changes occur which lead to the renin–angiotensin system and the sympathetic nervous system acting in an unopposed manner and give rise to signs of circulatory congestion and low output.

Many treatment strategies are similar regardless of the underlying cause of heart failure. Their aim is to protect the heart from the detrimental effects of the compensatory mechanisms which operate in chronic heart failure. Nevertheless, an understanding of the underlying disease process is important. In some cases this condition may be amenable to surgical correction (for example patent ductus arteriosus, pericardial effusion), but where this is not the case, diagnosis of the disease process will allow the most appropriate drug treatment to be prescribed, as described below. It is important to remember that medical therapy does not correct the ultimate underlying cause, but merely temporarily redresses the balance of neurohormonal mechanisms so that congestive signs are controlled and the patient's quality of life improves. As the underlying disease progresses (as often happens) this becomes more difficult to achieve and the animal eventually becomes refractory to treatment.

General medical strategies for the management of heart failure

It seems obvious that if an organ is failing, the work load it has to perform should be reduced. Rest should be an integral part of any treatment plan for a heart failure patient. Reducing the level of activity of the animal will reduce tissue perfusion requirements and therefore cardiac work load. Work load of the heart can also be reduced pharmacologically. Since most cases require a combination of drugs consideration should be given to any drug incompatibilities.

Diuretics

Diuretic therapy is fundamental to the medical management of congestive heart failure (Michell,

1988a). The basic aim of using these drugs is to oppose the compensatory mechanisms which, by stimulating retention of sodium and water, elevate central venous and cardiac filling pressures. By lowering cardiac filling pressure, diuretics reduce cardiac preload and thus the work of the heart muscle. It must be remembered, however, that reducing cardiac filling pressure could potentially reduce the force of cardiac muscle contraction. Judicious use of diuretics will be beneficial in those patients who are operating on the relatively flat portion of the cardiac function curve (Fig. 34.30) where the fall in cardiac filling pressure occurs with little or no decrease in cardiac output. It is also important to realize that dietary salt restriction and drugs with a venodilator action will also reduce cardiac filling pressure and will act synergistically with diuretics.

Other beneficial actions of diuretics include fluid mobilization from blood vessel walls which increases their compliance and their responsiveness to vasodilator drugs. In addition, some diuretic drugs (most notably frusemide) are thought to have a venodilator action of their own, particularly when administered by the intravenous route.

The site of action of the diuretic drugs used in the treatment of heart failure is the nephron where tubular transport processes for reabsorption of sodium are inhibited. The potency of these drugs as diuretics and the side effects (in terms of electrolyte and acid–base disturbances) which result from their use, depends on their site of action within the nephron.

Potassium-losing diuretics

Frusemide

Frusemide is the only loop diuretic which is licensed for veterinary use. By inhibiting the co-transport of sodium, potassium and chloride ions in the loop of Henle, loop diuretics are the most efficacious diuretics available, being capable of stimulating the loss of up to 20% of the filtered load of sodium ions. Loop diuretics also promote loss of potassium, magnesium and calcium in the urine. Excessive loss of potassium and magnesium may have detrimental consequences for other

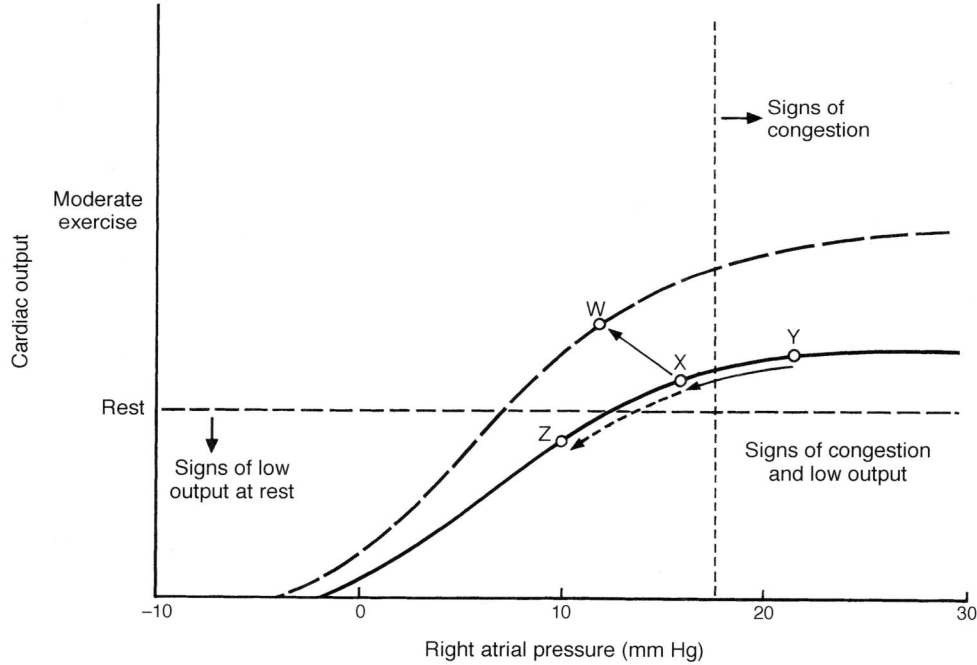

Figure 34.30 Schematic representation of the cardiac function curve of an animal in Stage 3 heart failure who is showing signs of circulatory congestion with normal activity (curve III, solid line). Therapeutic measures (diuretics, vasodilation) to reduce cardiac filling pressures, if used judiciously, may move the patient from point X to point Y and hence relieve signs of congestion without leading to problems of low output at rest. Indeed, the reduction in wall tension which results from treatment may allow the heart to function more efficiently at lower filling pressures, moving from point X to point W as the cardiac function curve shifts upwards and to the left. If diuretics and vasodilation are used in an overzealous fashion, filling pressures will be excessively reduced (moving to point Z) leading to problems of low output even at rest.

drug therapies, for example cardiac glycosides and certain antidysrhythmic drugs. Frusemide can be administered orally or parenterally. In cases of severe pulmonary oedema due to left-sided heart failure, the intravenous administration of frusemide (up to 4 mg kg^{-1}) is indicated. Frusemide is thought to have venodilator actions on the pulmonary vasculature which occur more rapidly than its natriuretic effects and these contribute to its therapeutic action in the management of cardiogenic pulmonary oedema. Following intravenous administration, the onset of action of frusemide peaks at 30 min and returns to baseline within 2–3 h. When administered orally, the absorption of frusemide from the intestine can be variable in terms of rate and extent. This may be affected by the formulation of the preparation, the individual animal and the degree of congestion in the intestinal circulation. It is important to recognize that the dose required varies for each individual patient according to its physiological state and to the pharmacological effects of concurrent therapies (vasodilators, dietary salt restriction and other diuretics) which may be employed (Fox, 1992). In general, cats are more sensitive to frusemide than are dogs and unless lower dosages are used in the cat serious side effects may result.

Hydrochlorothiazide

Hydrochlorothiazide is a thiazide diuretic which works by interfering with sodium transport in the early distal tubule and is capable of causing excretion of up to 10% of the filtered load of sodium in the urine. Excessive loss of both potassium and magnesium in the urine will occur with thiazide diuretics but they reduce urinary loss of calcium. Hydrochlorothiazide can be administered by intramuscular injection or orally (2–4 mg kg^{-1}). The absorption of orally administered drug will be affected by the state of the intestinal circulation and in cases of refractory right-sided heart failure, parenteral administration may be more successful. The duration of action of hydrochlorothiazide is longer than frusemide with effects being evident for up to 12 hours after administration.

Adverse effects of potassium-losing diuretics

Overzealous use of diuretic drugs will lead to a fall in cardiac output and arterial blood pressure due to excessive reduction in cardiac filling pressure. This will lead to clinical signs of dehydration, weakness due to poor muscle perfusion, and azotaemia due to reduced renal blood flow and a consequent decrease in glomerular filtration rate. In addition, particularly in animals which are anorectic, excessive potassium loss in the urine can result in hypokalaemia. This may contribute to the state of muscle weakness, cause gastrointestinal and renal problems, predispose to the development of cardiac arrhythmias and enhance the toxicity of cardiac glycosides (Brobst, 1986). Monitoring plasma potassium and urea concentrations in animals on diuretic therapy is good clinical practice as it allows early correction of hypokalaemia and prerenal azotaemia. Hypomagnesaemia may contribute to the adverse effects of loop and thiazide diuretics although less information is available from veterinary patients (Cobb and Michell, 1992). The animals most susceptible to these problems are cats which are often anorectic and azotaemic on presentation and become dehydrated very rapidly when challenged with potent diuretics (particularly frusemide). Provided appetite remains reasonably good, diuretic-induced hypokalaemia is less likely to be significant.

Potassium-sparing diuretics

These drugs are relatively weak diuretics when used alone as their site of action is in the late distal tubule of the nephron (they promote the loss of < 5% of the filtered load of sodium). If combined with frusemide or thiazide diuretics they will reduce potassium loss stimulated by such drugs. Spironolactone (an aldosterone receptor antagonist), amiloride and triamterene (which block sodium entry into distal tubular cells via aldosterone-mediated pathways) are potassium sparing diuretics used in human medicine. These drugs will also reduce magnesium loss in the urine. Combined preparations of thiazides and these drugs are available. It should be remembered that angiotensin converting enzyme (ACE) inhibitors (see vasodilator drug therapy) also reduce aldosterone secretion and so can be considered potassium-sparing diuretics. It is not recommended that conventional potassium-sparing diuretics are used with ACE inhibitors since hyperkalaemia could result. Dietary potassium supplementation is an alternative strategy to prevent hypokalaemia resulting from the use of potassium-losing diuretics.

Vasodilator drug therapy

The rationale behind using vasodilator drugs in the management of heart failure is to reduce the work load on the failing heart both by decreasing excessive cardiac filling pressures (by reducing preload; venodilation) and by reducing the resistance against which the heart has to work to pump the blood around the circulation (by reducing afterload; arterial vasodilation). The use of these drugs is an attempt to restore the balance between vasoconstrictor neurohormonal mechanisms activated by poor cardiac function and the natural vasodilator mechanisms which are reduced in chronic heart failure. The balance is delicate since excessive preload reduction may result in poor cardiac output once the cardiac filling pressure is reduced to the steep part of the cardiac function curve (see Fig. 34.30). Excessive afterload reduction may reduce arterial blood pressure to such a level that tissue perfusion is reduced and clinical signs of hypotension result. Vasodilator drugs are classified according to whether they act primarily on arterioles (arteriolar dilators), veins (venodilators) or on both sides of the circulation (balanced dilators).

Arteriolar dilators

Hydralazine has a spasmolytic effect on arteriolar vascular smooth muscle, the precise mechanism of action of which remains unknown. In veterinary medicine it has been most successfully used in the management of dogs with mitral regurgitation (Kittleson *et al.*, 1983). By lowering systemic vascular resistance (arterial dilation) with hydralazine, the aim is to encourage blood to follow the normal pathway from the left ventricle rather than regurgitating through the mitral valve, thus increasing the forward flow through the aorta. Ideally, dogs given hydralazine should be hospitalized and monitored closely. Following oral administration, the onset of action of hydralazine is 30–60 min with peak effect at 3–5 h and duration of effect for 11–13 h. The dose of hydralazine required varies between individual dogs and a starting dose of 0.5 mg kg^{-1} every 12 h is recommended and this can be increased to effect up to 3 mg kg^{-1}. Effective treatment will result in improvement of mucous membrane colour, capillary refill time and arterial pulse pressure in addition to resolving signs of circulatory congestion. The decrease in arterial blood pressure which occurs with effective treatment is subclinical but may cause reflex activation of the sympathetic nervous system and the renin–angiotensin–aldosterone systems. Combined use of hydralazine with diuretic therapy will prevent excessive sodium and water retention occurring in response to the small falls in arterial blood pressure which occur with effective doses of hydralazine. Weakness, lethargy and tachycardia indicate an excessive decrease in peripheral resistance resulting in clinical hypotension and these signs will occur with overdosage. Some 20–30% of dogs treated with hydralazine show signs of vomiting and anorexia which may be intractable, thus forcing withdrawal of the drug. These side effects may account for the unpopularity of this medication in veterinary medicine.

Venodilator drugs

Organic nitrates are routinely used in human medicine for the treatment of angina, where reduction of venous return and cardiac preload relieves angina attacks by reducing the work and therefore oxygen demand of the ischaemic myocardium. Glyceryl trinitrate (nitroglycerin) is taken sublingually in human patients to avoid the excessive first pass hepatic metabolism which follows gastrointestinal absorption of the drug. Alternatively, the percutaneous route of administration can be used. This is the route recommended for use in dogs and cats where the drug is applied in ointment form to shaved or hairless areas of skin (gloves should be worn when administering the drug). Dosing is empirical at a rate of 0.5–5 cm every 6–8 h. No pharmacokinetic studies have been performed in dogs or cats to determine the bioavailability of glyceryl trinitrate following percutaneous administration and the efficiency of absorption across dog skin has been questioned (DeLellis and Kittleson, 1992). Little information is available concerning the use of the orally active organic nitrate, isosorbide dinitrate in the dog and cat. Continuous use of these drugs in humans results in tolerance (Parker, 1992).

Balanced vasodilators

Sodium nitroprusside

Sodium nitroprusside is a potent arteriolar and venodilator drug with a similar mechanism of action to the organic nitrates. It has a very short duration of action and is administered by continuous intravenous infusion starting at an initial infusion rate of 1–5 µg kg^{-1} min^{-1}. It reduces pulmonary and systemic vascular resistance decreasing ventricular filling pressure and is most useful in the management of acute, life-threatening cardiogenic pulmonary oedema. The dose can be titrated upwards to effect whilst monitoring arterial blood pressure since excessive falls in arterial blood pressure are an indication of overdosage. The effects are reversed within 1–10 min of slowing the infusion rate allowing fine control of the drug's effects. Since delivery of the drug requires accurate control at a low rate of fluid administration, an infusion pump should be used. In dogs with severe cardiac failure resulting from poor systolic function (dilated cardiomyopathy), a drug providing positive inotropic support (for example dobutamine) is required in addition to sodium nitroprusside, otherwise the reduction in preload caused by venodilation may result in a precipitous fall in cardiac output. Intravenous infusion of sodium nitroprusside should not exceed 48 h since toxic metabolites (thiocyanate) build up in the circulation. Infusions should be stopped gradually rather than abruptly to prevent rebound increases in vascular resistance and cardiac filling pressures.

Prazosin

Prazosin is a balanced vasodilator drug which can be given orally to dogs. It is an alpha$_1$-selective adrenoceptor antagonist which blocks excessive sympathetic stimulation of vascular alpha$_1$-adrenoceptors without affecting the autoinhibition of noradrenaline release by presynaptic alpha$_2$-adrenoceptors. The recommended dosage is 1 mg tid for dogs weighing less than 15 kg and 2 mg tid for dogs weighing more than 15 kg. In humans and experimental animals, although prazosin is very effective initially, with repeated dosing its effects become attenuated, possibly as the renin–angiotensin system assumes greater importance in regulating vascular tone.

Angiotensin converting enzyme inhibitors

Given the effects of angiotensin II which are central to the pathophysiology of chronic heart failure, the effects of drugs which inhibit the formation of angiotensin II by inhibition of angiotensin converting enzyme (ACE) are predictable. They are balanced vasodilators and will enhance the excretion of sodium and water by reducing circulating levels of aldosterone and ADH; thus they have a potassium-sparing diuretic effect. Angiotensin converting enzyme is also responsible for the breakdown of the natural vasodilator, bradykinin and some of the effects of ACE inhibitors can be attributed to potentiating bradykinin. Their effects on the vasculature are less profound and slower to take effect when compared to hydralazine and nitroprusside (Kittleson et al., 1993), hence these drugs are preferred to the ACE inhibitors when dealing with cases of life-threatening pulmonary oedema due to left-sided heart failure. Indeed, clinical signs may continue to improve for several weeks in human heart failure patients on ACE inhibitors and multicentre controlled clinical trials in veterinary medicine suggest that the same is true in veterinary medicine. Small but significant effects have been demonstrated on survival time of dogs with dilated cardiomyopathy and mitral valvular heart disease treated with enalapril (COVE Study Group, 1995)

Captopril was the first ACE inhibitor to be produced. It contains a sulphydryl group which causes certain side effects which are common to sulphydryl compounds, namely alterations in taste perception, proteinuria and drug-induced blood dyscrasias (Jaffe, 1986). The recommended dosage is 0.5–2.0 mg kg^{-1} three times daily. Oral absorption is reduced by food. Exceeding the upper limit of this dose gives no further beneficial therapeutic effect but increases the drug's toxicity. Angiotensin II may maintain glomerular filtration pressures in the face of poor renal perfusion by constricting the efferent arteriole more than the afferent arteriole. Removal of this protective mechanism may precipitate acute renal failure in some patients with subclinical, pre-existing renal dysfunction. Hence blood plasma urea and creatinine should be determined in animals before and after they are put on ACE inhibitors. As with other vasodilator drugs, hypotension is a possible side effect, particularly if used in combination with high doses of diuretics. In humans, ACE inhibition has been associated with a drug-induced cough.

Enalapril is an ACE inhibitor with significant advantages over captopril (Allen et al., 1987). It does not possess a sulphydryl group and so lacks the associated side effects mentioned above. It is a pro-drug, the active form being a metabolite, enalaprilat, formed by the liver. The onset of action is slower than captopril and its duration of effect is longer (12–14 h). Recommended dosing in dogs is 0.5–1.0 mg kg^{-1} every 12–24 h and in cats is 0.25 mg kg^{-1} every 12 h. Side effects are those associated with ACE inhibition described above for captopril.

Benazepril is an ACE inhibitor recently licensed for veterinary use. It shares many properties with enalapril, lacking a sulphydryl group and being a pro-drug. In addition, the excretion of the active metabolite from the body occurs both in the bile and the urine. This contrasts with enalapril, which is eliminated in the urine only where dose adjustment may be necessary in animals with significant impairment of renal function. The recommended dose rate of benazepril for the dog is 0.25 to 0.5 mg kg^{-1} orally every 24 hours. Currently, there is no authorized dose rate for cats.

Drugs which alter the force of cardiac muscle contraction

In cardiac failure due to poor myocardial systolic function, administration of drugs which increase the force with which the cardiac muscle contracts seems a logical strategy to adopt. Such drugs should increase stroke volume, reduce end-systolic ventricular volume and reverse the neurohormonal reflexes which occur in response to poor cardiac output, thus allowing the heart to function more efficiently at lower filling pressures. A counter argument might, however, be that in myocardial systolic failure the heart muscle should be rested not stimulated to contract more forcefully (Michell, 1988b). In some cases of heart failure (for example during the early stages of valvular heart disease), myocardial systolic function is normal and the administration of positive inotropic agents would seem unnecessary. In other situations, disorders of myocardial relaxation are responsible for the failure of cardiac function (for example hypertrophic cardiomyopathy). Here, drugs which increase the force of contraction are inappropriate and drugs which enhance the ability of cardiac muscle to relax are indicated.

Positive inotropic agents

An ideal positive inotropic agent should increase the force of contraction of cardiac muscle at a given degree of end-diastolic stretch without reducing efficiency of energy use, increasing the heart rate or predisposing to cardiac arrhythmias. The drug should also lack vasoconstrictor action on peripheral blood vessels.

Drugs which enhance myocardial intracellular cyclic AMP concentration

Beta-adrenergic agonists and phosphodiesterase type III/IV inhibitors will both raise intracellular cyclic AMP and increase myocardial contractility. The synthetic catecholamine, dobutamine is the beta-adrenoceptor agonist of choice since it has selective action on beta$_1$ adrenoceptors and at dose rates which increase the force of contraction ($3–7$ µg kg^{-1} min^{-1}), it has minimal effects on heart rate and no vasoconstrictor effects. It is used in the intensive care of severe myocardial systolic failure. It is rapidly taken up and metabolized by the tissues and has to be given by continuous intravenous infusion, the rate of which should be accurately controlled by an infusion pump. Continuous ECG monitoring is required to detect increases in heart rate and the onset of arrhythmias which are indicative of toxicity. Some studies in human medicine have suggested long-term beneficial effects even following brief dobutamine infusions (Laing et al., 1984). Similar studies have not been reported in veterinary medicine and the cost of the drug may be prohibitive for many patients.

The bypyridine compounds amrinone and milrinone (phosphodiesterase type III/IV inhibitors) were heralded as having great promise on their introduction, being potent positive inotropes with little effect on heart rate and possessing mild arteriolar vasodilator activity (Colucci et al., 1986). Indeed, initial studies of the use of milrinone in dogs with systolic failure (which is orally active) proved promising (Kittleson et al., 1985b, 1987; Keister et al., 1990). Unfortunately, no placebo-controlled trials have been performed in veterinary medicine and human studies have shown a detrimental effect of milrinone on long-term survival in patients with chronic congestive heart failure (Packer et al., 1991). Such findings cast serious doubt on the future of such drugs. Indeed, it has been suggested that any drug which produces its positive inotropic effects by raising cyclic AMP in the myocardium will have long-term detrimental effects (Packer, 1992b) in the same way as chronic exposure of the myocardium to high concentrations of catecholamines is thought to be toxic (Mann et al., 1992).

Cardiac glycosides

Controversy over the use of this group of drugs in the management of heart failure has been present in the literature of both human and veterinary medicine for many years, yet their popularity among clinicians survives (Lewis, 1990; Snyder and Atkins, 1992). Most would agree that the primary indication for cardiac glycosides is in the management of supraventricular tachycardia, particularly where this co-exists with systolic myocardial dysfunction, as is often the case in dilated cardiomyopathy in dogs. The controversy surrounds their use in heart failure patients which are in normal sinus rhythm and results of large-scale controlled trials in human medicine are only beginning to be reported (Packer et al., 1991).

The classical actions of cardiac glycosides on the failing heart are to increase the force of contraction of the heart muscle and decrease the heart rate via a number of both central and peripheral effects which result in increased vagal tone to the heart. In addition, other reflex effects occur which inhibit both sympathetic nerve and renin–angiotensin system activity. The ability of the drugs to increase the sensitivity of cardiac and arterial baroreceptors so that they respond to lower pressures leading to a reduction in sympathetic tone may underlie these beneficial circulatory effects which are now thought to occur independently of any positive inotropic action (Ferguson et al., 1989). These effects give sound reasons for employing cardiac glycosides in heart failure patients where systolic muscle function is not affected (such as valvular heart disease) although alternative means of achieving these effects now exist (for example ACE inhibitors).

Digoxin is the only cardiac glycoside which currently is readily available for use by the veterinary practitioner. The narrow therapeutic index of glycosides means that the digoxin dosage should be accurately calculated for each animal. In dogs, less than 20 kg a dose of 0.005–0.01 mg kg^{-1} bid is recommended whereas dogs greater than 20 kg in weight should receive 0.22 mg m^{-2} bid (a total dose of 0.25 mg bid should not be exceeded). The dosages should theoretically be based on lean body weight. Dosing on a twice daily basis prevents large peaks and troughs in plasma concentration. The half-life of digoxin in the dog is reported to be 23–39 h. In the cat, a dose of 0.01 mg kg^{-1} every other day is recommended and a 30% reduction should be made if aspirin and frusemide are administered concurrently (Atkins et al., 1988). Renal excretion of digoxin is an important route of elimination and reduced renal function will lead to toxicity occurring at these dose rates. Food will reduce the rate of absorption of digoxin from the gastrointestinal tract and the absorption characteristics will vary from one formulation to another. Use of digoxin can be facilitated by monitoring serum levels of the drug which should fall between 1.0 and 2.5 ng ml^{-1}. This therapeutic range should be achieved within three to five half-lives of starting therapy (that is within 3–5 days). Rapid digitalization by giving loading doses is rarely necessary and is associated with a higher incidence of toxicity.

Signs of digoxin toxicity (anorexia and vomiting) are due to the effects of the drug on the chemoreceptor trigger zone in the medulla. In addition, myocardial toxicity will result in cardiac arrhythmias, particularly of ventricular origin. Unfortunately, myocardial toxicity can occur without gastrointestinal signs, particularly in dogs with myocardial systolic failure. Hypokalaemia and hypomagnesaemia caused by diuretic therapy will enhance the toxicity of digoxin so blood plasma electrolyte concentrations should be monitored. Concurrent use of other drugs such as quinidine and verapamil will also increase the risk of toxicity, therefore a reduction in digoxin dosage should be made if these drugs are given in combination. In managing digoxin toxicity, electrolyte abnormalities should be corrected and ventricular arrhythmias treated with lignocaine (see below).

Negative inotropes

It might seem somewhat illogical to suggest the use of drugs which reduce the force of cardiac muscle contractility in an animal suffering the consequences of inadequate cardiac performance. However, if the effects of chronic stimulation of the myocardium by catecholamines are indeed harmful to the myocardium (Mann et al., 1992), drugs which antagonize these effects (beta-blockers) may be beneficial. In addition, beta-blockers will reduce sympathetic stimulation of renin by renal nerves, thus inhibiting angiotensin II production. The danger, however, in the short term, is removal of positive inotropic support and a deterioration in heart failure signs (low output and congestion). Nevertheless, encouraging results have been produced from clinical studies in people with dilated cardiomyopathy where long-term use of beta-blockers has produced positive effects on exercise tolerance and survival (Englemeier et al., 1985; Gilbert et al., 1990). Their use in veterinary medicine in this disease has yet to be critically examined.

In cases of heart failure due to diastolic dysfunction (hypertrophic cardiomyopathy) the use of negative inotropes in the absence of signs of congestion is an accepted form of treatment. Here, beta-blockers have been the mainstay of treatment, reducing heart rate, systolic outflow tract gradients and myocardial oxygen demand and so controlling myocardial ischaemia and arrhythmias. Any documented beneficial effects that beta-blockers may have on diastolic function (relaxation of the ventricular muscle) are inconsistent and there are theoretical reasons why beta-blockers might impair relaxation of cardiac muscle. By contrast, the calcium channel blocker, diltiazem, has been shown to improve ventricular muscle relaxation time and is beneficial in the management of feline hypertrophic cardiomyopathy (Bright et al., 1991). The recommended dosage of 0.5–2.5 mg tid proves problematic in the UK since the smallest tablet size available is 60 mg.

In conclusion, the medical management of heart failure often involves the use of multiple drug therapy (particularly in the chronic stages) in an attempt to allow the heart to function adequately at lower filling pressures. Knowledge of the underlying disease process will assist in the selection of the most appropriate drug(s) and a basic understanding of the pharmacology of the drugs will allow drug interactions and toxicity to be predicted, monitored for and avoided.

MANAGEMENT OF CARDIAC ARRHYTHMIAS

Abnormalities in the generation and/or the conduction of electrical impulses in the heart can give rise to an overall reduction in the heart rate (bradydysrhythmias) or a rapid heart rate (tachydysrhythmias). In both circumstances, cardiac function may be compromised. Slow rates (<50 bpm) lead to inadequate output despite a very large stroke volume and fast irregular rhythms lead to insufficient time for adequate filling of the heart during diastole, thus giving rise to low stroke volume. In addition, tachycardias which encroach on diastole will reduce the time for myocardial blood flow and lead to ischaemia of the heart muscle. In any situation where cardiac function is already compromised, the development of an arrhythmia will tend to lead to decompensation and result in clinical signs of heart failure. Severe arrhythmias may give rise to an acute decrease in cardiac output and poor perfusion of the brain leading to loss of consciousness (syncope). It is important to remember that the presence of a cardiac arrhythmia does not necessarily indicate a primary cardiac problem; it may be an indication of a number of systemic problems (for example electrolyte, neurological, gastrointestinal disorders and circulatory shock of non-cardiac origin).

In some circumstances, the underlying cause of the arrhythmia will be amenable to specific treatment or will be self-limiting and the arrhythmia will resolve without anti-arrhythmic drug treatment. In other cases, the effects of the arrhythmia may be life-threatening or the underlying cause either cannot be diagnosed or is not amenable to treatment. Here, symptomatic anti-arrhythmic drug therapy is indicated. It is important to recognize those situations where cardiac arrhythmias may occur so that they can be detected early and the patient can be monitored to determine whether anti-arrhythmic therapy is necessary.

In the following discussion of the management of different cardiac arrhythmias, a brief overview of the possible underlying causes is given followed by practical decisions concerning therapy and the realistic goals of such therapy. The diagnostic electrocardiographic features of specific cardiac arrhythmias are described in Table 34.3.

Bradycardia

Symptomatic bradycardia results from problems of impulse generation in the sinus node and/or its conduction from the atria to the ventricles. Both of these processes are influenced by the autonomic nervous system with the parasympathetic system slowing and the sympathetic system accelerating impulse generation and conduction.

Table 34.9 Non-cardiac causes of symptomatic bradycardia and their management

Cause	Management
Hypothermia	Increase core temperature by administration of warm fluids
Hyperkalaemia	
Renal failure (oliguric)	Diagnose and treat the underlying cause
Hypoadrenocorticism	Promote urine output by giving potassium free intravenous fluids
Severe metabolic acidosis	Emergency treatment to protect the heart if necessary (calcium gluconate, sodium bicarbonate, insulin and glucose)
Neurological diseases	
Raised intracranial pressure	Diagnose and give specific treatment for the underlying cause
Meningoencephalitis	Antimuscarinic therapy (e.g. atropine) to increase heart rate.
Drugs	Specific therapy
Alpha$_2$ adrenoceptor agonist sedatives	Alpha$_2$ adrenoceptor antagonists
Beta-adrenoceptor antagonists	Beta-adrenoceptor agonists
Calcium channel blocking drugs	Intravenous calcium gluconate
Cardiac glycosides	Digoxin antibodies
Phenothiazines (especially acepromazine)	Atropine

Non-cardiac causes of bradycardia

Sinus bradycardia is often a normal finding in athletic dogs (50 bpm or below) and is rarely associated with clinical signs. Even in dogs showing signs of vague illness, such as lethargy, which demonstrate mild sinus bradycardia, use of drugs which increase the heart rate (for example atropine) does not usually improve their behaviour. Profound symptomatic bradycardia may be caused by a number of factors which do not involve organic cardiac disease, some of which are shown in Table 34.9. In many cases it is an alteration in the balance between parasympathetic and sympathetic tone to the heart which results in bradycardia so that therapy with antimuscarinic drugs (particularly where vagal tone is raised) or beta-adrenoceptor agonists is indicated to increase heart rate together with supportive therapy such as intravenous fluids and warmth. It is important to consider the underlying cause before using such symptomatic therapy as it may not always be indicated. For example, use of atropine to control bradycardia following the administration of an alpha$_2$-adrenoceptor agonist may potentiate the transient hypertension which results after administration of such drugs to dogs and cats. Administration of beta-adrenoceptor agonists to increase the heart rate in a dog with bradycardia due to digoxin toxicity would increase the potential for ventricular tachycardia to develop. Thus, where possible, specific therapy should be administered based on the diagnosis of the underlying cause. These extrinsic factors should be considered before diagnosing the cause of symptomatic bradycardia as being due to organic disease of the sinoatrial node or of the conducting pathways in the heart (see below).

Symptomatic bradycardia associated with organic cardiac disease

Sick sinus syndrome

This term is used to describe idiopathic disorders of the sinoatrial node, where the animals show signs of intermittent sinus arrest, sinoatrial block or sinus bradycardia. The subsidiary pacemakers fail to generate adequate escape rhythms. Some cases also show intermittent supraventricular tachyarrhythmias which may contribute to the clinical signs. This is a heterogeneous and imprecisely defined group of conditions rather than a single disease. Miniature schnauzers, pugs and dachshunds have been reported as presenting with this syndrome but it has also been seen in mixed breed dogs. In the management of this condition (see below), it is important to manage the bradycardia first before treatment of the tachycardic episodes can be undertaken safely.

Persistent atrial standstill ('silent atrium')

In persistent atrial standstill the sinus node fails to generate electrical impulses and the heart rate is governed by supraventricular, junctional or ventricular escape beats. This condition is rare in dogs and cats and should be distinguished from the potentially reversible sinoventricular rhythm which accompanies severe and life-threatening hyperkalaemia

Atrioventricular block

Failure or delay in the conduction of the sinoatrial impulse may be classified as first, second (Mobitz type I and II) or third degree atrioventricular (AV) block (Table 34.3). In some cases, heart block can be intermittent and therefore more difficult to diagnose without the use of a continuous ambulatory ECG. First degree AV block and Mobitz type I second-degree AV block are common in the dog and rarely signify intrinsic disease of the conducting system. They are easily abolished following exercise or atropine administration (0.02–0.04 mg kg^{-1} i.m. or i.v.). Atropine may cause an initial increase in the severity of the block (by a central action) but within 10–15 min sinus rhythm results. By contrast, in the cat even low-grade heart block is an abnormal finding and warrants further investigation.

Idiopathic persistent high-grade second-degree (Fig. 34.31) and complete (third degree) AV block (Fig. 34.32) occur in middle-aged or older dogs and are often associated with clinical signs. These may consist of weakness, exercise intolerance and syncope. In chronic cases signs of congestive heart failure may develop. In some cases, underlying causes such as infiltrative myocardial disease, hypertrophic cardiomyopathy or bacterial endocarditis may be present. Idiopathic third degree AV block has been reported in the dog in association with acquired myasthenia gravis (Hackett et al., 1995). If obvious organic heart disease can be identified, the prognosis is much worse than for idiopathic cases where no obvious pathological process can be detected. Drug toxicity (calcium channel blockers, digoxin, beta-adrenoceptor antagonists) or electrolyte disturbances (hyperkalaemia) should be ruled out as possible causes of AV block.

Medical management of symptomatic bradycardia due to organic heart disease

Pacemaker implantation is the only long-term solution to animals exhibiting high-grade second-

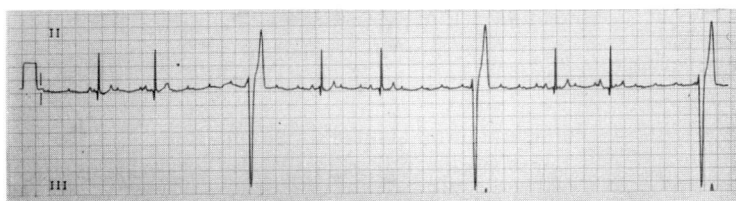

Figure 34.31 Second degree atrioventricular heart block. Note the non-conducted P waves and regular ventricular escape complexes.

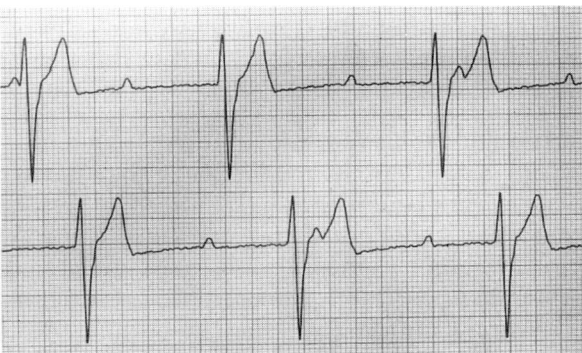

Figure 34.32 Complete (third degree) atrioventricular heart block. The P waves present are not related to the QRS complexes which are abnormal and represent an idioventricular escape rhythm.

degree or complete AV block, persistent atrial standstill, and many cases of sick sinus syndrome. In an emergency, heart rate can be best increased by using beta-adrenoceptor agonists such as isoprenaline (10 ng kg^{-1} min^{-1}) or dopamine (2–10 µg kg^{-1} min^{-1}), given by continuous intravenous infusion. An oral dose rate of isoprenaline has been described (5–10 mg three to four times daily) but there is less scope for the clinician to control the effects of the drug. Dopamine is the preferred choice since it lacks the profound peripheral vasodilatation in skeletal muscle which occurs following isoprenaline administration. Although these drugs can be life-saving in severe cases before pacemaker implantation, their use can be associated with the occurrence of ventricular tachyarrhythmias. These should be controlled by stopping the infusion of the drug and *not* by the administration of drugs which suppress ventricular arrhythmias (for example lignocaine) since such drugs will suppress the escape rhythms which maintain some cardiac output in these animals.

Antimuscarinic drugs often fail to increase the heart rate in animals with heart block and atrial standstill since high vagal tone is not involved in the pathogenesis of these arrhythmias. Junctional escape rhythms may sometimes increase in rate when antimuscarinic drugs are used and some dogs with sick-sinus syndrome can be managed chronically with such drugs. Test doses of atropine will demonstrate those cases where such therapy may be worth trying. Oral preparations of antimuscarinic agents include propantheline bromide (7.5–15 mg three times daily for dogs). In dogs with both bradycardia and tachycardia, administration of antimuscarinic drugs may worsen the episodes of tachycardia as these drugs increase conduction through the AV node. In these cases, the bradycardia should be managed by the use of a pacemaker and drugs which suppress the supraventricular tachycardia (see below) can then be safely employed. The use of pacemakers to treat symptomatic bradycardias has been extensively covered by others (Sisson, 1989; Darke *et al.*, 1989; Sisson *et al.*, 1991b).

Tachycardias

The sinus node can be driven by excessive stimulation of sympathetic tone to discharge at a rate which begins to compromise cardiac function leading to sinus tachycardia. Rapid heart rates may also result from abnormalities in automaticity and or conduction which lead to cardiac arrhythmias. Electrophysiological mechanisms involved in the pathogenesis of tachydysrhythmias include:

- *Ectopic foci*, which reach threshold before the sinus nodal tissue causing premature beats or sustained tachycardia.
- *Afterdepolarizations*, which occur in the repolarization phase of a normal beat (hence are described as triggered activity).
- *Re-entry* which occurs when an electrical impulse circulates around a conduction pathway, exciting the rest of the heart each time it does. If the circulation of a re-entrant rhythm is continuous, a sustained ectopic rhythm will develop (for example atrial fibrillation). Intermittent circulation will lead to paroxysmal episodes of tachycardia.

A surface ECG does not distinguish which electrophysiological mechanism predominates in the arrhythmia but consideration of the cellular mechanisms responsible for arrhythmogenesis does enable an appreciation of the mechanism of action of antidysrhythmic drugs. Fig. 34.33 shows a schematic diagram of the pathogenesis of tachydysrhythmias and the sites at which antidysrhythmic drugs act to suppress such arrhythmias. Hypoxic, damaged heart tissue has a less negative resting membrane potential and hence could reach threshold and fire more quickly than the sinoatrial node and so, potentially, could give rise to ectopic foci. Catecholamines will speed the rate at which the diastolic membrane potential drifts towards threshold and so can contribute to the generation of ectopic impulses. Triggered activity is thought to occur when cardiac muscle cells become overloaded with calcium in their cytoplasm. Hypoxia will reduce the efficiency with which calcium is extruded from the cytoplasm or pumped into intracellular stores. Drugs, such as digoxin, will lead to cellular overload with calcium, hence their arrhythmogenic potential. Conditions which favour re-entry include a long conduction pathway (stretched myocardium), slow conduction (a low safety margin for conduction leading to a unidirectional block as occurs in damaged, hypoxic tissue) and rapid repolarization (an effect of catecholamine stimulation).

Supraventricular tachydysrhythmias

Sinus tachycardia (heart rates greater than 160–180 bpm in the dog and 240 bpm in the cat respectively) can occur in response to pain, fright, fever, anaemia, circulatory shock and hyperthyroidism, all states where sympathetic tone to the heart increases and as a result, the rate of impulse generation and conduction is enhanced. Drugs such as levothyroxine and bronchodilators such as terbutaline, if given in excess, may produce sinus tachycardia as a side effect. Treatment of the underlying condition (or cessation of the offending drug) will be sufficient, in most cases, to reduce the heart rate and drug therapy is not usually necessary.

Supraventricular tachydysrhythmias (Fig. 34.34a–d) develop, most commonly, in animals where there is stretch of the atria (particularly the left atrium), for example, in dogs with dilated cardiomyopathy or mitral valvular insufficiency, and in cats with hypertrophic cardiomyopathy. Some

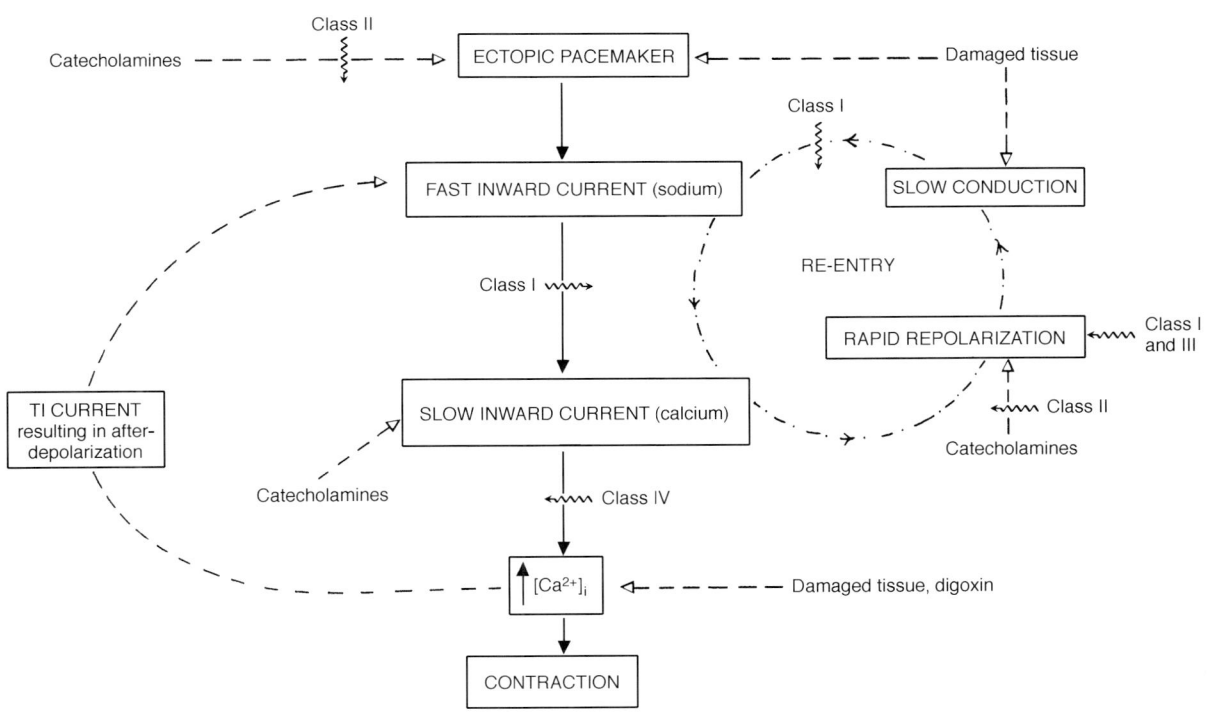

Figure 34.33 Diagram illustrating the electrophysiological mechanisms involved in cardiac arrhythmogenesis and the sites at which antidysrhythmic drugs exert their actions. TI, transient inward current (afterdepolarization).

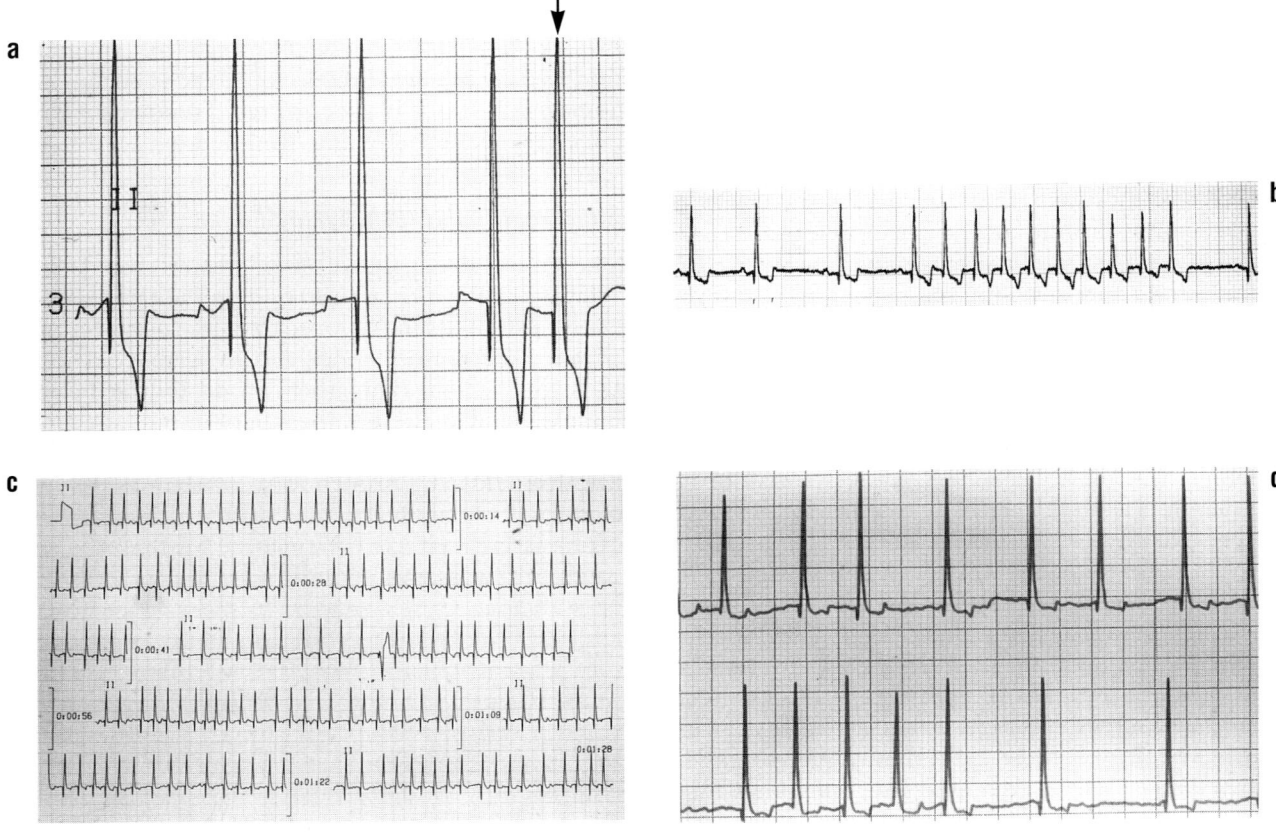

Figure 34.34 Paper speed 25 mm s⁻¹; 1 cm mV⁻¹. (a) Premature supraventricular contraction (arrow). The P wave associated with the premature QRS complex is absent and has been 'lost' in the preceding T wave. (b) Paroxysmal supraventricular tachycardia. (c) Atrial fibrillation. Note the irregular R–R intervals and rapid ventricular response rate. One ventricular premature complex is present. (d) Atrial fibrillation. The R–R intervals are irregular and no visible P waves are present.

congenital defects such as mitral and tricuspid dysplasia, patent ductus arteriosus and ventricular septal defect, which lead to atrial stretch, are also associated with supraventricular tachydysrhythmias. The larger the normal heart size of the animal, the more readily supraventricular arrhythmias (particularly atrial fibrillation) will be supported. Indeed, a recent survey has shown that in Irish wolfhounds the incidence of atrial fibrillation is about 10% in apparently healthy animals (Brownlie, 1991). Size, however, does not appear to be the only factor involved as the same survey found no cases of atrial fibrillation in normal Old English mastiffs.

Management of supraventricular tachydysrhythmias

Most commonly, paroxysmal or sustained atrial tachydysrhythmias (usually atrial fibrillation) are associated with animals showing signs of congestive heart failure. Management of these arrhythmias should be part of the treatment of the heart failure since an uncontrolled heart rate will lead to severe compromise of cardiac function. Digoxin is the drug of choice in the management of these cases (with the exception of re-entrant supraventricular tachycardia occurring in animals with ventricular pre-excitation syndrome, where it is contraindicated) since it is the only drug currently available which slows conduction through the AV node without reducing myocardial contractility. This is particularly important in animals with poor systolic function as is the case in dilated cardiomyopathy. In severe cases of congestive heart failure due to dilated cardiomyopathy, it may be desirable to give a more effective positive inotrope, such as dobutamine. Dobutamine, however, will tend to increase conduction through the AV node, thus accelerating the ventricular response rate in atrial fibrillation. Concurrent treatment with digoxin will tend to reduce the ventricular response rate. If possible, slow digitalization is recommended (see earlier for dose rates). High loading doses are dangerous, particularly in dogs which are hypoxic and have poor myocardial contractility.

Digoxin will not convert atrial arrhythmias into sinus rhythm but reduces the significance of the arrhythmia by slowing the ventricular response. The ideal ventricular rate which should be aimed for in the management of atrial arrhythmias has not been determined for the dog or cat. Most cardiologists would suggest that rates in excess of 160 bpm in the dog under examination conditions are too high. Some suggest training the owners to record the heart rate at home using a stethoscope and suggest a target rate of between 70 and 110 bpm in the dog and 80–140 bpm in the cat (Hamlin, 1992a). Such heart rates can rarely be achieved by the use of digoxin alone. Measurement of serum digoxin levels should be made after 5 days on maintenance therapy to ensure that the therapeutic serum concentration of digoxin has been achieved but not exceeded. Additional drug therapy may then be instituted in an attempt to reduce the heart rate further.

The second drug recommended for use in atrial arrhythmias is diltiazem (0.5 mg kg^{-1} three times daily for dogs, twice daily for cats). Diltiazem is a calcium channel blocker which has effects on both cardiac and vascular smooth muscle. Conduction of electrical impulses through the AV node relies on slow calcium channels and diltiazem slows conduction through the AV node. It has the potential to reduce cardiac muscle contractility, which partly depends on calcium entry during the cardiac action potential. Diltiazem is thought to have less of a negative inotropic effect when compared with verapamil, possibly because it also reduces afterload whereas verapamil is less effective in this respect. Both verapamil and diltiazem reduce the excretion of digoxin which may necessitate a reduction in the dose of digoxin if combined with a calcium channel blocker. Calcium channel blockers are the drugs of choice in the management of re-entrant supraventricular tachycardia in animals with ventricular pre-excitation syndrome. Conversion of atrial arrhythmias into a normal sinus rhythm has been reported following the use of calcium channel blockers (Johnson, 1984). The conversion is short-lived in animals with underlying cardiac disease unless therapy is maintained. The arterial vasodilator properties of diltiazem will also reduce afterload and enhance coronary blood flow during diastole.

Beta-adrenoceptor antagonists can also be used to reduce the ventricular response rate in cases of supraventricular tachydysrhythmia. Propranolol is a non-selective beta-adrenoceptor antagonist which can be used for this purpose at an oral dose rate of 0.5–1 mg kg^{-1} twice or three times daily. The negative inotropic effect of propranolol will be particularly marked in animals relying on sympathetic drive to compensate for poor myocardial contractility. Beta-blockers, therefore, should be used with caution in any animal with signs of congestive heart failure, particularly when poor systolic function is likely to be the underlying cause. Cardioselective beta-blockers have been produced, with the main advantage that they show less tendency, compared with propranolol, to precipitate asthmatic attacks by blocking the protective bronchodilator effect of circulating adrenaline. Dose rates are available for drugs such as atenolol and metoprolol but we currently lack experience with the use of such drugs in veterinary medicine.

It should be remembered that digoxin, calcium channel blockers and beta-blockers all decrease conduction through the AV node via different mechanisms and so will have a synergistic effect when administered together. When introducing a second drug, close monitoring of the patient is necessary to ensure that excessive reduction in the heart rate does not occur. Recently, adenosine has been used in human medicine to convert unstable supraventricular tachycardia into sinus rhythm (Melio et al., 1993) and the development of drugs with favourable pharmacokinetics which are selective for cardiac adenosine receptors may, in the future, add to the therapeutic alternatives available for the management of supraventricular tachydysrhythmias.

With atrial tachydysrhythmias of sudden onset following surgery or trauma, where there is no sign of cardiomegaly or congestive heart failure, it may be reasonable to attempt to convert the rhythm into normal sinus rhythm. This can be attempted by the use of quinidine or diltiazem. Quinidine has antimuscarinic properties and so may increase the ventricular rate initially before converting the rhythm back into sinus rhythm. For this reason, it is recommended to digitalize the animal before attempting conversion with quinidine. When administering quinidine with digoxin, it should be remembered that quinidine displaces digoxin from skeletal muscle binding sites so raising the serum concentration of digoxin. A 50% reduction in the digoxin dose is recommended under these circumstances.

Animals (usually large breed dogs) with atrial fibrillation where the ventricular response rate is relatively slow (<150 bpm) and where there is no evidence of heart failure are likely to develop problems eventually. When they are not showing clinical signs it is reasonable to follow them and give no therapy, particularly as the optimum heart rate for a dog with atrial fibrillation has not been established.

Ventricular arrhythmias

Table 34.10 shows some of the common clinical situations associated with ventricular arrhythmias. As can be seen, many cardiac and extra-cardiac conditions which compromise oxygen supply to cardiac muscle leading to ischaemia, or which increase sympathetic stimulation to the heart or generate factors which are toxic to the myocardium, commonly give rise to ventricular arrhythmias. If cardiac muscle is abnormal or diseased in some way the chances of arrhythmias developing and being sustained are greater when compared to animals with a normal myocardium.

It is important to distinguish between ventricular escape beats (Fig. 34.31) which occur due to failure of generation and or conduction of impulses from the sinoatrial node (which are preceded by a pause) and ventricular premature contractions (Fig. 34.35a,b) which occur prematurely after the preceding sinus beat. Escape complexes should never be suppressed by the use of antidysrhythmic drugs.

Having diagnosed the presence of ventricular premature contractions (VPCs) or bouts of ventricular tachycardia (Fig. 34.35c,d), the next decision to make is whether or not drug treatment is indicated to suppress that arrhythmia. Obviously, where there is an underlying predisposing condition for which there is appropriate treatment then this should be administered (for example fluid therapy to treat hypovolaemic shock and/or to correct acid–base and electrolyte disturbances, oxygen therapy to treat hypoxia, blood transfusion to increase oxygen-carrying capacity in severe anaemia). It is important that plasma electrolytes are measured in animals with cardiac arrhythmias since not only can abnormalities contribute to arrhythmogenesis but the efficacy and toxicity of antiarrhythmic drugs will be affected by electrolyte disturbances, particularly of potassium ion concentration. The danger with ventricular arrhythmias is that they may progress to ventricular fibrillation which leads to death very rapidly.

Table 34.10 Conditions affecting the myocardium which predispose to ventricular arrhythmias

Predisposing condition	Examples
Ischaemia	Hypotension of any cause (circulatory shock) Concentric cardiac muscle hypertrophy (aortic stenosis)
Hypoxia	Severe anaemia Compromised respiratory function leading to anoxia
Primary cardiac muscle disease	Dilated cardiomyopathy Hypertrophic cardiomyopathy Neoplastic infiltrative disease Myocarditis
Trauma	Chest trauma following road traffic accident giving rise to myocardial contusions Head trauma (changes autonomic balance to the heart)
Toxicity	Myocardial depressant factor produced in diseases which compromise blood flow to the pancreas (pancreatitis, gastric dilatation–volvulus syndrome, septic shock) Drugs such as halothane, digoxin, sympathomimetics, antidysrhythmic agents and doxorubicin.
Electrolyte and acid–base disturbances	Severe acidosis and hyperkalaemia

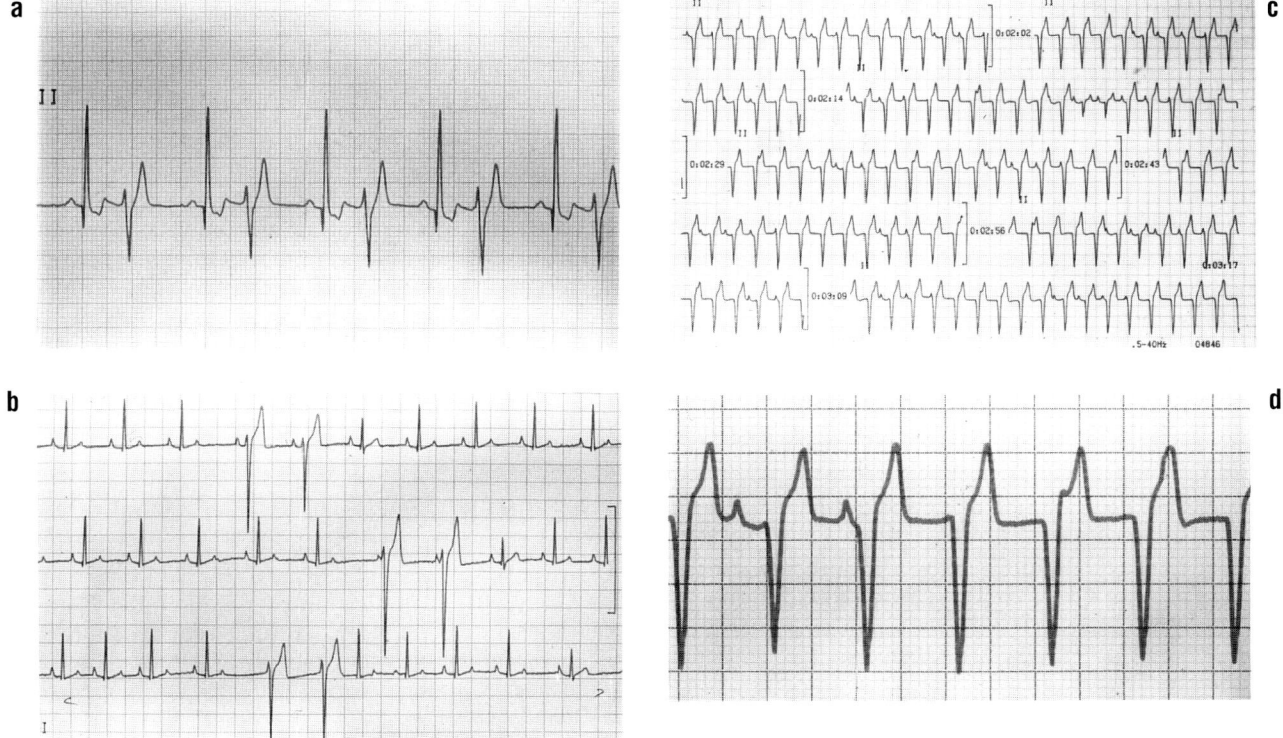

Figure 34.35 Paper speed 25 mm s^{-1}; 1 cm mV^{-1}. (a) Ventricular bigeminy. Every other complex is a ventricular premature complex. (b) Pairs of ventricular premature complexes interrupt the normal sinoatrial rhythm. (c) Continuous ventricular tachycardia. (d) Continuous ventricular tachycardia. P waves are superimposed on the abnormal QRS complexes.

When should a ventricular arrhythmia be treated?

It is not possible to predict which patterns of ventricular arrhythmia are most likely to progress to ventricular fibrillation. The recommendations for treating or not treating a specific ventricular arrhythmia are therefore not based on controlled scientific studies but more on intuition. The importance of this decision is that many of the antidysrhythmic drugs used to treat ventricular arrhythmias have pro-arrhythmogenic potential and so could make the situation worse.

The decision to give drugs to suppress a ventricular arrhythmia is probably best made by assessing whether or not the rhythm disturbance is resulting in haemodynamic abnormalities. Those animals with weak pulses, poor peripheral perfusion and signs of muscle weakness and mental depression which can be attributed to the arrhythmia, should be treated. In addition, it is thought that frequent ventricular premature contractions (more than 20 per minute), particularly if they are multiform and are characterized by beats which occur immediately after the previous repolarization phase (the so called 'vulnerable period') are more likely to progress to ventricular fibrillation.

Drugs used to treat ventricular arrhythmias

The drugs used most commonly in veterinary practice to treat ventricular arrhythmias are the Class I drugs (local anaesthetic agents) and the Class II drugs (beta-adrenoceptor antagonists). Fig. 34.33 shows the ways in which these drugs interfere with the pathological mechanisms involved in arrhythmogenesis. Since the mechanisms involved in the generation of most ventricular arrhythmias cannot be determined from the surface ECG, the choice of drug remains empirical and trial therapy is essentially the only way by which the efficacy of a particular drug can be assessed.

Lignocaine is a Class Ib anti-arrhythmic agent and seems to have the advantage of showing selective suppressant action on damaged and ischaemic cardiac muscle cells with a less negative resting membrane potential while having little or no effect on the automaticity of atrial and normal ventricular myocardial tissue. In most cases, therefore, it is the first drug of choice for treating serious ventricular arrhythmias. It is essential to ensure preparations of lignocaine *without* adrenaline are used. Lignocaine is administered as an intravenous bolus injection (given over 1–2 min) at a dose rate of 2 mg kg^{-1} in the dog and 0.5–1 mg kg^{-1} in the cat initially. Further boluses may be given (up to 6 mg kg^{-1} total dose in the dog) if no response is seen initially. Lignocaine toxicity can result in seizures which may be controlled with diazepam. If the plasma potassium concentration is normal, lignocaine will, in most cases, successfully suppress the arrhythmia or at least reduce the frequency of VPCs. A more sustained effect can be achieved by continuous intravenous infusion of lignocaine at a rate of 30–80 µg kg^{-1} min^{-1} in the dog and 10–20 µg kg^{-1} min^{-1} in the cat. Orally active Class 1b drugs are available and have been shown to be effective in longer-term therapy (tocainide at a dose of 10–20 mg kg^{-1} tid, for example).

If lignocaine is not successful, procainamide (Class 1a agent) would be the next drug to try at a dose rate of 5–15 mg kg^{-1} intravenously or intramuscularly. In an intensive care setting, procainamide can be given by continuous intravenous infusion at a dose of 25–40 µg kg^{-1} min^{-1}. Oral procainamide can be administered at 10–20 mg kg^{-1} every 6 h for longer-term therapy. In some cases, administration of propranolol (0.25–1 mg kg^{-1} orally or 0.1 mg kg^{-1} intravenously) with lignocaine or procainamide may provide a synergistic effect. Caution must be exercised when using these agents, particularly by the intravenous route, as they all possess the ability to reduce myocardial contractility. In addition, propranolol will reduce the clearance of lignocaine from the circulation, thus potentiating the toxicity of lignocaine, hence the need to reduce the dose of lignocaine if combined with propranolol.

The goals of drug therapy for ventricular arrhythmias should be an improvement of the animal's haemodynamic status and a reduction in the frequency of VPCs. If this can be achieved and if the underlying disease can be successfully resolved, the need for drug therapy should also disappear. If the underlying problem is not amenable to treatment, long-term drug therapy may be necessary. There is no evidence that anti-dysrhythmic drugs used under these circumstances will prolong the duration of the animal's life but the quality of life may improve if the frequency and duration of syncopal attacks are reduced. Unfortunately, it is equally possible that some arrhythmias can be worsened by long-term administration of anti-arrhythmic drugs. The significance and incidence of worsening of arrhythmias by the drugs used to treat them can only be assessed by studies which use continuous ambulatory ECG monitoring. The use of two drugs with different mechanisms of action (such as propranolol and procainamide) may produce a synergistic effect. This may allow a reduction in the dosage of the two agents used, which is beneficial since it should reduce the side effects of the drugs, including their pro-arrhythmogenic potential (Tilley, 1991, Hamlin, 1992b).

REFERENCES

Acevedo, R.A., Theis, J.H., Kraus, J.F. and Longhurst, W.M. (1981) Combination of filtration and histochemical stain for detection and differentiation of *Dirofilaria immitis* and *Dipetalonema reconditum* in the dog. *American Journal of Veterinary Research* **42**, 537–540.

Allen, T.A., Wilke, W.L. and Fettman, M.J. (1987) Captopril and enalapril: angiotensin converting enzyme inhibitors. *Journal of the American Veterinary Medical Association* **190**, 94–96.

Allert, J.A. (1990) Autonomic control of the cardiovascular system. *Seminars in Veterinary Medicine and Surgery (Small Animal)* **5**, 17–23.

Anantharaman, G. and Ballevre, O. (1993) The role of taurine in feline dilated cardiomyopathy. *Veterinary International* **5**, 24–27.

Anderson, C.A. and Dubielzig, R.R. (1984) Vegetative endocarditis in dogs. *Journal of the American Animal Hospital Association* **20**, 149–152.

Aronsohn, M. (1985) Cardiac haemangiosarcoma in the dog: A review of 38 cases. *Journal of the American Veterinary Medical Association* **187**, 922–926.

Atkins, C.E., Snyder, P.S. and Keene, B.W. (1988) Effect of aspirin, furosemide, and commercial low salt diet on digoxin pharmacokinetic properties in clinically normal cats. *Journal of the American Veterinary Medical Association* **193**, 1264–1268.

Atkins, C.E., Snyder, P.S, Keene, B.W. and Rush, J.E. (1989) Effects of compensated heart failure on digoxin pharmacokinetics in cats. *Journal of the American Veterinary Medical Association* **195**, 945–950.

Atkins, C.E., Snyder, P.S., Keene, B.W., Rush, J.E. and Eicker, S. (1990) Efficacy of digoxin for treatment of cats with dilated cardiomyopathy. *Journal of the American Veterinary Medical Association* **196**, 1463–1469.

Atkins, C.E., Gallo, A.M., Kurzman, I.D. and Cowen, P. (1992) Risk factors, clinical signs and survival in cats with a clinical diagnosis of idiopathic hypertrophic cardiomyopathy: 74 cases (1985–1989). *Journal of the American Veterinary Medical Association* **201**, 613–618.

Atwell, R.B. and Kelly, W.R. (1980) Canine parvovirus: a cause of chronic myocardial fibrosis and adolescent congestive heart failure. *Journal of Small Animal Practice* **21**, 609–620.

Baker, K.M., Booz, G.W. and Dostal, D.E. (1992) Cardiac actions of angiotensin II: Role of an intracardiac renin–angiotensin system. *Annual Review of Physiology* **54**, 227–241.

Beardow, A.W. and Buchanan, J.W. (1993) Chronic mitral valve disease in cavalier King Charles spaniels: 95 cases (1987–1991). *Journal of the American Veterinary Medical Association* **203**, 1023–1029.

Bennett, D., Gilbertson, E.M. and Grennan, D. (1978) Bacterial endocarditis with polyarthritis in two dogs associated with circulating autoantibodies. *Journal of Small Animal Practice* **19**, 185–196.

Berg, R.J, Wingfield, W.E. and Hoopes, P.J. (1984) Idiopathic haemorrhagic pericardial effusion in eight dogs. *Journal of the American Veterinary Medical Association* **185**, 988–992.

Berry, K., Lombard, C. and Reinhard, M.K. (1984) Bacterial endocarditis complicated by aortic valvular insufficiency and third degree atrioventricular block in a mixed breed dog. *The Compendium on Continuing Education* **6**, 396–402.

Bonagura, J. D. (1983) Bacterial endocarditis. In: *Textbook of Veterinary Internal Medicine* (Ed. S. J. Ettinger) 2nd edn. W.B. Saunders, Philadelphia, pp. 1052–1062.

Bonagura, J. D. (1989) Cardiovascular diseases. In: *The Cat: Diseases and Clinical Management* (Ed. R.G. Sherding). Churchill Livingstone, New York, pp. 649–753.

Bonagura, J.D. (1994) Echocardiography. *Journal of the American Veterinary Medical Association* **204**, 516–522.

Bond, B.R. and Fox, P.R. (1984) Advances in feline cardiomyopathy. *Veterinary Clinics of North America* **14**, 1021–1038.

Boudreaux, M.K., Dillon, A.R., Ravis, W.R., Sartin, E.A. and Spano, J.S. (1991) Effects of treatment with aspirin or aspirin/dipyridamole combination in heartworm-negative, heartworm infected, and embolised heartworm-infected dogs. *American Journal of Veterinary Research* **52**, 1992–1999.

Bouvagnet, P., Leger, J., Dechesne, C.A., Dureau, G., Anoal, M. and Leger, J.J. (1985) Local changes in myosin types in diseased human atrial myocardium: A quantitative immunofluorescence study. *Circulation* **72**, 272–279.

Bovee, K.C., Littman, M.P., Saleh, F., Beeuwkes, R., Mann, W., Koster, P.T. and Kinter, L.B. (1986) Essential hereditary hypertension in dogs: a new animal model. *Journal of Hypertension* **4** (supplement), S172–S173.

Brayley, K.A., Lunney, J. and Ettinger, S.J. (1994) Con triatriatum dexter in a dog. *Journal of American Animal Hospital Association* **30**, 153–156.

Bright, J.M. (1983) Controversies in veterinary medicine: is the long term use of digitalis for treatment of low output failure unwarranted? *Journal of the American Animal Hospital Association* **19**, 233–236.

Bright, J.M., Golden, A.L., Gompf, R.E., Walker, M.A. and Toal R.L. (1991) Evaluation of the calcium channel-blocking agents diltiazem and verapamil for treatment of feline hypertrophic cardiomyopathy. *Journal of Veterinary Internal Medicine* **5**, 272–282.

Bright, J.M., Golden, A.L. and Daniel, G.B. (1992) Feline hypertrophic cardiomyopathy: Variations on a theme. *Journal of Small Animal Practice* **33**, 266–274.

Brobst, D. (1986) Review of the pathophysiology of alterations in potassium homeostasis. *Journal of the American Veterinary Medical Association* **188**, 1019–1025.

Brown, N.O., Patnaik, A.K. and MacEwen, E.G. (1985) Canine haemangiosarcoma. *Journal of the American Veterinary Medical Association* **186**, 56–58.

Brownlie, S.E. (1991) An electrocardiographic survey of cardiac rhythm in Irish wolfhounds. *Veterinary Record* **129**, 470–471.

Brownlie, S.E., Cobb, M.A., Chambers, J., Jackson, G. and Thomas, S. (1991) Percutaneous balloon valvuloplasty in four dogs with pulmonic stenosis. *Journal of Small Animal Practice* **32**, 165–169.

Buchanan, J.W. (1977) Chronic valvular disease (endocardosis) in dogs. *Advances in Veterinary Science and Comparative Medicine* **21**, 75–106.

Buchanan, J.W. (1992) Causes and prevalence of cardiovascular disease. In: *Current Veterinary Therapy* (Eds R.W. Kirk and J.D. Bonagura). W.B. Saunders, Philadelphia, pp. 647–655.

Buoscio, D.A., Sisson, D., Zachery, J. F. and Luethy, M. (1994) Clinical and pathological characterisation of an unusual form of subvalvular aortic stenosis in four golden retriever puppies. *Journal of American Animal Hospital Association* **30**, 100–110.

Calvert, C.A. (1982) Valvular bacterial endocarditis in the dog. *Journal of the American Veterinary Medical Association* **180**, 1080–1084.

Calvert, C.A. (1986) Dilated congestive cardiomyopathy in Doberman Pinschers. *The Compendium on Continuing Education* **8**, 417–430.

Calvert, C.A., Greene, C.E. and Hardie, E.M. (1985) Cardiovascular infections in dogs: epizootiology, clinical manifestations and prognosis. *Journal of the American Veterinary Medical Association* **187**, 612–616.

Calvert, C.A. and Greene, C.E. (1986) Bacteraemia in dogs: diagnosis, treatment and prognosis. *The Compendium on Continuing Education* **8**, 179–186.

Calvert, C.A. and Rawlings, C.A. (1988) Canine heartworm disease. In: *Canine and Feline Cardiology* (Ed. P.R. Fox). Churchill Livingstone, New York, pp. 519–549.

Cobb, M.A. (1992) Idiopathic dilated cardiomyopathy:

advances in aetiology, pathogenesis and management. *Journal of Small Animal Practice* **33**, 113–118.

Cobb, M.A. and Brownlie, S.E. (1992) Intrapericardial neoplasia in 14 dogs. *Journal of Small Animal Practice* **33**, 309–316.

Cobb, M.A. and Michell, A.R. (1992) Plasma electrolyte concentrations in dogs receiving diuretic therapy for cardiac failure. *Journal of Small Animal Practice* **33**, 526–529.

Colucci, W.S., Wright, R.F. and Braunwald, E. (1986) New positive inotropic agents in the treatment of congestive heart failure. *New England Journal of Medicine* **314**, 349–358.

Coulter, D.B. and Keith, J.C. (1984) Blood pressures obtained by indirect measurement in conscious dogs. *Journal of the American Veterinary Medical Association* **184**, 1375–1378.

COVE Study Group (1995) Controlled clinical evaluation of enalapril in dogs with heart failure: results of the Cooperative Veterinary Enalapril Study group. *Journal of Veterinary Internal Medicine* **9**, 243–252.

Cowgill, L.D. and Kallet, A.J. (1983) Recognition and management of hypertension in the dog. In: *Current Veterinary Therapy: Small Animal Practice VIII* (Ed. R.W. Kirk). W.B. Saunders, Philadelphia, pp. 1025–1028.

Cowgill, L.D. and Kallet, A.J. (1986) Systemic hypertension. In: *Current Veterinary Therapy IX: Small Animal Practice* (Ed. R.W. Kirk). W.B. Saunders, Philadelphia, pp. 360–364.

Darke, P.G.G. (1986) Congenital heart defects in small animals. *British Veterinary Journal* **142**, 203–209.

Darke, P.G.G. (1987) Valvular incompetence in cavalier King Charles spaniels. *Veterinary Record* **120**, 365–366.

Darke, P.G.G., McAreavey, D. and Been, M. (1989) Transvenous cardiac pacing in 19 dogs and one cat. *Journal of Small Animal Practice* **30**, 491–499.

DeLellis, L.A. and Kittleson, M.D. (1992) Current uses and hazards of vasodilator therapy in heart failure. In: *Current Veterinary Therapy XI* (Eds R.W. Kirk and J.D. Bonagura), W. B. Saunders, Philadelphia, pp. 700–708.

Denniss, R.A., Marsh, J.D., Quigg, R.J., Gordon, J.B. and Colucci, W.S. (1989) Beta-adrenergic receptor number and adenylate cyclase function in denervated transplanted and cardiomyopathic human hearts. *Circulation* **79**, 1028–1034.

Detweiler, D.K., Riedesel, D.H. and Knight, D.H. (1993) Mechanical activity of the heart. In: *Duke's Physiology of Domestic Animals* (Eds M.J. Swenson and W.O. Reece), 11th edn. Cornell University Press, Ithaca, pp. 145–169.

Dillon, A.R. (1989) Pharmacology of heartworm therapeutics. *Californian Veterinarian* **43**, 23–25.

Dow, S.W. and Jones, R.L. (1989) Bacteraemia: pathogenesis and diagnosis. *The Compendium on Continuing Education* **11**, 432–443.

Dow, S.W., Fettman, M.J. and Smith, K.R. (1990). Effects of dietary acidification and potassium depletion on acid–base balance, mineral metabolism and renal function in adult cats. *Journal of Nutrition* **120**, 569–578.

Dow, S.W., Fettman, M.J., Smith, K.R., Ching, S.V., Hamer, D.W. and Rogers, Q.R. (1992) Taurine depletion and cardiovascular disease in adult cats fed a potassium-depleted acidified diet. *American Journal of Veterinary Research* **53**, 402–405.

Dubey, J.P. and Carpenter, J.L. (1993) Histologically confirmed clinical toxoplasmosis in cats: 100 cases (1952–1990). *Journal of the American Veterinary Medical Association* **203**, 1556–1565.

Dukes, J. (1992) Hypertension: a review of the mechanisms, manifestations and management. *Journal of Small Animal Practice* **33**, 119–129.

Dunn, J.K., Jefferies, A.R., Evans, R.J. and Herrtage, M.E. (1987) Chronic granulocytic leukaemia in a dog with associated bacterial endocarditis, thrombocytopenia and pre-retinal and retinal haemorrhages. *Journal of Small Animal Practice* **28**, 1079–1086.

Dzau, V.J. (1992) Autocrine and paracrine mechanisms in the pathophysiology of heart failure. *American Journal of Cardiology* **70**, 4C–11C.

Edwards, N.J. and Rebhun, W.C. (1979) Generalised cryptococcosis: a case report. *Journal of American Animal Hospital Association* **15**, 439–445.

Elwood, C.M., Cobb, M.A. and Stepien, R.L. (1993) Clinical and echocardiographic findings in ten dogs with vegetative bacterial endocarditis. *Journal of Small Animal Practice* **34**, 420–427.

Englemeier, R.S., O'Connell, J.B., Walsh, R., Rad, N., Scanlon, P.J. and Gunnar, R.M. (1985) Improvement in symptoms and exercise tolerance by metoprolol in patients with dilated cardiomyopathy: a double blind, randomised, placebo-controlled trial. *Circulation* **72**, 536–546.

Ettinger, S.J. and Suter, P.F. (1970) Heart sounds and phonocardiography. In: *Canine Cardiology*. W.B. Saunders, Philadelphia, pp. 12–39.

Evans, S.M. and Biery, D.N. (1980) Congenital peritoneopericardial diaphragmatic hernia in the dog and cat: a literature review and 17 additional case histories. *Veterinary Radiology* **21**, 108–116.

Ferguson, D.W., Berg, W.J., Sanders, J.S., Roach, P.J., Kempf, J.S. and Kienzle, M.G. (1989) Sympathoinhibitory responses to digitalis glycosides in heart failure patients: direct evidence from sympathetic neural recordings. *Circulation* **80**, 65–77.

Fingland, R.B, Bonagura, J.D. and Myer, C.W. (1986) Pulmonic stenosis in the dog: 29 cases. *Journal of the American Veterinary Medical Association* **189**, 218–226.

Flanders, J. A. (1986) Feline aortic thromboembolism. *The Compendium on Continuing Education* **8**, 473–484.

Forster, C. and Armstrong, P.W. (1990) Pacing-induced heart failure in the dog: evaluation of peripheral vascular alpha-adrenoceptor subtypes.

Journal of Cardiovascular Pharmacology **16**, 708–718.

Fossum, T.W., Miller, M.W., Rogers, K.S., Bonagura, J.D. and Meurs, K.M. (1994) Chylothorax associated with right-sided heart failure in five cats. *Journal of the American Veterinary Medical Association* **204**, 84–89.

Fox, P.R. (1988a) Canine myocardial disease. In: *Canine and Feline Cardiology* (Ed. P.R. Fox). Churchill Livingstone, New York, pp. 467–493.

Fox, P.R. (1988b) Feline myocardial disease. In: *Canine and Feline Cardiology* (Ed. P.R. Fox). Churchill Livingstone, New York, pp. 435–466.

Fox, P.R. (1992) Current uses and hazards of diuretic therapy. In: *Current Veterinary Therapy XI* (Eds R.W. Kirk and J.D. Bonagura). W.B. Saunders, Philadelphia, pp. 668–676.

Fox, P.R. and Bond, B.R. (1983) Non-selective and selective angiocardiography. *Veterinary Clinics of North America: Small Animal Practice* **13**, 259–272.

Fregin, G.F., Luginbuhl, H. and Guarda F. (1972) Myocardial infaction in a dog with bacterial endocarditis. *Journal of the American Veterinary Medical Association* **160**, 956–963.

Gibbs, C., Gaskell, C.J., Darke, P.G.G. and Wotton, P.R. (1982) Idiopathic pericardial haemorrhage in dogs: a review of fourteen cases. *Journal of Small Animal Practice* **23**, 483–500.

Gilbert, E.M., Anderson, J.L., Deitchman, D., Yanowitz, F.G., O'Connell, J.B., Renlund, D.G., Bartholomew, M., Mealey, P.C., Larrabee, P. and Bristow, M.R. (1990) Long term beta-blocker vasodilator therapy improves cardiac function in idiopathic dilated cardiomyopathy: a double blind, randomized study of bucindolol versus placebo. *American Journal of Medicine* **88**, 223–229.

Goetz, K.L. (1988) Physiology and pathophysiology of atrial peptides. *American Journal of Physiology* **254**, E1–E15.

Gompf, R.E. (1983) Physical examination of the cardiopulmonary system. *Veterinary Clinics of North America* **13**, 201–215.

Gompf, R.E. and Tilley, L.P. (1979) Comparison of lateral and sternal recumbent positions for electrocardiography in the cat. *American Journal of Veterinary Research* **40**, 1483–1486.

Gooding, J.P., Robinson, W.F., Wyburn, R.S. and Cullen, L.K. (1982) A cardiomyopathy in English Cocker Spaniels: a clinicopathological investigation. *Journal of Small Animal Practice* **23**, 133–149.

Gooding, J.P., Robinson, W.F. and Mews, G.L. (1986) Echocardiographic characterisation of dilatation cardiomyopathy in the English Cocker Spaniel. *American Journal of Veterinary Research* **47**, 1978–1983.

Goodwin, J.K. and Lombard, C.W. (1992) Patent ductus arteriosus in adult dogs: clinical features of 14 cases. *Journal of the American Animal Hospital Association* **28**, 349–354.

Gordon, D.B. and Goldblatt, H. (1967) Direct percutaneous determination of systemic blood pressure and production of renal hypertension in the cat. *Proceedings for the Society for Experimental Biology and Medicine* **125**, 177–180.

Hackett, T.B., Van Pelt, D.R., Willard, M.D., Martin, L.G., Shelton, G.D. and Wingfield, W.E. (1995). Third degree atrioventricular block and acquired myasthenia gravis in four dogs. *Journal of the American Veterinary Medical Association* **206**, 1173–1176.

Haggstrom, J., Kvart, C. and Hansson, K. (1995) Heart sounds and murmurs: changes related to severity of chronic valvular disease in the cavalier King Charles spaniel. *Journal of Veterinary Internal Medicine* **9**, 75–85.

Hall, L.W., Dunn, J.K., Delaney, M. and Shapiro, L.M. (1991) Ambulatory electrocardiography in dogs. *Veterinary Record* **129**, 213–216.

Hamlin, R.L. (1988) Pathophysiology of heart failure. In: *Canine and Feline Cardiology* (Ed. P.R. Fox), Churchill Livingstone, New York, pp. 159–170.

Hamlin, R.L. (1992a) Therapy of supraventricular tachycardia and atrial fibrillation. In: *Current Veterinary Therapy XI* (Eds R.W. Kirk and J.D. Bonagura). W.B. Saunders, Philadelphia, pp. 745–749.

Hamlin, R.L. (1992b) Current uses and hazards of ventricular antiarrhythmic therapy. In: *Current Veterinary Therapy XI* (Eds R.W. Kirk and J.D. Bonagura), W.B. Saunders, Philadelphia, pp. 694–700.

Harpster, N.K. (1983) Boxer cardiomyopathy. In: *Current Veterinary Therapy VIII: Small Animal Practice* (Ed. R.W. Kirk). W. B. Saunders Co, Philadelphia, pp. 329–337.

Harpster, N.K. (1986) Feline myocardial diseases. In: *Current Veterinary Therapy IX: Small Animal Practice* (Ed. R.W. Kirk). W. B. Saunders, Philadelphia, pp. 380–398.

Heilbrunn, S.M, Shah, P., Bristow, M.R., Valantino, H.A., Ginsberg, R. and Fowler, M.B. (1989) Increased beta-receptor density and improved haemodynamic response to catecholamine stimulation during long term metoprolol therapy in heart failure from dilated cardiomyopathy. *Circulation* **79**, 483–490.

Henry, C.J. and Dillon, R. (1994) Heartworm disease in dogs. *Journal of the American Veterinary Medical Association* **204**, 1148–1151.

Herrtage, M.E.H., Hall, L.W. and English, T.A.H. (1983) Surgical correction of tetralogy of Fallot in a dog. *Journal of Small Animal Practice* **24**, 51–62.

Higgens, R.J., Krakowka, S., Metzler, A.E. and Koestner, A. (1981) Canine distemper virus-associated cardiac necrosis in the dog. *Veterinary Pathology* **18**, 472–486.

Hoey, A., Marchant, C., Atwell, R., Brown, L. and Serina, C. (1991) Canine dilated cardiomyopathy – are there defects at the receptor level? *B.S.A.V.A. Congress Proceedings (Free Communications)* p. 142.

Hoskins, J.D., Hagstad, H.V., Hribernik, J.N. and Breitschwerdt, E.B. (1984) Heartworm disease in dogs from Louisiana: pretreatment clinical and laboratory evaluation. *Journal of American Animal Hospital Association* **20**, 205–210.

IMPROVE Study Group (1995) Acute and short-term hemodynamic, echocardiographic, and clinical effects of enalapril maleate in dogs with naturally acquired heart failure. Results of the Invasive Multicenter PROspective Veterinary Evaluation of Enalapril Study Group. *Journal of Veterinary Internal Medicine* **9**, 234–242.

International Small Animal Cardiac Health Council (1994) *Recommendations for the Diagnosis of Heart Disease and the Treatment of Heart Failure in Small Animals* p. 5.

Jacobs, D.E. and Prole, J.H.B. (1975) *Angiostrongylus vasorum* and other nematodes in British greyhounds. *Veterinary Record* **96**, 180.

Jaffe, I.A. (1986) Adverse effects profile of sulphydryl compounds in man. *American Journal of Medicine* **80**, 471–476.

Johnson, J.T. (1984) Conversion of atrial fibrillation in two dogs using verapamil and supportive therapy. *Journal of the American Animal Hospital Association* **21**, 429–434.

Johnsson, L. (1972) Coronary arterial lesions and myocardial infarcts in the dog: a pathologic and microangiopathic study. *Acta Veterinaria Scandinavica* **38** (suppl): 1–80.

Katz, A.M. (1990) Cardiomyopathy of overload. A major determinant of prognosis in congestive heart failure. *New England Journal of Medicine* **322**, 100–110.

Keene, B.W. (1988) Chronic Valvular Disease in Dogs. In: *Canine and Feline Cardiology* (Ed. P.R. Fox). Churchill Livingstone, New York, pp. 409–418.

Keene, B.W., Panciera, D.P., Atkins, C.E., Regitz, V., Schmidt, M.J. and Shug, A.L. (1991) Myocardial L-carnitine deficiency in a family of dogs with dilated cardiomyopathy. *Journal of the American Veterinary Medical Association* **198**, 647–650.

Keister, D.M., Kittleson, M.D., Bonagura, J.D., Pipers, F.S. and Knauer, K.W. (1990) Milrinone: a clinical trial in 29 dogs with moderate to severe congestive heart failure. *Journal of Veterinary Internal Medicine* **4**, 79–86.

Kienle, R.D., Thomas, W.P. and Pion, P.D. (1994). The natural clinical history of canine congenital subaortic stenosis. *Journal of Veterinary Internal Medicine* **8**, 423–431.

Kittleson, M.D., Eyster, G.E., Olivier, N.B. and Anderson L.K. (1983) Oral hydralazine therapy for chronic mitral regurgitation in the dog. *Journal of the American Veterinary Medical Association* **182**, 1205–1209.

Kittleson, M.D., Eyster, G.A., Knowlen, G.G., Olivier N.B. and Anderson, L.K. (1984) Myocardial function in small dogs with chronic mitral regurgitation and severe congestive heart failure. *Journal of the American Veterinary Medical Association* **184**, 455–459.

Kittleson, M.D., Eyster, G.E., Knowlen, G.G., Olivier, N.B. and Anderson, L.K. (1985a) Efficacy of digoxin administration in dogs with idiopathic congestive cardiomyopathy. *Journal of the American Veterinary Medical Association* **186**, 162–165.

Kittleson, M.D., Pipers, F.S., Knauer, K.W., Keister, D.M., Knowlen, G.G. and Miner, W.S. (1985b) Echocardiographic and clinical features of milrinone in dogs with myocardial failure. *American Journal of Veterinary Research* **46**, 1659–1664.

Kittleson, M.D., Johnson, L.E. and Pion, P.D. (1987) The acute haemodynamic effects of milrinone in dogs with severe idiopathic myocardial failure. *Journal of Veterinary Internal Medicine* **1**, 121–127.

Kittleson, M.D, Pion, P.D, Delellis, L.A, Mekhamer, Y., Dybdal, N. and Lothrop, C.D. (1992) Increased serum growth hormone concentration in feline hypertrophic cardiomyopathy. *Journal of Veterinary Internal Medicine* **6**, 320–324.

Kittleson, M.D., Johnson, L.E., Pion, P.D. and Mekhamer, Y.E. (1993) The acute haemodynamic effects of captopril in dogs with heart failure. *Journal of Veterinary Pharmacology and Therapeutics* **16**, 1–7.

Kleine, L.J, Zook, B.C. and Munson, T.O. (1970) Primary cardiac haemangiosarcoma in dogs. *Journal of the American Veterinary Medical Association* **157**, 326–337.

Knowlen, G.G., Kittleson M.D., Nachreiner R.F. and Eyster, G.E. (1983) Comparison of plasma aldosterone concentration among clinical status groups of dogs with chronic heart failure. *Journal of the American Veterinary Medical Association* **183**, 991–996.

Kobayashi, D.L., Peterson, M.E., Graves, T.K., Lesser, M. and Nichols, C.E. (1990) Hypertension in cats with chronic renal failure and hyperthyroidism. *Journal of Veterinary Internal Medicine* **4**, 58–62.

Kramer, G.A., Kittleson, M.D., Fox, P.R., Lewis, J. and Pion, P.D. (1995). Plasma taurine concentrations in normal dogs and in dogs with heart disease. *Journal of Veterinary Internal Medicine* **9**, 253–258.

Kubo, S.H., Rector, T.S., Bank, A.J., Williams, R.E. and Heifetz, S.M. (1991) Endothelium-dependent vasodilation is attenuated in patients with heart failure. *Circulation* **84**, 1589–1596.

Laing, C., Sherman, L.G., Doherty, J.V., Doherty, J.V., Wellington, K., Lee, V. and Hood, W.B. (1984) Sustained improvement of cardiac function in patients with congestive heart failure after short term infusion of dobutamine. *Circulation* **69**, 113.

Lawler, D.F., Templeton, A.J. and Monti, K.L. (1993) Evidence for genetic involvement in feline dilated cardiomyopathy. *Journal of Veterinary Internal Medicine* **7**, 383–387.

Lehmkuhl, L.B., Ware, W.A. and Bonagura, J.D. (1994) Mitral stenosis in 15 dogs. *Journal of Veterinary Internal Medicine* **8**, 2–17.

Lenghaus, C. and Studdert, M.J. (1982) Generalised parvovirus disease in neonatal pups. *Journal of the American Veterinary Medical Association* **181**, 41–45.

Lenghaus, C., Studdert, M.J. and Finnie, J.W. (1980) Acute and chronic canine parvovirus myocarditis following intrauterine innoculation. *Australian Veterinary Journal* **56**, 465–468.

Levy, S.A. and Duray, P.H. (1988) Complete heart block in a dog seropositive for *Borrelia burgdorferi*. *Journal of Veterinary Internal Medicine* **2**, 138–144.

Lewis, R.P. (1990) Digitalis: a drug that refuses to die. *Critical Care Medicine* **18**, S5–S13.

Littman, M.P. (1994). Spontaneous systemic hypertension in 24 cats. *Journal of Veterinary Internal Medicine* **8**, 79–86.

Littman, M.P., Robertson, J.L. and Bovee, K.C. (1988) Spontaneous systemic hypertension in dogs: five cases (1981–1983). *Journal of the American Veterinary Medical Association* **193**, 486–494.

Liu, S.K. (1977) Pathology of feline heart diseases. *Veterinary Clinics of North America* **7**, 323–339.

Liu, S.K., Tilley, L.P. and Lord, P.E. (1975) Feline cardiomyopathy. In: *Recent Advances in Studies on Cardiac Structure and Metabolism 10*, University Park Press, Baltimore, pp. 627–640.

Liu, S., Maron, B.J. and Tilley, L.P. (1979) Canine hypertrophic cardiomyopathy. *Journal of the American Veterinary Medical Association* **174**, 708–713.

Liu, S.K., Maron, B.J. and Tilley, L.P. (1981) Feline hypertrophic cardiomyopathy: gross anatomic and quantitative features. *American Journal of Pathology* **102**, 388–395.

Liu, S.K., Fox, P.R. and Tilley, L.P. (1982) Excessive moderator bands in the left ventricle of 21 cats. *Journal of the American Veterinary Medical Association* **180**, 1215–1219.

Liu, S.K., Tilley, L.P., Tappe, J.P. and Fox, P.R. (1986) Clinical and pathological findings in dogs with atherosclerosis: 21 cases (1970–1983). *Journal of the American Veterinary Medical Association* **189**, 227–232.

Lombard, C.W. and Buergelt, C.D. (1983) Vegetative bacterial endocarditis in dogs: echocardiographic diagnosis and clinical signs. *Journal of Small Animal Practice* **24**, 325–339.

Luis Fuentes, V. (1992) Feline heart disease: an update. *Journal of Small Animal Practice* **33**, 130–137.

Macintire, D.K. and Snider, T.G. (1984) Cardiac arrhythmias associated with multiple trauma in dogs. *Journal of the American Veterinary Medical Association* **184**, 541–545.

Maddy, K.T. (1958) Disseminated coccidioidomycosis of the dog. *Journal of the American Veterinary Medical Association* **132**, 483–489.

Mann, D.L., Kent, R.L., Parsons, B. and Cooper, G. (1992) Adrenergic effects on the biology of the adult cardiac myocyte. *Circulation* **85**, 790–804.

Margulies, K.B., Hildebrand, F.L., Lerman, A., Perrella, M.A. and Burnett, J.C. (1990) Increased endothelin in experimental heart failure. *Circulation* **82**, 2226–2230.

Marks, C.A. (1993) Hypertrophic cardiomyopathy in a dog. *Journal of the American Veterinary Medical Association* **203**, 1020–1022.

Martin, M.W.S. and Neal, C. (1992) Distribution of angiostrongylosis in Cornwall. *Journal of Small Animal Practice* **33**, 327–330.

Matic, S.E. and Herrtage, M.E. (1987) Diagnosis and treatment of occult dirofilariasis in an imported dog. *Journal of Small Animal Practice* **28**, 183–196.

Mauldin, G.E., Fox, P.R., Patnaik, A.K., Bond, B.R., Mooney, S.C. and Matus, R.E. (1992) Doxorubicin-induced cardiotoxicosis. *Journal of Veterinary Internal Medicine* **6**, 82–88.

Melio, F.R., Mallon, W.K. and Newton, E. (1993) Successful conversion of unstable supraventricular tachycardia to sinus rhythm with adenosine. *Annals of Emergency Medicine* **22**, 709–713.

Michell, A.R. (1988a) Diuretics and cardiovascular disease. *Journal of Veterinary Pharmacology and Therapeutics* **11**, 246–253.

Michell, A.R. (1988b) Pathophysiology of chronic heart failure. *Proceedings of the Association for Veterinary Clinical Pharmacology and Therapeutics* **12**, 1–8.

Miller, M.S. and Tilley, L.P. (eds) (1995) Treatment of cardiac arrhythmias and conduction disturbances. In: *Manual of Canine and Feline Cardiology*, 2nd edn. W.B. Saunders, Philadelphia, pp. 371–411.

Moe, G.W., Grima, E.A., Angus, C., Wong, N.L., Hu, D.C.K., Howard, R.J. and Armstrong, P.W. (1991) Responses of atrial natriuretic factor to acute and chronic increases of atrial pressure in experimental heart failure in dogs. *Circulation* **83**, 1780–1787.

Moise, N.S. and Gilmour, R.F. (1992) Inherited sudden cardiac death in German Shepherds. In: *Current Veterinary Therapy XI: Small Animal Practice* (Ed. R.W. Kirk), W.B. Saunders, Philadelphia, pp. 749–751.

Monnet, E., Orton, E.C., Salman, M. and Boon, J. (1995) Idiopathic dilated cardiomyopathy in dogs: survival and prognostic indicators. *Journal of Veterinary Internal Medicine* **9**, 12–17.

Morgan, R.V. (1986) Systemic hypertension in four cats: ocular and medical findings. *Journal of American Animal Hospital Association* **22**, 615–621.

Morris, J.G., Rogers, Q.R. and Pacioretty, L.M. (1990) Taurine: an essential nutrient for cats. *Journal of Small Animal Practice* **31**, 502–509.

Muir, W.W. and Weisbrode, S.E. (1982) Myocardial ischaemia in dogs with gastric dilatation – volvulus. *Journal of the American Veterinary Medical Association* **181**, 363–366.

Mullaney, T.P., Levin, S. and Indrieri, R.J. (1983) Disseminated aspergillosis in a dog. *Journal of the American Veterinary Medical Association* **182**, 516–518.

Mulvihill, J.J. and Priester, W.A. (1973) Congenital

heart disease in dogs: epidemiologic similarities to man. *Teratology* **7**, 73–78.

Muna, W.F.T., Ferrans, V.J., Pierce, J.E. and Roberts, W.C. (1978) Discrete subaortic stenosis in Newfoundland dogs: association of infective endocarditis. *American Journal of Cardiology* **41**, 746–754.

Nielson, S.W. and Nielson, L.B. (1954) Coronary embolism in valvular bacterial endocarditis in two dogs. *Journal of the American Veterinary Medical Association* **125**, 376–380

Norgaard, A., Bagger, J.P., Bjerregaard, P., Baandrup, U., Kjeldsen, K. and Thomsen, P.E.B. (1988) Regulation of left ventricular function and Na/K pump concentration in suspected idiopathic dilated cardiomyopathy. *American Journal of Cardiology* **61**, 1312–1315.

Novotny, M.J., Hogan, P.M. and Flannigan, G. (1994) Echocardiographic evidence for myocardial failure induced by taurine deficiency in domestic cats. *Canadian Journal of Veterinary Research* **58**, 6–12.

O'Grady, M.R., Holmberg, D.L., Miller, C.W. and Coskshutt, J.R. (1989) Canine congenital aortic stenosis: a review of the literature and commentary. *Canadian Veterinary Journal* **30**, 811–815.

Odin, M. and Dubey, J.P. (1993) Sudden death associated with *Neospora caninum* myocarditis in a dog. *Journal of the American Veterinary Medical Association* **203**, 831–833.

Olivier, N.B. (1988) Congenital heart disease in dogs. In: *Canine and Feline Cardiology* (Ed. P.R. Fox). Churchill Livingstone, New York, pp. 357–389.

Ortega-Mora, L.M., Gomez-Bautista, M. and Rojo-Vazquez, F.A. (1989) The acid phosphatase activity and morphological characteristics of *Dipetalonema dracunculoides* (Cobbold, 1870) microfilariae. *Veterinary Parasitology* **33**, 187–190.

Packer, M. (1992a) Pathophysiology of chronic heart failure. *Lancet* **340**, 88–92.

Packer, M. (1992b) Treatment of chronic heart failure. *Lancet* **340**, 92–95.

Packer, M., Carver, J.R., Rodeheffer, R.J. (1991) Effect of oral milrinone on mortality in severe chronic heart failure. *New England Journal of Medicine* **325**, 1468–1475.

Page, A., Edmunds, G. and Atwell, R.B. (1993) Echocardiographic values in the Greyhound. *Australian Veterinary Journal* **70**, 361–364.

Panciera, D.L. (1994) Hypothyroidism in dogs: 66 cases. *Journal of the American Veterinary Medical Association* **204**, 761–767.

Parker, J.O. (1992) Update on nitrate tolerance. *British Journal of Clinical Pharmacology* **34**, 11S–14S.

Patnaik, A.K., Liu, S.K., Hurvitz, A. and Clelland, A.J. (1975) Canine chemodectoma (extra-adrenal paragangliomas): a comparative study. *Journal of Small Animal Practice* **16**, 785–801.

Patterson, D.F. (1968) Epidemiologic and genetic studies of congenital heart disease in the dog. *Circulation Research* **23**, 171–202.

Patterson, D.F. (1984) Two hereditary forms of ventricular outflow obstruction in the dog: pulmonary valve dysplasia and discrete subaortic stenosis. In: *Congenital Heart Disease: Causes and Processes* (Eds J.J. Nora and A. Takao), Futura Publishing, Mount Kisco, pp. 43–64.

Patterson, D.F. (1989) Hereditary congenital heart defects in dogs. *Journal of Small Animal Practice* **30**, 153–165.

Patterson, D.F., Pyle, R.L., Van Mierop, L.H.S., Melbin, J. and Olson, M.M. (1974) Hereditary defects of the conotruncal septum in Keeshund dogs: pathologic and genetic studies. *American Journal of Cardiology* **38**, 187–205.

Patteson, M.W., Gibbs, C., Wotton, P.R. and Day, M.J. (1993) *Angiostrongylus vasorum* infection in seven dogs. *Veterinary Record* **133**, 565–570.

Paulsen, M.E., Allen, T.A., Jaenke, R.S., Ching, S., Severn, G.A. and Hammond, T. (1989) Arterial hypertension in two canine siblings: ocular and systemic manifestations. *Journal of the American Animal Hospital Association* **25**, 287–295.

Pearson, C.R. and Head, K.W. (1976) Malignant haemangioendothelioma (angiosarcoma) in the dog. *Journal of Small Animal Practice* **17**, 737–745.

Pedersen, H.D. (1996) Mitral valve prolapse in dogs. In: *Proceedings of the 6th Annual Congress of the European Society of Veterinary Internal Medicine*, Veldhoven, Holland.

Peterson, E.N., Moise, N.S., Brown, C.A., Hollis, N.E. and Slater, M.R. (1993) Heterogeneity of hypertrophy in feline hypertrophic disease. *Journal of Veterinary Internal Medicine* **7**, 183–189.

Peterson, M.E., Taylor, R.S. and Greco, D.S. (1990) Acromegaly in 14 cats. *Journal of Veterinary Internal Medicine* **4**, 192–201.

Pion, P.D. (1989) Taurine deficiency myocardial failure: new evidence for old theories. *Cornell Veterinarian* **79**, 5–9.

Pion, P.D., Kittleson, M.D., Rogers, Q.R. and Morris, J.G. (1987) Myocardial failure in cats associated with low plasma taurine: a reversible cardiomyopathy. *Science* **237**, 764–768.

Pion, P.D. and Kittleson, M.D. (1989) Therapy for feline aortic thromboembolism. In: *Current Veterinary Therapy X: Small Animal Practice* (Ed. R. W. Kirk). W.B. Saunders, Philadelphia, pp. 295–302.

Pion, P.D., Kittleson, M.D., Thomas, W.P., Skiles, M.L. and Rogers, Q.P. (1992a) Clinical findings in cats with dilated cardiomyopathy and relationship of findings to taurine deficiency. *Journal of the American Veterinary Medical Association* **201**, 267–274.

Pion, P.D., Kittleson, M.D., Thomas, W.P., Delellis, L.A. and Rogers, Q.R. (1992b) Response of cats with dilated cardiomyopathy to taurine supplementation. *Journal of the American Veterinary Medical Association* **201**, 275–284.

Pipers, F.S., Bonagura, J.D., Hamlin, R.L. and Kittleson, M. (1981) Echocardiographic abnormalities of the mitral valve associated with left-sided heart diseases in the dog. *Journal of the American Veterinary Medical Association* **179**, 580–586.

Pyle, R.L., Patterson, D.F. and Chacko, S. (1976) The genetics and pathology of discrete aortic stenosis in the Newfoundland dog. *American Heart Journal* **92**, 324–334.

Ramsey, I.K., Littlewood, J.D.L., Dunn, J.K. and Herrtage, M.E.H. (1996) The role of chronic disseminated intravascular coagulation in a case of canine angiostrongylosis. *Veterinary Record* **138**, 360–363.

Rawlings, C.A., Dawe, D.L., McCall, J.W., Keith, J.C. and Prestwood, A.K. (1982) Four types of occult *Dirofilaria immitis* infection in dogs. *Journal of the American Veterinary Medical Association* **180**, 1323–1326.

Remillard, R.L., Ross, J.N. and Eddy, J.B. (1991) Variance of indirect blood pressure measurements and prevalence of hypertension in clinically normal dogs. *American Journal of Veterinary Research* **52**, 561–565.

Ringwald, R.J. and Bonagura, J.D. (1988) Tetralogy of Fallot in the dog: clinical findings in 13 cases. *Journal of American Animal Hospital Association* **24**, 33–43.

Roth, L. (1994) Bacterial aortic endocarditis associated with subaortic stenosis. *Journal of Small Animal Practice* **35**, 169–172.

Rush, J.E., Keene, B.W. and Fox, P.R. (1990) Pericardial disease in the cat: a retrospective evaluation of 66 cases. *Journal of American Animal Hospital Association* **26**, 39–46.

Schaub, R.G., Gates, K.A. and Roberts, R.E. (1982) Effect of aspirin on collateral blood flow after experimental thrombosis of the feline aorta. *American Journal of Veterinary Research* **43**, 1647–1650.

Schelling, C.G., Greene, C.E., Prestwood, A.K. and Tsang, V.C.W. (1986) Coagulation abnormalities associated with acute *Angiostrongylus vasorum* infection in dogs. *American Journal of Veterinary Research* **47**, 2669–2673.

Sisson, D. (1989) Bradyarrhythmias and cardiac pacing. In: *Current Veterinary Therapy XI* (Eds. R.W. Kirk and J.D. Bonagura), W.B. Saunders, Philadelphia, pp. 286–294.

Sisson, D. and Thomas, W.P. (1984) Endocarditis of the aortic valve in the dog. *Journal of the American Veterinary Medical Association* **184**, 570–576.

Sisson, D., Thomas, W.P., Ruehl, W.W. and Zinkl, J.G. (1984) Diagnostic value of pericardial fluid analysis in the dog. *Journal of the American Veterinary Medical Association* **184**, 51–55.

Sisson, D., Luethy, M. and Thomas, W.P. (1991a) Ventricular septal defect accompanied by aortic regurgitation in five dogs. *Journal of American Animal Hospital Association* **27**, 441–448.

Sisson, D., Thomas, W.P., Woodfield, J., Pion, P.D., Leuthy, M. and DeLellis, L.A. (1991b) Permanent transvenous pacemaker implantation in forty dogs. *Journal of Veterinary Internal Medicine* **5**, 322–331.

Sisson, D., Thomas, W.P., Reed, J., Atkins, C.E. and Gelberg, H.B. (1993) Intrapericardial cysts in the dog. *Journal of Veterinary Internal Medicine* **7**, 364–369.

Snyder, P.S. and Atkins, C.E. (1992) Current uses and hazards of the digitalis glycosides. In: *Current Veterinary Therapy XI: Small Animal Practice* (Ed. R.W. Kirk), W.B. Saunders, Philadelphia, pp. 689–693.

Soll, M.D. (1992) Recommended procedures for the diagnosis and management of heartworm (*Dirofilaria immitis*) infection. In: *Proceedings of the Heartworm Symposium*, 1992, American Heartworm Society, pp. 289–294.

Spaulding, G.L. and Owens, J.M. (1985) Cor pulmonale In: *Manual of Small Animal Cardiology* (Eds L.P. Tilley and J.M. Owens). Churchill Livingstone, New York, pp. 167–180.

Staaden, R.V. (1981) Cardiomyopathy of English cocker spaniels. *Journal of the American Veterinary Medical Association* **178**, 1289–1292.

Swensen, L., Haggstrom, J., Kvart, C. and Juneja, R.K. (1996). Relationship between parenteral cardiac status in cavalier King Charles spaniels and prevalence and severity of chronic valvular disease in offspring. *Journal of the American Veterinary Medical Association* **208**, 2009–2112.

Thomas, R.E. (1985) Case of canine heartworm disease (*Dirofilaria immitis*) in the U.K. *Veterinary Record* **117**, 14–15.

Thomas, R.E. (1987) Congestive heart failure in young cocker spaniels (a form of cardiomyopathy?): details of eight cases. *Journal of Small Animal Practice* **28**, 265–279.

Thomas, W.P., Mathewson, J.W., Suter, P.F., Reed, J.R. and Meierheury, E.F. (1984a) Hypertrophic obstructive cardiomyopathy in a dog: clinical, haemodynamic, angiographic and pathologic studies. *Journal of the American Animal Hospital Association* **20**, 253–260.

Thomas, W.P., Reed, J.R., Bauer, T.G. and Breznock, E.M. (1984b) Constrictive pericardial disease in the dog. *Journal of the American Veterinary Medical Association* **184**, 546–553.

Thomas, W.P., Reed, J.R. and Gomez, J.A. (1984c) Diagnostic pericardiography in dogs with spontaneous pericardial effusion. *Veterinary Radiology* **25**, 2–16.

Thomas, W.P., Gaber, C.E., Jacobs, G.J., Kaplan, P.M., Lombard, C.W., Moise, N.S. and Moses, B.L. (1993) Recommendations for standards in transthoracic two-dimensional echocardiography in the dog and cat. *Journal of Veterinary Internal Medicine* **7**, 247–252.

Thrusfield, M.V, Aitken, C.G.G. and Darke, P.G.G. (1985) Observations on breed and sex in relation to canine heart valve incompetence. *Journal of Small Animal Practice* **26**, 709–717.

Tilley, L.P. (1991) Pro-Con: should ventricular arrhythmias be treated in dogs? *Proceedings of the 9th American College of Veterinary Internal Medicine Forum*, New Orleans, pp. 681–683.

Tilley, L.P. (1992) In: *Essentials of Canine and Feline Electrocardiography*. Lea and Febiger, Philadelphia, p. 175.

Tilley, L.P., Liu, S.K., Gilbertson, S.R., Wagner, M.D. and Lord, P.F. (1977) Primary myocardial disease in the cat. *American Journal of Pathology* **87**, 493–522.

Tilley, L.P., Bond, B.R., Patnaik, A.K. and Liu, S.K. (1981) Cardiovascular tumours in the cat. *Journal of American Animal Hospital Association* **17**, 1009–1021.

Turner, J.L., Broddon, J.D., Lees, G.E. and Greco, D.S. (1990) Idiopathic hypertension in a cat with secondary hypertensive retinopathy associated with a high salt diet. *Journal of American Animal Hospital Association* **26**, 647–651.

Van Fleet, J.F. and Ferrans, V.J. (1986) Myocardial diseases of animals. *American Journal of Pathology* **124**, 98–178.

Vollmar, A.M., Reusch, C., Kraft, W. and Schulz R (1991) Atrial natriuretic peptide concentration in dogs with congestive heart failure, chronic renal failure and hyperadrenocorticism. *American Journal of Veterinary Research* **52**, 1831–1834.

Ware, W.A. and Bonagura, J.D. (1986) Canine myocardial diseases. In: *Current Veterinary Therapy IX: Small Animal Practice* (Ed. R.W. Kirk), W.B. Saunders, Philadelphia, pp. 370–380.

Ware, W.A., Lund, D.D., Subieta, A.R. and Schmid, P.G. (1990) Sympathetic activation in dogs with congestive heart failure caused by chronic mitral valve disease and dilated cardiomyopathy. *Journal of the American Veterinary Medical Association* **197**, 1475–1481.

White, R.N., Stepien, R.L., Hammond, R.A., Holden, D.J., Torrington, A.M., Millner, H.R., Cobb, M.A. and Hellen, S.H. (1995) Mitral valve replacement for the treatment of congenital mitral dysplasia in a bull terrier. *Journal of Small Animal Practice* **36**, 407–410.

Whitney, J.C. (1974) Observations on the effect of age on the severity of heart valve lesions in the dog. *Journal of Small Animal Practice* **15**, 511–522.

Williams, G.D., Adams, L.G., Yaeger, R.G., McGrath, R.K., Read, W.K. and Bilderback, W.R. (1977) Naturally occurring trypanosomiasis (Chagas' disease) in dogs. *Journal of the American Veterinary Medical Association* **171**, 171–177.

Wood, G.L., Hirsch, D.C., Selcer, R.R., Rinaldi, M.G. and Boorman, G.A. (1978) Disseminated aspergillosis in a dog. *Journal of the American Veterinary Medical Association* **172**, 704–707.

Zucker, I.H., Earle, A.M. and Gilmore, J.P. (1977) The mechanism of adaptation of left atrial stretch receptors in dogs with chronic congestive heart failure. *Journal of Clinical Investigation* **60**, 323–331.

35

Diseases of the Respiratory System

W. T. Clark

Introduction	345	Nasal cavity and nasopharynx	347
History and presenting signs	345	Larynx	351
Physical examination	345	Trachea, bronchi and lungs	353
The approach to the investigation of a respiratory problem	347	Mediastinum and pleural cavity	362

INTRODUCTION

In dogs and cats the respiratory system has several functions. The most important function is to transfer oxygen and carbon dioxide between blood and the atmosphere outside the animal and thus regulate the homeostasis of oxygenation and acid–base balance. In dogs the respiratory system has a significant role in thermoregulation by means of heat loss which occurs due to evaporation from the surfaces of the airways and the mouth when the animal is panting. Vocalization is another function of the respiratory system in both dogs and cats.

Respiratory failure and death may be the outcome of some progressive diseases affecting the respiratory system, for example laryngeal obstruction, whereas other conditions may cause obvious clinical signs and discomfort to the animal but pose no danger of respiratory failure. Chronic sinusitis is an example of such a condition.

As a generalization it can be said that diseases of the respiratory system usually produce clinical signs which are readily apparent to the owner and to the veterinarian. It is not usually necessary to do extensive investigation to confirm that a dog or cat has a respiratory problem but it is quite often necessary to do considerable testing to identify the nature, extent and cause of the disease process.

HISTORY AND PRESENTING SIGNS

A complete and careful history is the essential first step in the investigation of a respiratory problem but the principles involved in collecting the historical information are largely the same as for other body systems and do not require extensive discussion here.

Specific inquiry regarding possible exposure to infectious agents should be made. Dogs which have recently been in kennels may have been exposed to the agents which cause infectious tracheobronchitis whereas cats in a boarding cattery may have come in contact with viruses which cause upper respiratory tract infections. The vaccination status of the animals is also relevant in this regard.

Yeast and fungal infections often have specific geographical distributions and should be suspected if the animals have visited or lived in areas where diseases caused by these organisms are endemic.

The major presenting signs of respiratory diseases in dogs and cats are set out in Table 35.1.

PHYSICAL EXAMINATION

It is very important to stand back and observe the whole animal before performing a detailed examination of the respiratory system. At this stage abnormal behaviours such as coughing or sneezing may be seen or the sound of stridor may be heard. With the animal at rest dyspnoea may be evident and the rate and character of respiration should be noted. The respiratory system should then be examined in detail in a systematic way.

Table 35.1 Presenting signs of respiratory disease

Sneeze	Sneezing is caused by irritation within the nasal cavity and localizes the problem to the nose.
Nasal discharge	This may come from one nostril or both and may be serous, purulent or haemorrhagic or any combination. Problems causing nasal discharge largely arise from the nasal cavity, nasopharynx or frontal sinuses.
Haemoptysis	Bleeding from the lungs or bronchi is an unusual presenting sign in dogs or cats. It usually indicates a serious problem involving the lung.
Cough	The receptors for the cough reflex are situated in the larynx, trachea and bronchi so coughing is a feature of diseases involving these structures. In dogs coughing is often a feature of left-sided heart enlargement where the enlarged left atrium presses on the bronchi.
Tachypnoea	Unusually rapid respiration is a feature of diseases which restrict lung expansion. This may be due to pulmonary fibrosis or to diseases involving the pleural cavity. In dogs tachypnoea must be differentiated from panting which is a physiological response brought on by hyperthermia, exercise and excitement.
Dyspnoea	This term is used when an animal shows a degree of breathing effort which is inappropriate for the amount of exercise the animal has recently taken. Dyspnoea is recognized and assessed by noting changes in the rate, rhythm or character of respiration. Dyspnoea can be a presenting feature of many respiratory diseases and is a measure of the animal's attempts to maintain gas exchange in a situation where respiratory function is failing.
Orthopnoea	This term describes the situation where an animal can only breathe easily when it is standing.
Stridor	This is a loud and usually high-pitched noise produced when air moves rapidly through a narrow opening. Stridor is most commonly caused by lesions which narrow the laryngeal opening but it can occur with tracheal stenosis.

Inspection of the nose and face will reveal lesions involving the bones of the nose although these are fairly uncommon. The presence and character of any nasal discharge should be noted and whether it involves one nostril or both. The patency of the nasal cavity can be determined by noting whether there is sufficient air movement to displace a wisp of cotton held near the nostril.

Inspection of the pharynx and larynx can only be carefully carried out when the animal is heavily sedated or anaesthetized. A laryngoscope is a useful instrument for depressing the tongue and epiglottis and illuminating the opening to the larynx. Palpation of the larynx and cervical trachea forms part of the examination but rarely detects significant abnormality. Palpation of the thoracic wall sometimes detects rib fractures or neoplastic masses but in many cases is not informative.

Percussion of the chest detects changes in resonance and inferences can be made concerning the contents of the thorax. An increase in resonance is associated with an increased amount of air in the chest as happens in pneumothorax whereas dullness on percussion indicates the presence of denser substances such as fluid or solid organs. Dogs vary so much in size, shape and degree of subcutaneous fat that there is no standard measure of resonance so the chest should be percussed dorsally and ventrally, left and right listening for asymmetry in the resonant sounds.

Auscultation, using a stethoscope, allows recognition and characterization of sounds arising from the respiratory system. In general the sound is loudest when the head of the stethoscope is placed close to the origin of the sound. A stethoscope can be used to listen to abnormal sounds arising from the larynx but it is mainly used to examine sounds arising within the airways of the chest. The terminology used to describe the findings on auscultation has recently been much simplified and old terms have been discarded.

Normal breath sounds are produced by air moving through the conducting airways and in healthy dogs and cats at rest these sounds may be so quiet as to be inaudible. In the examination room dogs often pant due to excitement, high ambient temperature, pyrexia and some diseases. In these animals the increased air flow causes quite loud, harsh breath sounds clearly audible all over the chest. Animals with some respiratory diseases may have an increased rate and depth of respiration and again breath sounds may be clearly heard. In dogs and cats with diseases involving the airways and lungs, abnormal sounds may be detected although they are certainly not present in the majority of animals with diseases in these areas. The abnormal sounds are described as crackles and wheezes. Crackles are clicking, popping, bubbling sounds which are usually discontinuous and best heard during inspiration. The crackles are thought to be produced by the sudden opening of small airways which were previously blocked or occluded. Wheezes are whistling or squeaking sounds which are long and drawn out and produced by air passing through narrow airways.

For cats and most dogs the area for auscultation of the respiratory system is fairly small and the information obtained by auscultation is largely limited to recognizing that an abnormality exists. The nature and the extent of the abnormality is better determined by other tests.

Abnormal respiratory signs can be produced by disease processes which originate in other parts of the body and only indirectly affect the respiratory system. Examples include cardiac enlargement causing coughing, diabetic ketoacidosis producing metabolic acidosis with compensatory hyperventilation, and gross abdominal distension causing dyspnoea. A complete physical examination and review of the history will usually reveal whether the disease primarily involves the respiratory system or whether it originates elsewhere.

Dogs and cats have substantial reserves of respiratory function. Many pets live very quiet and sedentary lives so the disease process is often very advanced by the time the animal shows signs which are recognized by its owner. If the animal is dyspnoeic at rest it has almost exhausted all its reserves and very little stress in the nature of restraint or positioning for diagnostic procedures may precipitate fatal respiratory failure.

THE APPROACH TO THE INVESTIGATION OF A RESPIRATORY PROBLEM

There are so many diagnostic procedures which can be carried out on the respiratory system that it is essential, for cost and efficiency, to localize the problem before resorting to detailed investigations. Fortunately, in most cases, using information from the history and physical examination it is possible to narrow the dysfunction to one of four areas (Table 35.2).

NASAL CAVITY AND NASOPHARYNX

Diagnostic procedures for the nasal cavity and nasopharynx

Radiology

This is a most useful technique for examining the nasal cavity and the nasal sinuses as air provides good contrast for outlining the turbinates and surrounding bones. Correct positioning is very important to avoid superimposition of the mandibles. For the nasal cavity the dorsoventral exposure with an intraoral film or a ventrodorsal projection with the mouth opened wide give the most diagnostic films. Lateral views are usually less informative although they do show whether the disease process extends to the frontal sinuses. If the frontal sinuses are involved it may be necessary to take skyline views so that left and right sides can be compared.

Changes noted on radiography include loss of turbinate detail, increased radiopacity, septal deviation, vomer erosion and mineralization within the nasal cavity. Destruction of the maxillary and palatine bones sometimes occurs and extranasal soft tissue masses may be seen. Turbinate destruction and increased radiolucency are features of chronic infections, such as aspergillosis, whereas increased radiodensity occurs when the nasal passages become filled with discharge or tumour (Gibbs *et al.*, 1979; Sullivan *et al.*, 1986, 1987).

Computed tomography is an excellent technique for demonstrating proliferative and destructive lesions within the nasal cavity but at the present time this technology is not widely available for small animals (Codner *et al.*, 1993).

Table 35.2 Localizing features of respiratory disease

Site	History and clinical signs
Nasal cavity and nasopharynx	Sneezing, nasal discharge, obstructed air flow, sometimes facial deformity
Larynx	Airway obstruction, stridor, coughing
Trachea, bronchi, lungs	Coughing, sometimes dyspnoea, tachypnoea or obstruction. Sometimes abnormal airway sounds
Mediastinum and pleural cavity	Dyspnoea, tachypnoea, sometimes coughing

Endoscopy

The rostral part of the nasal cavity can be examined with an otoscope and this instrument may allow identification and removal of a recently inhaled foreign body. Most neoplasms arise from the ethmoturbinate region in the caudal part of the nose beyond the reach of an otoscope. The nasal cavity can be thoroughly examined using a rigid endoscope of the type used for arthroscopy, however there are some difficulties with the technique. Diseased nasal chambers almost always contain mucopurulent discharge which has to be flushed away before the nasal cavity and mucosa can be seen. Irrigating saline can be infused alongside the endoscope or a Foley catheter can be passed through the mouth into the caudal nares and used to flush the nose. The presence of more than a very small amount of discharge indicates some disease process in the nose. The nasal mucosa is easily damaged and this leads to copious haemorrhage making endoscopy difficult. Foreign bodies and fungal plaques are usually easily recognized but neoplastic and chronic inflammatory lesions are often hard to recognize especially if the mucosa is still intact (Sullivan, 1987).

Tumours sometimes involve the caudal nares and this area can be examined using a dental mirror after pulling the soft palate rostrally. Alternatively a fibreoptic bronchoscope may be used in large dogs. The instrument is inserted through the mouth and the tip is turned behind the soft palate to view the nasopharyngeal opening.

Microbiology

Examinations for bacteria are often performed on nasal discharges but the organisms isolated are usually secondary invaders and rarely of pathogenic significance. Cryptococcal organisms can be easily recognized on smears and can be cultured. Fungal infections are usually due to *Aspergillus* or *Penicillium* species. Smears and cultures are not very reliable tests for fungal infections in the nose as they sometimes fail to find the organisms and positive culture of these common environmental organisms may occur in dogs without the disease. Serological tests are useful as affected dogs usually give positive reactions whereas healthy dogs have no *Aspergillus* or *Penicillium* antigens or antibodies (Sharp *et al.*, 1991).

Cytology

Samples for cytology are usually obtained by inserting a cytology brush or swab into the nose and then rolling the cells on to a slide. Cytology is particularly useful for diagnosing neoplasia although in some cases the test may be negative if the lesion is not exfoliating cells. Inflammatory changes are commonly seen but are usually non-specific and therefore of limited assistance in diagnosis (French, 1987).

Biopsy

Tissues may be obtained for histology via the nares or by exploratory rhinotomy. However, rhinotomy involves major surgery and is to be avoided unless there is a good chance that it can help the patient. Several biopsy techniques have been described using cutting needles such as the Tru-cut biopsy needle or aspiration of pieces of tissue using rigid or soft catheters. When using rigid needles or catheters it is important to avoid penetrating the cribriform plate so the distance from the nares to the mass is measured on a radiograph and used as a guide for the distance the needle should be inserted (Withrow *et al.*, 1985; Love *et al.*, 1987a).

Disease conditions of the nasal cavity and nasopharynx

Acute rhinitis

Acute onset of a nasal discharge may be due to trauma, foreign material in the nasal cavity or infection with distemper or the feline respiratory viruses. However, in these cases diagnosis is usually fairly easily made on history and physical examination and the discharge resolves spontaneously or in response to treatment of the underlying cause. Nursing care is important so that the external nares do not become blocked with dry discharge.

Foreign body rhinitis

Dogs with foreign bodies in the nasal cavity are usually presented with acute sneezing and nasal irritation. Foreign bodies are rarely the cause of a longstanding nasal discharge in the dog and almost never in the cat. Foreign bodies are usually composed of plant material and are similar in radiodensity to surrounding tissues. They usually occupy the rostral part of the nasal cavity and are best diagnosed by endoscopy and removed with forceps.

Cryptococcal rhinitis

Infection with the yeast organism *Cryptococcus neoformans* can involve a number of tissues of the body but the nasal cavity is a common site in the cat although less so in the dog. Nasal infection may extend to involve the bones and subcutaneous tissue so that in addition to nasal discharge affected animals sometimes have swelling and distortion of the face. The organisms are usually present in large numbers and can be readily found on smears from the nose or material aspirated from the swellings (Fig. 35.1).

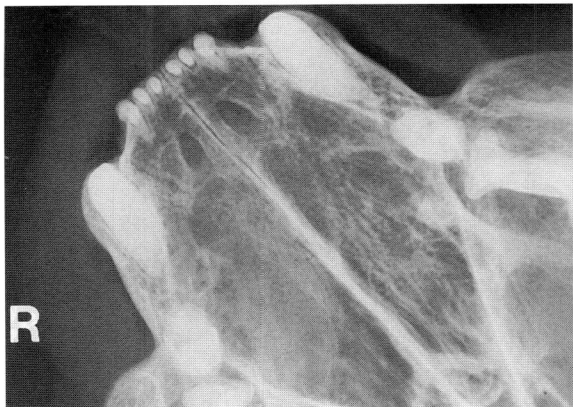

Figure 35.1 Nasal cryptococcus infection in a cat. The right side of the nasal cavity shows increased radiodensity and some loss of turbinate detail.

Treatment with antifungal drugs has produced encouraging results although, as yet, there is no agreed protocol for choice of drug, dosage or duration. Ketoconazole is usually effective in cats and dogs with minimal side effects but treatment has to be continued for several months. It has been suggested that combination therapy with ketoconazole and flucytosine may give better results but flucytosine is expensive and sometimes provokes skin reactions in dogs although this does not seem to be a problem in cats (Shaw, 1988). Clinical studies have shown that itraconazole is also effective with fewer side effects than ketoconazole (Medleau *et al.*, 1995).

Healthy cats and dogs are serologically negative for cryptococcus antigen (Medleau *et al.*, 1990) so antigen levels can be used to monitor the progress of therapy. Therapy has to be continued for months and recurrence may still happen after all signs have cleared up and antigen levels have fallen to zero.

Fungal rhinitis

Fungal infections develop in the nasal cavities of dogs but not in cats. The disease has been reported from many parts of the world but there does seem to be some geographical variation in the prevalence of the disease. The principal organisms involved are *Aspergillus fumigatus* and *Penicillium* species.

Adults of the long-nosed breeds are usually involved and present with a copious purulent discharge which is sometimes haemorrhagic. The organisms cannot always be isolated from the discharge and furthermore *Aspergillus* and *Penicillium* species are commonly present in the environment and can sometimes be isolated from the noses of healthy dogs. Radiographic changes, although not completely specific, are suggestive as there is usually turbinate destruction accompanied by increased radiolucency in the rostral part of the nasal cavity. Diagnosis is confirmed by viewing a mycelial plaque on endoscopy or by positive serological test (Fig. 35.2).

Success or partial success has been claimed for a number of treatments including local therapy

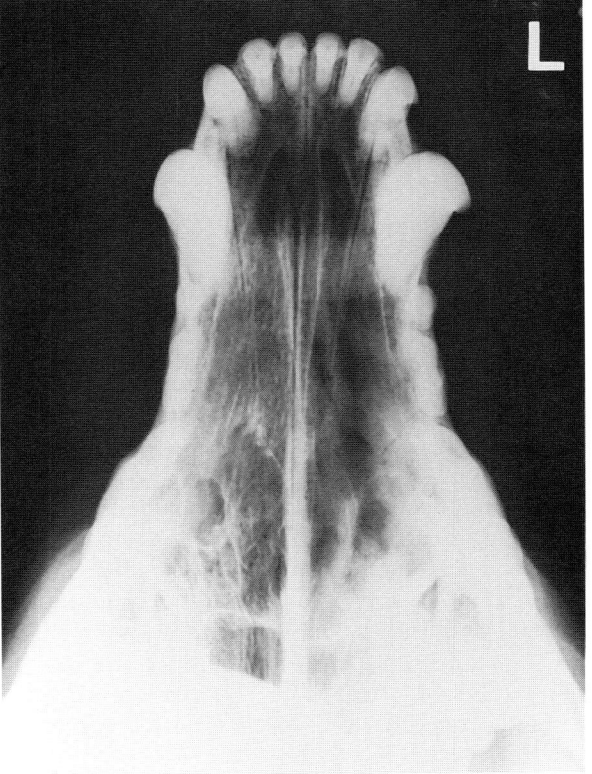

Figure 35.2 Nasal aspergillosis in a dog. The left nasal cavity shows turbinate destruction as increased radiolucency and absence of turbinate pattern in the mid-section of the radiograph. There is increased radiodensity in the caudal part of the left nasal cavity due to displacement of air by fungus or exudate.

such as surgery or flushing with enilconazole or clotrimazole or systemic therapy with antifungal drugs such as thiabendazole, ketoconazole, itraconazole and fluconazole. From a number of reports on clinical cases it seems that systemic therapy is successful in about 50% of cases whereas local irrigation of the nose can be successful in up to 90% of cases (Sharp et al., 1992).

Mycotic infection of the nasal mucosa with *Rhinosporidium seeba* has been reported in a small number of dogs in North America. Affected animals develop proliferative lesions which arise from within the nasal cavity. Recurrence may follow surgical removal and there is little information on medical therapy (Allison et al., 1986).

Parasitic rhinitis

Infestation with nasal parasites is not a problem in cats and occurs only very rarely in dogs. The parasite *Linguatula serrata* is well described in dogs but appears to be extremely rare. The nasal mite *Pneumonyssoides* (formerly *Pneumonyssus*) *caninum* occasionally infects dogs and causes signs of nasal irritation. Successful treatment has been reported using ivermectin at a dose rate of 0.2 mg kg^{-1}, orally or by subcutaneous injection (Marks et al., 1994).

Neoplasia

In the cat the nasal cavity is an uncommon site for neoplasia. A report on 16 cases of neoplasia involving the feline nasal passages and nasal sinuses described five animals with adenocarcinomas and five with undifferentiated carcinomas (Cox et al., 1991). The small number of cases examined by the author have been mainly of lymphoid origin. Canine nasal tumours usually affect middle-aged or elderly animals, especially those with long noses. The presenting signs include sneezing, epistaxis, respiratory noise, nasal and ocular discharge (Morrison et al., 1989). In a minority of cases the lesion involves the bones of the face and leads to deformity. The tumour usually remains in the primary site until a late stage in the disease but extension into the cranium and distant metastasis have been reported (Smith et al., 1989; Hahn and Matlock, 1990).

Radiography is a useful step in diagnosis. The lesion usually involves one side of the nose more than the other so there is a lack of symmetry on the radiograph. Radiodensity is usually increased as air is replaced by tumour and discharge and there is usually an obvious loss of bone detail in the areas of the turbinates (Fig. 35.3). Endoscopy

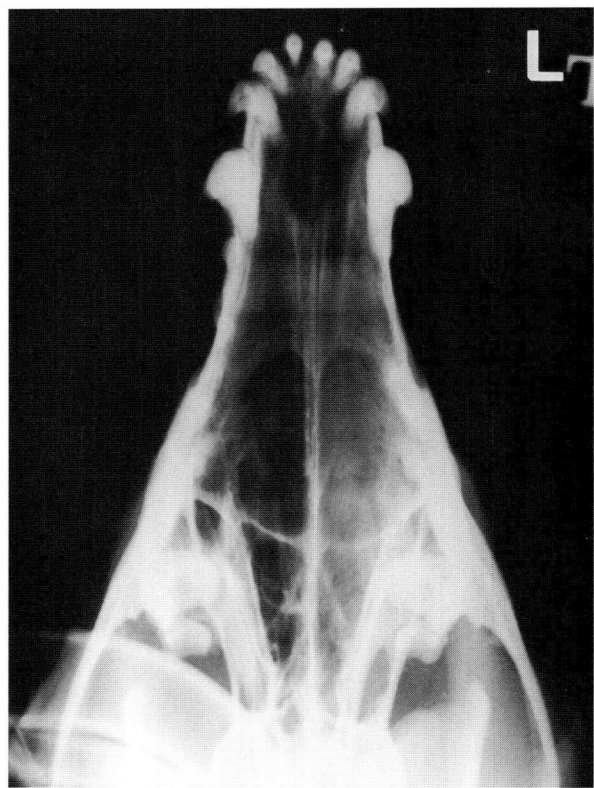

Figure 35.3 Nasal adenocarcinoma in a dog. The mid and caudal parts of the left nasal chamber show increased radiodensity and loss of the turbinate pattern due to the presence of tumour tissue.

is often of little value as blood and discharge restricts the view and even when the nose is cleared a mucous membrane-covered tumour may be hard to differentiate from normal structures in the nose.

Diagnosis depends on identifying neoplastic processes by cytology or histopathology. Cytology specimens are easily obtained but are not always diagnostic whereas histopathology will usually give a clear answer provided the correct tissue has been sampled. Most canine tumours develop in the ethmoturbinate region which makes them less accessible for accurate biopsy and in a small number of cases exploratory rhinotomy may be required to examine the lesion and collect samples.

Adenocarcinoma is probably the most common type of nasal tumour but chondrosarcoma and osteosarcoma are also fairly common. Unfortunately most of the nasal neoplasms carry a poor prognosis. The published results of cases treated surgically show that the median survival is

Table 35.3 Drugs for nasal diseases

Drug	Species	Dose and route (mg kg⁻¹)	Frequency	Duration	Indications
Ketoconazole	C,D	10, p.o.	12 h	3–6 months	Cryptococcal rhinitis
Itraconazole	C,D	10, p.o.	24 h	3–6 months	Cryptococcal rhinitis
Enilconazole	D	10, as a 5% solution for nasal irrigation	12 h	7–10 days	Nasal aspergillosis
Ivermectin	D	0.2, s.c. or p.o. (not used in Collie dogs)	Once		*Pneumonyssoides caninum*

C, cat; D, dog.

very short and current chemotherapeutic agents have little effect on these tumours. Orthovoltage and megavoltage radiotherapy has been used following surgical debulking with some reasonable survival rates. Computed tomography gives a good indication of the extent of the neoplasm and helps plan therapy. One series of 77 cases reported an overall survival of 60% at one year and 38% at two years (Theon *et al.*, 1993). Brachytherapy using intracavitary iridium isotope after surgery also produced some reasonable survival times. However, these treatments are not without difficulties and complications.

Chronic rhinitis

A number of conditions can lead to chronic non-specific inflammatory changes in the nasal mucosa. In animals which have dysphagia due to a pharyngeal disorder food material may enter the nose from the nasopharynx and cause sneezing and a purulent discharge. Similar complications usually follow oronasal fistula where there is a defect in the palate due to trauma or neoplasia. If the underlying problem can be corrected the signs of rhinitis usually clear up quickly.

Nasopharyngeal polyps can cause dyspnoea and nasal discharge in young cats. The lesions arise in the middle ear or eustachian tube and can be detected on radiography or by inspection of the nasopharynx. Although the lesions can be easily withdrawn from the eustachian tube recurrence is quite likely and much better results are achieved if a bulla osteotomy is also carried out (Kapatkin *et al.*, 1990).

It is quite common to find dogs with radiographic changes involving the turbinates and chronic inflammatory changes on biopsy of the mucosa and turbinates but no aetiology can be determined. These cases are simply classified as chronic rhinitis. Lymphoplasmacytic rhinitis has been described in a small series of dogs and corticosteroid therapy controlled the clinical signs (Burgener *et al.*, 1987).

Sinusitis

The frontal sinuses in cats and dogs are often involved in disease processes as an extension of conditions in the nasal cavity. However, cats are sometimes presented with a chronic purulent discharge and radiography shows that the most significant changes are in the frontal sinuses which are full of pus. It has been postulated that secondary bacterial infection follows upper respiratory tract viral infection, but these cats often do not have a very convincing history of viral infection. Studies have shown that these cats do not have a high prevalence of feline leukaemia or feline immunodeficiency virus infection (Norsworthy, 1993). Antibiotic therapy usually reduces the discharge while the cat is on treatment but the signs recur when treatment ends. These animals often improve considerably after surgery to remove pus from the frontal sinuses, curette the diseased mucosa and enlarge the opening between the sinuses and the nasal cavity.

LARYNX

The larynx is a complex structure of cartilages, muscles, nerves and mucosal folds. It functions as a valve controlling air flow into and out of the trachea and also prevents the aspiration of material during eating and drinking. The entrance to the larynx, known as the glottis, is formed by the arytenoid cartilages and vocal folds on either side and when the glottis is closed these structures meet in the midline. Further protection of the airway is provided by the backward repositioning of the epiglottis during swallowing. The sound waves of phonation are produced in the larynx and change in bark or meow may be an early sign of laryngeal disease.

Abduction of the arytenoid cartilages and vocal folds to increase the airway diameter is produced by contraction of the dorsal cricoarytenoid muscles. These muscles are innervated by the caudal laryngeal nerves which are branches of the vagus nerves.

■ Diagnostic procedures for the larynx

Radiology

Radiography can provide good images of the structures of the neck and larynx but the complexity of the laryngeal cartilages and the adjacent hyoid apparatus sometimes makes interpretation difficult. Although mass lesions will be seen on radiography they can usually be identified more easily on endoscopy or palpation.

Endoscopy

Endoscopy provides useful information in laryngeal disease but has to be carried out under general anaesthesia or deep sedation which can have some risks in animals with airway obstruction. A laryngoscope can be used to depress the tongue and epiglottis and illuminate the opening to the larynx.

Structural abnormalities can be recognized easily but functional abnormalities are more difficult to identify. Anaesthesia depresses respiratory function and laryngeal movement so that animals which are breathing quietly often show little or no laryngeal movement. As anaesthesia lightens and the animal starts to swallow, cough or hyperventilate abduction and adduction of the folds and arytenoid cartilages becomes obvious in normal animals but asymmetrical or depressed in laryngeal paralysis. At this stage the animal may be so lightly anaesthetized that swallowing and chewing movements make examination difficult. Positioning is important when comparing movement of the right and left arytenoids and the animal should be in sternal recumbency. The major functional abnormality is laryngeal paralysis where the abductor muscles fail to open the larynx during inspiration.

Other tests of laryngeal function

Mild degrees of airway obstruction have little effect on blood gas tensions but severe obstructions lead to lowered oxygen tensions and raised carbon dioxide tensions. This test is not necessary for diagnosis as severely affected animals are easily recognized on clinical examination but changes in blood gas values have been used to evaluate improvement in respiratory function following surgical procedures (Love et al., 1987b). Assessment of air flow can be made by tidal breathing flow–volume loop analysis. In this technique, tidal air flow in conscious animals is measured and, by electronic processing, produces loop patterns which are distinctively distorted in animals with airway obstructions. The technique has been used to document laryngeal obstructions and improvement following surgery on the airways (Amis et al., 1986; Burbidge et al., 1991).

Electromyography of the dorsal cricoarytenoid muscle usually detects evidence of neurogenic atrophy in cases of laryngeal paralysis. The cost of the equipment and difficulty in placing the recording electrode in severely atrophied muscles are limitations of the technique (Greenfield, 1987).

■ Disease conditions of the larynx

Laryngitis

Primary and localized inflammatory disease of the larynx is unusual but the mucosa of the larynx is often inflamed when the animal has an infection involving the respiratory tract such as tracheobronchitis or the animal is coughing from whatever cause. Inflammation of the mucosa may cause a change in the tone of the animal's bark and on laryngoscopic examination the mucosa, particularly round the arytenoids, is redder than normal. The mucosal changes reverse quickly when the underlying problems resolve.

Laryngeal paralysis

This condition is quite common in dogs but has been described rarely in cats. In some countries the problem occurs in young dogs of the Siberian Husky and Bouvier des Flandres breeds and there is evidence of a familial distribution. However, the problem is most often seen in middle-aged or old dogs of the larger breeds. The aetiology is unknown but the pathological changes of neurogenic atrophy of laryngeal muscles and Wallerian degeneration of the recurrent laryngeal nerves have been described. In the literature there have been suggestions that affected animals may have a generalized neuropathy or may be hypothyroid. Evidence from several published case studies now shows that few dogs have these complications.

Bilateral paralysis of the abductor muscles is

usually gradual in onset and the dog develops stridor associated with inspiration, diminished exercise tolerance and sometimes signs of hypoxia. Diagnosis is made by endoscopy when the arytenoid cartilages and the vocal folds fail to abduct during inspiration and in severe cases they may be drawn towards the midline during inspiration (Greenfield, 1987).

Treatment of laryngeal paralysis aims to increase the laryngeal opening without destroying its function in protecting the airway. Partial laryngectomy which involves removing the vocal folds and part of one arytenoid cartilage has been widely used (Ross et al., 1990). The technique is reasonably successful but does have a number of failures due to aspiration of food or water or due to recurrence of obstruction. The technique currently favoured is arytenoid lateralization (White, 1989) where one arytenoid is fixed in an abducted position. Although good results have been reported there are still some problems with aspiration.

Laryngeal stenosis and laryngeal collapse

The aetiology of these conditions is not entirely clear. In laryngeal stenosis, fibrous tissue narrows the entrance to the larynx and the arytenoids cannot be even passively abducted. Endotracheal intubation via the larynx is difficult or impossible in these animals.

In laryngeal collapse, the arytenoid cartilages lose their rigid structure so that the cuneiform processes become drawn into the laryngeal lumen and the corniculate processes which normally maintain the dorsal arch of the glottis collapse toward the midline thus completely obstructing the airway. These changes are probably secondary in brachycephalic breeds where high negative pressures are generated when the dog tries to draw air through restricted nasal passages. When collapse occurs in dogs without obvious nasal obstruction the lesion may be due to laryngeal paralysis or, perhaps, there may be some degenerative change in the cartilage itself. Laryngeal collapse is a difficult problem to deal with as the loss of cartilage rigidity makes it hard to reconstruct a free airway.

Partial laryngeal obstruction may be caused by eversion of the mucosa of the lateral ventricles and by displacement of the glosso-epiglottic mucosa but these conditions can be treated surgically (Bedford, 1983).

Stenosis of the larynx due to neoplasia is uncommon in dogs but cats occasionally have diffuse infiltration of the laryngeal mucosa with lymphoid neoplasms.

TRACHEA, BRONCHI AND LUNGS

Diagnostic procedures for the trachea, bronchi and lungs

Radiology

Radiography is a very useful technique for identifying and defining lower respiratory tract disease but attention to positioning and exposure is necessary to obtain diagnostic films. General anaesthesia, even of short duration, results in decreased aeration and increased blood flow in the dependent lung which can then appear to be abnormally radiodense. This can be partly corrected by positive pressure ventilation prior to exposing the film. In order to examine the lungs fully it is necessary to obtain both left and right lateral views as well as ventrodorsal or dorsoventral views.

The volume of the dependent lung in lateral recumbency is half the volume of the lung when the patient is in sternal recumbency. Non-visualization of a moderately radiodense lesion in a dependent lung is due to the combined effects of reduced aeration, compression and increased blood flow in normal lung surrounding the lesion (Biller and Myer, 1987; Steyn and Green, 1990).

Fluoroscopy using an image intensifier is a good method for diagnosing tracheal and bronchial collapse provided sedative drugs which suppress the cough centre are not used. Contrast techniques can be used to outline the trachea and the bronchial tree but are seldom used as more information can be obtained by bronchoscopy.

Endoscopy

Endoscopy can provide useful information on the lumen and lining of the trachea and bronchi and can identify areas to sample for cytology or histopathology. The conducting airways are easy to examine with an endoscope as they are air filled and have rigid walls. Rigid and flexible endoscopes both give good views in the dog but it can be difficult to find an endoscope long enough and fine enough to use in the cat. General anaesthesia is essential for bronchoscopy and care must be taken to prevent hypoxia when the endoscope fills a large proportion of the trachea. In large dogs the bronchoscope is passed through the endotracheal tube which has a T-connection allowing anaesthetic gas to pass alongside the scope.

With rigid bronchoscopes the carina and parts of both major bronchi can be seen but flexible endoscopes can be advanced further into the bronchial tree and are more useful for sample collection. The endobronchial anatomy is described by Amis and McKiernan (1986) and the flexible bronchoscope can be directed into the bronchi of specific lung lobes. Standard human bronchoscopes are too short to reach far into the bronchial tree of large dogs and they are usually too large to pass down the tracheas of cats. The lining of the airways is smooth and pink and there is normally little or no discharge or exudate within the lumen. Diseased animals have thickening and reddening of the mucosa and often considerable amounts of discharge coming from the more distal bronchi. On occasion parasitic nodules, foreign bodies or tumours may be seen.

Tracheal, bronchial and alveolar cytology

Microscopic examination of exfoliated cells and discharges can be helpful when dealing with animals with a history of chronic cough. Samples may be obtained from the tracheobronchial mucosa or from the bronchoalveolar lining. The choice depends on where the disease process is thought to be located. Samples from the trachea and bronchi may be obtained using a guarded sterile cytology brush passed through a bronchoscope or may be obtained by tracheobronchial lavage; the latter technique may be carried out under general anaesthesia or in a conscious animal if it is cooperative. Bronchoalveolar lavage involves passing a catheter or bronchoscope much further into the bronchial tree and then using saline to flush and aspirate cells from the alveoli and distal bronchi (Hawkins et al., 1990).

Cytology sometimes establishes the cause of the problem, for example when neoplastic cells or fungal organisms are found but this is relatively uncommon. Changes in the numbers and morphology of the cell types give useful information on the underlying pathological processes and help to narrow down the list of likely causes (Hoffmann and Wellman, 1986). Fungal organisms were identified in bronchoalveolar lavage fluids from six out of nine dogs with pulmonary blastomycosis, histoplasmosis or coccidioidomycosis (Hawkins and DeNicola, 1990).

Transthoracic fine needle aspiration cytology is possible for large lung lesions lying near the chest wall but most lung lesions are small, multiple and diffuse and in these cases aspiration cytology is usually disappointing.

The value of cytology samples obtained from lungs by using Menghini aspiration biopsy needles was assessed in a series of 41 dogs and two cats (Teske et al., 1991). The cytological diagnosis was accurate in 83% of cases but 31% of the animals developed pneumothorax after the procedure and five animals died.

Histopathology

Samples of bronchial mucosa may be obtained with fine biopsy forceps passed through a bronchoscope. The samples are very small and difficult for a pathologist to orientate but they can give information on the nature of inflammatory changes in the mucosa. Samples of diseased lung may be obtained at thoracotomy but it is sometimes hard to justify the risk and expense of this procedure. Lung biopsies can be obtained with forceps through a bronchoscope but there is a risk of perforating the lung and causing pneumothorax.

Microbiology

A study on 33 normal dogs showed that swabs from the lower trachea failed to isolate bacteria from 63% of the animals (McKiernan et al., 1984). In animals with chronic diseases of the lower respiratory tract it is unusual to find bacteria which could be considered to be primary respiratory tract pathogens and it is likely that most of the organisms are secondary invaders. *Bordetella bronchiseptica*, canine adenovirus and canine parainfluenza virus can be isolated from dogs with acute tracheobronchitis and feline herpesvirus and feline calicivirus can cause similar problems in cats. However, microbiology is rarely needed to diagnose these conditions.

Parasitology

Certain parasitological tests are useful when investigating diseases of the lower respiratory tract. Respiratory signs are common in heartworm disease and this possibility should be checked out early in the investigation.

Examination of bronchial discharges can also be carried out but it is usually easier although less sensitive to look for swallowed larvae in faeces. Lungworm infection in cats is usually diagnosed in this way.

Haematology

Most of the haematological changes in animals with bronchial or pulmonary diseases are non-specific. Occasionally a marked rise in circulating eosinophils occurs in a dog or cat with respiratory signs and suggests an allergic or parasitic cause for the problem. Chronic respiratory disease with low oxygen tension may induce secondary polycythaemia.

Blood gas tensions

Blood gas tensions remain at fairly normal levels until the animal goes into serious respiratory failure and from this point the fall in oxygen tension parallels the decline in respiratory function. However, clinical signs alone are enough to indicate that the animal is in serious difficulties. It is fairly unusual to find elevated carbon dioxide levels in a conscious dog even if it has quite severe lung disease but raised carbon dioxide levels are common in animals with respiratory depression due to illness or anaesthesia.

Pulmonary function tests

A range of function tests measuring flows, compliance and volumes are widely used to monitor respiratory diseases in humans. Many of them require patient cooperation and are not easily adapted to small animal patients.

Values for respiratory compliance and pulmonary compliance have been published for dogs (Corcoran, 1991) but the necessity to make the measurements under anaesthesia and the variability in the normal values due to variation in the size and chest shape of different canine breeds limits the application of this measurement.

Pulmonary scintigraphy

Scanning techniques can be used to measure the distribution of radioisotopes in the lungs. Using special techniques, measurements of air flow and blood flow can be made. These techniques require expensive equipment and the use of radioisotopes and are limited to only a few specialist centres (Bauer and Thomas, 1983).

Disease conditions of the trachea, bronchi and lungs

Infectious tracheobronchitis in dogs

This condition, which is often referred to by its common name of kennel cough, spreads readily in kennels or pounds where numbers of dogs are kept together. Affected animals suddenly develop a harsh hacking cough but in most cases the dogs show no systemic illness and the cough resolves in a few days. Diagnostic tests are rarely indicated for this self-limiting condition but it is important that affected animals are recognized and isolated as the disease can spread readily in hospital wards or via anaesthetic equipment. Several infectious agents are involved and there is still some debate as to which are the most significant. Routine canine vaccines often include canine parainfluenza virus and canine adenovirus 2 and a vaccine for *Bordetella bronchiseptica* is also available. An epidemiological study on the effectiveness of the vaccines indicated that vaccination reduces the risk of contracting infectious tracheobronchitis (Thrusfield *et al.*, 1989).

Tracheal and bronchial collapse

Tracheal collapse is a common condition affecting dogs but not cats. Affected dogs are middle-aged or old and belong to the toy breeds. The aetiology of the condition is unclear but grossly and histologically there are degenerative changes in the cartilaginous rings and the dorsal tracheal ligament which leads to dorsoventral flattening and reduction in the cross-sectional area of the trachea (Fig. 35.4). Secondary inflammatory changes occur in the tracheal mucosa. The cervical or thoracic trachea or commonly parts of both may be involved and sometimes the mainstem bronchi may also collapse. Affected dogs are usually presented with a long history of harsh paroxysmal coughing but the animal is usually otherwise bright and well. Exercise and excitement often brings on the clinical signs.

Plain radiographs may show a narrowed tracheal lumen but may also fail to demonstrate collapse as it only occurs during certain stages of the respiratory cycle. Over-extension and over-flexion of the neck can produce apparently abnormal tracheal outlines in normal animals. Definitive diagnosis can be made by endoscopy where the loose dorsal ligament folds into the airway and instead of a circular cross-section the trachea has an elliptical shape. Fluoroscopy is also a good method of diagnosing tracheal collapse. The occlusion of the airway is very obvious when the dog coughs and fluoroscopy reveals the location and extent of the abnormality. The cervical trachea collapses during the inspiratory phase of the respiratory cycle whereas the thoracic trachea and bronchi collapse during expiration.

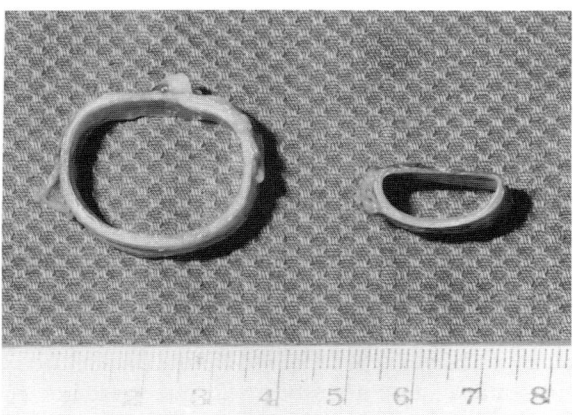

Figure 35.4 The specimen on the left shows the shape of a normal canine tracheal ring. On the right the dorsal tracheal ligament is excessively stretched. The change in shape leads to occlusion of the airway.

Many of the dogs with tracheal collapse also have other chest pathology such as bronchial thickening, obesity or left atrial dilation. It is not really clear what role these factors play in the aetiology of tracheal collapse or indeed which factors are causing the dog to cough.

The disease is usually progressive and the signs get worse with time. Medical treatment to control the signs includes bronchodilators, sedatives, antitussives and short courses of corticosteroids and these usually produce improvement. In the author's view glucocorticoids are much more effective than the other drugs but side effects may be a problem on long-term therapy. In a series of 100 cases reported by White and Williams (1994) 71 dogs on medical treatment showed resolution of clinical signs for longer then one year.

The role of surgery in this condition is still subject to some debate. Good results were claimed for a technique using a spiral prosthesis applied around the trachea and sutured to the rings to restore rigidity (Fingland, 1989). However, further study has shown that in some animals the trachea becomes devitalized due to damage to segmental blood vessels which supply the trachea. In a modification of the original technique care is taken to preserve the blood supply on one side of the trachea (Coyne *et al.*, 1993). An alternative technique uses a number of separate ring prostheses carefully placed to avoid damage to too much of the vascular supply. The technique is not applicable to collapse of the thoracic trachea and in practical terms many of the cases are not suitable surgical candidates and should be managed medically.

Tracheal and bronchial foreign bodies

Foreign bodies in the conducting airways are uncommon in dogs and very rare in cats. The most common foreign bodies are grass, wheat or barley awns. In some parts of the world there are species of grasses which are particularly likely to cause this problem. A variety of other objects, many of them radiodense, have also been reported. The foreign objects commonly lodge at the carina or in a branch of the bronchial tree.

Affected animals typically have a history of a very sudden onset of severe coughing. Sometimes this stage is missed or no action is taken and the dog develops a very chronic cough. Halitosis is often a feature of chronic cases but in general the dogs are quite well. Radiography will reveal radiodense foreign bodies lying in the caudal part of the trachea but will not reveal grass awns which have a radiodensity similar to surrounding tissues. Grass awns usually lodge in a caudal lobe bronchus and on radiography there is often a focal ill-defined increase in radiodensity round one of the caudal lobe bronchi. Bronchoscopy will often allow visualization of part of a foreign body but it may be necessary to first flush and aspirate surrounding exudate. The foreign body is removed using suitable forceps guided by endoscopy or by fluoroscopy if the object is radiodense. These cases usually have a good prognosis (Dobbie *et al.*, 1986; Lotti and Niebauer, 1992).

Canine chronic bronchial disease

This is a rather ill-defined condition or series of conditions affecting the bronchi. Other authors have used the terms chronic bronchitis, eosinophilic bronchitis and allergic bronchitis but at this stage little is known about the aetiology and it is not clear whether there are several diseases or variable manifestations of one condition. The presenting signs are similar regardless of the underlying aetiology.

Affected dogs are middle aged to elderly and, although some authors say small breeds are more commonly affected, it can occur in all sizes of dogs. The history of these cases includes a long period of coughing sometimes with periods of remission but there is a tendency for the cough to become more troublesome. Sometimes there are signs of airway obstruction but apart from these signs the dogs are usually well. The findings on chest auscultation are variable but in some cases crackles and wheezes are pronounced. On radiography the lungs often show increased interstitial density and pronounced peribronchial density but in milder form these changes resemble the pattern commonly attributed to ageing (Fig. 35.5). Patrid and Amis (1992) question the attribution of bronchial changes to ageing as they believe that these animals have true bronchial pathology. Cytology on bronchial washings from a series of 16 cases revealed that neutrophils were the predominant cells in 14 dogs whereas eosinophils were the main cells present in two animals (Patrid *et al.*, 1990).

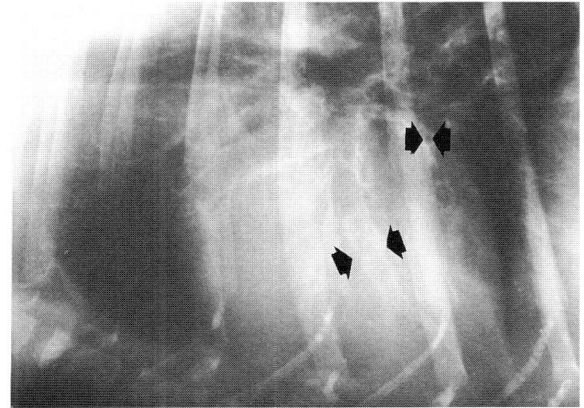

Figure 35.5 Chronic bronchitis in a dog. The arrows indicate thickened bronchial walls which show as distinct parallel lines in longitudinal projection and as circles in transverse projection.

On endoscopic examination the bronchial mucosa appears thickened and inflamed and there is a considerable amount of a thick mucopurulent exudate. There is some discussion in the literature about the prevalence of secondary bacterial infection but in one study bacteria were isolated from only a small proportion of dogs with chronic bronchial disease (Patrid *et al.*, 1990). The pathological changes include thickening of the bronchial mucosa with inflammatory cell infiltration and increased mucus production (Pirie and Wheeldon, 1976).

Respiratory function studies on a series of dogs with chronic bronchial disease showed that some of the animals had low blood oxygen tensions but all had normal carbon dioxide tensions. Changes in expiratory air flow pattern and in the regional distribution of an inhaled radioaerosol were also found in some dogs. The findings are compatible with obstructive disease in the airways. Following bronchodilator therapy the expiratory flow improved but there was no improvement in blood oxygen tension (Patrid *et al.*, 1990).

Bronchiectasis is a term used for irreversible bronchial dilation caused by the destruction of the elastic and muscular components of the bronchial wall. The cause of these changes is unclear and it is unknown whether bronchiectasis is an extension of the disease process in chronic bronchitis or whether there is some other aetiology. The dilated segments of bronchi fill with secretion resulting in a chronic cough. Diagnosis is made by contrast radiography of the bronchial tree and as this technique is infrequently performed the true prevalence of bronchiectasis is unknown. In the dog the cranial and middle lobes are more frequently involved and it is usual for several lobes to be involved. Unless the lesion is very restricted and can be excised the outlook for treatment is poor.

Congenital abnormalities in the structure and function of epithelial cilia have been reported in dogs. The term ciliary dyskinesia has been used to describe the dysfunction which results in poor clearance of respiratory secretions. Young dogs are affected and have chronic accumulation of nasal and bronchial discharges. Diagnosis is made on recognizing the abnormalities in cilia obtained by bronchial biopsy and examined by electron microscopy. However, it has been said that abnormal ciliary ultrastructure can be produced by acquired respiratory diseases. Dogs with primary ciliary dyskinesia may have other congenital abnormalities such as immotile sperm and situs inversus where there is transposition of the heart and abdominal organs (Crager, 1992).

The long-term prognosis for chronic bronchial disease is not good as the disease process is rarely reversible. However, medical therapy can often relieve the signs to a considerable extent. Therapy may include bronchodilation, corticosteroids to reduce airway inflammation and antibiotics to control infection but it should be noted that the majority of cases probably do not have significant bacterial infection. Obese dogs have large accumulations of fat within the mediastinum and a weight reduction programme often improves respiratory function in these cases. Mucolytic and expectorant drugs may help to clear bronchial secretions but there is some debate on the effectiveness of drugs currently available for this purpose. The use of cough suppressants may be criticized on the grounds that retention of excess secretions may enhance the damage to the airways but in some cases symptomatic relief from almost continual coughing is essential for the dog and its owners.

Feline bronchial disease

Bronchial disease in the cat is not particularly common and differs in many respects from the disease in dogs. The condition has some similarities to human asthma and the terms feline asthma and feline allergic bronchitis have been used. Young adult animals are usually involved and the clinical signs are often intermittent with normal respiration in between. The main presenting signs are periods of coughing and airway obstruction. On physical examination no abnormality may be found but during attacks the cat may show obvious expiratory difficulty and on auscultation wheezes may be heard during expiration. On radiology the lungs may appear over-inflated due to air trapped by bronchial constriction.

Bronchial wash cytology often reveals increased numbers of eosinophils, macrophages, neutrophils and lymphocytes but only in a small proportion of cats are eosinophils the predominant cell type (Corcoran et al., 1995).

The aetiology of the condition is unclear but a hypersensitivity response is thought to be responsible for causing intermittent bronchospasm, although the inciting agents have not so far been identified.

Treatment involves corticosteroids and bronchodilators to control the condition but for some cats long-term treatment is needed (Moise et al., 1989).

Bacterial bronchopneumonia

Acute bacterial bronchopneumonia is uncommon in cats and dogs which are vaccinated against respiratory viral infections and have warm dry housing. A report on 42 canine cases found that sporting and working dogs were more likely to be involved and 47% of the dogs were less than one year of age. The clinical presentation can be quite variable. Coughing is common but not a feature of every case. Pyrexia and signs of systemic illness are also common. Radiographic changes in the lungs are variable in extent and include interstitial and alveolar radiodensities. The white cell picture typically shows a neutrophilia with a left shift and bronchial cytology reveals a septic mucopurulent exudate. Gram-negative organisms predominate (Thayer and Robinson, 1984).

Acute necrotizing pneumonia due to streptococcal infection has been reported in mixed breed dogs admitted to a research establishment (Garnett et al., 1982). A similar outbreak with a high mortality caused by streptococci has been seen by the author in a greyhound kennel. Acute cases of bacterial bronchopneumonia may die before therapy can be instigated but less acute cases can be expected to respond to antibiotic therapy and supportive therapy aimed at improving respiration.

Chronic bacterial bronchopneumonia is not common in dogs or cats although cases are occasionally seen. Unusual organisms such as actinomyces may be found in the lesions. The pathological processes may be reasonably restricted to one or more lobes and will be seen as consolidated areas on radiography. On bronchoscopy pus will be seen coming from the bronchi of affected lobes. Treatment of this type of pneumonia is difficult and may not be very rewarding. The animal may improve while on antibiotics only to relapse when treatment stops. If medical treatment is to be successful it will have to be continued for several months so a non-toxic drug must be chosen. If the lesion is confined to one lobe surgical excision may be useful but it is likely that at thoracotomy the presence of additional small focal lesions shows that the disease is more widespread than indicated by radiography.

Aspiration pneumonia

Aspiration pneumonia can present as an acute or chronic problem. The acute form is more dramatic but the chronic form is probably more common. Acute aspiration occurs when an animal vomits and inhales food and gastric secretions while recovering from anaesthesia. Veterinarians are well aware of this risk and the measures to be taken to prevent it. Another cause of acute aspiration is near drowning where water is inhaled. This is not a common accident and in the author's experience it usually involves young dogs falling into swimming pools.

Chronic aspiration occurs in animals which have swallowing difficulties due to dysfunction of the pharynx or oesophagus or abnormal laryngeal function due to disease or following surgery. The pneumonia is often limited and mild but the animals have a cough. Diagnosis of inhalation pneumonia is usually made on history and clinical signs. On radiography there are one or more large areas of consolidation usually involving the dependent parts of the lungs but the radiographic findings are not pathognomonic although they do give a good indication of the extent of the disease.

For chronic aspiration the prognosis is quite good for the small number of cases where the underlying problem can be corrected. Acute aspiration is often a serious situation where extensive lung destruction will occur despite vigorous corrective and supportive therapy.

Parasitic infection

Heartworm disease caused by *Dirofilaria immitis* is prevalent in many parts of the world. The presence of adult worms in the pulmonary arteries leads to inflammatory changes in the arteries and the lung parenchyma and severely affected dogs are often presented with a history of coughing and poor exercise tolerance. Heartworm disease must always be included as a possible cause of disease of the lower respiratory tract in dogs which have lived in areas where the disease is endemic. The diagnosis and treatment of *Dirofilaria* infection is discussed in Chapter 48.

Angiostrongylus vasorum is a nematode parasite which appears to be increasing in prevalence in a number of European countries. The life cycle of this parasite involves an intermediate host and several species of snails and slugs are known to be involved. Adult parasites reside in the right ventricle and branches of the pulmonary artery. Eggs hatch in the pulmonary vessels and first stage larvae pass into the alveoli and then via the bronchi and alimentary tract to the faeces. Common presenting signs in infected dogs are coughing, dyspnoea and reduced exercise tolerance. Radiographic changes commonly found in dogs with clinical signs are numerous ill-defined focal areas of increased radiodensity throughout the lung fields. Specific changes associated with right ventricle or pulmonary artery involvement are less common.

Studies on infected dogs have recognized a number of clinical signs not directly attributable to respiratory disease. It is known that the parasite can occasionally be found in the systemic circulation and it is postulated that unusual signs may be produced by inflammation or thrombosis due to parasites which have lodged in systemic arteries. Diagnosis is best confirmed by finding larvae in faeces or bronchial wash specimens. Successful treatment has been reported using oral fenbendazole at a dose rate of 20 mg kg^{-1} day^{-1} for three weeks or 0.2 mg k^{-1} ivermectin by subcutaneous injection on one occasion or on two occasions a week apart (Martin *et al.*, 1993).

Aelurostrongylus abstrusus is a common parasite in cats in many areas of the world (Fig. 35.6). The parasite has a somewhat complicated life cycle involving an intermediate host (slugs and snails) and sometimes a transport host (bird, frog

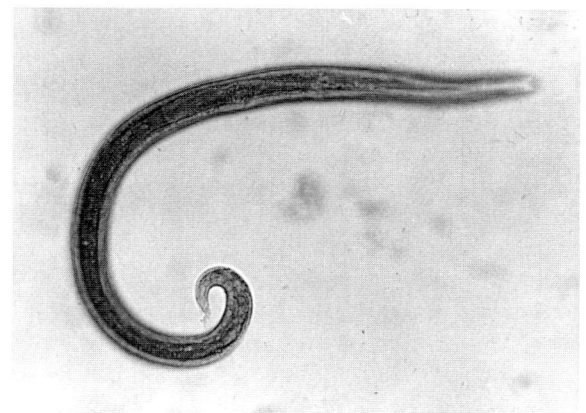

Figure 35.6 *Aelurostrongylus* larva in cat faeces.

or rodent). The adult parasite develops in the terminal bronchioles setting up bronchiolitis and interstitial pneumonia. Although infection is very common most cats are asymptomatic. However, cats are occasionally presented with severe dyspnoea and a marked cough. On radiographs of the chest there are multiple, ill-defined opacities 2–3 mm in diameter widely disseminated throughout the lung fields. There are alveolar, bronchial and interstitial changes but the bronchial and interstitial changes may become more obvious when the alveolar changes clear (Losonsky *et al.*, 1978) (Fig. 35.7). Diagnosis can be confirmed by finding larvae in bronchial washings or in faeces (Willard *et al.*, 1988). Treatment with fenbendazole must be carried out for several days to kill the adult parasites and corticosteroids and bronchodilators may be required for severely dyspnoeic cats.

Filaroides osleri is a canine parasite which has a wide geographical distribution but a low prevalence of disease. The parasites produce multiple granulomas, several millimetres in diameter, in the trachea and bronchi near the carina. A common mode of transmission is from mother to pups and it is suggested that this occurs when the mother feeds the pups on regurgitated food. Affected dogs have a loud and persistent cough and very severe cases may have a degree of airway obstruction. Diagnosis is easily made on endoscopy but the granulomas are sometimes seen on radiographs and the larvae may be found in faeces or bronchial washings. In the literature there are case reports of successful treatment with a number of anthelmintics but no carefully followed-up trials to establish the effectiveness of treatment for this parasite.

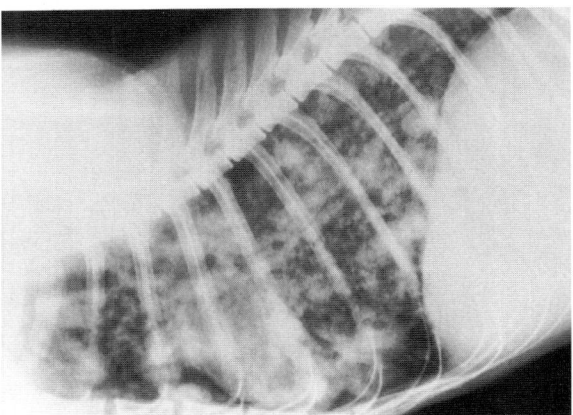

Figure 35.7 Severe *Aelurostrongylus* infection in a cat. There are numerous ill-defined radiodense foci throughout the lungs.

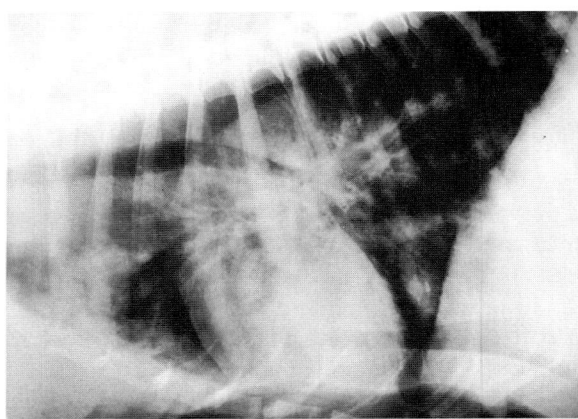

Figure 35.8 Eosinophilic pneumonia in a dog. There is marked peribronchial thickening seen as circular radiodensities round the end-on bronchi. There is also considerable interstitial radiodensity.

Eosinophilic pneumonia

At the present time the disease or complex of diseases associated with hypersensitivity reactions in the lower respiratory tract are not clearly understood. The main features are inflammatory changes in the bronchi or lung parenchyma associated with substantial eosinophil infiltration and quite often an elevation in the number of circulating eosinophils. A number of names have been used for this condition including eosinophilic bronchitis, allergic bronchitis, pulmonary eosinophilia and pulmonary infiltration with eosinophils. The disease process is thought to involve an IgE-mediated allergic reaction to as yet unidentified allergens.

Dogs with this condition have a history of persistent coughing, sometimes with evidence of dyspnoea and airway obstruction on chest auscultation. Bronchoscopy shows inflammatory changes in the airways with numerous eosinophils present in bronchial wash samples. A circulating eosinophilia is common but not invariably present. The radiographic changes are variable but usually include peribronchial thickening and increased interstitial radiodensity but alveolar changes are also sometimes present (Fig. 35.8). At an early stage of the disease investigation it is important to rule out parasitic infection as heartworm cases often have eosinophilia and a history of coughing and other parasites may also cause eosinophilia.

Treatment with prednisolone usually produces a good clinical response and some degree of resolution of the lung pathology as assessed by radiology. In a series of 14 cases 12 dogs went into complete remission on prednisolone therapy although six dogs required continuous or repeated medication (Corcoran *et al.*, 1991).

Pulmonary haemorrhage

Radiographic studies on injured dogs have shown that a high proportion have some degree of pulmonary haemorrhage shortly after the accident. On radiography there are patchy alveolar densities with air bronchograms and in some cases whole lobes may be consolidated. These haemorrhages are usually not, in themselves, life-threatening and many dogs show no clinical signs of pulmonary injury. The damage normally resolves in a few days without active treatment.

The importance of lung contusion lies in the risk it adds to animals which have anaesthesia and surgery for other injuries. Unless there is a compelling necessity for immediate surgery it is best to delay repair of injuries for 24–48 h to allow full evaluation of the injured animal including assessment of respiratory function.

Pulmonary oedema

Veterinarians are very familiar with left-sided heart failure in dogs where the animals have a history of coughing and radiographs of the chest show left atrial enlargement and pulmonary oedema. However, it seems likely that in many cases the cough is due to the dilated left atrium pressing on the left mainstem bronchus. Dyspnoea is usually a more obvious sign of pulmonary oedema than coughing especially in the cat.

The pathogenesis of pulmonary oedema is fairly complex but the most important factors are increased capillary hydrostatic pressure and changes in alveolar and vessel wall permeability. Pulmonary oedema can be classified into hydrostatic oedema and permeability oedema although some aetiologies cause both types of change.

Hydrostatic oedema is a common cause of respiratory signs and respiratory failure in small animals. It is usually produced by left-sided heart failure resulting from mitral valve insufficiency in dogs and cardiomyopathy in dogs and cats. Hydrostatic oedema can be iatrogenic due to overtransfusion of colloids but dogs with healthy kidneys are fairly resistant to overtransfusion although more care may be necessary in cats. Textbooks describe a number of causes of permeability oedema such as near drowning, smoke inhalation and electrocution but all of these are uncommon.

It is often impossible to make a diagnosis of pulmonary oedema on history and physical examination alone as the signs are variable in presentation and not sufficiently specific. Dyspnoea with rapid shallow respiration is seen in severe cases. On chest auscultation there may be abnormal airway sounds and in cases with cardiac disease heart murmurs or arrhythmias may be detected. Radiography of the lungs is very helpful in establishing a diagnosis of pulmonary oedema but distressed animals must be handled carefully and radiography may have to be delayed until respiratory failure is controlled. Radiographic changes include coalescing fluffy densities and air bronchograms and the lesions have a perihilar, dorsal and bilateral distribution. If the oedema is due to cardiovascular disease changes in cardiac outline may also be noted (Allen and Kruth, 1988).

It is important to recognize that the clinical signs of dyspnoea and sometimes coughing develop late in the process when the animal's respiratory reserve is all but exhausted. In severe cases emergency resuscitation may be required. A number of measures can be helpful.

Administration of oxygen can relieve hypoxia provided the animal does not struggle too much. Exercise restriction by cage rest often produces a marked improvement and sedatives can be used but must not cause respiratory depression if the animal is near respiratory failure or vasodilation if this is contraindicated by the animal's clinical condition.

Diuretics such as frusemide are usually very effective in relieving pulmonary oedema in the initial stages but they will become less effective as the underlying disease causing oedema progresses. Overuse of diuretics by reducing extracellular fluid can lead to inadequate circulating blood volume.

Pulmonary oedema can reflexly induce bronchoconstriction so bronchodilator drugs may be helpful. In cases where the oedema is due to changes in permeability glucocorticoid drugs may be indicated.

The prognosis for animals with pulmonary oedema is generally not very good. The immediate therapy for the oedema is usually effective but many of the underlying diseases such as cardiomyopathy and valvular disease are progressive so the aim of treatment is to improve the animal's condition and extend its life by therapy which assists cardiac function and controls oedema.

Paraquat toxicity

Acute respiratory distress and renal failure a few days after accidental ingestion of the herbicide paraquat has been reported in dogs. Affected animals show signs of progressive respiratory failure associated with alveolar haemorrhage, oedema, necrosis of the bronchial and alveolar epithelium and pulmonary fibrosis (Darke et al., 1977). The prognosis is extremely poor but there is a report of one case treated successfully with supportive therapy (O'Sullivan, 1989).

Pulmonary neoplasia

Secondary tumours which develop after metastatic spread from a neoplasm elsewhere are common in small animals. Common canine tumours which readily spread to the lungs include mammary gland carcinoma, fibrosarcoma, melanoma, osteosarcoma and haemangiosarcoma. Secondary tumours rarely produce clinical signs of respiratory disease, unless miliary in nature.

Primary tumours arising from bronchial or pulmonary tissues are rare in cats but are found occasionally in old dogs. The clinical radiographic and pathological features of 17 feline cases have been described (Barr et al., 1987). In a survey of 210 canine cases 75% were adenocarcinomas and 20% were alveolar carcinomas (Ogilvie et al., 1989a).

Dogs with primary pulmonary neoplasms have variable presenting signs which may include coughing, dyspnoea, lethargy, weight loss and diminished exercise tolerance. The radiographic appearance of the lesions can be variable and sometimes quite confusing. In some cases there are single well-circumscribed masses and occasionally there are multiple masses. Other cases

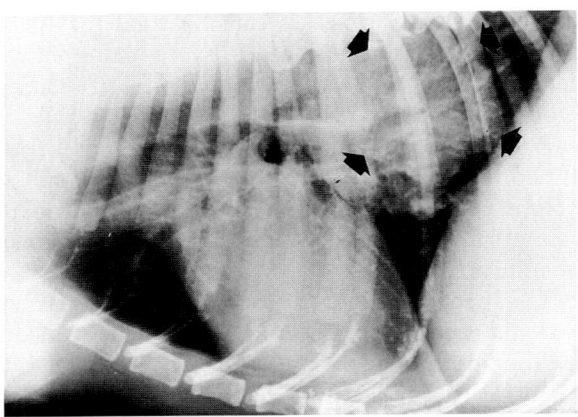

Figure 35.9 Bronchial carcinoma in a dog. The large radiodense lesion is fairly well circumscribed in the caudal lung lobe.

show lobar consolidation or diffuse infiltration throughout most of the lung (Fig. 35.9). These variable radiographic changes mimic those produced by many non-neoplastic conditions so that final diagnosis depends on finding neoplastic cells in samples obtained by fine needle aspiration or bronchial wash or biopsy at thoracotomy.

On rare occasions dogs with lung neoplasms develop paraneoplastic syndromes of which the most common is hypertrophic osteopathy in the bones of the distal parts of the limbs. In the series of 210 cases mentioned above hypertrophic osteopathy was found in six dogs and other paraneoplastic syndromes were even less common.

The results of surgical excision of primary lung neoplasms in dogs has been assessed in a series of 76 cases. When all macroscopic tumour was removed and there was no obvious lymph node enlargement the median survival was 330 days. However, animals with widespread tumours or lymph node enlargement had a much shorter survival (Ogilvie et al., 1989b).

Pulmonary thromboembolism

Acute thrombosis of the pulmonary arteries can cause severe illness and death in dogs. The condition is not easy to diagnose and most of the information comes from necropsy surveys. Affected dogs are usually middle aged or old and are affected with underlying conditions such as cardiac disease, neoplasia, hyperadrenocorticism, disseminated intravascular coagulation or sepsis (LaRue and Murtaugh, 1990). In a series of 31 dogs treated for immune-mediated haemolytic anaemia 10 animals developed pulmonary thromboembolism (Klein et al., 1989).

The clinical signs of respiratory distress and the changes on plain radiographs are not diagnostic. Pulmonary arteriography or combined ventilation and perfusion scintigraphy will demonstrate the vascular occlusion but these facilities are not readily available and the dogs are often very ill. At the present time the prognosis is very poor.

MEDIASTINUM AND PLEURAL CAVITY

Changes within the mediastinal and pleural spaces occur in a number of disease conditions in dogs and cats. The mediastinum connects cranially with the deep fascial planes of the neck through the thoracic inlet and the mediastinum also communicates with the perivascular and peribronchial interstitial spaces of the lung. There is normally no communication between the mediastinal and

Table 35.4 Drugs for diseases of the trachea, bronchi and lungs

Drug	Species	Dose and route (mg kg^{-1})	Frequency	Duration	Indications
Theophylline	D	9, p.o.	6 h	as required	Bronchodilation
Theophylline	C	4, p.o.	8 h	as required	Bronchodilation
Terbutaline	C	0.6, mg/cat p.o., s.c.	12 h	as required	Bronchodilation
Codeine	D	0.2, p.o.	6 h	as required	Cough suppression
Dextromethorphan	D	1.5, p.o.	8 h	as required	Cough suppression
Butorphanol	D	0.5, p.o.	12 h	as required	Cough suppression
Fenbendazole	C	50, p.o.	24 h	5 days	*Aelurostrongylus abstrusus*

C, cat; D, dog.

pleural spaces but lesions developing in the mediastinum, for example tumours, often cause changes in the pleural cavity such as effusion.

In most dogs and cats there is not a tight air or fluid seal between the left and right pleural cavities. Ventral perforations in the mediastinum make it likely that a disease process will involve both sides although occasionally unilateral changes are seen.

Dyspnoea is a common clinical sign in animals with mediastinal or pleural diseases. These animals develop constrictive respiratory failure when fluid or solid structures limit lung expansion. Mediastinal masses may constrict veins and lymphatics and may interfere with the function of the oesophagus, trachea and vagus nerves producing a wide range of possible clinical signs. In normal cats the anterior part of the chest is quite pliable and can be easily compressed but in cats with mediastinal neoplasms, for example lymphosarcoma, the chest feels solid and resists compression.

Diagnostic procedures for the mediastinum and pleural cavity

Radiology and ultrasonography

Radiology is often helpful in identifying mediastinal or pleural lesions. Air within these spaces produces an increase in radiolucency and fluid or solid lesions or organs are radiodense and conceal many of the normal structures of the chest. Removal of a major part of the fluid may be necessary before diagnostic films are obtained. Fluid is, however, useful for ultrasound examination of the chest as fluid conducts sound much better than air-filled lungs. Occasionally solid organs such as the liver may be identified in animals with effusion following diaphragmatic rupture.

Examination of pleural fluid and tissue aspirates

Thoracocentesis is indicated in cases where there is fluid in the pleural cavity. Samples are normally obtained by inserting a needle through the seventh or eighth intercostal space a little higher than mid way between the sternum and the spine. Most information is obtained from the protein content of the fluid, the number and type of cells in the fluid and the presence or absence of bacteria. Fine needle aspiration cytology of large mediastinal masses will often confirm that the lesion is neoplastic.

Exploratory surgery and endoscopy

In a small number of cases a definitive diagnosis cannot be established and exploratory thoracotomy may be required but this is probably only justified in cases where there is some prospect of removing the lesion. Endoscopic techniques have been described for the mediastinum and pleura but as anaesthesia and full asepsis is required they seem to have little advantage over thoracotomy.

Disease conditions of the mediastinum and pleural cavity

Pneumomediastinum

This condition usually arises after a motor vehicle accident but it can arise from an injury at the base of the neck extending into the trachea. In most cases the origin of the air in the mediastinum is unknown but is thought to arise from a small rupture of lung tissue at the hilus of the lung. The air tracks along the connective tissue to the mediastinum and then to the subcutaneous tissue via the entrance to the chest between the first ribs.

Considerable amounts of air can accumulate causing quite marked distension of the subcutaneous tissue of the head, neck and thorax. The condition is easily recognized on palpation of the distended subcutaneous tissue where there is crepitation or a crackling sensation. On chest radiography several normal structures which are not normally visible are clearly delineated by air in the mediastinum. Both inner and outer aspects of the trachea will be seen plus major branches of the aorta, the cranial vena cava and the azygos vein. Gas shadows may be seen extending from the thoracic inlet into the tissues of the neck (Fagin, 1988).

Although the clinical presentation of subcutaneous emphysema looks quite dramatic the animals do not appear sick unless they have other injuries. In a series of 17 cases 14 of the dogs also had pneumothorax (Van den Broek, 1986). The condition is usually self-limiting and the subcutaneous air is re-absorbed in a few days.

Mediastinal neoplasia

Primary mediastinal neoplasms may arise from lymph nodes, thymus, aortic body chemoreceptors or ectopic thyroid or parathyroid tissue. Lymphatic tumours involving thymus or lymph node are by far the most common. Mediastinal tumours cause clinical signs by restricting lung expansion or by compressing and sometimes invading the vena cava, thoracic duct, oesophagus, trachea or heart. The disease process often leads to fluid collecting in the pleural cavity. The lesion is usually identified on radiography as a large mass in the cranial mediastinum although in some cases fluid will have to be drained before the tumour can be demonstrated. On a ventrodorsal view it is often noted that the air-filled trachea is clearly deviated to one side by the mass. Confirmation of the disease is made on finding neoplastic cells in pleural fluid or on fine needle aspiration cytology of the mass.

The prognosis for these neoplasms is not very good. Chemotherapy may be considered for lymphatic neoplasms. Some success has been claimed for surgically resecting some mediastinal tumours but in general most of these tumours are too malignant or too extensive for surgery.

Pneumothorax

Pneumothorax can arise from a penetrating wound in the thoracic wall or from perforation of the thoracic oesophagus or trachea or from lesions in the lung such as bullae, foreign bodies or tumours. However, these are uncommon causes. In most cases pneumothorax follows a motor vehicle accident and the air is presumed to come from a small tear in the lung. As the pleural space fills with air, lung expansion becomes much reduced and the animal becomes obviously dyspnoeic. An experimental study on healthy dogs found that they could tolerate a volume of air in the thorax equal to 150% of lung volume without overt distress. Increasing the pneumothorax to over 175% of lung volume caused distress (Bennett *et al.*, 1989). Increased resonance may be detected on chest percussion and the diagnosis is easily made by radiography when the collapsed lungs are seen to be surrounded by radiolucent areas with no bronchial pattern. Usually the air extends to both sides of the chest.

Animals with pneumothorax often have other injuries such as pulmonary haemorrhage, haemothorax or diaphragmatic hernia. The lung tears tend to seal after the lung collapses. Animals with moderate dyspnoea will recover in 3–4 days with cage rest alone. For animals with severe respiratory problems provision should be made for continuous drainage until leakage of air stops. If the problem cannot be controlled this way thoracotomy to identify and close the leak may be considered but fortunately is rarely required.

Haemothorax

A degree of haemothorax often accompanies other traumatic injuries to the chest. In the absence of any history of trauma warfarin poisoning is probably the most likely cause of severe intrapleural haemorrhage. A prolonged activated clotting time in a sample of circulating blood suggests further investigation of a coagulation disorder.

Signs of haemorrhagic shock become obvious when a dog loses 30 ml blood kg^{-1} body weight from the circulation (20 ml kg^{-1} for a cat). Severe shock occurs when a dog loses 40 ml kg^{-1} or a cat loses 30 ml kg^{-1}. About 30 ml kg^{-1} of fluid must accumulate in the pleural space before a dog shows any signs of respiratory difficulty at rest and at least 50–60 ml kg^{-1} must accumulate before a dog shows severe dyspnoea (Crowe, 1988). Thus the absence of dyspnoea cannot be taken to rule out thoracic haemorrhage and the increase in respiratory rate which occurs with haemothorax is largely due to hypovolaemic shock.

Radiography and ultrasonography will confirm that there is fluid in the thorax and an aspirated sample will establish a diagnosis of haemothorax. Blood lost into the pleural space usually does not clot. This is due to rapid defibrination and activation of fibrinolytic mechanisms. If a sample obtained by thoracocentesis clots this suggests that the sample has been obtained by traumatic damage to another structure.

A substantial proportion of red cells shed into the pleural space are eventually re-absorbed into the circulation so haemothorax is usually managed conservatively without chest drainage. If the animal shows severe shock or severe dyspnoea autotransfusion may be useful particularly in cases with anticoagulant poisoning. Here blood is aspirated from the chest and re-introduced into a vein. There may be some risk of release of inflammatory factors from damaged platelets but the risk may be justified when dealing with an acute emergency situation.

There is some controversy in the literature about the complications of haemothorax. It is suggested that on some occasions fibrin deposited on the pleura of the lung leads to contracting fibrous tissue and restricted lung expansion. It is unclear whether this complication occurs to a significant extent in dogs and cats.

Pleural effusion

The pleural cavity in a normal cat or dog contains 2–10 ml fluid. Pleural fluid formation is controlled by the balance of Starling's forces; namely colloid oncotic pressure and capillary hydrostatic pressure.

The hydrostatic pressure in the capillaries which supply the parietal pleura is higher than the pressure in the pulmonary capillaries which supply the visceral pleura. Hence, fluid is produced on the parietal pleura and absorbed on the visceral pleura. Some absorption also occurs via lymphatics on the parietal pleura. Accumulation of fluid in the pleural space comes about due to decreased absorption or increased production (Forrester, 1988).

The mechanisms causing pleural fluid to accumulate are:

1. Increased capillary hydrostatic pressure, for example congestive heart failure;
2. Decreased capillary oncotic pressure, for example hypoalbuminaemia;
3. Increased capillary permeability, for example inflammation or neoplasia;
4. Lymphatic obstruction, for example neoplasia.

The presence of pleural fluid is normally recognized on thoracic radiographs. Dogs and cats which have dyspnoea at rest have very large amounts of fluid in the pleural space and this is easily seen on radiographs. The presence of large amounts of fluid will obscure the radiographic details of structures such as the heart and lungs and removal of much of the fluid may be necessary in order to look for other thoracic lesions, particularly neoplasms. However, before removing the fluid ultrasound examination may be worthwhile.

Examination of a sample of fluid is an important step in the diagnostic process. Most information is obtained from the protein content of the fluid, the number and type of cells present and the presence or absence of bacteria (Forrester *et al.*, 1988).

Pleural effusions can be classified as transudates, exudates or chylous effusions. Pure transudates have a protein content of less than 25 g l^{-1} and a nucleated cell count of less than 1000 ml^{-1}. The presence of fluid in the pleural cavity can set up an inflammatory response with an increase in protein above 25 g l^{-1} and an increase in cells up to 5000 ml^{-1}. The fluid is then usually described as a modified transudate. Exudates have a protein concentration over 30 g l^{-1} and in excess of 7000 nucleated cells per ml (French, 1990). Chylous effusions have a milky colour and contain large numbers of chylomicrons.

The common causes of pleural effusion are listed in Table 35.5.

Pleural transudates

The term hydrothorax is sometimes used for the condition where transudate accumulates in the pleural cavity. Pure transudates are not very common in cats or dogs and when they do occur they are most likely associated with low oncotic pressure due to hypoalbuminaemia. Modified transudates are quite common in both species due to a number of causes which include right-sided heart failure, neoplastic obstruction of venous or lymphatic drainage and diaphragmatic hernia with occlusion of venous drainage from herniated liver lobes. Sometimes neoplastic cells are obvious on cytology but in other cases the cause of the pleural transudate must be sought by using other diagnostic techniques.

Thoracic drainage is indicated to relieve immediate respiratory distress and to allow further radiographic investigation of the thorax, but is unlikely to prevent further effusion. Diuretics and increasing the serum albumin concentration may give short-term relief but are not of much value unless the underlying cause of the hydrothorax can be corrected.

Pleural exudates

The term pyothorax is sometimes used for the condition where exudate accumulates in the pleural cavity. Exudates may be classified as septic or non-septic. Septic exudates contain bacteria and signs of neutrophil degeneration in response to the bacterial infection whereas non-septic exudates have no bacteria and few degenerative neutrophils.

Dogs and cats with pleural exudates may have systemic signs such as pyrexia and anorexia but it is surprising how often an animal is presented with only a short history of dyspnoea yet on examination a very large amount of exudate is

Table 35.5 Common causes of pleural effusion

Dogs	Cats
Congestive heart failure	Bacterial infection
Neoplasia	Feline infectious peritonitis
Diaphragmatic hernia	Neoplasia
Lymphangiectasia	Congestive heart failure
Trauma	
Anticoagulant toxicity	
Bacterial infection	
Hypoalbuminaemia	
Oesophageal perforation	

present in the thorax. The condition usually involves both sides of the chest but is occasionally confined to one side (Fig. 35.10).

In the author's experience bacterial pyothorax is more common in the cat than in the dog and in the cat a mixed infection is usually involved including anaerobes. Infections with *Nocardia* and *Actinomyces* species are more likely to occur in the dog than in the cat (Fooshee, 1988).

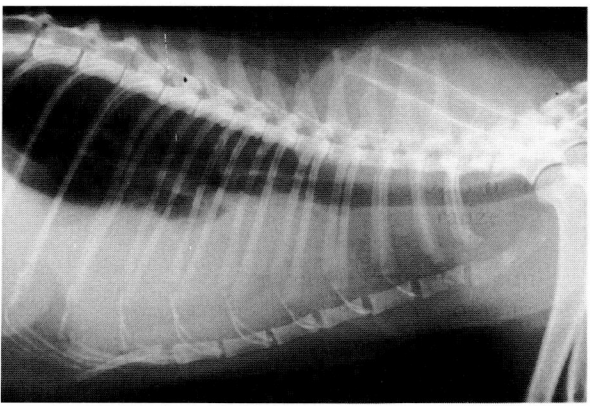

Figure 35.10 Septic pleurisy in a cat. Fluid in the pleural cavity has reduced the air filled lung and completely masks the cardiac outline.

Although there are several routes by which organisms might reach the pleural cavity in most cases it is impossible to find out how the infection got there.

Treatment is along the same lines as a septic lesion anywhere else, namely drainage and antibiotics. Immediate drainage should be carried out through a thoracostomy tube. This allows improvement in respiratory function. Good results have been reported using continuous chest drainage for several days until the chest is radiographically clear. Intermittent drainage and pleural lavage may be less successful in clearing the exudate. Continuous chest drainage requires 24 h supervision so the alternative is thoracotomy to remove all the pus and clean up the pleural cavity. The mediastinum may need to be broken down to drain both sides of the chest or thoracostomy tubes placed in both sides.

Antibiotic therapy is continued for 3 months. In a series of 22 canine cases treated by aspiration, drainage or thoracotomy 14 dogs made a long-term recovery (Robertson *et al.*, 1983). In another series of 12 dogs treated by continuous tube drainage there were eight long-term recoveries (Turner and Breznock, 1988).

Neoplasia and feline infectious peritonitis are causes of non-septic pleural effusion (Fig. 35.11). In cases with tumours the neoplastic cells may sometimes be seen in the fluid but they have to be differentiated from reactive mesothelial cells. The exudate in cats with feline infectious peritonitis has a high protein content in the order of 40–60 g l^{-1} with gamma globulins making up a higher than normal proportion of the protein content (French, 1990).

A series of 82 feline cases of pleural effusion were reported by Davies and Forrester (1996). These cats were commonly suffering from mediastinal lymphoma, pyothorax, cardiomyopathy or feline infectious peritonitis. Cats with pyothorax or effusion secondary to trauma had the best prognosis but for the other conditions the prognosis was guarded to poor.

The criteria for determining the nature of pleural fluids were assessed in a study on samples from 22 cats (Stewart *et al.*, 1990). Exudates had a ratio of pleural fluid protein concentration to serum protein concentration in excess of 0.5. Exudates had lactate dehydrogenase levels in excess of 200 IU l^{-1}. Three cats with septic pleural effusion had glucose concentrations less than 0.6 mmol l^{-1}, pH less than 6.9 and neutrophils forming over 85% of the nucleated cells. Eight cats with pleural effusion due to malignancy had fluid with a pH greater than 7.2 and neutrophils comprising less than 45% of the cells.

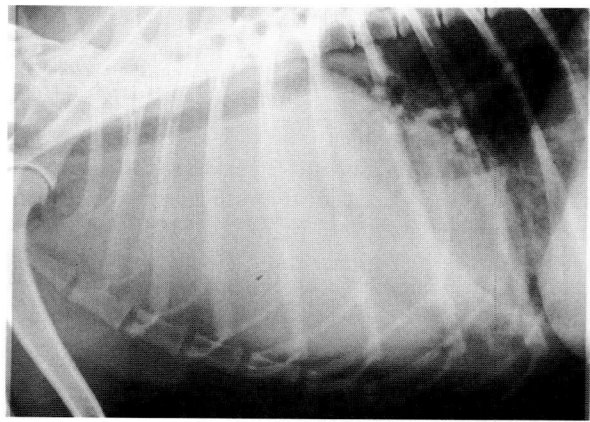

Figure 35.11 Lymphosarcoma in a dog. A large neoplasm in the mediastinal lymph node is displacing the trachea upwards. The thorax also contains a considerable amount of fluid which is masking the cardiac outline.

Chylothorax

Chyle is lymphatic fluid which originates in the intestine and is conveyed to the cranial vena cava via the thoracic duct. The fluid contains a high concentration of fat in the form of chylomicrons which gives the fluid its white opaque colour although chyle can have a pinkish tinge if it contains some blood. Chyle often contains large numbers of lymphocytes. Not all white fluids aspirated from the thorax contain chylomicrons. Some contain cholesterol and are often called pseudochylous effusions.

The best method for determining the nature of the fluid is to measure the triglyceride and cholesterol concentrations relative to plasma (Fossum *et al.*, 1986a).

Chylous effusions contain concentrations of triglycerides in excess of 1.2 mmol l^{-1}. A simple test often used is to add ether to the fluid which clears if it contains chylomicrons.

Confusion has occurred in the veterinary literature where the term pseudochylous effusion has been used for fluids which appear chylous from cases where no rupture of the thoracic duct can be demonstrated. Pseudochylous effusions are really modified transudates and perhaps the term pseudochylous should be dropped as it tends to confuse the identity of these fluids.

For many years chylothorax was thought to be mainly due to rupture of the thoracic duct but a study of 34 canine cases found that five were associated with trauma, five were caused by neoplastic obstruction and 24 were idiopathic associated with lymphangiectasia of the rostral part of the thoracic duct (Fossum *et al.*, 1986b). Obstruction or laceration of the thoracic duct was experimentally induced in six dogs. All the dogs developed chylothorax but the condition was of short duration and resolved spontaneously within two weeks. This result does not support the idea that rupture of the thoracic duct is a cause of chylothorax (Hodges *et al.*, 1993). Chylothorax has been reported in cats associated with thoracic duct lymphangiectasia, cardiomyopathy and neoplasia (Fossum, 1988).

Medical treatment and repeated chest drainage are of limited value for long-term management of cases of chylothorax. The outlook is very poor if the underlying cause such as neoplasia or cardiomyopathy cannot be controlled. Thoracic duct ligation has been quite widely used for cases with rupture or lymphangiectasia of the thoracic duct but the published results have been variable. In a series of 15 canine cases there were eight long-term, disease-free survivors (Birchard *et al.*, 1988). In a report on 37 cats with chylothorax 15 animals were treated by ligation of the thoracic duct or cysterna chyli but this resulted in complete resolution of pleural fluid in only 20% of the cases (Fossum *et al.*, 1991).

Obliteration of the pleural space by provoking a fibrous reaction is termed pleurodesis and has been used for chylothorax and other pleural effusions. The technique was used successfully in five out of nine dogs with chylothorax (Orsher and Harvey, 1990) although less successful results have been reported by others. Two techniques have been used to allow the fluid to enter the abdomen where it is absorbed. One technique makes a mesh-covered hole in the diaphragm and the other uses a silastic tube and pump to push fluid from the chest to the abdomen. Success has been claimed for both techniques but there are as yet insufficient cases to assess whether they offer a practical solution to the problems caused by pleural effusion.

REFERENCES

Allen, D.G. and Kruth, S.A. (1988) Pulmonary edema. In: *Small Animal Cardiopulmonary Medicine*. B.C. Decker, Toronto, pp. 183–190.

Allison, N., Willard, M.D., Bentinck-Smith, J. and Davis, K. (1986) Nasal rhinosperidiosis in two dogs. *Journal of the American Veterinary Medical Association* **188**, 869–871.

Amis, T.C. and McKiernan, B.C. (1986) Systematic identification of endobronchial anatomy during bronchoscopy in the dog. *American Journal of Veterinary Research* **47**, 2649–2657.

Amis, T.C., Smith, M.M., Gaber, E. and Kurpershoek, C.J. (1986) Upper airway obstruction in canine laryngeal paralysis. *American Journal of Veterinary Research* **47**, 1007–1010.

Barr, F., Gruffydd-Jones, T.J., Brown, P.J. and Gibbs, C. (1987) Primary lung tumours in the cat. *Journal of Small Animal Practice* **28**, 1115–1125.

Bauer, T. and Thomas, W.P. (1983) Pulmonary diagnostic techniques. *Veterinary Clinics of North America* **13**, 273–298.

Bedford, P.G.C. (1983) Displacement of the glosso-epiglottic mucosa in canine asphyxiate disease. *Journal of Small Animal Practice* **24**, 199–207.

Bennett, R.A., Orton, E.C., Tucker, A. and Heiller, C.L. (1989) Cardiopulmonary changes in conscious dogs with induced progressive pneumothorax. *American Journal of Veterinary Research* **50**, 280–284.

Biller, D.S. and Myer, C.W. (1987) Case examples demonstrating the clinical utility of obtaining both right and left thoracic radiographs in small animals. *Journal of the American Animal Hospital Association* **23**, 381–386.

Birchard, S.J., Smeak, D.D. and Fossum, T.W. (1988) Results of thoracic duct ligation in dogs with chylothorax. *Journal of the American Veterinary Medical Association* **193**, 68–71.

Burbidge, H.M., Goulden, B.E. and Jones, B.R. (1991) An experimental evaluation of castellated laryngofissure and bilateral arytenoid lateralisation for the relief of laryngeal paralysis in dogs. *Australian Veterinary Journal* **68**, 268–272.

Burgener, D.C., Slocombe, R.F. and Zerbe, C.A. (1987) Lymphoplasmacytic rhinitis in five dogs. *Journal of the American Animal Hospital Association* **23**, 565–568.

Codner, E.C., Lurus, A.G., Miller, J.B., Gavin, P.R., Gallina, A. and Barbee, D.D. (1993) Comparison of computed tomography with radiography as a noninvasive diagnostic technique for chronic nasal disease in dogs. *Journal of the American Veterinary Medical Association* **202**, 1106–1110.

Corcoran, B.M. (1991) Static respiratory compliance in normal dogs. *Journal of Small Animal Practice* **32**, 438–442.

Corcoran, B.M., Thoday, K.L., Henfrey, J.I., Simpson, J.W., Burnie, A.G. and Mooney, C.T. (1991) Pulmonary infiltration with eosinophils in 14 dogs. *Journal of Small Animal Practice* **32**, 494–502.

Corcoran, B.M., Foster, D.J. and Luis Fluentes, V. (1995) Feline asthma syndrome: a retrospective study of the clinical presentation in 29 cats. *Journal of Small Animal Practice* **36**, 481–488.

Cox, N.R., Brawner, W.R., Powers, R.D. and Wright, J.C. (1991) Tumors of the nose and paranasal sinuses in cats: 32 cases with comparison to a national data base (1977 through 1987). *Journal of the American Animal Hospital Association* **27**, 339–347.

Coyne, B.E., Fingland, R.B., Kennedy, G.A. and Debowes, R.M. (1993) Spiral prosthesis of the cervical trachea. *Veterinary Surgery* **22**, 269–275.

Crager, C.S. (1992) Canine primary ciliary dyskinesia. *Compendium on Continuing Education* **14**, 1440–1445.

Crowe, D.T. (1988) Help for the patient with thoracic haemorrhage. *Veterinary Medicine* **83**, 578–588.

Darke, P.G.G., Gibbs, C., Kelly, D.F., Morgan, D.G., Pearson, H. and Weaver, B.M.Q. (1977) Acute respiratory distress in the dog associated with paraquat poisoning. *Veterinary Record* **100**, 275–277.

Davies, C. and Forrester, S.D. (1996) Pleural effusion in cats – 82 cases (1987–1995). *Journal of Small Animal Practice* **37**, 217–224.

Dobbie, G.R., Darke, P.G.G. and Head, K.W. (1986) Intrabronchial foreign bodies in dogs. *Journal of Small Animal Practice* **27**, 227–234.

Fagin, B.D. (1988) A radiographic approach to diagnosing pneumomediastinum. *Veterinary Medicine* **83**, 571–577.

Fingland, R.B. (1989) Tracheal collapse. In: *Current Veterinary Therapy X* (Ed. R.W. Kirk). W.B. Saunders, Philadelphia, pp. 353–360.

Fooshee, S.K. (1988) Managing the cat with septic pleural effusion. *Veterinary Medicine* **83**, 907–913.

Forrester, S.D. (1988) The categories and causes of pleural effusion in cats. *Veterinary Medicine* **83**, 894–906.

Forrester, S.D., Troy, G.C. and Fossum, T.W. (1988) Pleural effusions: pathophysiology and diagnostic considerations. *Compendium on Continuing Education* **10**, 121–136.

Fossum, T.W. (1988) The characteristics and treatment of feline chylothorax. *Veterinary Medicine* **83**, 914–928.

Fossum, T.W., Jacobs, R.M. and Birchard, S.J. (1986a) Evaluation of cholesterol and triglyceride concentrations in differentiating chylous and nonchylous pleural effusions in dogs and cats. *Journal of the American Veterinary Medical Association* **188**, 49–51.

Fossum, T.W., Birchard, S.J. and Jacobs, R.M. (1986b) Chylothorax in 34 dogs. *Journal of the American Veterinary Medical Association* **188**, 1315–1318.

Fossum, T.W., Forrester, S.D., Swenson, C.L., Miller, M.W., Cohen, N.D., Boothe, H.W. and Birchard, S.J. (1991) Chylothorax in cats: 37 cases (1969–1989). *Journal of the American Veterinary Medical Association* **198**, 672–678.

French, T.W. (1987) The use of cytology in the diagnosis of chronic nasal disorders. *Compendium on Continuing Education* **9**, 115–120.

French, T.W. (1990) Effusions in serous cavities. *Proceedings of the 8th ACVIM Forum*, pp. 19–22.

Garnett, N.L., Eydelloth, R.S., Swindle, M.M., Vonderfecht, S.L., Strandberg, J.D. and Luzarrage, M.B. (1982) Haemorrhagic streptococcal pneumonia in newly procured research dogs. *Journal of the American Veterinary Medical Association* **181**, 1371–1374.

Gibbs, C., Lane, J.G. and Denny, H.R. (1979) Radiological features of intra-nasal lesions in the dog: a review of 100 cases. *Journal of Small Animal Practice* **20**, 515–535.

Greenfield, C.L. (1987) Canine laryngeal paralysis. *Compendium on Continuing Education* **9**, 1011–1017.

Hahn, K.A. and Matlock, C.L. (1990) Nasal carcinoma metastatic to bone in two dogs. *Journal of the American Veterinary Medical Association* **197**, 491–494.

Hawkins, E.C. and DeNicola, D.B. (1990) Cytologic analysis of tracheal wash specimens and bronchoalveolar lavage fluid in the diagnosis of mycotic infections in dogs. *Journal of the American Veterinary Medical Association* **197**, 79–83.

Hawkins, E.C., DeNicola, D.B. and Kuehn, N.F. (1990) Bronchoalveolar lavage in the evaluation of pulmonary disease in the dog and cat. *Journal of Veterinary Internal Medicine* **4**, 267–274.

Hodges, C.C., Fossum, T.W. and Evering, W. (1993) Evaluation of thoracic duct healing after experimental laceration and transection. *Veterinary Surgery* **22**, 431–435.

Hoffmann, W.E. and Wellman, M.L. (1986) Tracheobronchial cytology. In: *Current Veterinary Therapy IX* (Ed. R.W. Kirk). W.B. Saunders, Philadelphia, pp. 243–247.

Kapatkin, A.S., Mattiesen, D.T., Noone, K.E., Church, E.M., Scavelli, T.E. and Patnaik, A.K. (1990) Results of surgery and long-term follow-up in 31 cats with nasopharyngeal polyps. *Journal of the American Animal Hospital Association* **26**, 387–392.

Klein, M.K., Dow, S.W. and Rosychuk, R.A.W. (1989) Pulmonary thromboembolism associated with immune-mediated hemolytic anaemia in dogs: ten cases (1982–1987). *Journal of the American Veterinary Medical Association* **195**, 246–250.

LaRue, M.J. and Murtaugh, R.J. (1990) Pulmonary thromboembolism in dogs: 47 cases (1986–1987). *Journal of the American Veterinary Medical Association* **197**, 1368–1372.

Losonsky, J.M., Smith, F.G. and Lewis, R.E. (1978) Radiographic findings of *Aelurostrongylus abstrussus* infection in cats. *Journal of the American Animal Hospital Association* **14**, 348–355.

Lotti, U. and Niebauer, G.W. (1992) Tracheobronchial foreign bodies of plant origin in 153 Hunting Dogs. *Compendium on Continuing Education* **14**, 900–905.

Love, S., Barr, A., Lucke, V.M. and Lane, J.G. (1987a) A catheter technique for biopsy of dogs with chronic nasal disease. *Journal of Small Animal Practice* **28**, 417–424.

Love, S., Waterman, A.E. and Lane, J.G. (1987b) The assessment of corrective surgery for canine laryngeal paralysis by blood gas analysis: a review of 35 cases. *Journal of Small Animal Practice* **28**, 597–604.

Marks, S.L., Moore, M.P. and Rishniw, M. (1994) *Pneumonyssoides caninum*: the canine nasal mite. *Compendium on Continuing Education* **16**, 577–582.

Martin, M.W.S., Ashton, G., Simpson, V.R. and Neal, C. (1993) Angiostrongylosis in Cornwall: clinical presentations of eight cases. *Journal of Small Animal Practice* **34**, 20–25.

McKiernan, B.C., Smith, A.R. and Kissil, M. (1984) Bacterial isolates from the lower trachea in clinically healthy dogs. *Journal of the American Animal Hospital Association* **20**, 139–142.

Medleau, L., Marks, A., Brown, J. and Borges, W.L. (1990) Clinical evaluation of cryptococcal antigen latex agglutination test for diagnosis of cryptococcosis in cats. *Journal of the American Veterinary Medical Association* **196**, 1470–1473.

Medleau, L., Jacobs, G.J. and Marks, M.A. (1995) Itraconazole for the treatment of cryptococcus in cats. *Journal of Veterinary Internal Medicine* **9**, 39–42.

Moise, N.S., Wiedenkeller, D., Yeager, A.E., Blue, J.T. and Scarlett, J. (1989) Clinical, radiographic and bronchial cytologic features of cats with bronchial disease: 65 cases (1980–1986). *Journal of the American Veterinary Medical Association* **194**, 1467–1473.

Morrison, T., Read, R. and Eger, C. (1989) A retrospective study of nasal tumours in 37 dogs. *Australian Veterinary Practitioner* **19**, 130–134.

Norsworthy, G.D. (1993) Surgical treatment of chronic nasal discharge in 17 cats. *Veterinary Medicine* **88**, 526–537.

Ogilvie, G.K., Haschek, W.M., Withrow, S.J., Richardson, R.C., Harvey, H.J., Henderson, R.A., Fowler, J.D., Norris, A.M., Tomlinson, J., McCaw, D., Klausner, J.S., Reschke, R.W. and McKiernan, B.C. (1989a) Classification of primary lung tumors in dogs: 210 cases (1975–1985). *Journal of the American Veterinary Medical Association* **195**, 106–108.

Ogilvie, G.K., Weigel, R.M., Haschek, W.M., Withrow, S.J., Richardson, R.C., Harvey, H.J., Henderson, R.A., Fowler, J.D., Norris, A.M., Tomlinson, J., McCaw, D., Klausner, J.S., Reschke, R.W. and McKiernan, B.C. (1989b) Prognostic factors for tumor remission and survival in dogs after surgery for primary lung tumor: 76 cases (1975–1985). *Journal of the American Veterinary Medical Association* **195**, 109–112.

Orsher, R.J. and Harvey, C.E. (1990) Tetracycline sclerotherapy (pleurodesis) for the treatment of chylothorax in dogs. *Veterinary Surgery* **19**, 72–73.

O'Sullivan, S.P. (1989) Paraquat poisoning in the dog. *Journal of Small Animal Practice* **30**, 361–364.

Patrid, P. and Amis, T.C. (1992) Chronic tracheobronchial disease in the dog. *Veterinary Clinics of North America* **22**, 1203–1229.

Patrid, P.A., Hornof, W.J., Kurpershoek, C.J. and Cross, C.E. (1990) Canine chronic bronchitis: a pathophysiologic evaluation of 18 cases. *Journal of Veterinary Internal Medicine* **4**, 172–180.

Pirie, H.M. and Wheeldon, E.B. (1976) Chronic bronchitis in the dog. *Advances in Veterinary Science and Comparative Medicine* **20**, 253–276.

Robertson, S.A., Stoddart, M.E., Evans, R.J., Gaskell, C.J. and Gibbs, C. (1983) Thoracic empyema in the dog; a report of twenty-two cases. *Journal of Small Animal Practice* **24**, 103–119.

Ross, J.T., Matthiesen, D.T., Scavelli, T.J. and Noone, K. (1990) Treatment of laryngeal paralysis in the dog by partial laryngectomy: a critical evaluation of the technique, description of complications and long term results in 45 cases. *Veterinary Surgery* **19**, 75

Sharp, N.J.H., Harvey, C.E. and Sullivan, M. (1991) Canine nasal aspergillosis and penicilliosis. *Compendium on Continuing Education* **13**, 41–48.

Sharp, N., Sullivan, M. and Harvey, C.E. (1992) Treatment of canine nasal aspergillosis. *In Practice* January 1992, 27–31.

Shaw, S.E. (1988) Successful treatment of 11 cases of feline cryptococcosis. *Australian Veterinary Practitioner* **18**, 135–139.

Smith, M.O., Turrel, J.M., Bailey, C.S. and Cain, G.R. (1989) Neurologic abnormalities as the predominant signs of neoplasia of the nasal cavity in dogs and cats: seven cases (1973–1986). *Journal of the American Veterinary Medical Association* **195**, 242–245.

Stewart, A., Padrid, P. and Lobingler, R. (1990) Feline pleural fluid analysis. Diagnostic utility of pH, glucose, LDH, total protein and differential cell count. *Proceedings of the 8th Annual ACVIM Forum*, p. 1121.

Steyn, P.F. and Green, R.W. (1990) How patient positioning affects radiographic signs of canine lung disease. *Veterinary Medicine* **85**, 796–805.

Sullivan, M. (1987) Rhinoscopy: a diagnostic aid. *Journal of Small Animal Practice* **28**, 839–844.

Sullivan, M., Lee, R., Jakovljevic, S. and Sharp, N.J.H. (1986) The radiological features of aspergillosis of the nasal cavity and frontal sinuses in the dog. *Journal of Small Animal Practice* **27**, 167–180.

Sullivan, M., Lee, R. and Skae, C.A. (1987) The radiological features of sixty cases of intra-nasal neoplasia in the dog. *Journal of Small Animal Practice* **28**, 575–585.

Teske, E., Stokhof, A.A., van den Ingh, T.S.G.A.M., Wolvekamp, W.Th.C., Slappendal, R.J. and de Vries H.W. (1991) Transthoracic needle aspiration biopsy of the lung in dogs with pulmonic diseases. *Journal of the American Animal Hospital Association* **27**, 289–294.

Thayer, G.W. and Robinson, S.K. (1984) Bacterial bronchopneumonia in the dog. *Journal of the American Animal Hospital Association* **20**, 731–735.

Theon, A.P., Madewell, B.R., Hart, M.F. and Dungworth, D.L. (1993) Megavoltage irradiation of neoplasms of the nasal and paranasal cavities in 77 dogs. *Journal of the American Veterinary Medical Association* **202**, 1469–1475.

Thrusfield, M.V., Aitken, C.G.G. and Muirhead, R.H. (1989) A field investigation of kennel cough: efficacy of vaccination. *Journal of Small Animal Practice* **30**, 550–560.

Turner, W.D. and Breznock, E.M. (1988) Continuous suction drainage for management of canine pyothorax. *Journal of the American Animal Hospital Association* **24**, 485–494.

Van den Broek, A. (1986) Pneumomediastinum in seventeen dogs: aetiology and radiographic signs. *Journal of Small Animal Practice* **27**, 747–757.

White, R.A.S. (1989) Unilateral arytenoid lateralisation: an assessment of the technique and long term results in 62 dogs with laryngeal paralysis. *Journal of Small Animal Practice* **30**, 543–549.

White, R.A.S. and Williams, J.M. (1994) Tracheal collapse in the dog – is there really a role for surgery? A survey of 100 cases. *Journal of Small Animal Practice* **35**, 191–196.

Willard, M.D., Roberts, R.E., Allison, N., Grieve, R.B. and Escher, K. (1988) Diagnosis of *Aelurostrongylus abstrusus* and *Dirofilaria immitis* infections in cats from a humane shelter. *Journal of the American Veterinary Medical Association* **192**, 913–916.

Withrow, S.J., Susaneck, S.J., Macey, D.W. and Shectz, J. (1985) Aspiration and punch biopsy techniques for nasal tumors. *Journal of the American Animal Hospital Association* **21**, 551–554.

36

Diseases of the Alimentary Tract

C. P. Sturgess

Introduction	371	Oesophageal disease	389
History	371	Gastric disease	398
Physical examination	372	Small intestinal disease	416
Clinical investigation	372	Colonic disease	432
Oropharyngeal disease	382	Diseases of the anorectal region	438
Dysphagia	387		

INTRODUCTION

The alimentary tract may be described as the hollow, often tubular, organs of the digestive system extending from the lips to the anus (Concise Veterinary Dictionary, 1988).

Together with the associated salivary glands and pancreas the alimentary tract is involved in the acquisition of water, macro- and micronutrients and the elimination of waste. The gastrointestinal tract (GIT) has also an important immunological role being the largest lymphoid organ in the body and is involved in the dual processes of protection against disease and tolerance to food allergens. Failure of this immunological function is responsible for many of the chronic alimentary diseases that are seen.

Alimentary tract dysfunction is extremely common and a major reason for clients to seek veterinary advice and assistance. Although vomiting and diarrhoea are classically associated with alimentary disease this is not an exclusive relationship. A significant proportion of gastrointestinal (GI) cases do not present with these signs. Moreover, vomiting and diarrhoea can be associated with non-GIT disease.

Good historical detail is vitally important in the investigation of GI disease as, in many cases, physical examination and basic laboratory data are unrewarding.

HISTORY

The classification of GI disease into acute and chronic conditions can be helpful. Acute disease presents a real diagnostic challenge since, although the majority are self-limiting and require little if any treatment, acute life-threatening conditions such as parvovirus infection, intussusceptions, gastric dilation/volvulus (GDV) need to be identified and treated promptly and aggressively. Chronic disease is less likely to respond to symptomatic therapy and frequently requires specific therapy after a definitive diagnosis has been made.

Historical details are important when making the initial decision in a case that presents with GI signs as to whether this indeed reflects primary disease of the alimentary tract or is secondary to systemic disease.

The following historical information is helpful in reaching this decision and planning any necessary investigation:

- Age – congenital, acquired, infectious and neoplastic conditions tend to be age-linked;
- Breed – genetic and predisposing factors, e.g. GDV in deep chested dogs, adenocarcinoma in Siamese cats;
- Sex – few GI diseases show a sex predilection although other conditions that can cause vomiting and diarrhoea do, e.g. pyometra;

- Previous history of intestinal disease (N.B. this can be misleading);
- Duration of signs;
- Major presenting signs – vomiting, diarrhoea, dysphagia etc.;
- Associated systemic signs – depression, lethargy, inappetance, weight loss;
- Indications for involvement of other organs – respiratory signs, polydypsia;
- Health of other animals in the group;
- Diet;
- Lifestyle, e.g. access to toxins, scavenger;
- Current medication – prescribed and non-prescribed.

Vomiting

The following should be ascertained in relation to vomiting:

- Relationship to feeding;
- Frequency;
- Progression;
- Nature of vomit:
  undigested / partially digested food
  unproductive
  froth
  bile
  projectile
  smell, e.g. fetid
  blood – fresh or 'coffee grounds'
- Changes in body weight.

Diarrhoea

The following should be considered:

- Frequency;
- Consistency and colour;
- Volume;
- Presence of mucus or blood including distribution of blood within the faeces, i.e. fresh blood, on surface or mixed throughout stool, or tarry melaena;
- Pain or difficulty in passing faeces;
- Changes in body weight;
- Continence;
- Urgency.

Having obtained a good history it is essential that the information is interpreted in the correct manner as this can have major implications in diagnostic planning. The following distinctions are extremely helpful in drawing up an initial diagnostic plan. (See relevant Chapters in Section I for a more in-depth discussion.)

- Dysphagic or anorexic?
- Vomiting, regurgitation or retching?
- Large or small bowel diarrhoea?
- Tenesmus (straining to pass faeces) or dyschezia (pain and/or difficulty in passing faeces)?

PHYSICAL EXAMINATION

A complete physical examination should be performed in all cases to confirm the abnormalities described by the owners and to evaluate the major body systems in order to differentiate between alimentary and systemic disease. In geriatric cases it is also important as intercurrent disease may adversely affect the prognosis and limit the range of treatments available.

In many cases, the clinician should be in a position to make a diagnosis or, in the case of acute disease, be confident that the process is self-limiting. If a diagnosis is not apparent it should be possible to direct the investigation and treatment by answering the following questions.

- Is the condition life-threatening requiring immediate investigation and treatment?
- Are signs of systemic disease present?
- If so which body system(s) is (are) affected?
- Do the history and clinical examination support a primary alimentary problem?
- Which part(s) of the alimentary tract appear(s) to be involved?
- Is the patient retching, regurgitating or vomiting?
- Is the diarrhoea likely to be of large or small bowel origin?

CLINICAL INVESTIGATION

An enormous variety of diagnostic procedures can be used to investigate alimentary disease. The results of the history and physical examination should indicate in which direction the investigation should proceed and which tests are likely to be of high diagnostic value.

It is particularly important in alimentary disease that a logical progression for the investigation is adopted as 'going back' to a test that should have been performed earlier can sometimes be made very difficult by subsequent investigations and treatments.

Haematology and biochemistry

Routine blood sampling tends to be a low yield diagnostic procedure in alimentary disease but is helpful in ruling out systemic causes of GI signs, to screen geriatric patients for intercurrent disease and to assess the status of patients with acute, life-threatening intestinal conditions.

Anaemia

GI bleeding can be a major cause of unexplained anaemia. The presence of blood in the faeces is not always recognized by the client and, if the bleed is acute, it may take some time before blood appears in the stool. Intestinal bleeding usually results in a regenerative anaemia and is associated with haematemesis, melaena or haematochezia. Non-regenerative anaemia will also occur with chronic GI haemorrhage secondary to iron deficiency or in acute haemorrhage (less than two days) where a regenerative response has yet to occur.

White blood cell changes

Changes in white cell indices are more frequently detected in GI disease but are often non-specific. Eosinophilia is perhaps the most helpful and can suggest eosinophilic gastroenteritis or parasitism.

Leucopenia is commonly observed during the acute phase of viral infections particularly parvovirus and distemper.

Biochemistry

Changes in routine biochemical parameters are uncommon in chronic alimentary disease but, when they occur, can be of value (Table 36.1).

Serology

Feline leukaemia virus (FeLV) and feline immunodeficiency virus (FIV) testing should be carried out on all cats with chronic or recurrent disease. This is particularly important in cases of gingivitis and stomatitis and alimentary lymphosarcoma. FIV-associated large and small bowel diarrhoeas are also seen. Thyroid hormone levels are a valuable screening test in older cats (greater than 6–7 years) with weight loss (particularly in the face of polyphagia) and/or chronic diarrhoea.

Trypsin-like immunoreactivity (TLI), folate and cobalamin

These tests have become firmly established to assess exocrine pancreatic and small intestinal function, and small intestinal bacterial overgrowth in dogs (Table 36.2). The value of folate and cobalamin in feline intestinal disease is less well established as the reference range is very wide.

TLI measures the combined activity of trypsin and trypsinogen in a serum sample and is both highly sensitive and specific for the diagnosis of canine exocrine pancreatic insufficiency (EPI). Blood should be taken after a fast of several hours. The result is unaffected by administration of oral pancreatic supplements. Dogs that have an equivocal result usually have a normal result or one consistent with EPI on retesting. Feline TLI testing is not currently available in the UK but is performed in the USA. Exocrine pancreatic insufficiency is, however, rare in cats.

Faecal analysis

Faecal analysis should be performed as part of baseline data collection in cases of chronic vomiting and/or diarrhoea. Microscopic examination for evidence of undigested food as an indication of small intestinal disease tends to be subjective and imprecise since it is influenced by diet and faecal

Table 36.1 Associations between biochemical changes and alimentary disease

Biochemical change	Occurrence in GI disease
Hypocalcaemia	Dietary imbalance, intestinal malabsorption, necrotizing pancreatitis
Hypochloraemia	Vomiting
Hypercholesterolaemia	Pancreatitis
Hypocholesterolaemia	Maldigestion/malabsorption, protein-losing enteropathy, exocrine pancreatic insufficiency
Hyperglycaemia	Acute pancreatitis
Hypoglycaemia	Intestinal malabsorption, insulinoma
Hypokalaemia	Vomiting, diarrhoea, laxatives, anorexia
Hyperglobulinaemia	Chronic intestinal inflammation, especially inflammatory bowel disease and neoplasia
Hypoalbuminaemia	Maldigestion, malabsorption, malnutrition, protein-losing enteropathy (also hypoglobulinaemia)
Hyponatraemia	Severe diarrhoea, vomiting
Uraemia	Intestinal bleeding

Table 36.2 Sites of absorption of folate and cobalamin and interpretation of abnormal results

	Folate	Cobalamin
Site of absorption	Duodenum and proximal jejunum	Distal jejunum and ileum
Increased serum levels	SIBO EPI Vitamin supplementation	Vitamin supplementation
Decreased serum levels	Severe disease of proximal small intestine ? certain drugs (phenytoin, sulphasalazine, sulphonamides)	Severe disease of distal small intestine SIBO EPI Absorption defects (giant schnauzers, Shar pei (USA))

EPI, exocrine pancreatic insufficiency; SIBO, small intestinal bacterial overgrowth.

transit time, although the presence of undigested starch granules, which can be stained with Lugol's iodine, are suggestive of EPI. The presence of *Clostridium perfringens* spores in a faecal smear is highly suggestive of diarrhoea due to *C. perfringens*-associated endotoxicosis. If GI haemorrhage is suspected then examination for occult blood can be performed but false positives are common and may be due to the ingestion of oral iron, aspirin, cimetidine or significant quantities of vegetable haem-protein or red meat.

A single, negative, direct smear, flotation or sedimentation analysis does not reliably rule out the presence of endoparasites or protozoans particularly *Giardia lamblia*. In such cases prospective treatment with benzimidazoles or metronidazole in the face of a negative faecal sample may be warranted.

Faecal culture should also be carried out for the presence of *Campylobacter* or *Salmonella* species. The interpretation of the significance of a faecal bacterial load, especially if these organisms are part of the 'normal' gut flora, is very difficult and the diagnosis of bacterial overgrowth can rarely be made in this manner.

Faecal examination using electron microscopy (EM) or immune-based techniques for the presence of enteric viruses is of value in specific cases. It is important that a faecal sample rather than a swab is submitted for examination.

Fat and carbohydrate malabsorption

A variety of tests have been described for evaluation of fat and carbohydrate absorption in small intestinal disease. Few, if any, have been shown to be practical and of diagnostic value in clinical practice.

Enteropathogenic Escherichia coli (EPEC)

Considerable recent interest has been focused on the importance of EPEC in chronic diarrhoea. These coliforms produce a variety of different toxins which are capable of initiating diarrhoea. Diagnosis is based on using polymerase chain reaction techniques on coliform colonies isolated from a faecal sample. The significance of EPEC in cats is less clear as EPEC can be isolated from many normal cats.

Breath hydrogen testing

Breath hydrogen testing can be used to evaluate small intestinal carbohydrate malabsorption and bacterial overgrowth (Washabau *et al.*, 1986; Muir *et al.*, 1994). The test relies on there being few bacteria in the small intestine to ferment food and little carbohydrate escapes the small intestine to be broken down by colonic bacteria. Where small intestinal bacterial overgrowth (SIBO) exists carbohydrate fermentation occurs in the small intestine resulting in production of increased amounts of hydrogen. Carbohydrate malabsorption, on the other hand, permits undigested carbohydrate to pass through to the colonic bacteria where fermentation occurs. The hydrogen released is absorbed into the circulation and liberated in the exhaled breath. Standardization of the test to permit its clinical use in dogs involves fasting followed by the oral administration of lactulose, a complex sugar which is poorly absorbed in the small intestine and normally metabolized by the colonic flora. This test aids the diagnosis of SIBO (Fig. 36.1) but is of no value in the diagnosis of carbohydrate malabsorption.

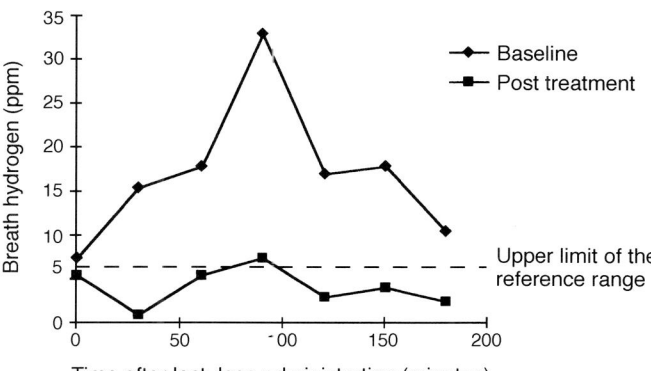

Figure 36.1 Breath hydrogen test results after administration of lactulose from an 8-year-old, neutered, male, standard poodle with a 4-year history of intermittent diarrhoea before and after antibiotic treatment (oxytetracycline 20 mg kg^{-1} tid for one month).

Exhaled breath is collected in a latex anaesthetic bag via a one way valve and face mask in dogs and by placing cats in a perspex chamber. Samples are collected at 15–30 minute intervals and an aliquot immediately analysed. The perspex chamber technique allows automated continuous monitoring. Clinically this technique has so far proven more useful in dogs than cats.

Small intestinal permeability testing

Small intestinal permeability testing is a new and potentially valuable function test. Substances, without specific carrier systems, move from the gut lumen into the body by two basic methods. A transcellular route for small molecules (less than 0.4 nm) and an intercellular route, across the tight junctions between enterocytes, for larger molecules (greater than 0.4 nm). Intercellular transport is not normally a major route of access to the submucosa. Damage to the small intestinal mucosa frequently results in the reduction in transcellular transport capacity due to villus blunting and atrophy and an increase in intercellular transport as the tight junctions between enterocytes become more 'leaky' (Fig. 36.2).

By selecting suitable probes that are not digested or degraded and are excreted intact by the kidney, intestinal function can be assessed. Early methods used chromium-51 (^{51}Cr) EDTA, polyethylene glycol and xylose (Maxton et al., 1986; Hall, 1989). However, radioisotopes are not easily handled and single sugars can be influenced by gastric emptying, intestinal transit time and renal excretion rates. For these reasons a two probe system was developed using probes of different sizes one of which was absorbed by a transcellular route and the other via an intercellular route. Cellubiose/mannitol (Hall and Batt, 1991), lactulose/mannitol (Papasouliotis et al., 1993a) and lactulose/rhamnose (Quigg et al., 1994) have been used.

Measuring differential recovery in the urine allows a better evaluation of small intestinal function, as both probes should be similarly influenced by gastric emptying, intestinal transit time and glomerular filtration rate. The final data are expressed as a ratio of the percentage of the large to small probe recovered in the urine (Table 36.3)

Table 36.3 Mean normal lactulose (large sugar) and rhamnose (small sugar) excretion with lactulose:rhamnose ratios together with examples from clinical cases with abnormal permeabilities

Pathology	% rhamnose excretion	% lactulose excretion	lactulose:rhamnose ratio
Mean (normal dogs)	16.0	1.8	0.12
Eosinophilic enteritis	25.2	3.4	0.13
Alimentary lymphosarcoma	3.0	1.0	0.33
Alimentary lymphosarcoma	40.3	36.5	0.91
Lymphocytic/plasmacytic enteritis	12.3	13.3	0.92
Eosinophilic enteritis and villus atrophy	7.5	1.8	0.24
Inflammatory bowel disease	6.4	5.9	0.92
Lymphangiectasia	9.8	7.3	0.7
Lymphangiectasia	6.3	1.7	0.27
Lymphangiectasia	15.4	7.2	0.42

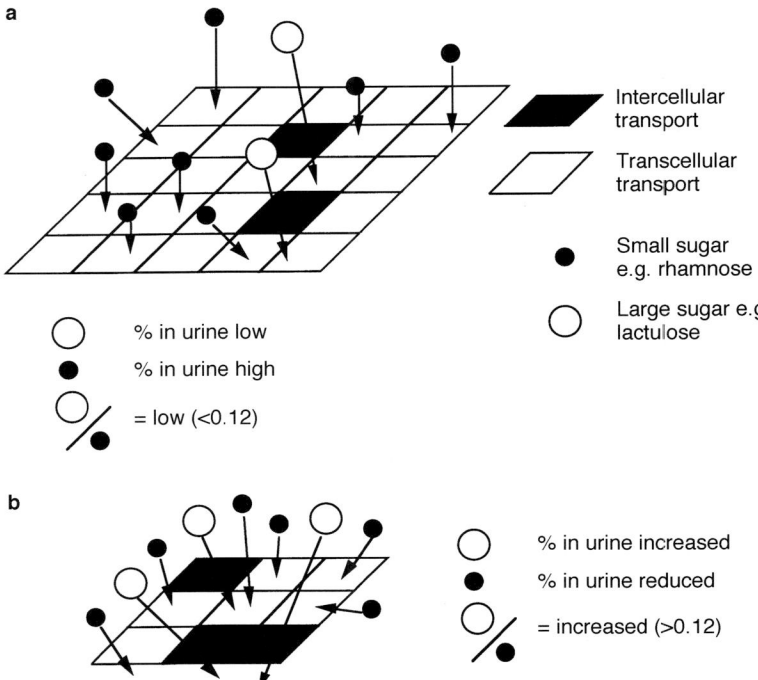

Figure 36.2 Diagram of the passage of small and large sugars through (a) normal and (b) diseased small intestinal wall. Note the diseased small intestine has a reduced surface area and therefore there is less transcellular transport. Intercellular junctions are more leaky increasing absorption of larger molecules.

measured by high performance liquid chromatography (HPLC).

The lactulose/rhamnose test requires overnight fasting and an empty urinary bladder. The lactulose/rhamnose solution is administered orally and the dog is kennelled. After 5 hours, 10 ml of urine is collected into thiomersal and the sugars are assayed. As lactulose has been given, a breath hydrogen test can also be conducted over the same time period.

Diagnostic imaging

Diagnostic imaging can be of major value in the investigation of oropharyngeal disease, dysphagia, some motility disorders, and in the detection of tumours, foreign bodies and intussusceptions. In cases of chronic vomiting and diarrhoea, it tends to be a low yield diagnostic procedure. As with all radiography, plain survey films should always be obtained before contrast studies are performed.

Ultrasonography of the alimentary tract generally requires an experienced ultrasonographer but can be of particular value for assessing the pancreas, intestinal wall thickness and the detection of GIT-associated masses. The ability to perform ultrasound-guided fine needle aspirates or tru-cut biopsies of masses enables a diagnosis to be reached without the need for a laparotomy and, where appropriate, chemotherapy can be instigated immediately the diagnosis is obtained.

Following plain survey radiographs, contrast studies provide further information about the structure and function of the GIT. In most instances liquid barium or a barium meal are the most appropriate techniques. If there is a possibility of alimentary perforation an iodine-based contrast medium is preferred as, unlike barium, it is rapidly removed from body cavities.

Evaluation of the oral cavity

Adequate evaluation of the oropharynx generally requires heavy sedation or general anaesthesia except in the most cooperative patients. Standard dorsoventral and lateral views of the skull and pharyngeal area are required. Good positioning is essential as artefacts associated with rotation are easily created. Oblique views of the mandibles and maxilla are of value in specific conditions. For a detailed discussion of dental radiography the reader is referred to specialist texts (Douglas *et al.*, 1987).

Evaluation of swallowing

Fluoroscopy is the technique of choice for imaging the swallowing reflex. Paste, liquid and barium mixed with food given in small amounts to the conscious patient can be followed as they are collected as a bolus at the base of the tongue before initiating the swallowing reflex. The bolus can then be followed along the oesophagus and into the stomach. The presence of gastric reflux can also be detected. If sedation is necessary then low dose acepromazine has minimal effects on the swallowing process.

Evaluation of the oesophagus

Megaoesophagus can be frequently diagnosed on plain radiographs. A conscious or lightly sedated patient is necessary for oesophageal evaluation as heavy sedation or anaesthesia can create an artefactual megaoesophagus. A 'herring bone' pattern in the caudal third of the oesophagus following administration of contrast is a normal finding in cats. If partial obstruction of the oesophagus is suspected then mixing barium with food provides a more effective contrast study.

Evaluation of the stomach

Gastric morphology

Positive contrast gastrography or double contrast procedures require large volumes of dilute barium (30% w/v barium; 10–20 ml kg^{-1}) to cause mild gastric distension. Dosing can usually be best achieved by stomach tubing rather than force feeding the animal. Barium will normally begin to move into the duodenum within 30 min. Ideally four views of the stomach are required (both laterals, a ventrodorsal and dorsoventral) following administration and then at intervals thereafter depending on the speed of gastric emptying. It is easy to create an artefactual lesion and care must be taken not to over-interpret the films. For a lesion to be regarded as pathological it should be present on more than one view and preferably at more than one time point (see Chapter 5).

Double contrast gastrograms can be performed by administering 2 ml/kg^{-1} of barium and then insufflating the stomach with air. Alternatively the stomach can be inflated after a positive contrast study once the majority of barium has entered the small intestine.

Gastric motility and emptying

Fluid and solid material adopt different routes of travel through the stomach and use different physiological mechanisms for gastric emptying. In general, the gastric emptying of fluids is of less clinical value hence it is difficult to combine a morphological and functional study of the stomach as one procedure. Moreover, gastric emptying times are very variable and have been quoted at 0.5–2 h (Miyabayashi et al., 1986) and 1–7 h (Jakovljevic, 1988) in dogs and 15–120 min in cats (Morgan, 1981).

A more reliable method of examining gastric emptying involves a barium meal or barium impregnated polyspheres (see later). For a barium meal 5–7 ml kg^{-1} of 60% w/v barium is added to 8 g kg^{-1} of ground kibble. Normal emptying times of 7–15 h (mean 11 h) have been reported in dogs (Burns and Fox, 1986) and 9.5–13.7 h (mean 11.6 h) in cats (Steyn and Twedt, 1994). Emptying times are affected by caloric density, nutrient composition, osmolality and particle size of the test meal so should be standardized wherever possible. Emptying times can also be affected by physiological factors such as stress, pain or sedation as well as metabolic factors such as hypokalaemia.

Evaluation of the small intestine

Small intestinal morphology and transit times can be assessed following administration of liquid barium. Similar care should be adopted when interpreting the results as for the stomach and normal anatomic variations disregarded. Normal transit times of around 3–5 h in dogs (Miyabayashi et al., 1986) and 30–60 min in cats (Hogan and Aronson, 1988) are quoted.

Evaluation of the large intestine

The large intestine can not be evaluated in a follow-through study but requires a barium enema. Patient preparation is crucial to avoid artefacts and achieve complete filling of the colon. The patient should be starved and given warm water enemas and bowel cleansing solutions (e.g. Klean Prep – Norgine). The colon is filled with 30% w/v barium to give a positive contrast study via a balloon-tipped catheter. The barium is then drained and air introduced to provide double contrast.

Barium impregnated polyspheres (BIPS)

BIPS are of two sizes (5 mm and 1.5 mm diameter) presented in gelatine capsules and are designed to mimic the passage of food through the GIT. BIPS can be helpful in detecting physical obstructions (including partial obstructions) (Fig. 36.3) and intestinal motility disorders such as delayed gastric emptying. They have potential advantages over barium contrast studies in these areas as the BIPS are of consistent size and formulation, are

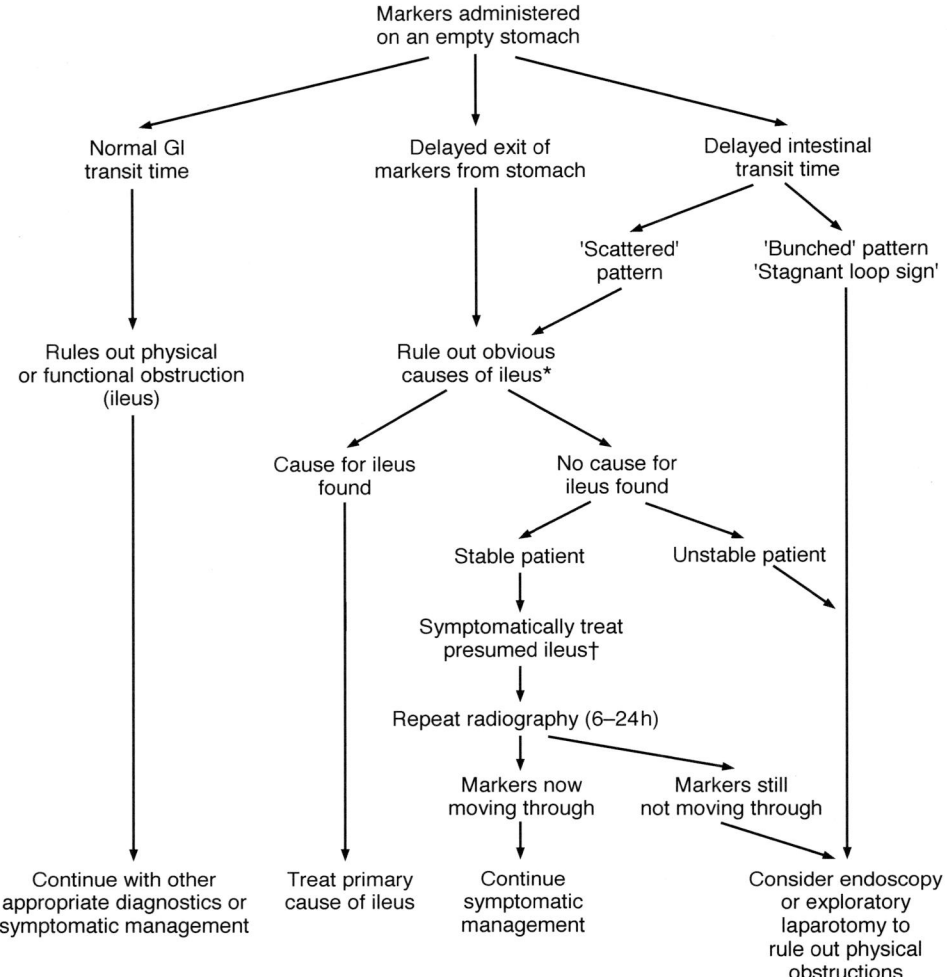

Figure 36.3 Algorithm showing the use of barium impregnated polyspheres on an empty stomach in the diagnosis of alimentary tract obstructions. *Hypokalaemia, acute pancreatitis, severe acute gastroenteritis, acute hepatitis, anticholinergics, previous abdominal surgery. †Lactated Ringers + KCl, metoclopramide, cisapride, antibiotics.

easier and cleaner to administer and require fewer radiographs to be taken. If surgical intervention is required leakage into the abdomen is less likely. They are of limited value in animals that are vomiting and in critically ill patients as the time taken to reach a diagnosis may be too long. BIPS can be administered to animals after fasting or in conjunction with a standard meal. Interpretation is based on the position, scattering and relationship between the small and large BIPS, e.g. persistent bunching in the small intestine is suggestive of a physical obstruction whereas wide scattering suggests poor motility. Passage of the small BIPS but retention of the large spheres is suggestive of a partial obstruction.

Endoscopy

In the majority of cases of chronic alimentary disease, a definitive diagnosis can only be obtained by histological examination of the GIT. Material can be obtained by fine needle aspirate or tru-cut biopsy under ultrasound guidance where there is an identifiable mass. Otherwise, endoscopy or exploratory coeliotomy is required.

Flexible endoscopy has several distinct advantages over exploratory coeliotomy and has revolutionized veterinary gastroenterology over the past few years. However, the limitations of endoscopy must always be borne in mind (Table 36.4) when deciding on the most appropriate

Table 36.4 Limitations of flexible endoscopy

- Requires general anaesthesia
- Requires a wide range of scope sizes to enable all patients to be examined
- Distal jejunum and ileum not accessible to examination
- Poor assessment of intestinal function
- Only detects mucosal/submucosal lesions
- Only small biopsies can be obtained which may not be representative and can be difficult to orientate
- Considerable 'start-up' and maintenance costs involved

Table 36.6 Potential complications following GI endoscopy

- GI perforation either by overinsufflation or following biopsy, especially of ulcerated areas
- Decreased venous return following overinflation of the stomach
- Mucosal haemorrhage
- Transmission of enteropathogenic organisms to other patients
- Acute bradycardia
- Damage to major blood vessels or adjacent organs
- Postendoscopy gastric dilatation–volvulus
- ? bacteraemia due to increased bacterial translocation following insufflation of the small intestine increasing its permeability

diagnostic test. Endoscopy circumvents the need for invasive surgery which can be a particular problem in some patients which may be immunosuppressed and have poor wound healing capacity such as dogs with protein-losing enteropathy. It also allows direct visualization of the mucosal surface and multiple biopsies can be taken. Immunosuppressive treatment, if required can commence as soon as the biopsy results are available without the delay necessary to allow wound healing following laparotomy. Endoscopy is indicated in many alimentary conditions (Table 36.5) and is associated with a relatively low complication rate (Table 36.6).

Endoscopic examination of the upper GIT requires an overnight fast and water should be withheld on the day of endoscopy. Lower GI endoscopy can be carried out under sedation but in most cases general anaesthesia is preferred. Thorough patient preparation is required, the patient should be starved for at least 24 h and an oral laxative, e.g. Klean-prep (Norgine) 30 ml kg^{-1} given twice one hour apart the night before. On the day of endoscopy two warm water enemas should be given.

Endoscopy is of limited value unless facilities for taking biopsies are available. Many diseases do not cause gross changes in the intestines and of those that do, very few have pathognomonic features. Multiple biopsies (6–10) should be taken from both the stomach and the duodenum. Serial biopsies taken every 5–10 cm along the length of the colon should be obtained.

Successful endoscopy requires dexterity in manipulating the endoscope, particularly when passing the scope through the pylorus, and an appreciation of the normal anatomic appearance of the intestinal system.

Patients should be placed in left lateral recumbency as, in this position, the pylorus is suspended making passage into the duodenum easier. During large bowel endoscopy left lateral recumbency facilitates drainage of fluid into the descending colon from where it can be aspirated more easily.

Upper GI endoscopy

The endoscope is lubricated and introduced into the proximal oesophagus with the neck extended. The oesophagus is distended with air and the

Table 36.5 Principal indications/contraindications for endoscopy

Upper GI endoscopy	Lower GI endoscopy	Contraindications
Evaluation of dysphagia	Evaluation of persistent haematochezia	Patient unfit for anaesthesia
Evaluation of regurgitation	Evaluation of persistent tenesmus	Patient too small
Evaluation of chronic vomiting	Evaluation of faecal incontinence	Perforation of the bowel suspected
Evaluation of haematemesis	Evaluation of chronic diarrhoea	Patient inadequately prepared
Evaluation of melaena	Evaluation of persistent mucoid stools	Patient has a severe bleeding tendency
Evaluation of chronic diarrhoea	Evaluation of dyschezia	
Retrieval of oesophageal foreign body		
Bougienage of oesophageal stricture		
Placement of perendoscopic gastrostomy tubes		

scope is advanced towards the cardia; there should be little resistance. Biopsies of the oesophagus are not easily obtained and in most cases unnecessary. The cardia is slit-like and often has a reddened appearance representing the transition from oesophageal to gastric mucosa. The endoscope normally passes easily into the stomach which should be examined in a systematic way. As prolonged inflation of the stomach can make passage into the duodenum more difficult, visual inspection of the stomach can be carried out at this stage and biopsies taken after examination of the duodenum. Examination of the area around the cardia requires retroflexion of the endoscope as a 'J' manoeuvre (Fig. 36.4). The endoscope is then advanced into the pylorus which lies ventral to the incisura angularis. The pylorus can be identified as a sphincter lying centrally in the antrum. Passage of the endoscope through the pylorus requires practice. The endoscope should be advanced keeping the pylorus central which may require torquing of the endoscope. It is often helpful to have one operator applying gentle forward pressure as required while the endoscopist keeps the tip of the scope in the pylorus. As the tip of the endoscope contacts the pylorus, vision will be lost to be replaced by a dark space (the pyloric canal) surrounded by a blurred red mucosa. Intermittent insufflation should be continued but care must be taken not to overinflate the stomach particularly when passage through the pylorus takes some time. In most instances the pylorus will yield and the endoscope can be easily advanced into the duodenum. In cases where passage is difficult, the pylorus can be relaxed with glucagon (0.05 mg kg^{-1} i.v. (maximum dose 1 mg)). The use of metoclopramide is controversial as it can enhance antral contraction (Matz et al., 1991). Once the duodenum has been entered, duodenal juice can be collected if necessary. Washing of the tip of the endoscope should be avoided until after the juice has been collected as this will dilute the sample by an unknown amount. The endoscope should be advanced to use the majority of its functional length which in most cases will be past the duodenal flexure. In some cats and small dogs passage into the proximal jejunum is possible. Once the duodenum has been inspected multiple biopsies of the duodenum can be taken as the endoscope is withdrawn into the stomach where

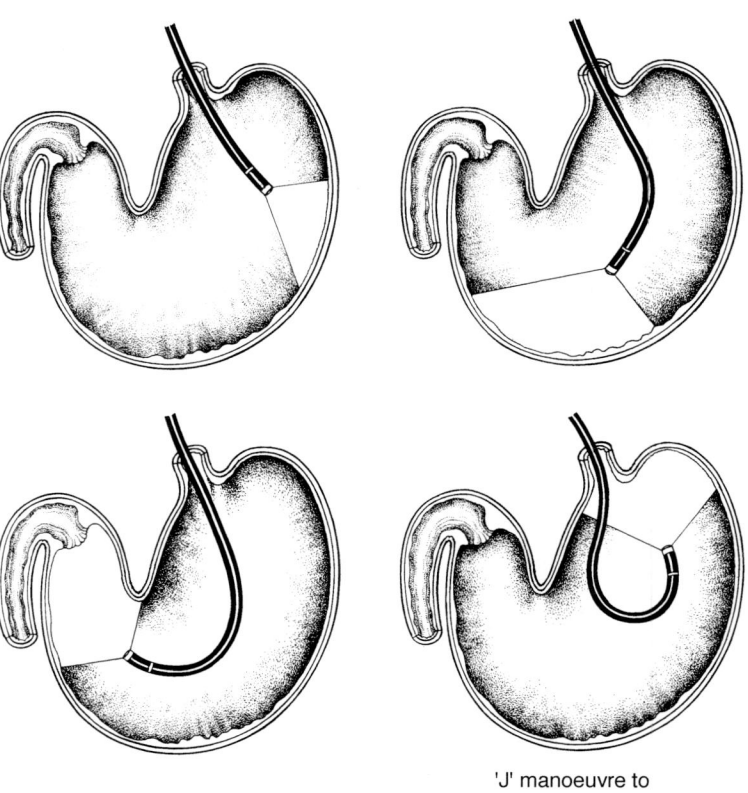

Figure 36.4 Endoscopic examination of the stomach.

'J' manoeuvre to examine cardia

biopsies of the pylorus, antrum, body and fundus can then be obtained. As the endoscope is being withdrawn into the oesophagus, air within the stomach should be removed by suction. If aggressive lesions are apparent within the stomach and/or duodenum a rapid diagnosis can sometimes be made by preparing a squash preparation of a suitable biopsy. This may allow treatment to be instigated earlier.

Colonoscopy

Before colonoscopy, a digital examination of the anus should have been carried out as very distal lesions can be easily missed. Colonoscopy can be performed using a rigid proctoscope or a flexible endoscope. Flexible endoscopy has the advantage of allowing examination of the whole colon to the ileocolic valve. The endoscope is introduced into the rectum and the colon insufflated. It is usually necessary to have an assistant clamp the anal sphincter around the scope to prevent the air from escaping. The endoscope is advanced to the left colonic flexure, along the transverse colon to the right flexure (often inapparent) and into the ascending colon where the ileocolic valve can be viewed as a button-like protuberance in the wall of the colon and the caecum is seen as a dark passage directly ahead. The endoscope is then withdrawn, biopsying at intervals along the length of the colon if no specific lesion has been identified.

▪ Duodenal fluid examination

Duodenal fluid can be collected using sterile polypropylene tubing introduced via the instrument channel of the endoscope and is an accurate technique for the diagnosis of giardiasis. Neoplastic cells, particularly in cases of lymphosarcoma can also be collected using this technique.

Duodenal fluid collection and quantitative culture is used as a definitive diagnosis of SIBO. Colony counts greater than 10^5 ml^{-1} in dogs (Batt *et al.*, 1983) and greater than 10^7–10^8 ml^{-1} in cats (Johnston *et al.*, 1993) are considered abnormal. Unfortunately, in order to accurately quantify bacterial numbers, particularly anaerobes, immediate culture is required.

▪ Evaluation of brush border enzymes

Evaluation of brush border enzymes can be used as a sensitive indicator of acquired small intestinal pathology which can occur in the absence of marked histopathological changes (Batt, 1986). Dying or damaged intestinal epithelial cells leak their contents or are sloughed into the lumen, hence appreciable rises in serum brush border enzyme levels do not occur.

▪ Urease activity

The role of *Helicobacter* spp. in human intestinal disease is well established. The presence of these spiral organisms in the gastric mucosa of dogs and cats has been demonstrated and the association between their presence and gastric disease is becoming increasingly probable (Lee *et al.*, 1992). Although a variety of tests for helicobacteriosis are available for use in humans, diagnosis in dogs and cats relies either on direct visualization of the bacteria in biopsy specimens or on their ability to split urea. A urease test can be simply performed by embedding a biopsy in a urea containing gel (Clotest – Bripharm Ltd, Surrey, UK) containing a pH-sensitive dye which turns pink as urea is split into ammonia.

▪ Gastric allergy testing

Challenging patients with suspected food allergies can be a potentially dangerous procedure which can lead to fatal anaphylaxis. Gastroscopic food sensitivity testing involves small amounts of food extracts being dripped onto the gastric mucosa. The site is then observed for 2–3 minutes for evidence of erythema, blanching, oedema or petechiation (Guilford *et al.*, 1991). Gastric allergy testing only assesses IgE-mediated immediate type hypersensitivity and not delayed-type hypersensitivity which occurs in some animals.

▪ Abdominocentesis

Abdominocentesis can be a rapid and valuable technique in dogs and cats that present with an acute abdominal crisis or in cases where abdominal fluid has been detected clinically or using diagnostic imaging. Samples should be submitted for cytology, culture, protein estimation and cholesterol and triglyceride concentrations where appropriate.

If only small quantities of fluid are present, a sample can be obtained by peritoneal lavage. Warmed saline (20 ml kg^{-1}) is introduced into the abdomen and distributed by gentle manipulation. After several minutes a sample is withdrawn which can be submitted for cytological examination and culture.

Exploratory coeliotomy

Abdominal surgery is a frequently performed procedure in general practice in animals with both acute and chronic intestinal disease. Results of exploratory surgeries are often disappointing both for the owner and surgeon as 'everything appeared normal'. Improved diagnostic rates can be achieved by:

- More extensive initial investigation to give a better idea of the pathology likely to be present;
- Greater surgical exposure allowing complete inspection of the alimentary system and its associated structures;
- Increased sampling; all organs that are suspected to be involved in the pathological process should be biopsied and the biopsies submitted for histopathology.

Exploratory coeliotomy is sometimes required even where extensive, alternate diagnostic techniques are available (Table 36.7). Proper technique is essential for obtaining full thickness intestinal biopsies particularly in patients where there is increased risk of dehiscence.

OROPHARYNGEAL DISEASE

Oropharyngeal disease is very common in dogs and cats especially as they grow older. It is more frequently clinically significant in cats.

Clinical signs

Primary clinical signs include inappetance, halitosis, ptyalism, oral haemorrhage and oropharyngeal dysphagia. Patients with oral disease frequently have good appetites and ask for food but refuse to eat or take only a few mouthfuls when food is presented to them. Some cats will back away from food as though bitten. Patients may adopt bizarre head positions when eating and drinking. Pyrexia, pawing or rubbing the face, difficulty in opening or closing the jaws, nasal discharge and paroxysmal jaw chattering are also seen. Dehydration can be a significant problem, especially in cats, who derive most of their fluid intake from food.

Physical examination

A complete physical examination is essential to rule out more generalized disease as a cause of the clinical signs, for example animals with chronic renal failure may present with 'rubber jaw' or oral ulceration. The mucocutaneous junctions should be carefully examined for evidence of autoimmune disease or exposure to caustic chemicals. Other mucosal surfaces should be inspected if there is evidence of buccal mucosal haemorrhage. A neurological examination is required if there are problems with prehension and swallowing of food, or if there is evidence of facial asymmetry or ptyalism.

Examination of the oral cavity frequently requires general anaesthesia as many patients resent having their mouths forced open and many lesions of the oral cavity are very painful. Even with the most cooperative of patients examination of the oro- and nasopharynx is not possible.

Table 36.7 Indications, contraindications and major complications of exploratory coeliotomy

Indications	Contraindications and complications
Rapid decline in patient condition	Diagnosis can be obtained non-invasively
Suspected intestinal perforation	Wound dehiscence
Lesion likely to be in jejunum/ileum	Unacceptable anaesthetic risk
Lesions not involving the mucosal surface	Delay in commencing immunosuppressive therapy
Disease of associated lymph nodes	Poor wound healing likely, e.g. recent glucocorticoid administration, protein-losing enteropathy
Suspected intestinal obstruction	
Chronic pancreatic disease	

Diagnosis

In cases where the cause of the problem is not obvious, a diagnostic investigation should be carried out. This may require routine haematology and biochemistry, serology (FeLV, FIV), fungal (*Candida* spp., *Cryptococcus* spp.) and viral (FCV, FHV-1) cultures, assays for antinuclear antibody, radiography and biopsy. Examination of the nasopharynx can be carried out under general anaesthesia using a small flexible endoscope or alternatively curved forceps, a light source and dental mirror. It is important to examine all areas of the mouth including the base of the tongue where string foreign bodies can lodge. Multiple biopsies of oral lesions should be taken. Frequently it is only at the edge of a lesion that diagnostic material is present, more centrally a mixture of inflammatory cells and necrotic tissue is found regardless of the cause of the lesion.

Stomatitis

Stomatitis together with gingivitis, pharyngitis and glossitis can result from local and systemic disease (Table 36.8) and is a commonly encountered problem particularly in cats. Clinical signs are rarely helpful in suggesting the aetiology. It is useful to ascertain from the history whether the stomatitis is acute or chronic. Acute disease is most frequently associated with the ingestion of caustic or irritant chemicals which can include household plants, e.g. poinsettia, pine needles, *Philodendron*. Electrical burns associated with cable chewing tend to cause acute, linear lesions of the hard palate, gingivae and commissures of the lips (Wolf 1992) and may be associated with cardiac arrhythmias and pulmonary oedema. Dental, immune-mediated and metabolic diseases, nutritional deficiencies, neoplasia and microorganisms tend to be associated with chronic progressive disease.

Chronic feline gingivitis-stomatitis-pharyngitis

The gingivitis/stomatitis complex is a frustrating condition for the owner and the veterinarian to deal with and can be very painful for the cat. The aetiology is unknown but is likely to be the end result of a variety of disease processes which cause infiltration of the mucosa with lymphocytes and plasma cells. Less commonly an eosinophilic infiltrate is seen. Gingivitis/stomatitis can affect cats of any age. A relatively mild gingivitis is commonly seen in young pedigree cats and is frequently self-limiting.

Feline leukaemia virus (FeLV), feline immunodeficiency virus (FIV) and feline calicivirus (FCV) have all been implicated in the pathogenesis of the disease. Around 10–15% of cases are FeLV/FIV positive. It is unlikely that these viruses cause direct damage to the mucosal surface but the gingivitis/stomatitis arises secondary to immunosuppression. The role of FCV in chronic disease is uncertain. The virus can undoubtedly cause severe oral ulceration during acute infection but whether this sets up sufficient mucosal damage to initiate chronic progression is unclear. FCV can be isolated from the gingiva of many cats with gingivitis and stomatitis but it has also been isolated from about 25% of healthy cats at shows (Coutts *et al.*, 1994). Dental decay frequently accompanies gingivitis and stomatitis

Table 36.8 Stomatitis – potential causes and disease associations

Cause	Disease associations
Dental disease	
Immune-mediated disease	Pemphigus, systemic or discoid lupus erythematosus, idiopathic, immunodeficiency, food sensitivity, drug reactions
Microorganisms	Primarily viral especially FCV, FHV-1, FIV, FeLV, CAV-1, distemper virus. Rarely fungal
Metabolic	Uraemia, diabetes mellitus
Neoplasia	e.g. squamous cell carcinoma, fibrosarcoma, lymphosarcoma, haemangiosarcoma
Traumatic	Road traffic accident, persistent over-grooming
Caustic, toxic or irritant	Including antineoplastic therapy
Nutritional imbalance	Hypervitaminosis A, niacin or riboflavin deficiencies
Chronic disease	Predisposed to stomatitis and ulceration particularly with protein-calorie malnutrition

and many cases respond favourably to dental hygiene in the short term. A hypersensitivity to plaque bacteria has been suggested as a possible aetiology.

Treatment options

1. Initially, oral hygiene procedures should be performed. This involves full prophylaxis including subgingival curettage and polishing. Teeth with significant resorptive lesions and retained roots should be extracted. Regular cleaning is then required every 6–12 months. The importance of owner compliance can not be overemphasized and good tooth cleaning at home should be instituted using oral rinses, gels or pastes.
2. Antibiotics alone rarely produce more than a temporary improvement, but may aid control of oral flora where tooth cleaning is difficult (such cats are also frequently difficult to medicate). Regular intermittent regimes can be successful in some cases. Suitable antibiotics include amoxycillin/clavulanate (Synulox; Pfizer Ltd), metronidazole/spiramycin (Stormogyl; Rhône Mérieux Ltd), clindamycin (Antirobe; Upjohn Ltd).
3. Corticosteroids are most useful in cases where there is a marked inflammatory cell infiltrate and hypergammaglobulinaemia. Prior screening for retrovirus should be performed. Glucocorticoids are contraindicated in acute cases of FCV or feline herpes virus (FHV-1) infection. An immunosuppressive dose (prednisolone 2–4 mg kg^{-1} divided bid) for one to three weeks followed by a gradual tapering of the dose is preferred but in cats that resent oral medication or in cases where the mouth is particularly painful parenteral or intralesional preparations are indicated. Methylprednisolone acetate (Depomedrone V; Upjohn Ltd) can be given initially at 2 mg kg^{-1} every two to three weeks for three to five doses and thereafter at intervals of six to eight weeks. Triamcinolone (Vetalog; Ciba Animal Health) at a dose of 0.6 mg injected into each lesion (maximum of 6 mg).
4. Gold salt therapy has been suggested but its efficacy and toxicity in cats has not been evaluated.
5. Diathermy and cryosurgery have been successful in some cases. There is a risk, however, of causing exacerbation of the hyperplasia and damaging the submucosal tissues.
6. Radical tooth extraction has been advocated and good success rate reported by some clinicians. Success is not guaranteed and full dental extraction is an expensive and time consuming procedure. Pre- and postextraction radiographs should be obtained to ensure all tooth fragments have been removed. Initially the canines are left *in situ* to maintain mouth shape and hold the tongue in place but these may also require removal.
7. Megestrol acetate (Ovarid; Mallinckrodt Vet Ltd) has been used in many cases of chronic gingivitis/stomatitis but offers no clinical advantage over corticosteroids and is associated with undesirable side effects including lethargy, obesity and diabetes mellitus.

Regardless of the treatment chosen, the prognosis for recovery is poor. Many cases can, however, be adequately controlled for long periods.

■ Oral trauma

Traumatic lesions are most commonly seen in cats following road traffic accidents and 'high rise' syndrome. Separation of the mandibular symphysis is most frequently encountered and is easily corrected surgically. Splitting of the hard palate following rotational forces on the skull or impact from a fall may not require surgical intervention if there is no communication with the nasal passages. Larger lesions require mucoperiosteal flaps. For repair of more complex oral defects and fractures the reader is referred to suitable orthopaedic or surgical texts.

■ Oral neoplasia

Tumours of the oral cavity are frequently seen, with melanomas and squamous cell carcinomas being most common in dogs and squamous cell carcinomas and fibrosarcomas in cats (Cotter, 1981).

Patients usually present when the mass is quite large and is causing anorexia, dysphagia, drooling or halitosis. Diagnosis is based on histological examination of multiple biopsies taken from the edge of the lesion. Radiographs to evaluate bone involvement are helpful although it is noteworthy that squamous cell carcinomas involving bone in cats carry a slightly better prognosis than those that do not. Survey films are also indicated to check for pulmonary metastases.

A wide variety of tumours have been found affecting the oral cavity including plasmacytomas, osteosarcomas, haemangiosarcomas, lymphosarcomas, myeloblastomas, rhabdomyomas and papillomas.

Squamous cell carcinoma

These tumours can affect any part of the oral cavity and tongue and can mimic many other oral conditions. They range from slowly progressive, superficial, localized, erythematous, ulcerative plaques to aggressive proliferative mass-like lesions. Squamous cell carcinomas of the oral cavity invade locally but are slow to metastasize whereas tongue and tonsillar lesions appear more aggressive and often metastasize.

Radical surgical excision, where possible, with adjunctive radiation or chemotherapy is recommended. Cisplatin is the chemotherapeutic agent of choice in dogs, but should only be used intralesionally in cats as it is highly toxic if given systemically.

Malignant melanoma

Typically melanomas present as pigmented, friable masses of the gingival or buccal mucosa but amelanotic tumours do occur. Radical surgery with adjunctive radiation therapy is required, however the prognosis remains poor.

Fibrosarcoma

Fibrosarcomas are most commonly found originating from the hard palate or maxilla and are usually firm masses. Local invasion and local and distant metastasis are common. Median survival time following radical surgical excision is approximately 11 months (Kosovsky *et al.*, 1991).

Epulides

Epulides are generally benign tumours of the gingival margin. They are primarily seen in dogs, but have been reported in cats (Stebbins *et al.*, 1989). Classification of epulides is controversial, but it is important that they are differentiated from more malignant neoplasms. Acanthomatous epulides are the most aggressive type. All forms can be treated with surgical excision. Metastasis is rare.

Eosinophilic granuloma complex

Eosinophilic granuloma is seen frequently in cats and has been recorded in the Siberian husky (Madewell *et al.*, 1980). In cats, ulcers, granulomas and plaques occur. Ulcers most frequently affect the upper lip of adult cats and appear as firm, well circumscribed erosive lesions (so called rodent ulcers). The aetiology of these ulcers is unknown and eosinophils are not always seen on histopathological examination. Granulomas and plaques occur in the mouth as well-circumscribed, erythematous raised areas often associated with a circulating eosinophilia. Squamous cell carcinoma is an important differential diagnosis for these lesions.

Treatment with systemic or intralesional corticosteroids (see Treatment of gingivitis/stomatitis) usually causes remission. Some cases respond more favourably to progestogen therapy but care must be taken if long-term use is envisaged. Surgical excision, cryosurgery or radiation therapy has been suggested for refractory lesions. The use of antibiotics (amoxycillin/clavulanate and trimethoprim sulphadiazine) for lip ulcers has been advocated and reported to be successful (Scott, 1980).

Oropharyngeal foreign bodies

Foreign bodies are usually self-evident but string foreign bodies can loop around the base of the tongue and may not be obvious on a cursory inspection of the oral cavity. Long blades of barbed grass can become lodged dorsal to the soft palate in the nasopharynx and cause coughing, retching and dysphagia. Foreign bodies in the gingival sulci, tonsillar crypts and tongue have also been reported.

Nasopharyngeal polyps

Polyps involving the nasopharynx are thought to be the result of chronic inflammation. They are usually attached to narrow stalks extending from the middle ear via the eustachian tube. In the nasopharynx they cause stertorous breathing, sneezing and dysphagia. The majority of the mass can easily be removed by traction but attention should be paid to the underlying cause (usually otitis media) and more radical surgery of the middle ear may be required to prevent recurrence.

Disorders of the palate

Cleft palate is seen as a congenital disorder in dogs and cats and in some cases may also be heritable

(Shih Tzu, Siamese, pointers and bulldogs) (Harvey, 1987). Clinical signs are usually apparent from a young age with milk appearing at the nostrils during suckling. Treatment is surgical.

Elongation of the soft palate, as part of the brachycephalic airway syndrome, primarily affects the respiratory tract rather than the GIT.

Congenitally short soft palates are seen in both cats and dogs. The palate fails to contact with the epiglottis and thus does not protect the airway resulting in a chronic nasal discharge.

Pharyngitis

'Pharyngitis' is commonly diagnosed in cats and dogs with vague signs of inappetance, dysphagia and retching or vomiting. Primary disease is rare and usually associated with trauma or the ingestion of toxic or caustic substances. The condition is more frequently seen secondary to widespread oral, respiratory or systemic disease.

Tonsillar disease

Primary tonsillitis is comparatively rare and appears most commonly in young toy breed dogs. A variety of bacteria have been cultured but may not represent primary agents. Affected dogs cough and gag and then retch or expectorate small quantities of white foamy mucus. Patients can be depressed, pyrexic and inappetant. Examination of the tonsils under general anaesthesia is usually required. The tonsils appear hyperaemic and mottled and may have petechiae and small focal abscesses (visualized as white specks) on the surface. Protrusion of the tonsils is difficult to assess as there is great variation between individuals. The condition is usually responsive to antimicrobials but tends to recur. Most animals will, however, recover spontaneously with age. Tonsillectomy is rarely necessary and can cause severe, potentially life-threatening, haemorrhage.

Neoplasia generally causes massive enlargement of the tonsils resulting in gagging and dysphagia. Lymphosarcoma (bilateral enlargement) and squamous cell carcinoma (unilateral enlargement) are most commonly seen. Diagnosis is based on the clinical picture and the results of fine needle aspiration cytology or histopathological examination of grab biopsies. Lymphosarcoma can be treated with standard chemotherapy protocols. Squamous cell carcinoma is usually highly malignant and aggressive. Treatment is rarely successful.

Salivary gland disease

Salivary mucocele

Sialoceles result from leakage of the saliva into the subcutis of the neck, pharyngeal wall or sublingual tissue (ranula). The cause is not always apparent but trauma e.g. road traffic accident in cats is likely. Cervical sialoceles result in unilateral swelling below the mandibles. Pharyngeal sialoceles can significantly compromise the patient's ability to eat or drink. Ranulae appear under the tongue. Diagnosis is by aspiration of a sample of mucoid brown fluid of low cellularity. Surgical drainage, marsupialization and removal of the affected gland(s) are curative.

Sialoadenitis

Trauma to the salivary glands can result in a painful swollen gland with associated anorexia, pyrexia and pain on opening the mouth. Diagnosis is based on the results of fine needle aspiration cytology. Treatment with antibacterial therapy and, occasionally, surgical drainage is effective.

Salivary gland necrosis

Necrosis is a rare disease of unknown pathogenesis most commonly reported in terriers particularly Jack Russells (Kelly et al., 1979). The salivary gland becomes enlarged and firm and affected animals develop persistent anorexia, depression, ptyalism, gagging, vomiting and frequent swallowing. Diagnosis requires biopsy. Surgical resection is sometimes palliative.

Salivary gland neoplasia

Neoplasia is usually seen in old cats and dogs as malignant tumours of epithelial origin. Disease is frequently advanced at presentation having already infiltrated the local area. The prognosis is therefore poor.

Ptyalism

Ptyalism can result from both hypersalivation and an inability to swallow normal saliva production. It can be seen associated with a variety of salivary, oropharyngeal and oesophageal diseases. It can also be associated with systemic diseases particularly hepatic encephalopathy in cats. Phenobarbitone responsive (3–4 mg kg^{-1} bid) hypersalivation has been reported in two dogs (Chapman and Malik, 1992).

Miscellaneous diseases

Salivary gland foreign bodies, sialoliths, autoimmune disease (Sjögren's syndrome) and salivary gland fistula are rare conditions in cats and dogs.

DYSPHAGIA

Dysphagia is defined as difficulty in swallowing and should be differentiated from anorexia and inappetance which may appear similar to the owner.

Aetiology

Swallowing requires the coordination of five cranial nerves (trigeminal, facial, glossopharyngeal, vagus and hypoglossal) mediated through the swallowing centre (Suter and Watrous, 1980). The tongue, hard and soft palates, pharynx and oesophagus are intimately involved in this process.

Swallowing is initiated by the voluntary movement of a food bolus into the pharynx by caudodorsal movement of the tongue pressing the food bolus against the hard palate (Watrous, 1983). The bolus is detected by pharyngeal receptors which initiate an involuntary closure of the nasopharynx by elevating the soft palate and closing the palatopharyngeal folds. The airway is protected by closure of the glottis and tipping the epiglottis during which time the cricopharyngeal sphincter relaxes. Pharyngeal muscle contraction then moves the bolus into the oesophagus where peristalsis carries it into the stomach (Zawie, 1987).

Dysphagia is more commonly described in dogs than cats which may reflect lifestyle as dogs are more likely to chase and chew sticks and scavenge resulting in an increased incidence of oropharyngeal trauma and foreign bodies. Dysphagias can be classified as functional or mechanical (Table 36.9) or according to the structures involved namely oral, pharyngeal or oesophageal.

Table 36.9 Functional and mechanical causes of dysphagia. See Table 36.11 for causes of megaoesophagus which can lead to oesophageal dysphagia

Functional disorders	Congenital – cricopharyngeal dysphagia CNS lesions – masses, trauma, inflammation Paresis of cranial nerves V, VII, IX, X or XII Microbial – botulism, rabies, toxoplasmosis Toxic – lead Neuromuscular dysfunction – polymyositis, myopathies
Mechanical disorders	Oropharyngeal masses – elongated soft palate, neoplasia or abscessation of epiglottis, tonsils, pharyngeal wall or soft palate Pharyngeal oedema – insect bites/stings, caustic chemicals, excessively hot food, trauma, allergy Trauma – mandibular or hyoid fractures, bite wounds Temporomandibular joint dysfunction – malformation, degenerative joint disease, craniomandibular osteopathy Tongue dysfunction – neoplasia, trauma Extra-oral masses causing obstruction – retropharyngeal lymphadenopathy, salivary gland enlargement, trauma/abscessation of peripharyngeal tissue Eosinophilic granuloma complex

Clinical findings

Typically, dysphagic patients show weight loss, increased appetite and often appear to be messy feeders. When food is given they tend to have difficulties in prehending or swallowing food although with time many animals will adapt to overcome a functional or mechanical problem. Pain may eventually lead to reluctance to eat with patients continually demanding food but then only taking a few mouthfuls or not eating at all when it is presented to them.

Modifications in eating behaviour, poor coordination of swallowing or neurological deficits that accompany dysphagia greatly increase the risk of aspiration pneumonia. Aspiration pneumonia is characterized by a dramatic deterioration in the patient's condition, coughing, tachypnoea, pyrexia and depression.

Oral dysphagia

The patient is unable to prehend food or form a bolus which exhibits as an inability to pick up food, excessive chewing, throwing the head about whilst eating, food falling out of the mouth or being held in the cheeks, facial asymmetry, inability to lap fluids, drooling saliva and an inability to control the tongue. Retching or gagging are rare as the bolus does not reach the pharynx.

Pharyngeal dysphagia

These animals are able to prehend food and form a bolus but show repeated attempts to swallow with gagging, retching and coughing. Food may return into the mouth, appear at the nostrils or be inhaled. Inhalation results in paroxysmal coughing. Pharyngeal dysphagia occurs due to defective sensory or motor function. There is asynchrony in protection of the airway, failure of the cricopharyngeal sphincter to relax or failure of the pharyngeal muscles to contract (Watrous, 1983). Eating is associated with discomfort and such patients tend to become anorexic.

Cricopharyngeal dysphagia (achalasia) is a specific condition associated with either failure of the oesophageal sphincter to dilate or, more commonly, asynchrony of sphincter dilation with swallowing. Suggested aetiologies include neurological deficits, atrophy, fibrosis or hypertrophy of the sphincter muscle, trauma, neuromuscular deficits and neoplasia. Rarely cricopharyngeal dysphagia is associated with generalized neuromuscular disease such as myasthenia gravis. Cricopharyngeal dysphagia is very uncommon in the cat.

Most cases are congenital and become apparent post-weaning (Rosin and Hanlon, 1972) but acquired cases do occur. An hereditary predisposition has been suggested in cocker spaniels (Weaver, 1983) and poodles. Clinical signs are similar to other pharyngeal dysphagias.

Oesophageal dysphagia

Oesophageal dysphagia is seen relatively frequently (Watrous, 1983) and is associated with passive regurgitation of undigested food after feeding. Aspiration pneumonia is common.

Diagnosis

Recognition of dysphagia is based on a good clinical history, distinguishing dysphagia from anorexia, regurgitation and vomiting. Physical examination should include a neurological evaluation. It is often helpful to observe the patient eating rather than rely on an owner's description. A distinction between vomit (acid) and regurgitated or retched (alkaline) material can be made by measuring the pH of the sample (Shelton, 1982). Adequate examination of the oral cavity may require sedation or anaesthesia which can be combined with survey radiographs of the head, neck and thorax. Where there is evidence of more generalized systemic disease such as hypothyroidism or myasthenia gravis then specific tests should be carried out.

Contrast studies, particularly if performed in association with fluoroscopy (Suter and Watrous, 1980), allow a detailed study of the swallowing process to be performed (Table 36.10).

Treatment

The prognosis for swallowing disorders is generally guarded and unless a specific, treatable underlying cause can be identified, the response to symptomatic therapy tends to be poor. Aspiration pneumonia should be treated with aggressive antibiosis but is liable to recur. Feeding can be improved by varying the consistency of the diet to one that the patient can cope with best. Long-term feeding through a gastrostomy tube is appropriate in some cases but requires dedicated and informed owners and good veterinary support.

Table 36.10 Clinical and fluoroscopic localization of disease in the dysphagic animal

Clinical sign	Type of dysphagia		
	Oral	Pharyngeal	Oesophageal
Defective bolus formation	+	+/-	–
Retention of food	+	–	–
Food falls out of mouth	+	–	–
Nasal egress of food	–	+	+/-
Failure of pharynx to contract	–	+	–
Retention of food in the pharynx	–	+	–
Cricopharyngeal achalasia	–	+	+
Retention of food in the oesophagus	–	–	+
Retching	–	+	–
Regurgitation	–	–	+

Cricopharyngeal dysphagia can be successfully treated in around 70% of cases by partial cricopharyngeal myotomy. Accurate diagnosis is essential as a myotomy performed for other causes of dysphagia will worsen the condition (Elkins, 1987).

OESOPHAGEAL DISEASE

Oesophageal disease tends to be underdiagnosed as most owners perceive the regurgitation that occurs as vomiting so that subsequent investigations tend to be directed towards the stomach and small intestines.

Megaoesophagus

Aetiology

Megaoesophagus or oesophageal dilation is a common cause of regurgitation (Clifford *et al.*, 1971; Simpson, 1994). The condition may be congenital or acquired and hereditary predispositions have been reported in dogs. Idiopathic megaoesophagus is inherited in the wire-haired fox terrier (Osborne *et al.*, 1967) and miniature schnauzer (Cox *et al.*, 1980) and breed predispositions have been reported in the Great Dane, Irish setter, German shepherd dog and shar pei. It is relatively rare in the cat (Harvey *et al.*, 1974) although it may also be inherited (Clifford *et al.*, 1971) with Siamese-related breeds being predisposed. The difference in the prevalence of the condition between dogs and cats may reflect the predominance of smooth muscle fibres in the feline oesophagus.

Megaoesophagus in dogs under six months of age may be due to immaturity of the oesophageal muscle and animals can recover spontaneously by one year of age (Simpson and Else, 1991a). A number of causes and disease associations of megaoesophagus have been documented (Zook and Gilmore 1967; Mason, 1976; Sharp *et al.*, 1984; Leib, 1986; Zawie, 1987; Hoenig *et al.*, 1990; Maddison and Allan, 1990) (Table 36.11).

The aetiology of congenital megaoesophagus is unknown. However, current opinion suggests that oesophageal motor function remains intact and the disease is associated with a sensory failure or a lesion in the swallowing centre (medial part of the lateral reticular formation of the brainstem) (Zawie, 1987). Failure of the high pressure zone of the distal oesophagus to open is not a primary problem but occurs due to lack of peristalsis.

Table 36.11 Causes and disease associations of megaoesophagus

Neuromuscular	Oesophageal obstruction
Idiopathic megaoesophagus	Neoplasia
Myasthenia gravis – focal and generalized	Vascular ring anomaly
Systemic lupus erythematosus	Extra-oesophageal compression
Polymyositis/polymyopathy	Strictures (see Table 36.14)
Dystrophin deficiency	Granulomas
Glycogen storage disease type II	Foreign bodies
Dermatomyositis	**Toxic**
Feline dysautonomia	Thallium
Giant cell axonal neuropathy	Lead
Immune-mediated polyneuritis	Organophosphates and anticholinesterases
Ganglioradiculitis	Acrylamide
Spinal muscle atrophy	**Other**
Bilateral vagal damage	Mediastinitis/mediastinal mass
Familial reflex myoclonus	Broncho-oesophageal fistula
Cervical vertebral instability	Gastric heterotopia
Brainstem trauma, neoplasia or vascular disease	Hypoadrenocorticism
Polyradiculoneuritis	Hypothyroidism
Botulism	Pituitary dwarfism
Distemper	*Trypanosoma cruzi* infection (not UK)
Tetanus	Thymoma
	Postviral disease in cats

Clinical findings

The majority of cases present with regurgitation of undigested food shortly after eating but some animals will retain food in the dilated oesophagus for a considerable period of time before regurgitation. Less commonly, patients will only regurgitate liquids, especially saliva, which is unassociated with feeding. Some cases of megaoesophagus will present with aspiration pneumonia as the primary sign. Appetite is usually increased initially, but becomes depressed if aspiration pneumonia develops. Congenital cases fail to thrive and gain weight whereas adult animals tend to lose condition.

Diagnosis

History and clinical signs will often suggest megaoesophagus which can be confirmed, in the majority of cases, by a plain, conscious, lateral radiograph (Figs 36.5 and 36.6). Typically the dilated oesophagus is gas filled which helps to outline the dorsal and ventral walls of the oesophagus and the dorsal wall of the trachea. Evidence of an aspiration pneumonia is frequently present in the dependent areas of the caudal part of the left cranial, right middle, accessory and caudal lung lobes. Contrast studies are usually unnecessary and aspiration of barium is a risk. In subtle cases contrast studies preferably with fluoroscopy may be required.

Following confirmation of a megaoesophagus every effort should be made to define a primary cause. Some or all of the following tests may be required; adrenocorticotrophic hormone (ACTH) stimulation test, thyroid stimulating hormone (TSH) stimulation test, a complete bio-

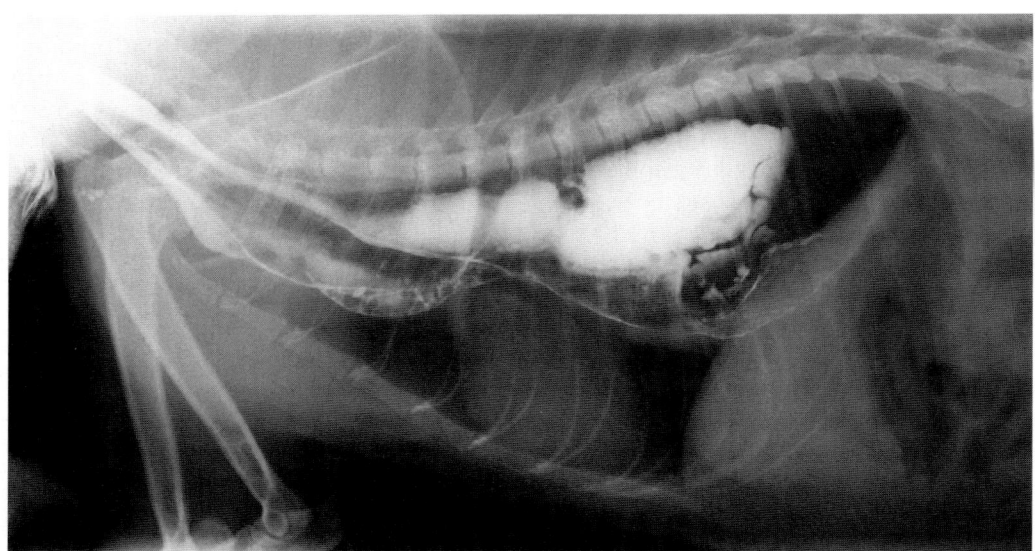

Figure 36.5 Idiopathic megaoesophagus in a 6-year-old, female Burmese cat with a two-month history of regurgitation and dyspnoea.

Figure 36.6 Megaoesophagus secondary to myasthenia gravis in an 11-year-old, neutered, female Hungarian vizla dog. Note the gas-filled oesophagus allowing the dorsal and ventral wall of the oesophagus (small arrows) and the dorsal wall of the trachea (large arrows) to be seen.

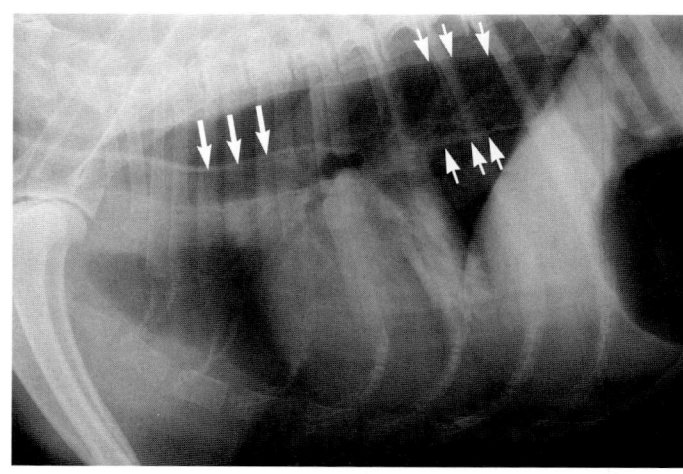

chemical screen, assays for antinuclear antibodies and acetylcholine receptor antibodies, endoscopy, electromyography, nerve conduction velocities, muscle biopsy, serum lead, thallium and botulinum toxin concentrations, acetylcholinesterase activity (Shelton, 1992; Simpson, 1994). If an animal is to be anaesthetized for diagnostic testing, great care must be taken to prevent aspiration of oesophageal fluid particularly during induction and the recovery phase.

Treatment

Treatment of megaoesophagus, even when a primary cause has been defined, can be frustrating and expensive. Therapy for the underlying disease may help but even when the primary condition is controlled the megaoesophagus does not always resolve. Surgical techniques have been described for the reduction of oesophageal size but success rates are generally very poor.

Symptomatic management should centre on providing adequate nutrition in the form of a low volume, high energy diet. Patients should be fed from an elevated position and encouraged to sit for 15 min after feeding. For small dogs or cats it is often more appropriate to carry them as though 'burping' a baby. Solid food is generally preferred to liquid diets. Long-term gastrostomy feeding is suitable for some patients, but aspiration pneumonia may still occur due to pooling of saliva in the oesophagus which is then regurgitated and aspirated. Where aspiration pneumonia is present, broad spectrum antibacterials such as clavulanic acid potentiated amoxycillin, fluoroquinolones or cephalosporins should be given for at least two weeks.

Cholinergic drugs such as bethanechol have little beneficial effect in dogs as the oesophagus consists primarily of skeletal muscle. Metoclopramide is contraindicated as it increases distal oesophageal tone which can reduce passage of food into the stomach. Due to the increased smooth muscle content of the feline oesophagus, cholinergic and prokinetics such as metoclopramide or cisapride may be more effective. The value of cisapride in the treatment of canine megaoesophagus has yet to be evaluated.

Care needs to be taken when immunosuppressive doses of glucocorticoids are used to treat immune-mediated diseases such as myasthenia gravis, systemic lupus erythematosus (SLE), polymyositis or polyneuritis as acute exacerbation of aspiration pneumonia can occur.

Prognosis

The prognosis in most cases of megaoesophagus is guarded. Oesophageal function in young animals will improve as they mature and recovery rates of 20–40% are reported in young dogs. Occasional cases of transient, adult onset, megaoesophagus have been reported (Hendricks *et al.*, 1984). Megaoesophagus secondary to appropriately treated polymyositis, polyradiculoneuritis, SLE, focal myasthenia gravis, hypoadrenocorticism, botulism, mediastinitis and broncho-oesophageal fistula may carry a more favourable prognosis.

■ Vascular ring anomalies

Vascular ring anomalies are relatively common in the dog (Fundquist, 1970) but are rare in the cat (Uzuka and Nakama, 1988). The condition appears to be more common in German shepherd dogs (Zawie, 1987), Irish setters and Boston terriers.

During normal embryonic development, the pulmonary artery and aorta develop in the left side of the thorax and are connected by the ductus arteriosus. A number of different congenital vascular anomalies have been described (Woods *et al.*, 1978; van der Linde-Sipman, 1981; Hurley *et al.*, 1993) although the most common is a persistent right aortic arch. The persistent right aortic arch results in the oesophagus becoming entrapped between the aorta (on the right), the pulmonary artery (on the left), the ductus (ligamentum) arteriosum (dorsally) and the heart base (ventrally) (Fig. 36.7). This ring prevents adequate dilation of the oesophagus during swallowing so food but not fluid is retained in the oesophagus cranial to the heart base. With time a prestenotic dilation of the oesophagus occurs.

Another, clinically significant, anomaly occurs when the left subclavian artery originates from the right aortic arch. The vessel follows a course to the left and passes over the top of the oesophagus causing constriction.

Clinical signs

Classically, regurgitation occurs after weaning onto solid food. The undigested food is usually regurgitated shortly after feeding and is frequently re-eaten. As the oesophageal dilation progresses regurgitation can become delayed. Affected puppies and kittens usually present before six months of age with regurgitation, failure to gain weight and frequently aspiration

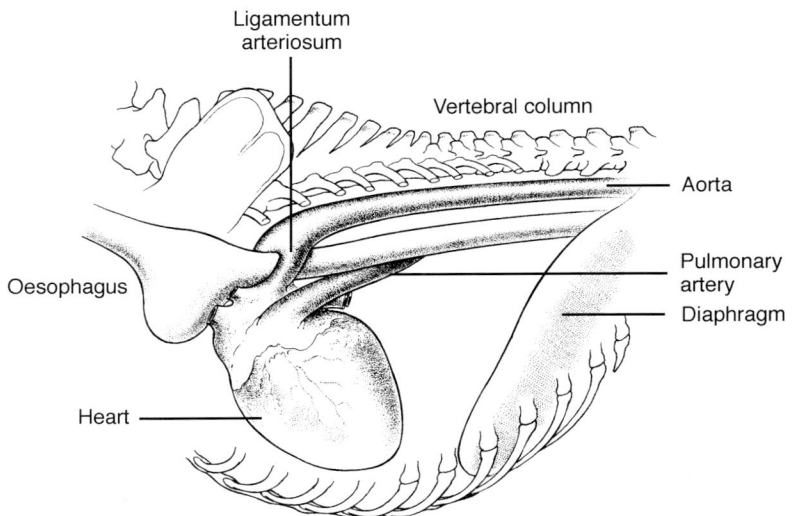

Figure 36.7 Diagram of the thoracic structures in a patient with a persistent right aortic arch that can lead to constriction of the oesophagus.

pneumonia. Occasionally a bulge may appear at the thoracic inlet after feeding due to the oesophagus becoming distended with food.

Diagnosis

Differentiation from other causes of regurgitation is important. This can usually be achieved with contrast radiography, endoscopy or fluoroscopy. Endoscopy is useful in distinguishing extra- from intramural lesions causing stricture. Fluoroscopy allows assessment of oesophageal motility caudal to the stricture which can be abnormal in some dogs. Angiography is required to establish the type and location of the anomaly.

Treatment

Early treatment is essential in order to reduce the risks of the stricture and dilation becoming permanent. A lateral thoracotomy and transection of the constricting band forming the vascular ring is required. Where possible the nutritional status of the patient should be improved prior to transection which may require the surgical placement of a gastrostomy tube. Aspiration pneumonia, if present, should also be controlled before surgery. The prognosis for complete recovery is guarded with up to 50% of dogs still exhibiting signs and as many as 40% being euthanased following surgery.

Oesophageal foreign bodies and oesophageal perforation

The oesophagus is an incredibly distensible structure and is able to accommodate most objects that are swallowed. Foreign body obstructions do, however, occur (Spielman *et al.*, 1992) and are more frequently encountered in dogs than cats (Ryan and Green, 1975), probably due to their scavenging nature, and are prevalent in small breed dogs particularly West Highland white terriers (Houlton *et al.*, 1985). The most common foreign bodies are bones in dogs and fish hooks or needles in cats. Foreign bodies are usually located at the thoracic inlet, heart base or diaphragmatic hiatus where the oesophagus is least distensible.

Foreign bodies can be complicated by oesophagitis (and secondary stricture) and oesophageal perforation leading to mediastinitis or broncho-oesophageal fistula formation. Recurrent smooth oesophageal foreign bodies such as hairballs in a cat should prompt the clinician to look for an underlying motility disorder.

Clinical findings

Patients usually present with an acute onset of salivation, gagging, retching, dysphagia, regurgitation or repeated attempts to swallow. Physical examination is often unhelpful but the pharynx and base of the tongue should be examined carefully for the presence of linear foreign bodies.

The development of coughing, respiratory signs, depression, lethargy, pyrexia and dehydration a few days after the initial signs indicates that aspiration pneumonia or oesophageal perforation may have already occurred.

Diagnosis

A diagnosis can generally be made from the history and plain radiographs as the majority of foreign bodies are radio-opaque. Occasionally endoscopy or contrast studies are required. If there is a possibility that oesophageal perforation has already occurred then an iodine-based contrast medium should be used. Oesophageal perforation is associated with the accumulation of gas, fluid or food in the cervical area, mediastinum or pleural cavity but is not a consistent sign.

Treatment

Oesophageal foreign bodies should be viewed as emergency cases as the longer they are present the greater the risk of mucosal damage and therefore the likelihood of perforation or stricture. Removal can be accomplished in one of four ways:

1. Endoscopic retrieval per os;
2. Fluoroscopic-guided retrieval per os;
3. Manipulation of the foreign body into the stomach ± gastrotomy and removal;
4. Thoracotomy.

In most cases, foreign bodies can be successfully removed using a rigid endoscopic retrieval and large crocodile forceps as the endoscope dilates and protects the oesophagus during the procedure. Retrieval with a flexible endoscope is appropriate for small penetrating objects such as needles, but can be difficult with larger objects as the grab forceps available are often too small and basket retrieval is difficult as it can not be passed over the foreign body. Whichever method is used, only gentle traction should be employed. If the foreign body is firmly wedged in the lumen oesophageal necrosis may have already occurred and surgical treatment may be more appropriate.

Where the foreign body is lying close to the cardia, gentle pressure to push it into the stomach is often preferable rather than trying to drag it along the entire length of the oesophagus where it may become lodged in a less accessible area.

Thoracotomy and surgical removal is required if the foreign body is tightly wedged or significant perforation has already occurred. Oesophageal surgery should not be undertaken lightly as complication rates are high and postoperative management complex (Houlton et al., 1985). Urgent referral may be the most appropriate way to manage such cases.

After removal of a foreign body the oesophagus should be carefully inspected for damage. Hyperaemia and ulceration are common findings. Survey radiographs and contrast studies may also be appropriate to detect minor perforations. Small tears and lacerations (less than 1 cm) can be managed conservatively with broad-spectrum antibacterials, mucosal protectants, such as sucralfate, and resting the oesophagus by feeding via a gastrostomy tube.

Prognosis

Initial prognosis following removal is guarded as perforation of devitalized tissue may occur and strictures can develop some days later. Local motility deficits can also occur days to a week or more after removal.

Oesophagitis

Clinically significant oesophagitis is uncommon in veterinary practice, however, the prevalence of low grade oesophagitis is probably quite high.

Aetiopathogenesis

Inflammation of the oesophagus may occur for a number of reasons (Table 36.12) but can be broadly divided into two categories: reflux oesophagitis and oesophagitis caused by direct damage to the

Table 36.12 Aetiopathogenesis of oesophagitis

Reflux oesophagitis	Direct mucosal injury
Incompetent gastro-oesophageal sphincter	Thermal injury
Reflux of irritant substances – gastric acid, pepsin, bile, pancreatic enzymes	Swallowing strong acids, alkalis or corrosives
Abnormal oesophageal clearance – decreased peristalsis, salivary bicarbonate or mucosal resistance	Foreign body obstruction
Delayed gastric emptying	Acute and persistent vomiting
	Drugs lodging in oesophagus after administration – doxycycline, tetracycline, NSAID, potassium chloride, ferrosulphate/succinate, ascorbic acid, alprenolol
	Infectious agents – feline calicivirus, papillomatosis

oesophageal mucosa. Gastro-oesophageal reflux is a normal phenomenon in dogs and cats but is mild and transient. Oesophagitis is unlikely to develop because of neutralization of the acid by saliva and the low contact time as the material quickly re-enters the stomach following normal oesophageal peristalsis.

Following the onset of oesophagitis, the distal high pressure zone of the cardia fails allowing further reflux of gastric acid and pepsin to enter the oesophagus and the development of a vicious cycle (August, 1983).

Clinical signs

Clinical signs will vary according to the extent of the injury which can range from mild mucosal damage to deep ulceration involving the muscle layers. Oesophagitis is a painful condition and patients show repeated swallowing behaviour, regurgitation of food, reluctance to eat, salivation and haematemesis. Depression and polydypsia may also be seen, together with weight loss and regurgitation of viscous, often blood-tinged, saliva-like fluid.

Diagnosis

A history of recent general anaesthesia is a common feature in many cases. Laboratory and radiographic studies are usually unhelpful although segmental oesophageal narrowing may be seen on plain radiographs. Fluoroscopic studies can be used to show gastro-oesophageal reflux and oesophageal dysmotility. The most sensitive diagnostic procedure, however, is endoscopy.

Treatment

Treatments involve correction of the underlying disease, where known, and symptomatic therapy of the inflammation. Oesophageal rest for 24–48 h is helpful followed by feeding a low fat diet. Prolonged fasting is not recommended as this may increase the risks of stricture formation. Reduction in gastric acidity can be achieved with H_2 blockers such as cimetidine, ranitidine or famotidine or using proton pump inhibitors (Table 36.13). Gastro-oesophageal reflux can be reduced using prokinetics such as metoclopramide or cisapride. Mucosal protection is achieved using sucralfate or colloidal bismuth suspensions. Anti-inflammatory doses of prednisolone may reduce the risk of stricture. Drugs that reduce lower oesophageal tone such as anticholinergics and sedatives should be avoided.

Prognosis

The prognosis depends on the severity of the inflammation but is guarded in severe or chronic cases. Aggressive therapy is required but oesophageal stricturing may still occur.

■ Oesophageal stricture

Oesophageal stricture is usually the end product of a previous oesophageal insult (Pearson et al., 1978a) (Table 36.14) which results in fibrosis reducing the oesophageal diameter and preventing normal oesophageal dilation and peristalsis. Strictures can be single and localized or multiple and involve a significant length of the oesophagus. They can occur at any level of the oesophagus. Dilation of the oesophagus cranial to the stricture will occur with time.

Clinical signs

The clinical signs are similar to those seen with all other oesophageal problems. Liquids tend to be tolerated better than solids.

Table 36.13 Suggested dose rates of drugs used to treat canine and feline oesophagitis

Therapy	Dose rate/route in dogs	Dose rate/route in cats
Metoclopramide[a]	0.5–1.0 mg kg^{-1} p.o./i.v./s.c./i.m. sid–bid; 1–2 mg kg^{-1} day^{-1} i.v. by continuous infusion	As dog
Cisapride	0.1–0.5 mg kg^{-1} p.o. bid–tid	2.5 mg cat^{-1} p.o. bid
Cimetidine	4–10 mg kg^{-1} p.o./i.v. tid–qid	4–10 mg kg^{-1} p.o./i.v. tid–qid
Ranitidine	2 mg kg^{-1} p.o./i.v. tid	2.5 mg kg^{-1} i.v. bid or 3.5 mg kg^{-1} p.o. bid
Famotidine	0.5 mg kg^{-1} p.o. sid–bid	0.5–1 mg kg^{-1} p.o./i.v. sid–bid
Omeprazole	0.7 mg kg^{-1} p.o. sid	0.75–1.0 mg kg^{-1} p.o. sid
Sucralfate	0.5–1 g dog^{-1} p.o. bid–tid	0.25 g cat^{-1} p.o. bid–tid
Prednisolone[a]	0.5 mg kg^{-1} day^{-1}	0.5–1.0 mg kg^{-1} day^{-1}

[a] Licensed preparations

Table 36.14 Predisposing factors which may result in oesophageal stricture formation

Oesophageal foreign body
Vascular ring anomalies
Oesophagitis
One- to three-weeks postanaesthetia (secondary to oesophagitis)
Following surgical intervention
Iatrogenic following endoscopy, stomach tubing

Diagnosis

Contrast radiography or endoscopy can be used. In cases where the stricture is severe, contrast studies especially if performed in conjunction with fluoroscopy help to evaluate the extent of the stricture.

Management

Treatment of strictures can be difficult, frustrating and expensive. Most cases are treated with bougienage or, preferably, balloon catheter dilation (Burk et al., 1987; Sooy et al., 1987) (Figure 36.8). The fibrotic tissue is broken down by the passage of increasingly large bougies or by gentle inflation of a balloon catheter. Care must be taken not to attempt overly aggressive dilation as oesophageal tearing can result. After dilation, the patient should be encouraged to eat and prednisolone can be given at a dose of 1 mg kg^{-1} day^{-1} to reduce the extent of the re-stricturing that inevitably occurs. Repeated dilation every 3–4 days is required which means frequent anaesthetics.

Surgical techniques have been described involving resection of the affected portion of the oesophagus (Johnson et al., 1992) but have a poor success rate and are associated with many post-surgical complications.

Regardless of the technique employed the prognosis for patients with oesophageal stricture is guarded.

Peri-oesophageal masses

External compression of the oesophagus may result in varying degrees of obstruction (c.f. vascular ring anomalies). Oesophageal compression can occur secondary to enlarged bronchial or mediastinal lymph nodes, peri-oesophageal abscesses and tumours of thoracic structures, such as lymphosarcoma, thymomas, heart base masses (Zawie, 1987). Obstruction can be caused by neoplasms affecting the retropharyngeal and cervical areas, for example thyroid tumours which can also be associated with bulging of the cervical oesophagus following feeding (Gruffydd-Jones et al., 1979).

Clinical signs

The clinical signs are similar to those seen with all other oesophageal problems. The onset of signs is usually slow with liquids being tolerated better than solids. Other clinical signs associated with the mass may also be apparent.

Diagnosis

Survey radiographs usually demonstrate the presence of a mass with contrast studies determining the site and extent of the obstruction. Ultrasound-guided biopsies can be helpful in making a diagnosis but in some cases a thoracotomy is required in order to obtain suitable biopsy material.

Treatment

Treatment is highly dependent on the cause of the mass. In many cases, the masses have become large before signs of oesophageal obstruction are apparent and hence the prognosis is often poor.

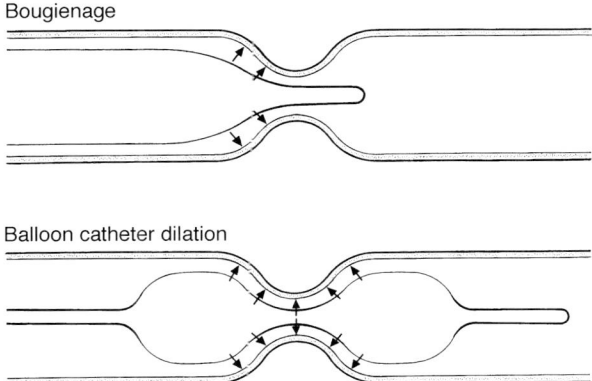

Figure 36.8 Diagram showing the forces exerted on an oesophageal stricture by a bougie compared to a balloon catheter. The radial forces created by a balloon catheter are a superior method of stricture dilation.

Oesophageal diverticuli

Oesophageal diverticuli are rarely diagnosed in dogs and cats and may be congenital or acquired

(Pearson et al., 1978b). The diverticulum is usually located at either the thoracic inlet or just cranial to the diaphragm (Simpson and Else, 1991a).

Aetiology

Acquired (pulsion) diverticuli (Fig. 36.9) are thought to occur secondary to increased oesophageal intraluminal pressure associated with food accumulation and deep oesophageal inflammation which leads to the mucosa and submucosa herniating through the muscularis. Foreign bodies are a common predisposing cause (Pearson et al., 1978b). Traction diverticuli occur when inflammation causes adhesions with surrounding tissue. As the fibrous tissue contracts, the oesophagus is distorted and the diverticulum forms.

Congenital diverticuli are thought to arise due to weakness in the oesophageal wall or abnormal separation of the oesophagus and trachea during embryological development.

Clinical signs

Regurgitation, often unassociated with feeding, retching, gagging, and slow weight gain are commonly observed. Impaction of the diverticulum with food may lead to secondary infection and oesophagitis resulting in pain on eating and pyrexia. Ulceration and perforation of the diverticulum may result in mediastinitis.

Diagnosis

Diagnosis relies on radiography including contrast studies and/or endoscopy. Unlike oesophageal dilation, oesophageal diverticuli tend to be pouch like in appearance with a narrow opening into the normal oesophagus.

Management

Small diverticuli can be managed conservatively with a bland diet. Larger structures require surgical resection, which as with other oesophageal surgery carries a guarded prognosis.

Oesophageal neoplasia

Primary and metastatic neoplasia affecting the oesophagus is rare in cats and dogs. Metastatic tumours are more common and include bronchial carcinoma, thymic lymphoma, thyroid carcinoma and mammary carcinoma (Ridgeway and Suter, 1979). Squamous cell carcinomas are the most common primary tumours but neuroendocrine carcinoma (Patnaik et al., 1990), leiomyomas, osteosarcoma and undifferentiated sarcomas and carcinomas are described. Fibrosarcomas secondary to *Spirocerca lupi* (Fox et al., 1988) are seen in the USA and Africa.

Clinical findings

Initially few clinical signs are evident but as the mass grows it interferes with oesophageal function producing similar clinical signs to those seen with oesophageal stricture or obstruction.

Diagnosis

Radiographs will frequently detect the presence of a mass but confirmation relies on obtaining biopsy material which is most easily achieved during endoscopy.

Management

Surgical resection of benign tumours is possible. Malignant tumours carry a poor prognosis as few are likely to be responsive to chemotherapy. Radiation therapy is possible but there are associated risks of radiation-induced oesophagitis. In some cases palliation can be achieved with bougienage but needs to be performed with great care as the oesophagus can rupture easily.

Oesophageal motility abnormalities

Oesophageal motility abnormalities can occur without megaoesophagus. In many cases this is

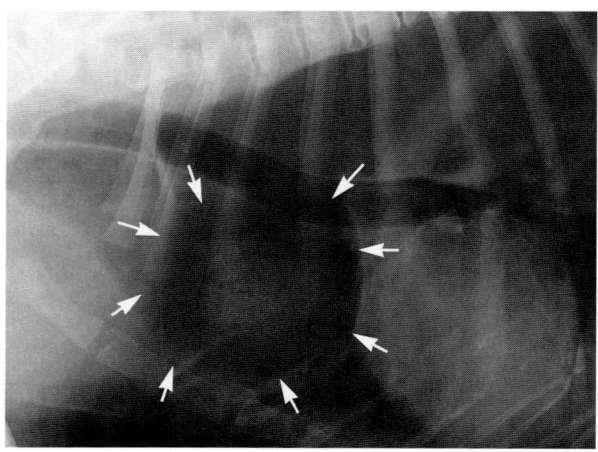

Figure 36.9 Oesophageal diverticulum (arrows) and chronic bronchitis in an 8-year-old, male, German shepherd dog with a three-year history of regurgitation, vomiting and pyrexia.

subclinical, particularly in Shar peis. Bouviers can develop abnormal motility secondary to muscular dystrophy. Clinical signs are similar to, but less severe than, those of megaoesophagus. Eating may be painful due to oesophageal spasm associated with the passage of a food bolus and aspiration pneumonia may occur. The pathogenesis of these mobility abnormalities is unclear but it is thought they may represent an early stage of disease prior to the development of megaoesophagus. Dysperistalsis can also occur secondary to oesophagitis and mediastinitis (Eastwood et al., 1975).

Diagnosis is made fluoroscopically where coordinated oesophageal peristalsis is replaced by random contractions. Treatment is similar to that for megaoesophagus with cisapride appearing to be a promising therapy.

Oesophageal fistulae

Fistulae between the oesophagus and the airways are occasionally reported in dogs. Broncho-oesophageal fistulae (right caudal bronchus) are most common usually developing secondary to a foreign body. Congenital fistulae have been reported and Cairn terriers may be predisposed (Basher et al., 1991).

Clinical signs include regurgitation and dysphagia. Coughing associated with eating and drinking is frequently seen together with signs associated with aspiration pneumonia.

Diagnosis is based on thoracic radiography where localized lung pathology associated with an oesophageal foreign body is common. Contrast studies should be undertaken with care due to the communication with the airways and false negative studies occur. Bronchoscopy and endoscopy do not always identify the fistulous tract.

Treatment is surgical with lobectomy often being required. The prognosis, providing the animal survives the immediate postoperative period, is good.

Hiatal hernia

Although rare, both hiatal hernias and gastro-oesophageal intussusception have been reported

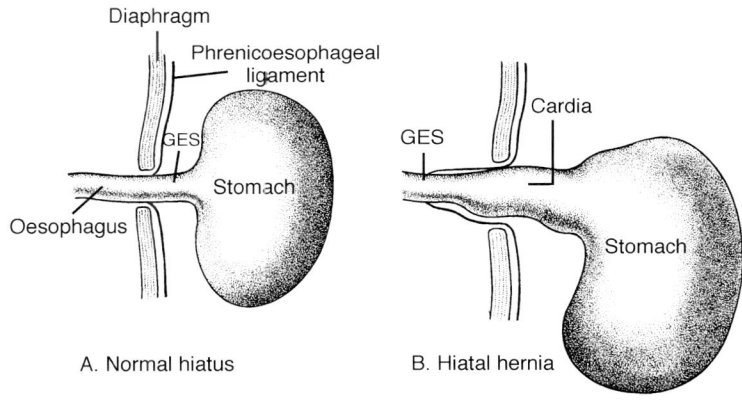

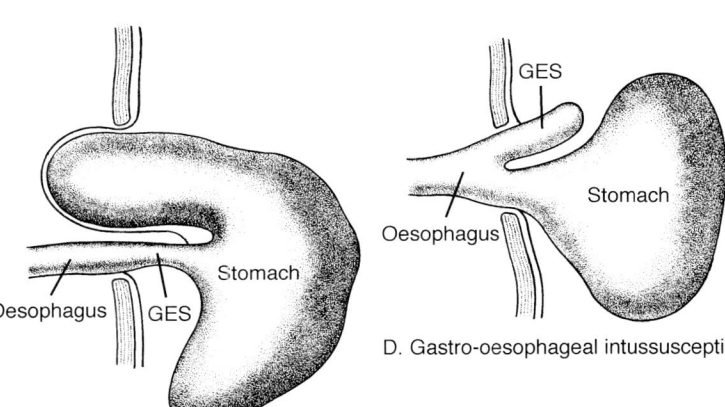

Figure 36.10 Classification of hiatal disease (Modified from Williams, 1990). GES, gastro-oesophageal sphincter.

in dogs and cats and can be intermittent or persistent (Fig. 36.10). Congenital defects in the diaphragmatic hiatus (Gaskell et al., 1974), laryngeal stridor (Burnie et al., 1989) and an incompetent lower oesophageal sphincter (van Sluijs and Happe, 1985) have been implicated. The conditions appear more common in large breed dogs, Shar peis and animals less than one year old (Ellison et al., 1987).

Paraoesophageal hiatal hernias (Fig. 36.10) are rarely reported in dogs and have not been reported in cats. Because lower oesophageal pressure is unaffected they are frequently subclinical.

Clinical findings

Intermittent regurgitation, pain on eating and occasionally haematemesis are most commonly reported (Simpson and Else, 1991a). Occasionally respiratory distress may occur especially with coexisting laryngeal paralysis. Many cases, in dogs, have secondary oesophageal dilation and aspiration pneumonia.

Diagnosis

Fluoroscopic examination of the oesophagus and cardia provides a more effective method of diagnosis than standard contrast radiographs. However, the diagnosis of an intermittent condition can be particularly difficult.

Treatment

Surgical treatments used have included fundopexy, gastropexy and repair of the oesophageal hiatus. If underlying laryngeal/soft palate disease is present then this should be corrected first. Symptomatic medical management of the reflux oesophagitis that occurs should also be undertaken.

GASTRIC DISEASE

Gastric anatomy and physiology

The stomach has four major functions:

1. Temporary storage of food;
2. Digestion (by secretion of acid and enzymes);
3. Mixing and grinding of ingesta;
4. Controlling the rate of entry of ingesta to the small intestines.

Gross anatomy

The stomach is divided into five regions (Fig. 36.11) but functionally the proximal part stores food and secretes digestive juices whereas the distal part regulates the release of hydrochloric acid and grinds food. The flow of ingesta from the stomach to the duodenum is controlled by the pylorus and antrum. The stomach lies to the left of the mid-line and is fixed at the gastro-oesophageal sphincter, as it passes through the diaphragm, and the hepatogastric and hepatoduodenal ligaments of the lesser omentum which are attached to the pylorus. Movement of the pylorus is further restricted by the mesoduodenum and bile duct.

The wall of the stomach consists of serosal, muscular, submucosal and mucosal layers. The submucosa and mucosa are thrown into folds, the gastric plicae or rugae, which run parallel to the greater curvature.

Although the pylorus is considered a distinct area due to the increase in muscle mass, muscle fibres are continuous with the antrum. The pylorus of the cat is unique in that it is narrow and has a constant high resistance even when the pyloric muscle is paralysed.

Vascular supply is via the coeliac trunk where the hepatic and splenic arteries give rise to the left

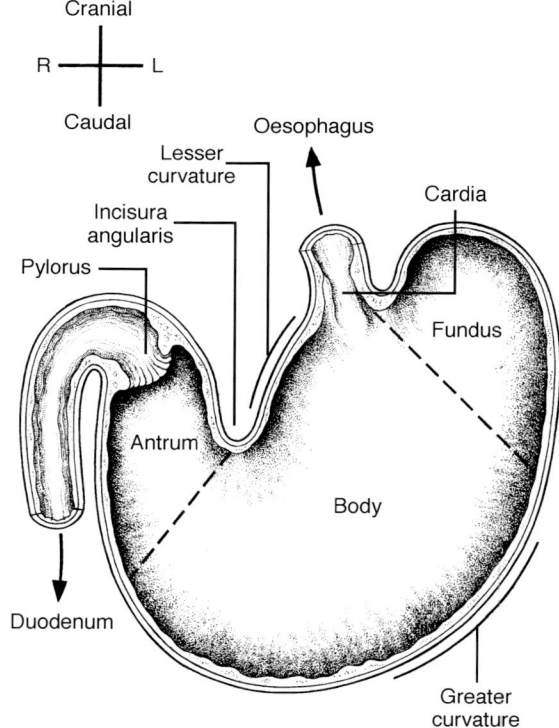

Figure 36.11 Gross anatomy of the stomach.

and right gastroepiploic arteries and left and right gastric arteries running along the greater and lesser curvatures. Venous drainage is via the gastrosplenic and gastroduodenal veins which flow into the portal circulation.

Innervation is supplied by the vagus nerve which contains sensory and parasympathetic fibres and is involved in contractility and secretory activities. The splanchnic nerve contains predominantly sympathetic, motor fibres which regulate gastric blood flow and modulate gastric motility and bicarbonate secretion. The sensory fibres present in the splanchnic nerve are involved in the transmission of visceral pain.

Microscopic anatomy and the gastric mucosal barrier

The stomach is lined with a single layer of epithelial cells which invaginates to form gastric pits containing mucus-secreting cells (Fig. 36.12). Gastric glands also contain specialized secretory cells. In the proximal stomach these cells consist of oxyntic (parietal), chief and endocrine cells. In the distal stomach the glands contain primarily endocrine cells which secrete biogenic amines, e.g. serotonin, and peptide hormones, e.g. gastrin. Oxyntic cells are responsible for secretion of hydrochloric acid whereas chief cells produce pepsinogen. The gastric mucosa has to protect the stomach from damage by abrasive foods, proteolytic enzymes, low pH, foreign bodies, drugs and toxins. Rapid turnover of the gastric mucosa is therefore essential. Mucus is continually being produced acting as a barrier between the hostile luminal environment and the epithelial cells. Hydrophobic phospholipid membranes and cytoplasmic bicarbonate provide the epithelial cells with some innate resistance. Epithelial cells possess the ability to alter their shape and can slide along the basement membrane rapidly to close small mucosal deficits.

Prostaglandins in the gastric mucosa play an important cytoprotective role, inhibiting gastric acid production, stimulating bicarbonate secretion and increasing mucosal blood flow.

Gastric arterioles pick up bicarbonate, a by-product of hydrogen ion production, as they pass the gastric pits. The bicarbonate is carried to the mucosa and submucosa where it can rapidly remove free hydrogen ions from ulcerated areas.

■ Motility

The fundus of the stomach acts as a reservoir relaxing initially in response to swallowing.

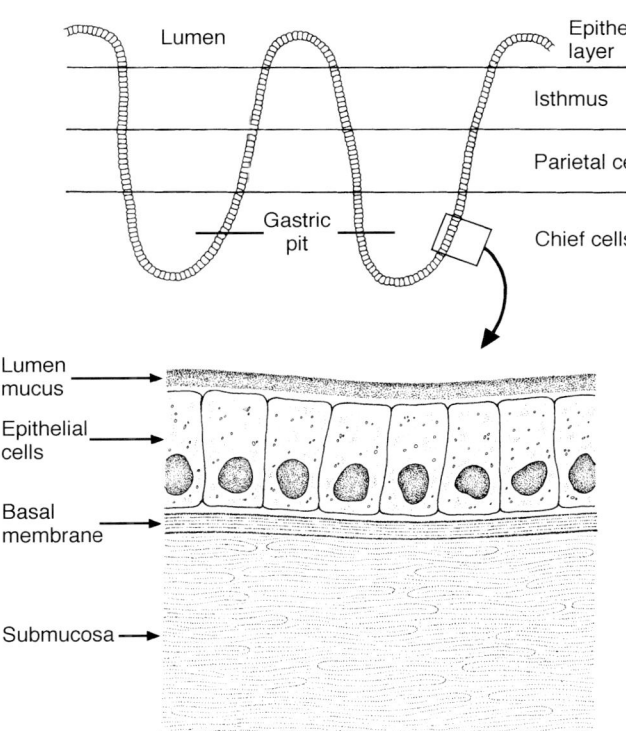

Figure 36.12 Diagram of a proximal gastric gland showing the layers forming the mucosal barrier.

Further relaxation occurs due to pressure caused by the fundus filling with food (receptive relaxation). Fundic activity is controlled by the vagus nerve and the neurotransmitter vasoactive intestinal peptide (VIP) and nitric oxide. Fundic activity is important in regulating the gastric emptying rate of fluids. The distal stomach and in particular the pylorus and antrum are involved in mixing and grinding food and thereby control gastric emptying of solids (Winans, 1976).

Gastric motility occurs in the absence of innervation. An electrically active area of muscle, 'the pacemaker', is located along the greater curvature of the stomach which provides the basic electrical rhythm. Superimposed on this background are spikes of activity which, when they coincide with a pacemaker peak, initiate muscular contraction. Rates of contraction are increased by vagal activity, gastrin and cholecystokinin (CCK) and decreased by sympathetic activity, secretin, glucagon, somatostatin, VIP and gastrointestinal inhibitory peptide. Distension of the stomach results in relaxation of the gastro-oesophageal sphincter and the body of the stomach, and contraction of the pylorus to prevent dumping of stomach contents into the duodenum. Overdistension of the stomach with air during endoscopy has a similar effect making passage through the pylorus difficult. The presence of nutrients and acid in the upper small intestine inhibits gastric emptying as do nutrients in the ileum and colon as well as colonic distension.

Interdigestive motility, housekeeper contractions, occur when the stomach is empty. These are sweeping contractions which move any residual contents of the stomach into the duodenum. Intermediate motility is seen in the transition phase between digestive and interdigestive motility (Itoh *et al.*, 1977).

Gastric contents are normally emptied in an orderly fashion with liquids (primarily under fundic control) preceding solids (Hinder, 1983). Carbohydrates and proteins precede fats. Fibre is retained in the stomach until the remainder of the nutrients have entered the duodenum (Hinder and Kelly, 1977). High calorie and high viscosity diets are emptied more slowly than low calorie or low viscosity diets. The pH, osmolality, fat and protein content of the chyme entering the duodenum also affects the rate of gastric emptying (Hall *et al.*, 1988; Sidery *et al.*, 1994).

■ Gastric secretions

Gastric secretions have an important role in the initiation of protein digestion, absorption of calcium, iron, trace minerals and cobalamin, in the sterilization of food, maintenance of the bacterial flora and protection of the gastric mucosa.

Pepsin

Cleavage of pepsinogen by hydrochloric acid produces pepsin which degrades proteins by splitting peptide bonds to produce polypeptides. Pepsin itself can also catalyse the cleavage of pepsinogen. Optimal activity occurs at a pH of 2.0, irreversible inactivation by neutral pH occurring in the duodenum. The primary activity of pepsin is against collagen and therefore its activity is directed towards digestion of meat rather than vegetable matter. It is not, however, an essential part of digestion. Pepsin also acts to release gastrin and CCK. Secretion of pepsinogen is stimulated by neural (vagus nerves), hormonal and paracrine (histamine, cholinergic agonists, CCK, secretin, gastrin and VIP) activity and is inhibited by somatostatin, peptide Y and neuropeptide YY (Raufman, 1992). The increase in pepsinogen secretion following mucosal damage may have an important role in the development of gastric ulceration.

Intrinsic factor

Mucoprotein that binds to cobalamin (B_{12}) is essential for its subsequent absorption in the distal small intestine. Humans with gastric atrophy have secondary cobalamin deficiencies.

Mucus

Mucus, which is a mixture of mucopolysaccharides and glycoprotein, forms a protective coating over the surface of the stomach (Fig. 36.12). Its essential properties of viscosity, adhesiveness and gelation are determined by the composition which is disrupted at low pH. The pH at the mucosal surface of the stomach is, however, neutral but mucus is continually being degraded at the luminal surface. Luminal degradation is slowed by a surface active phospholipid layer (similar to alveolar surfactant) which is hydrophobic, repelling aqueous solutions such as hydrochloric acid and pepsin (Hills and Kirkwood, 1992). Mucus retards the passage of macromolecules but permits the movement of electrolytes and small molecules. It also acts to aggregate microorganisms, bind enterotoxins and interact with secreted IgA. Mucus production is stimulated by cholinergic nerve activity, some prostaglandins and gastric inflammation.

Electrolyte secretion

Hydrogen, chloride, sodium, potassium and bicarbonate ions are present in gastric secretions. Hydrochloric acid is secreted from the oxyntic cells which absorb carbon dioxide and produce hydrogen ions and bicarbonate. This energy-dependent process is catalysed by carbonic anhydrase. The bicarbonate produced is returned to the plasma and constitutes the postprandial 'alkaline tide'. Chloride is actively transported from the plasma via the oxyntic cell to the gastric lumen.

The potassium concentration in gastric secretions is 10–20 mmol l^{-1} (2–5 times the plasma concentration). This is primarily derived from oxyntic cellular potassium. The sodium found in gastric secretion is derived from the mucosal surface cells and the passive secretion of interstitial fluid.

The surface mucosal cells secrete bicarbonate into the mucus layer, with the rate of secretion being related to the rate of acid production. Prostaglandins, calcium, CCK, gastrin, peptide hormones and cholinergic agents stimulate bicarbonate secretion whereas non-steroidal anti-inflammatory drugs (NSAIDs) inhibit this process.

Regulation of acid secretion

Acid secretion is regulated by an integrated mechanism involving neurotransmitters, peptide hormones and paracrine activity. The effects of these substances are mediated by the release of histamine, possibly from enterochromaffin cells, which acts via H_2 receptors on the oxyntic cells. Gastrin and acetylcholine are also important mediators of acid production. Selectively blocking any one of the three receptors markedly reduces the secretory response. Acetylcholine receptors are of the M_3 muscarinic type which can be blocked by atropine. Gastrin appears to act by stimulating the release of histamine from enterochromaffin cells. CCK is a competitive inhibitor of gastrin at its receptor site. Acid secretion by the oxyntic cell is mediated via cAMP and protein kinases which act to increase the activity of an ATPase at the luminal border which secretes hydrogen ions. It is this ATPase which is blocked by proton pump inhibitors such as omeprazole.

Acid secretion is down-regulated by secretin, CCK, prostaglandins (produced by CNS and local mechanisms) and dopamine. Acid secretion is increased by dopaminergic antagonists such as metoclopramide. Background acid secretion, in dogs, is approximately 1% of maximal capacity.

Feeding stimulates acid production in three separate phases. The *cephalic phase,* initiated by the anticipation of feeding and hypoglycaemia is followed by the *gastric phase* which is the most important determinant of acid production. Release of gastrin by mechanical distension of the antrum causes acid production. Finally, the *intestinal phase,* leads to acid secretion and is mediated by food in the small intestines. Acid, fat and hyperosmolar solutions in the small intestine inhibit acid secretion (Debas, 1987).

Acute gastritis

Acute gastritis is commonly seen in cats and dogs and is usually manifest by a sudden onset of anorexia and vomiting. It is important to differentiate acute gastritis from other causes of non-gastric vomiting (Table 36.15, Fig. 36.13). The difference between acute and chronic gastritis is related to the duration of vomiting.

Vomiting that occurs immediately after the consumption of food or water is associated with loss of receptive relaxation and therefore an increase in intragastric pressure. Vomiting of undigested food many hours after ingestion is associated with inflammation and subsequent gastric atony. Inflammation can also directly stimulate the vomiting centre (Table 36.16).

Aetiology

Acute gastritis occurs as a result of loss of the integrity of the gastric mucosal barrier resulting in increased permeability, erosions and in some cases ulceration of the mucosa (Burrows, 1986a). Once the mucosal barrier is breached pepsin and gastric acid provoke further inflammation and damage establishing a vicious cycle. Histamine released from mast cells in the submucosa causes vasodilation and stimulates additional acid production

Table 36.15 Some non-gastric conditions that may be associated with true vomiting in dogs and cats

• Intestinal obstruction	• Pyometra
• Acute pancreatitis	• Diabetes mellitus
• Hepatitis/hepatic failure	• Hypoadrenocorticism
• Renal failure	• Vestibular disease
• Peritonitis	• CNS lesions
• Colitis	Tumours
• Constipation	Trauma
• Toxaemia	Inflammation
	Hydrocephalus

402 DISEASES OF THE ALIMENTARY TRACT

Table 36.16 Aetiology of acute gastritis

Primary gastritis	Secondary gastritis
Dietary indiscretion / sensitivity	Renal failure (uraemic gastritis)
Foreign bodies	Infectious disease and sepsis
Poisons, e.g. thallium, ethylene glycol, heavy metals, herbicides (organophosphates/chlorides)	Hypoadrenocorticism
	'Stress' and trauma
Drugs especially NSAIDs, glucocorticoids	CNS lesions
Toxic plants	Acute and chronic liver disease
Bacterial and fungal toxins	Vascular compromise
Bacteria, e.g. *Salmonella*	Disseminated intravascular coagulation
Viruses, e.g. parvovirus, coronavirus, distemper virus, rotavirus	

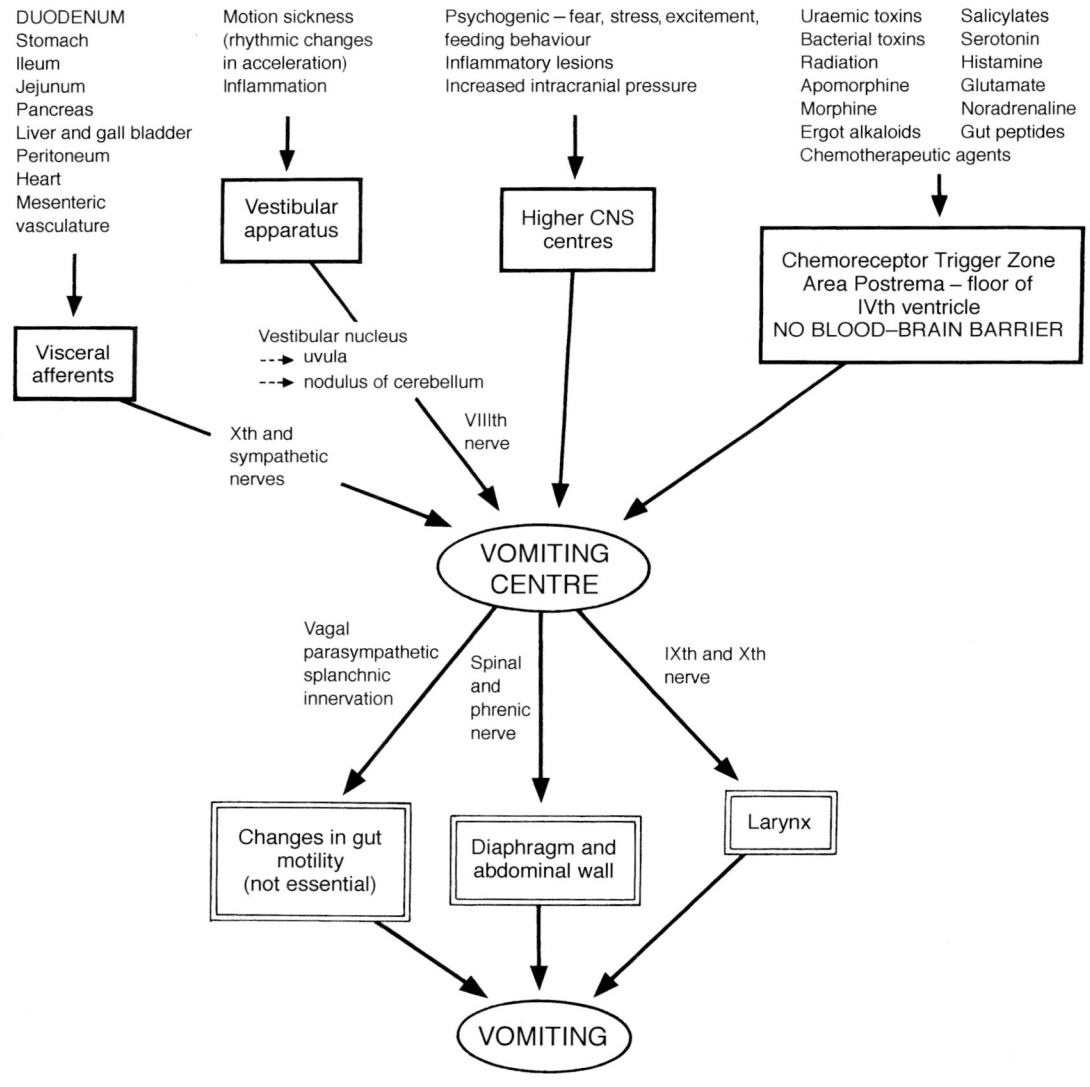

Figure 36.13 Pathophysiology of vomiting.

(Dunn, 1989). Cellular infiltration of the mucosa may occur which increases disruption of mucosal function and decreases the ability to heal. The pain associated with gastritis is thought to be due to gastric muscular spasm due to the back-diffusion of hydrochloric acid (Burrows, 1986a). Extravasation of plasma into the gastric lumen occurs via the intercellular junctions or through denuded areas of epithelium leading to a protein-losing gastropathy.

Gastritis can result from a wide variety of causes (Table 36.16). Due to its acidity, few bacteria are able to survive in the stomach with the exception of spiral bacteria such as *Helicobacter* spp. Established gastritis causes a rise in gastric pH towards neutral due to back-diffusion of acid. At more neutral pH bacterial colonization can occur thus exacerbating the gastritis. Enterotoxins from contaminated food can cause acute gastritis more commonly in dogs due to their feeding habits. Toxins produced by staphylococci, *Clostridium perfringens, E. coli* and *Klebsiella* spp. have been implicated.

The mucosal surface can be damaged physically by foreign bodies, which can also stimulate excess acid production by distending the antrum and obstructing the pyloric outflow causing retention of gastric contents and gastritis. Excessive heat and radiation-induced injury as well as a wide variety of chemicals and plants have been associated with gastritis in dogs and cats (Guilford and Strombeck, 1996).

NSAIDs

Dogs and cats are particularly sensitive to NSAIDs which have a number of adverse effects on the GIT including mucosal ulceration, perforation and haemorrhage. Cats have low levels of glucuronyl transferase in the liver leading to a prolonged half-life of NSAIDs such as aspirin. There also appears to be breed differences in NSAID half-lives. In dogs lesions are most common in the antrum and pylorus but can occur anywhere in the GIT. NSAIDs damage the mucosal surface in a variety of ways including: direct toxicity to epithelial cells, increased back-diffusion of acids, decreased synthesis of cytoprotective prostaglandins, bicarbonate and mucus, reduced mucosal blood flow and microvascular injury.

The adverse effects of NSAIDs can be reduced by giving them with food, using buffered products or the concurrent administration of misoprostol (1–3 µg kg^{-1} p.o. tid–qid).

Secondary gastritis

A wide variety of systemic disorders or dysfunction of other parts of the GIT can cause gastritis (Table 36.15).

1. Hyperacidity disorders secondary to gastrin secreting tumours (amine precursor uptake and decarboxylation (APUD) tumours) e.g. gastrinomas, insulinomas, phaeochromocytomas, mast cell tumours releasing histamine or head injuries.
2. Decreased gastric mucosal blood flow in hypovolaemic shock, portal hypertension or disseminated intravascular coagulation.
3. Erosions and ulcers secondary to severe systemic disease causing reduced mucosal blood flow, reduced mucus and prostaglandin secretion and increased gastric acid secretion.
4. Renal disease causes gastric erosions and ulceration primarily by decreased mucosal blood flow caused by diffuse vascular injury, reduced renal gastrin metabolism, gastric hypersecretion and acidosis.
5. Hepatic disease can cause gastric lesions by reducing blood flow secondary to the formation of thrombi and gastric hypersecretion. It is unlikely that hyperammoniaemia achieves toxic levels.
6. Gastroduodenal reflux; reflux of bile from the duodenum has been suggested as a cause of gastritis but this is not well supported experimentally (Fontolliet *et al.*, 1984).

Clinical findings

There is a sudden onset of acute vomiting and depression. Initially food may be present in the vomit but as anorexia develops small amounts of bile or blood-stained fluid are produced. Palpation of the abdomen frequently produces cranial abdominal pain and dogs may adopt a praying position whereas cats adopt a crouched or tucked-up posture. Dehydration and hypokalaemia can lead to weakness and collapse. Acid–base disturbances occur in approximately 50% of cases with the majority of animals paradoxically becoming *acidotic*.

Diagnosis

Most cases of acute vomiting, especially those involving dietary indiscretion, are self-limiting so a definitive diagnosis is not made. However, it is important to rule out other causes of acute vomiting such as pancreatitis, pyloric or intestinal obstruction, acute hepatitis, systemic disease or poisoning.

Treatment

Treatment usually involves symptomatic management with intravenous fluids, antiemetics and mucosal protection. Once recovery has begun dietary management is important. If the gastritis is secondary then treatment or management of the primary cause is required.

Intravenous fluids should support maintenance requirements as well as correcting pre-existing dehydration. An additional 2–4 ml kg^{-1} should be given each time the animal vomits to cover the increased fluid loss. Hartmann's solution (lactated Ringer's) with added potassium (20 mmol l^{-1} of fluids for maintenance) is ideal. Once vomiting is controlled oral fluids can be introduced.

Antiemetics

Metoclopramide (Emequell – Pfizer) (0.2–0.5 mg kg^{-1} tid–qid i.v., i.m., s.c. or p.o.; 1–2 mg kg^{-1} day^{-1} as continuous i.v. infusion). Metoclopramide's dopaminergic activity is responsible for the neurological side effects that seem to be more common in cats than dogs. Metoclopramide also has a peripheral action mediated by 5HT$_4$ and D$_2$ receptors accounting for its wider spectrum of activity. Metoclopramide has only a peripheral action in cats as central receptors are lacking. There is evidence to suggest that metoclopramide may not be the most appropriate antiemetic for the treatment of gastritis as it may predispose the patient to gastric and duodenal mucosal ulceration.

Cisapride (Prepulsid – Jansen) (0.1–0.5 mg kg^{-1} tid–qid in dogs; 2.5 mg cat^{-1} bid) has a similar peripheral action to metoclopramide without the central effects and may be particularly useful in cats which cannot tolerate metoclopramide but it is only available in tablet form.

Chlorpromazine (Largactil – May & Baker) (0.5 mg kg^{-1} sid–tid)
Prochlorpromazine (Stemetil – Rhone-Poulenc Rorer) (gastritis 0.1 mg kg^{-1} tid–qid i.m.) These are broad spectrum α$_2$ adrenergic antagonists which prevent vomiting associated with stimulation of the chemoreceptor trigger zone at low doses and the vomiting centre at higher doses. They are associated with a number of side effects including hypotension and epileptogenesis. Prochlorpromazine also has the advantage of being available as suppositories allowing vomiting animals to be treated at home.

Motilin agonists These act to increase gastric emptying, e.g. erythromycin at a low dose (1–5 mg kg^{-1}) has been shown to be helpful in dogs.

Ondansetron (Zofran – Glaxo) (0.15 mg kg^{-1} h^{-1} i.v.) This belongs to a new group of 5HT$_3$ serotonergic, antagonist, antiemetic drugs which may help to prevent chemotherapy-induced vomiting. They are, however, expensive and need to be given by intravenous infusion. They have little depressant effect on the CNS as their effects appear to be primarily peripheral. They are particularly indicated in the treatment of chemotherapy-induced vomiting rather than gastritis.

Antacids and mucosal protectants

Antacids In order to be effective for the treatment of gastric ulceration, antacids need to be given 2–4 hourly and acid rebound may occur if they are given less frequently. There is little correlation in humans between healing rate of ulcers and the acid neutralization capability of an antacid. Antacids will raise gastric pH without systemic effect and will also bind bile acids and inactivate pepsin (Moreland, 1988). Sodium bicarbonate, magnesium or calcium-based salts and aluminium hydroxide have all been used alone and in combination to try and reduce potential adverse effects. Magnesium-based compounds increase motility whereas aluminium reduces motility and may potentially cause constipation (Forrester et al., 1989). Aluminium may have a cytoprotective role by inducing prostaglandin synthesis (Papich, 1989). Potential adverse consequences related to giving large quantities of unbalanced ions, particularly magnesium, have to be considered.

Mucosal protectants Kaolin is of limited value in acute gastritis as it has no effect on protecting or soothing inflamed gastric mucosa. It may, however, bind bacterial and other toxins. Colloidal bismuth subcitrate (1–3 mg kg^{-1} tid–qid) has valuable cytoprotective and demulcent effects and is safer than bismuth subsalicylate in cats (due to the release of salicylic acid). Long-term use has been associated with bismuth toxicity in humans. Bismuth causes blackening of the faeces and should not be mistaken for melaena.

Sucralfate This is a disaccharide complex which is dissociated in an acid environment to negatively charged sucrose octasulphate and aluminium hydroxide that bind to the positively charged proteins of ulcers and necrotic tissue five times more strongly than to normal mucosa acting as a gastric 'bandage' (Hardin et al., 1987). Sucralfate acts to stimulate prostaglandin release (increasing local blood flow and mucosal repair), increase mucus viscosity, increase mucus output and increase bicarbonate secretion by the gastric mucosa. It will also absorb bile acids and inactivate pepsin. Sucralfate is most effective if given prior to feeding.

H$_2$ antagonists

Cimetidine (Tagamet – Smith Kline and French) (5–10 mg kg^{-1} tid–qid, p.o., i.m. or i.v.) This is available as tablets, syrup or injection. Cimetidine acts to inhibit histamine release by blocking the H$_2$ receptors. It will also inhibit certain liver enzymes affecting drug metabolism especially theophylline, warfarin, calcium channel blockers and possibly propranolol and lidocaine. Cimetidine may also act as an immunostimulant and increase luminal bicarbonate and mucus production. Side effects are rarely apparent in dogs and cats but, in humans, include gynaecomastia, androgen effects, reduced parathyroid hormone production, fits, lethargy and vomiting.

Ranitidine (Zantac – Glaxo) (2 mg kg^{-1} tid p.o. dogs; 3.5 mg kg^{-1} bid p.o. cats) This is also a potent H$_2$ blocker but has a longer duration of activity and less inhibition of drug metabolism. It is available as tablets or syrup.

Famotidine (Pepcid – Morson) (0.5 mg kg^{-1} sid–bid p.o. in dogs) This acts on the H$_2$ receptors and has the longest duration of action.

All three compounds appear equipotent in terms of decreasing acid output.

Omeprazole (Losec – Astra) This is a proton pump inhibitor which is extremely effective at preventing acid secretion. It is not recommended for long-term use due to the profound hyposecretion of acid and high gastrin levels that this causes, which can result in hypertrophic changes to the gastric mucosa.

Misoprostol (Cytotec – Searle) This is a synthetic prostaglandin E$_1$ derivative which is used in humans in the treatment of gastric ulcers following the use of NSAIDs. It has also been effective in dogs (Murtaugh *et al.*, 1993) and has been given at 1–5 µg kg^{-1} every 8 h. Unfortunately it is only available in 200 µg tablets which makes dosing of small dogs and cats a problem. Its use in non-NSAID-associated ulceration has not been evaluated. Side effects include diarrhoea and abdominal pain (Papich, 1989).

Dietary management

Initially strict dietary rest is required to allow restoration of the gastric mucosal barrier. Once vomiting has ceased, a low fat (less than 6% on a dry matter basis) highly digestible diet should be used. The diet should be fed as frequent small meals followed by a slow return to the normal type and frequency of feeding.

■ Chronic gastritis

Chronic vomiting is defined as intermittent or persistent vomiting that has failed to respond to symptomatic therapy and has been present for more than three weeks. It is not uncommon for animals with chronic vomiting to have little or no gastric mucosal changes on biopsy, whereas other animals which are not vomiting show histological evidence of mucosal damage (Twedt and Magne, 1986). The reason for the disparity between clinical and histological changes is unclear.

Chronic gastritis can be classified in a number of ways (Table 36.17). Non-ulcerative gastritis is most frequently seen. Ulceration indicates advanced disease and is most commonly associated with gastric neoplasia.

Table 36.17 Classifications of chronic gastritis in dogs and cats

Aetiological classification	Histological classification	Breed associations
Allergic	Eosinophilic	Basenji
Drug-associated	Granulomatous	Drentse partrijshond
Foreign body-induced	Lymphocytic/plasmacytic	Norwegian Lundehund
Parasitic	Non-specific, superficial, diffuse, atrophic or hypertrophic gastritis	
Toxic		
Uraemic		
(Mycotic)		
? Spiral bacteria-associated		
? Reflux – duodenal		

Chronic idiopathic gastritis

Aetiology
This is the most common form of chronic gastritis in dogs and cats. Although the aetiology is rarely determined, it is likely that the gastric mucosa is subjected to persistent antigenic insult. Histopathological examination of biopsy samples reveals a non-ulcerative chronic inflammatory process with varying degrees of infiltration by lymphocytes and plasma cells. An associated lymphocytic/plasmacytic enteritis is present in some cases.

Clinical findings
Patients frequently have a long history of intermittent vomiting, which often responds, temporarily, to a variety of symptomatic therapies. Some weight loss may occur but, in general, patients are bright, adequately hydrated and in reasonable body condition.

Endoscopic and histopathological changes
The mucosa of the stomach can appear grossly normal or reddened with excessive mucus, oedema and sometimes small erosions. Histological changes include patchy, degenerative changes of the glands and an inflammatory cell infiltrate. With time the surface epithelium may be destroyed and replaced by fibrotic tissue. The process can be divided into chronic superficial gastritis and chronic simple diffuse gastritis which tends to be more extensive and involve the full thickness of the mucosa. Diffuse gastritis may represent a progression of a non-resolving superficial gastritis (van Der Gaag and Happe, 1989).

Atrophic gastritis

Aetiology
Atrophic gastritis is a rare condition of older dogs of unknown aetiology (Burrows, 1986a) associated with loss in gastric secretory capacity. In humans it can occur with *Helicobacter* infection where it is associated with an increased risk of development of gastric neoplasia.

The condition may represent the end stage of chronic gastritis. However, it is possible that this is an immune-mediated disease as the condition can be reproduced experimentally by immunizing dogs against their own gastric secretions (Twedt and Magne, 1986). A lack of acid production may develop and predispose the patient to bacterial overgrowth (Strombeck et al., 1981). A failure of the negative feedback mechanisms results in elevated plasma gastrin and gastric ulceration may occur.

Atrophic gastritis can also result from the prolonged use of powerful inhibitors of gastric acid secretion, such as omeprazole.

Clinical findings
Typically there is a history of chronic vomiting of months duration which has failed to respond to symptomatic therapy. The vomiting is rarely associated with feeding and the vomitus may contain food, bile or mucus. Blood in the vomitus, gastric pain and weight loss are rare.

Endoscopic and histopathological changes
The gastric mucosa appears thin and discoloured with the submucosal blood vessels becoming more prominent. The gastric mucus is reduced and inflammatory cells are present. The epithelium is flattened and metaplastic cells are frequent. The gastric pits are deformed and contain abnormal mucus. Following removal of the cause most of these histological changes will resolve.

Hypertrophic gastritis

Hypertrophic gastritis shows similarities to Ménétrièr's disease in humans (van Der Gaag et al., 1976; Van Kruiningen, 1977) and can be classified as focal, polypoid or diffuse. It is more frequently seen in older and male dogs. Basenjis and boxers are more commonly affected by the diffuse form (Burrows, 1986a) whereas toy breeds, especially Lhaso apsos, Shih tzus, miniature poodles and Maltese terriers, tend to develop the focal form (Bellinger et al., 1990) which gives rise to pyloric stenosis. Focal disease involving the fundus is also recorded in the dog (Kipnis, 1978). Hypertrophic gastritis has been rarely reported in the cat (Dennis et al., 1987). A variety of potential aetiologies have been suggested including immune-mediated disease (Twedt and Magne, 1986), systemic mastocytosis with histamine release and hypergastrinaemia (Dunn, 1989), parasitic and toxic conditions (Van Kruiningen, 1977) and secondary to renal tubular disease and gastrin retention in Basenjis (Twedt and Magne, 1986).

Clinical findings
Diffuse weight loss, diarrhoea, anaemia and intermittent vomiting are common. Anorexia, melaena, polydipsia, haematemesis, abdominal pain and depression have also been reported (Clark, 1985; Bellinger et al., 1990; Sikes et al., 1986). Gaseous distension of the stomach and intestines is often associated with the diffuse form (Van Kruiningen, 1977) whereas persistent vomiting secondary to pyloric obstruction is a feature of the focal form.

Endoscopic and histopathological changes

Diffuse or focal mucosal thickening is seen. Focal lesions can appear polypoid or as discrete areas of mucosal hypertrophy. Gastric ulceration can also be present. Histologically, hypertrophy and metaplasia of the mucosa and epithelium is seen with increased mucus-forming cells and mucus cysts. Variable amounts of fibrosis and inflammatory cell infiltration accompany the hypertrophic changes.

Eosinophilic gastritis

Aetiology

Eosinophilic infiltrates of the stomach are rare and can be focal or diffuse (Twedt and Magne, 1986). Although the aetiology is unknown, immune-mediated disease, food allergy or parasitism have been postulated. Eosinophilic gastritis may form part of a generalized eosinophilic gastroenteritis (Burrows, 1986a) or hypereosinophilic syndrome in cats (Hendricks, 1981; Neer, 1991).

Clinical findings

Chronic vomiting with haematemesis, melaena, anorexia, depression and weight loss are commonly observed. With advanced ulceration cranial abdominal pain may be present. Obstruction of the pylorus by a focal eosinophilic granuloma can cause more persistent vomiting.

Endoscopic and histopathological changes

Grossly, there is rugal hypertrophy and mucosal ulceration in the diffuse form. The mucosa assumes a granular thickened with a 'cobblestone' appearance. Focal granulomas are associated with necrosis, oedema and fibrosis. Histologically there is a marked eosinophilic infiltrate and fibrosis involving the mucosa which may extend into the muscularis and serosa. Eosinophilic gastritis is characterized by schirrhous thickening of the gastric wall resembling neoplasia (Hayden and Fleischman, 1977).

Granulomatous/histiocytic gastritis

Histiocytic gastritis is clinically similar to eosinophilic gastritis, and has been associated with amyloidosis (McLeod et al., 1981). Histologically there is a granulomatous infiltrate (macrophages and neutrophils) but significant numbers of eosinophils can be present. A number of causes have been identified including neoplasia, parasites, fungal diseases, feline infectious peritonitis and foreign material (van Der Gaag et al., 1991).

Spiral organisms

The role of spiral organisms in chronic gastritis is still a subject of debate in cats and dogs. Undoubtedly, cases of gastritis where they are the only defined aetiology agent, do occur and these animals frequently respond to treatment for helicobacteriosis. However, *Helicobacter* spp. are common inhabitants of the stomach in cats and dogs (Geyer et al., 1993) without any obvious associated pathology. This situation is similar to that encountered in humans. A number of species have been identified including *H. pylori*, *H. felis*, and *H. heilmanii* (formerly *Gastrospirillium hominis*) (Geyer et al., 1993). Diagnosis is based on their presence in gastric biopsies or on their ability to split urea (see earlier).

Parasitic gastritis

Parasitic infection of the stomach is not consistently associated with clinical disease. A number of parasites have been described including, *Ollulanus tricuspis*, *Physaloptera* spp., *Gnathostoma* spp. in cats, *Spirocerca lupi* (not in the UK) and *Aonchotheca putorii*. Diagnosis is based on the presence of adult worms in the vomit or their eggs/larvae in the faeces. All except *Spirocerca* are nematodes and can be treated with benzimidazole or pyrantel-based products.

Gastric ulceration

Benign gastric ulceration occurring as a sequel to damage to the gastromucosal barrier (GMB) is relatively rare. More commonly ulceration is secondary to another disease process (Table 36.18).

Ulceration occurs as a result of external factors upsetting the balance between normal acid and pepsin secretion and the mucosal protection system. The most common sites for ulcer formation are the non-acid-producing areas of the stomach, i.e. the fundus, incisura angularis, antrum and pylorus. The reason for this is unclear but it may reflect local vascular factors (Moreland, 1988). There is no known age or breed predisposition to gastric ulceration but females are more commonly affected than males.

NSAIDs are potent ulcerogenic drugs due to their ability to suppress the synthesis of cytoprotective mucosal prostaglandins via inhibition of cyclo-oxygenase and arachidonic acid pathways (Wallace et al., 1990; Taha and Russell, 1993). In addition they inhibit mucus secretion and may increase pepsin-mediated mucolysis and decrease

Table 36.18 Causes of gastroduodenal ulceration in dogs and cats

Primary GIT disease	Gastric hyperacidity	Drug induced	Systemic disease
Neoplasia	Gastrinomas	**NSAID**	**Disseminated intravascular coagulation**
Gastric dilatation–volvulus	Mast cell tumours	**Corticosteroids**	**Renal failure**
Chronic gastritis	Other APUD tumours		**Liver failure**
Pyloric outflow obstruction			**Hypovolaemic shock**
Eosinophilic gastritis			Trauma
Inflammatory bowel disease			Acute pancreatitis
Chemical damage			Hypoadrenocorticism
			Neurological disease
			Cyclic haematopoiesis
			Trauma

The most common causes are in bold type. APUD, amine precursor uptake and decarboxylation.

mucus viscosity (Rees et al., 1983). Loss of the mucus barrier plays an important role in the ability of hydrogen ions to penetrate and damage the GMB. Corticosteroids appear to cause ulceration in a similar manner (Moreland, 1988; Twedt, 1983). Great care must be taken when administering both classes of drug at the same time as the risk of gastric ulceration developing is very high. Prophylactic mucosal protection should be instituted.

The role of *Helicobacter* spp. in canine and feline gastric ulceration is not known. In humans they have been shown to actively digest the GMB, in particular the surface active layer, which results in the mucus becoming less hydrophobic thereby increasing the rate of luminal degradation (Hills, 1993).

Hypovolaemic, septic or toxic shock can lead to gastric ulceration (Johnson and Willard, 1990). Ulcers also occur secondary to medical or surgical management of spinal injuries which is thought to relate to disruption of the sympathetic/parasympathetic drive leading to decreased blood flow and increased acid and pepsin production. The frequent use of glucocorticoids and/or NSAIDs in this condition further exacerbates the problems. Ulceration is reported in 2% of dogs with intravertebral disc lesions (Moore and Withrow, 1982).

Chronic liver disease especially cirrhosis may lead to gastric and duodenal ulceration. The precise mechanism by which this occurs is unclear (Twedt, 1985; Johnson and Willard, 1990) but may involve:

1. Failure of the liver to remove histamine and gastrin from the circulation;
2. Failure to clear bile acids which stimulates gastrin release;
3. Portal hypertension reducing mucosal blood flow;
4. Hypoproteinaemia and negative nitrogen balance reducing epithelial cell turnover.

Acute liver disease associated with DIC will cause gastric mucosal damage secondary to thrombus formation.

Gastric ulceration and bleeding can occur in acute pancreatitis as a result of an extension of the inflammatory process and reflux of pancreatic enzymes and bile into the stomach.

Chronic renal disease and uraemia is a well recognized cause of gastric and oral ulceration. Although the pathogenesis is unclear, local irritation of the mucosal surfaces by ammonia and urea, vasculitis and interference with the GMB are thought to be involved. Other factors may include reduced gastrin clearance, increased histamine release and an altered calcium:phosphorus ratio (Breitschwerdt et al., 1986; Moreland, 1988; Johnson and Willard, 1990). Calcification of the rugal folds in chronic renal disease will also predispose to ulceration.

Mast cell tumours can occur anywhere along the GIT and may infiltrate the liver and spleen (Tams and Macy, 1981). They are also prevalent in many non-alimentary sites especially the skin. Degranulation leads to histamine release, gastric hyperacidity and ulceration.

Gastrin is produced by the G cells in the gastric antrum and duodenum but can also be produced by pancreatic tissue APUDomas leading to hypergastrinaemia and Zollinger–Ellison syndrome (Happe et al., 1980; Breitschwerdt et al., 1986). Hypergastrinaemia leads to gastric acid production and changes in the GMB resulting in ulceration. Circulating gastrin can be assayed and is normally below 100 µg ml^{-1} (Johnson and Willard, 1990).

Ulcer pain is associated with exposure of nerve endings to gastric acid and to motility disturbances. There appears to be a correlation between the size of the ulcer and the degree of pain. Bleeding is associated with acid erosion of superficial blood vessels, severe bleeding occurring when there is arterial erosion.

There is a strong correlation between gastric ulceration and neoplasia. For this reason all ulcers should be biopsied (Simpson and Else, 1991b). Biopsies should be obtained from the ulcer edge as samples taken from the centre often contain degenerative inflammatory cells and are associated with an increased risk of perforation.

Clinical findings

Gastric ulceration should be suspected when there is haematemesis. Blood may be fresh or partially degraded (coffee grounds) and may also be present as melaena in the stool. Polydipsia, weight loss, salivation, anorexia and gastric pain may also be seen. Other GI signs may be present. A lack of haematemesis or melaena does not rule out gastric ulceration.

Diagnosis of chronic gastritis

Laboratory findings are non-specific and include leukocytosis, eosinophilia and anaemia. The anaemia is usually regenerative but can be normocytic and normochromic (associated with chronic disease) or microcytic and hypochromic (associated with iron deficiency (Huxtable et al., 1982)) and non-regenerative. Anaemia in association with GI signs, and in the absence of other causes of blood loss, is suggestive of ulceration. Hypoproteinaemia, electrolyte and acid/base disturbances are also seen. Hypoproteinaemia is thought to be the result of a protein-losing gastropathy and will affect both albumin and globulin fractions.

Diagnostic imaging is rarely helpful. Double contrast gastrography may identify mucosal abnormalities in cases of hypertrophic gastritis, ulceration, focal granulomatous lesions associated with pyloric obstruction and delayed gastric emptying. Ultrasonographic measurement of stomach wall thickness can be indicative of pathology.

Diagnosis generally requires endoscopy and biopsy or exploratory coeliotomy and biopsy. Acute ulcers tend to be shallow, friable and bleed easily. Chronic ulcers have raised margins and an area of central fibrosis. Irregularly shaped ulcers are indicative of neoplasia. Normal histopathology in the face of endoscopic changes may indicate disease predominantly affecting the deeper layers of the stomach (Clark, 1985; Walter et al., 1985). Under these circumstances surgical, full thickness biopsies are required in order to obtain a definitive diagnosis.

High serum gastrin levels associated with a rugal hypertrophy in a non-azotaemic patient, are suggestive of hypergastrinaemia secondary to a pancreatic gastrinoma.

Management and treatment of chronic gastritis

Where the underlying cause of the gastritis is determined, this should be specifically treated. In the majority of cases no primary cause is evident and symptomatic therapy should be initiated. Diet plays a major role in the management of gastritis as there is a tendency for gastric motility to be disturbed resulting in retention of food within the stomach. A highly digestible low fat diet can significantly improve gastric emptying and reduce vomiting. In cases of eosinophilic or atrophic gastritis where dietary sensitivity has been implicated in the pathogenesis an elimination diet should be used.

Sucralfate or colloidal bismuth is often helpful in the treatment of chronic gastritis. Acid inhibition is rarely necessary unless there is evidence of mucosal erosion or ulceration. Acid inhibitors are contraindicated in cases of atrophic gastritis where there is already hypo- or achlorhydria. Their use in cases of hypertrophic gastritis can be of value.

Antiemetics are rarely necessary in chronic gastritis as vomiting is usually low grade and intermittent. Prokinetic drugs (metoclopramide, cisapride or erythromycin) may be helpful where there is delayed gastric emptying secondary to hypomotility. Such drugs are contraindicated where the delayed gastric emptying is secondary to pyloric obstruction associated with mucosal hypertrophy.

Antibacterial agents are only indicated when bacterial overgrowth occurs secondary to hypoacidity or in the treatment of helicobacteriosis.

Corticosteroids are indicated in chronic non-responsive gastritis or when there is histological evidence of a severe inflammatory infiltrate, e.g. lymphocytic/plasmacytic or eosinophilic gastritis. Prednisolone is given at immunosuppressive doses (1–2 mg kg^{-1} p.o. bid) for one to two weeks after which time the dose is gradually reduced over two to three months. In refractory cases, azathioprine may be required in addition to corticosteroids.

Surgical resection of focal areas of mucosal

hypertrophy is usually successful. Pyloroplasty techniques are often required where there is evidence of pyloric outflow obstruction (Sikes et al., 1986; Dennis et al., 1987).

Recently, emphasis in the treatment of gastric ulceration has changed from the use of antisecretory drugs towards drugs that promote gastric mucosal healing and improve gastric protective mechanisms such as sucralfate and misoprostol. Where possible the underlying cause(s) of the ulceration should be addressed.

■ Gastric foreign bodies

Gastric foreign bodies are common, particularly in dogs (Fig. 36.14). Many remain asymptomatic for long periods only causing clinical signs when the pylorus becomes obstructed. This usually occurs when the interdigestive 'housekeeper' contractions try to force the foreign body through the pylorus. The majority of foreign bodies cause little gastric mucosal damage although erosion, ulceration and even perforation can occur. Occasionally gastric foreign bodies are potentially harmful due to their contents which can be liberated by the gastric acidity, e.g. mercury-containing batteries.

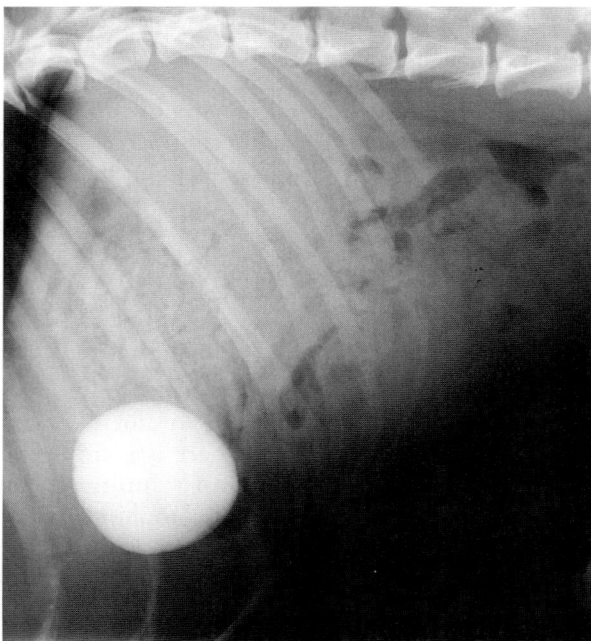

Figure 36.14 Gastric foreign body (a stone) in a 5-year-old, neutered, male, Boxer dog with a 7-month history of intermittent vomiting and depression

Clinical signs

Foreign bodies can be clinically silent, cause acute vomiting or be associated with persistent or intermittent vomiting. Abdominal palpation can be painful if there is pyloric obstruction. Other clinical signs are usually due to the effects of vomiting or mucosal damage.

Diagnosis

Diagnosis can normally be made radiographically although radiolucent foreign bodies may not be detected. In these cases contrast studies or endoscopy is required.

Treatment

Gastrotomy is required for removal of large foreign bodies. Smaller items can be removed endoscopically with basket forceps and needles or pins with grab forceps. Adequate patient preparation, particularly correction of dehydration, acid/base and electrolyte disturbances prior to anaesthesia is essential.

Hairballs in cats

Vomiting of hairballs is common in cats and is a consequence of grooming behaviour particularly in long-haired breeds. Cats lack significant interdigestive motility hence the hair does not move on from the stomach. Hairball concretions (trichobezoars) which impact the pyloric outflow occasionally become clinically significant. Similar mats can be found in wool-sucking cats. In cases where hairballs become a clinical problem there is usually an underlying alimentary disease which needs to be addressed to prevent the recurrence of the hairball following surgical removal.

■ Gastric neoplasia

Gastric neoplasia is rare in dogs (less than 1% of all canine tumours) and is even less common in cats.

Aetiology

Both primary and secondary neoplasia affects the stomach. Older dogs (mean age 9 years) (Sullivan et al., 1987), males (65% of cases) and especially rough collies, setters and terriers are most commonly affected. Carcinomas/adenocarcinomas are more common in dogs and lymphomas in cats (Brodey, 1966). Various other neoplasms have

GASTRIC DISEASE

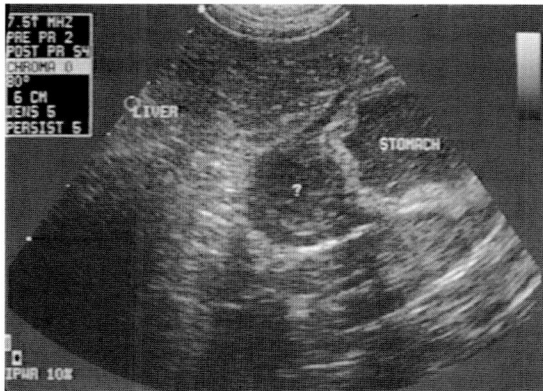

Figure 36.15 Mass lesion (?) in the gastric wall caused by a leiomyosarcoma in a 10-year-old, neutered, female, English cocker spaniel which presented with a two-week history of vomiting.

been recorded including leiomyomas, leiomyosarcomas (Fig. 36.15), carcinoid tumours (arising from the endochromaffin cells), fibromas, fibrosarcomas, squamous cell carcinomas, plasmacytomas and adenomatous polyps. Approximately 30% of canine gastric tumours are benign. Malignant tumours usually metastasize to the draining lymph nodes, pancreas and liver. They occur most frequently along the lesser curvature, at the cardia and pylorus. Predisposing factors have been suggested in the pathogenesis of gastric tumours (Table 36.19).

Clinical findings

Cases commonly present with signs typical of chronic gastritis. As the tumour develops vomiting becomes more persistent and weight loss, polydipsia and haematemesis/melaena may occur (Sullivan et al., 1987). Anorexia, ptyalism, depression and anaemia develop with advanced neoplasia. Sudden death may occur if the neoplasm erodes a major blood vessel or associated ulceration leads to gastric rupture.

Table 36.19 Potential predisposing factors associated with gastric neoplasia

Helicobacter spp. infections
Diet
High carbohydrate, low fat, low protein diets
Dietary carcinogens
Atrophic gastritis and gastric hypoacidity
Reflux gastritis
Gastric polyps

Diagnosis

Plain radiographs are rarely diagnostic and ultrasonography is relatively insensitive giving both false positive and false negative findings. Diagnosis is based on the presence of consistent filling abnormalities on contrast, preferably double contrast, radiography. Even with these techniques, plaque-like masses can be difficult to visualize and a similar picture can be seen in non-neoplastic gastric ulceration.

Diagnosis is based on histopathological examination of endoscopic or surgical biopsies. Not all gastric tumours involve the mucosal surface (e.g. leiomyomas/myosarcomas) hence a normal endoscopic biopsy result does not necessarily preclude gastric neoplasia. Gastrinomas may be diagnosed by measuring basal gastrin levels or gastrin levels before and after an intravenous calcium gluconate challenge test. High gastrin levels are also seen in non-neoplastic conditions such as renal failure (Shaw, 1988).

Treatment

Where possible surgical resection is recommended. This may require complex procedures particularly if the tumour involves the pyloric region, e.g. gastroduodenostomy or partial gastrectomy. Chemotherapy of gastric lymphoma in cats using standard protocols has been reported to give remission times of 3–13 months (Couto, 1984). Treatment with cimetidine improves survival time in humans with gastric neoplasia and may be of value in cats and dogs.

Gastric motility disorders

Gastric motility disorders may occur as a result of primary alimentary disease or may be secondary to systemic disorders (Table 36.20). Primary motility disorders in cats are anecdotal as some cats with chronic vomiting respond to prokinetic therapy.

Clinical signs

Patients may vomit large volumes of food long after ingestion (usually greater than 12 h post-feeding). Food can appear undigested or partially digested and may have a faecal odour which can also be seen in intestinal obstruction. Abdominal discomfort and palpable gastric distension may also be evident. Before vomiting, animals are uncomfortable and anorexic, although weight loss is not inevitable. Melaena or haematemesis may occur.

Table 36.20 Causes of abnormal gastric motility

Primary alimentary disease	Systemic disorders
Gastroenteritis	Electrolyte disturbance – hypokalaemia, hypo- and hypercalcaemia
Pancreatitis	Acidosis
Gastric over-distension	Endocrinopathy – hypoadrenocorticism, hyper- and possibly hypothyroidism, diabetes mellitus
Gastric dilation–volvulus	
Chronic gastritis/ulceration	Pain
Inflammatory bowel disease	Peritonitis
Gastric neoplasia	Stress / fear
Primary gastric dysmotility	Dysautonomia
Constipation	Liver failure
Malabsorption	Uraemia
? pylorospasm	Postsurgical
	Trauma, especially to abdomen or CNS
	Drugs, especially atropine, narcotics, e.g. pethidine, clenbuterol

Diagnosis

A complete biochemical profile, including electrolytes and bile acids, can be helpful in ruling out systemic diseases. Cortisol and thyroid hormone concentrations and ACTH, and TSH/TRH stimulation tests should be performed where appropriate. The blood sample frequently appears lipaemic due to gastric retention of food despite starvation.

Plain radiographs are often suggestive of gastric retention as large quantities of food are present following an appropriate period of starvation. Barium meal or BIPS studies can also be used to demonstrate delayed emptying. However, neither of the procedures is particularly valuable in identifying the aetiology. Barium should be avoided if subsequent endoscopy is planned.

Ultimately, diagnosis is based on endoscopy or coeliotomy and biopsy. Ultrasonography is of some value in assessing gastric wall thickness and in the diagnosis of neoplastic disease. It is, however, most useful in the diagnosis of pancreatic lesions. Coeliotomy is the technique of choice as it allows full thickness biopsies to be obtained, examination of the gastric muscle and pancreas and, where appropriate, surgical correction or placement of a jejunostomy tube.

Management

Wherever possible attempts should be made to define the primary cause. If this is not possible or there appears to be primary motility disorder then symptomatic therapy is indicated.

Diet

Feeding small, frequent, low fat meals will stimulate gastric emptying. Liquidizing the food may also be helpful.

Prokinetic drugs

These drugs are contraindicated if there is gastric outflow obstruction which can also present with signs of delayed gastric emptying with secondary dysmotility due to chronic gastric distension. Cisapride and metoclopramide act to increase the amplitude of antral contractions, inhibit relaxation of the fundus and coordinate gastric, pyloric and duodenal motility all of which lead to accelerated emptying (Hall *et al.*, 1990). There are some indications that cisapride may be more effective.

Erythromycin acts as a motilin agonist at low doses and also has a direct action on cholinergic neurones. Motilin acts to stimulate smooth muscle activity. A postprandial dose of 5 mg kg^{-1} has been used in dogs.

Rapid gastric emptying

Rapid emptying is usually a result of surgical intervention affecting the pylorus but has been recorded in dogs with myenteric ganglionitis and may well occur in hyperthyroid cats which have decreased orocaecal transit times (Papasouliotis *et al.*, 1993b). Frequent feeding of small meals with high levels of soluble fibre to reduce gastric dumping is recommended.

Gastric outflow obstruction

There are a number of causes of gastric outflow obstruction (Table 36.21). The clinical signs of gastric outflow obstruction are similar to gastric motility disorders, i.e. food fails to proceed into the small intestine resulting in delayed vomiting. Anorexia and weight loss are also commonly seen. Projectile vomiting is not pathognomonic for pyloric obstruction.

Table 36.21 Causes of gastric outflow obstruction

Pyloric stenosis (chronic hypertrophic pyloric gastropathy)	
Pyloric dysfunction	
Obstruction secondary to	foreign bodies
	gastric neoplasia
	polyps
	pancreatic neoplasia
Pyloric fibrosis	
?? pylorospasm	

Pylorospasm leading to outflow obstruction is described in toy breeds and particularly in excitable or nervous animals (Burrows, 1986a; Dunn, 1989). However, the existence of pylorospasm as an entity has been recently questioned since gastric emptying is a result of coordinated movement of the antrum, pylorus and duodenum thus 'pylorospasm' probably represents a motility disorder affecting several areas of the GIT leading to delayed gastric emptying and should be treated as described above.

Congenital pyloric stenosis, seen in puppies and kittens postweaning (Pearson et al., 1974; Dunn, 1989) is described but is unlikely to be a distinct entity. Some cases are a result of mucosal hypertrophy whereas others may be due to inadequate innervation and failure of the pylorus to relax.

Pyloric obstruction is seen as a consequence of hypertrophy of the antral mucosa and/or the muscularis. Muscular hypertrophy is most commonly seen in brachycephalic breeds such as boxers and Boston terriers. In adult animals, generalized, multifocal or focal (polypoid) hypertrophy of the mucosa is more common. Small breeds such as Lhaso apsos, Maltese, Pekinese and Shih tzus are over-represented as are male dogs (Bellinger et al., 1990). The aetiopathogenesis is unclear but increased gastrin levels leading to mucosal hypertrophy have been implicated.

Diagnosis

Mass lesions or foreign bodies causing pyloric obstruction should be ruled out using appropriate imaging techniques, endoscopy or coeliotomy. Diagnosis is based on the demonstration of hyperplastic pyloric mucosa or a protuberant muscular pylorus making passage of an endoscope into the duodenum difficult. Muscular hypertrophy is difficult to appreciate on endoscopy. Histological changes range from normal to mucosal erosions, oedema and cystic or hyperplastic glandular changes. An inflammatory infiltrate may be present. The presence of *Campylobacter*-like organisms associated with hyperplastic gastritis has been described (Leblanc et al., 1993).

Treatment

Pyloromyotomy is usually sufficient for mucosal hypertrophy but more extensive gastric involvement may require pyloroplasty techniques. In the most extreme cases gastroduodenostomy may be necessary. These procedures can be associated with serious postoperative complications but generally the prognosis is good.

Pyloric dysfunction in cats

Pyloric stenosis or dysfunction is a condition seen almost exclusively in young Siamese cats (less than one-year old) (Pearson et al., 1974). A number of these cases had concurrent megaoesophagus and/or chronic oesophagitis. Grossly the pylorus appears normal and autonomic dysfunction is postulated. Treatment involves pyloric surgery and management of the megaoesophagus and oesophagitis.

Gastric dilatation and volvulus

Gastric dilatation and volvulus (GDV) covers a group of conditions which can involve gastric dilatation, gastric dilatation and volvulus or, more rarely, chronic gastric volvulus. Gastric dilatation, usually accompanied by volvulus, is a dramatic, peracute, life-threatening condition of dogs. GDV is most prevalent in large breed, deep chested dogs such as Great Danes, German Shepherds, Saint Bernards, Irish setters, dobermans, weimeraners and basset hounds. It has occasionally been reported in cats and in smaller breed dogs with dachshunds being over-represented (Burrows, 1986a). The reported age range is 2 months to 15 years (Muir, 1982).

Gastric dilatation

Gastric dilatation alone is a relatively rare condition which can eventually result in gastric atony and persistent gastric distension. Affected dogs usually have abdominal enlargement and are depressed, uncomfortable, eructating and show intermittent, usually ineffectual, vomiting/retching. Patients are usually haemodynamically stable unless they progress to volvulus.

Cases are managed by induction of emesis unless there is evidence of ingestion of caustic or sharp material. Prophylactic gastropexy is advisable if there is no obvious history of gluttony.

The author and colleagues have seen a few cases of repeated, frequent gastric dilatation which continues to occur even after gastropexy. Investigation has failed to reveal a primary cause and response to symptomatic management such as prokinetics has been disappointing. These animals carry a guarded prognosis.

Predisposing causes for GDV

Whether the stomach dilates and rotates in a given animal at any given time is the result of the combination of a series of predisposing factors:

- Dilatation of the stomach secondary to ingestion of gas, food or fluid;
- Splenic engorgement following displacement by gastric dilatation may prevent spontaneous recovery;
- Gastric volvulus, which is generally thought to occur following dilatation;
- Conformation; deep chested dogs have an increased tendency to twist, possibly due to defective eructation;
- Postprandial exercise (though mean time post-feeding reported as 7 h, range 1–40 h);
- Composition of diet, e.g. swelling of dried food has been implicated in some studies (Van Kruiningen et al., 1987) but not others (Burrows and Ignaszewski, 1990);
- Rapid intake of large volumes of food/fluid;
- Increased production or intake of gas, e.g. ingestion of highly fermentable food (Van Kruiningen et al., 1987). Aerophagia in nervous, excited or dyspnoeic animals is likely to be more important (Caywood et al., 1977; Brockman 1994);
- Defective eructation (neural or anatomic causes);
- Delayed gastric motility and gastric emptying disorders (for causes see earlier) (Hall, 1989; Burrows and Ignaszewski, 1990);
- Genetics; GDV appears to be more common in certain lines of certain breeds;
- Non-specific GI disease; many cases have displacement of pylorus and fundus (Frendin et al., 1988);
- ? Elevated gastrin levels increasing gastro-oesophageal sphincter pressure and inhibiting eructation;
- ?? Laxity of gastric ligaments (Orton, 1986).

Pathophysiology

When the stomach distends, the gastro-oesophageal sphincter is prevented from opening and this effectively prevents eructation or vomiting which could relieve the intragastric pressure. An increased level of gastrin, initiated by distension, further increases gastro-oesophageal sphincter pressure, delays gastric emptying and predisposes to aerophagia, thus creating a vicious cycle.

Distension of the stomach interferes with venous return to the heart, reducing cardiac output and leading to hypovolaemic shock. Lactic acidosis can become marked, eventually leading to multiple organ failure. Cardiac arrhythmias occur as a consequence of cardiac ischaemia and release of myocardial depressant factors by the pancreas and spleen (Brockman, 1994). Local blood supply to the stomach is reduced further by microvascular infarction and gastric oedema results in mucosal ischaemia and necrosis. Mucosal damage is worsened by the build up and penetration of gastric acid through the mucosal barrier. Distension of the stomach prevents normal diaphragmatic function thereby interfering with breathing and reducing oxygenation, which in turn accelerates lactic acid build up and further impairs tissue perfusion. Unless these changes are rapidly corrected, disseminated intravascular coagulation and irreversible shock develops causing death (Simpson and Else, 1991b). Even when

Table 36.22 Changes in serum chemistry during development and following initial treatment of GDV

Parameter	Change
Packed cell volume	Gradual ↑; ↓↓ with treatment
Albumin and total protein	Mild ↑; ↓↓ with treatment
Potassium	Gradual ↑; ↑↑ with treatment progressing to ↓
Phosphorus	↑
Sodium, chloride and calcium	no change
Glucose	↑; ↓ with treatment
Creatine kinase	↑↑
Acid–base	Acidosis, ↓ pH and bicarbonate; worsens during immediate post-treatment
P_{O_2}	↓↓

the GDV is resolved, further, severe damage to the tissue can occur due to reperfusion injuries. Electrolyte and acid–base disturbances are summarized in Table 36.22.

Clinical signs

The history reveals a sudden increase in abdominal size, frequent attempts to vomit and salivate. This may be preceded by a period of restlessness. Without treatment, collapse and death occur rapidly. Examination reveals pallor, tachycardia, poor pulse quality and poor capillary refill time, dehydration, abdominal discomfort, grunting respiration, weakness and abdominal tympany.

Diagnosis

Diagnosis can usually be made on clinical presentation although the differentiation between dilatation alone and dilatation–volvulus can be difficult. Passage of a stomach tube may not reliably differentiate between the two conditions. Torsion results in a gas-filled pylorus lying dorsal to a gas-filled fundus creating a soft tissue fold across the stomach on a right lateral radiograph (Hathcock, 1984; Brockman, 1994).

Treatment and management (Leib and Martin, 1987)

GDVs are true medical emergencies. Treatment should follow three basic rules:

1. Decompression;
2. Treatment of shock;
3. Surgical correction (if there is volvulus).

Fluid therapy

Fluids should precede/accompany decompression. Fluids (lactated Ringers) should be given at shock rates of 90 ml h^{-1} which can be a problem in large breed dogs as this can represent 3–4 l h^{-1}. It is essential, therefore, that a wide-bore catheter(s) is (are) placed. An inflatable bag compressor is a valuable addition to emergency facilities in a practice since it enables very rapid fluid administration. If possible at least 15 min of fluid therapy should be given before decompression.

Decompression

Initially, partial decompression is best achieved by trocharization using a 14–16G needle rather than stomach tubing the animal which is more stressful and can precipitate sudden death. Less rapid decompression also reduces the rate of reperfusion and the release of large amounts of free oxygen radicals and toxic metabolites into the circulation. After partial decompression a stomach tube can be more easily and safely passed allowing gastric lavage. The presence of blood and mucosa in the lavage is a poor prognostic sign.

Adjunctive treatment

- Corticosteroids; shock doses of methylprednisolone have not been shown to increase long-term survival. They should not be given until 30 min after fluid administration has commenced.
- H$_2$ blockers given intravenously may be valuable.
- Antibacterials: broad spectrum cover is routinely administered as GDV cases are predisposed to septicaemia due to bacterial translocation from the GIT and reduced reticuloendothelial function. Antibacterials should be given intravenously, e.g. ampicillin (10–20 mg kg^{-1} tid) and enrofloxacin (2.5 mg kg^{-1} bid–tid, Baytril; Bayer) or cefuroxime (10–20 mg kg^{-1} tid, Zinacef; Glaxo).
- NSAIDs: flunixin meglumine may have valuable anti-endotoxic activity but it should be given with extreme care, especially if the animal has been given corticosteroids as gastric mucosal integrity is likely to be already compromised. Flunixin, in common with other NSAIDs also inhibits prostaglandin-mediated protection of renal perfusion. Flunixin has not been shown to be beneficial in one small study (Davidson et al., 1992).
- Free radical scavengers: desferrioxamine mesylate (25 mg kg^{-1} i.m.) given 30 min into treatment has been shown to increase survival and decrease reperfusion injuries (Lantz and Badylak, 1992) in experimental models. Clinical experience is limited.

Surgery

Surgical intervention is required to reposition the stomach, manage areas of necrosis and to prevent recurrence (75–80% of GDVs will recur without gastropexy).

Management of gastric necrosis is most rapidly achieved by invagination of the affected area rather than excision. The technique also has a reduced risk of abdominal contamination from gastric contents.

A wide variety of gastropexy techniques are described. Fundopexy and circumcostal, incisional and muscular flap gastropexies are associated with the lowest recurrence rates (0–3.3%) (Ellison, 1993). In critically ill patients, tube gastrostomy may be preferred as it is a more rapid technique and allows continual decompression. However, this technique results in a higher recurrence rate (3–11%) (Ellison, 1993) and may require revision when the patient is more stable. Splenectomy may be required if there has been marked vascular compromise and the spleen fails to contract following derotation.

It is essential that the surgical anatomy is understood so that the stomach can be fully derotated prior to fixation. This can be achieved by standing on the right side of the abdomen, lifting the pylorus and moving it to the right side while the fundus is pushed to the left side of the abdomen.

Management of complications

Complications are common following GDV surgery (Fig. 36.16) hence good postoperative monitoring is essential for surgery to be successful.

Cardiac arrhythmias occur in 40–50% of cases 12–72 h postsurgery as multiple ventricular premature (VPC) complexes, or as paroxysmal or persistent ventricular tachycardia. Electrolyte and acid–base status should be checked and corrected if necessary. VPCs should be treated if there is R on T, they are multifocal or the heart rate is above 150 bpm. Lignocaine (2–4 mg kg^{-1}), usually given as a slow intravenous bolus, should be followed by continuous infusion at 50–100 µg kg^{-1} min^{-1}. If this is ineffective then procainamide hydrochloride or quinidine sulphate may be required. Care needs to be exercised when using these drugs as their hepatic metabolism and renal excretion may be compromised.

Paralytic ileus occurs in as many as 30% of patients and there may be delayed gastric emptying. Metoclopramide or cisapride are appropriate drugs to use in such cases.

Disseminated intravascular coagulation occurs in a significant number of cases, and may require heparin therapy (10–75 u kg^{-1} s.c. tid) in conjunction with a plasma transfusion.

Prognosis

Prognosis is highly dependent on the state of systemic collapse at presentation and whether there is gastric necrosis. Mortality rates of 23–60% are quoted (Meyer-Lindenberg *et al.*, 1993).

Chronic gastric volvulus

Some dogs present with a recurrent history of chronic, usually self-relieving mild to moderate gastric distension, anorexia and/or vomiting. Borborygmi, eructation and weight loss are also reported. Radiographs show evidence of a torsed but not necessarily dilated stomach. There may be evidence of liver damage due to congestive hepatopathy on biochemical examination. Treatment requires surgical gastropexy.

SMALL INTESTINAL DISEASE

Introduction

The small intestine carries out the processes of digestion and absorption of food. It also has a major immunological role in controlling small intestinal flora and initiating tolerance to food antigens. Failure of this immunological role is a common precursor to many, chronic, small intestinal diseases. The surface area of the small intestine is greatly increased by the presence of folds and finger-like villi. Additional surface area is created by the microvilli present on each enterocyte.

Carrier proteins are present on the microvilli specialized for the transport of glucose, amino acids, fatty acids and other nutrients. Absorbed material is carried to the liver via rich capillary beds which connect with the portal vein. Dietary fat and fat-soluble vitamins are absorbed into a central lacteal. The small intestine is innervated by vagal parasympathetic and paravertebral sympathetic efferent fibres. The parasympathetic fibres are important for the regulation of motility. Afferent sympathetic and parasympathetic fibres relay sensory information.

The epithelium of the small intestine is composed of a variety of cells and is delineated by a basement membrane (Fig. 36.17). Enterocytes are continually being desquamated from the tip of the

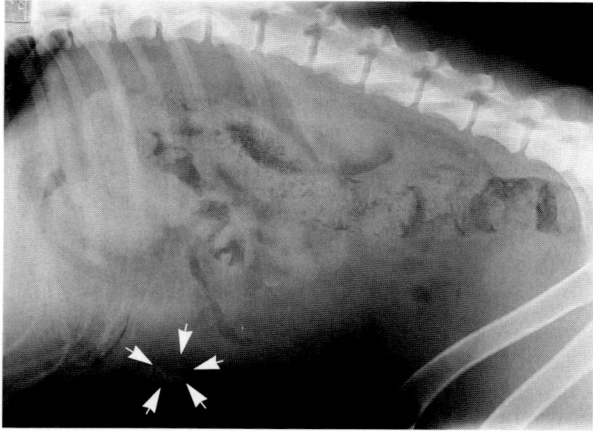

Figure 36.16 Gastric rupture postsurgery for a gastric volvulus in a 6-year-old, neutered, female, Weimeraner dog. Note the poor serosal detail and free faecal material in the ventral abdomen (arrows).

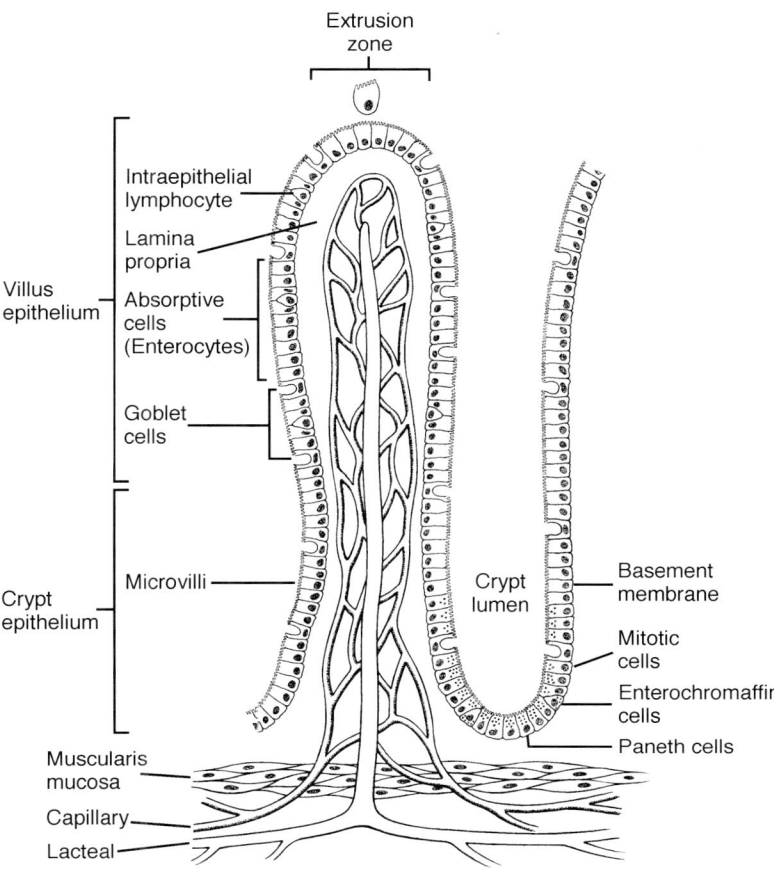

Figure 36.17 Diagram showing the anatomy of a villus–crypt unit of the small intestine.

villus and replaced by rapidly dividing crypt cells. Migration of enterocytes from crypt to villus tip occurs over three to five days (Eastwood, 1977). Lymphoid material is accumulated in distinct areas (Peyer's patches) where specialized epithelial cells (M-cells) are thought to be responsible for sampling the antigenic milieu. The lamina propria lies below the epithelium and is composed primarily of B and T lymphocytes, plasma cells, eosinophils and macrophages. At the base of the villus–crypt unit lies the muscularis mucosa which separates the mucosa from the submucosa. Below the submucosa lie the circular and then longitudinal smooth muscle layers and finally the serosa.

Small intestinal motility mixes chyme from the stomach with pancreatic and biliary secretions to ensure efficient digestion of nutrients and slows the passage of contents through the tubular lumen. Passage through the small intestine is a mixture of braking segmentation motility and forward moving peristalsis. Neurological control is mediated by cholinergic, adrenergic and serotoninergic activity. Passage of intestinal contents from the ileum into the colon is via the ileocolic junction which opens in response to food entering the stomach and prevents reflux from the colon into the small intestine.

Enteritis

Enteritis can be divided into acute and chronic disease but this is somewhat artificial and of limited practical value. Enteritis typically presents as diarrhoea which may be accompanied by other abdominal and systemic signs.

Diarrhoea is defined as increased frequency and/or fluidity and/or volume of faeces thus frequent passage of bulky but well-formed stools should still be considered as diarrhoea. Diarrhoea can be divided into:

- Osmotic diarrhoea associated with a failure of digestion leading to nutrient retention and therefore increased fluid is held in the lumen;
- Secretory diarrhoea results from exaggerated villus response leading to large volumes of isotonic fluid entering the lumen. This may be activated by bacterial toxins, e.g. enteropatho-

genic *E. coli* (EPEC) or *Salmonella* spp. or it may be associated with an osmotic diarrhoea where the presence of undigested nutrients in the lumen leads to bacterial degradation to organic acids, amines, ammonia and hydroxy fats.
- Increased permeability; large volumes of fluid normally move across the intestinal epithelium into the lumen (up to 2700 ml day^{-1} in a 20 kg dog), of which 95% is resorbed in the ileum and colon (Drazner, 1983). Inflammation, neoplasia, ulceration and cardiac disease can increase this loss and, in severe cases, be accompanied by macromolecules resulting in a protein-losing enteropathy.
- Motility diarrhoea occurs due to a loss of segmentation motility but normal peristalsis (Murdoch, 1986) presenting the colon with sudden large volumes of fluid which it is unable to resorb adequately.

Sudden onset diarrhoea in clinically healthy animals, like acute vomiting, is usually self-limiting. But, acute, life-threatening diarrhoea associated with viral enteritis, e.g. parvovirus can occur (Table 36.23).

Chronic diarrhoea may be defined as diarrhoea that is not self-limiting or fails to respond to symptomatic therapy and is of more than three weeks standing. It can be persistent or intermittent and is rarely life-threatening. It can, however, reflect serious underlying disease (Table 36.24).

Differentiating diarrhoea into essentially large or small bowel in origin (see Chapter 7) and associating it with intestinal or systemic disease is of practical value in planning appropriate investigations.

Table 36.23 Aetiology of sudden onset diarrhoea in dogs and cats

Dietary	Overeating
	Scavenging
	Soiled food
	Sudden dietary change
	Dietary intolerance, e.g. lactase deficiency
Viral	Canine — Parvovirus
	Distemper
	Rotavirus
	Coronavirus
	Feline — Parvovirus (panleukopenia)
	Rotavirus
	Leukaemia virus
	Astrovirus
	? Torovirus
Parasitic	*Uncinaria* spp.
	Ancylostoma spp.
	Trichuris spp.
	Cryptosporidia spp.
	Giardiasis
Bacterial	*Salmonella* spp.
	Campylobacter spp.
	Clostridium difficile
	C. perfringens
	Tyzzer's disease
Miscellaneous	Haemorrhagic gastroenteritis
	Intestinal obstruction
	Intussusception
	Severe systemic disease

Treatment of diarrhoea

Treatment of diarrhoea is dependent on defining its cause. A variety of non-specific therapies are also available which can be of value in ameliorating the effects of diarrhoea whatever its origin.

Table 36.24 Aetiology of chronic diarrhoea in dogs and cats

Primary diarrhoea	Diarrhoea secondary to systemic disease
Giardiasis	Hyperthyroidism
Exocrine pancreatic insufficiency	Feline leukaemia virus
Inflammatory bowel disease	Feline immunodeficiency virus
Eosinophilic enteritis	Feline coronavirus
Dietary hypersensitivity	Hypoadrenocorticism
Lymphangiectasia	Hepatic failure
Small intestinal bacterial overgrowth	Renal failure
Intestinal neoplasia	Congestive cardiac disease
Partial obstruction	
Villous atrophy (secondary to acute diarrhoea)	
Motility disorders	

Intestinal protectants

These drugs are generally of very little value as, although faecal character improves, water content remains abnormal. Bismuth subsalicylate is useful as it also has anti-inflammatory, antibacterial and antisecretory activity.

Motility modifiers

Opiate-based compounds such as codeine, loperamide and diphenoxylate (Table 36.25) promote segmentation motility of the intestine slowing transit time and increasing the opportunity for electrolytes and water absorption. They are *contraindicated* if toxigenic diarrhoea is suspected as absorption of toxins and bacteria will be increased.

Dietary diarrhoea

Aetiology

Dietary diarrhoea may arise for a number of reasons:

- dietary indiscretion;
- excessive intake;
- dietary hypersensitivity, intolerance or allergy;
- sudden dietary change;
- diet contains preformed toxins;
- diet contains pathogenic bacteria.

Dietary indiscretion and excessive intake is most commonly seen in dogs which may well scavenge without the owner's knowledge. Similarly, cats may be receiving inappropriate foods from another source. Overfeeding is particularly common in puppies and kittens and some diet sheets that accompany new puppies and kittens suggest that entirely inappropriate volumes of food should be given. Sudden dietary change can cause diarrhoea and is often made worse as the owner then abruptly changes the diet back to the original product. High carbohydrate diets may cause diarrhoea (particularly in cats) as can predominantly meat based diets (Murdoch, 1986).

True dietary allergies are *rare* in dogs and cats, although a variety of foods have been implicated in individual cases including beef, milk, wheat, egg and horse meat (Merchant and Taboada, 1991). Milk 'allergy' is more likely to reflect intolerance to lactose due to a lack of the intestinal lactase enzyme and is more common in cats.

Clinical findings

Dietary diarrhoea is typified by a bright, active, appetant patient with large volume, small intestinal diarrhoea.

Diagnosis

Diagnosis is usually circumstantial when the animal recovers following dietary rest and the subsequent introduction of a bland diet. Animals that are suspected to scavenge can be investigated by strict supervision at home and whilst out walking. This may require muzzling of dogs during exercise. Alternatively the dogs can be hospitalized or kennelled. Cats which may be receiving inappropriate diets from other sources may require kennelling or hospitalization.

Where dietary sensitivity is suspected the animal should be fed a protein source to which it has not previously been exposed together with a gluten-free carbohydrate component, e.g. rice or potatoes. Ideally, once the animal has recovered it should be re-challenged with the original diet to confirm that diarrhoea recurs. Owners are understandably reluctant to pursue this last phase in many cases. In refractory cases, home-cooked elimination diets are sometimes more effective than commercially available 'hypoallergenic' diets.

Table 36.25 Suggested dose rates for opiate motility modifying drugs in cats and dogs

Drug	Dose rate (mg kg^{-1})	Frequency	Route
Dogs			
Codeine	0.5–2.0	bid	p.o.
Loperamide	0.1–0.2	bid–tid	p.o.
Diphenoxylate	0.1–0.2	bid–tid	p.o.
Cats			
Loperamide	0.08–0.16	bid	p.o.
Diphenoxylate	0.05–0.1	bid	p.o.

Such diets should be fed for up to 6–8 weeks before this line of therapy is abandoned as unsuccessful.

Viral enteritis

A wide range of viruses have been implicated in the aetiology of acute and chronic diarrhoea in dogs and cats (Tables 36.23 and 36.24).

Coronaviruses and rotaviruses cause relatively mild diarrhoea associated with invasion of the enterocytes of the villus tip leading to a varying degree of villus atrophy. This reduces the small intestinal surface area and thus can lead to malabsorption. Crypt structure remains intact and new enterocytes will be rapidly produced and migrate to the villus tip, hence malabsorption is only temporary.

In contrast, canine and feline parvovirus (panleukopenia or infectious enteritis) attack the rapidly dividing cells in the villus crypt. This results in much more profound villus atrophy which is less able to resolve as new enterocytes are not being produced. The immunosuppression that also accompanies parvovirus infection predisposes these cases to secondary bacterial infection. Chronic diarrhoea and weight loss may develop due to malabsorption.

Clinical findings

The majority of coronavirus infections are asymptomatic or associated with mild depression, anorexia and diarrhoea in young puppies and kittens. Vomiting is rare and the signs are self-limiting. Coronavirus causing feline infectious peritonitis can also be associated with chronic diarrhoea in cases where there is granulomatous inflammation of the intestinal tract.

Rotavirus infections in adults usually result in a low-grade self-limiting enteritis with anorexia and mucoid diarrhoea lasting up to ten days. In neonates, a more acute disease is seen with vomiting and diarrhoea leading to dehydration and collapse if left untreated.

Parvovirus represents a life-threatening disease particularly in puppies and kittens. It is characterized by a period of anorexia, depression and inappetence which is followed by acute vomiting. Diarrhoea may not develop for up to 48 h after the onset of vomiting. Abdominal pain can be marked and diarrhoea has the typical, though not pathognomonic, smell associated with the presence of blood. Sloughed intestinal mucosa may also be present. A similar clinical syndrome has been reported in cats with feline leukaemia virus.

Protrusion of the nictitating membrane–diarrhoea complex in cats

The cause of this syndrome is still unclear but a torovirus has been implicated (Muir *et al.*, 1990; Rutgers, 1991). The diarrhoea is chronic and can be long-standing, lasting several months. It appears to be infectious in nature as it tends to spread through a household although the degree to which individuals are affected can be very variable. The virus is thought to cause an autonomic ganglionopathy and hence the diarrhoea is due to altered intestinal motility. This may explain its poor response to treatments used for other viral diarrhoeas which are associated with villus damage.

Diagnosis

Diagnosis of viral diarrhoea is based on the demonstration of the virus in a faecal sample or the presence of viral antigen or antibodies to the virus in blood. Parvovirus infection can be difficult to prove in immunized animals but generally the antibody titre following natural infection is significantly higher than vaccinal titres. A profound leukopenia in a diarrhoeic puppy or kitten is also highly suggestive of parvovirus. Demonstration of the virus by faecal haemagglutination, ELISA or microscopy can give false negative results as viral levels are often very low when there is severe diarrhoea. Parvoviruses are also seen in the faeces of clinically healthy individuals. Definitive diagnosis may require histopathology of the intestine.

Treatment

Treatment is symptomatic and supportive with fluid, electrolyte and acid–base balance being the most important initial considerations. Broad-spectrum antibacterial agents, antiemetics and vitamin supplements are also of value. Hyperimmune serum in the face of established disease has not been shown to be of use and intestinal protectants such as kaolin are also of little value. Motility modifiers, such as anticholinergics or opiates, and glucocorticoids are contraindicated.

Bacterial infections

Primary bacterial enteritis is rare in dogs and cats. Infections involving *Campylobacter* spp.

and *Salmonella* spp. are usually opportunistic as both bacteria may be recovered from healthy individuals. *Clostridium perfringens*-associated diarrhoea is caused by the organism elaborating a toxin which results in acute mucoid or haemorrhagic diarrhoea but chronic intermittent problems are also reported. *Clostridium difficile* has been associated with antibiotic-induced diarrhoea (Berry and Levett, 1986). Yersiniosis is a rare cause of chronic diarrhoea in dogs and cats associated with *Yersinia pseudotuberculosis* which is potentially zoonotic and *Y. enterocolitica*. Tyzzer's disease due to *Bacillus piliformis* is also occasionally seen in puppies and kittens causing a severe life-threatening gastroenteritis. Mycobacterial-associated diarrhoea has also been reported.

Enteropathogenic E. coli

There is mounting evidence to support the role of EPEC in the aetiology of canine diarrhoea. Their role in feline cases is less clear as significant numbers of healthy cats harbour EPEC. EPEC cause diarrhoea due to their ability to produce toxins or to attach and invade the mucosa. Diagnosis is based on polymerase chain reaction techniques on colonies isolated from faecal samples in suspected cases. Treatment is with a suitable antibacterial agent but cases do recur suggesting that there may be underlying immune deficiencies in some dogs. The use of autogenous vaccines is being investigated.

Clinical findings

With bacterial-associated diarrhoea a full spectrum of disease from acute, life-threatening diarrhoea, e.g. Tyzzer's disease in puppies or kittens (Jones *et al.*, 1985), to chronic, intermittent problems, to clinically asymptomatic cases is encountered. *Yersinia* has been associated with mesenteric lymphadenopathy in cats (Obwolo and Gruffydd-Jones, 1977).

Diagnosis

Diagnosis is based on the demonstration of pathogenic bacteria on faecal culture. Selective media and repeat cultures may be required in some cases. Pathogenic bacteria are also associated with diarrhoea secondary to other disease processes affecting the normal regulation of bowel flora hence treatment of the pathogenic bacteria alone may not resolve the clinical signs.

Parasitic infections

Nematodes (roundworms)

Parasitic disease is usually only clinically significant in young puppies and kittens where heavy burdens of *Toxocara* spp. or *Toxascaris leonina* can induce vomiting and diarrhoea. On rare occasions these parasites can cause bowel obstruction.

Diarrhoea caused by hookworms (*Ancylostoma caninum* or *Uncinaria stenocephala*) are most important in young dogs. Whipworm (*Trichuris vulpis*) can be associated with chronic enterocolitis in dogs; the diarrhoea may vary from blood-tinged and mucoid to profuse and watery. Whipworm infection is rare in cats. Larvae from both hook- and whipworms can invade and damage the intestinal mucosa. Heavy *Ancylostoma* infections can cause severe mucosal damage, acute diarrhoea and melaena. Anaemia and ascites secondary to hypoproteinaemia may occur. Pedal dermatitis and anal ulceration and pruritus due to migrating larvae is also seen.

Diagnosis is based on faecal worm egg counts. A single negative faecal does not rule-out these infections as intermittent excretion of ova occurs. Worming with a benzimidazole, pyrantel or a nitroscanate-based product is highly effective in the treatment of nematode infestations, though severe mucosal damage caused by *Ancylostoma* may be slow to heal. Balls of dead ascarids can potentially cause obstruction. Piperazine-based products have lower efficacy especially against larval forms and can be neurotoxic especially in small puppies and kittens where overdosage is frequent.

Cestodes (tapeworm)

Echinococcus spp., *Taenia* spp. and *Dipylidium caninum* infections are rarely associated with GI disease in dogs and cats.

Protozoan infections

Coccidia

Cystoisospora (formerly *Isospora* spp.) infection causes diarrhoea with mucus and blood in young animals. *Cryptosporidia* infections are usually asymptomatic but chronic and severe diarrhoea may be seen in kittens, puppies and immunosuppressed adults. Occasionally, apparently immune competent adults are infected. *Toxoplasma gondii* usually causes very mild diarrhoea in cats but reactivation has been implicated in cats with IBD that appear to fail to respond to immunosuppressive therapy.

Cystoisospora and *Cryptosporidia* infections are diagnosed by sugar flotation or formol–ether sedimentation. *Toxoplasma* oocysts are only excreted for around ten days (4–14 days following infection). Diagnosis is based on high or rising, preferably IgM, antibody titres.

Trimethoprin sulphur is effective in the treatment of *Cystoisospora* by reducing oocyst production and allowing natural immunity to develop. Treatment of *Cryptosporidia* is often unsuccessful as clinically affected animals are usually immunosuppressed. Clindamycin has been recommended but its efficacy is questionable. Clindamycin is, however, the treatment of choice for toxoplasmosis at a dose rate of 25 mg kg^{-1} divided bid/tid in cats.

Giardiasis

Giardia lamblia is a pear-shaped protozoan parasite usually found in the duodenum (Pitts, 1983) and occasionally the colon (Ewing and Aldrete, 1973) of dogs. In cats the parasite is most commonly found in the jejunum and ileum (Kirkpatrick, 1986). The prevalence of giardiasis in chronic diarrhoea varies from 4 to 33% (Burnie *et al.*, 1983; Burrows and Lillis, 1967). This wide range probably reflects difficulties in diagnosis due to the trophozoites remaining attached to the mucosal surface and only being excreted intermittently. Giardiasis is likely to be a significantly underdiagnosed cause of chronic diarrhoea in cats and dogs. Infection usually occurs via the ingestion of contaminated water.

Clinical signs

Disease associated with giardiasis is thought to be due to physical damage to the mucosa resulting in malabsorption, decreased bile salt deconjugation and interference with lipase activity causing steatorrhoea (Kirkpatrick and Farrell, 1982). It has also been suggested that giardiasis may be associated with immunosuppression (Pitts, 1983). Giardiasis most commonly results in intermittent or persistent chronic diarrhoea in puppies and kittens although asymptomatic infections can occur. Diarrhoea tends to have an 'oatmeal' or 'frothy' appearance and is usually steatorrhoeic. Occasionally tenesmus, mucus and increased frequency, suggesting large bowel involvement, are seen in dogs. Most cases remain appetant but lose weight.

Diagnosis

Definitive diagnosis is difficult; flotation and concentration techniques for the detection of faecal cysts is recommended as identification of trophozoites in saline faecal smears is less reliable (Ridley and Hawgood, 1956; Kirkpatrick, 1986). Even so, excretion of cysts or trophozoites is intermittent and detection requires multiple faecal samples to be taken. More recently diagnosis has been based on duodenal fluid aspirates or biopsies in dogs. An ELISA test for *Giardia* trophozoite antigens in the faeces has been developed but has not proven to be more sensitive than faecal examination (Barr and Bowman, 1994).

Treatment

Around two-thirds of cases are responsive to metronidazole at a dose rate of 25 mg kg^{-1} bid for 5 days followed by 10 mg kg^{-1} bid for 5 days. At the higher dose rates neurological side effects are seen in some cats. Alternatively, fenbendazole (Panacur; Hoechst Roussel Vet) at 50 mg kg^{-1} day^{-1} for 3 days is licensed for the treatment of giardiasas. Giardiasas is a zoonotic disease so strict hygiene standards should be maintained. *Giardia* cysts can remain viable in a moist environment for several weeks.

Haemorrhagic gastroenteritis

Aetiology

This is a relatively rare condition of small breed dogs, especially poodles, miniature schnauzers, Shetland sheepdogs, cavalier King Charles spaniels. There is no sex predisposition but cases are most frequently observed in dogs between two and four years of age. Haemorrhagic gastroenteritis (HGE) has been seen in greyhounds.

The condition may result from intestinal anaphylaxis which can be triggered by food allergens, bacterial enterotoxins or intestinal parasites resulting in a marked increase in intestinal permeability, however there is little evidence to support this hypothesis. Some evidence exists that HGE may be an immune-mediated disease as it can be created experimentally by injecting anticolon antibodies (Bicks and Walker, 1962). HGE should be differentiated from other causes of haemorrhagic diarrhoea (Table 36.26).

Clinical signs

HGE results in an acute onset of vomiting and diarrhoea containing large amounts of blood. Affected animals may present with pale mucous membranes, tachycardia, tachypnoea and a subnormal temperature.

Table 36.26 Differential diagnosis of haemorrhagic diarrhoea (excluding haemorrhagic gastroenteritis)

Infectious	Parvovirus
	Salmonella
	Canine adenovirus
	Clostridium perfringens
	Leptospirosis
	Campylobacter spp.
Toxic	Corrosive or irritant chemicals
	Warfarin
	Thallium
	Arsenic
Metabolic	Hypoadrenocorticism
	Uraemia
	Acute pancreatitis
	Acute hepatitis
Ischaemic	Intestinal obstruction, e.g. foreign bodies, intussusceptions, volvulus
	Hypovolaemic shock
	Endotoxic shock
	Disseminated intravascular coagulation
Neoplastic	e.g. Lymphosarcoma, polyps

Diagnosis

Diagnosis of HGE is based on the age, breed, clinical signs and having excluded other causes of haemorrhagic diarrhoea (Table 36.26).

Management

Aggressive fluid therapy and correction of electrolyte and acid–base abnormalities are essential. Antibacterial agents should be used due to the increased rate of bacterial translocation from the intestinal lumen. If necessary, DIC should be treated with plasma and heparinization. Food should be withheld for 24–48 h after which the animal should be fed a diet based on novel protein sources.

Prognosis is favourable providing treatment is rapid and aggressive. A mortality rate of about 10% has been reported and 10–15% of cases recur (Simpson and Else, 1991b).

Intestinal obstruction

Intestinal obstruction usually involves the small intestine or ileocolic valve. The lumen can be obstructed by foreign bodies, neoplasms, intussusceptions (Fig. 36.18) or stricture formation. Rarely, obstruction occurs secondary to hypertrophy of the mucosa. Foreign bodies are by far the most common cause in dogs. In cats, foreign bodies are more likely to be linear and cause partial obstruction. Intestinal pseudo-obstruction is caused by a lack of contraction and an inability to maintain tone in the smooth muscle of a segment(s) of bowel resulting in distended loop(s). The lack of contraction results in an interruption in the flow of ingesta and has been associated with sclerosing enteropathy in dogs and diffuse lymphoma in cats.

Clinical findings

Clinical presentation is dependent on the location of the obstruction, whether it causes a total or partial blockage, the length of bowel that is involved (linear versus non-linear) and whether

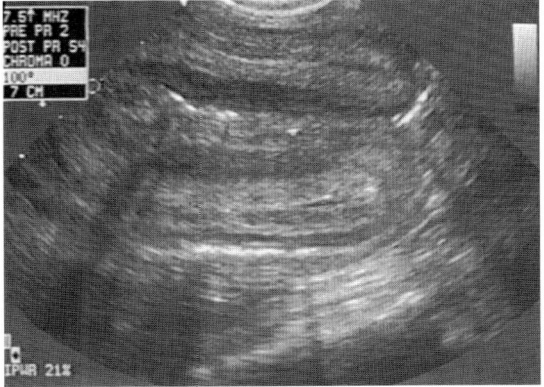
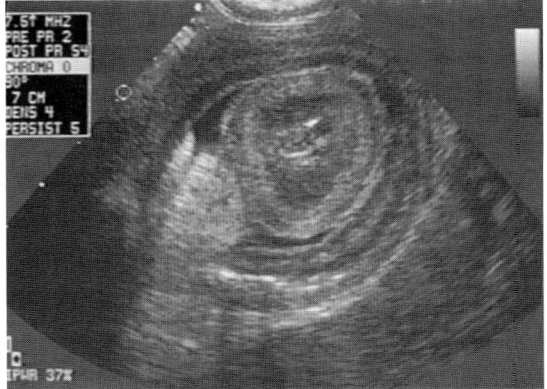

Figure 36.18 (a) Longitudinal and (b) transverse ultrasound images of an intussusception in a 2-year-old, male great Dane. Note the multilayered appearance on the longitudinal view and the typical 'onion-like' arrangement in the transverse view.

perforation has occurred. Upper small intestinal obstruction tends to cause persistent vomiting which may have a faecal appearance and initial diarrhoea followed by a lack of defecation. Distal obstructions cause less persistent vomiting and faeces are rarely passed. Intussusceptions cause vomiting and the passage of faeces containing variable amounts of jelly-like blood.

Partial obstructions and linear foreign bodies can cause vague signs and intermittent vomiting, diarrhoea and inappetance which is apparently responsive to a variety of treatments.

A palpable, often non-painful mass can be felt in many co-operative animals particularly cats with foreign bodies or tumours. Intussusceptions have a 'sausage' shaped feel and are frequently painful. Cranial to the obstruction the bowel loops become stagnant and dilated which can also be appreciated on abdominal palpation.

Diagnosis

Radiography is particularly effective for diagnosing radiodense foreign bodies. Radiolucent foreign bodies, tumours and intussusceptions are often recognizable due to stacking of stagnant loops of intestine proximal to the obstruction, the presence of radiodense sediment (gravel sign) and as soft tissue masses displacing other loops of intestine.

Barium studies or BIPS are required to identify some obstructions but if urgent surgery is contemplated then barium is inadvisable and BIPS can be too slow in providing an answer. In such cases exploratory coeliotomy may be more appropriate. Contrast studies are most valuable in the diagnosis of partial obstructions or linear foreign bodies. Linear foreign bodies sometimes produce subtle changes on plain radiographs with the small intestine appearing clumped into a ball with poor serosal detail and multiple gas bubbles. Contrast studies reveal eccentric pleating, convolution and foreshortening of the duodenum and jejunum. If a linear foreign body is suspected then an oral examination should be performed to check for thread, elastic etc. looped around the base of the tongue as, unless anchored, most linear foreign bodies pass uneventfully through the alimentary tract.

Ultrasonography can be valuable in the diagnosis of intestinal masses or intussusceptions; the latter have an onion ring appearance (see Fig. 36.18b). The presence of abdominal fluid will also be readily apparent in cases where there is peritonitis associated with intestinal rupture due to sharp foreign bodies or necrosis following intussusception. Long-standing linear foreign bodies will eventually 'cheesewire' through the intestinal wall.

Treatment

Stabilization of the patient for surgery is the main aim of therapy. This usually involves fluid therapy and antibacterial agents to reduce bacterial translocation from the stagnant loops of intestine. Intravenous antibacterial therapy may be required in some cases. Surgical relief of the obstruction can then be performed. Enterectomy is advisable if there is compromise of the intestinal wall. Plication of the intestines following an intussusception may also be necessary to reduce the likelihood of recurrence. Wound dehiscence and peritonitis is a recognized complication, typically occurring 3–5 days postsurgery. Adynamic ileus in response to chronic obstruction can also occur. Following surgery, fluids should be given intravenously for 12–24 h and food withheld for 24–48 h. In the long term, stricture can occur at the site of surgery resulting in recurrence of the clinical signs.

Small intestinal bacterial overgrowth (SIBO)

SIBO is a recognized cause of chronic diarrhoea in dogs and humans. In normal cats duodenal bacterial numbers are much higher (10^5–10^8 ml^{-1} of duodenal juice) and the fluid commonly contains obligate anaerobic bacteria hence SIBO in a cat can be difficult to demonstrate and its existence as a clinical entity in cats has not been well proven.

SIBO is not a diagnosis *per se* but a reflection of inadequate control of the intestinal bacterial flora. SIBO may occur for a variety of reasons:

- Achlorhydria and elevation of gastric pH which allows bacteria to survive passage through the stomach (Hoenig, 1980);
- Extensive use of broad spectrum antibacterials which allows proliferation of individual bacterial subpopulations;
- Paralytic ileus, pseudo-obstruction or intestinal obstruction which permits bacterial proliferation (Simpson, 1982);
- Impaired intestinal immunity associated with deficiency in intestinal IgA secretion (Whitbread *et al.*, 1984); German shepherd dogs and golden retrievers seem to be over-represented;

- The presence of undigested nutrients in the lumen permitting proliferation of bacteria secondary to maldigestion, e.g. exocrine pancreatic insufficiency or malabsorption, e.g. inflammatory bowel disease (IBD), lymphangiectasia.

Both aerobic and anaerobic bacteria may be involved resulting in damage to the jejunal mucosa. Organisms reported include *Pseudomonas aeruginosa* (Simpson, 1982), *Bacteroides* spp. (Reife *et al.*, 1980), *E. coli*, *enterococci*, and *Clostridium* spp. (Batt and Hall, 1989). Morphological changes can be seen on histopathological examination as a degree of villus atrophy and lymphocytic/plasmacytic infiltration (Rutgers *et al.*, 1988). Aerobic overgrowth causes loss of brush-border enzyme activity especially alkaline phosphatase. Anaerobic overgrowth can result in marked changes in the glycocalyx, interfering with mucosal protection which can lead to increased intestinal permeability (Leib, 1987; Batt and Hall, 1989). SIBO can result in deconjugation of bile salts and steatorrhoea. The increased luminal fat levels are converted by the bacteria into hydroxy fatty acids which, together with the deconjugated bile salts, result in a secretory diarrhoea (Simpson *et al.*, 1996). Carbohydrate may be utilized by the bacteria with production of metabolites which further exacerbate the diarrhoea (Batt, 1987). Increased hydroxy fatty acids can also result in large bowel signs with mucoid diarrhoea, blood and tenesmus.

Clinical findings

Dogs with SIBO frequently present with intermittent chronic diarrhoea which may or may not be associated with weight loss. In our clinic, a significant number of dogs also present with signs of large bowel diarrhoea which may be accompanied by weight loss. In some cases appetite will be reduced (secondary to cobalamin deficiency) although polyphagia and coprophagia are also seen. If weight loss is significant then the possibility of EPI or other causes of malabsorption should be considered. Over 70% of dogs with EPI have concurrent SIBO (Williams *et al.*, 1987). Historically, diarrhoea associated with SIBO is sensitive to antibacterial agents but recurs after therapy has ceased.

Diagnosis

SIBO is suggested by increased serum folate (50% of cases) and decreased serum cobalamin (25% of cases). Increased baseline levels of breath hydrogen and elevated breath hydrogen (above 6 ppm) within 2 h of feeding or the administration of lactulose are seen in 80% of cases (Washabau *et al.*, 1986). Definitive diagnosis is based on quantitative cultures of duodenal juice samples obtained during endoscopy. SIBO can also cause decreased xylose absorption which should be borne in mind when performing this test where malabsorption is suspected (Washabau *et al.*, 1986). Biopsy of the small intestine may reveal inflammatory bowel disease but this finding should be interpreted with care because although it can be a predisposing factor it can also occur as a result of chronic SIBO.

Treatment

Where possible the underlying cause, such as EPI, should be treated but many cases appear to be associated with defective immunoregulation. In this instance symptomatic therapy is required. This involves the use of antibacterial agents (Hall, 1989) and dietary management. Antibacterial agents should initially be given for one month but in refractory cases a two-month course followed by a gradual reduction in dose may produce remission. Appropriate treatment regimes would include:

- Oxytetracycline – 15–20 mg kg^{-1} tid
- Metronidazole – 10 mg kg^{-1} bid
- Tylosin – 20 mg kg^{-1} bid
- Low fat highly digestible diet
- ? diets containing fructo-oligosaccharides may be useful in controlling intestinal flora.

Prognosis

In cases where treatment of the underlying cause is not possible, therapy is aimed at controlling the clinical signs rather than curing the animal.

Eosinophilic enteritis

Aetiology

Eosinophilic enteritis is an uncommon diagnosis and may be associated with infiltration of the colon (eosinophilic enterocolitis) and stomach (eosinophilic gastroenteritis). In cats it can form part of a hypereosinophilic syndrome (HES) (Fig. 36.19) where there is also involvement of the bone marrow, kidney, liver, spleen, lymph nodes, heart and skin (Neer, 1991; Huibregtse and Turner, 1994). The relationship of HES to the eosinophilic variant of chronic myeloid leukaemia is unclear but eosinophilic leukaemia can also involve the small intestine.

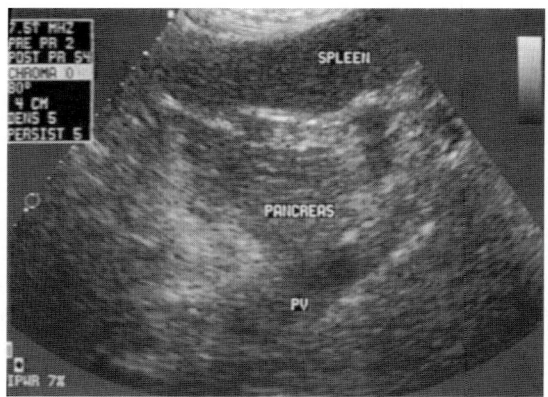

Figure 36.19 Ultrasound images of hypereosinophilic syndrome in a 10-year-old, neutered, male Russian blue cat which presented with a four-month history of weight loss and small intestinal diarrhoea. Note the thickening of the small intestinal wall (a) and the prominent echogenic pancreas (b).

The presence of eosinophils suggests an allergic aetiology but this has not been proven. The type of diet (Quigley and Henry, 1981), heavy burdens of *Toxocara canis* larvae (Hayden and Van Kruiningen, 1973) and mast cell tumours have been implicated in the pathogenesis. In the majority of cases there is no obvious aetiological agent and these cases are labelled 'idiopathic'.

Middle aged cats (average eight years) (Moore 1983) and young dogs (Quigley and Henry, 1981) are usually affected. German shepherd dogs and dobermann pinschers may be over-represented.

Clinical signs

Typically, patients present with weight loss and chronic small bowel diarrhoea. The severity of the disease depends on the degree and extent of the infiltration. Advanced disease causes severe weight loss, depression, anorexia, melaena or fresh blood. Hypoproteinaemia and occasionally ascites and subcutaneous oedema due to severe protein losing enteropathy occurs during the terminal-stages due to the extent of the intestinal mucosal damage and resultant increased permeability. On physical examination the intestines can feel thickened. Vomiting occurs more commonly in cats and in dogs if there is gastric involvement. Tenesmus, haematochezia and dyschezia suggests colonic involvement.

Diagnosis

Circulating eosinophilia greater than 1500×10^9 l^{-1} which in some cases may be as high as $70\,000 \times 10^9$ l^{-1} together with signs of intestinal disease are highly suggestive. Hypoproteinaemia with low serum albumin and globulin concentrations occurs in advanced cases. Definitive diagnosis is based on histological examination of biopsies obtained during endoscopy or laparotomy or cytological examination of ultrasound-guided fine needle aspirates of thickened intestinal loops. Worm egg counts should be performed on faecal samples.

Treatment

Eosinophilic infiltrates in cats tend to be less responsive to corticosteroid medication compared to dogs. Immunosuppressive doses of prednisolone (1–2 mg kg^{-1} divided bid in dogs; 3–4 mg kg^{-1} bid in cats) should be given for 2–4 weeks followed by a gradual dosage reduction over several months. Azathioprine (1–2 mg kg^{-1}) can be used to treat intractable cases in dogs but it may take between one and four weeks before a significant effect is appreciated. Hydroxyurea (12.5–15 mg kg^{-1} bid) has been used successfully in cats.

As diet may be a factor, a hypoallergenic diet containing a novel protein source should be provided. Ideally two diets should be available. The first, given during initial treatment, is a sacrifice diet to which the patient may become intolerant due to the ongoing inflammatory changes in the lamina propria. Once inflammation is controlled by treatment, a second (maintenance) diet is introduced.

Inflammatory bowel disease (IBD)

Aetiology

IBD is a description of an infiltrative condition of the lamina propria which can extend to involve the submucosa. A variety of inflammatory cells can be involved leading to the subclassification of IBD into lymphocytic/plasmacytic (most common), granulocytic, neutrophilic, histiocytic, necrotic, ulcerative and angiopathic (Jergens *et al.*, 1992; Wilcock, 1992).

Lymphocytic/plasmacytic IBD has been associated with giardiasis, lymphosarcoma, lymphangiectasia, SIBO and dietary hypersensitivity (DiBartola *et al.*, 1982; Franklin *et al.*, 1986; Rutgers 1989). Infiltration by lymphocytes and plasma cells may also occur in the stomach and colon. In the majority of cases of lymphocytic/plasmacytic IBD there is malabsorption and in advanced disease PLE can develop. In some cases lymphocytic/plasmacytic IBD may reflect the early stages of alimentary lymphosarcoma.

More recently a breakdown in tolerance to the normal bowel flora has been implicated in the pathogenesis of disease (Duchmann *et al.*, 1995) which can follow a minor inflammatory insult, e.g. diet change.

Lymphocytic/plasmacytic IBD is seen most frequently in middle-aged dogs with no sex or breed disposition other than in basenjis and lundehunds. In basenjis, PLE secondary to IBD is considered hereditary but the mode of inheritance is not known (Breitschwerdt *et al.*, 1980). Some basenjis have histological changes without overt disease (Maclauchlan *et al.*, 1988). IBD is one of the commonest causes of small intestinal disease in cats (Rutgers *et al.*, 1988).

Clinical signs

Dogs may present with vomiting and diarrhoea as the main clinical sign. Where vomiting is present, it is slowly progressive and usually contains bile or undigested food. The diarrhoea is usually typical of small intestinal disease and tends to be soft rather than liquid. Blood is rarely present. Clinical signs often wax and wane with acute 'flare-ups' which are associated with anorexia, depression and abdominal pain. Between episodes, appetite is variable and polyphagia may be present. There is progressive weight loss and in advanced cases PLE develops.

Cats tend to present with vomiting as a predominant clinical sign although this may, in part, reflect their natural reticence to defecate in front of the owner and the fact that they bury there faeces. Even so, diarrhoea is not consistently seen in all cases of feline IBD. Some cases show no GI signs and present with unexplained weight loss despite a good or sometimes increased appetite. Significant PLE is less common in cats.

Diagnosis

As IBD can occur either as a primary condition (idiopathic IBD) and secondary to a variety of other diseases (Table 36.27) a full gastrointestinal work-up needs to be performed in order to identify and treat the underlying cause. Diagnosis of IBD is based on histological examination of intestinal biopsies. Various attempts have been made to classify the severity of disease on a histological basis. As lymphocytes and plasma cells are normal residents of the lamina propria, subtle increases in their numbers may be of questionable significance as this is a subjective assessment and will depend on the pathologist concerned. At the other end of the spectrum severe infiltration can be difficult to differentiate from early lymphosarcoma. Varying degrees of villous atrophy are commonly present.

Classification of IBD into mild, moderate or severe should be based on the combination of clinical signs, e.g. degree of weight loss, frequency of acute episodes, presence of PLE as well as the histological findings.

Treatment

Client education is important when treating IBD as therapy is aimed at control rather than cure and

Table 36.27 Potential causes of inflammatory bowel disease in cats and dogs

Food allergy
Gluten sensitivity
Nematode parasites
Cryptosporidiosis
Giardiasis
Small intestinal bacterial overgrowth
Clostridium perfringens infection
Campylobacteriosis
? Salmonellosis
Hyperthyroidism
FeLV infection
FIV infection
Neoplasia

relapses will occur. Where possible dietary therapy alone should be tried. A low fat, highly digestible, gluten-free diet with a defined protein source is ideal. Diets with increased levels of potassium, water and fat-soluble vitamins are desirable. Strict adherence to a dietary trial for four to six weeks is essential.

In more severely affected animals concurrent drug therapy is required and an initial sacrifice diet followed by a second therapeutic diet may be appropriate (see under eosinophilic enteritis). Drug therapy for IBD may include:

- Prednisolone initially at immunosuppressive doses (1 mg kg^{-1} bid for dogs; 2–4 mg kg^{-1} bid for cats) for two to four weeks followed by gradual dose reduction over two to three months;
- Metronidazole may also be effective and may act by inhibiting cell-mediated immunity as well as controlling anaerobic overgrowth (dose 10 mg kg^{-1} bid) (Tams, 1987; Rutgers, 1989).
- Tylosin has also proved effective in the management of IBD (Van Kruiningen, 1976).
- Azathioprine (1–2 mg kg^{-1} for two weeks followed by alternate day therapy) for refractory cases in dogs. There is a lag effect of about seven days before full efficacy is attained.
- Azathioprine should be used with great care in cats (dose rates of 0.3–0.5 mg kg^{-1} on alternate days have been used). Cyclophosphamide (200 mg m^{-2}) once weekly may be a better alternative in cats.
- Cyclosporin has proved useful in the management of IBD in humans. Dose rates of 10 mg kg^{-1} p.o. bid for five days (repeated on a five days on, two days off basis) have been used in dogs and cats.
- Motility modifiers, e.g. short courses of opiate such as loperamide (0.1 mg kg^{-1} p.o. tid) or diphenoxylate (0.1–0.2 mg kg^{-1} p.o. tid) are of value in treating acute episodes of severe watery diarrhoea.

Adverse reactions to food

Adverse reactions to food are frequently seen in cats and dogs and may simply reflect dietary indiscretion or the feeding of a new diet that is substantially different from the animal's current food. Foods may also contain preformed toxins (food poisoning) which produces a rapid onset (within hours) of clinical signs or potentially pathogenic bacteria which are able to colonize the intestines of certain individuals and produce clinical signs some days later.

Dietary hypersensitivity

Aetiology

Hypersensitivity implies an immunological mechanism as distinct from food intolerance that does not. Food hypersensitivity can present as an acute, potentially life-threatening anaphylactic reaction (very rare), e.g. peanut allergy in children. More commonly immediate-type hypersensitivity is seen within several hours of feeding. Delayed-type hypersensitivity is thought to be the most prevalent type of food allergy in humans but is poorly characterized. Hypersensitivity occurs almost exclusively to dietary proteins or glycoproteins and may not always result in intestinal signs. It is estimated that around 10% of allergic skin disease is dietary based (Johnson, 1987). Food hypersensitivity can also affect the nervous, urinary or respiratory systems (White, 1986).

In the normal animal, the mucosal immune system is presented with small amounts of dietary protein absorbed by enterocyte endocytosis or via the M cells overlying the Peyer's patches. This type of presentation leads to tolerance to that protein by initiating a 'suppressor' T cell response. IgA antibodies are produced against potentially harmful antigens and excreted into the lumen where they prevent absorption of the antigen. Should the antigen enter the lamina propria it is complexed with IgA (which is not complement fixing) and transported to the liver for degradation and excretion in the bile.

Damage to the mucosal barrier leading to increased mucosal permeability may allow antigens to bypass these mucosal responses and initiate an inflammatory reaction involving the production of IgG or IgE antibodies (Batt and Hall, 1989).

As dietary hypersensitivity has an immunological pathogenesis, clinical signs are usually not associated with a sudden change of diet but occur towards antigens to which the patient has been exposed for some time (Johnson, 1987).

There appears to be no age, breed or sex predisposition to dietary hypersensitivity although a familial gluten sensitive enteropathy is described in Irish setters (Batt *et al.*, 1984). Dietary hypersensitivity towards milk, beef, mutton, chicken, rabbit, horse, fish, eggs, canned food, cod liver oil and mice have been described in cats (Wills, 1991). Milk, beef, cheese, dry and semi-moist diets and cereals account for 80% of cases in dogs (August, 1985). Hypersensitivity to pork, chicken, egg and fish is, at present, comparatively rare.

Clinical findings

Asthma, seizures and cystitis have been reported to be associated with food hypersensitivity but vomiting, diarrhoea and skin lesions are considerably more common (Merchant and Taboada, 1991).

A number of chronic enteropathies have been associated with food hypersensitivity including lymphocytic/plasmacytic IBD, eosinophilic enteritis and hypereosinophilic syndrome, idiopathic colitis, HGE and gluten sensitive enteropathy (Hayden and Van Kruiningen, 1982; Batt et al., 1984; Nelson et al., 1984; Franklin et al., 1986; Simpson, 1994). Dermatological signs include pruritus (which tends to be poorly responsive to corticosteroid medication), papular eruptions, alopecia, self-trauma and secondary bacterial infections (August, 1985). Skin lesions appear most frequently on the face, neck, ears, feet, axilla and ventral abdomen (Johnson, 1987).

Diagnosis

In addition to the clinical signs described above dietary hypersensitivity is suggested by:

- circulating eosinophilia;
- depressed folate and cobalamin levels;
- increased intestinal permeability (may be present when the only clinical signs are related to the skin and not the GIT);
- histopathological changes suggesting IBD, eosinophilic enteritis or gluten-sensitive enteropathy.

Definitive diagnosis is based on response to dietary trials. This involves resolution of clinical signs on a suitable exclusion diet followed by recurrence on provocation with the original food. Ideal diets contain single source proteins and non-gluten-containing carbohydrate. These can be given as preformed 'veterinary diets' or where possible home-made diets. As dietary therapy is becoming more widely used it is becoming increasingly difficult to find novel protein sources. For the majority of patients cottage cheese, chicken, rabbit or lamb are suitable.

In order for therapy to be effective, exclusion of other foods needs to be total which can be extremely difficult in cats that roam outside. It should be emphasized to clients that the diet and water should be fed to the exclusion of everything else. Exclusion should continue for at least three weeks and some cases may require up to 8–10 weeks before an improvement is seen. Provocative challenge is helpful in proving dietary involvement but many clients are understandably reluctant to do this.

Prognosis and management

Management relies on exclusion of the offending antigen(s) from the diet. In many cases dietary hypersensitivity may be the result of underlying permeability problems, in which case patients eventually develop sensitivity to the new diet. The prognosis for such cases is much poorer.

In the short term, corticosteroids and antihistamines may be beneficial in some animals but are rarely practical for long-term management (August, 1985).

Food intolerance

Dietary intolerance is suggested by an historical association between a particular food or food type and diarrhoea/vomiting, e.g. lactose intolerance in lactase-deficient animals. There is no documented evidence of an immunological mechanism and avoidance of that food prevents recurrence.

Food idiosyncrasy

Adverse reactions to certain food additives may produce a reaction similar to that associated with food hypersensitivity. Home cooked diets usually prevent recurrence.

Gluten-sensitive enteropathy

A familial gluten-sensitive enteropathy has been defined in Irish setters (Hall and Batt, 1990) but gluten sensitivity is likely to affect a wider number of dogs and cats. Clinical signs relate to the malassimilation of nutrients. In Irish setters the disease is seen between 4 to 7 months of age as a failure to gain weight accompanied by chronic diarrhoea. Histopathology of intestinal biopsies shows villus atrophy and crypt hyperplasia with an inflammatory infiltrate in the lamina propria.

Diagnosis is based on resolution of signs when the animal is fed a gluten-free diet and recurrence of clinical signs when the diet is withdrawn. The prognosis is generally good so long as the enteropathy is not advanced.

Protein losing enteropathy (PLE)

PLE refers to group of conditions in which there is leakage of plasma proteins into the intestines. The leakage allows loss of both albumin and

Table 36.28 Potential causes of protein-losing enteropathy

Gastric disease	Chronic gastritis
	Gastric ulceration
	Neoplasia
Small intestinal disease	Inflammatory bowel disease
	Eosinophilic enteritis
	Parasitic enteritis
	Neoplasia
	Lymphangiectasia
	Haemorrhagic gastroenteritis
Large intestinal disease	Colitis (idiopathic, ulcerative, histiocytic, granulomatous)
	Neoplasia

globulin into the intestinal lumen leading to the development of hypoproteinaemia. In the long-term, protein loss may result in ascites, pleural effusion and peripheral oedema (this usually occurs when the albumin concentration is less than 15 g l^{-1}).

PLE represents a progression of many intestinal diseases (Table 36.28) and generally worsens the prognosis for their successful management. Diagnosis of the underlying disease is essential for successful therapy.

In contrast, hypoproteinaemia secondary to liver failure or glomerulonephropathy results in the preferential loss of albumin. Globulin levels are usually normal or raised.

Lymphangiectasia

Lymphangiectasia is a chronic disease of the intestines associated with dilation and rupture of the lymphatic vessels in the villi, mucosa, submucosa and serosa which results in significant loss of plasma proteins (Burns, 1982; Sherding, 1986). In individual cases the aetiology is unknown but it may arise as a result of primary lymphatic disease or secondary to other systemic diseases (Table 36.29). Norwegian lundehund, Yorkshire terriers and Basenjis are predisposed but there is no age or sex predisposition. Lymphangiectasia is a significant PLE. Hypoproteinaemia, hypocholesterolaemia, lymphopenia and reduced secretion of IgA predispose to bacterial overgrowth and secondary bacterial infections (Suter *et al.*, 1985; Fossum, 1989). Significant loss of specific proteins may occur such as antithrombin III which may result in thromboembolism.

Clinical findings

The clinical presentation is usually typical of a PLE but chronic malabsorption of fat and fat soluble vitamins may be of significance. The majority of cases present with diarrhoea and weight loss. Initially animals can be polyphagic but they become inappetant with advancing disease. Occasionally an animal presents without a history of diarrhoea but with marked weight loss, anaemia and fluid effusions.

Diagnosis

History and clinical signs strongly suggest a PLE. Plasma concentrations of folate and cobalamin are usually low. SIBO is common. Hypocalcaemia may be present, even when correction for the hypoalbuminaemia is made, due to hypovitaminosis D. Permeability testing is abnormal (Table 36.3). Ultrasonography reveals thickening of the small intestinal wall with values greater than 5 mm in dogs and 3 mm in cats. A definitive diagnosis is based on histological examination of biopsy material. At endoscopy the small intestine may appear more granular and patches of white, lipid-filled dilated villi may be present. Biopsy reveals dilation of the lacteals, a degree of villus atrophy and crypt hyperplasia (Batt and Hall, 1989). In some cases diagnosis can only be made from full thickness biopsies which demonstrate submucosal lymphatic obstruction. Surgical biopsies carry an increased risk of dehiscence as most patients are debilitated and markedly hypoalbuminaemic.

Treatment

Regardless of cause, lymphangiectasia carries a guarded prognosis since the individual response to treatment is unpredictable and very variable.

Prednisolone at 1 mg kg^{-1} bid in combination with tylosin may be of value in reducing inflam-

Table 36.29 Aetiology of lymphangiectasia

Hereditary	Norwegian lundehund
	Yorkshire terrier
	Basenji
Primary lymphatic disease	Congenital abnormality of intestinal lymphatics
	Extraintestinal lymphatic abnormality
	Lymphangitis
	Lymphatic obstruction (inflammation, neoplasia, extralymphatic mass)
Secondary to systemic disease	Congestive heart failure
	Constrictive pericarditis
	Portal hypertension

mation and controlling secondary bacterial overgrowth. A low fat, highly digestible diet is essential. Caloric intake can be increased with careful addition of medium chain triglycerides (e.g. 1–2 ml kg^{-1} coconut oil) as medium-chain triglycerides are absorbed directly into the portal circulation (Sherding, 1986; Fossum, 1989). Protein intake can be increased with low fat cottage cheese. Any dietary change needs to be introduced slowly.

Volvulus and strangulation of the small intestine

Volvulus, torsion or strangulation of the bowel results in rapid ischaemia and an acute abdominal crisis. If tissue becomes transiently ischaemic, significant reperfusion injury may occur following surgical correction. Small intestinal volvulus is rare and is more common in German shepherd dogs (EPI may be a possible predisposing factor in this breed). Clinical signs, consistent with intestinal obstruction, include vomiting, anorexia, pain and defecation of small amounts of bloody faeces. Radiographically there are gas-filled distended loops of bowel. Mortality rates are high and efforts should be made to reduce the risk of reperfusion injury by allowing a gradual return of the blood supply to the affected loops of bowel. Treatment consists of surgical correction and/or resection.

Small intestinal strangulation can occur following abdominal tears, hernias or adhesions. The umbilical and inguinal regions are common sites after abdominal trauma.

Short bowel syndrome

Short bowel syndrome in dogs and cats is generally iatrogenic. It is a sequel to radical bowel resection in cases of intussusception, volvulus or strangulation where more than 85% of the small bowel is removed. Malabsorption results in chronic diarrhoea, weight loss, SIBO and foul-smelling faeces. Following radical bowel resection mucosal hyperplasia attempts to replace the lost surface area but this may take several weeks to months. Highly digestible, low fat diets are indicated and small quantities of gel-forming fibre may help. Parenteral cobalamin or folate supplementation may be required if the specific absorptive sites have been lost. Broad-spectrum antibacterial agents can be given to treat the SIBO and H$_2$ blockers to treat gastric hyperacidity if necessary. Cholestyramine may help to bind malabsorbed bile acids but can lead to taurine depletion in cats. Loperamide may reduce the severity of the diarrhoea.

Motility disorders of the small intestine

Adynamic ileus

A transient lack of small intestinal peristalsis results in pooling of intestinal contents in the dependent areas of the GIT. A variety of causes of adynamic ileus are described including abdominal surgery, electrolyte imbalance, inflammation of the intestinal tract, pancreas, peritoneum or other abdominal organs. Canine parvovirus, autonomic neuropathies and anticholinergic drugs may also cause adynamic ileus. Clinical signs include anorexia, vomiting, depression, mild abdominal distension and pain due to the accumulation of gas in the hypomotile bowel.

Auscultation reveals a lack of gut sounds and abdominal radiographs usually show distended loops of gas- and fluid-filled intestine. GI transit time is delayed with a tendency to retain BIPS in the stomach or to scatter them along the length of the GIT.

Treatment relies on identification of the primary cause. Prokinetic drugs such as metoclopramide or cisapride may be helpful.

Intestinal neoplasia

A variety of tumours may be associated with the small intestine. The majority are primary tumours and, of these, adenocarcinoma (Fig. 36.20), lymphosarcoma (Fig. 36.21), adenoma, adenomatous polyps and leiomyosarcoma are most commonly reported (Head and Else, 1981). The tumour may cause partial or total obstruction, or mucosal invasion may result in maldigestion and malabsorption. Siamese cats appear to be predisposed to adenocarcinoma.

Adenocarcinomas are most frequently seen as mass lesions in middle aged to older animals. They present as obstructive lesions and are frequently ulcerated leading to melaena. The clinical signs are typically insidious in onset with increasing frequency of vomiting, diarrhoea and weight loss. Diagnosis is based on abdominal palpation, radiographic abnormalities and the results of fine

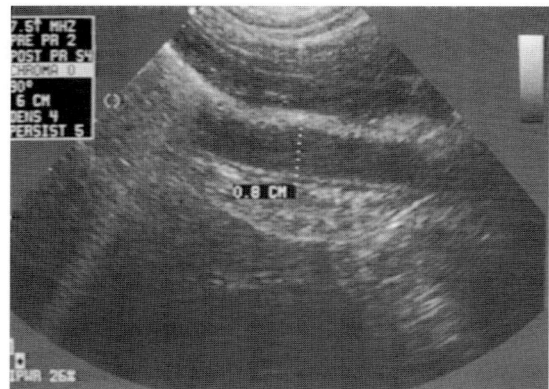 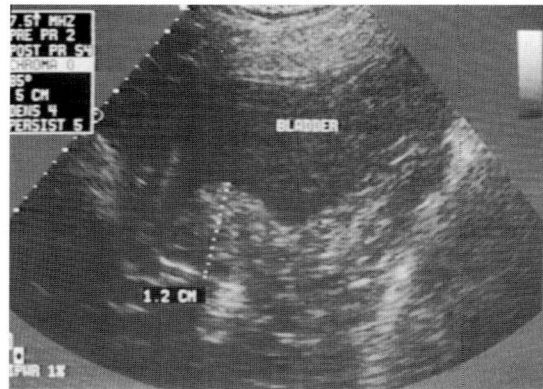

Figure 36.20 Ultrasound images of diffuse thickening of the small intestinal wall (a) and the presence of a mass within the bladder wall (b) in an 8-year-old, neutered, female Staffordshire bull terrier which presented with a four-month history of vomiting, diarrhoea and weight loss. A diagnosis of a metastatic intestinal adenocarcinoma was made on histopathological examination of biopsies obtained at coeliotomy.

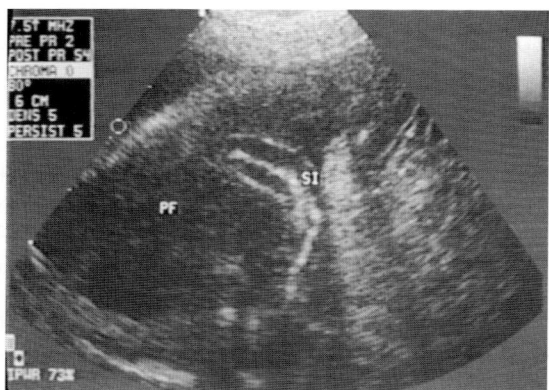

Figure 36.21 Diffuse thickening of the small intestinal (SI) wall and free peritoneal fluid (PF) in an 8-year-old, male Rottweiler dog which presented with a one-month history of weight loss and diarrhoea. A diagnosis of lymphosarcoma was made on cytological examination of ultrasound-guided fine needle aspirates of the thickened intestinal wall. The peritoneal fluid was a septic exudate.

needle aspiration cytology or histological examination of biopsy material obtained percutaneously or at exploratory laparotomy. Many cases have already metastasized to the regional lymph nodes and more distant tissues by the time of presentation. Where appropriate, surgical removal with adjunctive chemotherapy offers the best prognosis.

Lymphosarcomas are more common in young adult dogs and cats. They can present as an obstructive mass lesion but more commonly diffusely invade the mucosa causing chronic diarrhoea, weight loss and PLE in advanced cases. Approximately 30% of cats are FeLV positive and FIV-associated tumours have also been described. Palpable thickening of the small intestines occurs and usually there is evidence of malabsorption and, in some cases, bacterial overgrowth. Diagnosis is based on fine-needle aspiration cytology or histological examination of biopsy material taken either endoscopically or during surgery. Alimentary lymphosarcoma carries a grave prognosis. Solitary nodular masses can be resected and the animal can be given adjunctive chemotherapy. Standard chemotherapy protocols have been used for the treatment of diffuse lymphosarcoma but the results have generally been disappointing.

COLONIC DISEASE

Introduction

Food residues normally reach the colon 4–6 h after food is ingested and remain in the colon for 24–48 h. The colon acts to conserve water by absorbing fluid and electrolytes from the ileal residues. The majority of absorption occurs in the ascending and transverse colon where segmented contractions and retrograde peristalsis retain and mix the ileal residue (Burrows and Merritt, 1983). The colon has a functional reserve which can assist in water absorption in the presence of small intestinal disease.

Once adequate water absorption has occurred,

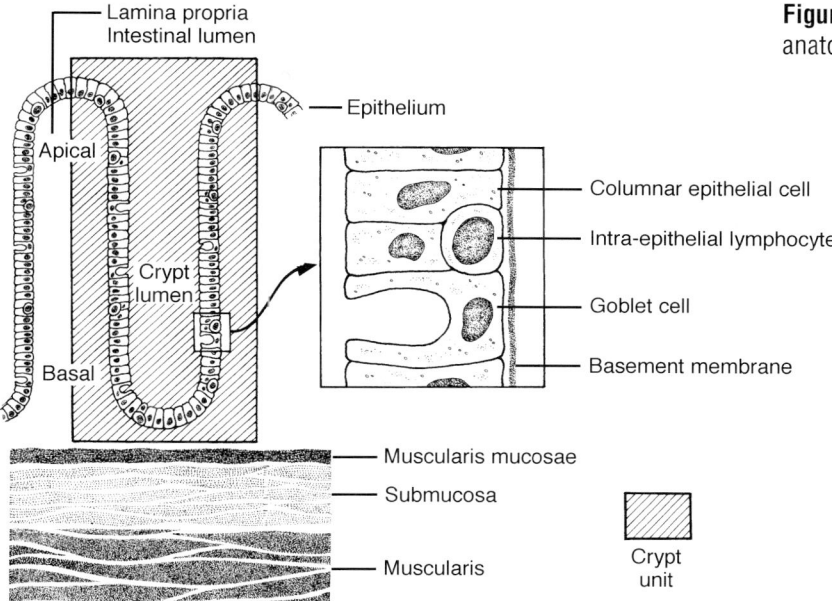

Figure 36.22 Diagram of the microscopic anatomy of the colon.

peristalsis sweeps the colonic residue into the descending colon for storage prior to defecation. Faecal material is normally not present in the post-pelvic colon. The passage of faeces along the colon is facilitated by the large amounts of mucus produced by the goblet cells. The main stimulus for colonic contraction is distension of the lumen.

The colonic mucosa is folded into a series of crypts which contain many mucus-secreting cells but no villi (Fig. 36.22). Unlike the small intestine, the lymphoid tissue is not arranged in a series of patches but is spread throughout the colon as lymphoid aggregates.

Colonic disease results in a disruption of the normal absorptive capacity, lubrication and motility of the colon and is characterized by watery diarrhoea, haematochezia, dyschezia, tenesmus, excess mucus production, constipation and megacolon.

Colitis

Aetiology

Inflammatory disease of the colon can be seen alone or as part of a more generalized gastroenterocolitis. If signs of colitis persist for more than three weeks duration it is generally considered to be chronic.

Colitis has generally been classified according to the predominant cellular infiltrate rather than by aetiology (Table 36.30). The pathogenesis of colitis is poorly understood and it is not known whether the histological changes represent different clinical conditions or different stages of the same condition or variations in expression of a few conditions.

Various aetiological agents have been suggested including viruses, fungi and bacteria, *Trichuris vulpis*, renal failure and dietary hypersensitivity (Bolton and Brown, 1972; Nelson *et al.*, 1984; Simpson and Else, 1991c). An ulcerative colitis has been described in FIV-positive specific pathogen free cats (Sturgess, 1997). The involvement of the immune system is clear and many forms of colitis respond to metronidazole which may act by suppressing cell-mediated immunity (Tams, 1987). Dietary hypersensitivity may also play a significant role as clinical improvement has been seen with 'hypoallergenic' diets (Nelson *et*

Table 36.30 Classification of canine and feline colitis

- Idiopathic, non-ulcerative colitis
- Eosinophilic colitis
- Histiocytic colitis
- Granulomatous colitis
- Parasitic colitis
- (Mycotic colitis)

al., 1984; Simpson *et al.*, 1994). However, the colon is unlikely to be a major site for the development of dietary sensitivity.

Idiopathic colitis

Non-ulcerative idiopathic colitis is relatively common in dogs (Bush, 1985) but rare in cats (Rutgers, 1989). It is characterized by a lymphocytic/plasmacytic infiltrate of the mucosa and submucosa. As the disease progresses fibrosis occurs which can lead to stricture formation.

In general, colitis appears to be more common in young, adult dogs. There is no sex predisposition but German shepherds, golden retrievers and rough collies are to be over-represented.

Eosinophilic colitis

Eosinophilic colitis may occur alone or as part of a more generalized eosinophilic (gastro)enterocolitis or hypereosinophilic syndrome. An accompanying circulating eosinophilia is common. This condition can result in colonic ulceration and diarrhoea containing fresh blood.

Histiocytic colitis

Histiocytic colitis is characterized by ulceration and infiltration of the mucosa and submucosa with periodic acid–Schiff-positive macrophages or histiocytes. Boxers are predisposed to histiocytic colitis but there have also been reports in French bulldog (Bush, 1985) and in a cat (Van Kruiningen and Dobbins, 1979).

Granulomatous colitis

Granulomatous colitis tends to cause focal, proliferative lesions characterized by infiltration with macrophages, giant cells, lymphocytes and plasma cells. It probably represents a distinct entity although some workers feel that it shows similar features to cases of histiocytic and eosinophilic colitis (Van Kruiningen *et al.*, 1983). Granulomatous colitis shows similarities to Crohn's disease in humans (Ewing and Gomez, 1973).

Clinical signs

The onset of signs is typically associated with stress or excitement (Bush, 1985). Dogs and cats remain bright and alert, have a normal appetite and do not lose weight. The diarrhoea can vary from watery to mucoid and jelly-like with fresh blood. The blood is typically mixed with the stool in contrast to rectal or anal lesions when the blood lies on the surface of formed faeces (haematochezia). Vomiting may occur in approximately 30% of cases and is due to vagal stimulation of the vomiting centre rather than transmural spread of the inflammation causing concurrent gastritis. Many animals exhibit tenesmus (Simpson, 1996), dyschezia, and increased urgency and frequency of defecation.

Ulceration may be associated with eosinophilic, histiocytic or granulomatous colitis (it is rare in lymphocytic/plasmacytic disease) and results in significant haematochezia and dyschezia. Pyrexia is seen in some cases of granulomatous colitis.

Diagnosis

Faecal examination for endoparasites and bacteria, particularly *Salmonella* spp., *Campylobacter* spp. and *Trichuris vulpis*, should be carried out. Shedding of oocysts in *T. vulpis* infections is intermittent and therefore the condition may not be readily diagnosed.

Breath hydrogen studies and measurement of plasma folate and cobalamin concentrations may help to rule out cases of SIBO presenting with large bowel signs. Plain radiography is rarely rewarding. A double contrast enema may identify the presence of a stricture or consistent mural lesion.

Definitive diagnosis of colonic disease requires endoscopy and biopsy. Endoscopy will reveal the presence of ulcerative changes and mucosal thickening which is seen as a granular or cobblestone appearance with poor visibility of the submucosal blood vessels. The mucosa may be friable and bleed easily when touched by the endoscope. Multiple biopsies should be taken from regions where there is obvious pathology. If no macroscopic lesions are evident serial biopsies should be obtained from the entire length of the colon.

Histological changes include inflammatory cell infiltration of the lamina propria, goblet cell hyperplasia and increased numbers of intraepithelial lymphocytes (a non-specific response to inflammation). Occasional mixed infiltrates are observed (van Der Gaag *et al.*, 1990) which may support a common aetiology for colitis. Mucosal whipworm larvae may be present in cases of parasitic colitis.

Treatment

Initially, control of colitis should be attempted using sulphasalazine and dietary therapy (Ridgeway, 1984). The dose for sulphasalazine is as follows:

- Dogs 12.5 mg kg^{-1} p.o. qid for 14 days then 12.5 mg kg^{-1} p.o. bid for 28 days;
- Cats 10–20 mg kg^{-1} p.o. sid for 14 days.

Keratoconjunctivitis sicca (KCS) is a major potential complication of sulphasalazine therapy and tear production should be checked before and at regular intervals during treatment in dogs. If tear production decreases drug therapy should be withdrawn.

Newer aminosalicylates, mesalazine and olsalazine which contain 5-aminosalicylate are reported to have a reduced risk of causing KCS (Barnett and Joseph, 1987) but tear production should still be monitored. Tablets are enteric coated so are unsuitable for smaller dogs and cats. Sulphasalazine is unlikely to be effective in eosinophilic or granulomatous colitis.

If the response to sulphasalazine is poor, or in cases of eosinophilic or granulomatous colitis, then immunosuppressive doses of corticosteroids can be used alone or as an adjunctive therapy. In the most severe cases azathioprine may be required (contraindicated in cats).

Chronic corticosteroid therapy can also be given rectally as enema or foam preparations. Enemas are generally better tolerated by the patients and allow topical administration of corticosteroids and reduction of the total dose. Tylosin has proven useful in the management of granulomatous colitis.

Diet plays an important part in the therapy of colitis. Currently, select protein 'hypoallergenic' diets are favoured in the treatment of colitis rather than low residue or high fibre diets due to the possible role of dietary hypersensitivity. Hypoallergenic diets also tend to be low residue. A protein source to which the patient has not previously been exposed (Nelson et al., 1984) should be fed. The use of such diets has improved periods of drug-free remission (Simpson et al., 1994) in cases of chronic colitis.

Despite treatment, relapses are common and the aim is to manage rather than cure the condition. In general the lymphocytic/plasmacytic and eosinophilic forms of colitis in dogs respond well to treatment whereas granulomatous and histiocytic colitis is less responsive.

■ Irritable bowel syndrome (IBS)

Aetiology

A significant minority (up to about 17%) of cases of large bowel diarrhoea (Henroteaux, 1990) will show no histological evidence of inflammatory disease. This group may have a motility disorder causing a functional diarrhoea with clinical signs being worsened or initiated by stress. Most affected individuals do not have an overtly abnormal environment, rather IBS appears to reflect an abnormal stress response to common events.

The disorder is seen in all ages and breeds of dog but appears to be more common in working dogs or highly excitable or nervous animals. Many dogs may have the potential to develop IBS but because of their sedentary lifestyle problems never become apparent.

Clinical presentation

Typically cases have a long history of intermittent, non-responsive diarrhoea (soft stools) with episodes of acute exacerbation. Despite this there is little or no deterioration in physical condition and the animal remains appetant, bright and alert. During acute episodes, the diarrhoea tends to be watery and mucoid but rarely bloody. Excessive borborygmi, flatulence, tenesmus and abdominal discomfort may be seen.

Rarely, dogs may present with dyschezia or constipation associated with colonic spasm. The history may also reveal some alteration to the dog's lifestyle such as moving house, the arrival of a baby or a working dog undergoing training.

Diagnosis

Diagnosis is based on exclusion of other causes of the clinical signs and identifying an association with a change in lifestyle. If removal of that change results in clinical improvement then a diagnosis of IBS is supported.

Treatment

Where possible environmental change should be minimized. Dietary change to a low allergen, low fat, highly digestible, low fermentability diet achieves the most promising results. The traditional high fibre diets used in IBS may exacerbate the signs in some dogs.

Various types of pharmacological management have been used. Motility modifiers such as cisapride or mebeverine hydrochloride (an antispasmodic; 2 mg kg^{-1} p.o. tid) have variable success. Diphenoxylate and loperamide are sometimes helpful in the short term (Chiapella, 1986). The use of anxiolytic drugs such as diazepam may also be helpful in restoring normal faecal consistency during a period of acute disease. Many cases will improve as the dog gets older but the prognosis remains guarded unless the underlying cause can be identified and removed.

Constipation

Aetiology

Constipation can be defined as the absence of defaecation (obstipation is intractable constipation). It is important to differentiate an enlarged colon due to constipation from an enlarged colon due to megacolon that subsequently becomes impacted. Constipation occurs when there is interference with the passage of faeces through the rectum and anus (Fig. 36.23).

Retention of faeces in the colon results in further water absorption making the faeces harder and less deformable and thus more difficult to pass. Initially there will be considerable efforts to defaecate but with time these efforts will diminish which must not be interpreted as improvement. With time colonic motility diminishes, intrinsic neurones degenerate and megacolon develops.

Clinical findings

Dogs are usually presented earlier in the course of disease as the owner notices their attempts to defecate. Animals will occasionally vomit and may produce ribbon-like faeces if there is partial obstruction caused by pelvic lesions or prostatic disease. Some cases present with apparent diarrhoea as a small amount of watery mucoid material is all that is produced. Cats tend to present with more advanced disease as their constipation tends to remain unobserved as they attempt to defecate outside.

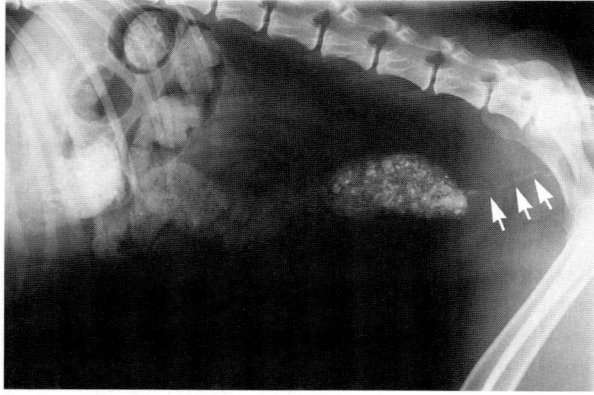

Figure 36.23 Constipation in a 10-year-old female crossbred dog which presented with a one-year history of faecal tenesmus. Note the mineral density of the faeces indicating the chronicity of the constipation and the thin line of faeces (arrows) in the terminal colon caused by an obstructive adenocarcinoma.

Constipated animals may become anorexic and depressed and may show evidence of abdominal pain.

Diagnosis

A diagnosis of constipation can usually be made on physical examination but further efforts should then be made to define the underlying cause. This should include a neurological examination, pelvic and lumbosacral radiographs, a serum biochemistry profile including electrolytes, assessment of hydration status and rectal examination (if possible).

Treatment

Rehydration of the patient is an essential first step. Severely constipated animals may have to be anaesthetized to allow lubricated warm water enemas to be given and for the faecal mass to be gently broken down by manual fragmentation. Lactulose, liquid paraffin, docusate sodium (Sherding, 1990) or saline will aid the softening and lubrication process. Soapy enemas should be avoided as they will irritate the colon (Hoskins, 1990). Phosphate enemas and large volumes of glycerine are toxic in cats and should not be used. On rare occasions a coeliotomy and colotomy may be required to remove very hardened concretions particularly in cats.

Prevention of constipation involves correction of the underlying cause, increasing exercise levels, providing a high fibre (>10% dry matter) diet and minimizing predisposing causes by regular grooming and removal of ectoparasites.

Continuous long-term use of laxatives should be avoided as they can cause increased intestinal fluid loss. A wide variety of laxatives are available (Sherding, 1994); bulk-forming laxatives are preferable for longer-term use.

Pseudocoprostasis is most common in long-haired dogs and cats. Careful removal of the faecal mass under sedation general anaesthetic should be performed. Trapped faeces may then be expelled with some force! The hair covering the perianal region should subsequently be kept short and any faecal soiling of the perineum cleaned away immediately.

Megacolon

Aetiology

Congenital and acquired megacolon are seen in both dogs and cats. Cats appear to be more frequently affected than dogs. The condition is characterized by a dilated hypomotile colon.

Congenital disease is associated with the absence of the myenteric plexus and an agangliosis of the distal colon or rectum (Webb, 1985). This results in a state of constant tone and pseudo-obstruction leading to dilation of the colon proximally, chronic constipation and then development of a megacolon (Burrows, 1986b). Loss of enteric hormones such as VIP and substance P may also lead to megacolon. Interference with the normal defecation reflex may occur in animals with sacral spinal cord defects.

Acquired megacolon may follow a variety of causes which result in chronic constipation and ultimately loss of tone within the colonic musculature (Table 36.31).

Clinical findings

Clinically, megacolon presents identically to constipation. In some cases, where the megacolon is due to dysautonomia, other systemic signs may be evident, e.g. megaoesophagus, prominent third eyelids, lack of tear and saliva production. A careful neurological examination should be performed to identify any associated deficits in bladder or hind limb function.

Diagnosis

A diagnosis of constipation is made if the colon remains flaccid and fails to contract after removal of the faecal material. Congenital megacolon requires excisional biopsy to demonstrate agangliosis.

Treatment

It is rarely possible to restore colonic motility and constipation rapidly recurs. Bulking agents and prokinetic drugs, such as cisapride and bethanechol (Davis and Baggot, 1980), may help but frequently fail to elicit a response. Bethanechol can be given at 0.25 mg kg^{-1} p.o. tid to dogs and 1–5 mg cat^{-1} p.o. tid. Ultimately many cases require subtotal colectomy (Webb, 1985; Bright et al.,

Table 36.31 Causes of constipation in cats and dogs

Dietary	Indigestible material, e.g. bone, fur, wool Low residue diets
Inactivity	Obesity Kennelling/hospitalization
Psychological	Territorial competition Dirty litter tray
Difficulty in posturing to defecate	Neurological deficits Orthopaedic disease, e.g. hip dysplasia, spinal pain, pelvic fractures
Painful anorectal conditions	Anal sac disease Anorectal stricture Perianal bite wounds Pseudocoprostasis (faeces impacted around anus)
Anorectal obstruction	Extraluminal, e.g. fractures, pelvic, intrapelvic or perineal masses Intraluminal, e.g. perineal hernia, rectal prolapse, faecolith
Megacolon	Idiopathic Dysautonomia Lumbosacral neurological disease Hypothyroidism
Fluid/electrolyte imbalance	Dehydration Hypokalaemia Hyper- or hypocalcaemia
Drug-related	Anticholinergics Opioids Sucralfate Barium Aluminium hydroxide antacids Calcium channel blockers Antihistamines

1986). A decision regarding surgery should not be delayed too long as a megacolon of greater than six months standing responds less well to surgery. Chronic diarrhoea may follow surgery but usually resolves. Where possible the ileocolic valve should be left in place to prevent ascending infection. Surgery in dogs tends to be less successful than in cats.

■ Colonic neoplasia

Adenocarcinoma, lymphosarcoma and polyps are the most common colonic tumours in cats and dogs (Head and Else, 1981). In one study, there appeared an association between neoplasia and low fibre diets, steatorrhoea and colitis (Crow, 1985). FeLV and FIV can be involved in the pathogenesis in cats.

Adenocarcinomas (Fig. 36.24) tend to be focal lesions which frequently ulcerate becoming secondarily infected and causing obstruction of the colon. The majority of lesions are found in the terminal colon and rectum. Metastatic spread to the sublumbar lymph nodes and beyond is common.

Lymphosarcomas are generally diffuse and may involve the entire colon. They rarely ulcerate or cause obstruction but they interfere with water and electrolyte reabsorption from the faeces.

Polyps are benign and only significant if they cause obstruction or bleed. They are commonly found in the rectum.

Clinical findings

Clinical signs especially of obstruction and constipation can appear suddenly even though the growth of the tumour has been slow. Adenocarcinomas and polyps cause obstructive signs, e.g. tenesmus and dyschezia whereas lymphosarcoma is more likely to cause watery diarrhoea. Lymphosarcomas and adenocarcinomas are associated with marked wasting and progressive loss of colonic function.

Diagnosis

Neoplasia is suggested based on physical examination, contrast radiography (adenocarcinomas typically produce an apple core filling defect), ultrasonography and endoscopic appearance. Definitive diagnosis relies on cytology of ultrasound-guided fine needle aspirates or histological examination of percutaneous tru-cut or endoscopic biopsies. Adenocarcinomas appear as discrete often ulcerated lesions whereas lymphosarcomas impart a more granular appearance to the colonic mucosa. Polyps appear as pedunculate lesions extending from the rectal wall.

Treatment

Polyps can be removed surgically though they occasionally regrow. Neither lymphosarcomas nor adenocarcinomas respond well to surgical or chemotherapeutic management.

■ DISEASES OF THE ANORECTAL REGION

■ Faecal incontinence

Faecal incontinence is a serious problem with 50% of pets being euthanased within a few days of its onset. The majority of animals are elderly. True faecal incontinence is caused by anal sphincter failure. Reservoir incontinence where animals have a poor capacity to store faeces is characterized by frequent conscious voiding rather than the passive dribbling of faeces.

Aetiology

Faecal incontinence can be caused by local problems associated with primary sphincter dysfunction, e.g. inflammatory lesions, post-anal surgery, or secondary to neoplasia. Sphincter dysfunction may also occur due to neuromuscular disease, e.g.

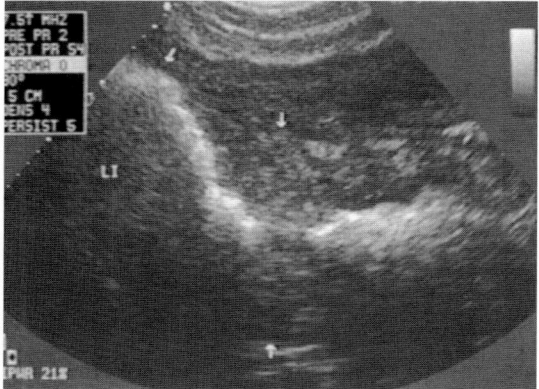

Figure 36.24 Localized thickening of the colon due to a well-differentiated adenocarcinoma in a 10-year-old female crossbred dog which presented with a one-year history of faecal tenesmus and fresh blood in the stool. LI, large intestine; arrows indicate the margins of the large intestinal wall.

neuropathies, myopathies, CNS disease and cauda equina syndromes. In old animals sphincter tone is poor and animals with diarrhoea are more likely to become incontinent.

Diagnosis

It is important to try and define the primary cause of the incontinence. This may require extensive medical and neurological investigations.

Treatment

Where possible this should be directed towards the primary disease. Where the cause is inapparent or untreatable, surgical implantation of a perianal silastic sling has been shown to be of value. Medical therapy should be aimed at reducing faecal water and faecal bulk, slowing transit time and increasing sphincter tone. This can be achieved with opiate motility modifiers (Table 36.25) or alpha-adrenergic agonists, e.g. phenylpropanolamine.

Rectal stricture

Rectal strictures are relatively common in dogs but rare in cats. They can be congenital or acquired. The most common cause of acquired stricture formation is post-anorectal surgery, but trauma, severe inflammatory disease of the large bowel and tumours are also reported (Seim, 1986). The tenesmus that the stricture causes induces further inflammation and fibrosis.

Clinical findings

Dogs present with a history of episodic tenesmus, dyschezia, haematochezia and the passage of ribbon-like faeces. Pain may be marked with the animal crying as it attempts to defecate.

Diagnosis

Strictures can usually be identified on rectal examination as a narrow band of tissue encompassing the rectum. Colonoscopy should be performed to rule out neoplasia.

Treatment

In the absence of neoplasia the fibrous band can be broken down under general anaesthesia and prednisolone at 1 mg kg^{-1} day^{-1} given to minimize the chances of recurrence. Bulking agents should be used to produce soft well-formed faeces.

Many strictures do, unfortunately, reform and surgical resection may be required which predisposes the animal to faecal incontinence. Surgery is also indicated if there is neoplasia.

Proctitis

Inflammation of the rectum usually accompanies colitis but it occasionally occurs in isolation. Clinically the animal may present with tenesmus and dyschezia without diarrhoea. Biopsy usually reveals a lymphocytic/plasmacytic infiltrate but eosinophilic infiltrates and focal suppurative lesions are occasionally seen. Treatment consists of feeding a low allergy diet containing fermentable fibre, and sulphasalazine. Severe cases may require intrarectal corticosteroid enemas.

Perineal hernia

Perineal hernias are relatively common in older, particularly male, dogs and are occasionally seen in cats. The pelvic diaphragm fails and the rectum and in some cases also the bladder prolapses through the defect causing tenesmus, dyschezia, constipation and urinary obstruction. Rectal examination reveals dilatation or deviation of the rectum. Atrophy of the pelvic muscles may also be appreciated. Perineal herniation may be a sequel to any cause of chronic tenesmus which should be addressed before repair to reduce the risk of recurrence. Idiopathic, degenerative hernias also occur. Surgical fixation may require the use of mesh implants.

Rectal prolapse

Rectal prolapse is most common in young animals following persistent diarrhoea and tenesmus. The prolapse may be just mucosal or involve the whole rectal wall as a tubular mass which needs to be differentiated from a colonic intussusception. Small prolapses can be manually reduced and a purse-string suture applied together with intrarectal administration of local anaesthetic or corticosteroid ointment or enemas. Extensive or chronic prolapses may require surgical resection. Recurrent prolapses need colopexy.

Anal sac disease

Anal sac disease presents as 'scooting' in dogs and excessive licking in cats where it is less common.

When the anal sac becomes severely inflamed dyschezia and haematochezia may develop. Impacted glands will occasionally abscess. Management is by gentle evacuation. Recurrent cases can be treated by instillation of antibiotic/corticosteroid cream into the sacs. If this fails chemical cautery with tincture of iodine or removal is appropriate. Apocrine adenocarcinomas of the anal sacs are malignant tumours which often produce parathyroid hormone-like substances leading to hypercalcaemia. Metastasis is common as is local recurrence following removal.

Perianal fistula

Perianal fistulas are chronic inflammatory lesions of the perianal tissue. They are particularly common in middle-aged to older German shepherds and to a lesser extent Irish setters and labradors but all breeds as well as cats can be affected. Clinical signs include licking and 'scooting', and advanced cases may show dyschezia and tenesmus. The fistulas usually discharge a foul-smelling, purulent and/or bloody discharge. Lesions begin as small ulcers and can eventually develop to extend into the pelvis. Successful treatment usually involves radical, frequently repeated, surgery. Faecal incontinence is the most frequent postoperative complication.

Imperforate anus and rectal agenesis

These deformities are usually recognized within days of birth. Occasionally they become obvious when constipation leads to marked abdominal distension. Imperforate ani can be easily dealt with by perforation. Atresi ani also carries a good prognosis. Rectal agenesis requires major surgery and careful examination for other anorectovaginal deformities should be carried out before attempting surgical correction.

REFERENCES

August, J.R. (1983) Gastrointestinal disorders in the cat. *Veterinary Clinics of North America* **13**, 585–597.

August, J.R. (1985) Dietary hypersensitivity in dogs: cutaneous manifestations, diagnosis and management. *Compendium of Continuing Education* **7**, 469–477.

Barnett, K.C. and Joseph, E.C. (1987) Keratonconjunctivitis sicca in the dog following 5-aminosalicylic acid administration. *Human Toxicology* **6**, 377–383.

Barr, S.C. and Bowman, D.D. (1994) Giardiasis in dogs and cats. *Compendium of Continuing Education* **16**, 603–610.

Basher, A.W.P., Hogan, P.M., Hanna, P.E., Runyon, C.L. and Shaw, D.H. (1991) Surgical correction of a congenital bronchoesophageal fistula in a dog. *Journal of the American Veterinary Association* **199**, 479–482.

Batt, R.M. (1986) New approaches to malabsorption in dogs. *Compendium of Continuing Education* **8**, 783–795.

Batt, R.M. (1987) The effects of intestinal bacterial overgrowth on mucosal enzymes and absorption in the dog. *Veterinary Annual* **27**, 188–195.

Batt, R.M. and Hall, E.J. (1989) Chronic enteropathies in the dog. *Journal of Small Animal Practice* **30**, 3–12.

Batt, R.M., Medham, J.R. and Carter, M.W. (1983) Bacterial overgrowth associated with a naturally occurring enteropathy in the German Shepherd dog. *Research in Veterinary Science* **35**, 42–46.

Batt, R.M., Carter, M.W. and McLean, L. (1984) Morphological and biochemical studies of a naturally occurring enteropathy in the Irish setter: a comparison with coeliac disease in man. *Research in Veterinary Science* **37**, 339–346.

Bellinger, C.R., Maddison, J.E., Macpherson, G.C. and Ilkiw, J.E. (1990) Chronic hypertrophic pyloric gastropathy in 14 dogs. *Australian Veterinary Journal* **67**, 317–320.

Berry, A.P. and Levett, P.N. (1986) Chronic diarrhoea in dogs associated with *Clostridium difficile* infection. *Veterinary Record* **118**, 102–103.

Bicks, R.O. and Walker, R.H. (1962) Immunologic colitis in dogs. *American Journal of Digestive Diseases* **7**, 574–584.

Bolton, G.R. and Brown, T.T. (1972) Mycotic colitis in a cat. *Veterinary Medicine, Small Animal Clinic* **63**, 978–981.

Breitschwerdt, E.B., Halliwell, W.H., Foley, C.W., Stark, D.R. and Carwin, L.A. (1980) A hereditary diarrhoeic syndrome in the Basenji characterised by malabsorption, protein-losing enteropathy and hypergammaglobulinaemia. *Journal of the American Animal Hospital Association* **16**, 551–560.

Breitschwerdt, E.B., Turk, M.A.M., Glaze, M.B., Crawford, M.P., Littlefield, M.A. and Roussel, A.J. (1986) Chronic azotemia and hypertension in two Bluetick Coonhound siblings. *Compendium of Continuing Education* **8**, 487–491.

Bright, R.M., Burrows, C.F., Goring, R., Fox, S. and Tilmant, L. (1986) Subtotal colectomy for treatment of acquired megacolon in the dog and cat. *Journal of the American Veterinary Medical Association* **188**, 1412–1416.

Brockman, D. (1994) Management of gastric dilatation–volvulus syndrome in the dog. *In Practice* **16**, 63–69.

Brodey, R.S. (1966) Alimentary tract neoplasms in the cat: a clinicopathologic survey of 46 cases. *American Journal of Veterinary Research* **27**, 74–80.

Burk, R.L., Zawie, D.A. and Garvey, M.S. (1987) Balloon catheter dilation of intramural esophageal strictures in the dog and cat: a description of the procedure and a report of six cases. *Seminars in Veterinary Medicine and Surgery* **2**, 241–247.

Burnie, A.G., Simpson, J.W., Lindsay, B. and Miles, R.S. (1983) Excretion of Campylobacters, Salmonellae and *Giardia lamblia* in the faeces of stray dogs. *Veterinary Research Communications* **6**, 133–138.

Burnie, A.G., Simpson, J.W. and Corcoran, B.M. (1989) Gastro-oesophageal reflux and hiatus hernia associated with laryngeal paralysis in a dog. *Journal of Small Animal Practice* **30**, 414–416.

Burns, J. and Fox, S. (1986) The use of barium meal to evaluate total gastric emptying times in the dog. *Veterinary Radiology* **27** 169–172.

Burns, M.G. (1982) Intestinal lymphangiectasia in the dog: a case report and review. *Journal of the American Animal Hospital Association* **18**, 97–105.

Burrows, C.F. (1986a) Diseases of the canine stomach. *Veterinary Annual* **26**, 270–282.

Burrows, C.F. (1986b) Constipation. In: *Current Veterinary Therapy IX* (Ed. R.W. Kirk). W.B. Saunders, Philadelphia, pp. 904–908.

Burrows, C.F. and Ignaszewski, L.A. (1990) Canine gastric dilatation–volvulus. *Journal of Small Animal Practice* **31**, 495–501.

Burrows, C.F. and Merritt, A.M. (1983) The influence of alpha cellulose on the myoelectrical activity of the proximal canine colon. *American Journal of Physiology* **245**, G301–G306.

Burrows, R.B. and Lillis, W.G. (1967) Intestinal protozoan infections in the dog. *Journal of the American Veterinary Association* **150**, 880–887.

Bush, B.M. (1985) Colitis in the dog. *The Veterinary Annual* **25**, 337–347.

Caywood, D., Teague, H.D., Jackson, D.A., Levitt, M.D. and Bond, J.H. (1977) Gastric gas analysis in the canine gastric dilatation–volvulus syndrome. *Journal of the American Animal Hospital Association* **13**, 459–462.

Chapman, B.L. and Malik, R. (1992) Phenobarbitone-responsive hypersalivation in two dogs. *Journal of Small Animal Practice* **33**, 549–552.

Chiapella, A. (1986) Diagnosis and management of chronic colitis in the dog and cat. *Current Veterinary Therapy IX* (Ed. R.W. Kirk). W.B. Saunders, Philadelphia, pp. 896–903.

Clark, W.A. (1985) Canine gastric hyperplasia. *The Veterinary Annual* **25**, 245–247.

Clifford, D.H., Soifer, F.K., Wilson, C.F., Waddell, E.D. and Guilloud, G.L. (1971) Congenital achalasia of the esophagus in four cats of common ancestry. *Journal of the American Veterinary Medical Association* **158**, 1554–1560.

Concise Veterinary Dictionary (1988) (Ed. R.S. Hine). Oxford University Press, Oxford, p. 20.

Cotter, S.M. (1981) Oral pharyngeal neoplasms in the cat. *Journal of the American Animal Hospital Association* **17**, 917–920.

Couto, C.G. (1984) Gastrointestinal neoplasia. In: *Proceedings of the Eighth Annual Kal Kan Symposium*, Columbus, Ohio, p. 17.

Coutts, A.J., Dawson, S., Willoughby, K. and Gaskell, R.M. (1994) Isolation of feline respiratory viruses from clinically healthy cats at UK cat shows. *Veterinary Record* **135**, 555–556.

Cox, V.S., Wallace, L.J., Anderson, V.E. and Rushmer, R.A. (1980) Hereditary esophageal dysfunction in the miniature Schnauzer dog. *American Journal of Veterinary Research* **41**, 326–330.

Crow, S.E. (1985) Tumours of the alimentary tract. *Veterinary Clinics of North America* **15**, 577–596.

Davidson, J.R., Lantz, G.C., Salisbury, S.K. *et al.* (1992) Effects of flunixin meglumine on dogs with experimental gastric dilatation–volvulus. *Veterinary Surgery* **21**, 113–120.

Davis, L.R. and Baggot, J.D. (1980) Gastrointestinal pharmacology. In: *Veterinary Gastroenterology* (Ed. N.V. Anderson). Lea Febiger, Philadelphia, pp. 277–281.

Debas, H.T. (1987) Peripheral regulation of gastric acid secretion. In: *Physiology of the Gastrointestinal Tract* (Ed. L.R. Johnson). Raven Press, New York, pp. 911–930.

Dennis, R., Herrtage, M.E., Jefferies, A.R., Matic, S.E. and White, R.A.S. (1987) A case of hypertrophic gastropathy in a cat. *Journal of Small Animal Practice* **28**, 491–504.

DiBartola, S.P., Rogers, W.A., Boyce, J.T. and Grimm, J.P. (1982) Regional enteritis in two dogs. *Journal of the American Veterinary Medical Association* **181**, 904–908.

Douglas, S.W., Herrtage, M.E. and Williamson, H.D. (1987) *Principles of Veterinary Radiography*, 4th edn. Baillière Tindall, London, pp. 193–198.

Drazner, F.H. (1983) Mechanisms of diarrhoeal disease. In: *Current Veterinary Therapy VII* (Ed. R.W. Kirk). W.B. Saunders, Philadelphia, pp. 773–783.

Duchmann, R., Kaiser, I., Hermann, E., Mayet, W., Ewe, K. and Meyer, K-H. (1995) Tolerance exists towards resident bacterial flora but is broken in active inflammatory bowel disease (IBD). *Clinical and Experimental Immunology* **102**, 448–455.

Dunn, J.K. (1989) The vomiting dog. *In Practice* **11**, 184–192.

Eastwood, G.L. (1977) Gastrointestinal epithelial renewal. *Gastroenterology* **72**, 962–975.

Eastwood, G.L., Castell, D.O. and Higgs, R.H. (1975) Experimental oesophagitis in cats impairs lower oesophageal pressure. *Gastroenterology* **69**, 146–153.

Elkins, A.D. (1987) Correcting cricopharyngeal achalasia in a puppy. *Pet Practice* **82**, 1241–1242.

Ellison, G.W. (1993) Gastric dilatation volvulus. Surgical prevention. *Veterinary Clinics of North America* **23**, 513–530.

Ellison, G.W., Lewis, O.D., Philips, L. and Jarvin, G.B.

(1987) Oesophageal hiatus hernia in small animals: literature review and a modified surgical technique. *Journal of the American Animal Hospital Association* **23**, 391–399.

Ewing, G.O. and Aldrete, A.V. (1973) Canine giardiasis presenting as chronic ulcerative colitis: a case report. *Journal of the American Animal Hospital Association* **9**, 52–55.

Ewing, G.D. and Gomez, J.A. (1973) Canine ulcerative colitis. *Journal of the American Animal Hospital Association* **9**, 395–406.

Fontolliet, C., Mossimann, F., Diserens, H., Burri, B., Loup, P.W. and Mosimann, R. (1984) Modifications of the gastric mucosal barrier induced by experimental duodenogastric reflux: an electron microscopic study. *Scandinavian Journal of Gastroenterology* **19** (Suppl. 92), 75–77.

Forrester, S.D., Boothe, D.M. and Willard, M.D. (1989) Clinical pharmacology of antiemetic antiulcer drugs. *Seminars in Veterinary and Medical Surgery* **4**, 194–201.

Fossum, T.W. (1989) Protein-losing enteropathy. *Seminars in Veterinary and Medical Surgery* **4**, 219–225.

Fox, S.M., Burns, J. and Hawkins, J. (1988) Spirocercosis in the dog. *Compendium of Continuing Education* **10**, 807–822.

Franklin, R.T., Jones, B.D. and Fledman, B.F. (1986) Medical conditions of the small intestine. In: *Canine and Feline Gastroenterology* (Ed. B.D. Jones). W.B. Saunders, Philadelphia, pp. 161–202.

Frendin, J., Fundquist, B. and Stavenborn, M. (1988) Gastric displacement in dogs without clinical signs of acute dilatation. *Journal of Small Animal Practice* **29**, 775–779.

Fundquist, B. (1970) Oesophageal plasty as a supporting measure in the operation for oesophageal constriction following vascular malformation. *Journal of Small Animal Practice* **11**, 421–427.

Gaskell, C.O., Gibb, C. and Pearson, H. (1974) Sliding hiatus hernia with reflux oesophagitis in two dogs. *Journal of Small Animal Practice* **15**, 503–509.

Geyer, C., Colbatzky, F., Lechner, J. and Hermanns, W. (1993) Occurrence of spiral-shaped bacteria in gastric biopsies of dogs and cats. *Veterinary Record* **133**, 18–19.

Gruffydd-Jones, T.J., Gaskell, C.J. and Gibb, C. (1979) Clinical and radiographical features of anterior mediastinal lymphosarcoma in the cat: a review of 30 cases. *Veterinary Record* **104**, 304–307.

Guilford, W.G. and Strombeck, D.R. (1996) Acute gastritis. In: *Strombeck's Small Animal Gastroenterology* (Eds W.G. Guilford, S.A. Center, D.R. Strombeck *et al.*), 3rd edn. W.B. Saunders, Philadelphia, pp. 263–274.

Guilford, W.G., Olsen, J., Reid, D., *et al.* (1991) Gastroscopic food sensitivity testing in the dog. *Journal of Veterinary Internal Medicine* **5**, 132.

Hall, E.J. (1989) Primary treatment of small intestinal diseases. *Veterinary Annual* **29**, 226–231.

Hall, E.J. and Batt, R.M. (1990) Enhanced intestinal permeability to Cr-labelled EDTA in dogs with small intestinal disease. *Journal of the American Veterinary Medical Association* **196**, 91–95.

Hall, E.J. and Batt, R.M. (1991) Differential sugar absorption for the assessment of intestinal permeability: the cellobiose/mannitol test in gluten sensitive enteropathy of Irish setters. *Research in Veterinary Science* **51**, 83–87.

Hall, J.A. (1989) Canine gastric dilatation–volvulus update. *Seminars in Veterinary and Medical Surgery* **4**, 188–193.

Hall, J.A., Burrows, C.F. and Twedt, D.C. (1988) Gastric motility in dogs. Part 1. Normal gastric function. *Compendium of Continuing Education* **10**, 1282–1293.

Hall, J.A., Twedt, D.C. and Burrows, C.F. (1990) Gastric motility in dogs: Part II. Disorders of gastric motility. *Compendium of Continuing Education* **12**, 1373–1390.

Happe, R.P., van der Gaag, I. and Lamers, C.B. (1980) Zollinger–Ellison syndrome in the dog. *Veterinary Pathology* **17**, 177–182.

Hardin, C.K., Sexton, C.R. and Peoples, J.B. (1987) Efficiency of sucralphate in preventing peptic ulceration induced by nonsteroidal anti-inflammatory drugs. *American Surgery* **53**, 373–376.

Harvey, C.E. (1987) Palate defects in dogs and cats. *Compendium of Continuing Education* **9**, 404–418.

Harvey, C.E., O'Brien, J.A., Durie, V.R. *et al.* (1974) Megaoesophagus in the dog: a clinical survey of 79 cases. *Journal of the American Veterinary Medical Association* **165**, 443–446.

Hathcock, J.T. (1984) Radiographic view of choice for the diagnosis of gastric volvulus: the right lateral view. *Journal of the American Animal Hospital Association* **20**, 967–969.

Hayden, D.W. and Fleischman, R.W. (1977) Scirrhous eosinophilic gastritis in dogs with gastric arteritis. *Veterinary Pathology* **14**, 441–448.

Hayden, D.W. and Van Kruiningen, H.J. (1973) Eosinophilic gastroenteritis in German Shepherd dogs and its relationship to visceral larva migrans. *Journal of the American Veterinary Medical Association* **162**, 379–384.

Hayden, D.W. and Van Kruiningen, H.J. (1982) Lymphocytic–plasmacytic enteritis in German Shepherd dogs. *Journal of the American Animal Hospital Association* **18**, 89–96.

Head, K.W. and Else, R.W. (1981) Neoplasia and other allied conditions of the canine and feline intestine. *Veterinary Annual* **21**, 190–208.

Hendricks, J.C., Maggio-Price, L. and Dougherty, J.F. (1984) Transient esophageal dysfunction mimicking megaoesophagus in three dogs. *Journal of the American Veterinary Medical Association* **185**, 90–92.

Hendricks, M. (1981) A spectrum of hypereosinophilic syndromes exemplified by 6 cats with eosinophilic enteritis. *Veterinary Pathology* **18**, 188–200.

Henroteaux, M. (1990) Results of an endosopic study

of colitis in dogs: predominance of idiopathic colitis. *Annales de Médecine Vétérinaire* **134**, 389–392.

Hills, B.A. (1993) Gastric mucosal barrier: evidence for *H. pylori* ingesting gastric surfactant and deriving protection from it. *Gut* **34**, 588–593.

Hills, B.A. and Kirkwood, L.S. (1992) Gastric mucosal barrier: barrier to hydrogen ions imparted by gastric surfactant in vitro. *Gut* **33**, 1039–1041.

Hinder, R.A. (1983) Individual and combined roles of the pylorus and the antrum in the gastric emptying of a liquid and a digestible solid. *Gastroenterology* **84**, 281–286.

Hinder, R.A. and Kelly, K.A. (1977) Canine gastric emptying of solids and liquids. *American Journal of Physiology* **233**, E335.

Hoenig, M. (1980) Intestinal malabsorption attributed to bacterial overgrowth in a dog. *Journal of the American Veterinary Medical Association* **176**, 533–535.

Hoenig, M., Mahaffey, M.B., Parnell, P.G. and Styles, M.E. (1990) Megaoesophagus in two cats. *Journal of the American Veterinary Medical Association* **196**, 763–765.

Hogan, P.M. and Aronson, E. (1988) The effect of sedation on transit time of feline gastrointestinal contrast studies. *Veterinary Radiology* **29**, 85–88.

Hoskins, J.D. (1990) Management of faecal impaction. *Compendium of Continuing Education* **12**, 1579–1585.

Houlton, J.E.F., Herrtage, M.E., Taylor, P.M. and Watkins, S.B. (1985) Thoracic oesophageal foreign bodies in the dog: a review of ninety cases. *Journal of Small Animal Practice* **26**, 521–536.

Huibregtse, B.A. and Turner, J.L. (1994) Hypereosinophilic syndrome and eosinopilic leukemia: a comparison of 22 hypereosinophilic cats. *Journal of the American Animal Hospital Association* **30**, 591–599.

Hurley, K., Miller, M.W., Willard, M.D. and Boothe, H.W. (1993) Left aortic arch and right ligamentum arteriosum causing esophageal obstruction in a dog. *Journal of the American Veterinary Medical Association* **203**, 410–412.

Huxtable, C.R., Mills, J.N., Clark, W.T. and Thompson, R. (1982) Chronic hypertrophic gastritis in a dog: successful treatment by partial gastrectomy. *Journal of Small Animal Practice* **23**, 639–647.

Itoh, Z., Aizawa, I., Takeuchi, S. and Takayanagi, R. (1977) Diurnal changes in gastric motor activity in conscious dogs. *American Journal of Digestive Diseases* **22**, 117–124.

Jakoljevic, S. (1988) Gastric radiology and gastroscopy in the dog. *Veterinary Annual* **28**, 172–182.

Jergens, A.E., Moore, F.M., Haynes, J.S. and Miles, K.G. (1992) Idiopathic inflammatory bowel disease in dogs and cats: 84 cases (1987–1990). *Journal of the American Veterinary Medical Association* **201**, 1603–1608.

Johnson, K.A., Maddison, J.E. and Allan, J.E. (1992) Correction of cervical oesophageal stricture in a dog by creation of a traction diverticulum. *Journal of the American Veterinary Medical Association* **201**, 1045–1048.

Johnston, K., Lamport, A. and Batt, R.M. (1993) An unexpected bacterial flora in the proximal small intestine of normal cats. *Veterinary Record* **132**, 362–363.

Johnson, L.W. (1987) Food allergy in a dog: diagnosis by dietary management. *Modern Veterinary Practice* **68**, 236–239.

Johnson, S.E. and Willard, M.D. (1990) Haematemesis, erosion and ulceration. In: *Proceedings 8th ACVIM*, Washington DC, pp. 441–444.

Jones, B.R., Johnstone, A.C. and Hathcock, W.S. (1985) Tyzzers' disease in kittens with familial primary hyperlipoproteinaemia. *Journal of Small Animal Practice* **26**, 411–419.

Kelly, D.F., Lucke, V.M., Denny, H.R. and Lane, J.G. (1979) Histology of salivary gland infarction in the dog. *Veterinary Pathology* **16**, 438–443.

Kipnis, R.M. (1978) Focal cystic hypertrophic gastropathy in a dog. *Journal of the American Veterinary Medical Association* **173**, 182–184.

Kirkpatrick, C.E. (1986) Feline giardiasis: a review. *Journal of Small Animal Practice* **27**, 69–80.

Kirkpatrick, C.E. and Farrell, J.P. (1982) Giardiasis. *Compendium of Continuing Education* **4**, 4367–4378.

Kosovsky, J.K., Mathiesen, D.T., Marretta, S.M. and Patnaik, A.K. (1991) Results of partial mandibulectomy for the treatment of oral tumours in 142 dogs. *Veterinary Surgery* **20**, 397–401.

Lantz, G.C. and Badylak, S.F. (1992) Treatment of reperfusion injuries in dogs with experimentally induced gastric dilatation–volvulus. *American Journal of Veterinary Research* **53**, 1594–1598.

Leblanc, B., Fox, J.G., Le Net, J.L., Masson, M.T. and Picard, A. (1993) Hyperplastic gastritis with intraepithelial *Campylobacter*-like organisms in a beagle dog. *Veterinary Pathology* **30**, 391–392.

Lee, A., Krakowka, S., Fox, J.G., Otto, G., Eaton, K.A. and Murphy, J.C. (1992) The role of *Helicobacter felis* in chronic canine gastritis. *Veterinary Pathology* **29**, 487–494.

Leib, M.S. (1986) Megaoesophagus in the dog. In: *Current Veterinary Therapy IX* (Ed. R.W. Kirk). W.B. Saunders, Philadelphia, pp. 848–852.

Leib, M.S. (1987) Stagnant loop syndrome in the dog and cat. *Seminars in Veterinary Medicine and Surgery* **2**, 257–265.

Leib, M.S. and Martin, R.A. (1987) Therapy of gastric dilatation–volvulus in dogs. *Compendium of Continuing Education* **9**, 1155–1163.

Maclauchlan, N.J., Breitschwerdt, E.B., Chalmers, J.M., Argenzio, R.A. and De Buyascher, E.V. (1988) Gastroenteritis of Basenji dogs. *Veterinary Pathology* **25**, 26–41.

McLeod, C.G., Langlinais, P.C. and Brown, J.C. (1981) Ulcerative histiocytic gastritis and amyloidosis in a dog. *Veterinary Pathology* **18**, 117–120.

Maddison, J.E. and Allan, G.S. (1990) Megaoesophagus

attributable to lead toxicosis in a cat. *Journal of the American Veterinary Association* **197**, 1357–1358.

Madewell, B.R., Stannard, A.A., Pulley, L.T. and Nelson, V.G. (1980) Oral eosinophilic granuloma in Siberian husky dogs. *Journal of the American Veterinary Medical Association* **177**, 701–703.

Mason, K.V. (1976) A case of myasthenia gravis in a cat. *Journal of Small Animal Practice* **17**, 467–472.

Matz, M.E., Leib, M.S., Monroe, W.E., Davenport, D.J., Nelson, L.P. and Kenny, J.E. (1991) Evaluation of atropine, glucagon and metoclopramide for facilitation of endoscopic intubation of the duodenum of dogs. *American Journal of Veterinary Research* **52**, 1948–1950.

Maxton, D.G., Bjarson, I., Reynolds, A.P., Catt, S.D., Peters, T. and Menzies, I.S. (1986) Lactulose, ^{51}Cr-labelled ethylenediaminetetra-acetate, L-rhamnose and polyethylene glycol 400 as probe markers for assessment in vivo of human intestinal permeability. *Clinical Science* **71**, 71–80.

Merchant, S.R. and Taboada, J. (1991) Food allergy and immunologic diseases of the gastrointestinal tract. *Seminars in Veterinary Medicine and Surgery* **6**, 316–321.

Meyer-Lindenberg, A., Harder, A., Fehr, M., Lüerssen, D. and Brunnberg, L. (1993) Treatment of gastric dilation–volvulus and a rapid method of prevention of relapse in dogs: 134 cases (1988–1991). *Journal of the American Veterinary Medical Association* **203**, 1303–1307.

Miyabayashi, T., Morgan, J.P., Atilola, A.O. and Muhumuza, L. (1986) Small intestinal emptying times in normal Beagle dogs. *Veterinary Radiology* **27**, 164–168.

Moore RP (1983) Feline eosinophilic enteritis. In: *Current Veterinary Therapy VIII* (Ed. R.W. Kirk). W.B. Saunders, Philadelphia, pp. 791–793.

Moore, R.W. and Withrow, S.J. (1982) Gastrointestinal haemorrhage and pancreatitis associated with intervertebral disc disease in the dog. *Journal of the American Veterinary Medical Association* **180**, 1443–1447.

Moreland, K.J. (1988) Ulcer disease of the upper gastrointestinal tract in small animals: pathophysiology, diagnosis and management. *Compendium of Continuing Education* **10**, 1265–1279.

Morgan, J.P. (1981) The upper gastrointestinal examination in the cat: normal radiographic appearance using positive contrast medium. *Veterinary Radiology* **22**, 159–169.

Muir, P., Harbour, D.A., Gruffydd-Jones, T.J. et al. (1990) A clinical and microbiological study of cats with protruding nictitating membrane and diarrhoea: isolation of a novel virus. *Veterinary Record* **127**, 324–330.

Muir, P., Gruffydd-Jones, T.J., Cripps, P., Papsouliotis, K. and Brown, P.J. (1994) Breath hydrogen excretion after oral administration of xylose to cats. *Journal of Small Animal Practice* **35**, 86–92.

Muir, W.W. (1982) Acid base and electrolyte disturbances in dogs with gastric dilation volvulus. *Journal of the American Veterinary Medical Association* **181**, 229–231.

Murdoch, D.B. (1986) Diarrhoea in the dog and cat: 1. Acute diarrhoea. *British Veterinary Journal* **142**, 307–316.

Murtaugh, R.J., Matz, M.E., Labato, M.A. and Boudrieau, R.J. (1993) Use of synthetic prostaglandin E1 (misoprostol) for protection of aspirin-induced gastroduodenal ulceration in arthritic dogs. *Journal of the American Veterinary Medical Association* **202**, 251–256.

Neer, T.M. (1991) Hypereosinophilic syndrome in cats. *Compendium of Continuing Education* **17**, 549–555.

Nelson, R.W., Dimperio, M.E. and Long, G.G. (1984) Lymphocytic–plasmacytic enteritis in the cat. *Journal of the American Veterinary Medical Association* **184**, 1133–1140.

Obwolo, M. and Gruffydd-Jones, T.J. (1977) *Yersinia pseudotuberculosis* in the cat. *Veterinary Record* **100**, 424–425.

Orton, E.C. (1986) Gastric dilatation–volvulus. In: *Current Veterinary Therapy IX* (Ed. R.W. Kirk). W.B. Saunders, Philadelphia, pp. 856–862.

Osborne, C.A., Clifford, D.H. and Jessen, C. (1967) Hereditary esophageal achalasia in dogs. *Journal of the American Veterinary Medical Association* **151**, 572–581.

Papasouliotis, K., Gruffydd-Jones, T.J., Sparkes, A.H., Cripps, P.J. and Millard, W.G. (1993a) Lactulose and mannitol as probe markers for *in vivo* assessment of passive intestinal permeability in healthy cats. *American Journal of Veterinary Research* **58**, 840–844.

Papasouliotis, K., Muir, P., Gruffydd-Jones, T.J., Galloway, P., Smerdon, T. and Cripps, P.J. (1993b) Decreased orocecal transit time as measured by the exhalation of breath hydrogen in hyperthyroid cats. *Research in Veterinary Science* **55**, 115–118.

Papich, M.G. (1989) Medical therapy for gastrointestinal ulcers. In: *Current Veterinary Therapy X* (Ed. R.W. Kirk). W.B. Saunders, Philadelphia, pp. 911–918.

Patnaik, A.K., Erlandson, R.A. and Liberman, P.H. (1990) Esophageal neuroendocrine carcinoma in a cat. *Veterinary Pathology* **27**, 128.

Pearson, H., Gaskell, C.J., Gibb, C. and Waterman, A. (1974) Pyloric and oesophageal dysfunction in the cat. *Journal of Small Animal Practice* **15**, 487–501.

Pearson, H., Darke, P.G.G., Gibbs, C., Kelly, D.F. and Orr, C.M. (1978a) Reflux oesophagitis and stricture formation after anaesthesia: a review of seven cases in dogs and cats. *Journal of Small Animal Practice* **19**, 507–519.

Pearson, H., Gibbs, C. and Kelly, D.F. (1978b) Oesophageal diverticulum formation in the dog. *Journal of Small Animal Practice* **19**, 341–356.

Pitts, R.P. (1983) Giardiasis. In: *Current Veterinary*

Therapy VIII (Ed. R.W. Kirk). W.B. Saunders, Philadelphia, pp. 796–797.

Quigg, J., Bryden, G., Ferguson, A. et al. (1994) Evaluation of canine small intestinal permeability using the lactulose/rhamnose urinary excretion test. *Research in Veterinary Science* **55**, 326–332.

Quigley, P.J. and Henry, K. (1981) Eosinophilic enteritis in the dog: a case report with a brief review of the literature. *Journal of Comparative Pathology* **91**, 387–392.

Raufman, J.P. (1992) Regulation of pepsinogen secretion. *Current Opinions in Gastroenterology* **8**, 907–910.

Rees, W.D.W., Bribbons, I.C. and Turnberg, L.A. (1983) Effects of NSAID and prostaglandins on alkaline secretion by rabbit gastric fundus in vitro. *Gut* **24**, 784–789.

Reife, S.P., Goldstein, J. and Alpo, D.H. (1980) Effects of secreted *Bacterioides* proteases on the human intestinal brush border hydrolysis. *Journal of Clinical Investigation* **66**, 314–322.

Ridgeway, M.D. (1984) Management of chronic colitis in the dog. *Journal of the American Veterinary Medical Association* **185**, 804–806.

Ridgeway, R.L. and Suter, P.F. (1979) Clinical and radiographic signs in primary and metastatic oesophageal neoplasms of the dog. *Journal of the American Veterinary Medical Association* **174**, 700–704.

Ridley, D.S. and Hawgood, B.C. (1956) The value of formol ether concentration of faecal cysts and ova. *Journal of Clinical Pathology* **9**, 74–76.

Rosin, E. and Hanlon, G.F. (1972) Canine cricopharyngeal achalasia. *Journal of the American Veterinary Medical Association* **160**, 1496–1499.

Rutgers, H.C. (1989) Diarrhoea in the cat. *In Practice* **11**, 139–148.

Rutgers, H.C. (1991) Diarrhoea in the cat: a monograph. Waltham Centre for Pet Nutrition, Melton Mowbray.

Rutgers, H.C., Batt, R.M. and Kelly, D.F. (1988) Lymphocytic-plasmacytic enteritis associated with bacterial overgrowth in a dog. *Journal of the American Veterinary Medical Association* **192**, 1739–1740.

Ryan, W.W. and Green, R.W. (1975) The conservative management of oesophageal foreign bodies and their complications: a review of 66 cases in dogs and cats. *Journal of the American Animal Hospital Association* **11**, 243–249.

Scott, D.W. (1980) Feline dermatology 1900–1978: a monograph. *Journal of the American Animal Hospital Association* **16**, 331.

Seim, H.B. (1986) Diseases of the anus and rectum. In: *Current Veterinary Therapy IX* (Ed. R.W. Kirk). W.B. Saunders, Philadelphia, pp. 916–921.

Sharp, N.J.H., Nash, A.G. and Griffiths, I.R. (1984) Feline dysautonomia (Key–Gaskell syndrome): a clinical and pathological study of forty cases. *Journal of Small Animal Practice* **25**, 599–615.

Shaw, D.H. (1988) Gastrinoma (Zollinger–Ellison syndrome) in the dog and cat. *Canadian Veterinary Journal* **29**, 448–452.

Shelton, G.D. (1982) Swallowing disorders in the dog. *Compendium of Continuing Education* **4**, 607–614.

Shelton, D.H. (1992) Megaoesophagus secondary to acquired myasthenia gravis. In: *Current Veterinary Therapy XI* (Ed. R.W. Kirk). W.B. Saunders, Philadelphia, pp. 580–583.

Sherding, R.G. (1986) Intestinal lymphangiectasia. In: *Current Veterinary Therapy IX* (Ed. R.W. Kirk). W.B. Saunders, Philadelphia, pp. 885–888.

Sherding, R.G. (1990) Management of constipation and dyschezia. *Compendium of Continuing Education* **12**, 677–680.

Sherding, R.G. (1994) Diseases of the intestines. In: *The Cat: Diseases and Clinical Management* (Ed. R.G. Sherding) 2nd edn. Chuchill Livingstone, New York, pp. 1271.

Sidery, M.B., Macdonald, I.A. and Blackshaw, P.E. (1994) Superior mesenteric artery blood flow and gastric emptying in humans and the differential effects of high fat and carbohydrate meals. *Gut* **35**, 186–190.

Sikes, R.I., Birchard, S., Patnaik, A. and Bradley, R. (1986) Chronic hypertrophic pyloric gastropathy: a review of 16 cases. *Journal of the American Animal Hospital Association* **22**, 99–104.

Simpson, J.W. (1982) Bacterial overgrowth causing intestinal malabsorption in a dog. *Veterinary Record* **110**, 335–336.

Simpson, J.W. (1994) Management of megaoesophagus in the dog. *In Practice* **16**, 14–16.

Simpson, J.W. (1996) Differential diagnosis of faecal tenesmus in dogs. *In Practice* **18**, 283–287.

Simpson, J.W. and Else, R.W. (1991a) Conditions of the oesophagus. In: *Digestive Disease in the Dog and Cat*. Blackwell Scientific Publications, Oxford, p. 39.

Simpson, J.W. and Else, R.W. (1991b) Conditions of the stomach. In: *Digestive Disease of the Dog and Cat*. Blackwell Scientific Publications, Oxford, p. 60.

Simpson, J.W. and Else, R.W. (1991c) Diseases of the large intestine. In: *Digestive Disease of the Dog and Cat*. Blackwell Scientific Publications, Oxford, p. 140.

Simpson, J.W., Maskell, I.E. and Markwell, P.J. (1994) Use of a restricted antigen diet in the management of idiopathic canine colitis. *Journal of Small Animal Practice* **35**, 233–238.

Simpson, K.W., Simpson, J.W. and Thomas, D. (1996) Small intestinal disease. In: *Manual of Canine and Feline Gastroenterology*. BSAVA, Cheltenham, pp. 114–150.

Sooy, T.E., Adams, W.M., Pitts, R. et al. (1987) Balloon catheter dilation of alimentary tract strictures in the dog and cat. *Veterinary Radiology* **28**, 131–137.

Spielman, B.L., Shaker, E.H. and Garvey, M.S. (1992) Esophageal foreign body in dogs: a retrospective study of 23 cases. *Journal of the American Animal Hospital Association* **28**, 570–574.

Stebbins, K.E., Morse, C.C. and Goldschmidt, M.H. (1989) Feline oral neoplasia: a ten year survey. *Veterinary Pathology* **26**, 121–128.

Steyn, P.F. and Twedt, D.C. (1994) Gastric emptying in the normal cat: a radiographic study. *Journal of the American Animal Hospital Association* **30**, 78–80.

Strombeck, D.R., Doe, M. and Jang, S. (1981) Maldigestion and malabsorption in a dog with chronic gastritis. *Journal of the American Veterinary Medical Association* **179**, 801–805.

Sturgess, C.P. (1997) Studies on mucosal effector mechanisms in feline immunodeficiency virus (FIV) infection in cats. PhD thesis, University of Bristol, pp. 94–96.

Sullivan, M., Lee, R., Fisher, E.W., Nash, A.S. and McCandlish, I.A.P. (1987) A study of 31 cases of gastric carcinoma in dogs. *Veterinary Record* **120**, 79–83.

Suter, P.F. and Watrous, B.J. (1980) Oropharyngeal dysphagias in the dog: a cinefluorographic analysis of experimentally induced and spontaneously occurring swallowing disorders. *Veterinary Radiology* **21**, 24–39.

Suter, M.M., Plamer, D.G. and Schen, K.H. (1985) Primary intestinal lymphangiectasia in three dogs. A morphological and immunological investigation. *Veterinary Pathology* **22**, 123–130.

Taha, A.S. and Russell, R.I. (1993) *Helicobacter pylori* and NSAID: incompatible partners in peptic ulcer disease. *Gut* **34**, 580–583.

Tams, T.R. (1987) Chronic canine lymphocytic plasmacytic enteritis. *Compendium of Continuing Education* **9**, 1184–1194.

Tams, T.R. and Macy, D.W. (1981) Canine mast cell tumours. *Compendium of Continuing Education* **3**, 869–882.

Twedt, D.C. (1983) Disorders of gastric retention. In: *Current Veterinary Therapy VIII* (Ed. R.W. Kirk). W.B. Saunders, Philadelphia, pp. 761–765.

Twedt, D.C. (1985) Cirrhosis: a consequence of chronic liver disease. *Veterinary Clinics of North America* **15**, 166–167.

Twedt, D.C. and Magne, M.L. (1986) Chronic gastritis. In: *Current Veterinary Therapy IX* (Ed. R.W. Kirk). W.B. Saunders, Philadelphia, pp. 852–856.

Uzuka, Y. and Nakama, S. (1988) Persistent right aortic arch in a cat. *Comparative Animal Practice* **2**, 14–16.

van Der Gaag, I. and Happe, R.P. (1989) Follow-up studies by peroral gastric biopsy and necropsy in vomiting dogs. *Canadian Journal of Veterinary Research* **53**, 468–472.

van Der Gaag, I., Happe, R.P. and Wolvekamp, W.Th.C. (1976) A Boxer dog with chronic hypertrophic gastritis resembling Menetrier's disease in man. *Veterinary Pathology* **13**, 172–185.

van Der Gaag, I., van der Linde-Sipman, J.S., Van Sluijs, F.J. and Wolvekamp, W.Th.C. (1990) Regional eosinophilic coloproctitis, typhlitis and ileitis in a dog. *Veterinary Quarterly* **12**, 1–6.

van Der Gaag, I., Niel, M.H.F., Belshaw, B.E. and Wolvekamp, W.Th.C. (1991) Gastric granulomatous cryptococcosis mimicking gastric carcinoma in a dog. *Veterinary Quarterly* **13**, 185–189.

van der Linde-Sipman (1981) Vascular ring caused by a left aortic arch, right ligamentum arteriosum and part of the right dorsal aorta in a cat. *Zentralblatt fur Veterinarmedizin A* **28**, 569–573.

Van Kruiningen, H.J. (1976) Clinical efficacy of tylosin in canine inflammatory bowel disease. *Journal of the American Animal Hospital Association* **12**, 498–501.

Van Kruiningen, H.J. (1977) Giant hypertrophic gastritis of Basenji dogs. *Veterinary Pathology* **14**, 19–28.

Van Kruiningen, H.J. and Dobbins, W.O. (1979) Feline histiocytic colitis. *Veterinary Pathology* **16**, 215–222.

Van Kruiningen, H.J., Ryan, M.J. and Shindel, N.M. (1983) The classification of feline colitis. *Journal of Comparative Pathology* **93**, 275–294.

Van Kruiningen, H.J., Wotan, L.D., Stake, P.E. and Lord, P.F. (1987) The influence of diet and feeding frequency on gastric function in the dog. *Journal of the American Animal Hospital Association* **23**, 145–153.

Van Sluijs, F.J. and Happe, R.P. (1985) Surgical diseases of the stomach. In: *Textbook of Small Animal Surgery* (Ed. D.J. Slatter). W.B. Saunders, Philadelphia, pp. 684–712.

Wallace, M.S., Zawie, D.A. and Garvey, M.S. (1990) Gastric ulceration in the dog secondary to the use of non-steroidal anti-inflammatory drugs. *Journal of the American Veterinary Medical Association* **26**, 467–472.

Walter, M.C., Goldschmidt, M.H., Stone, E.A., Dougherty, J.F. and Matthiesen, D.T. (1985) Chronic hypertrophic pyloric gastropathy as a cause of pyloric obstruction in the dog. *Journal of the American Veterinary Medical Association* **186**, 157–161.

Washabau, R.J., Strombeck, D.R., Buffington, C.A. *et al.* (1986) Use of pulmonary hydrogen gas excretion to detect carbohydrate malabsorption in dogs. *Journal of the American Veterinary Medical Association* **189**, 674–679.

Watrous, B.J. (1983) Clinical presentation and diagnosis of dysphagia. *Veterinary Clinics of North America* **13**, 437–459.

Watrous, B.J. and Suter, P.F. (1979) Normal swallowing in the dog: a cineradiographic study. *Veterinary Radiology* **20**, 99–109.

Weaver, A.D. (1983) Cricopharyngeal achalasia in cocker spaniels. *Journal of Small Animal Practice* **24**, 209–214.

Webb, S.M. (1985) Surgical management of acquired megacolon in the cat. *Journal of Small Animal Practice* **26**, 399–405.

Whitbread, T.J., Batt, R.M. and Gaithwaite, G. (1984) Relative deficiency in IgA in the German shepherd dog: a breed abnormality. *Reserach in Veterinary Science* **37**, 350–352.

White, S.D. (1986) Food hypersensitivity in 30 dogs. *Journal of the American Veterinary Medical Association* **188**, 695–698.

Wilcock, B. (1992) Endoscopic biopsy interpretation in

canine and feline enterocolitis. *Seminars in Veterinary and Medical Surgery* **7**, 162–171.

Williams, D.A., Batt, R.M. and McLean, L. (1987) Bacterial overgrowth in the duodenum of dogs with exocrine pancreatic insufficiency. *Journal of the American Veterinary Medical Association* **191**, 201–206.

Williams, J.M. (1990) Hiatal hernia in a Shar-pei. *Journal of Small Animal Practice* **31**, 251–254.

Wills, J. (1991) Dietary hypersensitivity in cats. *In Practice* **13**, 87–93.

Winans, C.S. (1976) The fickle pylorus. *Gastroenterology* **70**, 622–623.

Wolf, A.M. (1992) Feline gingivitis, stomatitis and pharyngitis. In: *Current Veterinary Therapy XI* (Eds R.W. Kirk and J.D. Bonagura). WB Saunders, Philadelphia, pp. 568–572.

Woods, C.B., Rawlings, L., Barber, D. and Walker, M. (1978) Oesophageal deviation in four English bulldogs. *Journal of the American Veterinary Medical Association* **172**, 934–939.

Zawie, D.A. (1987) Medical diseases of the oesophagus. *Compendium of Continuing Education* **9**, 1146–1152.

Zook, B.C. and Gilmore, C.E. (1967) Thallium poisoning in dogs. *Journal of the American Veterinary Medical Association* **151**, 206–217.

37

Diseases of the Liver and Biliary Tract

J. Rothuizen

Functional anatomy of the liver	448
Liver physiology	450
Pathophysiology of clinically important syndromes	451
History taking in hepatobiliary diseases	461
Physical examination	461
Laboratory examination	462
Investigative techniques	465
HEPATOBILIARY DISEASES OF DOGS	**467**
Hepatitis and cirrhosis	467
Circulatory disorders of the liver	471
Congenital metabolic diseases of the liver	475
Tumours of the liver	477
Liver dysfunction resulting from systemic disease	479
Diseases of the biliary tract	483
FELINE LIVER DISEASES	**486**
Specific aspects of feline liver physiology	487
Cholangitis	487
Congenital portosystemic shunts	489
Feline liver dysfunction resulting from systemic disease	489
Tumours of the liver	491

FUNCTIONAL ANATOMY OF THE LIVER

The liver is the largest parenchymal organ weighing around 3% of the body weight in adults and 5% in young animals. In dogs and cats it is divided into six lobes that are deeply separated up to the hilus, which permits the liver to fold and unfold during respiration. The liver lies in the middle and right part of the cranial abdomen. The gallbladder lies in the right side of the liver between the quadrate and the right medial lobes at the diaphragmatic side. The liver is surrounded by the rib cage and is therefore normally not palpable. The stomach lies closely to the visceral side of the liver and its position is very much determined by the size of the liver.

Bile system

One of the main functions of the liver is detoxification or catabolism of exogenous and endogenous compounds, most of which are excreted into the bile. The biliary tree consists of small bile ducts which unite to form the larger intrahepatic ducts that leave the liver lobes to form the large extrahepatic common bile duct. The common bile duct enters the duodenum 3–6 cm from the pylorus. The sphincter of Oddi controls the release of bile into the duodenum. In cats the pancreatic duct joins the common bile duct at the duodenal papilla, whereas dogs have a separate enteric opening for the pancreatic duct. The gallbladder is connected to the common bile duct via the short cystic duct. It is the main reservoir in which bile is stored and concentrated.

Blood supply

The blood is supplied to the liver by both the hepatic artery and the portal vein and is drained by a number of hepatic veins that enter the caudal vena cava near the diaphragm. The total blood flow to the liver accounts for about 20–25% of the cardiac output, of which 70–80% comes from the portal vein. The ratio between portal and arterial blood supply is dynamic: the portal flow increases following ingestion of food, whereas the arterial blood supply increases when the portal flow is insufficient and decreases in the presence of hepatic venous congestion (Greenway and Oshiro, 1972). In cases of complete deprivation of portal blood flow to the liver (for example, congenital portosystemic shunts or portal vein thrombosis), the arterial flow increases by 50–100%, but despite this adaptation the total hepatic blood supply remains subnormal. Changes in the arterial flow do not influence portal flow. In the fasting state, the portal vein and hepatic artery each supply roughly half the oxygen used by the liver.

The great compliance of the hepatic vascular bed makes the organ a reservoir of blood. The liver normally contains around 10–15% of the total blood volume of the body, which can be doubled in severe cardiac failure. In case of moderate blood loss about 25% of the reduced circulating blood volume can be released from the liver.

Microanatomy

The liver contains different cell types, of which the parenchymal cells or hepatocytes predominate. Other cell types include endothelial cells, bile duct epithelium, Kupffer cells and fat-storing cells. The hepatocytes are arranged in cell plates one layer thick, radiating around the terminal hepatic vein, formerly called central veins (Fig. 37.1). The free sinusoidal membranes at both sides of the hepatocytes are separated from the sinusoids by a one cell layer of sinusoidal cells (endothelial and Kupffer cells); between the hepatocyte and the sinusoidal cell layers is the perisinusoidal space of Disse. The endothelial cells have many sieve-like openings permitting even large molecules, but not cells, to move from the sinusoids into and out of the space of Disse. The perisinusoidal space is the beginning of the hepatic lymphatic system. Lymph flows in the opposite direction to that of the blood, as does bile in the canaliculi. The sinusoidal cells are very efficient in removing endotoxins and particles such as bacteria.

The membranes of adjacent hepatocytes form the bile canaliculi sealed by tight junctions. The canalicular membrane has a specialized excretory function. The bile flows from the canaliculi into short collecting ducts, which drain into the bile ductule of the portal area. The ductules and the larger bile ducts are lined with cuboidal epithelial cells.

For understanding the pathophysiology, it is important to realize that the liver at the microanatomical level consists of functional haemodynamic units or acini different from the lobules that are a mere anatomical description (Fig. 37.2). An acinus is a unit of liver tissue which receives its blood from one pair of terminal branches of the portal vein and the hepatic artery

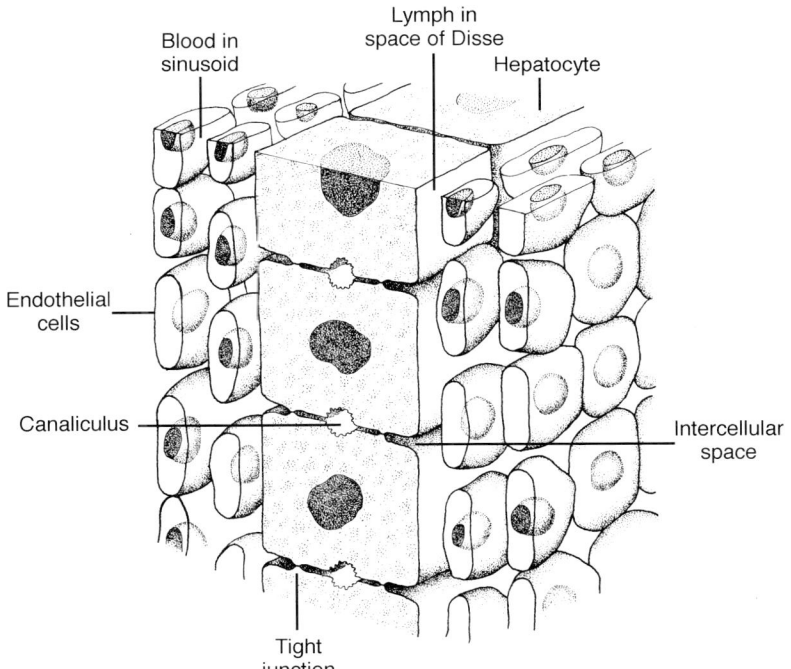

Figure 37.1 Microanatomy of the normal liver. Plates of hepatocytes are surrounded by the perisinusoidal lymphatic space of Disse and the sinusoidal blood. Bile flow in the canaliculi is opposite to the blood flow.

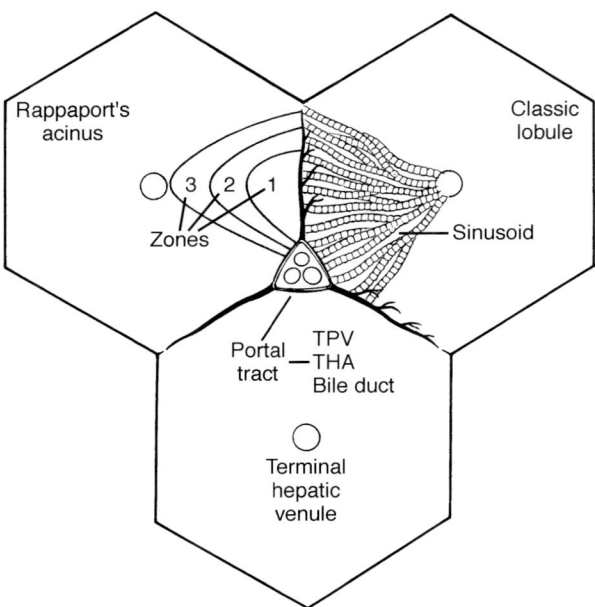

Figure 37.2 Schematic representation of the smallest functional unit of the liver, the acinus. The acini are divided into three zones. Zone 1 receives blood rich in growth factors and oxygen; zone 3 gets the poorest blood. Terminal branch of the portal vein (TPV); terminal branch of the hepatic artery (THA); terminal hepatic vein, or central vein in the old nomenclature (THV).

(McCuskey, 1994). The efferent blood flow is through several terminal hepatic veins at the periphery of an acinus.

In an acinus the zone around the portal vein gets blood with the highest content of oxygen, growth factors (mainly insulin) and nutrients and cells around the terminal veins get the poorest type of blood. In cases of hypoxia and shock, adaptation may come too late and the peripheral cells in the acini may become necrotic. Signs of liver dysfunction are, therefore, common after an episode of circulatory collapse or acute haemolysis.

Although all hepatocytes are similar and capable of performing a range of metabolic functions, some functions are confined to certain areas (Gumucio et al., 1994). The urea cycle enzymes are predominantly active in the portal zone, whereas the other ammonia capturing system, forming glutamine, resides exclusively in cells around the terminal hepatic veins. Gluconeogenesis occurs predominantly in the portal zone and glycolysis near the terminal hepatic veins. All zones are engaged in protein and lipid metabolism. Drug metabolism via the cytochrome $P450$ system is located primarily around the terminal veins.

LIVER PHYSIOLOGY

The liver has an enormous reserve capacity with respect to most of its functions. Removal of 70–80% of the normal liver is possible without any noticeable clinical effect. Another unique feature of the liver is its great regenerative capacity following loss of hepatocytes which is regulated by growth factors such as insulin and insulin-like growth factor. It is essential for maintenance of liver mass and regeneration that portal blood with these factors reaches the liver. Animals with a congenital portosystemic shunt have an undersized liver which can grow and reaches its normal weight in about four weeks after surgical closure of the shunt. Liver metabolism is regulated by hormones. In general, insulin is inhibitory in the mobilization of fatty acids and glucose, whereas glucagon, glucocorticoids and to a lesser extent thyroid hormone, growth hormone and catecholamines are stimulatory.

The liver plays a key role in many metabolic processes (Fig. 37.3). It regulates the concentration of glucose and many proteins in plasma. Triglycerides from adipose tissue or intestinal chylomicrons are converted into lipoproteins by the liver, which can be released into the circulation for use by other tissues. Biotransformation of endogenous products, for example ammonia and steroid hormones, and of exogenous toxic products, for example toxic chemicals and endotoxins from intestinal bacteria, is performed by the liver. Heavy metals are directly excreted into the bile. Large molecules are preferentially excreted into bile after conjugation which makes them sufficiently hydrophilic. Smaller molecules are transformed and then released into the circulation to be excreted by the kidneys. The liver also stores glycogen, metals and vitamins. The capacity to store and release a large volume of blood has already been mentioned. The liver produces blood cells in embryonal life. Hepatic extramedullary haematopoiesis may be regained in adulthood in cases of anaemia.

Features of liver physiology are important to understand the clinical presentation of liver diseases. The huge reserve capacity of the liver implies that hepatobiliary diseases often only become apparent clinically at a late stage when the reserve is lost. Acute or subacute diseases are

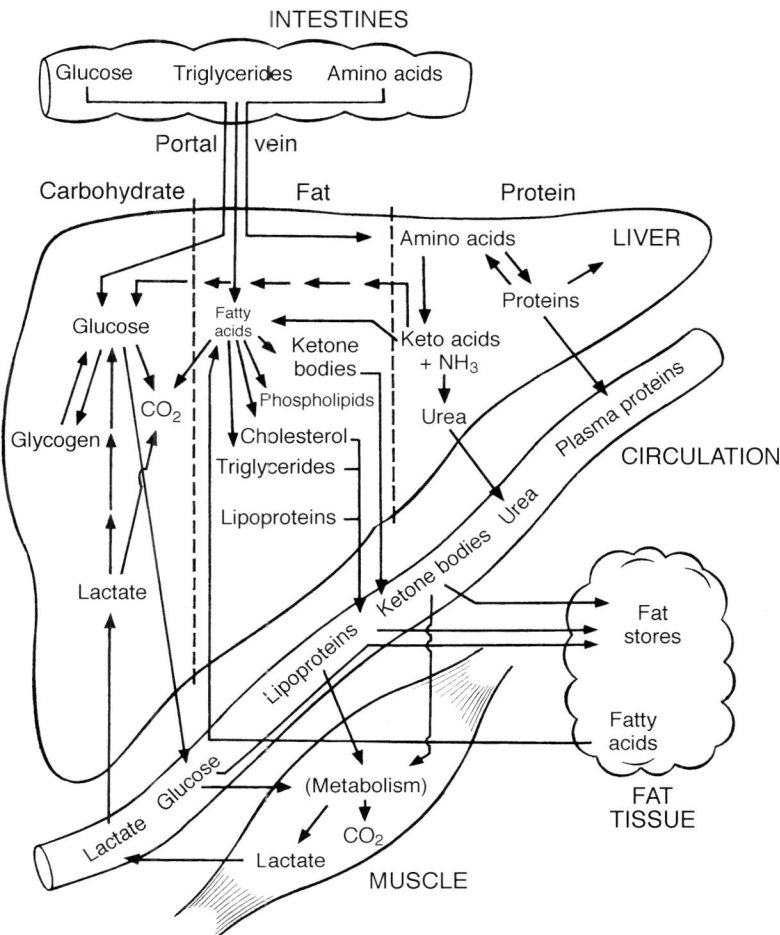

Figure 37.3 Diagram showing the interrelations between the metabolism of carbohydrates, fats, and proteins and the central role of the liver in metabolism.

often subclinical. The central role of the liver in metabolism explains why dysfunction of extrahepatic organs often occurs in liver disease with signs not primarily indicating involvement of the liver. Conversely, the central place in detoxification and metabolism implies that the liver is very often secondarily involved in metabolic diseases (for example diabetes mellitus or Cushing's disease) and in toxic diseases (due to endotoxins or chemical toxins).

PATHOPHYSIOLOGY OF CLINICALLY IMPORTANT SYNDROMES

A number of clinical syndromes may develop in different liver diseases. They are discussed here because they are important for understanding the clinical manifestations of hepatobiliary diseases and are referred to when signs, diagnostic procedures and specific diseases are being discussed.

Cholestasis and icterus

Bile production

Normally, bile flow results from bile production in the proximal part of the biliary system and concentration in the distal part. Active excretion of bile acids is responsible for about half the bile production. Bile acids are produced by the liver from cholesterol as a major route of cholesterol excretion (Fig. 37.4). The two acids formed are cholic acid and chenodeoxycholic acid (the primary bile acids). Bile acids are conjugated with glycine and taurine before excretion which makes them hydrophilic. Active excretion creates an osmotic gradient, which results in passive excretion of water into the canaliculi. Colonic bacteria transform part of the conjugated bile acids by deconjugation and 7α-hydroxylation. The latter reaction produces the secondary bile acids, deoxycholate from cholic acid and lithocholate

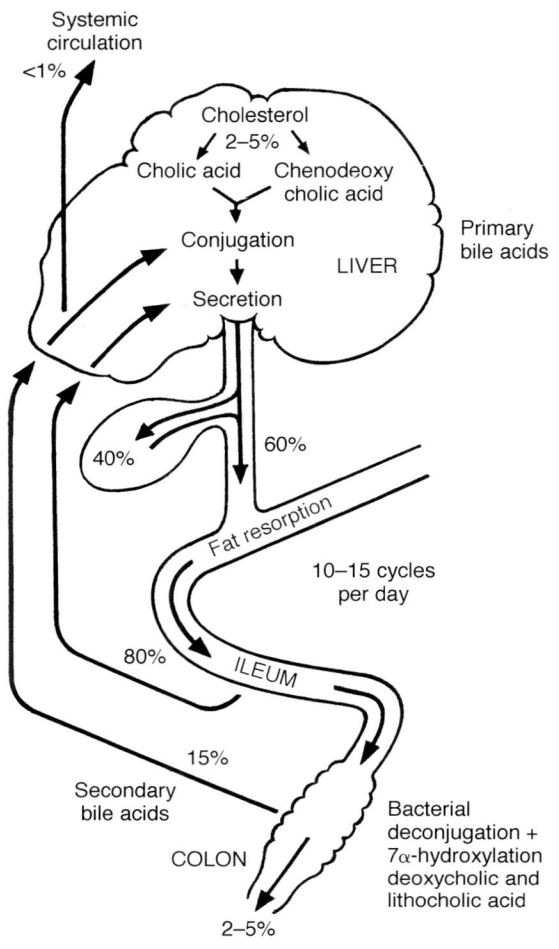

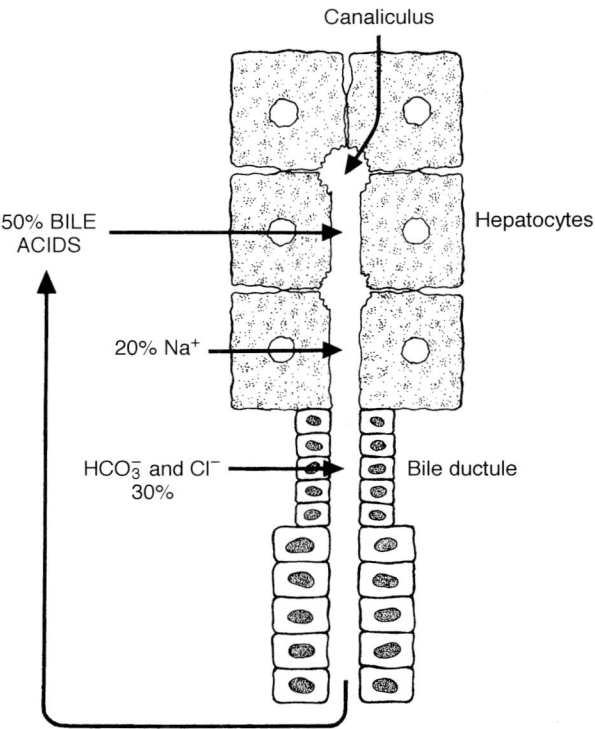

Figure 37.5 Sites of active bile secretion in the liver lobule and their relative contributions.

Figure 37.4 Normal metabolism of bile acids and their enterohepatic cycle. The percentages represent the fractions of the total bile acid pool.

from chenodeoxycholic acid. The unconjugated bile acids can be absorbed throughout the intestinal tract by passive diffusion, whereas the conjugates are actively absorbed in the ileum. Lithocholic acid, which is hepatotoxic and may induce severe cholestasis, is poorly absorbed. The reabsorbed bile acids are very efficiently cleared by the liver from the portal blood and re-excreted. About 95% of excreted bile acids is reabsorbed in the intestinal tract. Hence only a small fraction is lost from the enterohepatic circulation that cycles 10–15 times per day. The lost fraction is replenished by *de novo* synthesis in the liver.

The remaining bile production occurs through active secretion of sodium into the canaliculi (Fig. 37.5). This is stimulated by barbiturates and insulin and inhibited by oestrogens, deficient thyroxine and derivatives of chlorpromazine. The last 30% of bile is not produced by the hepatocytes but by the bile duct epithelium by active excretion of bicarbonate and chloride. This secretion is induced by the gastrointestinal hormones pentagastrin and secretin.

Apart from the gallbladder and the sphincter of Oddi there is no active transport of bile by peristalsis. About 60% of the bile is released directly into the duodenum, the rest being stored in the gallbladder. Contraction of the gallbladder is mainly induced by cholecystokinin secreted by the duodenal mucosa under influence of fat or protein ingestion (Rothuizen *et al.*, 1990; Abiru *et al.*, 1994). Gall bladder contraction may also be provoked by magnesium chloride (Sterczer *et al.*, 1996). Contraction of the gallbladder is gradual over 1–2 hours and the gallbladder is often incompletely emptied following a meal. Bile becomes concentrated about tenfold in the gallbladder and in the larger bile ducts by active absorption of sodium, bicarbonate and water.

Cholestasis

Cholestasis is a reduced bile flow. The obstruction may be intrahepatic or extrahepatic. Most clinical cases are intrahepatic and signs only develop when the pathology is present throughout the liver since obstruction of bile flow in part of the liver is easily compensated for by the other lobes. Extrahepatic cholestasis only gives clinical signs when the bile flow is almost completely obstructed at the level of the common bile duct. Cholestasis may cause accumulation of bile constituents in plasma, such as bilirubin, alkaline phosphatase and γ-glutamyl transpeptidase. However, it is not possible to differentiate between extrahepatic and intrahepatic cholestasis by these assays (Van den Ingh et al., 1986). All forms of cholestasis are detected in liver biopsies as accumulations of brown bile pigment in hepatocytes and Kupffer cells and bile plugs in the canaliculi. In severe cholestasis copper accumulates in the hepatocytes due to inadequate excretion into the bile.

Intrahepatic cholestasis

This form may occur due to leakage through the tight junctions that separate canaliculi from sinusoids and transcellular regurgitation into the intercellular space and the space of Disse (Fig. 37.6). This can occur in endotoxaemia, sepsis and in cases of adverse drug reactions. *Leptospira* produces enzymes which destroy the tight junctions giving severe intrahepatic cholestasis without other liver functions being affected greatly. Swelling of hepatocytes due to fat accumulation can occlude the canaliculi. Necrosis of liver cells for whatever reason may provide a direct connection between canaliculi and the sinusoidal/perisinusoidal bed for back flow of bile. Pathology in the portal areas such as infiltration of inflammatory or tumour cells or deposition of fibrous tissue may block the flow of bile out of the acini.

In cholestasis, the hepatocytes may become overloaded with substances to be excreted and back diffusion into the space of Disse and then to the circulation may also contribute to the cholestasis.

Extrahepatic cholestasis

Extrahepatic cholestasis is relatively rare in dogs and cats. It is caused by complete blockage of bile flow at the level of the common bile duct (Van den Ingh et al., 1986; Fahie and Martin, 1995). The bile ducts proximal to the obstruction dilate and become tortuous, which is characteristic (Nyland and Gillett, 1982). The gallbladder may be distended but in chronic cases only a small quantity of highly concentrated mucinous bile may be present. The size of the gallbladder is, therefore, not a reliable indicator of extrahepatic cholestasis. Bile leakage in the portal areas causes necrosis and an inflammatory reaction. In acute cases there is also periportal oedema, which is replaced by periportal fibrosis after several weeks. The portal bile ducts may also proliferate and become tortuous (Fig. 37.7).

Impaired fat absorption from a lack of intestinal bile acids may induce a deficiency of fat-soluble vitamins D and K (Neer and Hedlund, 1989). Coagulopathy due to non-functioning vitamin K-dependent clotting factors may give a prolonged prothrombin time which is corrected within hours of parenteral vitamin K administration. Rarely in chronic cases, vitamin D deficiency may cause skeletal decalcification.

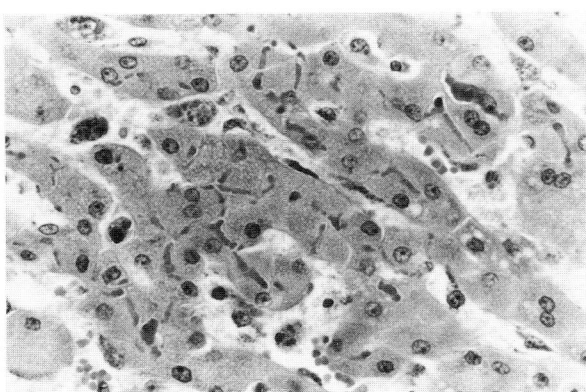

Figure 37.6 Intrahepatic cholestasis with bile thrombi in the canaliculi and bile pigment in the Kupffer cells and hepatocytes.

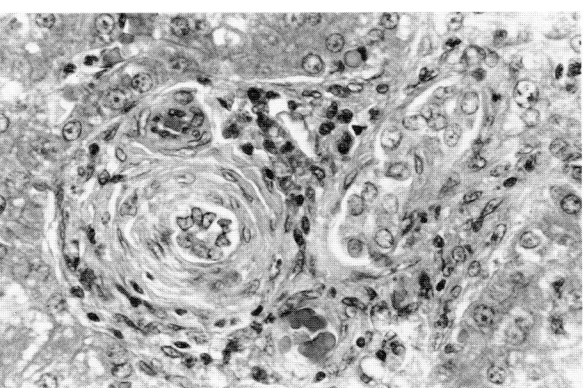

Figure 37.7 Chronic extrahepatic bile duct obstruction in a dog. There are concentric rings of fibrosis around the bile duct and mononuclear inflammatory cells in the portal area.

Bilirubin metabolism and icterus

Bilirubin is the pigment which gives bile its yellow–brown colour. It is the normal end-product of the catabolism of haem. The healthy liver clears bilirubin very effectively from plasma and normal plasma concentrations in dogs and cats are very low (<3.5 µmol l^{-1}). Bilirubin is excreted into the bile and in cases of cholestasis, plasma levels may increase. If concentrations exceed 15 µmol l^{-1}, the pigment diffusing into tissues becomes clinically apparent as icterus. Haem is present mainly in red cell haemoglobin, but also in hepatic haemoproteins. Although the pool size of hepatic haemoproteins is small in comparison to haemoglobin, their turnover is faster and their degradation accounts for 25% of the normal bilirubin production (Rothuizen *et al.*, 1992).

Bilirubin must be conjugated before excretion because of its hydrophobic characteristics (Fig. 37.8). The insoluble unconjugated pigment is bound to albumin in the circulation. Conjugated bilirubin is excreted into bile and is not reabsorbed from the intestines. In cases of bacterial overgrowth, bilirubin may become deconjugated by bacterial enzymes and the pigment may enter an enterohepatic cycle. In the colon, bilirubin is degraded by bacteria into black and brown pigments (stercobilins) that give faeces their normal colour. Lightly coloured faeces due to absence of pigments may be seen in severe cholestasis. Such 'acholic faeces' almost always indicates complete extrahepatic bile duct obstruction. A colourless product, urobilinogen, is also produced some of which is absorbed into the portal circulation. Most of it is cleared by the liver, but a little reaches the systemic circulation and can be excreted in the urine by glomerular filtration and tubular secretion.

It has been practice to measure urobilinogen and bilirubin in urine in order to differentiate cholestatic and haemolytic causes of icterus. Urobilinogen and bilirubin production would be expected to decrease in cases of cholestasis and increase with haemolysis. However, measurement of urobilinogen is of little clinical value, because its concentration in urine is so variable and it is rapidly oxidized in light into urobilin, which is not measured in the Ehrlich reaction.

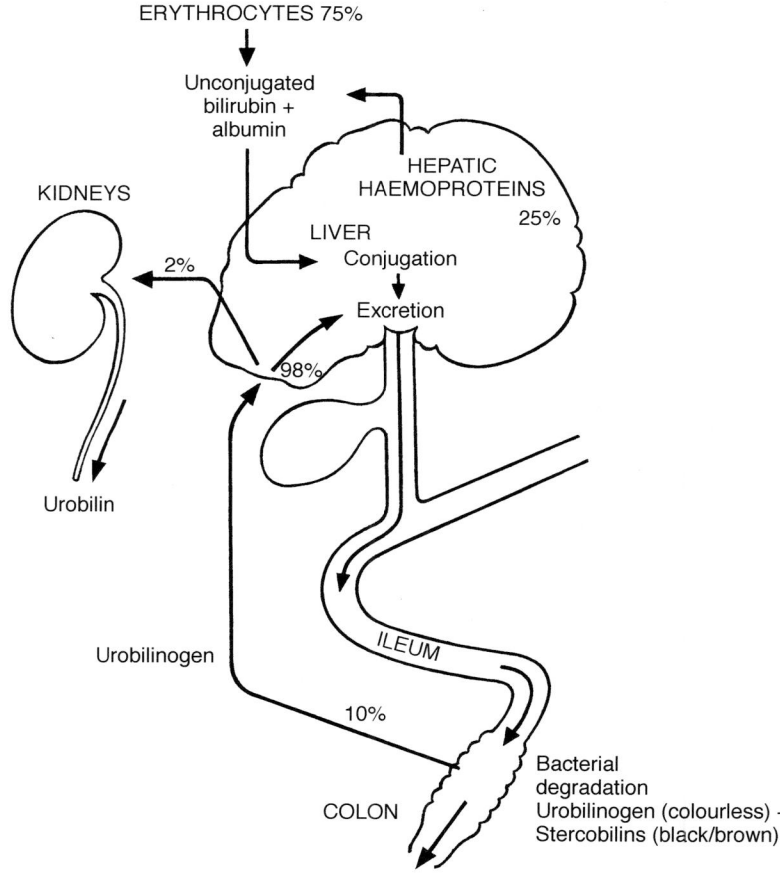

Figure 37.8 Normal production and metabolism of bilirubin. The percentages give the fraction of the total production of bilirubin.

Conjugated bilirubin may be excreted in urine as the renal threshold in dogs and cats is relatively low. Bilirubin in feline urine is abnormal and indicates liver disease. However, canine kidneys, particularly males and less so females (Piens *et al.*, 1996), are capable of forming bilirubin out of haem and can also conjugate and excrete it. Therefore urine of healthy dogs often contains detectable concentrations of bilirubin.

Bilirubin in plasma is usually measured with a diazo reaction in which the conjugates react quickly (direct) and unconjugated (indirect) bilirubin only after addition of an accelerator. Conjugated bilirubin in plasma is always pathological and indicates cholestasis. However, the measurement of direct and indirect reacting bilirubin is of limited value in differentiating cholestatic and haemolytic causes of hyperbilirubinaemia. There are a number of reasons for this. In cases of cholestasis an inconsistent mixture of different conjugates is formed which makes the distinction between direct and indirect reaction arbitrary. In liver disease there is increased production of unconjugated bilirubin and in severe acute haemolysis the liver is secondarily damaged by hypoxia resulting in a decreased bilirubin clearance and cholestasis. In primary liver disease there is considerable haemolysis, presumably due to instability of the erythrocyte membranes caused by high bile acid levels in plasma and prolonged trapping of red blood cells in the spleen in cases of portal hypertension. Animals with liver disease may also have increased bilirubin production from hepatocyte haemoproteins. Consequently, hepatobiliary and haemolytic diseases can be similar with respect to the production and clearance of bilirubin and the presence of cholestasis (Rothuizen and van den Brom, 1987).

Animals with mild or gradually developing anaemia have no liver damage and due to the great reserve capacity of the liver, they do not develop icterus. Careful clinical investigation is much more important than measurement of bilirubin in plasma. Only in severe acute haemolysis is the primary disease extrahepatic. If the mucous membranes are not very pale, an underlying hepatobiliary disease must be suspected.

Conjugated bilirubin in plasma tends to bind covalently and irreversibly to albumin (Rothuizen and van den Ingh, 1988). This biliprotein complex can only escape the circulation when albumin is catabolized; its half-life is about two weeks. Therefore, after recovery from the cholestatic disease, icterus may remain for several weeks. Icterus does not necessarily reflect the actual situation and this should be borne in mind when interpreting clinical findings or evaluating therapy.

Portal hypertension, ascites and acquired portosystemic collateral circulation

Portal hypertension

Portal hypertension is an abnormally high pressure in the portal circulation. The normal pressure in the portal vein is 0–5 mmHg. Portal hypertension can be caused by increased delivery of blood to the portal system or by increased resistance to blood drainage from the portal system. Increased delivery of blood occurs with arteriovenous fistulae in the splanchnic circulation or in the liver, although these are rare. Portal hypertension is usually caused by increased resistance to portal blood flow, which may be prehepatic (in the portal vein), intrahepatic or posthepatic (in the hepatic veins, caudal vena cava or heart). Intrahepatic diseases only cause portal hypertension when the liver is diffusely affected.

With intrahepatic obstruction to the portal circulation, the liver is not congested and is usually small rather than enlarged. The most frequent cause of portal hypertension is cirrhosis, followed by chronic hepatitis, lymphoma, fibrosis, neonatal hepatitis and congenital hypoplasia of the intrahepatic portal vein branches (van den Ingh *et al.*, 1995). However, some portal hypertension can also occur with fatty infiltration of the liver, tumour metastases, reactive hepatitis and extrahepatic cholestasis.

The main prehepatic cause of portal hypertension is portal vein thrombosis (van Winkle and Bruce, 1993). Posthepatic causes may be localized in the caudal vena cava and the heart. Cardiac insufficiency is the most common cause and is usually easy to recognize on physical examination. Thrombosis of the caudal vena cava is unusual.

Portal hypertension may cause ascites and portosystemic collateral formation (Boothe *et al.*, 1996) leading to hepatic encephalopathy. Hepatic encephalopathy is dealt with in another section. Congestion of the intestines in portal hypertension may reduce intestinal absorption and cause diarrhoea, which is a common sign of chronic liver disease.

Ascites

Accumulation of free abdominal fluid may result from portal hypertension alone or from a combination of increased portal blood pressure and reduced oncotic pressure due to hypoproteinaemia. In pre- and posthepatic causes, the plasma albumin concentration is normal and portal hypertension is the only cause of ascites formation. In which case, the hydrostatic pressure is high and causes severe congestion of the splanchnic organs. The resultant free abdominal fluid contains lymph, plasma and erythrocytes and is therefore a clear but slightly serosanguineous transudate. Intrahepatic causes are always chronic and thus hypoalbuminaemia also contributes to decreased intravascular fluid retention and there is only a moderate degree of hypertension. In these cases increased hepatic and splanchnic lymph production exceeds the capacity of the lymphatic system giving a clear transudate which is colourless or in cases of icterus, yellowish.

The diagnosis of ascites in which congestive heart failure has been excluded, should involve an abdominal tap. Clear colourless or yellowish transudate indicates an intrahepatic disease requiring liver biopsy for diagnosis and a serosanguineous transudate indicates either portal vein or vena caval thrombosis. Clear colourless transudate may also occur in non-hepatic diseases associated with severe hypoalbuminaemia, such as nephrotic syndrome and protein-losing enteropathy.

The ascitic fluid can contain a significant amount of albumin as a result of diffusion of this small protein out of the circulation. Complete removal of the ascitic fluid in portal hypertension is not only pointless as the cause remains and hence the ascites quickly recurs, but also undesirable because part of the albumin stores are removed, which in turn leads to an even more rapid recurrence of ascites. Furthermore, the reformation of ascites leads to hypovolaemia, which stimulates compensatory aldosterone production with sodium retention and potassium excretion. Loss of potassium often causes an exacerbation of hepatic encephalopathy. Ascites can be treated more effectively with a low-sodium diet and diuretics that do not increase potassium excretion. However, ascites is merely a sign and not a disease and therapeutic efforts should aim at curing the underlying disease.

Portosystemic collaterals

These are small, non-functional blood vessels in the omentum and mesentery, which become functional as a result of high portal pressure, thereby allowing portal blood to bypass the liver to the caudal and cranial vena cava. Acquired portosystemic collateral vessels only develop when there is a high pressure gradient between the portal vein and the vena cava and therefore only when the cause is pre- or intrahepatic. High pressure in both the vena cava and the portal vein does not induce shunting (Boothe et al., 1996). The degree of shunting may vary from normal to 100%, depending on the cause and the stage of the process. Acquired portosystemic shunts are always multiple and typically localized in the mesorectum, in the omentum where it is attached near the left kidney and along the gastric cardia and in the oesophageal wall. Intraluminal bleeding from oesophageal varices is a serious complication of portal hypertension in humans, but does not occur in companion animals because the vessels lie on the serosal side and not under the mucosa.

The collateral circulation can lead to hepatic encephalopathy. In addition, toxins from the gastrointestinal tract are inadequately removed from the portal blood, which can lead to vomiting and other problems.

■ Hepatic encephalopathy

Hepatic encephalopathy (HE) is defined as dysfunction of the brain secondary to liver dysfunction. HE, like portal hypertension and cholestasis, is not a diagnosis but a common clinical syndrome that can develop in a number of liver diseases in the dog and cat.

There are two forms of HE: an acute and a chronic form. The acute form is rare and only seen in fulminant hepatic failure. It is a severe disorder caused by a sudden and almost complete loss of liver function due to hepatic necrosis. These cases are comatose and develop icterus, vomiting and diffuse intravascular coagulation. They usually die within a few days. The causes of fulminant hepatitis will be given in the section on specific diseases.

The most common form of HE in companion animals is the chronic form. The underlying liver dysfunction causes portosystemic collateral circulation, which may be acquired due to portal hypertension or congenital in case of a single shunt (Rothuizen, 1993). The chronic form is sometimes referred to as portosystemic encephalopathy (PSE). The reserve capacity of the liver in dogs even with severe parenchymal damage, prevents the development of HE in the absence of portosystemic shunting (Rothuizen and van den Ingh, 1982a,b). Therefore in dogs, as in humans, HE should be considered a syndrome in which the liver function is reduced though still adequate, but fails to exert its role as a guardian between the intestine and the rest of the body.

In cats, the hepatic reserve is not as large and thus cats can develop chronic HE with parenchymal liver disease in the absence of portosystemic shunting. The main reason for this is that cats can not adequately synthesize arginine, which is important in the urea cycle. Inadequate ammonia detoxification may cause anorexia and induce HE. Fasting cats may also develop hepatic fat accumulation which further reduces liver function and enhances protein catabolism. This begins earlier in cats than dogs. All of these factors may trigger HE in cats in the absence of shunting. Nevertheless HE is usually associated with shunting.

The presence of portosystemic shunting alone is not sufficient to cause HE; hepatic functions must also be compromised. This is true for all pre- and posthepatic causes of portal hypertension that induce shunting and also for congenital shunts. In the latter condition the liver has been deprived of growth factors from birth and is therefore abnormally small with a low functional parenchymal mass. The causal relation between portosystemic shunting and HE implies that in conditions where shunting is expected to develop (i.e. portal hypertension) precautions must be taken to avoid the triggering of HE.

Clinical signs

The clinical signs of HE are variable (Tyler, 1990). Initial neurological signs are non-specific and are often only recognized retrospectively, when more specific signs have developed. These may include apathy, listlessness, excessive sleepiness and decreased mental alertness. In more advanced cases ataxia, circling, head pressing, salivation, stupor and coma may be seen. Seizures are uncommon except in cats. The episodic nature of HE is characteristic and usually one or two days of severe signs alternate with more or less normal periods of between several days to weeks. Apart from the neurological signs of HE, other signs related to the underlying disease may be seen, such as polyuria, vomiting, diarrhoea, weight loss, decreased exercise tolerance, lethargy, dysuria and haematuria and in case of congenital diseases sometimes poor or retarded growth.

Pathogenesis

The pathogenesis of HE is multifactorial and not yet completely understood. Only the most important and clinically relevant factors will be dealt with here. Chronic HE is essentially a neurotransmitter dysfunction involving several transmitter systems in the brain. Once the underlying liver disease is cured, the encephalopathy disappears completely without any permanent brain damage. Only in cases where haemodynamic derangements due to surgery or anaesthesia have occurred, may permanent cerebrocortical necrosis remain. The most important neurotransmitter systems involved are the glutamate, the gamma-aminobutyric acid and benzodiazepine (GABA/BZ) and the dopamine/noradrenaline pathways (Maddison, 1992; Ferenci et al., 1992).

Glutamate neurotransmission and ammonia metabolism

Glutamate is one of the most abundant excitatory neurotransmitters. In hyperammoniaemia it becomes depleted resulting in impaired brain function (Fig. 37.9).

Ammonia is produced mainly in the intestinal tract, both in the colon by bacterial degradation of nitrogenous compounds (proteins, amines, urea) and by glutamine metabolism liberating ammonia in the intestinal mucosa. Most of the intestinal ammonia is resorbed and enters the portal vein. The healthy liver is extremely efficient in removing ammonia and converting it into urea in the urea cycle. Urea formation occurs exclusively in the liver. It is released into the blood and removed from the body by renal excretion. Some of the urea enters the saliva and recirculates in an enterohepatic cycle. The plasma ammonia concentration is normally very low (< 45 µmol l^{-1}).

In cases of portosystemic shunting, ammonia bypasses the liver and systemic concentrations become increased and neurotoxic. Neurons are separated from the blood by a layer of astrocytes and substances in the circulation have to pass through the astrocytes before reaching the neurones. The astrocytes incorporate ammonia into glutamine by glutamine synthetase. This enzyme has little reserve capacity and can not handle much more than physiological concentrations. Glutamine diffuses into the adjacent neurone and is converted into glutamate by glutaminase. Glutamate is then partly converted into GABA. The excitatory neurotransmitter glutamate and inhibitory GABA form a finely tuned equilibrium determining the excitability of postsynaptic neurones. In hyperammoniaemia the capacity of

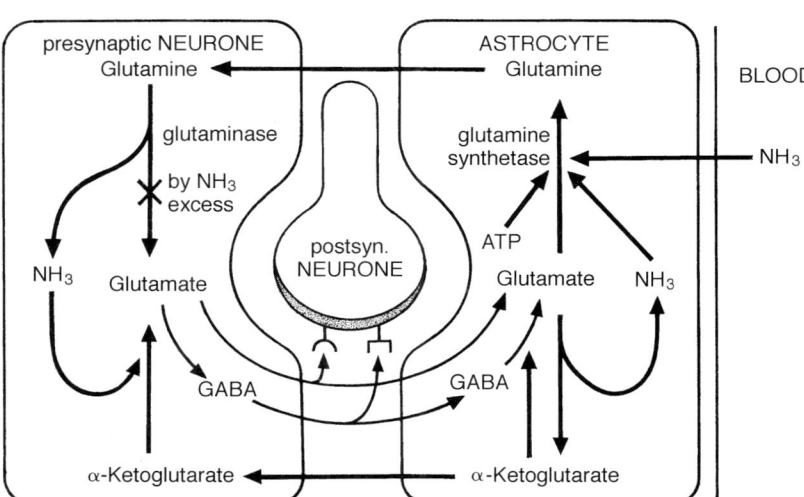

Figure 37.9 The glutamine–glutamate shuttle between astrocytes and neurones in the brain. The capacity of glutamine synthetase in astrocytes is limited and in hyperammoniaemia, ammonia instead of glutamine can diffuse into the neurones. Excess ammonia inhibits glutaminase, resulting in hampered glutamate production and accumulation of glutamine. Glutamate is a stimulatory neurotransmitter which becomes deficient causing hepatic encephalopathy.

astrocytic glutamine synthetase becomes overloaded and excess ammonia diffuses into neurones. High neuronal ammonia concentrations inhibit glutaminase activity resulting in accumulation of glutamine and depletion of the neurotransmitter glutamate. The disturbed glutamate–glutamine–ammonia shuttle between astrocytes and neurones is an important factor in the pathogenesis of HE (Deutz et al., 1988).

GABA/BZ receptor complex

GABA neurotransmission is the most abundant inhibitory system in the brain. In HE the GABA tone is abnormally high inducing suppression of normal brain functions. The origin of the increased GABA activity is not known, but treatment with receptor antagonists may dramatically improve HE. There are, however, no long-acting drugs available to exploit this clinically. The GABA/BZ receptor complex binds many different ligands like GABA, benzodiazepine and barbiturates. The clinical consequence is that one should be extremely careful in using benzodiazepines or barbiturates in anaesthesia and avoid them as far as possible since they potentiate HE and can be fatal! Seizures may be a manifestation of HE and it is important to be certain that HE is not involved before an epileptic animal is treated with these anticonvulsants.

Deranged catecholaminergic neurotransmission

Dopamine and noradrenaline also play a role in the pathogenesis of HE. This is related to the role the liver plays in amino acid metabolism. Normally, the aromatic amino acids tryptophan, tyrosine and phenylalanine are almost completely cleared by the liver from the portal circulation and only very low concentrations reach the systemic blood and the brain. The neurones require low levels of these aromatic amino acids (AAA) because they are precursors of dopamine and noradrenaline. In this catecholamine pathway the capacity of the enzyme, tyrosine-3-hydroxylase, is rate limiting (Fig. 37.10). In HE, excess AAA are processed via alternative metabolic pathways in the brain producing octopamine, ß-phenylethanolamine and tyramine which are structurally similar to the physiological catecholamines and occupy their receptors. They are called 'false neurotransmitters' since they have only very weak intrinsic activities and block normal dopaminergic and noradrenergic neurotransmission and thus contribute to the pathogenesis of HE.

Branched chained amino acids (BCAA) valine, leucine and isoleucine are passively involved in this process. Together with the AAA they form neutral amino acids and use the same carrier system to enter the brain through the blood–brain barrier. Plasma BCAA levels are reduced in chronic liver dysfunction because they are exploited as an alternative energy source in muscles and other tissues. The low ratio of BCAA to AAA in plasma gives the aromatics easier access to the brain since there is less competition for the common carrier.

Clinical implications

Ammonia

To understand clinical implications in ammonia metabolism it is important to appreciate that only the molecular, non-ionized form (NH_3) passes

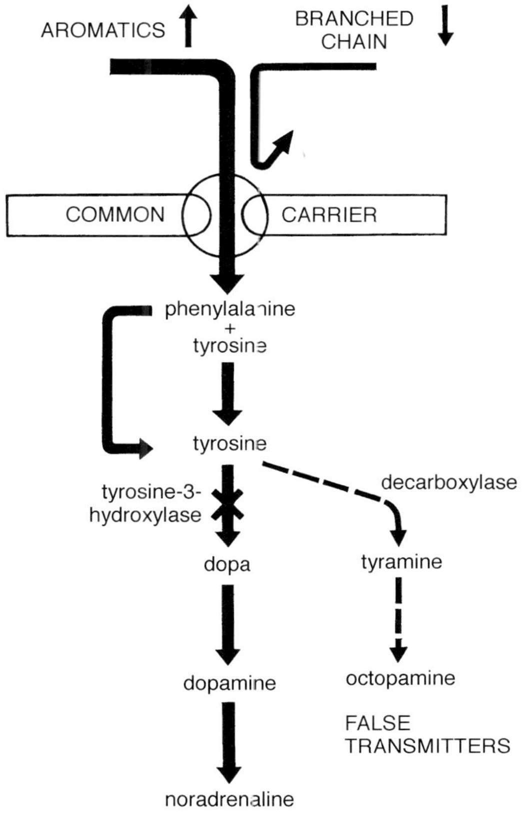

Figure 37.10 The role of neutral amino acids in the pathogenesis of hepatic encephalopathy. Aromatic and branched chain amino acids compete for a common carrier over the blood–brain barrier. Portosystemic shunting causes an excess of aromatic and a reduction of branched chain amino acids in the circulation and in the brain. The aromatic amino acid tyrosine reaches levels exceeding the capacity of the converting enzyme tyrosine-3-hydroxylase and the excess is decarboxylated to form non-functional neurotransmitters which displace dopamine and noradrenaline from the receptors.

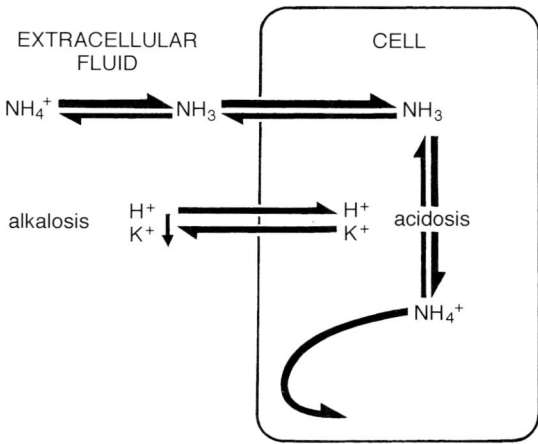

Figure 37.11 Hypokalaemia causes a shift of potassium ions from cells into the extracellular fluid, in exchange for hydrogen (and sodium). This causes intracellular acidosis and extracellular alkalosis. Molecular ammonia from the circulation can easily penetrate the cells. There it becomes ionized which prevents its back-diffusion out of the cell. This may result in ammonia toxicity.

cell membranes easily, whereas NH_4^+ does not. Intracellularly, both forms have equal metabolic effects. In alkalosis there is more NH_3, which may aggravate the neurotoxic effect of ammonia and should be prevented or corrected in any patient with chronic liver disease. Alkalosis also results in the formation of alkaline urine from which the non-ionized ammonia is readily reabsorbed. This changes the kidney from an ammonia excreting into an ammonia generating organ. The most serious form of alkalosis is induced by hypokalaemia (Fig. 37.11). Low plasma potassium is replenished by exchanging intracellular potassium for sodium and hydrogen; the hydrogen shift induces extracellular alkalosis and intracellular acidosis. Ammonia penetrates the cell membrane easily but intracellularly it becomes ionized and cannot leave the cell, thus acting as a one-way scavenger of ammonia.

Hypokalaemia can occur in chronic liver disease. Potassium may be lost in cases of diarrhoea or when potassium-losing diuretics are used to treat ascites. In cases of dehydration, activation of the renin–angiotensin–aldosterone system induces renal sodium and water retention and potassium loss, for example as occurs when portal hypertension causes ascites formation.

Catabolic conditions are common in advanced liver disease and may contribute to the onset of HE. Increased breakdown of peripheral proteins liberates glutamine which gives rise to ammonia formation. The neurotoxic action of ammonia is further enhanced by mercaptans produced by intestinal flora out of methionine (Merino *et al.*, 1975). Methionine is part of many so called 'liver supporting' medications that are clinically useless and in any event, should not be given orally.

Ammonia measurement in plasma is the only practical way to diagnose HE. Due to the incorporation of ammonia into glutamine the mean arterial concentration may exceed that in venous blood and moderate increases can be missed in venous samples (Rothuizen and van den Ingh,

1982a). In cases of doubt an ammonia tolerance test always gives a clear result. About 40% of dogs with HE have ammonium biurate crystals in the urine sediment. If present, these are highly specific for conditions causing HE in dogs other than Dalmatians. These crystals result from inadequate hepatic metabolism and excessive urinary excretion of both ammonia and uric acid (Maretta et al., 1981). Some animals are presented with signs of haematuria or dysuria due to these uroliths.

Increased GABA/BZ receptor tone

Anaesthesia with benzodiazepines, acepromazine and barbiturates should be avoided if possible in patients with HE. The best anaesthetic regimen for animals with liver dysfunction used in the author's clinic is premedication with a low dose of fentanyl and droperidol followed by induction of anaesthesia with intravenous sufentanyl (an opiate) dosed to effect. Anaesthesia is maintained by a combination of slow infusion of sufentanyl and low dose inhalation of isoflurane with oxygen and nitrous oxide by mechanical ventilation to ensure adequate oxygenation. Monitoring the blood pressure may be important because haemodynamic instabilities may result in irreversible cerebral necrosis.

Impaired catecholaminergic neurotransmission

The deranged neutral amino acid metabolism has a few consequences. Firstly, catabolism due to anorexia should be prevented or treated. In severe cases intravenous feeding support can be of importance and if so glucose and amino acid infusions are indicated (Laflamme, 1988). The type of amino acids chosen for infusion should be aimed at normalizing the BCAA:AAA ratio.

The deranged catecholamine metabolism also helps to explain the cause of polyuria which occurs in about half the patients with chronic liver disease. Catecholamines inhibit the release of adrenocorticotrophin (ACTH), the hormone which stimulates cortisol secretion from the adrenals. Failure of this inhibition results in an increased ACTH release and hypercortisolism (Rothuizen and Mol, 1987; Meyer and Rothuizen, 1994). Chronic cortisol excess and deranged GABA neurotransmission induce inadequate pituitary secretion of antidiuretic hormone (vasopressin) and hence impaired urine concentration by the kidneys (Rothuizen et al., 1995a,b).

Treatment of HE

HE may occur in a variety of liver diseases and it is of prime importance to diagnose and if possible, treat the underlying disease. Symptomatic support of HE may gain time for treatment of the underlying disease, preparation of a patient for surgery, or provide life-long support when liver functions are permanently damaged. HE can be treated by feeding a low-protein high-carbohydrate diet to reduce intestinal ammonia and AAA production (Laflamme, 1988; Bauer and Schenck, 1989). The caloric requirement must be fulfilled to prevent catabolism. The degree of protein restriction depends on the condition. In cases of chronic active hepatitis and cirrhosis, the inflammation can be cured but the fibrosis and often the portosystemic collaterals remain. Such animals need life-long protein restriction at a level just sufficient to prevent HE and yet not to compromise hepatic protein synthesis which could induce ascites formation. In contrast, very strict protein reduction is needed for short-term preparation of patients with congenital shunts for surgery, since anaesthesia is more complicated in case of overt HE. Cats require about twice as much protein as dogs, but otherwise similar recommendations should be followed.

In cases requiring long-term treatment of HE oral administration of disaccharides such as lactulose ($1-3$ ml kg^{-1} day^{-1} in divided doses) may be helpful. Lactulose is not absorbed in the small intestines and is degraded into volatile free fatty acids by colonic bacteria (Conn and Bircher, 1989). The resulting acidification gives a shift to non-absorbable ionized ammonia, increased colon motility and an altered and less ammoniagenic flora. In animals with advanced HE, forced intravenous diuresis (100 ml kg^{-1} day^{-1}) to excrete as much ammonia as possible and intravenous feeding (glucose and amino acids with a favourable BCAA:AAA ratio) is essential. Furthermore, conditions that aggravate HE, like hypovolaemia, hypokalaemia and alkalosis should be corrected and drugs like benzodiazepines, barbiturates and methionine avoided. Glucocorticoid medication which induces catabolism should be avoided if possible, although it remains the drug of choice in chronic active hepatitis.

■ Blood coagulopathy in liver disease

All of the clotting factors except the Von Willebrand subtype of factor VIII are synthesized in the liver. The activation of factors II, VII, IX and X depends on the availability of vitamin K, which may be poorly absorbed in cases with extrahepatic cholestasis (Neer and Hedlund, 1989). The equilibrium between activation and inactivation of the coagulation cascade depends also on clotting inhibiting proteins, mainly antithrombin III, which is synthesized in the liver. In addition, the clearance of activated clotting factors and of antithrombin depends on the reticuloendothelial system which is largely localized in the liver. The liver may also affect the primary haemostasis by prolonged retention of thrombocytes at their site of degradation, the spleen, due to portal hypertension. This may induce abnormally low thrombocyte counts.

Although the liver may affect blood coagulation in many ways, disseminated intravascular coagulation (DIC) is the most frequent and serious coagulopathy (Badylak, 1988; Badylak et al., 1983). This occurs especially in cases with diffuse liver cell necrosis such as some forms of hepatitis, lymphosarcoma or metastatic tumours. The coagulopathy may be subclinical. For this reason it is essential to measure blood coagulation and plasma fibrinogen before taking a liver biopsy. Fibrinogen levels below 1 g l^{-1} are an absolute contraindication for liver biopsy.

There is little point in treating coagulopathy due to liver disease. DIC will disappear spontaneously if the underlying disease can be successfully treated.

HISTORY TAKING IN HEPATOBILIARY DISEASES

The recognition of liver disorders based on history and clinical signs is usually difficult. Most of the signs are non-specific and thus liver disorders are often overlooked. The incidence of liver and biliary tract diseases is around 1–2% of all clinical cases in dogs and cats, but this figure depends on the breed and country (Andersson and Sevelius, 1991). For example, the incidence of inherited portosystemic shunts alone in the Irish wolfhound and Cairn terrier population in the Netherlands is 4 and 2%, respectively (Meyer et al., 1995).

The difficulty in interpreting clinical signs may occur for several reasons. The liver plays an essential role in numerous metabolic processes and disturbances in these can affect the function of other organ systems, which often leads to the impression that dysfunction of the other system is the primary disease. Hepatic encephalopathy and polydipsia are good examples. The liver may also be affected secondarily by diseases of other organ systems, with the result that the same clinical signs and abnormal laboratory findings can occur as in a primary liver disease. For example, primary liver disorders often cause vomiting and diarrhoea, while at the same time a primary gastrointestinal disorder often results in a secondary (reactive) hepatitis. In both cases the signs are the same and laboratory tests indicate liver damage. In addition, dogs with polyuria and polydipsia may have markedly elevated alkaline phosphatase (AP) and moderately elevated alanine aminotransferase (ALT) in plasma. These findings are consistent with hyperadrenocorticism, but also with many primary liver diseases.

The most important signs and the frequency with which they occur in primary liver diseases referred to a university clinic are given below. The pattern in a first opinion population is probably similar. These signs occur in a variety of combinations in many liver diseases: apathy and listlessness (60%), reduced appetite (59%), vomiting (58%), weight loss (50%), polydipsia (45%), diarrhoea (27%), reduced exercise tolerance sometimes associated with weakness (27%), ascites (21%), neurological signs such as ataxia and compulsive walking and sometimes epilepsy (12%), icterus (12%), abnormally light coloured (acholic) faeces (7%), abnormal bleeding tendency (1%) and painful, frequent micturition (0.5%). Abdominal pain is very rare, but is sometimes seen with cholecystitis.

The pathophysiology of these signs is explained in the preceding part of this chapter. It is important to realize that the entire spectrum of signs may occur in most hepatobiliary diseases and it is impossible in most cases to relate them to a specific liver disease.

PHYSICAL EXAMINATION

Physical examination related to hepatobiliary diseases should concentrate on the mucous membranes and abdominal palpation. In case of hepatomegaly or ascites, examination of the cardiovascular system is indicated to rule out cardiac disease.

Abnormalities of the mucous membranes may include icterus, pallor and indications of coagulopathy. Mild anaemia is common in hepatic diseases due to reduced erythrocyte survival time and inadequate erythropoiesis, but is non-specific since it occurs in many other disorders. The degree of pallor of the mucous membranes is important in cases of icterus, since only in acute and massive haemolysis, for example autoimmune haemolysis, does the liver become secondarily damaged. In all other cases icterus indicates hepatobiliary disease. Icterus is most easily detected by yellow-coloured sclerae. In case of doubt centrifugation of plasma always reveals the readily visible colour of bilirubin even in slightly increased concentrations. Coagulopathy in liver disease is almost always due to DIC, which may be visible in rare cases as petechiae in mucous membranes or the skin. Of course, petechiae are not specific for hepatic disease.

Hepatomegaly may be palpable on abdominal examination. In general, hepatomegaly is rare in liver diseases of dogs. It occurs only in case of tumours and secondary involvement of the liver in systemic diseases, such as venous congestion, fatty infiltration in diabetes mellitus, glycogen accumulation in hyperadrenocorticism, amyloidosis, lymphoma and metastatic tumours. In contrast, hepatobiliary diseases in cats are commonly associated with hepatomegaly. The anatomical relations between diaphragm, liver and thoracic wall in cats permit easier detection of liver enlargement than in dogs. As a rule of thumb, all hepatobiliary diseases except congenital portosystemic shunts may induce hepatomegaly in cats. Cats may also have liver enlargement due to systemic diseases.

Abdominal palpation may also reveal splenomegaly in cases of portal hypertension. This is not always so and an enlarged spleen may occur with other conditions. Ascites due to portal hypertension and/or hypoproteinaemia may also indicate liver disease. Although there are many other diseases that can induce ascites formation.

Non-specific findings associated with liver dysfunction include some degree of emaciation and an indication of hyperadrenocorticism which may be secondary to liver disease (see hepatic encephalopathy) with muscle atrophy, abdominal distension and symmetric alopecia.

LABORATORY EXAMINATION

There are a number of different categories of laboratory blood tests which can be used in the diagnosis of hepatobiliary diseases. These include enzyme activities in plasma, bile acid concentrations, serum proteins, blood coagulation tests, ammonia and ammonia tolerance tests and a miscellaneous group. There is a tendency in many clinics to use 'liver profiles' incorporating as many parameters as possible to characterize hepatic disease. Thorough consideration of these parameters has introduced another philosophy to use only those parameters that really aid in the assessment of the disease.

Plasma enzymes

The measurement of enzyme activities in plasma is based on the assumption that changes in the liver or bile ducts cause more enzyme than normal to be released resulting in increased activity in the blood (Abdelkader and Hauge, 1986). Enzymes may be released due to necrosis of the cell or increased permeability of the cell membrane. The latter condition may be transient and completely reversible with only cytoplasmic or cell membrane-bound enzymes released. The enzyme activity in plasma depends on the number of cells involved per unit time, the cellular concentration of the enzyme and its subcellular location. In the circulation the enzyme is catabolized at a rate measured by the half-life, which is specific for each enzyme. This degradation occurs predominantly in the reticuloendothelial system in the liver. As a result of these factors, the plasma activity is different for different enzymes in the same sample. High concentration in the cell and a long half-life in plasma make an enzyme a sensitive indicator of liver damage.

It is important to appreciate that enzymes indicate the degree of liver cell damage and not the function of the liver. High enzyme activities can occur in acute liver degeneration which may be transient, reversible and because of the large reserve capacity of the liver, of no significant influence to liver function. In contrast, chronic liver disease may take months or years to reach the symptomatic stage; the enzyme release per time unit is low giving normal or slightly elevated levels. However, at the same time liver function may be dramatically impaired. In other words, liver enzymes tend to lose diagnostic sensitivity in chronic, advanced liver disease.

Enzymes are not only present in the liver but may be found in many other tissues (Sutherland, 1989). The same type of enzyme present in different tissues may, despite being detected in the same way in the plasma sample, be physically different with respect to plasma half-life and molecular charge (pK_a); so called isoenzymes. Differences of isoenzymes in half-life and relative concentrations in the liver and other tissues determine the specificity of the enzyme in the diagnosis of hepatobiliary diseases. The most important enzymes in the dog and cat are discussed below.

Alkaline phosphatase

Alkaline phosphatase (AP) occurs in most organs but primarily in bone, liver, kidney, small bowel mucosa and placenta (Wellman et al., 1982). Hepatic AP resides mainly in the hepatocytes lining the canaliculi and in bile duct epithelium. The enzyme is present in the microsomal membranes of the cell. AP from the kidney and intestinal mucosa is mostly released into the urine and intestinal lumen, respectively. The half-life of the intestinal, kidney and placental AP is only a few minutes, so the contribution of AP from these organs is negligible. The half-life of AP from liver and bone is about 70 h and AP from these sources can cause elevated AP activity in plasma. In cholestasis there is also back-diffusion of bile into the circulation. Extrahepatic cholestasis usually causes very high plasma AP activity.

In addition, glucocorticoids, either endogenous or exogenous, can induce a hepatic isoenzyme of AP, leading to increased AP activity (Sanecki et al., 1987). This isoenzyme can be recognized, because after heating plasma to 65°C for 2 min, the liver and bone AP are almost completely inactivated whereas glucocorticoid-induced AP is not (Teske et al., 1986). In the cat AP is of less importance in diagnosis because the half-life is very short (5.8 h). There is no heat-stable isoenzyme induced by glucocorticoids in cats.

In young growing dogs, the high osteoblastic activity gives normal AP values 2–3 times higher than in mature dogs. In the absence of skeletal disease (osteomyelitis, osteosarcoma, fractures) increased plasma AP is always of hepatic origin, either due to hepatobiliary disease or to induction by steroids. AP is the most sensitive enzyme in dogs for the detection of hepatobiliary diseases. In the absence of skeletal disease it is also highly liver specific.

Gamma-glutamyl transpeptidase

Gamma glutamyl transpeptidase (γGT) is very liver specific and is localized in cell membranes of the bile duct epithelium. It is also found in the kidney, intestine and brain, but these do not contribute to plasma γGT. In dogs and cats elevated γGT indicates cholestasis. It is released into the blood from damaged bile duct epithelium and by back-diffusion of γGT-containing bile into the circulation. In the cat, in which AP has less clinical importance, γGT is a slightly more sensitive parameter (Center et al., 1986b). In the dog, it is sometimes possible on the basis of γGT measurements to say whether or not an elevated AP is associated with cholestasis, but it is still not possible to determine the underlying cause. In the dog, γGT is elevated in 80% of liver disorders and is therefore not very sensitive. During recovery from a hepatobiliary disease the plasma γGT remains elevated for longer than other enzymes.

Transaminases

Alanine aminotransferase (ALT) and aspartate aminotransferase (AST) were known in the older nomenclature as GPT and GOT, respectively. The biological half life of both ALT and AST is 3–5 h. ALT is liver specific in dogs and cats with relatively little activity in other tissues. It is localized in the cytoplasm of hepatocytes and released by damage to the cell membrane (Aminlari et al., 1994). The cell does not have to be irreversibly damaged. ALT is elevated in nearly 90% of dogs with liver disorders. In both the dog and the cat, ALT is fairly sensitive and specific and thus a good parameter for use in screening for the presence of liver disease.

AST is not liver specific. In the dog it is mainly present in cardiac and skeletal muscle and other tissues with less in the liver. In the cat it is more limited to the liver. AST is chiefly located in the mitochondria and thus only released by cell death. AST is increased in 74% of dogs with liver diseases and is thus less sensitive and specific.

Other enzymes

Other enzymes have been used to evaluate liver diseases. Examples include lactate dehydrogenase (LDH), sorbitol dehydrogenase (SDH), glutamate dehydrogenase (GLDH), choline esterase (CHE) and 5'-nucleotidase. These enzymes are less useful than those already discussed due to a lack of sensitivity and/or specificity.

Bile acids

Bile acids in plasma are very specific for detecting hepatobiliary disease. The plasma concentration depends on a number of liver functions and on intestinal absorption. Reduced hepatic functions such as clearance from plasma (parenchymal disease or portosystemic collateral circulation), conjugation, biliary excretion and bile transport may all give rise to increased bile acid concentrations. In most hepatobiliary diseases one or more of these dysfunctions is present and hence bile acids are not useful for differentiating between different types of liver disease. For example, very high levels may be detected in both portosystemic shunting and in extrahepatic cholestasis.

Bile acids are more sensitive and specific than AP and ALT and unlike the enzymes, bile acids indicate hepatobiliary function rather than actual cellular damage (Center et al., 1985a, 1986a; Rutgers et al., 1988). Bile acids are therefore often very raised in animals with chronic disease and severely impaired liver function, in which the enzymes tend to be relatively low (Johnson et al., 1985). In some cases with equivocal fasting bile acid concentrations, it is necessary to take an additional measurement two hours after feeding (Center et al., 1991).

Bile acids in plasma are a mixture of the different bile acid metabolites which are all measured by the same enzymatic reaction. It is possible to measure the individual bile acid metabolites, but this requires elaborate procedures and there is no proven additional clinical value. Theoretically, abnormally low bile acid levels could occur in cases of inadequate production in the liver or when in intestinal loss due to inadequate absorption is not compensated for by hepatic synthesis. However, the normal bile acid concentration in plasma is so low that decreased values are below the detection limit.

Blood examination in the diagnostic screening for hepatobiliary disease

In general, blood examination does not permit the discrimination of one liver disease from another. The same spectrum of changes may be present in different diseases of the liver or biliary tract. Therefore extended liver profiles including more parameters do not increase the diagnostic value of blood examination. Blood parameters are commonly evaluated for diagnostic value by their tendency to be increased in liver disease (sensitivity), which is in fact a comparison of animals with liver disease and healthy individuals. In practice, however, the choice is not between liver disease and health, but between liver disease and any other disease with similar signs and physical findings. Hence, the specificity in the relevant patient population is of prime importance. Multivariate analysis of a large number of parameters measured in our clinic in a patient population in which the presence of hepatobiliary disease was one of the differential diagnoses (based on history and physical examination) revealed that total bile acids, AP and ALT had the best specificity and sensitivity. The combinations of bile acids with AP and of bile acids with ALT were very efficient in screening for hepatobiliary disease, with at least one parameter increased indicating disease. Addition of more parameters did not improve the specificity or sensitivity. The next best combination was AP with ALT, which is also specific but less sensitive than a combination including bile acids. AP in cats is quite insensitive to detect hepatobiliary diseases; in this species ALT with bile acids is the best combination for screening.

For animals with neurological signs in which hepatic encephalopathy is suspected, measurement of ammonia or an ammonia tolerance test is the most direct approach. Normal ammonia values lead to the diagnosis of a primary neurological disorder; hyperammoniaemia should be followed by further diagnosis of the underlying liver disease.

It may be useful to measure parameters indicating relevant aspects of the liver function, such as serum proteins or plasma ammonia in specific cases. A good example is chronic active hepatitis in which hypoalbuminaemia and portal hypertension may induce complications such as ascites, portosystemic collaterals and hepatic encephalopathy. Such a diagnosis may be followed by measurement of ammonia, serum proteins or the degree of shunting to evaluate the risk of complications that may be prevented by specific measures. Such extended measurements do not contribute to the diagnosis but serve to improve the clinical management of a patient with a known diagnosis.

Other blood examinations

Chronic dysfunction of the liver can cause hypoalbuminaemia (Meyer and Center, 1986). Albumin and most of the protein factors in coagulation are produced exclusively in the liver. Hypoalbuminaemia rarely reaches the oedema limit (about 15 g l^{-1}). The biological half-life of albumin is 12 days.

In hepatobiliary diseases, blood coagulation may be abnormal usually as a result of DIC. Measurement of fibrinogen is required before the liver is biopsied to be sure that there is no severe coagulopathy (fibrinogen <1 g l^{-1}).

Ammonia is an important parameter when hepatic encephalopathy is suspected, as is the ammonia tolerance test (ATT). An ATT should be performed in all cases in which the fasting ammonia is only slightly elevated. Ammonia measurements easily give erroneous results.

Ammonia forms quickly from proteins, amines and urea in blood at room temperature and therefore samples should be placed immediately on ice and centrifuged in a cooled centrifuge. Measurements should be performed as quickly as possible. Plasma may be kept at 0–4°C for 4 h, or frozen at −20°C for 24 h until analysis. Other sources for errors are saliva, sweat or cigarette smoke. Therefore, the inner side of the tube stopper should not be touched and smoking prohibited in the clinic and laboratory. It is also essential to avoid contamination with traces of the ammonium chloride test solution during an ATT.

In the ATT, an ammonia-containing solution may be administered rectally or orally. The rectal ammonia administration is well tolerated whereas oral ammonia may induce vomiting. Two ml of a 5% ammonium chloride solution per kg body weight is given rectally using a soft catheter introduced to a depth of 10–20 cm depending on the size of the animal. Blood is sampled just before and 20 and 40 min after the challenge (Rothuizen and van den Ingh, 1982b). Animals with liver disease but without portosystemic collateral circulation show no increase of the plasma ammonia concentration during the test; in all animals with shunting there is at least doubling of ammonia when basal values are only moderately increased. In cases with very high basal concentrations the rise may not be significant. Worsening of the HE due to the ammonia load is not seen with this dosage.

INVESTIGATIVE TECHNIQUES

Liver biopsy procedures

Menghini technique

In most diseases of the liver and biliary tract the histological changes are specific and the diagnosis can be made by histological examination of a liver biopsy. The simplest technique is percutaneous (so-called 'blind') liver biopsy which can be obtained under local anaesthesia. The biopsy is obtained from the left side of the liver to prevent rupture of the gallbladder, which lies on the right side, and also of large blood vessels and bile ducts in the hilus. The liver makes large excursions with the diaphragm and therefore it is important to choose a biopsy technique where the needle enters the liver for as short a time as possible to prevent trauma to the liver. This is possible with the Menghini cannula; other biopsy devices may require several seconds in the liver. For dogs the best cannula size is 18 cm long and 1.4 mm outer diameter; the typical biopsy weight is 20 mg. For cats a 14 cm/1.2 mm device is appropriate. Liver tissue should be immediately fixed in 5% buffered formaldehyde.

With the dog lying on its right side, the Menghini needle is introduced in the midline 1–2 cm behind the xiphoid process. After disinfection of the skin and injection of local anaesthetic, a small stab incision is made through the abdominal wall, to permit introduction of the Menghini cannula which is attached to a 5 ml syringe filled with saline. The blunt tip of the cannula may be used to carefully 'palpate' intraabdominal structures without immediately penetrating them. This is important because one must be certain to puncture the liver and not other structures such as the stomach, which is painful, or the diaphragm. The animal must be fasted for at least 6 h, since it can be difficult to find the liver beyond a full stomach. 'Palpation' of the liver with the cannula requires experience obtained on cadavers. The site of the left lateral and medial lobes depends very much on the shape of the animal; in dogs with a deep chest the cannula has to be advanced underneath the stomach to reach the liver, whereas in brachycephalic breeds the liver is immediately within reach. The diseased liver may be small or enlarged, thus altering the anatomical relationships. With the tip of the cannula on the liver surface, the actual biopsy is performed within a second by penetrating the liver 2–3 cm and gently aspirating tissue into the tip of the needle, which is kept there by maintaining suction whilst withdrawing it. The cannula contains a mandrin 3 cm shorter than the needle which prevents liver tissue being aspirated into the syringe and broken into pieces. It is preferable to take two biopsies, since this considerably increases the diagnostic accuracy. It should be remembered that a biopsy obtained in this manner is a blind sample of the liver and that a local process could be missed which should be borne in mind if the histological report does not agree with the clinical or biochemical abnormalities. In cases of ascites the abdominal wall and the skin must be closed with a few sutures to prevent leakage of fluid.

The contraindications for a liver biopsy are

severe congestion of the liver and abnormal coagulation (fibrinogen below 1 g l^{-1}). Percutaneous liver biopsy may be impossible in an animal with ascites with a small, hard and fibrotic liver, which moves away in the ascitic fluid when touched by the needle. In such cases laparoscopy or laparotomy may be required to obtain liver tissue for histological examination.

The major disadvantage of the blind procedure is that focal lesions may be missed. This is prevented by performing ultrasonography of the liver before puncture. Ultrasonography visualizes the structure of the liver and focal processes as small as 5 mm may be sampled under ultrasound guidance (Hager et al., 1985).

Possible complications of liver biopsy are prolonged bleeding from the liver, gallbladder or bile duct rupture and trauma to the stomach or diaphragm and thoracic structures. Liver biopsy is a relatively simple and safe procedure in experienced hands, but it should not be attempted on an occasional basis by an inexperienced person. The author has performed many thousands of blind biopsies and seen only a few complications.

Fine needle biopsy

Liver puncture may also be performed to obtain liver cells for cytological instead of histological examination. Fine needle aspiration biopsy using a 22G needle (a disposable injection needle is long enough in most cases) provides enough liver cells to make a smear which can be examined cytologically. The smear is air dried and can be kept in that condition before staining. Since the histological structure is lost, only changes that may be recognized in individual cells are detectable, such as fat, glycogen, or copper accumulation in hepatocytes or the presence of tumour cells (Kristensen et al., 1990; Teske et al., 1992). The advantage of fine needle aspiration is that it is simple, safe and the staining and examination may be completed within a day. Fine needle biopsy may also be performed in cases with coagulopathy and therefore measurement of coagulation parameters is not essential. The author prefers a right intercostal approach, because the right part of the liver lies in close contact with the abdominal wall. The needle is connected to an air-filled syringe and the liver is punctured and aspirated in the right 10th intercostal space at the chondrocostal junction after local disinfection of the skin. Local anaesthesia is not required.

For all biopsies it is important to realize that the clinician depends very much on the experience of the pathologist or cytologist.

■ Laparoscopy

Laparoscopy is the examination of the abdominal cavity with a rigid endoscope. It allows inspection of organs and guided biopsy. Laparoscopy can be performed when local processes are suspected in the liver or when the percutaneous technique fails to obtain a biopsy (Rothuizen, 1985). The technique is of less importance since the introduction of ultrasonography. The equipment is expensive and complications may occur.

■ Ultrasonography

Ultrasonography has become widely available and may be used to visualize the liver, gallbladder and portal and hepatic veins. An experienced investigator can detect local structural changes such as tumours, abscesses or hyperplasia as well as diffuse processes. Gallstones, distended bile ducts and abnormal vascular structures such as congenital portosystemic shunts may also be seen. It is advisable to perform ultrasonography routinely before taking a percutaneous liver biopsy. It is possible to puncture localized structures under ultrasound guidance and this considerably improves the diagnostic accuracy of liver biopsies.

■ Portography

The course of the portal vein and the presence of acquired portal collateral vessels can be visualized by portography (Suter, 1982). The simplest method is by the injection of a contrast material into an intestinal vein via a small laparotomy incision (portal venography). Catheterization of the coeliac or the cranial mesenteric artery via the femoral artery is indicated in cases in which arteriovenous shunts are suspected.

■ Radioisotope imaging of the liver

These methods are only available in specialized centres, but can provide very precise, often quantitative data concerning specific aspects of the liver function (Kerr and Hornof, 1986; van den Brom and Rothuizen, 1990; Daniel et al., 1991; Meyer et al., 1994; Koblik et al., 1995; Bahr et al., 1996; Foster-van Hijfte et al., 1996).

Hepatobiliary Diseases of Dogs

HEPATITIS AND CIRRHOSIS

Acute hepatitis

Aetiology

Acute hepatitis can be caused by chemicals such as organic solvents (Aguilera et al., 1988), phosphorus (Burnell et al., 1976), drugs including nalidixine acid, paracetamol and mebendazole (Thornburg, 1988), viral infection (infectious canine hepatitis) and mycotoxins (Bastianello et al., 1987; Little et al., 1991). Hepatitis resulting from sepsis (reactive hepatitis), leptospirosis and haemolysis are discussed in other sections. Drugs containing sulphonamides may induce a severe type of hepatitis which presents mainly as a chronic disease, destructive cholangiolitis.

Pathogenesis

Depending on the extent of the liver cell necrosis, intracellular enzymes will be released and bile will leak back into the circulation. In acute hepatitis all of the enzymes are usually elevated. Fever may occur as a result of pyrogens from necrotic tissue or reduced removal of endotoxins and bacteria from the portal blood. DIC often occurs. Extensive liver cell necrosis with severe loss of liver function is referred to as *fulminant hepatitis* and leads to the development of hepatic encephalopathy, DIC and hypoglycaemia. This severe form progresses rapidly to coma and death.

Acute hepatitis is characterized by liver necrosis and the accompanying inflammatory reaction (Fig. 37.12). Depending on the severity of the hepatitis, there may be acidophilic bodies, focal necrosis and confluent or bridging necrosis, beginning in the centre of the acinus, or there may even be massive liver necrosis. The necrosis is usually liquefying with collapse of the reticular framework, but coagulation necrosis can also be found. The inflammatory infiltrate consists of round cells and neutrophils with ceroid-filled macrophages called 'scavenger cells'. Infectious canine hepatitis (ICH) is usually characterized by confluent and bridging necrosis in the centrilobular zone and by the presence of intranuclear inclusions in hepatocytes and Kupffer cells. The virus can also be demonstrated by immunofluorescence.

Clinical signs

Signs are acute and include general malaise, anorexia, vomiting, dehydration, icterus and sometimes fever and bleeding. In fulminant hepatitis there is rapidly worsening HE. The clinical picture is entirely dependent on the severity of the liver damage and may vary from insignificant to fulminant lethal disease.

Diagnosis

Blood examination reveals marked elevation of all liver enzymes and in most cases bilirubin. The diagnosis is confirmed by percutaneous liver biopsy after checking blood clotting. Hepatic encephalopathy in fulminant hepatitis is characterized by excessively high blood ammonia values. It is often difficult to find the cause, but the history may be of great value.

Management

Only symptomatic treatment is possible using intravenous fluid therapy to correct hypovolaemia, shock, acidosis or alkalosis, hypoglycaemia and electrolyte disturbances. Avoid glucocorticoids; they are unhelpful and contraindicated in acute infections. In severe liver damage an antibiotic, for example ampicillin, is indicated because bacteria in the portal circulation are no longer effectively removed. The management of hepatic encephalopathy has been discussed earlier in this chapter. Experimental studies have suggested that administration of

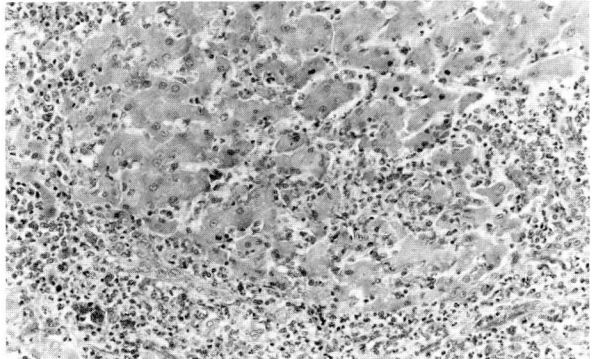

Figure 37.12 Acute hepatitis with confluent lytic necrosis at the periphery of the acinus.

insulin and glucagon increases the survival rate but this treatment has not been developed for clinical use. The prognosis is entirely dependent on the degree and amount of liver damage.

Leptospirosis (see Chapter 48)

Chronic active hepatitis (CAH) and cirrhosis in the dog

These two subjects are discussed together because they have the same pathogenesis and the clinical and pathological changes often overlap. CAH is a chronic hepatitis, characterized by periportal fibrosis, infiltration of lymphocytes and plasma cells and periportal liver necrosis. The liver is diffusely affected and hence a blind biopsy is sufficient to make the diagnosis. Cirrhosis is a process with fibrosis and regeneration, in which the fibrous tissue originating in the portal areas of different acini make connections. The normal acini are than dissected by fibrous tissue and the normal architecture becomes disturbed, with smaller or larger hyperplastic nodules (micro- and macronodular cirrhosis, respectively). Cirrhosis is the end-stage of CAH.

Aetiology

Chronic active hepatitis is presumably the result of a viral infection in most cases. Infectious canine hepatitis (ICH) is thought to be one of the causes. The author has found antibody titres unrelated to vaccination against ICH in many cases. However, there may be other as yet unidentified viruses which cause CAH. In the case of ICH virus, infection in non-vaccinated animals gives a very acute disease which may progress rapidly to fulminant hepatic failure. With previous vaccination which has not been boosted regularly, inadequate immune protection presumably leads to subclinical, on going and progressive hepatitis (Gocke *et al.*, 1967, 1970). It is known that after experimental infection with ICH in partially immune dogs, the virus only remains detectable for a few weeks, after which CAH develops. The disease is slowly progressive over a period of months or years. The virus itself is not detectable in the chronic stage when clinical signs develop and the type of inflammatory reaction and good response to immunosuppressive drugs suggest that the first injury brought about by the infection leads to an adverse immune response with a self-perpetuating autoimmune type of liver cell necrosis. CAH and cirrhosis may also result from other causes of chronic on-going liver cell damage caused by anticonvulsant drugs (Bunch, 1985, 1987; Dayrell-Hart *et al.*, 1991), chemicals or toxins (aflatoxin). Inherited copper accumulation in Bedlington terriers and West Highland white terriers also leads to damage of hepatocytes with secondary hepatitis and fibrosis. The reaction, however, begins in zone 3 of the acini instead of the portal areas. Although inherited copper toxicosis eventually leads to cirrhosis, the disease should not be classified as CAH but as a distinct entity due to an inherited metabolic error. In Doberman pinschers there is a very aggressive form of CAH which does not respond to therapy; this is a sex-linked disorder of females and the underlying cause may well be an inherited immune defect (Thornburg *et al.*, 1984; Crawford *et al.*, 1985; van den Ingh *et al.*, 1988a; Franklin and Saunders, 1988) (Fig. 37.13). However, there also appear to be many more subclinical cases in Dobermanns (Speety *et al.*, 1996).

Pathogenesis

CAH is not a chronic extension of an acute hepatitis. The gradually progressive liver cell necrosis may cause a constant elevation of all liver enzymes and the bile acids. However, in less active hepatitis and in end-stage cirrhosis, the release of enzymes into the plasma may be insignificant and then the liver enzymes may be normal or only slightly elevated. Icterus does not always develop. CAH is always a diffuse process

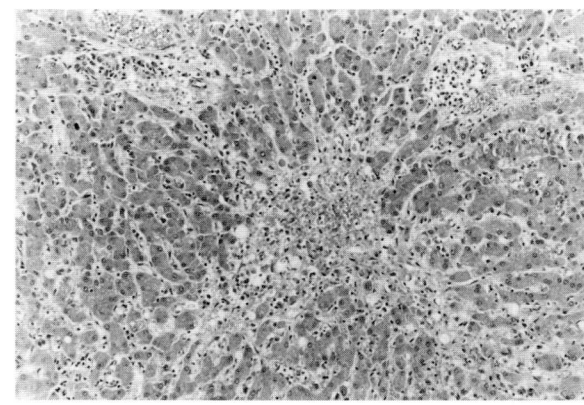

Figure 37.13 Chronic active hepatitis in a dog with infiltrates of lymphocytes and plasma cells in the portal areas, from where it extends into the acinus (piecemeal necrosis). There is little fibrous tissue and the acinar structure is intact.

throughout the liver. Liver function is diminished by the loss of functional tissue and reduced portal blood flow resulting from fibrosis (Kreuzer et al., 1972). There are often low albumin and fibrinogen levels. The conversion of ammonia remains adequate. Hepatic encephalopathy can only develop if portosystemic collaterals develop as a result of portal hypertension. At this stage there is usually cirrhosis and the liver is small. The associated hypoalbuminaemia and portal hypertension eventually lead to ascites. The ascitic fluid is clear and colourless, or yellow if there is icterus.

CAH may occur at any age and in any breed, although there is a predisposition in some breeds as indicated above. The incidence of CAH is relatively high and it is one of the most common liver diseases (Strombeck and Gribble, 1978).

CAH is characterized histologically by fibrosis, inflammation (mainly lymphocytes and plasma cells) and loss of liver cells, mainly in the form of piecemeal necrosis in the portal areas. In cirrhosis formation of portoportal bridging fibrosis and of hyperplastic nodules of liver parenchyma induces rebuilding of the original structure (Fig. 37.14). The inflammatory infiltration and loss of liver cells (especially with piecemeal necrosis and acidophilic bodies) vary considerably, depending on the activity of the process (Hardy, 1986; Jarrett et al., 1987). In both cirrhosis and CAH there is usually hepatocellular cholestasis. Depending on the pathogenesis, the cirrhosis will be macronodular or micronodular. In the dog cirrhosis is mostly macronodular. In the Doberman pinscher, however, there is a chronic active hepatitis that develops into a micronodular cirrhosis, with copper accumulation as a result of a severe cholestasis.

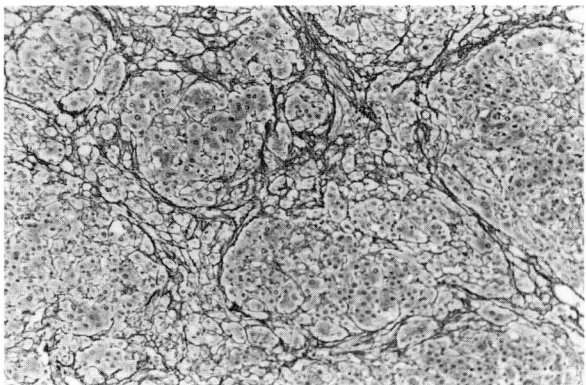

Figure 37.14 Chronic active hepatitis and cirrhosis in a Doberman pinscher. The liver is divided into hypofunctional hyperplastic nodules by fibrous tissue strands.

Clinical signs

The most frequent signs, only a few of which may occur in any one patient, include apathy, reduced appetite, vomiting, poor exercise tolerance, polydipsia, sometimes icterus, ascites, diarrhoea, weight loss and hepatic encephalopathy.

Diagnosis

Polydipsia occurs remarkably often (about 75% of cases). Physical examination usually reveals no specific findings. The liver enzymes are usually increased and there is often hypoalbuminaemia. The diagnosis can only be made by liver biopsy. In case of macronodular cirrhosis blind puncture of a hyperplastic nodule gives normal tissue. At least two different biopsies should, therefore, be taken. Ultrasonography prior to biopsy is advised and cirrhosis may be suspected by the appearance of a small liver with an irregular surface (Fig. 37.15).

Management

Prednisolone at a dose of 1 mg kg^{-1} day^{-1} is required for a prolonged period, preceded by a dose of 2 mg kg^{-1} day^{-1} for one week. Prednisone is also useful but has to be made active by conversion in the liver into prednisolone. If the hepatitis does not respond adequately, then a combination of 0.5 mg prednisone kg^{-1} day^{-1} and 1.0 mg azathioprine kg^{-1} day^{-1} should be used (Magne and Chiapella, 1986). It is important to evaluate the response to treatment by liver biopsy (for example, every 6 weeks). Glucocorticoids themselves give liver changes and increased activities of liver enzymes and bile acids in plasma, hence blood examination is not suitable to evaluate the response to treatment. Medication must be continued until there is histological resolution of the hepatitis. If therapy is stopped too soon the hepatitis will recur. Treatment must be continued for at least 6 weeks and sometimes more than six months. Without treatment, CAH progresses to cirrhosis. Apart from specific treatment directed at the hepatitis, many patients need supportive care directed at dehydration and management of HE (see under that section).

The prognosis of CAH is favourable. Treatment is often successful and the disease can be cured completely. Sometimes there are later recurrences but these respond well when the treatment is repeated. Only in the female Dobermann is the disease non-responsive and usually lethal.

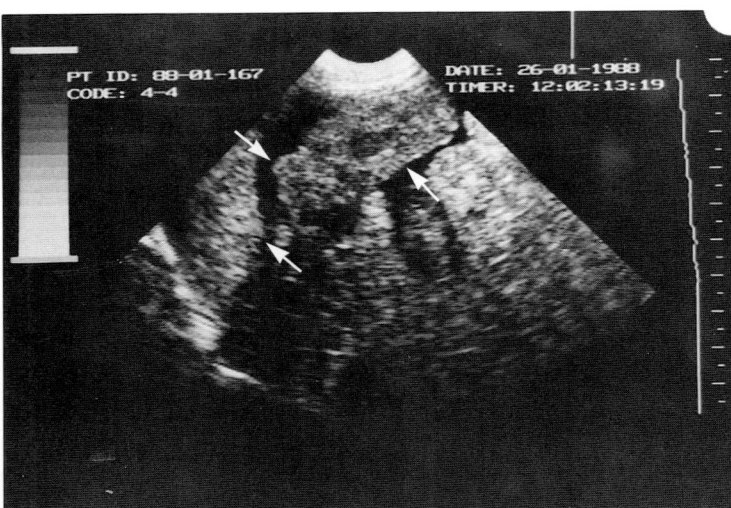

Figure 37.15 Ultrasonogram of a bobtail with liver cirrhosis and ascites. The arrows indicate the irregular surface of the liver lobes; the black areas in between represent free abdominal fluid.

In cases of cirrhosis the prognosis depends on the activity of the on going hepatitis and the degree of liver regeneration. If the hepatitis is still active (judged by the number of inflammatory cells) there is a good chance that significant improvement can be achieved. With the disappearance of the inflammatory infiltrates in the portal areas, liver perfusion may normalize and portal hypertension may decrease. The author has seen cases with HE and ascites due to cirrhosis and CAH, in which medication resulted in disappearance of the ascites, the signs of HE, reduction of the collaterals visualized by angiography and improvement of the ammonia tolerance test. Such cases require permanent precautions to avoid HE, by giving a reduced protein diet and lactulose. Complete resolution of the hepatic lesions in cirrhosis is not possible and the liver will remain functionally subnormal. Nevertheless, non-working dogs can be maintained at a satisfactory level for a long period. In cirrhosis there are no parameters by which the final outcome can be predicted and thus every case should be given a chance on therapy.

For prevention it is important that dogs obtain regular booster vaccination against ICH.

Congenital hepatoportal fibrosis and portal vein hypoplasia

Pathogenesis

Although an increase in connective tissue develops in many disorders of the liver, it is seldom the only abnormality. Hepatoportal fibrosis is a disorder that occurs in young dogs of a few months of age. In view of the age and the fact that it is already a chronic change, the condition is likely to be congenital and seems to be inherited (van den Ingh and Rothuizen, 1983; Rand et al., 1988; Rutgers et al., 1993). Such a disease seems to be quite prevalent in Cairn terriers, at least in the USA (Schermerhorn et al., 1996). The fibrosis causes portal hypertension, leading to ascites and portosystemic collaterals develop, which can lead to hepatic encephalopathy. Portal hypoplasia is a congenital disease in which the small terminal branches of the portal veins are partially or completely absent. There are cases in which portal fibrosis and portal vein hypoplasia co-exist and the conditions are likely to be different forms of one disease entity.

The liver is small and hard. Large hyperplastic nodules are uncommon. Histologically there is either fibrous tissue in the portal areas or hypoplasia of the branches of the portal veins, or both. In response to reduced portal liver perfusion there can be proliferation of the arterioles in the portal areas. There is little or no inflammation.

Clinical signs

Signs include weight loss, abdominal distension due to ascites, hepatic encephalopathy, polydipsia and occasionally vomiting or diarrhoea.

Diagnosis

Blood examination reveals hypoalbuminaemia. Liver enzymes may be elevated but bile acids are increased, ammonia elevated and ammonia tolerance test abnormal. Differentiation from cirrhosis can only be made by histological examination of a liver biopsy. In cases with only portal vein hypoplasia histology does not permit differentiation from congenital portosystemic shunts or portal vein thrombosis, in which low portal perfusion also gives very small or invisible portal vein branches. In these cases additional investigations such as ultrasonography or portography are required. Abdominal distension due to ascites is rare in portosystemic shunts, but is present in most cases of portal fibrosis or portal vein hypoplasia. Ascites in portal vein thrombosis occurs at any age and the fluid is serosanguineous instead of colourless.

Management

The condition is incurable. Only symptomatic treatment can be given to reduce HE and ascites. These patients tend to deteriorate quickly once clinical signs develop. Euthanasia may therefore be encouraged.

Neonatal (lobular dissecting) hepatitis

Pathogenesis

This is a diffuse fibrosis most often in puppies 1–6 months old, with pericellular fibrosis around all hepatocytes. The disease has also been called lobular dissecting hepatitis (Bennett *et al.*, 1983; Jennsen and Nielsen, 1991; van den Ingh and Rothuizen, 1994). The cause is not known, although there are indications that it is congenital and possibly hereditary. The diffuse fibrosis causes portal hypertension. Ascites always develops because albumin synthesis is decreased. The ascitic fluid is similar to that in cirrhosis, i.e. clear and colourless, or yellow if there is icterus. Portal hypertension leads to portosystemic collaterals and hence hepatic encephalopathy. Reduced removal of endotoxins and bacteria from the portal blood can result in vomiting. The clinical picture closely resembles that of cirrhosis and congenital portal fibrosis or portal vein hypoplasia.

The liver is small and has a smooth or finely granular surface. Eventually hyperplastic nodules can develop. Microscopically there is very diffuse fibrosis, pericellular and around small groups of cells and mainly mononuclear inflammation. The liver cells are hypertrophied and liver cells with more than one nucleus are found, a characteristic of regeneration in the fetal and neonatal period. There is usually hepatocellular cholestasis.

Clinical signs

Signs include weight loss, ascites, hepatic encephalopathy, polyuria and sometimes vomiting or diarrhoea.

Diagnosis

Abdominal fluid is clear, colourless or yellow in cases of icterus. Blood examination reveals hypoalbuminaemia; liver enzymes may or may not be elevated, but bile acids are increased. Ammonia may be elevated and the ammonia tolerance test is abnormal.

Liver biopsy is diagnostic and reveals the characteristic histological changes. Percutaneous liver biopsy may be difficult because the small, firm liver in the ascitic fluid keeps moving away from the biopsy needle.

Management

The condition is incurable and is in this respect similar to congenital portal fibrosis or portal vein hypoplasia.

CIRCULATORY DISORDERS OF THE LIVER

Congenital portosystemic shunts (PSS)

Pathogenesis

These are congenital short-circuits between the portal vein and a large vein outside the portal drainage area, usually via a single large vessel that is not normally functional after birth. These shunts are inherited at least in some breeds (Meyer *et al.*, 1995). Congenital shunts are persisting veins that develop during the normal embryonal development but normally disappear in a later stage. Shunts occur in both dogs and cats. Portosystemic shunts are large diameter vessels which therefore offer little resistance to the portal blood flow. Since the portal capillary bed in the liver has a much higher resistance to flow, most of the portal blood bypasses the liver via the shunt. Normally about 80% of the blood flow to the liver is via the portal flow and this provides about 50% of the oxygen requirement. In addition, the portal blood contains various hepatotropic factors such as insulin that are necessary for the growth and metabolic function of the liver. Portosystemic shunts thus result in a poorly developed and poorly functional liver. Of much greater importance, however, is the fact that many substances absorbed from the intestine are almost completely removed from a normal portal circulation. Even if liver function remained adequate in the presence of a portosystemic shunt, the concentrations of these materials in the systemic circulation would remain high, because they would only be delivered to the liver by recirculation via the hepatic arteries. In particular, ammonia and the aromatic amino acids which are not removed can cause hepatic encephalopathy. Circulation of endotoxins can cause vomiting. Histologically, there is usually primary atrophy of the hepatocytes. The portal vein is poorly developed proximal to the shunt and not readily detectable in the portal areas and there is compensatory proliferation of portal arterioles (Fig. 37.16).

In many cases the kidneys are enlarged, but histologically they remain normal. Enlargement may be the result of compensatory hypertrophy, since the kidneys handle a large number of compounds which are normally being excreted or metabolized in the liver.

Poor liver function often results in hypoalbuminaemia, but it is seldom severe enough to cause ascites in the absence of portal hypertension. The animal is usually underweight and may become stunted because of poor liver function and gastrointestinal problems. There is also inadequate conversion of uric acid into allantoin and so uric acid is excreted in the urine together with ammonia. This often leads to poorly soluble ammonium urate crystals, which can form bladder, kidney, or

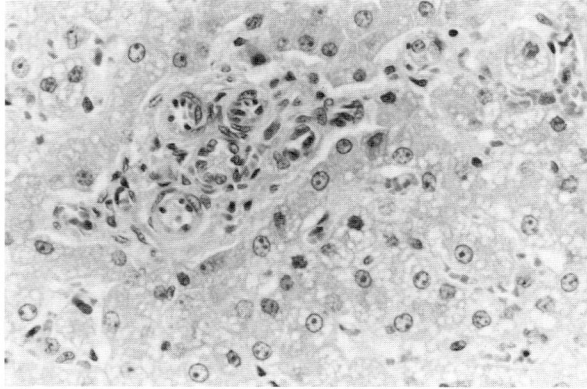

Figure 37.16 Reduced portal perfusion of the liver in a Yorkshire terrier with a congenital portosystemic shunt results in proliferation of hepatic arterioles and undetectable portal veins in the portal areas. There is also microvescicular steatosis of hepatocytes due to hypoperfusion.

urethral calculi (Maretta et al., 1981). These are small, rough and yellow and are radiolucent.

Portosystemic shunts can be classified as intrahepatic (two types) or extrahepatic (thus far five types). The intrahepatic shunts may originate from the left (persistent ductus venosus) or right branch of the portal vein (Fig. 37.17). Extrahepatic portocaval shunts may originate from the gastroduodenal, gastrosplenic or mesenteric vein. In addition, there are also extrahepatic shunts from the portal system to either the azygos or hemiazygos vein. In rare cases the portal vein is only connected with another systemic vein, without a normal connection to the liver. In these cases there is no adequate therapy. The clinical signs are the same in all cases. Intrahepatic shunts are usually found in large breeds, whereas the extrahepatic shunts have only been found in small and medium-sized breeds (Bostwick and Twedt, 1995). The inherited nature has been proven in Irish wolfhounds and Cairn terriers. The incidence of shunts in these breeds is 2–4% in the Netherlands. Shunts occur in nearly all breeds and males and females are equally represented. Cats may have either intra- or extrahepatic shunts, although extrahepatic shunts predominate.

Clinical signs

In most cases there is apathy, excessive sleeping and rapid fatigue, but there can be short intervening periods of normal activity. Usually the animal is underweight, but growth need not be retarded (Rothuizen et al., 1982). Polydipsia usually occurs, as well as vomiting, anorexia and sometimes diarrhoea. Ascites seldom occurs. Usually there are neurological abnormalities which can be extremely variable. Signs can vary from slight apathy to compulsive movements, ataxia and even coma. Periodic blindness often occurs. The syndrome of HE has been explained previously. There may be acute micturition problems caused by ammonium urate calculi. Clinical signs may be non-specific for a long period and although this is typically a disease of young animals, some cases are presented later in middle-age (Cape et al., 1992), especially dogs with portoazygos shunts (Johnson et al., 1989).

Diagnosis

The clinical signs are not pathognomonic. Physical examination reveals no specific findings. Blood ammonia concentrations are greatly elevated in most cases and ammonia tolerance test results are always abnormal (Rothuizen and van

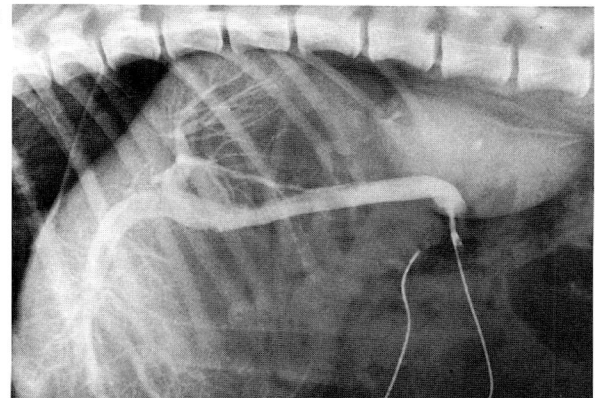 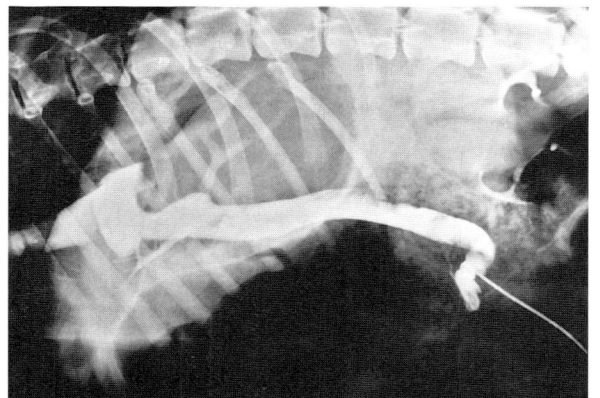

Figure 37.17 (a) Portal venogram of a normal dog taken after catheterization of the portal vein during abdominal surgery. (b) Portal venogram of a Bouvier with an intrahepatic portosystemic shunt arising from the left branch of the portal vein (persistent ductus venosus).

den Ingh, 1982a,b). Abnormal ammonia values do not discriminate single congenital from multiple acquired shunts. Bile acids are increased in most cases, but this is a less-sensitive parameter than ammonia (Center et al., 1985b; Meyer, 1986; Tisdall et al., 1995). Moreover, increased bile acids are not specific for portosystemic shunting, since they may be increased by liver dysfunction without shunting. Moderate microcytic anaemia (Meyer and Harvey, 1994) and leucocytosis are frequent findings in animals with shunts, but these findings are also not specific. Liver enzymes and albumin may or may not be in the abnormal range.

It is advisable to localize the shunt before surgery. Ultrasonography may directly visualize the shunt (Wrigley et al., 1987; Tiemessen et al., 1995). Ultrasonography has become the method of choice to directly visualize and specify the type of shunt (Holt et al., 1995; Lamb, 1996; Lamb et al., 1996a) (Fig. 37.18). If ultrasonography is not conclusive, the only way to confirm the diagnosis is by portography (Suter, 1982; Birchard et al., 1989). The fraction of blood bypassing the liver may be quantified using radioisotope imaging (van Vechten et al., 1994; Meyer et al., 1994; Foster-van Hijfte et al., 1996). Liver biopsies may be indicative of congenital shunts, but they are not diagnostic (see under portal vein hypoplasia). Plain radiographs usually reveal a small liver and sometimes large kidneys. Ammonium biurate crystals in the urine of dogs other than Dalmatians indicate hepatic encephalopathy (present in about 40% of the cases). Patients with congenital portosystemic shunts do not develop icterus.

Management

Surgical closure of the shunt is the only specific treatment (Martin et al., 1986; Lawrence et al., 1992; Tobias et al., 1996; Vogt et al., 1996). Good results with remission of signs without supportive care may be possible in about 80% of the cases with extrahepatic shunts and in about 50% of animals with intrahepatic shunts. Similar results may be obtained in cats (Holt et al., 1995; White et al., 1996). It is important to have the patient in good condition before surgery as the chance of intraoperative or early postoperative complications is much reduced. Supportive measures for encephalopathy including those for anaesthesia have been explained in that section. It is important to evaluate blood glucose before, during and after surgery, since impaired carbohydrate metabolism can lead to hypoglycaemia, which is one of the major postoperative causes of death. Coagulation should also be checked before surgery.

Complete recovery usually occurs within a few weeks. Even severe neurological signs are completely reversible. The prognosis of surgical intervention depends on the type of shunt. Without surgery, supportive care may be insufficient to maintain normal life permanently. The mode of inheritance is not known and thus it is not possible to offer advice on breeding selection.

Hepatic congestion

Pathogenesis

Congestion of the liver is caused by postsinusoidal obstruction to venous drainage. It is usually

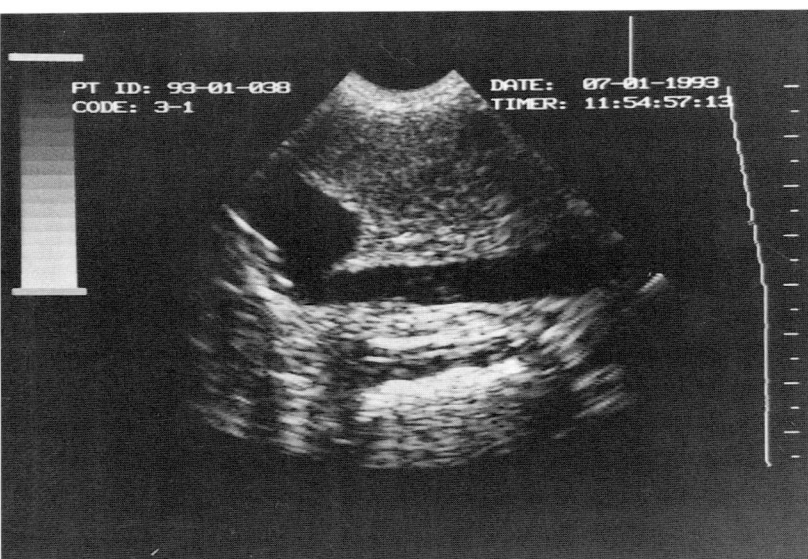

Figure 37.18 Ultrasonogram of a large intrahepatic portocaval shunt in an Irish wolfhound.

caused by congestive heart disease. An obstruction of the thoracic part of the caudal vena cava by tumour or thrombus can also cause hepatic congestion. The most frequent example is an adrenocortical tumour that invades into the vena cava via the adrenal vein and continues to grow in the direction of blood flow. In all cases there is not only portal hypertension but also congestion of the caudal part of the body. In addition to hepatomegaly there may be splenomegaly, ascites and oedema of the caudal part of the body. Ascites caused by hepatic congestion is always serosanguineous, because erythrocytes also escape from the congested capillary bed. The abdominal fluid aspirate can therefore look similar to the ascitic fluid associated with neoplasia or peritonitis.

The hepatic congestion rarely has important consequences for liver function. There may be mild elevations of liver enzyme levels in plasma. Sometimes there is slight hypoalbuminaemia, but this is caused by the diffusion of albumin in the ascitic fluid rather than reduced production in the liver.

An acutely congested liver is enlarged, darkly coloured and usually has a layer of fibrin on the capsule. If the congestion is chronic, fibrous tissue forms around the central veins, while in the periportal areas there is hyperplasia and regeneration of liver parenchyma. The fibrin on the capsule becomes organized. Rarely in chronic congestion micronodular cirrhosis (called cardiac cirrhosis) may develop. This results in a surface pattern of islands of tissue surrounded by vascular spaces, which is the reverse of the normal pattern of liver parenchyma surrounding central veins.

Clinical signs

The signs are those of the primary disease. As liver function remains largely normal there are no typical signs of liver disease.

Diagnosis

For cardiac diseases refer to Chapter 34. Obstruction localized in the vena cava is not associated with signs of cardiac disease. In these rare cases there is high pressure in the vena cava, measured via the saphenous vein, compared with a normal central venous pressure, measured via the jugular vein. Ultrasonography will demonstrate hepatic congestion and may help elucidate the cause.

Management

Tumours or thrombi growing into the vena cava can sometimes be removed surgically. The management of cardiac disease is discussed elsewhere.

■ Thrombosis of the portal vein

Pathogenesis

Thrombosis of the portal vein only occurs in dogs and is fairly uncommon. It is seen with hypercoagulability of the blood such as occurs in the nephrotic syndrome, or in case of abnormal intima of the portal vein. Depending on the rate and degree of closure of the portal vein, there may be acute portal hypertension or portal hypertension with the formation of collaterals. Sometimes the thrombosis of the portal vein occurs in one of its branches, for example in the left branch as a result of an ascending infection via the umbilical vein. With unilateral obstruction of the portal vein there is atrophy of one side of the liver and compensatory hyperplasia of the other, which may result in displacement of the stomach. The part of the liver deprived of portal blood develops compensatory hypertrophy of arterioles, which is histologically visible in the portal areas, as in congenital shunts and congenital portal vein hypoplasia. Chronic cases with acquired portosystemic collaterals may have hepatic encephalopathy.

Clinical signs

Signs include abdominal distension due to ascites, which may be haemorrhagic, sometimes hepatic encephalopathy and occasionally vomiting.

Diagnosis

Abdominal fluid aspiration usually reveals serosanguineous ascitic fluid. If cardiac causes can be excluded, then obstruction of the cranial vena cava and thrombosis of the portal vein remain as differentials. Measurement of the pressure in the caudal vena cava via a catheter in the saphenous vein will differentiate between these two. If the pressure in the vena cava is normal, then the diagnosis is made by exclusion. Liver biopsy, ultrasonography and portography can confirm the diagnosis (Willard *et al.*, 1989; van Winkle and Bruce, 1993; Lamb *et al.*, 1996b).

Unilateral hepatomegaly with displacement of the stomach can be detected by abdominal palpation, but is easily recognized by ultrasonography or radiography. There is no ascites in this case because of adequate function of the other half of the liver. The diagnosis can only be confirmed by angiography and laparotomy.

Management

Therapy depends on the primary disorder, for example nephrotic syndrome. Acute thrombosis may be relieved surgically. In chronic cases with hepatic encephalopathy, symptomatic support may be required.

Arteriovenous fistula

Pathogenesis

Shunts between an artery and the portal venous system give rise to arterial pressure in the portal system, hence portal hypertension. These fistulae are rare and in most reported cases they were congenital, but they may also result from trauma or abdominal surgery. The connection may reside in the liver, or in the extrahepatic splanchnic system. Portal hypertension leads to formation of multiple portosystemic collaterals and ascites (Moore and Whiting, 1986; Whiting *et al.*, 1986; Bailey *et al.*, 1988). Intrahepatic fistulae may cause a reversal of the blood flow in the portal system known as hepatofugal (away from the liver, instead of hepatopetal) flow.

The fistulae are often multiple and are distinctly visible as wide, tortuous and pulsating vessels. Intrahepatic fistulae result in an enlarged lobe of the liver containing many cavernous vessels. Histologically the portal areas have many arterioles and wide portal vein branches with a thickened wall.

Clinical signs

The signs are those of portal hypertension, hepatic encephalopathy, ascites, diarrhoea, depression, anorexia and vomiting.

Diagnosis

Abdominal palpation may reveal local enlargement of a liver lobe. Laboratory examination gives increased plasma concentrations of the liver enzymes, bile acids and in case of portosystemic shunting, ammonia. None of these are diagnostic. Ultrasonography may indicate the presence of the wide tortuous vessels. The diagnosis is confirmed by angiography of the coeliac or the cranial mesenteric artery.

Management

Surgical removal of the affected liver lobe or ligation of the extrahepatic fistula can relieve the clinical signs completely. Pre-anaesthetic care is important in cases of hepatic encephalopathy.

CONGENITAL METABOLIC DISEASES OF THE LIVER

Copper toxicosis in Bedlington terriers

Aetiology

This disease occurs in Bedlington terriers and is an accumulation of copper in the liver, as the result of an autosomally recessive hereditary disorder (Johnson *et al*., 1980). West Highland white terriers may have a similar disease, but the pathogenesis and inheritance are not known (Thornburg *et al*., 1986).

Pathogenesis

Normally, part of the copper taken in with the food is absorbed in the intestine and transported to the liver in the portal blood loosely bound to albumin. Most is taken up by the hepatocytes and excreted into the bile via the liver cell lysosomes. In the liver, a small amount is incorporated in the protein, ceruloplasmin, which is released into the plasma. Copper in ceruloplasmin is used in a number of enzymes and proteins in which it is essential for normal function. Most of the copper is bound to the protein metallothionein. Copper is excreted into the bile bound to an unidentified protein and leaves the body with the faeces.

In Bedlington terriers that have copper storage disease, the hepatocytes are almost completely unable to excrete copper in the bile and hence there is an accumulation of copper in the liver (Brewer *et al*., 1992). The exact nature of the defect is not known, but it appears to be a lysosomal disorder. Because the copper accumulation begins gradually, signs usually only appear after the age of 4 years (Hultgren *et al*., 1986). The increased copper concentration in the liver can be confirmed after 1 year of age. Before that age some dogs with the disease have stored insufficient copper to distinguish them from normal animals.

The disease appears in two forms. There is a chronic form in which the copper accumulation leads to liver cell necrosis, secondary hepatitis and cirrhosis. Some dogs have an acute or peracute form with haemolytic anaemia. The haemolysis is probably the result of a sudden release of a large amount of copper from the liver into the blood. The mechanism for this is not clear. The high copper concentrations cause acute haemolysis and because liver function is already reduced, this leads to severe icterus. Tubulonephrosis may occur and can lead to uraemia. Haemolysis leads to centrilobular liver necrosis (see section on secondary liver disorders). In dogs surviving the haemolytic crisis, cirrhosis occurs more frequently than in other animals.

Copper accumulation begins in hepatocytes around the central veins and gradually spreads outward toward the portal areas (Thornburg *et al*., 1990). The copper is stored in the liver cell in granules which by electron microscopy and by enzyme histochemistry appear to be lysosomes. The copper is stored in such a way that it is of little toxicity for the liver cell. Liver cell damage only occurs when a certain level is exceeded. The damage leads to ongoing liver cell necrosis and secondary inflammation which can eventually lead to cirrhosis. The normal concentration of copper in the canine liver is between 50 and 300 $\mu g\ g^{-1}$ of dried tissue. Dogs with copper accumulation have levels exceeding 1000 $\mu g\ g^{-1}$ at one year of age, but most cases have higher concentrations. With time levels of 12 000 $\mu g\ g^{-1}$ may be reached. At one year a few dogs have concentrations between 300 and 1000 $\mu g\ g^{-1}$ and most of them appear not to accumulate when re-examined later.

Laboratory examination may reveal any deviation seen in chronic hepatitis and cirrhosis. There are no specific blood parameters which are specific for copper accumulation. Ceruloplasmin and free copper concentrations are not different from healthy dogs, whereas Wilson's disease in humans is associated with decreased ceruloplasmin levels.

Affected animals can also be asymptomatic. Heterozygote carriers cannot be distinguished from homozygote healthy animals with liver biopsy. A DNA marker closely linked to the disease has recently been published (Yuzbasiyan-Gurkan *et al*., 1997). We have evaluated the diagnostic value of the DNA test and found it to be at least 95% accurate. In countries where the incidence has been measured, about 30–50% of the population of all Bedlington terriers had the disease.

Clinical signs

In the chronic form signs are similar to those seen with chronic active hepatitis and cirrhosis. In the acute form there is acute haemolysis, anaemia, severe icterus, sometimes uraemia. The acute form is often lethal within a few days.

Diagnosis

On the basis of physical and blood examinations it is not possible to differentiate this disease from hepatitis/cirrhosis or haemolysis due to other causes. The diagnosis can only be made by demonstrating copper accumulation in a liver biopsy in animals older than one year.

Histologically, copper in a liver biopsy may be detected with histochemistry using staining with rubeanic acid. The same staining may be used in smears of material obtained with fine needle biopsy. There is good correlation between the results of sensitive copper analysis and those of semiquantitative judgement of rubeanic acid staining for copper (Fig. 37.19). The author prefers the reliable and easy method of staining a fine needle biopsy smear (Johnson et al., 1984; Teske et al., 1992). It is important that an experienced cytologist or pathologist judges the amount of copper using a standard protocol.

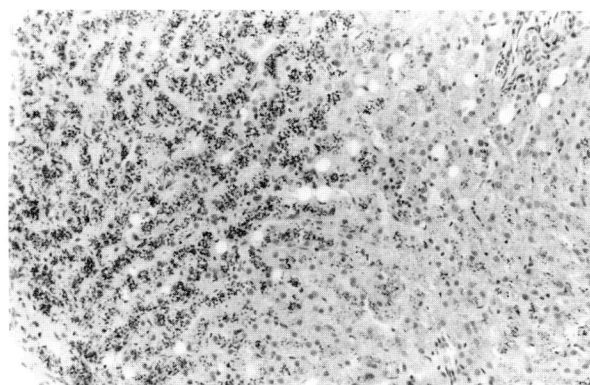

Figure 37.19 Copper accumulation stained with rubeanic acid in the liver of a Bedlington terrier. Copper has preferentially accumulated in the area around the terminal hepatic veins.

Management

Once signs of chronic hepatitis or cirrhosis, or those of an acute haemolytic crisis have developed it is often difficult to improve the patient. Supportive care is important. The management of hepatic encephalopathy, portal hypertension and ascites has been discussed previously. Haemolytic crisis is a very serious event. Administration of penicillamine which chelates metals, particularly copper, is indicated (Twedt et al., 1988; Allen et al., 1987). The penicillamine/copper complex is excreted by the kidneys into the urine thus removing free copper from the circulation. Intravenous infusion with forced diuresis is helpful to enhance urinary excretion.

It is important to try to prevent clinical signs of copper accumulation. Hence, asymptomatic dogs should be examined at a young age and if there is copper accumulation, life-long medication with drugs that prevent further accumulation of copper is essential. There are two drugs available and both are given orally. Penicillamine may be given 30 min before each meal in a total daily dose of 25 mg kg^{-1}. Penicillamine binds copper entering the circulation after feeding and the bound complex is excreted in the urine. Zinc is also used, given as zinc gluconate in a dosage of 30 mg kg^{-1} day^{-1} in divided doses immediately before each meal. Other zinc salts irritate the gastric mucosa and induce vomiting. Zinc induces the formation of copper binding metallothionein at the level of the intestinal mucosa, thus preventing the absorption of copper (Sternlieb, 1994). The two drugs should not be combined since they form complexes and inactivate each other. These medications are unable to reduce hepatic copper levels in most cases, but they prevent further accumulation and the development of the symptomatic stage. Another measure to prevent further accumulation is to reduce the copper content of the food. Commercial foods may differ by a factor three with respect to the copper concentration as indicated in the specification. Home-made food should not contain ox liver which contains high quantities of copper. Rice, bread and cereals are practically free of copper.

It is now possible to detect heterozygote carriers as well as homozygous free and sick dogs with a DNA test. This permits breeders to select breeding stock so that the disease gets completely eradicated.

TUMOURS OF THE LIVER

Primary neoplasia

Hepatocellular carcinoma

Among epithelial tumours hepatic cell carcinoma occurs more frequently than hepatic cell adenoma (Strombeck, 1978). Both tumours are usually solitary arising from one lobe and may become very large. Hepatic cell carcinomas grow slowly and have little tendency to metastasize. These tumours can be present for a long time without signs, but with increasing size they can displace the stomach and cause vomiting. They seldom have consequences for liver function since they grow out of one lobe leaving the rest of the liver intact. The liver enzymes are usually only slightly elevated and may be normal. Liver cell carcinomas produce signs only when very large at which stage they are usually palpable. Hypoglycaemia occurs in 20–40% of cases (Leifer et al., 1985). The cause is unknown but is possibly a paraneoplastic syndrome due to formation of insulin-like growth factors. In some cases hypoglycaemia induces exercise intolerance or episodic weakness. Liver cell carcinoma is associated with chronic hepatitis and cirrhosis in humans but such a relation does not exist in dogs. It is typically a disease of old dogs.

Histologically, these tumours are well-differentiated and it can be very hard to distinguish them histologically from normal liver.

Clinical signs

Signs include chronic vomiting and sometimes weakness or exercise intolerance. The tumour may be so large that the abdomen is extended.

Diagnosis

Abdominal palpation usually reveals a mass in the liver, but it may be difficult to distinguish such masses from those arising in the spleen. Ultrasonography reveals a large mass with an echodensity similar to that of normal liver. Localized enlargement of the liver often combined with displacement of the stomach is identified on radiography (Evans, 1987). Histology of a liver biopsy may be diagnostic, but sometimes the liver architecture and differentiation are so normal that a histological diagnosis cannot be made. Hence, the diagnosis is based on a combination of these methods. Liver enzymes or bile acids may not be elevated.

Management

Surgical removal of the affected liver lobe is the only definitive treatment (Kosovsky et al., 1989; Lewis et al., 1990). This may be successful if the tumour is not localized near the hilus or the large vessels or bile ducts. Peripherally localized carcinomas are well resectable and in most cases there is no metastasis. It is important to monitor blood glucose concentration to prevent cerebral damage from hypoglycaemia during or directly following surgery.

Haemangiosarcoma

Haemangiosarcoma is the most common mesenchymal hepatic tumour (Hammer and Sikkema, 1995). They are usually smaller (up to a few centimetres) and multiple. Because of their multiple character there can be a more extensive liver cell loss and cholestasis than with the epithelial tumours. There can be a pronounced elevation of liver enzymes and also icterus. Haemangiosarcomas occur mainly in older animals. Apart from originating in the liver, they may have metastasized from other organs, particularly the spleen.

Clinical signs

Mesenchymal tumours usually have a severe and rapid course, with anorexia, vomiting, weight loss and sometimes icterus. Abdominal distension and haemorrhagic ascites due to rupture of the tumour may be present.

Diagnosis

There may be palpable liver enlargement but this is not always the case. Blood examination usually reveals high liver enzymes and bile acids but this is not specific. Ultrasonography visualizes the tumours that appear as dark echolucent masses due to their rich vascularization. The diagnosis may be confirmed by laparotomy. Ultrasound-guided biopsy is possible but these tumours can be hard to recognize for the pathologist or cytologist. The diagnosis may easily be missed by a blind biopsy.

Mesenchymal tumours are usually inoperable and rapidly progressive. Survival times are usually not more than a few weeks or months.

Secondary (metastatic) neoplasia

Tumours of organs in the portal drainage area metastasize first to the liver. Haemangiosarcomas of the spleen are by far the most frequent, followed by pancreas carcinomas and gastrointestinal tumours (Hammer and Sikkema, 1995). Tumours from outside the portal drainage area can also metastasize to the liver rather than in the lungs.

Tumour metastases are almost always multiple and distributed throughout the liver. Depending on their size, there can be severe liver damage and often cholestasis.

Clinical signs

The signs may originate mainly from the primary organ, for example vomiting in the case of gastric tumours, extrahepatic cholestasis with pancreas tumours, or ascites resulting from haemorrhage from haemangiosarcoma in the spleen. The main signs caused by the liver damage are general malaise, anorexia, vomiting and icterus. There may be palpable hepatomegaly.

Diagnosis

Physical and laboratory signs of liver damage and/or cholestasis are not specific (McConnell and Lumsden, 1983). The diagnosis is made by histology of the tumour which can easily be missed by a percutaneous liver biopsy. This is prevented by ultrasonography (Fig. 37.20) which permits the guided puncture of a tumour in the liver or at the primary site.

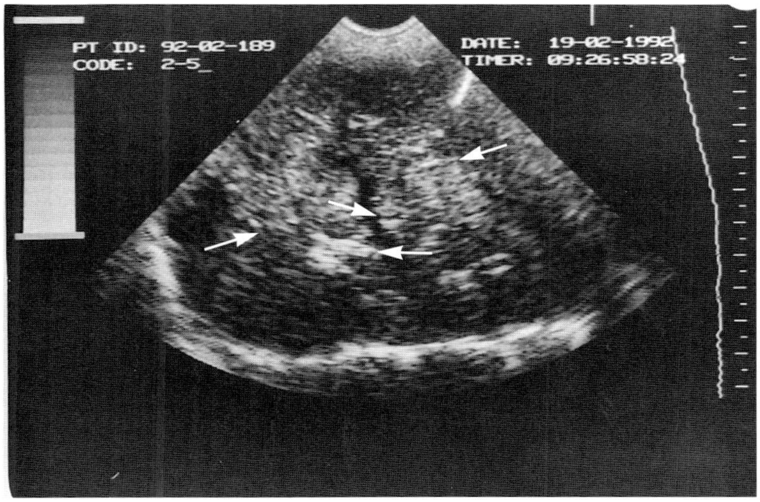

Figure 37.20 Metastic tumours in the liver visualized by ultrasound. The enlarged liver lobe shows an irregular echodensity (arrows).

Surgery is virtually never possible because of multiple metastases and the prognosis is hopeless.

Generalized neoplasia (malignant lymphoma)

Pathogenesis

Lymphoma occurs frequently in the liver (Hammer and Sikkema, 1995). Clinical signs often arise because of liver damage and infiltration of tumour cells causes hepatomegaly and may cause intrahepatic cholestasis. There is often severe liver dysfunction due to diffuse and widespread damage. Tumour infiltration is usually most severe in the portal areas and around the central veins. Sometimes this causes severe portal hypertension with ascites and collateral formation. In such cases hepatic encephalopathy may develop.

In most cases the liver involvement is part of a generalized neoplasia, but in some cases malignant lymphoma may exclusively involve the liver. If the lymphoma is not found by blood or bone marrow examination and there is no enlargement of lymph nodes, the diagnosis will easily be made by liver biopsy if the liver is involved.

Histiocytomas can also involve the liver and frequently affect Bernese Mountain dogs in which there may be an inherited basis. Myeloid tumours may also occur in the liver.

Clinical signs

The signs are highly variable depending on the organ systems involved. With respect to the liver, signs of icterus, malaise, anorexia and vomiting may occur. Sometimes there is ascites and hepatic encephalopathy. Hepatomegaly and splenomegaly may give abdominal distension.

Diagnosis

Ultrasonography can be helpful (Nyland, 1984) and the diagnosis can always be confirmed by a percutaneous liver biopsy. In lymphoma, blood coagulation is often abnormal. The diffuse involvement of the liver makes the tumour readily detectable in fine needle cytological smears. Fine needle biopsy may be used safely in cases of coagulopathy.

Management

Chemotherapy for lymphoma is discussed in Chapter 50.

LIVER DYSFUNCTION RESULTING FROM SYSTEMIC DISEASE

The liver plays a central role in the metabolism of proteins, fats and carbohydrates. In systemic diseases in which fat and carbohydrate metabolism are changed, the liver can become involved in the illness. In addition, the liver is an important buffer between the outside world (for example against bacteria and toxins from the gastrointestinal tract) and the rest of the body. Finally, secondary liver damage can occur in different forms of acute hypoxia such as haemolytic anaemia or shock.

Non-specific reactive hepatitis

Pathogenesis

Non-specific reactive hepatitis is a diffuse or focal liver damage with secondary inflammatory reaction resulting from toxaemia or sepsis. Reactive hepatitis can occur in any toxaemic, septic, inflammatory, or necrotizing process. When the process is in the portal drainage area all of the toxins are transported exclusively to the liver, whereas toxins and bacteria from processes elsewhere are first diluted in the general circulation before reaching the liver. It is thus understandable that reactive hepatitis is most often caused by processes in the abdominal cavity.

Reactive hepatitis develops in most cases of gastroenteritis and extensive gastric or intestinal tumours (for example lymphoma), as a result of increased toxin absorption. It also develops in peritonitis (including local peritonitis resulting from abdominal surgery) and other inflammatory processes in the organs drained by the portal vein. Reactive hepatitis is thus most often caused by gastrointestinal disorders (Dillon, 1985). However, vomiting and/or diarrhoea often occur with primary liver disorders. Hence, when a patient with gastrointestinal problems is found to have high liver enzyme levels, the classic chicken-or-egg situation is encountered and may only be resolved by liver biopsy.

The circulating toxins, inflammatory mediators and microbes cause a reticuloendothelial proliferation and infiltration of neutrophils in the liver. There may also be focal liver necrosis. In chronic cases there is also lymphocytic and plasmacytic inflammation. There can be mild to severe cholestasis in the canaliculi. In some cases of sepsis there may be diffuse foci of necrosis, microabscesses, or granulomas, for example with canine herpesvirus, toxoplasmosis, brucellosis, tuberculosis, *Escherichia coli*, migrating *Toxocara canis* larvae (Chapman *et al.*, 1993; Iwanaka *et al.*, 1993).

Adult dogs exposed to *Toxocara* infection can develop a focal hepatitis as a result of the migrating larvae that are killed in the liver by the normal defence mechanisms. These dogs have a diffusely spread granulomatous eosinophilic inflammatory reaction. Haematologically there is also eosinophilia.

Reactive hepatitis is different from the primary chronic active form in that the type of inflammatory cells differ with a predominance of neutrophils and sometimes eosinophils instead of lymphocytes and plasma cells and the location of the inflammation in the liver acini is diffuse rather than portal or periportal (Fig. 37.21).

ALT, AST and bile acids are often elevated because of liver cell damage and canalicular cholestasis but there is little change in other liver functions because there is adequate remaining functioning liver tissue. Blood coagulation and serum albumin concentrations are also not usually affected. There may, however, be severe hypoalbuminaemia if the gastrointestinal problem is a protein-losing enteropathy.

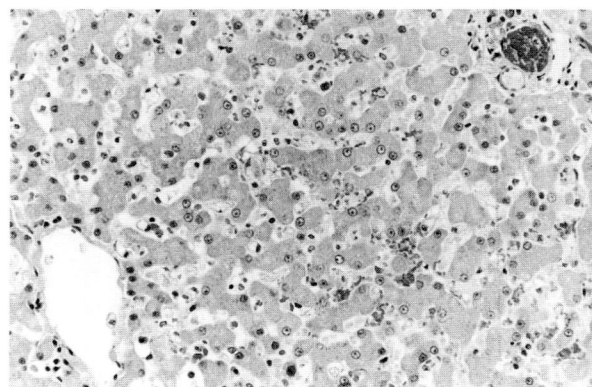

Figure 37.21 Non-specific reactive hepatitis in a dog. This common liver abnormality is characterized by increased leucocytes and Kupffer cells and often intrahepatic cholestasis.

Clinical signs

The clinical signs are often determined by the primary disorder. Hence there is often vomiting and/or diarrhoea. There is sometimes fever. When reactive hepatitis is severe, there can be icterus, general malaise and sometimes reduced exercise tolerance.

Diagnosis

Differentiation between primary liver diseases and reactive hepatitis is only possible by histological examination of a liver biopsy. Focal hepatitis is usually so diffusely distributed that a blind liver biopsy is adequate. The abnormalities described under pathogenesis are characteristic. Once the diagnosis of reactive hepatitis is made, it can be very difficult to localize the primary process. Further gastrointestinal examination is often indicated. It is sometimes necessary to search for the cause by exploratory laparotomy, but inflammatory processes outside the abdomen can also cause reactive hepatitis. In these cases the diagnosis can be pursued in the same way as for fever of unknown origin.

Management

The therapy and prognosis depend completely on the primary disorder. Reactive hepatitis itself requires no treatment, since it resolves spontaneously after removal of the cause. If the cause cannot be found, long-term treatment with antibiotics may be worthwhile. When there has been *Toxocara* infection, avoidance of further contact is essential.

■ Steroid hepatopathy

Pathogenesis

Both spontaneous hyperadrenocorticism and the administration of glucocorticoids cause specific abnormalities in the liver (Fig. 37.22). There is glycogen accumulation in the hepatocytes which results in large vacuoles. Hepatocytes display cell membrane-bound and subcellular organelle changes (Rutgers *et al.*, 1995). This leads to varying degrees of hepatomegaly (Badylak and van Vleet, 1981, 1982; Fittschen and Bellamy, 1984). These changes can cause elevation of the plasma levels of transaminases, especially ALT, and there is always a marked elevation of AP. The latter is caused not only by liver damage but also by induction of an isoenzyme of AP by glucocorticoids. These steroid-induced changes in the liver almost never cause clinical signs. It is, however, of great importance to know whether the patient has been treated recently with glucocorticoids if liver enzymes are measured.

Clinical signs

The signs are those of hyperadrenocorticism. The changes in the liver can result in hepatomegaly, which may be detected by abdominal palpation. It is important to remember that a number of signs that occur in hyperadrenocorticism also occur in primary liver disease for example apathy, reduced exercise tolerance, polydipsia, hepatomegaly and elevated AP, ALT and bile acids in plasma.

Diagnosis

It is often helpful to know whether elevated liver enzyme levels and bile acids are due to glucocorticoid use. This can be determined by a percutaneous liver biopsy, as the histological changes are specific. These diffuse changes are even detectable in cytological smears from fine needle biopsies. The glucocorticoid-induced AP can be distinguished because most of it is still active after heating the plasma to 65° for 2 min. The diagnosis of hyperadrenocorticism is discussed elsewhere.

Management

The glucocorticoid-induced changes in the liver are reversible within a few weeks to months after removal of the cause. The prognosis depends on the cause of the glucocorticoid excess.

■ Liver changes in diabetes mellitus

Pathogenesis

The liver plays a central role in fat metabolism. In diabetes mellitus there is increased lipolysis in adipose tissue and therefore increased delivery of fatty acids to the liver, while the production of triglycerides is also increased. Fat accumulates in the liver cells beginning around the central veins and progressing toward the periphery of the lobule (Dillon, 1985). Hepatomegaly develops. Sometimes there is cholestasis, which can be quite severe. There is more severe liver dysfunction with fatty change than with glycogen accumulation. In humans the chronic fatty change can lead to hypertrophic liver cirrhosis, but in dogs and cats this is very rare.

Clinical signs

Fatty change in the liver is usually present in diabetes mellitus and may cause mild to severe

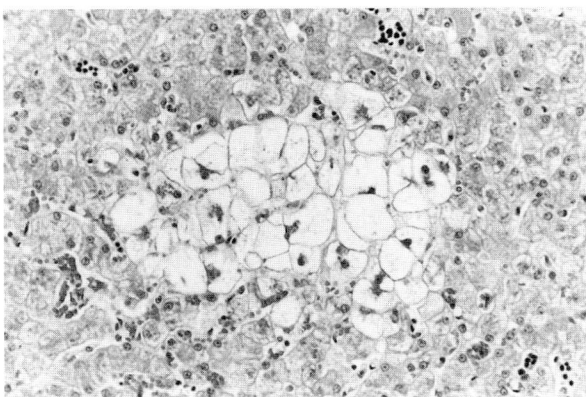

Figure 37.22 Hepatopathy induced by glucocorticoids, with accumulation of glycogen in the hepatocytes. There are also some foci of extramedullary haematopoiesis; the dog had been treated with prednisolone for autoimmune haemolytic anaemia.

intrahepatic cholestasis, in which case, physical examination reveals hepatomegaly and icterus. All the liver enzymes in plasma can be mildly to severely increased. Transient hepatic fat accumulation not related to diabetes may occur in fasting pups of toy breeds.

Diagnosis

Histological demonstration of the fatty change in a liver biopsy confirms the diagnosis in combination with persistent hyperglycaemia.

Management

Treatment of the fatty change is not necessary, since with good regulation of the diabetes, it gradually disappears.

■ Hypoxic liver damage

Pathogenesis

Liver degeneration or necrosis can occur with any cause of acute hypoxia. In this context it is important to remember that the blood supply of the liver is predominantly venous and therefore relatively low in oxygen content and adaptation to hypoxia requires time. Possible causes include acute haemolysis as in cases of autoimmune haemolysis and shock. Histologically there is necrosis of the centrilobular zone 3 (the oxygen-poor part of the liver lobule). Extensive necrosis may occur with confluent and bridging necrosis leading to disturbed architecture of the liver acini. Necrosis induces a secondary inflammatory reaction of polymorphonuclear cells. There is usually widespread cholestasis. In case of haemolysis there is erythrophagocytosis and/or accumulation of iron pigment in the reticuloendothelial system. Sometimes extramedullary haematopoiesis is seen in the liver. In addition to the general illness and icterus, hepatic encephalopathy can also occur in severely affected cases.

These changes explain why haemolytic anaemia is so often accompanied by an increase, sometimes marked, in conjugated bilirubin. It is the cholestasis rather than the haemolysis that determines the icterus and hence bilirubin is predominantly of the conjugated direct reacting type. ALT, AST, AP and γGT can be severely elevated. Sometimes the liver dysfunction is so severe that this, in spite of an adequate treatment of the haemolysis, leads to death.

Clinical signs

The onset is acute with signs of shock or anaemia. The mucous membranes with anaemia are jaundiced and very pale. Signs resulting from liver dysfunction depend on the extent of liver necrosis and may vary from general illness and malaise to hepatic encephalopathy. Anorexia and vomiting may occur as result of impaired detoxifying function of the liver.

Diagnosis

The presence and severity of the liver changes can only be confirmed by histological examination of a liver biopsy. These changes are specific and therefore confirmatory. An impression of the severity and course of the liver necrosis is provided by measurements of the liver enzymes and bile acids in plasma, but they may also be elevated in any other hepatobiliary diseases. Hepatic encephalopathy can be confirmed by measuring blood ammonia or by an ammonia tolerance test.

The diagnosis of the underlying disease causing anaemia or shock is not discussed here.

Management

Management primarily involves treatment of the underlying cause of the liver damage. There is no specific treatment for the liver lesions and the liver will recover spontaneously in most cases. In case of severe damage the impaired liver functions may become life-threatening. Only symptomatic supportive therapy for the liver dysfunction can be given to gain time for regeneration of the liver. Specific measures to control hepatic encephalopathy may be important. Remember that the course of the liver regeneration cannot be evaluated by the degree of the icterus. The prognosis is good to hopeless, depending on the severity of the liver damage.

■ Amyloidosis

Amyloidosis of the liver is rare in dogs or cats and almost invariably involves the secondary form which may develop in the course of chronic inflammatory processes or tumours. In cases of generalized secondary amyloidosis there is usually some deposition of amyloid in the liver, but this seldom leads to clinical signs referable to the liver (Thornburg and Moody, 1981). Deposits of amyloid in the liver are visible as an amorphous hyaline and eosinophilic material in the space of Disse. Depending on the amount of amyloid the liver may be enlarged on abdominal palpation, but this is unusual. Liver enzymes and bile acids in plasma may be increased but may remain normal. Amyloidosis is a systemic disease involving a number of organs. The kidneys are the most commonly affected site with amyloid deposition in the glomeruli. There is severe proteinuria and in advanced cases also uraemia. Amyloidosis of the kidneys usually determines the clinical picture.

Management

There is no specific treatment available for amyloidosis. The deposition of amyloid is progressive and the prognosis is hopeless.

DISEASES OF THE BILIARY TRACT

Congenital abnormalities

Double gallbladder

In the dog and more often in the cat, there is sometimes a double gallbladder. Although the emptying of the gallbladder is not optimal and there is a local stasis of bile, this disorder rarely leads to clinical problems. The condition may be detected at surgery or ultrasonography.

Atresia of the bile ducts

Pathogenesis
Although a neonatal inflammation of the bile ducts could also result in atresia, this rare disorder is probably congenital but not hereditary. There can also be complete absence (agenesis) of the bile ducts. Secondary liver changes, such as biliary fibrosis or cirrhosis, can cause reduced liver function. Maldigestion and malabsorption develop as a result of the absence of bile in the duodenum.

Clinical signs
The most prominent signs are neonatal icterus, retarded growth and acholic faeces.

Diagnosis
Jaundice and increased plasma AP, γGT and bile acids indicate cholestasis. Histology of a liver biopsy reveals the typical signs of chronic extrahepatic cholestasis but it does not suggest an underlying cause. The definitive diagnosis is made at laparotomy.

Management
The only possible treatment is surgical. One may relieve the cholestasis by a cholecystoduodenostomy.

Cysts arising from the bile ducts

Hepatic cysts are in fact cysts of the bile ducts and are congenital. They consist of spaces filled with watery or mucous fluid lined by a single layer of biliary epithelium. They vary in size from a few millimetres to about 10 cm. There are two forms: in one form one or a few cysts occur and in the other form there are multiple small cysts frequently associated with renal cysts (McKenna and Carpenter, 1980; van den Ingh and Rothuizen, 1985). Both forms occur in both the dog and the cat (Stebbins, 1989). Congenital dilatation of the bile ducts can consist of a local dilatation of the larger intrahepatic bile ducts or a diffuse or local dilatation of both the intrahepatic and extrahepatic bile ducts. Gallstones may develop in the dilated bile system. These can be seen with ultrasonography, but are usually radiolucent. When there are multiple cysts the liver is sometimes fibrotic and consequently there may be portal hypertension. This can lead to formation of collaterals and sometimes also ascites and hepatic encephalopathy. Multiple biliary cysts may occur in combination with multiple renal cysts arising from the tubules. In this case uraemia can also develop. In cats there can be relatively large solitary cysts, which displace the stomach and cause vomiting. This rare condition probably remains asymptomatic in most cases. Only large space-occupying cysts, multiple cysts and secondarily infected cysts will give rise to clinical signs. Icterus occurs only in case of cysts diffusely spread throughout the biliary system.

Diagnosis
The diagnosis is easily made with ultrasonography. The cysts are seen as echolucent fluid-filled space-occupying lesions.

Management
Solitary cysts can be removed surgically, which often requires resection of the entire liver lobe involved (Washizu et al., 1996). Infected cysts need antibiotic treatment with ampicillin or amoxycillin. Multiple cysts cannot be treated. Symptomatic management of portal hypertension and hepatic encephalopathy may be required.

Acquired biliary disorders

Cholangitis–cholecystitis

Pathogenesis
In the dog, infection of the common bile duct by reflux from the duodenum is possible but the

infection is usually haematogenous. Infection is always caused by bacteria, often *E. coli*, but sometimes *Streptococcus* or *Staphylococcus* spp. (Taboada and Meyer, 1989). Anaerobes such as *Clostridium* which normally occur in the gallbladder can become pathogens. Predisposing factors are gallstones and extrahepatic cholestasis (Matthiesen and Lammerding, 1984). In the dog cholangitis or cholecystis almost never occur without these predisposing factors. Sometimes an acute emphysematous cholecystitis occurs. If there is cholangitis, extrahepatic cholestasis is a consequence, which induces the most prominent signs. In cases in which only the gallbladder is involved there is no cholestasis. In these cases signs of cranial abdominal pain, sometimes with fever, may prevail. There are cases in which severe bleeding from an affected blood vessel in the wall of the gallbladder occurs resulting in anaemia with a haemogram typical for blood loss. The inflammation may result in spontaneous (non-traumatic) perforation of the gallbladder, giving ascites and an aseptic peritonitis.

Clinical signs
The most prominent signs are usually those of extrahepatic cholestasis with icterus. Vomiting, fever and sometimes pain in the epigastric region may occur. There may occasionally be gallbladder rupture or bleeding giving ascites or anaemia, respectively.

Diagnosis
Icterus and elevation of cholestasis-indicating enzymes (AP and γGT) and bile acids are not specific, as are inflammatory changes in leucocytes. Examination of a liver biopsy reveals the typical changes of acute extrahepatic cholestasis with neutrophils in the lumen of the bile ducts. Ultrasonography demonstrates calculi which may be radiolucent and therefore missed by radiography. Differentiation between cholangitis/cholecystitis and primary extrahepatic cholestasis is only possible during laparotomy, when other causes of extrahepatic cholestasis can be excluded. Occult bleeding from the gallbladder can be visualized during gastroduodenoscopy. Anaesthesia should not include morphine analogues since these induce closure of the sphincter of Oddi which would prevent the efflux of blood into the duodenum.

Management
Antibiotics that are effectively excreted in the bile (ampicillin, chloramphenicol) should be administered for several weeks. Ampicillin is usually very effective (50 mg kg^{-1} day^{-1} in divided doses for 4 weeks). In cases of biliary calculi or gallbladder bleeding, surgical intervention is required for cholecystectomy and removal of calculi.

Gallstones

Pathogenesis
Gallstones seldom occur in dogs and cats and then mostly in the dog. The gallstones consist mostly of bile pigment (calcium bilirubinate) and/or cholesterol and hence they are usually radiolucent (Mullowney and Tennant, 1982). The pathogenesis is not well understood. Gallstones can be produced experimentally in dogs fed a diet rich in carbohydrate and low in protein and fat. The pathogenesis is probably different from that in humans, in which gallstones occur mainly in women from relative oversaturation of the bile with cholesterol. Gallstones are formed in the gallbladder and can damage the mucosa and induce cholecystitis. In many apparently healthy dogs multiple very tiny calculi are present forming a sludge of crystals. They appear not to be clinically relevant and it is not known whether bile sludge formation has any relationship with cholelithiasis. Gallstones may enter the common bile duct and occlude it to cause extrahepatic cholestasis and bile duct rupture (Harris *et al.*, 1984).

Clinical signs
The signs are usually those of extrahepatic cholestasis from obstruction of the common bile duct (Kirpensteijn *et al.*, 1993). Sometimes there are more acute signs of epigastric pain and vomiting. Occasionally secondary cholangitis or cholecystitis results in perforation. Gallstones are, however, usually asymptomatic.

Diagnosis
If extrahepatic cholestasis causes the signs, the characteristic abnormalities will be found in the liver biopsy. The presence of calculi are best demonstrated by ultrasonography (Fig. 37.23). Gallstones are seldom detected by radiography. The excretion of radiographic contrast media is markedly reduced in cholestasis, so that cholecystography may not be possible. If there is no extrahepatic cholestasis, cholecystography can be used and the stones will be seen as filling defects.

Management
The gallstones can be removed surgically, during which the gallbladder and common bile duct must be flushed out to prevent leaving any stones behind. If there is severe cholecystitis, chole-

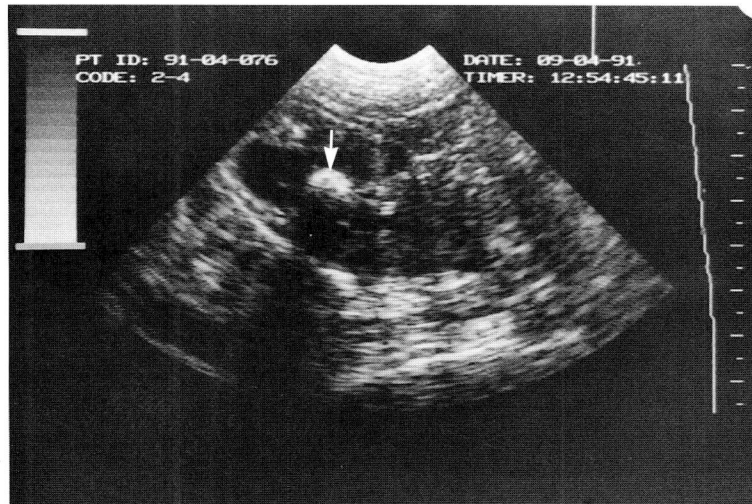

Figure 37.23 Ultrasonogram of a cat with chronic cholangiohepatitis and a stone in the gallbladder. The echodense stone (arrow) is clearly depicted in the dark fluid in the gallbladder.

cystectomy should be performed. In all cases it is necessary to begin antibiotic therapy based on culture of the bile. Medical treatment with chenodeoxycholic acid, as used in humans, to enlarge the bile acid pool and relieve the relative oversaturation with cholesterol, is contraindicated in the dog. The intestinal flora in the dog convert this drug into the extremely hepatotoxic lithocholic acid. Ursodeoxycholic acid does not have this side effect and can be safely used in dogs. Oral administration of bile acids has the beneficial effect of enhancing the bile flow which, in the absence of complete bile duct obstruction, may help to prevent infection and to remove small calculi.

Hyperplasia of the biliary epithelium

This disorder can develop after long-term administration of high doses of progestins, usually to suppress oestrus. The cystic hyperplasia of the mucosa is found mainly in the gallbladder without clinical signs. Occasionally the abnormality is so extensive that the large bile ducts are also affected and become obstructed causing extrahepatic cholestasis.

In clinical cases the history is important, but the diagnosis can only be made at laparotomy. There is no specific therapy available and the administration of progestins should be discontinued.

Bile duct carcinoma

Pathogenesis

Tumours of the biliary epithelium occur infrequently. In the dog they usually arise from intrahepatic bile ducts and readily metastasize to the liver and other organs. Multiple metastases throughout the biliary system gives signs of cholestasis in most cases. In the cat they occur more often in the large bile ducts and result in obstruction (Haines et al., 1996). The disease is rapidly progressive (Patnaik et al., 1981).

Clinical signs

Icterus is the most common sign. There is often widespread infiltration of the tumour in the liver and thus hepatomegaly.

Diagnosis

Physical and laboratory examination only indicate extrahepatic cholestasis. The diagnosis can easily be missed with a blind liver biopsy, but the tumours are detectable with ultrasonography and guided biopsy is diagnostic.

Management

The tumour is usually very infiltrative. It can sometimes be completely removed by lobectomy, but in most cases no treatment is possible by the time clinical signs occur. In view of the rapid progression of the disease euthanasia should be considered following this diagnosis.

Biliary tract rupture

Pathogenesis

The gallbladder or bile duct can rupture following trauma or perforation due to ulcerative inflammation. The latter is often associated with cholelithiasis. In the majority of cases the cause is trauma, usually caused by an automobile, which tears a lobular bile duct from its junction with the hepatic duct or common bile duct (Watkins et al., 1983; Parchman and Flanders, 1990). Because of the deep separations between the lobes in the canine and feline liver, only the duct from one lobe is usually torn. The leakage of bile causes clinically detectable ascites. The high concentration of bile acids causes chemical peritonitis and absorption of bile pigments from the abdomen causes severe icterus. Both peritonitis and the absorption of bile acids can cause vomiting. The peritonitis causes impaired fluid resorption from the abdominal cavity, hence the rapid accumulation of ascites within a few days of the perforation. Since *Clostridium* is often present in the normal gallbladder, there is a risk of clostridial infection. Occasionally spontaneous rupture of the gallbladder occurs as a result of cholecystitis, usually due to gallstones.

Clinical signs
Severe icterus and ascites develop within a few days. Vomiting is usual and there may be general malaise and anorexia. Fever and general illness are remarkably rare given the severe peritonitis.

Diagnosis
A history of recent trauma may be a strong indication. Aspiration of the ascitic fluid reveals free bile in the abdominal cavity, which is diagnostic.

Management
Surgical repair is required following correction of the dehydration, electrolyte and pH abnormalities. The tear in the large bile duct can easily be found by pressing some bile out of the gallbladder. When there is rupture of the gallbladder due to local cholecystitis, cholecystectomy is indicated and any gallstones removed. Vigorous peritoneal lavage is indicated. Postoperative treatment for a few weeks with penicillin or ampicillin is advisable because of the risk of clostridial infection. The prognosis is good. Even very ill animals with severe chemical peritonitis recover rapidly (Martin *et al.*, 1988).

Destructive cholangiolitis

Pathogenesis
This is total absence of bile flow mimicking extrahepatic bile duct obstruction but caused by destruction of intrahepatic bile ducts in the smaller portal areas. The cause is an adverse reaction to sulphonamide drugs such as trimethoprim/sulpha (van den Ingh *et al.*, 1988b; Rowland *et al.*, 1992). The small bile ducts in the portal areas become completely necrotic, which results in bile flow obstruction. The dogs become very icteric and have extremely high AP, γGT, bile acids and transaminases in plasma. Not only clinically but also histologically the liver disease is very similar to extrahepatic bile duct obstruction. Signs usually develop a few days after repeated medication with a sulphur-containing drug.

Clinical signs
Signs occur at any age and include sudden onset anorexia, depression, vomiting, polyuria and sometimes acholic stool, in combination with marked icterus. The liver may be moderately enlarged.

Diagnosis
The history is very important. With ultrasonography the expected findings of enlarged, tortuous extrahepatic bile ducts which may be found in extrahepatic cholestasis, are not present. The diagnosis is made on the basis of the characteristic histological findings.

Management
There is no specific therapy, apart from immediate cessation of the drug administered. Supportive care consists of prevention of dehydration and antiemetic drugs. It may be helpful to give bile salts (ursodeoxycholic acid) which can increase bile flow, but there are few data about this therapy. The prognosis is very poor; most dogs do not survive.

Feline Liver Diseases

The general part of this chapter on functional anatomy, physiology and clinically important syndromes is relevant to both dogs and cats. The same holds for the sections on history taking, physical examination, laboratory examination and other investigative techniques. The section on diseases of the biliary tract is also applicable for cats. However, there are a number of specific diseases of cats that are different from dogs. The physiology of the liver differs from that of dogs in some specific aspects. Clinically relevant differences in feline physiology will be dealt with, followed by a number of specific liver diseases of cats.

SPECIFIC ASPECTS OF FELINE LIVER PHYSIOLOGY

One important difference between dogs and cats is the low capacity of the liver enzymes responsible for conjugation of cholephilic substances to make them more polar as a prerequisite for biliary or urinary excretion. The low glucuronosyl transferase capacity is important for the metabolism of endogenous products such as bilirubin and exogenous compounds, either drugs or toxins. The elimination of drugs like chloramphenicol, non-steroidal anti-inflammatory drugs and anticonvulsants depends on this function of the liver. Hence, toxic side effects develop more easily in cats in cases of overdosage or reduced liver function.

Cats also have different amino acid requirements than dogs, because they can not synthesize sufficient quantities of a number of amino acids. Thus arginine, taurine and carnitine are essential amino acids for cats. Arginine is an important intermediate metabolite in the hepatic urea cycle in which ammonia is being converted into urea. This causes a relatively high susceptibility to hyperammoniaemia and hepatic encephalopathy when protein intake is inadequate, for example from anorexia. Cats, unlike dogs, may develop hepatic encephalopathy in cases of parenchymal liver disease without portosystemic collateral circulation. Arginine and taurine are involved in the hepatic production of apoproteins which are used to form the very low density lipoproteins. These lipoproteins are the form in which the liver can secrete triglycerides into the circulation for further metabolization. Insufficient availability of arginine and taurine may lead to accumulation of triglycerides in the liver, for example during fasting. Taurine also plays a role in detoxification, since it is being used by the liver as a conjugating group to make substances such as bile acids more hydrophilic. Taurine is also involved in glutathione metabolism which is one of the major routes in the detoxification of many toxins. Carnitine is an intermediate enabling β-oxidation of long chain fatty acids in mitochondria which may be impaired in anorexia.

CHOLANGITIS

Acute cholangitis

Pathogenesis

Cats may have two different forms of cholangitis, an acute and a chronic form. It is not certain whether they are different stages of the same disease. However, the chronic form is usually not preceded by a recognizable acute episode and the type of the inflammatory process is different in both forms. Hence the author considers the acute and chronic forms as different entities and they are discussed separately.

Acute cholangitis is most likely due to an ascending infection from the intestinal tract, but haematogenous infection may also occur. It is a bacterial infection and *E. coli* can be cultured from the bile in most cases. The result is a suppurative inflammation. Histologically, the reaction is that of acute extrahepatic cholestasis, with portal oedema and polymorphonuclear inflammatory cells. Inflammatory cells are also present in the lumens of the bile ducts, which differentiates it from simple extrahepatic cholestasis (Fig. 37.24). Due to the diffuse obstruction throughout the biliary tree, bile flow is hampered at the level of the proximal intrahepatic tributaries. Hence the extrahepatic biliary tree is not distended as in simple extrahepatic cholestasis.

Clinical signs

The signs are those of acute or subacute (1–3 weeks) inflammatory disease with general illness and often fever, together with those of extrahepatic cholestasis, mainly icterus. The degree of icterus is variable and depends on the severity of the inflammation (Hirsch and Doige, 1983; Shaker et al., 1991).

Diagnosis

The bile acids and in many cases also the activity of ALT in plasma is elevated, but this only

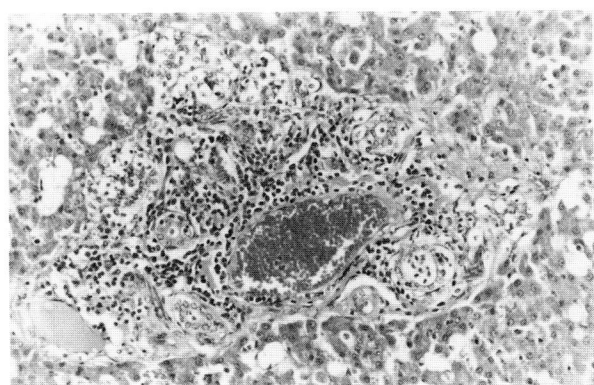

Figure 37.24 Acute cholangiohepatitis in a cat. There is infiltration of neutrophils and some lymphocytes in the lumen of the bile ducts and in the portal area of the acinus.

indicates hepatobiliary disease in general. Ultrasonography does not give the changes expected in extrahepatic cholestasis, since the extrahepatic bile ducts are not dilated and tortuous. In cases with severe cholestasis the gallbladder tends to be empty since the intrahepatic bile ducts are also obstructed; normally the gallbladder is always visible. The diagnosis can only be confirmed with histological examination of a liver biopsy. It is possible to sample bile from the gallbladder with a fine needle using ultrasound guidance, for bacterial culture and antibiotic sensitivity testing. This may be especially helpful in cases that are resistant to antibiotic therapy.

Management

Antibiotics which are well excreted into bile are indicated (Jackson et al., 1994). The author prefers a 3–4-week course of amoxycillin and clavulanic acid. Chloramphenicol, although well excreted into bile, is not advisable since it may be toxic due to impaired detoxification and reduced bile flow. Treatment is successful in most cases, but results should be evaluated with a repeated liver biopsy before cessation of medication.

■ Chronic cholangiohepatitis

Pathogenesis

This form of cholangitis is different from the acute form and in many respects is comparable with chronic active hepatitis in dogs. There is no acute onset of the disease and when patients develop clinical signs they are already in the chronic stage. The bile is sterile in animals with chronic cholangiohepatitis, which does not preclude possible infection at an earlier stage. In some cases liver flukes are detected as a primary cause of cholangitis. Whatever the cause, the type of inflammatory reaction in chronic cases is not suppurative but mononuclear (lymphocytes and plasma cells) and the inflammation extends from the portal areas into the parenchyma in a similar way to canine chronic active hepatitis. The difference is that in cats there is diffuse intra- and extrahepatic cholestasis with mononuclear inflammatory cells in the bile ducts, which suggests an autoimmune destruction of biliary and liver cell epithelium. Without treatment the disease progresses to cirrhosis (Fig. 37.25). The liver tends to be enlarged and is therefore palpable. Only in advanced cirrhosis is the organ small.

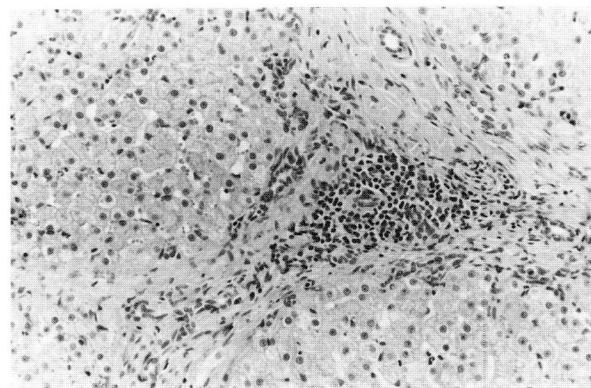

Figure 37.25 Chronic cholangiohepatitis in a cat with bile duct proliferation in the portal area, infiltration with lymphocytes and disturbance of the normal acinar structure with fibrous tissue bridging between portal areas. This is the beginning of cirrhosis.

The results of the disease are impaired liver functions, cholestasis and portal hypertension. Acquired portosystemic collaterals may develop and both parenchymal dysfunction and collaterals may induce hepatic encephalopathy. Ascites may occur, but this is rare in comparison to dogs with chronic active hepatitis (Prasse et al., 1982).

Clinical signs

Signs of general illness with decreased appetite, weight loss and malaise are seen. The cholestasis gives a variable degree of icterus which tends to diminish in chronic cases, possibly because the kidneys take over many excretory functions. Hepatomegaly occurs in most cases and in advanced cases there is hepatic encephalopathy and sometimes ascites. Fever is uncommon.

Diagnosis

There may be palpable enlargement of the liver and blood examination reveals high bile acid levels with variable increment of the ALT activity (Zawie and Garvey, 1984; Center, 1986). These findings are not specific to differentiate this disease from other hepatobiliary disorders. Ultrasonography indicates a diffusely enlarged liver, often with increased echodensity which is also not specific. An empty gallbladder may occasionally indicate the disease. The diagnosis depends on the specific histology of the liver, hence a biopsy is required. If there is no response to medication, liver fluke infection should be suspected and confirmed by examination of multiple faecal samples (Bielsa and Greiner, 1985; Lewis et al., 1991).

Management

The disease responds well to medication with prednisolone which suppresses the inflammation. Long-term treatment is mandatory, comparable to that in chronic active hepatitis in dogs. Prednisolone (1 mg kg^{-1} day^{-1}) is given an initial dose of 2 mg kg^{-1} day^{-1} for one week. It is important to evaluate the response by liver biopsies after six weeks of treatment since the liver changes resulting from chronic glucocorticoid administration induce elevated liver enzymes and bile acids in plasma which makes blood examination unreliable to evaluate the condition of the liver. Medication must be continued until there is no doubt about the cessation of the inflammation histologically. Supportive care may be required during the initial period to control dehydration and hepatic encephalopathy. If histological examination indicates the development of fat accumulation in the liver, this requires specific supportive care as discussed under hepatic lipidosis. The prognosis is favourable, as treatment is often successful and the disease can be cured completely. Liver fluke infection may be treated with praziquantel.

CONGENITAL PORTOSYSTEMIC SHUNTS

Most of the remarks made on pathogenesis, clinical signs, diagnosis and management also apply to cats. The types of shunts seen in dogs may also occur in cats. Cats tend to have more extrahepatic shunts. There is no breed predisposition for cats and consequently, there is no indication that it is an inherited disease (Rothuizen et al., 1982; Berger et al., 1986).

In cats it is not only important to monitor the blood glucose level during and following surgery, but one should also be aware of the risk of insufficient intake of the essential amino acids for cats as mentioned in the introduction. Supplementation may be given intravenously or orally.

FELINE LIVER DYSFUNCTION RESULTING FROM SYSTEMIC DISEASE

Cats, like dogs, display liver changes in multicentric diseases such as hypoxia (anaemia or shock), diabetes mellitus, hyperadrenocorticism (spontaneous or iatrogenic) and amyloidosis. Amyloidosis is more common in cats than in dogs (Blunden and Smith, 1992). Non-specific reactive hepatitis may also occur in cats, but is much less frequently diagnosed than in dogs. The remarks made for dogs also apply to cats. A few comments should be made for liver lesions in feline infectious peritonitis and in hyperthyroidism.

The liver in feline infectious peritonitis (FIP)

Infectious peritonitis is an infectious viral disease. The manifestations may be variable depending on the organs involved. Ascites and pleural effusion are not always present. In many cases, the liver is a major site of inflammation. In FIP there is a granulomatous inflammatory reaction in the liver with multiple small granulomas throughout the parenchyma. The granulomas are too small to be detected with ultrasonography, but are visible microscopically in a percutaneous liver biopsy. Although these granulomas are not entirely specific for FIP, they give a very strong indication for this diagnosis.

For further details on the disease refer to Chapter 49.

The liver in feline hyperthyroidism

Hyperthyroidism is associated with fatty infiltration of the hepatocytes. This does not cause clinical signs of liver dysfunction, but explains the abnormally high liver enzymes and bile acid levels seen in many cases. The fatty changes are not severe and there is no liver enlargement. A number of signs associated with hyperthyroidism mimic those of primary liver diseases, for example polyuria, vomiting, diarrhoea and weight loss. Hence one may elect to measure blood parameters to screen for liver disease and a subsequent liver biopsy may reveal the histological changes. Hyperthyroidism is discussed in detail in Chapter 39.

Hepatic lipidosis

Pathogenesis

Fat accumulation in the liver generally occurs as a result of metabolic conditions in which there is increased deposition or impaired removal of triglycerides in the liver. Clinically, this may be important in diabetes mellitus as discussed for dogs. Subclinical fat accumulation only detectable on histological examination, occurs in many other conditions such as high caloric intake, hypoxia and induction by a number of toxic substances. Cats, however, may display an idiopathic form of liver lipidosis which may become life-threatening. This form is referred to as feline hepatic lipidosis.

Accumulation of triglycerides results from a disturbed balance between triglyceride uptake by the liver and its removal. The latter is normally achieved by formation of lipoproteins (especially very low density lipoprotein, VLDL) which is the way the liver can secrete fatty acids into the circulation for metabolism in other tissues. Another route for the liver to metabolize fatty acids is by β-oxidation.

Obese cats seem to be predisposed but lean cats may also develop lipidosis. It is generally appreciated that prolonged fasting is a most important factor inducing lipidosis (Biourge et al., 1993). Fasting may affect the hepatic fatty acid metabolism in three ways (Biourge et al., 1990; Cantafora et al., 1991). First, fasting induces peripheral lipolysis and increased delivery of fatty acids to the liver. Second, the intake of essential amino acids may be inadequate. Deficiency of arginine and taurine may inhibit the apoprotein formation necessary to produce VLDLs in which the liver can secrete the fatty acids, hence further hepatic accumulation of triglycerides occurs. Finally, carnitine deficiency may give impairment of the β-oxidation which is a major pathway for fatty acid catabolism in the liver (Jacobs et al., 1989, 1990).

Most cats with lipidosis have slight hyperglycaemia which is not due to stress, since they also have impaired glucose tolerance (Center et al., 1993). The mechanism underlying the deranged glucose metabolism is not known. There is no tendency to develop overt diabetes mellitus and therefore the condition is not a form of prediabetes. Both high and low levels of insulin and glucagon have been reported. However, high doses of insulin are required to lower the blood glucose in these cats suggesting insulin resistance. High growth hormone concentrations have been recorded in a few patients, which could explain the insulin resistance. However, this could not be related to progestin administration or other factors known to induce growth hormone excess. Whatever the cause, hyperglycaemia is a possible factor contributing to the accumulation of triglycerides.

Lipidosis results in hepatomegaly with yellow discoloration and a friable texture. As in all types of hepatomegaly the margins of the lobes become rounded. Swelling of cells can give rise to intrahepatic cholestasis and reduced liver function and fasting may trigger hepatic encephalopathy.

Lipidosis may occur at any age in either sex. There seems to be an increased incidence around middle age. Individual susceptibility plays a part in that some cats sustain prolonged fasting without developing lipidosis whereas others get recurrences with every episode of prolonged fasting. It is remarkable that hepatic lipidosis occurs regularly in the United States but less frequently in Europe and more on the continent than in Britain. It is not known whether these regional differences reflect genetic differences or differences in diet.

Clinical signs

Cats are presented with anorexia and malaise. There may be occasional vomiting. Icterus is a regular finding and hepatic encephalopathy may occur.

Diagnosis

The clinical signs and findings at physical examination (icterus and hepatomegaly) are not specific and neither are elevated bile acids and liver enzymes in plasma. Slight or moderate hyperglycaemia and prolonged increment of plasma glucose in a glucose tolerance test may indicate lipidosis, but is not diagnostic. It should be remembered that stress during blood sampling often gives hyperglycaemia in cats. The diagnosis can only be made by liver biopsy and because of the diffuse nature of the disease a blind procedure is always diagnostic (Fig. 37.26).

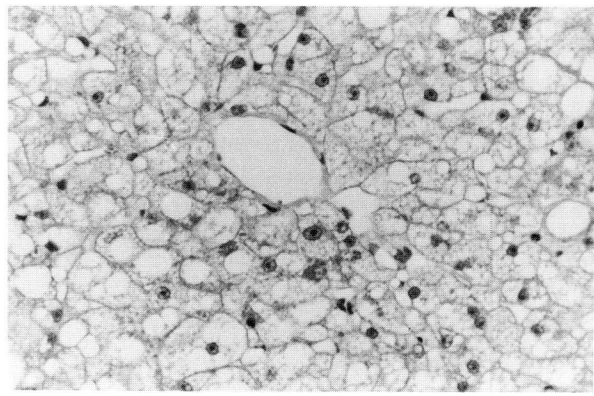

Figure 37.26 Fatty liver in a cat. There is micro- and macrovesicular steatosis of the hepatocytes.

Management

It is important to get the cat out of its catabolic state and to supply the amino acids essential to prevent further fat accumulation and development of hepatic encephalopathy. Force feeding of fluid food is required and this can be achieved in most cases by slow oral injection from a syringe (Cornelius and Rogers, 1985; Biourge et al., 1991; Center et al., 1993). Feeding via a nasogastric tube is necessary if the cat is unable to be force fed. Baby milk or veterinary milk formulations with a similar composition are usually adequate. It may be advisable to give vitamin B supplementation. There is little point in giving glucose as an energy source, since these animals tend to have glucose intolerance and can not adequately utilize it. So-called lipotrophic compounds like methionine are not recommended (see section on hepatic encephalopathy). Insulin administration is not recommended, because of the risk of life-threatening hypoglycaemia. Hyperglycaemia seems to be a secondary phenomenon. These measures often have to be continued for a long period, which the owner can do at home. Nevertheless, the prognosis is guarded and roughly half of the cats survive.

Supportive care includes restoration of fluid and electrolyte balance. Ammonia, electrolytes and pH should be monitored and supportive care directed at hepatic encephalopathy if required.

TUMOURS OF THE LIVER

All tumour types described for dogs may also occur in cats (Post and Patnaik, 1992; Patnaik, 1992). The most common tumour in cats is malignant lymphoma. The liver is involved in most cases with the multicentric form of the disease and can be diagnosed by cytology of aspirates from lymph nodes. Alternatively, liver biopsy is a sensitive way to make the diagnosis and a smear from a fine needle biopsy is adequate. Chemotherapy is discussed in Chapter 50.

REFERENCES

Abdelkader, S.V. and Hauge, J.G. (1986) Serum enzyme determination in the study of liver disease in dogs. *Acta Veterinaria Scandinavia* **27**, 59–70.

Abiru, H., Sarna, S.K. and Condon, R.E. (1994) Contractile mechanisms of gallbladder filling and emptying in dogs. *Gastroenterology* **106**, 1652–1661.

Aguilera, T.E., Mayer, V.R. and Gomez, C.G. (1988) Plasma bile acids, lactate dehydrogenase, and sulphobromophthalein retention test in carbon tetrachloride intoxication. *Journal of Small Animal Practice* **29**, 711–717.

Allen, K.G.D., Twedt, D.C. and Hunsaker, H.A. (1987) Tetramine cupruretic agents: a comparison in dogs. *American Journal of Veterinary Research* **48**, 28–30.

Aminlari, M., Vaseghi, T., Sajedianfard, M.J. and Samsami, M. (1994) Changes in arginase, aminotransferases and rhodanese in sera of domestic animals with experimentally induced liver necrosis. *Journal of Comparative Pathology* **110**, 1–9.

Andersson, M. and Sevelius, E. (1991) Breed, sex and age distribution in dogs with chronic liver disease: a demographic study. *Journal of Small Animal Practice* **32**, 1–5.

Badylak, S.F. (1988) Coagulation disorders and liver disease. *Veterinary Clinics of North America, Small Animal Practice* **18**, 87–93.

Badylak, S.F. and van Vleet, J.F. (1981) Sequential morphologic and clinicopathologic alterations in dogs with experimentally induced glucocorticoid hepatopathy. *American Journal of Veterinary Research* **42**, 1310–1318.

Badylak, S.F. and van Vleet, J.F. (1982) Tissue gamma glutamyl transpeptidase activity and hepatic ultrastructural alterations in dogs with experimentally induced glucocorticoid hepatopathy. *American Journal of Veterinary Research* **43**, 649–655.

Badylak, S.F., Dodds, W.J. and van Vleet, J.F. (1983) Plasma coagulation factor abnormalities in dogs with naturally occurring hepatic disease. *American Journal of Veterinary Research* **44**, 2336–2340.

Bahr, A., Daniel, G.B., DeNovo, R., Young, K. and Merryman, J.L. (1996) Quantitative hepatobiliary scintigraphy with deconvolutional analysis for the measurement of hepatic function in dogs. *Veterinary Radiology and Ultrasound* **37**, 214–220.

Bailey, M.Q., Willard, M.D., McLoughlin, M.A., Gaber, C. and Hauptman, J. (1988) Ultrasonographic findings associated with congenital hepatic arteriovenous fistula in three dogs. *Journal of the American Veterinary Medical Association* **192**, 1099–1101.

Bastianello, S.S., Nesbit, J.W., Williams, M.C. and Lange, A.L. (1987) Pathological findings in a natural outbreak of aflatoxicosis in dogs. *Onderstepoort Journal of Veterinary Research* **54**, 635–640.

Bauer, J.E. and Schenck, P.A. (1989) Nutritional management of hepatic disease. *Veterinary Clinics of North America, Small Animal Practice* **19**, 513–526.

Bennett, A.M., Davies, C.J. and Lucke, V.M. (1983) Lobular dissecting hepatitis in the dog. *Veterinary Pathology* **20**, 179–188.

Berger, B., Whiting, P.G., Breznock, E.M., Bruhl-Day, R. and Moore, P.F. (1986) Congenital feline portosystemic shunts. *Journal of the American Veterinary Medical Association* **188**, 517–521.

Bielsa, L.M. and Greiner, E.C. (1985) Liver flukes

(*Platynosomum concinnum*) in cats. *Journal of the American Animal Hospital Association* **21**, 269–274.

Biourge, V., MacDonald, M.J. and King, L. (1990) Feline hepatic lipidosis: pathogenesis and nutritional management. *Compendium of Continuing Education* **12**, 1244–1258.

Biourge, V., Pion, P., Lewis, J., Morris, J.G. and Rogers, Q.R. (1991) Dietary management of idiopathic feline hepatic lipidosis with a liquid diet supplemented with citrulline and choline. *Journal of Nutrition* **121**, S155–156.

Biourge, V., Pion, P., Lewis, J., Morris, J.G. and Rogers, Q.R. (1993) Spontaneous occurrence of hepatic lipidosis in a group of laboratory cats. *Journal of Veterinary Internal Medicine* **7**, 194–197.

Birchard, S.J., Biller, D.S. and Johnson, S.E. (1989) Differentiation of intrahepatic versus extrahepatic portosystemic shunts in dogs using positive-contrast portography. *Journal of the American Animal Hospital Association* **25**, 13–17.

Blunden, A.S. and Smith, K.C. (1992) Generalised amyloidosis and acute liver haemorrhage in 4 cats. *Journal of Small Animal Practice* **33**, 566–570.

Boothe, H.W., Howe, L.M., Edwards, J.F. and Slater, M.R. (1996) Multiple extrahepatic portosystemic shunts in dogs: 30 cases (1981–1993). *Journal of the American Veterinary Medical Association* **208**, 1849–1854.

Bostwick, D.R. and Twedt, D. (1995) Intrahepatic and extrahepatic portal venous anomalies in dogs: 52 cases (1982–1992). *Journal of the American Veterinary Medical Association* **206**, 1181–1185.

Brewer, G.J., Schall, W., Dick, R., Yuzbasiyangurkan, V., Thomas, M. and Padgett, G. (1992) Use of copper-64 measurements to diagnose canine copper toxicosis. *Journal of Veterinary Internal Medicine* **6**, 41–43.

Bunch, S.E., Castleman, W.L., Baldwin, B.H., Hornbuckle, W.E. and Tennant, B.C. (1985) Effects of long term primidone and phenytoin administration on canine hepatic function and morphology. *American Journal of Veterinary Research* **46**, 105–115.

Bunch, S.E., Conway, M.B. and Center, S.A. (1987) Toxic hepatopathy and intrahepatic cholestasis associated with phenytoin administration in combination with other anticonvulsant drugs in three dogs. *Journal of the American Veterinary Medical Association* **190**, 194–198.

Burnell, J.M., Dennis, M.B., Clayson, M.S., Smuckler, E.A. and Cift, R.A. (1976) Evaluation in dogs of cross-circulation in the treatment of acute hepatic necrosis induced by yellow phosphorus. *Gastroenterology* **71**, 827–831.

Cantafora, A., Blotta, I., Rossi, S.S, Hoffamann, A.F. and Sturman, J.A. (1991) Dietary taurine content changes liver lipids in cats. *Journal of Nutrition* **121**, 1522–1528.

Cape, L., Panciera, D.L., Partington, B., Bjorling, D.E. and Dubielzig, R.R. (1992) Glomerulonephritis and a congenital portocaval shunt in a seven-year-old dog. *Journal of the American Animal Hospital Association* **28**, 419–423.

Center, S.A. (1986) Feline liver disorders and their management. *Compendium of Continuing Education* **8**, 889–903.

Center, S.A., Baldwin, B.H., Erb, H.N. and Tennant, B.C. (1985a) Bile acid concentrations in the diagnosis of hepatobiliary disease of the dog. *Journal of the American Veterinary Medical Association* **187**, 935–940

Center, S.A., Baldwin, B.H., de Lahunta, A., Dietze, A.E. and Tennant, B.C. (1985b) Evaluation of serum bile acid concentrations for the diagnosis of portosystemic venous anomalies in the dog and cat. *Journal of the American Veterinary Medical Association* **186**, 1090–1094.

Center, S.A., Baldwin, B.H, Erb, H. and Tennant, B.C. (1986a) Bile acid concentrations in the diagnosis of hepatobiliary disease in the cat. *Journal of the American Veterinary Medical Association* **189**, 891–896.

Center, S.A., Baldwin, B.H., Dillingham, S., Erb, H.N. and Tennant, B.C. (1986b) Diagnostic value of serum gamma glutamyl transferase and alkaline phosphatase activities in hepatobiliary disease in the cat. *Journal of the American Veterinary Medical Association* **188**, 507–510.

Center, S.A., ManWarren, T., Slater, M.R. and Wilentz, E. (1991) Evaluation of twelve hour preprandial and two hour postprandial serum bile acids concentrations for diagnosis of hepatobiliary disease in dogs. *Journal of the American Veterinary Medical Association* **199**, 217–226.

Center, S.A., Crawford, M.A., Guida, L., Erb, H.N. and King, J. (1993) A retrospective study of 77 cats with severe hepatic lipidosis: 1975–1990. *Journal of Veterinary Internal Medicine* **7**, 49–59.

Chapman, B.L., Hendrick, M.J. and Washabau, R.J. (1993) Granulomatous hepatitis in dogs: nine cases (1987–1990). *Journal of the American Veterinary Medical Association* **203**, 680–684.

Conn, H.O. and Bircher, J. (1989) *Hepatic Encephalopathy: Management with Lactulose and Other Related Carbohydrates.* Medi-Ed Press, East Lansing.

Cornelius, L.M. and Rogers, K.S. (1985) Idiopathic hepatic lipidosis in cats. *Modern Veterinary Practice* **66**, 377–380.

Crawford, M.A., Schall, W.D., Jensen, R.K. and Tasker, J.B. (1985) Chronic active hepatitis in 26 Doberman Pinschers. *Journal of the American Veterinary Medical Association* **187**, 1343–1352.

Daniel, G.B., Bright, R., Ollis, P. and Shull, R. (1991) Per rectal portal scintigraphy using 99mTechnetium pertechnetate to diagnose portosystemic shunts in dogs and cats. *Journal of Veterinary Internal Medicine* **5**, 23–27.

Dayrell-Hart, B., Steinberg, S.A., Van Winkle, T.J. and Farnbach, G.C. (1991) Hepatotoxicity of phenobarbital in dogs: 18 cases (1985–1989). *Journal of the American Veterinary Medical Association* **199**, 1060–1066.

Deutz, N.E.P., Bovee, W.M.M.J., Chamuleau, R.A.F.M., De Haan, J.G., De Graaf, A.A. and De Beer, R. (1988) *In Vivo* brain ¹H-NMR spectroscopy during acute hepatic encephalopathy (HE). In: *Advances in Ammonia Metabolism and Hepatic Encephalopathy* (Eds P.B. Soeters, J.H.P. Wilson, A.J. Meijer and E. Holm). Elsevier, Amsterdam, pp 439–446.

Dillon, R. (1985) The liver in systemic disease. An innocent bystander. *Veterinary Clinics of North America Small Animal Practice* **15**, 97–117.

Evans, S.M. (1987) The radiographic appearance of primary liver neoplasia in dogs. *Veterinary Radiology* **28**, 192–196.

Fahie, M.A. and Martin, R.A. (1995) Extrahepatic biliary tract obstruction: a retrospective study of 45 cases (1983–1993). *Journal of the American Animal Hospital Association* **31**, 478–482.

Ferenci, P., Puspok, A. and Steindl, P. (1992) Current concepts in the pathophysiology of hepatic encephalopathy. *European Journal of Clinical Investigation* **22**, 573–581.

Fittschen, C. and Bellamy, J.E.C. (1984) Prednisone induced morphologic and chemical changes in the liver of dogs. *Veterinary Pathology* **21**, 399–406.

Foster-van Hijfte, M.A., McEvoy, F.J., White, R.N., Lamb, C.R. and Rutgers, H.C. (1996) Per rectal portal scintigraphy in the diagnosis and management of feline congenital portosystemic shunts. *Journal of Small Animal Practice* **37**, 7–11.

Franklin, J.E. and Saunders, G.K. (1988) Chronic active hepatitis in Doberman pinschers. *Compendium of Continuing Education* **10**, 1247–1255.

Gocke, D.J., Preisig, R., Morris, T.Q., McKay, D.G. and Bradley, S.E. (1967) Experimental viral hepatitis in the dog: production of persistent disease in partially immune animals. *Journal of Clinical Investigation* **46**, 1506–1517.

Gocke, D.J., Morris, T.Q. and Bradley, S.E. (1970) Chronic hepatitis in the dog: the role of immune factors. *Journal of the American Veterinary Medical Association* **156**, 1700–1705.

Greenway, C.V. and Oshiro, G. (1972) Intrahepatic distribution of portal and hepatic arterial blood flows in anesthetized cats and dogs and the effect of portal occlusion, raised venous pressure and histamine. *Journal of Physiology* **227**, 472–485.

Gumucio J.G., Bilir, B.M., Moseley, R.H. and Berkowitz, C.M. (1994) The biology of the liver cell plate. In: *The Lver: Biology and Pathobiology*, 3rd edn (Eds Arias, I.M. *et al.*). Raven Press, New York, pp. 1143–1163.

Hager, D.A., Nyland, T.G. and Fisher, P. (1985) Ultrasound-guided biopsy of the canine liver, kidney, and prostate. *Veterinary Radiology* **26**, 82–88.

Haines, V.L., Brown, P.R., Hruban, R.H. and Huso, D.L. (1996) Adenocarcinoma of the hepatopancreatic ampulla in a domestic cat. *Veterinary Pathology* **33**, 439–441.

Hammer, A.S. and Sikkema, D.A. (1995) Hepatic neoplasia in the dog and the cat. *Veterinary Clinics of North America Small Animal Practice* **25**, 419–435.

Hardy, R. (1986) Chronic hepatitis in dogs: a syndrome. *Compendium of Continuing Education* **8**, 904–914.

Harris, S.J., Simpson, J.W. and Thoday, K.L. (1984) Obstructive cholelithiasis and gall bladder rupture in a dog. *Journal of Small Animal Practice* **25**, 661–667.

Hirsch, V.M. and Doige, C.E. (1983) Suppurative cholangitis in cats. *Journal of the American Veterinary Medical Association* **182**, 1223–1226.

Holt, D.E., Schelling, C.G., Saunders, H.M. and Orsher, R.J. (1995) Correlation of ultrasonographic findings with surgical, portographic, and necropsy findings in dogs and cats with portosystemic shunts: 63 cases (1987–1993). *Journal of the American Veterinary Medical Association* **207**, 1190–1193.

Hultgren B.D., Stevens, J.B. and Hardy, R.M. (1986) Inherited, chronic, progressive hepatic degeneration in Bedlington Terriers with increased liver copper concentrations: clinical and pathologic observations and comparison with other copper associated liver diseases. *American Journal of Veterinary Research* **47**, 365–377.

Iwanaka, M., Orita, S. and Mokuno (1993) Tyzzer's disease complicated with distemper in a puppy. *Journal of Veterinary Medical Science* **55**, 337–339.

Jackson, M.W., Panciera, D.L. and Hartmann, F. (1994) Administration of vancomycin for treatment of ascending bacterial cholangiohepatitis in a cat. *Journal of the American Veterinary Medical Association* **204**, 602–605.

Jacobs, G., Cornelius, L., Allen, S. and Greene, C. (1989) Treatment of idiopathic hepatic lipidosis in cats: 11 cases (1986–1987). *Journal of the American Veterinary Medical Association* **195**, 635–638.

Jacobs, G., Cornelius, L., Keene, B., Rakich, P. and Shug, A. (1990) Comparison of plasma, liver, and skeletal muscle carnitine concentrations in cats with idiopathic hepatic lipidosis and in healthy cats. *American Journal of Veterinary Research* **51**, 1349–1351.

Jarrett, W.F.H., O'Neil, B.W. and Lindholm, I. (1987) Persistent hepatitis and chronic fibrosis induced by canine acidophil cell hepatitis virus. *Veterinary Record* **120**, 234–235.

Jenssen, A.L. and Nielsen, O.L. (1991) Chronic hepatitis in three young standard poodles. *Journal of Veterinary Medicine* **38**, 194–197.

Johnson, G.F., Sternlieb, I. and Twedt, D.C. (1980) Inheritance of copper toxicosis in Bedlington terriers. *American Journal of Veterinary Research* **41**, 1865–1866.

Johnson, G.F., Gilbertson, S.R., Goldfischer, S., Grunshoff, P.S. and Sternlieb, I. (1984) Cytochemical detection of inherited copper toxicosis of Bedlington terriers. *Veterinary Pathology* **21**, 57–60.

Johnson, S.E., Rogers, W.A., Bonagura, J.D. and Caldwell, J.H. (1985) Determination of serum bile acids in fasting dogs with hepatobiliary disease. *American Journal of Veterinary Research* **46**, 2048–2053.

Johnson, S.E., Crisp, S.M., Smeak, D.D. and Fingeroth, J.M. (1989) Hepatic encephalopathy in two aged dogs secondary to a presumed congenital portal azygous shunt. *Journal of the American Animal Hospital Association* **25**, 129–137.

Kerr, L.Y. and Hornof, W.J. (1986) Quantitative hepatobiliary scintigraphy using 99mTc DISIDA in the dog. *Veterinary Radiology* **27**, 173–177.

Kirpensteijn, J., Fingland, R.B., Ulrich, T., Sikkema, D.A. and Allen, S.W. (1993) Cholelithiasis in dogs: 29 cases (1980–1990). *Journal of the American Veterinary Medical Association* **202**, 1137–1142.

Koblik, P.D., Hornof, W.J., Yen, C.-K., Fisher, P.E. and Komtebedde, J. (1995) Use of technetium 99m sulfur colloid scintigraphy to evaluate changes in reticuloendothelial function in dogs with experimentally induced chronic biliary cirrhosis and portosystemic shunting. *American Journal of Veterinary Research* **56**, 688–693.

Kosovsky, J.E., Manfra-Marretta, S., Matthiesen, D.T. and Patnaik, A.K. (1989) Results of partial hepatectomy in 18 dogs with hepatocellular carcinoma. *Journal of the American Animal Hospital Association* **25**, 203–206.

Kreuzer, W., Schueller, E.F., Worthington, G. and Schenk, J.R. (1972) Hemodynamic studies of cirrhosis in the dog. *Surgery, Gynecology and Obstetrics* **135**, 89–93.

Kristensen, A.T., Weiss, D.J., Klausner, J.S. and Hardy, R.M. (1990) Liver cytology in cases of canine and feline hepatic disease. *Compendium of Continuing Education* **12**, 797–808.

Laflamme, D.P. (1988) Dietary management of canine hepatic encephalopathy. *Compendium of Continuing Education* **10**, 1258–1263.

Lamb, C.R. (1996) Ultrasonographic diagnosis of congenital portosystemic shunts in dogs: results of a retrospective study. *Veterinary Radiology and Ultrasound* **37**, 281–288.

Lamb, C.R., Foster-van Hijfte, M.A., White, R.N., McEvory, F.J. and Rutgers, H.C. (1996a) Ultrasonographic diagnosis of congenital portosystemic shunt in 14 cats. *Journal of Small Animal Practice* **37**, 205–209.

Lamb, C.R., Wrigley, R.H., Simpson, K.W., Forster-van Hijter, M., Garden, O.A., Smyth, J.B., Rutgers, H.C. and White, R.N. (1996b) Ultrasonographic diagnosis of portal vein thrombosis in four dogs. *Veterinary Radiology and Ultrasound* **37**, 121–129.

Lawrence, D., Bellah, J.R. and Diaz, R. (1992) Results of surgical management of portosystemic shunts in dogs: 20 cases (1985–1990). *Journal of the American Veterinary Medical Association* **201**, 1750–1753.

Leifer, C.E., Peterson, M.E., Matus, R.E. and Patnaik, A.K. (1985) Hypoglycemia associated with nonislet cell tumor in 13 dogs. *Journal of the American Veterinary Medical Association* **186**, 53–55.

Lewis, D.D., Bellenger, C.R., Lewis, D.T. and Latter, M.R. (1990) Hepatic lobectomy in the dog: a comparison of stapling and ligation techniques. *Veterinary Surgery* **19**, 221–225.

Lewis, D.T., Malone, J.B., Taboada, J., Hribernik, T.N., Pechman, R.D. and Dean, P.W. (1991) Cholangiohepatitis and choledochectasia associated with *Amphimerus pseudofelineus* in a cat. *Journal of the American Animal Hospital Association* **27**, 156–162.

Little, C.J.L., McNeil, P.E. and Robb, J. (1991) Hepatopathy and dermatitis in a dog associated with the ingestion of mycotoxins. *Journal of Small Animal Practice* **32**, 23–26.

Maddison, J.E. (1992) Hepatic encephalopathy. Current concepts of the pathogenesis. *Journal of Veterinary Internal Medicine* **6**, 341–353.

Magne, M.L. and Chiapella, A.M. (1986) Medical management of canine chronic hepatitis. *Compendium of Continuing Education* **8**, 915–921.

Maretta, S.M., Pask, A.J., Greene, R.W. and Liu, S-K. (1981) Urinary calculi associated with portosystemic shunts in six dogs. *Journal of the American Veterinary Medical Association* **187**, 133–137.

Martin, R.A., August, J.R., Barber, D.L. and Luther, F. (1986) Left hepatic vein attenuation for treatment of patent ductus venosus in a dog. *Journal of the American Veterinary Medical Association* **189**, 1465–1468.

Martin, R.A., MacCoy, D.M. and Harvey, H.J. (1988) Surgical management of extrahepatic biliary tract disease: a report of eleven cases. *Journal of the American Animal Hospital Association* **22**, 301–307.

Matthiesen, D.T. and Lammerding, J. (1984) Gallbladder rupture and bile peritonitis secondary to cholelithiasis and cholecystitis in a dog. *Journal of the American Veterinary Medical Association* **184**, 1282–1283.

McConnell, M.F. and Lumsden, J.H. (1983) Biochemical evaluation of metastatic liver disease in the dog. *Journal of the American Animal Hospital Association* **19**, 173–178.

McCuskey, R.S.M. (1994) The hepatic microvascular system. In: *The Liver: Biology and Pathobiology*, 3rd edn (Ed. I.M. Arias). Raven Press, New York, pp. 1089–1106.

McKenna, S.C. and Carpenter, J.L. (1980) Polycystic disease of the kidney and liver in the Cairn Terrier. *Veterinary Pathology* **17**, 436–442.

Merino, G.E., Jetzer, T., Doizaki, W.M.D. and Najarian, J.S. (1975) Methionine-induced hepatic coma in dogs. *American Journal of Surgery* **130**, 41–46.

Meyer, D.J. (1986) Liver function tests in dogs with portosystemic shunts: measurement of serum bile acid concentration. *Journal of the American Veterinary Medical Association* **188**, 168–169.

Meyer, D.J. and Center, S.A. (1986) Approach to the diagnosis of liver disorders in dogs and cats. *Compendium of Continuing Education* **8**, 880–888.

Meyer, D.J. and Harvey, J.W. (1994) Hematologic changes associated with serum and hepatic iron alterations in dogs with congenital portosystemic vascular anomalies. *Journal of Veterinary Internal Medicine* **8**, 55–56.

Meyer, H.P. and Rothuizen, J. (1994) Increased free cortisol in plasma in dogs with portosystemic encapalopathy (PSE). *Domestic Animal Endocrinology* **11**, 317–322.

Meyer, H.P., Rothuizen, J., Van den Brom, W.E., Voorhout, G., Van Slijs, F.J., How, K.L. and Pollak, Y.W.E.A. (1994) Quantitation of portosystemic shunting in dogs by ultrasound-guided injection of ^{99M}Tc-macroaggregates into a splenic vein. *Research in Veterinary Science* **57**, 58–62.

Meyer, H.P., Rothuizen, J. and Ubbink, G.J. (1995) Increasing incidence rate of hereditary intrahepatic portosystemic shunts (PSS) in Irish wolfhounds in the Netherlands (1984–1992). *Veterinary Record* **136**, 13–16.

Moore, P.F. and Whiting, P. (1986) Hepatic lesions associated with intrahepatic arterioportal fistulae in dogs. *Veterinary Pathology* **23**, 57–62.

Mullowney, P.C. and Tennant, B.C. (1982) Choledocholithiasis in the dog; a review and a report of a case with rupture of the common bile duct. *Journal of Small Animal Practice* **23**, 631–638.

Neer, T.M. and Hedlund, C.S. (1989) Vitamin K dependent coagulopathy in a dog with bile and cystic duct obstructions. *Journal of the American Animal Hospital Association* **25**, 461–464.

Nyland, T.G. (1984) Ultrasonic patterns of canine hepatic lymphosarcoma. *Veterinary Radiology* **25**, 167–172.

Nyland, T.G. and Gillett, N.A. (1982) Sonographic evaluation of experimental bile duct ligation in the dog. *Veterinary Radiology* **23**, 252–260.

Parchman, M.B. and Flanders, J.A. (1990) Extrahepatic biliary tract rupture: evaluation of the relationship between the site of rupture and the cause of rupture in 15 dogs. *Cornell Veterinarian* **80**, 267–272.

Patnaik, A.K. (1992) A morphologic and immunocytochemical study of hepatic neoplasms in cats. *Veterinary Pathology* **29**, 405–415.

Patnaik, A.K., Hurvitz, A.I., Lieberman, P.H. and Johnson, G.F. (1981) Canine bile duct carcinoma. *Veterinary Pathology* **18**, 439–444.

Piens, K., DeSchepper, J. and De Pelsmaker, K. (1996) Bilirubinuria without hyperbilirubinaemia in bitches with pyometra. *Vlaams Diergeneeskundig Tijdschrift* **65**, 31–33.

Post, G. and Patnaik, A.K. (1992) Nonhematopoietic hepatic neoplasms in cats: 21 cases (1983–1988). *Journal of the American Veterinary Medical Association* **201**, 1080–1082.

Prasse, K.W., Mahaffey, E.A., DeNovo, R. and Cornelius, L. (1982) Chronic lymphocytic cholangitis in three cats. *Veterinary Pathology* **19**, 99–108.

Rand, J.S., Best, S.J. and Mathews, K.A. (1988) Portosystemic vascular shunts in a family of American cocker spaniels. *Journal of the American Animal Hospital Association* **24**, 265–272.

Rothuizen, J. (1985) Laparoscopy in small animal medicine. *Veterinary Quarterly* **7**, 225–228.

Rothuizen, J. (1993) Portosystemic hepatic encephalopathy related. In: *Animal Models in Liver Research with Congenital and Acquired Disorders in the Dog* (Ed. C.E. Cornelius). Academic Press, New York, pp. 403–416.

Rothuizen, J. and Mol, J.A. (1987) The pituitary-adrenocortical system in canine hepatic encephalopathy. *Frontiers in Hormone Research* **17**, 28–36.

Rothuizen, J. and van den Brom, W.E. (1987) Bilirubin metabolism in canine hepatobiliary and haemolytic disease. *Veterinary Quarterly* **9**, 235–240.

Rothuizen, J. and van den Ingh, T.S.G.A.M. (1982a) Arterial and venous ammonia concentrations in the diagnosis of canine hepatoencephalopathy. *Research in Veterinary Science* **33**, 17–21.

Rothuizen, J. and van den Ingh, T.S.G.A.M. (1982b) Rectal ammonia tolerance test in the evaluation of portal circulation in dogs with liver disease. *Research in Veterinary Sciences* **33**, 22–25.

Rothuizen, J., van den Ingh, T.S.G.A.M., Voorhout, G., van der Luer, R.J.T. and Wouda, W. (1982) Congenital porto-systemic shunts in sixteen dogs and three cats. *Journal of Small Animal Practice* **23**, 67–81.

Rothuizen, J. and van den Ingh, T.S.G.A.M. (1988) Covalently protein-bound bilirubin conjugates in cholestatic disease of dogs. *American Journal of Veterinary Research* **49**, 702–704.

Rothuizen, J., Vries-Chalmers Hoynck van Papendrecht, R.D. and van den Brom, W.E. (1990) Post prandial and cholecystokinin induced emptying of the gall bladder in dogs. *Veterinary Record* **126**, 505–507.

Rothuizen, J., van den Brom, W.E. and Fevery, J.M.J. (1992) The origins and kinetics of bilirubin in dogs with hepatobiliary and haemolytic diseases. *Journal of Hepatology* **15**, 17–24.

Rothuizen, J., Biewenga, W.J. and Mol, J.A. (1995a) Chronic glucocorticoid excess and impaired osmoregulation of vasopressin release in dogs with hepatic encephalopathy. *Domestic Animal Endocrinology* **12**, 13–24.

Rothuizen, J., De Kok, I., Slob, A. and Mol, J.A. (1995b) GABAergic inhibition of the pituitary release of ACTH and MSH is impaired in dogs with hepatic encephalopathy. *Domestic Animal Endocrinology* **3**, 59–68.

Rowland, P.H., Center, S.A. and Dougherty, S.A. (1992) Presumptive trimethoprim-sulfadiazine-related hepatotoxicosis in a dog. *Journal of the American Veterinary Medical Association* **200**, 348–350.

Rutgers, H.C., Stradley, R.P. and Johnson, S.E. (1988) Serum bile acid analysis in dogs with experimentally induced cholestatic jaundice. *American Journal of Veterinary Research* **49**, 317–320.

Rutgers, H.C., Haywood, S. and Kelly, D.F. (1993) Idiopathic hepatic fibrosis in 15 dogs. *Veterinary Record* **133**, 115–118.

Rutgers, H.C., Batt, R.M., Vaillant, C. and Riley, J.E. (1995) Subcellular pathologic features of glucocorticoid-induced hepatopathy in dogs. *American Journal of Veterinary Research* **56**, 899–907.

Sanecki, R.K., Hoffmann, W.E., Gelberg, H.B. and Dorner, J.L. (1987) Subcellular location of corticosteroid induced alkaline phosphatase in canine hepatocytes. *Veterinary Pathology* **24**, 296–301.

Shaker, E.H., Zawie, D.A., Garvey, M.S. and Gilbertson, S.R. (1991) Suppurative cholangiohepatitis in a cat. *Journal of the American Animal Hospital Association* **27**, 148–150.

Schermerhorn, T., Center, S.A., Dykes, N.L., Rowland, P.H., Yeager, A.E., Erb, H.N., Oberhansley, K. and Bonda, M. (1996) Characterization of hepatoportal microvascular dysplasia in a kindred of Cairn terriers. *Journal of Veterinary Internal Medicine* **10**, 219–230.

Speety, M., Ihantola, M. and Westermark, E. (1996) Subclinical versus clinical hepatitis in the dobermann: evaluation of changes in blood parameters. *Journal of Small Animal Practice* **37**, 465–470.

Stebbins, K.E. (1989) Polycystic disease of the kidney and liver in an adult Persian cat. *Journal of Comparative Pathology* **100**, 327–330.

Sterczer, A., Vörös, K. and Karsai, F. (1996) Effect of cholagogues on the volume of the gallbladder of dogs. *Research in Veterinary Science* **60**, 44–47.

Sternlieb, I. (1994) Copper and zinc. In: *The Liver: Biology and Pathobiology*, 3rd edn (Eds I.M. Arias *et al.*). Raven Press, New York, pp. 585–596.

Strombeck, D.R. (1978) Clinicopathologic features of primary and metastatic neoplastic disease of the liver in dogs. *Journal of the American Veterinary Medical Association* **173**, 267–269.

Strombeck, D.R. and Gribble, D. (1978) Chronic active hepatitis in the dog. *Journal of the American Veterinary Medical Association* **173**, 380–386.

Suter, P.F. (1982) Radiographic diagnosis of liver disease in dogs and cats. *Veterinary Clinics of North America, Small Animal Practice* **12**, 153–173.

Sutherland, R.J. (1989) Biochemical evaluation of the hepatobiliary system in dogs and cats. *Veterinary Clinics of North America, Small Animal Practice* **19**(5), 899–927.

Taboada, J. and Meyer, D.J. (1989) Cholestasis associated with extrahepatic bacterial infection in five dogs. *Journal of Veterinary Internal Medical* **3**, 216–221.

Teske, E., Rothuizen, J., de Bruijne, J.J. and Mol, J.A. (1986) Separation and heat stability of the corticosteroid-induced and hepatic alkaline phosphatase isoenzymes in canine plasma. *Journal of Chromatography* **369**, 349–356.

Teske, E, Brinkhuis, B.G., Bode, P., van den Ingh, T.S.G.A.M. and Rothuizen, J. (1992) Cytological detection of copper for the diagnosis of inherited copper toxicosis in Bedlington terriers. *Veterinary Record* **131**, 30–32.

Thornburg, L.P. (1988) A study of canine hepatobiliary diseases. 5. Drug-induced hepatopathies. *Companion Animal Practice* **2**(8), 17–21.

Thornburg, L.P. and Moody, G.M. (1981) Hepatic amyloidosis in a dog. *Journal of the American Animal Hospital Association* **17**, 721–723.

Thornburg, L.P., Rottinghaus, G., Koch, J. and Hause, W.R. (1984) High copper levels in two dobermann pinschers with subacute hepatitis. *Journal of the American Animal Hospital Association* **20**, 1003–1005.

Thornburg, L.P., Shaw, D., Dolan, M., Raisbeck, M., Crawford, S., Dennis, G.L. and Olwin, D.B. (1986) Hereditary copper toxicosis in West Highland White Terriers. *Veterinary Pathology* **23**, 148–154.

Thornburg, L.P, Rottinghaus, G., McGowan, M.M, Kupka, K., Crawford, S. and Forbes, S. (1990) Hepatic copper concentrations in purebred and mixed-breed dogs. *Veterinary Pathology* **27**, 81–88.

Tiemessen, I., Rothuizen, J. and Voorhout, G. (1995) Ultrasonography in the diagnosis of congenital portosystemic shunts in dogs. *Veterinary Quarterly* **17**, 50–53.

Tisdall, P.L.C., Hunt, G.B., Tsoukalas, G. and Malik, R. (1995) Post-prandial serum bile acid concentrations and ammonia tolerance in Maltese dogs with and without hepatic vascular anomalies. *Australian Veterinary Journal* **72**, 121–126.

Tobias, K.S., Barbee, D. and Pluhar, G.E. (1996) Intraoperative use of subtraction angiography and an ultrasonic aspirator to improve identification and isolation of an intrahepatic portosystemic shunt in a dog. *Journal of the American Veterinary Medical Association* **208**, 888–890.

Twedt, D.C., Hunsaker, H.A. and Allen, K.G.D. (1988) Use of 2,3,2-tetramine as a hepatic copper chelating agent for treatment of copper hepatotoxicosis in Bedlington Terriers. *Journal of the American Veterinary Medical Association* **192**, 52–56.

Tyler, J.W. (1990) Hepatoencephalopathy. Part I. Clinical signs and diagnosis. *Compendium of Continuing Education* **8**, 1069–1073.

Van den Brom, W. and Rothuizen J. (1990) Quantitation of the hepatobiliary dynamics in clinically normal dogs by use of 99mTc iminodiacetate excretory scintigraphy. *American Journal of Veterinary Research* **51**, 249–252.

Van den Ingh, T.S.G.A.M and Rothuizen, J. (1983) Hepatoportal fibrosis in three young dogs. *Veterinary Record* **19**, 575–577.

Van den Ingh, T.S.G.A.M and Rothuizen, J. (1985) Congenital cystic disease of the liver in seven dogs. *Journal of Comparative Pathology* **95**, 405–414.

Van den Ingh, T.S.G.A.M., Rothuizen, J. and van den Brom, W.E. (1986) Extrahepatic cholestasis in the dog and the differentiation of extrahepatic and intrahepatic cholestasis. *Veterinary Quarterly* **8**, 150–157.

Van den Ingh, T.S.G.A.M., Rothuizen, J. and Cupery, R. (1988a) Chronic active hepatitis with cirrhosis in the Doberman Pinscher. *Veterinary Quarterly* **10**, 84–89.

Van den Ingh, T.S.G.A.M., Rothuizen, J. and van Zinnicq Bergman, H.M. (1988b) Destructive cholangiolitis in seven dogs. *Veterinary Quarterly* **10**, 240–245.

Van den Ingh, T.S.G.A.M. and Rothuizen, J. (1994) Lobular dissecting hepatitis in juvenile and adult dogs. *Veterinary Pathology* **8**, 217–220.

Van den Ingh, T.S.G.A.M., Rothuizen, J. and Meyer, H.M. (1995) Circulatory disorders of the liver in dogs and cats. *Veterinary Quarterly* **17**, 70–75.

Van Vechten, B.J., Komtebedde, J. and Koblik, P.D. (1994) Use of transcolonic portal scintigraphy to monitor blood flow and progressive postoperative attenuation of partially ligated single extrahepatic portosystemic shunts in dogs. *Journal of the American Veterinary Medical Association* **204**, 1770–1774.

Van Winkle, T.J. and Bruce, E. (1993) Thrombosis of the portal vein in 11 dogs. *Veterinary Pathology* **30**, 28–35.

Vogt, J.C., Krahwinkel, D.J., Bright, R.M., Daniel, G.B., Toal, R.L. and Rohrbach, B. (1996) Gradual occlusion of extrahepatic portosystemic shunts in dogs and cats using the Ameroid constrictor. *Veterinary Surgery* **25**, 495–502.

Washizu, M., Kobayashi, K., Misaka, K., Hyashi, T., Kinoshita, G., Kondo, M., Aoki, S., Orima, H. and Washizu, T. (1996) Surgery of hepatic cysts in a cat. *Journal of Veterinary Medical Science* **54**, 1051–1053.

Watkins, P.E., Pearson, H. and Denny, H.R. (1983) Traumatic rupture of the bile duct in the dog: a report of seven cases. *Journal of Small Animal Practice* **24**, 731–740.

Wellman, M.L., Hoffmann, W.E., Dorner, J.L. and Mock, R.E. (1982) Comparison of the steroid induced, intestinal, and hepatic isoenzymes of alkaline phosphatase in the dog. *American Journal of Veterinary Research* **43**, 1204–1207.

White, R.N., Foster van Hijfte, M.A., Petrie, G., Lamb, C.R. and Hammond, R.A. (1996) Surgical treatment of intrahepatic portosystemic shunts in six cats. *Veterinary Record* **139**, 314–317.

Whiting, P.G., Breznock, E.M., Moore, P., Kerr, L., Berger, B. and Gregory, C. (1986) Partial hepatectomy with temporary hepatic vascular occlusion in dogs with hepatic arteriovenous fistulas. *Veterinary Surgery* **15**, 171–180.

Willard, M.D., Bailey, M.Q., Hauptman, J. and Mullaney, T. (1989) Obstructed portal venous flow and portal vein thrombus in a dog. *Journal of the American Veterinary Medical Association* **194**, 1449–1451.

Wrigley, R.H., Konde, L.J., Park, R.D. and Lebel, J.L. (1987) Ultrasonographic diagnosis of portacaval shunts in young dogs. *Journal of the American Veterinary Medical Association* **191**, 421–424.

Yuzbasiyan-Gurkan, V., Blanton, S.H., Cao, Y., Ferguson, P., Venta, P.J. and Brewer, G.J. (1997) Linkage of a microsatellite marker to the canine copper toxicosis locus for Bedlington terriers. *American Journal of Veterinary Research* **58**, 23–27.

Zawie, D.A. and Garvey, M.S. (1984) Feline hepatic disease. *Veterinary Clinics of North America, Small Animal Practice* **14**, 1201–1230.

38

Diseases of the Exocrine Pancreas

D. A. Williams

Introduction	498	Pancreatitis	501
Anatomy	498	Exocrine pancreatic insufficiency	509
Biochemistry	499	Neoplasia of the exocrine pancreas	518
Physiology	501	Pancreatic flukes in cats	519

INTRODUCTION

The major function of the exocrine pancreas is to secrete digestive enzymes and coenzymes as well as factors that play a role in the absorption of specific nutrients such as cobalamin (vitamin B_{12}) and zinc. Antibacterial factors present in pancreatic juice inhibit bacterial proliferation in the proximal small intestine, and pancreatic secretions also influence the function of the small intestine by contributing to the normal degradation of exposed brush border enzymes, and by exerting a trophic effect on the mucosa.

ANATOMY

The pancreas of dogs and cats consists primarily of right and left lobes with a small central body where the lobes join together (Fig. 38.1). It develops from bud-like primordia arising from the embryonic small intestine, and therefore represents an extension of the glandular mucosa of the duodenum, to which it remains connected by secretory ducts. In the dog, two ducts are usually present. The pancreatic duct opens adjacent to the bile duct on the major duodenal papilla, and the accessory pancreatic duct opens on the minor duodenal papilla a few centimetres distal to the major duodenal papilla. These two duct systems usually communicate within the gland. In some dogs only the accessory pancreatic duct (the larger of the two) is present and all pancreatic juice enters the duodenum through the minor duodenal papilla. In the cat, only the pancreatic duct is generally present, and it fuses with the bile duct before opening at the major duodenal papilla. However, in approximately 20% of cats

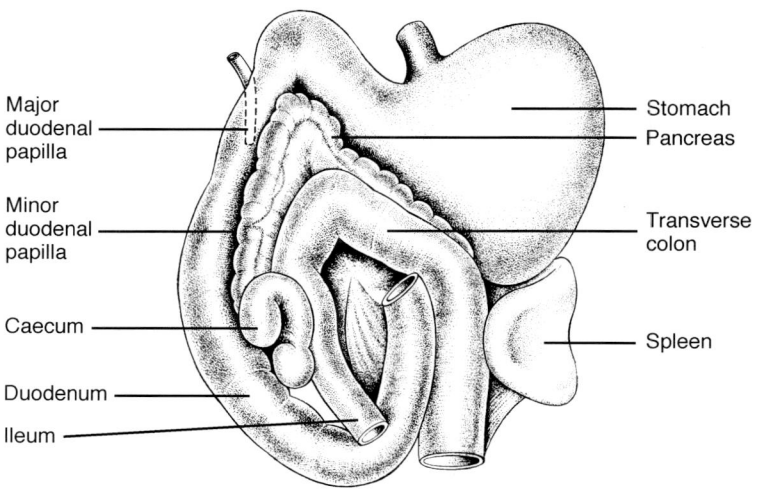

Figure 38.1 Anatomical associations of the canine pancreas.

the accessory pancreatic duct is also present. Additional accessory pancreatic tissue may be present sporadically in some individuals (Schummer et al., 1979).

Anatomically the pancreas is closely associated with the stomach, liver and duodenum (Fig. 38.1). The body lies in the bend of the cranial part of the duodenum, the right lobe lies in the mesoduodenum and accompanies the descending duodenum, and the left lobe lies in the deep wall of the greater omentum and accompanies the pyloric part of the stomach to the left. The pancreas is well supplied with blood by branches of the coeliac and cranial mesenteric arteries. Venous drainage terminates in the portal vein.

Each microscopic pancreatic lobule is composed mainly of cells that synthesize the digestive enzymes (acinar cells), and a smaller number of cells that make up the branching duct system (Bockman, 1978). The cells lining the tubular segments of the gland into which acinar cells secrete (centroacinar cells) are the major site of pancreatic bicarbonate and fluid secretion. The pancreas also contains endocrine tissue, the islets of Langerhans, but this accounts for only 1–2% of the gland.

In many species, including dogs and cats, an islet–acinar portal system communicates between the endocrine and the exocrine tissue. Essentially all of the blood leaving the islets goes into acinar capillaries before leaving the pancreas, and the acinar cells, particularly those surrounding the islets, are therefore exposed to high concentrations of islet hormones. This is thought to be an important mechanism by which insulin and other regulatory peptides exert regulatory roles on the exocrine pancreas (Williams and Goldfine, 1993).

Although the pancreas is not supplied by well-defined extrinsic nerves it is richly supplied with myelinated and unmyelinated nerve fibres, derived from the vagus and splanchnic nerves. In addition to the traditional cholinergic (parasympathetic) and adrenergic (sympathetic) transmitters it is now apparent that serotonin, dopamine, and a variety of regulatory peptides including vasoactive intestinal polypeptide (VIP), gastrin releasing peptide (GRP), substance P, neuropeptide Y, and enkephalin-related peptides are also present in these nerve fibres (Holst, 1993).

BIOCHEMISTRY

The acinar cells secrete a fluid rich in enzymes that degrade proteins, lipids and polysaccharides (Table 38.1). This protein-rich secretion is diluted and carried along the duct system by the profuse, watery, bicarbonate-rich secretion of the centroacinar and duct cells (Case and Argent, 1993). Although this bicarbonate contributes to the neutralization of gastric acid emptied into the duodenum, it is probably not indispensable for the maintenance of a neutral pH since secretion of bicarbonate and absorption of hydrogen ions by the intestinal mucosa itself provides a tremendous capacity to dispose of acid.

Several mechanisms exist that discourage autodigestion of the pancreas by the enzymes that it secretes (Rinderknecht, 1993). First, proteolytic and phospholipolytic enzymes are synthesized, stored and secreted by the pancreas in the form of inactive zymogens (indicated by the addition of the prefix pro- or the suffix -ogen to the enzyme name (Table 38.1). Enzymes from several sources, including some lysosomal proteases, are capable of activating pancreatic zymogens, but ordinarily activation of zymogens does not occur until they

Table 38.1 Major secretory proteins of the exocrine pancreas of the dog

Enzymes secreted as inactive zymogens			
	Trypsinogens	→	trypsins
	Chymotrypsinogens	→	chymotrypsins
	Proelastases	→	elastases
	Procarboxypeptidases	→	carboxypeptidases
	Prophospholipase A_2	→	phospholipase A_2
Coenzyme			
	Procolipase	→	colipase
Enzymes			
	α-amylase		
	Lipase		
Inhibitor			
	Pancreatic secretory trypsin inhibitor		

DISEASES OF THE EXOCRINE PANCREAS

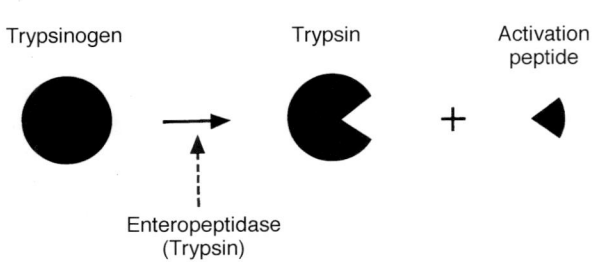

Figure 38.2 Diagrammatic representation of zymogen activation (activation of trypsinogen to trypsin by enteropeptidase). Modified from Williams (1989), p. 1530.

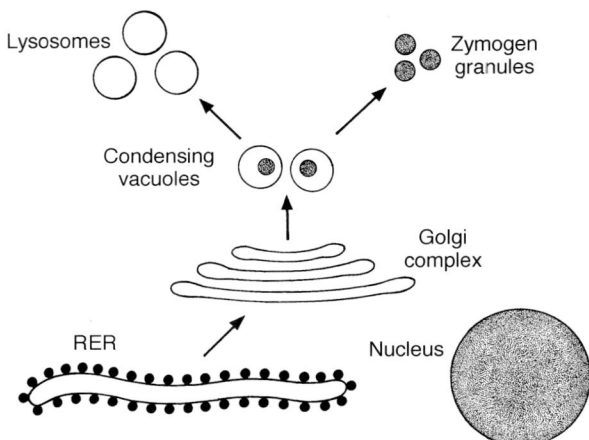

Figure 38.4 Normal intracellular routing of digestive and lysosomal enzymes to separate compartments within the pancreatic acinar cell. Modified from Williams (1989), p. 1531.

are secreted into the small intestine. The enzyme enteropeptidase, synthesized by duodenal enterocytes, is particularly effective at cleaving the activation peptides from trypsinogens to form trypsins (Fig 38.2). Active trypsins subsequently cleave activation peptides from other digestive zymogens (Fig. 38.3).

Secondly, from the moment that synthesis of digestive enzymes begins they are segregated, along with potentially damaging lysosomal enzymes, into the lumen of the rough endoplasmic reticulum. Segregation of enzymes in the cisternal space is continued as they are processed through the Golgi apparatus, where lysosomal enzymes are selectively routed to lysosomes. The digestive enzymes are incorporated into condensing vacuoles and ultimately zymogen granules, in which they are stored prior to secretion (Fig. 38.4) (Scheele and Kern, 1993).

Finally, the acinar cells contain a specific trypsin inhibitor that is synthesized, stored and secreted together with the digestive enzymes (Laskowski and Kato, 1980; Rinderknecht, 1993). This pancreatic secretory trypsin inhibitor immediately inhibits any trypsin produced should there be activation of trace amounts of trypsinogen within the acinar cell or duct system, and therefore blocks further intrapancreatic activation of the digestive enzymes (Fig. 38.5) (Laskowski and Kato, 1980; Rinderknecht, 1993).

PHYSIOLOGY

The exocrine pancreas secretes juice into the duodenum both in the absence of food (basal or interdigestive secretion) and in response to a meal. The response following feeding is biphasic: an initial phase that peaks at about two hours and is rich in enzymes, and a second more voluminous phase that peaks at about eleven hours and is rich in bicarbonate (Itoh et al., 1980).

Pancreatic secretion occurs as a response to cephalic stimulation, such as the anticipation and smell of food, as well as gastric and intestinal stimulation due to the presence of food in the stomach and small intestine. The response to these stimuli is mediated by a complex interplay of excitatory and inhibitory nervous and hormonal mechanisms; in dogs and cats the endocrine mechanisms

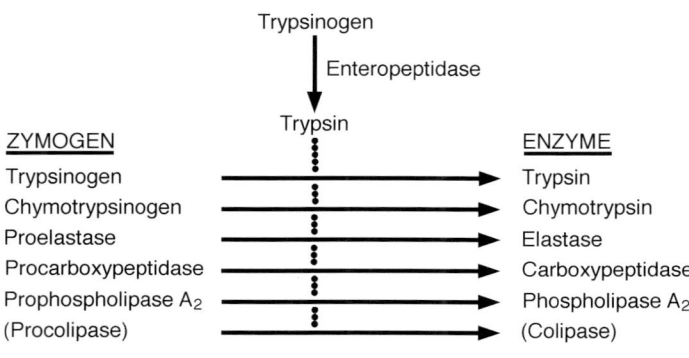

Figure 38.3 Activation of pancreatic proteases and phospholipase.

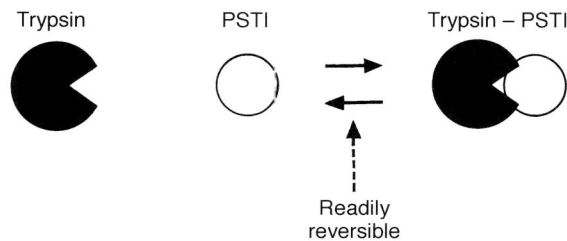

Figure 38.5 Pancreatic secretory trypsin inhibitor (PSTI) is a low-molecular-weight (6000) trypsin-specific inhibitor protein present in pancreatic zymogen granules and pancreatic juice. It prevents intrapancreatic cascade activation of pancreatic enzymes following spontaneous autoactivation of trace amounts of trypsin within the pancreas. A transient inhibitor only, it is eventually digested in the duodenum by the trypsin that it temporarily inhibits. Modified from Williams (1989), p. 1530.

are probably of particular importance (Singer, 1993). Secretin and cholecystokinin, released into the blood from the proximal small intestine when acid and partly digested food are emptied from the stomach into the duodenum, stimulate the secretion of bicarbonate-rich and enzyme-rich components of pancreatic juice, respectively (Williams and Yule, 1993).

PANCREATITIS

Inflammatory disease of the pancreas in humans is usually divided into acute and chronic types based on a combination of diagnostic criteria that may be loosely applied to cats and dogs (Table 38.2) (Sarner, 1993). Acute pancreatitis may be defined as inflammation of the pancreas with a sudden onset. Recurrent acute disease refers to repeated bouts of inflammation with little or no permanent pathological changes. Chronic pancreatitis is a continuing inflammatory disease characterized by irreversible morphological change and possibly leading to permanent impairment of function. Both acute and chronic pancreatitis may be further subdivided based on the aetiology, if known, and the degree of severity. Diagnostic limitations often preclude the strict application of these criteria in veterinary medicine, and the true prevalence of each is not known, but acute and recurrent acute disease are more commonly diagnosed than chronic pancreatitis.

Acquisition of knowledge about naturally occurring pancreatitis in dogs and cats has been hindered by the lack of specific laboratory tests, the inaccessibility of the gland, and reluctance to biopsy pancreatic tissue. When examined at exploratory laparotomy or necropsy the acutely inflamed pancreas is oedematous, and there may be fibrinous adhesions to adjacent organs. Severely affected areas of pancreas may be liquified, sterile pseudocysts may form, and secondary infection with enteric organisms may produce abscesses. Histologically there is extensive multifocal infiltration by neutrophils, and varying degrees of haemorrhage, necrosis, oedema and vessel thrombosis. Haemorrhages may be present in the omentum and in the pancreas, and there are often chalky areas of fat necrosis both adjacent to the pancreas and elsewhere. The peritoneal cavity may contain a small amount of bloodstained fluid containing fat droplets (Jubb *et al.*, 1985).

Table 38.2 Classification of pancreatitis

Acute		
	Aetiology	Various
	Severity	Mild
		no multisystem failure
		uncomplicated recovery
		Severe
		multisystem failure
		complication, e.g. pseudocyst, abscess
Chronic		
	Aetiology	Various
	Severity	Mild
		minimal morphological change
		subclinical loss of exocrine or exocrine function
		Severe
		severe morphological damage
		clinical exocrine pancreatic insufficiency or diabetes mellitus

After an acute episode, there may be complete resolution, or the inflammatory process may continue to smoulder asymptomatically. Chronic pancreatitis may lead to fibrosis and atrophy such that only a few distorted lobules remain (Jubb et al., 1985).

Although recent reports have described acute necrotizing pancreatitis in cats similar to that seen in dogs (Schaer and Holloway, 1991; Hill and Van Winkle, 1993; Simpson et al., 1994) as well as a histologically distinct suppurative form (Hill and Van Winkle, 1993), chronic mild interstitial pancreatitis characterized by inflammation of interstitial tissue apparently spreading from the ducts, is the type of pancreatic inflammation traditionally reported in cats (Duffell, 1975; Kelly et al., 1975; Jubb et al., 1985; Williams, 1989). This latter type of pancreatitis is often accompanied by cholangiohepatitis, inflammatory bowel disease, and sometimes by interstitial nephritis, each of which may be of greater clinical significance than the pancreatitis.

Pathophysiology

It is generally believed that pancreatitis develops when there is activation of digestive enzymes within the gland with resultant pancreatic autodigestion. The site of initiation of enzyme activation has been assumed to be the intercellular space or duct system, but recent studies have indicated an intracellular basis for abnormal zymogen activation. It has been shown that before the development of overt pancreatitis in several experimental models, abnormal fusion of lysosomes and zymogen granules occurs, probably due to failure of normal intracellular transport, storage or exocytosis of zymogen granule contents (Fig. 38.6). Lysosomal proteases are capable of activating trypsinogen, and pancreatic secretory trypsin inhibitor is ineffective at the acid pH present in lysosomes. Failure of the normal subcellular mechanisms for effective segregation of zymogens and lysosomal proteases (Fig. 38.4) may be a common underlying mechanism in the development of pancreatitis due to a variety of otherwise dissimilar causes (Steer and Meldolesi, 1987; Steer and Saluja, 1993).

Once intracellular activation of trypsinogens to trypsins takes place, further activation of all enzymes, particularly proelastase and prophospholipase, will amplify pancreatic damage. Experimental and clinical studies indicate that activation of progressively larger amounts of protease and phospholipase within the gland is associated with transformation of mild oedematous pancreatic inflammation to haemorrhagic or necrotic pancreatitis with multisystem involvement (Fig. 38.7, Table 38.3) (Lasson, 1984; Steer and Meldolesi, 1987).

Once enzyme activation is initiated, oxygen-derived free radicals may be important in the progression of pancreatitis. These radicals can damage cell membranes directly by peroxidation of lipids within the membrane. Under normal

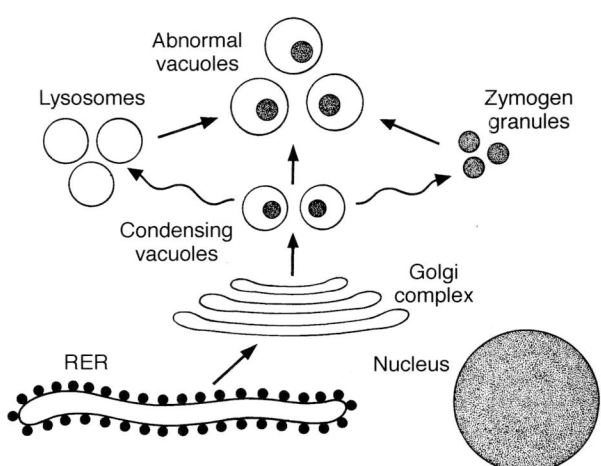

Figure 38.6 Experimental disruption of protein transport by acinar cells. Abnormal accumulation of secretory proteins within the cisternal compartment stimulates lysosomal degradation pathways with resultant mixing of zymogens and lysosomal proteases. Subsequent activation of zymogens by lysosomal proteases at the acid pH in these vacuoles may result in pancreatitis. Modified from Williams (1989), p. 1531.

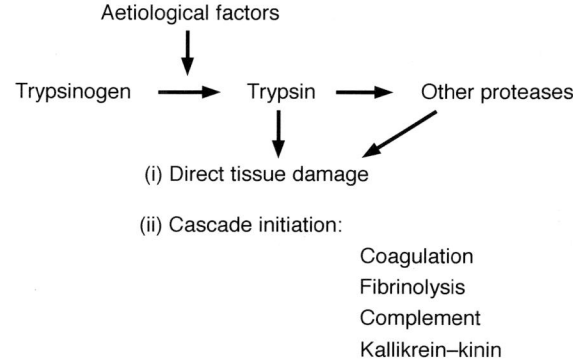

Figure 38.7 Local and systemic effects of trypsin in pancreatitis. Modified from Williams (1989), p. 1533.

Table 38.3 The role of enzymes in the pathophysiology of pancreatitis

Enzyme	Pathophysiological action
Trypsin	Activation of other proteases
	Coagulation and fibrinolysis
	(disseminated intravascular coagulation)
Phospholipase A_2	Hydrolysis of cell membrane phospholipids
	Pulmonary surfactant degradation
	Demyelination
	(cell necrosis and liberation of toxic substances such as myocardial depressant factor)
	(respiratory distress)
	(neurological signs – pancreatic encephalopathy)
Elastase	Degradation of elastin in blood vessel walls
	(haemorrhage, oedema, respiratory distress)
Chymotrypsin	Activation of xanthine oxidase and subsequent generation of oxygen-derived free radicals
	(membrane damage)
Kallikrein	Kinin generation from kininogens
Kinins	Vasodilation, pancreatic oedema
	(hypotension, shock)
Complement	Cell membrane damage, aggregation of leucocytes
	(local inflammation)
Lipase	Fat hydrolysis
	(local fat necrosis, hypocalcaemia)

circumstances, the small amounts of free radical which form are detoxified by scavenger enzymes such as superoxide dismutase and catalase, but when the capacity of the defence mechanisms is exceeded tissue injury ensues. Perfusion of the pancreas with free-radical scavengers ameliorates the severity of pancreatitis induced by a variety of experimental manipulations (Sanfey et al., 1984).

Plasma protease inhibitors, especially α-macroglobulins (Fig. 38.8), are vital in protecting against the otherwise fatal effects of proteolytic enzymes in the vascular space. Dogs tolerate intravenous injection of trypsin or chymotrypsin without showing adverse effects providing free α-macroglobulins are available to bind these proteases. Once α-macroglobulins are no longer available death ensues rapidly from acute disseminated intravascular coagulation and shock as the free proteases activate the kinin, coagulation, fibrinolytic and complement cascade systems (Fig. 38.7) (Ohlsson et al., 1971).

Binding of proteases by α-macroglobulin results in a change in conformation which allows the complex to be recognized and rapidly cleared from the plasma by the reticuloendothelial system. This removal is important since α-macroglobulin-bound proteases retain catalytic activity, particularly against low-molecular-weight substrates (Fig. 38.8); normal functioning of the reticuloendothelial system is an important factor determining survival in experimental pancreatitis (Kark et al., 1974; Marcoullis and Rothenberg, 1981).

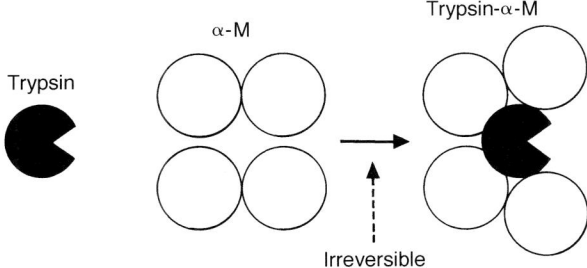

Figure 38.8 α-Macroglobulins (α-M_1 and α-M_2) are high-molecular-weight (750 000) plasma proteins. These are highly effective 'life-saving' inhibitors when large amounts of almost any proteolytic enzymes, including pancreatic digestive proteases, are released into the vascular space. Complexes of enzyme and inhibitor are rapidly cleared by the reticuloendothelial system. Modified from Williams (1989), p. 1530.

Plasma α_1-protease inhibitor (Fig. 38.9) is still available to bind proteases when α-macroglobulins are saturated with trypsin, but binding to α_1-protease inhibitor does not protect against life-threatening complications. Although pancreatic proteases bound to α_1-protease inhibitor are effectively inhibited, the binding is reversible (Fig.

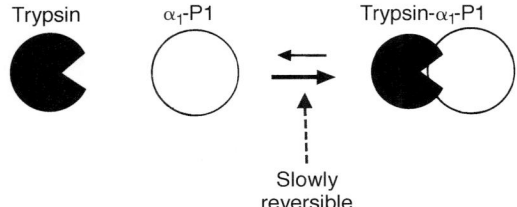

Figure 38.9 Alpha$_1$-protease inhibitor (α_1 antitrypsin, α_1-PI) is an albumin-sized (molecular weight 55 000) protein present in plasma and intercellular fluid. It probably functions primarily as an inhibitor of neutrophil elastase and other proteolytic enzymes released during inflammation, thus localizing the inflammatory response. It may also act as a temporary inhibitor of proteases released into the intercellular fluid and blood during acute pancreatitis, but is not 'life-saving' in this disease. Modified from Williams (1989), p. 1530.

38.9). Alpha$_1$-protease inhibitor probably functions largely as a transient inhibitor and an intermediary in the transport of protease to the protective α-macroglobulins, particularly in the extravascular spaces into which the large α-macroglobulin molecules cannot permeate (Ohlsson et al., 1971; Lasson, 1984).

Aetiology

The cause of spontaneous canine and feline pancreatitis is usually unknown, but the following have been implicated as possible aetiological factors.

Nutrition

The exocrine pancreas is highly responsive to changes in nutritional substrates present in the diet. It has been reported that pancreatitis is more prevalent in obese animals, and difficult to induce experimentally in malnourished dogs (Goodhead, 1971). However, malnutrition has also been reported to cause pancreatic inflammation and atrophy in human patients, and pancreatitis has been observed after refeeding following a prolonged fast (Pitchumoni and Scheele, 1993).

Hyperlipoproteinaemia

Some familial hyperlipoproteinaemias in humans are associated with frequent episodes of pancreatitis that respond to control of serum triglyceride levels (Steer and Saluja, 1993). There is anecdotal evidence that pancreatitis in dogs often develops following a fatty meal, and may be particularly prevalent in miniature schnauzers with idiopathic hyperlipoproteinaemia. It is not known why hyperlipidaemia might cause pancreatitis, but it has been suggested that toxic fatty acids are generated within the pancreas by the action of lipase on abnormally high concentrations of triglycerides in pancreatic capillaries.

Drugs

A number of drugs have been associated with the development of pancreatitis, although absolute proof of a causal relationship is often unavailable (Mallory and Kern, 1980; Hansen and Carpenter, 1983). Suspect drugs commonly used in veterinary medicine include thiazide diuretics, frusemide, azathioprine, L-asparaginase, sulphonamides and tetracycline. Considerable controversy exists as to whether or not corticosteroids may induce pancreatitis, a particular problem since they may be of value in the treatment of pancreatitis.

Infection

Viral and parasitic infections may be associated with pancreatitis, but only as part of a more generalized disease (Rothenbacher and Lindquist, 1963; Smart et al., 1973). Bacterial infection increases the severity of experimental pancreatitis, and it may act similarly in spontaneous disease (Keynes, 1980).

Duct obstruction

Experimental obstruction of the pancreatic ducts produces inflammation, particularly when the gland is stimulated to secrete. The pathology in this model is characterized by oedema, chronic inflammation, atrophy and fibrosis rather than fulminating acute pancreatitis (Steer and Saluja, 1993). Clinical conditions that may lead to obstruction of the pancreatic ducts include biliary calculi, sphincter spasm, oedema of the duct or duodenal wall, tumour, parasites and surgical interference (Steer and Saluja, 1993). Biliary calculi are a major cause of pancreatitis in humans, but this has not been reported in dogs and cats, presumably because of the low incidence of gallstones in these species, and in dogs, the separation of the pancreatic and bile ducts. Convergence of the feline biliary and pancreatic ducts may be a factor in the prevalence of coexistent chronic interstitial pancreatitis and cholangiohepatitis in that species (Duffell, 1975; Kelly *et al.*, 1975; Jubb *et al.*, 1985).

Duodenal reflux

Surgically induced reflux of duodenal juice into the pancreatic ducts causes severe acute pancreatitis. Enteropeptidase, activated pancreatic enzymes, bacteria and bile present in the refluxed juice may all contribute to development of pancreatitis (Steer and Saluja, 1993). Under normal circumstances such reflux is unlikely to occur since the duct opening is surrounded by a specialized compact, smooth mucosa over the duodenal papilla, and is equipped with an independent sphincter muscle (Keane *et al.*, 1981). These protective mechanisms may fail in the face of abnormally high duodenal pressure, such as may occur with vomiting (Steer and Saluja, 1993).

Hypercalcaemia

Pancreatitis is considered a complication of hypercalcaemia in human patients (Geokas *et al.*, 1985), but the validity of this association has been questioned (Steer and Saluja, 1993). Pancreatitis has been reported in a dog with primary hyperparathyroidism, and following induction of iatrogenic hypercalcaemia in a dog (Neuman, 1975; Schaer, 1979).

Trauma

Surgical manipulation, automobile accidents, and falling from high buildings are potential causes of pancreatic trauma, but reports of pancreatitis following such insults are rare, and in most cases of abdominal trauma, injury to the pancreas is probably mild or unrecognized (Suter and Olsson, 1969; Steer and Saluja, 1993). Pancreatitis is a rare complication of pancreatic biopsy using either wedge or needle techniques, and is also uncommon following resection of pancreatic neoplasms (Dalton and Hill, 1972; Moossa and Altorki, 1983).

Uraemia

Morphological changes in the pancreas have been associated with renal failure in a number of species, although severe acute pancreatitis is clearly not a common complication of renal failure in dogs and cats (Polzin *et al.*, 1983). It is likely that renal failure secondary to acute pancreatitis is encountered more frequently (Goldstein *et al.*, 1976).

Ischaemia

Ischaemia may be important in the pathogenesis of acute pancreatitis, either as a primary cause or as an exacerbating influence. Pancreatic ischaemia may develop during shock or secondary to hypotension during general anaesthesia, and may explain some instances of postoperative pancreatitis in which areas remote from the pancreas are operated upon (Sanfey *et al.*, 1985; Steer and Saluja, 1993).

Hereditary

Hereditary factors are important in some forms of pancreatitis in human patients, such as those associated with familial hyperlipoproteinaemia and developmental abnormalities of the duct system (Geokas *et al.*, 1985; Steer and Saluja, 1993; Westermarck *et al.*, 1993a). Similar mechanisms may explain the anecdotal high prevalence of pancreatitis in some animal breeds such as miniature schnauzers.

Miscellaneous

Scorpion stings are frequent causes of pancreatitis in human beings in Trinidad, and experimental administration of scorpion venom to dogs also induces pancreatitis (Steer and Saluja, 1993). Administration of cholinesterase inhibitor insecticides and cholinergic agonists have also been associated with the development of pancreatitis (Dressel *et al.*, 1979; Geokas *et al.*, 1985). Pancreatitis and gastrointestinal haemorrhage have been reported in association with intervertebral disc disease in dogs, although it is not known if this arises as a direct consequence of spinal cord trauma or corticosteroid therapy, or a combination of these factors (Moore and Withrow, 1982).

Diagnosis

History and clinical signs

Animals with acute pancreatitis are usually presented because of depression, anorexia, vomiting and, in some cases, diarrhoea. Severe acute disease may be associated with shock and collapse, whereas other cases may have a history of less dramatic signs of several weeks duration. Some dogs demonstrate abdominal pain by assuming a 'prayer' position with the forelimbs outstretched, the sternum on the floor, and the hindlimbs raised. Signs of pain are usually, but not always, elicited on abdominal palpation. A cranial abdominal mass is palpable in some cases, and occasionally there is mild ascites. Most affected animals are mildly to moderately dehydrated and febrile. Uncommon systemic complications of pancreatitis that may be apparent on physical examination include jaundice, respiratory distress, bleeding disorders, and cardiac arrhythmias. Although dogs of any age may develop pancreatitis, affected animals are usually middle aged or older, sometimes obese, and the onset of signs may have followed ingestion of a large amount of fatty food (Holroyd, 1968; Anderson, 1972; Lees et al., 1978; Schaer, 1979; Garvey and Zawie, 1984; Pidgeon, 1987). The clinical signs of chronic pancreatitis are poorly documented, but are probably extremely variable and non-specific.

Radiographic signs

Radiographic signs reported with pancreatitis include: increased density, diminished contrast and granularity in the right cranial abdomen, displacement of the stomach to the left, widening of the angle between the pyloric antrum and the proximal duodenum, displacement of the descending duodenum to the right, presence of a mass medial to the descending duodenum, static gas pattern in or thickened walls of the descending duodenum, static gas pattern in or caudal displacement of the transverse colon, gastric distension suggestive of gastric outlet obstruction, and delayed passage of barium through the stomach and duodenum with corrugation of the duodenal wall indicating abnormal peristalsis. Unfortunately definitive radiographic evidence supporting a diagnosis of pancreatitis is usually not present, the most common finding being a somewhat subjective loss of visceral detail ('ground glass appearance') in the anterior abdomen (Suter and Olsson, 1969; Gibbs et al., 1972; Kleine and Hornbuckle, 1978).

Ultrasonic imaging is a promising approach to visualization of the diseased pancreas. Non-homogeneous masses and loss of echodensity have been observed in dogs with experimental pancreatitis, and ultrasonography confirmed the presence of a complex cystic mass in the cranial abdomen of a dog that had a pancreatic pseudocyst associated with acute pancreatitis (Nyland et al., 1983; Murtaugh et al., 1985; Rutgers et al., 1985). Similar findings have been reported in cats (Simpson et al., 1994).

Laboratory aids to diagnosis

Leucocytosis is a common haematological finding in acute pancreatitis. The packed cell volume may be increased as a result of dehydration, although in some cases anaemia is observed (Schaer, 1979; Feldman et al., 1981; Mulvany et al., 1982; Jacobs et al., 1985; Kitchell et al., 1986).

Azotaemia is frequently present, and usually reflects dehydration, but sometimes there may be acute renal failure secondary to hypovolaemia, or to other mechanisms such as circulating vasotoxic agents and plugging of the renal microvasculature by either fat deposits or microthrombi from the sites of disseminated intravascular coagulation (Goldstein et al., 1976; Feldman et al., 1981; Mulvany et al., 1982; Jacobs et al., 1985; Kitchell et al., 1986).

Liver enzyme activities are often increased, reflecting hepatocellular injury as a result of either hepatic ischaemia or exposure of the liver to high concentrations of toxic products delivered from the pancreas in portal blood (Andrzejewska et al., 1985). In some cases there is marked hyperbilirubinaemia with clinically apparent icterus, which may indicate severe hepatocellular damage and/or intrahepatic and extrahepatic obstruction to bile flow.

Hyperglycaemia is also common, probably as a result of hyperglucagonaemia and stress-related increases in the concentrations of catecholamines and cortisol. Some affected animals are diabetic following recovery from acute episodes of pancreatitis.

Hypocalcaemia has often been reported, but is usually mild to moderate and not associated with clinical signs of tetany. The mechanism leading to development of hypocalcaemia is not clear, but deposition of calcium as soaps following excessive breakdown of fat by released pancreatic lipase is one potential explanation (Anderson, 1972; Schaer, 1979; Kornegay, 1982).

Hypercholesterolaemia and hypertriglyceridaemia are very common and hyperlipaemia is often grossly apparent even though food has not been ingested for many hours (Anderson, 1972; Schaer, 1979). Extreme hyperlipaemia may prevent accurate determination of other serum biochemical values.

Serum concentrations of pancreatic enzymes are usually increased. Clinical and experimental observations have involved primarily amylase and lipase, but recently phospholipase A_2 and serum trypsin-like immunoreactivity have been investigated (Mia et al., 1978; Borgström and Ohlsson, 1980; Stickle et al., 1980; Feldman et al., 1981; Geokas et al., 1981; Mulvany et al., 1982; Wagner and Macy, 1982; Westermarck and Rimaila-Pärnänen, 1983; Izquierdo et al., 1984; Jacobs et

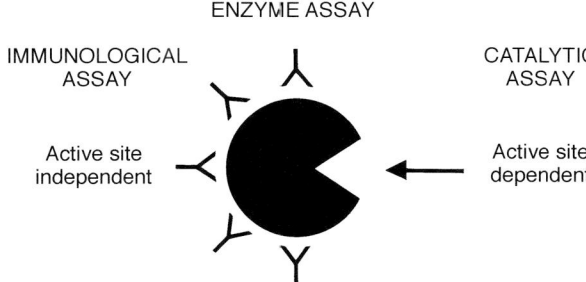

Figure 38.10 Immunoassays (such as that used to assay trypsin-like immunoreactivity) measure the concentration of antigenic determinants on the surface of enzyme molecules and therefore usually detect both zymogens and active enzymes. In contrast, catalytic assays (such as those commonly used to assay amylase and lipase) measure substrate degrading activity of the enzyme and therefore do not detect inactive zymogen. Modified from Williams (1989), p. 1536.

al., 1985; Kitchell et al., 1986; Simpson et al., 1989a). Numerous different assay methods for these substances exist, including conventional catalytic assays and newer highly specific immunoassays (Fig. 38.10), and it is important that an appropriate method for each species be utilized.

Parallel changes in the concentrations of the various enzymes and zymogens have been observed in experimental studies, however this is not always the case in clinical situations. Marked elevations of one enzyme may be accompanied by minimal elevations of another, furthermore, normal enzyme activities may be present in some affected dogs (Schaer, 1979; Strombeck et al., 1981; Westermarck and Rimaila-Pärnänen, 1983). It is possible that by the time some clinical cases are investigated, the inflamed pancreas has been depleted of enzymes, due to their previous release into the bloodstream. Similar reasoning may explain the lack of correlation between the magnitude of the increases in enzyme activities and the clinically perceived severity of disease and eventual outcome.

Increased concentrations of circulating pancreatic enzymes also occur secondary to reduced clearance from the plasma, as happens in renal failure (Polzin et al., 1983). Since azotaemia is common in acute pancreatitis it is sometimes difficult to determine whether increased levels of pancreatic enzymes are due to pancreatic inflammation or renal disease. It is generally believed that increases more than two to three times above the upper limit of normal are unlikely to result from renal dysfunction alone, although there are exceptions (Wagner and Macy, 1982; Polzin et al., 1983).

Amylase and lipase also originate from extrapancreatic sources, and activities of both enzymes may be increased in dogs with hepatic, or neoplastic disease in the absence of pancreatitis (Blum and Linscheer, 1970; Stickle et al., 1980; Strombeck et al., 1981; Jacobs et al., 1982). Lipase activity has been reported to be a more reliable marker for the diagnosis of pancreatitis than that of amylase. However, dexamethasone administration has been shown to increase canine serum lipase activity up to fivefold without histological evidence of pancreatitis, although parallel increases in amylase activity do not occur (Parent, 1982). Moderate elevations of serum lipase in dogs receiving dexamethasone should therefore not be taken as strong evidence for pancreatitis unless amylase is also increased.

Attempts to identify a pancreas-specific isoenzyme of canine amylase, as has been possible in human beings, have produced contradictory findings but have failed to identify a pancreas-specific isoamylase (Stickle et al., 1980; Jacobs et al., 1982; Simpson et al., 1984, 1991; Murtaugh and Jacobs, 1985a; Williams et al., 1986).

The presence of either trypsin complexed with the plasma protease inhibitor α_1-protease inhibitor (Fig. 38.9) or of trypsinogen activation peptides (Fig 38.2) are specific markers for pancreatitis, since trypsin and its activation peptide are only released into the bloodstream in pancreatitis. Furthermore, there is evidence that the concentration of these molecules correlates with the severity and clinical course of the disease (Brodrick et al., 1979; Borgström and Ohlsson, 1980; Geokas et al., 1981, 1982, 1985; Borgström and Lasson, 1984; Lasson, 1984; Durie et al., 1985; Largman et al., 1986; Gudgeon et al., 1990; Fernández-del Castillo et al., 1992; Schmidt et al., 1992; Karanjia et al., 1993). However, technical complexities may limit the clinical application of these assays.

Elevations of serum amylase and lipase in cats with acute pancreatitis are less than in dogs, as are normal activities of these enzymes (Suter and Olsson, 1969; Duffell, 1975; Owens et al., 1975; Schaer, 1979; Garvey and Zawie, 1984). An experimental study demonstrated that whereas serum lipase increased significantly in cats after induction of pancreatitis, amylase activity never increased above normal, and actually decreased significantly during the course of the disease (Kitchell *et al.*, 1986).

Clearly there is no widely available ideal test or combination of tests for the diagnosis of acute pancreatitis, and in the absence of direct examination of pancreatic tissue, the diagnosis can only be tentative. Nonetheless, careful evaluation of the entire clinical picture will in many instances give a high degree of confidence in the presumptive diagnosis. If gross or histopathological confirmation of the diagnosis is required, or the possibility of other abdominal disease is to be eliminated, it is important that attention be given to stabilization of fluid and electrolyte status before general anaesthesia and surgical exploration of the abdomen.

■ Treatment

The basis for therapy of acute pancreatitis is maintenance of fluid and electrolyte balance while the pancreas is 'rested' by withholding food, and thereby allowed to recover from the inflammatory episode (Lankisch, 1984). If drug-induced pancreatitis is suspected then any incriminated agents should be withdrawn and replaced by an unrelated alternative drug if necessary. Sufficient balanced electrolyte solution should be given parenterally to replace fluid deficits and provide maintenance requirements while all oral intake is suspended for three or four days. Mild cases of pancreatitis may spontaneously improve after one or two days. Other patients require aggressive fluid therapy over several days to treat severe dehydration and ongoing fluid electrolyte loss due to vomiting and diarrhoea. Many animals become hypokalaemic during such therapy and serum potassium should be monitored and supplemented as needed by addition of potassium chloride to the intravenous fluids. Serum creatinine or blood urea nitrogen should also be followed to document resolution of azotaemia. Although metabolic acidosis is probably common in acute pancreatitis, this may not always be the case and vomiting patients may be alkalotic. Blind correction of suspected acid–base abnormalities should therefore not be attempted unless documented by appropriate tests. Excessive bicarbonate administration may precipitate signs of hypocalcaemia in individuals with subclinical hypocalcaemia. It is common practice to give antibiotics during this supportive period, particularly when toxic changes are evident in the haemogram or when the patient is febrile (Lankisch, 1984). Trimethoprim–sulphonamide combination therapy is a reasonable choice since this combination attains therapeutic levels in canine pancreas (Bradley, 1989).

If abdominal pain is severe then analgesic therapy (pethidine) should be given to provide relief. Hyperglycaemia is often mild and transient, but in some cases frank diabetes mellitus may develop and require treatment with insulin. Respiratory distress, neurological problems, cardiac abnormalities, bleeding disorders, and acute renal failure are all poor prognostic signs. Attempts should be made to manage these complications by appropriate supportive measures, but recovery is unlikely unless the underlying pancreatitis resolves.

Some affected animals do not improve, or continue to deteriorate, in spite of supportive care. Recent observations have indicated that in severe pancreatitis, there is marked consumption of plasma protease inhibitors as activated pancreatic proteases are cleared from the circulation, and that saturation of available α-macroglobulins is rapidly followed by acute disseminated intravascular coagulation, shock and death (Ohlsson *et al.*, 1971; Borgström and Ohlsson, 1980; Geokas *et al.*, 1981; Lasson, 1984; McMahon *et al.*, 1984; Wendt *et al.*, 1984; Durie *et al.*, 1985; Murtaugh and Jacobs, 1985b; Largman *et al.*, 1986). Transfusion of plasma or whole blood to replace α-macroglobulins may be life-saving in these circumstances, and has the additional benefit of maintaining plasma albumin concentrations (Cuschieri *et al.*, 1983; Wendt *et al.*, 1984). Low-molecular-weight dextrans have also been used to expand plasma volume, but they may aggravate bleeding tendencies, contain no protease inhibitor and provide no major advantages over plasma administration (Lankisch, 1984).

The use of corticosteroids in pancreatitis has been recommended because they stabilize lysosomal membranes, reduce inflammation and alleviate shock, but they have not been shown to be of value in experimental acute studies (Attix *et al.*, 1981). They should be given only on a short-term basis to animals in shock, and then in concert with fluids and plasma as described above. Longer periods of administration may impair removal of α-macroglobulin-bound proteases from the plasma by the reticuloendothelial system, with resultant complications due to reduced enzyme clearance (Adham *et al.*, 1983).

The use of peritoneal dialysis to remove toxic material accumulated in the peritoneal cavity is beneficial experimentally, and is thought by many to be useful in human patients (Lankisch, 1984). Although peritoneal dialysis is impractical in most veterinary hospitals, in those patients in which acute pancreatitis is confirmed at exploratory laparotomy, removal of as much free fluid as possible by abdominal lavage is advisable. In some cases pancreatitis may be localized to one lobe of the gland, and surgical resection of the affected area may be followed by complete recovery (Denny and Lucke, 1972; Salisbury et al., 1988).

Inhibition of pancreatic secretion through nasogastric suction of gastric secretions, and by the use of drugs such as antacids, cimetidine and direct inhibitors of pancreatic secretion such as atropine, acetazolamide, glucagon, calcitonin and somatostatin or its analogues have also not yet been proved to be more effective than simply withholding food and water (Attix et al., 1981; Lankisch, 1984). Administration of a variety of naturally occurring and synthetic enzyme inhibitors with selective actions against individual pancreatic digestive enzymes has shown promise in experimental studies, but their value remains to be demonstrated in clinical trials (Balldin and Ohlsson, 1979; Balldin et al., 1984; Lankisch, 1984; Hermon-Taylor and Heywood, 1985).

One to two days after cessation of vomiting, small amounts of water should be offered, and if there is no recurrence of clinical signs, food may be gradually re-introduced. The diet should have a high carbohydrate content (rice, pasta, potatoes) since protein and fat are more potent stimulants of pancreatic secretion. If there is continued improvement, gradual introduction of a low-fat maintenance diet should be attempted. Another period of food deprivation should be instituted if signs of pancreatitis recur (Pidgeon, 1987).

In many patients a single episode of pancreatitis occurs, and all that is necessary in the way of long-term therapy is to avoid feeding meals with an excessively high fat content. In other patients repeated bouts of pancreatitis occur and it may be beneficial to feed a moderately or severely fat-restricted diet permanently. In spite of this, some animals experience recurrent disease (Pidgeon, 1987).

Oral pancreatic enzyme supplements have been shown to decrease the pain that accompanies chronic pancreatitis in human beings, probably by feedback inhibition of endogenous pancreatic enzyme secretion (Slaff et al., 1984). It is not known if they are of similar value in dogs or cats, but in individuals with chronic or recurrent signs attributed to pancreatitis a trial period of enzyme therapy may be warranted.

Prognosis

Pancreatitis is an unpredictable disease of widely varying severity, and it is difficult to give a prognosis even when a diagnosis is definitively established. Acute fulminating pancreatitis may be fatal despite early and aggressive supportive measures, but some dogs recover fully after an isolated severe episode. In other cases, relatively mild or moderate chronic or recurrent pancreatitis persists despite all therapy, and either the patient dies in an acute severe exacerbation of the disease, or is euthanatized because of failure to recover and the expense of long-term supportive care.

EXOCRINE PANCREATIC INSUFFICIENCY

Progressive loss of exocrine pancreatic acinar cells ultimately leads to failure of nutrient absorption due to inadequate production of digestive enzymes. The functional reserve of the pancreas is considerable, however, and signs of exocrine pancreatic insufficiency (EPI) do not occur until a large proportion of the gland has been destroyed.

The most common cause of EPI in the dog is pancreatic acinar atrophy (PAA). Pancreatic insufficiency is caused less commonly by chronic pancreatitis, and rarely by pancreatic neoplasia (Hill, 1972; Pfister et al., 1980; Rimaila-Pärnänen and Westermarck, 1982; Bright, 1985). Although not yet documented, it is likely that congenital abnormalities of canine pancreatic exocrine function such as pancreatic hypoplasia, isolated deficiencies of individual pancreatic enzymes, and deficiency of enteropeptidase also occur (Jubb et al., 1985; Lerner and Lebenthal, 1993).

Aetiology

Pancreatic acinar atrophy

Atrophy of the acinar cells of the pancreas in the absence of a pronounced inflammatory response may occur in a variety of experimental circumstances. Spontaneous development of severe PAA in previously healthy adult animals appears to be uniquely common in the dog, although reports indicate that similar conditions occur sporadically in other species (Hasholt, 1972; Balk et al., 1975; Eppig and Leiter, 1977; Port et al., 1981).

The underlying cause of canine PAA is unknown, but numerous nutritional deficiencies such as amino acid imbalance and copper deficiency in the rat, and protein-calorie malnutrition in humans, cause atrophy of exocrine tissue (Barbezat and Hansen, 1968; Levenson et al., 1971; Fell et al., 1982; Mizunuma et al., 1984; Geokas et al., 1985). Other possible aetiologies include: (1) pancreatic duct obstruction, (2) primary congenital abnormalities of the pancreas; (3) toxicosis; (4) ischaemia; (5) viral infection; (6) immune-mediated disease and (7) defective secretory and/or trophic stimuli, but there is no evidence to support the role of any of these in the pathogenesis of naturally occurring canine PAA (Van Kruiningen, 1982). Although PAA may occur at any age in a wide variety of breeds, a high prevalence in the young German shepherd dog is recognized (Anderson and Low, 1965; Hill et al., 1971; Sateri, 1975; Weber and Freudiger, 1977; Westermarck, 1980; Van Kruiningen, 1982; Hall et al., 1991). Investigations of family histories have suggested that predisposition to development of the disease is inherited in an autosomal recessive fashion in this breed (Weber and Freudiger, 1977; Westermarck, 1980).

The pancreatic atrophy of CBA/J mice is the only naturally occurring disorder that resembles canine PAA (Eppig and Leiter, 1977). Morphological study of pancreas from affected mice has implicated destabilization of zymogen granules as one of the earliest ultrastructural abnormalities, whereas biochemical studies indicate that premature activation of trypsinogen and chymotrypsinogen occurs within the zymogen granules, with subsequent mild inflammatory cell infiltration (Eppig and Leiter, 1977; Leiter and Cunliff-Beamer, 1977).

Chronic pancreatitis

Although chronic pancreatitis is a common cause of EPI in humans, it appears to be uncommon in dogs (Anderson and Low, 1965; Hill et al., 1971; Rimaila-Pärnänen and Westermarck, 1982). There are no well-documented reports of dogs with either chronic relapsing pancreatitis or severe acute pancreatitis resulting in EPI, but those animals with EPI and coexistent diabetes mellitus probably fall into this category. A similar combination of clinical signs is seen in association with chronic pancreatitis in humans, in contrast to PAA in which endocrine tissue is spared (Andriulli et al., 1981; Grendell and Cello, 1983). Exocrine pancreatic insufficiency is much less commonly diagnosed in cats. Chronic pancreatitis has been the underlying cause in most reported cases (Holzworth and Coffin, 1953; Anderson and Strafuss, 1971; Watson et al., 1981; Hoskins et al., 1982).

Miscellaneous causes of EPI

In children, cystic fibrosis and congenital hypoplasia (Schwachman syndrome) are common causes of EPI. Less common causes include congenital deficiencies of individual pancreatic digestive enzymes or of intestinal enteropeptidase, but none of these have been described in dogs or cats. Occasionally young dogs are seen that have signs of EPI and perhaps diabetes mellitus from a very early age, and congenital pancreatic hypoplasia or aplasia may be the underlying causes (Jubb et al., 1985; Boari et al., 1994).

EPI has been reported as a complication of proximal duodenal resection and cholecystoduodenostomy in cats, a finding which probably reflects the absence of dual pancreatic ducts in this species such that damage to the major duodenal papilla blocks pancreatic secretion (Tangner et al., 1982).

Pathophysiology

Nutrient malabsorption in canine EPI probably does not arise solely as a consequence of failure of intraluminal digestion. Morphological changes in the small intestine of dogs with EPI have occasionally been reported, and studies of naturally occurring and experimental EPI in several species have revealed abnormal activities of mucosal enzymes. Impaired function as indicated by abnormal transport of sugars, amino acids and fatty acids has also been documented. The cause of this mucosal pathology is unknown, but the absence of the trophic influence of pancreatic secretions, bacterial overgrowth in the small intestine, and endocrine and nutritional factors may all be contributory (Williams, 1989).

Small intestinal mucosa

Exocrine pancreatic insufficiency is associated with increased activities of jejunal brush border maltase and sucrase (Arvanitakis and Olsen, 1974; Batt et al., 1979; Simpson et al., 1989c). These increased activities have been attributed to reduced degradation of exposed brush border proteins due to decreased pancreatic protease activity within the gut lumen (Fig. 38.11) (Arvanitakis and Olsen, 1974), an explanation supported by the normalization of these enzyme

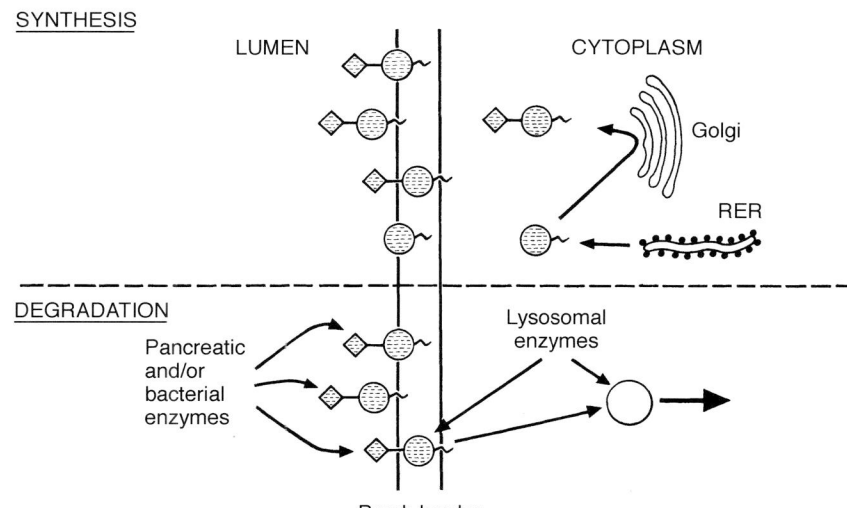

Figure 38.11 Factors influencing activities of jejunal brush border enzymes. The importance of degradation by intraluminal proteases depends at least in part on the location of the enzyme in the membrane, and hence its susceptibility to proteolytic attack. Modified from Alpers and Seetharam (1977).

activities in response to treatment with pancreatic enzymes (Kwong et al., 1978; Williams et al., 1985a). The abnormal accumulation of these enzymes and perhaps other proteins on the surface of the brush border membrane may interfere with normal absorption.

The activity of alkaline phosphatase, an enzyme relatively resistant to degradation by intraluminal proteases, is decreased in dogs with EPI, as is jejunal protein synthesis. Both protein synthesis and alkaline phosphatase activity normalize after treatment (Batt et al., 1979; Kenny and Maroux, 1982; Williams et al., 1985a). The mechanism for the defect in protein synthesis is not known, but several factors may contribute including malnutrition and intraluminal or humoral factors. Pancreatic secretions and the products of digestion exert a trophic effect on the small intestine, an effect clearly absent or diminished in untreated dogs. Insulinopenia, present in untreated animals, may be an additional factor since insulin has a stimulatory effect on DNA synthesis in the gastrointestinal tract.

Small intestinal microflora

Bacterial overgrowth ($>1 \times 10^5$ organisms ml^{-1} duodenal juice) is common in dogs with EPI. Changes in the intestinal microflora may arise secondary to loss of the antibacterial properties of pancreatic juice, or as a consequence of as yet undefined abnormalities of intestinal immunity or motility. Achlorhydria, a factor predisposing to development of bacterial overgrowth, has been commonly reported in human patients with chronic disease of the exocrine pancreas, but has been shown not to occur in canine EPI (Williams et al., 1987).

The pathological changes associated with bacterial overgrowth depend on the type of bacteria involved. In those dogs with increases in aerobic and facultative anaerobic bacteria, changes in the activities of brush border enzymes are similar to those observed in dogs with EPI that do not have bacterial overgrowth. In contrast, when the overgrowth includes obligate anaerobic bacteria there is often an associated decrease in many enzyme activities, and in some cases, partial villous atrophy. These findings are consistent with the known ability of some strains of obligate anaerobic bacteria to produce enzymes that release or destroy exposed brush border enzymes. Even when bacterial overgrowth does not include large numbers of obligate anaerobes, the abnormal microflora may be of clinical significance since bacteria may indirectly impair absorption by competing for nutrients and by changing intraluminal factors such as the concentration of conjugated bile salts (Williams et al., 1987).

Pancreatic regulatory peptides

Histopathological examination of pancreas from dogs with PAA reveals almost total atrophy of acinar tissue, but plentiful, disorganized islet tissue, accompanied by numerous ganglia and patent exocrine ducts. Immunohistochemical staining shows many insulin-, glucagon-, somatostatin- and pancreatic polypeptide-immunoreactive cells scattered haphazardly throughout residual islet tissue. This differs from the more organized arrangement of cells in normal canine pancreas, in which a central core of insulin- and scattered somatostatin-immunoreactive cells is surrounded by a halo of glucagon- (left lobe) or pancreatic polypeptide- (right lobe), immunoreactive cells.

Disturbance of the morphological relationships between islet cells may impair intra-islet and/or entero-islet homeostatic mechanisms and might account for subnormal basal plasma insulin concentrations in dogs with PAA. The aetiology of these neuronal regulatory peptide abnormalities is unknown, though perhaps they arise as a result of neuronal overgrowth in response to loss of target tissue (Vaillant et al., 1983, 1984; Orci, 1984).

Glucose intolerance

In dogs with EPI secondary to pancreatitis there may be frank diabetes mellitus due to islet cell destruction. Oral and intravenous glucose tolerance are also abnormal in untreated dogs with PAA, although diabetes mellitus has not been reported in these dogs (Hill and Kidder, 1972; Greve and Anderson, 1973; Williams and Batt, 1986).

The 'incretin' effect is reduced in dogs with experimental pancreatic atrophy. 'Incretin' refers to insulinotrophic factors released from the gut which are responsible for the augmentation of insulin secretion in response to orally administered glucose compared to that stimulated by the same dosage of intravenously administered glucose. Gastric inhibitory polypeptide (GIP) is probably an important factor contributing to 'incretin' activity and feeding does not stimulate GIP release from the small bowel of dogs with PAA unless pancreatic enzymes are added to the food. The failure of GIP secretion appears to arise because products of digestion (glucose, amino acids, fatty acids) are the stimuli for GIP release rather than the act of feeding or the undigested constituents of food itself (Rogers et al., 1983). Intravenous glucose tolerance in untreated dogs with PAA is associated with subnormal resting and stimulated insulin concentrations. Treatment of PAA is followed by normalization of intravenous glucose tolerance, although basal plasma insulin concentrations remain subnormal (Williams and Batt, 1986).

It is probable that the abnormalities in glucose homeostasis are related at least in part to metabolic changes associated with the catabolic state of many untreated dogs with EPI. Withholding food from dogs for a period of 2 weeks produces a decrease in circulating insulin concentrations. Such lower insulin levels facilitate enhanced lipolysis increasing the concentrations of plasma free fatty acids available as an energy source (de Bruijne et al., 1981).

Nutritional status

Many dogs with EPI have been suffering from malabsorption for a considerable period of time before a diagnosis is made. Long-term protein calorie malnutrition results in altered circulating concentrations of insulin and other hormones contributing to changes in glucose homeostasis and intestinal mucosal function. Severe protein-calorie malnutrition may impair mucosal protein synthesis as well as normal immune response, which may in turn contribute to the development of changes in the intestinal microflora. Furthermore, malnutrition has been shown to impair the capacity to maintain protective mucosal mucin content, and accelerates the development of brush border enzyme deficiency in intraluminal bacterial overgrowth (Salazar de Sousa, 1984; Sherman et al., 1985a,b).

Absorption of trace elements in EPI may be promoted or inhibited, however preliminary investigations have not revealed any trace element deficiencies in dogs with EPI, though only serum copper and zinc levels have been assessed (Williams, 1985).

Mild to severe decreases in serum cobalamin levels have been observed in dogs and cats with EPI (Batt and Morgan, 1982). The mechanism for malabsorption of cobalamin in canine EPI is not known, but overgrowth of cobalamin-binding bacteria in the proximal small bowel may be responsible. In addition, deficiency of pancreatic proteases may prevent the normal release of cobalamin from salivary and/or gastric R proteins. These proteins bind ingested cobalamin in the stomach, where the low pH prevents binding to gastric intrinsic factor, and subsequent degradation in the proximal small bowel by pancreatic proteases is an important factor in the successful transfer of cobalamin from R proteins to intrinsic factor. A deficiency intrinsic factor in canine pancreatic juice may also directly contribute to cobalamin malabsorption in EPI (Simpson et al., 1989b; Batt et al., 1989; Fyfe, 1993).

Serum concentrations often do not normalize after otherwise effective treatment (Williams, 1993). Cobalamin is essential for DNA synthesis and severely subnormal serum cobalamin concentrations may adversely affect the normal proliferation of crypt cells in the intestinal mucosa, and hence the specific activities of jejunal mucosal enzymes. It is, therefore, possible that persistent cobalamin deficiency may be a contributory factor in those cases where response to treatment is suboptimal.

Serum folate concentrations may be increased in dogs with EPI, both before and after treatment. These high serum folate levels may reflect overgrowth of bacteria in the small intestine, since intraluminal bacteria commonly synthesize and release folate. The elevations of serum folate associated with canine EPI are probably of little functional significance (Batt and Morgan, 1982; Williams et al., 1987).

Fat malabsorption, which may be exacerbated by bacterial overgrowth, results in malabsorption of fat-soluble vitamins. Serum tocopherol (vitamin E) concentrations are often severely subnormal in canine EPI, and they do not increase in response to treatment, perhaps because treatment does not completely normalize fat absorption, or perhaps because intraluminal bacterial overgrowth persists (Williams, 1985).

Tocopherol deficiency decreases the proliferative response of canine lymphocytes to mitogenic stimulants and if this reflects an *in vivo* defect in immune function, tocopherol deficiency may be an additional factor predisposing to overgrowth of intestinal bacteria in dogs with EPI (Langweiler et al., 1981). Tocopherol deficiency may cause pathological changes in smooth muscle, central nervous system, skeletal muscle and retina, although such changes have not yet been documented in dogs with chronic EPI.

Subnormal serum concentrations of vitamin A have also been observed in dogs with EPI, but no associated signs of deficiency were reported (Coffin and Thordal-Christensen, 1953). Vitamin K-responsive coagulopathy arises occasionally in patients with EPI (Perry et al., 1991).

Diagnosis

History and clinical signs

Animals with EPI usually have a history of weight loss in the face of a normal or increased appetite. Polyphagia is often severe, but this is by no means always the case and some dogs may even have periods of inappetence. Coprophagia and pica are also common. Water intake may also increase in some dogs, and in chronic pancreatitis there may be polyuria and polydipsia due to diabetes mellitus (Raiha and Westermarck, 1989).

Diarrhoea often accompanies EPI, but can be very variable in character. Most owners report frequent passage of large volumes of semiformed faeces, although some dogs have intermittent or continuous watery diarrhoea, and in other instances diarrhoea is infrequent and is not considered a problem. Diarrhoea generally improves or resolves in response to fasting. Introduction of a low fat diet may also decrease or eliminate diarrhoea. There may be a history of vomiting, and commonly there is marked borborygmis and flatulence. Owners sometimes believe that the dog suffers from episodes of abdominal discomfort (Raiha and Westermarck, 1989).

In some dogs there has been a protracted history of gastrointestinal disturbances before the final diagnosis of EPI, the significance of which is not clear, but which may merely represent initial failure to diagnose EPI. Appropriate testing early in the course of the disease before the 'classic signs' have appeared will allow the diagnosis to be made before severe deterioration of body condition occurs.

Pancreatic acinar atrophy is very prevalent in young German shepherd dogs, thus EPI is often initially suspected because of the age and breed of the affected dog. It must be emphasized, however, that even in young German shepherd dogs small intestinal disease is more prevalent than EPI, and that PAA may occur in a wide variety of breeds at any age. Chronic pancreatitis is probably more common in older dogs, but the true prevalence of EPI due to chronic pancreatitis is not known.

Mild to marked weight loss is usually seen in association with EPI. In extreme cases dogs may be physically weak owing to loss of muscle mass. The hair coat is often in poor condition and there may be a foul odour due to soiling of the coat with fatty faecal material or passage of excessive flatus.

Laboratory aids to diagnosis

The history and clinical signs of EPI are non-specific, vary in severity, and do not distinguish the condition from other causes of malabsorption. Although replacement therapy with oral pancreatic enzymes is generally successful, response to treatment is not a reliable diagnostic approach. Not all dogs with EPI respond to treatment, and dogs with self-limiting small intestinal disease might improve spontaneously, giving the false impression of responding to enzyme supplementation. Furthermore, veterinarians often advise a change in diet when treating dogs with EPI, and this in itself can lead to clinical improvement in some with small intestinal diseases.

In dogs with PAA, atrophy of the pancreas is readily observed on gross inspection at exploratory laparotomy or laparoscopy, although in dogs with chronic pancreatitis it may be impossible to gauge accurately the amount of residual exocrine pancreatic tissue because of severe adhesions and fibrosis. These procedures involve unnecessary anaesthetic and surgical risks and therefore cannot be recommended as a means of diagnosing EPI.

Routine laboratory test results are generally not helpful in establishing a diagnosis of EPI. Serum alanine aminotransferase is often mildly to moderately increased and may reflect hepatocyte damage secondary to increased uptake of hepatotoxic substances through an abnormally permeable small intestinal mucosa. Other routine serum biochemical test results are unremarkable, except that total lipid, cholesterol and polyunsaturated fatty acid concentrations are often reduced. Mild lymphopenia and eosinophilia are occasionally seen in dogs with EPI, but complete blood count results are usually within normal limits, and major abnormalities should be perused as evidence of additional or alternative underlying disorders (Hill, 1972; Sateri, 1975; Van Kruiningen, 1982).

Many specific laboratory tests have been described for the diagnosis of EPI, including examination of faeces for undigested food particles and/or steatorrhoea, assessment of postprandial plasma turbidity with and without the addition of pancreatic enzymes to the food, and evaluation of blood glucose concentration following the oral administration of starch. The sensitivities and specificities of these tests are highly questionable, and none have been shown to reliably distinguish dogs with small intestinal disease from those with EPI. The most reliable tests currently available include assay of serum trypsin-like immunoreactivity (TLI), assay of faecal proteolytic activity using a casein-based substrate, and the bentiromide (N-benzoyl-L-tyrosyl-p-aminobenzoic acid or BT-PABA) absorption test (Williams and Batt, 1988).

Serum trypsin-like immunoreactivity

Trypsinogen is synthesized exclusively by the pancreas and measurement of the serum concentration of this zymogen by radioimmunoassay (Canine TLI Assay Kit, Diagnostic Products Corporation, 5700 West 96th Street, Los Angeles, CA 90045) provides a good indirect index of pancreatic function. This immunoassay detects both trypsinogen and trypsin, hence the use of the term trypsin-like immunoreactivity (TLI) to describe the total concentration of these two immunoreactive elements. Radioimmunoassays for trypsin are species specific, and assays for human TLI do not detect canine TLI. Measurement of serum TLI is much simpler than most of the other tests for EPI in that analysis of just a single serum sample obtained after food has been withheld for several hours is all that is required. Serum TLI is quite stable under normal conditions and samples can therefore be mailed to an appropriate laboratory. Administration of oral pancreatic extracts does not affect serum TLI concentration in either normal dogs or dogs with EPI (Williams and Batt, 1988).

Measurement of serum TLI has been shown to be a highly sensitive and specific test for the diagnosis of canine EPI. Serum TLI concentrations are dramatically reduced in dogs with EPI whereas TLI concentrations in dogs with small intestinal disease are not significantly different from normal (Fig. 38.12).

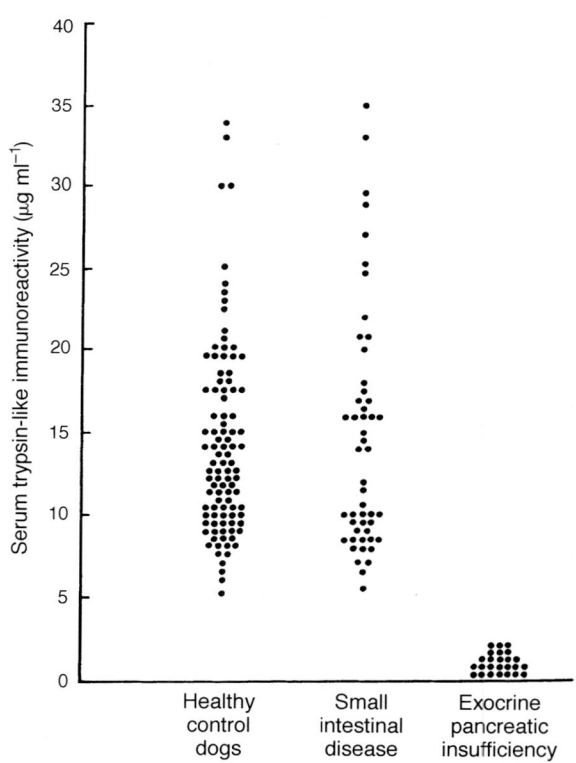

Figure 38.12 Serum trypsin-like immunoreactivity in 100 healthy dogs, 50 dogs with small intestinal disease and 25 dogs with exocrine pancreatic insufficiency. Reproduced from Williams and Batt (1988), with permission.

It can be predicted that serum TLI concentrations will be normal in those cases where EPI is due to tumours obstructing the pancreatic ducts, or to congenital deficiencies of enzymes other than trypsinogen. A very small proportion of samples submitted to the author's laboratory for analysis have subnormal serum TLI concentrations (5.0 mg l^{-1}) that are greater than those observed in dogs with EPI (2.5 mg l^{-1}). In such cases, subsequent retesting usually reveals serum TLI concentrations that are either clearly consistent with EPI or normal. Failure to withhold food before blood sampling or recovery of pancreatic function following an episode of pancreatitis may explain these 'grey zone' results. A few dogs have consistent equivocal serum TLI concentrations, but these individuals rarely appear to benefit from enzyme therapy. It is likely that they have some reduction of pancreatic secretory capacity that is not sufficient to cause clinical signs.

Serum amylase, isoamylases, lipase and phospholipase A$_2$ activities are generally normal or only slightly reduced in EPI. Non-pancreatic sources of these enzymes are present in dogs and although their activities may increase in inflammatory disease of the pancreas, unlike trypsinogen they do not decrease proportionally as the mass of functional exocrine pancreatic tissue declines (Simpson et al., 1991).

Bentiromide absorption test

Chymotrypsin activity in the proximal small intestine may be assayed *in vivo* by the oral administration of the synthetic substrate bentiromide (*N*-benzoyl-L-tyrosyl-*p*-aminobenzoic acid or BT-PABA). Free PABA is released from this substrate by chymotrypsin, absorbed from the gut lumen, and subsequently excreted in the urine. Absorption may be assessed by measuring PABA in either plasma or urine. The relatively high cost of the substrate, the requirement for either multiple blood sampling or collection of urine in a metabolism cage, and the technical expertise required for the PABA assay have largely restricted its use to referral practices and institutions. Moreover, there is overlap between the results from dogs with EPI and those with small intestinal disease (Fig. 38.13). Test results in healthy cats vary considerably, but a clearly abnormal result was obtained in one cat with EPI (Sherding *et al.*, 1982; Hawkins *et al.*, 1986; Perry *et al.*, 1991).

An advantage of the bentiromide absorption test over the serum TLI assay is that it should

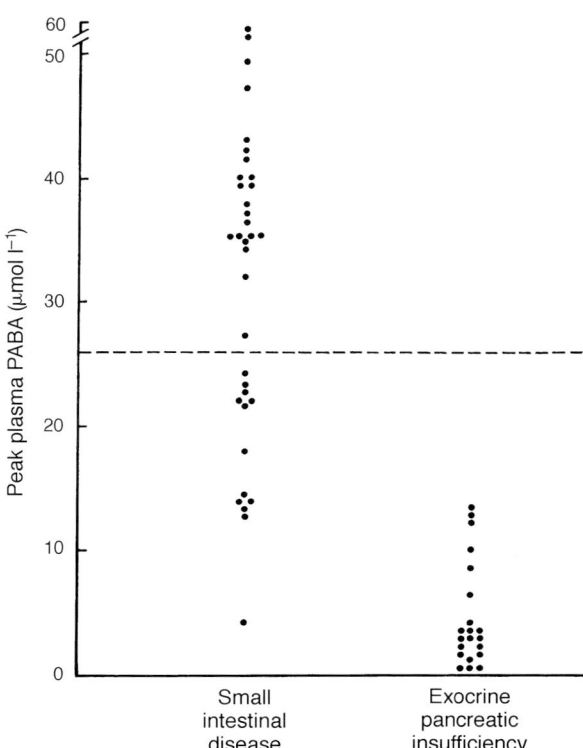

Figure 38.13 Peak plasma *p*-aminobenzoic acid (PABA) concentration after combined bentiromide/xylose absorption testing of 35 dogs with small intestinal disease and 22 dogs with exocrine pancreatic insufficiency. The dashed line indicates the lower limit of the range of peak plasma PABA values in healthy dogs. Reproduced from Williams and Batt (1988), with permission.

detect EPI in those cases caused by obstruction to the flow of pancreatic juice; in these animals release of trypsinogen into the blood, and hence the concentration of TLI, may not be abnormal.

Faecal proteolytic activity

Faecal proteolytic activity has been used as an index of pancreatic enzyme activity for many years, but the reliability of the test varies widely depending on the assay method employed. The widely used X-ray film digestion test is unreliable, and gives many false negative and false positive results. Proteolytic activity can be measured more precisely using protein substrates such as casein. Faecal proteolytic activity as assessed by such methods is consistently low in most dogs with EPI, but because dogs with normal pancreatic function occasionally pass faeces with low proteolytic activity, a minimum of three faecal samples must be tested. Some dogs with EPI have normal faecal proteolytic activity as assessed by this assay, but this is rare (Fig. 38.14). This type of test is suitable for use in the cat, but similar caution should be exercised in the interpretation of results since healthy cats may also pass faeces with negligible proteolytic activity (Strombeck, 1978; Hill, 1972; Westermarck and Sandholm, 1980; Westermarck, 1982; Canfield et al., 1983; Williams and Reed, 1990; Williams et al., 1990).

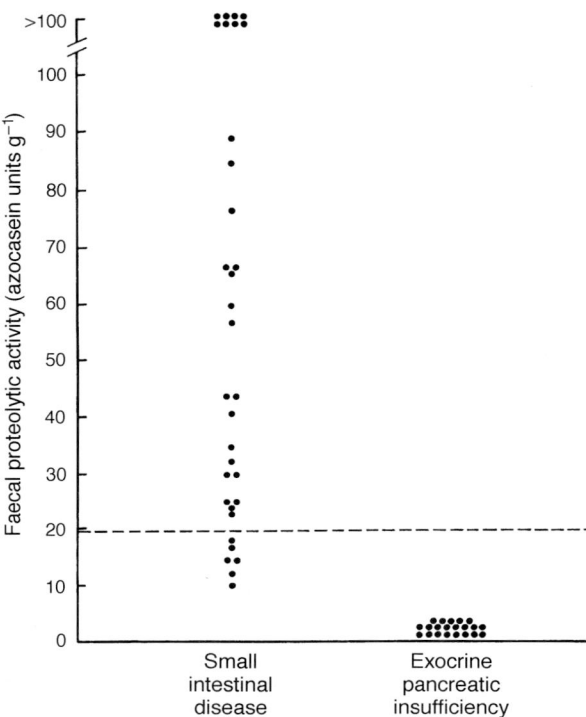

Figure 38.14 Faecal proteolytic activity determined by azocasein assay of 3 day collections from 34 dogs with small intestinal disease and 22 dogs with exocrine pancreatic insufficiency. The dashed line indicates the lower limit of the range of values in healthy dogs. Reproduced from Williams and Batt (1988), with permission.

■ Treatment

Enzyme replacement

Most dogs with EPI can be successfully managed by supplementing each meal with pancreatic enzymes from ox or pig pancreas. This can be accomplished using commercially available dried pancreatic extracts. Numerous formulations of these extracts are available (tablets, capsules, powders, granules) and their enzyme content and bioavailability varies widely (Niessen et al., 1983). The addition of two teaspoons of powdered non-enteric-coated preparation with each meal per 20 kg of body weight is generally an effective starting dose. This can be mixed with a maintenance dog food immediately before feeding. Two meals a day are usually sufficient to promote weight gain. Dogs will generally gain 0.5–1.0 kg per week, and diarrhoea will resolve within 4–5 days. In some cases the reduction in frequency of defecation is dramatic, and other signs such as coprophagia and polyphagia often disappear within a few days. As soon as clinical improvement is apparent owners can determine a minimum effective dose of enzyme supplement that prevents return of clinical signs. This varies slightly between batches of extract, and also from dog to dog. Most affected animals require at least one teaspoonful of enzyme supplement per meal. One meal per day is sufficient in some dogs, whereas others continue to require two. Commercial dried pancreatic extracts are expensive and when available, substitution of 3–4 ounces (75–100 g) per 20 kg of body weight of chopped raw ox or pig pancreas obtained from animals certified as healthy following appropriate post-mortem inspection is a more economical alternative. Pancreas can be stored frozen at –20°C for at least 3 months and enzyme activity will be adequately maintained.

Measures to increase the effectiveness of enzyme supplementation

Only a small proportion of the oral dose of each enzyme is delivered functionally intact to the small intestine. Pancreatic lipase is rapidly inactivated at the acid pH encountered in the stomach, whereas trypsin and other pancreatic proteases, although relatively acid resistant, are susceptible to degradation by gastric pepsins. In human beings with EPI, as much as 90% of ingested lipase and 80% of ingested trypsin are inactivated before delivery to the jejunum (Dimagno, 1979). In view of the expense of pancreatic enzyme preparations, attempts have been made to increase the effectiveness of enzyme supplementation. These include use of enteric-coated preparations, neutralization or inhibition of secretion of gastric acid, preincubation of enzymes with food prior to feeding, and supplementation with bile salts.

Enteric-coated preparations have been formulated in an attempt to protect orally administered enzymes from gastric acid. In studies in humans these preparations have generally proved to be no more effective than non-enteric-coated extracts. In the author's experience enteric-coated preparations have been either ineffective or less effective than powdered pancreatic extract in treating dogs with EPI. Uncrushed pancreatic enzyme tablets are also ineffective whereas the same formulation was effective when crushed before feeding. In those few dogs with suboptimal weight gain in response to pancreatic enzymes alone the author has found no advantage in increasing the dose of enzymes above two teaspoonfuls per meal.

Gastric acid secretion may be reduced by administration of the histamine type 2 receptor antagonist cimetidine. When given at a dosage of 300 mg/20 kg body weight with oral pancreatic enzymes to dogs with ligated pancreatic ducts, this drug does improve fat absorption, but does not decrease faecal wet or dry weight (Pidgeon and Strombeck, 1982). The routine use of cimetidine in the treatment of EPI is not recommended given the expense of the drug and the fact that so many dogs respond well to enzymes alone. Moreover, the drug has not proved beneficial in those dogs who do not respond optimally to enzymes alone. The use of oral antacids (sodium bicarbonate, aluminium and magnesium hydroxide) to decrease intragastric lipase destruction does not increase the effectiveness of enzyme therapy in experimental EPI (Pidgeon and Strombeck, 1982). Indeed, although antacids may increase the quantity of orally administered pancreatic lipase reaching the small intestine, lingual and/or gastric lipase activity, which probably accounts for the considerable residual fat absorption in dogs with EPI, may be inhibited since an acid pH is optimal for intragastric lipolysis (Abrams et al., 1984).

Preincubation of food with enzyme powder for 30 min before feeding does not improve the effectiveness of oral enzyme treatment in promoting fat absorption in dogs with ligated pancreatic ducts (Pidgeon and Strombeck, 1982). This is not surprising since optimal activity will not be achieved unless lipase is in solution at the appropriate pH and temperature and in the presence of appropriate concentrations of colipase and bile acids; conditions which are unlikely to be encountered in the feeding bowl.

There is no evidence that bile release is deficient in naturally occurring EPI, and addition of bile salts to enzyme supplements does not improve fat absorption over that obtained when enzymes alone are given with food to dogs with ligated pancreatic ducts (Pidgeon and Strombeck, 1982).

Dietary modification

Numerous studies show that fat absorption does not return to normal despite appropriate enzyme therapy (Pidgeon and Strombeck, 1982). Dogs appear to compensate by eating slightly more than usual, and as with any individual dog it is necessary to regulate the amount of food given in order to maintain ideal body weight.

Although therapy with regular maintenance dog food and appropriate enzyme replacement is usually effective, feeding of a highly digestible, low fibre diet may be advantageous (Westermarck et al., 1990). Dietary fibre impairs pancreatic enzyme activity, and high fibre diets should probably be avoided (Dutta and Hlasko, 1985). Highly digestible diets may be of particular value in promoting caloric uptake in those dogs with EPI that do not regain normal body weight when fed regular food with enzyme replacement. These patients may also benefit from addition of medium-chain triglycerides to the food. Some medium-chain triglycerides are absorbed intact, and their hydrolysis by lipase proceeds much faster than that of long-chain triglycerides, so that fat absorption is facilitated (Grendell, 1983).

Vitamin supplementation

Dogs with EPI may have severely subnormal concentrations of serum cobalamin and tocopherol which do not necessarily increase in response to treatment with oral pancreatic enzymes, even when the clinical response is otherwise excellent (Williams, 1985). Clinical signs associated with naturally occurring deficiencies of these vitamins in the dog have not been documented, but both may contribute to intestinal mucosal changes and perhaps cause systemic signs of deficiency including either myopathy or myelopathy and other abnormalities of nervous tissue as has been reported in other species. It therefore seems prudent to supplement with these vitamins if serum concentrations are subnormal. In the author's experience, supplementation with large oral doses of tocopherol (400–500 IU given once daily with food for one month) is effective in returning serum concentrations to normal. In contrast cobalamin must be give parenterally (250 mg by intramuscular or subcutaneous injection once a week for several weeks) to normalize serum concentrations.

Potential deficiencies of other vitamins in canine EPI have not been investigated in detail. Malabsorption of other fat-soluble vitamins is to be expected, but malabsorption of vitamins A, D and K may not be as marked as with tocopherol, since tocopherol appears to be particularly sensitive to abnormalities in the intestinal lumen (Sokol et al., 1983). It should be noted that doses of individual vitamins in multivitamin preparations may be insufficient to normalize serum concentrations and that parenteral or very high oral doses may be required for adequate supplementation.

Antibiotic therapy

Dogs with PAA commonly have overgrowth of bacteria in the small intestine but in most cases this is a subclinical abnormality and affected individuals respond very well to treatment with oral enzyme replacement alone (Williams et al., 1987). Bacterial overgrowth can cause malabsorption and diarrhoea, however, and in those individuals that do not respond to oral enzymes alone antibiotic therapy may be of value (King and Toskes, 1979). Oral oxytetracycline, metronidazole or tylosin may be effective in improving the clinical response in some of these dogs (Westermarck et al., 1993b). Long-lasting untreated bacterial overgrowth may cause mucosal damage that is only partially reversible following even prolonged antibiotic therapy, and this may explain why some dogs fail to return to normal body weight (King and Toskes, 1981). Whether a predisposition to recurrent development of overgrowth exists after antibiotic therapy is not known.

Glucocorticoid therapy

In those dogs that respond poorly to the above treatments, oral prednisolone (or prednisone) at an initial dose of 2–4 mg kg^{-1} for 7–14 days is often beneficial. Some such cases have lymphocytic–plasmacytic or eosinophilic enteritis. Long-term administration is generally unnecessary, and the drug can be withdrawn over a 1–2 month period.

Prognosis

EPI is generally irreversible and lifelong treatment is required. It has been suggested that enzyme therapy may be withdrawn without return of clinical signs in some affected dogs (Van Kruiningen, 1982). This must be a very rare event judging by the infrequency with which such claims are made, and in such cases the possibility of an initial misdiagnosis must be considered. Nonetheless, given the expense of treatment, it is reasonable to withdraw enzyme supplement for a trial period every six months or so and observe the dog for recurrence of polyphagia and diarrhoea. Pancreatic acinar tissue does have some capacity to regenerate and it is not inconceivable that following either pancreatitis or PAA residual acinar tissue might regenerate sufficiently to prevent clinical signs of EPI. Although treatment will be required for life in most cases, the prognosis is generally good. Some dogs may fail to regain normal body weight, but these animals usually have total resolution of diarrhoea and polyphagia and are quite acceptable as pets.

Treatment of dogs with diabetes mellitus and EPI due to chronic pancreatitis is likely to be more troublesome and expensive. Diabetes mellitus may be particularly difficult to regulate in view of a probable coexistent derangement in the secretion of glucagon and somatostatin. Inflammation in residual pancreatic tissue may cause anorexia and vomiting further complicating regulation of diabetes mellitus.

NEOPLASIA OF THE EXOCRINE PANCREAS

Pancreatic adenocarcinomas occur primarily in older animals and may be acinar or duct cell in origin. Both are uncommon and are particularly rare in cats. Pancreatic carcinoma may be more common in Airedale terriers than other breeds (Anderson and Johnson, 1967; Priester, 1974; Banner et al., 1979; Jubb et al., 1985).

Adenocarcinomas are usually highly malignant tumours, and have often metastasized to the liver and local lymph nodes, or less commonly to the lungs, at the time of presentation. Clinical signs are usually non-specific: weight loss, anorexia, depression, and vomiting. Affected animals are often icteric due to associated obstruction of the bile ducts or widespread hepatic metastasis. Occasionally dogs will present with characteristic signs of diabetes mellitus or EPI due to obstruction of the pancreatic ducts or beta cell destruction (Anderson and Johnson, 1967; Cornelius, 1976; Bright, 1985).

There are usually no specific findings on physical examination but there may be abdominal tenderness and occasionally a cranial abdominal mass is palpable. Abdominal radiographs may suggest pancreatitis or indicate the presence of an anterior mass, whereas thoracic radiographs may reveal pulmonary metastasis.

Ultrasonographic examination may help further define pancreatic abnormalities, and cytological examination of abdominal fluid or of material aspirated from suspect areas may reveal neoplastic cells.

There are no specific laboratory tests for pancreatic carcinoma, and results of routine tests may be misleading. Elevated activities of amylase and lipase are seen in some dogs with pancreatic carcinoma. Hepatic involvement is usually indicated by marked elevations of alkaline phosphatase and bilirubin, with lesser increases in alanine aminotransferase, suggestive of an obstructive hepatopathy (Anderson and Johnson, 1967; Cornelius, 1976). In most cases definitive diagnosis requires exploratory laparotomy. Chronic pancreatitis may grossly resemble pancreatic carcinoma, therefore visual inspection alone may be misleading.

Given the frequency of metastasis at the time of diagnosis the prognosis for animals with carcinomas of the exocrine pancreas is extremely poor. There are no reports of curative therapy, but surgical excision of localized lesions, perhaps in combination with chemotherapy, may be palliative. Therapy with insulin and pancreatic enzymes may be required to treat associated diabetes mellitus and EPI (Anderson and Johnson, 1967; Bright, 1985).

PANCREATIC FLUKES IN CATS

There are several reports of infection with the pancreatic fluke, *Eurytrema procyonis*, in cats (Fox *et al.*, 1981; Roudebush and Schmidt, 1982; Anderson *et al.*, 1987). Associated pathology generally includes pancreatic atrophy and fibrosis that in some cases, together with duct obstruction, may severely decrease exocrine pancreatic secretory capacity. In spite of marked loss of exocrine tissue, however, weight loss and diarrhoea have not been reported, and the infection is usually subclinical.

Infection is often an incidental finding based on observation of characteristic eggs in the faeces. However, one report described an infected cat that had marked inflammatory infiltrates in association with the parasites, and a 2-year history of weight loss and intermittent vomiting, consistent with pancreatitis perhaps progressing to clinical EPI (Anderson *et al.*, 1987). Treatment with fenbendazole has been reported to be effective.

REFERENCES

Abrams, C.K., Hamosh, M., Hubbard, V.S., Dutta, S.K. and Hamosh, P. (1984) Lingual lipase in cystic fibrosis. Quantitation of enzyme activity in the upper small intestine of patients with exocrine pancreatic insufficiency. *Journal of Clinical Investigation* **73**, 374–382.

Adham, N.F., Song, M.K. and Haberfelde, G.C. (1983) Relationship between the functional status of the reticuloendothelial system and the outcome of experimentally induced pancreatitis in young mice. *Gastroenerology* **84**, 461–469.

Alpers, D.H. and Seetharam, B. (1977) Pathophysiology of diseases involving intestinal brush border proteins. *New England Journal of Medicine* **296**, 1047–1050.

Anderson, N.V. (1972) Pancreatitis in dogs. *Veterinary Clinics of North America* **2**, 79–97.

Anderson, N.V. and Johnson, K.H. (1967) Pancreatic carcinoma in the dog. *Journal of the American Veterinary Medical Association* **150**, 286–295.

Anderson, N.V. and Low, D.G. (1965) Juvenile atrophy of the canine pancreas. *Animal Hospital* **1**, 101–109.

Anderson, N.V. and Strafuss, A.C. (1971) Pancreatic disease in dogs and cats. *Journal of the American Veterinary Medical Association* **159**, 885–891.

Anderson, W.I., Georgi, M.E. and Car, B.D. (1987) Pancreatic atrophy and fibrosis associated with *Eurytrema procyonis* in a domestic cat. *Veterinary Record* **120**, 235–236.

Andriulli, A., Masoero, G., Felder, M., Vantini, I., Petrillo, M., Cavallini, G., Bianchi Porro, G., Dobrilla, G. and Verme, G. (1981) Circulating trypsin-like immunoreactivity in chronic pancreatitis. *Digestive Diseases and Sciences* **26**, 532–537.

Andrzejewska, A., Dlugosz, J. and Kurasz, S. (1985) The ultrastructure of the liver in acute experimental pancreatitis in dogs. *Experimental Pathology* **28**, 167–176.

Arvanitakis, C. and Olsen, W.A. (1974) Intestinal mucosal disaccharidases in chronic pancreatitis. *American Journal of Digestive Diseases* **19**, 417–421.

Attix, E., Strombeck, D.R., Wheeldon, E.B. and Sterns, J.S. (1981) Effects of an anticholinergic and a corticosteroid on acute pancreatitis in experimental dogs. *American Journal of Veterinary Research* **42**, 1668–1674.

Balk, M.W., Lang, C.M., White, W.J. and Munger, B.L. (1975) Exocrine pancreatic dysfunction in guinea pigs with diabetes mellitus. *Laboratory Investigation* **32**, 28–32.

Balldin, G. and Ohlsson, K. (1979) Trasylol prevents trypsin-induced shock in dogs. *Hoppe-Seyler's Zeitschrift für Physiologische Chemie* **360**, 651–656.

Balldin, G., Lasson, Å. and Ohlsson, K. (1984) Aprotinin turn-over studies in dog and in man with severe acute pancreatitis. *Hoppe-Seyler's Zeitschrift für Physiologische Chemie* **365**, 1417–1423.

Banner, B.F., Alroy, J. and Kipnis, R.M. (1979) Acinar cell carcinoma of the pancreas in a cat. *Veterinary Pathology* **16**, 543–547.

Barbezat, G.O. and Hansen, J.D.L. (1968) The exocrine pancreas and protein-calorie malnutrition. *Pediatrics* **42**, 77–92.

Batt, R.M. and Morgan, J.O. (1982) Role of serum folate and vitamin B_{12} concentrations in the differentiation of small intestinal abnormalities in the dog. *Research in Veterinary Science* **32**, 17–22.

Batt, R.M., Bush, B.M. and Peters, T.J. (1979) Biochemical changes in the jejunal mucosa of dogs with naturally occurring exocrine pancreatic insufficiency. *Gut* **20**, 709–715.

Batt, R.M., Horadagoda, N.U., McLean, L., Morton, D.B. and Simpson, K.W. (1989) Identification and characterization of a pancreatic intrinsic factor in the dog. *American Journal of Physiology* **256**, G517–G523.

Blum, A.L. and Linscheer, W.G. (1970) Lipase in canine gastric juice. *Proceedings of the Society for Experimental Biology and Medicine* **135**, 565–568.

Boari, A., Williams, D.A. and Famigli-Bergamini, P. (1994) Observations on exocrine pancreatic insufficiency in a family of English setter dogs. *Journal of Small Animal Practice* **34**, 247–250.

Bockman, D.E. (1978) Anastomosing tubular arrangement of dog exocrine pancreas. *Cell and Tissue Research* **189**, 497–500.

Borgström, A. and Lasson, Å (1984) Trypsin–alpha$_1$-protease inhibitor complexes in serum and clinical course of acute pancreatitis. *Scandinavian Journal of Gastroenterology* **19**, 1119–1122.

Borgström, A. and Ohlsson, K. (1980) Immunoreactive trypsins in sera from dogs before and after induction of experimental pancreatitis. *Hoppe-Seyler's Zeitschrift für Physiologische Chemie* **361**, 625–631.

Bradley, E.L. (1989) Antibiotics in acute pancreatitis. Current status and future directions. *American Journal of Surgery* **158**, 472–477.

Bright, J.M. (1985) Pancreatic adenocarcinoma in a dog with maldigestion syndrome. *Journal of the American Veterinary Medical Association* **187**, 420–421.

Brodrick, J.W., Geokas, M.C., Largman, C., Fassett, M. and Johnson, J.H. (1979) Molecular forms of immunoreactive pancreatic cationic trypsin in pancreatitis patient sera. *American Journal of Physiology* **237**, E474–E480.

Canfield, P.J., Fairburn, A.J. and Church, D.B. (1983) Effect of various diets on fecal analysis in normal dogs. *Research in Veterinary Science* **34**, 24–27.

Case, R.M. and Argent, B.E. (1993) Pancreatic duct cell secretion: control and mechanisms of transport. In: *The Pancreas: Biology, Pathobiology and Disease*, 2nd edn (eds V.L.W. Go, E.P. DiMagno, J.D. Gardner, E. Lebenthal, H.A. Reber and G.A. Scheele). Raven Press, New York, pp. 301–350.

Coffin, D.L. and Thordal-Christensen, A. (1953) The clinical and some pathological aspects of pancreatic disease in dogs. *Veterinary Medicine* **48**, 193–198.

Cornelius, L.M. (1976) Laboratory diagnosis of acute pancreatitis and pancreatic adenocarcinoma. *Veterinary Clinics of North America: Small Animal Practice* **6**, 671–678.

Cuschieri, A., Cumming, J.R.G., Meehan, S.E and Mackie, C.R. (1983) Treatment of acute pancreatitis with fresh frozen plasma. *British Journal of Surgery* **70**, 710–712.

Dalton, J.R.F. and Hill, F.W.G. (1972) A procedure for the examination of the liver and pancreas in dogs. *Journal of Small Animal Practice* **13**, 527–530.

de Bruijne, J.J., Altszuler, N., Hampshire, J., Visser, T.J. and Hackeng, W.H.L. (1981) Fat mobilization and plasma hormone levels in fasted dogs. *Metabolism* **30**, 190–194.

Denny, H.R. and Lucke, J.N. (1972) A case of acute pancreatic necrosis in the dog. *Journal of Small Animal Practice* **13**, 545–551.

Dimagno, E.P. (1979) Medical treatment of pancreatic insufficiency. *Mayo Clinic Proceedings* **54**, 435–442.

Dressel, T.D., Goodale, R.L., Arneson, M.A. and Borner, J.W. (1979) Pancreatitis as a complication of anticholinesterase insecticide intoxication. *Annals of Surgery* **189**, 199–204.

Duffell, S.J. (1975) Some aspects of pancreatic disease in the cat. *Journal of Small Animal Practice* **16**, 365–374.

Durie, P.R., Gaskin, K.J., Ogilvie, J.E., Smith, C.R., Forstner, G.G. and Largman, C. (1985) Serial alterations in the forms of immunoreactive pancreatic cationic trypsin in plasma from patients with acute pancreatitis. *Journal of Pediatric Gastroenterology and Nutrition* **4**, 199–207.

Dutta, S.K. and Hlasko, J. (1985) Dietary fiber in pancreatic disease: effect of high fiber diet on fat malabsorption in pancreatic insufficiency and *in vitro* study of the interaction of dietary fibers with pancreatic enzymes. *American Journal of Clinical Nutrition* **41**, 517–525.

Eppig, J.J. and Leiter, E.H. (1977) Exocrine pancreatic insufficiency syndrome in CBA/J mice. Ultrastructural study. *American Journal of Pathology* **86**, 17–30.

Feldman, B.F., Attix, E.A., Strombeck, D.R. and O'Neill, S. (1981) Biochemical and coagulation changes in a canine model of acute necrotizing pancreatitis. *American Journal of Veterinary Research* **42**, 805–808.

Fell, B.F., King, T.P. and Davies, N.T. (1982) Pancreatic atrophy in copper-deficient rats: histochemical and ultrastructural evidence of a selective effect on acinar cells. *Histochemical Journal* **14**, 665–680.

Fernández-del Castillo, C., Schmidt, J., Rattner, D.W., Lewandrowski, K., Compton, C.C., Jehanli, A., Patel, G., Hermon-Taylor, J. and Warshaw, A.L. (1992) Generation and possible significance of trypsinogen activation peptides in experimental acute pancreatitis in the rat. *Pancreas* **7**, 263–270.

Fox, J.N., Mosley, J.G., Vogler, G.A., Austin, J.L. and Reber, H.A. (1981) Pancreatic function in domestic cats with pancreatic fluke infection. *Journal of the American Veterinary Medical Association* **178**, 58–60

Fyfe, J.C. (1993) Feline intrinsic factor (IF) is pancreatic in origin and mediates ileal cobalamin (CBL) absorption. *Journal of Veterinary Internal Medicine* **7**, 133.

Garvey, M.S. and Zawie, D.A. (1984) Feline pancreatic disease. *Veterinary Clinics of North America: Small Animal Practice* **14**, 1231–1246.

Geokas, M.C., Largman, C., Durie, P.R., Brodrick, J.W., Ray, S.B., O'Rourke, M. and Vollmer, J. (1981) Immunoreactive forms of cationic trypsin in plasma and ascitic fluid of dogs with experimental pancreatitis. *American Journal of Pathology* **105**, 31–39.

Geokas, M.C., Reidelberger, R., O'Rourke, M., Passaro, E. and Largman, C. (1982) Plasma pancreatic trypsinogens in chronic renal failure and after nephrectomy. *American Journal of Physiology* **242**, 177–182.

Geokas, M.C., Baltaxe, H.A., Banks, P.A., Silva, J. and Frey, C.F. (1985) Acute pancreatitis. *Annals of Internal Medicine* **103**, 86–100.

Gibbs, C., Denny, H.R., Minter, H.M. and Pearson, H. (1972) Radiological features of inflammatory conditions of the canine pancreas. *Journal of Small Animal Practice* **13**, 531–544.

Goldstein, D.A., Llach, F. and Massry, S.G. (1976) Acute renal failure in patients with acute pancreatitis. *Archives of Internal Medicine* **136**, 1363–1365.

Goodhead, B. (1971) Importance of nutrition in the pathogenesis of experimental pancreatitis in the dog. *Archives of Surgery* **103**, 724–727.

Grendell, J.H. (1983) Nutrition and absorption in diseases of the pancreas. *Clinics in Gastroenterology* **12**, 551–562.

Grendell, J.H. and Cello, J.P. (1983) Chronic pancreatitis. In: *Gastrointestinal Disease*, 3rd edn (eds M.H. Sleisenger and J.S. Fordtran). W.B. Saunders, Philadelphia, pp. 1485–1514.

Greve, T. and Anderson, N.V. (1973) The high-dose, intravenous glucose tolerance test (H-IVGTT) in dogs. *Nordisk Veterinaermedicin* **25**, 436–445.

Gudgeon, A.M., Heath, D.I., Hurley, P., Jehanli, A., Patel, G., Wilson, C., Shenkin, A., Austen, B.M., Imrie, C.W. and Hermon-Taylor, J. (1990) Trypsinogen activation peptide assay in the early prediction of severity of acute pancreatitis. *Lancet* **335**, 4.

Hall, E.J., Bond, P.M., McLean, C., Batt, R.M. and McLean, L. (1991) A survey of the diagnosis and treatment of canine exocrine pancreatic insufficiency. *Journal of Small Animal Practice* **32**, 613–619.

Hansen, J.F. and Carpenter, R.H. (1983) Fatal acute systemic anaphylaxis and hemorrhagic pancreatitis following asparaginase treatment in a dog. *Journal of the American Animal Hospital Association* **19**, 977–980.

Hasholt, J. (1972) Atrophy of the pancreas in budgerigars. *Nordisk Veterinaermedicin* **24**, 458–461.

Hawkins, E.C., Meric, S.M., Washabau, R.J., Feldman, E.C. and Turrel, J.M. (1986) Digestion of bentiromide and absorption of xylose in healthy cats and absorption of xylose in cats with infiltrative intestinal disease. *American Journal of Veterinary Research* **47**, 567–569.

Hermon-Taylor, J. and Heywood, G.D. (1985) A rational approach to the specific chemotherapy of pancreatitis. *Scandinavian Journal of Gastroenterology* **117**, 39–46.

Hill, F.W.G. (1972) Malabsorption syndrome in the dog: a study of thirty-eight cases. *Journal of Small Animal Practice* **13**, 575–594.

Hill, F.W.G. and Kidder, D.E. (1972) The oral glucose tolerance test in canine pancreatic malabsorption. *British Veterinary Journal* **128**, 207–214.

Hill, F.W.G., Osborne, A.D. and Kidder, D.E. (1971) Pancreatic degenerative atrophy in dogs. *Journal of Comparative Pathology* **81**, 321–330.

Hill, R.C. and Van Winkle, T.J. (1993) Acute necrotizing pancreatitis and acute suppurative pancreatitis in the cat. A retrospective study of 40 cases (1976–1989). *Journal of Veterinary Internal Medicine* **7**, 25–33.

Holroyd, J.B. (1968) Canine exocrine pancreatic disease. *Journal of Small Animal Practice* **9**, 269–281.

Holst, J.J. (1993) Neural regulation of pancreatic exocrine function. In: *The Pancreas: Biology, Pathobiology and Disease*, 2nd edn (Eds V.L.W. Go, E.P. DiMagno, J.D. Gardner, E. Lebenthal, H.A. Reber and G.A. Scheele). Raven Press, New York, pp. 381–402.

Holzworth, J. and Coffin, D.L. (1953) Pancreatic insufficiency and diabetes mellitus in a cat. *Cornell Veterinarian* **43**, 502–512.

Hoskins, J.D., Turk, J.R. and Turk, M.A. (1982) Feline pancreatic insufficiency. *Veterinary Medicine/Small Animal Clinician* **77**, 1745–1748.

Itoh, Z., Ryuichi, H. and Katsutoshi, M. (1980) Biphasic secretory response of exocrine pancreas to feeding. *American Journal of Physiology* **238**, G332–G337.

Izquierdo, R., Sandberg, L., Nora, M.O., Squillaci, G., Hoppensteadt, D., Walenga, J., Fareed, J. and Prinz, R.A. (1984) Comparative study of protease inhibitors on coagulation abnormalities in canine pancreatitis. *Journal of Surgical Research* **36**, 606–613.

Jacobs, R.M., Hall, R.L. and Rogers, W.A. (1982) Isoamylases in clinically normal and diseased dogs. *Veterinary Clinical Pathology* **11**, 26–32.

Jacobs, R.M., Murtaugh, R.J. and DeHoff, W.D. (1985) Review of the clinicopathological findings of acute pancreatitis in the dog: use of an experimental model. *Journal of the American Animal Hospital Association* **21**, 795–800.

Jubb, K.V.F., Kennedy, P.C. and Palmer, N. (1985) The pancreas. In: *Pathology of Domestic Animals*, 3rd edn (Eds K.V.F. Jubb, P.C. Kennedy and N. Palmer). Harcourt Brace Jovanovich, Orlando, pp. 313–327.

Karanjia, N.D., Widdison, A.L., Jehanli, A., Hermon-

Taylor, J. and Reber, H.A. (1993) Assay of trypsinogen activation in the cat experimental model of acute pancreatitis. *Pancreas* **8**, 189–195.

Kark, J.A., Victor, M., Hines, J.D. and Harris, J.W. (1974) Nutritional vitamin B_{12} deficiency in rhesus monkeys. *American Journal of Clinical Nutrition* **27**, 470–478.

Keane, F.B., Dozois, R.R., Go, V.L.W. and Dimagno, E.P. (1981) Interdigestive canine pancreatic juice composition and pancreatic reflux and pancreatic sphincter anatomy. *Digestive Diseases and Sciences* **26**, 577–584.

Kelly, D.F., Baggot, D.G. and Gaskell, C.J. (1975) Jaundice in the cat associated with inflammation of the biliary tract and pancreas. *Journal of Small Animal Practice* **16**, 163–172.

Kenny, J.A. and Maroux, S. (1982) Topology of microvillar membrane hydrolases of kidney and intestine. *Physiological Reviews* **62**, 91–128.

Keynes, M.W. (1980) A nonpancreatic source of the proteolytic enzyme amidase and bacteriology in experimental acute pancreatitis. *Annals of Surgery* **191**, 187–199.

King, C.E. and Toskes, P.P. (1979) Small intestine bacterial overgrowth. *Gastroenterology* **76**, 1035–1055.

King, C.E. and Toskes, P.P. (1981) Protein-losing enteropathy in the human and experimental rat blind loop syndrome. *Gastroenterology* **80**, 504–509.

Kitchell, B.E., Strombeck, D.R., Cullen, J. and Harrold, D. (1986) Clinical and pathologic changes in experimentally induced acute pancreatitis in cats. *American Journal of Veterinary Research* **47**, 1170–1173.

Kleine, L.J. and Hornbuckle, W.E. (1978) Acute pancreatitis: the radiographic findings in 182 dogs. *Journal of American Veterinary Radiological Society* **19**, 102–106.

Kornegay, J.N. (1982) Hypocalcemia in dogs. *Compendium on Continuing Education for the Practicing Veterinarian* **4**, 103–112.

Kwong, W.K.L., Seetharam, B. and Alpers, D.H. (1978) Effect of exocrine pancreatic insufficiency on small intestine in the mouse. *Gastroenterology* **74**, 1277–1282.

Langweiler, M., Schultz, R.D. and Sheffy, B.E. (1981) Effect of vitamin E deficiency on the proliferative response of canine lymphocytes. *American Journal of Veterinary Research* **42**, 1681–1685.

Lankisch, P.G. (1984) Acute and chronic pancreatitis: an update on management. *Drugs* **28**, 554–564.

Largman, C., Reidelberger, R.D. and Tsukamoto, H. (1986) Correlation of trypsin–plasma inhibitor complexes with mortality in experimental pancreatitis in rats. *Digestive Diseases and Sciences* **31**, 961–969.

Laskowski, M. and Kato, I. (1980) Protein inhibitors of proteinases. *Annual Review of Biochemistry* **49**, 593–626.

Lasson, Å. (1984) Acute pancreatitis in man. A clinical and biochemical study of pathophysiology and treatment. *Scandinavian Journal of Gastroenterology* [Supplement] **99**, 1–57.

Lees, G.E., Suter, P.F. and Johnson, G.C. (1978) Pulmonary edema in a dog with acute pancreatitis and cardiac disease. *Journal of the American Veterinary Medical Association* **172**, 690–696.

Leiter, E.H. and Cunliff-Beamer, T. (1977) Exocrine pancreatic insufficiency syndrome in CBA/J mice. *Gastroenterology* **73**, 260–266.

Lerner, A. and Lebenthal, E. (1993) Hereditary diseases of the pancreas. In: *The Pancreas: Biology, Pathobiology and Disease*, 2nd edn (Eds V.L.W. Go, E.P. DiMagno, J.D. Gardner, E. Lebenthal, H.A. Reber and G.A. Scheele). Raven Press, New York, pp. 1083–1094.

Levenson, S.M., Kan, D., Gruber, C., Crowley, L., Jaffe, E., Nakao, K., Geever, E. and Seifter, E. (1971) Strange hemolytic anemia and pancreatic acinar atrophy and fibrosis. *Federation Proceedings* **30**, 1785–1802.

Mallory, A. and Kern, F. (1980) Drug-induced pancreatitis: a critical review. *Gastroenterology* **78**, 813–820.

Marcoullis, G. and Rothenberg, S.P. (1981) Intrinsic factor-mediated intestinal absorption of cobalamin in the dog. *American Journal of Physiology* **241**, G294–299.

McMahon, M.J., Bowen, M., Mayer, A.D. and Cooper, E.H. (1984) Relation of α_2 macroglobulin and other antiproteases to the clinical features of acute pancreatitis. *American Journal of Surgery* **147**, 164–170.

Mia, A.S., Koger, H.D. and Tierney, M.M. (1978) Serum values of amylase and pancreatic lipase in health mature dogs and dogs with experimental pancreatitis. *American Journal of Veterinary Research* **39**, 965–969.

Mizunuma, T., Kawamura, S. and Kismino, Y. (1984) Effects of injecting excess arginine on rat pancreas. *Journal of Nutrition* **114**, 467–471.

Moore, R.W. and Withrow, S.J. (1982) Gastrointestinal hemorrhage and pancreatitis associated with intervertebral disk disease in the dog. *Journal of the American Veterinary Medical Association* **180**, 1443–1447.

Moossa, A.R. and Altorki, N. (1983) Pancreatic biopsy. *Surgical Clinics of North America* **63**, 1205–1214.

Mulvany, M.H., Feinberg, C.K. and Tilson, D.L. (1982) Clinical characterization of acute necrotizing pancreatitis. *Compendium on Continuing Education for the Practicing Veterinarian* **4**, 394–405.

Murtaugh, R.J. and Jacobs, R.M. (1985a) Serum amylase and isoamylases and their origins in healthy dogs and dogs with experimentally induced acute pancreatitis. *American Journal of Veterinary Research* **46**, 742–747.

Murtaugh, R.J. and Jacobs, R.M. (1985b) Serum antiprotease concentrations in dogs with spontaneous and experimentally induced acute pancreatitis. *American Journal of Veterinary Research* **46**, 80–83.

Murtaugh, R.J., Herring, D.S., Jacobs, R.M. and DeHoff, W.D. (1985) Pancreatic ultrasonography in dogs with experimentally induced acute pancreatitis. *Veterinary Radiology* **26**, 27–32.

Neuman, N.B. (1975) Acute hemorrhagic pancreatitis associated with iatrogenic hypercalcemia in a dog. *Journal of the American Veterinary Medical Association* **166**, 381–382.

Niessen, K.H., Konig, J., Molitor, M. and Neef, B. (1983) Studies on the quality of pancreatic preparations: enzyme content, prospective bioavailability, bile acid pattern, and contamination with purines. *European Journal of Pediatrics* **141**, 23–29.

Nyland, T.G., Mulvany, M.H. and Strombeck, D.R. (1983) Ultrasonic features of experimentally induced acute pancreatitis in the dog. *Veterinary Radiology* **24**, 260–266.

Ohlsson, K., Ganrot, P.O. and Laurell, C.B. (1971) In vivo interaction between trypsin and some plasma proteins in relation to tolerance to intravenous infusion of trypsin in dogs. *Acta Chirurgica Scandinavica* **137**, 113–121.

Orci, L. (1984) Patterns of cellular and subcellular organization in the endocrine pancreas. *Journal of Endocrinology* **102**, 3–11.

Owens, J.M., Drazner, F.H. and Gilbertson, S.R. (1975) Pancreatic disease in the cat. *Journal of the American Animal Hospital Association* **11**, 83–89.

Parent, J. (1982) Effects of dexamethasone on pancreatic tissue and on serum amylase and lipase activities in dogs. *Journal of the American Veterinary Medical Association* **180**, 743–746.

Perry, L.A., Williams, D.A., Pidgeon, G. and Boosinger, T.R. (1991) Exocrine pancreatic insufficiency with associated coagulopathy in a cat. *Journal of the American Animal Hospital Association.* **27**, 109–114.

Pfister, K., Rossi, G.L., Freudiger, U. and Bigler, B. (1980) Morphological studies in dogs with chronic pancreatic insufficiency. *Virchows Archiv. A, Pathological Anatomy and Histopathology* **386**, 91–105.

Pidgeon, G. (1987) Exocrine pancreatic disease in the dog and cat. *Companion Animal Practice* **1**, 67–71.

Pidgeon, G. and Strombeck, D.R. (1982) Evaluation of treatment for pancreatic exocrine insufficiency in dogs with ligated pancreatic ducts. *American Journal of Veterinary Research* **43**, 461–464.

Pitchumoni, C.S. and Scheele, G.A. (1993) Interdependence of nutrition and exocrine pancreatic function. In: *The Pancreas: Biology, Pathobiology and Disease*, 2nd edn (Eds V.L.W. Go, E.P. DiMagno, J.D. Gardner, E. Lebenthal, H.A. Reber, and G.A. Scheele). Raven Press, New York, pp. 449–473.

Polzin, D.J., Osborne, C.A., Stevens, J.B. and Hayden, D.W. (1983) Serum amylase and lipase activities in dogs with chronic primary renal failure. *American Journal of Veterinary Research* **44**, 404–410.

Port, C.D., Maschgan, E.R., Pond, J., Kirschner, B., Poticha, S. and Scarpelli, D.G. (1981) Chronic exocrine pancreatic insufficiency in 2 Indian lions (*Panthera leo persica*). *Journal of Comparative Pathology* **91**, 483–491.

Priester, W.A. (1974) Data from eleven United States and Canadian colleges of veterinary medicine on pancreatic carcinoma in domestic animals. *Cancer Research* **34**, 1372–1375.

Raiha, M. and Westermarck, E. (1989) The signs of pancreatic degenerative atrophy in dogs and the role of external factors in the etiology of the disease. *Acta Veterinaria Scandinavica* **30**, 447–452.

Rimaila-Pärnänen, E. and Westermarck, E. (1982) Pancreatic degenerative atrophy and chronic pancreatitis in dogs: a comparative study of 60 cases. *Acta Veterinaria Scandinavica* **23**, 400–406.

Rinderknecht, H. (1993) Pancreatic secretory enzymes. In: *The Pancreas: Biology, Pathobiology and Disease*, 2nd edn (Eds V.L.W. Go, E.P. DiMagno, J.D. Gardner, E. Lebenthal, H.A. Reber and G.A. Scheele). Raven Press, New York, pp. 219–251.

Rogers, W.A., O'Dorisio, T.M., Johnson, S.E., Cataland, S., Stradley, R.P. and Sherding, R.G. (1983) Postprandial release of gastric inhibitory polypeptide (GIP) and pancreatic polypeptide in dogs with pancreatic acinar atrophy. *Digestive Diseases and Sciences* **28**, 345–349.

Rothenbacher, H. and Lindquist, W.D. (1963) Liver cirrhosis and pancreatitis in a cat infected with *Amplimerus pseudofeliseus*. *Journal of the American Veterinary Medical Association* **143**, 1099–1102.

Roudebush, P. and Schmidt, D.A. (1982) Fenbendazole for treatment of pancreatic fluke infection in a cat. *Journal of the American Veterinary Medical Association* **180**, 545–546.

Rutgers, H.C., Herring, D.S. and Orton, E.C. (1985) Pancreatic pseudocyst associated with acute pancreatitis in a dog: ultrasonographic diagnosis. *Journal of the American Animal Hospital Association* **21**, 411–416.

Salazar de Sousa, J. (1984) Malnutrition and small intestinal mucosa. *Journal of Pediatric Gastroenterology and Nutrition* **3**, 321–322.

Salisbury, S.K., Lantz, G.C., Nelson, R.W. and Kazacos, E.A. (1988) Pancreatic abscess in dogs: six cases (1978–1986). *Journal of the American Veterinary Medical Association* **193**, 1104–1108.

Sanfey, H., Bulkley, G.B. and Cameron, J.L. (1984) The role of oxygen-derived free radicals in the pathogenesis of acute pancreatitis. *Annals of Surgery* **200**, 405–413.

Sanfey, H., Broe, P.J. and Cameron, J.L. (1985) Experimental ischemic pancreatitis: treatment with albumin. *American Journal of Surgery* **150**, 297–300.

Sarner, M. (1993) Pancreatitis definitions and classification. In: *The Pancreas: Biology, Pathobiology and Disease*, 2nd edn (Eds V.L.W. Go, E.P. DiMagno, J.D. Gardner, E. Lebenthal, H.A. Reber and G.A. Scheele). Raven Press, New York, pp. 575–580.

Sateri, H. (1975) Investigations on the exocrine pancreatic function in dogs suffering from chronic exocrine pancreatic insufficiency. *Acta Veterinaria Scandinavica Supplementum* **53**, 1–86.

Schaer, M. (1979) A clinicopathologic survey of acute

pancreatitis in 30 dogs and 5 cats. *Journal of the American Animal Hospital Association* **15**, 681–687

Schaer, M. and Holloway, S. (1991) Diagnosing acute pancreatitis in the cat. *Veterinary Medicine* **1986**, 782–795.

Scheele, G.A. and Kern, H.F. (1993) Cellular compartmentation, protein processing, and secretion in the exocrine pancreas. In: *The Pancreas: Biology, Pathobiology and Diseases*, 2nd edn (Eds V.L.W. Go, E.P. DiMagno, J.D. Gardner, E. Lebenthal, H.A. Reber and G.A. Scheele). Raven Press, New York, pp. 121–150.

Schmidt, J., Fernandez-Del Castillo, C., Rattner, D.W., Lewandrowski, K., Compton, C.C. and Warshaw, A.L. (1992) Trypsinogen-activation peptides in experimental rat pancreatitis: prognostic implications and histopathologic correlates. *Gastroenterology* **103**, 1009–1016.

Schummer, A., Nickel, R. and Sack, W.O. (1979) The alimentary canal general and comparative. In: *The Viscera of the Domestic Mammals*. Springer-Verlag, New York, Heidelberg, Berlin, pp. 119–136.

Sherding, R.G., Stradley, R.P., Rogers, W.A. and Johnson, S.E. (1982) Bentiromide:xylose test in healthy cats. *American Journal of Veterinary Research* **43**, 2272–2273.

Sherman, P., Forstner, J., Roomi, N., Khatri, I. and Forstner, G. (1985a) Mucin depletion in the intestine of malnourished rats. *American Journal of Physiology* **248**, G418–G423.

Sherman, P., Wesley, A. and Forstner, G. (1985b) Sequential disaccharidase loss in rat intestinal blind loops: impact of malnutrition. *American Journal of Physiology* **248**, G626–G632.

Simpson, J.W., Doxey, D.L. and Brown, R. (1984) Serum isoamylase values in normal dogs and dogs with exocrine pancreatic insufficiency. *Veterinary Research Communications* **8**, 303–308.

Simpson, K.W., Batt, R.M., McLean, L. and Morton, D.B. (1989a) Circulating concentrations of trypsin-like immunoreactivity and activities of lipase and amylase after pancreatic duct ligation in dogs. *American Journal of Veterinary Research* **50**, 629–632.

Simpson, K.W., Morton, D.B. and Batt, R.M. (1989b) Effect of exocrine pancreatic insufficiency on cobalamin absorption in dogs. *American Journal of Veterinary Research* **50**, 1233–1236.

Simpson, K.W., Morton, D.B., Sorensen, S.H., McLean, L., Riley, J.E. and Batt, R.M. (1989c) Biochemical changes in the jejunal mucosa of dogs with exocrine pancreatic insufficiency following pancreatic duct ligation. *Research in Veterinary Science* **47**, 338–345.

Simpson, K.W., Simpson, J.W., Lake, S., Morton, D.B. and Batt, R.M. (1991) Effect of pancreatectomy on plasma activities of amylase, isoamylase, lipase and trypsin-like immunoreactivity in dogs. *Research in Veterinary Science* **51**, 78–82.

Simpson, K.W., Shiroma, J.T., Biller, D.S., Wicks, J., Johnson, S.E., Dimski, D. and Chew, D. (1994) Ante mortem diagnosis of pancreatitis in four cats. *Journal of Small Animal Practice* **35**, 93–99.

Singer, M.V. (1993) Neurohormonal control of pancreatic enzyme secretion in animals. In: *The Pancreas: Biology, Pathobiology and Disease*, 2nd edn (eds V.L.W. Go, E.P. DiMagno, J.D. Gardner, E. Lebenthal, H.A. Reber and G.A. Scheele). Raven Press, New York, pp. 425–448.

Slaff, J., Jacobson, D., Tillman, C.R., Curington, C. and Toskes, P. (1984) Protease-specific suppression of pancreatic exocrine secretion. *Gastroenterology* **87**, 44–52.

Smart, M.E., Downey, R.S. and Stockdale, P.H.G. (1973) Toxoplasmosis in a cat associated with cholangitis and progressive pancreatitis. *Canadian Veterinary Journal* **14**, 313–316.

Sokol, R.J., Farrell, M.K., Heubi, J.E., Tsang, R.C. and Balistreri, W.F. (1983) Comparison of vitamin E and 25-hydroxyvitamin D absorption during childhood cholestasis. *Journal of Pediatrics* **103**, 712–717.

Steer, M.L. and Meldolesi, J. (1987) The cell biology of experimental pancreatitis. *New England Journal of Medicine* **316**, 144–150.

Steer, M.L. and Saluja, A.K. (1993) Experimental acute pancreatitis: studies of the early events that lead to cell injury. In: *The Pancreas: Biology, Pathobiology and Disease*, 2nd edn (Eds V.L.W. Go, E.P. DiMagno, J.D. Gardner, E. Lebenthal, H.A. Reber and G.A. Scheele). Raven Press, New York, pp. 489–500.

Stickle, J.E., Carlton, W.W. and Boon, G.D. (1980) Isoamylases in clinically normal dogs. *American Journal of Veterinary Research* **41**, 506–509.

Strombeck, D.R. (1978) New method for evaluation of chymotrypsin deficiency in dogs. *Journal of the American Veterinary Medical Association* **173**, 1319–1323.

Strombeck, D.R., Farver, T. and Kaneko, J.J. (1981) Serum amylase and lipase activities in the diagnosis of pancreatitis in dogs. *American Journal of Veterinary Research* **42**, 1966–1970.

Suter, P.F. and Olsson, S.E. (1969) Traumatic hemorrhagic pancreatitis in the cat: a report with emphasis on the radiological diagnosis. *Journal of the American Veterinary Radiology Society* **10**, 4–11.

Tangner, C.H., Turrell, J.M. and Hobson, H.P. (1982) Complications associated with proximal duodenal resection and cholecystoduodenostomy in two cats. *Veterinary Surgery* **11**, 60–64.

Vaillant, C., Batt, R.M. and Williams, D.A. (1983) Regulatory peptide abnormalities in dogs with pancreatic acinar atrophy. *Regulatory Peptide* **7**, 304.

Vaillant, C., Giraud, A. and Williams, D.A. (1984) Pancreatic enkephalin immunoreactivity in canine pancreatic acinar atropy. *Digestive Diseases and Sciences* **29**, 92S.

Van Kruiningen, H.J. (1982) Pancreatic atrophy. In: *Comparative Gastroenterology*. Charles C. Thomas, Springfield, Illinois, pp. 42–64.

Wagner, A.E. and Macy, D.W. (1982) Nephelometric determination of serum amylase and lipase in naturally occurring azotemia in the dog. *American Journal of Veterinary Research* **43**, 697–699.

Watson, A.D.J., Church, D.B., Middleton, D.J. and Rothwell, T.L.W. (1981) Weight loss in cats which eat well. *Journal of Small Animal Practice* **22**, 473–482.

Weber, V. and Freudiger, U. (1977) Erbanalytische untersuchungen uber die chronische exokrine pankreasinsuffizienz geim deutschen schafermund. *Schweizer Archiv für Tierheilkunde* **119**, 157–163.

Wendt, P., Fritsh, A., Schulz, F., Wunderlich, G. and Blumel, G. (1984) Proteinases and inhibitors in plasma and peritoneal exudate in acute pancreatitis. *Hepato-Gastroenterology* **31**, 277–281.

Westermarck, E. (1980) The hereditary nature of canine pancreatic degenerative atrophy in the German Shepherd dog. *Acta Veterinaria Scandinavica* **21**, 389–394.

Westermarck, E. (1982) The diagnosis of pancreatic degenerative atrophy in dogs: a practical method. *Acta Veterinaria Scandinavica* **23**, 197–203.

Westermarck, E. and Rimaila-Pärnänen, E. (1983) Serum phospholipase A$_2$ in canine acute pancreatitis. *Acta Veterinaria Scandinavica* **24**, 477–487.

Westermarck, E. and Sandholm, M. (1980) Fecal hydrolase activity as determined by radial enzyme diffusion: a new method for detecting pancreatic dysfunction in the dog. *Research in Veterinary Science* **28**, 341–346.

Westermarck, E., Wiberg, M. and Junttila, J. (1990) Role of feeding in the treatment of dogs with pancreatic degenerative atrophy. *Acta Veterinaria Scandinavica* **31**, 325–331.

Westermarck, E., Batt, R.M., Vaillant, C. and Wiberg, M. (1993a) Sequential study of pancreatic structure and function during development of pancreatic acinar atrophy in a German Shepherd dog. *American Journal of Veterinary Research* **54**, 1088–1094.

Westermarck, E., Myllys, V. and Aho, M. (1993b) Effect of treatment on the jejunal and colonic bacterial flora of dogs with exocrine pancreatic insufficiency. *Pancreas* **8**, 559–562.

Williams, D.A. (1985) Studies on the diagnosis and pathophysiology of canine exocrine pancreatic insufficiency. PhD Thesis, University of Liverpool, UK.

Williams, D.A. (1989) Exocrine pancreatic disease. In: *Textbook of Veterinary Internal Medicine*, 3rd edn (Ed. S.J. Ettinger). W.B. Saunders, Philadelphia, pp. 1528–1554.

Williams, D.A. (1993) Exocrine pancreatic insufficiency. *Waltham Focus* **2**, 9–14.

Williams, D.A. and Batt, R.M. (1986) Reversible intravenous glucose intolerance in canine exocrine pancreatic insufficiency. *Proceedings of the Fourth Annual Veterinary Medicine Forum of the ACVIM*, Washington, DC, pp. 14–19.

Williams, D.A. and Batt, R.M. (1988) Sensitivity and specificity of radioimmunoassay of serum trypsin-like immunoreactivity for the diagnosis of canine exocrine pancreatic insufficiency. *Journal of the American Veterinary Medical Association* **192**, 195–201.

Williams, D.A. and Reed, S.D. (1990) Comparison of methods for assay of fecal proteolytic activity. *Veterinary Clinical Pathology* **19**, 20–24.

Williams, D.A., Batt, R.M. and McLean, L. (1985a) Reversible impairment of protein synthesis may contribute to jejunal abnormalities in exocrine pancreatic insufficiency. *Clinical Science* **68**, 37P

Williams, D.A., Jacobs, R.M. and Murtaugh, R.J. (1985b) Comments on isoamylases (letters). *American Journal of Veterinary Research* **46**, 1598–1599.

Williams, D.A., Batt, R.M. and McLean, L. (1987) Bacterial overgrowth in the duodenum of dogs with exocrine pancreatic insufficiency. *Journal of the American Veterinary Medical Association* **191**, 201–206.

Williams, D.A., Reed, S.D. and Perry, L.A. (1990) Fecal proteolytic activity in clinically normal cats and in a cat with exocrine pancreatic insufficiency. *Journal of the American Veterinary Medical Association* **197**, 210–212.

Williams, J.A. and Goldfine, I.D. (1993) The insulin–acinar relationship. In: *The Pancreas: Biology, Pathobiology and Disease*, 2nd edn (Eds V.L.W. Go, E.P. DiMagno, J.D. Gardner, E. Lebenthal, H.A. Reber and G.A. Scheele). Raven Press, New York, pp. 789–802.

Williams, J.A. and Yule, D.I. (1993) Stimulus-secretion coupling in pancreatic acinar cells. In: *The Pancreas: Biology, Pathobiology and Disease*, 2nd edn (Eds V.L.W. Go, E.P. DiMagno, J.D. Gardner, E. Lebenthal, H.A. Reber and G.A. Scheele). Raven Press, New York, pp. 167–189.

39

Diseases of the Endocrine System

M. E. Herrtage

Disorders of the pituitary gland	526	Disorders of the adrenal glands	544
Disorders of the thyroid gland	534	Disorders of the endocrine pancreas	561
Disorders of the parathyroid glands	541		

DISORDERS OF THE PITUITARY GLAND

Anatomy and physiology

The hypothalamus and pituitary form a complex functional unit that controls much of the endocrine system. The pituitary gland is a small ovoid structure which lies in a distinct fossa, the sella turcica, within the sphenoid bone just ventral to the hypothalamus. The pituitary consists of two functional and morphological parts which have separate origins; the anterior lobe of the pituitary develops from Rathke's pouch, which arises from the roof of the oral cavity, and the posterior lobe of pituitary or neurohypophysis which is a ventral extension of the hypothalamus.

The hypothalamus is important in the regulation of anterior and posterior pituitary function. The release of hormones from the anterior lobe of the pituitary is controlled by hypothalamic peptides which are transported to the anterior pituitary by the capillaries of the hypothalamic–hypophyseal portal circulation (Table 39.1). The hypothalamus contains a number of autonomic centres that control thirst, satiety, body temperature, emotional reactions and sympathetic responses and serves as an important link between the brain and the endocrine system.

The anterior pituitary produces and releases a number of trophic hormones which control many of the endocrine glands (Fig. 39.1). It consists of three cell types: acidophils, basophils and chro-

Table 39.1 Hypothalamic control of hormone release from the anterior lobe of the pituitary

Anterior lobe hormone	Hypothalamic hormone (stimulatory action)	Hypothalamic hormone (inhibitory action)
TSH – thyroid-stimulating hormone	TRH – thyrotrophin releasing hormone	
ACTH – adrenocorticotrophic hormone	CRH – corticotrophin releasing hormone	
GH – growth hormone	GHRH – growth hormone releasing hormone (somatocrinin)	GHRIH – growth hormone release inhibitory hormone (somatostatin)
FSH – follicle-stimulating hormone	GnRH – gonadotrophin releasing hormone	
LH – luteinizing hormone	GnRH – gonadotrophin releasing hormone	
PRL – Prolactin	PRH – prolactin releasing hormone	PRIH – prolactin release inhibitory hormone (dopamine)
MSH – melanocyte-stimulating hormone	MSHRH – MSH releasing hormone	MSH-RIH – MSH release inhibitory hormone

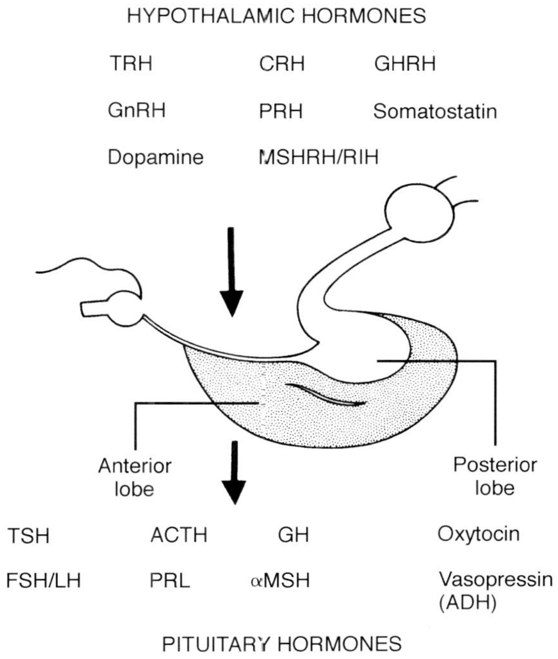

DISORDERS OF THE PITUITARY GLAND | 527

HYPOTHALAMIC HORMONES

TRH	CRH	GHRH
GnRH	PRH	Somatostatin
Dopamine	MSHRH/RIH	

Anterior lobe — **Posterior lobe**

| TSH | ACTH | GH | Oxytocin |
| FSH/LH | PRL | αMSH | Vasopressin (ADH) |

PITUITARY HORMONES

Figure 39.1 Hypothalamic-pituitary hormone production and release. TRH, thyrotrophin releasing hormone; CRH, corticotrophin releasing hormone; GHRH, growth hormone releasing hormone; GnRH, gonadotrophin releasing hormone; PRH, prolactin releasing hormone; MSHRH, melanocyte stimulating hormone releasing hormone; MSHRIH, melanocyte stimulating hormone releasing inhibitor hormone; TSH, thyroid stimulating hormone; ACTH, adrenocorticotrophic hormone; GH, growth hormone; FSH, follicle stimulating hormone; LH, luteinizing hormone; PRL, prolactin; αMSH, α-melanocyte stimulating hormone; ADH, antidiuretic hormone.

mophobes. The acidophils include somatotrophs which secrete growth hormone and lactotrophs which secrete prolactin; basophils include gonadotrophs which secrete follicle-stimulating hormone and luteinizing hormone, and thyrotrophs which secrete thyroid-stimulating hormone; chromophobes include corticotrophs which secrete adrenocorticotrophic hormone and cells which secrete melanocyte-stimulating hormone (MSH). The actions of these hormones are summarized in Table 39.2.

The release of hormones which control a specific endocrine gland, for example the thyroid and adrenal glands, is regulated by a negative feedback mechanism whereby the hormone of the target gland affects the secretion of the relevant releasing factor from the hypothalamus and/or the trophic hormone from the anterior pituitary (see Figs 39.6 and 39.9).

The release of hormones which do not act through a target endocrine gland, i.e. growth hormone, prolactin and MSH, are controlled through a balance of effects of the relevant stimulatory and inhibitory factors, produced by the hypothalamus, on the anterior pituitary (Fig. 39.2).

The posterior pituitary releases stored vasopressin (antidiuretic hormone, ADH) and oxytocin which have been synthesized in the supraoptic and paraventricular nuclei of the hypothalamus. ADH increases the permeability of the distal convoluted tubules and collecting ducts of the kidney and thus controls water excretion. Oxytocin stimulates uterine contractions and milk ejection.

Table 39.2 Actions of the hormones released from the anterior lobe of the pituitary

TSH	Thyroid stimulating hormone stimulates the biosynthesis of thyroid hormones and the release of thyroxine into the circulation.
ACTH	Adrenocorticotrophic hormone maintains adrenocortical size and stimulates the adrenal glands to secrete glucocorticoids.
GH	Growth hormone stimulates growth of the long bones provided the epiphyses are open. It also enhances protein anabolism and has marked anti-insulin activity.
FSH	Follicle-stimulating hormone stimulates ovarian follicular growth and maturation in the female. In the male, it stimulates testicular growth, spermatogenesis and testosterone production.
LH	Luteinizing hormone is required for ovulation and stimulates the formation of the corpus luteum. With FSH it stimulates maximum oestrogen secretion. In the male, LH (ICSH) stimulates the interstitial cells to produce and release testosterone.
PRL	Prolactin, in conjunction with other hormones, induces mammary development and lactation. Prolactin also maintains lactation in the female. In the male it has a stimulatory effect on prostate growth.
MSH	Melanocyte stimulating hormone is produced primarily in the pars intermedia as part of the prohormone

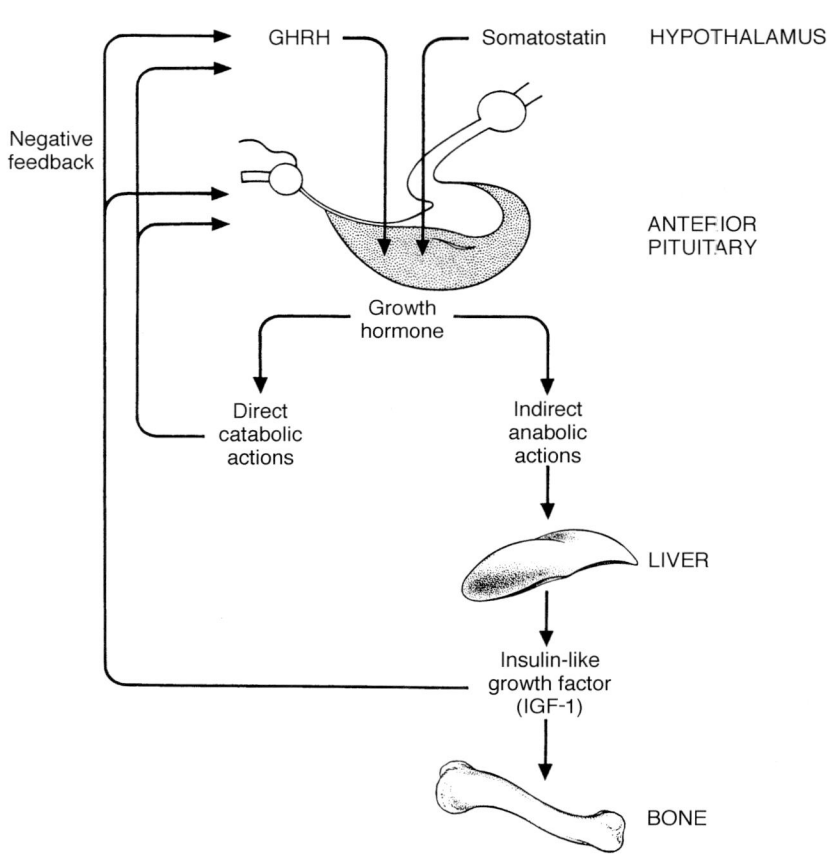

Figure 39.2 Regulation of growth hormone release.

■ Congenital hypopituitarism

Congenital hypopituitarism results from inadequate secretion of growth hormone with resultant retardation of growth (pituitary dwarfism). This rare condition has been reported in a number of breeds of dog, but is most commonly seen in German shepherd dogs, where it has been shown to be inherited as an autosomal recessive trait (Andresen and Willeberg, 1976). In the dog, pituitary dwarfism is most commonly associated with cystic dilation of Rathke's pouch which is thought to cause pressure atrophy of the pituitary resulting in reduced secretion of anterior pituitary hormones. Hypoplasia of the pituitary has been reported in the cat, but appears to be rare.

Clinical signs

Affected animals appear normal at birth, but growth retardation is usually evident by weaning. A deficiency of growth hormone produces proportionate dwarfism. The degree of stunting is variable and probably depends on the extent of pituitary damage. Delayed growth plate closure and dental eruption have been reported, but in most cases these delays appear to be minimal.

Growth hormone is required to produce a normal adult hair coat in the dog. In pituitary dwarfism the fine puppy coat is retained and becomes matted and woolly in appearance. The hair coat is slowly lost from the trunk, leading to the development of bilaterally symmetrical, non-pruritic alopecia by a year of age. The hair loss is mainly from areas of friction such as the flanks, neck and ventral abdomen and where hair is lost the skin usually becomes hyperpigmented. Other areas such as the head and feet are generally spared and affected dogs retain the facial characteristics of a puppy (Fig. 39.3). Hair loss does not appear to be a feature of congenital hypopituitarism in the cat.

The function of other endocrine systems controlled by the anterior pituitary is often normal or near normal. However, in more severe cases signs of secondary hypothyroidism and/or secondary hypoadrenocorticism may develop. Gonadal involvement may result in testicular

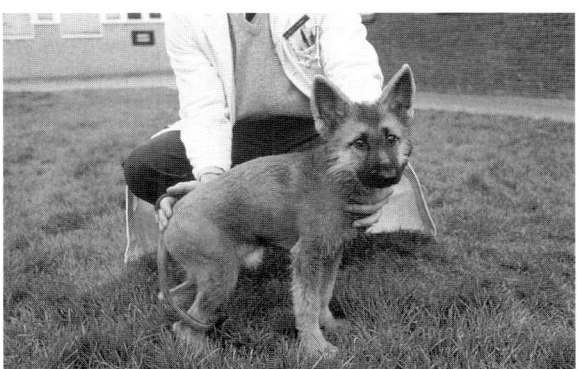

Figure 39.3 A 7-month-old German shepherd dog with congenital hypopituitarism illustrating the immature facial features, small stature and symmetrical truncal alopecia.

atrophy in the male and abnormal oestrus cycles in the bitch.

Diagnosis

The differential diagnosis of stunting is given in Table 39.3. The diagnosis of congenital hypopituitarism can be made by measurement of plasma growth hormone concentrations. Since basal plasma growth hormone concentrations may be low in healthy animals, a stimulation test using clonidine and xylazine should be performed (Eigenmann *et al.*, 1984a). Growth hormone concentration can be assessed indirectly by measuring insulin-like growth factor (IGF-1). Pituitary dwarfs also have abnormally low serum IGF-1 concentrations (Eigenmann *et al.*, 1984a).

Thyroid function tests and adrenal function tests should be performed to assess thyroidal and adrenal function.

Treatment

Canine growth hormone is not available for therapeutic use, but bovine, porcine and human growth hormone preparations have been used for treatment. The diagnosis of hypopituitarism is usually made too late in development to influence growth significantly and affected animals remain permanent dwarfs. Growth hormone administration, however, has been shown to be effective in producing regrowth of hair at a dose of 0.1 iu kg^{-1} subcutaneously three times a week for four to six weeks. Treatment with exogenous growth hormone can be associated with the development of antibodies, which could interfere with its subsequent action (van Herpen *et al.*, 1994). Growth hormone is expensive and its repeated use may result in the development of diabetes mellitus.

Thyroid hormone replacement should be used in cases of secondary hypothyroidism (see under Hypothyroidism). Thyroid hormone therapy has been used in an attempt to stimulate hair growth in pituitary dwarfs with normal thyroid function with variable success. In these cases, half the normal replacement dose of thyroxine is administered for several months to produce a response.

Growth hormone-responsive alopecia in mature dogs

An endocrine alopecia which responds to exogenous growth hormone administration has been described, however, the aetiology of this condition remains unclear and its relationship with insufficient growth hormone secretion unproven (see Chapter 47).

Table 39.3 Differential diagnosis of poor growth or stunting

Endocrine causes	Congenital panhypopituitarism (pituitary dwarf) Congenital hypothyroidism (disproportionate dwarf) Juvenile-onset diabetes mellitus Hyperadrenocorticism Hypoadrenocorticism
Non-endocrine causes	Malnutrition, maldigestion (e.g. exocrine pancreatic insufficiency) and malabsorption. Severe metabolic disorders associated with major organ dysfunction, e.g. portosystemic shunting, congenital renal dysplasia, congenital heart defects (e.g. tetralogy of Fallot) and mucopolysaccharidoses. Skeletal dysplasias will produce disproportionate dwarfs, e.g. enchondrodystrophy in the English pointer and chondrodysplasia of the Alaskan malamute.

Clinical signs

The condition is seen in several breeds including poodles, pomeranians, chow chows, keeshonds and Airedale terriers and is more common in males. Affected animals show progressive hair loss leading to bilaterally symmetrical, non-pruritic alopecia with hyperpigmentation of the skin from two years of age onwards. The hair loss is usually confined to the trunk (Fig. 39.4). Animals are otherwise in good health with normal thyroid and adrenal function.

It is essential to rule out other causes of endocrine alopecia before considering a diagnosis of growth hormone-responsive alopecia (Table 39.4).

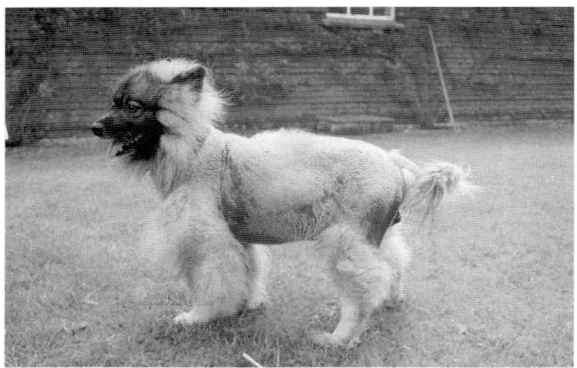

Figure 39.4 A 5-year old male keeshond with so-called growth hormone-responsive alopecia.

Table 39.4 Differential diagnosis of bilaterally symmetrical truncal alopecia

Hypothyroidism
Hyperadrenocorticism
Sertoli cell tumour
Ovarian imbalance
Congenital hypopituitarism
Growth hormone responsive alopecia in mature dogs
Adrenal sex hormone imbalance
Follicular dysplasia[a]

[a] Follicular dysplasia should be ruled out by skin biopsy.

Diagnosis and treatment

Observations suggest that many dogs with this condition have normal plasma growth hormone concentrations and a normal response to stimulation with clonidine or xylazine. Despite normal growth hormone concentrations, some of these cases will respond to exogenous growth hormone administration. It is known that endogenous and exogenous glucocorticoids are potent inhibitors of growth hormone secretion, an effect mediated through enhanced somatostatin release, and some animals with growth hormone-responsive alopecia may have mild or fluctuating hyperadrenocorticism (Rijnberk et al., 1993). Other cases have appeared to respond to seemingly unrelated treatments such as castration and this has led to the term castration-responsive alopecia being used. A study in pomeranians both with and without alopecia showed that growth hormone concentrations did not increase significantly after stimulation irrespective of whether the dogs had alopecia or not (Schmeitzel and Lothrop, 1990). These authors suggested that at least in the pomeranian, there might be an adrenal sex hormone imbalance due to a partial deficiency of 21-hydroxylase enzyme resulting in hyperprogesteronism and/or hyperandrogenism. This deficiency would reduce cortisol production and thereby increase adrenocorticotrophic hormone (ACTH) secretion causing adrenal hyperplasia and excess adrenocortical androgen production, which inhibits new hair growth.

Until the cause of this disorder is known, it is difficult to recommend rational treatment. Growth hormone therapy using a similar protocol to that given for congenital hypopituitarism has been used successfully in some cases. Careful monitoring is important because growth hormone is diabetogenic. If adrenal sex hormone imbalance is suspected neutering or therapy with mitotane or ketoconazole may be effective. However the side effects and risks of mitotane and ketoconazole treatment need to be considered (see section on Hyperadrenocorticism).

■ Acromegaly

Chronic hypersecretion of growth hormone in the adult results in acromegaly, an insidious condition associated with connective tissue and bone overgrowth. In the dog, acromegaly is caused by progestogen therapy or by endogenous progesterone produced during the metoestrus phase of the oestrus cycle. The progesterone-induced growth hormone excess originates from hyperplastic ductular epithelium in the mammary gland and not from the pituitary (Selman et al., 1994). In the cat, acromegaly is caused by a pituitary tumour that secretes excess growth hormone. This cause has not been reported in the dog.

Clinical signs

Clinical signs of acromegaly develop slowly in middle-aged to older intact bitches, which are either cycling normally or being given regular treatment with progestogens to prevent oestrus. Initially there is increased soft tissue swelling around the head and neck and this may result in excessive panting, inspiratory stridor and exercise intolerance. There may be excessive skin folds and thickened skin around the head, neck and distal extremities and increased interdental spacing particularly of the incisor teeth (Fig. 39.5). Since growth hormone antagonizes the effects of insulin, mild glucose intolerance or overt diabetes mellitus develop which can lead to polyuria and polydipsia. Diabetes mellitus induced by growth hormone may be reversible or permanent depending on the circulating concentration and duration of the excessive growth hormone secretion. Initially, hyperglycaemia is associated with increased insulin concentrations, but as the disease progresses beta cell exhaustion may result in lowered insulin secretion. Most cases of acromegaly present with insulin-resistant diabetes mellitus and patients require abnormally high doses of exogenous insulin to control blood glucose concentrations.

Diagnosis

Laboratory findings of uncontrolled or poorly regulated diabetes mellitus with hyperglycaemia and glycosuria are found in most cases. A definitive diagnosis of acromegaly can be made by demonstrating elevated concentrations of growth hormone or IGF-1 in serum (Eigenmann, 1981; Eigenmann et al., 1984b).

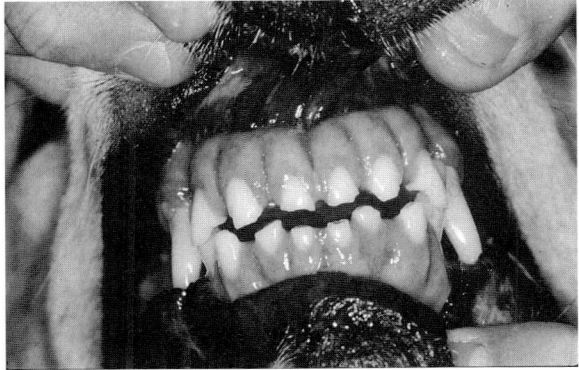

Figure 39.5 Increased interdental spaces in a 12-year old Labrador retriever bitch with acromegaly and associated insulin-resistant diabetes.

Treatment

Successful treatment of acromegaly in the bitch involves the withdrawal of progestogen therapy and ovariohysterectomy for oestrus control. Insulin requirements may decrease dramatically or even cease completely following the withdrawal of progestogen therapy or after ovariohysterectomy. Patients should therefore be monitored very closely to avoid insulin overdosage and the development of hypoglycaemia. In the cat, pituitary irradiation using a linear accelerator or cobalt-60 source has been successful in reducing the growth hormone secretion.

Pituitary tumours

Primary and secondary tumours can involve the pituitary gland. Primary tumours may be functional or non-functional. Adenomas of the anterior lobe of the pituitary are the most common and these may secrete ACTH resulting in pituitary-dependent hyperadrenocorticism. Other tumours may compress and destroy pituitary tissue by expansion causing a reduction in the secretion of trophic hormones which may result in clinical signs of hormone deficiency. There are a number of clinical signs, such as polyuria and polydipsia due to impaired ADH synthesis or release, lethargy and weight gain due to secondary hypothyroidism, and atrophy of the sex organs due to reduced gonadotrophin release. Pressure by a pituitary mass on the osmoreceptors of the hypothalamus may induce alterations in water intake ranging from polydipsia to adipsia.

Clinical signs associated with a pituitary tumour include listlessness, depression, anorexia, vomiting, aimless wandering, head pressing, staring, apparent blindness, ataxia, incoordination, head tilt, circling and seizures. The diagnosis of a pituitary mass can be confirmed by computed tomography or magnetic resonance imaging. Endocrine function tests will help to demonstrate whether the tumour is functional or if hypopituitarism is present.

If neurological signs are apparent, radiotherapy using megavoltage radiation is the treatment of choice and has been successful in reducing the size of the pituitary mass. Pituitary-dependent hyperadrenocorticism can be treated with mitotane (see section on Hyperadrenocorticism).

Diabetes insipidus

Diabetes insipidus is characterized by severe polyuria, with the passage of large quantities of dilute urine and resultant polydipsia. Diabetes insipidus can be caused by either a partial or total failure to synthesize or release ADH (central diabetes insipidus) or a partial or total failure of the renal tubules to respond to ADH (nephrogenic diabetes insipidus).

Both forms of diabetes insipidus may be congenital or acquired. Central diabetes insipidus may result from neoplasia or head trauma, but is usually idiopathic in the dog and cat. Rarely, inflammatory and parasitic lesions have been associated with central diabetes insipidus. Nephrogenic diabetes insipidus may be secondary to a variety of renal and metabolic disorders, including chronic renal failure, renal medullary fibrosis, tubular necrosis, hyperadrenocorticism, pyometra and hypercalcaemia, or may be idiopathic.

Diabetes insipidus must be differentiated from primary polydipsia with resultant polyuria, so-called psychogenic polydipsia, where there is a relative lack of ADH due to overhydration and frequently reduced renal concentrating power due to a decrease in medullary hypertonicity from the wash-out effect of handling large quantities of fluid.

Clinical signs

Clinical signs of diabetes insipidus include marked polyuria, frequently with nocturia and incontinence, and severe polydipsia with the animal usually consuming more than 200 ml kg^{-1} 24 h^{-1}. The differential diagnosis of polyuria and polydipsia is given in Table 39.5. In acquired cases, the onset of clinical signs is usually sudden. Affected dogs start searching for water and may become anorexic and lose weight as a result. Despite their increased thirst, affected animals remain mildly to moderately dehydrated. Affected animals generally show no other clinical signs, although neurological signs may be noted, particularly if diabetes insipidus is associated with a pituitary tumour.

Diagnosis

Haematological, biochemical and electrolyte profiles are generally unremarkable in animals with central or idiopathic nephrogenic diabetes insipidus. When abnormalities are noted, they are

Table 39.5 Differential diagnosis of polydipsia/polyuria

Polyuria with compensatory polydipsia
Osmotic diuresis
Diabetes mellitus
Primary renal glycosuria/Fanconi's syndrome
Polyuric renal failure/post-obstructive diuresis
Interference with ADH release and/or renal response to ADH
Chronic renal failure
Glomerulopathy/nephrotic syndrome
Pyelonephritis
Pyometra
Hyperadrenocorticism
Chronic liver disease
Hypercalcaemia
Hypoadrenocorticism
Central diabetes insipidus
Nephrogenic diabetes insipidus
Hypokalaemia
Hyperthyroidism
Drugs/diet
Primary polydipsia
Psychogenic polydipsia

ADH, antidiuretic hormone.

usually secondary to dehydration. The most significant finding is very dilute urine of low specific gravity, usually between 1.001 and 1.005. The urine specific gravity is almost invariably less than glomerular filtrate, i.e. <1.010, indicating good renal tubular function with resorption of solute in excess of water. Urine osmolality is low and typically below that of plasma, which is often mildly or moderately elevated due to the concomitant dehydration (Table 39.6). In psychogenic polydipsia, the plasma osmolality is usually decreased due to the overhydration.

A carefully monitored water deprivation test will confirm the animal's inability to concentrate its urine in diabetes insipidus, despite becoming dehydrated. Renal function must be assessed before undertaking this test and the test must always be discontinued if the patient loses more than 5% of its body weight. Urine and plasma osmolality measurements provide more definitive information than urine specific gravity alone (Table 39.6, see also Chapter 9).

The ADH response test is used to distinguish central diabetes insipidus from nephrogenic diabetes insipidus. Dogs and cats with central diabetes insipidus will concentrate their urine in response to the administration of exogenous ADH whereas dogs with nephrogenic diabetes insipidus will show no response.

Treatment

Successful treatment of central diabetes insipidus requires long-term replacement therapy using desmopressin (DDAVP, Ferring), a vasopressin analogue. Desmopressin is available as an injection and as nasal drops, which provide antidiuretic activity for about 8 h. One to four drops of the nasal preparation placed in the conjunctival sac twice daily will control the polydipsia and polyuria in most dogs and cats with central diabetes insipidus.

Chlorpropamide, an oral sulphonylurea hypoglycaemic agent, potentiates the effects of ADH on the renal tubules and therefore requires the presence of at least some endogenous ADH. Although chlorpropamide has been shown to be effective in partial central diabetes insipidus in humans, the results in dogs have been inconsistent and variable. It may take several weeks to obtain an effect and hypoglycaemia is a potential adverse effect. A dose of 10–40 mg kg^{-1} orally once daily has been suggested in dogs. Chlorpropamide is not recommended for use in cats.

Thiazide diuretics such as hydrochlorothiazide and chlorothiazide have a paradoxical effect in both central and nephrogenic diabetes insipidus. Urine output may be decreased by up to 50%, although the urine is still not isothenuric. The suggested doses for hydrochlorothiazide and chlorothiazide are 2–4 mg kg^{-1} twice daily and 20–40 mg kg^{-1} twice daily, respectively. The precise dose should be tailored to each patient and the effect may be enhanced by concurrent use of a sodium-restricted diet. Patients should be monitored periodically for electrolyte disturbances, particularly hypokalaemia.

Idiopathic central diabetes insipidus has a

Table 39.6 Differentiation of central diabetes insipidus (CDI), nephrogenic diabetes insipidus (NDI) and psychogenic polydipsia (PP)

Parameter	Before water deprivation	After water deprivation		
		CDI	NDI	PP
Urine				
U specific gravity	<1.010	<1.010	<1.010	<1.025
U osmolality	<300	<300	<300	<700
Plasma				
P osmolality	>300 CDI or NDI <295 PP	>310	>310	±310
U:P osmolality	<1.0	<1.0	<1.0	2–3
ADH response test				
U specific gravity	<1.010	>1.015	<1.010	<1.025
U:P osmolality	<1.0	>1.0	<1.0	>1.0

Osmolality measured in mOsm kg^{-1}. U, urine; P, plasma.

favourable prognosis with treatment. Animals with an expanding hypothalamic or pituitary tumour have a more guarded prognosis, especially if neurological signs are present. Central diabetes insipidus following head trauma carries a variable prognosis; spontaneous recovery may occur within a few days or weeks in some cases, but in others the damage is permanent. Nephrogenic diabetes insipidus tends to have a more guarded prognosis.

DISORDERS OF THE THYROID GLAND

Anatomy and physiology

The thyroid gland lies within the cervical fascia between the sternothyroideus muscles and the trachea and consists of two lobes which are only rarely connected by an isthmus. The glands are not palpable in healthy dogs or cats. Palpable enlargements are referred to as goitre.

Two parathyroid glands are normally associated with each thyroid lobe. The internal parathyroids usually lie within the thyroid capsule at the caudal pole of each lobe.

The thyroid gland actively takes up inorganic iodide, resulting in levels that are 10–200 times that of serum. The inorganic iodide enters the thyroid follicular cells and is transformed into metabolically active thyroid hormones, thyroxine (T4) and triiodothyronine (T3). The synthesis and secretion of T4 and T3 is controlled by thyroid-stimulating hormone (TSH), a glycoprotein secreted by the thyrotroph cells of the anterior pituitary. Secretion of TSH is stimulated by thyrotrophin-releasing hormone (TRH), a hypothalamic tripeptide. A classic negative feedback system operates to maintain the plasma concentrations of T4 and T3 within close limits (Fig. 39.6).

In plasma, more than 99% of T3 and T4 is bound to plasma proteins, mainly albumin and

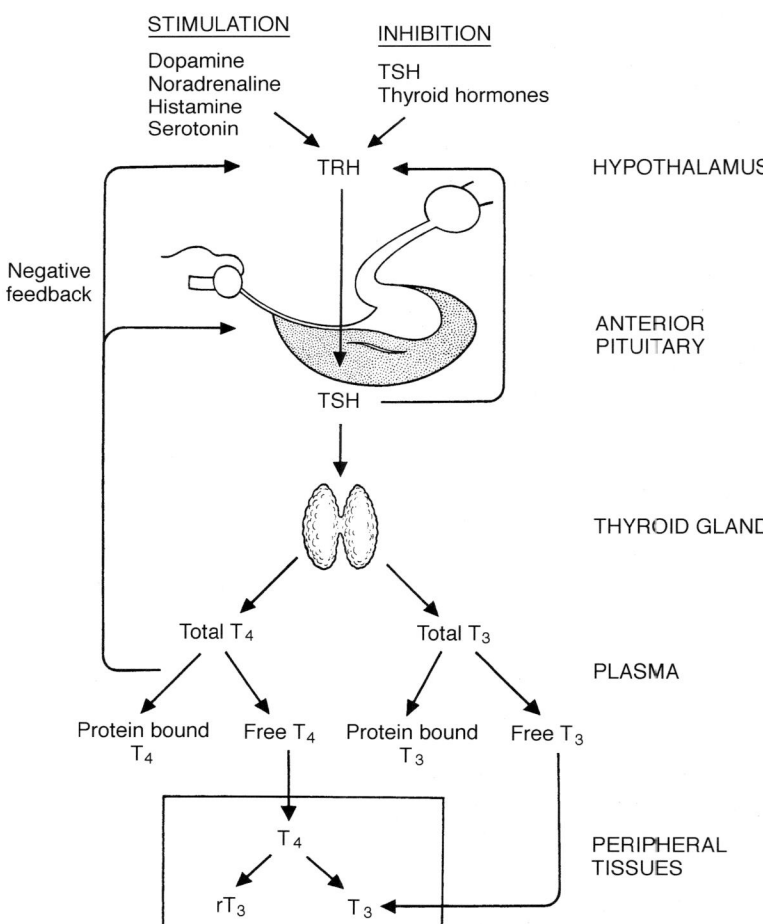

Figure 39.6 Regulation of thyroid function.

globulins. It is the free (unbound) hormones which are metabolically active. Although T4 is the major secretory product of the thyroid gland, the metabolic activity of T3 is much greater. About 80% of the plasma T3 concentration is produced by deiodination of T4 in peripheral tissues, mainly the liver and kidneys.

In catabolic states such as those produced by starvation, anorexia or debilitating disease, T4 is deiodinated to reverse T3 (rT3), an inactive metabolite, at the expense of T3 production.

Thyroid hormones play a dominant role in controlling metabolism. They increase basal metabolic rate, stimulate cellular oxygen consumption, promote carbohydrate absorption from the intestine and regulate lipid metabolism. Thyroid hormones are also essential for normal growth and development and they activate the anagen (growth) phase of the hair cycle. Some effects of thyroid hormones, such as stimulation of the nervous and cardiovascular systems, are mediated by an increased sensitivity to catecholamines.

Hypothyroidism

Hypothyroidism is the most commonly diagnosed endocrinopathy in the dog and estimates of incidence range from 1 in 156 to 1 in 500 depending on the criteria for diagnosis (Chastain and Panciera, 1995). Naturally occurring hypothyroidism is an extremely rare clinical disorder in cats (Rand et al., 1993).

Primary hypothyroidism is the most common type of hypothyroidism in the dog and usually results from lymphocytic thyroiditis or thyroid atrophy. Thyroid atrophy can be the end result of lymphocytic thyroiditis. Thyroid neoplasia may occasionally be associated with hypothyroidism. Congenital hypothyroidism (cretinism) is rare and may be caused by thyroid agenesis, dysgenesis or dyshormonogenesis.

Secondary hypothyroidism is usually associated with pituitary neoplasia but may also occur with congenital panhypopituitarism. Tertiary hypothyroidism due to hypothalamic dysfunction, iodine deficiency and serum transport defects are all rare causes of hypothyroidism.

The most common cause of feline hypothyroidism is iatrogenic destruction or removal of the thyroid gland following radioactive iodine therapy or surgery for treatment of hyperthyroidism. Spontaneous acquired hypothyroidism has been reported in a cat with lymphocytic thyroiditis (Rand et al., 1993). Congenital hypothyroidism has been reported in the cat and may be associated with goitre (Arnold et al., 1984; Jones et al., 1992).

Clinical signs

The clinical signs with hypothyroidism are very variable and often vague. Some cases present with a classic combination of clinical signs whereas others may exhibit only one sign. Hypothyroidism usually affects young to middle-aged dogs of the larger breeds. Golden retrievers, Doberman pinschers and Irish setters appear to be over-represented.

Lethargy, mental dullness, bradycardia, poor exercise tolerance, weight gain without an increase in food intake, intolerance to cold and hypothermia are the most common clinical signs associated with hypothyroidism (Panciera, 1994).

Bilaterally symmetrical, non-pruritic alopecia affecting the flanks, thorax, ventral trunk and neck is associated with inhibition of the hair cycle (Fig. 39.7). The remaining hair coat is dry and dull. The skin is often thickened (myxoedematous) and hyperpigmented. Myxoedema of the skin is most evident on the head resulting in a tragic facial expression. The skin, particularly on the ventral abdomen, may be cold and clammy to the touch. Comedones, seborrhoea and recurrent pyoderma may also be noted (Nesbitt et al., 1980).

Intact females often have abnormal oestrous cycles and males may show a lack of libido and infertility. Constipation and corneal lipidosis may occasionally be noted.

Neurological signs may be seen in some dogs with hypothyroidism and include neuromuscular dysfunction with cranial nerve abnormalities, laryngeal paralysis, megaoesophagus, lower motor neurone disease and encephalopathy

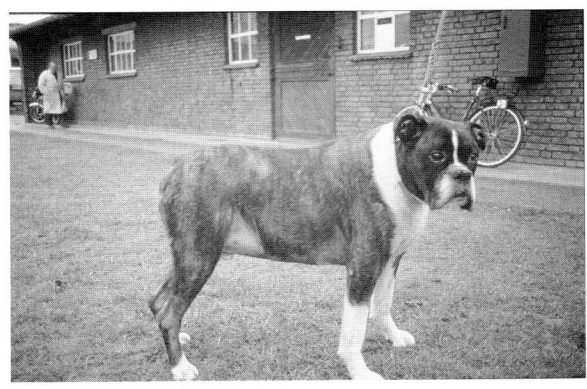

Figure 39.7 An 8-year-old boxer dog with hypothyroidism showing symmetrical alopecia.

(Bischel et al., 1988; Jaggy et al., 1994). Clinical signs of lameness, dragging of the feet, quadriparesis, hearing impairment and nystagmus have also been reported. Electromyography may reveal fibrillation potentials and positive sharp waves. Motor nerve conduction velocities may be decreased and tendon reflexes appear sluggish.

Congenital hypothyroidism has been reported in a number of breeds including the boxer (Mooney and Anderson, 1993) and the giant schnauzer (Greco et al., 1991). Clinical signs of congenital hypothyroidism include hypothermia, lethargy, disproportionate dwarfism with a short, broad skull, short thick limbs and kyphosis, delayed dental eruption, thickened skin and a dry hair coat. Radiographic changes include delayed epiphyseal ossification and epiphyseal dysgenesis (Saunders and Jezyk, 1991).

Laboratory findings

Hypercholesterolaemia is found in about 70% of hypothyroid dogs. Thyroid hormones stimulate biliary excretion of cholesterol and a deficiency of these hormones results in an increase in the cholesterol content of the liver. To prevent overloading the liver with cholesterol, the low-density lipoprotein receptors are down-regulated to limit low-density and high-density lipoprotein uptake from the circulation. Plasma levels of these lipoproteins rise causing hypercholesterolaemia (Watson and Barrie, 1993).

Hypercholesterolaemia may also occur with high-fat diets, hyperadrenocorticism, diabetes mellitus, nephrotic syndrome, chronic liver disease and primary hyperlipoproteinaemia.

Mild normocytic, normochromic, non-regenerative anaemia occurs in about 30% of hypothyroid dogs and represents a physiological response to the lowered basal metabolic rate.

Mild to moderate increases in serum activity of alanine aminotransferase, aspartate aminotransferase, alkaline phosphatase and creatine kinase may be noted. Increased creatine kinase activity is particularly associated with myopathy in cases of hypothyroidism.

Thyroid function tests

Serum total T4 and free T4

Baseline serum T4 concentration using a validated assay is more accurate than serum T3 in assessing the status of thyroid gland function and is recommended for initial evaluation of the thyroid gland. Random fluctuations in serum T4 concentrations occur, but a true circadian rhythm has not been identified.

Serum T4 concentrations can be affected by breed, age, illness and drug administration. Certain breeds particularly the sight hounds have lower serum T4 concentrations than other breeds and this is important when interpreting results from greyhounds or Afghan hounds. Serum T4 concentrations tend to be higher in young growing puppies and lower in old dogs when compared to normal adult concentrations. Concurrent illness can suppress serum thyroid hormone concentrations (sick euthyroid syndrome). The degree of suppression is dependent on the severity of the illness or catabolic state rather than the specific disorder. Various drugs can alter thyroid hormone metabolism and serum binding particularly glucocorticoids, anticonvulsants, nonsteroidal anti-inflammatory drugs, frusemide and anaesthetic agents (Ferguson, 1988).

Serum free T4 concentrations measure metabolically active T4 and should not be influenced by the effects of serum binding. However, measurement of serum free T4 by most assays has not proved to be any more reliable than total T4 concentrations in the diagnosis of hypothyroidism.

A low baseline serum T4 concentration with a history and clinical signs compatible with hypothyroidism may be sufficient evidence to warrant a therapeutic trial. In one study, the predictive value of a positive test result was 0.75 and of a negative test result was 0.87 using T4 concentrations to diagnose hypothyroidism (Miller et al., 1992). Serum T4 concentrations in the low normal or below normal range should have further tests performed such as a canine TSH concentration and/or a TSH or TRH stimulation test if the index of suspicion is still high for hypothyroidism.

Serum T4 concentrations in the normal range are unlikely to be associated with hypothyroidism. However, antibodies to thyroid hormone can cause discordance between measured thyroid hormone concentrations and clinical status of the dog. Depending on their concentration, binding affinity and the assay method used, thyroid antibodies can result in either falsely elevated or falsely low thyroid hormone concentrations. Autoantibodies to T4 and T3 can be measured in these cases.

Serum total T3 and free T3

Baseline serum T3 concentrations are less accurate for predicting hypothyroidism than serum T4. Random fluctuations in serum T3 concentrations are greater than with serum T4 and have a greater tendency to be misleading with respect to the status of thyroid gland function. Possible explanations for this discrepancy include the preference of the normal thyroid gland for secreting T4, the intracellular formation and location of most T3, the preferential secretion of T3 compared to T4 as thyroid function progressively fails and the development of anti-T3 antibodies. The diagnostic value of serum T3 concentrations in hypothyroidism is therefore inferior to serum T4.

TSH stimulation test

The administration of exogenous bovine TSH to measure thyroid secretory reserve is the most definitive method currently available for the diagnosis of hypothyroidism. The protocol and interpretation criteria are given in Table 39.7. The use of this test is limited by the expense of the TSH injection and its inconsistent availability.

Peak serum T4 responses are decreased by non-thyroidal illness and drug administration in the same way as basal T4 concentrations. Thyroid function testing is thus best performed after resolution of non-thyroidal illness and, if possible, with the patient off all mediation.

TRH stimulation test

TRH is readily available and less expensive than TSH. However the T4 response to TRH is less predictable and peak concentrations tend to be lower than with TSH stimulation. Increasing the dose of TRH increases the duration but not the magnitude of the T4 response. TRH administration may cause cholinergic signs such as salivation, vomiting and defecation. Responses are also affected by non-thyroidal illness and drug administration.

Reverse T3 (rT3)

The measurement of serum rT3 concentration can be useful in identifying cases with significant non-thyroidal illness and should be reserved for those cases with discordant or equivocal T4 concentrations. If the serum rT3 concentration is high in a dog with low or low-normal T4, hypothyroidism is unlikely to be the cause of the animal's clinical signs.

Endogenous canine TSH (c-TSH)

A reliable assay for canine TSH should be a valuable aid to diagnosis particularly in primary hypothyroidism where the concentrations should be high. However, a validated c-TSH assay has only recently become available and its use in the diagnosis of hypothyroidism is still being evaluated. In one study, it was concluded that cTSH measurements were a useful additional diagnostic test to serum T4 concentrations in the diagnosis of

Table 39.7 Protocol and interpretation of the TSH and TRH stimulation tests

TSH stimulation test
Protocol
- Collect plasma or serum sample for basal T4 concentration.
- Administer bovine TSH intravenously at a dose rate of 0.1 iu kg^{-1} up to a maximum dose of 5 iu.
- Collect second sample for T4 concentration 6 h later.

Interpretation
- A diagnosis of primary hypothyroidism can be confirmed if both the pre and post T4 samples are below the reference range for basal T4 concentration.
- In normal animals, the T4 concentration should stimulate to well within or above the normal reference range for T4. In most animals, the T4 concentration should increase by at least 1.5 times the basal concentration.
- Interpretation of intermediate results is more difficult and may occur in association with non-thyroidal illness, treatment with certain drugs, secondary hypothyroidism or possibly during the early stages of primary hypothyroidism.

TRH stimulation test
Protocol
- Collect plasma or serum sample for basal T4 concentration.
- Administer 200 µg protirelin (TRH-Cambridge, Cambridge) per dog intravenously. Injection may cause salivation, vomiting and tachycardia.
- Collect second sample for T4 concentration 4 h later.

Interpretation
- Similar to TSH stimulation test although stimulation of T4 concentrations is less than with TSH and the response to TRH shows greater individual variation.

cases of suspected hypothyroidism, but that the sensitivity of the test was insufficient to obviate the need for a dynamic test (TSH or TRH stimulation test) to confirm the diagnosis in some cases of hypothyroidism (Ramsey et al., 1998).

Thyroid biopsy

Although not commonly performed, the histological examination of a thyroid gland biopsy provides an accurate method of differentiating between primary and secondary hypothyroidism. In primary hypothyroidism, there is loss of thyroid follicles resulting from either lymphocytic thyroiditis or thyroid atrophy. In secondary hypothyroidism, the thyroid follicles become distended with colloid and the follicular epithelial cells are flattened. Testing thyroid function is still required to make a diagnosis of hypothyroidism, since the degree of histological change does not always relate to reduced hormone production and release.

Treatment

Thyroid hormone replacement is required for the treatment of hypothyroidism. Synthetic forms of T4 and T3 are available. Sodium levothyroxine (L-thyroxine) is the treatment of choice because it most closely resembles the preferential secretion of T4 by the normal thyroid gland. Synthetic T4 is readily deiodinated to T3 in peripheral tissues and therefore does not by-pass the normal cellular regulatory processes that control the production of the more potent T3 in those tissues.

An initial replacement dose of L-thyroxine is 20–40 µg kg^{-1} daily in divided doses. Although it has been suggested that once daily dosing is sufficient in many cases (Nachreiner and Refsal, 1992), the author has documented several cases where once daily administration has failed to maintain adequate serum concentrations throughout the day with a consequent failure of the clinical signs to resolve fully. Poor absorption and a short half-life for T4 explain why dogs require higher doses and more frequent administration than human patients with hypothyroidism.

Therapy should always be continued for a minimum of three months. Improved activity and mental alertness is usually seen within two weeks, but skin and hair coat changes may take up to 6 months to resolve. Improved left ventricular function demonstrated by echocardiography and increased amplitude of the P and R waves on ECG is detectable within two months (Panciera, 1994).

The effect of treatment can be monitored by measurement of post-pill serum T4 concentrations. Sampling at 4–6 h after dosing will give a peak serum T4 concentration and a sample taken just prior to dosing will give the lowest serum T4 concentration. The dose and frequency of administration should be adjusted to maintain the serum T4 concentration within the normal range throughout the day. Underdosage may lead to treatment failure and overdosage can lead to iatrogenic hyperthyroidism. Replacement therapy is required for life.

Cases of congenital hypothyroidism should be treated as early as possible to achieve normal growth and development. The dose may require adjustment as the patient grows and gets older.

L-triiodothyronine must be administered every 8 h at a dose of 4–6 µg kg^{-1}. The disadvantages of this drug are its short half-life, expense and difficulty in monitoring. Treatment with synthetic T3 is rarely justified.

Possible causes for cases failing to respond to replacement therapy include misdiagnosis, inadequate dose or frequency of administration, poor gastrointestinal absorption and peripheral tissue resistance.

Hyperthyroidism

Hyperthyroidism (thyrotoxicosis) is a multisystemic disorder resulting from excessive circulating concentrations of T4 and/or, T3. Hyperthyroidism is the most common endocrine disorder of the domestic cat, but is rare in the dog.

Functional adenomatous hyperplasia (adenoma) affecting one or both thyroid lobes is the most common cause of feline hyperthyroidism. The pathogenesis is unknown but the frequent involvement of both thyroid lobes would suggest a circulating factor may be involved. Thyroid carcinoma is a rare cause of hyperthyroidism in the cat (Turrel et al., 1988). Although thyroid carcinoma is the major thyroid tumour of the dog, it is rarely functional (Peterson et al., 1989).

Iatrogenic hyperthyroidism caused by excessive thyroid hormone supplementation is recognized occasionally.

Clinical signs

Hyperthyroidism is a disease of middle-aged to older cats, with a mean age of 13 years and range of 6–21 years (Thoday and Mooney, 1992). Only 6% of hyperthyroid cats are younger than 10 years of age at the time of diagnosis. There is no breed or sex predisposition.

The clinical signs of hyperthyroidism relate to the excessive secretion of thyroid hormones and their general stimulatory effect on different body systems. The frequency and severity of the clinical signs are highly variable in cats with hyperthyroidism and are influenced by the duration of hyperthyroidism, the ability of the body systems to cope with the demands imposed by thyroid hormone excess and the presence of concomitant disease in the older animal. In most cases, the clinical signs of hypothyroidism are slowly progressive with an insidious onset. Since most cats maintain a good appetite and remain active for their age, owners frequently feel the cat is in good health until weight loss or other signs develop. The major presenting sign is therefore progressive weight loss frequently accompanied by polyphagia (Fig. 39.8). Affected cats are often hyperactive and become irritable or aggressive which can make clinical examination difficult. Polydipsia, polyuria and intermittent gastrointestinal signs such as vomiting, diarrhoea and the passage of voluminous fatty faeces are also common signs.

Cardiac abnormalities are frequently recognized in hyperthyroid cats. There is usually a tachycardia with a heart rate in excess of 240 beats per minute and systolic murmurs, gallop rhythms or dysrhythmias are frequently detected on auscultation. In severe cases, clinical signs of congestive heart failure may develop and these may include dyspnoea, resulting from pulmonary oedema or accumulation of pleural fluid, and ascites. The cardiac signs are associated with cardiomyopathy, usually the hypertrophic form, which develops secondarily to excessive thyroid hormone secretion. Electrocardiographic abnormalities may include tachycardia, increased R wave amplitude particularly in lead II and various atrial and ventricular dysrhythmias and conduction disturbances.

Although there are no specific skin lesions, the coat of cats with hyperthyroidism is often matted and unkempt. Affected cats may also develop heat intolerance with panting and dysphonia.

Although most hyperthyroid cats are polyphagic and hyperactive, about 10% of cases are presented with severe depression and muscle weakness which may result in ventroflexion of the neck. Weight loss remains a feature but is usually associated with anorexia rather than increased appetite. This clinical presentation is referred to as 'apathetic' hyperthyroidism.

In most cases, there is palpable enlargement of one or both thyroid lobes. Thyroid palpation requires both skill and practice. The thyroid gland is not usually palpable in the normal cat. Enlarged lobes of the thyroid are usually located just distal to the larynx but can be quite mobile and descend down the neck and occasionally pass into the thoracic inlet.

Laboratory findings

Routine haematological and biochemical screening tests are useful not only because results may show alterations that support a diagnosis of hyperthyroidism but may also indicate evidence of concurrent disease in the older cat.

The most frequent haematological change is a relative polycythaemia with a mild to moderate increase in red cell parameters (red blood cell count, packed cell volume and haemoglobin concentration). A mature neutrophilia with lymphopenia and eosinopenia is also common and probably reflects a stress response. However, eosinophilia and lymphocytosis are found in some cats with hyperthyroidism.

An increase in serum activity of the enzymes alanine aminotransferase (ALT), aspartate aminotransferase (AST), alkaline phosphatase (AP) and lactate dehydrogenase (LDH) is a frequent but non-specific finding. The reason for the increase is not clear. Evidence of concurrent renal dysfunction in hyperthyroidism is common with mild to moderate elevations in serum creatinine and urea. These increases may be related to increased protein catabolism and prerenal azotaemia. Careful consideration should be given to the method of treatment selected for hyperthyroid cats with concomitant azotaemia since at least some of these cats will develop clinical signs of renal failure

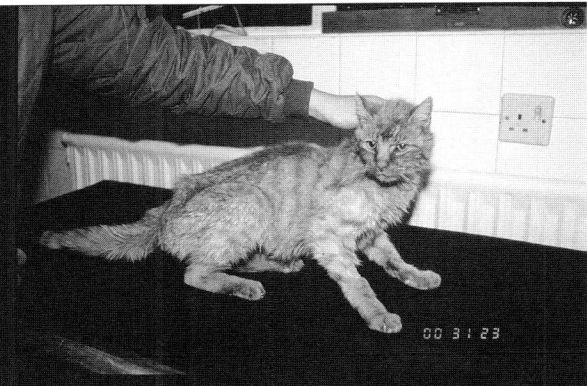

Figure 39.8 A 14-year-old domestic shorthair cat with hyperthyroidism illustrating weight loss, unkempt hair coat and reluctance to being restrained.

caused by a deterioration in renal function when the hyperthyroid state is corrected.

Thyroid function tests

Increased serum basal thyroid hormone concentrations are diagnostic of hyperthyroidism. In the majority of cases, both serum T4 and T3 concentrations are increased, often markedly, however in a few cases serum T3 concentrations are in the normal range despite obvious elevation of the serum T4 concentration. There is, therefore, usually no advantage in determining serum T3 concentrations and serum total or free T4 concentrations provide a reliable indication of hyperthyroidism.

About 5% of cases of hyperthyroidism have normal serum thyroid hormone concentrations at the time of examination and this may be due to an early stage of the disease, significant daily fluctuations of thyroid hormone concentrations (Peterson et al., 1987) or the effect of concurrent non-thyroidal illness (Peterson and Gamble, 1990). In such cases where hyperthyroidism is still suspected on clinical grounds, a diagnostic T4 concentration may be obtained by re-testing in 3–6 weeks.

Alternative diagnostic tests for equivocal cases of hyperthyroidism include the TRH stimulation test and the T3 suppression test. For the TRH stimulation test, TRH is administered at a dose of 0.1 mg kg^{-1} intravenously with blood samples taken before and 4 h after injection. Serum total T4 concentrations increase by more than 60% in healthy cats whereas most hyperthyroid cats stimulate by less than 50% (Peterson et al., 1994). For the T3 suppression test, a morning sample is collected for serum total T4 estimation and 25 mg of triiodothyronine is given orally and the same dose repeated every 8 h for a total of seven doses. A second blood sample is collected for serum total T4 estimation at 2–6 h after the final dose. Serum T4 concentrations show at least a 50% suppression of basal T4 following T3 suppression whereas little or no suppression of T4 concentration occurs in hyperthyroid cats (Peterson et al., 1990).

Diagnostic imaging

Hyperthyroid cats with secondary cardiomyopathy usually show cardiac enlargement which is evident on both radiographic and echocardiographic examinations. However, it is important to recognize that significant concentric hypertrophy can occur without affecting the appearance of the cardiac silhouette on thoracic radiographs and the diagnosis of cardiomyopathy in these cases can only be made from echocardiographic findings.

Thyroid imaging using radioactive iodine or technetium-99m is a useful diagnostic technique if gamma camera facilities are available. The technique determines whether there is unilateral or bilateral lobe involvement which is valuable if surgical thyroidectomy is to be performed. The technique also determines any alteration in the position of the thyroid gland, the rare case of abnormal ectopic thyroid tissue within the thorax, or the presence of distant metastases from a functional thyroid carcinoma.

Treatment

There are three options for treatment of hyperthyroidism; antithyroid medication, surgical thryoidectomy and radioactive iodine.

Medical management of hyperthyroidism using antithyroid drugs is indicated to prepare hyperthyroid cats for surgical thyroidectomy in order to improve their general condition and reduce the risk of complications arising during surgery. Antithyroid drugs are also recommended for the initial treatment of hyperthyroid cats with concurrent azotaemia in order to ascertain whether significant deterioration in renal function is likely to occur after medical control of the hyperthyroid state. If there is no deterioration in renal function after 3–4 weeks of treatment, then surgical thyroidectomy or radioactive iodine therapy for hyperthyroidism can be considered. Antithyroid drugs can also be used for long-term management of hyperthyroidism particularly in cases where owners refuse surgical treatment.

Carbimazole inhibits thyroid hormone synthesis and is the antithyroid drug most widely used in the United Kingdom. It is a safe and effective form of treatment and is undoubtedly the treatment of choice for aged cats and those with concurrent disease. Carbimazole is rapidly converted into methimazole after oral administration and methimazole is the most widely used antithyroid drug in the USA (Peterson et al., 1988).

Carbimazole is initially administered at a dose of 5 mg orally three times daily. Serum total thyroxine concentrations decrease to within the reference range after 3–15 days (Mooney et al., 1992). Within two weeks, the dose can be reduced in most cats to 5 mg of carbimazole administered twice daily and this is continued for the remainder of the cat's life. Periodic assessment of thyroid hormone is necessary to confirm that the hyperthyroid state is being adequately controlled. Adjustment of the dosage is required in some cases to maintain the euthyroid state. Adverse reactions to carbimazole include anorexia, vomiting and lethargy which are usually transient, but more serious reactions such as pruritus, self-induced excoriation, hepatopathy, jaundice, and bleeding diatheses have been reported and may necessitate withdrawal of this drug.

The aim of surgical thyroidectomy is to remove all of the abnormally functioning thyroid tissue. Surgical thyroidectomy is a highly effective treatment for feline hyperthyroidism but can be associated with significant morbidity and mortality if cats are not carefully assessed and stabilized prior to surgery. Preoperative treatment with carbimazole and propranolol will control the excessive thyroid hormone production and protect the heart against the effects of excess thyroid hormone. The dose of propranolol is 2.5–5 mg administered orally every 8 h for 7–14 days before surgery.

The anaesthetic protocol for the hyperthyroid cat should be carefully considered using agents which have the minimum effect on cardiac rhythm. Techniques for unilateral and bilateral thyroidectomy have been reported for cats with hyperthyroidism. Both intracapsular and extracapsular techniques have been designed to preserve parathyroid function after removal of the abnormal thyroid tissue.

The potential complications associated with thyroidectomy include hypoparathyroidism, Horner's syndrome and laryngeal paralysis. The most serious complication is hypocalcaemia associated with damage or removal of the parathyroid glands. Since only one parathyroid gland is required for maintenance of normocalcaemia, hypoparathyroidism is mostly identified in cats treated by bilateral thyroidectomy. Hypocalcaemia is usually transient and may manifest anorexia, vocalization, lethargy, muscular tremors, tetany and convulsions. The treatment of postoperative hypocalcaemia is outlined in Table 39.8.

Radioactive iodine therapy is a safe and effective method of treating hyperthyroidism but requires the cat to be housed in licensed premises with restricted access until the radiation dose rate has decreased to an acceptable level. This usually requires hospitalization for around four weeks. The radioisotope used most commonly is iodine-131 (^{131}I) which has a half-life of 8 days and emits both β-particles and γ-radiation. The β-particles cause most tissue damage. Radioactive iodine can be administered subcutaneously and has not been associated with any adverse reactions (Mooney, 1994).

DISORDERS OF THE PARATHYROID GLANDS

Anatomy and physiology

The normal dog and cat usually have four small parathyroid glands. One pair of glands are generally found in the fascia cranial to each of the thyroid lobes. The caudal pair of parathyroid glands are embedded in the parenchyma of each thyroid lobe. The location and number of the parathyroid glands can vary. Each parathyroid gland contains chief cells which synthesize and secrete parathyroid hormone (PTH).

PTH secretion is controlled by the serum ionized calcium concentration and maintains the serum ionized calcium within narrow limits. If the serum ionized calcium concentration falls below the set point, PTH release is enhanced.

Table 39.8 Management of postoperative hypocalcaemia

Immediate therapy
Administer 1.0–1.5 ml of 10% calcium gluconate or calcium glubionate by slow intravenous injection. Stop injection if bradycardia develops. Repeat as necessary.

Maintenance therapy
Begin oral supplementation as soon as possible using 50–75 mg kg^{-1} day^{-1} of elemental calcium in three or four divided doses (equivalent to 500–750 mg kg^{-1} day^{-1} of calcium gluconate or 400–600 mg kg^{-1} day^{-1} of calcium lactate) and 0.03 mg kg^{-1} dihydrotachysterol orally once daily.

Monitor the serum calcium concentration and decrease the dihydrotachysterol by 0.01 mg kg^{-1} every other day once serum calcium is within the reference range. Adjust doses of dihydrotachysterol and calcium supplementation according to subsequent serum calcium concentrations. In most cases, hypocalcaemia is temporary.

Concentrations of serum ionized calcium above the set point inhibit PTH secretion. Total serum calcium consists of both ionized and protein-bound fractions. Although serum protein-bound calcium is affected by several factors including the circulating albumin concentration and acid–base status, it is only the ionized calcium which is physiologically active. It is important to appreciate this, since most laboratories only measure total serum calcium.

PTH tends to increase serum ionized calcium concentrations through a number of integrated actions. In the kidney, PTH increases tubular reabsorption of calcium and enhances renal excretion of phosphate. PTH also activates 1α-hydroxylase, the renal enzyme which converts 25-hydroxycholecalciferol into the active form of vitamin D, 1,25-dihydroxycholecalciferol (calcitriol). Increased circulating 1,25-dihydroxycholecalciferol enhances calcium and phosphate absorption by the intestine. In bone, PTH promotes the release of calcium and phosphate into the extracellular fluid by stimulating osteoclast and osteocyte activity and by suppressing osteoblastic activity. The combination of calcium mobilization from bone and retention of calcium by the kidneys causes the serum ionized calcium concentration to rise.

Calcium plays an important role in neuromuscular excitability, membrane permeability, muscle contraction, enzyme activity, hormone release and blood coagulation as well as acting as an essential structural component of the skeleton.

Hypoparathyroidism

Hypoparathyroidism is caused by inadequate production and secretion of PTH (primary hypoparathyroidism) or, more rarely, by deficient end-organ responsiveness to circulatory PTH (pseudohypoparathyroidism). The two most common causes of primary hypoparathyroidism are iatrogenic injury or removal of the parathyroid glands during thyroidectomy (see under treatment of hyperthyroidism) and idiopathic hypoparathyroidism due to destruction and atrophy of the parathyroid glands. Idiopathic hypoparathyroidism probably results from immune-mediated destruction of the parathyroid glands and this is supported by the diffuse lymphocytic infiltrations found in the parathyroid glands of some affected animals.

Clinical signs

Idiopathic hypoparathyroidism is rare but has been reported in the dog and cat (Bruyette and Feldman, 1988; Peterson et al., 1991). The disease affects young to middle-aged animals of various breeds. A female bias has been reported in dogs.

The clinical signs of hypoparathyroidism relate to neuromuscular abnormalities that develop secondary to hypocalcaemia and include seizures, convulsions, focal trembling or twitching, generalized muscle fasciculations, ataxia, stiff gait, weakness, panting, anorexia and lethargy. The fact that clinical signs tend to be intermittent and are often precipitated by exercise, excitement or stress, suggests a physiological adaptation to severe hypocalcaemia.

Posterior lenticular cataract formation can occur secondary to hypocalcaemia in dogs and cats. Electrocardiography has shown prolongation of QT interval in some cases of hypoparathyroidism.

Laboratory findings

Profound hypocalcaemia (serum total calcium less than 2.0 mmol l^{-1}) and severe hyperphosphataemia (serum phosphate greater than 1.3 mmol l^{-1}) with normal renal function (blood urea and serum creatinine) are found in cases of primary hypoparathyroidism. The differential diagnosis of hypocalcaemia is given in Table 39.9.

PTH assays are available and have been validated for use in the dog and cat (Torrance and Nachreiner, 1989; Barber et al., 1993). An inappropriately low plasma PTH concentration in a hypocalcaemic animal is diagnostic of primary hypoparathyroidism. Careful sample handling is essential to avoid erroneous results since PTH is heat labile.

Table 39.9 Differential diagnosis of hypocalcaemia

Primary hypoparathyroidism
Chronic renal failure[a]
Hypoalbuminaemia[a]
Intestinal malabsorption[a]
Acute pancreatitis[a]
Eclampsia
Acute renal failure
Ethylene glycol toxicity
Phosphate-containing enemas

[a] Not usually associated with clinical signs of tetany

Treatment

The treatment protocol for hypocalcaemia is outlined in Table 39.8; similar principles are used when treating dogs and cats. Parenteral calcium preparations should be used as emergency therapy to correct hypocalcaemic tetany. Maintenance therapy using calcium and vitamin D supplementation must be tailored to the individual patient and the dose adjusted according to the serum calcium concentration. Dihydrotachysterol supplementation can prove expensive in larger dogs. Vitamin D_2 at a dose of 1000–6000 iu kg^{-1} day^{-1} or calcitriol at a dose of 0.03–0.06 µg kg^{-1} day^{-1} may be used as alternatives.

With adequate monitoring of the serum calcium concentration, the prognosis in cases of primary hypoparathyroidism is usually excellent.

Hyperparathyroidism

Hyperparathyroidism can be primary or secondary. Primary hyperparathyroidism is a disorder resulting from autonomous and excessive secretion of PTH by one or more of the parathyroid glands. Secondary hyperparathyroidism is an adaptive increase in PTH secretion as a result of a chronic stimulation from a tendency to reduced concentration of ionized calcium in plasma. Secondary hyperparathyroidism may occur as a result of chronic renal failure (see Chapter 41) and calcium deficiency during growth (see Chapter 44).

Primary hyperparathyroidism is most commonly caused by a small solitary parathyroid adenoma. PTH excess may also be caused by nodular hyperplasia in one or more of the parathyroid glands (DeVries et al., 1993). Very rarely the disease is caused by a parathyroid carcinoma (Berger and Feldman, 1987).

Clinical signs

Primary hyperparathyroidism is an uncommon disease of older dogs and cats (Berger and Feldman, 1987; Kallet et al., 1991). There is no sex or breed predilection.

The clinical signs in hyperparathyroidism are variable. The disease may be asymptomatic or may result in mild to severe systemic illness. The clinical signs relate to hypercalcaemia and include polyuria, polydipsia, anorexia, vomiting, depression, muscle weakness, constipation and weight loss.

Clinical examination may reveal bradycardia. The small size of the parathyroid lesions mean that the nodules are rarely palpable.

Laboratory findings

Hypercalcaemia (serum total calcium greater than 3.0 mmol l^{-1}) and hyperphosphataemia (serum phosphate concentration less than 1.3 mmol l^{-1}) are found in cases of primary hyperparathyroidism provided renal function is normal. Prolonged increases in the circulating calcium concentration will facilitate calcium deposition in the kidneys causing renal function to deteriorate and serum phosphate concentrations to rise. If renal failure develops, primary hyperparathyroidism is difficult to differentiate from secondary renal hyperparathyroidism.

The differential diagnosis of hypercalcaemia is given in Table 39.10. Primary hyperparathyroidism is an uncommon cause of hypercalcaemia (Elliott et al., 1991).

Circulating PTH concentrations are inappropriately increased in animals with primary hyperparathyroidism. The PTH assay provides a useful differentiation in hypercalcaemic patients because plasma PTH concentrations are low in dogs with cancer-associated hypercalcaemia. Careful handling of the sample is essential to avoid erroneous results since PTH is heat labile.

Diagnostic imaging

Ultrasonographic examination of the parathyroid glands has been shown to be useful in the evaluation of hypercalcaemic dogs and can be used to identify hyperplastic parathyroid glands and parathyroid adenomas (Wisner et al., 1993). Ultrasound examination of the kidneys may also reveal the hyperechoic medullary band characteristic of nephrocalcinosis in the dog. The medullary band may be seen in normal cats.

Table 39.10 Differential diagnosis of hypercalcaemia

Cancer-associated hypercalcaemia
Lymphoproliferative disease
Apocrine cell adenocarcinoma of the anal sac
Multiple myeloma
Other solid tumours
Hypoadrenocorticism
Chronic renal failure
Primary hyperparathyroidism
Granulomatous diseases, e.g. the systemic mycoses
Vitamin D intoxication

Treatment

The hypercalcaemic crisis should be treated by aggressive intravenous fluid therapy using 0.9% sodium chloride solution (see also Chapter 50). Saline will restore the circulating fluid volume and promote calcium excretion. Frusemide at a dose of 2–4 mg kg^{-1} may also be administered intravenously twice daily to enhance calcium excretion. Bisphosphonates have also been used in dogs to control hypercalcaemia.

Primary hyperparathyroidism should be resolved following parathyroidectomy. Parathyroid adenomas are usually easily identified and removed. Postoperative complications include hypocalcaemia since the remaining parathyroid glands may be atrophic and require a period of adaptation before control of circulating calcium is regained.

DISORDERS OF THE ADRENAL GLANDS

Anatomy and physiology

The adrenal glands are located craniomedially to each kidney in retroperitoneal fat. On cross-section, the adrenal cortex appears pale yellow whereas the medulla is dark brown. The cortex completely surrounds the medulla and consists of three distinct zones: the outer zona glomerulosa (arcuata) comprising about 25% of the cortex, the middle zona fasciculata comprising approximately 60% and the inner zona reticularis, which accounts for the remaining 15% of the cortex. The zona reticularis is adjacent to the medulla, which comprises 10–20% of the total volume of the adrenal gland.

The adrenal cortex produces about 30 different hormones, many of which have little or no clinical significance. The hormones can be divided into three groups based on their predominant actions: mineralocorticoids, which are important in electrolyte and water homeostasis, glucocorticoids, which promote gluconeogenesis, and small quantities of sex hormones, particularly male hormones that have weak androgenic activity. Aldosterone is the most important mineralocorticoid and is produced by the zona glomerulosa. The principal glucocorticoid, cortisol, and the sex hormones are produced in the zonas fasciculata and reticularis.

Glucocorticoid and mineralocorticoid release are controlled by different mechanisms. Glucocorticoid release is controlled almost entirely by ACTH secreted by the anterior pituitary, which in turn, is regulated by corticotrophin releasing hormone (CRH) from the hypothalamus (Fig. 39.9). CRH is secreted by the neurones in the anterior portion of the paraventricular nuclei within the hypothalamus and is transported to the anterior pituitary by the portal circulation, where it stimulates ACTH release. There is probably an internal or 'short loop' negative feedback control by ACTH on CRH. ACTH secreted into the systemic circulation causes cortisol release with concentrations rising almost immediately. Cortisol has direct negative feedback effects on (1) the hypothalamus to decrease formation of CRH and (2) the anterior pituitary gland to decrease the formation of ACTH. These feedback mechanisms help regulate the plasma concentration of cortisol.

Secretion of CRH and ACTH is normally episodic and pulsatile, which results in fluctuating cortisol concentrations during the day. Diurnal variation is superimposed on this type of release. It is usually stated that in the dog CRH, ACTH and thus cortisol levels are highest in the early hours of the morning and that in the cat, they are greatest in the evening. However, a true circadian rhythm of cortisol concentrations has been difficult to confirm in the dog and cat. The episodic release of CRH and ACTH is perpetuated by the reciprocal effect of cortisol acting through negative feedback control. This reciprocal arrangement does not hold during periods of stress when both ACTH and cortisol are maintained at high levels, because the effects of stress tend to override the normal negative feedback control.

Aldosterone release is influenced primarily by the renin–angiotensin system and by plasma potassium concentrations (Fig. 39.9). Renin is secreted into the blood by the cells of the juxtaglomerular apparatus, which consists of specialized cells in the wall of the afferent arteriole immediately proximal to the glomerulus and the specialized epithelial cells of the distal convoluted tubule adjacent to that arteriole, the macula densa. Renin release may be stimulated by stretch receptors in the juxtaglomerular apparatus in response to hypotension or reduced renal blood flow, or by sodium and chloride receptors in the macula densa. Renin is also released by sympathetic nerve stimulation and is inhibited by angiotensin II, antidiuretic hormone, hypertension and increased reabsorption of sodium by the renal tubules.

DISORDERS OF THE ADRENAL GLANDS 545

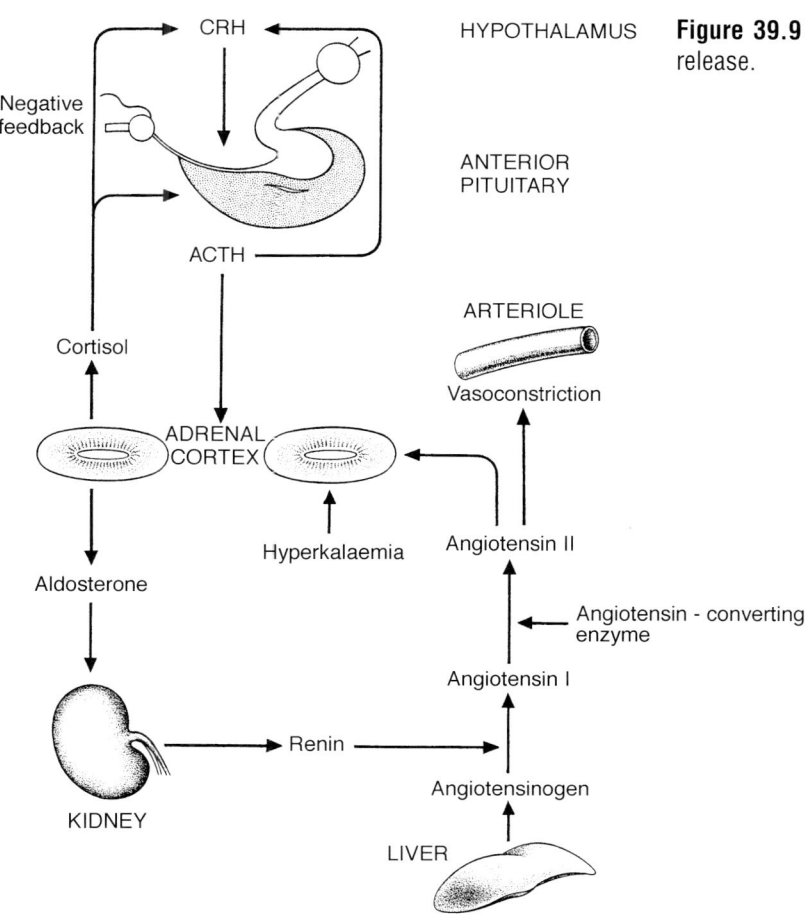

Figure 39.9 Regulation of adrenocortical hormone release.

Renin is an enzyme which splits circulating angiotensinogen, produced by the liver, into angiotensin I. Angiotensin I is converted into angiotensin II by angiotensin converting enzyme, which is located almost entirely in the pulmonary capillary endothelium. Angiotensin II is a powerful vasoconstrictor and stimulates aldosterone secretion from the zona glomerulosa. Through its action on the distal convoluted tubule, aldosterone has a negative feedback effect on the juxtaglomerular apparatus.

Potassium has a direct stimulatory effect on the zona glomerulosa cells to release aldosterone. ACTH and sodium play a less significant role in aldosterone secretion. ACTH is necessary to maintain normal aldosterone output. In the absence of ACTH, the zona glomerulosa partially atrophies, causing mild to moderate aldosterone deficiency, whereas there is almost total loss of glucocorticoid synthesis and release.

The main function of aldosterone is to protect against hypotension and potassium intoxication.

Aldosterone promotes sodium, chloride and water reabsorption as well as potassium excretion in many epithelial tissues including the intestinal mucosa, salivary glands, sweat glands and kidneys. Its main site of action is the renal tubule where it promotes sodium and chloride reabsorption in the proximal convoluted tubule and sodium reabsorption by exchange with potassium in the distal convoluted tubule. It is one of the complex regulatory systems for the regulation of extracellular fluid electrolyte concentrations, extracellular fluid volume, blood volume and arterial pressure.

■ Hypoadrenocorticism

Hypoadrenocorticism is a syndrome that results from a deficiency of both glucocorticoid and mineralocorticoid secretion from the adrenal cortices. Destruction of more than 95% of both adrenal cortices causes a clinical deficiency of all adrenocortical hormones and is termed primary hypoadrenocorticism (Addison's disease). Secondary hypoadrenocorticism is caused by a deficiency in ACTH which leads to atrophy of the adrenal cortices and impaired secretion of glucocorticoids. The production of mineralocorticoids, however, usually remains adequate.

Primary hypoadrenocorticism (Addison's disease)

Primary hypoadrenocorticism occurs more frequently in the dog than is recognized but it is much less common than hyperadrenocorticism (Cushing's disease). Hypoadrenocorticism is rare in the cat and only eight cases have been reported (Peterson and Greco, 1989). The clinical signs, diagnosis and treatment of hypoadrenocorticism in the dog and cat are similar.

Primary hypoadrenocorticism in the dog has been associated with the following conditions.

Idiopathic adrenocortical insufficiency is the commonest cause in the dog and is thought to result from immune-mediated destruction of the adrenal cortex. The presence of antiadrenal antibodies in two dogs and characteristic histopathological findings in another support this hypothesis (Schaer et al., 1986). In humans, hypoadrenocorticism has been found to be associated with other immune-mediated endocrine disorders such as thyroiditis, diabetes mellitus, hypoparathyroidism, primary gonadal failure and atrophic gastritis. A similar autoimmune polyglandular disease has also been recognized in dogs.

Mitotane-induced adrenocortical necrosis occurs occasionally. Although mitotane usually spares the zona glomerulosa and therefore mineralocorticoid secretion, cases of complete adrenocortical failure can occasionally occur (see under treatment of hyperadrenocorticism).

Bilateral adrenalectomy, haemorrhage or infarction of the adrenal cortex or mycotic or neoplastic involvement of the adrenal gland can also lead to adrenal insufficiency, but these are rare causes.

The loss or damage to the adrenal cortex leads to mineralocorticoid and glucocorticoid deficiency. Aldosterone is the major mineralocorticoid and deficiency causes impaired ability to conserve sodium and water and failure to excrete potassium leading to hyponatraemia and hyperkalaemia. Hyponatraemia induces lethargy, depression and nausea and leads to the development of hypovolaemia, hypotension, reduced cardiac output and decreased renal perfusion. Hyperkalaemia causes muscle weakness, hyporeflexia and impaired cardiac conduction. Glucocorticoid deficiency causes decreased tolerance of stress, loss of appetite and a mild normocytic, normochromic anaemia.

Clinical signs

There are no breed predilections but the possibility of a hereditary factor has been suggested in some breeds, for example standard poodles (Shaker et al., 1988). Hypoadrenocorticism appears to be a disease of the young and middle-aged dog with an age range of 3 months to 9 years and a median age of 4–5 years. Approximately 70% of reported cases are female (Peterson and Kintzer, 1996).

The progression of adrenocortical insufficiency may be acute or chronic. Chronic hypoadrenocorticism is far more common than the acute disease in the dog.

Acute primary hypoadrenocorticism

The clinical appearance of the acute form is that of hypovolaemic shock (adrenocortical crisis). The animal is usually found in a state of collapse or collapses when stressed. Other signs include weak pulse, profound bradycardia, abdominal pain, vomiting, diarrhoea, dehydration and hypothermia. The condition is rapidly progressive and life threatening. Aggressive fluid therapy will help most patients and allow more time to make a diagnosis.

Chronic primary hypoadrenocorticism

The clinical signs in the chronic form are often vague and non-specific (Table 39.11). The diagnosis should be considered in any dog with a waxing and waning type of illness or that shows episodic weakness and collapse (Herrtage and McKerrell, 1995). The most consistent clinical signs include anorexia, vomiting, lethargy depression and/or weakness. The severity of each sign can vary during the course of the disease and may be interspersed with periods of apparent good health often following non-specific veterinary therapy, usually consisting of corticosteroid medication and/or fluid administration. Other common clinical signs include dehydration, bradycardia and weak femoral pulses. In a few cases, severe gastrointestinal haemorrhage can occur resulting in profound anaemia (Medinger et al., 1993). Hypoadrenocorticism can easily be mistaken for chronic renal insufficiency, primary neuromuscu-

Table 39.11 Clinical signs of primary hypoadrenocorticism (in approximate decreasing order of frequency)

Anorexia
Lethargy/depression
Vomiting
Weakness
Weight loss
Waxing/waning course
Dehydration
Diarrhoea
Previous response to therapy
Collapse
Hypothermia
Slow capillary refill time
Shaking
Polyuria/polydipsia
Melaena
Weak pulse
Bradycardia (< 60 bpm)

lar disorders and diseases which cause weight loss, weakness, anorexia, vomiting and diarrhoea.

Laboratory findings

The most common laboratory findings are listed in Table 39.12.

Table 39.12 Laboratory findings in primary hypoadrenocorticism

Haematology
Lymphocytosis
Eosinophilia
Relative neutropenia
Anaemia: usually a normocytic, normochromic, non-regenerative anaemia, but can be blood loss anaemia associated with gastrointestinal haemorrhage
Biochemistry
Azotaemia
Hyponatraemia (< 135 mmol l^{-1})
Hyperkalaemia (> 5.5 mmol l^{-1})
Reduced sodium:potassium ratio (< 25:1)
Reduced bicarbonate and total CO_2 concentrations
Hypochloraemia
Hypercalcaemia
Hypoglycaemia
Urinalysis
Specific gravity variable (usually 1.015–1.030)
Endocrine testing
Low basal serum cortisol concentration with a failure to stimulate in response to ACTH administration
Raised plasma ACTH concentration

Haematological changes may include lymphocytosis, eosinophilia and mild normocytic, normochromic, non-regenerative anaemia. However, these findings are not as consistent as those changes seen in hyperadrenocorticism. Normal or elevated eosinophil and lymphocyte counts in an ill animal with signs compatible with hypoadrenocorticism are significant, because the expected response to stress is eosinopenia and lymphopenia. The mild anaemia may not be obvious until the dog has been rehydrated since dehydration may mask the anaemia.

The most consistent laboratory findings in hypoadrenocorticism are prerenal azotaemia, hyponatraemia and hyperkalaemia. Blood urea and serum creatinine are increased as a result of reduced renal perfusion and decreased glomerular filtration rate. Reduced renal perfusion results from hypovolaemia, reduced cardiac output and hypotension, which in turn result from chronic fluid loss through the kidneys, acute fluid loss through vomiting and/or diarrhoea, and inadequate fluid intake.

Prerenal azotaemia is usually associated with concentrated urine (specific gravity >1.030) whereas the urine in primary renal failure is often isosthenuric or only mildly concentrated (1.008–1.025). Some severe cases of hypoadrenocorticism, however, may develop impaired concentrating ability because the chronic sodium loss reduces the renal medullary concentration gradient. Therefore, the laboratory findings may resemble those of chronic renal failure. With adequate fluid therapy, the blood urea will return to normal in cases of hypoadrenocorticism.

Sodium is usually less than 135 mmol l^{-1} and potassium greater than 5.5 mmol l^{-1}. The ratio of sodium to potassium may be more reliable than the absolute values. The normal ratio of sodium to potassium varies between 27:1 and 40:1, whereas in patients with hypoadrenocorticism, the ratio is commonly less than 25:1 and may be below 20:1. Blood samples must be collected before intravenous fluids are administered otherwise the electrolyte concentrations may quickly return to normal. Even so, approximately 10% of cases may have normal electrolyte concentrations at the time of presentation and these are usually thought to be early cases of hypoadrenocorticism.

Mild to moderate hypercalcaemia is seen in about a third of cases of hypoadrenocorticism, usually those dogs which are most severely affected by the disease. Hypercalcaemia is caused by haemoconcentration, increased renal tubular reabsorption and decreased glomerular filtration.

Cases of hypoadrenocorticism have a tendency to develop hypoglycaemia because glucocorticoid deficiency reduces glucose production by the liver and peripheral cell receptors become more sensitive to insulin. Severe hypoglycaemia is uncommon (Willard et al., 1982) but the potential should remain a concern for the clinician.

Electrocardiographic findings

Hyperkalaemia impairs cardiac conduction which can be assessed by electrocardiography (ECG) (Fig. 39.10). Although the ECG changes do not

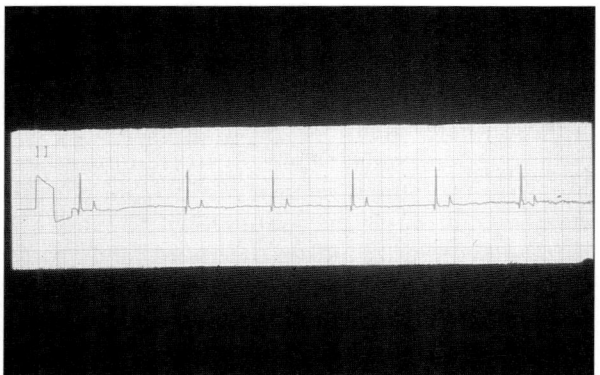

Figure 39.10 An ECG recording from a bearded collie dog with hypoadrenocorticism demonstrating absent P waves, marked bradycardia and peaked T waves. Plasma sodium was 136 mmol l^{-1} and plasma potassium 9.3 mmol l^{-1}.

correlate directly with serum potassium levels, the following guidelines have proved helpful:

> 5.5 mmol l^{-1}	peaking of the T wave shortening of the Q-T interval
> 6.5 mmol l^{-1}	increased QRS duration
> 7.0 mmol l^{-1}	P wave amplitude decreased P-R interval prolonged
> 8.5 mmol l^{-1}	P wave absent severe bradycardia (sinoventricular rhythm)

Electrocardiography can also be used for monitoring the patient during treatment.

Radiographic findings

Dogs with hypoadrenocorticism may show radiographic signs of hypovolaemia which include microcardia, decreased size of pulmonary vessels and reduced size of the caudal vena cava. The changes are not specific and only represent changes associated with hypovolaemia and dehydration irrespective of the cause. A few dogs with hypoadrenocorticism develop oesophageal dilatation as a result of generalized muscle weakness and this can be seen on thoracic radiographs (Burrows, 1987).

Endocrine testing

The ACTH stimulation test is commonly used to confirm the presence of hypoadrenocorticism and the protocol is described in Table 39.16. The intravenous preparation of ACTH (tetracosactin) should be used as absorption by other routes can not be relied on if the patient is collapsed or severely hypotensive. In hypoadrenocorticism, the resting cortisol level will be low with a subnormal or negligible response to ACTH (see Fig. 39.15). The ACTH stimulation test, however, does not distinguish between primary and secondary hypoadrenocorticism.

Plasma ACTH concentrations are required to differentiate primary and secondary hypoadrenocorticism. Plasma ACTH concentrations are low in secondary hypoadrenocorticism and markedly raised in primary hypoadrenocorticism.

Treatment

Acute primary hypoadrenocorticism

Aggressive intravenous fluid therapy using normal saline should be used in the acute crisis to treat the hyperkalaemia, which is life-threatening. The response to treatment is predictable and often dramatic. Glucose and insulin therapy or calcium administration are therefore not usually required for the treatment of hyperkalaemia due to hypoadrenocorticism. The serum potassium falls because of the dilution effect of the saline and the improvement in renal perfusion. The increased renal blood flow allows further excretion of potassium into the urine.

Glucocorticoid therapy should be used early in the treatment of the acute crisis. Once the animal has improved with saline and glucocorticoids, maintenance therapy with mineralocorticoids can be instigated (see below). Glucocorticoids of choice in the acute crisis include:

- hydrocortisone sodium succinate — 10 mg kg^{-1} i.v. repeated every 3–6 h
- prednisolone sodium succinate — 5 mg kg^{-1} i.v. repeated every 3–6 h
- dexamethasone sodium phosphate — 0.5–1.0 mg kg^{-1} i.v. given once

If plasma cortisol concentrations are to be measured for the diagnosis of hypoadrenocorticism, then dexamethasone should be used as the other preparations cross-react with cortisol in the assay.

Chronic primary hypoadrenocorticism (maintenance therapy)

Fludrocortisone acetate (Florinef, Squibb) is an oral synthetic adrenocortical steroid with mineralocorticoid effects and is the treatment of choice for maintenance therapy in the dog. An initial dose of 15 µg kg^{-1} day^{-1} of fludrocortisone is given and serum electrolytes measured after 5–7 days. The dose rate should then be adjusted until the sodium and potassium levels are within the normal range. The daily maintenance dose required is usually between 15 and 30 µg kg^{-1} day^{-1} (Kintzer and Peterson, 1997). The dose often has to be increased during the first 6–18 months of therapy and the drug may need to be administered twice daily in a few cases.

Daily glucocorticoid supplementation is not required after initial treatment in the majority of cases. However, the owners of animals with hypoadrenocorticism should be given a supply of prednisolone tablets to be administered if the patient appears unwell. Prednisolone at a dose of 0.1–0.2 mg kg^{-1} daily should be sufficient as a physiological replacement for those cases that do require glucocorticoid medication.

Salt supplementation using salt tablets or salting the food should be instigated initially to help correct hyponatraemia but can be gradually reduced and phased out as it is not usually required long term. Dogs requiring unusually high doses of fludrocortisone, however, may respond to oral salt and fewer fludrocortisone tablets.

The prognosis for hypoadrenocorticism is generally excellent providing owner education is adequate.

Secondary hypoadrenocorticism

Secondary hypoadrenocorticism is associated with a deficiency of glucocorticoids caused by a deficiency in ACTH production and/or release. The production of mineralocorticoids, although reduced, generally remains adequate. Secondary hypoadrenocorticism occurs in both dogs and cats.

Secondary hypoadrenocorticism can be associated with destructive lesions, for example nonfunctional tumours, in the hypothalamus or anterior pituitary. More commonly, however, the condition is iatrogenic with clinical signs occurring after cessation of glucocorticoid therapy. In these cases, secondary hypoadrenocorticism is caused by prolonged suppression of ACTH secretion from glucocorticoid therapy. In the cat, secondary hypoadrenocorticism is seen following prolonged megoestrol acetate therapy.

Clinical signs

The clinical signs are variable and may include depression, anorexia, occasional vomiting or diarrhoea, weak pulse and sudden collapse when stressed. If the secondary hypoadrenocorticism is associated with cessation of glucocorticoid therapy, then clinical signs of iatrogenic hyperadrenocorticism (Cushing's disease) are usually present.

Diagnosis and treatment

The diagnosis is based on a failure of the animal's cortisol levels to respond to ACTH stimulation (see Fig. 39.15). Glucocorticoid replacement, using prednisolone at a dose of 0.1–0.2 mg kg^{-1} daily is indicated for immediate correction of the clinical signs. Further treatment and the prognosis depend on the cause and whether it can be eliminated.

Hyperadrenocorticism (Cushing's disease)

Hyperadrenocorticism is associated with excessive production or administration of glucocorticoids and is one of the most commonly diagnosed endocrinopathies in the dog. Hyperadrenocorticism is rare in the cat (Watson and Herrtage, 1998).

Hyperadrenocorticism can be spontaneous or iatrogenic. Spontaneously occurring hyperadrenocorticism may be associated with inappropriate secretion of ACTH by the pituitary (pituitary-dependent hyperadrenocorticism) or associated with a primary adrenal disorder (adrenal-dependent hyperadrenocorticism) (see Fig. 39.11).

Pituitary-dependent hyperadrenocorticism

Pituitary-dependent hyperadrenocorticism accounts for 80% of dogs and the majority of cats with naturally occurring hyperadrenocorticism. Excessive ACTH secretion results in bilateral adrenocortical hyperplasia and increased cortisol secretion. There is a failure of the negative feedback mechanism of cortisol on ACTH. However, episodic secretion of ACTH results in fluctuating cortisol levels that may at times be within the normal range. The presence of excessive cortisol secretion can be confirmed by measuring urine cortisol excretion over a 24-hour period.

Figure 39.11 The hypothalamic–pituitary adrenal axis in (a) pituitary-dependent and (b) adrenal-dependent hyperadrenocorticism

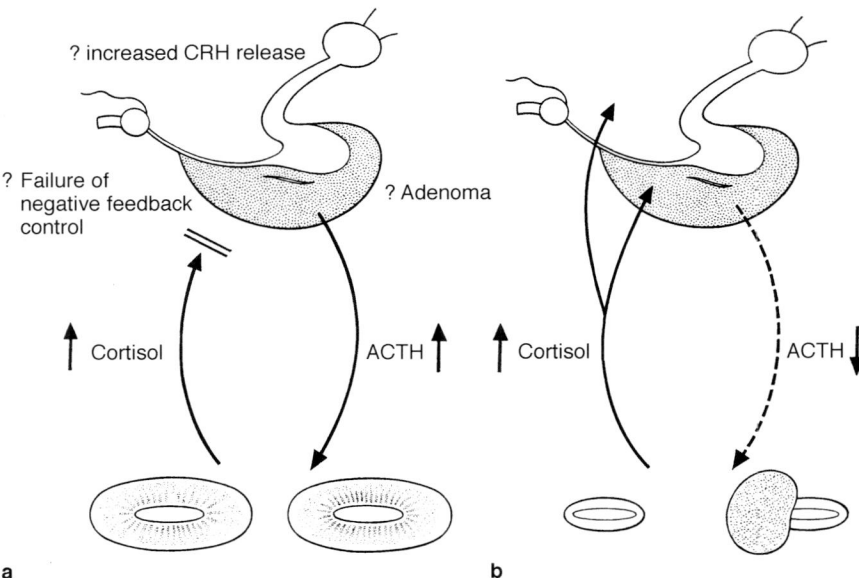

Pathological changes in pituitary-dependent hyperadrenocorticism include microadenomas and macroadenomas of the corticotroph cells.

Microadenomas are less than 1 cm in diameter. The incidence of corticotroph adenomas associated with pituitary-dependent hyperadrenocorticism varies widely probably because detection of small tumours requires careful microdissection, experience and special stains. In one study using immunocytochemical staining, more than 80% of dogs with pituitary-dependent hyperadrenocorticism were positive for pituitary adenomas (Peterson et al., 1982a).

Macroadenomas are larger than 1 cm in diameter and only a small percentage of dogs have large corticotroph adenomas (Duesberg et al., 1995). These may compress the remaining pituitary gland and extend dorsally into the hypothalamus. However, they are generally slow growing and do not always produce neurological signs. Malignant pituitary tumours are rare.

Primary failure of the negative feedback response. The defect responsible for pituitary-dependent hyperadrenocorticism unassociated with pituitary neoplasia is unknown. A primary failure of the negative feedback response by cortisol has been proposed. Others suspect an overproduction of CRH from the hypothalamus, which may cause diffuse hyperplasia of ACTH-producing cells in the anterior pituitary.

From a clinical point of view the precise pituitary pathology is not of great importance unless neurological signs are present at the time of diagnosis or become apparent during the initial treatment.

Adrenal-dependent hyperadrenocorticism

The remaining 15–20% of spontaneous cases of hyperadrenocorticism in dogs and cats are caused by unilateral or bilateral adrenal tumours, which can be benign or malignant.

Adrenocortical adenomas are small, well-circumscribed tumours that do not metastasize and are not locally invasive. Approximately 50% are partially calcified (Reusch and Feldman, 1991).

Adrenocortical carcinomas are usually large, locally invasive, haemorrhagic and necrotic. Tumour calcification also occurs in about 50% of dogs. The tumours frequently invade the phrenicoabdominal vein and caudal vena cava and metastasize to the liver, lung and kidney.

In dogs, adrenocortical adenomas and carcinomas occur in approximately equal proportions. The cortex contiguous to the tumour and that of the contralateral gland become atrophied in the presence of functional adenomas and carcinomas (Fig. 39.11b). This is important if the tumour is removed surgically as postoperatively the animal may not be able to secrete sufficient glucocorticoids. Function of the zona glomerulosa should not be affected.

Clinical signs

Any breed of dog can develop hyperadrenocorticism but poodles, dachshunds and small terriers, for example the Yorkshire terrier, Jack Russell terrier and Staffordshire bull terrier, appear more at risk of developing pituitary-dependent hyperadrenocorticism. Adrenocortical tumours occur more frequently in larger breeds of dog. No breed predisposition has been recorded in cats.

Pituitary-dependent hyperadrenocorticism is usually a disease of the middle-aged to older dog, with an age range of 2–16 years and a median age of 7–9 years. Dogs with adrenal-dependent hyperadrenocorticism tend to be older with a range of between 6 and 16 years and a median age of 10–11 years (Reusch and Feldman, 1991).

There is no significant difference in sex distribution in pituitary-dependent hyperadrenocorticism, however, female dogs are three times more likely to develop adrenal tumours than males.

Affected dogs usually develop a classic combination of clinical signs associated with increased glucocorticoid levels and these are listed in Table 39.13 in approximate decreasing order of frequency. Larger breeds of dogs, however, may not show all the classic signs.

Hyperadrenocorticism has an insidious onset and is slowly progressive over many months or even years. Many owners consider the early signs as part of the normal ageing process of their dog. In a few cases, clinical signs may be intermittent, with periods of remission and relapse (Peterson et al., 1982b) and in other cases there may be rapid onset and progression of clinical signs.

Polydipsia, defined as water intake in excess of 100 ml kg^{-1} body weight day^{-1} and polyuria, defined as urine production in excess of 50 ml kg^{-1} body weight day^{-1}, are seen in virtually all cases of hyperadrenocorticism. Excessive thirst, nocturia and/or urination in the house are usually noted by owners. The polydipsia occurs secondary to the polyuria, which is only partially responsive to water deprivation. The precise cause of the polyuria remains obscure, but may be due to increased glomerular filtration rate, inhibition of the release of ADH, inhibition of the action of ADH on the renal tubules or possibly accelerated inactivation of ADH.

Increased appetite is common but most owners often assess this as a sign of good health. A voracious appetite, scavenging or stealing food, however, may give rise to concern especially if the dog previously had a poor appetite. Polyphagia is assumed to be a direct effect of glucocorticoids.

The pot-bellied appearance is very common in hyperadrenocorticism but may be so gradual that owners fail to recognize its significance (Fig. 39.12). The abdominal distension is associated with redistribution of fat to the abdomen, liver enlargement and abdominal muscle wasting and weakness. The weakness of the abdominal muscles make palpation of the pendulous abdomen easier and more rewarding.

The gradual onset of lethargy and poor exercise tolerance are usually considered by most owners to be compatible with ageing. Only when muscle weakness is severe as reflected by an inability to climb stairs or jump into the car does the owner become concerned. Lethargy, excessive panting and poor exercise tolerance are probably an expression of muscle wasting and weakness. Apart from the development of a pendulous abdomen, decreased muscle mass may be noted around the limbs, over the spine or over the temporal region. Muscle weakness is the result of muscle wasting caused by protein catabolism.

Occasionally, dogs with hyperadrenocorticism develop myotonia, characterized by persistent active muscle contractions that continue after voluntary or involuntary stimuli. All limbs may be affected, but the signs are usually more severe in the hindlegs. The animals with myotonia walk with a stiff stilted gait. The affected limbs are rigid and rapidly return to extension after being passively flexed. Spinal reflexes are difficult to elicit because of the rigidity, but pain sensation is

Table 39.13 Clinical signs of hyperadrenocorticism (in approximate decreasing order of frequency)

Polydipsia and polyuria
Polyphagia
Abdominal distension
Liver enlargement
Muscle wasting/weakness
Lethargy, poor exercise tolerance
Skin changes
Alopecia
Persistent anoestrus or testicular atrophy
Calcinosis cutis
Myotonia
Neurological signs

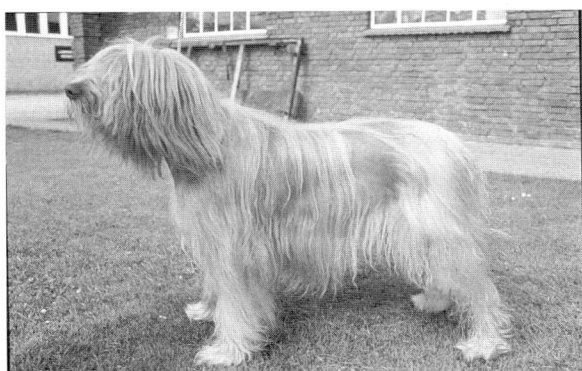

Figure 39.12 A 10-year-old bearded collie dog with hyperadrenocorticism illustrating symmetrical alopecia and a distended abdomen.

normal. The muscles are usually slightly hypertrophied rather than being atrophied and a myotonic dimple can be elicited by percussion of the affected muscle. Bizarre high frequency discharges are noted on electromyography (Duncan et al., 1977).

The skin particularly over the ventral abdomen becomes thin and inelastic. Elasticity can be assessed clinically by tenting the skin between the thumb and forefinger. In the normal dog the skin will flow back to a smooth contour but in hyperadrenocorticism it remains tented. Striae can form as a result of this inelasticity. The abdominal veins are prominent and easily visible through the thin skin. There is often excessive surface scale and comedomes, caused by follicular plugging, are seen especially around the nipples (Fig. 39.13). Hyperpigmentation of the skin is rare in canine hyperadrenocorticism.

Protein catabolism causing atrophic collagen also leads to excessive bruising either following venepuncture or other minor trauma. Wound healing is extraordinarily slow, presumably because of inhibition of fibroblast proliferation and collagen synthesis. Healing wounds often undergo dehiscence and even old scars may start to break down (Fig. 39.13).

Calcinosis cutis is a frequent finding in biopsy material from the skin, however clinical evidence of calcinosis cutis is less common. The gross appearance can vary but the predilection sites are the neck, axilla, ventral abdomen and inguinal areas (Fig. 39.13). Calcinosis cutis usually appears as a firm, slightly elevated, white or cream plaque surrounded by a ring of erythema. Large plaques tend to crack, become secondarily infected and develop a crust containing white powdery material. The exact pathogenesis is unknown but plasma calcium and phosphorus concentrations are usually normal. Mineralization of the soft tissues may be seen at other sites, for example the bronchial walls and kidneys on radiographic examination (see below).

Thinning of the haircoat, leading to bilaterally symmetric alopecia, is frequently seen with hyperadrenocorticism and occurs because of the inhibitory effect of cortisol on the anagen or growth phase of the hair cycle. The remaining hair is dull and dry because it is in the telogen or resting phase of the hair cycle. The alopecia is non-pruritic and affects mainly the flanks, ventral abdomen and chest, perineum and neck. The head, feet and tail are usually the last areas to be affected (Fig. 39.12). The coat colour is often lighter than normal.

Entire bitches with hyperadrenocorticism usually cease to cycle. The length of anoestrus, often years, indicates the duration of the disease process. In the intact male both testes become soft and flabby. Anoestrus and testicular atrophy occur due to the negative feedback effect of high concentrations of cortisol on the pituitary which also suppresses secretion of gonadotrophic hormones.

Although uncommon at the time of presentation, a few cases develop neurological signs in association with large expanding functional pituitary tumours. The most common clinical signs are dullness, depression, loss of learned behaviour, anorexia, aimless wandering, head pressing, circling, ataxia, blindness, anisocoria and seizures. More often, however, neurological signs develop during initial treatment of pituitary-dependent hyperadrenocorticism with mitotane. This is thought to involve removal of the negative feedback of cortisol, which can cause some pituitary tumours to enlarge rapidly.

Laboratory findings

The main haematological, biochemical and urinalysis findings are listed in Table 39.14.

The most consistent haematological finding is a stress leucogram with a relative and absolute lymphopenia ($< 1.5 \times 10^9$ l^{-1}) and eosinopenia ($< 0.2 \times 10^9$ l^{-1}). Lymphopenia is most likely the result of steroid lymphocytolysis and/or redistribution of T cells to lymphoid tissues and eosinopenia results from bone marrow sequestration of eosinophils. A mild to moderate neutrophilia and monocytosis may be present and it is

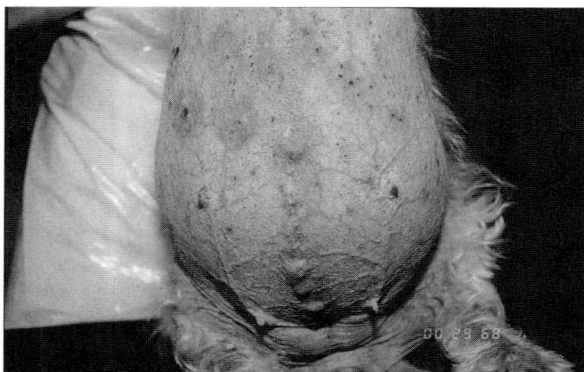

Figure 39.13 An 11-year-old neutered female dachshund with hyperadrenocorticism illustrating the symmetrical alopecia, distended abdomen, thin skin, comedomes, calcinosis cutis and partial breakdown of a laparotomy wound. See colour plate.

Table 39.14 Laboratory findings in hyperadrenocorticism

Haematology
Lymphopenia ($< 1.5 \times 10^9$ l^{-1})
Eosinopenia ($< 0.2 \times 10^9$ l^{-1})
Neutrophilia
Monocytosis
Erythrocytosis

Biochemistry
Increased alkaline phosphatase (often markedly elevated) **Dog only**
Increased ALT
High normal fasting blood glucose. Rarely diabetic except for the cat.
Decreased blood urea
Increased cholesterol (>8 mmol l^{-1})
Lipaemia
Increased bile acid concentrations

Urinalysis
Urine specific gravity <1.015
Glycosuria (<10% of canine cases)
Urinary tract infection

Other findings
Low T4 concentrations
Subnormal T4 response to TSH or TRH stimulation

thought that excessive glucocorticoids result in decreased capillary margination and diapedesis and increased release from the bone marrow. The red cell count is usually normal, although mild polycythaemia may occasionally be noted. Platelet counts may also be elevated. These findings are thought to result from stimulatory effects of glucocorticoids on the bone marrow.

Glucocorticoids, both endogenous or exogenous, induce a specific hepatic isoenzyme of alkaline phosphatase in the dog. The increase in serum alkaline phosphatase is commonly 5–40 times the normal level and is perhaps one of the most reliable indicators of hyperadrenocorticism. Measurement of the specific steroid-induced isoenzyme of alkaline phosphatase has been used for more accurate assessment of elevated serum alkaline phosphatase activity (Oluju et al., 1984). A marked increase in serum alkaline phosphatase is rarely seen in cats with hyperadrenocorticism, because they do not possess a steroid-induced isoenzyme and have the ability to clear serum of excess alkaline phosphatase.

Alanine aminotransferase (ALT) is commonly elevated in hyperadrenocorticism, but the increase is usually only mild and is believed to result from liver damage caused by swollen hepatocytes due to glycogen storage.

Blood glucose is usually in the high normal range, but about 10% of canine cases will develop overt diabetes mellitus. The gluconeogenic effect of glucocorticoids results in insulin antagonism and subsequent development of pancreatic islet cell exhaustion. The cat appears more prone to developing hyperglycaemia and overt diabetes. In contrast to the dog where polydipsia and polyuria are among the earliest clinical signs of hyperadrenocorticism, the onset of polydipsia and polyuria is delayed in the cat and coincides with the development of moderate to severe hyperglycaemia and glycosuria. Hyperadrenocorticism should be suspected in any cat which requires high daily insulin doses to control the hyperglycaemia and glycosuria.

Blood urea is usually below normal due to the continual urinary loss associated with glucocorticoid-induced diuresis. Serum creatinine concentration also tends to be in the low to normal range.

Cholesterol and lipid concentrations are usually increased due to glucocorticoid stimulation of lipolysis. Cholesterol is usually greater than 8 mmol l^{-1} but this is not a specific finding as cholesterol is also raised in hypothyroidism, diabetes mellitus, chronic liver disease and chronic renal disease, all of which may be differential diagnoses. Lipaemia is important as it can interfere with the accurate assessment of a number of laboratory parameters.

The specific gravity of the urine is usually less than 1.015 and is often hyposthenuric (< 1.010) provided water has not been withheld. Dogs with hyperadrenocorticism can concentrate their urine if water is deprived, but their concentrating ability is usually reduced. Glycosuria is present in the 10% of cases with diabetes mellitus. Urinary tract infection is common and occurs in about half the cases of hyperadrenocorticism.

Basal thyroxine concentrations are decreased in about 70% of dogs with hyperadrenocorticism (Peterson et al., 1984). This is, in part, due to inhibition of thyrotrophin-releasing hormone (TRH) and reduced pituitary secretion of thyroid-stimulating hormone (TSH). Excess cortisol, however, may also alter thyroid hormone binding to plasma proteins and enhance the metabolism of thyroid hormone. The response to stimulation by TSH usually parallels normal dogs but thyroxine concentrations both before and after stimulation with TSH are subnormal (Peterson et al., 1984).

Diagnostic imaging

Radiographic examination of the thorax and abdomen is advisable in all cases of suspected or proven hyperadrenocorticism. Although positive diagnostic information is only obtained in the small number of cases in which adrenal enlargement can be detected, the number and frequency of radiological changes consistent with hyperadrenocorticism provide a useful aid to diagnosis. In addition, survey radiographs may reveal significant intercurrent disease. The radiological signs of hyperadrenocorticism have been reviewed (Huntley et al., 1982) and the common changes are listed in Table 39.15.

Hepatomegaly is the most consistent radiographic finding in hyperadrenocorticism. Good radiographic contrast permits easy identification of the abdominal structures because of the large deposits of intra-abdominal fat. Hepatomegaly may be mild to severe and the ventral lobe borders vary in shape between being distinctly rounded and sharply wedge-shaped. The pot-bellied appearance is usually very obvious on the recumbent lateral projection (Fig. 39.14). Hepatomegaly and a pendulous abdomen are the most consistent radiographic findings in cats with hyperadrenocorticism.

Adrenal enlargement is the least common finding on abdominal radiographs. Gross enlargement is suggestive, though not diagnostic, of an adrenocortical carcinoma. Unilateral mineralization in the region of an adrenal gland suggests the possibility of an adrenal tumour. Both adrenocortical adenomas and carcinomas can become mineral-

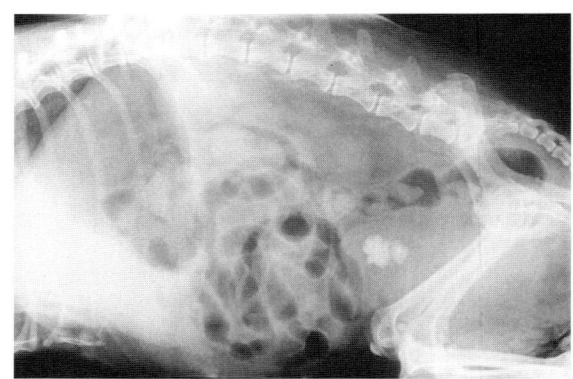

Figure 39.14 Abdominal radiograph of a Shih tzu bitch with hyperadrenocorticism showing a distended abdomen, enlarged liver and the presence of cystic calculi.

Table 39.15 Radiological signs of hyperadrenocorticism

Abdominal radiographs
Liver enlargement
Good radiographic contrast
Pot-bellied appearance
Calcinosis cutis/soft tissue mineralization
Distended bladder
Cystic or renal calculi
Adrenal enlargement/mineralization
Osteopenia

Thoracic radiographs
Tracheal and bronchial wall mineralization
Pulmonary metastasis from adrenocortical carcinoma
Osteopenia
Congestive heart failure (rare)
Pulmonary thromboembolism (rare)

ized. Radiography of the abdomen not infrequently demonstrates calcification of the adrenal glands in normal older cats and is not associated with any functional abnormality.

Calcinosis cutis tends to have a nodular mineralization pattern, whereas calcification in the fascial planes, for example just dorsal to the thoracolumbar spine, tends to be linear. Mineralization may also be seen in the renal pelvis, liver, gastric mucosa and abdominal aorta.

A grossly distended urinary bladder may be seen radiographically even when the animal has been allowed to urinate prior to radiographic examination. Cystic calculi may also be present and are usually associated with urinary tract infection. Occasionally the impression of osteopenia is gained from a distinct reduction in radiographic density of the lumbar vertebral bodies relative to the vertebral end plates.

Tracheal and bronchial wall calcification is frequently seen radiographically in cases of hyperadrenocorticism. Calcification of these structures, however, can be seen in animals as part of the normal ageing process and is not considered to be a highly significant finding (Huntley et al., 1982).

The thoracic radiographs should also be examined for evidence of pulmonary metastases from an adrenocortical carcinoma, congestive heart failure, osteopenia of the thoracic spine and pulmonary thromboembolism. The latter is a rare complication of hyperadrenocorticism and may be suspected when the radiographic signs include pleural effusion, increased diameter and blunting of pulmonary arteries, decreased vascularity of the affected lobes and overperfusion of the unobstructed pulmonary vasculature (Fluckiger and Gomez, 1984). However in some cases of pulmonary thromboembolism, the radiographs may reveal no abnormalities.

Abdominal ultrasonography has been used to examine the adrenal glands. It is a challenge for the ultrasonographer to consistently distinguish between normal and hyperplastic adrenal glands since the diagnosis of adrenal hyperplasia is somewhat subjective. The measurement of the thickness (ventrodorsal dimension) of the adrenal gland has been shown to be more sensitive than either the length or width of the gland. A thickness of greater than 7.5 mm for the left adrenal gland is considered to provide the best sensitivity and specificity as a diagnostic test for canine pituitary-dependent hyperadrenocorticism (Bartez et al., 1995).

Abdominal ultrasonography can also detect large adrenocortical tumours (Kantrowitz et al., 1986). Adrenal masses are diagnosed by the location of the mass and clinical signs exhibited by the animal. There is a propensity for adrenal tumours to invade nearby vessels and surrounding tissues, therefore a thorough ultrasonographic examination of adjacent vessels and tissues should be performed. Mineralization is frequently associated with benign and malignant adrenocortical tumours in the dog and acoustic shadowing may aid in localizing the adrenal tumour. If an adrenal mass is identified, the liver should also be examined ultrasonographically for evidence of hepatic metastases.

Computed tomography (CT) and magnetic resonance imaging (MRI) have proved helpful in the diagnosis of adrenal tumours, adrenal hyperplasia and large pituitary tumours but these techniques are expensive and not widely available (Voorhout et al., 1988; Bertoy et al., 1995).

Endocrine screening tests

A presumptive diagnosis of hyperadrenocorticism can be made from clinical signs, physical examination, routine laboratory tests and radiographic findings, but the diagnosis must be confirmed by either ACTH stimulation test or a low-dose dexamethasone suppression test.

ACTH stimulation test

The protocol for the ACTH stimulation test is shown in Table 39.16. It is the best screening test for distinguishing spontaneous from iatrogenic hyperadrenocorticism and reliably identifies more than 50% of dogs with adrenal-dependent hyperadrenocorticism and about 85% of dogs with pituitary-dependent hyperadrenocorticism. It is a simple test to perform and the only one that documents excessive production of glucocorticoids by the adrenal cortex. The information gained also provides a baseline for monitoring mitotane therapy.

However, the ACTH stimulation test does not reliably differentiate adrenal-dependent from pituitary-dependent hyperadrenocorticism. A

Table 39.16 Protocols for endocrine screening tests for hyper- and hypoadrenocorticism

The ACTH stimulation test
- Collect 3 ml plasma or serum sample for basal cortisol concentration.[a]
- Inject 0.25 mg of synthetic ACTH (tetracosactrin; Synacthen, Ciba) intravenously to dogs over 5 kg. Use only 0.125 mg in dogs less than 5 kg and in cats.
- Collect a second sample for cortisol concentration 30–60 min later.

[a] The recent administration of glucocorticoids such as hydrocortisone, prednisolone or prednisone may result in elevated cortisol concentrations due to cross-reactivity in many cortisol assays. For this reason glucocorticoids should be withheld for at least 24 hours before testing. There is no cross-reactivity with dexamethasone, but dexamethasone will suppress cortisol concentrations in patients with an intact hypothalamic–pituitary adrenal axis.

The low-dose dexamethasone screening test
- Collect 3 ml plasma or serum sample for cortisol determination.
- Inject 0.01 mg kg^{-1} of dexamethasone intravenously.
- Collect a second sample for cortisol concentration 4 h later and a third sample 8 h after dexamethasone administration.

The urine corticoid:creatinine ratio
- Urine (5 ml) is collected in the morning for cortisol and creatinine measurements. It is preferable for the dog to be at home for this test so that it is as little stressed as possible. The urine corticoid:creatinine ratio is determined by dividing the urine cortisol concentration (in µmol l^{-1}) by the urine creatinine concentration (in µmol l^{-1}).

diagnosis of hyperadrenocorticism should not be excluded on the basis of a normal ACTH response if the clinical signs are compatible with the disease. Occasionally, an animal under chronic stress may develop some degree of adrenal hyperplasia, which produces an abnormal or equivocal ACTH response result. The author has seen this in a number of severe systemic diseases, for example uncontrolled diabetes mellitus and pyometra and has documented a normal ACTH response after treatment in each case.

For interpretation it is essential to use absolute values for plasma cortisol concentrations both before and after ACTH stimulation rather than a ratio or percentage increase in post-ACTH cortisol concentration over the basal concentration. Regardless of the pre-ACTH cortisol value, diagnosis of hyperadrenocorticism depends on the demonstration of a post-ACTH cortisol concentration higher than 600 nmol l^{-1} (Fig. 39.15).

Low-dose dexamethasone suppression test

The protocol for the low-dose dexamethasone suppression test is shown in Table 39.16. It is more reliable than the ACTH stimulation test in confirming hyperadrenocorticism, since the results are diagnostic in all adrenal-dependent cases and in 90–95% of dogs with pituitary-dependent hyperadrenocorticism. However, it is not as useful as the ACTH stimulation test for the detection of iatrogenic hyperadrenocorticism. It is also affected by more variables, takes 8 hours to complete, and does not provide pretreatment information that may aid in monitoring the effects of mitotane therapy. The low-dose dexamethasone suppression test, like the ACTH stimulation test, does not reliably differentiate pituitary-dependent from adrenal-dependent hyperadrenocorticism.

Interpretation of the results of a low-dose dexamethasone suppression test must be based on the laboratory's normal range of cortisol values for the dose and preparation of dexamethasone administered. If the dose of dexamethasone fails to adequately suppress circulating cortisol concentrations in a dog with compatible clinical signs, a diagnosis of hyperadrenocorticism is confirmed. Although basal and 8-h postdexamethasone samples are most important for interpretation of the test (Fig. 39.16), one or more samples taken at intermediate times (for example, 2, 4 or 6 h) during the test period may also prove helpful. If a plasma cortisol concentration determined 2–6 h after dexamethasone injection is suppressed to below 40 mmol l^{-1}, whereas the 8-h sample shows escape from cortisol suppression, then a diagnosis of pituitary-dependent hyperadrenocorticism can be made.

Other screening tests

Evaluation of urinary corticoid/creatinine ratio (Table 39.16) rather than the more laborious 24-h urinary corticoid excretion has been shown to be a simple and valuable screening test (Rijnberk et al., 1988).

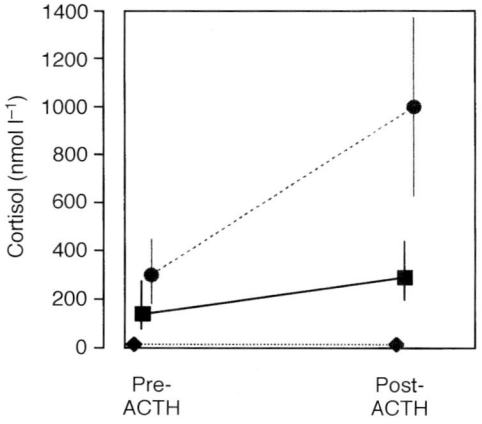

Figure 39.15 Interpretation of the ACTH stimulation test. ♦, Iatrogenic hyperadrenocorticism or primary hypoadrenocorticism; ■, normal; ●, hyperadrenocorticism.

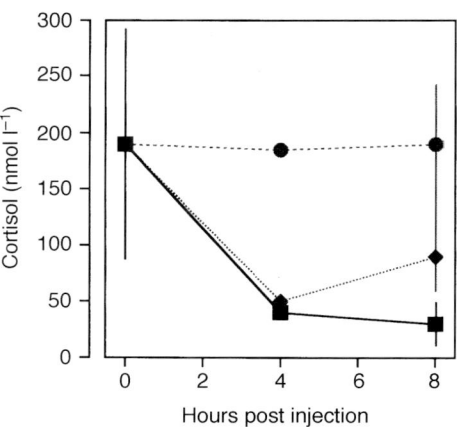

Figure 39.16 Interpretation of the low-dose dexamethasone screening test. ■, Normal; ♦, hyperadrenocorticism – possible pituitary-dependent hyperadrenocorticism response; ●, hyperadrenocorticism – possible adrenal-dependent hyperadrenocorticism response.

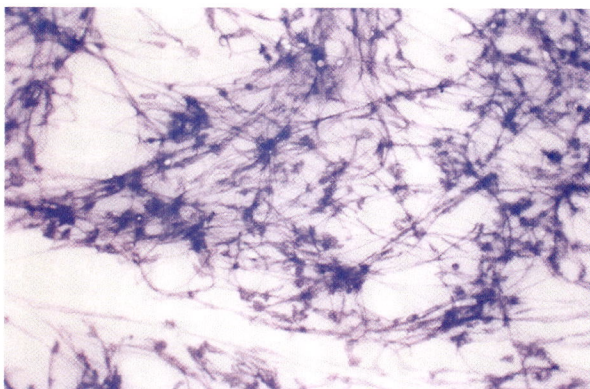

Figure 20.2 A non-diagnostic lymph node aspirate. Poor technique during smear preparation has resulted in severe cellular and nuclear disruption. May–Grünwald Giemsa; original magnification ×125.

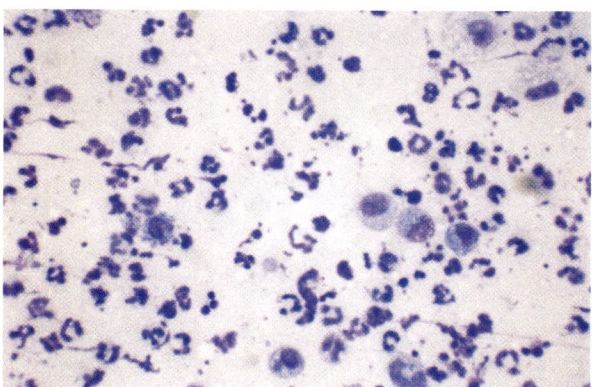

Figure 20.3 Fine-needle aspirate taken from the necrotic centre of an enlarged submandibular lymph node. This aspirate consisted of a large number of degenerate neutrophils and fewer macrophages. There was no clear indication that this node was neoplastic although subsequent histopathological examination showed that this was the case (lymphoma). May–Grünwald Giemsa ×50.

a

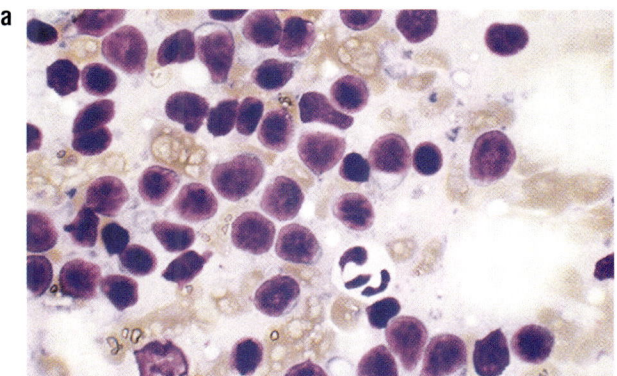

b

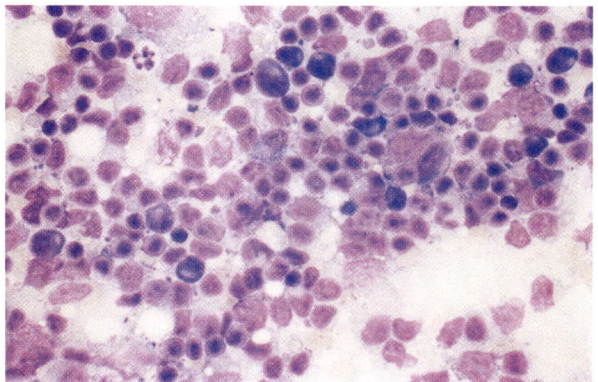

Figure 20.4 (a) Fine needle aspirate of a reactive lymph node showing lymphoid hyperplasia. The aspirate is moderately haemodiluted. The nucleated cells present, with the exception of the single neutrophil, are small or medium-sized lymphocytes showing clumping of nuclear chromatin. (b) Fine needle aspirate of a lymph node from a dog with immune-mediated polyarthritis. This consists of a mixed population of small and medium-sized lymphocytes, plasma cells, neutrophils and macrophages. The number of lymphoblasts comprised less than 10% of the nucleated cells counted. The increased number of plasma cells present suggests a degree of antigenic stimulation. May–Grünwald Giemsa, (a) ×250; (b) ×50.

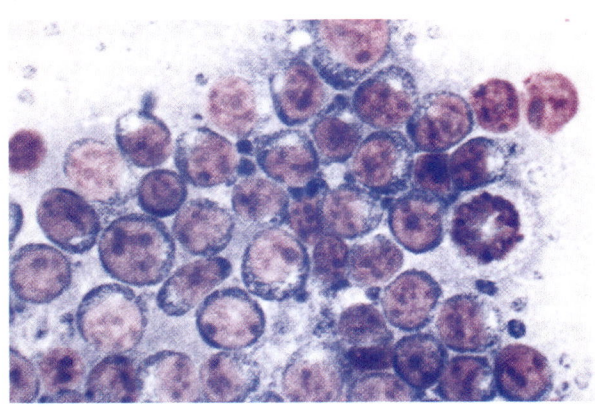

Figure 20.5 Fine needle aspirate of the submandibular lymph node of a dog showing unequivocal evidence of lymphoid malignancy (lymphoma). A monomorphic population of pleomorphic lymphoblasts is present. Note the extreme variation in nucleolar size, shape and number. The cytology in this case is consistent with a diagnosis of lymphoblastic lymphoma. May-Grünwald Giemsa ×250.

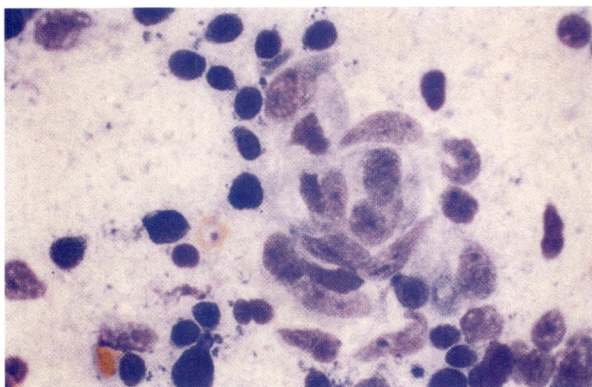

Figure 20.6 Fine needle aspirate of a submandibular lymph node showing a central cluster of non-lymphoid, spindle-shaped cells. These cells represented a metastatic tumour deposit from a fibrosarcoma. May–Grünwald Giemsa ×250.

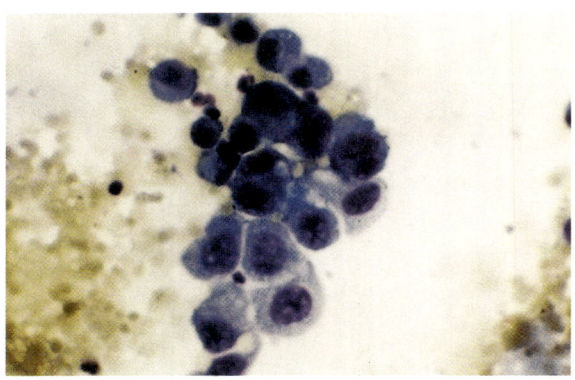

Figure 23.1 A cluster of neoplastic urothelial cells in a Giemsa-stained preparation of urine sediment from a dog with a transitional cell carcinoma of the bladder wall. Note the irregular way in which the cells are arranged and the variable nuclear:cytoplasmic ratio May–Grünwald Giemsa ×125.

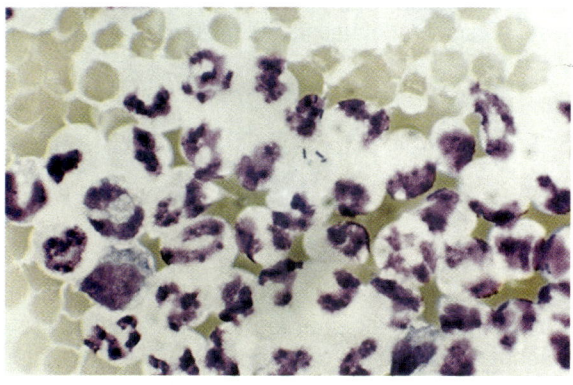

Figure 23.2 Prostatic wash from a dog with acute prostatitis. Note the degenerate appearance of the neutrophils, a few of which contained intracellular bacteria. May–Grünwald Giemsa ×250.

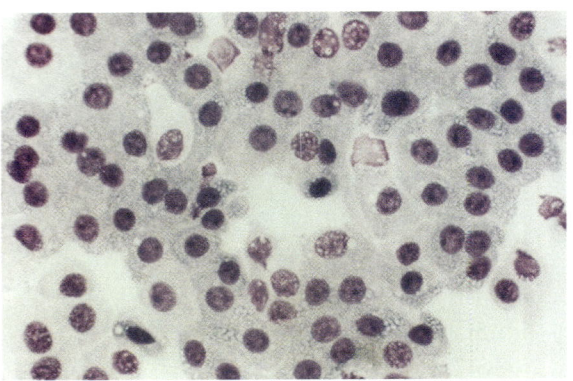

Figure 23.3 Prostatic wash from a dog with benign hyperplasia of the prostate gland. Large sheets of epithelial cells are present. The cells appear uniform with respect to size and shape. May–Grünwald Giemsa ×125.

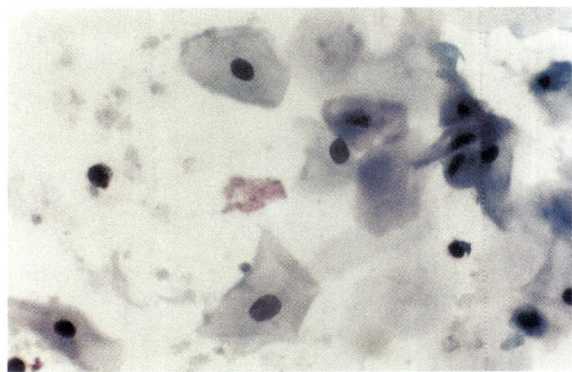

Figure 23.4 This prostatic wash contains large numbers of keratinized or partially keratinized urothelial cells consistent with squamous metaplasia of the prostate gland. Squamous metaplasia may be seen with functional Sertoli cell tumours in response to high circulating oestrogen levels. May–Grünwald Giemsa ×125.

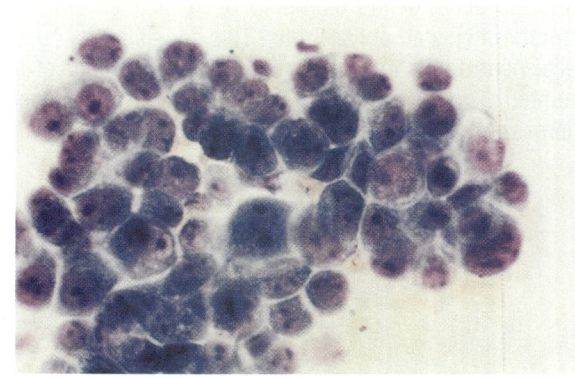

Figure 23.5 This fine needle aspirate of the prostate gland from a dog with a large prostatic carcinoma was taken under ultrasound guidance. An irregular cluster of urothelial cells is present. The cells are showing marked variation in cell size, nuclear:cytoplasmic ratio, and nucleolar number, size and shape. May–Grünwald Giemsa ×125.

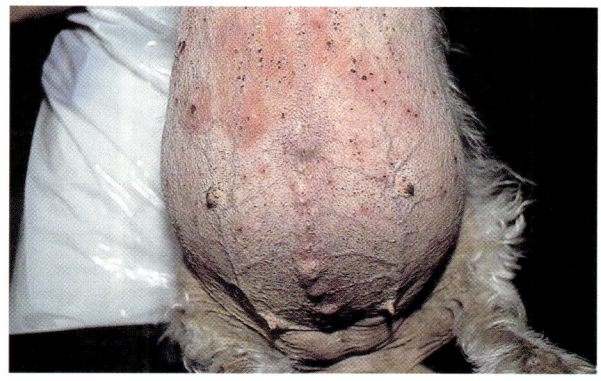

Figure 39.13 An 11-year-old neutered female dachshund with hyperadrenocorticism illustrating the symmetrical alopecia, distended abdomen, thin skin, comedomes, calcinosis cutis and partial breakdown of a laparotomy wound.

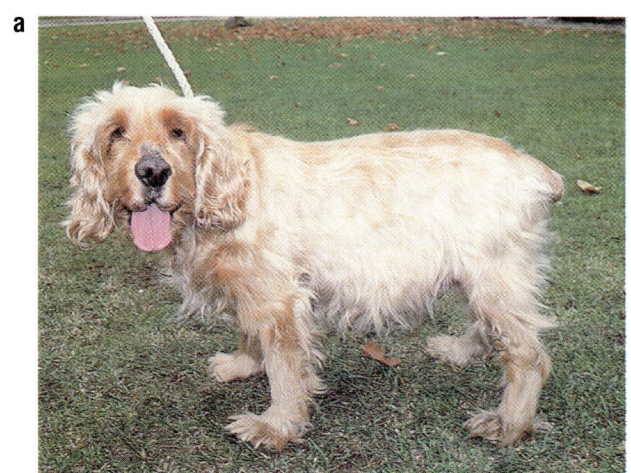

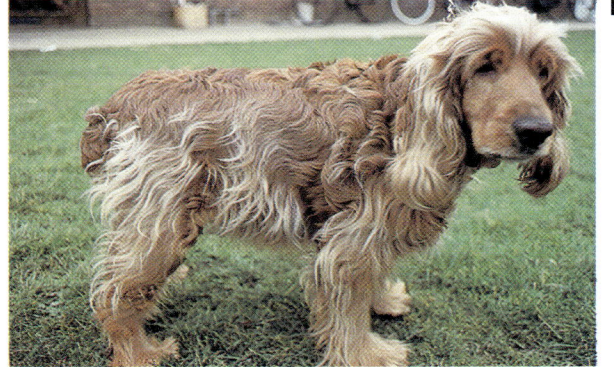

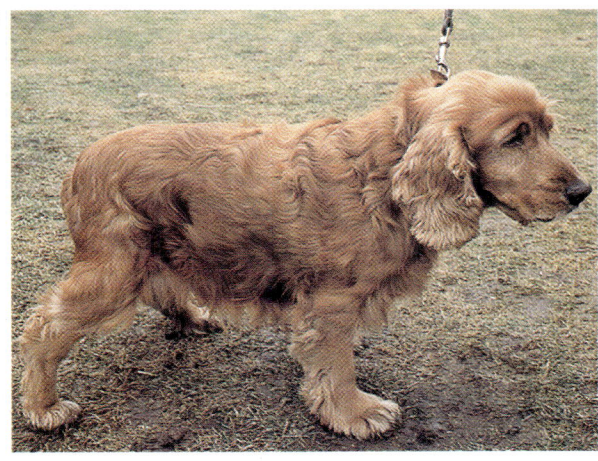

Figure 39.17 Photographs of a 9-year old cocker spaniel bitch taken (a) before treatment of hyperadrenocorticism, (b) 16 weeks after commencing therapy and (c) one year later. Note the improvement in the hair coat and the increased muscle tone.

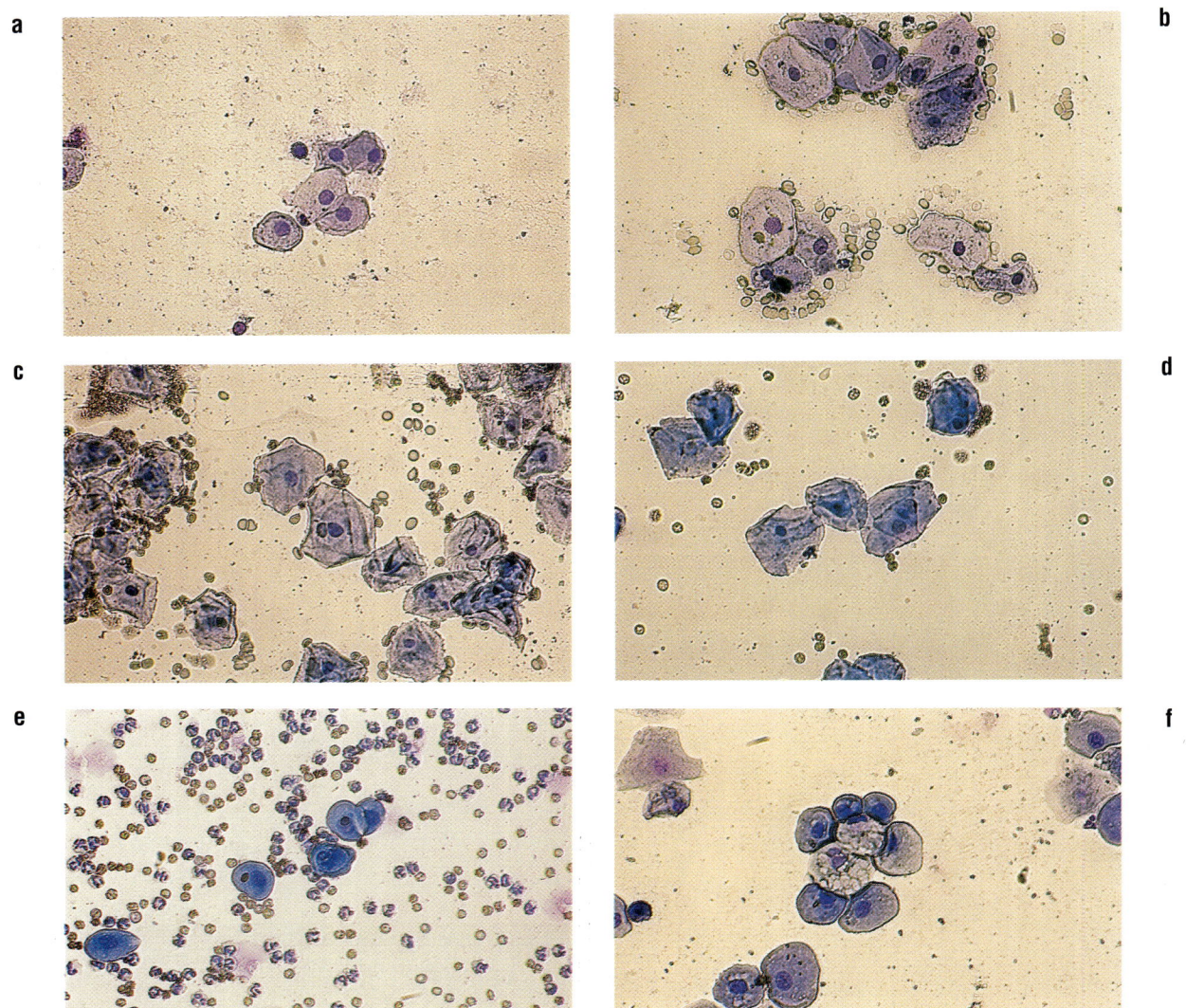

Figure 40.1 Photomicrographs of vaginal smears collected from bitches during various stages of the oestrous cycle. (a) Anoestrus; the smear comprises parabasal and small intermediate epithelial cells. Cells which have lost their cytoplasm can also be seen. Polymorphonuclear leucocytes are often present during anoestrus although they are not shown here. (b) Proestrus; the smear comprises small intermediate epithelial cells, large intermediate epithelial cells, and erythrocytes. A few polymorphonuclear leucocytes are also present. Bacteria can also be seen adherent to epithelial cells. (c) Early oestrus; the smear comprises large intermediate epithelial cells and erythrocytes. Polymorphonuclear leucocytes are no longer present. (d) Oestrus; the smear comprises anuclear epithelial cells, large intermediate epithelial cells and erythrocytes. The amount of background debris (including bacteria) is often reduced. (e) Metoestrus; the smear comprises large numbers of polymorphonuclear leucocytes, small intermediate epithelial cells and parabasal cells. Erythrocytes are also present in variable numbers. (f) Late metoestrus; the smear comprises parabasal cells and vacuolated small intermediate epithelial cells (higher magnification than figures a to e). The number of polymorphonuclear leucocytes is generally reduced.

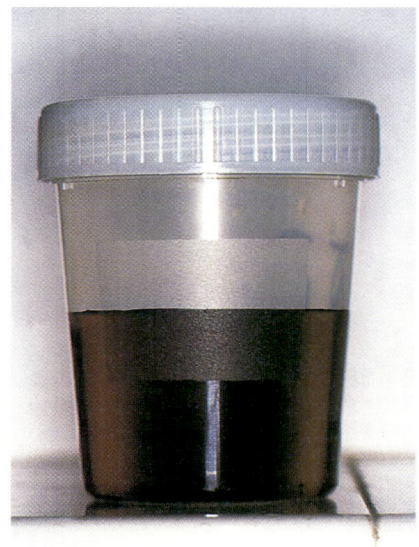

Figure 45.7 Haemoglobinuria resulting from acute intravascular haemolysis. Courtesy of J.K. Dunn.

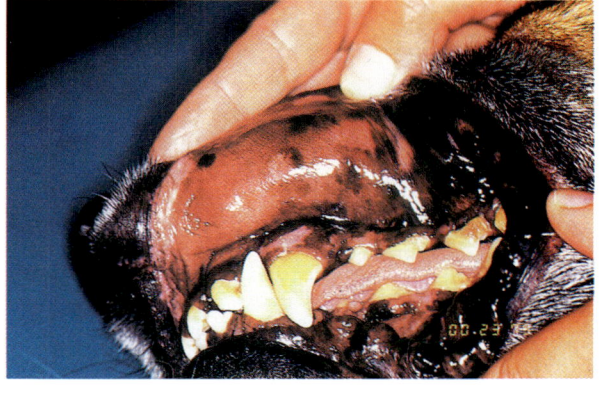

Figure 45.9 Marked congestion of the buccal mucosa in a German shepherd dog with polycythaemia secondary to bilateral renal lymphoma. Courtesy of J.K. Dunn.

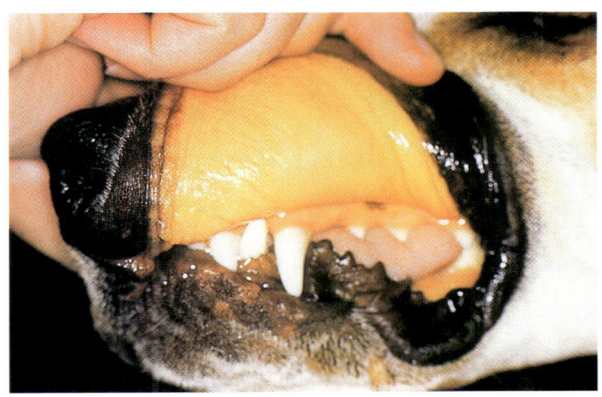

Figure 45.8 Icteric oral mucous membranes in a 1-year-old German short-haired pointer with acute autoimmune haemolytic anaemia. Courtesy of J.K. Dunn.

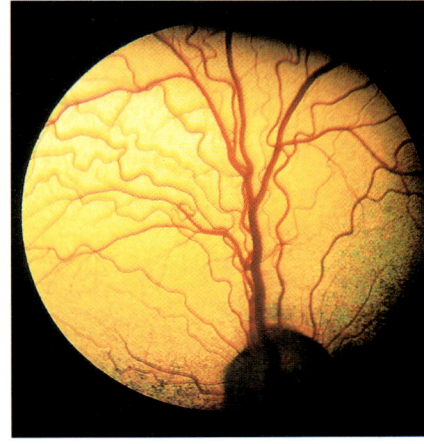

Figure 45.10 Distended and tortuous retinal blood vessels of a dog with polycythaemia vera. Courtesy of Mosby Year Book Europe Ltd.

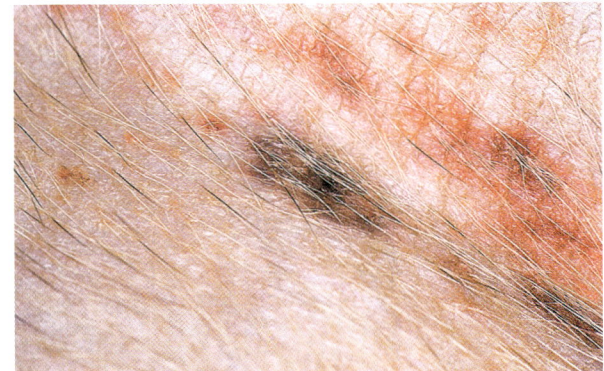
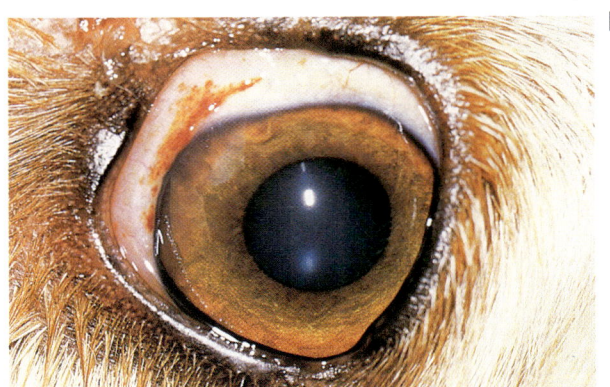

Figure 45.11 Clinical signs of thrombocytopenic purpura. (a) Petechial and ecchymotic haemorrhages on the skin of the ventral abdomen; (b) small petechial conjunctival haemorrhages. Courtesy of J.K. Dunn.

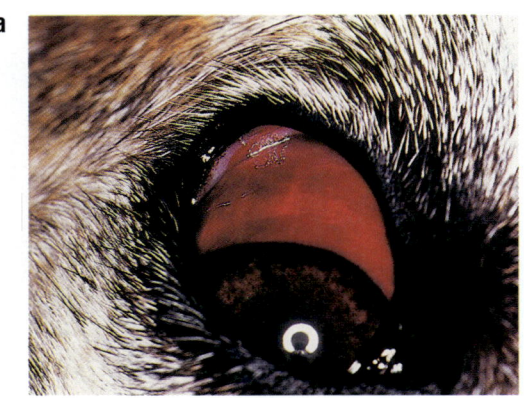
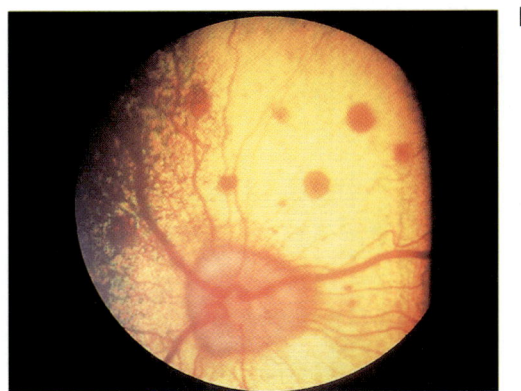

Figure 45.12 Clinical signs of thrombocytopenic purpura. (a) Extensive scleral haemorrhage. Courtesy of J.K. Dunn. (b) Retinal haemorrhages. Courtesy of the *Journal of Small Animal Practice*.

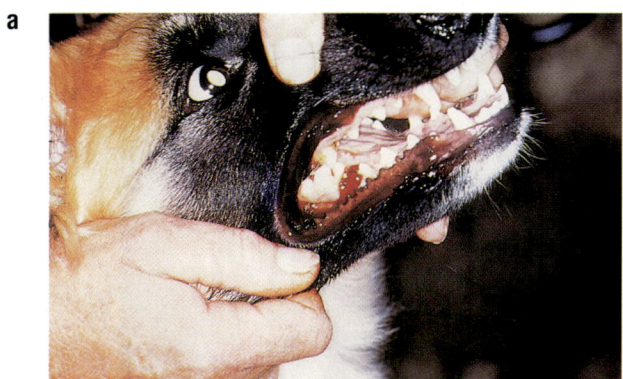

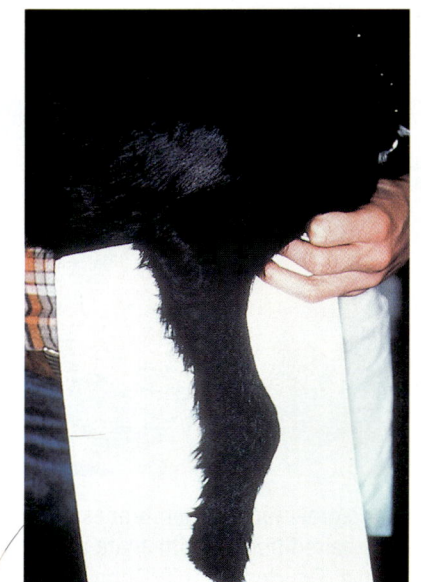

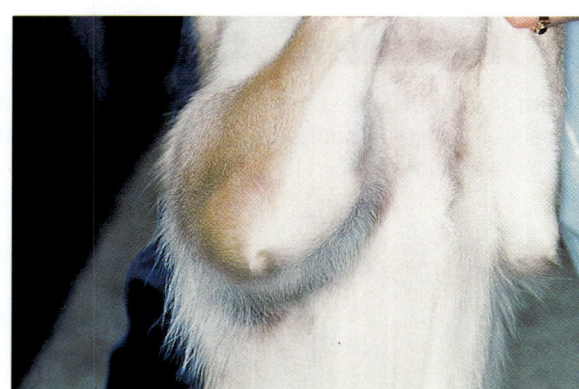

Figure 45.15 Bleeding manifestations of Factor VIII deficiency (haemophilia A). (a) Excessive bleeding after loss of deciduous teeth; (b) carpal haemarthrosis (photograph courtesy of Dr R.A.S. White); (c) haematoma in the soft tissues around the elbow.

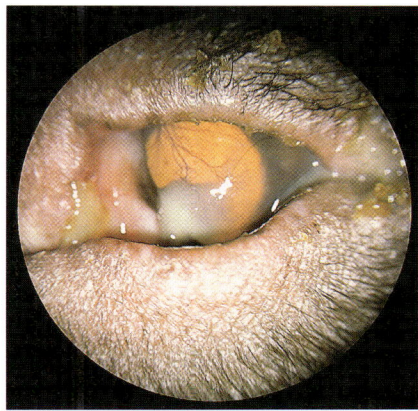

Figure 46.9 Keratoconjunctivitis sicca in a 6-year-old Irish water spaniel. Note the typical tenaceous mucopurulent ocular discharge and the resulting superficial keratitis.

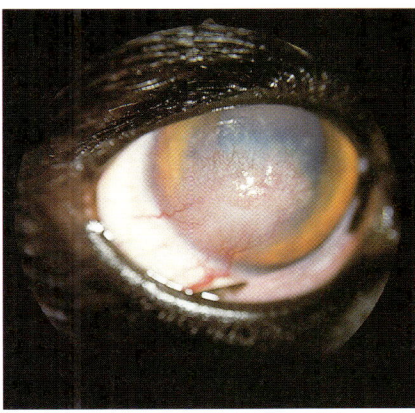

Figure 46.16 Chronic superficial keratitis (pannus) in a cross-bred dog.

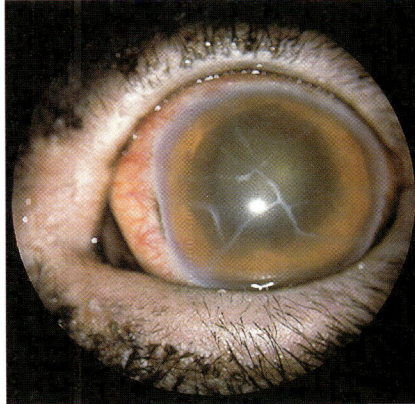

Figure 46.18 A St Bernard suffering from the uveodermatological syndrome. There is some loss of pigmentation in the eyelids. Uncontrolled uveitis has resulted in a secondary glaucoma with globe enlargement, splits in Descemet's membrane (corneal striae) and episcleral and conjunctival congestion.

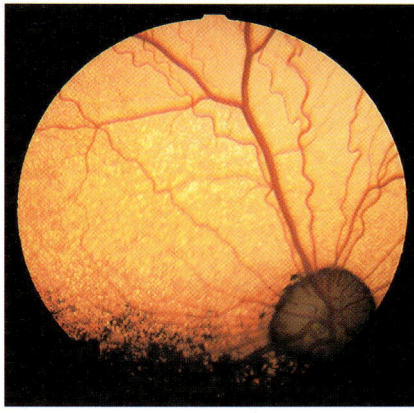

Figure 46.27 Normal fundus in an English springer spaniel.

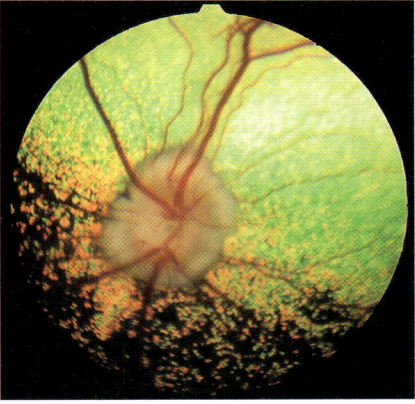

Figure 46.28 Normal fundus in a golden retriever. The retinal nerve fibres gain a myelin sheath just adjacent to the site that they join to form the optic nerve. This gives the optic disc an irregular, swollen appearance (pseudopapilloedema).

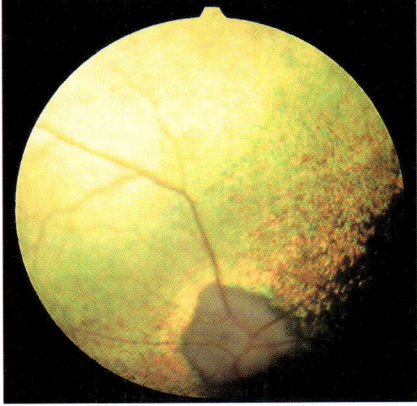

Figure 46.31 Generalized progressive retinal atrophy in a miniature poodle. There is marked retinal thinning manifested by tapetal hyperreflectivity and also attenuation of retinal blood vessels.

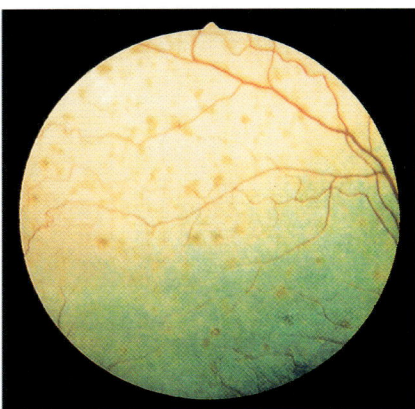

Figure 46.32 Pigmentary retinopathy in a Staffordshire bull terrier. This has the appearance of retinal pigment epithelial dystrophy, which has been seen in some dogs of this breed. Numerous light brown pigment spots can be seen across the tapetal fundus.

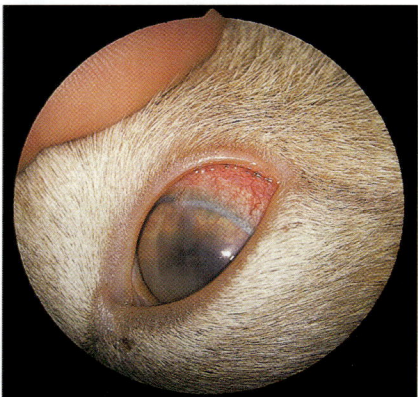

Figure 46.39 Anterior uveitis in a cat following a penetrating corneal wound. There is marked conjunctival and episceral blood vessel congestion and a large mass of inflammatory material can be seen ventrally in the anterior chamber.

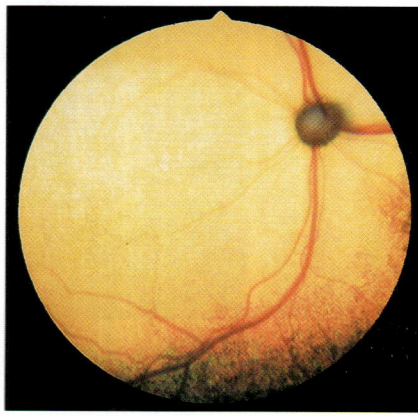

Figure 46.40 Normal feline fundus. Note the small and dark optic disc in comparison with that of the dog.

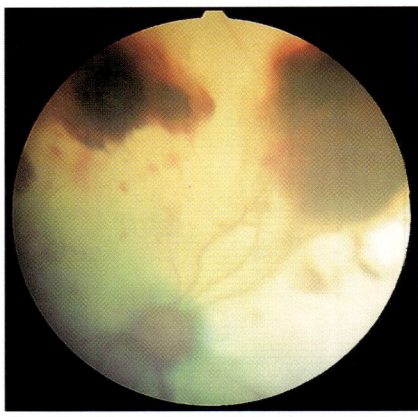

Figure 46.41 Large retinal and preretinal haemorrhages and partial retinal detachment in a cat with hypertension.

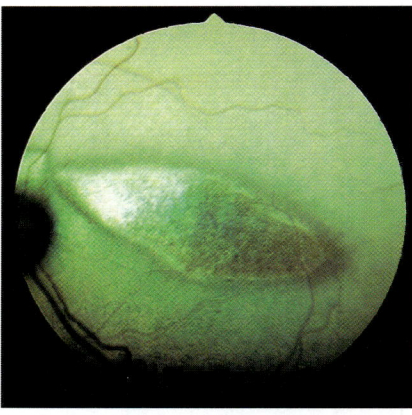

Figure 46.42 Feline central retinal degeneration due to dietary taurine deficiency. A large lozenge-shaped area of retinal thinning is seen dorsolateral to the optic disc encompassing the area centralis (area of greatest cone density).

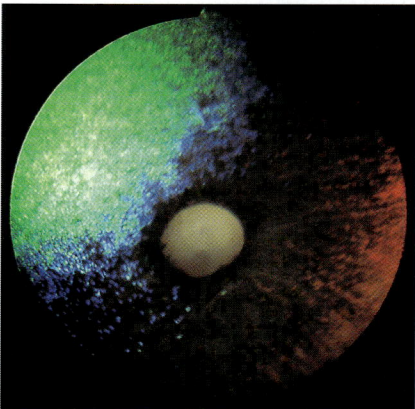

Figure 46.43 The fundus of one member of a litter of kittens with a generalised retinal atrophy of unknown aetiology. The optic disc has a small coloboma ventrally. No superficial retinal blood vessels are visible.

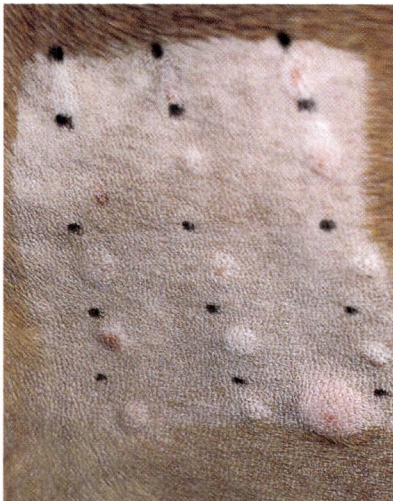

Figure 47.3 An intradermal skin test in a boxer, showing a number of positive reactions. The negative control is top left and the positive control is bottom right.

a

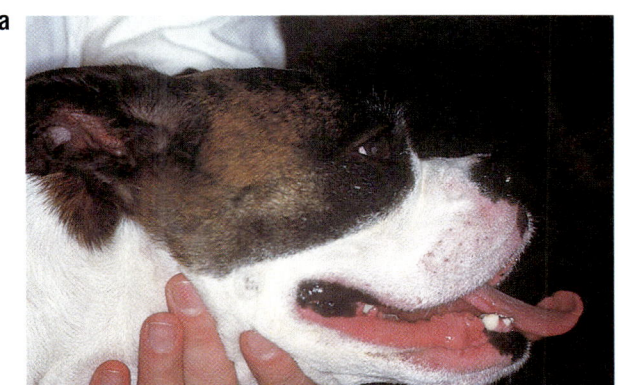

b

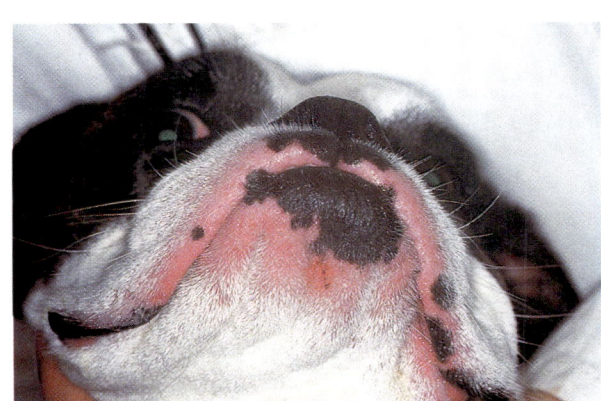

Figure 47.4 (a and b) Alopecia and erythema around the lips, muzzle, eyes and ears in a boxer with atopy.

All photographs on this page are courtesy of Michael Herrtage.

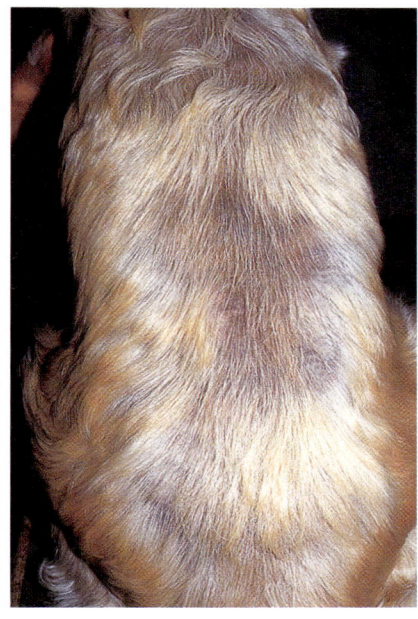

Figure 47.5 Alopecia and hyperpigmentation of the skin on the dorsum of a golden retriever with flea allergy dermatitis.

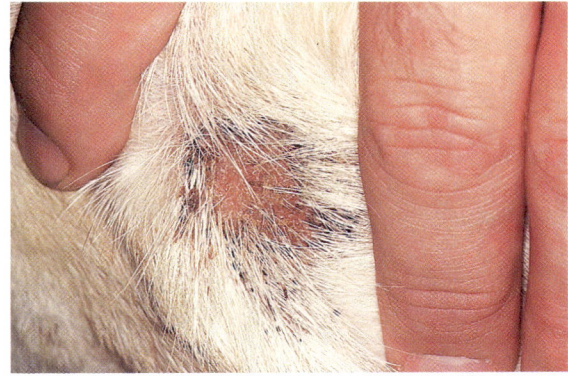

Figure 47.6 An area of acute moist dermatitis on the side of the face of a Labrador retriever with otitis externa.

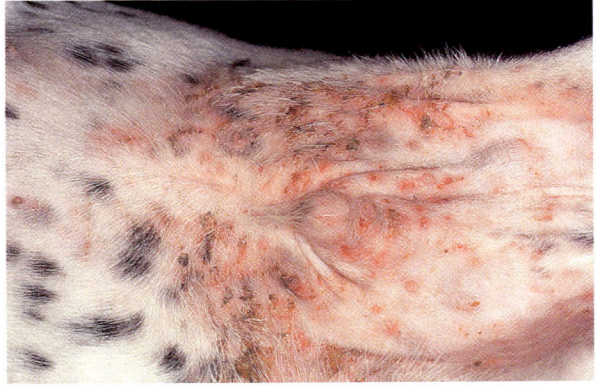

Figure 47.7 Superficial pustular dermatitis on the ventral abdomen of a 6-week-old pointer puppy.

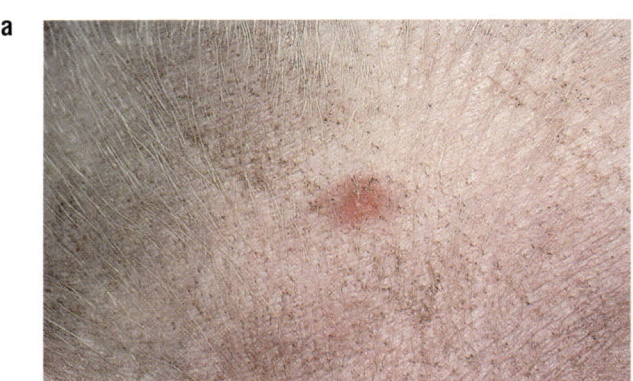
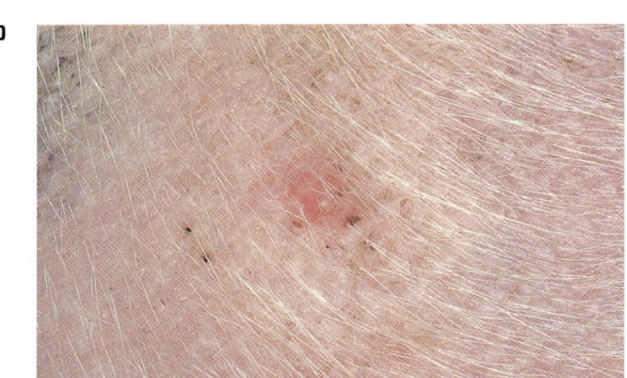
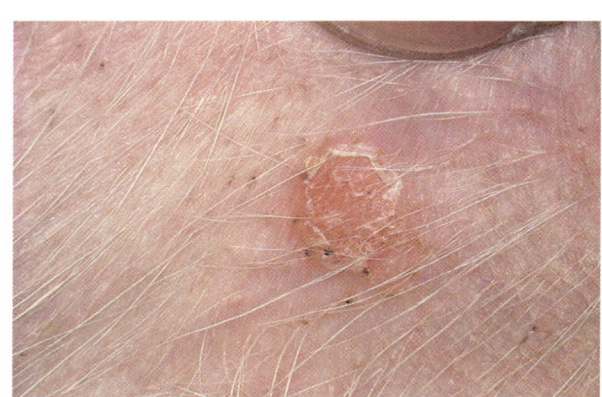
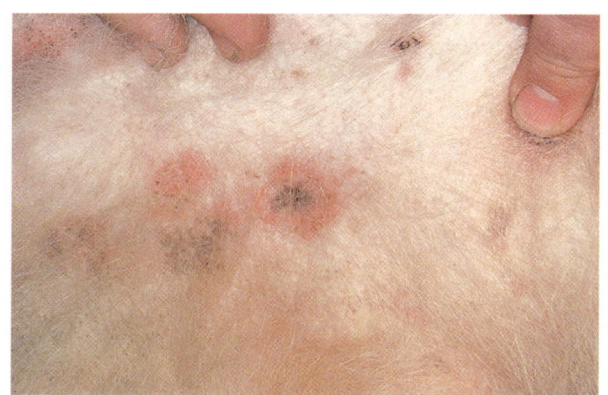

Figure 47.8 A papule (a), a pustule (b), an epidermal collarette (c) and pigmentation and crusting (d) in a dog with superficial bacterial folliculitis.

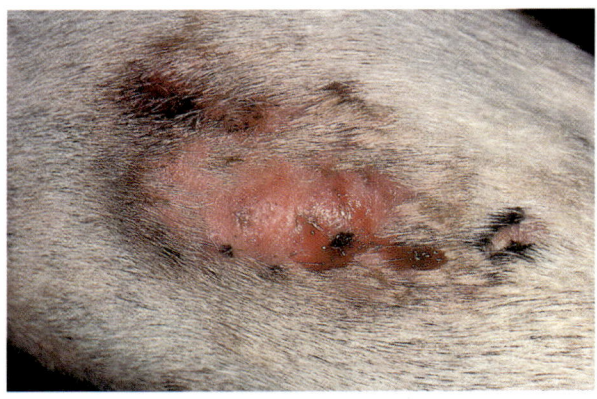

Figure 47.9 Localized area of deep pyoderma on the lateral aspect of the hindleg of a boxer.

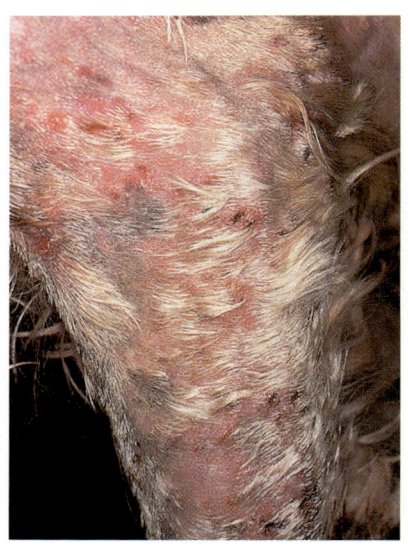

Figure 47.10 Generalized deep pyoderma in an Afghan hound. The hair on the forelimb has been clipped to show the discharging sinuses.

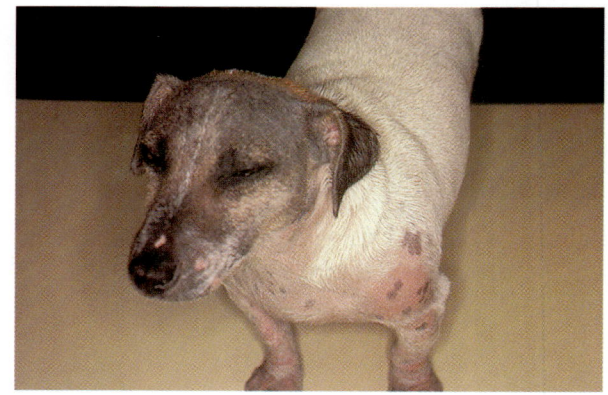

Figure 47.11 Generalized squamous demodicosis in a Jack Russell terrier.

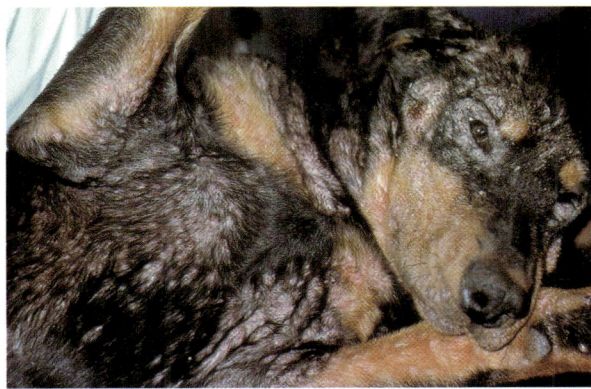

Figure 47.12 Generalized demodicosis with secondary bacterial furunculosis in a Doberman pinscher.

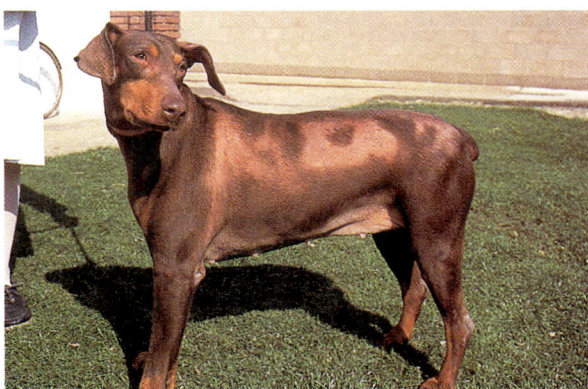

Figure 47.15 Bilaterally symmetrical, non-pruritic alopecia in a Doberman pinscher with hypothyroidism. The pattern of alopecia is typical for an endocrinopathy.

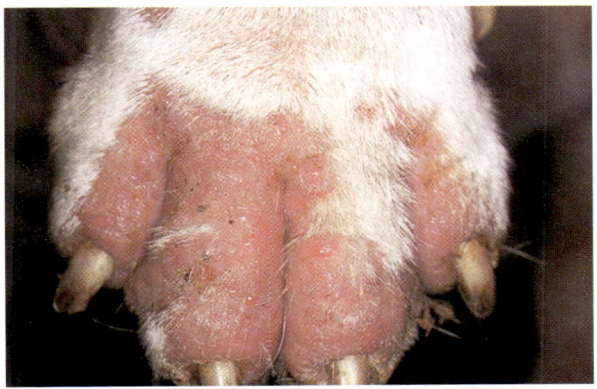

Figure 47.13 Demodicosis confined to the feet of an English bull terrier.

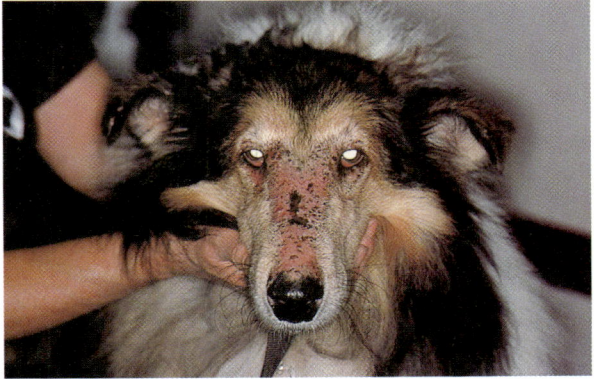

Figure 47.16 Alopecia, crusting and erosions on the bridge of the nose in a rough collie with pemphigus foliaceous.

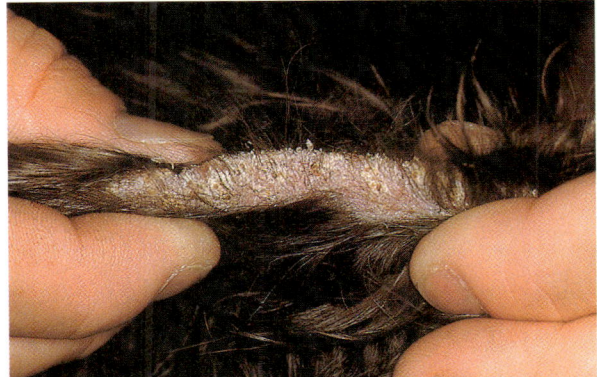

Figure 47.14 Alopecia and crusting of the edge of the pinna in an English springer spaniel with sarcoptic mange.

All photographs on this page and the facing page are courtesy of Michael Herrtage.

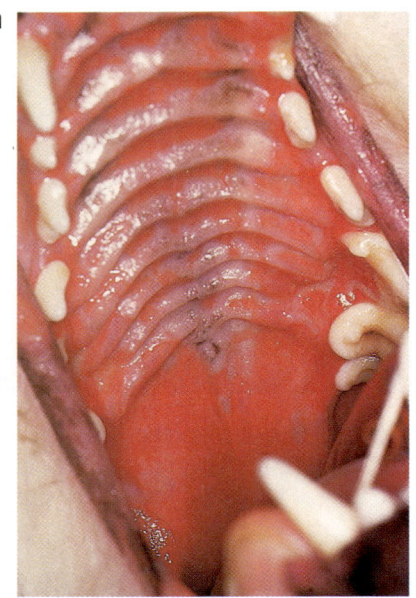
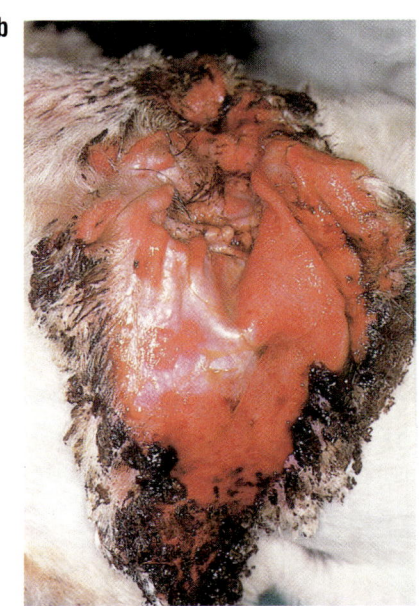

Figure 47.17 Ulceration of the oral cavity (a) and ear (b) of an Old English sheepdog with bullous pemphigoid.

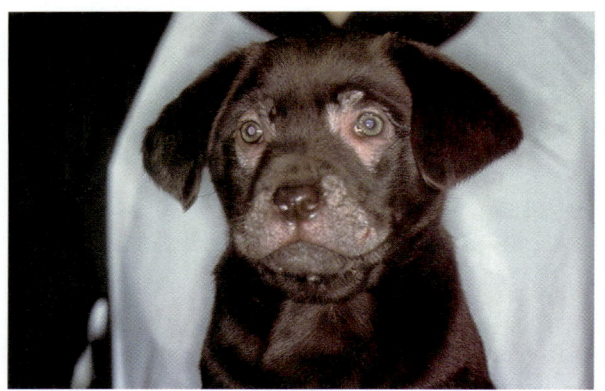

Figure 47.18 Juvenile cellulitis in a 10-week-old Labrador puppy.

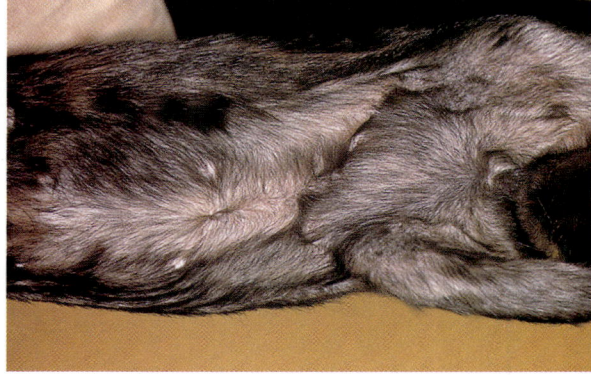

Figure 47.20 Diffuse symmetrical alopecia affecting the ventral abdomen and medial and caudal aspects of the hindlimbs in a domestic short-haired cat with flea allergy dermatitis.

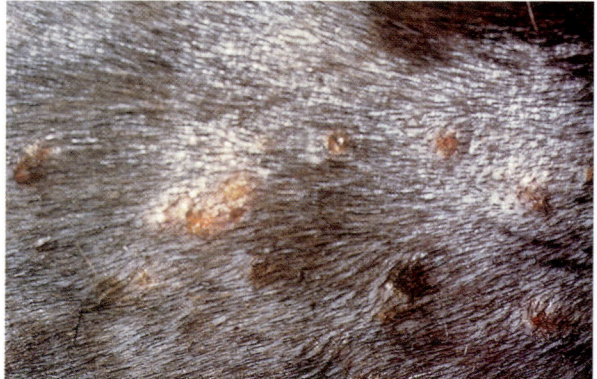

Figure 47.19 Papulocrustaceous reactions on the dorsum of a domestic short-haired cat with flea allergy dermatitis. The hair has been clipped to show the lesions.

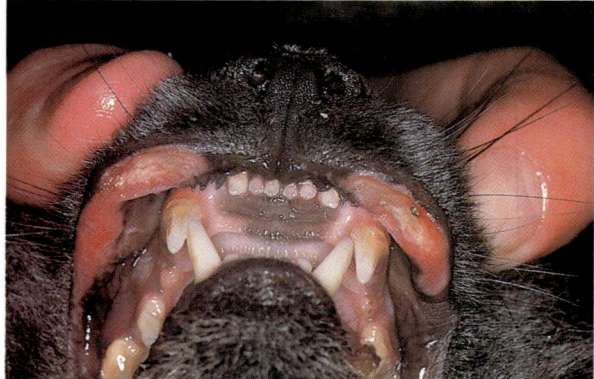

Figure 47.21 Eosinophilic ulcers affecting the upper lip of a domestic short-haired cat.

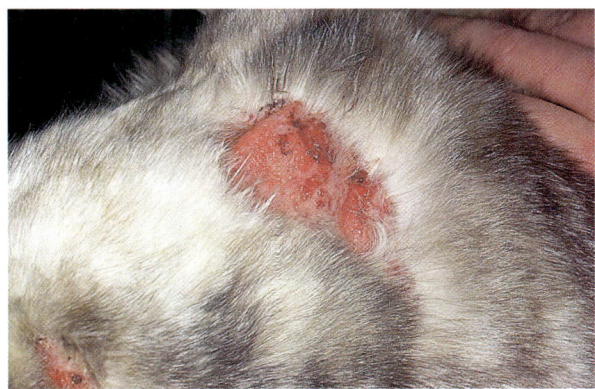

Figure 47.22 Eosinophilic plaque on the flank of a long-haired cat.

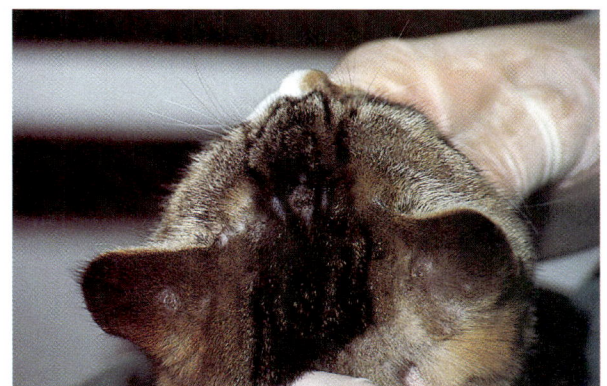

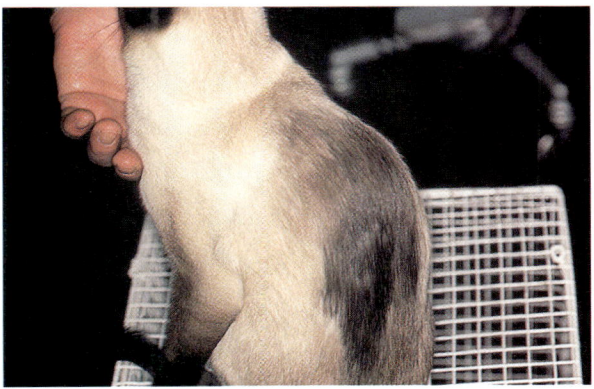

Figure 47.23 Psychogenic alopecia in a Siamese. There is diffuse alopecia along the back and the new hair has grown back with the point colour. Fleas etc. have been ruled out.

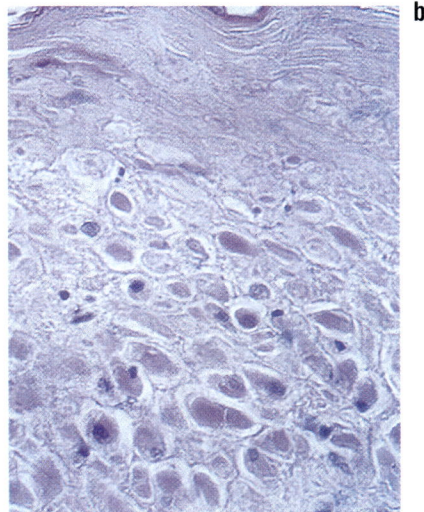

Figure 47.25 (a) Typical skin lesions of feline cowpox; (b) multiple intracytoplasmic eosinophilic inclusions in the epidermis of a cat with feline cowpox.

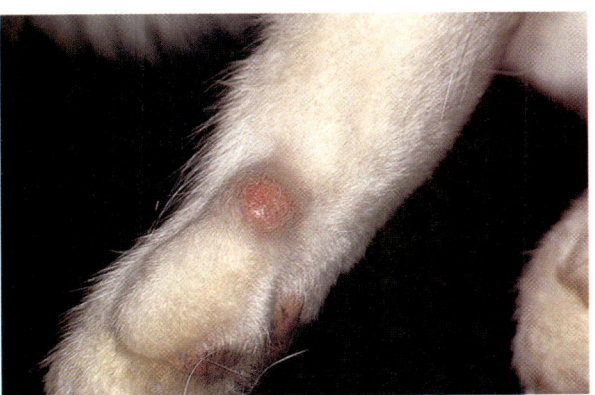

Figure 47.24 One of a number of nodules affecting a domestic short-haired cat with feline leprosy.

All photographs on this page and the facing page, apart from Figure 47.25(a), are courtesy of Michael Herrtage.

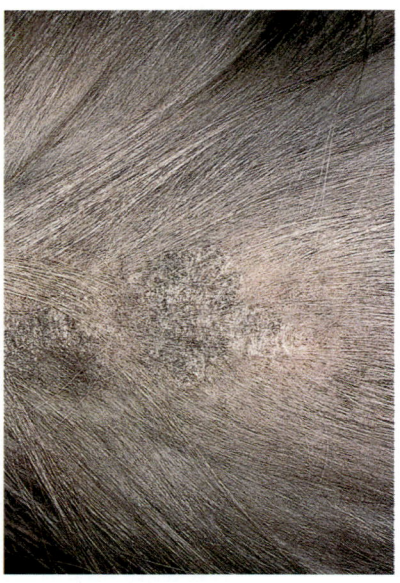

Figure 47.26 Diffuse alopecia along the dorsum in a Persian cat with *Microsporum canis* infection. Courtesy of Michael Herrtage.

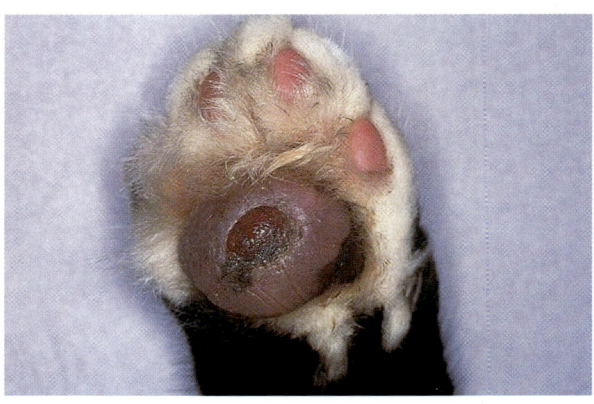

Figure 47.28 Plasma cell pododermatitis in a domestic short-haired cat. Courtesy of Michael Herrtage.

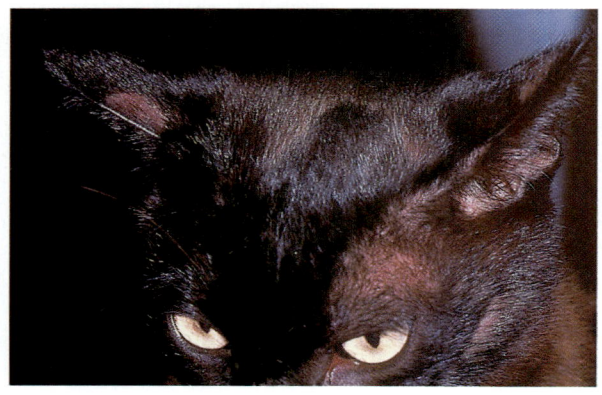

Figure 47.27 Focal lesions on the ears and face of a Burmese cat with *Trichophyton mentagrophytes* infection. The diffuse hair loss over the temporal region is normal in this breed. Courtesy of Michael Herrtage.

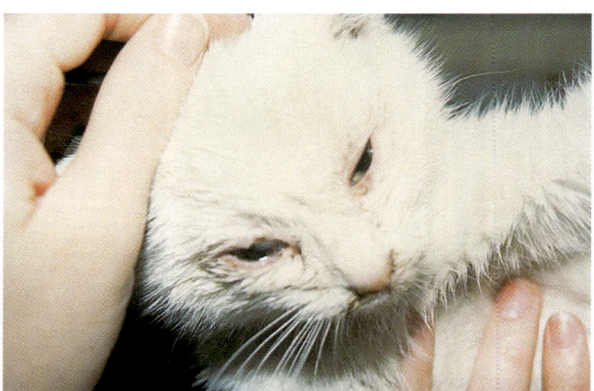

Figure 49.1 Oculonasal discharge in a cat infected with feline herpesvirus. Courtesy of Michael Herrtage.

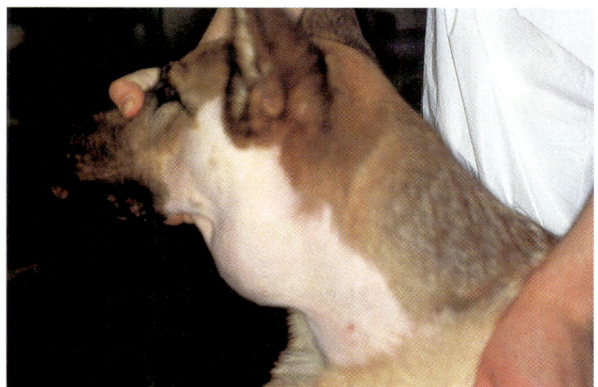

Figure 50.5 German shepherd bitch, presented with a grossly enlarged submandibular lymph node due to nodal metastasis of a mast cell tumour. The primary (poorly differentiated) mast cell tumour was located on the lower lip.

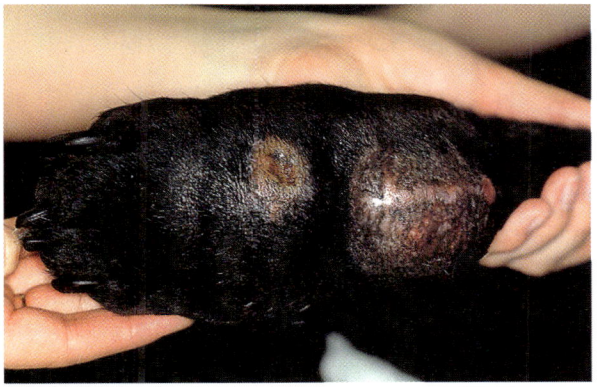

Figure 50.8 Mast cell tumour of foot associated with oedematous swelling and erythema.

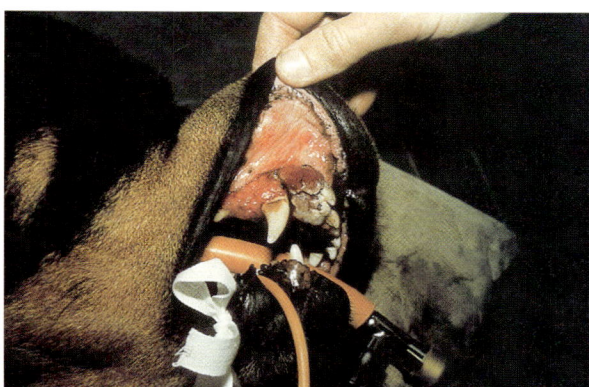

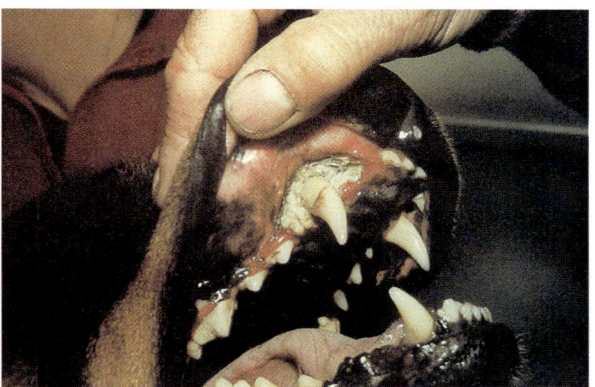

Figure 50.15 The typical response of an oral tumour to radiation therapy. Rottweiler with an osteosarcoma of the premaxilla, before treatment (a). The same dog at the end of a 4-week course of radiation therapy (b). The tumour has completely regressed but there remains necrotic bone at the tumour site which may require surgical debridement at a later date.

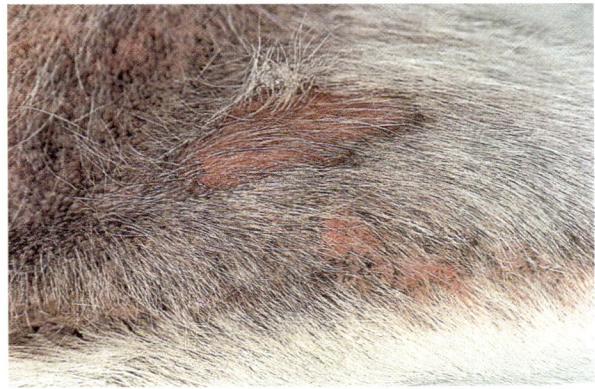

Figure 50.16 Acute radiation skin reaction: erythema and superficial desquamation of the skin may occur towards the end of a course of radiation treatment and in the immediate post-treatment period. These effects may cause temporary discomfort but usually resolve spontaneously as the normal tissues regenerate.

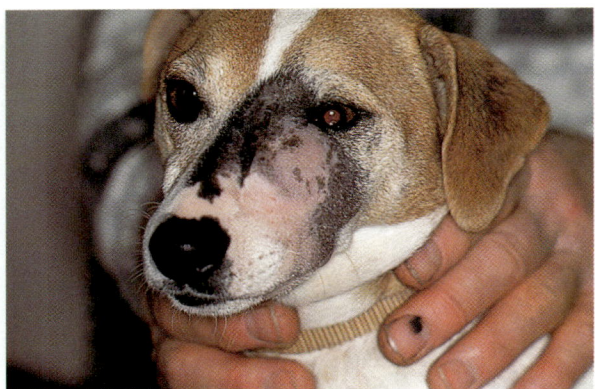

Figure 50.17 Post-radiation hair loss: alopecia is common in irradiated skin occurring weeks to months after radiation exposure.

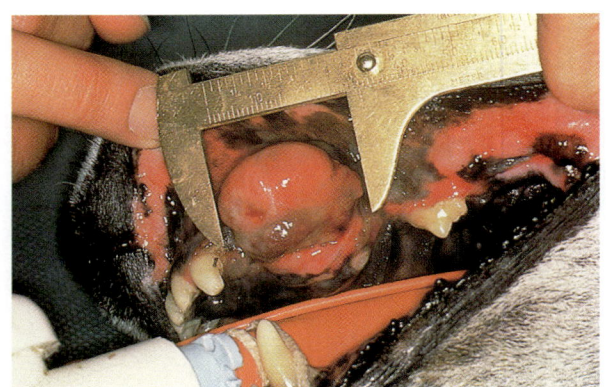

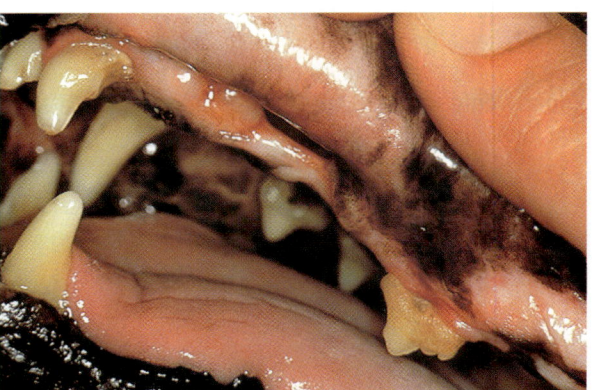

Figure 50.19 Radiation response. (a) Maxillary squamous cell carcinoma with extension into the nasal chamber preventing surgical management. (b) A complete regression of the tumour is achieved following 3600 cGy radiation delivered in 4 × weekly fractions. (This is the same dog as shown in Fig. 50.18)

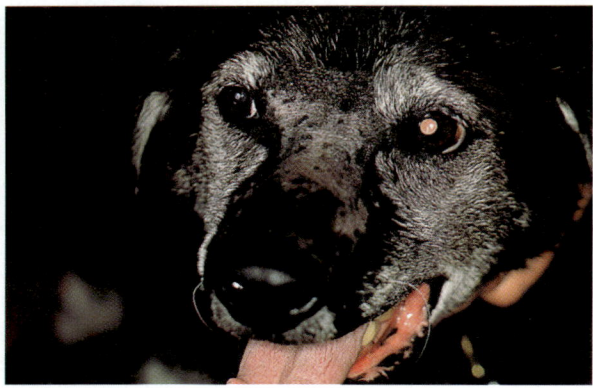

Figure 50.18 Patchy regrowth of hair: in many cases the hair will eventually regrow but this regrowth may be patchy and, as in the example shown, the hair may be grey/white.

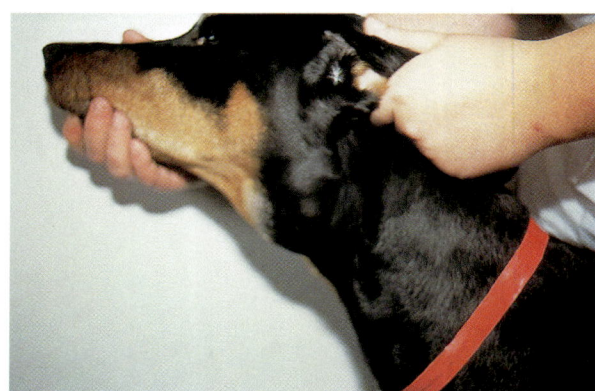

Figure 50.22 Canine multicentric lymphoma. This Dobermann was presented with generalized lymph adenopathy. The gross enlargement of submandibular lymph nodes is typical of that commonly seen in canine multicentric lymphoma.

Endocrine tests to differentiate the cause of hyperadrenocorticism

The ability to differentiate between pituitary- and adrenal-dependent hyperadrenocorticism is important in order to provide the most effective method of management for the disease. An accurate test is therefore required to differentiate pituitary from adrenal causes of hyperadrenocorticism. The determination of plasma ACTH concentrations in the dog provides a reliable test for differentiating pituitary and adrenal causes of hyperadrenocorticism providing sample handling is meticulous. Dogs with adrenal tumours have very low endogenous ACTH concentrations whereas cases of pituitary-dependent hyperadrenocorticism have high normal or high concentrations. Diagnostic imaging techniques, particularly abdominal ultrasonography, have also proved sensitive in distinguishing animals with pituitary-dependent hyperadrenocorticism from those with adrenocortical tumours.

The high-dose dexamethasone suppression test was the most commonly used test for differentiating the cause of hyperadrenocorticism, but is less accurate than abdominal ultrasonography or plasma ACTH measurements.

High-dose dexamethasone suppression test

This test is indicated in those cases where the diagnosis of hyperadrenocorticism has been established by a screening test, but the differentiation of adrenal-dependent and pituitary-dependent hyperadrenocorticism has not been determined. The high-dose of dexamethasone (0.1 mg kg^{-1} administered intravenously) inhibits pituitary ACTH secretion through negative feedback in pituitary-dependent hyperadrenocorticism thus suppressing serum cortisol concentrations by 50% or more by 4 h. Adrenocortical tumours are autonomous and thus serum cortisol is not suppressed at 4 h. Approximately 20–30% of pituitary-dependent cases, however, will not suppress with this test. The test does not differentiate adrenocortical adenomas from adrenocortical carcinomas.

Treatment of pituitary-dependent hyperadrenocorticism

Mitotane therapy

Mitotane (*op'*-DDD; Lysodren, Bristol Laboratories) is the treatment of choice for pituitary-dependent hyperadrenocorticism. During its evaluation as an insecticide, mitotane was discovered to have adrenocorticolytic effects. It selectively destroys the zona fasciculata and zona reticularis while tending to preserve the zona glomerulosa.

Mitotane therapy should only be considered once the diagnosis of hyperadrenocorticism has been confirmed. Because of its powerful effects, it should never be used empirically. Before treatment is instigated, the patient's daily water consumption should be measured over at least two consecutive 24-h periods. If the water intake and appetite are not increased then baseline lymphocyte and eosinophil counts and an ACTH stimulation test are required to monitor the response to therapy.

Initial treatment

The author prefers to hospitalize the patient for the initial course of treatment, although many clinicians have dogs treated by their owners at home, with the owners doing the necessary monitoring.

Mitotane is given orally at a dose rate of 50 mg kg^{-1} day^{-1} and should be administered with food. Concomitant glucocorticoid treatment is not advised, although if the dog is being treated at home, the owner should be given a small supply of prednisolone tablets. Daily mitotane therapy should be continued until any of the following changes are noted: the water intake of a polydipsic dog drops to below 60 ml kg^{-1} day^{-1}, the dog takes longer to consume its meal than before treatment or stops eating completely, the dog vomits or has diarrhoea, or the dog becomes listless and depressed.

The initial course of mitotane is then stopped and the dog put on maintenance therapy (see below). The importance of close monitoring of the patient during this period cannot be overemphasized.

Mitotane therapy is comparatively safe and the side-effects which commonly occur, for example, anorexia, vomiting or diarrhoea, are rarely serious providing they are noticed early so that the mitotane can be withheld. Some of the problems occasionally encountered during treatment are summarized in Table 39.17 with their suggested management.

The majority of dogs with pituitary-dependent hyperadrenocorticism require between 7 and 14 days treatment with an average of 10 days before water consumption drops below 60 ml kg^{-1} day^{-1}. If the dog is not polydipsic or polyphagic then treatment should continue until the lymphocyte

Table 39.17 Possible problems that may be encountered during mitotane therapy and their management

Problem	Management
Vomiting or anorexia within the first 3 days of treatment (gastric irritation)	Discontinue mitotane and reassess patient. Divide dose and give 2 to 4 times day
Profound weakness, depression and anorexia usually around day 4 or 5 of treatment	Discontinue mitotane and reassess patient. Check sodium and potassium levels and institute prednisolone (0.2 mg kg^{-1} day^{-1}) Reassess ACTH stimulation test. Start maintenance therapy with mitotane
Acute onset of neurological signs (due to sudden expansion of the pituitary tumour)	Reassess patient. Continue mitotane unless the dog is anorexic, vomiting or depressed. Give prednisolone 2.0 mg kg^{-1} day^{-1} or dexamethasone 0.1 mg kg^{-1} day^{-1} and decrease dose slowly once neurological signs have resolved
Failure to resume normal water intake	Recheck urinalysis and blood urea. Reassess ACTH stimulation test. Increase mitotane by 50% if post ACTH cortisol level is greater than 200 nmol l^{-1}
Failure to regrow hair	Reassess ACTH stimulation test. Determine baseline T4. Increase mitotane by 50% if post ACTH cortisol level is greater than 200 nmol l^{-1}. (If < 120 nmol l^{-1} perform a TRH/TSH stimulation test)
Excessive depression or weakness related to weekly maintenance therapy	Reassess patient. Check sodium and potassium levels. Repeat ACTH stimulation test. If cortisol level post-ACTH is less than 15 nmol l^{-1} reduce maintenance dose or give every other week.

count is above 1.0×10^9 cells l^{-1} or the eosinophil count is above 0.3×10^9 cells l^{-1}. However, the best method of evaluating treatment is by use of the ACTH stimulation test. In adequately treated cases, the basal and ACTH stimulated serum cortisol concentrations should be below 120 nmol l^{-1} (Dunn et al., 1995). If the serum cortisol concentrations exceed 200 nmol l^{-1} with ACTH stimulation, then further mitotane should be administered until the cortisol concentrations are adequately suppressed. A few dogs respond in 2–3 days, and occasionally others require more than 60 consecutive days of treatment. It is important to emphasize that each dog must be treated as an individual if treatment is to be successful.

Maintenance therapy

Having produced sufficient adrenocortical damage with daily mitotane treatment, it is important to continue therapy, albeit at a lower dose, otherwise the zona glomerulosa will regenerate a hyperplastic zona fasciculata and zona reticularis and the clinical signs will recur.

Mitotane is given at a dose of 50 mg kg^{-1} week^{-1} with food. Cases that are well controlled may sleep for a few hours after the weekly dose and for that reason it is often recommended that the treatment is given in the evening. More profound depression or weakness requires re-evaluation and possibly a reduction of the maintenance dose. Failure to control the polydipsia may require an increased dose of mitotane (Table 39.17).

Re-examination

Treated dogs should be re-examined 6 to 8 weeks after completion of the initial therapy, unless there are any problems. Marked improvement should be noted at this time. The most obvious and rapid response is a reduction in water intake, urine output and appetite and this is usually obvious at the end of the initial course of therapy. Muscle strength and exercise tolerance improve over the first 3–4 weeks. Skin and hair coat changes take longer and the progress is variable. The skin and alopecia may deteriorate markedly before improving; alternatively there may be gradual and noticeable resolution of the dermatological signs. Although improvement should be noted by 8 weeks, the skin and haircoat may not return to normal for 3–6 months (Fig. 39.17). A few dogs have dramatic changes in coat colour following successful therapy.

Re-examination every 3–6 months is recommended for the remainder of the animal's life. Relapses and episodes of overdosage do occur and re-assessment of adrenal reserve by ACTH stimulation testing is indicated. Relapses may require a short course of daily mitotane therapy or an increase in the maintenance dosage. Overdosage requires reassessment by an ACTH stimulation test and a reduction of the maintenance dose.

In one study, the mean survival time of treated dogs was 30 months with a range of a few days to over 7 years (Dunn et al., 1995). Other studies have shown similar survival times (Kintzer and Peterson, 1991).

Other therapeutic options for pituitary-dependent hyperadrenocorticism

Hypophysectomy has been successfully performed in the dog for the treatment of pituitary-dependent hyperadrenocorticism, but the operation is technically difficult.

Bilateral adrenalectomy has been employed successfully but involves the risk of putting an ill animal with a compromised immune system and poor wound healing through a difficult surgical procedure. Currently, bilateral adrenalectomy appears to be the most successful means of treating feline hyperadrenocorticism. Patients treated by this approach require life-long treatment for hypoadrenocorticism.

Ketoconazole has a reversible inhibitory effect on glucocorticoid synthesis while having minimal effects on mineralocorticoid production.

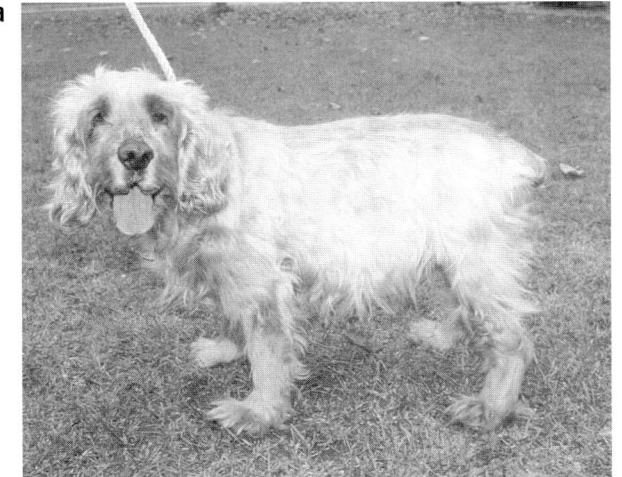
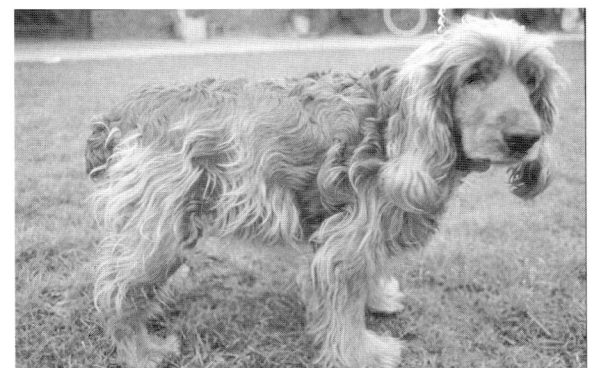
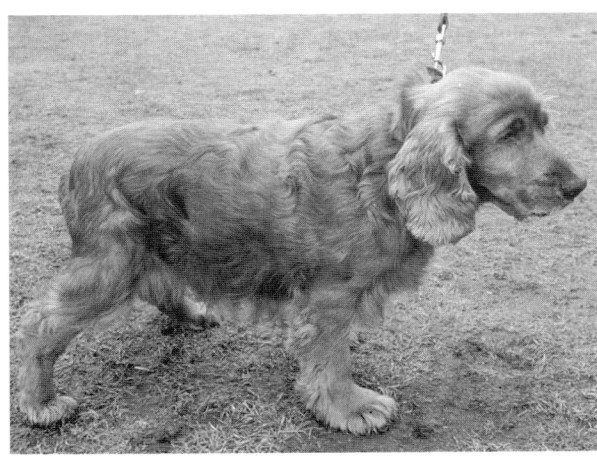

Figure 39.17 Photographs of a 9-year old cocker spaniel bitch taken (a) before treatment of hyperadrenocorticism, (b) 16 weeks after commencing therapy and (c) one year later. Note the improvement in the hair coat and the increased muscle tone. See colour plate.

Ketoconazole has been used effectively to control hyperadrenocorticism in dogs, but it is not effective in cats. However, ketoconazole is not uniformly efficacious in dogs and between one-third to one-half of all dogs treated fail to respond adequately.

The initial recommended dosage of ketoconazole is 10 mg kg^{-1} twice daily for 14 days. Alternatively, treatment is initiated at 5 mg kg^{-1} twice daily for the first seven days to assess drug tolerance, then increased to 10 mg kg^{-1}. The efficacy of the initial 14-day course of treatment is determined by an ACTH stimulation test. To ensure adequate control of hyperadrenocorticism, both the basal and post-ACTH serum cortisol concentrations must be lowered to the basal reference range. If the serum cortisol concentrations remain above this range, the dosage is increased to 15 mg kg^{-1} twice daily, and an ACTH response test repeated in 14 days (Feldman and Nelson, 1996).

L-*Deprenyl* (selegiline hydrochloride) is a monoamine oxidase inhibitor that inhibits ACTH secretion by increasing dopaminergic tone to the hypothalamic–pituitary axis. The use of L-deprenyl for treatment of hyperadrenocorticism has been evaluated in dogs. Although the effectiveness of treatment is variable, one major advantage of L-deprenyl is the lack of any severe adverse effects, including iatrogenic hypoadrenocorticism.

Treatment is initiated at a dosage of 1 mg kg^{-1} daily. If an inadequate response is seen after two months, the dosage is increased to 2 mg kg^{-1} day^{-1}. If this dosage also proves ineffective, alternative treatment is required. If this is effective, daily treatment should be continued for the remainder of the dog's life. Response to treatment is evaluated by the resolution of clinical signs. About 50% of dogs fail to respond adequately to this treatment.

Treatment of adrenal-dependent hyperadrenocorticism

Dogs diagnosed as having adrenal-dependent hyperadrenocorticism carry the best prognosis if the tumour can be removed surgically, although mitotane therapy has also been recommended (Kintzer and Peterson, 1994).

Unilateral adrenalectomy requires considerable experience and expertise because of the complex anatomy. The technique is well-described using the paracostal, flank approach (Johnston, 1977, 1983). It should only be performed by experienced surgeons as perioperative mortality is high. Postoperative support is important as the contralateral adrenal cortex will be atrophic and unable to respond to the stress of surgery. Replacement glucocorticoid therapy may therefore be required for 7–10 days postoperatively. Unilateral adrenalectomy is the recommended treatment for cats with adrenocortical tumours.

Phaeochromocytoma

Tumours of the adrenal medulla (phaeochromocytomas) are rare in dogs and have not been reported in cats. Phaeochromocytomas are usually unilateral, benign, slow-growing tumours that may reach a considerable size. Rarely, they are malignant and may invade the caudal vena cava or metastasize to lung, liver or bone. Phaeochromocytomas may secrete excessive amounts of catecholamines.

Clinical signs

Clinical signs of a phaeochromocytoma may relate to an abdominal mass compressing adjacent structures or to the secretion of catecholamines (Gilson *et al.*, 1994).

Clinical signs related to tumour size might include a palpable abdominal mass, ascites and hindlimb weakness. Secretion of catecholamines may be intermittent or persistent and can cause hypotension or hypertension, tachycardia, tachydysrhythmias with weakness and trembling, head pressing or seizures. Epistaxis and retinal haemorrhages may also be noted. The clinical signs vary depending on whether an excess of adrenaline or noradrenaline is predominant.

Diagnosis and treatment

A diagnosis of phaeochromocytoma should be suspected in any unexplained case of episodic weakness (Herrtage and McKerrell, 1995). Radiographic and ultrasonographic examinations will often reveal a mass in the adrenal area. Confirmation, however, requires quantification of the urinary excretion of catecholamines and their metabolites, which are not widely available.

Surgical removal is the treatment of choice, but should only be performed by experienced surgeons since excessive handling of the tumour during surgery may provoke massive secretion of catecholamines and the tumours tend to be invasive. Pentolamine (Rogitine, Ciba), an alpha-blocker for intravenous use, can be used at a dose of 0.02–0.1 mg kg^{-1} to lower blood pressure while manipulating the tumour and lignocaine or propranolol can be administered intravenously as necessary during surgery to control tachycardia or tachyarrhythmias.

DISORDERS OF THE ENDOCRINE PANCREAS

Anatomy and physiology

Functionally the pancreas comprises two separate glands; an exocrine portion and an endocrine portion. The exocrine pancreatic secretions contain digestive enzymes which are excreted into the intestinal lumen. The endocrine pancreas is composed of the islets of Langerhans, which secrete at least four hormones. Four cell types have been identified in the pancreatic islets with light microscopy on the basis of staining properties and histochemistry; the alpha cells which secrete glucagon, the beta cells which secrete insulin, the delta cells which secrete somatostatin and the F cells which secrete pancreatic polypeptide. A number of other peptides, for example gastric inhibitory polypeptide (GIP) and cholecystokinin (CCK), are also found in the islet cells.

Insulin and glucagon are involved in the control of carbohydrate, lipid and protein metabolism and are particularly important in blood glucose homeostasis. Glucose is the most potent stimulus for insulin secretion, although some other sugars and amino acids may also stimulate insulin release. The release of glucagon is inhibited by glucose, whereas the release of glucagon is stimulated by ingestion of protein, acute hypoglycaemia, catecholamines and glucocorticoids.

Diabetes mellitus

Diabetes mellitus is a heterogeneous condition in the dog and cat rather than a single disease entity. It is characterized by a relative or absolute deficiency of insulin secretion by the beta cells of the islets of Langerhans in the pancreas. Carbohydrate metabolism and in particular blood glucose concentration is controlled by the balance between the action of catabolic hormones, for example glucagon, cortisol, catecholamines and growth hormone on the one hand, and the principal anabolic hormone, insulin, on the other. A relative or absolute deficiency of insulin results in decreased utilization of glucose, amino acids and fatty acids by peripheral tissues, particularly liver, muscle and adipose tissue. Failure of glucose uptake by these cells leads to hyperglycaemia. Once the renal threshold for glucose reabsorption is exceeded, an osmotic diuresis ensues with loss of glucose, electrolytes and water in the urine. Compensatory polydipsia prevents the animal becoming dehydrated. The loss of glucose leads to catabolism of the body's reserves, especially of fat. Excessive fat catabolism leads to the production and accumulation of ketone bodies (acetoacetic acid, β-hydroxybutyric acid and acetone) and the onset of diabetic ketoacidosis. In diabetic ketoacidosis, the dog is unable to maintain an adequate fluid intake and becomes rapidly dehydrated due to the uncontrolled osmotic diuresis. The dehydration and acidosis requires emergency care if the animal is to survive.

In humans, diabetes is classified as type I, insulin-dependent diabetes mellitus (IDDM) and type II, non-insulin-dependent diabetes mellitus (NIDDM). This classification has not proved very useful in veterinary medicine since nearly all dogs and the majority of cats with diabetes mellitus require insulin therapy regardless of the underlying aetiology. Classifying diabetes mellitus into primary and secondary causes is of more use clinically in the dog (Table 39.18). In secondary diabetes which is caused by peripheral insulin resistance there is initially a compensatory increase in insulin secretion, but after a period of time the islet cells become exhausted, the beta cells are destroyed and their function is permanently lost.

Table 39.18 Aetiology of diabetes mellitus in the dog and cat

Primary islet cell degeneration
  Islet cell destruction (?autoimmune)
  Chronic pancreatitis
  Amyloidosis

Secondary diabetes mellitus
  obesity - causing down-regulation of insulin receptors
  antagonism to insulin
    by counter-regulatory hormones
      hyperadrenocorticism
      progesterone-induced growth hormone excess (dogs only)
      acromegaly
      hypothyroidism
      hyperthyroidism
    by drug therapy
      glucocorticoids
      progestogens

Clinical signs

Diabetes mellitus is a disease of middle-aged dogs with a peak incidence around 8 years of age. Genetic predisposition to diabetes has been found in keeshunds and samoyeds. Cairn terriers, poodles and dachshunds may also be over-represented. Entire females are more frequently affected than males and this is due mainly to the induction of growth hormone secretion by progesterone and other progestogens. Diabetes mellitus is recognized in middle-aged to older cats of any breed, but the disease appears to be more common in male cats.

Polyuria, polydipsia, increased appetite and weight loss develop over a few weeks in uncomplicated cases. In entire bitches, this usually occurs during the metoestrus phase of the oestrus cycle.

Hepatomegaly, muscle wasting and infections of the urinary or respiratory tracts may be noted on clinical examination. Ulcerative skin lesions and cutaneous xanthomas have occasionally been reported. If the diabetes remains uncontrolled, an accumulation of ketone bodies may occur which causes metabolic acidosis and leads to depression, anorexia, vomiting and rapid dehydration. Coma and death may result from severe hypovolaemia and circulatory collapse.

Diagnosis

Urine analysis reveals persistent glycosuria and often ketonuria. Despite the high solute load in the urine which would tend to increase the specific gravity of the urine, many older dogs may have impaired renal concentrating power and thus the specific gravity of the urine is variable, typically ranging between 1.015 and 1.045. Bacterial cystitis is common and occasionally may involve gas-producing organisms which can cause emphysematous cystitis.

Plasma biochemistry reveals a fasting hyperglycaemia (> 10 mmol l^{-1}) and hyperlipidaemia. In some patients the blood will be lactescent due to lipaemia. Liver enzymes are usually raised and liver function tests such as bile acid concentrations may be abnormal. In cases where diabetes is associated with pancreatitis, amylase and lipase concentrations may be elevated.

In diabetic ketoacidosis, there are serious derangements in fluid, electrolyte and acid–base status. The most frequent abnormalities are prerenal azotaemia, hyponatraemia and metabolic acidosis. The cat appears to be less prone to developing diabetic ketoacidosis.

Treatment

Treatment can be divided into the acute management of diabetic ketoacidosis and the stabilization of the uncomplicated diabetic. The ketoacidotic dog can be stabilized as for the uncomplicated case, once it has started to feed normally.

Management of diabetic ketoacidosis

Although the healthy ketotic diabetic can usually be managed conservatively without fluid therapy or intensive care, diabetic ketoacidosis characterized by hyperglycaemia, ketonaemia, metabolic acidosis, dehydration and electrolyte imbalance is a medical emergency that is associated with a high mortality rate (Macintire, 1993). Treatment should consist of fluid and electrolyte replacement, reduction of blood glucose concentration, correction of acidosis and identification of precipitating causes. A treatment protocol is given in Table 39.19.

Fluid therapy

Intravenous replacement of fluid and electrolytes is essential for the successful management of diabetic ketoacidosis. Unless serum electrolytes suggest otherwise, 0.9% sodium chloride is the initial fluid of choice. The fluid deficit is usually about 10% of body weight and this should be replaced over a period of 24–48 h.

Sodium chloride may be alternated with lactated Ringer's solution or, if the blood glucose falls below 10 mmol l^{-1}, a solution containing 0.18% sodium chloride and 4% glucose. Urine output should be measured and if possible, a central venous catheter used to monitor central venous pressure during fluid therapy.

Insulin therapy

Soluble insulin should be used in the treatment of diabetic ketoacidosis. Although intermittent administration using the intravenous and intramuscular routes has been used, low-dose intravenous insulin infusion using 0.1 units kg^{-1} h^{-1} is effective and appears to be associated with fewer side effects such as hypokalaemia and hypoglycaemia. Low-dose intravenous insulin infusion provides a steady, gradual reduction of blood glucose and ketone concentrations and is less likely to cause increases in glucagon, cortisol and growth hormone that can occur with intermittent bolus administration of insulin.

Blood glucose should be monitored every 2 h. Glucose-containing fluids should be introduced when the blood glucose concentration falls below 10 mmol l^{-1} and the insulin infusion should be stopped when the blood glucose reaches

Table 39.19 Treatment protocol for diabetic ketoacidosis in the dog

1. **Intravenous fluid and electrolyte replacement**
   0.9% sodium chloride initially then alternate with lactated Ringer's solution.
   Monitor urine output and if possible, central venous pressure.

2. **Insulin therapy**
   (a) **Low-dose insulin infusion** – add 5 units soluble insulin to 500 ml lactated Ringer's solution and infuse at a rate of 0.1 units kg^{-1} h^{-1} through a separate intravenous catheter. Use of an infusion pump or paediatric burette is helpful in controlling the rate of infusion. Monitor blood glucose concentration every 2 h.
   (b) **Soluble insulin injection** – a dose of 1 unit kg^{-1} is divided and a quarter of the dose given intravenously and three-quarters intramuscularly. The dose is repeated every 4–6 h. Monitor blood glucose concentration every 2 h.

3. **Continue intravenous fluid and electrolyte replacement**
   Continue alternating 0.9% sodium chloride with lactated Ringer's solution while blood glucose remains above 10 mmol l^{-1}. Use 0.18% sodium chloride with 4% glucose solution when blood glucose falls below 10 mmol l^{-1}.

4. **Potassium supplementation**
   Ideally supplementation with potassium should be based on serum potassium concentrations. In the absence of serum potassium measurements, add 20 mmol of potassium chloride to each 500 ml bag of intravenous fluid solution. The rate of administration should not exceed 0.5 mmol kg^{-1} h^{-1}. This treatment will be safe providing the patient has adequate urine production.

5. **Phosphate supplementation**
   Phosphate shifts in the same way as potassium. Hypophosphataemia is only likely to occur in severe diabetic ketoacidosis, but can be severe (< 0.5 mmol l^{-1}). Dose of 0.01–0.03 mmol kg^{-1} h^{-1} of potassium phosphate in calcium free fluid, e.g. normal saline is required if hypophosphataemia is suspected.

6. **Correction of acidosis**
   Bicarbonate therapy is not necessary provided renal function has been re-established. It is only indicated in life-threatening acidosis and only one third of the calculated replacement dose should be used to prevent excessive blood HCO_3 concentrations.

7. **Antibiotic therapy**

6 mmol l^{-1}. Once the insulin infusion is halted, blood glucose concentrations will increase so that further infusion of insulin may be required if the patient is not eating or a longer-acting insulin preparation may be introduced if its appetite has returned.

Potassium supplementation
Initially a deficit in total body potassium is usually masked by the acidosis which causes potassium to move extracellularly. Serum potassium concentration can decrease rapidly as renal function improves and as insulin therapy causes potassium to move back into the cells. Although hypokalaemia is less likely to occur with low dose insulin infusion, replacement therapy should be started within a few hours of instigating fluid and insulin therapy.

In the absence of serum potassium measurements, 20 mmol of potassium chloride should be added to every 500 ml of intravenous fluid solution given after insulin therapy has commenced.

Phosphate supplementation
Phosphate moves between the intracellular and extracellular compartments in the same way as potassium. Hypophosphataemia, which more commonly occurs in cats, can cause haemolytic anaemia, weakness, ataxia and seizures. Phosphate supplementation is only usually required in animals with severe diabetic ketoacidosis. Potassium phosphate at a dose of 0.01–0.03 mmol kg^{-1} h^{-1} i.v. is recommended to correct hypophosphataemia.

Bicarbonate therapy
The use of sodium bicarbonate to correct the acidosis in diabetic ketoacidosis is controversial. Rapid correction of the acidosis with bicarbonate can lead to metabolic alkalosis, tissue anoxia due to a shift to the left of the haemoglobin–oxygen dissociation curve, and paradoxical cerebral acidosis because CO_2 crosses the blood–brain barrier more rapidly than bicarbonate ions. For these reasons bicarbonate should be used only in life-

threatening acidosis (arterial pH < 7.0). Provided normal renal function is restored and adequate fluid therapy is given, the acidosis will resolve without bicarbonate administration.

Antibiotic therapy
Broad-spectrum antibiotic therapy is required because bacterial infection is often a common precipitating factor for diabetic ketoacidosis and the use of intravenous and urinary catheters may predispose the patient to infection.

Other common concurrent illnesses in the dog with diabetic ketoacidosis include pancreatitis, renal failure, congestive heart failure, hyperadrenocorticism and pyometra. Entire bitches may be resistant to insulin therapy during the metoestus phase of their oestrus cycle.

Management of uncomplicated diabetes mellitus
The primary goal of diabetes therapy is to maintain normoglycaemia and thereby control the signs that occur secondary to hyperglycaemia and glycosuria which result in the development of complications (Table 39.20). The essentials of good stabilization of diabetes mellitus in the dog requires understanding by the owner, and adherence to a regular daily routine that involves diet, insulin administration and regular, controlled exercise.

Stabilization can be carried out satisfactorily at home, but particularly if the dog is ketotic, it may be preferable to hospitalize the animal during stabilization since it is easier to monitor blood glucose more closely.

Most diabetic dogs are presented with severe islet cell degeneration and atrophy. Therefore diabetes mellitus in dogs is insulin-dependent. Rarely, bitches may be presented during the metoestus phase of the oestrus cycle before islet cell exhaustion has occurred. If ovariohysterectomy is performed immediately the signs of diabetes become apparent in these patients, there may be complete remission of clinical signs. However, in the majority of bitches this opportunity is missed or goes unnoticed and permanent damage to the islet cells occurs.

Dietary therapy
Appropriate dietary therapy is an essential part of the management of diabetes. The diet must be well-balanced and constant in both composition and amount fed at each meal. It is, therefore, most convenient to use a commercial diet. Canned or dry foods which contain complex carbohydrates should be fed as slow digestion and absorption minimizes the fluctuations in postprandial blood glucose concentrations. Semi-moist foods which contain a predominance of easily assimilated carbohydrates in the form of disaccharides and propylene glycol should be avoided because of marked postprandial hyperglycaemia (Holste et al., 1989). There is evidence that diets with a high fibre content improve glycaemic control by delaying starch hydrolysis and glucose absorption thereby reducing postprandial fluctuations in blood glucose (Nelson et al., 1991). High fibre diets are also beneficial in correcting obesity. However, there may be disadvantages in using high fibre diets such as reduced palatability and the fact that low caloric density may cause the patient to lose excessive weight or fail to gain weight if the patient is already below ideal body weight. The author tends to reserve high fibre diets for those patients that are difficult to stabilize and/or are obese.

Finally, the feeding schedule should be designed to enhance the action of insulin and minimize postprandial hyperglycaemia. The daily caloric intake should occur when insulin is present in the circulation and is capable of handling glucose absorbed from the intestine. Several small meals are preferable to one large feed as these will help minimize postprandial hyperglycaemia and thus help to control fluctuations in blood glucose. The author routinely recommends two equal meals fed at times to coincide with insulin activity. In cases that prove difficult to stabilize three or four smaller meals are fed during the day.

Titbits and scavenging must be avoided as they tend to destabilize diabetic patients.

Insulin therapy
For routine stabilization in the dog insulin zinc suspension (lente) which contains a mixture of 30% insulin zinc suspension (amorphous) and 70% insulin zinc suspension (crystalline) is the preparation of choice. When given by subcutaneous

Table 39.20 Complications associated with diabetes mellitus

Hypoglycaemia
Ketoacidosis
Cataract formation
Hepatic lipidosis
Pancreatitis
Infections
Retinopathy
Diabetic nephropathy
Diabetic neuropathy
Skin disease

injection, it is an intermediate acting insulin with an onset of activity at 1–2 h, peak activity around 6–12 h and a duration of action of between 18 and 26 h in the dog. The times for peak activity and duration of action vary with the individual, but in most dogs once daily administration is adequate.

Lente insulin is usually given as a single morning injection at the same time or just before the first meal, with the second meal given 6–8 h later to coincide with peak insulin activity. An initial dose of 0.5–1.0 unit kg^{-1} is given. Insulin is probably best dosed on body surface area rather than on a simple body weight basis. Thus small dogs (<15 kg) tend to require 1.0 unit kg^{-1} and larger dogs (>25 kg) receive 0.5 unit kg^{-1}. Although the subcutaneous route is ideal for long-term use, the intramuscular route may be used initially, especially in moderately dehydrated or ketotic animals, because absorption from subcutaneous depots in these patients may be slow and erratic.

In general, cats appear to metabolize insulin more rapidly than dogs, therefore in order to avoid the complications of twice daily insulin injections, it is best to use a protamine zinc insulin preparation. A similar initial dose of 0.5–1.0 unit kg^{-1} is recommended.

Insulin should be administered using specific 0.5 ml or 1.0 ml syringes calibrated in units (100 units ml^{-1}). Insulin preparations should be stored in a refrigerator at 2–8°C because they are adversely affected by heat or freezing. Preparations should be rolled gently to re-suspend the particles before use.

A patient will usually take 2–4 days to respond fully to a dose of insulin or a change in preparation. It is important to avoid increasing the dose too quickly before equilibration has occurred as this can lead to a sudden and precipitous fall in blood glucose due to overdosage with insulin. In most cases, adjustments in the insulin dose should be made in small changes of not more than 2–4 units per injection.

The type of preparation and frequency of administration may require alteration in those patients that prove difficult to stabilize with this standard routine. However, it is good for the clinician to become familiar with one type of insulin preparation and only change from that preparation if the insulin is the cause of the instability.

The standard daily routine is as follows:

8.00 am   Give lente insulin injection subcutaneously.
8.30 am   Feed half of the measured daily ration.
2.30 pm   Feed second half of the daily ration.
           Keep daily routine constant including exercise.
           Avoid titbits and scavenging.

Monitoring therapy

Ideally, monitoring should consist of serial blood glucose measurements taken throughout the day as tighter diabetic control can be gained than with urine glucose estimations. Initially at least two blood glucose estimations should be made, one before insulin is administered and the second just before the second feed. Once the dog appears fairly stable more frequent blood samples should be taken (every 2–3 h) throughout the day to assess the degree of stabilization. An assessment of daily water intake can also provide useful information about the degree of diabetic control.

Blood glucose concentrations should ideally be maintained between 5 and 9 mmol l^{-1}. The blood glucose concentration will usually be highest in the morning before insulin is administered and lowest just before the second feed. A trace of glucose in the morning urine sample may be acceptable but the urine should be negative at other times in the day. However, it is important to remember that urine glucose may not reflect the blood glucose concentration at the same point in time and if the urine glucose is negative, the blood glucose concentration could be hypoglycaemic (< 3.0 mmol l^{-1}), normoglycaemic or hyperglycaemic (> 5.5 mmol l^{-1}).

Although the author's clients monitor urine for glucose and ketones regularly, he does not advocate adjusting daily insulin dosages on the basis of morning urine glucose measurements. Instead, he prefers to continue with a fixed insulin dosage unless the patient remains unstable for more than several days.

Measurement of glycated proteins such as fructosamine and glycosylated haemoglobin, are used increasingly in the dog and cat to monitor the response to treatment. The irreversible, non-enzymatic glycation process occurs throughout the life span of the protein, mainly albumin in the case of fructosamine, and is proportional to the glucose concentration over that time. These measurements reflect the average blood glucose concentration over the preceding one to two weeks in the case of serum fructosamine and two to three months in the case of glycosylated haemoglobin (Jensen, 1995). Fructosamine concentrations less than 400 mmol l^{-1} indicate good glycaemic control whereas concentrations above 500 mmol l^{-1} are found in newly diagnosed or poorly controlled diabetics (Reusch et al., 1993). Glycosylated haemoglobin is less routinely available as an assay. Well controlled diabetic dogs have between 4 and 6% glycosylated haemoglobin, whereas poorly controlled diabetics have concentrations greater than 7% (Nelson, 1995).

Diabetic records (Fig. 39.18) should be kept by the owner for each patient as alterations to stability can be assessed more easily over a period of time. Insulin requirements will be increased by infection, oestrus particularly the metoestrus phase of the cycle, pregnancy and ketoacidosis. It is recommended that entire bitches should undergo ovariohysterectomy to avoid insulin resistance during subsequent seasons.

Investigation of instability

If a patient appears to be poorly stabilized at home despite repeated attempts to provide adequate glycaemic control, check the diabetic record and examine the patient for signs of disease that could cause insulin resistance, for example infection, oestrus, pregnancy, ketoacidosis or hyperadrenocorticism. Go through the daily routine with the owner to make sure that the diet is constant and measured and that there is no access to titbits or scavenging. Check the insulin preparation for type, expiry date and storage, and also the ability of the owner to administer insulin (adequate mixing, correct dosage and injection technique).

If an obvious cause cannot be determined, the dog should be hospitalized on its daily routine and serial blood glucose determinations made every 1–2 h throughout the day. Determinations made with glucose reagent strips and a glucose meter are simple, fast and sufficiently accurate for this purpose. The results should then be plotted on a graph against time, although it is important to realize that precise glucose curves may vary from day to day in any diabetic patient.

Three major causes of instability can be determined from the graph of serial blood glucose determinations. The first is insulin-induced hyperglycaemia, also called the Somogyi overswing, where excessive insulin dosage leads to paradoxical hyperglycaemia (Fig. 39.19). The blood glucose concentration is high in the morning before insulin is given, but falls sharply to hypoglycaemic concentrations (<3.5 mmol l^{-1}) after insulin administration. The hypoglycaemic period is short in duration and is not associated with signs of hypoglycaemia. In fact, the nadir can easily be missed if frequent sampling is not performed. The low blood glucose concentration stimulates the release of hormones antagonistic to insulin, such as glucagon, cortisol and catecholamines, and these cause the glucose concentration to rebound quickly to high levels. If blood glucose and/or urine glucose concentrations were measured only before insulin and before the second feed, the concentrations would be high and this could easily be misinterpreted as a reason for increasing the daily insulin dose, when in fact, the dog is already being overdosed. The treatment for insulin-induced hyperglycaemia is to reduce the daily dose of insulin to prevent the hypoglycaemia that causes the dramatic swing in blood glucose concentrations.

The second cause of instability is due to rapid metabolism of insulin which means that an intermediate acting insulin preparation does not last for a full 24 hours (Fig. 39.20). In such cases, the blood glucose concentration is high in the morning before insulin is given, but falls to normal

Figure 39.18 Diabetic record

Date	Urine exam	Insulin time & dose	Food	Drink	Body weight	Blood results	Notes
15 March	am glucose -ve ketones -ve	18 units lente insulin s.c. 8.00 am	3/4 tin Doggo 8.30 am 2.30 pm	0.9 L	24 kg	2.00 pm Blood glucose 4.6 mmol/l	Bright and alert

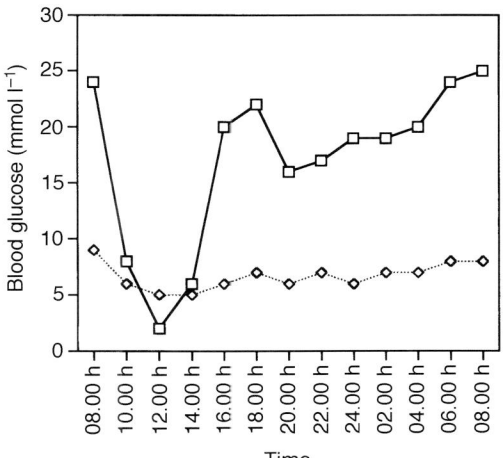

Figure 39.19 A 24-hour blood glucose curve from a dog with insulin-induced hyperglycaemia (Somogyi overswing). □, Patient; ◇, ideal diabetic curve.

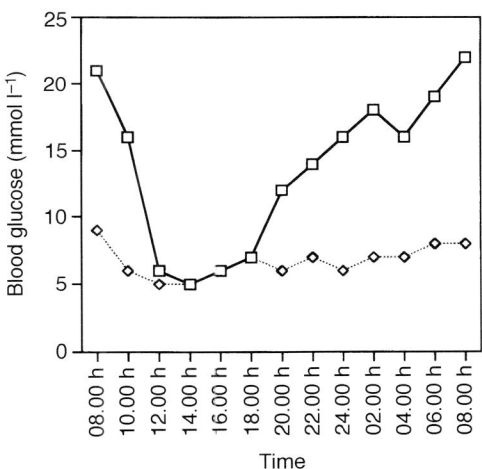

Figure 39.20 A 24-hour blood glucose curve from a dog with rapid metabolism of insulin. □, Patient; ◇, ideal diabetic curve.

concentrations for much of the day. However after the second feed the blood glucose concentration rises and remains high for the remainder of the day. This results in a considerable period of hyperglycaemia and results in glycosuria in the morning and often nocturnal polydipsia and polyuria. The treatment of rapid insulin metabolism is either to try a longer-acting insulin preparation, for example protamine zinc insulin or ultralente, or to administer two doses of lente insulin 12 h apart with four small meals given approximately at six-h intervals.

The third cause of instability is associated with insulin resistance. In these cases, the animal remains persistently hyperglycaemic despite an insulin dosage of more than 2.2 units kg^{-1} day^{-1} (Fig. 39.21). Although some patients can be stabilized satisfactorily at doses higher than this, peripheral antagonism to insulin activity is likely to be present. In those cases where adequate

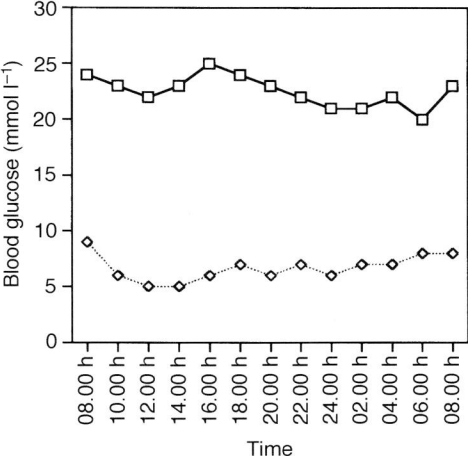

Figure 39.21 A 24-hour blood glucose curve from a dog receiving more than 2.2 units of insulin kg^{-1} bodyweight indicating insulin resistance. □, Patient; ◇, ideal diabetic curve.

stabilization is not possible, thorough investigation of the patient is required to try and identify the precise cause of insulin resistance. Some of the causes of insulin resistance are listed in Table 39.21. Correction or treatment of the underlying cause will usually enable the patient to be stabilized at a lower dose of insulin with improved glycaemic control.

Table 39.21 Causes of insulin resistance

Obesity
Hyperadrenocorticism
Exogenous glucocorticoid administration
Metoestrus phase of the oestrus cycle
Exogenous progestagen administration
Acromegaly
Hypothyroidism
Hyperthyroidism
Impaired absorption of insulin
Excessive insulin antibody formation
Phaeochromocytoma
Glucagonoma

Insulinoma

Functional islet cell tumours (insulinomas) are the most frequently occurring tumours of the endocrine pancreas in dogs. Most insulin-secreting tumours are malignant islet cell carcinomas which metastasize to regional lymph nodes and/or the liver. Early diagnosis is important as dogs with metastases have significantly reduced survival times.

Insulinomas are composed of neoplastic β-cells which continue to release insulin despite the presence of hypoglycaemia. Hypoglycaemia is normally the major inhibitory stimulus for insulin secretion. As a result of hyperinsulinism, tissue utilization of glucose continues, the hypoglycaemia worsens and, ultimately, clinical signs develop. The onset and severity of clinical signs is determined by the degree of hypoglycaemia and the rate at which the plasma concentration of glucose falls. A rapid decline in plasma glucose concentration may occur with fasting, exercise or excitement in dogs with insulinomas.

The brain is an obligate consumer of glucose. Cerebral cells have limited stores of glycogen and a limited ability to utilize protein and amino acids for energy. These cells will be the first affected by hypoglycaemia. Prolonged and profound hypoglycaemia causes ischaemic neuronal cell damage identical to that caused by cerebral hypoxia.

Hypoglycaemia is a potent stimulus for the release of hormones which have an antagonistic action to insulin. These include glucagon, growth hormone, glucocorticoids, catecholamines and possibly thyroid hormones. These hormones act in concert to raise the plasma glucose concentration. Some of the clinical manifestations of hypoglycaemia such as muscle tremors, nervousness, restlessness and hunger may result from stimulation of the sympathetic nervous system and increased levels of circulating catecholamines.

Clinical signs

Insulinomas usually occur in middle-aged to older dogs (mean age of 8.7 years) of any breed, although medium to large breeds appear to be predisposed. No sex predisposition has been reported. Insulinomas appear to be very rare in cats (Hawks et al., 1992).

A tentative diagnosis of hyperinsulinism is generally based on fulfilment of the criteria from Whipple's triad: (1) the presence of neurological signs typical of hypoglycaemia, which may be precipitated by exercise or excitement; (2) hypoglycaemia (plasma glucose less than 3 mmol l^{-1}) at the time of the clinical signs; and (3) resolution of clinical signs following feeding or administration of glucose.

Clinical signs associated with hypoglycaemia include fatigue, generalized weakness, collapse, muscle tremors, altered behaviour, confusion/disorientation, apparent blindness, ataxia, incoordination, stupor and seizures (Dunn et al., 1993). These signs are usually episodic in nature and may occur with fasting, exercise or excitement in dogs with insulinomas. Provocative stimuli such as the intravenous administration of glucagon or glucose, results in excessive secretion of insulin from neoplastic β-cells. This response may be even greater if glucose is administered orally as numerous intestinal hormones (glucagon, secretin, cholecystokinin, gastrin and gastric inhibitory peptide) are secreted in response to oral glucose and these in turn increase insulin secretion. It is by this mechanism that feeding has been reported to initiate clinical signs in dogs with insulinomas.

Seizure activity is one of the most common clinical manifestations of hypoglycaemia. The seizures may be grand mal or focal in nature and are normally self-limiting, lasting between 30 s and 5 min. Peripheral neuropathy with nerve degeneration and demyelination has also been associated with canine insulinoma in a few cases (Schrauwen, 1991).

Insulinomas are generally small tumours and do not lead to malignant cachexia. Thus weight loss is not usually a feature of this disease.

Laboratory findings

A presumptive diagnosis of insulinoma is based on the presence of typical clinical signs in association with persistent hypoglycaemia and an inappropriately high plasma insulin concentration.

A fasting plasma glucose concentration of 3 mmol l^{-1} or less is found in most cases. Some dogs with insulinoma show no clinical signs despite having extremely low blood glucose concentrations (< 2 mmol l^{-1}) because they are able to adapt to these low concentrations over a prolonged period of time. Differential diagnosis of hypoglycaemia in adult dogs includes insulinoma, liver disease, extrapancreatic neoplasia, septicaemia and hypoadrenocorticism (Table 39.22).

Plasma insulin concentrations greater than 20 mU l^{-1} in association with hypoglycaemia are inappropriate and an insulin glucose ratio greater than 4.2 U mol^{-1} is considered diagnostic (Dunn et al., 1992). In normal dogs, insulin levels fall as glucose concentrations decrease.

Table 39.22 Differential diagnosis of hypoglycaemia in adult dogs

Incorrect anticoagulant/delayed separation of serum from red blood cells
Functional islet cell tumour (insulinoma)
Excessive insulin administration
Extra-pancreatic tumours, particularly hepatic tumours
Liver disease
Septicaemic or endotoxic shock
Hypoadrenocorticism
Idiopathic in working dogs
Severe polycythaemia

In borderline cases, an intravenous glucose tolerance test using 0.5 g glucose kg^{-1} body weight has proved useful. Insulin-secreting tumours retain a degree of responsiveness to the glucose challenge and a glucose half-life of less than 20 min and/or a fractional clearance rate of more than 3% min^{-1} is highly suggestive of insulinoma in the dog.

Although hypoalbuminaemia, hypokalaemia and increases in alkaline phosphatase and alanine aminotransferase have occasionally been reported, these findings are not specific or helpful in achieving a definitive diagnosis.

Ultrasonography

Abdominal ultrasonography using a high quality diagnostic ultrasound machine has been used to examine the pancreas of dogs with suspected insulinomas. In one study a pancreatic mass was identified as a spherical or lobular hypoechoic nodule in 75% of dogs with insulinomas (Lamb et al., 1995). Tumours as small as 7 mm have been identified in the pancreas. However, ultrasonography has proved less sensitive for the detection of hepatic or lymphatic metastases.

Pathology

Insulinomas are located in the left lobe of the pancreas most commonly, followed by the right lobe and the body of the pancreas. Tumours are usually solitary but multiple masses may occur. Rarely, there is a diffuse islet cell tumour with no discrete nodule. There does not appear to be a difference in survival in relation to tumour location within the pancreas, but there is a suggestion that tumours with a high mitotic count carry a worse prognosis (Dunn et al., 1993).

Insulinomas in dogs are highly malignant and there is often gross evidence of metastasis at the time of diagnosis.

Treatment

Management of insulinomas should be directed at specific treatment of the tumour, reduction of insulin secretion and correction of hypoglycaemia.

Surgical resection of the pancreatic tumour and metastatic tumour masses should be the first approach to therapy. Postoperative recovery is routine in many cases, but postoperative complications including pancreatitis, hyperglycaemia, overt diabetes mellitus and hypoglycaemia can occur. In nearly all cases, hypoglycaemia will recur eventually due to metastases.

Medical management should be used if widespread metastasis is present or if hypoglycaemia recurs following surgery. This should consist of dietary manipulation with frequent small meals of a diet high in proteins, fats and complex carbohydrates. Prednisolone, which inhibits insulin and stimulates glycogenolysis, is useful in raising blood glucose concentration and is given at a dose of 0.5–1.0 mg kg^{-1} daily in divided doses. Diazoxide, a non-diuretic, benzothiazine antihypertensive drug which inhibits insulin secretion, has also been used successfully at a dose of 10 mg kg^{-1} daily in divided doses increasing to 60 mg kg^{-1} daily if necessary to control hypoglycaemia. More recently octreotide, a somatostatin analogue which inhibits insulin synthesis and secretion, has been tried with variable success (Simpson et al., 1995).

The prognosis is guarded due to the malignant nature of the disease. However, many dogs do well with medical and surgical management. The median time to recurrence of clinical signs after surgery is 12 months (range 4–16 months) and the median postoperative survival time was 14 months (range 10–33 months) in one study (Dunn et al., 1993).

REFERENCES

Andresen, E. and Willeberg, P. (1976) Pituitary dwarfism in German Shepherd dogs: additional evidence of simple autosomal recessive inheritance. *Nord Vet Med* **28**, 481–486.

Arnold, U., Opitz, M., Grosser, I., Bader, R. and Eigenmann, J.E. (1984) Goitrous hypothyroidism and dwarfism in a kitten. *Journal of the American Animal Hospital Association* **20**, 753–758.

Barber, P.J., Elliott, J. and Torrance, A.G. (1993) Measurement of feline intact parathyroid hormone: assay validation and sample handling studies. *Journal of Small Animal Practice* **34**, 614–620.

Bartez, P.Y., Nyland, T.G. and Feldman, E.C. (1995) Ultrasonographic evaluation of the adrenal glands in dogs. *Journal of the American Veterinary Medical Association* **207**, 1180–1183.

Berger, B. and Feldman, E.C. (1987) Primary hyperparathyroidism in dogs: 21 cases (1976–1986). *Journal of the American Veterinary Medical Association* **191**, 350–356.

Bertoy, E.H., Feldman, E.C., Nelson, R.W., Duesberg, C.A., Kass, P.H., Reid, M.H. and Dublin, A.B. (1995) Magnetic resonance imaging of the brain in dogs with recently diagnosed but untreated pituitary-dependent hyperadrenocorticism. *Journal of the American Veterinary Medical Association* **206**, 651–656.

Bischel, P., Jacobs, G. and Oliver, J.E. (1988) Neurological manifestations associated with hypothyroidism in four dogs. *Journal of the American Veterinary Medical Association* **192**, 1745–1747.

Bruyette, D.S. and Feldman, E.C. (1988) Primary hypoparathyroidism in the dog: report of 15 cases and review of 13 previously reported cases. *Journal of Veterinary Internal Medicine* **2**, 7–14.

Burrows, C.F. (1987) Reversible mega-oesophagus in a dog with hypoadrenocorticism. *Journal of Small Animal Practice* **28**, 1073–1078.

Chastain, C.B. and Panciera, D.L. (1995) Hypothyroid diseases. In: *Textbook of Veterinary Internal Medicine: Diseases of the Dog and Cat*, 4th edn (Eds S.J. Ettinger and E.C. Feldman). W.B. Saunders, Philadelphia, pp. 1487–1501.

DeVries, S.E., Feldman, E.C., Nelson, R.W. and Kennedy, P.C. (1993) Primary parathyroid gland hyperplasia in dogs: six cases (1982–1991). *Journal of the American Veterinary Medical Association* **202**, 1132–1136.

Duesberg, C.A., Feldman, E.C., Nelson, R.W., Bertoy, E.H., Dublin, A.B. and Reid, M.H. (1995) Brain magnetic resonance imaging for the diagnosis of pituitary macrotumours. *Journal of the American Veterinary Medical Association* **206**, 675–662.

Duncan, I.D., Griffiths, I.R. and Nash, A.S. (1977) Myotonia in canine Cushing's disease. *Veterinary Record* **100**, 30–31.

Dunn, J.K., Heath, M.F., Herrtage, M.E., Jackson, K.F. and Walker, M.J. (1992) Diagnosis of insulinoma in the dog: a study of 11 cases. *Journal of Small Animal Practice* **33**, 514–520.

Dunn, J.K., Bostock, D.E., Herrtage, M.E., Jackson, K.F. and Walker, M.J. (1993) Insulin-secreting tumours of the canine pancreas: clinical and pathological features of 11 cases. *Journal of Small Animal Practice* **34**, 325–331.

Dunn, K.J., Herrtage, M.E. and Dunn, J.K. (1995) Use of ACTH stimulation tests to monitor the treatment of canine hyperadrenocorticism. *Veterinary Record* **137**, 161–165.

Eigenmann, J.E. (1981) Diabetes mellitus in elderly female dogs: recent findings on pathogenesis and clinical implications. *Journal of the American Animal Hospital Association* **17**, 805–812.

Eigenmann, J.E., Zanesco, S., Arnold, U. and Froesch, E.R. (1984a) Growth hormone and insulin-like growth factor 1 in German Shepherd dwarf dogs. *Acta Endocrinologica* **105**, 289–293.

Eigenmann, J.E., Patterson, D.F., Zapf, J. and Froesch, E.R. (1984b) Insulin-like growth factor 1 in the dog: a study in different dog breeds and in dogs with growth hormone elevation. *Acta Endocrinologica* **105**, 294–301.

Elliott, J., Dobson, J.M., Dunn, J.K., Herrtage, M.E. and Jackson, K.F. (1991) Hypercalcaemia in the dog: a study of 40 cases. *Journal of Small Animal Practice* **32**, 564–571.

Feldman, E.C. and Nelson, R.W. (1996) Hyperadrenocorticism In: *Canine and Feline Endocrinology and Reproduction*. 2nd edn. W.B. Saunders, Philadelphia, pp. 187–265.

Ferguson, D.C. (1988) The effect of nonthyroidal factors on thyroid function tests in dogs. *Compendium of Continuing Education for the Practicing Veterinarian* **10**, 1365–1376.

Fluckiger, M.A. and Gomez, J.A. (1984) Radiographic findings in dogs with spontaneous pulmonary thrombosis or embolism. *Veterinary Radiology* **25**, 124–131.

Gilson, S.D., Withrow, S.J., Wheeler, S.L. and Twedt, D.C. (1994) Pheochromocytoma in 50 dogs. *Journal of Veterinary Internal Medicine* **8**, 228–232.

Greco, D.S., Feldman, E.C., Peterson, M.E., Turner, J.L., Hodges, C.M. and Shipman, L.W. (1991) Congenital hypothyroid dwarfism in a family of giant schnauzers. *Journal of Veterinary Internal Medicine* **5**, 57–65.

Hawks, D., Peterson, M.E., Hawkins, K.L. and Rosebury, W.S. (1992) Insulin-secreting pancreatic (islet cell) carcinoma in a cat. *Journal of Veterinary Internal Medicine* **6**, 193–196.

Herrtage, M.E. and McKerrell, R.E. (1995) Episodic weakness. In: *Manual of Dog and Cat Neurology*, 2nd edn. (Ed. S.L. Wheeler). British Small Animal Veterinary Association, Cheltenham, pp. 189–207.

Holste, L.C., Nelson, R.W., Feldman, E.C. and Bottoms, G.D. (1989) Effect of dry, soft moist, and canned dog food on postprandial blood glucose and insulin concentrations in healthy dogs. *American Journal of Veterinary Research* **50**, 984–989.

Huntley, K., Frazer, J., Gibbs, C. and Gaskell C.J. (1982) The radiological features of canine Cushing's syndrome: a review of forty-eight cases. *Journal of Small Animal Practice* **23**, 369–380.

Jaggy, A., Oliver, J.E., Ferguson, D.C., Mahaffey, E.A. and Glaus, T. (1994) Neurological manifestations of hypothyroidism: a retrospective study of 29 dogs. *Journal of Veterinary Internal Medicine* **8**, 328–336.

Jensen, A.L. (1995) Glycated blood proteins in canine diabetes mellitus. *Veterinary Record* **137**, 401–405.

Johnston, D.E. (1977) Adrenalectomy via retroperitoneal approach in dogs. *Journal of the American Veterinary Medical Association* **170**, 1092.

Johnston, D.E. (1983) Adrenalectomy in the dog. In: *Current Techniques in Small Animal Surgery* (Ed. M.J. Bojrab). Lea and Febiger, Philadelphia, pp. 386–388.

Jones, B.R., Gruffydd-Jones, T.J., Sparkes, A.H. and Lucke, V.M. (1992) Preliminary studies on congenital hypothyroidism in a family of Abyssinian cats. *Veterinary Record* **131**, 145–148.

Kallet, A.J., Richter, K.P., Feldman, E.C. and Brum, D.E. (1991) Primary hyperparathyroidism in cats: seven cases (1984–1989). *Journal of the American Veterinary Medical Association* **199**, 1767–1771.

Kantrowitz, C.M., Nyland, T.G. and Feldman, E.C. (1986) Adrenal ultrasonography in the dog: detection of tumours and hyperplasia in hyperadrenocorticism. *Veterinary Radiology* **27**, 91–96.

Kintzer, P.P. and Peterson, M.E. (1991) Mitotane (o,p′-DDD) treatment of 200 dogs with pituitary-dependent hyperadrenocorticism. *Journal of Veterinary Internal Medicine* **5**, 182–190.

Kintzer, P.P. and Peterson, M.E. (1994) Mitotane treatment of 32 dogs with cortisol-secreting adrenocortical neoplasms. *Journal of the American Veterinary Medical Association* **205**, 54–60.

Kintzer, P.P. and Peterson, M.E. (1997) Treatment and long-term follow-up of 205 dogs with hypoadrenocorticism. *Journal of Veterinary Internal Medicine* **11**, 43–49.

Lamb, C.R., Simpson, K.W., Boswood, A. and Matthewman, L.A. (1995) Ultrasonography of pancreatic neoplasia in the dog: a review of 16 cases. *Veterinary Record* **137**, 65–68.

Macintire, D.K. (1993) Treatment of diabetic ketoacidosis in dogs by continuous low-dose intravenous infusion of insulin. *Journal of the American Veterinary Medical Association* **202**, 1266–1272.

Medinger, T.L., Williams, D.A. and Bruyette, D.S. (1993) Severe gastrointestinal tract haemorrhage in three dogs with hypoadrenocorticism. *Journal of the American Veterinary Medical Association* **202**, 1869–1872.

Miller, A.B., Nelson, R.W., Scott-Moncrieff, J.C., Neal, L. and Bottoms, G.D. (1992) Serial thyroid hormone concentrations in healthy euthyroid dogs, dogs with hypothyroidism, and euthyroid dogs with atopic dermatitis. *British Veterinary Journal* **148**, 451–458.

Mooney, C.T. (1994) Radioactive iodine therapy for feline hyperthyroidism: efficacy and administration. *Journal of Small Animal Practice* **35**, 289–294.

Mooney, C.T. and Anderson, T.J. (1993) Congenital hypothyroidism in a boxer dog. *Journal of Small Animal Practice* **34**, 31–35.

Mooney, C.T., Thoday, K.L. and Doxey, D.L. (1992) Carbimazole therapy of feline hyperthyroidism. *Journal of Small Animal Practice* **33**, 228–235.

Nachreiner, R.F. and Refsal, K.R. (1992) Radioimmunoassay monitoring of thyroid hormone concentrations in dogs on thyroid replacement therapy: 2674 cases (1985–1987). *Journal of the American Veterinary Medical Association* **201**, 623–629.

Nelson, R.W. (1995) Diabetes mellitus. In: *Textbook of Veterinary Internal Medicine*, 4th edn. (Eds S.J. Ettinger and E.C. Feldman). W.B. Saunders, Philadelphia, pp. 1529–1530.

Nelson, R.W., Ihle, S.L., Lewis, L.D., Salisbury, S.K., Miller, T., Bergdall, V. and Bottoms G.D. (1991) Effects of dietary fibre supplementation on glycemic control in dogs with alloxan-induced diabetes mellitus. *American Journal of Veterinary Research* **52**, 2060–2066.

Nesbitt, G. H., Izzo, J., Peterson, L. and Wilkins, R.J. (1980) Canine hypothyroidism: a retrospective study of 108 cases. *Journal of the American Veterinary Medical Association* **177**, 1117–1122.

Oluju, M.P., Eckersall, P.D. and Douglas, T.A. (1984) Simple quantitative assay for canine steroid-induced alkaline phosphatase. *Veterinary Record* **115**, 17.

Panciera, D.L. (1994) Hypothyroidism in dogs: 66 cases (1987–1992). *Journal of the American Veterinary Medical Association* **204**, 761–767.

Peterson, M.E. and Greco, D.S. (1989) Primary hypoadrenocorticism in ten cats. *Journal of Veterinary Internal Medicine* **3**, 55–58.

Peterson, M.E. and Gamble, D.A. (1990) Effect of nonthyroidal illness on serum thyroxine concentrations in cats: 494 cases (1988). *Journal of the American Veterinary Medical Association* **197**, 1203–1208.

Peterson, M.E. & Kintzer, P.P. (1996) Pretreatment clinical and laboratory findings in dogs with hypoadrenocorticism: 225 cases (1979–1993). *Journal of the American Veterinary Medical Association* **208**, 85–91.

Peterson, M.E., Krieger, D.T., Drucker, W.D. and Halmi, N.S. (1982a) Immunocytochemical study of the hypophysis in 25 dogs with pituitary-dependent hyperadrenocorticism. *Acta Endocrinologica* **101**, 15–24.

Peterson, M.E., Gilbertson, S.R. and Drucker, W.D. (1982b) Plasma cortisol response to exogenous ACTH in 22 dogs with hyperadrenocorticism caused by an adrenocortical neoplasia. *Journal of the American Veterinary Medical Association* **180**, 542–544.

Peterson, M.E., Ferguson, D.C., Kintzer, P.P. and Drucker, W.D. (1984) Effects of spontaneous hyperadrenocorticism on serum thyroid hormone concentrations in the dog. *American Journal of Veterinary Research* **45**, 2034–2038.

Peterson, M.E., Graves, T.K. and Cavanagh, I. (1987) Serum thyroid hormone concentrations fluctuate in cats with hyperthyroidism. *Journal of Veterinary Internal Medicine* **1**, 142–146.

Peterson, M.E., Kintzer, P.P. and Hurvitz A.I. (1988) Methimazole treatment of 262 cats with hyperthyroidism. *Journal of Veterinary Internal Medicine* **2**, 150–157.

Peterson, M.E., Kintzer, P.P., Hurley, J.R. and Becker, D.V. (1989) Radioactive iodine treatment of a functional thyroid carcinoma producing hyperthyroidism in a dog. *Journal of Veterinary Internal Medicine* **3**, 20–25.

Peterson, M.E., Graves, T.K. and Gamble, D.A. (1990) Triiodothyronine (T3) suppression test: an aid in the diagnosis of mild hyperthyroidism in cats. *Journal of Veterinary Internal Medicine* **4**, 233–238.

Peterson, M.E., James, K.W., Wallace, M., Timothy, S.D. and Joseph, R.J. (1991) Idiopathic hypoparathyroidism in five cats. *Journal of Veterinary Internal Medicine* **5**, 47–51.

Peterson, M.E., Broussard, J.D. and Gamble, D.A. (1994) Use of the thyrotropin releasing hormone stimulation test to diagnose mild hyperthyroidism in cats. *Journal of Veterinary Internal Medicine* **8**, 279–286.

Ramsey, I.K., Evans, H. and Herrtage, M.E. (1998) Thyroid stimulating hormone and total thyroxine concentrations in euthyroid, sick euthyroid and hypothyroid dogs. *Journal of Small Animal Practice* **38**, 540–545.

Rand, J.S., Levine, J., Best, S.J. and Parker, W. (1993) Spontaneous adult-onset hypothyroidism in a cat. *Journal of Veterinary Internal Medicine* **7**, 272–276.

Reusch, C.E. and Feldman, E.C. (1991) Canine hyperadrenocorticism due to adrenocortical neoplasia: pretreatment evaluation in 41 dogs. *Journal of Veterinary Internal Medicine* **5**, 3–10.

Reusch, C.E., Liehs, M.R., Hoyer, M and Vochezer, R. (1993) Fructosamine: a new parameter for diagnosis and metabolic control in diabetic dogs and cats. *Journal of Veterinary Internal Medicine* **7**, 177–182.

Rijnberk, A., van Herpen, H., Mol, J.A. and Rutteman, G.R. (1993) Disturbed release of growth hormone in mature dogs: a comparison with congenital growth hormone deficiency. *Veterinary Record* **133**, 542–545.

Rijnberk, A., Van Wees, A. and Mol, J.A. (1988) Assessment of two tests for the diagnosis of canine hyperadrenocorticism. *Veterinary Record* **122**, 178–180.

Saunders, H.M. and Jezyk, P.K. (1991) The radiographic appearance of canine congenital hypothyroidism: skeletal changes with delayed treatement. *Veterinary Radiology* **32**, 171–177

Schaer, M., Riley, W.J., Buergelt, C.D., Bowen, D.J., Senior D.F., Burrows, C.F. and Campbell, G.A. (1986) Autoimmunity and Addison's disease in the dog. *Journal of the American Animal Hospital Association* **22**, 789–794.

Schmeitzel, L.P. and Lothrop, C.D. (1990) Hormonal abnormalities in Pomeranians with normal coat and in Pomeranians with growth hormone-responsive dermatosis. *Journal of the American Veterinary Medical Association* **197**, 1333–1341.

Schrauwen, E. (1991) Clinical peripheral polyneuropathy associated with canine insulinoma in the dog. *Veterinary Record* **128**, 211–212.

Selman, P.J., Mol, J.A., Rutteman, G.R., Van Garderen, E. and Rijnberk, A. (1994) Progestin-induced growth hormone excess in the dog originates in the mammary gland. *Endocrinology* **134**, 287–292.

Shaker, E., Hurvitz, A.J. and Peterson, M.E. (1988) Hypoadrenocorticism in a family of standard poodles. *Journal of the American Veterinary Medical Association* **192**, 1091–1092.

Simpson, K.W., Stepien, R.L., Elwood, C.M., Boswood, A. and Vailliant, C.R. (1995) Evaluation of the long-standing somatostatin analogue octreotide in the management of insulinoma in three dogs. *Journal of Small Animal Practice* **36**, 161–165.

Thoday, K.L. and Mooney, C.T. (1992) Historical, clinical and laboratory features of 126 hyperthyroid cats. *Veterinary Record* **131**, 257–264.

Torrance, A.G. and Nachreiner, R (1989) Intact parathyroid hormone assay and total calcium concentration in the diagnosis of disorders of calcium metabolism in dogs. *Journal of Veterinary Internal Medicine* **3**, 86–89.

Turrel, J.M., Feldman, E.C., Nelson, R.W. and Cain, G.R. (1988) Thyroid carcinoma causing hyperthyroidism in cats: 14 cases (1981–1986). *Journal of the American Veterinary Medical Association* **193**, 359–364.

van Herpen, H., Rinjberk, A. and Mol, J.A. (1994) Production of antibodies to biosynthetic human growth hormone in the dog. *Veterinary Record* **134**, 171.

Voorhout, G., Stolp, R., Lubberink, A.A.M.E. and Van Waes, P.F.G.M. (1988). Computed tomography in the diagnosis of canine hyperadrenocorticism not suppressible by dexamethasone. *Journal of the American Veterinary Medical Association* **192**, 641–646.

Watson, P.J. and Herrtage, M.E. (1998) Hyperadrenocorticism in six cats. *Journal of Small Animal Practice* **39**, 175–184.

Watson, T.D.G. and Barrie, J. (1993) Lipoprotein metabolism and hyperlipidaemia in the dog and cat: a review. *Journal of Small Animal Practice* **34**, 479–487.

Willard, M.D., Schall, W.D., McCaw, D.E. and Nachreiner, R.F. (1982) Canine hypoadrenocorticism: report of 37 cases and review of 39 previously reported cases. *Journal of the American Veterinary Medical Association* **180**, 59–62.

Wisner, E.R., Nyland, T.G., Feldman, E.C., Nelson, R.W. and Griffey, S.M. (1993) Ultrasonographic evaluation of the parathyroid glands in hypercalcemic dogs. *Veterinary Radiology and Ultrasound* **34**, 108–111.

40

Diseases of the Reproductive System

G. C. W. England

DISEASES OF THE FEMALE REPRODUCTIVE SYSTEM	574	DISEASES OF THE MALE REPRODUCTIVE SYSTEM	594
Introduction	574	Introduction	594
Clinical history	574	Clinical history	594
Physical examination	574	Physical examination	594
Investigative techniques	575	Investigative techniques	595
The bitch	577	The dog	595
The queen	589	The tom	602

Diseases of the Female Reproductive System

INTRODUCTION

The bitch and queen differ from each other in both their reproductive physiology and anatomy. Whilst the bitch is a monoestrous, non-seasonal, polytocous animal which ovulates spontaneously, the queen is a seasonally polyoestrous, polytocous animal in which ovulation must be induced. The arrangement of the internal genitalia is similar although in the queen the ovarian bursa only partly covers the ovary, and the queen possesses tubular cervical glands, major vestibular glands and a retractor clitoris muscle.

CLINICAL HISTORY

The collection of data from an animal's owner should help to construct a list of differential diagnoses. Many cases of 'infertility' are caused by a lack of understanding of the normal reproductive physiology on behalf of the owner, and careful questioning may reveal this to be the cause of apparent reproductive failure.

The previous breeding history, including parity and litter size, together with information regarding the stud animal are probably the most important factors to consider, although additional information concerning the timing of the onset of puberty, present cyclicity, general medical history and the administration of pharmaceutical compounds may also be useful.

PHYSICAL EXAMINATION

Following a complete clinical examination to rule out systemic disease, specific examination of the reproductive tract may be undertaken. In the bitch the vulva becomes progressively enlarged throughout proestrus, and frequently becomes distinctly softened and less swollen following the surge in plasma luteinizing hormone (LH). The vaginal fluid changes in colour from serosanguineous to serous during oestrus, however there are many normal variations; in addition a mucoid vaginal discharge is commonly present in pregnant bitches and in non-pregnant bitches during early metoestrus (dioestrus). In the queen, vulval oedema is usually absent and there is no vaginal discharge during oestrus.

Digital examination of the vestibule and caudal vagina is a useful procedure; in the queen sedation and the use of an otoscope may be necessary. When examining bitches for the optimum mating time, material for examination of exfoliative vaginal cytology, and mucus arborization should be collected before digital examination.

The mammary glands should be examined for size, texture and presence of secretion. Detection of mammary enlargement is a useful indicator of the late luteal phase of the cycle in both pregnant and non-pregnant bitches (Concannon, 1986).

The uterus may be palpated in the caudal abdomen dorsal to the bladder in cases of uterine pathology or during oestrus; examination may be helped by initially identifying the cervix which is large during oestrus.

INVESTIGATIVE TECHNIQUES

Several techniques can be used for the investigation of reproductive disease in the bitch and queen. Indirect methods designed to differentiate the oestrogenic (follicular) phase from the progestational (luteal) phase of the cycle include exfoliative vaginal cytology (Christie et al., 1972; Linde and Karlsson, 1984), cervicovaginal mucus arborization examination (England and Allen, 1989a) and vaginoscopy (Lindsay, 1983). Similar changes in vaginal cytology are found in the queen but these techniques are not particularly useful since sample collection may induce ovulation and because little is known about the normal variation.

Vaginal cytology relies on the principle that cells of the vaginal mucosa change in shape, size and staining characteristics in relation to the endocrine environment. During anoestrus the vaginal epithelium is two or three cell layers in thickness and the surface cells are small and round with an obvious nucleus; these are termed parabasal cells. The vaginal smear during anoestrus is therefore dominated by parabasal cells whilst a small number of polymorphonuclear leucocytes may also be present. The vaginal mucosa proliferates under the influence of the hormone oestrogen; the number of cell layers increases and the surface cells become progressively larger. These cells are termed small intermediate epithelial cells and are seen predominantly during proestrus. Larger epithelial cells become irregular in outline and may accumulate keratin; these cells are termed large intermediate epithelial cells and are found within the smear during oestrus. Very large cells may lose their nuclei and are termed anuclear cells. These cells are found in large numbers during the fertile period. Specific stains may be used to demonstrate the presence of keratin. Erythrocytes are also present during proestrus and oestrus, whereas polymorphonuclear leucocytes are generally absent. The vaginal mucosa returns to its original thickness during metoestrus (dioestrus) when plasma progesterone concentrations increase. The vaginal smear at this time is characterized by the return of small intermediate epithelial cells and parabasal cells, some of which are vacuolated (termed metoestrous cells). There is a large influx of polymorphonuclear leucocytes at the beginning of metoestrus; the return of these cells is a good indicator of the end of the fertile period.

Standard classification of the cell types is now in general use (Christie et al., 1972; Christiansen, 1984) and examination of vaginal cytology is commonly used to monitor the bitch's oestrous cycle and to suggest the optimal time for mating or insemination (Olson, 1989; Wright, 1990). The use of the anuclear cell index appears to be particularly valuable (England, 1992a). The appearance of the vaginal smear during the oestrous cycle is shown in Figs. 40.1 and 40.2.

Vaginal endoscopy, laparoscopy and laparotomy (Lindsay, 1983; Hadley, 1975; Wildt et al., 1979) are also useful for examination of pathological as well as cyclical changes within the reproductive tract. These techniques facilitate the collection of biopsy material for histopathological examination. The measurement of circulating hormone concentrations may be of value for confirming the presence of gonadal tissue, the detection of hormone secreting neoplasms and cystic structures, the prediction and confirmation of ovulation and for monitoring variations from the normal.

The internal reproductive organs may also be examined radiographically (Ackerman, 1981; Feeney and Johnston, 1986) or using real-time B-mode ultrasonography (Poffenbarger and Feeney, 1986; England and Allen, 1989b; England et al., 1990; Wallace et al., 1992; Yeager et al., 1992). The use of these imaging modalities has recently been reviewed (Rivers and Johnston, 1991); their main advantages being that they may reveal the shape, size and internal architecture of organs.

Recently a method of transcervical uterine cannulation using an endoscope has been developed for the collection of uterine samples for microbiology and cytology (Watts and Wright, 1995; Watts et al., 1996).

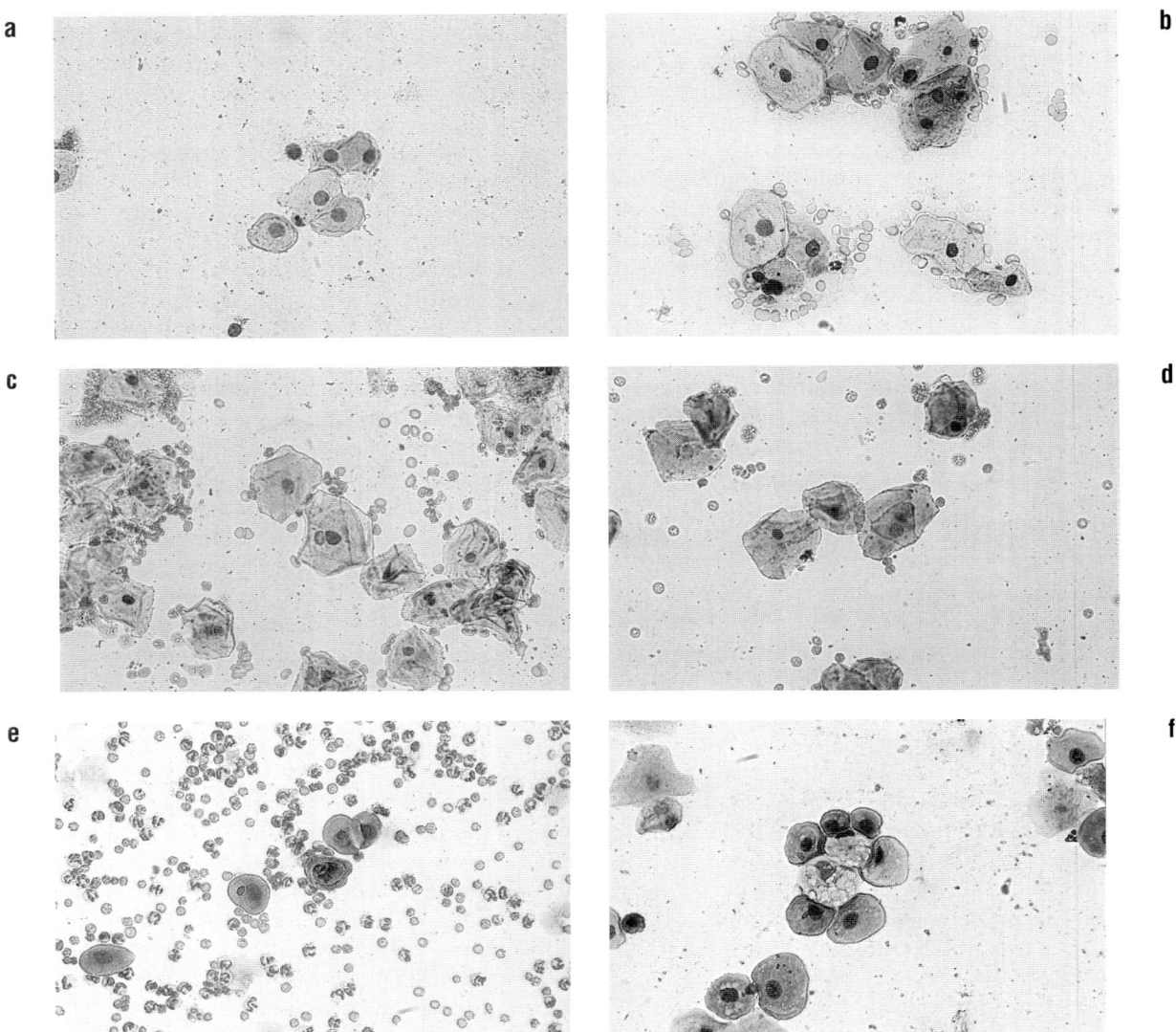

Figure 40.1 Photomicrographs of vaginal smears collected from bitches during various stages of the oestrous cycle. (a) Anoestrus; the smear comprises parabasal and small intermediate epithelial cells. Cells which have lost their cytoplasm can also be seen. Polymorphonuclear leucocytes are often present during anoestrus although they are not shown here. (b) Proestrus; the smear comprises small intermediate epithelial cells, large intermediate epithelial cells, and erythrocytes. A few polymorphonuclear leucocytes are also present. Bacteria can also be seen adherent to epithelial cells. (c) Early oestrus; the smear comprises large intermediate epithelial cells and erythrocytes. Polymorphonuclear leucocytes are no longer present. (d) Oestrus; the smear comprises anuclear epithelial cells, large intermediate epithelial cells and erythrocytes. The amount of background debris (including bacteria) is often reduced. (e) Metoestrus; the smear comprises large numbers of polymorphonuclear leucocytes, small intermediate epithelial cells and parabasal cells. Erythrocytes are also present in variable numbers. (f) Late metoestrus; the smear comprises parabasal cells and vacuolated small intermediate epithelial cells (higher magnification than figures a to e). The number of polymorphonuclear leucocytes is generally reduced. See colour plate.

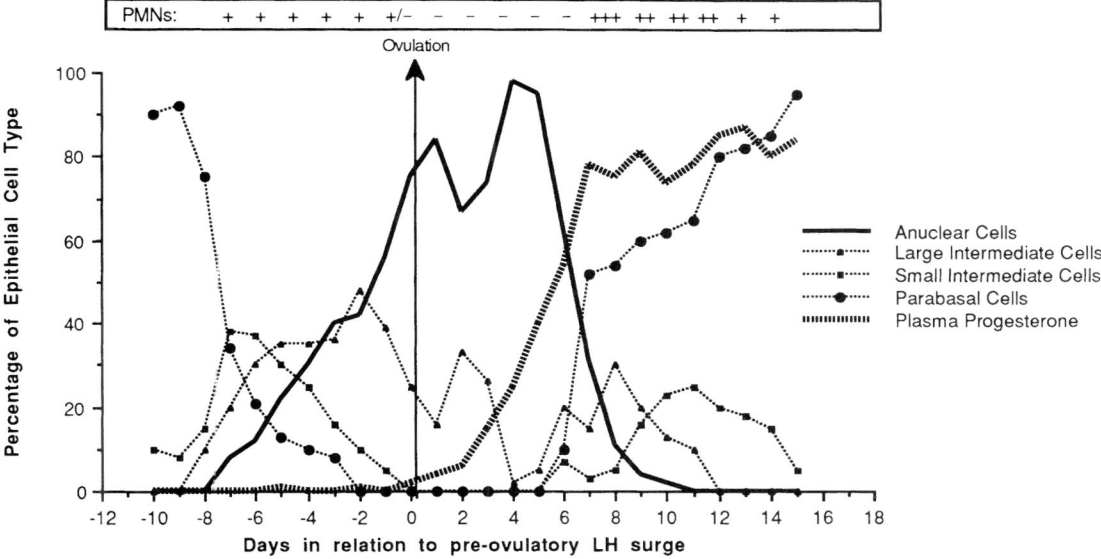

Figure 40.2 Schematic representation of the changes of exfoliative vaginal epithelial cells and peripheral plasma progesterone concentration during proestrus, oestrus and early metoestrus in the bitch. The number of polymorphonuclear leucocytes (PMNs) are represented as being absent (−), present in low number (+) or present in large numbers (+++).

THE BITCH

Reproductive endocrinology

The bitch is a monoestrous, non-seasonal, polytocous animal which ovulates spontaneously at the end of a variable follicular phase lasting from 4 to 28 days. The development of the ovarian follicle is initiated by the production of gonadotrophin releasing hormone (GnRH) which induces the release of follicle stimulating hormone (FSH) and luteinizing hormone (LH). Oestradiol concentrations reach a peak in late proestrus approximately 2 days before the preovulatory surge of LH and decline following the LH surge throughout most of oestrus (Concannon et al., 1975; Olson et al., 1982).

During proestrus progesterone concentrations are low (<1.5 ng ml^{-1}) but gradually increase at the time of the preovulatory LH surge (Concannon et al., 1975), and continue to increase throughout oestrus to reach peak values of 15–90 ng ml^{-1} by 15–30 days after the LH peak (Concannon, 1983). During proestrus and oestrus, LH concentrations are reduced compared with late anoestrus (Olson et al., 1982). The preovulatory surge in plasma LH occurs after the decline in plasma oestrogen and appears to be facilitated by the simultaneous increase in progesterone (Concannon et al., 1979) (Fig. 40.3).

There is little difference in progesterone concentrations between pregnant and non-pregnant bitches (Austad et al., 1976), although a broadening of the progesterone plateau has been noted during pregnancy, and the luteal phase is slightly longer in non-pregnant bitches (Concannon et al., 1977b) (Fig. 40.4). Oestrogen concentrations do not differ between pregnant and non-pregnant bitches; they consistently increase during the luteal phase of the cycle (Concannon et al., 1989).

During the period of declining plasma progesterone, plasma prolactin concentrations increase (Knight et al., 1977). Prolactin concentrations have been shown to be four times greater in pregnant bitches compared with non-pregnant bitches 55–60 days after the LH surge (McCann et al., 1988).

Abnormal endocrinological events

Delayed puberty

The onset of puberty is normally at between 6 and 23 months of age (Andersen and Wooten, 1959; Rogers et al., 1970). Smaller breeds generally

578 DISEASES OF THE REPRODUCTIVE SYSTEM

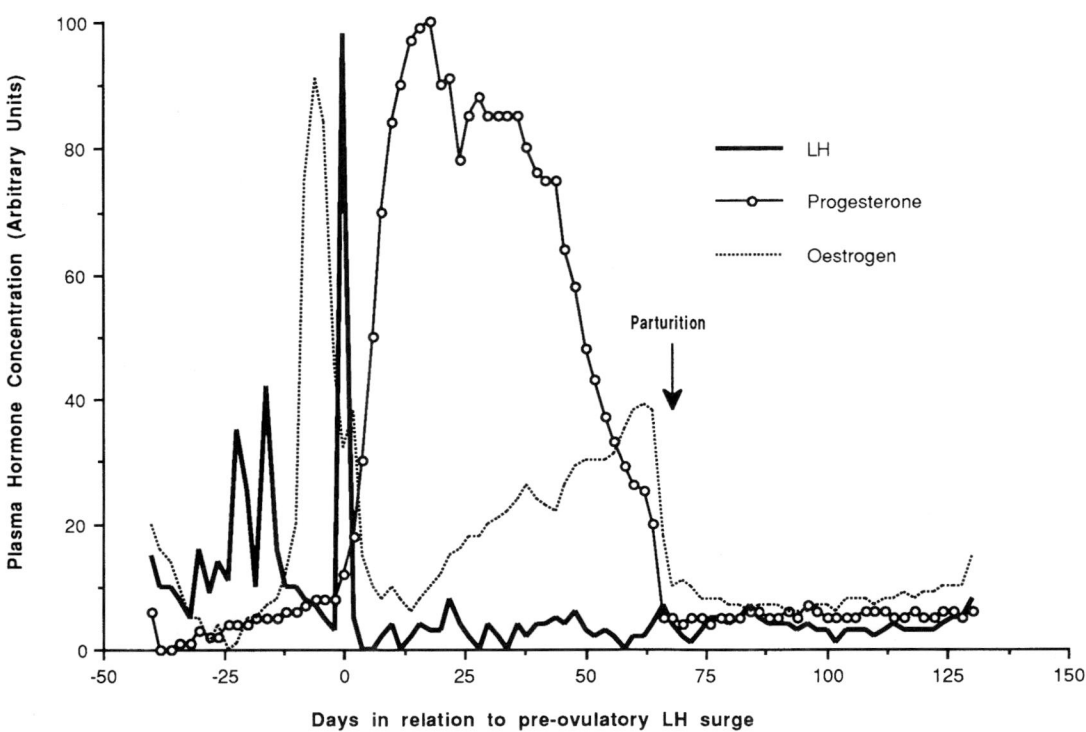

Figure 40.3 Schematic representation of the changes in peripheral plasma oestrogen, LH and progesterone concentration during the pregnant oestrous cycle of the bitch.

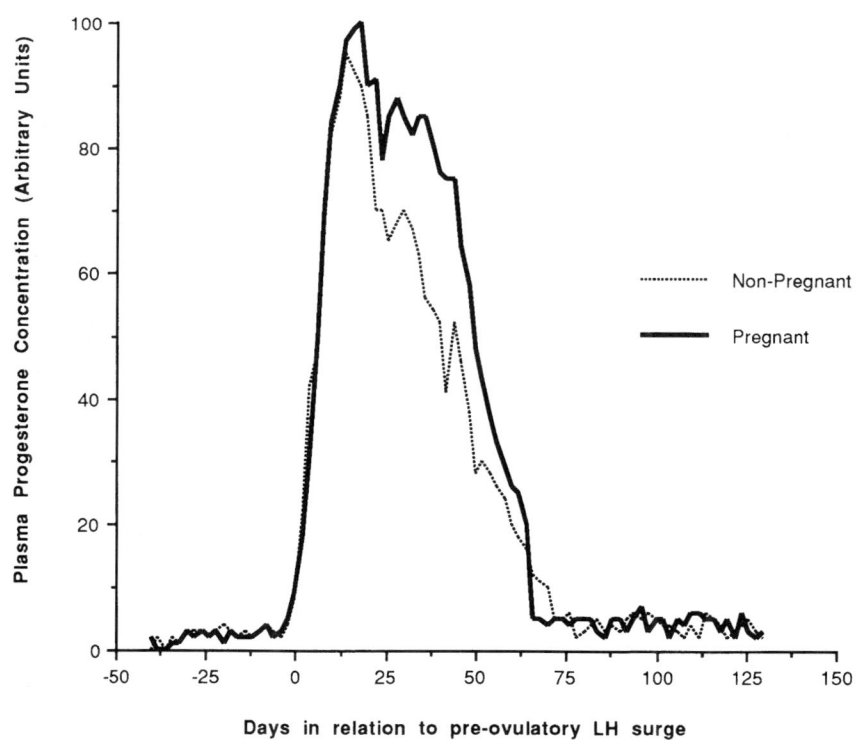

Figure 40.4 Schematic representation of peripheral plasma progesterone concentrations during metoestrus (dioestrus) and pregnancy of the bitch.

reach puberty at an earlier age than large or giant breeds. Bitches that do not demonstrate oestrus behaviour at the anticipated age are considered to have delayed puberty. However, investigation of such cases should not commence until the bitch has reached 24 months of age, and has been carefully observed for signs of oestrus and if possible has been housed with another bitch in oestrus (Johnston, 1991). The investigation of delayed puberty involves collection of information on housing and diet since poor environmental conditions and nutrition may be associated with failure to cycle (Christiansen, 1984), and a thorough clinical examination to rule out chronic debilitating disease. It has been suggested that bitches cycle within 1 to 6 months of attaining adult height and weight (Feldman and Nelson, 1987a). Plasma progesterone concentration should be measured to ensure that the bitch has not recently ovulated at an unobserved oestrus.

There has been increasing interest in the relationship between thyroid hormone insufficiency and abnormalities of the oestrous cycle (Manning, 1979; Johnston, 1989a). The potential mechanism of this abnormality has not been fully established, however prolactin is released after the injection of thyrotrophin releasing hormone (TRH) (Reimers et al., 1978), therefore factors which affect endogenous TRH release probably affect prolactin and thyroid function (Concannon, 1986). Hypothyroidism has been associated with prolonged anoestrus and infertility. Low concentrations of plasma thyroid hormones and failure to respond to a stimulation test may be used to confirm the condition, although clinically these animals usually have classical clinical signs associated with hypothyroidism (see Chapter 39). After correct replacement therapy most bitches will cycle within 6 months. Hypothyroidism in greyhounds has been shown not to be related to poor reproductive function (Beale et al., 1992).

Prolonged anoestrus

There are several causes of failure of normal reproductive cyclicity. However, a common problem is the failure of observation of the signs of oestrus. This may occur in fastidious bitches which quickly remove any vaginal discharge, or when the discharge is scant. In bitches examined for abnormal cyclicity, plasma progesterone concentrations should be established. Elevated concentrations (greater than 2 ng ml^{-1}) will indicate missed ovarian activity within the previous 2 months.

The average interoestrus interval is 31 weeks (Rowlands, 1950) and although there is some variation around this mean value this has no apparent effect on fertility. Certain breeds, for example the basenji, cycle only once per year. The reason for these variations is unclear. Prolonged anoestrus therefore represents an interoestrus interval greater than anticipated for that particular animal. Investigation of thyroid function as described above is indicated in these cases.

Progesterone-producing ovarian cysts have been described in the bitch, producing prolonged interoestrus intervals and cystic endometrial hyperplasia (Burke, 1986). The cysts can be identified using ultrasonography or radiology and the diagnosis confirmed by serial measurement of plasma progesterone concentration.

Drug-induced anoestrus should also be considered when the interoestral interval is prolonged. Pharmaceutical preparations that have the ability to prevent oestrus include glucocorticoids, anabolic steroids as well as androgens and progestogens.

Oestrus induction may be attempted if there is no underlying disease and if breeding is essential. This has been attempted using oral oestrogens alone (5 mg diethylstilboestrol daily) given orally until 2 days after the signs of oestrus (Bouchard et al., 1993) or combined with LH and FSH (Moses and Shille, 1988). The latter method is not always successful (Shille et al., 1989). Pharmacological doses of gonadotrophins may stimulate oestrus and ovulation. Arnold et al. (1989) used 20 IU kg^{-1} equine chorionic gonadotrophin (eCG) daily intramuscularly for 5 days and a single intramuscular injection of 500 IU human chorionic gonadotrophin (hCG) on the fifth day. This gave good results although plasma oestrogen concentrations were high and might therefore interfere with gamete transport (England and Allen, 1991a). Oestrus induction has also been attempted using pulsatile intravenous administration of GnRH (Vanderlip et al., 1987), GnRH superagonists (Concannon, 1989) and prolactin antagonists such as cabergoline, bromocriptine and metergoline (Auskova et al., 1974; Handaja Kusuma and Tainurier, 1993; Jeukenne and Verstegen, 1997).

Silent oestrus

Some bitches have normal cyclical activity, including follicular growth and ovulation, without any external signs of proestrus or oestrus. Certain breeds, for example the greyhound, may have only slight serosangineous discharge and minimal vulval swelling during oestrus.

Ovulation may be confirmed by examination of plasma progesterone concentration. Alternatively, the weekly collection of cells from the bitch's vagina will allow anticipation of oestrus.

Split oestrus

This occurs most frequently at the first oestrus, but can occur at any stage in the reproductive life of the bitch. An initial phase of follicular growth and oestrogen secretion occurs, resulting in the clinical signs of proestrus. However, ovulation does not follow; follicles regress and the signs of proestrus disappear. Subsequently a second follicular phase appears (2–12 weeks later) and the bitch develops proestrus, oestrus and then ovulates normally. This syndrome is confusing since it may be thought that the bitch has failed to ovulate or that fertilization with subsequent fetal resorption/abortion has occurred.

The recognition of split oestrus syndrome is important to ensure that future mating is achieved at the correct time.

Prolonged proestrus or oestrus

The normal interval to ovulation from the onset of vulval bleeding is between 6 and 20 days (England *et al.*, 1989a). For the 'average' bitch, the surge in plasma LH occurs on day 10 and ovulation follows two days later. There are, however, many normal bitches that do not ovulate at this time, and many bitches with prolonged proestrus are at the extremes of normality; they simply ovulate later in the cycle than anticipated. These animals do not require treatment but careful assessment of the optimum mating time. It is unlikely that the administration of hCG will produce normal ovulation earlier in the cycle, however few data are available on the use of this agent.

Oestrogen-secreting follicular cysts may produce persistent oestrus in the bitch. However, they are very rare and treatment which involves ovariectomy should not be undertaken lightly since the bitch may have a normal but prolonged period of proestrus, or a persistent vaginitis (which causes local pheromone production causing males to be attracted). The persistent elevation of plasma oestrogen may lead to bone marrow suppression with anaemia and thrombocytopenia.

Ovulation failure

Until the advent of routine monitoring of plasma progesterone concentration, a diagnosis of ovulation failure was made on the basis of an interoestrus interval shortened by approximately two months (Johnston, 1988). The frequency of ovulation failure is approximately 1% of oestrous cycles (Arbeiter, 1993) and the diagnosis is commonly made by serial monitoring of plasma progesterone concentration. Attempts to induce ovulation during oestrus using 500 IU kg^{-1} hCG between one day before to one day after the first mating may be successful (Johnston, 1991).

Pseudopregnancy

The incidence of clinical false pregnancy in the bitch is not known. Clinical signs develop a few weeks after the end of oestrus and may persist for several months. Behavioural changes may include anorexia, nest making and nursing of inanimate objects. Lactation may result in mastitis.

The mechanisms involved in the development of clinical false pregnancy are not known. It was thought previously to have been due either to an overproduction of progesterone or abnormal persistence of the corpora lutea (Marshall and Halnan, 1917; Mallo, 1971). However, this was subsequently shown not to be the case (Smith and McDonald, 1971; Hadley, 1975). Serum prolactin concentrations are elevated during late pregnancy and are associated with behavioural changes and lactation, and a similar rise in prolactin has been reported in non-pregnant bitches (Reimers *et al.*, 1978; DeCoster *et al.*, 1983). Prolactin release is potentiated by declining plasma progesterone concentrations during the late luteal phase (Concannon *et al.*, 1978). False pregnancy can be initiated by removal of corporal lutea (ovariohysterectomy) during the luteal phase. Such cases of iatrogenic pseudopregnancy may be persistent, therefore ovariohysterectomy should not be planned until at least 3 months after the end of oestrus. Conservative therapy may be sufficient in many cases (Whitney, 1967) although this may be supplemented by the administration of diuretic and sedative agents. If further treatment is necessary, pregnancy and pyometra must be eliminated as differential diagnoses before administration of exogenous reproductive steroids. Progestogens, androgens, oestrogens and combinations of these may be used for treatment (Allen and England, 1990). Depot or daily oral progestogen therapy is commonly advocated in the UK, although oral androgen/oestrogen products are also available. An orally active androgen (mibolerone) is available in other countries but not the UK. The use of oestrogens alone has not been evaluated. Long treatment periods may be required for complete remission, and it is frequently necessary to use reducing dose regimes, to prevent recurrence. The use of dopamine agonists (bromocriptine, carbergolamine), which produce a rapid and prolonged inhibition of prolactin secretion, may be used in persistent cases. Bromocriptine is available in the UK and has been shown to be effective for the control of pseudopregnancy at doses of 5 µg kg^{-1} day^{-1} (Spicer, 1979; Allen, 1986), although the drug causes vomiting and has therefore not found wide acceptance (Jochle et al., 1989). Carbergoline and metergoline have a higher level of activity, longer duration of action and better tolerance than bromocriptine (Jochle et al., 1987; Handaja Kusuma and Tainturier, 1993). Hysterectomy after the clinical signs have disappeared will prevent subsequent recurrence. It is unwise to perform surgery while signs persist.

Acromegaly

The chronic oversecretion of growth hormone may be induced by endogenous progesterone or exogenous progestogens (Concannon et al., 1980a; Eigenmann and Venker-van Haagen, 1981). This may cause an overgrowth of connective tissue in the oral, pharyngeal and laryngeal regions, producing inspiratory stridor and widened interdental spaces. Bitches may also be polydipsic/polyuric, have distended abdomens and excessive skin folding in the facial area. The polydipsia is associated with a secondary diabetes mellitus (see below).

Progesterone-induced acromegaly is not uncommon in the bitch during the luteal phase, and signs regress as progesterone concentrations decline. Treatment of these cases is by ovariohysterectomy although this may induce pseudopregnancy.

Diabetes mellitus

During the luteal phase of the cycle increased secretion of growth hormone is responsible for peripheral insulin antagonism resulting in a transient reversible Type II diabetes (although the clinical signs may be severe). Diabetes may also occur during pregnancy; the sensitivity to insulin is reduced as early as 35 days after ovulation (McCann and Concannon, 1983). Ovariohysterectomy of known diabetic bitches reduces the period of instability associated with the luteal phase.

Reproductive organs

The normal ovaries are positioned in the dorsal abdominal cavity immediately caudal to the kidneys in close association with the abdominal wall. Each ovary is surrounded by a fatty bursa which prevents examination of the ovarian surface. During proestrus the ovary increases in size due to the development of multiple follicles. The follicles, which may reach 1 cm in diameter, undergo extensive luteinization during the preovulatory surge of LH; progesterone is therefore produced before ovulation. A central fluid cavity persisits in young mature corpora lutea (Concannon et al., 1977a; England and Allen, 1989b).

The narrow uterine tubes are confluent with the uterine horns. These are relatively long and join caudally to form the uterine body. The vagina is long and is narrowed cranially by a dorsomedian postcervical fold, which may be confused with the cervix.

■ Diseases of the ovary

Ovarian agenesis

Failure of ovarian development is an uncommon and frequently unilateral defect that may be associated with agenesis of the ipsilateral uterine tube and horn. It does not cause infertility unless the changes are bilateral in which case there is a continued state of anoestrus, which fails to respond to exogenous gonadotrophin administration.

Ovarian cysts

Cyst-like structures are frequently identified on ovaries at routine surgery. These are often parabursal in origin, and have no significance on cyclicity or fertility.

Follicular and luteal cysts have also been identified (Dow, 1960). There is little clear information on the definitive diagnosis and treatment of these cysts although surgical removal has been reported in one bitch with polycystic ovaries (Vaden, 1978). Oestrogen-secreting follicular cysts may produce persistent oestrus (Burke, 1986). However, cases of persistent oestrus may spontaneously regress, presumably as a result of ovulation since a normal elevation of plasma progesterone follows. Oestrus lasting longer than 4 weeks is rare and may be associated with anaemia and thrombocytopenia. Ovulation may be induced using exogenous hormones (hCG, 500 IU kg^{-1}, GnRH, 50 µg total dose), although ovariohysterectomy may be required in unresponsive cases. It is not known if these cases represent ovarian follicular cysts. Solitary cysts lined by luteal tissue have also been identified (Dow, 1960), however the significance of these is unclear. Burke (1986) suggested that progesterone-producing cysts produced prolonged anoestrus (sic) and cystic endometrial hyperplasia.

Ovarian tumours

These are not common in the bitch, accounting for approximately 1.0% of all neoplasms (Cotchin, 1961; Hayes and Harvey, 1979); the mean age of occurrence is 8 years (Withrow and Susaneck, 1986). The tumours may be germ cell, epithelial or sex-cord stromal in origin. Ovarian tumours do not commonly metastasize and are frequently endocrinologically inactive. The clinical signs are usually related to a mass effect or ascites. Tumours which produce hormones may produce signs of persistent oestrus and bone marrow suppression (oestrogen secreting) or cystic endometrial hypoplasia and pyometra (progesterone secreting).

Diagnosis may be made on the basis of clinical signs, palpation, radiography and ultrasonography. Ovariohysterectomy is the treatment of choice; care should be taken not to rupture neoplasms since metastatic spread is often by transcoelomic seeding.

Intersexuality

Intersexuality is usually recognized because of abnormal phenotypic sex appearance. Intersex animals may be classified into those with abnormalities of chromosomal, gonadal or phenotypic sex. The recognition of abnormalities of chromosomal sex requires the construction of a karyotype. Generally these animals are phenotypic female or males with underdeveloped genitalia. In the dog, abnormalities in chromosomal number (XXY, XXX, XO), chimeras and mosaics have been reported (Meyers-Wallen and Patterson, 1986, 1989). Animals with abnormalities of gonadal sex are those in which chromosomal and gonadal sex do not agree. This has been shown to be an autosomal recessive trait in the American cocker spaniel, and to be familial in other breeds (Meyers-Wallen and Patterson, 1988). These animals may be categorized as (a) true hermaphrodites with one ovotestis, oviducts and external female genitalia, (b) true hermaphrodites with ovotestis and/or epididymides and masculinized external genitalia and (c) XX males. Females with abnormalities of phenotypic sex (female pseudohermaphrodites) have ovaries and XX chromosomes. These are masculinized due to exposure to exogenous or endogenous androgens *in utero*.

Intersexual animals may be sterile depending on the underlying abnormality. Common reasons for presentation of these females are associated with clitoral hypertrophy (see later). The removal of the reproductive tract including gonads is usually necessary, following which the clitoris may reduce in size, although subsequent clitoridectomy may be necessary.

Diseases of the uterus

Aplasia of the tubular genital tract

Aplasia of one segment of the uterine horn and/or uterine tube may not influence fertility if the contralateral side is normal. Bilateral agenesis is associated with infertility although the bitch may cycle, ovulate and mate normally. The condition is most frequently noted during routine ovariohysterectomy. An unusual case of fibrosis of the uterine body has been described associated with dystocia (Dover, 1965).

Radiographic diagnosis may be made by injection of radio-opaque contrast medium into the cranial vagina during oestrus (Lagerstedt, 1993), however, poor filling of the uterine horns may normally occur. Laparotomy and laparoscopy are more valuable diagnostic tools.

Cystic endometrial hyperplasia – pyometra

During metoestrus (dioestrus) plasma progesterone concentrations are high, promoting endometrial growth and glandular secretion; changes which regress at the end of the luteal phase. However, with continuing cycles, the endometrium becomes thickened due to an increase in the size and number of endometrial glands, this is referred to as cystic endometrial hyperplasia (Fig. 40.5). The endometrial gland secretion may lead to the accumulation of fluid within the uterine lumen; termed mucometra or hydrometra (Nelson and Feldman, 1986a). Bacterial contamination may occur during oestrus, when the cervix is relaxed, and be involved in the development of pyometra during the following luteal phase. The aetiology is poorly understood, but this explanation is favoured since the bacteria commonly isolated in cases of pyometra are commensal species normally isolated from the anus or urinary tract (von Baier *et al.*, 1958; Sandholm *et al.*, 1975). However, experimental infection of the uterus has failed to produce pyometra. The clinical disease may be induced by the therapeutic administration of

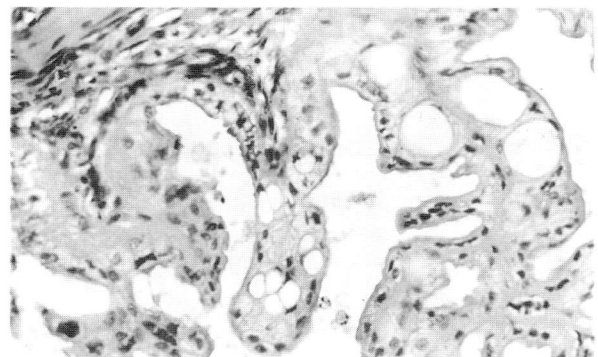

Figure 40.5 Histological appearance of uterine tissue in a bitch with cystic endometrial hyperplasia. There is hyperplasia of the endometrium and cystic distension of the glandular regions. The section was stained with haematoxylin and eosin; magnification, × 100.

progestogens (Pettit, 1965) and oestrogens (for example for the treatment of unwanted matings) which enhance the stimulatory effects of progesterone on the uterus (Nelson and Feldman, 1986b), and may result in prolonged opening of the cervix.

Pyometra commonly affects middle-aged and elderly bitches, although with the increased therapeutic use of progestogens and oestrogens, earlier presentation is not uncommon. There is no relation to parity or previous history of reproductive disease.

The clinical signs may include vaginal discharge, lethargy, inappetance, polydipsia and polyuria, vomiting, nocturia, diarrhoea and abdominal enlargement. In approximately one third of cases there is no vaginal discharge and fluid is retained within the uterus (Renton and Aughey, 1971). These cases of closed-cervix pyometra generally have an absolute neutrophilia, which is not necessarily present in cases of open-cervix pyometra. Diagnosis can be made on the basis of clinical findings together with the identification of an enlarged fluid-filled uterus using radiography or ultrasound examination.

The treatment of choice is ovariohysterectomy combined with appropriate fluid therapy and administration of antimicrobial preparations. Some bitches have been successfully treated following the insertion of uterine drains (Gourley, 1975). Medical treatment with prostaglandin $F_{2\alpha}$ has also been successful by causing cervical relaxation, myometrial contraction, lysis of corpora lutea and a reduction in plasma progesterone concentration (Sokolowski, 1980). Naturally occurring prostaglandins must be used at relatively low doses (0.25 mg kg^{-1} daily or 0.125 mg kg^{-1} twice daily for 5 days) to reduce their side effects of salivation, vomiting, diarrhoea, dyspnoea, abdominal pain and tachycardia (Lein, 1983; Feldman and Nelson, 1986). Synthetic prostaglandins are more potent and should be used with care. Longer treatment periods are necessary in some cases, and death during therapy has been reported (Gilbert et al., 1989). Prostaglandins are not recommended for use in cases of closed-cervix pyometra because of the risk of uterine rupture (Renton et al., 1993). Broad-spectrum antimicrobial therapy should always be administered since 10% of bitches with pyometra are bacteraemic (Nelson et al., 1982). Gilbert and et al. (1989) cured 82% of bitches using prostaglandin and 22% subsequently whelped. The long-term complications were recurrent metritis, anoestrus, failure to conceive and abortion. Surgical drainage of the uterus has been attempted to retain reproductive ability (Gourley, 1975). The success rates have been variable and the technique is not recommended. Progesterone receptor antagonists such as RU486 should be useful for the treatment of bitches with pyometra. A new antagonist RU46534 has been shown to be clinically efficacious (Breitkopf et al., 1996); this product is commercially available in France.

Methorragie

The occurrence of a mucohaemorrhagic vaginal discharge during the luteal phase of the cycle in elderly bitches has been associated with histological lesions within the ovaries and endometrium. Usually the bitches are clinically well. The treatment of choice is ovariohysterectomy.

Uterine tumours

Uterine tumours are uncommon (Brodey and Roszel, 1967) although leiomyomata are seen most frequently in older bitches. These tumours are rarely associated with clinical signs and are frequently incidental findings at post mortem.

Intersexuality

Intersex animals may present with a range of abnormalities of the tubular genitalia including hypoplastic uterine horns alongside vasa deferentia. The aetiology of intersexuality is discussed above.

Diseases of the vagina and vestibule

Vaginal hypoplasia/aplasia

Segmental aplasia of the mullerian duct system may be partial and produce vaginal hypoplasia, or be complete and result in vaginal aplasia. The latter will result in infertility (Wadsworth et al., 1978; Hawe and Loeb, 1984), and cause the retention of uterine fluid with similar signs to pyometra.

Radiographic diagnosis may be made using a positive contrast vaginogram.

Hymenal or vestibular constrictions

Strictures of the lower reproductive tract are common in bitches. Circular strictures are usually found at the junction of the vestibule and the vagina, although vestibulovulvar strictures and cranially positioned transverse fibrous bands are sometimes present (Wykes and Soderberg, 1983).

Vestibulovaginal strictures may be associated with signs of vulval pruritus (Holt and Sayle, 1981) or chronic vaginitis (Soderberg, 1986a) although they are often only noted during attempted mating. Under general anaesthesia small constrictions and fibrous bands may be manually broken down, although surgical exploration via an episiotomy may be required for larger transverse bands. Surgery may be performed early in oestrus before mating.

Prepubertal vaginitis

A purulent vaginal discharge is sometimes seen in bitches from 2 months of age. Clinical signs include frequent licking, perivulval dermatitis and attractiveness to male dogs. Significant numbers of coagulase-positive staphylococci can be isolated, and the condition will respond temporarily to antimicrobial therapy. Clinical signs usually regress after the first oestrus (Burke, 1986) and treatment is not usually required; some control may be achieved by the daily administration of 0.5 mg diethylstilboestrol for 5 days.

Vaginitis

Many bacterial species are present in the vagina of clinically normal bitches (Allen and Dagnall, 1982; Baba et al., 1983). The aerobic commensals commonly isolated include *Escherichia coli*, staphylococci and streptococci (Olson and Mather, 1978; Allen and Dagnall, 1982), the majority of which probably originate from the skin and the digestive tract. Although the bacterial flora changes after mating these changes are not permanent (Allen and Dagnall, 1982).

The bacteria commonly isolated from bitches with vaginitis are also usually commensals (Hirsh and Wiger, 1977; van Duijkeren, 1992). Bitches with vaginal discharge do not necessarily have vaginitis; the differential diagnoses for vaginitis include: proestrus and oestrus, cystitis, pyometra, metritis, parturition, subinvolution of placental sites and juvenile vaginitis. Neutrophils are frequently present within the discharge of bitches with vaginitis, although they are also normally seen in the vaginal smear of any non-oestral bitch. Male dogs are frequently attracted to a bitch with a vaginal discharge regardless of its cause.

The aetiology of many cases of vaginitis often remains obscure. Specific causes include certain bacterial or viral infections (see below), chemical irritation (e.g. urine), mechanical irritation (foreign bodies), neoplasia or anatomical abnormalities of the vagina (Johnson, 1991). Diagnosis of the specific cause requires manual, endoscopic and contrast radiographic examination of the caudal genitourinary tract. Removal of the underlying cause rapidly results in a cure. However, in one study no causal factor was identified in 32% of cases (Johnson, 1991). The empirical treatment with systemic and topical antimicrobial agents may be of some value.

Specific infectious causes of vaginitis include *Brucella canis* and herpes virus. *Brucella* is not found in the UK and is the only specific bacterial cause of infertility. Occasionally pure growths of a single bacterial species may be considered significant, however pure growths may be isolated from normal dogs (Bjurstrom and Linde-Forsberg, 1992). It is, therefore, not rational to exclude animals from mating on the basis of vaginal culture of commensal bacteria such as beta-haemolytic streptococci.

Canine herpes virus may cause genital lesions; bitches may develop vesicular vaginal or vestibular lesions, with severe vaginitis being reported after experimental infection (Hill and Mare, 1974). Infection of the pregnant bitch may produce small litters, late abortion, stillbirths and the birth of underdeveloped pups (Poste and King, 1971). Neonatal infection may occur during passage of the pup through the birth canal (Hashimoto and Hirai, 1986).

Vaginal hyperplasia

Vaginal hyperplasia (commonly termed prolapse) reflects an accentuated response of the caudal

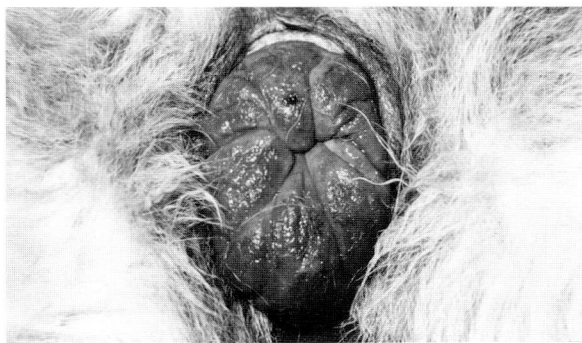

Figure 40.6 Protrusion of hyperplastic vaginal tissue through the vulva of a boxer bitch during oestrus. The changes in this case involve the entire circumference of the vagina.

vaginal floor to normal circulating oestrogen concentrations. Usually the vaginal mucosa cranial to the external urethral orifice is involved, becoming oedematous and thickened. This rapidly increases in size and a large smooth pink mass protrudes from the vulva. Occasionally the circumference of the vagina may be involved (Fig. 40.6). In most bitches the mass decreases in size at the end of oestrus, therefore conservative management with local cleansing and lubrication are sufficient. Ovariohysterectomy during the subsequent anoestrus will prevent recurrence. Artificial insemination may be necessary in bitches that are required for breeding, or submucosal resection of the tissue may be performed during early oestrus before mating. A minority of surgically treated cases will recur, however the use of surgery has been questioned since a familial tendency has been reported in certain breeds (Jones and Joshua, 1982).

Vaginal prolapse

Although rare, true prolapse of the vagina has been reported during oestrus (Schutte, 1967) when it may prevent mating. Chronic prolapse requiring hysteropexy has also been reported during pregnancy (Memon et al., 1993).

Vaginal cysts

Vaginal cysts are rare in bitches and it has been suggested that they are dilations of embryonic remnants of the vaginal floor. Cysts usually cause no clinical signs although tenesmus has been reported (Cauvin et al., 1995).

Vaginal tumours

The incidence of vaginal and vestibular tumours is low (Brodey and Roszel, 1967); the majority are benign leiomyomata, fibromas and polyps (Withrow and Susaneck, 1986). These often develop from the ventral vaginal floor cranial to the urethral orifice. Bitches may have few clinical signs until a mass is noted protruding from the vulva. Signs of vaginitis may occur, although blood spotting and dysuria are more often associated with malignant tumours especially those involving the caudal bladder and urethra. The surgical removal of benign neoplasms via an episiotomy, combined with ovariohysterectomy ensures a low rate of recurrence, although the role of circulating hormones on tumour growth has not been established. The prognosis for malignant neoplasms, commonly leiomyosarcomas, is good following surgery in the absence of metastases. Local metastasis is most common.

Diseases of the external genitalia

Congenital anomalies

Hypoplasia of the vulva has been described and may be associated with perivulval dermatitis (Christiansen, 1984). There is considerable breed variation in the normal vulval anatomy; the greyhound for example has small external genitalia. Congenital abnormalities including vulvar atresia and vulvar agenesis are rare, and commonly result in chronic vaginitis. The congenital absence of the dorsal vulvar commissure allows direct visualization of the vestibular floor and clitoris. An inverted 'U' episioplasty may be used to correct the defect and reverse the clitoritis and vaginitis (Burke and Smith, 1975).

Clitoral hypertrophy

True hermaphrodites, male pseudohermaphrodites and animals with abnormalities of chromosomal sex may have external female genitalia and develop clitoral hypertrophy from about 6 months of age onwards. The clitoris, which may contain an os, frequently protrudes from the vulva and may become inflamed (Fig. 40.7). Removal of the source of androgens (gonads) produces resolution of the signs. However, if the clitoris contains bone, enlargement may persist and surgical resection may be necessary.

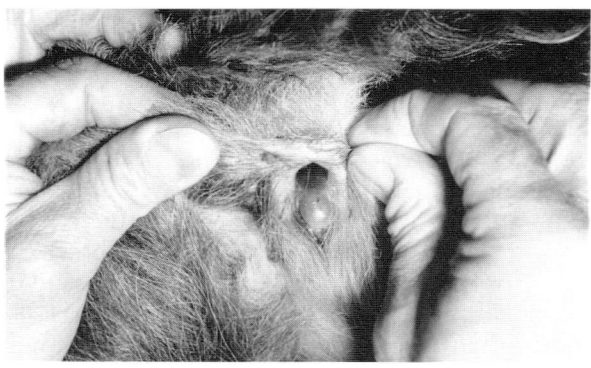

Figure 40.7 Hypertrophy, ossification and protrusion of the clitoris in a bitch secondary to intersexuality. Top is the dorsal vulval commissure.

Vulval hypoplasia

A small or infantile vulva is said to occur most commonly in bitches which have been neutered before puberty, although there is controversy regarding this relationship. A moist perivulval dermatitis may result, especially if the bitch is overweight and there are excessive perineal skin folds (Fig. 40.8). Medical management of these lesions with topical antimicrobial and corticosteroid preparations is often unsuccessful, although parenteral oestrogen therapy may be useful temporarily. Radical episioplasty to remove the diseased tissue is necessary in many of these cases.

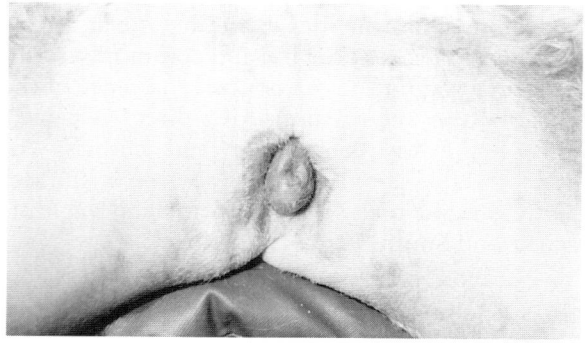

Figure 40.8 Perivulval skin inflammation subsequent to a recessed position of the vulva and excessive perineal skin folding. Top is the dorsal vulval commissure.

Transmissible venereal tumour

This is a coitally transmitted neoplasm that affects the external genitalia of either sex. It is not identified in the UK except in dogs which have been imported (Booth, 1994). Transmission of the tumour occurs at coitus when cells from the infected individual 'seeds' the genital mucosa of the recipient (Cohen, 1974). The lesions are found on the external and internal genitalia and are often friable and multilobulated, and may be solitary or multiple. There is frequent ulceration and serosanguineous discharge. Biopsy of the lesion is required for definitive diagnosis. Spontaneous regression of the tumour may occur especially after surgical debulking, although various chemotherapeutic regimes have been suggested, including the use of cyclophosphamide and vincristine (Calvert et al., 1982). Radiation therapy is also valuable (Thrall, 1982).

Diseases of pregnancy

Conception or implantation failure

The most common reason for failure of conception is inappropriate timing of mating. The fertile period of the bitch is between days 4 and 8 after the surge of plasma luteinizing hormone, since ovulation occurs between 24 and 44 hours after the LH peak (Smith and McDonald, 1971; Concannon et al., 1977b; Wildt et al., 1978) and ova are released as primary oocytes and do not mature until 2–3 days later (Andersen and Simpson, 1973; Phemister et al., 1973). Problems may occur because the behavioural signs of oestrus do not always correlate with the changes in peripheral plasma hormones (Mellin et al., 1976; Wildt et al., 1978) and frequently dog breeders insist on mating a set number of days from the onset of proestrus, even though the interval between this event and the LH surge is very variable (England et al., 1989a).

Other causes for failure of conception may be related to endocrinological and physical abnormalities previously discussed.

Abortion/resorption

The incidence of fetal death followed by resorption is not known (Freak, 1977), although Andersen and Simpson (1973) suggested that the frequency of resorption was 11% when the number of fetuses and corpora lutea were compared. Fetal abortion and resorption may have many causes including fetal defects, abnormal maternal environment, infectious agents and trauma (Feldman and Nelson, 1987a). *Brucella canis* can cause early embryonic death or abortion late in pregnancy followed by a vaginal discharge

(Carmichael, 1966; Carmichael and Kenney, 1968). Other specific infectious causes of abortion include canine distemper virus, canine herpes virus and *Toxoplasma gondii* infection (Cole *et al.*, 1954). In each case the bitch is usually systemically ill and has a vaginal discharge. Fetal death can be confirmed using real-time ultrasonography, when loss of fetal fluid and absence of heart beats are noted. Radiography may be useful for the detection of fetal or uterine gas, overlapping of the cranial bones and abnormal fetal posture. Treatment of the dam at the time of abortion may involve the administration of ecbolic agents such as oxytocin, combined with parenteral fluid therapy and antimicrobial preparations.

The cause of an abortion may be established by serological examination of the dam and bacterial isolation from the fetal membranes and stomach, however in many cases non-specific bacteria including *E. coli*, streptococci, proteus and pseudomonas are identified.

If has been suggested that the administration of progestogens during pregnancy may prevent recurrent resorption/abortion by suppressing myometrial contractions and increasing uterine protein secretion. However, no data are available to support the use of these compounds, which may increase the incidence of pyometra and result in the birth of masculinized female and cryptorchid male pups, and possibly impair or delay parturition resulting in fetal death.

Isolated spontaneous embryonic resorption may occur in the bitch during early pregnancy (up to 35 days) and is usually unsuspected since it produces few clinical signs, although resorption can be detected ultrasonographically (England, 1992b). Resorption of single conceptuses may be followed by continuation of the pregnancy and the birth of normal pups. Allen (1982) suggested that a high incidence of fetal death noted in one bitch could have been due to competition for uterine space.

Pregnancy hypoglycaemia

A reduction in blood glucose concentration associated with ketosis has been reported during pregnancy in the bitch (Jackson *et al.*, 1980; Hotston-Moore and Wotton, 1993); bitches are weak and may become comatose. Diagnosis is based on the measurement of plasma glucose concentration, and the rapid recovery following intravenous glucose administration. These rare cases are interesting since normally during the progestogenic phase of the oestrous cycle, bitches are likely to become hyperglycaemic (see section on diabetes mellitus above).

The postparturient period

Following parturition the uterus undergoes a process of involution that requires approximately 12 weeks to complete (Al-Bassam *et al.*, 1981a). A normal vaginal discharge which may be haemorrhagic, persists for up to 6 days, although a mucoid discharge may be present for up to 6 weeks postpartum.

Postparturient diseases

Placental retention

Despite many concerns, placental retention is uncommon in the bitch. The placenta is usually passed within 20 min of the birth of each pup, although occasionally fetuses are delivered without their placentae and these are expelled later, often together with a subsequent pup. If placentae are retained there may be a persistent green vaginal discharge, although diagnosis requires ultrasound examination, since palpation of the involuting uterus can be misleading. Placental retention may lead to metritis (see below), however frequently there are no adverse effects. Treatment should be restricted to the administration of oxytocin (1.0–2.0 IU kg^{-1}).

Postpartum haemorrhage

Haemorrhage after parturition may be due to physical injuries or placental necrosis. Severe haemorrhage is uncommon and coagulopathies should be suspected if bleeding persists. The parenteral administration of oxytocin (1.0–2.0 IU kg^{-1}) or ergometrine (0.2–0.5 mg depending on body weight) usually provides control.

Postpartum metritis

Metritis is associated with bacterial infection of the uterus following abortion, parturition, fetal and/or placental retention and obstetrical manipulation. Clinical signs of depression, pyrexia, anorexia and purulent vaginal discharge are usually noted 2–3 days after parturition. A neutrophilia with a left shift is common and enlargement of the uterus may be identified by radiography, palpation or using ultrasound. Since metritis is a bacterial disorder without the underlying hormonal component seen in pyometra, conservative medical management is feasible (Magne, 1986). Broad-spectrum antimicrobial therapy is required and both oxytocin and ergometrine have been used to stimulate myometrial activity and induce uterine drainage. The twice daily administration of low doses of naturally occurring prostaglandin (0.25 mg kg^{-1} daily) may also stimulate uterine evacuation. Oestrogens are contraindicated because of the possibility of increasing the absorption of toxins.

Uterine prolapse

Prolapse of the uterus in the bitch is rare (Wood, 1986). It occurs during the periparturient period when the cervix is open, although no specific cause or predisposing factors have been established. Physical examination confirms the diagnosis and allows differentiation from vaginal hyperplasia and leiomyomata. Laporotomy is usually required for correct replacement, although hysterectomy or amputation may be required if the uterus or broad ligaments are traumatized.

Subinvolution of placental sites

A serosangineous discharge may persist for longer than the normal 4–6 weeks postpartum in some bitches (Beck and McEntee, 1966; Al-Bassam *et al.*, 1981b) and this is suggestive of subinvolution of placental sites. Affected bitches are usually less than one year old, and are clinically normal with the exception of the vaginal discharge (Glenn, 1968). Palpation and ultrasonography may reveal discrete areas of uterine enlargement. The aetiology is uncertain but the migration of fetal trophoblasts into the endometrium and myometrium appears to be important (Al-Bassam *et al.*, 1981b).

Although spontaneous recovery has been reported this is rare (Shall *et al.*, 1971). Treatment may not be necessary but ovariohysterectomy may be considered if the bitch becomes anaemic or is not required for breeding. Recently the use of antimicrobial and progestogenic agents have proved successful (Dickie and Arbeiter, 1993); ecbolic agents provide no control of the clinical signs.

Hypocalcaemia

Eclampsia or puerperal tetany occurs most commonly during late pregnancy or early lactation in small to medium sized bitches (Austad and Bjerkas, 1976). The aetiology of hypocalcaemia is probably related to calcium loss in the milk combined with poor dietary availability. Hypocalcaemia causes loss of cell membrane bound calcium and subsequent changes in membrane potential. Early clinical signs are restlessness, panting, increased salivation and a stiff gait which progress to muscle fasciculations and pyrexi. If untreated, tetany and death result. The slow intravenous administration of a 10% calcium gluconate solution to effect (5–10 ml) produces a rapid response. Cardiac rate and rhythm should be monitored during administration. Further supplementation may be given subcutaneously and orally to prevent recurrence. Prevention of hypocalcaemia may be achieved by oral calcium supplementation in the last few days of pregnancy and during lactation. Excessive oral calcium administration reduces intestinal absorption of calcium and inhibits the secretion of parathyroid hormone, and although this is clinically significant in several species this does not appear to be the case in the bitch.

Diseases of the mammary glands

Pseudopregnancy

The clinical signs of pseudopregnancy include inappropriate lactation and behavioural changes which have previously been discussed. Frequently treatment is not warranted, however suppression of prolactin release can be achieved using exogenous androgens, oestrogens or progestogens, or using dopamine agonists such as bromocriptine (Allen and England, 1990).

Mastitis

Bacterial mastitis may be the result of ascending infection, direct trauma or haematogenous spread. The mammary glands are tender, warm and firm upon palpation and the bitch may become systemically ill. Milk may become contaminated with blood and inflammatory cells so that it thickens and turns yellow, pink or brown. Staphylococci, streptococci and *E. coli* are frequently isolated. Broad-spectrum antimicrobial preparations and the regular removal of milk are effective treatments. Ideally antimicrobial agents should be chosen on the basis of bacterial sensitivity, however this is not always feasible.

Galactostasis

Mammary congestion with milk combined with oedema of the gland may be seen during pseudopregnancy and late pregnancy. The engorged glands are warm and painful but bitches are generally not systemically ill, and bacteria are not isolated from the milk.

The inflammation may respond to milk removal, although this encourages further production. Therapy using diuretics may be required.

Agalactia

A lack of milk production in the bitch is rare, but an absence of milk letdown occurs more frequently especially in young nervous bitches, or bitches that have undergone an early elective caesarean operation. Inadequate nutrition may also result in decreased milk production. Failure of milk letdown may be treated with a single intramuscular injection of oxytocin (0.2–1.0 IU kg^{-1}). This does not increase milk production, and pups should be encouraged to suck to stimulate milk letdown.

Mammary tumours

Mammary tumours account for the largest proportion of neoplasms affecting the bitch. Two thirds of the tumours occur in glands 4 and 5, and in many bitches several other glands are also involved (Withrow and Susaneck, 1986). The incidence of neoplasia is significantly reduced following ovariohysterectomy before puberty (Schneider et al., 1969). Benign tumours (fibroadenomas) cause no clinical signs and there is no conclusive evidence that these are premalignant (Withrow and Susaneck, 1986). Malignant adenocarcinomas are usually adherent to the underlying musculature or to the skin, they increase in size rapidly and may ulcerate. A highly malignant inflammatory adenocarcinoma may cause clinical signs similar to mastitis. Occasionally clinical signs are related to the respiratory system since metastasis to the lungs is common.

Radical surgical removal is the treatment of choice. Both oestrogen and progesterone receptors have been identified in malignant and benign tumours (Donnay et al., 1993), for this reason both androgens and progestogens have been advocated to reduce tumour size before surgery. The antioestrogen, tamoxifen has been used for the control of mammary neoplasia in the bitch (Morris et al., 1993; Ruben, 1993), however the incidence of side effects which include vulval swelling and the presence of a vulval discharge, attractivness to male dogs and nesting behaviour may preclude the widespread use of this agent (Morris et al., 1993).

THE QUEEN

Reproductive endocrinology

The queen is a seasonally polyoestrus induced ovulator; eggs are only ovulated after mating or artificial stimulation (Greulich, 1934). There is no proestrus phase and oestral behaviour occurs with few changes of the external genitalia. During the follicular phase oestradiol concentrations are generally high although there is considerable variation (Verhage et al., 1976; Shille et al., 1979). Copulation produces a rapid pituitary-mediated release of LH (Robinson and Sawyer, 1987); usually multiple copulations are required to induce ovulation (Concannon et al., 1980b).

Progesterone concentrations remain basal until after the mating-induced LH surge, and increase coincidentally with ovulation (Schmidt et al., 1983); peak values are reached after 1 month (Fig. 40.9). From this time, progesterone concentrations in non-pregnant queens decline whereas they are maintained for a further 25–28 days during pregnancy. Queens that have ovulated but are not pregnant (pseudopregnant) do not return to oestrus until after the decline in plasma progesterone concentration.

Prolactin concentrations are elevated in the last third of pregnancy and during lactation (Banks and Stabenfeldt, 1983). There are no significant changes in prolactin concentration during pseudopregnancy (Christiansen, 1984).

Abnormal endocrinological events

Delayed puberty

The onset of the first oestrus is usually at 6–10 months of age, however this is influenced by body weight and season of birth. Puberty frequently occurs during the spring, therefore females born in autumn or winter may not reach puberty until the subsequent spring when they are at least 12 months old. Queens which do not demonstrate oestrus behaviour after this age may be investigated similarly to those with prolonged anoestrus (see below).

Prolonged anoestrus

The queen is seasonally polyoestrus and cyclicity is dependent on the photoperiod (Herron, 1977). In the northern hemisphere queens cycle from January or February, although the first oestrus may be irregular. In healthy queens 14 hours of

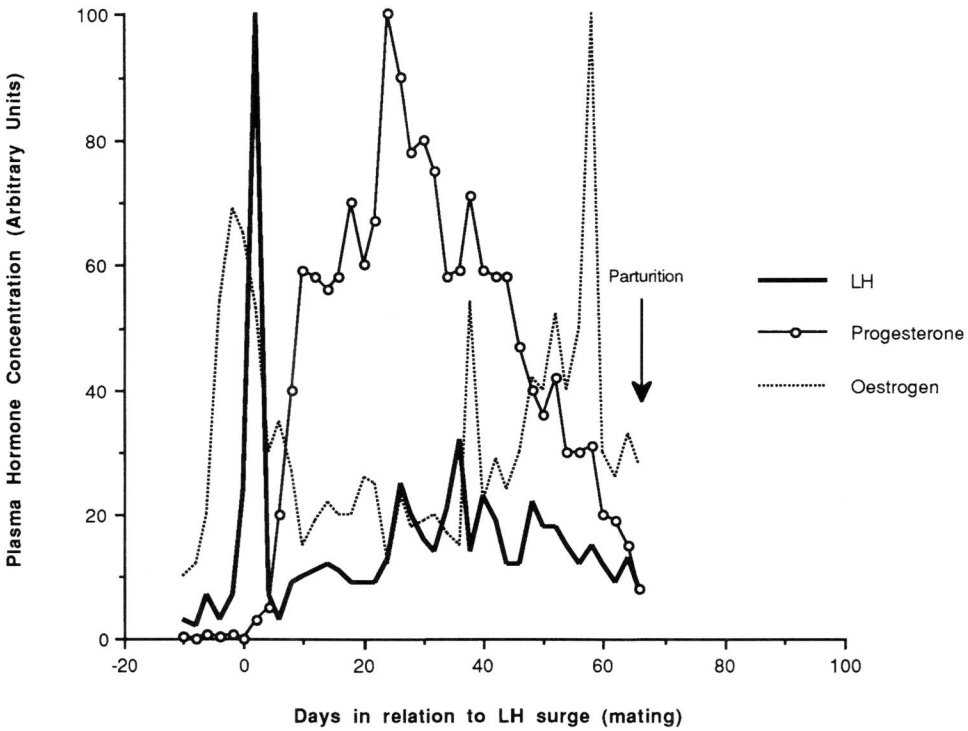

Figure 40.9 Schematic representation of the changes in peripheral plasma oestrogen, LH and progesterone during the pregnant oestrous cycle of the queen.

lighting per day will abolish anoestrus (Gruffydd-Jones, 1990), and the presence of an oestrous queen may stimulate cyclicity. Prolonged anoestrus may be associated with systemic disease, poor nutrition or parasite burden (Mosier, 1975). Abnormal ovarian development has also been suggested as a cause (Johnston *et al.*, 1983). Consideration should be given to the past use of progestogenic medication for dermatological or behavioural problems since this will postpone oestrus.

Induction of oestrus may be attempted using daily administration of gonadotrophins, although in young queens this produces ovarian overstimulation (Wildt *et al.*, 1978). Single doses (100 IU) of eCG followed 5 to 7 days later by 50 IU of hCG has produced ovulation with pregnancy rates similar to natural mating (Cline *et al.*, 1980). Other methods for the induction of oestrus have been recently reviewed (Goodrowe *et al.*, 1989).

Prolonged oestrus

Some unmated queens may have an oestrus which persists for two follicular cycles, even though the endocrinological events are normal. In these cases there are usually two peaks of plasma oestrogen concentration despite the persistent behavioural oestrus, however, persistently elevated oestrogen concentrations have also been identified (Feldman and Nelson, 1987b). The fertility of such cycles is not known; they are sporadic in occurrence and do not warrant treatment.

Ovulation failure

Each copulation causes a release of LH which may or may not be sufficient to cause ovulation. Less than 50% of queens in full oestrus ovulate after a single mating (Feldman and Nelson, 1987b), however more than 90% of females ovulate if mated three times at 4 h intervals for the first 3 days of oestrus (Schmidt, 1986). The release of LH occurs within 5 min after mating (Johnson and Gray, 1981), therefore a major determinant is the mating frequency. It is therefore important to ensure that multiple matings occur, although a single injection of 500 IU hCG on day 1 of oestrus will often induce ovulation (Wildt and Seager, 1978). Failure of ovulation can be demonstrated by low plasma progesterone concentrations.

Pseudopregnancy

Pseudopregnancy usually follows a sterile mating, although it may occur after a spontaneous ovulation (Lawler et al., 1993). After ovulation, plasma progesterone concentrations increase, and there is no return to oestrus; the interoestrus interval is approximately 37 days (Paape et al., 1975). There is no change in plasma prolactin concentration. The clinical signs of pseudopregnancy are therefore an absence of oestrus rather than lactation.

Reproductive organs

The reproductive organs of the queen are similar to those of the bitch. The ovaries are positioned in the dorsal abdomen ventral to the fourth lumbar vertebra and are partially surrounded by a bursa. During proestrus and oestrus there is growth and development of several follicles which protrude above the surface of the ovary. The uterus is morphologically similar to that of the bitch, although the cervix contains tubular glandular tissue. The vagina is relatively short, and Bartholian glands are present within the vestibule.

Diseases of the ovary

Ovarian agenesis

Ovarian hypoplasia and ovarian agenesis are rare but both result in permanent anoestrus and infertility if the changes are bilateral. At laparotomy or laparoscopy, small ovarian remnants containing fibrous tissue are usually identified (Schmidt, 1986). Chromosomal abnormalities have been reported in phenotypically normal females (Nicholas et al., 1980; Johnston et al., 1983).

Ovarian cysts

Similar to the bitch, many cysts noted at ovariohysterectomy and necropsy are not of ovarian origin but are frequently remnants of mesonephric and rete tubules, although true follicular cysts associated with hyperoestrogenism have been reported (Herron, 1986). Clinical signs include excessive and prolonged sexual behaviour. Attempts to induce ovulation using hCG may be successful, otherwise control may be achieved using progestogens (Christiansen, 1984) or ovariohysterectomy.

Premature ovarian failure

Queens may stop cycling from 8 years of age onwards. The aetiology of the premature termination of cyclicity is unknown. The investigation of these cases should be similar to those with prolonged anoestrus. High circulating concentrations of FSH and LH may be diagnostic (Feldman and Nelson, 1987b).

Ovarian tumours

Ovarian tumours generally reach a large size before diagnosis and are not frequently metastatic, commonly being granulosa–theca cell tumours (Herron, 1986). These tumours may secrete sex steroids and produce clinical signs of persistent oestrus, cystic endometrial hyperplasia and bilaterally symmetrical alopecia (Barrett and Theilen, 1977). Ovariohysterectomy is the treatment of choice.

Intersexuality

Hermaphrodite and male pseudohermaphrodite cats have been identified (Herron and Boehringer, 1975; Felts, 1982). The latter have external female genitalia with internal gonads containing testicular tissue. Affected queens may fail to cycle.

Diseases of the uterus

Aplasia of the tubular genital tract

Absence of a single uterine horn (uterus unicornis) does not often interfere with fertility although litter size may be reduced. Frequently in such cases there may also be absence of the ipsilateral ovary and kidney.

Segmental aplasia of the uterus may produce infertility if the condition is bilateral. Diagnosis is difficult; this is best achieved at laparotomy or laparoscopy.

Cystic endometrial hyperplasia – pyometra

The pathophysiology of this condition is similar to the bitch, although the long progestogenic period is only present in queens which have ovulated. However, spontaneous ovulations (Colby, 1980; Lawler et al., 1993) and the common use of exogenous progestogens may both allow the development of cystic endometrial hyperplasia (Thornton, 1967). Clinical signs include anorexia, lethargy, vomiting, polydipsia and a vaginal discharge which may be intermittent. Cases of both open and closed cervix pyometra may occur. Diagnosis is made in a similar manner to the bitch using palpation, radiography, ultrasonography and haematological examination. The treatment of choice is ovariohysterectomy combined with the administration of intravenous fluids and appropriate antimicrobial preparations. Surgical drainage has also been described (Vasseur and Feldman, 1982), as has the use of prostaglandins for promoting uterine evacuation (Henderson, 1984). The naturally occurring prostaglandin (dinoprost) administered at a dose of 0.1 mg kg^{-1} daily for 5 days has been successful (Feldman and Nelson, 1987b).

Uterine tumours

Malignant endometrial adenocarcinomas are the most common uterine neoplasm, but benign tumours have also been reported (Herron, 1986). These tumours may cause malaise and straining or a persistent haemorrhagic vaginal discharge. Radiography, ultrasonography or exploratory surgery may be diagnostic, and treatment is ovariohysterectomy.

Diseases of the vagina and vestibule

Vaginal aplasia

Segmental aplasia of the mullerian duct system may produce vaginal aplasia. This is rare in the cat, but as with the bitch it may result in infertility and produce retention of uterine fluid. Diagnosis may be made using positive contrast vaginography or exploratory surgery.

Vaginitis

Vaginitis is not common in the queen. It may occur secondarily to trauma at mating, to vaginal neoplasia or to uterine disease. Specific infectious causes are rare. Clinical signs include intensive licking and vaginal discharge. Successful treatment involves removal of the primary cause combined with appropriate systemic and local antimicrobial therapy.

Vaginal tumours

Pedunculated leiomyomata and fibromata may originate within the vagina. They are infrequent neoplasms which produce vaginitis and constipation due to dorsal impingement of the colon and rectum. Surgical removal via an episiotomy or laparotomy is usually curative.

Diseases of the external genitalia

Vulval aplasia

The presence of small labia with or without stenosis of the vestibule has been reported in the cat (Herron, 1986). This may result in a vaginitis and prevents normal intromission.

Intersexuality

Male pseudohermaphrodites have female external genitalia, although these are usually positioned more ventral than normal or are undersized, since intra-abdominal gonads contain testicular tissue. These animals are usually sterile; treatment is by removal of the reproductive tract and gonads.

Diseases of pregnancy

Conception or implantation failure

The most common reason for failure of conception is lack of sufficient LH stimulation to induce ovulation. Multiple matings are required to ensure the adequate release of LH, and a major determinant is the frequency of mating. Low plasma progesterone concentrations one week after mating demonstrate ovulation failure.

Other causes for failure of conception may be related to endocrinological, nutritional and physical abnormalities previously discussed.

Abortion/resorption

Abortion or resorption may be caused by environmental, nutritional, genetic, infectious or hormonal factors.

There are several viral agents that may induce abortion, resorption and stillbirths including feline herpesvirus I (Hoover and Griesemer, 1971), feline panleukopenia virus (Kilham et al., 1971), feline leukaemia virus (Herron, 1977; Hardy, 1981) and feline infectious peritonitis virus (Norsworthy, 1979). The diagnosis of these may be made on clinical signs, time of the abortion, examination of the aborted material and serological investigation (Troy and Herron, 1986).

Bacterial agents which have been isolated in cases of abortion include normal vaginal commensal bacteria such as E. coli, streptococci and staphylococci (Christiansen, 1984).

Treatment of the dam at the time of abortion may include the administration of broad-spectrum antimicrobial preparations, fluid therapy and drugs to stimulate uterine evacuation. The ecbolic effect of low doses of prostaglandin or ergometrine may be useful. In certain cases ovariohysterectomy may be warranted. Prevention involves serological screening of animals. Toxoplasmosis has also been associated with abortion, although congenital infections causing anorexia, dyspnoea, incoordination and death of kittens are more common (McKinney, 1973; Dubey and Johnstone, 1982).

Premature luteal regression has been suggested as a cause of habitual resorption or abortion. There are several hypothetical causes of this progesterone deficiency, however its existence has not been proven in the queen. Various treatments using exogenous progestogens have been suggested but these may increase the incidence of pyometra. Progestogen therapy during pregnancy may also produce masculinized female and cryptorchid male kittens, and may impair or delay parturition resulting in fetal death.

The postparturient period

Uterine involution may take up to 10 weeks in the queen. A vaginal discharge, which may be haemorrhagic and persist for up to 10 days after parturition is normal. A mucoid vaginal discharge may be present for up to 6 weeks postpartum.

Postparturient diseases

Placental retention

This is uncommon in the queen and does not consistently produce metritis. Diagnosis is difficult in the absence of real-time ultrasonography. Placentae may be passed normally several days after parturition. Treatment should be restricted to the administration of oxytocin.

Postpartum haemorrhage

Vaginal or uterine haemorrhage may follow parturition. If this persists for more than 5 days, control may be achieved using parentral administration of oxytocin, prostaglandin or ergometrine. Severe persistent haemorrhage may suggest a coagulopathy.

Subinvolution of placental sites

Persistent serosangineous discharge in an otherwise healthy cat may be the result of subinvolution of placental sites. The condition usually requires no treatment since the haemorrhage usually declines gradually. Queens should be monitored to ensure that anaemia does not develop, in which case ovariohysterectomy may be necessary. Ecbolic agents and antibiotics provide no control of the clinical signs.

Postpartum metritis

Bacterial infection of the uterus may follow abortion, parturition or placental retention. This produces depression, pyrexia and anorexia with a malodorous purulent vaginal discharge.

Diagnosis is based on clinical signs, the presence of a neutrophilia and uterine enlargement identified by radiography, palpation or ultrasonography. The treatment of choice is ovariohysterectomy combined with the administration of broad spectrum antimicrobials and fluid therapy. In queens required for breeding the twice daily administration of low doses of naturally occurring prostaglandin may help induce uterine evacuation.

Uterine prolapse

Prolapse of the uterus is rare but may occur immediately before or after parturition (Arnall, 1961). Replacement may be undertaken via laparotomy although hysterectomy may be required if the uterus or broad ligament are traumatized.

Hypocalcaemia

Eclampsia or puerperal tetany is rare in the queen but may occur during late pregnancy or early lactation. It is characterized by ataxia, tremors and pyrexia which if untreated may progress to tetany and death. The aetiology is thought to be similar to that in the bitch; occurring more commonly in queens with large litters.

The slow intravenous administration of a 10% calcium gluconate solution produces a rapid response; cardiac rate and rhythm should be monitored during administration. Additional supplementation may be given subcutaneously and orally to prevent recurrence. Prevention of hypocalcaemia may be achieved by oral calcium supplementation in the last few days of pregnancy and during lactation. Excessive oral administration of calcium reduces intestinal absorption of calcium and inhibits the secretion of parathyoid hormone, although this may not be a clinically significant effect in the queen.

Diseases of the mammary glands

Pseudopregnancy

Pseudopregnancy is not associated with lactation in the queen (see pseudopregnancy on pages 580 and 591).

Galactostasis

Oedematous mammary glands which are congested with milk may be seen following death of kittens, early weaning or teat inversion. Milk removal can be achieved by gentle massage of the nipple, although this encourages further milk production. Therapy using diuretics may be required.

Mastitis

Mastitis is rare in the queen; initial clinical signs include gastrointestinal disease or death of the kittens (Laliberte, 1986). Staphylococcal and streptococcal organisms are frequently isolated and the queen may be lethargic and pyrexic. Kittens should be removed to prevent further trauma and spread of infection (Gruffydd-Jones, 1985). Broad spectrum antimicrobial agents and poulticing of the glands should prevent the development of gangrenous mastitis (Gruffydd-Jones, 1980).

Mammary hyperplasia

Hyperplasia of mammary glandular tissue occurs during the first oestrus of young queens. The glands are enlarged and hyperaemic and may exude a dark brown secretion. Diuretics and corticosteroids cause resolution of the clinical signs, however these may recur at subsequent oestrous periods necessitating prevention by ovariohysterectomy. A degree of mammary hyperplasia follows the administration of progestogens, however the effect is reversible upon withdrawal of the drug.

Mammary hypertrophy

This is seen as a complication of progestogen therapy and usually regresses following withdrawal of the drug.

Diseases of the Male Reproductive System

INTRODUCTION

Although the dog and tom are similar to each other endocrinologically they are different anatomically. The dog possesses only a single accessory sex gland, the prostate, whereas the tom has a prostate gland and a pair of bulbourethral glands. The penis of the tom cat is directed caudally and is covered by cornified papilla.

CLINICAL HISTORY

The collection of a relevant clinical history is essential and may be useful for constructing a list of differential diagnoses. This should include previous breeding history, previous success as a sire, the administration of pharmaceutical compounds and general medical history. The onset of puberty is less easy to identify in the male than the female, but puberty is usually reached at nine months of age. However, the value of determining this in an individual is uncertain.

PHYSICAL EXAMINATION

As in the female a full clinical examination is mandatory to eliminate generalized systemic disease. Physical examination of the reproductive tract is limited in the tom to inspection and palpation of the external genitalia, whereas in the dog rectal palpation of the prostate gland is also possible. Testes should be examined and compared for their size and consistency. The epididymis should be evenly attached to the dorsolateral surface of the testis; particular note should be made of the epididymal tail which in the dog is usually 'pea-sized'.

The prostate gland should be symmetrical and globe shaped with a dorsal median furrow. The position of the prostate gland is variable, although it is usually intrapelvic. An increase in size occurs normally with advancing age. The prepuce should be examined for the presence of abnormal discharges and the penis exposed to allow inspection for any abnormalities.

INVESTIGATIVE TECHNIQUES

Several techniques can be used to investigate reproductive disease in the male animal. The collection of a semen sample may provide diagnostic information concerning testicular and prostatic function (Allen, 1992). Testicular biopsies may be obtained by incision or needle aspiration, although this is not advisable in breeding animals since it is followed by a marked inflammatory response (Larsen, 1977; James *et al.*, 1979a); incisional biopsies in particular may produce hypospermatogenesis, necrosis, tubular degeneration, fibrosis and inflammation (Lopate *et al.*, 1989). The measurement of circulating plasma hormones may be of value for the confirmation of testicular activity and for the diagnosis of testicular failure. Resting plasma concentrations of testosterone (James *et al.*, 1979b), LH (DePalatis *et al.*, 1978) and FSH (Feldman and Nelson, 1987a) may be diagnostic, however concentrations fluctuate markedly, and serial sampling or the response of plasma testosterone to the administration of hCG may be of more value (Mialot *et al.*, 1988; England *et al.*, 1989b). Imaging of the reproductive tract is possible radiographically, although more recently ultrasonography has been shown to be of considerable value for imaging the prostate (Feeney *et al.*, 1987) and testes (Pugh *et al.*, 1990; Miyabayashi *et al.*, 1990; England, 1991). Further evaluation of the prostate gland in the dog may be achieved by needle aspiration or biopsy of the gland, especially using ultrasound guiding. Cells may also be collected following prostatic massage and urethral washing (Barsanti and Finco, 1986). This technique involves passing a urethral catheter into the bladder to allow drainage of urine and flushing of the bladder with saline. Subsequently the catheter is partially withdrawn until its tip is within the prostatic urethra, as determined by rectal palpation. The prostate is then massaged per rectum or transabdominally for 1–2 min and the prostatic secretions are aspirated. A small volume of sterile saline (5–10 ml), flushed into the urethra, may aid recovery of cells for cytological examination.

THE DOG

Reproductive endocrinology

In all mammalian species the interstitial (Leydig) cells are the source of testosterone production; oestradiol is also produced in small quantities by aromatization of testosterone. The production of these hormones is stimulated by LH, whereas FSH appears to increase spermatogenesis directly via the Sertoli cells (Shille, 1989). Both testosterone and oestradiol provide a negative feedback mechanism for FSH and LH, the release of which is governed by GnRH. A schematic representation of these events is given in Fig. 40.10. Concentrations of testosterone, FSH and LH fluctuate markedly during a 24 h period (Amann, 1986) (Fig. 40.11).

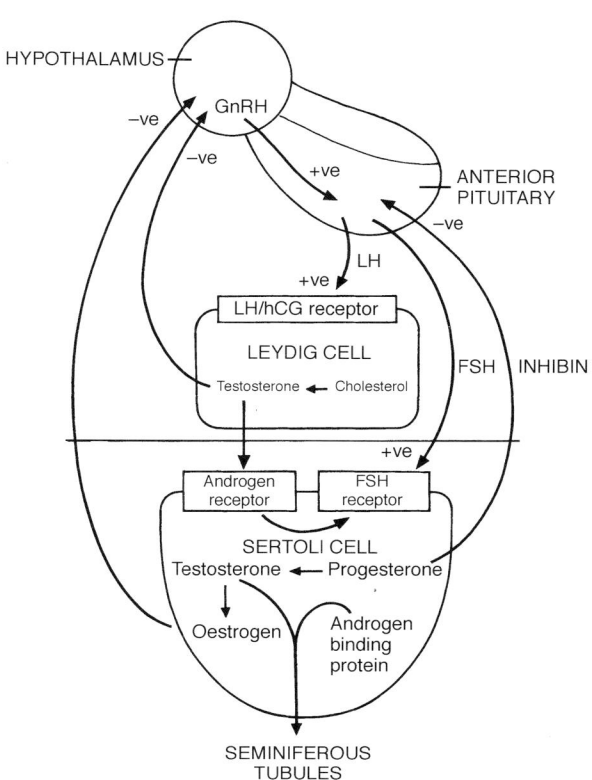

Figure 40.10 Schematic representation of gonadotrophin and testicular steroid production and regulation in the male.

Abnormal endocrinological events

Hypogonadism

Reduced secretion of FSH and LH may occur in cases of pituitary dysfunction and will result in impaired spermatogenesis (Feldman and Nelson, 1987a). In these cases serial sampling demonstrates that plasma LH, FSH and testosterone

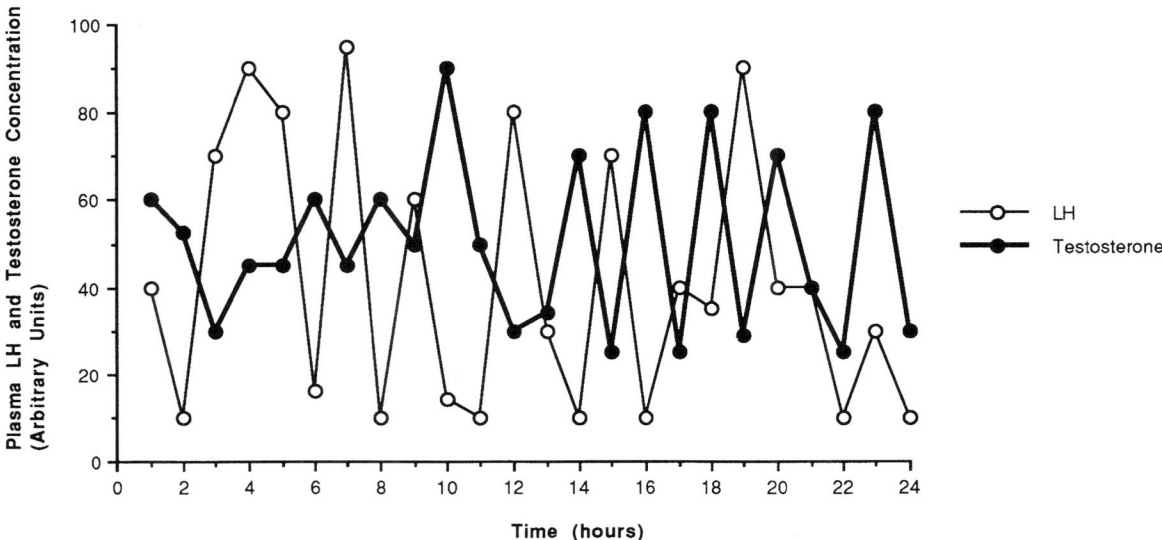

Figure 40.11 Schematic representation of the changes of peripheral plasma LH and testosterone concentration for a male dog during a 24-hour period.

concentrations are low. Testicular biopsy demonstrates an absence of spermatogenesis but no inflammation. The administration of FSH has been suggested to promote spermatogenesis (Larsen and Johnston, 1980) although the efficacy of this technique remains to be proven.

Poor libido

Frequently inability to copulate is the result of inexperience on behalf of the dog or poor breeding management. There is no evidence that reduced libido is the result of low plasma androgen concentrations. The administration of exogenous androgens is rarely curative, and can have an inhibitory effect upon pituitary function. In humans, exogenous androgens have been shown to reduce gonadotrophin secretion (Gordon et al., 1975) resulting in the suppression of endogenous testosterone secretion and testicular activity.

Impaired spermatogenesis

Differing terminology has been used to describe an absence of spermatogenesis including primary testicular failure, primary failure of spermatogenesis and Leydig cell failure (Feldman and Nelson, 1987a). Little is known about the occurrence and true aetiology of these conditions and inappropriate terminology has been frequently adapted from other species. Low plasma concentrations of FSH and LH indicate a hypothalamic or pituitary lesion, whereas normal or increased concentrations are suggestive of primary spermatogenic failure with loss of feedback inhibition (Feldman and Nelson, 1987a). Low concentrations of plasma LH, FSH and testosterone may also occur secondarily to thyroid hormone deficiency. Histologically the testes of many azoospermic dogs have tubular degeneration, with normal or sparse numbers of Leydig cells. There may be breed predispositions to some of these changes (Dahlbom et al., 1995).

Certain cases of oligospermia may respond to the administration of oestrogen analogues or antioestrogen compounds (clomiphene citrate and tamoxifen respectively); it has been suggested that these cases represent early stages of primary spermatogenic failure (Feldman and Nelson, 1987a). The use of the synthetic androgen, mesterolone, may also be useful (England and Allen, 1991b). Thyroid function should always be evaluated in cases of poor semen quality; cases of hypothyroidism may benefit from supplementation, however the prognosis for fertility is often poor.

Reproductive organs

The testes of the dog are ellipsoidal in shape and are composed of seminiferous tubules suspended by the mediastinum testis. The rete testis transports spermatozoa from the seminiferous tubules into the epididymis, the latter being a tightly coiled tubular structure adherent to the testicular capsule. The tail of the epididymis is positioned dorsocaudally.

Spermatozoa are transported from the epididymis, via the ductus deferens to enter the urethra in its prostatic portion. The prostate is the only accessory gland in the dog and is usually located in an intrapelvic position. Two corpora cavernosa comprise the penis, which in its cranial portion contains an os, extending from the tip of the glans to the bulbus glandis. The urethra runs in a ventral groove within the os penis. The penis is completely enclosed within the prepuce.

Diseases of the testes and scrotum

Anorchidism

Congenital absence of both testes has been reported in man (Silber, 1978). In the dog this is extremely rare; only one case has been described (England et al., 1989b). Most cases of absence of scrotal testicular tissue are bilateral cryptorchids. Diagnosis may be made by a lack of response of plasma testosterone to a single intravenous injection of 750 IU hCG (England et al., 1989b).

Monorchidism

By definition this means the presence of a single testicle in the body. Most cases are unilateral cryptorchids, with a single abdominal testicle.

Cryptorchidism

Cryptorchid means hidden testicles, a condition which may be unilateral or bilateral. The testes normally descend into the scrotum following contraction of the gubernaculum testis by 10 days after birth (Gier and Marion, 1969), although a diagnosis of cryptorchid is not usually made until 10 weeks of age. The condition is likely to have a genetic base, and although the mode of inheritance is unknown it follows the model of a sex-limited autosomal recessive trait (Meyers-Wallen and Patterson, 1989). Both female and male parents will carry the gene but only homozygous males will be cryptorchid. The retained abdominal testis is more likely to become neoplastic. Medical therapy is not ethical; treatment is by removal of both testes to prevent neoplasia and breeding.

Ectopic testes

Dogs with testes which do not occupy the normal scrotal position are likely to be part of the cryptorchid syndrome. Testes may pass through the inguinal ring and be found in the femoral triangle, in the caudal perineum or cranial to the scrotum. Treatment is as for cryptorchidism.

Orchitis

Inflammation of the testis may be traumatic or non-traumatic in origin. Traumatic cases may be complicated by infection and haemorrhage and these changes may be severe (Burke, 1986). Conservative therapy involving antimicrobial preparations may be successful, although surgical debridement or castration may be necessary.

Infective orchitis is rare in the UK since *Brucella canis* infection does not occur. *Brucella* may be a significant problem in other countries producing spermatozoal abnormalities and infertility (Carmichael and Kenney, 1968). Bacterial orchitis may occur after retrograde passage of urine (Lein, 1977), causing suppurative inflammation and abscess formation. These cases are usually severe and castration is frequently necessary.

Spermatogenic arrest

The cessation of spermatogenesis with resultant azoospermia has been reported in the dog (Renton and Aughey, 1971). The condition has been identified in related animals (Hadley, 1972; Allen and Longstaffe, 1982) and autoantibodies directed against spermatozoa were found in two cases (Allen and Patel, 1982). Affected dogs are initially fertile until middle age; they then become azoospermic and have small testes but are otherwise clinically healthy. The prognosis for fertility is usually poor although the use of immunosuppressive doses of glucocorticoids has been suggested as a treatment (Feldman and Nelson, 1987a).

Testicular cysts

The occurrence of testicular cysts in the dog has only recently been recorded (England, 1991) (Fig. 40.12). The incidence of testicular cysts and their influence on fertility is unknown; they produce no clinical signs and may only be detected with ultrasound if they are very large.

Spermatocoele

Cystic distension of the testicular duct system may lead to an inflammatory response resulting in

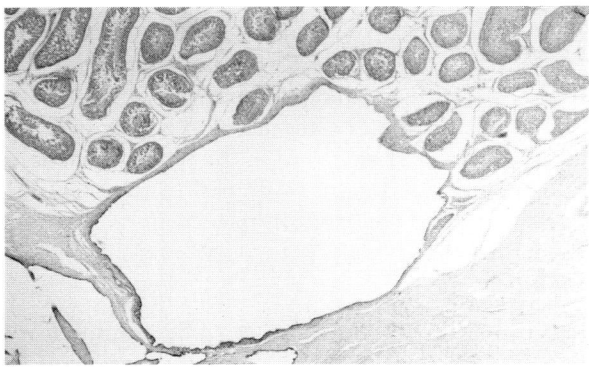

Figure 40.12 Cystic structure within the testes of a 6-year-old cross-bred dog. Section stained with haematoxylin and eosin; magnification × 104.

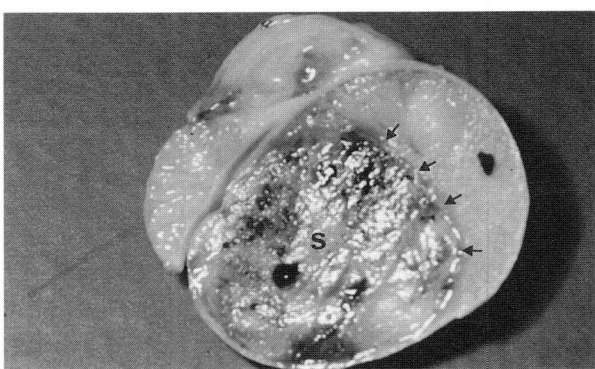

Figure 40.13 Sertoli cell tumour (S) located centrally within a canine testicle (arrows). The normal testicular tissue is compressed into a small peripheral region.

the formation of a sperm granuloma. These lesions are rare, although they may be detected by palpation. Obstruction of the testicular duct interferes with spermatozoal output.

Testicular tumours

Testicular tumours are the second most common tumour affecting the male dog (Cotchin, 1960; Susaneck and Withrow, 1986).

Interstitial cell tumours

Interstitial cell tumours arise from the Leydig cells, and may be single or multiple, occurring in one or both testes. They are usually 1–2 cm in diameter, yellow in colour and may occasionally have a necrotic core. They often produce no change in testicular size. Interstitial cell tumours are rarely malignant (Hayes and Pendergrass, 1976) and are generally endocrinologically inactive.

Sertoli cell tumours

Sertoli cell tumours are generally discrete unilateral slow-growing neoplasms. They have a nodular lobulated architecture (Fig. 40.13) and although the majority are initially benign up to 10% may be malignant (Crow, 1980). Not all Sertoli cell tumours are endocrinologically active, however the Sertoli cell tumour is the most common tumour associated with 'male feminizing syndrome', which may be due to increased production of oestrogen by the tumour, or increased conversion of androgen into oestrogen. Signs of feminization include mammary gland development, preputial swelling, male attractiveness with bilaterally symmetrical non-pruritic alopecia. In these cases the non-neoplastic testicle atrophies due to the negative feedback effect of oestrogen on the pituitary–hypothalamus. High oestrogen concentrations may produce bone marrow suppression (Sherding et al., 1981) and squamous metaplasia of the prostate gland. The diagnosis may be aided by the measurement of plasma oestrogen concentration.

Seminomas

Seminomas arise from spermatogenic tissue of the tubular epithelium, and are solitary unilateral tumours which may become very large. They are soft and usually benign, although metastasis has been noted (Crow, 1980; Tennant and Kelly, 1992). Feminization may also occur.

The ultrasonographic features of some non-palpable testicular neoplasms have been described (England, 1991). In all cases radiographic screening of the thorax and local lymph nodes should be undertaken. Castration is the treatment of choice.

Torsion of the spermatic cord

Rotation of one of the testes around the vertical axis causes occlusion of the pampiniform plexus, followed by swelling and necrosis of the testicle. The aetiology is unknown although it may be related to rupture of the scrotal ligament. Torsion is more common in enlarged neoplastic intra-abdominal testes (Pearson and Kelley, 1975). Prompt surgical removal of the affected testis is essential.

Diseases of the epididymides

Aplasia of the duct system

Unilateral and bilateral aplastic lesions of the testicular duct system have been reported in the dog (Copland and Maclachlan, 1976). Some workers have suggested that these lesions are not uncommon and are similar to those in other species (Feldman and Nelson, 1987a). In such cases azoospermia and oligospermia result, although histological examination of the testes is normal.

Epididymitis

Epididymitis may be the result of trauma and/or infection. Infectious agents may enter the epididymis via the vas deferens or seminiferous tubules, through the vaginal tunic or haematogenously (Soderberg, 1986b). The epididymis becomes enlarged and painful and the resulting inflammation can cause fibrosis and obstruction. Differential culture of the second and third fractions of the ejaculate may help to isolate bacterial causes. Histological examination of a testicular biopsy will be normal. Serology for brucellosis should be undertaken in dogs which have been imported. Appropriate antimicrobial therapy may be helpful in certain cases, although castration may be necessary.

Diseases of the prostate gland (see also Chapter 41)

Benign prostatic hyperplasia

Hyperplasia of the prostatic epithelium begins early in the dog's life. It is associated with altered androgen/oestrogen ratios and may be present without clinical signs. However, in some dogs the enlarged gland impinges on the pelvic viscera and causes faecal tenesmus and may result in haematuria and haemospermia. Usually the gland is symmetrically enlarged and non-painful and the large gland may be demonstrated radiographically and ultrasonographically (Fig. 40.14). Castration produces rapid resolution of clinical signs. Exogenous progestogens and oestrogens may also be successfully used, however oestrogens may induce prostatic squamous metaplasia resulting in increased size of the gland. Recently antiandrogens have been used (Iguer-Ovada and Verstegen, 1996), and drugs such as flucamide, formestane and finasteride are now widely available.

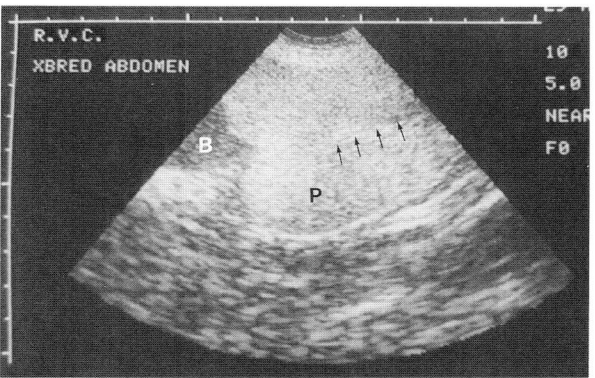

Figure 40.14 Ultrasound image of a 10-year-old dog with benign prostatic hyperplasia. The prostate gland is increased in echogenicity compared with normal. The gland is large but its margins are smooth. P, prostate; B, bladder. Arrows indicate the position of the more echogenic hilar region.

Bacterial prostatitis

Adult dogs may develop prostatitis following ascending infection of bacteria, commonly *E. coli*. Clinical signs include systemic illness, with vomiting and caudal abdominal pain (Barsanti and Finco, 1989). Animals are neutrophilic and the gland is painful and has an irregular contour on palpation. Urine culture and urethral washings may help with diagnosis.

Lesions may become chronic, and pockets of purulent exudate may form (prostatic abscessation) producing signs of recurrent cystitis. Treatment of these cases is difficult; antimicrobial therapy on the basis of the results of bacterial sensitivity may be required for up to 6 weeks. In certain cases surgical drainage is necessary.

Squamous prostatic metaplasia

A change in the prostatic glandular epithelium from cuboidal or columnar to squamous occurs secondarily to endogenous or exogenous hyperoestrogenism (Huggins and Clark, 1940). This predisposes to cyst formation, infection and abscessation (Johnston, 1985), but is not a preneoplastic change. A presumptive diagnosis may be made on the clinical signs and history. Treatment is directed towards removal of the source of oestrogen since the condition is reversible (Huggins and Clark, 1940).

Prostatic cysts

Two types of prostatic cyst have been identified. The least common are discrete retention cysts associated with blockage of the prostatic ducts. These occur within the parenchyma of the prostate, causing distortion of its outline. More commonly cysts are found adjacent to the prostate, attached by small stalk-like adhesions (Weaver, 1978). These are remnants of the uterus masculinus (vestigial Mullerian ducts). The clinical signs of both types of cyst are related to their size; they may produce pelvic canal obstruction, faecal tenesmus, dysuria and haematuria (Atilola and Pennock, 1986). Diagnosis may be made radiographically, although ultrasound examination can differentiate the internal architecture of the organ (Feeney *et al.*, 1987). Excision or marsupialization are the treatments of choice; castration and hormone therapy are of no value.

Prostatic tumours

Adenocarcinomas are the most common neoplasms affecting the prostate gland of the dog; approximately 5% of dogs with prostatic disease have neoplasia (Weaver, 1981). Tumours are firm upon palpation and tend to metastasize to iliac and sublumbar lymph nodes (Fig. 40.15), and to the vertebral bodies of caudal lumbar vertebrae. Clinical signs are associated with the increased size of the gland, although dogs may have a haemorrhagic urethral discharge and hindlimb pain (Durham and Dietze, 1986). Diagnosis may be made on the basis of clinical signs, radiographic findings, the presence of neoplastic cells collected by urethral washing following prostatic massage or semen collection (Barsanti and Finco, 1984). Needle aspiration under ultrasound guidance or biopsy are valuable diagnostic tools (Barsanti and Finco, 1986). Radiotherapy may be useful for treatment, however the animal should be carefully examined for metastatic spread before embarking on therapy. Antiandrogens may provide some control of the clinical signs.

■ Diseases of the penis and prepuce

Penile hypoplasia

Hypoplasia of the penis is rare but has been reported in several breeds of dog (Proescholdt and DeYoung, 1977) and may be due to sex chromosome abnormalities (Johnston, 1989a). The clinical signs are often related to pooling of urine within the prepuce, which may be prevented by surgical enlargement of the preputial opening and shortening the length of the prepuce.

Hypospadius

Failure of the genital folds to fuse during development may result in an abnormal termination of the urethra caudal and ventral to the glans penis. Hypospadius may be classified into six types relating to the position of the defect; the perineal form is the most common (Kipnis, 1974; Adler and Hobson, 1978). Affected dogs may also have a short and deviated penis. Treatment is related to the severity of the abnormality but may include reconstructive surgery or amputation.

Persistent penile frenulum

Normal rupture of the ventral penile frenulum occurs due to mechanical stress. Failure of rupture results in persistence of the frenulum, and causes ventral deviation of the penis during erection. Surgical correction involves incision of the avascular frenulum. However, a hereditable nature of the condition has been established in one breed (Hutchinson, 1973).

Congenital deformity of os penis

This may result in penile deviation and inability to move the penis into and out of the prepuce. Desiccation of the glans penis may result if it is persistently exposed. Conservative management, preputial surgery or amputation may be necessary.

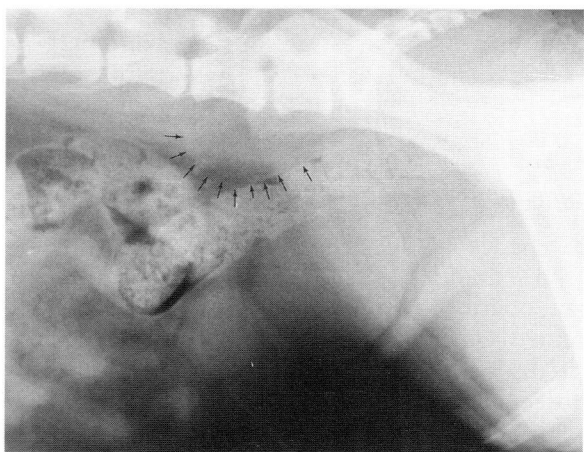

Figure 40.15 Caudal abdominal radiograph of dog with sublumbar lymphadenopathy (arrows) secondary to prostatic neoplasia.

Diphallia

Duplication of the penis is rare. It may result from anomalous duplication of the cloacal membrane and formation of two genital tubercules (Johnston, 1989b). Affected dogs may also have abnormalities of the urinary tract.

Phimosis

An abnormally small preputial orifice may occur either congenitally or as the result of trauma or inflammation. A narrow stream of urine during micturition and urine pooling within the prepuce result, and may cause balanoposthitis. Affected dogs are not able to copulate and shown signs of pain during erection. Surgical enlargement of the orifice is usually curative.

Paraphimosis

Failure of the glans penis to be retracted fully into the prepuce may be due to a small preputial orifice, inversion of the preputial skin and hair, a short prepuce or neurogenic factors affecting the preputial muscles. The penis may become dry and necrotic, and secondary urethral obstruction may result. Application of ice packs and lubricants, and enlargement of the urethral orifice may successfully allow retraction, although amputation may be necessary in persistent cases.

Priapism

Persistent enlargement of the penis in the absence of sexual excitement may be the result of neurogenic abnormalities such as lumbar spinal lesions or lumbosacral disease. Myelography is often necessary for an accurate diagnosis. Conservative management may be successful.

Fractured os penis

Fracture of the os penis may follow a traumatic incident, and usually causes swelling, urethral haemorrhage and dysuria (Stead, 1972; Jeffery, 1974). Radiographic examination is required, although palpation may be diagnostic after the swelling has reduced. Indwelling urethral catheters may be helpful during the initial healing phase. Occasionally large callus formation causes urethral constriction, warranting permanent urethrostomy or penile amputation.

Urethral prolapse

Excessive sexual excitement or urinary straining may produce prolapse of the terminal portion of

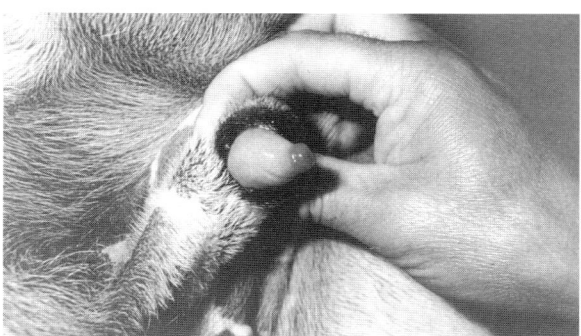

Figure 40.16 Prolapse of the urethral mucosa in a 2-year-old cross-bred dog.

the urethra (Fig. 40.16). The everted portion becomes oedematous and may bleed, although some dogs show no clinical signs. The urethra may be replaced if not damaged (Firestone, 1941), although amputation of the distal penis may be necessary (Copland, 1975). The condition has only been described in intact males (Johnston, 1989b) and castration should be considered to prevent recurrence.

Lymphoid hyperplasia

Small raised 1–2 mm nodules may be identified on the surface of the caudal glans in the region of the preputial reflection. These are not vesicles although the condition has been termed 'dog pox' (Joshua, 1975). Lesions are commonly noted at routine examination, their significance is unknown, although they may become traumatized and bleed during mating or semen collection.

Preputial discharge

Mucopurulent preputial discharge is normal in the male dog although excessive discharge may be associated with posthitis (inflammation of the prepuce). Many species of aerobic bacteria are frequently isolated both in normal dogs and in those with preputial discharge (Allen and Dagnall, 1982). Preputial trauma, foreign bodies and tumours must be eliminated as primary causative lesions. In many cases the aetiology remains unknown; mycoplasmas were isolated in 92% of cases of balanoposthitis in one study (Doig, 1981). Culture of mycoplasmas or pure growths of antimicrobial resistant bacteria such as

Pseudomonas aeruginosa may be significant, although these have been identified in normal dogs. Severe inflammation may produce spermatozoal abnormalities probably mediated by heat stress (Oettle and Soley, 1986); these changes are reversible (Larsen, 1980; Oettle and Soley, 1986).

Treatment involves the removal of the predisposing cause and flushing of the preputial cavity and penis with antimicrobial or weak antiseptic solutions. Parenteral drug administration is usually of little value.

Discharge noted at the prepuce may also be haemorrhagic in nature and commonly originates from the prostate gland, although urethral prolapse and urethral mucosal neoplasms may also bleed.

Penile neoplasms

Tumours of the penis are rare in the dog. Squamous cell carcinomas are the most common type and these commonly spread locally and metastasize to the inguinal lymph nodes. Haemorrhage from an ulcerated neoplasm may be the first clinical sign, although usually there is frequent penile licking. Radical surgical resection is warranted in the absence of metastases.

Transmissible venereal tumour

This is a coitally transmitted neoplasm affecting the external genitalia of either sex that is not identified in the UK (Booth, 1994). Transmission of cells from the infected individual 'seeds' the genital mucosa of the recipient (Cohen, 1974). Lesions are friable and there is frequently ulceration and a serosangineous discharge. Excisional biopsy is required for definitive diagnosis. Single neoplasms should be treated by amputation. Various chemotherapy regimes have been suggested, including the use of cyclophosphamide and vincristine (Calvert *et al.*, 1982).

THE TOM

Reproductive endocrinology

Although it is assumed that endocrinological events in the tom are similar to those in other species, there are many areas where basic data are not available. As in the dog, circulating testosterone concentrations have been shown to fluctuate markedly (Goodrowe *et al.*, 1985). The concentrations of FSH and LH are not well established, but the response of plasma LH and testosterone to the administration of GnRH has been studied in both entire and castrated animals and shown to be similar to other species (Johnson and Gray, 1981).

Abnormal endocrinological events

Hypogonadism

Little information is available on this condition in the cat. However, it may occur following pituitary dysfunction and has been reported following fetal or neonatal panleukopenia virus infection (Csiza *et al.*, 1971; De Lahunta, 1971). Testicular hypoplasia has also been noted in toms with chromosomal abnormalities (see below).

Poor libido

Male cats which have been recently introduced to a new environment may demonstrate poor libido, or aggression to queens. These problems are more frequently encountered with young or inexperienced animals and reflects poor breeding management rather than endocrinological abnormalities. The administration of exogenous androgens does not improve libido and the negative feedback effects may reduce endogenous testosterone secretion and semen quality (Michael, 1961).

Impaired spermatogenesis

There are no data available on the endocrinological investigation of reproductive function in male cats with abnormalities of spermatogenesis. Testicular hypoplasia and absence of spermatogenesis has been reported in tortoiseshell-coloured toms associated with chromosomal abnormalities (Centerwall and Benirschke, 1975).

Reproductive organs

The testes of the cat are similar to the dog although they are positioned ventral to the anus. The testes are composed of seminiferous tubules supported by the mediastinum testis. The bilobed prostate gland is small and intrapelvic. The tom also has a pair of bulbourethral glands lateral to the base of the penis. The penis contains a small ungrooved os and is directed caudally within the prepuce; the undivided glans penis is conical in shape and is covered by cornified papillae.

Diseases of the testes and scrotum

Absence of gonads

Anorchia has not been reported in the cat. Monorchidism has been rarely noted (Herron, 1986).

Cryptorchidism

In most kittens the testes have descended into the scrotum at birth (Shille, 1989). Unilateral and bilateral non-descent of the testes is usually noted during routine examination. Clinical signs may occur later in life when abdominal enlargement and discomfort are related to the increased size of the gonad. Feminization has not been reported (Stein, 1981). A genetic base for the condition has not been established, although this is likely to be similar to the dog. Medical therapy is not ethical; treatment is by removal of both testes to prevent neoplasia and breeding.

Orchitis

Testicular inflammation is most commonly associated with trauma (especially bite wounds) in the cat; specific infectious agents are rarely involved. Conservative therapy involving the administration of antimicrobial preparations may be successful, although the complications of infection and haemorrhage may necessitate surgical debridement or castration.

Testicular degeneration

Reversible testicular degeneration and azoospermia has been reported associated with hypervitaminosis A. This might occur in tom cats fed large amounts of raw liver (Seawright et al., 1970). Elimination of the vitamin imbalance is usually curative.

Testicular tumours

Testicular tumours are rare in the tom (Feldman and Nelson, 1987b). Sertoli cell tumours have been reported in aged animals (Herron, 1986).

Diseases of the epididymides

There have been no specific epididymal lesions identified in the cat, although inflammation associated with traumatic orchitis is not uncommon.

Diseases of the prostate gland

There are no reports of neoplasia or disease of the prostate gland in the tom (Herron, 1986).

Diseases of the penis and prepuce

Penile–preputial adhesions

The early castration of kittens before the common layer of stratified epithelium, which joins the prepuce to the penis, has separated may result in adhesion formation between these structures (Herron, 1971). These cases are not usually associated with clinical disease, although the changes may predispose to infection. Castration later than 6 months of age, after penile–preputial separation will prevent the problem.

Penile abnormalities

Few cases of abnormalities of the penis have been reported in the tom. Penile hypoplasia, hypospadius and abnormal os penis have not been reported.

Phimosis

An abnormally small preputial orifice is an uncommon finding, but has been reported in the domestic short hair tom (Elkins, 1983). This abnormality may occur congenitally or as the result of trauma or inflammation. The clinical signs are similar to those in the dog, and the condition may be treated surgically by enlargement of the preputial orifice.

Priapism

Priapism (persistent and painful erection) is rare in the tom but may follow attempted mating and trauma may play a role in the aetiology (Gunn-Moore et al., 1995). Penile amputation is usually necessary.

Paraphimosis

Failure of the glans penis to be retracted fully into the penis due to an abnormal preputial ring has been described (Kirk, 1931). Drying and necrosis of the penis and secondary urethral obstruction may result, therefore prompt surgical correction is necessary.

Hair ring

A ring of hair around the prepuce may produce signs of prolonged thrusting or pain during mating (Hart and Peterson, 1971). These rings may also compress the penis and cause urine retention (Wooldridge, 1908). Careful examination of the male should allow identification and removal of hair rings before they produce clinical signs.

Penile and preputial inflammation

Inflammation of the penis and prepuce is most commonly associated with trauma. Conservative therapy involving antimicrobial and anti-inflammatory preparations may be successful, although surgical debridement may be necessary if there are complications of infection and haemorrhage.

Penile neoplasms

Tumours of the cat penis have not been reported (Johnston, 1989b).

REFERENCES

Ackerman, N. (1981) Radiographic evaluation of the uterus. *Veterinary Radiology* 22, 252–259.

Adler, P.L. and Hobson, H.P. (1978) Hypospadius: a review of the veterinary literature and a report of three cases in the dog. *Journal of the American Animal Hospital Association* 14, 721–727.

Al-Bassam, M.A., Thompson, R.G. and O'Donnell, L. (1981a) Normal post-partum involution of the uterus in the dog. *Canadian Journal of Comparative Medicine* 45, 217–232.

Al-Bassam, M.A., Thompson, R.G. and O'Donnell, L. (1981b) Involution abnormalities in the post-partum uterus of the bitch. *Veterinary Pathology* 18, 208–218.

Allen, W.E. (1982) Attempted oestrus induction in four bitches using pregnant mare serum gonadotrophin. *Journal of Small Animal Practice* 23, 223–231.

Allen, W.E. (1986) Pseudopregnancy in the bitch: the current view on aetiology and treatment. *Journal of Small Animal Practice* 27, 419–424.

Allen, W.E. (1992) *Fertility and Obstetrics in the Dog*. Blackwell Scientific Publications London, pp. 43–55.

Allen, W.E. and Dagnall, G.R.J. (1982) Some observations on the aerobic bacterial flora of the genital tract of the dog and bitch. *Journal of Small Animal Practice* 23, 325–336.

Allen, W.E. and England, G.C.W. (1990) Reproductive endocrinology of the bitch. In: *Manual of Small Animal Endocrinology* (Ed. M. Hutchinson). British Small Animal Veterinary Association, Cheltenham, pp. 127–142.

Allen, W.E. and Longstaffe, J.A. (1982) Spermatozoal arrest associated with focal degenerative orchitis in related dogs. *Journal of Small Animal Practice* 23, 337–343.

Allen, W.E. and Patel, J.R. (1982) Autoimmune orchitis in two related dogs. *Journal of Small Animal Practice* 23, 713–718.

Amman, R.P. (1986) Reproductive physiology and endocrinology of the dog. In: *Current Therapy in Theriogenology*, 2nd edn (Ed. D.A. Morrow). W.B. Saunders, Philadelphia, pp. 532–538.

Andersen, A.C. and Simpson, M.E. (1973) *The Ovary and Reproductive Cycle of the Dog (Beagle)*. Geron-X Inc., California.

Andersen, A.C. and Wooten, E. (1959) The estrous cycle of the dog. In: *Reproduction in Domestic Animals* I. (Eds H.H. Cole and P.T. Cupps). Academic Press, New York, p. 359.

Arbeiter, K. (1993) Anovulatory ovarian cycles in dogs. *Journal of Reproduction and Fertility Supplement* 47, 453–456.

Arnall, L. (1961) Prolapse of the uterus in the cat. *Veterinary Record* 73, 750–753.

Arnold, S., Arnold, P., Concannon, P.W., Weilenmann, R., Hubler, M., Casal, M., Dobeli, M., Eggenberger, E. and Rusch, P. (1989) Effect of duration of PMSG treatment on induction of oestrus, pregnancy rates and the complications of hyperoestrogenism in dogs. *Journal of Reproduction and Fertility Supplement* 39, 115–122.

Atilola, M.A.O. and Pennock, P.W. (1986) Cystic uterus masculinus in the dog. *Veterinary Radiology* 27, 8–14.

Auskova, M., Rezabek, K., Zikan, V. and Semonsky, M. (1974) Induction of oestrus and ovulation with an ergoline derivative, substance VUFB 6638, an inhibitor of prolactin secretion. *Physiologia Bohemoslovenica* 23, 417–421.

Austad, R. and Bjerkas, E. (1976) Eclampsia in the bitch. *Journal of Small Animal Practice* 17, 793–798.

Austad, R., Lunde, A. and Sjaastad, O.V. (1976) Peripheral plasma levels of oestradiol-17β and progesterone in the bitch during the oestrous cycle, in normal pregnancy and after dexamethasone treatment. *Journal of Reproduction and Fertility* 46, 129–136.

Baba, E., Hata, H. and Fukata, T. (1983) Vaginal and uterine microflora of adult dogs. *American Journal of Veterinary Research* 44, 606–609.

Banks, D.R. and Stabenfeldt, G.H. (1983) Prolactin in the cat. II. Diurnal patterns and photoperiod effects. *Biology of Reproduction* 28, 933–939.

Barrett, R.E. and Theilen, G.H. (1977) Neoplasms of the canine and feline reproductive tracts. In: *Current Veterinary Therapy* VI (Ed. R.W. Kirk), W.B. Saunders, Philadelphia, pp. 1179–1183.

Barsanti, J.A. and Finco, D.R. (1984) Evaluation of techniques for diagnosis of canine prostatic diseases. *Journal of the American Veterinary Medical Association* 185, 198–200.

Barsanti, J.A. and Finco, D.R. (1986) Canine prostatic diseases. *Veterinary Clinics of North America: Small Animal Practice* 16, 587–599.

Barsanti, J.A. and Finco, D.R. (1989) Canine prostatic

disease. In: *Textbook of Veterinary Internal Medicine*, 3rd edn (Ed. S.J. Ettinger), W.B. Saunders, Philadelphia, pp. 1859–1880.

Beale, K.M., Bloomberg, M.S., Gilder, J.V., Wolfson, B.B. and Keising, K. (1992) Correlation of racing and reproductive performance in greyhounds with response to thyroid function testing. *Journal of the American Animal Hospital Association* **28**, 263–269.

Beck, A.M. and McEntee, K. (1966) Subinvolution of placental sites in a bitch. A case report. *Cornell Veterinarian* **56**, 269–277.

Bjurstrom, L. and Linde-Forsberg, C. (1992) Long term study of aerobic bacteria of the genital tract of breeding bitches. *American Journal of Veterinary Research* **53**, 665–669.

Booth, M.J. (1994) Canine transmissible venereal tumour and ovarian papillary cystadenoma–carcinoma in a bitch. *Journal of Small Animal Practice* **34**, 39–42.

Bouchard, G.F., Gross, S., Ganjam, V.K., Youngquist, R.S., Concannon, P.W., Krause, G.F. and Reddy, C.S. (1993) Oestrus induction in the bitch with the synthetic oestrogen diethylstilboestrol. *Journal of Reproduction and Fertility Supplement* **47**, 515–516.

Breitkopf, M., Tammer, I., Hoffmann, B. and Bostedt, M. (1996) Treatment of pyometra with antigestagens in the bitch. *Proceedings of the 3rd International Symposium on Reproduction of Dogs, Cats and Exotic Carnivores.* p. 10.

Brodey, R.S. and Roszel, J.F. (1967) Neoplasms of the canine uterus, vagina and vulva: a clinicopathologic survey of 90 cases. *Journal of the American Veterinary Medical Association* **149**, 1047–1053.

Burke, T.J. (1986) *Small Animal Reproduction and Infertility*. Lea and Febiger, Philadelphia.

Burke, T.J. and Smith, C.W. (1975) Vulvovaginal cleft in a dog. *Journal of the American Animal Hospital Association* **11**, 774–776.

Calvert, C., Leifer, C.E. and MacEwen, E.G. (1982) Vincristine for treatment of transmissible venereal tumor in the dog. *Journal of the American Veterinary Medical Association* **183**, 987–990.

Carmichael, L.E. (1966) Abortion in 200 beagles (news report). *Journal of the American Veterinary Medical Association* **149**, 1126.

Carmichael, L.E. and Kenney, R.M. (1968) Canine abortion caused by *Brucella canis*. *Journal of the American Veterinary Medical Association* **152**, 605–616.

Cauvin, A., Sullivan, M., Harvey, M.J. and Thompson, M. (1995) Vaginal cysts causing tenesmus in a bitch. *Journal of Small Animal Practice* **36**, 321–324.

Centerwall, W.R. and Benirschke, K. (1975) An animal model for the XXY Klinefelter's syndrome in man: tortoise-shell and calico male cats. *American Journal of Veterinary Research* **26**, 1275–1280.

Christiansen, Ib. J. (1984) *Reproduction in the Dog and Cat*. Baillière Tindall, London.

Christie D.W., Bailey, J.B. and Bell, E.T. (1972) Classification of cell types in vaginal smears during the canine oestrous cycle. *British Veterinary Journal* **128**, 301–309.

Cline, E.M., Jennings, L.L. and Sojka, N.J. (1980) Breeding laboratory cats during artificially induced estrus. *Laboratory Animal Science* **30**, 1003–1005.

Cohen, D. (1974) The mechanism of transmission of the transmissible venereal tumor of the dog. *Transplantation* **17**, 8–11.

Colby, E.D. (1980) The estrus cycle and pregnancy. In: *Current Therapy in Theriogenology*, 1st edn (Ed. D.A. Morrow). W.B. Saunders, Philadelphia, pp. 832–839.

Cole, C.R., Sanger, V.L., Farrell, R.L. and Kornder, J.D. (1954) The present status of toxoplasmosis in veterinary medicine. *North American Veterinarian* **35**, 265–270.

Concannon, P.W. (1983) Reproductive physiology and endocrine patterns of the bitch. In: *Current Veterinary Therapy. Small Animal Practice.* Vol VIII (Ed. R.W. Kirk). W.B. Saunders, Philadelphia, pp. 886–900.

Concannon, P.W. (1986) Canine physiology of reproduction. In *Small Animal Reproduction and Infertility* (Ed. T.J. Burke). Lea and Febiger, Philadelphia, pp. 23–78.

Concannon, P.W. (1989) Induction of fertile oestrus in anoestrus dogs by constant infusion of GnRH agonists. *Journal of Reproduction and Fertility Supplement* **39**, 149–160.

Concannon, P.W., Hansel, W. and Visek, W.J. (1975) The ovarian cycle of the bitch: plasma estrogen, LH and progesterone. *Biology of Reproduction* **13**, 112–121.

Concannon, P.W., Hansel, W. and McEntee, K. (1977a) Changes in LH, progesterone and sexual behavior associated with preovulatory luteinization in the bitch. *Biology of Reproduction* **17**, 604–613.

Concannon, P.W., Powers, M.E., Holder, W. and Hansel, W. (1977b) Pregnancy and parturition in the bitch. *Biology of Reproduction* **16**, 517–526.

Concannon, P.W., Knight, P.J. and Hamilton, J.M. (1978) Parturition and lactation in the bitch. Serum progesterone, cortisol and prolactin. *Biology of Reproduction* **18**, 28.

Concannon, P.W., Weigand, N., Wilson, S. and Hansel, W. (1979) Sexual behavior in ovariectomised bitches in response to estrogen and progesterone treatment. *Biology of Reproduction* **20**, 799–809.

Concannon, P.W., Altszuler, N. and Hampshire, J. (1980a) Growth hormone, prolactin, and cortisol in dogs developing mammary nodules and an acromegalic-like appearance during treatment with medroxyprogesterone acetate. *Endocrinology* **106**, 1173–1177.

Concannon, P.W., Hodson, B. and Lein, D. (1980b) Reflex LH release in estrous cats following single and multiple copulations. *Biology of Reproduction* **23**, 111–117.

Concannon, P.W., McCann, J.P. and Temple, M. (1989) Biology and endocrinology of ovulation, pregnancy and parturition in the dog. *Journal of Reproduction and Fertility Supplement* **39**, 3–25.

Copland, M.D. (1975) Prolapse of the penile urethra in a dog. *New Zealand Veterinary Journal* **23**, 180–183.

Copland, M.D. and Maclachlan, N.J. (1976) Aplasia of the epididymis and vas deferens in the dog. *Journal of Small Animal Practice* **17**, 443–449.

Cotchin, E. (1960) Testicular neoplasms in dogs. *Journal of Comparative Pathology* **70**, 408–416.

Cotchin, E. (1961) Canine ovarian neoplasms. *Research in Veterinary Science* **2**, 133–141.

Crow, S.E. (1980) Neoplasms of the reproductive organs and mammary glands of the dog. In: *Current Therapy in Theriogenology*, 1st edn (Ed. D.A. Morrow). W.B. Saunders, Philadelphia, 640–646.

Csiza, C.K., Scott, F.W., de Lahunta, A. and Gillespie, J.H. (1971) Feline viruses XIV. Transplacental infections in spontaneous panleukopenia of cats. *Cornell Veterinarian* **61**, 423–439.

Dahlbom, M., Andersson, M., Huszenicza, G. and Alanko, M. (1995) Poor semen quality in Irish wolfhounds: a clinical, hormonal and spermatological study. *Journal of Small Animal Practice* **36**, 547–552.

DeCoster, R., Beckers, J-F., Beerens, D. and DeMay, J. (1983) A homologous radioimmunoassay for canine prolactin plasma levels during the reproductive cycle. *Acta Endocrinologica* **103**, 473–478.

De Lahunta, A. (1971) Comments on cerebellar ataxia and its congenital transmission in cats by feline leukopenia virus. *Journal of the American Veterinary Medical Association* **158**, 901–906.

DePalatis, L., Moore, J. and Falvo, R.E. (1978) Plasma concentrations of testosterone and LH in the male dog. *Journal of Reproduction and Fertility* **52**, 201–207.

Dickie, M.B. and Arbeiter, K. (1993) Diagnosis and therapy of the subinvolution of placental sites in the bitch. *Journal of Reproduction and Fertility Supplement* **47**, 471–475.

Doig, P.A. (1981) The genital mycoplasma and ureoplasma flora of healthy and diseased dogs. *Canadian Journal of Comparative Medicine* **45**, 233–237.

Donnay, I., Rauis, J., Wouters-Ballman, P., Devleeschouwer, N., Leclercq, G. and Verstegen, J.P. (1993) Receptors for oestrogen, progesterone and epidernal growth factor in normal and tumorous canine mammary tissues. *Journal of Reproduction and Fertility Supplement* **47**, 501–512.

Dover, P.M. (1965) An unusual case of dystocia in a bitch. *New Zealand Veterinary Journal* **13**, 201.

Dow, C. (1960) Ovarian abnormalities in the bitch. *Journal of Comparative Pathology* **70**, 59–69.

Dubey, J.P. and Johnstone, I. (1982) Fatal neonatal toxoplasmosis in cats. *Journal of the American Animal Hospital Association* **18**, 461–469.

Durham, S.K. and Dietze, A.E. (1986) Prostatic adenocarcinoma with and without metastasis to bone in dogs. *Journal of the American Veterinary Medical Association* **188**, 1432–1435.

Eigenmann, J.E. and Venker-van Haagen, A.J. (1981) Progestagen-induced and spontaneous canine acromegaly due to reversible growth hormone over-production. *Journal of the American Animal Hospital Association* **17**, 813–822.

Elkins, A.D. (1983) Surgical correction of congenital stricture of the preputial orifice in the cat. *Feline Practice* **13**, 20–23.

England, G.C.W. (1991) The relationship between ultrasonographic appearance, testicular size, spermatozoal output and testicular lesions in the dog. *Journal of Small Animal Practice* **32**, 306–311.

England, G.C.W. (1992a) Vaginal cytology and cervicovaginal mucus arborisation in the breeding management of bitches. *Journal of Small Animal Practice* **33**, 577–582.

England, G.C.W. (1992b) Ultrasound evaluation of pregnancy and spontaneous embryonic resorption in the bitch. *Journal of Small Animal Practice* **33**, 430–436.

England, G.C.W. and Allen, W.E. (1989a) Crystallisation patterns in anterior vaginal fluid from bitches in oestrus. *Journal of Reproduction and Fertility* **86**, 335–339.

England, G.C.W. and Allen, W.E. (1989b) Real time ultrasonic imaging of the canine ovary and uterus. *Journal of Reproduction and Fertility Supplement* **39**, 91–100.

England, G.C.W. and Allen, W.E. (1991a) Repeatability of events during spontaneous and gonadotrophin-induced oestrus in bitches. *Journal of Reproduction and Fertility* **93**, 443–448.

England, G.C.W. and Allen, W.E. (1991b) The effect of the synthetic androgen mesterolone upon seminal characteristics of dogs. *Journal of Small Animal Practice* **32**, 271–274.

England, G.C.W., Allen, W.E. and Blythe, S.A. (1989a) Variability of the time of calculated LH release in 218 canine pregnancies. *Veterinary Record* **125**, 624–625.

England, G.C.W., Allen, W.E. and Porter, D.J. (1989b) Evaluation of the testosterone response to hCG and the identification of a presumed anorchid dog. *Journal of Small Animal Practice* **30**, 441–443.

England, G.C.W., Allen, W.E. and Porter, D.J. (1990) Studies on canine pregnancy using B-mode ultrasound; development of the conceptus and determination of gestational age. *Journal of Small Animal Practice* **31**, 324–329.

Feeney, D.A. and Johnston, G.R. (1986) The ovaries and testes. In: *Textbook of Veterinary Diagnostic Radiology* (Ed. D.E. Thrall). W.B. Saunders, Philadelphia, pp. 467–468.

Feeney, D.A., Johnston, G.R., Klausner, J.S., Perman, V., Leininger, J.R and Tomlinson, M.J. (1987) Canine prostatic disease – comparison of ultrasonographic appearance with morphologic and microbiologic findings: 30 cases (1981–1985). *Journal of the American Veterinary Medical Association* **190**, 1027–1034.

Feldman, E.C. and Nelson, R.W. (1986) Pyometra. *Veterinary Clinics of North America: Small Animal Practice* 16, 561–576.

Feldman, E.C. and Nelson, R.W. (1987a) Canine female reproduction. In: *Canine and Feline Endocrinology and Reproduction*. W.B. Saunders, Philadelphia, pp. 399–547.

Feldman, E.C. and Nelson, R.W. (1987b) Feline reproduction. In: *Canine and Feline Endocrinology and Reproduction*. W.B. Saunders, Philadelphia, pp. 525–548.

Felts, J. (1982) Hermaphroditism in the cat. *Journal of the American Veterinary Medical Association* 181, 925–928.

Firestone, W.M. (1941) Prolapse of the male urethra. *Journal of the American Veterinary Medical Association* 99, 135–139.

Freak, M.J. (1977) Foetal resorption. *Pedigree Digest* 4, 4.

Gier, H.T. and Marion, G.B. (1969) Development of mammalian testes and genital ducts. *Biology of Reproduction* 1, 1–23.

Gilbert, R.O., Nothling, J.O. and Oettle, E.E. (1989) A retrospective study of 40 cases of canine pyometra-metritis treated with prostaglandin F-2alpha and broad-spectrum antibacterial drugs. *Journal of Reproduction and Fertility Supplement* 39, 225–229.

Glenn, B.L. (1968) Subinvolution of placental sites in the bitch. *18th Gaines Veterinary Symposium*. White Plains, Gaines Dog Research Center, pp. 7–10.

Goodrowe, K.L., Chakraborty, P.K. and Wildt, D.E. (1985) Pituitary and gonadal response to exogenous LH-releasing hormone in the male domestic cat. *Journal of Endocrinology* 105, 175–181.

Goodrowe, K.L., Howard, J.G., Schmidt, P.M. and Wildt, D.E. (1989) Reproductive biology of the domestic cat with special reference to endocrinology, sperm function and in-vitro fertilization. *Journal of Reproduction and Fertility Supplement* 39, 73–90.

Gordon, R.D., Thomas, M.J., Poynting, J.M. and Stocks, A.E. (1975) Effect of mesterolone on plasma LH, FSH, and testosterone. *Andrologia* 7, 287–296.

Gourley, I.M. (1975) Treatment of canine pyometra without ovariohysterectomy. In: *Current Techniques in Small Animal Surgery* (Ed. M.J. Bojrab), Lea and Febiger, Philadelphia, pp. 244–246.

Greulich, W.W. (1934) Artificially induced ovulation in the cat (*Felis domesticus*). *Anatomical Record* 58, 217–224.

Gruffydd-Jones, T.J. (1980) Acute mastitis in a cat. *Feline Practice* 10, 41–45.

Gruffydd-Jones, T.J. (1985) The genital system. In: *Feline Medicine and Therapeutics* (Ed. E.A. Chandler, C.J. Gaskell and A.D.R. Hilbery). Blackwell Scientific Publications, Oxford, pp. 152–157.

Gruffydd-Jones, T.J. (1990) Reproductive endocrinology of the cat. In: *Manual of Small Animal Endocrinology* (Ed. M. Hutchinson). British Small Animal Veterinary Association, Cheltenham, pp. 143–152.

Gunn-Moore, D.A., Brown, P.J., Holt, P.E. and Gruffydd-Jones, T.J. (1995) Priapism in seven cats. *Journal of Small Animal Practice* 36, 262–266.

Hadley, J.C. (1972) Spermatogenic arrest with azoospermia in two Welsh Springer Spaniels. *Journal of Small Animal Practice* 13, 135–138.

Hadley, J.C. (1975) Unconjugated oestrogen and progesterone concentrations in the blood of bitches with false pregnancy and pyometra. *Veterinary Record* 96, 545–547.

Handaja Kusuma, P.S. and Tainurier, D. (1993) Comparison of induction of oestrus in dogs using metergoline, metergoline plus human chorionic gonadotrophin, or pregnant mares' serum gonadotrophin. *Journal of Reproduction and Fertility Supplement* 47, 363–370.

Hardy, W.D. (1981) Feline leukemia virus non-neoplastic diseases. *Journal of the American Animal Hospital Association* 17, 941–947.

Hart, B.L. and Peterson, D.M. (1971) Penile hair rings in male cats may prevent mating. *Laboratory Animal Science* 21, 422–423.

Hashimoto, A. and Hirai, K. (1986) Canine herpesvirus infection. In: *Current Therapy in Theriogenology*, 2nd edn. (Ed. D.A. Morrow). W.B. Saunders, Philadelphia, pp. 516–520.

Hawe, R.S. and Loeb, W.F. (1984) Caudal vaginal agenesis and progressive renal disease in a Shih Tzu. *Journal of the American Animal Hospital Association* 20, 123–130.

Hayes, A. and Harvey, H.J. (1979) Treatment of metastatic granulosa cell tumor in a dog. *Journal of the American Veterinary Medical Association* 174, 1304–1308.

Hayes, H.M. and Pendergrass, T.W. (1976) Canine testicular tumors: epidemiologic features of 410 dogs. *International Journal of Cancer* 18, 482–487.

Henderson, R.T. (1984) Prostaglandin therapeutics in the bitch and queen. *Australian Veterinary Journal* 61, 317–319.

Herron, M.A. (1971) A potential consequence of prepubertal feline castration. *Feline Practice* 1, 17–25.

Herron, M.A. (1977) Feline reproduction. *Veterinary Clinics of North America* 7, 715–722.

Herron, M.A. (1986) Infertility from noninfectious causes. In: *Current Therapy in Theriogenology*, 2nd edn (Ed. D.A. Morrow) W.B. Saunders, Philadelphia, pp. 829–834.

Herron, M.A. and Boehringer, B.T. (1975) Male pseudohermaphroditism in the cat. *Feline Practice* 5, 30–36.

Hill, H. and Mare, C.J. (1974) Genital disease in dogs caused by canine herpesvirus. *American Journal of Veterinary Research* 35, 669–675.

Hirsh, D.C. and Wiger, N. (1977) The bacterial flora of the normal canine vagina compared with that of vaginal exudates. *Journal of Small Animal Practice* 18, 25–32.

Holt, P.E. and Sayle, B. (1981) Congenital vestibulo-vaginal stenosis in the bitch. *Journal of Small Animal Practice* **22**, 67–75.

Hoover, E.A. and Griesemer, R.A. (1971) Experimental feline herpesvirus infection in the pregnant cat. *American Journal of Pathology* **65**, 172–178.

Hotston-Moore, A. and Wotton, P.R. (1973) Preparturient hypoglycaemia in two bitches. *Veterinary Record* **133**, 396–397.

Huggins, C. and Clark, P.G. (1940) Quantitative studies of prostatic secretion II. The effect of castration and of estrogen injection on the normal and on the hyperplastic prostate glands of dogs. *Journal of Experimental Medicine* **72**, 747–752.

Hutchinson, J.A. (1973) Persistence of the penile frenulum in dogs. *Canadian Veterinary Journal* **14**, 71–75.

Iguer-Ovada, M. and Verstegen, J. (1996) Effect of finasteride on sperm output and characteristics, prostate function and fertility in male dogs. *Proceedings of the Third International Symposium on Reproduction of Dogs, Cats, and Exotic Carnivores*, p. 48.

Jackson, R.F., Bruss, M.C. and Growney, P.J. (1980) Hypoglycemia-ketonemia in a pregnant bitch. *Journal of the American Veterinary Medical Association* **177**, 1123–1127.

James, R.W., Heywood, R. and Fowler, D.J. (1979a) Serial percutaneous testicular biopsy in the beagle dog. *Journal of Small Animal Practice* **20**, 219–228.

James, R.W., Crook, D. and Heywood, R. (1979b) Canine pituitary-testicular function in relation to toxicity testing. *Toxicology* **13**, 237–247.

Jeffery, K.L. (1974) Fracture of the os penis in a dog. *Journal of the American Animal Hospital Association* **10**, 41–45.

Jeukenne, P. and Verstegen, J. (1997) Termination of dioestrus and induction of oestrus in dioestrous non-pregnant bitches by the prolactin antagonist cabergoline. *Journal of Reproduction and Fertility* **51**(Supplement), 59–66.

Jochle, W., Ballabio, R. and Di Salle, E. (1987) Inhibition of lactation in the beagle bitch with the prolactin inhibitor cabergoline (FCE 21336): dose response and aspects of long term safety. *Theriogenology* **27**, 799–811.

Jochle, W., Arbeiter, K., Post, K., Ballabio, R. and D'Ver, A.S. (1989) Effects on pseudopregnancy, pregnancy and interoestrous intervals of pharmacological suppression of prolactin secretion in female dogs and cats. *Journal of Reproduction and Fertility Supplement* **39**, 199–207.

Johnson, C.A. (1991) Diagnosis and treatment of chronic vaginitis in the bitch. *Veterinary Clinics of North America: Small Animal Practice* **21**, 523–531.

Johnson, L.M. and Gray, V.L. (1981) Luteinizing hormone in the cat. II. Mating-induced secretion. *Theriogenology* **109**, 247–252.

Johnston, D.I. (1985) The prostate. In: *Textbook of Small Animal Surgery* (Ed. D.H. Slatter), W.B. Saunders, Philadelphia, p. 1635.

Johnston, S.D. (1988) Noninfectious causes of infertility in the dog and cat. In: *Fertility and Infertility in Veterinary Practice* (Eds J.A. Laing, W.J. Morgan and W.C. Wagtner) Baillière Tindall, London, pp. 160–172.

Johnston, S.D. (1989a) Premature gonadal failure in female dogs and cats. *Journal of Reproduction and Fertility*, Supplement **39**, 65–72.

Johnston, S.D. (1989b) Disorders of the external genitalia of the male. In: *Textbook of Veterinary Internal Medicine*, 3rd edn (Ed. S.J. Ettinger). W.B. Saunders, Philadelphia, pp. 1881–1889.

Johnston, S.D. (1991) Clinical approach to infertility in bitches with primary anestrus. *Veterinary Clinics of North America: Small Animal Practice* **21**, 421–425.

Johnston, S.D., Buoen, L.C., Madl, J.E., Weber, A.F. and Smith, F.O. (1983) X-chromosome monosomy (37, XO) in a Burmese cat with gonadal dysgenesis. *Journal of the American Veterinary Medical Association* **182**, 986–989.

Jones, D.E. and Joshua, J.O. (1982) *Reproductive Clinical Problems in the Dog*, 1st edn. Wright, London, p 25.

Joshua, J.O. (1975) Dog pox: some clinical aspects of an eruptive condition of certain mucous surfaces in dogs. *Veterinary Record* **96**, 300–302.

Kilham, L., Margolis, G. and Colby, E.D. (1971) Cerebellar ataxia and its congenital transmission in cats by feline panleukopenia virus. *Journal of the American Veterinary Medical Association* **158**, 888–901.

Kirk, H. (1931) Phimosis and paraphimosis in the cat. *Veterinary Record* **11**, 832–833.

Kipnis, R.M. (1974) Membranous penile urethra and prepucial abnormality in a dog. *Veterinary Medicine Small Animal Clinician* **69**, 750–751.

Knight, P.J., Hamilton, J.M. and Hiddleston, W.A. (1977) Serum prolactin during pregnancy and lactation in the beagle bitch. *Veterinary Record* **101**, 202.

Lagerstedt, A-S. (1993) A method for uterine catheterisation in the bitch and its use for hysterography and uterine drainage. Thesis. Veterinarmedicinska fakulteten, Uppsala, Sweden.

Laliberte, L. (1986) Pregnancy, obstetrics and postpartum management of the queen. In: *Current Therapy in Theriogenology*, 2nd edn (Ed. D.A. Morrow), W.B. Saunders, Philadelphia, pp. 812–821.

Larsen, R.E. (1977) Testicular biopsy in the dog. *Veterinary Clinics of North America* **7**, 747–755.

Larsen, R.E. (1980) Infertility in the male dog. In: *Current Therapy in Theriogenology*, 1st edn (ed. D.A. Morrow), W.B. Saunders, Philadelphia, pp. 646–654.

Larsen, R.E. and Johnston, S.D. (1980) Management of canine infertility. In: *Current Veterinary Therapy VII* (ed. R.W. Kirk) W.B. Saunders, Philadelphia, pp. 1226–1231.

Lawler, D.F., Johnston, S.D., Hegstad, R.L., Keltner, D.G. and Owens, S.F. (1993) Ovulation without cervical stimulation in domestic cats. *Journal of Reproduction and Fertility Supplement* **47**, 57–61.

Lein, D.H. (1977) Canine orchitis. In: *Current Veterinary Therapy* VI (ed. R.W. Kirk). W.B. Saunders, Philadelphia, pp. 1255–1259.

Lein, D.H. (1983) Pyometritis in the bitch and queen. In: *Current Veterinary Therapy*, 8th edn (ed. R.W. Kirk). W.B. Saunders, Philadelphia, pp. 942–944.

Linde, C. and Karlsson, I. (1984) The correlation between the cytology of the vaginal smear and the time of ovulation in the bitch. *Journal of Small Animal Practice* **22**, 77–82.

Lindsay, F.E.F. (1983) The normal endoscopic appearance of the caudal reproductive tract of the cyclic and non-cyclic bitch; post uterine endoscopy. *Journal of Small Animal Practice* **24**, 1–5.

Lopate, C., Threlfall, W.R. and Rosol, T.J. (1989) Histopathologic and gross effects of testicular biopsy in the dog. *Theriogenology* **32**, 585–602.

Magne, M.L. (1986) Acute metritis in the bitch. In: *Current Therapy in Theriogenology*, 2nd edn (Ed. D.A. Morrow). W.B. Saunders, Philadelphia, pp. 505–506.

Mallo, G.L. (1971) False pregnancy. In: *Current Veterinary Therapy, Small Animal Practice*, 4th edn (ed. R.W. Kirk). W.B. Saunders, Philadephia, pp. 756–757.

Manning, P.J. (1979) Thyroid gland and arterial lesions of beagles with familial hypothyroidism and hyperlipoproteinemia. *American Journal of Veterinary Research* **40**, 820–828.

Marshall, F.H.A. and Halnan, E.T. (1917) On the post-oestrous changes occurring in the generative organs and mammary glands of the non-pregnant dog. *Proceedings of the Royal Society of London* **89**, 546–559.

McCann, J.P. and Concannon, P.W. (1983) Effects of sex, ovarian cycles, pregnancy and lactation on insulin and glucose response to exogenous glucose and glucagon in dogs (abstract). *Biology of Reproduction* **18**, 41.

McCann, J.P., Temple, M. and Concannon, P.W. (1988) Pregnancy-specific alterations in the metabolic endocrinology of domestic dogs including insulin resistance and modified regulation of growth hormone secretion. *Proceedings of the 11th International Congress of Animal Reproduction and Artificial Insemination*, Dublin, 2, pp. 103–105.

McKinney, H.R. (1973) A study of *Toxoplasma* infections in cats as detected by indirect fluorescent antibody method. *Veterinary Medicine Small Animal Clinician* **68**, 493–495.

Mellin, T.N., Orczyk, G.P., Hichens, M. and Behrman, H.R. (1976) Serum profiles of luteinizing hormone, progesterone and total estrogens during the canine estrous cycle. *Theriogenology* **5**, 175–187.

Memon, M.A., Pavletic, M.M. and Kumar, M.S.A. (1993) Chronic vaginal prolapse during pregnancy in a bitch. *Journal of the American Veterinary Medical Association* **202**, 295–297.

Meyers-Wallen, V.N. and Patterson, D.F. (1986) Disorders of sexual development in the dog. In: *Current Therapy in Theriogenology*, 2nd edn (ed. D.A. Morrow). W.B. Saunders, Philadelphia, pp. 567–574.

Meyers-Wallen, V.N. and Patterson, D.F. (1988) XX sex reversal in the American cocker spaniel dog: phenotypic expression and inheritance. *Human Genetics* **80**, 23–30.

Meyers-Wallen, V.N. and Patterson, D.F. (1989) Sexual differentiation and inherited disorders of sexual development in the dog. *Journal of Reproduction and Fertility Supplement* **39**, 57–64.

Mialot, J.P., Thibier, M., Toublanc, J.E., Castanier, M. and Scholler, R. (1988) Plasma concentration of luteinizing hormone, testosterone, dehydroepiandrosterone, androstenedione between birth and one year in the male dog; longitudinal study and hCG stimulation. *Andrologia* **20**, 145–154.

Michael, R.P. (1961) Observations upon the sexual behaviour of the domestic cat (*Felis catus*) under laboratory conditions. *Behaviour* **18**, 1–24.

Miyabayashi, T., Biller, D.S. and Cooley, A.J. (1990) Ultrasonographic appearance of torsion of a testicular seminoma in a cryptorchid dog. *Journal of Small Animal Practice* **31**, 401–403.

Morris, J.S., Dobson, J. and Bostock, D.E. (1993) Use of tamoxifen in the control of canine mammary neoplasia. *Veterinary Record* **133**, 539–542.

Moses, D.L. and Shille, V.M. (1988) Induction of estrus in greyhound bitches with prolonged idiopathic anestrus or with suppression of estrus after testosterone administration. *Journal of the American Veterinary Medical Association* **192**, 1541–1545.

Mosier, J.E. (1975) Common medical and behavioral problems in the cat. *Modern Veterinary Practice* **56**, 699–703.

Nelson, R.W. and Feldman, E.C. (1986a) Pyometra in the bitch. In: *Current Therapy in Theriogenology*, 2nd edn (ed. D.A. Morrow). W.B. Saunders, Philadelphia, pp. 567–574.

Nelson, R.W. and Feldman, E.C. (1986b) Pyometra. *Veterinary Clinics of North America, Small Animal Practice* **16**, 561–576.

Nelson, R.W., Feldman, E.C. and Stabenfeldt, G.H. (1982) Treatment of canine pyometra and endometritis with prostaglandin F2alpha. *Journal of the American Veterinary Medical Association* **181**, 899–903.

Nicholas, F.W., Muir, P. and Toll, G.L. (1980) An XXY male Burmese cat. *Journal of Heredity* **71**, 52–54.

Norsworthy, G.D. (1979) Kitten mortality complex. *Feline Practice* **9**, 57–64.

Oettle, E.E. and Soley, J.T. (1986) Severe sperm abnormalities with subsequent recovery following scrotal oedema and posthitis in a bulldog. *Journal of Small Animal Practice* **27**, 477–484.

Olson, P.N. (1989) Exfoliative cytology of the canine reproductive tract. *Proceedings of the Annual Meeting of the Society of Theriogenology*, pp. 259–263.

Olson, P.N.S. and Mather, E.C. (1978) Canine vaginal

and uterine bacterial flora. *Journal of the American Veterinary Medical Association* **172**, 708–710.

Olson, P.N., Bowen, R.A., Behrendt, M., Olson, J.D. and Nett, T.M. (1982) Concentrations of reproductive hormones in canine serum throughout late anestrus, proestrus and estrus. *Biology of Reproduction* **27**, 1196–1206.

Paape, S.R., Shille, V.M., Seto, H. and Stabenfeldt, G.H. (1975) Luteal activity in the pseudopregnant cat. *Biology of Reproduction* **13**, 470–474.

Pearson, H. and Kelley, D.F. (1975) Testicular torsion in the dog: a review of 13 cases. *Veterinary Record* **97**, 200–204.

Pettit, G.D. (1965) Progesterone-induced pyometra in the bitch. *Animal Hospital* **1**, 151–158.

Phemister, R.D., Holst, P.A., Spano, J.S. and Hopwood, M.L. (1973) Time of ovulation in the beagle bitch. *Biology of Reproduction* **8**, 74–82.

Poffenbarger, E.M. and Feeney, D.A. (1986) Use of gray-scale ultrasonography in the diagnosis of reproductive disease in the bitch: 18 cases (1981–1984). *Journal of the American Veterinary Medical Association* **189**, 90–95.

Poste, G. and King, N. (1971) Isolation of a herpesvirus from the canine genital tract: association with infertility, abortion and stillbirths. *Veterinary Record* **88**, 229–234.

Proescholdt, T.A. and DeYoung, D. (1977) Infantile penis in the canine. *Iowa Veterinarian* **2**, 59–62.

Pugh, C.R., Konde, L.J. and Park, R.D. (1990) Testicular ultrasound in the normal dog. *Veterinary Radiology* **31**, 195–199.

Reimers, T.J., Phemister, R.D. and Niswender, G.D. (1978) Radioimmunological measurement of follicle stimulating hormone and prolactin in the dog. *Biology of Reproduction* **19**, 673–679.

Renton, J.P. and Aughey, E. (1971) Certain interesting aspects of infertility in two Shetland collies. *Veterinary Record* **88**, 408–410.

Renton, J.P., Boyd, J.S. and Harvey, M.J.A. (1993) Observations on the treatment and diagnosis of open pyometra in the bitch (*Canis familiaris*). *Journal of Reproduction and Fertility Supplement* **47**, 465–469.

Rivers, B. and Johnston, G.R. (1991) Diagnostic imaging of the reproductive organs of the bitch. *Veterinary Clinics of North America: Small Animal Practice* **21**, 437–466.

Robinson, B.L. and Sawyer, C.H. (1987) Hypothalamic control of ovulation and behavioral estrus in the cat. *Brain Research* **418**, 41–51.

Rogers, A.L., Templeton, J.W. and Stewart, A.P. (1970) Preliminary observations of estrous cycles in large, colony raised laboratory dogs. *Laboratory Animal Care* **20**, 1133–1136.

Rowlands, I.W. (1950) Some observations on the breeding of dogs. *Proceedings of the Conference for the Society of the Study of Fertility*, London 2, pp. 40–55.

Ruben, J. (1993) Use of tamoxifen in the control of canine mammary neoplasia. *Veterinary Record* **133**, 602.

Sandholm, M., Vasenius, H. and Kivisto, A-K. (1975) Pathogenesis of canine pyometra. *Journal of the American Veterinary Medical Association* **167**, 1006–1010.

Schmidt, P.M. (1986) Feline breeding management. *Veterinary Clinics of North America: Small Animal Practice* **16**, 435–451.

Schmidt, P.M., Chakraborty, P.K. and Wildt, D.E. (1983) Ovarian activity, circulating hormones and sexual behavior in the cat. II. Relationships during pregnancy, parturition, lactation and the postpartum estrus. *Biology of Reproduction* **28**, 657–671.

Schneider, R., Dorn, C.R. and Taylor, D.O.N. (1969) Factors influencing canine mammary cancer development and post-surgical survival. *Journal of the National Cancer Institute* **43**, 1249–1258.

Schutte, A.P. (1967) Vaginal prolapse in a bitch. *Journal of the South African Veterinary Medical Asociation* **38**, 197–203.

Seawright, A.A., English, P.B. and Gartner, R.J.W. (1970) Hypervitaminosis A of the cat. *Advances in Veterinary Science and Comparative Medicine* **14**, 1–27.

Shall, W.D., Duncan, J.R., Finco, O.R. and Knecht, C.D. (1971) Spontaneous recovery after subinvolution of placental sites in a bitch. *Journal of the American Veterinary Medical Association* **159**, 1780–1785.

Sherding, R.G., Wilson, G.P. and Kociba, G.J. (1981) Bone marrow hypoplasia in eight dogs with Sertoli cell tumor. *Journal of the American Veterinary Medical Association* **178**, 497–501.

Shille, V.M. (1989) Reproductive physiology and endocrinology of the female and male. In: *Textbook of Veterinary Internal Medicine*, 3rd edn (Ed. S.J. Ettinger) W.B. Saunders, Philadelphia, pp. 1777–1791.

Shille, V.M., Lundstrom, K.E. and Stabenfeldt, G.H. (1979) Follicular function in the domestic cat as determined by estradiol 17β concentrations in plasma: relation to estrous behavior and cornification of exfoliated vaginal epithelium. *Biology of Reproduction* **21**, 953–963.

Shille, V.M., Thatcher, M.J., Lloyd, M.L., Miller, D.D., Seyfert, D.F. and Sherrod, J.D. (1989) Gonadotrophic control of follicular development and the use of exogenous gonadotrophins for induction of oestrus and ovulation in the bitch. *Journal of Reproduction and Fertility Supplement* **39**, 103–113.

Silber, S.J. (1978) Transplantation of a human testis for anorchia. *Fertility and Sterility* **30**, 181–184.

Smith, M.S. and McDonald, L.E. (1971) Serum levels of luteinising hormone and progesterone during the estrous cycle, pseudopregnancy and pregnancy in the dog. *Endocrinology* **94**, 404–412.

Soderberg, S.F. (1986a) Vaginal disorders. *Veterinary Clinics of North America, Small Animal Practice* **16**, 543–559.

Soderberg, S.F. (1986b) Infertility in the male dog. In: *Current Therapy in Theriogenology*, 2nd edn

(Ed. D.A. Morrow). W.B. Saunders, Philadelphia, pp. 544–548.

Sokolowski, J.H. (1980) Prostaglandin F2 alpha-THAM for medical treatment of endometritis, metritis and pyometritis in the bitch. *Journal of the American Animal Hospital Association* **16**, 119–122.

Spicer, C.J. (1979) Pseudopregnancy in the bitch. *Veterinary Record* **104**, 442.

Stead, A.C. (1972) Fracture of the os penis in the dog – two case reports. *Journal of Small Animal Practice* **13**, 19–23.

Stein, B.S. (1981) Tumors of the feline genital tract. *Journal of the American Animal Hospital Association* **17**, 1022–1025.

Susaneck, S.J. and Withrow, S.J. (1986) Tumors of the canine male reproductive tract. In: *Current Therapy in Theriogenology*, 2nd edn (Ed. D.A. Morrow). W.B. Saunders, Philadelphia, pp. 561–563.

Tennant, B. and Kelly, D.F. (1992) Malignant seminoma with gross metastases in a dog. *Journal of Small Animal Practice* **33**, 242–246.

Thornton, D.A.K. (1967) Uterine cystic hyperplasia in a Siamese cat following treatment with medroxyprogesterone. *Veterinary Record* **80**, 380–381.

Thrall, D.E. (1982) Orthovoltage radiotherapy of canine transmissible venereal tumours. *Veterinary Radiology* **23**, 217.

Troy, G.C. and Herron, M.A. (1986) Infectious causes of abortion and stillbirth in cats. In: *Small Animal Reproduction and Infertility* (Ed. T.J. Burke). Lea and Febiger, Philadelphia, pp. 258–269.

Vaden, P. (1978) Surgical treatment of polycystic ovaries in the dog (a case report). *Veterinary Medicine/Small Animal Clinician* **73**, 1160.

Vanderlip, S.L., Wing, A.E., Felt, P., Linke, D., Rivier, J., Concannon, P.W. and Lasley, B.L. (1987) Ovulation induction in anestrous bitches by pulsatile administration of gonadotrophin releasing hormone. *Laboratory Animal Science* **37**, 459–464.

van Duijkeren, E. (1992) Significance of the vaginal bacterial flora in the bitch: a review. *Veterinary Record* **131**, 367.

Vasseur, P.D. and Feldman, E.C. (1982) Pyometra associated with extrauterine pregnancy in a cat. *Journal of the American Animal Hospital Association* **18**, 870–874.

Verhage, H.G., Beamer, N.B. and Brenner, R.M. (1976) Plasma levels of estradiol and progesterone in the cat during polyestrus, pregnancy and pseudopregnancy. *Biology of Reproduction* **14**, 579–585.

von Baier, W., Kalich, J. and Taxacher, J. (1958) Uber pathogenese und behandlung der endometritis bei hundinnen. *Tierazrtliche Wochenschrift* **66**, 397–399.

Wadsworth, P.F., Hall, J.C. and Prentice, D.E. (1978) Segmental aplasia of the vagina in the Beagle bitch. *Laboratory Animals* **12**, 165–166.

Wallace, S.S., Mahaffey, M.B., Miller, D.M., Thompson, F.N. and Chakraborty, P.K. (1992) Ultrasonographic appearance of the ovaries of dogs during the follicular and luteal phases of the estrous cycle. *American Journal of Veterinary Research* **53**, 209–215.

Watts, J.R. and Wright, P.J. (1995) Investigating uterine disease in the bitch: uterine cannulation for cytology, microbiology and hysteroscopy. *Journal of Small Animal Practice* **36**, 201–206.

Watts, J.R., Wright, P.J. and Whithear, K.C. (1996) Uterine cervical and vaginal microflora of the normal bitch throughout the reproductive cycle. *Journal of Small Animal Practice* **37**, 54–60.

Weaver, A.D. (1978) Discrete prostatic (paraprostatic) cysts in the dog. *Veterinary Record* **102**, 435–439.

Weaver, A.D. (1981) Fifteen cases of prostatic carcinoma in the dog. *Veterinary Record* **109**, 71–76.

Whitney, J.C. (1967) The pathology of the canine genital tract in false pregnancy. *Journal of Small Animal Practice* **8**, 247–263.

Wildt, D.E. and Seager, S.W.J. (1978) Ovarian response in the estrual cat receiving varying dosages of hCG. *Hormone Research* **9**, 144–150.

Wildt, D.E., Chakraborty, P.K., Panko, W.B. and Seager, S.W.J. (1978) Relationship of reproductive behavior, serum luteinizing hormone and time of ovulation in the bitch. *Biology of Reproduction* **17**, 561–570.

Wildt, D.E., Panko, W.B., Chakraborty, P.K. and Seager, S.W.J. (1979) Relationship of serum estrone, estradiol 17β and progesterone to LH, sexual behavior and time of ovulation in the bitch. *Biology of Reproduction* **20**, 648–658.

Withrow, S.J. and Susaneck, S.J. (1986) Tumors of the canine female reproductive tract. In: *Current Therapy in Theriogenology*, 2nd edn (edn. D.A. Morrow). W.B. Saunders, *Philadelphia*, pp. 521–528.

Wood, D.S. (1986) Canine uterine prolapse. In: *Current Therapy in Theriogenology*, 2nd edn (Ed. D.A. Morrow). W.B. Saunders, Philadelphia, pp. 510–511.

Wooldridge, G.H. (1908) Retention of urine in a cat, due to spontaneous ligature of the penis with fur. *British Veterinary Journal* **15**, 305–306.

Wright, P.J. (1990) Application of vaginal cytology and plasma progesterone determinations to the management of reproduction in the bitch. *Journal of Small Animal Practice* **31**, 335–340.

Wykes, P.M. and Soderberg, S.F. (1983) Congenital abnormalities of the canine vagina and vulva. *Journal of the American Animal Hospital Association* **19**, 995–1000.

Yeager, A.E., Mohammed, H.O., Meyers-Wallen, V., Vannerson, L. and Concannon, P.W. (1992) Ultrasonographic appearance of the uterus, placenta, fetus and fetal membranes throughout accurately timed pregnancy in beagles. *American Journal of Veterinary Research* **53**, 342–351.

41

Diseases of the Urinary System

D. F. Senior

Anatomy and physiology	612	Nephrogenic diabetes insipidus	634
History taking	613	Congenital renal defects	635
Physical examination	614	Urinary tract infection	636
Investigative techniques and procedures	614	Urolithiasis	639
Renal failure	619	Feline lower urinary tract disease	643
Acute renal failure	619	Diseases of the canine prostate	646
Chronic renal failure	623	Disorders of micturition	649
Glomerulonephropathy	631		

ANATOMY AND PHYSIOLOGY

In dogs, the right kidney is relatively fixed in position and located craniodorsally whereas the left kidney is more caudal, mobile and can adopt variable positions. The situation is the same in the cat but both kidneys are more mobile. Kidneys of dogs and cats are characteristically bean-shaped and the medial border is indented by an oval opening called the hilus through which the ureter, renal artery, renal vein, lymph vessels and nerves pass. The renal parenchyma is made up of the internal medulla and external cortex.

The kidney is an extremely vascular organ with renal blood flow about 20% of cardiac output. In the medulla, the renal arteries give rise to six to eight interlobar arteries which branch to form the arcuate arteries at the corticomedullary junction. Arcuate arteries give rise to interlobular arteries which radiate into the cortex and further branch to form the afferent arterioles. Afferent arterioles enter the glomerulus after coming into close proximation with the distal convoluted tubule in an area known as the juxtaglomerular apparatus. Within the glomerulus, the afferent arteriole branches many times to form the glomerular tuft. On leaving the glomerulus, the capillaries give rise to the efferent arteriole which then forms the peritubular capillary network. The efferent arterioles of juxtamedullary nephrons give rise to vasa recta which traverse deep into the medulla and back again. The blood flow through the vasa recta is relatively sluggish compared to that in the cortical peritubular capillary network. The afferent and efferent arteriolar sphincters located before and after the glomerular capillary tuft control renal blood flow, glomerular filtration rate, and filtration fraction.

Glomerular filtrate is protein free. About 60–70% of filtered sodium and water is reabsorbed in the proximal convoluted tubule by a low-gradient mechanism. A further 25% of the filtered sodium is reabsorbed in the thick ascending limb and a final 4–7% is reabsorbed in the distal convoluted tubule and collecting duct. Distal nephron reabsorption is a low-capacity, high-gradient process which allows for fine-tuning of the final excretory product. The loop of Henle develops medullary hypertonicity by acting as a countercurrent multiplier. Under the action of antidiuretic hormone (vasopressin) the distal convoluted tubule and collecting duct are permeable to water. Water is reabsorbed into the hypertonic interstitium and the final urine becomes concentrated. The ureters exit the kidney at the hilus and pass in a reflection of the peritoneum to the trigonal region of the bladder. The ureters follow an oblique course through the detrusor muscle wall and urine enters the bladder after a short submucosal passage. When empty, the bladder lies within the pelvis or just ahead of the pubis; when distended, the bladder assumes a more cranial and

Table 41.1 Daily renal turnover of water, sodium, chloride and bicarbonate in an adult 20 kg dog

	Filtered	Excreted	Reabsorbed	FR %	Total in ECF (mmol)
H_2O (l/day^{-1})	110	0.8	109.2	99.3	4
Na^+ (mmol/day^{-1})	16 500	70	16 430	99.6	600
Cl^- (mmol/day^{-1})	12 430	100	12 330	99.2	440
HCO_3^- (mmol/day^{-1})	2 000	1	2 199	99.9+	80

ventral position within the abdominal cavity. The detrusor muscle and proximal urethra are composed entirely of smooth muscle whereas the distal urethra has an additional striated muscle component. Bladder and urethral function is controlled by both parasympathetic and sympathetic innervation.

The kidneys are regulatory organs that help to maintain constancy of the internal environment with respect to both volume and composition. They accomplish this purpose through ultrafiltration of plasma by the glomerulus and selective tubular reabsorption and secretion of water and solutes. The kidneys of a 20 kg dog filter 110 litres of water every day and reabsorb more than 99% of the filtered load (Table 41.1). The total quantity of sodium in the extracellular fluid of a 20 kg dog is 600 mmol whereas the daily filtered load of sodium is 16 500 mmol, most of which is reabsorbed. Such massive fluid turnover is necessary to control body fluid volume and composition precisely in the face of various threats to homeostasis.

The kidneys also function as organs of excretion and metabolism of many endogenous and exogenous metabolites. Endocrine functions of the kidney include production of erythropoietin, renin, and calcitriol. Further functions include control of blood pressure mediated by angiotensin II, maintenance of the bradykinin–kinin system and production of a complex array of prostaglandins.

HISTORY TAKING

Some owner observations may relate specifically to diseases of the urinary tract whereas other observations are non-specific and can be associated with other organ systems (Table 41.2).

Polyuria and pollakiuria must be differentiated because confusion can lead to a misdirected diagnostic effort. Polyuria, increased urine volume, can be difficult to quantitate but finding a reduced urine specific gravity provides supportive evidence. Urine specific gravity less than 1.025 in dogs and less than 1.035 in cats suggests higher than normal urine volume. Normal urine output is less than 20–50 ml kg^{-1} day^{-1} and may vary with diet, climatic conditions, and individual variations in water intake (Finco et al., 1982). Nocturia, often accompanies polyuria because bladder capacity is exceeded during the night. The magnitude of polyuria is diagnostically important because there is only a mild increase in urine volume in chronic renal failure whereas in psychogenic water drinking and diabetes insipidus urine volumes are much greater.

Pollakiuria, frequent passage of small volumes of urine, suggests an inflammatory condition of the lower urinary tract. Careful questioning is necessary when owners describe 'accidents' in the house. Animals with pollakiuria often have urgency to urinate but adopt a normal stance for urination whereas incontinence results in passage of urine when the animal is not consciously

Table 41.2 Clinical signs associated with urinary tract disease

System specific	General or non-specific
Anuria	Polyuria
Oliguria	Polydipsia
Urgency	Nocturia
Pollakiuria	Depression
Dysuria	Anorexia
Stranguria	Poor growth
Haematuria	Weight loss
Reduced urine stream	Vomiting
Incontinence	Melaena
Malodourous urine	Diarrhoea
	Facial swelling
	Blindness
	Peripheral oedema
	Seizures
	Tremors
	Discoloured urine

attempting to urinate, for example lying down or walking.

Characterization of haematuria can help to locate the source of bleeding. When the source of blood is in the upper urinary tract, urine usually appears brown throughout urination. Bleeding from the bladder results in the urine appearing progressively more red toward the end of urination and the last few drops may appear to be whole blood. Bleeding between urination is characteristic of lesions in the urethra, prostate and genital tract.

The duration of clinical signs may assist in the differentiation of acute and chronic renal failure and knowledge of exposure to drugs and toxins is important in patients with acute renal failure.

PHYSICAL EXAMINATION

Direct physical examination of the urinary tract in dogs is limited to palpation of the left kidney, bladder, urethra and prostate. In cats, both kidneys are readily palpated.

A number of physical findings commonly associated with renal failure are non-specific and can be observed in other diseases (Table 41.3). However, fibrous osteodystrophy (rubber jaw) and uraemic breath odour are specific for renal failure. Other specific physical findings include pain or changes in the shape, size and consistency of the kidneys, bladder, prostate and urethra and crepitus associated with uroliths. Detection of uroliths in the bladder may require the bladder to be palpated both when empty and when partially full to properly differentiate a mobile urolith from a fixed tumour. Prostatic size should be correlated with the age, breed and sexual status (for example intact or castrated).

INVESTIGATIVE TECHNIQUES AND PROCEDURES

Urine collection

Urethral catheterization is necessary to perform contrast radiography of the lower urinary tract; to empty the bladder and collect urine during clearance studies, to empty the bladder during urine retention, to measure residual bladder volume and to perform prostatic and bladder washes for cytological evaluation. Cystocentesis is the preferred method of urine collection for routine urinalysis and to obtain urine for microbiological evaluation because contamination with cells, bacteria and debris from the genital tract is avoided.

Water deprivation combined with a vasopressin response test, if necessary, can define disorders of water metabolism (Fig. 41.1). A degree of dehydration may need to be prolonged for up to 2 days to allow sufficient time for the kidneys to overcome medullary washout and generate medullary hypertonicity. During prolonged water deprivation small amounts of water should be given frequently so that a degree of dehydration is maintained but severe dehydration must be avoided.

Twenty-four hour urine collection enables estimation of endogenous creatinine clearance and 24-hour protein excretion. Test patients are best kept in a metabolism cage where voided urine can be collected in a chilled container or a container with 1–2 ml of toluene added as a preservative (Bovée and Joyce, 1974). The bladder is emptied, usually by catheterization at the beginning and end of the collection. Urine volume is recorded and, after thorough mixing, aliquots are drawn off and stored for subsequent analysis.

Prostatic and bladder washes are used to obtain cells for cytological evaluation. The bladder is catheterized, drained of urine, then rinsed several times with physiological saline. The bladder or prostate is then massaged by abdominal palpation, rectal manipulation or both. Desquamated cells are recovered by rinsing one final time with 10–30 ml of physiological saline. To obtain prostatic cells, the catheter tip is withdrawn to just distal to the prostatic urethra; after prostatic massage, saline is instilled to backflush cells into the bladder, then the catheter is advanced retrograde into the bladder and the irrigant containing prostatic cells is aspirated.

Table 41.3 Non-specific physical findings observed in renal failure

Poor hair coat
Oedema/ascites
Pale mucous membranes
Stomatitis
Oral ulcers
Tongue tip necrosis
Detached retina
Chemosis
Cachexia
Small stature

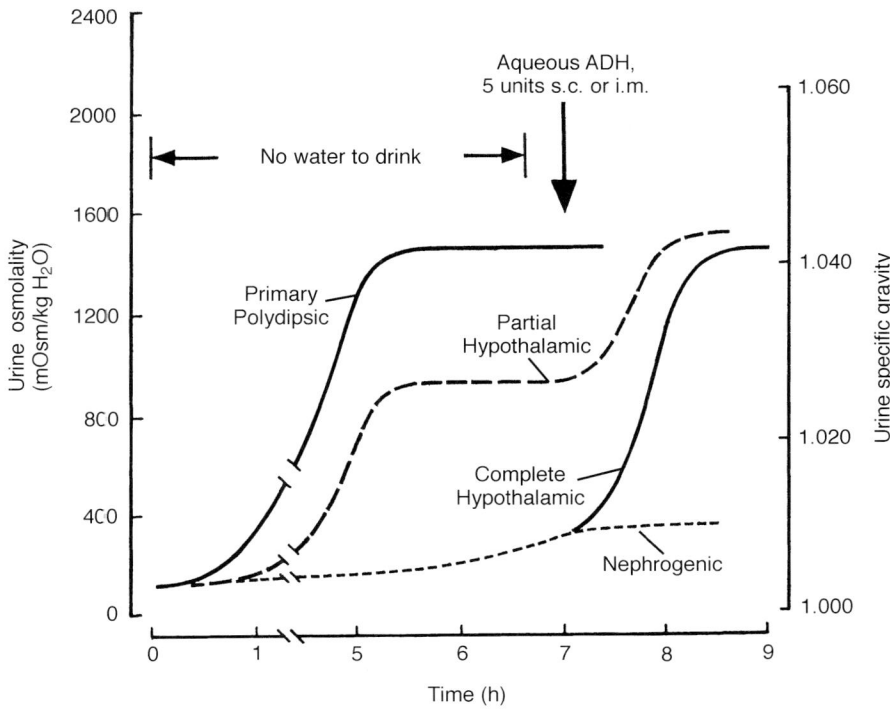

Figure 41.1 Expected urine osmolality and specific gravity after water deprivation and vasopressin administration in dogs with psychogenic water drinking, central diabetes insipidus, partial central diabetes insipidus and nephrogenic diabetes insipidus.

■ Imaging

Radiography and ultrasonography represent the cornerstones of urinary tract imaging. Computed tomography and magnetic resonance imaging provide excellent data but both techniques are not generally available. Patients should be prepared for radiography by evacuation of the bowels using oral salt solutions and enemas. The size, shape, location and radiographic density of the kidneys, bladder, prostate and parts of the urethra can be assessed on plain radiographs. Radio-opaque uroliths are visible. Intravenous urography better identifies the architecture and contents of the renal collection system, ureters, and the location of ureteral entry into the bladder. Nephropyelocentesis can be performed using fluoroscopic imaging during intravenous urography. Contrast cystography allows assessment of bladder shape and size, visualization of radiolucent calculi and identification of filling defects. Retrograde contrast urethrography allows identification of uroliths and strictures of the urethra.

Ultrasonography allows assessment of renal parenchymal architecture and identification of echogenic densities such as areas of tissue mineralization and uroliths (Walter et al., 1987). Tumours of the kidney and bladder are readily identified without the need for contrast radiography. Prostatic cysts, abscesses and tumours can be located and ultrasonography can assist in guidance for aspiration and biopsy of the kidney, bladder, bladder masses and prostate.

Scintigraphy can assist in detection of tumours but is best applied to estimation of renal function (Krawiec et al., 1986; Uribe et al., 1992).

Biopsy of the kidney can be performed under ultrasonic guidance or by manual fixation of the kidney via a keyhole laparotomy. Care must be taken to avoid the hilar area where rupture of the large vessels can cause profuse bleeding (Osborne, 1971). Biopsy of large bladder masses and specific areas of the prostate can also be performed using ultrasonic guidance (Feeney et al., 1987).

Cystoscopy allows visualization of the bladder, urethra and ureteral openings (Senior and Sundstrom, 1988; Brearley et al., 1988; McCarthy and McDermaid, 1990). Transabdominal cystoscopy can be performed in both male and female dogs of all sizes and cats whereas transurethral cystoscopy has been confined to female dogs larger than 7 kg. Biopsy, lithotripsy, tumour resection, ureteral catheterization and location of ectopic ureter can be performed via cystoscopy.

Urodynamic studies include urethral pressure profile and uroflowmetry to determine urethral competence and patency and cystometrography to assess bladder function (Holt, 1988; Oliver and Young, 1973 a, b; Rosin et al., 1980; Moreau et al., 1983a,b,c). All methods require special instrumentation not generally available in practice.

Laboratory investigation

Glomerular filtration rate

The most frequently used estimations of renal function are based on glomerular filtration rate (GFR) and include serum creatinine and blood urea nitrogen (BUN). Creatinine clearance, either exogenous or endogenous and inulin clearance are more accurate but are usually used only in experimental situations. Scintigraphy to estimate GFR of individual kidneys is available in a few referral centres.

The rate of production of creatinine from phosphocreatine in myocytes is proportional to muscle mass and thus remains relatively constant from day-to-day. Normal exercise does not affect creatinine production and although some diets cause a transient increase in serum creatinine in dogs, the fluctuations are minor (Watson et al., 1981). Creatinine is excreted by the kidney almost exclusively and the mechanism of renal handling in dogs and cats is by glomerular filtration only, with neither reabsorption nor significant secretion during passage through the tubules. Thus, serum creatinine levels are influenced by muscle mass and GFR. The standard test for creatinine is the Jaffe reaction which reacts to creatinine and a number of poorly identified substances in plasma known as non-creatinine chromagens (Finco et al., 1982). More recently a creatinine test that does not react with non-creatinine chromagens has been developed (Finco et al., 1992).

Urea is synthesized in the liver from portal blood ammonia, excess dietary amino acids and catabolism of endogenous protein. Renal excretion of urea involves glomerular filtration followed by reabsorption and secretion. The proportion of filtered urea that is subsequently excreted varies with fluid balance. Dehydration tends to cause urea retention and high fluid excretion enhances urea excretion. Thus, BUN levels vary with changes in GFR, dietary protein, body energy balance and body fluid status.

Normal values for serum creatinine and BUN vary widely because of variations in muscle mass, dietary protein and water throughput (Table 41.4). Animals may lose up to 60% of functional renal mass before a significant elevation occurs in either serum creatinine or BUN. More accurate clearance studies allow detection of reduced renal function and small changes in renal function when renal function is above 40% of normal, even when serum creatinine and BUN levels remain within the normal range.

Estimations of GFR based on clearance avoid inaccuracies associated with single serum creatinine and BUN measurement. Clearance is defined as the volume of plasma cleared of the measured substance per unit time.

$$C_X = \frac{U_X \times V}{P_X}$$

where C_X = clearance of X; U_X = urine concentration of X; P_X = plasma concentration of X; V = rate of urine production.

In order for renal clearance of a substance to reflect GFR accurately, several criteria must be met. The substance must not be bound to plasma protein, must be chemically inert in the kidney, and neither filtered nor reabsorbed in the renal tubule. Inulin satisfies all these criteria and provided allowance is made for non-creatinine chromagens, creatinine is a suitable alterative.

Several different methods of performing a clearance study have been described including 24-h endogenous creatinine clearance (Bovée and Joyce, 1974), exogenous creatinine clearance using intravenous infusion (Finco and Brown, 1991) or subcutaneous injection (Finco et al., 1982) and intravenous infusion of inulin (Finco and Brown, 1991) or iohexol (Brown et al., 1996). Measurement of the marker substance may be chemical or by scintillation counter (Rogers et al.,

Table 41.4 Normal values for serum creatinine and blood urea nitrogen

	Serum creatinine (μmol l^{-1})	Blood urea nitrogen (mg dl^{-1})
Dog	44–88–124[a]	8–16–24
Cat	62–106–160	19–29–39

[a] Low–mean–high.

1991). Normal values vary depending on the method used and whether the patient is anaesthetized. Clearance studies are time consuming, may require some animal training and are expensive so they are seldom performed in clinical veterinary medicine.

Scintigraphy allows rapid, accurate estimation of both GFR and the contribution of each kidney to total renal function (Finco and Brown, 1991). The need for expensive specialized equipment limits this method to referral centres.

Proteinuria

Normal urine contains little protein because the glomerular basement membrane excludes most plasma protein from the filtrate and the small quantity of filtered protein is subsequently reabsorbed and metabolized in the proximal tubule. A small amount of Tamm–Horsfall mucoprotein is added to tubular fluid in the thick ascending limb of the loop of Henle (Friedman et al., 1982).

Several disease states can increase proteinuria. Glomerulonephropathies can cause massive filtration of protein due to loss of normal glomerular permselectivity (Haraldsson et al., 1992). Less severe proteinuria develops when tubular damage lessens protein reabsorption or causes an inflammatory exudate. Infection and haemorrhage of the urinary tract can increase proteinuria (Table 41.5) (Bagley et al., 1991). Bence-Jones proteinuria is specifically associated with multiple myeloma. Tamm–Horsfall mucoprotein excretion may increase with many forms of systemic disease.

Urine protein can be measured by chemistry strip or sulphosalicylic acid turbidity.

Table 41.5 Values of urine protein in health and disease in dogs

	24-h protein excretion (mg/kg^{-1} day^{-1})	$U_{Pr/Cr}$[b]
Normal	< 30	< 1
Urinary tract infection (dog)[a]	30–100	1–3
Urinary tract haemorrhage (dog)[a]	30–100	
Glomerulonephritis	> 100	> 3

[a] Higher values can be observed if infection is extremely severe or if the PCV of erythrocytes in urine exceeds 10%.
[b] Convert both protein and creatinine values to mg dl^{-1} before making the ratio calculation.

Note: Urine protein analysis must use the Coomassie brilliant blue or trichloroacetic acid–Ponceau S method rather than the Biuret method.

Simultaneous consideration of urine volume based on urine specific gravity (SG) allows for more accurate estimation of the magnitude of proteinuria when protein is measured by the sulphosalicylic acid or chemistry strip methods. More dilute urine suggests greater daily protein loss. More accurate determination of proteinuria is based on measurement of protein in 24-h urine specimens. However, prolonged urine collection is not necessary because 24-h urine excretion can be calculated from urine protein/creatinine ratio ($U_{Pr/Cr}$) run on a single urine sample (White et al., 1984; McCaw et al., 1985; Grauer et al., 1985). For further analysis, urine can be concentrated by evaporation or dialysis. Subsequent electrophoretic separation of proteins allows examination of the molecular size of urine protein. More severe glomerular lesions result in a wide range of proteins, including large globulins, appearing in the urine.

Urinalysis

Routine urinalysis allows detection of abnormalities of the urinary tract and detection of systemic disease. The method of collection must be known because results vary between samples collected by voiding, catheterization and cystocentesis.

Analysis is best performed immediately after collection. Samples should be refrigerated if analysis is to be performed more than 1 h after collection and refrigerated urine yields satisfactory results up to 4–6 h after collection. Delay and refrigeration allow crystal precipitation and growth.

The colour of urine varies with urine concentration, and the presence of bilirubin, blood, haemoglobin, myoglobin, medications and their metabolites and bacterial pigments. Turbidity is produced by crystals, fat droplets, cells and bacteria. Odour is changed by diet and bacterial metabolites, particularly ammonia produced by bacterial urease.

Specific gravity

In the absence of abnormal amounts of large molecules in urine, for example protein and radiographic contrast agents, specific gravity correlates with urine osmolality and can be used to determine renal concentrating and dilating capacity. Animals are capable of producing dilute or concentrated urine if physiological demands require extremes but normal animals tend to produce relatively concentrated urine (Table 41.6). Patients with a defect of both concentration and dilution tend to produce urine in the isosthenuric

Table 41.6 Normal values for urine specific gravity and osmolality in dogs and cats

	Dog	Cat
Specific gravity		
Possible range	1.000–1.065	1.000–1.085
Usual range	1.035–1.045	1.045–1.065
Osmolality (mOsm/kg H_2O)		
Possible range	50–2400	50–3000
Usual range	1200–1600	1600–2400

range despite overhydration and dehydration, i.e. SG ~ 1.010. Very dilute urine (SG < 1.006) tends to be due to diabetes insipidus, psychogenic water drinking and rarely, hypoadrenocorticism.

pH

Dogs and cats normally produce urine with a pH of 5.5–7.5 but are capable of pH 5.0–9.0 in extremes. Low urine pH corresponds to excretion of an acid load whereas high urine pH corresponds to excretion of an alkaline load. However, paradoxical aciduria may develop during alkalaemia when concurrent dehydration and hypokalaemia exist. Urine pH tends to be alkaline when the animal consumes a diet with alkaline metabolites (for example vegetable protein, alkaline minerals), during the postprandial alkaline tide and with urease-producing urinary tract infection. In distal (or type I) renal tubular acidosis, urine pH is not maximally acidic even in the face of extreme metabolic acidosis and affected patients fail to acidify the urine when given test doses of ammonium chloride.

Glucose

Glucose is freely filtered at the glomerulus (not protein bound) then entirely reabsorbed in the proximal tubule so that normal urine contains undetectable levels of glucose. Glycosuria occurs when the filtered load of glucose exceeds the renal threshold for glucose reabsorption. In diabetes mellitus the renal threshold is exceeded by a massive increase in filtered glucose. In Fanconi-like syndrome and renal glycosuria the filtered load of glucose is normal but a tubular defect of glucose reabsorption results in a lowered renal threshold.

Haemoprotein

A positive haemoprotein reaction on chemistry test strip indicates the presence of erythrocytes, and free haemoglobin or myoglobin. Haematuria can be differentiated from haemoglobinuria by centrifugation of urine. With haematuria, erythrocytes undergo sedimentation. Usually the clinical presentation provides sufficient evidence to distinguish between haemoglobinuria and myoglobinuria. Precise analytical differentiation of haemoglobin from myoglobin in urine requires acrylamide gel electrophoresis or immunodiffusion.

Urine sediment

Excessive cellularity of the urine sediment is associated with urinary tract inflammation. The presence of bacteria and leucocytes indicates urinary tract infection. Cytological evaluation of freshly exfoliated cells can identify neoplasia. Crystalluria may be an incidental finding or may be associated with urolithiasis. Fat droplets are always present in feline urine and although they may indicate a disturbance of lipid metabolism in dogs, they are usually an incidental finding. Casts in urine are formed in the renal tubules from Tamm–Horsfall mucoprotein. Hyaline casts often appear in urine sediment when the kidneys are not directly involved in a disease process for example fever, whereas granular casts are observed during direct renal damage. Casts containing leucocytes indicate a pyogenic process in the renal parenchyma, for example pyelonephritis. Erythrocyte casts are rare in dogs and cats but may occur in patients with acute glomerular disease and haemorrhagic diathesis. Wide casts reflect the width of hypertrophied nephrons and are usually seen as an adaptation to reduced nephron numbers in chronic renal failure.

Tubular function

Measurement of fractional excretion of filtered substances allows an assessment of tubular function. Fractional excretion (FE) is calculated as follows from simultaneously drawn plasma and urine samples:

$$FE\% = \frac{U_X}{P_X} \times \frac{P_{cr}}{U_{cr}} \times 100$$

where U_X and P_X represent the urine and plasma concentrations of substance 'X', respectively and P_{cr} and U_{cr} represent the plama and urine concentrations of creatinine, respectively.

When prerenal azotaemia develops in animals with otherwise normal renal function, FE_{Na} is very low (usually less than 1%). By contrast, in acute renal failure, when tubular damage impairs tubular sodium reabsorption, FE_{Na} is high (usually > 3%).

Urine enzymes such as gamma-glutamyl-transpeptidase and *N*-acetylglucosaminidase can detect renal tubular epithelial cell damage, for example during aminoglycoside treatment.

Microbiology

Bacterial culture is best performed on urine samples collected by cystocentesis because results are not confused by contamination from the genital flora. Culture results from urine obtained by catheterization are usually accurate although low numbers of bacteria ($< 10^5$ ml^{-1}) may be due to genital contaminants. Culture of voided urine is unsatisfactory.

For antimicrobial drugs excreted in the urine, urine levels may exceed plasma levels 10 to 100 times. When infection is confined to the lower urinary tract in females, sensitivity tests are best run using a minimum inhibitory concentration (MIC) technique so that antimicrobial treatment options are based on drug levels achievable in urine. If infections involve the kidney or prostate, antimicrobial choice must be based on drug levels achievable in tissue. The weakly acidic pH of prostatic fluid in dogs suggests that weak bases achieve higher levels in the prostatic parenchyma than other drugs.

RENAL FAILURE

Azotaemia develops when loss of renal function causes serum creatinine and BUN to rise to abnormally high levels. Azotaemia may be due to prerenal, primary renal and postrenal causes. Prerenal azotaemia develops when renal perfusion is insufficient to maintain normal renal function but restoration of normal renal blood flow rapidly resolves azotaemia as renal function increases to normal. Primary renal azotaemia refers to loss of renal function due to renal parenchymal damage. Primary renal failure may be acute or chronic. Animals with acute renal failure suffer rapid loss of renal function and develop azotaemia acutely. In chronic renal failure (CRF), prolonged azotaemia leads to a combination of adaptive metabolic changes and clinical signs known as the uraemic syndrome and affected animals are said to be uraemic. Patients must be azotaemic for several weeks or longer for the uraemic syndrome to develop. Postrenal azotaemia refers to loss of kidney function due to urine outflow obstruction or rupture of the renal pelvis, ureters or lower urinary tract.

ACUTE RENAL FAILURE

History

Animals with acute renal failure (ARF) usually demonstrate sudden onset of depression, vomiting, anorexia and polydipsia. Oliguria is most common but polyuria may develop during recovery or may be present initially depending on the underlying cause of ARF. Seizures and muscle fasciculations may be observed and terminal patients can develop coma. Other clinical signs associated with the precipitating cause of ARF may be present.

Clinical findings

On physical examination, affected patients may be dehydrated. A characteristic 'uraemic breath' odour may be apparent and affected patients are often hypothermic if ARF is not due to bacterial infection. The kidneys may be larger than normal and painful on palpation. Postrenal causes of ARF are associated with a large distended bladder or fluid in the peritoneal cavity, retroperitoneal space or subcutaneous perineal tissue depending on the location of rupture. Lingual, palatine and gingival necrosis may develop. Anaemia is not usually present in the first few days of ARF unless there is some other cause of anaemia. However, if azotaemia persists, anaemia may develop after 10–14 days. Lymphopenia is common. Serum creatinine, BUN and serum phosphate levels rise rapidly and if renal damage is very severe they may continue to rise until death ensues or dialysis is commenced. Hypocalcaemia may accompany hyperphosphataemia. Hyperkalaemia and severe metabolic acidosis with a wide anion gap usually develop in patients with postrenal azotaemia or the oliguric form of ARF. Normokalaemia or even hypokalaemia often occur in the polyuric form. Blood glucose levels may be slightly elevated. Urine specific gravity is usually low (SG < 1.017) despite dehydration. Proteinuria, haematuria and glycosuria in the absence of severe hyperglycaemia are commonly found. The urine sediment is usually active revealing epithelial cells, erythrocytes, neutrophils, lymphocytes and hyaline, granular and cellular casts. On radiographic examination, the kidneys may be normal-sized or enlarged. Contrast studies may assist in determining the location of rupture or obstruction in the urinary tract. Ultrasonographic examination can be diagnostic, for example in hydronephrosis or with increased echogenicity in ethylene glycol intoxication (Adams *et al*., 1991).

Pathophysiological mechanisms

Many causes of ARF have been identified but all causes can be broadly divided into prerenal, primary renal or postrenal in origin (Table 41.7). The pathogenesis of ARF appears to be variable depending on the cause and no single mechanism can explain all observed phenomena in the variety of experimental models of ARF that have been studied. The initiation and maintenance of ARF may involve one or more of the following:

1. Decreased glomerular permeability;
2. Renal vasoconstriction;
3. Tubular backleak;
4. Tubular obstruction.

Decreased glomerular permeability may develop as a result of ischaemic or nephrotoxic insults. There may be a decrease in surface area or ultrafiltration coefficient of glomerular capillaries.

Reduced renal blood flow has been observed in all models of ARF. The renin–angiotensin system may play a role in initiation of vasoconstriction. As tubular cell damage allows poorly modified tubular fluid to reach the macula densa of the juxtaglomerular apparatus, renin–angiotensin activation is induced. In some instances there appears to be redistribution of blood away from superficial cortical nephrons with resultant cortical necrosis.

With reduced renal blood flow the outer medulla appears to be exquisitely sensitive to tissue anoxia because a relatively reduced vascularity (compared to the cortex) provides perfusion to an epithelium with very metabolically active cells, for example the S3 segment of the proximal convoluted tubule and the thick ascending limb of the loop of Henle. After the initial insult, renal blood flow can return to at least 50% of normal with no concurrent increase in GFR. In models of ARF where renal blood flow increases to or remains at 25–50% of normal while oliguria persists, efferent arteriolar dilation has been proposed as the cause of reduced GFR because reduced postglomerular resistance reduces glomerular hydrostatic pressure to below the level at which glomerular filtration can occur.

Tubular backleak refers to uncontrollable diffusion of filtrate back through the damaged tubular epithelium into the renal interstitium with subsequent oliguria. There is evidence that backleak plays a major role in maintenance of oliguria in some experimental models of ARF (Eknoyan *et al*., 1982). Tubular obstruction from cellular debris may initiate and sustain oliguria in experimental models of ischaemic ARF (Burke *et al*., 1982) but supportive evidence is lacking in nephrotoxic models except for ethylene glycol intoxication (Rowland, 1987).

Although the precise mechanisms of reduced renal function and persistent oliguria remain in question, common mechanisms appear to cause ischaemic cell injury. Loss of both normal cell

Table 41.7 Aetiology of acute renal failure

Prerenal causes	Hypovolaemia	Dehydration, haemorrhage, hypoadrenocorticoidism, hypoalbuminaemia, diuretic use
	Reduced 'effective' blood volume	Prolonged anaesthesia, congestive heart failure, antihypertensive agents, sepsis
	Renal haemodynamic changes	Adrenaline, prostaglandin synthesis inhibitors, haemolytic–uraemic syndrome
Primary renal causes	Nephrotoxic	Ethylene glycol, aminoglycoside antibiotics, heavy metals, radiographic contrast agents, thiacetarsemide, cisplatin, doxorubicin, amphotericin B, methoxyflurane, tetracyclines, sulphonamides, Easter lily ingestion, haemoglobin, myoglobin, non-steroidal anti-inflammatory drugs
	Infectious	Leptospirosis, ehrlichiosis, Lyme disease
	Other	Hypercalcaemia (lymphosarcoma, cholecalciferol rodenticide)
Postrenal causes	Obstruction	Urethral plugs (mucoid/cellular/crystalline), urethral urolithiasis, urethral stricture (neoplasia or trauma), bladder neoplasia with bilateral ureteral obstruction
	Rupture	Trauma, postobstruction

membrane permeability and active transmembrane electrolyte transport causes altered cytosolic composition and cell swelling (Humes, 1986).

'Reperfusion injury', resulting from generation of oxygen free radicals once blood flow is reestablished, may also significantly contribute to cellular damage. Calcium diffuses from the interstitium into the cystosol which normally has a very low concentration of calcium. Increased cytosolic calcium disrupts many cell processes including mitochondrial ATP production. In addition, ischaemia favours cellular conversion of ATP into AMP, adenosine, inosine and hypoxanthine (McCord, 1985). During subsequent reperfusion, hypoxanthine is converted into xanthine and uric acid with the generation of superoxide which is further metabolized to hydrogen peroxide, hydroxyl and other radicals. These highly reactive species cause peroxidation of lipid membranes and other lethal cell injury. The extent of reperfusion injury by this mechanism may depend to some extent on the level of xanthine oxidase in tissue. There are moderate quantities of xanthine oxidase in cat kidneys but very little in the dog.

Polyuric ARF appears to be a less severe form where GFR is reduced but combined glomerular and tubular disruption are insufficient to cause oliguria. Instead, impaired tubular handling of the reduced filtrate causes increased urine output.

After recovery from the oliguric phase of ARF a massive polyuria lasting for 24–72 h is common. Possible causes of polyuria include excretion of accumulated solutes, excretion of fluid volume overload from overzealous treatment and poor modification of the glomerular filtrate by damaged tubular cells.

Diagnosis

Patients with ARF typically exhibit sudden onset of depression, lethargy, anorexia, vomiting, diarrhoea, oliguria or polyuria, tremors, seizures and coma with the number and severity of signs depending on the primary cause and the extent of renal damage.

Once the presence of azotaemia is identified, differentiation between prerenal, primary renal and postrenal azotaemia must be made. In most patients with prerenal azotaemia, urine specific gravity is high and FE_{Na} is < 1. Correction of azotaemia by both rehydration and treatment of specific prerenal factors provides further evidence of prerenal azotaemia. Extreme bladder distension or rupture of urinary tract provide evidence of postrenal azotaemia. Following bladder rupture in dogs, hyponatraemia develops and the creatinine levels in the ascitic fluid are higher than in serum (Burrows and Bovée, 1974).

Once primary renal azotaemia is identified, differentiation between ARF and CRF is necessary to provide appropriate treatment and to give an accurate prognosis. Acute renal failure is readily recognized when a history of exposure to a nephrotoxin is associated with rapidly rising serum creatinine and BUN. However, azotaemia with relatively sudden onset of clinical signs may also be associated with CRF. Patients with ARF are usually oliguric but milder forms and some nephrotoxins are associated with polyuria, for example aminoglycosides, amphotericin B and hypercalcaemia. Major shifts in plasma sodium and potassium are more likely in ARF than in CRF. Patients with ARF tend not to be anaemic unless some other cause of anaemia exists concurrently. Urinalysis reveals mild proteinuria with an active urine sediment including many granular casts and exfoliated epithelial cells. Calcium oxalate dihydrate and/or monohydrate crystalluria is associated with ethylene glycol intoxication (Thrall *et al.*, 1985) and serum can be directly tested for recent ingestion of ethylene glycol. In some instances, renal biopsy is necessary to distinguish between ARF and CRF and to determine the severity of renal injury. Biopsy is not undertaken lightly in patients with ARF because of the high risk of haemorrhage. However, renal biopsy is usually performed if the patient is to be anaesthetized for placement of a dialysis catheter.

Management of ARF

In the management of ARF, recognition and correction of initiating factors must be prompt to minimize permanent renal damage. Likely initiating or predisposing factors should be identified and corrective or antidotal treatment provided as soon as possible to limit further renal damage. Treatment can be subdivided into non-specific management applicable to all patients with ARF and specific management which varies with the initiating cause.

Non-specific management

All prerenal factors should be rapidly corrected with an appropriate intravenous fluid. Usually balanced full strength, electrolyte solutions

Table 41.8 Management of hyperkalaemia in acute renal failure

Bicarbonate	
Amount of HCO$_3$ required (mmol) =	0.3 × BW kg × base deficit
OR	1–2 mmol/kg i.v.
Insulin/dextrose[a]	
Dextrose 50%	1.5 g kg^{-1} i.v.
Regular insulin	1 unit/3 g dextrose
Calcium gluconate[b]	
Calcium gluconate 10%	0.5–1 ml kg^{-1} i.v.

[a] Administration of exogenous insulin may not be necessary because glucose stimulates endogenous insulin release; however, the adequacy of insulin release is not known in cats with urethral obstruction.
[b] Counteracts the cardiotoxic effects of hyperkalaemia but does not reduce plasma K$^+$.

(sodium 130–154 mmol l^{-1}) are used with the precise composition chosen based on the particular haematological, colloidal, electrolyte and acid–base status of the patient. Anaemia should be corrected and hypoalbuminaemia treated with replacement plasma or alternative colloidal solutions. Hyperkalaemia should be corrected with specific treatment if values exceed 7.5 mmol l^{-1}. Specific treatments for hyperkalaemia include sodium bicarbonate, 50% dextrose with insulin and calcium gluconate (Table 41.8). These treatments reduce hyperkalaemia only transiently and dialysis may be necessary if hyperkalaemia persists.

Most dogs and cats with ARF develop metabolic acidosis with a wide anion gap but patients may be acidaemic or alkalaemic depending on respiratory compensation and the extent of vomiting. If the bicarbonate deficit is known, replacement bicarbonate can be given according to the formula:

$$\text{Replacement bicarbonate (mmol)} = 0.3 \times \text{body weight (kg)} \times \text{bicarbonate deficit (mmol/l)}$$

If bicarbonate measurement or blood gas values are unavailable, an estimate of bicarbonate deficit can be made: mild azotaemia, 5 mmol l^{-1} moderate azotaemia, 8 mmol l^{-1}; severe azotaemia, 12 mmol l^{-1}. Half the calculated bicarbonate deficit can be given in the first hour with the remainder given over the next 5–6 h. Frequent re-evaluation of bicarbonate deficit may be necessary in patients with severe azotaemia.

Once dehydration is corrected, patients may demonstrate oliguria or polyuria. If oliguria persists, rapid fluid and electrolyte administration must be curtailed otherwise excessive volume overload will lead to pulmonary oedema, respiratory distress and respiratory failure. In persistent oliguria, intravenous fluid administration rate should be calculated as follows: daily fluid volume = insensible losses (10–15 ml kg^{-1} day^{-1}) plus extraordinary losses (vomiting, diarrhoea, fever). Body weight should be measured at least daily to assess the adequacy of fluid volume administration. Insensible losses during oliguria must be replaced by fluids low in sodium (65.5–77 mmol^{-1}) or 5% dextrose in water.

Osmotic diuretics and loop diuretics combined with dopamine can be used in oliguric ARF once rehydration is achieved because establishment of adequate urine output simplifies fluid management of ARF patients. Treatment at or before the time of renal injury with both mannitol (Burke et al., 1982) and combined frusemide/dopamine (Lidner et al., 1979) ameliorated renal damage in experimental models of ARF but there is no evidence that renal function and survival are improved if these treatments are given after ARF is established.

Mannitol (20–25%) given at 0.25 g kg^{-1} i.v. over 3–5 min can be repeated once if diuresis is not established after 20–30 min. No further mannitol should be given if two doses fail to induce diuresis. If a brisk diuresis is established, 8–10% mannitol i.v. in water or in a balanced electrolyte solution can be continued to maintain the diuresis. Mannitol should not be given to patients that are already hypertonic (ethylene glycol intoxication). Also, patients with a high risk of congestive heart failure can develop volume overload, pulmonary oedema and respiratory failure when mannitol is given.

In one model of ARF, frusemide combined with dopamine was superior to either drug alone in ameliorating loss of renal function (Lidner et al., 1979). Frusemide alone is often sufficient to induce diuresis once ARF is established and it is not known if the combination of frusemide and dopamine is better than frusemide alone in this setting. Frusemide is given at 2 mg kg^{-1} i.v. with twice this dose repeated if diuresis is not induced by 30 min. Continuous dopamine infusion should be given at 3–5 µg kg^{-1} min^{-1} i.v. Dialysis is indicated if oliguria persists and the patient develops severe azotaemia, hyperkalaemia, acidaemia or volume overload.

Careful attention to fluid and electrolyte status is essential during the polyuric phase of ARF because patients tend to dehydrate and develop hypokalaemia (Brown et al., 1985). Frequent assessment of clinical fluid status and body weight are essential and regular serum sodium and potassium measurement may be necessary. The most appropriate fluids for the polyuric phase of ARF contain reduced sodium (65.5–77 mmol l^{-1}). Potassium supplementation may be necessary but on no account should the administration of potassium exceed 0.5 mmol kg^{-1} h^{-1} i.v.

Control of persistent vomiting is often necessary in ARF. Cimetidine hydrochloride 5–10 mg kg^{-1} i.v., i.m. or p.o. tid, ranitidine 2 mg kg^{-1} p.o. bid and the proton pump inhibitor, omeprazole given at 0.7–1.0 mg kg^{-1} p.o. sid (not in cats) are effective antiemetics (Thornhill, 1983). Metoclopramide 0.2–0.4 mg kg^{-1} p.o or s.q. tid may control abnormal motility and promote normal gastric emptying. When vomiting is severe and unrelenting, chlorpromazine 3 mg kg^{-1} p.o. sid to qid is a powerful centrally acting antiemetic. At higher doses chlorpromazine may lower blood pressure so the lowest effective dose should be given. Chlorpromazine also causes sedation which may complicate clinical assessment of the patient.

Peritoneal dialysis is indicated in patients with severe azotaemia, life-threatening hyperkalaemia, severe acidaemia, volume overload with congestive heart failure and drug intoxication. Peritoneal dialysis is expensive, time consuming and associated with high morbidity so the procedure is usually confined to patients with a reasonable chance of having kidney function restored and patients undergoing renal transplantation that require initial dialysis support. Results of peritoneal dialysis have been poor in veterinary medicine with less than 24% survival (Crisp et al., 1989). These discouraging results reflect complications of treatment, the extent of renal damage and poor survivability of patients with severe ARF.

Specific management

Specific treatment for the causes of ARF are available for ethylene glycol intoxication and leptospirosis. The lethal dose of ethylene glycol can be as low as 4.2–6.6 ml kg^{-1} in dogs and 1.5 ml kg^{-1} in cats. Intoxicated patients first develop vomiting and diarrhoea with hypovolaemia, metabolic acidosis with a wide anion gap, hypertonicity and neurological signs. After recovery from the initial phase, patients develop oliguric ARF. Specific treatment with the alcohol dehydrogenase inhibitors, ethanol or 4-methylpyrazole, should be given within 24 h of ethylene glycol ingestion (Table 41.9). Treatment with sodium bicarbonate to correct metabolic acidosis can also increase survival.

Leptospirosis is best treated with penicillin and streptomycin. Penicillin suppresses leptospiral growth but usually fails to eliminate the organism. Streptomycin is capable of eliminating leptospires from the urinary tract but is potentially nephrotoxic. During the acute phase of leptospirosis, patients are best treated with penicillin G 50 000 u kg^{-1} i.m. every 12 h for 10 days. Once renal function returns toward normal, streptomycin 10 mg kg^{-1} i.m. or s.q. qid for 7 days may be given to eliminate the carrier state.

CHRONIC RENAL FAILURE

History

Chronic renal failure, a state of stable or slowly progressive azotaemia occurs at a mean age of 7 years in dogs and 7.4 years in cats (Cowgill, 1973). However, in dogs there is a peak in the young because of congenital and developmental renal

Table 41.9 Treatment of ethylene glycol intoxication in dogs and cats

	Dogs	Cats
Ethanol 20%	5.5 ml kg^{-1} i.v. q 4 h × 5 then q 6 h × 4	5 ml kg^{-1} i.v. q 6 h × 5 then q 8 h × 4
4-methylpyrazole 5% (Grauer and Thrall, 1986)	20 mg kg^{-1} i.v. then 15 mg kg^{-1} i.v. at 12 and 24 h then 5 mg kg^{-1} i.v. at 36 h	No data
Sodium bicarbonate 5%[a] (empirical)	8.8 ml kg^{-1} i.p. or i.v. q 4 h × 5 then q 6 h × 4	6.6 ml kg^{-1} i.p. or i.v. q 4 h × 5 then q 6 h × 4

[a] Formula should be used when possible.
Bicarbonate deficit = 0.5 × BW (kg) × (20 − patient HCO$_3$)
(recheck serum bicarbonate and repeat administration q 6 h)

disease (Davenport, 1986). Prolonged azotaemia and altered renal function combine to give rise to the spectrum of clinical features known as the uraemic syndrome. Affected animals demonstrate reduced appetite, gradual weight loss and a poor hair coat. Both thirst and urine volume are increased with many patients needing to urinate during the night. Vomiting is common and in advanced cases melaena may develop. Exercise tolerance is reduced and, on occasion, affected animals develop muscle tremors and seizures.

Clinical signs

On physical examination, the signs mentioned above may be apparent and hypothermia is common. A characteristic halitosis known as 'uraemic breath' is often present. Oral mucous membranes are usually pale and shallow ulcers of the oral mucosa are often present. In long-standing patients, extreme flexibility of the mandible may be present (rubber jaw) but this is uncommon. In young dogs, both the mandible and maxilla may appear swollen and the teeth may be loose. Hypertension is common.

Pathophysiological mechanisms

The aetiology of CRF in dogs and cats is often obscure and the primary cause may be no longer present even though renal disease persists and progresses. Some of the known causes of CRF in dogs and cats are shown in Table 41.10.

Several factors contribute to the normocytic,

Table 41.10 Aetiology of CRF in the dog and cat

Dog	Cat
Idiopathic chronic interstitial nephritis	Idiopathic chronic interstitial nephritis
Irreversible ARF	Irreversible ARF
Familial renal dysplasia and aplasia	Renal lymphosarcoma
Norwegian elkhound	Pyogranulomatous nephritis of FIP
Lhasa apso	Polycystic kidney disease
Shih tzu	adult
Samoyed	familial in Persian cats
Cocker spaniel	congenital
Doberman pinscher	Glomerulonephritis[a]
Standard poodle	Bilateral hydronephrosis
Golden retriever	Amyloidosis
Soft-coated wheaten terrier	familial in Abyssinian cats
Congenital polycystic kidney disease	Pyelonephritis
Cairn terrier	Hypokalaemia (?)
Amyloidosis	Nephrolithiasis, bilateral
Familial	
Shar pei	
Beagle	
Other	
Glomerulonephritis[a]	
Hypercalcaemia	
Bilateral hydronephrosis	
Leptospirosis	
Pyelonephritis	
bacterial	
ascending	
haematogenous (SBE)	
fungal	
Nephrolithiasis, bilateral	
Fanconi-like syndrome	
Basenji	
Keeshond	
Hypertension (?)	

[a] See section on glomerulonephritis.

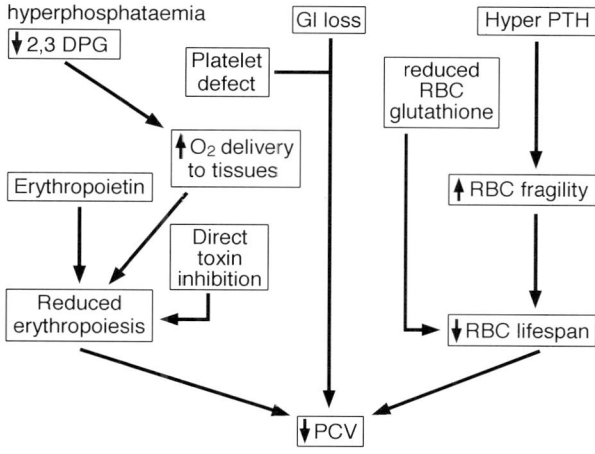

Figure 41.2 Pathogenesis of anaemia in chronic renal failure.

normochromic anaemia of CRF in dogs and cats (Fig. 41.2). The main cause of anaemia in CRF is reduced renal production of erythropoietin (Cowgill et al., 1990). Erythrocyte life span is reduced in part because of elevated PTH levels and reduced erythrocyte glutathione. Gastrointestinal blood loss may be enhanced because reduced platelet serotonin, ADP and thromboxane A_2 production and increased vessel wall PGI_2 production induce platelet dysfunction. Finally, elevated erythrocyte 2,3-diphosphoglycerate levels facilitate oxygen delivery to peripheral tissues so that a lower than normal haematocrit provides normal tissue oxygenation.

Animals with CRF are unable to produce urine concentration much above or below 300 mOsm kg^{-1} H$_2$O (SG = 1.010). Increased tubular fluid flow rate in the remaining functional nephrons and increased medullary blood flow through the vasa recta mediated by atrial natriuretic factor impair development of medullary hypertonicity. Also, collecting duct permeability in response to vasopressin may be impaired.

Oral ulcerations and shallow erosions of the stomach and small intestine develop in CRF (Cheville, 1979). Vomiting, anorexia and melaena are common. The cause of oral and gastrointestinal signs are obscure. Hydrolysis of urea to ammonia in saliva may play a role in oral ulceration and disruption of the protective integrity of gastrointestinal mucus by urea may induce anorexia, vomiting and melaena. Also, high gastrin levels in dogs with CRF may increase gastric acid production and contribute to gastritis (Thornhill, 1983).

Fibrous osteodystrophy develops in CRF because of renal secondary hyperparathyroidism, impaired renal production of 1,25-dihydroxycholecalciferol (calcitriol), impaired gastrointestinal calcium absorption and chronic metabolic acidosis (Fig. 41.3). As GFR decreases phosphorus tends to be retained. In early CRF, normal plasma phosphate levels are preserved by the phosphaturic effect of PTH which inhibits tubular phosphate reabsorption. As GFR declines further in advanced CRF, even maximal inhibition of phosphate reabsorption by elevated PTH fails to maintain normophosphataemia and serum phosphate levels rise. Loss of renal parenchymal mass and hyperphosphataemia impair renal

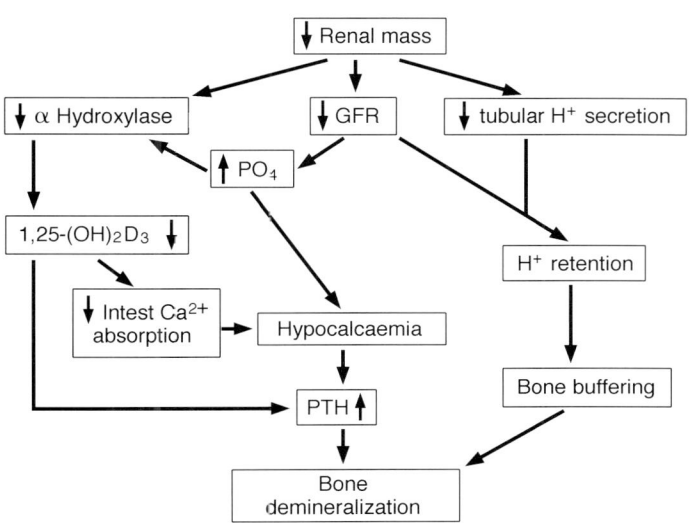

Figure 41.3 Pathogenesis of metabolic bone disease in chronic renal failure.

α-hydroxylase mediated conversion of 25-hydroxycholecalciferol into calcitriol. Reduced calcitriol levels allow uninhibited PTH production further exacerbating bone resorption and hyperphosphataemia. Dogs and cats fed normal diets tend to develop chronic metabolic acidosis because reduced renal mass limits renal excretion of ammonium, the main adaptive buffer for H^+ secretion. Excess H^+ is buffered in bone and the buffering effect renders calcium salts more available for resorption. The combined effect of low plasma calcitriol levels, high plasma PTH levels, and chronic metabolic acidosis causes impaired intestinal absorption of dietary calcium and severe demineralization of bone.

In more than half the dogs and cats with chronic renal disease there is also hypertension (Kallett and Cowgill, 1982; Ross and Labato, 1989; Kobayashi et al., 1990). The role of mild hypertension in the development and progression of CRF in dogs and cats is currently not clear. However, glomerulosclerosis and rapid progression of renal failure have been observed in severe hypertension (Morgan, 1986; Littman, 1990).

Human patients with CRF exhibit impaired neutrophil chemotaxis, lymphopenia, impaired cell-mediated immunity, and increased susceptibility to bacterial infections. Although uraemic dogs and cats are frequently lymphopenic, investigations of other aspects of immune function have not been reported.

Human patients with CRF have impaired glucose tolerance, fasting hyperinsulinaemia, reduced peripheral response to insulin and reduced degradation of insulin. A similar situation probably exists in dogs and cats, many of which exhibit mild hyperglycaemia.

Neurological disease in humans with CRF fall into two categories: uraemic encephalopathy and peripheral neuropathy. Depression, lethargy, weakness, twitching, tremors, head bobbing and seizures have been reported in dogs and cats with renal failure (Wolf, 1980), signs that may be analogous to disorders of consciousness, psychomotor behaviour, thinking, memory, speech, perception and emotion seen in humans. Increased cerebral calcium levels associated with hyperparathyroidism may play a role in uraemic encephalopathy in dogs (Akmal et al., 1984; Mahoney and Arieff, 1983). Although peripheral neuropathy has been associated with hyperparathyroidism and increased nerve calcium levels in dogs with experimental CRF, other studies have failed to support these early findings (Goldstein et al., 1978; Mahoney et al., 1984).

Hypokalaemia frequently accompanies CRF in cats (Dow et al., 1989). The main cause of hypokalaemia appears to be renal potassium loss (Dow et al., 1987) although diets that induce chronic metabolic acidosis may reduce gastrointestinal potassium absorption (Dow et al., 1990). Hypokalaemia may worsen renal function in cats with CRF and correction of hypokalaemia may result in improved renal function (Dow et al., 1987). Hypokalaemia could cause kidney damage by increasing tubular cell ammonium production although this mechanism is controversial (Tollins, 1985).

Progression of CRF

Renal function usually declines progressively in patients with CRF irrespective of the primary cause and even if the cause is no longer apparent. Factors that may contribute to spontaneous progression of CRF in mammals are shown in Table 41.11. Although glomerular hypertension has been documented in dogs with CRF (Brown et al., 1991a), its role in causing progression of CRF in dogs is not clear. Usual strategies to control glomerular hypertension do not appear to halt progression of CRF (Bovée et al., 1979c; Polzin et al., 1984, 1988). In addition, moderate dietary protein restriction does not appear to reduce glomerular hypertension as it does in other species (Brown et al., 1991a). Studies have not been performed in the cat. Dietary phosphate restriction has been reported to limit progressive loss of renal function in dogs (Brown et al., 1991b) and to prevent renal mineralization in cats (Ross, 1992). The effect of systemic hypertension and renal ammoniagenesis on progression of CRF have not been studied in dogs and cats.

Table 41.11 Factors that may contribute to progression of CRF in mammals

Factor	Clinical association
Glomerular hypertension	high protein diet
	high calorie diet
	high N=6 fatty acid diet
Renal mineralization	dietary phosphorus
	renal secondary hyperparathyroidism
Systemic hypertension	high sodium intake
Renal ammoniagenesis	metabolic acidosis
	hypokalaemia

Diagnosis of CRF

The presence of CRF is established based on clinical history, physical examination, and laboratory test results. The history usually includes chronically reduced appetite, vomiting, weight loss, increased water intake and increased urine volume. On physical examination, there may be hypothermia, poor hair coat, pale mucous membranes, uraemic breath odour, evidence of fibrous osteodystrophy and abnormal kidneys on palpation (for example small, firm, lumpy, large). Typical test results include normocytic, normochromic anaemia, lymphopenia, azotaemia, hyperphosphataemia and metabolic acidosis with increased anion gap. Both lipase and amylase may be increased 2.5–3 times normal without the presence of pancreatitis (Polzin et al., 1983a). Urinalysis shows isosthenuria, mild proteinuria (unless the disease process specifically involves the glomerulus) and a benign urine sediment. Occasional tubular casts may be wide. Renal size, shape and density may be abnormal on radiographic and ultrasonographic evaluation. Renal biopsy shows glomerular and tubular atrophy with variable degrees of glomerulosclerosis and mononuclear interstitial infiltrate with fibrosis. Tremendous variation exists with presenting signs and the degree of azotaemia at the time of presentation.

Management of chronic renal failure

Many animals first presented with CRF require stabilization of an acute crisis with appropriate fluid and electrolyte treatment. Causes of both renal damage and progression of renal failure must be identified and eliminated, if possible (Table 41.10). Owners should be advised of their pet's limited adaptability to sudden changes in environment and diet.

Dietary adjustment

Nutrition is the basis of management of CRF. Fresh, clean water must be available at all times and the diet should provide 70–110 kcal metabolizable energy kg^{-1} day^{-1}.

Protein

Recommended levels of protein feeding for dogs and cats with CRF are shown in Table 41.12. Every effort should be made to reduce BUN levels to less than 13.25 mmol l^{-1}. Low protein diets

Table 41.12 Protein restriction in dogs and cats with CRF

	Dog	Cat
Moderate restriction (BUN < 110 mg dl^{-1})		
g protein kg^{-1} BW day^{-1}	2–2.2	4.25
g protein 100 $kcal^{-1}$ ME	3.5	6.4
Severe restriction (BUN > 110 mg/d^{-1})		
g protein kg^{-1} BW day^{-1}	1.6	—
g protein 100 $kcal^{-1}$ ME	2.2	—

cause dogs with CRF to appear stronger, act more lively and have healthier hair coats (Polzin et al., 1984). In addition, urine volume is decreased. When dietary protein restriction is too severe in dogs with CRF, hypo-albuminaemia, anaemia and metabolic acidosis have been reported (Polzin, 1988). Dogs with CRF that were fed egg protein exclusively in a low-phosphate diet developed metabolic acidosis (Massry, 1989). Thus, when feeding a very low protein diet, patients should be checked routinely for anaemia, hypoproteinaemia and metabolic acidosis. Egg albumin should not be fed as the sole source of protein.

Phosphorus

When dietary phosphate intake is reduced commensurate with reduced GFR, renal secondary hyperparathyroidism can be controlled (Polzin et al., 1983b). Dietary levels of phosphate can be reduced to 30–60 mg 100 $kcal^{-1}$ ME in dogs and 100 mg 100 $kcal^{-1}$ ME in cats. The goal should be to reduce serum phosphorus levels to less than 1.75 mmol l^{-1}. Severe phosphate restriction predisposes dogs to metabolic acidosis (Hulter, 1984).

Sodium

Moderate dietary sodium restriction is recommended in dogs and cats with CRF: 50–60 mg 100 $kcal^{-1}$ ME. Even in advanced CRF, renal sodium excretion can accommodate a wide range of sodium intake provided dietary adjustment is made gradually over several days (Bricker et al., 1978). High sodium intake should be avoided because it can exacerbate hypertension and cause retinal detachment (Cowgill and Kallett, 1983).

Alkali treatment

Alkali treatment should be given when serum bicarbonate levels are less than 15 mmol l^{-1}. Doses required are variable but should start at 0.1 mmol kg^{-1} p.o. bid to tid in both dogs and cats. For sodium bicarbonate this corresponds to 10 mg kg^{-1} p.o. bid to tid. The sodium in sodium bicarbonate does not appear to exacerbate hypertension of CRF (Kurtz and Morris, 1983). Potassium citrate, potassium gluconate, calcium carbonate, calcium acetate and calcium citrate may also be used. However, calcium salts should not be administered in hyperphosphataemic patients because of the risk of soft tissue mineralization.

Vitamin supplementation

Dietary supplementation with B-complex and C vitamins is used in human uraemic patients because they tend to become deficient in folate, pyridoxine and ascorbate. Similar recommendations are made for dogs and cats but definitive data regarding requirements in these species are not available.

Control of renal secondary hyperparathyroidism

Renal secondary hyperparathyroidism can be controlled by: (a) low phosphate diet (see above); (b) phosphate binding agents given orally; and (c) low-dose calcitriol.

When dietary phosphate restriction alone fails to reduce serum phosphate levels to below 1.94 mmol l^{-1}, phosphate binders can assist in achieving this goal. Suitable phosphate binders include aluminium hydroxide gel and aluminium carbonate. Although the liquid forms may be more effective, tablet or capsule forms are more easily given and better accepted by dogs and cats.

The suggested dose for aluminium hydroxide or aluminium carbonate is 10–30 mg kg^{-1} p.o. tid with serum phosphate monitored every 10–14 days. Phosphate binders are more effective in lowering serum phosphate when given in conjunction with a low phosphate diet (Finco et al., 1985).

Calcium salts have been used as phosphate binders in human patients with CRF and they appear to be effective in the dog in reducing intestinal phosphate absorption (Lopez, 1984). Extreme care must be taken to normalize serum phosphate levels before administering calcium salts. Hypercalcaemia can develop during calcium salt administration and combined hypercalcaemia with persistent hyperphosphataemia causes soft tissue mineralization and rapid progression of renal failure.

Serum parathyroid hormone levels usually remain abnormally high even after the patient is fed a low phosphate diet and treated with phosphate binders. Direct inhibition of parathyroid hormone production can be provided by calcitriol given at 1.2–3.5 ng kg^{-1} p.o. sid, a dose that minimally effects intestinal calcium absorption (Nagode and Chew, 1991). Serum calcium and phosphorus levels must be monitored at regular intervals throughout calcitriol treatment because hyperphosphataemia and hypercalcaemia are absolute contraindications. Parathyroid hormone levels should be measured regularly to determine effectiveness of treatment. Hyperparathyroidism is known to be detrimental and anecdotal reports suggest that treated patients feel better, but the precise benefits of reducing parathyroid hormone levels using calcitriol in patients with CRF are yet to be determined.

Correction of anaemia

The anaemia of CRF in dogs and cats is best treated with epoetin alfa 50–100 U kg^{-1} s.q. twice weekly (Eschbach, 1989; Cowgill et al., 1990). Many patients with anaemia of CRF are iron depleted and this should be corrected by giving ferrous sulphate 100–200 mg p.o. sid for dogs and 50–100 mg p.o. bid for cats. Once serum iron concentration, total iron binding capacity and transferrin saturation are normal, treatment with epoetin alfa can begin (Cowgill, 1992). The patient's packed cell volume (PCV) should be measured regularly to determine the effectiveness of treatment and to prevent polycythaemia caused by overdoses. Once the anaemia is corrected, epoetin alfa can be given in lower doses and less often. Treatment with epoetin alfa is usually only reserved for CRF patients with severe anaemia (for example PCV < 0.25 l l^{-1} in dogs or < 0.20 l l^{-1} in cats) because the drug tends to be immunogenic in about 20–50% of dogs and cats (Cowgill, 1992). When patients develop antibodies to epoetin alfa, the drug is no longer effective and anaemia returns.

Before the development of epoetin alfa, anabolic steroids (for example nandrolone decanoate 1–1.5 mg kg^{-1} i.m. weekly) were recommended to correct the anaemia of CRF. This therapy is only minimally effective at correcting anaemia in human patients and efficacy in dogs and cats has not been demonstrated (Dainiak, 1985).

Appetite enhancement and antiemetics

Therapeutic diets may be made more palatable if food is warmed or the texture of the food is familiar to the patient. Improved appetite and decreased vomiting can be achieved in some patients with H$_2$-histamine receptor antagonists (Thornhill, 1983) such as cimetidine hydrochloride (5–10 mg kg^{-1} p.o. tid to qid in dogs; 2.5–5 mg kg^{-1} p.o. tid to bid in cats) or ranitidine hydrochloride (0.5 mg kg^{-1} p.o. bid in dogs and cats). In addition, the proton pump inhibitor, omeprazole given at 0.7–1.0 mg kg^{-1} p.o. sid (not in cats) can be effective. For gastric motility disturbances, metoclopramide 0.2–0.4 mg kg^{-1} p.o. tid in dogs and cats has also proved effective in the control of vomiting. For refractory vomiting, centrally acting antiemetics can be used as a choice of last resort (Borison and Hebertson, 1959), for example trimethobenzamide 3 mg kg^{-1} p.o. tid in dogs only; prochlorperazine 0.13 mg kg^{-1} p.o. tid to qid in dogs and cats; and chlorpromazine 0.5–2 mg kg^{-1} p.o. sid to qid in dogs and cats. Long-term use of centrally acting antiemetics is not recommended because they cause drowsiness.

Antihypertensives

Antihypertensives should be reserved for those patients with documented severe hypertension bearing in mind that even severe hypertension can be clinically silent (Cowgill and Kallet, 1986). Treatment for hypertension should be instituted in a stepwise manner, with re-evalaution of blood pressure after 2–4 weeks of treatment before adding the next level of treatment (Ross, 1992). The first step is to feed a low sodium diet that provides NaCl at 50–60 mg 100 kcal^{-1} ME day^{-1}. The second step is treatment with a diuretic such as hydrochlorothiazide 1–5 mg kg^{-1} p.o. bid for dogs and 2–4 mg kg^{-1} p.o. bid for cats. Animals in renal failure that do not respond to thiazide diuretics can be given frusemide 0.5–2 mg kg^{-1} p.o sid to bid for dogs and cats. Conservative doses should be given and patients checked regularly for dehydration which must be avoided. The third step uses beta-blockers. Atenolol 2 mg kg^{-1} p.o. sid for dogs and cats (Littman, 1992) or propranolol 0.2–1 mg kg^{-1} p.o. tid for dogs and 2.5–5 mg p.o. bid to tid for cats are the most commonly used. The fourth step uses vasodilators such as the alpha adrenergic antagonist prazosin 0.25–2 mg p.o. tid for dogs and cats or the angiotensin II converting enzyme (ACE) inhibitors enalapril 0.5–3 mg kg^{-1} p.o. sid to bid for dogs and 0.25–0.5 mg kg^{-1} p.o. sid to bid for cats and captopril 0.5–2 mg kg^{-1} p.o. tid for dogs and 6.25–12.5 mg p.o. bid to tid in cats. Calcium channel blockers such as diltiazem may be used for vasodilation but should not be used with propranolol as both are negative inotropes (Littman, 1992). When multiple drug regimens are required the potential for drug interactions becomes more likely particularly in CRF when drug retention and enhanced drug effects may occur.

Progression

The rate of progression of CRF can be monitored by serial measurement of GFR. With the exception of scintigraphy, which requires special expensive equipment, accurate measurement of GFR by clearance methods is tedious in the clinical setting. Plots of the reciprocal of serum creatinine against time have been suggested as a means to assess the rate of progression of renal disease and the effect of various therapeutic strategies to alter progression in both humans and dogs (Mitch et al., 1976; Allen et al., 1987). Unfortunately, such plots are relatively inaccurate and may have limited value (Walser et al. 1989). Special attention should be paid to those factors that are known to contribute to the progression of CRF in dogs and cats including high dietary phosphorus intake and severe hypertension in both dogs and cats and hypokalaemia in cats.

Dose adjustment in patients with renal failure

Adverse drug side effects are more common in animals with CRF (Senior, 1979; Riviere, 1984). Drugs excreted primarily by the kidneys tend to accumulate to higher than desired plasma levels when normal doses are given. Also, drug distribution and protein binding are altered in azotaemia so that side effects are enhanced.

Drugs primarily excreted by non-renal systems are less likely to cause a problem. Drugs primarily excreted by the kidneys may be (1) innocuous even at very high blood concentration; (2) toxic at high plasma concentration; or, even worse, (3) nephrotoxic at high plasma concentration. For drugs excreted primarily by the kidneys, dose adjustment should ideally be based on measured drug blood levels or by using an accurate measurement of the patient's GFR to estimate the dose fraction (K_f) (Riviere, 1984).

$$K_f = \text{patient GFR/normal GFR}$$

Dose modification can be made in two ways: (1) dose reduction, divide the normal dose by K_f, and

Table 41.13 Dose adjustments in renal failure

Antimicrobial agent	Nephrotoxic[a]	Route of elimination[b]	Adjustment[c]	Dose adjust[d] at per 3–5 mg dl^{-1}
Allopurinol	(?)	R	D/I	75%/1.5×
Amikacin	N	R	I	GFR*
Amoxicillin	–	R (H)	I	2×
Amphotericin B	N	Non-renal	A	–
Ampicillin	–	R (H)	I	2×
Aspirin	N	H (R)	I	1.5×
Atenolol	–	R	D/I	50%/2×
Azathioprine	–	H	N	N
Captopril	(?)	R (H)	N	N
Cefaclor	–	R	D	75%
Cefadroxil	–	R	I	2–4×
Cephalexin	–	R	I	2×
Cephalothin	–	R (H)	I	2×
Chloramphenicol	–	H (R)	N	N
Chlorpheniramine	–	H (R)	N	N
Chlorpromazine	–	G\H	N	N
Cimetidine	–	R	D	75%
Cisplatin	N	R (Non-renal)	D	75%
Clavulanic acid	–	R	N	N
Clindamycin	–	H (R)	N	N
Corticosteroids	–	H	N	N
Cyclophosphamide	–	H (R)	N	N
Cyclosporin	N	H	N	N
Diazepam	–	H (R GI)	N	N
Digoxin	–	R (Non-renal)	D/I	50%/3×*
Diltiazem	(?)	H	N	N
Diphenhydramine	–	H (R)	I	1.5×
Doxorubicin	N	H (R)	N	N
Doxycycline	(?)	R (H)	I	1.5×
D-penicillamine	N	R	Avoid	–
Erythromycin	–	H	N	N
Frusemide	–	R (H)	D	N
Gentamicin	N	R	I	GFR*
Heparin	–	Non-renal	N	N
Kanamycin	N	R	I	GFR*
Ketoconazole	–	H	N	–
Methimazole	–	H (R)	D	75%
Methotrexate	N	R	D	50%
Metoclopramide	–	R (H)	D	75%
Neomycin	N	R	A	–
Nifedipine	(?)	H	N	N
Penicillin G	–	R (H)	D, I	75%/2×
Phenobarbital	–	H (R)	I	N
Prazosin	–	H	N	N
Procainamide	–	R (H)	I	2–3×
Propranolol	–	H	N	N
Quinidine	–	H (R)	N	N
Ranitidine	–	R (H)	D	75%
Streptomycin	N	R	I	GFR*
Tetracycline	N	R (H)	I	2–3×
Ticarcillin	–	R	I	2–4×
Tobramycin	N	R	I	GFR*
Trimethoprim/sulphamethoxazole	–	R (H)	I	1.5×
Vinblastine	(?)	H	N	N
Vincristine	–	H	N	N
Warfarin	–	H (R)	N	N

[a] N = Nephrotoxic; (?) = nephrotoxicity reported in humans.
[b] R = Renal; H = hepatic; (R) or (H) = some minor renal or hepatic elimination.
[c] A = avoid; N = normal dose; D = dose adjustment; I = interval adjustment.
[d] GFR = base dose on measured GFR* = measure blood levels. 75% = use this percentage of the normal dose; 2× = increase interval between doses by this factor.

(2) interval adjustment, multiply the normal dose interval by K_f. As GFR estimations are not available in most clinical situations the reciprocal of serum creatinine can be used to estimate K_f provided the serum creatinine is less than 350 µmol l^{-1}. Aminoglycoside antimicrobials require precise dose adjustment calculated from K_f and increased interval, fixed dose adjustment appears to be less nephrotoxic than reduced dose, fixed interval adjustment (Riviere, 1984). A list of drugs that require dose adjustment in azotaemia is shown in Table 41.13.

Transplantation

Renal transplantation has proven reasonably successful between unrelated cats. Cyclosporine and prednisolone immunosuppression prevented acute allograft rejection. Only limited success has been achieved in dogs.

GLOMERULONEPHROPATHY

Glomerulonephropathy (GN) disrupts the permselectivity of the glomerular filtration mechanism so that large quantities of serum proteins are filtered. GN is caused by the accumulation of immune complexes or amyloid in the glomerulus (MacDougall et al., 1986; DiBartola and Benson, 1989). If proteinuria is sufficiently large, hypoalbuminaemia and peripheral oedema develop, i.e. the nephrotic syndrome (NS). Severe and persistent GN leads to CRF.

History

Historical findings and abnormalities on physical examination often relate more to underlying non-renal primary disease and complications of NS rather than to GN per se. Affected animals tend to be young adults (Wright et al., 1981; Wright and Nash, 1983; Arthur et al., 1986; Jaenke and Allen, 1986). Animals with heavy proteinuria lose weight, are lethargic and muscle wasted, and develop peripheral oedema and ascites. Signs associated with CRF develop once patients become azotaemic. Associated hypertension can cause sudden blindness because of retinal detachment (Cowgill and Kallet, 1986) and pulmonary thromboembolism can cause hyperpnoea, respiratory distress and sudden death (Slauson and Gribble, 1971; DiBartola and Meuten, 1980).

Clinical signs

Mild GN is often undetectable on physical examination. Peripheral oedema and mild ascites may be present. Affected kidneys may be uniformly enlarged, particularly in amyloidosis but normal sized and small kidneys can be observed, particularly in long-standing disease. Collected urine forms a foam when shaken due to the high protein content. Hypertension is present in 80% of dogs with GN (Cowgill and Kallet, 1986).

Pathophysiology

Glomerular disease with proteinuria is an extremely common accompaniment to many non-renal diseases where the proteinuria is never clinically significant and GN resolves once the primary cause is eliminated. Massive immune-complex deposition and amyloidosis causing heavy proteinuria, NS, and progression into CRF are much less common. The causes of GN in dogs and cats are shown in Table 41.14. Most cases of GN are secondary to a chronic non-renal disorder (Center et al., 1987). In glomerulonephritis the fundamental mechanism of injury involves activation of complement by antigen–antibody complexes located at various sites in the glomerulus. Although there may be instances where circulating immune complexes are deposited in the glomerulus, most antigens are 'planted' first before complexing with antibody. The source of antigen is often unknown but patients with diseases where circulating antigen is more common tend to develop glomerulonephritis, for example chronic inflammation and neoplasia. Complement activation plays a major role in inducing glomerular injury and proteinuria. Vascular endothelial damage causes activation of platelets and the coagulation cascade leading to further tissue damage and fibrin deposition. Thromboxane A_2 appears to be a mediator of platelet activation and leucocyte chemotaxis (Grauer et al., 1982). Immune-mediated damage alters glomerular permselectivity causing proteinuria and reduces basement membrane permeability causing reduced GFR. Antigen–antibody complexes may deposit in various locations: subendothelial, basement membrane, subepithelial or mesangial. Heavier cellular infiltration is associated with subendothelial deposition. Mesangioproliferative, membranoproliferative and membranous histological appearances all have

Table 41.14 Aetiology of glomerulonephropathy in dogs and cats

Dogs	Cats
Idiopathic	Idiopathic
membranous glomerulonephritis	
inherited or familial	
Doberman pinscher, Samoyed, Bernese mountain dog, English cocker spaniel	
Amyloidosis	Amyloidosis
Shar pei	Abyssinian
Beagle	
Other	
Non-renal primary disease	Non-renal primary disease
Infectious	Infectious
pyometra	FeLV
dirofilariasis	FIP
bacterial endocarditis	*Mycoplasma gatae* polyarthritis
ehrlichiosis	
borreliosis (Lyme disease)	
brucellosis	
Rocky Mountain spotted fever	
canine adenovirus-1	
leishmaniasis	
Inflammatory	Inflammatory
SLE	SLE
sulphonamide reaction	pancreatitis
pancreatitis	
Neoplastic	Neoplastic
lymphosarcoma	haemolymphatic neoplasia
other tumours	
Other	Other
hyperadrenocorticism	congestive heart failure
diabetes mellitus	mercury intoxication

been documented in dogs and cats. In most studies, IgG and C3 have been present on immunofluorescence and electron microscopy has revealed subendothelial, membranous, subepithelial and mesangial electron-dense deposits, thickening of the basement membrane and foot process fusion (Kurtz *et al.*, 1972; Wright *et al.*, 1981; MacDougall *et al.*, 1986). In human medicine, characteristic histological, immunofluorescent and electron microscopic appearances have been correlated with natural history of the disease, response to treatment and prognosis; however, such correlations have not been established in veterinary medicine.

Amyloidosis in dogs and cats is the reactive-systemic type usually secondary to chronic inflammation or neoplasia (DiBartola *et al.*, 1985; Benson *et al.*, 1985). Fragments of serum amyloid protein A (SAA), an acute-phase reactant produced in the liver, deposit in various tissues including the kidney (DiBartola and Benson, 1989). Although inflammatory conditions can predispose to chronically increased production of SAA, in 70% of dogs and most cats with amyloidosis, no underlying predisposing cause can be found (Clark and Seawright, 1969; Slauson *et al.*, 1970). Deposited amyloid adopts a β-pleated sheet biochemical conformation and stains green with Congo red under polarized light. There is seldom an inflammatory response to amyloid deposition but renal amyloid usually progresses to renal failure and massive proteinuria develops if glomerular deposition is significant.

The cause of sodium retention, hypertension, and oedema in most patients with NS is not clear but several mechanisms have been postulated including increased plasma renin activity due to hypovolaemia in the oedema development phase, increased distal nephron sodium reabsorption, and other as yet undefined sodium reabsorptive mechanisms which act independently of the renin–angiotensin–aldosterone axis. The classical explanation of oedema formation by sodium retention in response to hypovolaemia may not be valid in most human patients with NS because blood volume seems to be high, not low.

Many factors may contribute to the hypercoagulable state in NS including hepatic overproduction of factor VIII, renal loss of antithrombin III, platelet hyperaggregability and hyperfibrinogenaemia (Green and Kabel, 1982; Green et al., 1985; Rasadee and Feldman, 1985). Although pulmonary vessels are most commonly involved, thromboembolism can occur in other vascular beds (Slauson and Gribble, 1971).

Diagnosis

The hallmark of diagnosis for GN is proteinuria. The reaction of dipstick reagent pads must be interpreted bearing in mind urine specific gravity because dilute urine will cause a less strongly positive result. Sulphosalicylic acid turbidimetry is a more reliable screening test for proteinuria but the gold standard for detecting proteinuria is measurement of 24-h protein excretion. Whereas normal dogs and cats excrete less than 20 mg kg^{-1} day^{-1} protein, corresponding to a urine protein-to-creatinine ratio ($U_{Pr/Cr}$) of <1, proteinuria in GN exceeds 100 mg kg^{-1} day^{-1} corresponding to a $U_{Pr/Cr}$ of >3 (Table 41.5) (Barsanti and Finco, 1979b; White et al., 1984; Monroe et al., 1989). Extremely bloody urine and severe urinary tract infection may cause sufficient proteinuria to confuse the diagnosis of GN based on $U_{Pr/Cr}$ (Bagley et al., 1991). Proteinuria should be re-evaluated after such clinical conditions have been resolved.

Hypoalbuminaemia, hypercholesterolaemia and hyperfibrinogenaemia are usually present. The urine sediment often contains granular casts. Renal biopsy with examination under light microscopy, immunofluorescence and scanning electron microscopy is definitive.

Once GN is recognized, screening tests for the wide range of predisposing causes should be performed (Table 41.14). Baseline glomerular permselectivity and response to treatment can be assessed by estimating the sieving coefficient of albumin as follows:

$$\text{Sieving coefficient of albumin} = \frac{U_{alb}}{P_{alb}} \times \frac{P_{Cr}}{U_{Cr}} \times 100\%$$

where U_{alb} and P_{alb} are urine and plasma concentrations of albumin, respectively; and P_{Cr} and U_{Cr} are plasma and urine concentrations of creatinine, respectively.

Management of glomerulonephropathy

Identification and elimination of primary underlying causes of GN should be performed. Subsequent treatment can be divided into non-specific treatment applicable to all patients with GN and specific treatment for immune-mediated glomerulonephritis and amyloidosis.

Non-specific treatment

Diet

Moderate protein restriction with a diet containing 3–4 g protein 100 kcal^{-1} in dogs and 6.5 g protein 100 kcal^{-1} ME in cats has been recommended to reduce proteinuria (Polzin et al., 1989). Although hepatic albumin production may be diminished to some extent, amelioration of proteinuria allows a more positive albumin balance and serum albumin increases. Diets containing predominantly N3 fatty acids (for example linoleic acid, menhaden oil) may enhance prostacyclin activity and diminish platelet activity but efficacy in GN has yet to be documented (Rahman et al., 1987). Restriction of sodium chloride intake to 50 mg 100 kcal^{-1} ME may aid in control of oedema.

Diuretics

Frusemide 2–4 mg kg^{-1} p.o. bid to every other day is usually more effective than thiazide diuretics to control oedema but doses should always be conservative. Concurrent sodium restriction and vigorous diuretic treatment can cause severe hypotension in some individuals so symptomatic treatment for oedema should be confined to patients that develop severe oedema.

Anticoagulants

Patients with antithrombin III levels less than 75% of normal with serum fibrinogen greater than 3 g l^{-1} are thought to be at risk for thromboembolism and require preventive anticoagulant treatment (Green and Kabel, 1982). Low-dose aspirin 0.5 mg kg^{-1} p.o. bid in dogs and 75 mg p.o. twice weekly in cats to control platelet hyperactivity may selectively decrease platelet thromboxane A_2 production while leaving vessel wall PGI_2 production unaffected (Fitzgerald, 1988). Both direct platelet participation in glomerular damage and platelet contribution to hypercoagulation may be reduced by low-dose aspirin treatment but evidence of effectiveness in dogs and cats with GN is lacking. Anticoagulants such as heparin and coumarin and other platelet function inhibitors such as dipyridamole may be of benefit but guidelines for treatment have not been established in dogs and cats.

Antihypertensives
The discussion of treatment for hypertension on page 629 is relevant to patients with GN. Initial treatment should be at the low end of the dose range so that severe hypotension is avoided. The ACE inhibitors, for example captopril 0.5–2 mg kg^{-1} p.o. bid in dogs and 3.15–6.25 mg p.o. bid in cats or enalapril 0.1–0.5 mg kg^{-1} p.o. sid to bid in dogs may be better than other antihypertensive agents because they reduce efferent arteriolar sphincter tone and reduce glomerular capillary hydrostatic pressure (Heeg et al., 1987). However, a positive effect of ACE inhibitors in diminishing proteinuria and progression of glomerular disease has not been documented in dogs and cats.

Specific treatment
Immunosuppressive agents
Human patients with GN have been treated with corticosteroids, azathioprine, cyclophosphamide and cyclosporin A. Corticosteroids are beneficial in 'minimal change' disease and several other morphological forms of glomerulonephritis in humans and high dose 'pulse therapy' with methylprednisolone followed by long-term oral treatment has proven effective (Glassock, 1985). In dogs and cats, the beneficial effect of corticosteroids is not so clear and side effects such as increased azotaemia, increased proteinuria (Center et al., 1987) and enhanced risk of thromboembolism (Burns et al., 1981) may outweigh potential benefits. Corticosteroids may be effective in cats with membranous glomerulonephritis (Nash et al., 1979). Similarly beneficial effects of azathioprine, cyclophosphamide and cyclosporin A have yet to be documented in dogs and cats with glomerulonephritis.

Dimethyl sulphoxide (DMSO) and colchicine in amyloidosis
Administration of DMSO (80 mg kg^{-1} s.q. three times weekly) reduced proteinuria in two dogs with amyloidosis but other studies failed to demonstrate a beneficial effect (Gruys et al., 1981). Colchicine has been shown to be of benefit in certain forms of amyloidosis in humans but evidence of clinical effectiveness in dogs and cats is lacking.

Patients given specific and non-specific treatment for GN should be monitored regularly by measurement of serum albumin, GFR, $U_{Pr/Cr}$ seiving coefficient of albumin and blood pressure so that appropriate treatment changes may be made as necessary.

■ NEPHROGENIC DIABETES INSIPIDUS

Nephrogenic diabetes insipidus (NDI) causes polyuria and secondary polydipsia because of impaired renal tubular responsiveness to vasopressin. A rare congenital form has been described in dogs but most patients have an acquired form (Joles and Drays, 1979). Affected animals drink large volumes of water and pass 5–20 times the normal volume of urine. Nocturia, vomiting and abdominal distension can occur and, in congenital NDI, growth may be retarded. On physical examination, the urinary bladder is usually very large and urine specific gravity can be as low as 1.000–1.005. The defect responsible for the rare congenital form has not been elucidated in humans or dogs but in an experimental mouse model of congenital NDI, decreased intracellular cyclic AMP levels in response to vasopressin have been described which may have been partly due to high cyclic AMP phosphodiesterase in the medullary collecting duct (Jackson et al., 1980). Diagnosis of congenital NDI is based on life-long polyuria and polydipsia in a young animal, hypotonic urine, elimination of causes of acquired NDI, and inability to concentrate urine in response to water deprivation, hypertonic saline loading and ADH administration. Although specific treatment is not available for congenital NDI, urine volume can be decreased by feeding a low sodium diet and long-term treatment with a thiazide diuretic, for example chlorothiazide 20–40 mg kg^{-1} p.o. bid. This combination is thought to reduce urine volume by reducing ECF volume and therefore GFR. A greater proportion of filtered fluid is then reabsorbed proximally so that less fluid reaches the distal tubule and urine volume is decreased.

Many acquired causes of impaired renal concentrating capacity have been identified in dogs and cats (Table 41.15). However, in many patients, the precise cause of the concentrating defect remains obscure. Management of acquired NDI is based on elimination of the primary cause.

Table 41.15 Causes of impaired renal concentrating capacity in dogs and cats

Chronic renal failure
Hypokalaemia
Hypercalcaemia
Fanconi-like syndrome
Low protein diet
Medullary washout
Postobstructive diuresis
Polyuric phase of ARF
Amphotericin B treatment
Aminoglycoside treatment

CONGENITAL RENAL DEFECTS

Many congenital and familial renal defects have been identified in dogs and cats (Table 41.16). Azotaemia and the uraemic syndrome develop in immature animals with renal dysplasia, cortical hypoplasia, familial glomerulonephritis and tubulointerstital nephropathy. Chronic renal failure develops in young adult Abyssinian cats with amyloidosis and middle aged or older dogs with Fanconi-like syndrome and cats with polycystic kidney disease. Unilateral renal agenesis, primary renal glycosuria, and cystinuria do not cause CRF.

Renal dysplasia

Renal dysplasia has been reported in a wide range of dog breeds and cats (Table 41.16) and may develop in individuals of any breed and in mixbreeds. The history and clinical signs are those of CRF but patients tend to be very resistant to azotaemia, often exhibiting few clinical problems other than reduced growth until they are extremely azotaemic. Dramatic fibrous osteodystrophy is often observed in animals that have CRF during growth. Affected animals are often smaller than normal siblings. Progression towards end-stage renal disease is variable but long-term prognosis is usually poor. The pathogenesis of renal dysplasia is uncertain but a genetic basis for the disease is suspected (Bovée, 1984). Diagnosis of renal dysplasia is based on the appearance of CRF in an immature or young animal. The kidneys are usually small and irregular on palpation and radiographically but they can be normal sized. As the histological lesions tend to be segmental, a large wedge biopsy may be necessary to observe patchy areas of small and fetal glomeruli and dystrophic shrunken nephrons surrounded by fibrous tissue (O'Brien et al., 1982; Picutt and Lewis, 1987). Treatment for renal dysplasia is the same as that for CRF.

Polycystic kidney disease

The most common form of polycystic kidney disease (PCKD) develops in adult long-haired cats (Lulich et al., 1988; Biller et al., 1990). Bilateral renal enlargement caused by multiple large cysts is observed in cats with progressive CRF. Owners may report dark urine indicative of renal bleeding

Table 41.16 Congenital and familial renal diseases in dogs and cats

Dog	
Cortical hypoplasia	Alaskan malamute, cocker spaniel, keeshond, Irish wolfhound, King Charles spaniel, Lhasa apso, samoyed, Shih tzu
Dysplasia	Alaskan malamute, beagle, boxer, bulldog, great Dane, great Pyranees, soft-coated wheaten terrier, standard poodle, Yorkshire terrier
Agenesis (unilateral)	Beagle, Doberman pinscher
Tubulointerstitial nephropathy	Norwegian elkhound
Glomerulonephritis	Doberman pinscher, samoyed, English cocker spaniel
Amyloidosis	Shar pei
Fanconi-like syndrome	Basenji, Norwegian elkhound, schnauzer, Shetland sheepdog
Renal glycosuria	Norwegian elkhound, Scottish terrier, mongrels
Cystinuria	Dachshund, bulldog, basset hound, chihuahua, Yorkshire terrier, Irish terrier
Polycystic kidney disease	Cairn terrier
Cat	
Amyloidosis	Abyssinian
Polycystic kidney disease	DLH, Himalayan
Unilateral renal agenesis	DSH, Himalayan

and affected kidneys can be painful on palpation. The aetiology of PCKD in adult cats is not known but a familial pattern suggests a form of hereditary disease (Crowell and Hubbell, 1979). The location of the nephron from which the cysts arise has not been determined. General postulates of cyst formation include intratubular hypertension secondary to tubular obstruction from polyploid hyperplasia of the tubular epithelium, or metabolic defects of tubular wall integrity so that even normal intranephronic pressures cause bulges and outpouches that ultimately form cysts. These changes may be brought about experimentally by a variety of infectious and chemical agents. Diagnosis is based on renomegaly with CRF in an adult cat. Intravenous urography or ultrasound examination confirms the diagnosis. Specific treatment for PCKD is lacking. General treatment includes management of CRF and control of infection.

A rare form of PCKD has been observed in kittens and Cairn terrier puppies (McKenna and Carpenter, 1980). Renal enlargement becomes evident in the first few weeks after birth and affected animals become azotaemic. Multiple small cysts develop throughout the renal parenchyma so that the kidneys have the appearance of a sponge on gross inspection. This form of PCKD shares some of the characteristics of infantile PCKD in humans, a disease with autosomal recessive inheritance. Affected animals probably all die before adulthood. The cause of the condition is unknown. Diagnosis can be confirmed by ultrasound examination of the kidneys and at necropsy. Treatment is probably unwarranted.

Fanconi-like syndrome

Fanconi syndrome in humans is associated with tubular reabsorption defects for water, glucose, phosphate, sodium, potassium, amino acids and bicarbonate. A similar disease has been described in basenji's, Norwegian elkhounds, Shetland sheepdogs and schnauzers (Bovée et al., 1979a). In basenjis affected females outnumber males 3:1. Clinical signs tend to develop between 4 and 8 years of age and include polyuria, polydipsia, glycosuria and weight loss (Noonan and Kay, 1990). Plasma glucose levels are normal and urine specific gravity ranges from 1.000 to 1.018. Once clinical signs appear, some patients develop rapidly progressive CRF and die within a few months; others live for several years. Onset of severe metabolic acidosis often appears terminally. Kidneys may appear histologically normal at the onset of signs. Once azotaemia develops, mild to severe inflammatory changes and fibrosis become evident. Affected basenjis appear to have a transport defect of the luminal brush border membrane of the proximal tubule causing reabsorption defects for glucose, phosphate, sodium, bicarbonate, potassium, urate and amino acids (Bovée et al., 1978, 1979a).

Diagnosis is based on typical clinical presentation and documentation of glycosuria in the face of normoglycaemia and detection of multiple aminoaciduria by paper chromatography. There is no known specific treatment. Management of CRF may alleviate some clinical signs but probably does not change progression of the disease.

URINARY TRACT INFECTION

Urinary tract infection (UTI) is very common (Barsanti and Finco, 1979a; Ling, 1984; Osborne et al., 1989a) in dogs but relatively rare in cats (Kruger et al., 1991). A higher frequency of UTI is detected in female dogs compared with males (Bush, 1976; Kivisto et al., 1977). In most instances of UTI in dogs and cats the infection appears to be confined to the lower urinary tract. The true incidence of upper urinary tract infection remains unknown.

History

The hallmark clinical signs of UTI are those of acute lower urinary tract inflammation: haematuria, pollakiuria, dysuria and stranguria. However, the majority of infections are more chronic and clinically silent with little historical evidence of a problem other than malodorous urine.

Clinical signs

On physical examination of patients with acute UTI, the bladder is small with a thickened wall and even gentle palpation can be painful. In male dogs with acute prostatitis, rectal palpation of the prostate also can elicit a pain response. Prostatic abscessation causes the prostate to be asymmetric. Acute pyelonephritis may cause animals to develop lordosis and be painful when pressure is applied to the back and flank regions. Acute pyelonephritis, acute prostatitis and extremely severe acute cystitis can be associated with fever and leucocytosis. Most patients with UTI are afebrile. The majority of patients have a more chronic form of UTI with minimal clinical signs. The bladder wall may be slightly thickened but is usually not painful on palpation. Urine is malodorous and cloudy.

Pathophysiological mechanisms

Almost all UTI is caused by ascending infection. UTI develops when bacterial virulence is sufficient to overcome host defences. When host defences are normal, only virulent bacteria are capable of colonization but when host defences are reduced, more opportunistic bacteria can colonize. Seven species of bacteria account for most UTI in dogs (Table 41.17) (Ling and Ruby, 1978; Barsanti and Finco, 1979a; Ling, 1983). Bacterial virulence factors that enable colonization and penetration of tissue include expression of adhesins by which bacteria attach to uroepithelial cell binding sites, toxin production, urease production, expression of certain O:K:H serotypes, production of colicins to inhibit the growth of competing bacteria, and production of haemolysins and iron-chelating agents that enable bacteria to scavenge iron, an essential requirement for bacterial growth (Westerlund et al., 1987; Senior et al. 1992).

Host defences that serve to maintain a sterile urinary tract include frequent, complete voiding, increased urethral length and normal urethral pressure, properties of mucus and uroepithelial cells that prevent bacterial attachment, urinary secretion of immunoglobulin, acidic urine pH and high urine osmolality which can suppress bacterial growth and other as yet unidentified factors (Osborne and Klausner, 1979). Specific conditions that compromise one or more of the above defences include tumours and polyps, urolithiasis, atonic bladder, urethral obstruction, hyperadrenocorticoidism, persistent urachal diverticulum, indwelling urethral catheter and urethrostomy.

Diagnosis

Although history, clinical signs and urinalysis results may be suggestive of UTI, diagnosis is confirmed by finding microbes in the urine sediment and by isolation of microorganisms on urine culture. Urine should be collected by cystocentesis to avoid contamination of the specimen with genital microorganisms (Lees et al., 1984). The anatomical level of infection may be impossible to determine. Although most infections appear to be confined to the lower urinary tract, the prostate is frequently involved in intact male dogs. Pyelonephritis can be diagnosed in those rare instances when white blood cell casts appear in the urine sediment. Accurate determination of upper urinary tract infection requires collection of renal pelvic urine by retrograde ureteral catheterization (Senior and Newman, 1986) or by nephropyelocentesis (Ling et al., 1979) both of which are not usually practical in a clinical setting. Sublumbar pain, leucocytosis and characteristic findings on intravenous urography such as dilated renal pelvis and dilated ureters (Barber and Finco, 1979) can support but not confirm a diagnosis of pyelonephritis. Ultrasound findings can also be supportive of pyelonephritis but do not provide confirmation (Neuwirth et al., 1993). Fungal infections can be identified by recognition of characteristic fungal elements in the urine sediment and confirmed by fungal culture.

Management

For patients with a first episode of lower UTI, empirical treatment can be given based on the known antimicrobial sensitivity patterns of the major uropathogens (Table 41.18). Antimicrobial sensitivity tests are indicated when antimicrobial treatment has been given in the recent past because previously treated UTI is usually associated with more resistant strains of bacteria. Minimum inhibitory concentration (MIC) tests should be performed for each antimicrobial and drugs are likely to be successful if mean urinary concentration of the antimicrobial exceeds the

Table 41.17 Frequency of bacterial isolates from urinary tract infection in dogs

	Frequency (%)
Escherichia coli	26–67
Staphylococcus sp.	11–19
Proteus mirabilis	3–32
Streptococcus sp.	3–22
Klebsiella pneumoniae	2–8
Pseudomonas aeruginosa	2–4
Enterobacter cloacae	2–6

Table 41.18 Antimicrobials for empirical treatment of lower urinary tract infection[a]

	Escherichia coli	Staph. sp.	Proteus mirabilis	Strep. sp.	Klebsiella pneumoniae
Amoxicillin/clavulanic acid	80%[b]	>90%	80%	>90%	
Ampicillin		>90%		>90%	
Cephalexin		>90%		>90%	>90%
Enrofloxacin	>90%	>90%	>90%	>90%	>90%
Ormetoprim-sulpha	90%	>90%	80%	>90%	
Trimethoprim-sulpha	80%	>90%	80%	>90%	

[a] For doses see Table 41.19.
[b] Percentage of isolates expected to be sensitive.

MIC by a factor of four (Klatersky et al., 1974) (Table 41.19). For renal and prostatic infection, criteria for antimicrobial sensitivity should be based on drug concentrations in plasma rather than in urine (Klatersky et al., 1974). In addition, the acidic pH of prostatic fluid may limit penetration by some antimicrobials based on pK_a. Trimethoprim, ormetoprim and enrofloxacin appear to penetrate the prostate effectively based on pK_a whereas the lipid solubility of chloramphenicol also allows effective prostatic penetration. Follow-up urinalysis and urine culture are recommended to determine efficacy of treatment.

Persistent and recurrent UTI can be associated with incorrect drug, dose or duration of treatment which may be due to antimicrobial resistance or poor owner compliance. In persistent and recurrent UTI, antimicrobial sensitivity must be retested and the patient should be evaluated for the presence of an underlying predisposing condition that reduces resistance and predisposes the patient to UTI. Plain radiographs of the abdomen, intravenous urography, ultrasound examination of the kidneys, bladder and prostate, and prostatic aspirate, ejaculate and prostatic wash to obtain specimens for cytology and culture may be indicated (Barsanti et al., 1983; Ling et al., 1990a). Primary underlying causes such as concurrent corticosteroid treatment, urolithiasis, polyps and tumours should be eliminated if possible. Castration assists in eliminating the prostate as a residual site for infection (Cowan et al., 1991b). When the primary underlying cause of persistent and recurrent UTI cannot be identified or, if iden-

Table 41.19 Dose, minimum inhibitory concentration (MIC) and mean urinary concentration (MUC) of antimicrobials used in the treatment of urinary tract infection in dogs

	Dose (mg kg^{-1})	MIC break-point[a] (μg/ml)	MUC (μg/ml)
Amoxicillin	11 p.o. tid	64	202 ± 93
Ampicillin	25 p.o. tid	64	300 ± 55
Cephalexin	15 p.o. bid	120	500
Chloramphenicol	33 p.o. tid	32	124 ± 40
Enrofloxacin	2.5 p.o. bid	0.5	45 ± 15
Penicillin G	36 600 u/kg p.o. tid	74 (u/ml)	295 ± 211 (u/ml)
Penicillin V	26.4 p.o. tid	32	148 ± 99
Sulfasoxazole	10 p.o. tid	360	1466 ± 832
Trimethoprim-sulpha	15 p.o. tid	64	246/55
Amikacin	10 s.q. bid	85	342 ± 143
Gentamicin	2.2 s.q. tid	25	107 ± 33
Kanamycin	5.5 s.q. bid	132	530 ± 151
Tobramycin	2.2 s.q. tid	36	145 ± 86

[a] Bacteria with MIC levels above the break-point are unlikely to be effective
[b] Data developed by G.V. Ling, University of California, Davis, CA.

tified, cannot be eliminated, long-term low-dose antimicrobial treatment is indicated. Patients are given a full course of antimicrobial based on sensitivity test results for the initial 3–4 weeks of treatment. Treatment is then continued for at least 6 months by giving 50% of the regular daily dose at night after the patient has voided. Long-term treatment is often successful and development of resistant infection is seldom a problem.

Asymptomatic fungal infections confined to the lower urinary tract can be treated by eliminating the underlying predisposing cause and alkalinizing the urine to pH > 7.5 with sodium bicarbonate 12 mg kg^{-1} p.o. bid or potassium citrate 50 mg kg^{-1} p.o. bid (Lulich and Osborne, 1992). Symptomatic and renal infections should be treated with antifungal agents based on antifungal sensitivity tests. Amphotericin B can be given by direct bladder irrigation, flucytosine 50 mg kg^{-1} p.o. qid is also effective but development of fungal resistance can be rapid. Fluconazole is an effective antifungal agent for renal infections in humans. The human dose is 200–400 mg day^{-1} but veterinary doses have not been established.

UROLITHIASIS

History

The most common uroliths in dogs and cats are composed of struvite, calcium oxalate, ammonium urate and cystine; however, in both species, the proportional incidence of struvite uroliths appears to be decreasing while that of calcium oxalate uroliths is increasing (Table 41.20) (Osborne et al., 1996). Age, breed and sex distribution varies with urolith type (Table 41.21). Nephroliths may cause renal failure particularly if the uroliths are infected. Ureteral uroliths are rarely recognized. The majority of uroliths in dogs and cats are located in the bladder. Urethral uroliths are common in males and rare in females. In dogs, urethral uroliths tend to lodge proximal to the os penis and subsequent urethral outflow obstruction causes postrenal azotaemia and risk of eventual acute renal failure.

Clinical signs

Clinical signs vary with the location of uroliths. Nephroliths may cause sublumbar pain and haematuria but they are usually clinically silent. Cystic uroliths cause signs of lower urinary tract inflammation with haematuria, pollakiuria and stranguria. Physical examination of bladder uroliths reveals a thickened bladder wall with a solid movable mass in the lumen. Multiple cystic uroliths produce crepitus on palpation. Urethral uroliths in male dogs cause stranguria and intermittent incontinence with a full bladder. In cats, complete urethral obstruction may prevent urine dribbling. Urethral catheterization may be difficult with urethral uroliths.

Table 41.20 Analysis of uroliths from dogs and cats

	Reference	Total no. examined	Struvite	Urate	Cystine	Oxalate	Other
Dog	Brodey (1955)	52	42	10	–	–	–
	White (1966)	350	211	18	67	54	–
	Finco et al. (1970)	73	62	6	5	0	–
	Weaver (1970)	100	53	13	20	14	–
	Clark (1974)	110	49	2	24	35	–
	Brown et al. (1977)	438	307	21	95	12	3
	Hicking et al. (1981)	299[a]	151	16	37	4	18
	Bovée and McGuire (1984)	272[a]	187	19	9	27	30
	Osborne et al. (1989a)	2700[a]	1584	161	49	427	479
	Hesse (1990)	1731[a]	951	118	377	87	198
	Escolar (1990)	171[a]	79	13	44	28	7
Cat	Osborne et al. (1989a)	1200[a]	842	67	2	127	162
	Ling et al. (1990b)	150	121	5		11	13

[a] These surveys used accurate crystallographic, infrared spectroscopy or X-ray diffraction methods of urolith analysis.

Table 41.21 Criteria for determining the most likely mineral composition of uroliths in dogs

Age of dog	Immature animals (not Dalmatian) – usually struvite
Breed	Dalmatian: ammonium urate bulldog, dachshund, Basset hound, chihuahua, Irish and Yorkshire terrier (mature age males): cystine
Sex	Female dogs: struvite

Urinalysis	Crystalluria – same as urolith composition
	pH:
	  acid: cystine
	  alkaline: struvite
	  variable: calcium oxalate, ammonium urate
	Culture:
	  urease producers – *Staphylococcus intermedius*, *Proteus* spp.: struvite[a]
	Urolith analysis (if urolith passed): accurate quantitative crystallographic techniques are required

Serum chemistry	Hypercalcaemia[b]: calcium oxalate Metabolic acidosis (RTA): calcium phosphate[b] Pre- and postprandial bile acid elevation: ammonium urate
Radiographic appearance	Cystine: small, often multiple, rounded, mildly radiopaque Calcium oxalate: often spikey projections, very radiopaque Calcium phosphate: smooth, very radiopaque Struvite: smooth or spikey, multiple or single, mild to very radiopaque Ammonium urate: smooth, often multiple, poorly radiopaque

[a] Struvite uroliths can be formed in a sterile environment and uroliths composed of other minerals can become infected by urease-producing organisms.
[b] Extremely rare.

Pathophysiology

Uroliths are composed of a minor organic matrix component and a major crystalline component. Much of the phenomenon of urolith formation can be explained in terms of the physical chemistry of particles in solution. The role of organic matrix in urolith formation is currently not known.

Solutes in urine tend to precipitate at extreme supersaturation. Crystalline particles tend neither to grow nor dissolve in saturated solutions (Fig. 41.4). If the activity product (concentration) of solutes in solution is increased, crystalline particles grow; if the activity product of solutes in the solution is decreased, crystalline particles tend to dissolve. The rate of growth or dissolution of crystalline particles depends on the degree of supersaturation or undersaturation, respectively. The activity product in a saturated solution in equilibrium with crystalline particles equals the solubility product. In a solution devoid of crystalline particles, the activity product can exceed the solubility product (supersaturation) without spontaneous precipitation because more driving force for precipitation is required to initiate a new solid surface than to lay down precipitate on a pre-existing surface. Even with no pre-existing surface, when the activity product of the solution is increased even higher to the formation product, spontaneous precipitation will occur. The physi-

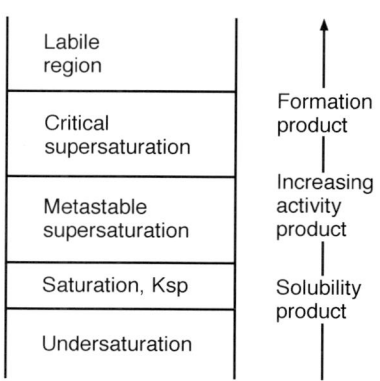

Figure 41.4 The effect of increasing activity product on solution saturation.

cal chemistry of urine is complicated by the interaction of ions and particles that make up uroliths with other ions in urine so that many organic and inorganic substances may act as inhibitors or promoters of crystal formation and growth.

Risk factors predisposing to struvite urolithiasis include high dietary magnesium and phosphorus, concentrated urine and most importantly, alkaline urine. The most important risk factor predisposing to struvite urolithiasis is increased urine pH (Taton et al., 1984; Buffington, 1989; Skoch et al., 1991). However, increased renal excretion of magnesium and phosphate and high urine osmolality also contribute. In dogs with struvite urolithiasis, increased urine pH is most often caused by urease-producing infections, e.g. *Staphylococcus intermedius* and *Proteus* spp. (Weaver and Pillinger, 1975). In cats, struvite uroliths are not usually associated with urease-producing infection. Risk factors for calcium oxalate urolithiasis in humans include hypercalciuria secondary to intestinal hyperabsorption of calcium, a renal 'leak' for calcium or excretion of calcium reabsorbed from bone at an increased rate. In addition, hyperoxaluria, hypocitraturia and defective macromolecular inhibitors of calcium oxalate crystal formation and growth have been described (Kok et al., 1990). Both intestinal hyperabsorption and renal 'leak' of calcium have been described in calcium oxalate urolith-forming miniature schnauzers but the precise cause of these metabolic alterations is not known (Lulich et al., 1991). Risk factors for ammonium urate urolithiasis include reduced hepatic uricase activity as observed in Dalmatian dogs (Porter, 1963) and congenital portosystemic vascular anastomosis (Marretta, 1981). In both conditions, urine urate excretion is increased. Formation of acidic urine and feeding of diets high in protein and purines are less important risk factors. The major risk factor for formation of cystine uroliths is a defect in tubular reabsorption of the amino acid cystine which is almost exclusively confined to male dogs (Case et al., 1992). A high protein diet and aciduria are contributory risk factors. Breeds with increased risk for cystine uroliths include the mastiff, Australian cattle dog, English bulldog, bull-mastiff, Newfoundland, pitbull terrier, Scottish deerhound, chihuahua and dachshund.

Diagnosis

Urolithiasis produces characteristic signs of lower urinary tract inflammation with cystic uroliths, urethral obstruction with urethral uroliths and loss of renal function with nephroliths. Abdominal and rectal palpation may reveal firm masses in the bladder and proximal urethra. Crepitus may be evident when palpating the bladder of animals with multiple cystic uroliths. Crystals typical of the mineral in the urolith may be evident in the urine sediment. Plain and contrast radiography including intravenous urography, cystography and retrograde urethrography can confirm the presence of uroliths and define their number, size and location. Urolithiasis can also be detected by ultrasonography. Determination of the mineral composition may be aided by the age, breed and sex of the patient, radiographic density of the uroliths, the mineral composition of crystals in the urine sediment, urine pH and urine bacterial culture, and quantitative analysis of surgically recovered or spontaneously passed uroliths by crystallographic analysis, infrared spectroscopy and X-ray diffraction (Table 41.21).

Management of uroliths

Struvite

Struvite uroliths can be dissolved medically, resected surgically and effectively prevented from recurrence in both dogs and cats (Abdullahi et al., 1984; Osborne et al., 1990). Preliminary tests before initiation of dietary dissolution in dogs allow identification of the most likely mineral composition of uroliths; establish a baseline of information concerning the number and size of uroliths, and identify any contraindications to the urolith dissolution protocol (Table 41.22). Dietary dissolution of struvite uroliths may be contraindicated in dogs with congestive heart failure, hypoalbuminaemia, hepatic failure, renal failure, ascites, oedema and hypertension.

Satisfactory rechecks (Table 41.22) should show smaller and less numerous uroliths at each visit and dogs eating the diet exclusively should have the following values: BUN 0.58 ± 0.44 mmol l^{-1}; serum magnesium 0.9 ± 0.1 mmol l^{-1}; serum phosphorus 1.2 ± 0.35 mmol l^{-1}; serum albumin 21 ± 3.0 g l^{-1}; serum alkaline phosphatase 147 ± 48 IU l^{-1} (Abdullahi et al., 1984). The urine culture should be sterile, urine specific gravity should be low (SG < 1.020), and urine pH should be acidic.

Prevention of struvite urolithiasis in dogs requires prevention of alkaline urine which in

Table 41.22 Dissolution protocol for struvite uroliths in dogs

1. Run preliminary check
   Physical examination, CBC, serum chemistry panel, urinalysis, urine culture and sensitivity, thoracic and abdominal radiographs, and blood pressure measurement.

2. Initiate protocol
   (a) Feed a low protein, low magnesium, low phosphate, high sodium diet exclusively.[a]
   (b) Treat with oral antimicrobial drugs based on urine culture and sensitivity results.
   (c) Treat with a urease inhibitor
   acetohydroxamic acid 12.5 mg kg^{-1} p.o. bid[b]

3. Monitor progress every 30 days
   Physical examination, serum chemistry panel, urinalysis, abdominal radiographs.

4. Continue dissolution protocol for 30 days after the first follow-up radiographs or ultrasound show no evidence of remaining uroliths.

[a] The only available commercial diet with proven efficacy in struvite urolith dissolution in dogs is Prescription Diet® Canine s/d® Hills Pet Nutrition.
[b] This strategy is optional and usually not required.

most cases requires prevention of UTI caused by a urease-producing infection. Once the urinary tract has been successfully cleared of all struvite uroliths, urine pH should be checked by the owners on a weekly basis. The dog should be investigated for UTI if alkaline urine is observed. Monitoring of urine pH is simplified by feeding a diet that unequivocally induces acid urine. Dogs that develop UTI repeatedly should be investigated to identify primary predisposing causes.

Dissolution of struvite uroliths in cats is usually different from the situation in dogs in that most cats form struvite uroliths in the absence of a urease-producing infection. Preliminary tests are still necessary. A specially formulated low magnesium, low phosphate diet that induces acidic urine must be fed and regular follow-up tests should be performed to ensure progress in urolith dissolution and to check for hypokalaemia and metabolic acidosis (Table 41.23).

Prevention of struvite urolithiasis and crystalluria in cats requires the urine pH to be maintained at less than 6.4 even at the peak of the postprandial alkaline tide at 4–6 h after each meal (Osborne et al., 1989b). Diets can also be low in both magnesium and phosphorus but the effect of urine pH on struvite activity product is much more important. Addition of acidifiers to normal diets by cat owners can achieve the same goal but toxic side effects include hypokalaemia, vomiting, diarrhoea and Heinz body anaemia (Maede et al., 1985). Fatal poisoning has been reported in kittens (Brown and Fox, 1984).

Table 41.23 Dissolution protocol for struvite uroliths in cats

1. Run preliminary check
   Physical examination, CBC, serum chemistry panel, urinalysis, urine culture and sensitivity and abdominal radiographs.

2. Initiate protocol
   (a) Feed a low magnesium, low phosphate acidifying diet.[a]
   (b) Treat with oral antimicrobial drugs based on urine culture and sensitivity results.[b]

3. Monitor progress every 30 days
   Physical examination, serum chemistry panel, urinalysis, abdominal radiographs.

4. Continue dissolution protocol for 30 days after the first follow-up radiographs or ultrasonographs show no evidence of remaining uroliths.

[a] The only available commercial diet with proven efficacy in struvite urolith dissolution in dogs is Prescription Diet® Canine s/d® Hills Pet Nutrition.
[b] This is seldom necessary because most uroliths are bacteriologically sterile.

Calcium oxalate

Calcium oxalate uroliths are resistant to current dissolution methods and must be removed surgically. Prevention of calcium oxalate urolith formation in dogs and cats has not been investigated but extrapolation from data in humans suggests that feeding a low protein (2.2 g 100 kcal^{-1} ME for dogs; 6.4 g 100 kcal^{-1} ME for cats), low sodium diet supplemented with potassium citrate 25–50 mg (0.07–0.14 mmol) kg^{-1} p.o. qid should be effective.

Ammonium urate

An effective protocol for dissolution of ammonium urate uroliths has been developed for Dalmatian dogs (Table 41.24). However, the safety and efficacy of this protocol in dogs with portosystemic vascular anastomosis is unknown. Little work has been done in cats.

High-dose allopurinol (30 mg kg^{-1} day^{-1} p.o.) combined with feeding a normal protein diet can induce xanthine urolith formation in ammonium urate urolith formers (Ling et al., 1991). Thus, allopurinol should only be given when concurrently feeding a low protein diet.

Prevention of ammonium urate uroliths in Dalmatian dogs can be achieved by feeding a low-protein diet, alkalinizing the urine and giving allopurinol so that the daily urate excretion is halved from the typical pretreatment level of 600–800 mg urate day^{-1} to 300–400 mg urate day^{-1}. Using spot urine specimens collected first thing in the morning before the animal is fed, urine urate/creatinine ratio should be reduced from the usual pretreatment value of 0.5–0.6 to a post-treatment value of 0.25–0.3 (Senior, unpublished).

Cystine

Dissolution and prevention of cystine uroliths has been documented in dogs. Dissolution in dogs can be achieved by feeding a diet low in protein and sodium, alkalinizing the urine with potassium citrate 100–200 mg (0.3–0.6 mmol) kg^{-1} day^{-1} to achieve a urine pH of 7.5, and giving the disulphide exchanger tiopronin 30–40 mg kg^{-1} day^{-1} p.o. divided into two or three daily doses (Hoppe et al., 1988). Prevention of recurrence of cystine uroliths may require the same dissolution protocol. Disulphide exchange treatment is always necessary to achieve success.

FELINE LOWER URINARY TRACT DISEASE

Diseases of the lower urinary tract are among the most common causes for cats to be presented for veterinary care. The non-obstructive form affects males and females with equal frequency whereas the obstructive form is confined to males almost exclusively.

History

Non-obstructive

Signs of feline lower urinary tract disease (FLUTD) are variable but usually include stranguria, pollakiuria, haematuria, and dysuria. Affected patients may vocalize during urination and urinate in inappropriate places. Clinical signs tend to spontaneously wax and wane in severity with periods of normalcy between episodes.

Obstructive

Urethral obstruction is almost exclusively confined to males with a peak of occurrence between 2 to 5 years of age. Obstructed cats unproductively strain to urinate and may cry out during the attempt. Licking of the genital region is frequently observed. Patients often hide in a secluded area. After 24–36 h of obstruction cats become very depressed and after 48 h they progress toward coma and die.

Table 41.24 Dissolution protocol for ammonium urate uroliths in Dalmatian dogs

1. Feed a low protein (2.2 g 100 kcal^{-1} ME), low sodium diet.
2. Alkalinize the urine:
   Potassium citrate 100–200 mg (0.3–0.6 mmol) kg^{-1} day^{-1} p.o.
   Sodium bicarbonate 80–160 mg (1–2 mmol) kg^{-1} day^{-1} p.o.
3. Treat with a xanthine oxidase inhibitor:
   Allopurinol 30 mg kg^{-1} day^{-1} divided into two or three daily doses.
4. Continue dissolution protocol for 30 days after the first follow-up radiographs or ultrasonographs show no evidence of remaining uroliths

Clinical signs

Non-obstructive

The bladder of cats with FLUTD is usually small and a thickened wall may be discernible. Bladder palpation appears to cause discomfort. The penis and preputial area may appear hyperaemic.

Obstructive

Patients examined soon after obstruction has developed may be fractious and may resist examination violently. After more prolonged obstruction, patients become progressively more depressed. An enlarged firm bladder is felt on abdominal palpation. The external genitalia are hyperaemic and manipulation of the penis and prepuce may cause intense pain. Mucocrystalline material may be observed protruding from the penile urethra.

Pathophysiological mechanisms

Non-obstructive

Among the identifiable causes of FLUTD, mineral precipitation appears to be associated with most whereas bacterial urinary tract infection is involved in less than 10% of cases (Table 41.25) (Osborne *et al.*, 1989c). However, cats with permanent perineal urethrostomy may be more prone to bacterial urinary tract infection (Osborne *et al.*, 1984; Kruger *et al.*, 1991). Neoplasia of the bladder is rare and is confined to cats older than 7 years. Most bladder neoplasms in cats are malignant (80%) (Gregory and Vasseur, 1983; Griffin and Gregory, 1992). Other rare causes of FLUTD include foreign bodies, fungi, parasites, anatomic defects and neurogenic disorders. After all known causes are ruled out there remains a large subset of patients for which the cause of FLUTD remains unknown. In a substantial proportion of these cats, haematuria with or without pyuria is observed. The bladder wall is thickened, the urine is sterile and uroliths are not detectable. Although the cause of this syndrome is obscure, various causes of idiopathic FLUTD have been postulated including viruses (Fabricant, 1977), food allergy, immune-mediated processes, deficiency of protective mucosal glycosaminoglycan and stress. Recently an analogy has been drawn between idiopathic FLUTD in cats and interstitial cystitis in humans, another idiopathic disorder (Buffington *et al.*, 1996).

Obstructive

Most cases of urethral obstruction are caused by occlusion of the urethra with mineral precipitates (Kruger *et al.*, 1991). The obstructive material can be composed of a proteinaceous plug with crystals or uroliths. There are rare reports of obstruction caused by a proteinaceous plug without crystals. Most crystals and uroliths are composed of struvite but other mineral types may also be involved (Osborne *et al.*, 1989c). The source of the mucoid proteinaceous material of urethral plugs is thought to be urethral mucus-secreting glands but the role of excessive or abnormal mucus production in obstructive FLUTD has yet to be clarified (Osborne *et al.*, 1984).

Prolonged urethral obstruction causes postrenal azotaemia, dehydration, hyperkalaemia and metabolic acidosis. After 2 days of complete obstruction, the cardiotoxic effects of hyperkalaemia become life-threatening. Typical electrocardiogram findings include bradycardia, absence of a P wave, wide sine-wave QRS complexes and a 'tented' T wave.

Diagnosis

Non-obstructive

Non-obstructive FLUTD should be assessed by urinalysis and with a urine culture and sensitivity

Table 41.25 Aetiology of feline lower urinary tract disease (P/O) (Kruger *et al.*, 1991)

	Mineral-related	Urinary tract infection	Idiopathic
Non-obstructive	28	3	80
Obstructive	780	1[a]	29

[a]Urease-producing infection associated with struvite urolithiasis.

test if bacterial infection is suspected. The mineral type of crystals in the urine sediment should be noted. Plain radiographs of the abdomen may reveal uroliths in the bladder but frequently pneumocystography, double-contrast cystography or ultrasonography are necessary to detect uroliths.

Obstructive

Obstructive FLUTD is identified by palpation of an enlarged firm bladder. Urinalysis and urine culture can be performed on urine collected by cystocentesis before catheterization or by catheterization after relief of the obstruction. Serum creatinine and BUN values allow assessment of the degree of azotaemia. Serum potassium levels and an ECG tracing should be performed in depressed cats to assess cardiotoxicity associated with hyperkalaemia.

Management

Non-obstructive

Struvite uroliths can be dissolved by feeding a low magnesium, low phosphorus, acidifying diet (Prescription Diet® Feline s/d®, Hills, Topeka, KS 66601) or by surgical resection. Calcium oxalate uroliths must be surgically resected because dietary dissolution is currently not possible. Medical dissolution of ammonium urate and cystine uroliths may be possible in cats but the safety and efficacy of dissolution protocols has not been established (see p. 643).

Urinary tract infection is treated with empirically chosen antimicrobials based on expected sensitivity patterns (see p. 638) or on culture and sensitivity results. Recurrent infections associated with perineal urethrostomy may require long-term low dose treatment (see p. 638–9).

Little is known about treatment of neoplasia of the lower urinary tract of cats. Surgical resection and follow-up chemotherapy of malignant tumours appear logical.

A wide variety of empirical remedies have been claimed to be successful in the treatment of idiopathic FLUTD. The waxing–waning nature of clinical signs makes evaluation of treatment modalities difficult unless clinical trials are properly controlled. Very few controlled trials have been performed. Diets that reduce the activity product of struvite in urine to a point where struvite precipitation is unlikely are recommended so that any possible inflammation caused by formation and passage of crystals is eliminated.

Table 41.26 Empirical treatment and hypothetical aetiology of idiopathic FLUTD

Treatment	To control
Diet (low struvite activity)	Crystalluria
Antimicrobials	Bacterial infection
Corticosteroids	Immune-mediated inflammation
Diuretics	Urine toxins
Anticholinergics	Detrusor hyperactivity
Glycosaminoglycans	Deficient mucus barrier
Elimination diet	Food allergy

However, simple crystalluria (not urolithiasis) does not appear to induce urinary tract inflammation in cats. Many empirical and symptomatic treatments have been given to control clinical signs (Table 41.26). This wide range of 'remedies' reflects the frustration felt by veterinarians when attempting to manage a condition where the aetiology and pathogenesis remain obscure. With the recent recognition of similarities between idiopathic FLUTD and interstitial cystitis in humans, intravesicular instillation of 50% dimethyl sulphoxide for 10 min on three consecutive days, distension of the bladder to a pressure of 80 cm H_2O for 10 min and administration of amitriptyline at 5–10 mg p.o. sid have been added to the armamentarium of empirical treatments (Kruger et al., 1996). So far, the absence of controlled clinical studies prevents recommendation of a particular course of action.

Obstructive

Affected cats must be handled very gently. Rehydration with intravenous fluids, preferably 2.5% dextrose in 0.45% saline, should be achieved in 4 h. Severe hyperkalaemia should be treated with sodium bicarbonate, insulin/dextrose, or calcium gluconate (Table 41.8). Metabolic acidosis can be corrected with sodium bicarbonate (Burrows and Bovée, 1978). Urethral obstruction can be relieved once cardiac stability is achieved. Deep tranquillization and analgesia or general anaesthesia is required so that the patient does not move during relief of obstruction and urethral trauma is minimized. The penis should be retracted caudoventrally. Saline is back flushed through an open-ended catheter as it is slowly advanced into the urethra. If urethral catheterization is impossible, the bladder can be decompressed by removing 20–30 ml of urine by cystocentesis. On occasion, emergency perineal urethrostomy may be required; however, this is only recommended as a salvage procedure because it may predispose to urinary tract infection (Griffin and Gregory, 1992). Urethral spasm may tend to cause urethral occlusion after the obstructing material is removed particularly if the urethra has been excessively traumatized. An indwelling urethral catheter can be placed for 24–48 h. Medications to control urethral spasm include phenoxybenzamine 5 mg p.o. sid for 3–5 days; diazepam 2.5 mg p.o. bid for 3–5 days and prednisone 2.5 mg p.o. bid for 3–5 days. Broad spectrum antimicrobial drugs should be administered particularly when an indwelling catheter is used. The antimicrobial may need to be changed after the indwelling urethral catheter is removed because the urinary tract tends to become colonized with resistant bacteria (Lees *et al.*, 1981).

Postobstructive diuresis may last up to 3 days and predisposes cats to dehydration and hypokalaemia. Intravenous fluids should be given to maintain hydration and normokalaemia. Intravenous potassium administration should not exceed 0.5 mmol kg^{-1} h^{-1}. Once the patient is able to eat and drink, the rate of intravenous fluid administration should be reduced gradually over 12–24 h with body weight monitored closely to see if the cat becomes dehydrated. If normal hydration is maintained, intravenous fluid administration can be withdrawn.

The mineral component of mucocrystalline plugs and uroliths causing obstruction should be analysed and appropriate dietary and treatment strategies adopted to prevent recurrence (see pp. 642–643).

DISEASES OF THE CANINE PROSTATE

The canine prostate is a bilobed organ located dorsally and wrapping around the urethra caudal to the bladder. In young adult dogs the prostate is usually within the pelvic canal. In older dogs, forward relocation into the abdomen usually occurs. The canine prostate becomes progressively larger with age under the influence of testicular androgens and the concurrent influence of oestrogen. Benign prostatic hyperplasia and prostatitis are common in dogs whereas prostatic abscesses, cysts and tumours are relatively uncommon.

Benign prostatic hyperplasia

History

Affected animals have no systemic signs of illness and may appear completely normal to the owner. A yellow to haemorrhagic urethral discharge may be evident between urination. Cloudy urine may be observed, and tenesmus may occur during defecation.

Clinical signs

On rectal examination the prostate is enlarged but remains mobile with normal consistency and bilateral symmetry. Faecal impaction may be present.

Pathophysiological mechanisms

A combination of testicular androgens and oestrogens induce hyperplasia of the prostatic epithelium (Lloyd *et al.*, 1975). Prostatic tissue may become more sensitive to androgenic stimulation with age (O'Shea, 1963). There is concurrent increased vascularity (Brendler *et al.*, 1983) and cysts tend to develop in dogs over 4 years of age (Huggins and Clark, 1940).

Diagnosis

An appropriate history with a symmetrically enlarged prostate of normal consistency on rectal examination is strong evidence of benign prostatic hyperplasia. Ultrasound examination reveals a normal or slightly hyperechoic prostatic parenchyma with small cysts evident in dogs older than 4 years of age. Prostatic fluid obtained by prostatic massage or ejaculation may be haemorrhagic but not purulent on cytological examination. Prostatic cells obtained by tissue aspirate appear normal. The leucogram is normal.

Treatment

The most effective treatment for clinical problems caused by benign prostatic hyperplasia is castration which causes rapid involution of the enlarged prostate (Schlotthauer, 1932; Berry *et al.*, 1978; Huggins and Clark, 1940). Low dose oestrogen treatment with diethylstilboestrol given at 0.1–0.2 mg p.o. sid for 5 days then twice weekly for 3 weeks depresses pituitary gonadotrophin secretion with consequently reduced testicular androgen secretion. The prostate atrophies when androgenic support of epithelial growth is lost (O'Shea, 1962). Oestrogen treatment can cause undesirable side effects. Prolonged treatment can cause squamous metaplasia of the prostatic epithelium with secretory stasis leading to cyst formation (Berg, 1958). High doses of oestrogen cause signs of oestrus and bone marrow aplasia with thrombocytopenia, leukopenia and anaemia which can be fatal (Tyslowitz and Dingemanse, 1941).

Luteinizing hormone releasing factor and the antiandrogen flutamide are used in humans to induce prostatic atrophy but they are expensive and there are no reports of their use in dogs. Ketoconazole is antiandrogenic and megoestrol acetate suppresses pituitary gonadotrophin release. Both may be useful in benign prostatic hyperplasia of dogs.

Paraprostatic cysts

Paraprostatic cysts arise from the prostatic capsule or bladder wall (Weaver, 1978). They can be very large and are usually located in the abdomen but may push caudally into the pelvic canal.

History

Affected dogs may have no clinical signs until the cysts are very large. Pressure on the urethra and displacement of the rectum and colon lead to dysuria and faecal tenesmus. Very large cysts can cause abdominal enlargement. Sudden fever and toxaemia develop if the cysts become infected. Haematuria and a yellow to bloody urethral discharge may be observed between urination.

Clinical signs

Large, sometimes firm masses are palpable on abdominal or rectal examination. The rectum may be displaced by the cyst.

Pathophysiology

The precise origin of most paraprostatic cysts is obscure. Some may arise from the remnant uterus masculinis on the dorsum of the prostate whereas others may be prostatic retention cysts (Weaver, 1978). The wall of the cyst may be thin or thick and some develop marked calcification (Sisson and Hoffer, 1977).

Diagnosis

Rectal examination may reveal cysts in the pelvic canal. Survey radiographs can show loss of detail in the caudal abdomen and the cyst wall may be calcified. Confusion between the location of cysts and the bladder on plain radiographs can be resolved with cystography or ultrasonography. Ultrasonography shows a thin-walled cyst with low echogenicity of the cyst fluid unless the cyst is infected. Aspiration fluid is usually yellow but can be serosanguineous, relatively acellular, and sterile.

Management

Surgical excision should be attempted and, if this is not possible, marsupialization should be performed. Concurrent castration is recommended.

Prostatitis

Bacterial infection of the prostate gland develops in almost all male dogs with urinary tract infection. In recurrent urinary tract infection the prostate gland may serve as a residual focus of infection leading to recolonization of the urinary tract once antimicrobial treatment is discontinued. Both acute and chronic prostatitis may develop but the chronic form is much more common.

History

Dogs with acute bacterial prostatitis develop anorexia and depression. Vomiting can develop if inflammation extends to the peritoneum. A yellow to serosanguineous discharge may or may not be present and a small proportion of dogs walk with a stiff stilted gait. Most dogs with chronic bacterial prostatitis show no signs. A constant or intermittent urethral discharge may be present between voiding.

Clinical signs

In acute bacterial prostatitis, dogs can develop a fever and the caudal abdomen and prostate can be painful and enlarged on palpation. Dogs with chronic bacterial prostatitis are usually normal on physical examination but some may have a urethral discharge.

Pathophysiological mechanisms

Prostatic cysts, neoplasia and impaired flow of prostatic secretions due to squamous metaplasia of the epithelium may predispose dogs to bacterial prostatitis. Bacterial colonization of the prostate usually extends from ascending infection of the urinary tract although haematogenous spread is possible (Greene and George, 1984; Ling et al., 1987). The most common causative microorganism is *E. coli* but the usual range of Gram-negative and Gram-positive microorganisms causing urinary tract infection can be involved and mycoplasmas have been implicated on occasion (Branam et al., 1984). *Brucella canis* also colonizes the prostate most likely by haematogenous spread. The normal canine prostate produces a zinc-complexed polypeptide with antibacterial properties called prostatic antibacterial factor (PAF) (Fair and Parrish, 1981). It is not known whether the presence or absence of normal levels of PAF production has an effect on the incidence of bacterial prostatitis in dogs.

Diagnosis

Acute bacterial prostatitis can be identified in patients with typical history and clinical signs. The prostate is generally uniformly symmetrical and may be slightly enlarged. Neutrophilia may be present in peripheral blood. Urinalysis shows evidence of urinary tract infection and bacterial culture and sensitivity should be performed. Prostatic fluid must usually be obtained by prostatic massage or direct fine-needle aspirate because affected dogs will not ejaculate. Cytological evaluation of prostatic fluid or aspirates show neutrophilic infiltrates and bacterial phagocytosis. Bacterial culture identifies the organism involved but special culture techniques may be necessary to isolate mycoplasmas. The prostate may appear hyperechoic on ultrasonography. Chronic bacterial prostatitis requires the same diagnostic methods but systemic signs of illness are absent. The prostate may appear variably sized based on the degree of prostatic hyperplasia and the consistency may be variable when chronic inflammation has caused areas of fibrosis. Prostatic fluid cytology is critical to diagnosis and neutrophils and macrophages should be present. Culture and histopathology of prostatic tissue is definitive but seldom necessary.

Management

In acute bacterial prostatitis the blood–prostatic fluid barrier is usually not intact. Thus, a wide range of antimicrobial agents may be used based on culture and sensitivity results. In chronic bacterial prostatitis, the pH of prostatic fluid is generally maintained at around 6.4 so that only weak bases and lipid-soluble antimicrobial agents can penetrate the prostate to achieve effective antimicrobial concentrations. For Gram-positive organisms erythromycin, clindamycin, chloramphenicol, sulfa/trimethoprim and enrofloxacin are likely to give best results and for Gram-negative organisms chloramphenicol, sulfa/trimethoprim, carbenicillin and enrofloxacin are preferred.

Antimicrobial treatment should be continued for 6 weeks. Castration assists in early resolution of prostatitis (Cowan et al., 1991a). If re-evaluation of prostatic fluid after the cessation of treatment indicates persistence of infection, long-term low-dose treatment can be given for 3–6 months at 50% of the normal daily dose. Sulfa/trimethoprim, cephalosporins and enrofloxacin have been used for long-term low-dose treatment. Although prostatectomy eliminates the possibility of prostatitis, this measure is seldom necessary or indicated. Furthermore, a high incidence of urinary incontinence follows prostatectomy in dogs (Hardie et al., 1984; Goldsmid and Bellenger, 1991).

Prostatic abscesses

Prostatic abscessation is a serious life-threatening disease. Even with vigorous treatment up to 50% of affected patients may die (Hardie et al., 1984).

History

Affected dogs often have a history of chronic bacterial prostatitis and may show faecal tenesmus, dysuria and overflow urinary incontinence. A mucopurulent or haemorrhagic urethral discharge may be present. Vomiting is frequently observed.

Clinical signs

Physical examination reveals a fever, dehydration and signs of endotoxaemia. The prostate gland may feel normal on palpation but is usually asymmetrically enlarged and painful with a fluctuant or firm region.

Pathophysiological mechanisms

Chronic bacterial prostatitis may lead to abscessation when infected areas coalesce. Alternatively, cysts that develop from benign prostatic hyperplasia, squamous metaplasia with stasis of secretions or paraprostatic cysts may become infected.

Diagnosis

Typical history and clinical signs suggest prostatic disease. Neutrophilia with a left shift is usually present in peripheral blood. Ultrasonic evaluation of the prostate reveals single or multiple fluid-filled cavities within the prostate. Cytological examination of prostatic fluid obtained by prostatic massage or fluid obtained by fine needle aspirate shows a purulent exudate. Culture of fluid usually yields aerobic bacteria but anaerobes may be involved (Barsanti *et al.*, 1983; Ling *et al.*, 1983).

Management

Vigorous treatment for septic shock followed by surgical drainage using penrose drains or marsupialization is the treatment of choice (Mullen *et al.*, 1990).

Prostatic adenocarcinoma

Prostatic adenocarcinoma mostly affects both intact and castrated medium to large breed dogs with a mean age of 9–10 years (Leav and Ling, 1968; Weaver, 1981; Dube *et al.*, 1984; Evans, 1985).

History

Affected dogs often show weight loss with weakness and stiffness of the hindlegs (Leav and Ling, 1968; Durham and Dietze, 1986). Faecal tenesmus and dysuria may be apparent and there can be a haemorrhagic urethral discharge (Leav and Ling, 1968; Durham and Dietz, 1986).

Clinical signs

In early cases, firm nodules may be apparent within the prostatic parenchyma on digital rectal examination. Usually the prostate is enlarged, asymmetric, firm and non-movable (Weaver, 1981). Transabdominal or rectal manipulation may illicit a pain response. Depending on the pattern of metastasis, signs of azotaemia and urethral obstruction also may be present.

Pathophysiological mechanisms

Metastases most commonly spread to the external and internal iliac lymph nodes and the lumbar vertebral bodies and pelvic bones (Leav and Ling, 1968; Durham and Dietz, 1986). Bony metastases may be responsible for much of the apparent pain and stiffness. Metastatic spread may also develop in the colonic and pelvic musculature and the lung (Leav and Ling, 1968). Extension into the bladder may cause signs of lower urinary tract inflammation and ureteral obstruction can lead to hydronephrosis and azotaemia (Leav and Ling, 1968). Urethral occlusion may cause urine retention and overflow incontinence (Weaver, 1981). Prostatic enlargement often displaces the colon dorsally leading to faecal tenesmus and obstipation. On rare occasions other tumours such as transitional cell carcinoma and metastatic cancer may develop in the prostate.

Diagnosis

The history and physical examination findings are highly suggestive and the probability of prostatic adenocarcinoma is very high when prostatic enlargement develops in castrated dogs (Krawiec and Heflin, 1992). Plain and contrast radiography reveal prostatic enlargement and asymmetry (Stone *et al.*, 1978). Poorly defined parenchymal mineralization may be apparent. The internal iliac lymph nodes are usually enlarged. Hydronephrosis, hydroureter and intravesicular and intraurethral filling defects may be observed. Metastatic lesions are often observed in the lumbar vertebrae and pelvic bones (Leav and Ling, 1968; Weaver, 1981). Thoracic metastasis can occur. Ultrasound examination reveals single or multiple regions of increased echogenicity within the prostatic parenchyma and the prostate is enlarged and asymmetric (Feeney *et al.*, 1987) often with an irregular capsular surface. Aspiration or biopsy with cytological and histopathological examination of prostatic tissue are definitive diagnostic tools but even aspirates may be confusing because of concurrent cysts, abscesses and haemorrhage (O'Shea, 1963; Taylor, 1973; Weaver, 1981).

Management

In early cases with no evidence of distant metastases, orthovoltage irradiation and prostatectomy have been used although complications and survival times have not been good (Taylor, 1973; Hardie *et al.*, 1984). Effective chemotherapy protocols have not yet been established. Castration and oestrogen treatment do not appear to affect the course of the disease (Weaver, 1981).

DISORDERS OF MICTURITION

Abnormal passage of urine includes incontinence, urination in inappropriate places and inability to empty the bladder completely with uninterrupted urine flow.

History

The patient's age and reproductive status must be known. With ectopic ureter, constant urine dripping is observed and normal urination may or may not occur depending on whether urine enters the bladder. Patent urachus is associated with passage of urine from the umbilicus. Conscious urination in inappropriate places can be due to poor cerebral cortical control as in puppies or senile dementia. Sudden need to urinate is most commonly due to lower urinary tract inflammation but may be caused by hyperreflexia of the detrusor muscle. Dribbling urine soon after urination with pollakiuria, stranguria and haematuria is usually associated with urinary tract infection, urolithiasis and in older animals bladder and urethral tumours. Stranguria and urine dribbling with a full bladder denotes urethral obstruction most often associated with urethral urolithiasis, urethral tumours and obstructive granulomatous urethritis. Incomplete urination interrupted repeatedly by urethral spasms is seen in patients with spinal cord lesions. Passage of urine in stress situations, when sleeping or coughing indicates urethral sphincter incompetence. Often this condition appears or is worsened in female dogs after ovariohysterectomy.

■ Physical findings

Urination should be observed so the problem is observed first hand. Urine stains or wetness on the hair coat should be noted. Bladder distension is seen with atonic bladder and urethral obstruction whereas a small firm bladder is associated with bladder irritation. Masses such as uroliths or tumours may be palpable within the bladder. The ease with which urine can be expressed from the bladder may give an indication of urethral competence but excessive force should not be used. Neurological examination is necessary to detect evidence of CNS lesions causing disordered micturition.

■ Pathophysiological mechanisms

Disturbances of micturition can be subdivided based on neurogenic and non-neurogenic causes (Table 41.27). A knowledge of the innervation of the lower urinary tract and the distribution of autonomic receptors can aid in understanding

Table 41.27 Aetiology of disturbances of micturition

Neurogenic	Non-neurogenic

Cerebral cortex
  youth, dementia, tumour
	Lower urinary tract inflammation
	  urinary tract infection
	  urolithiasis
	  tumour

Cord lesion, upper motor neurone
  disc disease
  trauma, tumour
	Urethral obstruction
	  urolithiasis
	  tumour
	  granulomatous urethritis

Cord lesion, lower motor neurone
  disc disease
  trauma, tumour	

Peripheral nerve lesions
  pelvic, pudendal
	Congenital anomalies
	  ectopic ureter
	  patent urachus
	  hypoplastic bladder
	  urethral incompetence
	  pseudohermaphroditism

Atonic bladder
  congenital
  acquired
    outflow obstruction
    dysautonomia (feline)
    idiopathic
	Adult onset urethral incompetence
	
	Miscellaneous
	  vaginal pooling
	  prostatic cyst
	  stress incontinence
	  urge incontinence

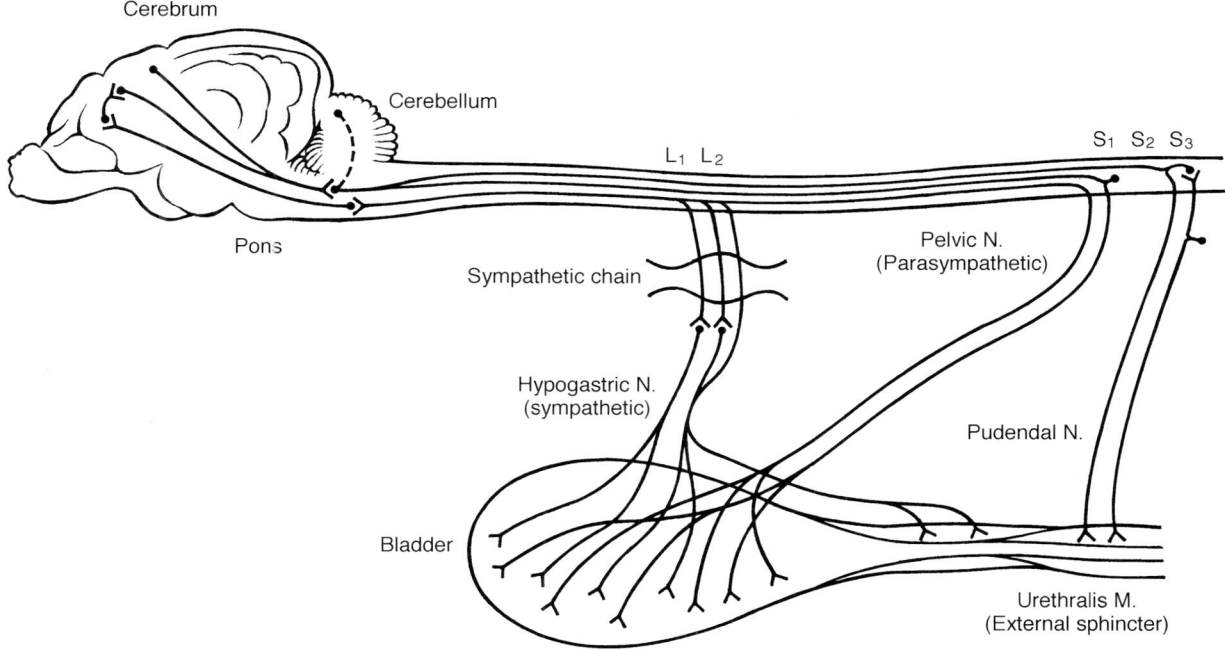

Figure 41.5 Innervation of the bladder.

neurogenic causes of incontinence and in formulating appropriate symptomatic treatment (Fig. 41.5). Cholinergic and beta-adrenergic receptors are concentrated in the detrusor muscle whereas alpha-adrenergic receptors are concentrated in the trigone, bladder neck and urethra (Moreau, 1982).

Lack of cortical control of urination prior to house training or litter training or in senile dementia causes normal complete urination but in inappropriate places. Upper motor neurone cord lesions often cause bladder spasticity so that voiding is initiated at a relatively low volume. The detrusor contraction is not very strong so the bladder is not completely emptied. Lack of coordination of urethral relaxation with urination causes spastic contraction of the urethra during urination, i.e. reflex dyssynergia. Lower motor neurone cord lesions cause bladder atony. If hypogastric innervation is preserved, the bladder may be difficult to express because alpha-adrenergic tone in the bladder neck and urethra is preserved. However, in most dogs, urethral tone is reduced. Usually the bladder fills, overdistension with atonic bladder may occur and overflow incontinence develops. Urinary tract infection is a common complication of neurogenic disturbances of micturition.

Atonic bladder may be congenital or acquired. The acquired form may be idiopathic or caused by urethral obstruction with overdistension and disruption of tight junctions between detrusor muscle cells. In feline dysautonomia, a disease affecting autonomic ganglia, cholinergic tone is diminished leading to bladder atony and overflow incontinence (Key and Gaskell, 1982; Sharp et al., 1984).

Lower urinary tract inflammation causes disruption and exaggeration of normal afferent stretch receptor activity and loss of normal coordination of bladder and urethral function. Urethral obstruction by uroliths causes urethral spasm adjacent to the urolith leading to urine retention and overflow incontinence. The cause of incontinence due to granulomatous urethritis and urethral tumour is similar and in all instances urethral obstruction may become complete with no passage of urine (Moroff et al., 1991).

Ectopic ureters are most common in female dogs. Golden retrievers, Siberian huskies, miniature and toy poodles, West Highland white terriers, collies, Labrador retrievers and Welsh corgis appear to be predisposed. During embryological development the urogenital sinus fails to migrate cranially to the trigonal position in the bladder. Short, incompetent urethra may occur with or without a hypoplastic bladder (Holt, 1990b). The cause of this malformation is unknown. When the neck of the bladder is positioned inside the pelvis even normal intra-abdominal pressure tends to force urine out of the urethra (Adams and Dibartola, 1983). Female dogs are often affected by urethral incompetence which may develop or worsen after ovariohysterectomy (Arnold *et al*., 1992). The number and sensitivity of alpha-adrenergic receptors in the neck of the bladder and the urethra are reduced after ovariectomy and restored after oestrogen replacement treatment in rabbits (Levin *et al*., 1980). A similar mechanism may be responsible for urethral incompetence in spayed female dogs (Batra and Iosif, 1983).

Vaginal pooling causes urine to accumulate in the proximal vagina during urination with subsequent passage after urination. A similar process causes passage of urine between urinations in dogs with large prostatic cysts that communicate with the urethra.

Stress incontinence occurs when fear or emotion causes abdominal muscle contraction with increased intra-abdominal pressure to a point where urethral sphincter tone is overcome. Urge incontinence usually develops with lower urinary tract inflammation but an idiopathic form where uncontrolled detrusor contraction occurred in the absence of detectable lower urinary tract inflammation has been described (Lappin and Barsanti, 1987).

Diagnosis

An accurate history that allows complete understanding of the patient's disturbance is probably the most valuable diagnostic tool. Physical examination and direct observance of urination are also necessary. Neurological examination should be performed to detect neurogenic causes. Urinalysis to determine the presence of urinary tract inflammation is essential. Catheterization of the urethra to detect urethral obstruction and to measure residual urine volume after micturition may be helpful. Radiographic evaluation including plain radiographs, cystography, intravenous pyelography and retrograde and voiding urethrography may be necessary. Urodynamic studies such as urethral pressure profilometry, uroflowmetry and

Table 41.28 Medications for disturbances of micturition

Classification	Mode of action	Dose	
		Dog	Cat
Detrusor relaxation			
propantheline	parasympatholytic	15–30 mg p.o. tid	7.5 mg p.o. q2d
	antispasmodic – smooth muscle	5 mg p.o. bid or tid	—
oxybutinin	weak parasympatholytic		
flavoxate	antispasmodic – smooth muscle	100–200 mg p.o. tid-qid	—
Detrusor contraction:			
bethanechol	parasympathomimetic	1–15 mg p.o. tid	1.25–2.5 mg p.o. tid
propranolol	beta-blocker	0.25–0.5 mg kg^{-1} p.o. tid	—
Urethral relaxation:			
diazepam	somatic muscle relaxation	2–10 mg p.o. tid	—
dantrolene	somatic muscle relaxation	safe dose not established in dog and cat	—
phenoxybenzamine	alpha-antagonist	5–15 mg p.o. tid	2.5–5.0 mg p.o. tid
baclofen	unknown	5–10 mg p.o. tid	
Urethral contraction:			
ephedrine	alpha-agonist	5–15 mg p.o.	2–5 mg p.o.
phenylephrine	alpha-agonist	—	—
phenylpropanolamine	alpha-agonist	1.5 mg kg^{-1} p.o. tid	—
imipramine	unknown	0.5–1.0 mg kg^{-1} p.o. tid	—
diethylstilbestrol	alpha-receptor enhancer	0.1–1.0 mg p.o. sid 5 days then 0.1–1.0 mg p.o. q 3–4 days	—
testosterone cypionate	unknown	2.2 mg kg^{-1} i.m. q 30 days	—
testosterone propionate		2.2 mg kg^{-1} i.m. q 2–7 days	

cystometrography to assess bladder and urethral function may be helpful (Moreau et al., 1983 a, b, c; Rosin and Barsanti, 1981) Cystoscopy can assist in the location and treatment of ectopic ureters (Senior and Sundstrom, 1988; Stone and Mason, 1990).

Management

Specific lesions that are correctable by surgery should be addressed. Ectopic ureters can be translocated into the bladder (Stone and Mason, 1990). Urethral pressure profilometry performed before surgical correction of ectopic ureter can predict the likelihood of postoperative incontinence due to concurrent urethral sphincter incompetence (Lane et al., 1992). Patent urachus should be ablated. Both surgical culposuspension and periurethral injection of Teflon® paste or glutaraldehyde cross-linked bovine collagen via cytoscopy have been described to prevent incontinence due to urethral sphincter incompetence (Holt, 1990a; Arnold et al., 1989; Wan et al., 1992). Ablation of the proximal vagina can prevent urine pooling. Trigonal–colonic anastomosis with bladder resection has been used for atonic bladder but the results are disappointing (Bovée et al., 1979b). Urethral uroliths must be removed or if that is not possible a urethrostomy must be established. Although bladder tumours are often refractory to chemotherapy, some transitional cell carcinomas in dogs (the most common form) respond quite well to treatment with piroxicam at 0.3 mg kg^{-1} p.o. sid (Knapp et al., 1994).

In many animals with disturbances of micturition, the cause of the disturbance cannot be identified or, more likely, can be identified but cannot be corrected. Medications to alter micturition so that more normal function is achieved are often necessary on a long-term basis. The therapeutic action of these drugs is based on their effect on autonomic receptor function (Table 41.28). Symptomatic administration of appropriate medication can often control disorders of micturition that are unacceptable to the owner. Diethylstilboestrol and methyltestosterone have been used in female and male dogs, respectively, to treat urethral incompetence. A synergistic action between diethylstilboestrol and alpha-agonists such as phenylpropanolamine has been observed in female dogs with incontinence. Treatment of concurrent urinary tract infection and control of disorders that induce polyuria can also assist in normalizing micturition.

REFERENCES

Abdullahi, S., Osborne, C.A., Leininger, J.R., Fletcher, T.F. and Griffith, D.P. (1984) Evaluation of a calculytic diet in female dogs with induced struvite urolithiasis. *American Journal of Veterinary Research* **45**, 1508–1519.

Adams, W.M. and Dibartola, S.P. (1983) Radiographic and clinical features of pelvic bladder in the dog. *Journal of the American Veterinary Medical Association* **182**, 1212–1217.

Adams, W.H., Toal, R.L. and Breider, M.A. (1991) Ultrasonographic findings in ethylene glycol (antifreeze) poisoning in a pregnant queen and 4 fetal kittens. *Veterinary Radiology* **32**, 60–62.

Akmal, M., Goldstein, D.A., Multani, S. and Massry, C.B. (1984) Role of uremia, brain calcium, and parathyroid hormone on changes in electro-encephalogram in chronic renal failure. *American Journal of Physiology* **246**, F575–F579.

Allen, T.A., Jaenke, R.S. and Fettman, M.J. (1987) A technique for estimating progression of chronic renal failure in the dog. *Journal of the American Veterinary Medical Association* **190**, 866–868.

Arnold, S., Jager, P., Dibartola, S.P., Lott-Stolz, G., Hauser, B., Hubler, M., Casal, M., Fairburn, A. and Rusch P. (1989) Treatment of urinary incontinence in dogs by endoscopic injection of teflon. *Journal of the American Veterinary Medical Association* **195**, 1369–1374.

Arnold, S., Arnold, P., Hubler, M. and Rusch, P. (1992) Urinary incontinence in spayed bitches: prevalence and breed predisposition. *European Journal of Companion Animal Practice* **2**, 65–68.

Arthur, J.E., Lucke, V.M., Newby, T.J. and Bourne, F.J. (1986) The long-term prognosis of feline idiopathic membranous glomerulonephropathy. *Journal of the American Animal Hospital Association* **22**, 731–737.

Bagley, R.S., Center, S.A., Lewis, R.M., Shin, S., Dougherty, S.A., Randolph, J.F. and Erb, H. (1991) The effect of experimental cystitis and iatrogenic blood contamination on the urine protein/creatinine ratio in the dog. *Journal of Veterinary Internal Medicine* **5**, 66–70.

Barber, D.L. and Finco, D.R. (1979) Radiographic findings in induced bacterial pyelonephritis in dogs. *Journal of the American Veterinary Medical Association* **175**, 1183–1190.

Barsanti, J.A. and Finco, D.R. (1979a) Laboratory findings in urinary tract infections. *Veterinary Clinics of North America* **9**, 729–748.

Barsanti, J.A. and Finco, D.R. (1979b) Protein concentration of urine in normal dogs. *American Journal of Veterinary Research* **40**, 1583–1588.

Barsanti, J.A. and Finco, D.R. (1989) Canine prostatic diseases. In: *Textbook of Veterinary Medicine*, 3rd edn (Ed. S.J. Ettinger). W.B. Saunders, Philadelphia, pp. 1859–1880.

Barsanti, J.A., Prasse, K.W., Crowell, W.A., Shotts,

E.B. and Finco, D.R. (1983) Evaluation of various techniques for diagnosis of chronic bacterial prostatitis in the dog. *Journal of the American Veterinary Medical Association* **183**, 219–224.

Batra, S.C. and Iosif, C.S. (1983) Female urethra: a target for estrogen action. *Journal of Urology* **129**, 418–420.

Benson, M.D., Dwulet, F.E. and DiBartola, S.P. (1985) Identification and characterization of amyloid protein AA in spontaneous canine amyloidosis. *Laboratory Investigation* **52**, 448–452.

Berg, O.A. (1958) Effect of stilbestrol on the prostate gland in normal puppies and adult dogs. *Acta Endocrinology* **27**, 155–164.

Berry, S.J., Strandberg, J.D., Saunders, W.J. and Coffey, D.S. (1978) Development of canine benign prostatic hyperplasia with age. *Prostate* **9**, 363–373.

Biller, D.S., Chew, D.J. and DiBartola, S.P. (1990) Polycystic kidney disease in a family of Persian cats. *Journal of the American Veterinary Medical Association* **196**, 1288–1290.

Borison, H.L. and Hebertson, L.M. (1959) Role of medullary emetic chemoreceptor trigger zone in post-nephrectomy vomiting dogs. *American Journal of Physiology* **197**, 850–852.

Bovée, K.C. (1984) Genetic and metabolic diseases of the kidney. In: *Canine Nephrology* (Eds K.C. Bovée, C.R. Bower and H. Bower). Harwal Publishing Co., pp. 339–354.

Bovée, K.C. and Joyce, T. (1974) Critical evaluation of glomerular function: 24-hour creatinine clearance in dogs. *Journal of the American Veterinary Medical Association* **174**, 488–491.

Bovée, K.C. and McGuire, T. (1984) Qualitative and quantitative analysis of uroliths in dogs. Definitive determination of chemical type. *Journal of the American Veterinary Medical Association* **185**, 983–987.

Bovée, K.C., Joyce, T., Reynolds, R. and Segal, S. (1978) The Fanconi syndrome in basenji dogs: a new model for renal transport defects. *Science* **201**, 1129–1131.

Bovée, K.C., Joyce, T., Blazer-Yost, B., Goldschmidt, M.S. and Segal, S. (1979a) Characterization of renal defects in dogs with a syndrome similar to Fanconi syndrome in man. *Journal of the American Veterinary Medical Association* **174**, 1094–1099.

Bovée, K.C., Pass, M.A., Wardley, R., Biery, D. and Allen, H.L. (1979b) Trigonal–colonic anastamosis. A urinary diversion procedure in dogs. *Journal of the American Veterinary Medical Association* **174**, 184–191.

Bovée, K.C., Kronfeld, D.S., Ramberg, C. and Goldschmidt, M. (1979c) Long-term measurement of renal function in partially nephrectomized dogs fed 56, 27, or 19% protein. *Investigative Urology* **16**, 378–384.

Branam, J.E., Keen, C.L., Ling, G.V. and Franti, C.E. (1984) Selected physical and chemical characteristics of prostatic fluid collected by ejaculation from healthy dogs and from dogs with bacterial prostatitis. *American Journal of Veterinary Research* **45**, 825–798.

Brearley, M.J., Milroy, E.J.G. and Rickards, D. (1988) A percutaneous approach for cystoscopy in male dogs. *Research in Veterinary Science* **44**, 380–382.

Brendler, C.B., Berry, S.J., Ewing, L.L., McCullough, A.R. and Cochran, R.C. (1983) Spontaneous benign prostatic hyperplasia in the beagle. *Journal of Clinical Investigation* **71**, 1114–1123.

Bricker, N.S., Fine, L.G., Kaplan, M.A., Epstein, M., Bourgoignie, J.J. and Licht, A. (1978) 'Magnification phenomenon' in chronic renal disease. *New England Journal of Medicine* **299**, 1287–1293.

Brodey, R.S. (1955) Canine urolithiasis. *Journal of the American Veterinary Medical Association* **126**, 1–9.

Brown, J.E. and Fox, L.M. (1984) Ammonium chloride/methionine toxicity in kittens. *Feline Practice* **14**, 16–19.

Brown, N.O., Parks, J.L. and Greene, R.W. (1977) Canine urolithiasis: retrospective analysis of 438 cases. *Journal of the American Veterinary Medical Association* **170**, 414–418.

Brown, S.A., Barsanti, J.A. and Crowell, W.A. (1985) Gentamicin-associated acute renal failure in the dog. *Journal of the American Veterinary Medical Association* **186**, 686–690.

Brown, S.A., Finco, D.R., Crowell, W.A. and Navar, L.G. (1991a) Dietary protein intake and the glomerular adaptations to partial nephrectomy in dogs. *Journal of Nutrition* **121**, 125–127.

Brown, S.A., Crowell, W.A., Barsanti, J.A., White, J.V. and Finco, D.R. (1991b) Beneficial effects of dietary mineral restriction in 15/16 nephrectomized dogs. *Journal of the American Society of Nephrology* **1**, 1169–1179.

Brown, S.A., Finco, D.R., Boudinot, F.D., Wright, J., Tarver, S.L. and Cooper, T. (1996) Evaluation of a single injection method using iohexol, for estimating glomerular filtration rate in dogs and cats. *American Journal of Veterinary Research* **57**, 105–110.

Buffington, C.A. (1989) Nutrition and struvite urolithiasis in cats. *Veterinary International Spring Conference*, pp. 3–15.

Buffington, C.A.T., Chew, D.J. and DiBartola, S.P. (1996) Interstitial cystitis in cats. *Veterinary Clinics of North America* **26**, 317–326.

Burke, T.J., Cronin, R.E., Duchin, K.L., Peterson, L.N. and Schrier, R.W. (1982) Ischemia and tubule obstruction during acute renal failure in dogs: mannitol in protection. *American Journal of Physiology* **238**, F305–F314.

Burns, M.G., Kelly, A.B., Hornof, W.J. and Howerth, E.W. (1981) Pulmonary artery thrombosis in three dogs with hyperadrenocorticism. *Journal of the American Veterinary Medical Association* **178**, 388–393.

Burrows, C.F. and Bovée, K.C. (1974) Metabolic changes due to experimental rupture of the canine urinary bladder. *American Journal of Veterinary Research* **35**, 1083–1088.

Burrows, C.F. and Bovée, K.C. (1978) Characterization and treatment of acid–base and renal defects due to urethral obstruction in cats. *Journal of the American Veterinary Medical Association* **172**, 801–805.

Bush, B.M. (1976) A review of the etiology and consequences of urinary tract infections in the dog. *British Veterinary Journal* **132**, 632–641.

Case, L.C., Ling, G.V., Franti, C.E., Ruby, A.L., Stevens, F. and Johnson, D.L. (1992) Cystine-containing urinary calculi in dogs: 102 cases (1981–1989). *Journal of the American Veterinary Medical Association* **201**, 129–133.

Center, S.A., Smith, C.A., Wilkinson, E., Erb, H.N. and Lewis, R.M. (1987) Clinicopathologic, renal immunofluorescent, and light microscopic features of glomerulonephritis in the dog: 41 cases (1975–1985). *Journal of the American Veterinary Medical Association* **190**, 81–90.

Cheville, N.F. (1979) Uremic gastropathy in the dog. *Veterinary Pathology* **16**, 292–309.

Clark, L.D. and Seawright, A.A. (1969) Generalized amyloidosis in seven cats. *Veterinaria Pathologia* **6**, 117–134.

Clark, W.T. (1974) The distribution of canine urinary calculi and their reoccurrence following treatment. *Journal of Small Animal Practice* **15**, 437–442.

Cowan, L.A., Barsanti, J.A., Brown, J. and Jain, A. (1991a) Effects of bacterial infection and castration on prostatic tissue zinc concentration in dogs. *American Journal of Veterinary Research* **52**, 1262–1264.

Cowan, L.A., Barsanti, J.A., Crowell, W. and Brown, J. (1991b) Effects of castration on chronic bacterial prostatitis in dogs. *Journal of the American Veterinary Medical Association* **199**, 346–350.

Cowgill, L.D. (1973) Diseases of the kidney. In: *Textbook of Veterinary Internal Medicine*, 2nd edn (Ed. S.J. Ettinger). W.B. Saunders, Philadelphia, pp. 1983.

Cowgill, L.D. (1992) Application of recombinant human erythropoietin in dogs and cats. In: *Current Veterinary Therapy* XI (Ed. R.W. Kirk). W.B. Saunders, Philadelphia, pp. 484–487.

Cowgill, L.D. and Kallet, A.J. (1983) Recognition and management of hypertension in the dog. In: *Current Veterinary Therapy* VIII (Ed. R.W. Kirk). W.B. Saunders, Philadelphia, pp. 1025–1028.

Cowgill, L.D. and Kallet, A.J. (1986) Systemic hypertension. In: *Current Veterinary Therapy* IX (Ed. R.W. Kirk). W.B. Saunders, Philadelphia, pp. 360–364.

Cowgill, L.D., Feldman, B., Levy, J. and James, K. (1990) Efficacy of recombinant human erythropoietin (r-HuEPO) for anemia in dogs and cats with renal failure. *Journal of Veterinary Internal Medicine* **4**, 126.

Crisp, M.S., Chew, D.J., DiBartola, S.P. and Birchard, S.J. (1989) Peritoneal dialysis in dogs and cats: 27 cases (1976–1987) *Journal of the American Veterinary Medical Association* **195**, 1262–1266.

Crowell, W.A. and Hubbell, J.J. (1979) Polycystic renal disease in related cats. *Journal of the American Veterinary Medical Association* **175**, 286–288.

Dainiak, N. (1985) The role of androgens in the treatment of chronic renal failure. *Seminars in Nephrology* **5**, 147–154.

Davenport, D.J. (1986) Familial renal disease in the dog and cat. In: *Nephrology and Urology* (Ed. E.B. Breitschwerdt). Churchill Livingstone, New York, p. 137.

DiBartola, S.P. and Benson, M.D. (1989) The pathogenesis of reactive systemic amyloidosis. *Journal of Veterinary Internal Medicine* **3**, 31–41.

DiBartola, S.P. and Meuten, D.J. (1980) Renal amyloidosis in two dogs presented for thromboembolic phenomena. *Journal of the American Animal Hospital Association* **16**, 129–135.

DiBartola, S.P., Benson, M.D., Dwulet, F.E. and Coracoff. (1985) Isolation and characterization of amyloid protein AA in the Abyssinian cat. *Laboratory Investigation* **52**, 485–489.

Dow, S.W., Fettman, M.J., LeCouteur, R.A. and Hamar, D.W. (1987) Potassium depletion in cats: renal and dietary influences. *Journal of the American Veterinary Medical Association* **191**, 1569–1575.

Dow, S.W., Fettman, M.J., Curtis, and LeCouteur, R.A. (1989) Hypokalemia in cats: 186 cases (1984–1987). *Journal of the American Veterinary Medical Association* **194**, 1604–1608.

Dow, S.W., Fettman, M.J., Smith, K.R., Hamar, D.W., Nagode, L.A., Fefsal, K.R. and Wilke, W.L. (1990) Effect of dietary acidification and potassium depletion on acid–base balance, mineral metabolism, and renal function in adult cats. *Journal of Nutrition* **120**, 569–578.

Dube, J.Y., Frenette, G., Tremblay, Y., Belanger, A. and Tremblay, R.R. (1984) Single case report of prostate adenocarcinoma in a dog castrated 3 months previously. Morphological, biochemical and endocrine determinations. *Prostate* **5**, 495–501.

Durham, S.K. and Dietze, A.E. (1986) Prostatic adenocarcinoma with and without metastasis to bone in dogs. *Journal of the American Veterinary Medical Association* **188**, 432–436.

Eknoyan, G., Bulger, R.E. and Dobyan, D.C. (1982) Mercuric chloride-induced acute renal failure in the rat. *Laboratory Investigation* **46**, 613–620.

Eschbach, J.W. (1989) The anemia of chronic renal failure: pathophysiology and the effects of recombinant erythropoietin. *Kidney International* **35**, 134–148.

Escolar, E. (1990) Structure and composition of canine urinary calculi. *Research in Veterinary Science* **49**, 327–333.

Evans, J.E. (1985) Prostatic adenocarcinoma in a castrated dog. *Journal of the American Veterinary Medical Association* **186**, 78–80.

Fabricant, C.G. (1977) Herpesvirus-induced urolithiasis in specific-pathogen-free male cats. *American Journal of Veterinary Research* **38**, 1837–1842.

Fair, W.R. and Parrish, R.F. (1981) Antibacterial substances in prostatic fluid. *Progress in Clinical Biological Research* **75**, 247–264.

Feeney, D.A., Johnston, G.R., Klausner, J.S., Perman, V., Leininger, J.R. and Tomlinson, M.J. (1987) Canine prostatic disease – comparison of ultrasonographic appearance with morphologic and microbiologic findings: 30 cases (1981–1985). *Journal of the American Veterinary Medical Association* **190**, 1027–1034.

Finco, D.R. and Brown, S.A. (1991) Exogenous creatinine clearance reliably measures glomerular filtration rate in dogs with reduced renal mass. *Journal of Veterinary Internal Medicine* **4**, 125 (Abstract).

Finco, D.R., Rosen, E. and Greene, R.W. (1970) Canine urolithiasis: a review of 133 clinical and necropsy cases. *American Journal of Veterinary Research* **157**, 1225–1228.

Finco, D.R., Coulter, D.B. and Barsanti, J.A. (1982) Procedure for a simple method of measuring glomerular filtration rate in the dog. *Journal of the American Animal Hospital Association* **18**, 804–806.

Finco, D.R., Crowell, W.A. and Barsanti, J.A. (1985) Effects of three diets on dogs with induced chronic renal failure. *American Journal of Veterinary Research* **46**, 646–653.

Finco, D.R., Brown, S.A. and Barsanti, J.A. (1992) Measurement of GFR in dogs using endogenous creatinine clearance (abstr). *American College of Veterinary Internal Medicine Proceedings*, p. 803.

Fitzgerald, G.A. (1988) Prostaglandins and related compounds. In: *Cecil Textbook of Medicine*, 18th edn (Eds J.B. Wyngaarden and C.H. Smith). W.B. Saunders Co., Philadelphia, p. 1275.

Friedman, J., Hoyer, J.R. and Seiler, M.W. (1982) Formation and clearance of tubulointerstitial immune complexes in kidneys of rats immunized with heterologous antisera to Tamm–Horsfall protein. *Kidney International* **21**, 575–582.

Glassock, R.J. (1985) Natural history and treatment of primary proliferative glomerulonephritis: a review. *Kidney International* **28**(S17), S136–S142.

Goldsmid, S.E. and Bellenger, C.R. (1991) Urinary incontinence after prostatectomy in dogs. *Veterinary Surgery* **20**, 253–256.

Goldstein, D.A., Chui, L.A. and Massry, S.G. (1978) Effect of parathyroid hormone and uremia on peripheral nerve calcium and motor nerve conduction velocity. *Journal of Clinical Investigation* **62**, 88–93.

Grauer, G.F. and Thrall, M.A.H. (1986) Ethylene glycol (antifreeze) poisoning. In: *Current Veterinary Therapy* IX (Ed. R.W. Kirk). W.B. Saunders, Philadelphia, pp. 206–212.

Grauer, G.F., Thomas, C.B. and Eicker, S.W. (1985) Estimation of quantitative proteinuria in the dog, using the urine protein-to-creatinine ratio from a random, voided sample. *American Journal of Veterinary Research* **46**, 2116–2119.

Grauer, G.F., Frisbie, D.D., Longhofer, S.L. and Cooley, A.J. (1992) Effects of a thromboxane synthetase inhibitor on established immune complex glomerulonephritis in dogs. *American Journal of Veterinary Research* **53**, 808–813.

Green, R.A. and Kabel, A.L. (1982) Hypercoagulable state in three dogs with nephrotic syndrome: role of acquired antithrombin III deficiency. *Journal of the American Veterinary Medical Association* **181**, 914–917.

Green, R.A., Russo, E.A., Green, R.T. and Kabel, A.L. (1985) Hypoalbuminemia-related platelet hypersensitivity in two dogs with nephrotic syndrome. *Journal of the American Veterinary Medical Association* **186**, 485–488.

Greene, C.E. and George, L.W. (1984) Canine brucellosis. In: *Clinical Microbiology and Infectious Diseases of the Dog and Cat* (Ed. C.E. Green). W.B. Saunders, Philadelphia, pp. 646–652.

Gregory, C.R. and Vasseur, P.B. (1983) Long-term examination of cats with perineal urethrostomy. *Veterinary Surgery* **12**, 210–212.

Griffin, D.W. and Gregory, C.R. (1992) Prevalence of bacterial urinary tract infection after perineal urethrostomy in cats. *Journal of the American Veterinary Medical Association* **200**, 681–684.

Gruys, E., Sijens, R.J. and Biewenga, W.J. (1981) Dubious effect of dimethylsulphoxide (DMSO) therapy on amyloid deposits and amyloidosis. *Veterinary Research Communications* **5**, 21–32.

Haraldsson, B.S., Johnsson, E.K.A. and Rippe, B. (1992) Glomerular permselectivity is dependent on adequate serum concentrations of orosomucoid. *Kidney International* **41**, 310–316.

Hardie, E.M., Barsanti, J.A. and Rawlings, C.A. (1984) Complications of prostatic surgery. *Journal of the American Animal Hospital Association* **20**, 50–56.

Heeg, J.E., deJang, P.E., van der Hem, G.K. and de Zeeuw, D. (1987) Reduction of proteinuria by angiotensin converting enzyme inhibition. *Kidney International* **32**, 78–83.

Hesse, A. (1990) Canine urolithiasis: epidemiology and analysis of urinary calculi. *Journal of Small Animal Practice* **31**, 599–604.

Hicking, W., Hesse, A., Gebhardt, M. and Vahlensieck, W. (1981) Analytich untersuchungen an harnsteinen von saugeetieren. In: *Analytiche Untersuchungen an symposien Bonn-Wien* (Ed. W. Vahlensieck). Darmstadt Steinkopff Verlag, p. 40.

Holt, P.E. (1990a) Long-term evaluation of colposuspension in the treatment of urinary incontinence due to incompetence of the urethral sphincter mechanism in the bitch. *Veterinary Record* **127**, 537–542.

Holt, P.E. (1990b) Urinary incontinence in dogs and cats. *Veterinary Record* **127**, 347–350.

Holt, P.E. (1988) Simultaneous urethral pressure profilometry: comparisons between continent and incontinent bitches. *Journal of Small Animal Practice* **29**, 761–769.

Hoppe, A., Denneberg, T. and Kagedal, B. (1988) Treatment of clinically normal and cystinuric dogs with 2-mercaptopropionylglycine. *American Journal of Veterinary Research* **49**, 923–928.

Huggins, C. and Clark, P.G. (1940) Quantitative studies of prostatic secretion II. The effect of castration and of estrogen injection on the normal and on the hyperplastic prostate glands of dogs. *Journal of Experimental Medicine* **72**, 747–750.

Hulter, H.N. (1984) Hypophosphaturia impairs the renal defense against metabolic acidosis. *Kidney International* **26**, 302–307.

Humes, H.D. (1986) Role of calcium in pathogenesis of acute renal failure. *American Journal of Physiology* **250**, F579–F589.

Jackson, B.R., Edwards, R.M. and Valtin, R.W. (1980) Evidence of vasopressin in medullary tubule of mice with hereditary nephrogenic diabetes insipidus. *Journal of Clinical Investigation* **55**, 110–115.

Jaenke, R.S. and Allen, T.A. (1986) Membranous nephropathy in the dog. *Veterinary Pathology* **23**, 718–733.

Joles, J.A. and Drays, S. (1979) Nephrogenic diabetes insipidus in a dog with renal medullary lesions. *Journal of the American Veterinary Medical Association* **174**, 830–835.

Kallett, A.J. and Cowgill, L.D. (1982) Hypertensive states in the dog. *American College of Veterinary Internal Medicine Scientific Proceedings*, p. 79.

Key, T.J.A. and Gaskell, C.J. (1982) Puzzling syndrome in cats associated with pupillary dilation. *Veterinary Record* **110**, 160.

Kivisto, A.K., Vasenius, H. and Sandholm, M. (1977) Canine bacteriuria. *Journal of Small Animal Practice* **18**, 707–712.

Klatersky, J., Danier, D., Swings, and Weerts, D. (1974) Antibacterial activity in serum and urine as a therapeutic guide in bacterial infections. *Journal of Infectous Diseases* **129**, 187–193.

Knapp, D.W., Richardson, R.C., Chan, T.C.K., Bottoms, G.D., Widmer, W.R., DeNicola, D.B., Teclaw, R., Bonney, P.L. and Kuczek, T. (1994) Piroxicam therapy in 34 dogs with transitional cell carcinoma of the urinary bladder. *Journal of Veterinary Internal Medicine* **8**, 273–278.

Kobayashi, D.L., Peterson, M.E., Graves, T.K., Lesser, M. and Nichols, C.E. (1990) Hypertension in cats with chronic renal failure or hyperthyroidism. *Journal of Veterinary Internal Medicine* **4**, 58–62.

Kok, D.J., Papapoulos, S.E. and Bijvoet, O.L.M. (1990) Crystal agglomeration is a major element in calcium oxalate urinary stone formation. *Kidney International* **37**, 51–56.

Krawiec, D.R. and Heflin, D. (1992) Study of prostatic disease in dogs: 177 cases (1981–1986). *Journal of the American Veterinary Medical Association* **200**, 1119–1122.

Krawiec, D.R., Badertscher, R.R., II, Twardock, A.R., Rubin, S.I. and Gelberg, H.B. (1986) Evaluation of ^{99m}Tc-diethylenetriaminepentaacetic acid nuclear imaging for quantitative determination of the glomerular filtration rate of dogs. *American Journal of Veterinary Research* **47**, 2175–2179.

Kruger, J.M., Osborne, C.A., Goyal, S.M., Wickstrom, S.L., Johnston, G.R., Fletcher, T.F. and Brown, P.A. (1991) Clinical evaluation of cats with lower urinary tract disease. *Journal of the American Veterinary Medical Association* **199**, 211–216.

Kruger, J.M., Osborne, C.A. and Iulich, J.P. (1996) Management of nonobstructive idiopathic feline lower urinary tract disease. *Veterinary Clinics of North America* **26**, 571–588.

Kurtz, T.W. and Morris, R.C., Jr (1983) Dietary chloride as a determinant of 'sodium-dependent' hypertension. *Science* **222**, 1139–1141.

Kurtz, J.M., Russell, S.W., Lee, J.C., Slauson, D.O. and Schechter, R.D. (1972) Naturally occurring canine glomerulonephritis. *American Journal of Pathology* **67**, 471–482.

Lane, I.F., Lappin, M.R. and Seim, H.B. (1992) Predictive value of urodynamic measurements in the management of ectopic ureters in the dog (abstr). *American College of Veterinary Internal Medicine Proceedings*, p. 802.

Lappin, M.R. and Barsanti, J.A. (1987) Urinary incontinence secondary to idiopathic detrusor instability: cystometrographic diagnosis and pharmacologic management in two dogs and a cat. *Journal of the American Veterinary Medical Association* **191**, 1439–1442.

Leav, I. and Ling, G.V. (1968) Adenocarcinoma of the canine prostate. *Cancer* **22**, 1329–1245.

Lees, G.E., Osborne, C.A., Stevens, J.B. and Ward, G.E. (1981) Adverse effects of open indwelling urethral catheterization in clinically normal male cats. *American Journal of Veterinary Research* **42**, 825–833.

Lees, G.E., Simpson, R.B. and Green, R.A. (1984) Results of analyses and bacterial cultures of urine specimens obtained from clinically normal cats by three methods. *Journal of the American Veterinary Medical Association* **184**, 449–454.

Levin, R.M., Shofer, F.S. and Wein, A.J. (1980) Estrogen induced alterations of autonomic receptor distribution in the rabbit urinary bladder (abstr). *Federation Proceedings* **39**, 296.

Lidner, A., Cutler, R.E. and Goodman, W.G. (1979) Synergism of dopamine plus furosemide in preventing acute renal failure in the dog. *Kidney International* **16**, 158–166.

Ling, G.V. (1983) Treatment of urinary tract infections with antimicrobial agents. In: *Current Veterinary Therapy* VIII (Ed. R.W. Kirk). W.B. Saunders, Philadelphia, pp. 1051–1055.

Ling, G.V. (1984) Therapeutic strategies involving antimicrobial treatment of the canine urinary tract. *Journal of the American Veterinary Medical Association* **185**, 1162–1164.

Ling, G.V. and Ruby, A.L. (1978) Aerobic bacterial flora of the prepuce, urethra and vagina of normal dogs. *American Journal of Veterinary Research* **39**, 695–698.

Ling, G.V., Ackerman, N., Lowenstine, L.J. and Cowgill, L.D. (1979) Percutaneous nephropyelocentesis and nephropyelostomy in the dog: a description of the technique. *American Journal of Veterinary Research* **40**, 1605–1612.

Ling, G.V., Branam, J.E., Ruby, A.L. and Johnson, D.L. (1983) Canine prostatic fluid: techniques of collection, quantitative bacterial culture, and interpretation of results. *Journal of the American Veterinary Medical Association* **183**, 201–206.

Ling, G.V., Lowenstine, L.J., Cullen, J.M., Ackerman, N. and Ruby, A.L. (1987) Chronic urinary tract infection in dogs: induction by inoculation with bacteria via percutaneous nephropyelostomy. *American Journal of Veterinary Research* **48**, 794–798.

Ling, G.V., Nyland, T.G., Kennedy, P.C., Hager, D.A. and Johnson, D.L. (1990a) Comparison of two sample collection methods for quantitative bacteriologic culture of canine prostatic fluid. *Journal of the American Veterinary Medical Association* **196**, 1479–1482.

Ling, G.V., Franti, C.E. and Ruby, A.L. (1990b) Epizootiologic evaluation and quantitative analysis of urinary calculi from 150 cats. *Journal of the American Veterinary Medical Association* **196**, 1459–1462.

Ling, G.V., Ruby, A.L., Harrold, D. and Johnson, D.L. (1991) Xanthine-containing urinary calculi in dogs given allopurinol. *Journal of the American Veterinary Medical Association* **198**, 1935–1940.

Littman, M.P. (1990) Spontaneous systemic hypertension in cats. American College of Veterinary Internal Medicine Abstract 82, *Journal of Veterinary Internal Medicine* **4**, 126.

Littman, M.P. (1992) Update: treatment of hypertension in dogs and cats. In: *Current Veterinary Therapy* XI (Ed. R.W. Kirk). W.B. Saunders, Philadelphia, pp. 838–841.

Lloyd, J.W., Thomas, J.A. and Mawhinney, M.G. (1975) Androgens and estrogens in the plasma and prostatic tissue of normal dogs and dogs with benign prostatic hypertrophy. *Investigative Urology* **13**, 220–222.

Lopez, S. (1984) Evaluation of calcium carbonate as an effective phosphorus binder in the dog. *Clinical Research* **32**, 452–459.

Lulich, J.P. and Osborne, C.A. (1992) Fungal urinary tract infections. In: *Current Veterinary Therapy* XI (Ed. R.W. Kirk). W.B. Saunders, Philadelphia, pp. 914–919.

Lulich, J.P., Osborne, C.A., Walter, P.A. and O'Brien, T.D. (1988) Feline idiopathic polycystic kidney disease. *Compendium of Continuing Education* **10**, 1030–1040.

Lulich, J.P., Osborne, C.A., Nagode, L.A., Polzin, D.J. and Parke, M.L. (1991) Evaluation of urine and serum analytes in miniature schnauzers with calcium oxalate urolithiasis. *American Journal of Veterinary Research* **52**, 1583–1590.

MacDougall, D.F., Cook, T., Steward, A.P. and Cattell, V. (1986) Canine chronic renal disease: prevalence and types of glomerulonephritis in the dog. *Kidney International* **29**, 1144–1151.

Maede, Y., Inaba, M. and Kashiwazaki, Y. (1985) Methionine-induced hemolytic anemia with methemoglobinemia and Heinz body formation in erythrocytes in cats. *Journal Japan Veterinary Medical Association* **38**, 568–571.

Mahoney, C.A. and Arieff, A.I. (1983) Central and peripheral nervous system effects of chronic renal failure. *Kidney International* **24**, 170–177.

Mahoney, C.A., Sarnacki, P. and Arieff, A.I. (1984) Uremic encephalopathy: role of brain energy metabolism. *American Journal of Physiology* **247**, F527–F532.

Marretta, S.M. (1981) Urinary calculi associated with portosystemic shunts in six dogs. *Journal of the American Veterinary Medical Association* **178**, 133–139.

Massry, S.G. (1989) Divalent ion metabolism and renal osteodystrophy. In: *Textbook of Nephrology*, 2nd edn. (Eds S.G. Massry and R.J. Glasscok). Williams and Wilkins, Baltimore, pp. 1278–1311.

McCarthy, T.C. and McDermaid, S.L. (1990) Cystoscopy. *Veterinary Clinics of North America* **20**, 1315–1339.

McCaw, D.L., Knapp, D.W. and Hewett, J.E. (1985) Effect of collection time and exercise restriction on the prediction of urine protein excretion, using urine protein/creatinine ratio in dogs. *American Journal of Veterinary Research* **46**, 1665–1669.

McCord, J.M. (1985) Oxygen-derived free radicals in post-ischemic tissue injury. *New England Journal of Medicine* **3**, 159–163.

McKenna, S.C. and Carpenter, J.L. (1980) Polycystic kidney disease of the kidney and liver in the Cairn terrier. *Veterinary Pathology* **17**, 436–442.

Mitch, W.E., Walser, M., Buffington, G.A. and Lemann, J., Jr (1976) A simple method for estimating progression of chronic renal failure. *Lancet* **ii**, 1326–1328.

Monroe, W.E., Davenport, D.J. and Saunders, G.K. (1989) Twenty-four hour urinary protein loss in healthy cats and the urinary protein–creatinine ratio as an estimate. *American Journal of Veterinary Research* **50**, 1906–1909.

Moreau, P.M. (1982) Neurogenic disorders of micturition in the dog and cat. *Compendium of Continuing Education* **4**, 12–22.

Moreau, P.M., Lees, G.E. and Gross, D.R. (1983a) Simultaneous cystometry and uro-flowmetry (micturition study) for evaluation of the caudal part of the urinary tract in dogs: reference values for healthy animals sedated with xylazine. *American Journal of Veterinary Research* **44**, 1774–1781.

Moreau, P.M., Lees, G.E. and Gross, D.R. (1983b) Simultaneous cystometry and uroflowmetry (micturition study) for evaluation of the caudal part of the urinary tract in dogs: studies of the technique. *American Journal of Veterinary Research* **44**, 1769–1773.

Moreau, P.M., Lees, G.E. and Hobson, H.P. (1983c) Simultaneous cystometry and uro-flowmetry for evaluation of micturition in two dogs. *Journal of the American Veterinary Medical Association* **183**, 1084–1088.

Morgan, R.V. (1986) Systemic hypertension in four cats: ocular and medical findings. *Journal of the American Animal Hospital Association* **22**, 615–621.

Moroff, S.D., Brown, B.A., Matthiesen, D.T. and Scott, R.C. (1991) Infiltrative urethral disease in female dogs: 41 cases (1980–1987). *Journal of the American Veterinary Medical Association* **199**, 247–251.

Mullen, H.S., Matthiesen, D.T. and Scavelli, T.D. (1990) Results of surgery and postoperative complications in 92 dogs treated for prostatic abscessation by a multiple penrose drain technique. *Journal of the American Animal Hospital Association* **26**, 369–379.

Nagode, L.A. and Chew, D.J. (1991) The use of calcitriol in treatment of renal disease of the dog and cat. *Purina International Symposium*, pp. 39–49.

Nash, A.S., Wright, N.G., Spencer, A.J., Thompson, H. and Fisher, E.W. (1979) Membranous nephropathy in the cat: a clinical and pathological study. *Veterinary Record* **105**, 71–77.

Neuwirth, L., Mahaffey, M., Crowell, W., Selcer, B., Barsanti, J., Cooper, R. and Brown, J. (1993) Comparison of excretory urography and ultrasonography for detection of experimentally induced pyelonephritis in dogs. *American Journal of Veterinary Research* **54**, 660–669.

Noonan, C.H.B. and Kay, J.M. (1990) Prevalence and geographic distribution of Fanconi syndrome in Basenjis in the United States. *Journal of the American Veterinary Medical Association* **197**, 345–349.

O'Brien, T.D., Osborne, C.A., Yano, B.L. and Barnes, D.M. (1982) Clinicopathologic manifestations of progressive renal disease in Lhasa Apso and Shih Tzu dogs. *Journal of the American Veterinary Medical Association* **180**, 658–664.

O'Shea, J.D. (1963) Studies on the canine prostate gland. *Journal of Comparative Patholology* **73**, 244–256.

Oliver, J.E. and Young, W.O. (1973a) Air cystometry in dogs under xylazine-induced restraint. *American Journal of Veterinary Research* **34**, 1433–1435.

Oliver, J.E. and Young, W.O. (1973b) Evaluation of pharmacologic agents for restraint in cystometry in the dog and cat. *American Journal of Veterinary Research* **34**, 665–668.

Osborne, C.A. (1971) Clinical evaluation of needle biopsy of the kidney and its complications in the dog and cat. *Journal of the American Veterinary Medical Association* **158**, 1213–1228.

Osborne, C.A. and Klausner, J.S. (1979) A problem specific data base for urinary tract infections. *Veterinary Clinics of North America* **9**, 783–794.

Osborne, C.A., Johnston, G.R., Polzin, D.J., Kruger, J.M., Poffenbarger, E.M., Goyal, S., Fletcher, T.F., Newman, J.A., Stevens, J.B. and McMenomy, M.F. (1984) Redefinition of the feline urologic syndrome: feline lower urinary tract disease with heterogenous causes. *Veterinary Clinics of North America* **14**, 409–438.

Osborne, C.A., Lulich, J.P., Unger, L.K., Sanna, J.J., Clinton, C.W. and Davenport, M.P. (1989a) Detection of uroliths and identification of their mineral composition. In: *Managing Canine and Feline Urolithiasis*. Veterinary Medicine Publishing Co., pp. 11–19.

Osborne, C.A., Polzin, D.J., Kruger, J.M., Lulich, J.P., Johnston, G.R. and O'Brien, T.D. (1989b) Relationship of nutritional factors to the cause, dissolution, and prevention of feline uroliths and urethral plugs. *Veterinary Clinics of North America* **19**, 561–581.

Osborne, C.A., Kruger, J.M., Johnston, G.R. and Polzin, D.J. (1989c) Feline lower urinary tract disorders. In: *Textbook of Veterinary Medicine*, 3rd edn (Ed. S.J. Ettinger). W.B. Saunders, Philadelphia, pp. 2057–2082.

Osborne, C.A., Lulich, J.P., Kruger, J.M., Polzin, D.J., Johnston, G.R. and Kroll, R.A. (1990) Medical dissolution of feline struvite urocystoliths. *Journal of the American Veterinary Medical Association* **196**, 1053–1063.

Osborne, C.A., Lulich, J.P., Ulrich, L.K., Koeler, L.A., Bird, K.A. and Bartges, J.W. (1996) Feline urolithiasis. *Veterinary Clinics of North America* **26**, 217–232.

Picut, C.A. and Lewis, R.M. (1987) Microscopic features of canine renal dysplasia. *Veterinary Pathology* **24**, 156–163.

Polzin, D.J. (1988) The importance of egg protein in reduced protein diets designed for dogs with renal failure. *Journal of Veterinary Internal Medicine* **2**, 15–21.

Polzin, D.J., Osborne, C.A., Stevens, J.B. and Hayden, D.W. (1983a) Serum amylase and lipase activities in dogs with chronic primary renal failure. *American Journal of Veterinary Research* **44**, 404–410.

Polzin, D.J., Osborne, C.A., Stevens, J.B. and Hayden, D.W. (1983b) Effects of modified protein diets on the nutritional status of dogs with induced chronic renal failure. *American Journal of Veterinary Research* **44**, 1694–1702.

Polzin, D.J., Osborne, C.A., Hayden, D.W. and Stevens, J.B. (1984) Influence of reduced protein diets on morbidity, mortality, and renal function in dogs with induced chronic renal failure. *American Journal of Veterinary Research* **45**, 506–517.

Polzin, D.J., Leininger, J.R., Osborne, C.A. and Jerai, K. (1988) Development of renal lesions in dogs after 11/12 reduction of renal mass. *Laboratory Investigation* **58**, 172–183.

Polzin, D., Osborne, C.A. and O'Brien, T. (1989) Diseases of the kidneys and ureters. In: *Textbook of Veterinary Internal Medicine* (Ed. S.J. Ettinger). W.B. Saunders, Philadelphia, pp. 1962–2046.

Porter, P. (1963) Urinary calculi in the dog. II. Urate stones and purine metabolism. *Journal of Comparative Pathology* **73**, 119–129.

Rahman, M.A., Stork, J.E. and Dunn, M.J. (1987) The

roles of eicosanoids in experimental glomerulonephritis. *Kidney International* 32 (S22), S40–S48.

Rasadee, A. and Feldman, B.F. (1985) Nephrotic syndrome: a platelet hyperaggregability state. *Veterinary Research Communications* 9, 199–211.

Riviere, J.E. (1984) Calculation of dosage regimens of antimicrobial drugs in animals with renal and hepatic dysfunction. *Journal of the American Veterinary Medical Association* 185, 1094–1097.

Rogers, K.S., Komkov, A., Brown, S.A., Lees, G.E., Hightower, D. and Russo, E.A. (1991) Comparison of four methods of estimating glomeruar filtration rate in cats. *American Journal of Veterinary Research* 52, 961–964.

Rosin, A., Rosin, E. and Oliver, J. (1980) Canine urethral pressure profile. *American Journal of Veterinary Research* 41, 1113–1116.

Rosin, A.E. and Barsanti, J.A. (1981) Diagnosis of urinary incontinence in dogs: role of the urethral pressure profile. *Journal of the American Veterinary Medical Association* 178, 814–822.

Ross, L.A. (1992) Endocrine hypertension. In: *Current Veterinary Therapy* XI (Ed. R.W. Kirk) W.B. Saunders, Philadelphia, pp. 309–313.

Ross, L.A. and Labato, M.A. (1989) Use of drugs to control hypertension in renal failure. In: *Current Veterinary Therapy* X (Ed. R.W. Kirk). W.B. Saunders, Philadelphia, p. 1201.

Rowland, J. (1987) Incidence of ethylene glycol intoxication in dogs and cats seen at Colorado State University veterinary teaching hospital. *Veterinary and Human Toxicology* 29, 41–44.

Schlotthauer, C.F. (1932) Observations on the prostate gland of the dog. *Journal of the American Veterinary Medical Association* 81, 645–652.

Senior, D.F. (1979) Drug therapy in renal failure. *Veterinary Clinics of North America* 9, 805–817.

Senior, D.F. and Newman, R. (1986) Retrograde ureteral catheterization in the dog. *Journal of the American Animal Hospital Association* 22, 831–834.

Senior, D.F. and Sundstrom, D.A. (1988) Cystoscopy in female dogs. *Compendium of Continuing Education* 10, 879–895.

Senior, D.F., DeMan, P. and Svanborg, C. (1992) Serotype, hemolysis production, and adherence characteristics of strains of *Escherichia coli* causing urinary tract infection in dogs. *American Journal of Veterinary Research* 53, 494–498.

Sharp, N.J.H., Nash, A.S. and Griffiths, I.R.G. (1984) Feline dysautonomia (the Key Gaskell syndrome): a clinical and pathological study of forty cases. *Journal of Small Animal Practice* 25, 599–615.

Sisson, D.D. and Hoffer, R.E. (1977) Osteocollagenous prostatic retention cyst: report of a canine case. *Journal of the American Animal Hospital Association* 13, 61–64.

Skoch, E.R., Chandler, E.A., Douglas, G.M. and Richardson, D.P. (1991) Influence of diet on urine pH and the feline urological syndrome. *Journal of Small Animal Practice* 32, 413–419.

Slauson, D.O. and Gribble, D.H. (1971) Thrombosis complicating renal amyloidosis in dogs. *Veterinary Pathology* 8, 352–355.

Slauson, D.O., Gribble, D.H. and Russell, S.W. (1970) A clinicopathologic study of renal amyloidosis in dogs. *Journal of Comparative Patholology* 80, 335–843.

Stone, E.A. and Mason, L.K. (1990) Surgery of ectopic ureters: types, method of correction, and postoperative results. *Journal of the American Animal Hospital Association* 26, 81–88.

Stone, E.A., Thrall, D.E. and Barber, D.L. (1978) Radiographic interpretation of prostatic disease in the dog. *Journal of the American Animal Hospital Association* 14, 115–118.

Taton, G.F., Hamar, D.W. and Lewis, L.D. (1984) Urinary acidification in the prevention and treatment of feline struvite urolithiasis. *Journal of the American Veterinary Medical Association* 184, 437–443.

Taylor, P.A. (1973) Prostatic adenocarcinoma in a dog with a summary of 10 cases. *Canadian Veterinary Journal* 14, 162–166.

Thornhill, J.A. (1983) Control of vomiting in the uremic patient. In: *Current Veterinary Therapy* VIII (Ed. R.W. Kirk). W.B. Saunders, Philadelphia, pp. 1022–1025.

Thrall, M.A., Dial, S.M. and Winder, D.R. (1985) Identification of calcium oxalate monohydrate crystals by x-ray diffraction in urine of ethylene glycol-intoxicated dogs. *Veterinary Pathology* 22, 625–628.

Tollins, J.P. (1985) Hypokalemic nephropathy in the rat. *Journal of Clinical Investigation* 79, 1447–1452.

Tyslowitz, R. and Dingemanse, E. (1941) Effect of large doses of estrogens on the blood picture of dogs. *Endocrinology* 29, 817–818.

Uribe, D., Krawiec, D.R., Twardock, A.R. and Gelberg, H.B. (1992) Quantitative renal scintigraphy determination of the glomerular filtration rate of cats with normal and abnormal kidney function using ^{99m}Tc-diethylenetriaminepentaacetic acid. *American Journal of Veterinary Research* 53, 1101–1107.

Walser, M., Drew, H.H. and LaFrance, N.D. (1989) Reciprocal creatinine slopes often give erroneous estimates of progression of chronic renal failure. *Kidney International* 36 (Suppl 27), 581–585.

Walter, P.A., Feeney, D.A., Johnston, G.R. and O'Leary, T.P. (1987) Ultrasonographic evaluation of renal parenchymal diseases in dogs: 32 cases (1981–1986). *Journal of the American Veterinary Medical Association* 191, 999–1012.

Wan, J., McGuire, E.J., Bloom, D.A. and Ritchey, M.I. (1992) The treatment of urinary incontinence in children using glutaraldehyde cross-linked collagen. *Journal of Urology* 148, 127–130.

Watson, A.D.J., Church, D.B. and Fairburn, A.J. (1981) Post-prandial changes in plasma urea and creatinine concentrations in dogs. *American Journal of Veterinary Research* 42, 1878–1880.

Weaver, A.D. (1970) Canine urolithiasis. Incidence, chemical composition and outcome of 100 cases. *Journal of Small Animal Practice* 11, 93–107.

Weaver, A.D. (1978) Discrete prostatic (paraprostatic) cysts in the dog. *Veterinary Record* **102**, 435–440.

Weaver, A.D. (1981) Fifteen cases of prostatic carcinoma in the dog. *Veterinary Record* **109**, 71–75.

Weaver, A.D and Pillinger, R. (1975) Relationship of bacterial infection in urine and calculi to canine urolithiasis. *Veterinary Record* **97**, 48–50.

Westerlund, W.T., Pere, A., Korhonen, T.K., Jarvinen, A.K., Sitonen, A. and Williams, P.H. (1987) Characterization of *Escherichia coli* strains associated with canine urinary tract infections. *Research in Veterinary Science* **42**, 404–406.

White, J.V., Oliver, N.B., Reimann, K. and Johnson, C. (1984) Use of protein-to-creatinine ratio in a single urine specimen for quantitative estimation of canine proteinuria. *Journal of the American Veterinary Medical Association* **185**, 882–885.

White, E.G. (1966) Symposium on urolithiasis. I. Introduction and incidences. *Journal of Small Animal Practice* **7**, 529–534.

Wolf, A.M. (1980) Canine uremic encephalopathy. *Journal of the American Animal Hospital Association* **16**, 735–738.

Wright, N.G., Nash, A.S., Thompson, H. and Fisher, E.W. (1981) Membranous nephropathy in the cat and dog: a renal biopsy and follow-up study of sixteen cases. *Kidney International* **45**, 269–277.

Wright, N.G. and Nash, A.S. (1983) Glomerulonephritis in the dog and cat. *Irish Veterinary Journal* **37**, 4–8.

42

Diseases of the Nervous System

R. S. Bagley and S. J. Wheeler

Introduction	662	Diseases of the spinal cord	681
Neurological syndromes	664	Diseases of the peripheral nervous system,	
Diagnosis	668	neuromuscular junction and muscle	686
Neurological diseases	674	Multifocal diseases of the nervous system	691
Diseases of the brain	674		

INTRODUCTION

Neurological lesions of the head, spine and neuromuscular system are localized by the physical and neurological examinations. Identification of the aetiology is by the use of various diagnostic aids. Most neurological problems fall into clear syndromes which reflect the site of the lesion.

Diagnostic approach

A complete physical examination must be performed prior to a neurological examination. This aims to provide information on two aspects of the case. First, an attempt must be made to establish whether the clinical signs present are truly neurological in origin, as diseases of other body systems may mimic neurological presentations. Secondly, neurological disorders may have their basis in systemic disease or may have systemic manifestations. Thus, a full evaluation of the general health of the dog should be made, both by clinical examination and by evaluation of haematology and blood biochemistry.

The neurological examination

Detailed descriptions of the neurological examination and the neuroanatomical basis of the

Table 42.1 Screening neurological examination

	General	Head	Eyes	Limbs
Observation	Gait Posture Mental status	Position (+/− tilt) Jaw function Lips (+/− droop) Tongue mobility Temporal muscles (+/− atrophy)	Position Movements Pupil size	Scuffing Knuckling Muscle atrophy

Testing	Hyperaesthesia
	Panniculus reflex
	Anal tone
	Tail tone
		Jaw tone
		Swallowing
		Gagging
		Facial sensation
		Palpebral reflex
			Menace response
			Pupilary light reflexes
			Oculovestibular reflexes
			Fundic examination
				Proprioception
				Hopping
				Reflexes:
				  withdrawal
				  patellar

Table 42.2 Cranial nerve tests

	Nerve	Clinical test	Normal response	Abnormal response
I	Olfactory	Smelling a non-irritant substance	Animal sniffs or licks nose	
II	Optic	1. Throw a piece of cotton wool in front of animal	Attention attracted	Attention not attracted
		2. Menace test	Eyelids close	Eyelids do not close
		3. Observe animal's movements in reduced light		Animal bumps into obstacles or wall
		4. Pupillary light reflex	Both pupils constrict, i.e. direct and consensual responses	Pupils do not constrict, i.e. direct and consensual responses absent)
III	Oculomotor	1. Evaluation of pupillary light reflexes	Pupils constrict	No response in affected eye; pupil constricts in normal eye (with bilateral lesions direct and consensual responses absent in *both* eyes)
		2. Oculocephalic reflex (observe eye movements when head moved laterally)	Induced horizontal nystagmus in both eyes	No induced nystagmus
IV	Trochlear	Observe eye position	Normal eye position	Rotary strabismus
V	Trigeminal	1. Pinch skin of face: ears, lips, muzzle to evaluate mandibular and maxillary branches; around eyes for ophthalmic branch	Skin moves, painful response	No response
		2. Nasal sensation for mandibular branch	Behavioural response	No response
		3. Corneal reflex for ophthalmic branch	Blink and retraction of globe	No response
		4. Palpebral reflex	Blink	No blink
		5. Jaw tone	Resistance to jaw opening	Jaw flaccid
VI	Abducens	Corneal reflex	Globe retracts	No response
VII	Facial	1. Pinch skin	Blink	No blink, but intact sensation
		2. Corneal reflex	Blink	No blink, but intact sensation
		3. Palpebral reflex	Blink	No blink, but intact sensation
		4. Schirmer tear test	Normal tear production	Reduced tear production
VIII	Vestibulocochlear	1. Auditory response (hand clap)	Behavioural response	No response
		2. Oculocephalic reflex	Induced nystagmus	No induced nystagmus
IX	Glossopharyngeal	Gag or swallowing reflex	Swallows	No swallowing
X	Vagus	1. Gag or swallowing reflex	Swallows	No swallowing
		2. Oculocardiac reflex	Cardiac rate slows	No rate reduction
XI	Accessory	Palpation of neck muscles	Normal muscle mass	Reduced muscle mass
XII	Hypoglossal	Retract tongue	Animal resists	Tongue paresis

From Moreau, P.M. (1989) Neurological examination of the cranial nerves. In: *Manual of Small Animal Neurology* (Ed. S.J. Wheeler), BSAVA Publications, Cheltenham.

functions of the central nervous system are given elsewhere (deLahunta, 1983; Oliver *et al.*, 1987; Wheeler, 1989).

In practice, an abbreviated form of neurological examination is useful as a screening procedure and can be carried out as a component of the routine physical examination. Regular performance of such an examination is to be encouraged as this will enhance the ability of the clinician to identify relatively subtle neurological deficits. The elements of this abbreviated examination are given in Table 42.1. If all the findings on this examination are normal, it is unlikely that further evaluation will reveal neurological deficits. However, if abnormalities are apparent, then a more detailed examination should be performed. Clearly, if the dog has an obvious neurological problem, the examination is addressed to meet that problem. Thus, in a paraplegic dog, a more thorough evaluation of limb reflexes may be appropriate, but in all cases the screening examination should be performed, or deficits will be missed.

Cranial nerve tests are summarized in Table 42.2. Other components of the neurological examination which relate specifically to the localization and assessment of the severity and extent of spinal cord lesions are described later.

There are a number of features with which the examiner must be familiar. The normal responses to some of the tests should be recognized, for example, the physiological nystagmus produced in the oculovestibular test. When localizing spinal lesions, the features of lower motor neurone (LMN) and upper motor neurone (UMN) deficits must be distinguished. Although both may result in paralysis, LMN lesions show an absence of local reflexes, marked neurogenic muscle atrophy and loss of muscle tone. This contrasts with UMN lesions where reflexes are intact or hyperactive, muscle atrophy is of the mild, disuse type, and muscle tone is normal or increased. The different types of urinary incontinence that may be seen with various nervous system lesions are quite different (see later and also Chapter 22).

Once the location of the lesion has been determined, an attempt to identify the nature of the disease process is made. The list of potential differential diagnoses may be modified on the basis of the breed or age of the dog and the appropriate history. However, this information cannot be used as the sole basis for diagnosis as many exceptions exist. It is important to realize that very few absolute rules apply to the occurrence of neurological disorders, and age can rarely be used to rule out a particular condition. For example, there may be a higher index of suspicion for tumours in older dogs, but neoplasia can also occur in young individuals. Confirmation of the nature of the lesion is achieved by the use of appropriate ancillary diagnostic aids.

NEUROLOGICAL SYNDROMES

Head

Localization of brain lesions

Brain disorders are localized on the basis of groups of signs encountered with lesions at different locations (Fig. 42.1).

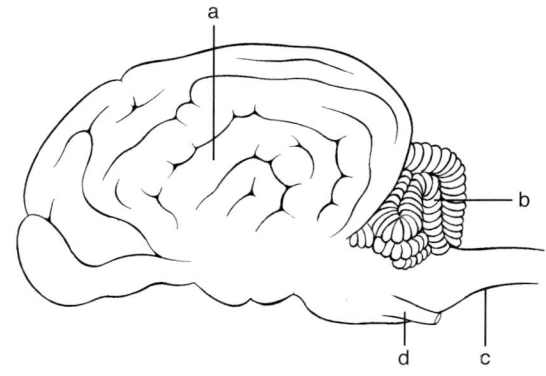

Figure 42.1 Brain localization. Four areas for localization of brain lesions. a, forebrain; b, cerebellum; c, brainstem; d, vestibular.

Forebrain

The classification 'forebrain' includes the cerebral cortex, and the diencephalon (thalamus and hypothalamus). Neurological signs referable to the forebrain can be classified broadly into two groups: those indicative of general cerebral dysfunction, and those indicating a focal lesion. Seizures, behavioural change and altered mental attitude are general, non-localizing signs. Hemiparesis, postural deficits, visual and menace deficits are indicative of a focal lesion, and these signs are contralateral to the lesion (Table 42.3).

Brainstem

Lesions of the brainstem produce a fairly characteristic clinical picture, with upper motor neurone-type (UMN) locomotor signs, deficits of

Table 42.3 Clinical signs of forebrain disease

Seizures
Behavioural change
Reduced level of awareness
Circling (generally towards the side of the lesion)
Pacing
Head pressing
Miotic pupils
Contralateral: Menace deficits
Postural reaction deficits
Mild cranial nerve deficits (V and VII)

cranial nerves (usually V–XII) and altered mental status. Lesions vary in their severity. Patients may show anything from a mild gait abnormality to tetraplegia; marked asymmetry is common. Major cranial nerve dysfunction occurs on the same side of the body as the lesion. Hemiparesis is also generally ipsilateral (Table 42.4).

Table 42.4 Clinical signs of brainstem disease

Ipsilateral hemiparesis
Sensorium alterations
Cranial nerve deficits (mainly V and VII–XII)

Vestibular system

The vestibular system controls the position of the limbs, body and eyes of the animal, and allows adjustments for alterations in the position of the head. Thus, it is responsible for maintaining balance and gait. Diseases of the vestibular system cause derangement of these functions. Head tilt, ataxia, nystagmus and circling are seen in affected animals. The important differentiation in a patient with a vestibular syndrome is between central and peripheral lesions. Peripheral vestibular syndromes result from lesions of the peripheral receptors in the inner ear and of the vestibular branch of cranial nerve VIII. Central vestibular disease is caused by lesions of the vestibular nuclei in the brainstem and their cerebellar connections. The importance of differentiating the two types of vestibular disease lies in the type of disease processes encountered at each location; most central lesions carry a poor prognosis. The most important differential feature is the presence of conscious proprioceptive deficits in central lesions; with peripheral lesions, conscious proprioception is normal (Table 42.5).

Table 42.5 Differentiating features of peripheral and central vestibular disease

	Peripheral	Central
Headtilt	Yes	Yes
Ataxia	Yes	Yes
Proprioceptive deficits	No	Ipsilateral
Paresis	No	Ipsilateral
Nystagmus	Yes	Yes
Variable nystagmus[a]	No	Yes
Other cranial nerve deficits	VII	Multiple
Horner's syndrome	Possible	Very rare

[a]Direction or character of nystagmus changes when head position is altered.

Cerebellum

The cerebellum is responsible for 'fine-tuning' of the movements of the body and head. Diseases of the cerebellum lead to loss of this function, with the resultant clinical signs of cerebellar ataxia, intention tremor and hypermetria. The menace response may also be absent.

■ Spine

It is usually apparent if an animal has spinal disease, either from the history or the physical findings. Less obvious circumstances where spinal disease should be suspected include poorly localized pain, and lameness that is not orthopaedic in origin.

Localization of spinal lesions

The neurological examination is carried out with the aim of determining the location of the spinal lesion to one of the following four areas of spinal cord (Fig. 42.2). The numbers refer to spinal cord segments, not vertebrae.

- A: C1–C5
- B: C6–T2   Brachial outflow
- C: T3–L3
- D: L4–S3   Lumbosacral outflow

Each limb is evaluated with the aim of placing it into one of the following categories:

- Normal
- Lower motor neurone type abnormality
- Upper motor neurone type abnormality

The effect of lesions on the LMN and UMN systems can be considered in terms of motor function, muscle atrophy, muscle tone and local

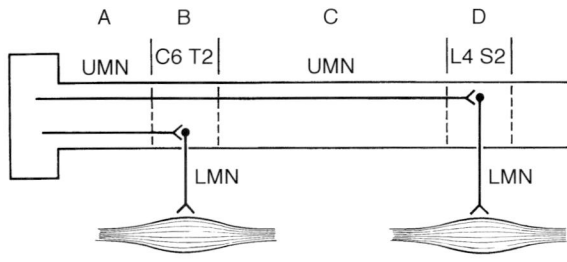

Figure 42.2 Upper and lower motor neurones.

reflexes. The clinical signs that allow differentiation between UMN and LMN abnormalities are summarized in Table 42.6.

LMN-type deficits are characterized by paresis or more usually flaccid paralysis, severe (neurogenic) muscle atrophy, reduced muscle tone and loss of local reflexes.

Table 42.6 Differentiation of upper and lower motor neurone-type deficits

Function	UMN	LMN
Locomotion	Paresis – paralysis	Flaccid paralysis
Reflexes	Intact – increased	Absent
Muscle atrophy	Disuse (mild)	Neurogenic (severe)
Muscle tone	Normal – increased	Decreased

In contrast, lesions causing UMN-type deficits show paresis or paralysis, mild (disuse) muscle atrophy, normal or increased muscle tone, and intact or hyperactive reflexes.

There are some variations in mild cases, but from the neurological examination, it should be possible to categorize each limb as being 'normal', 'UMN' or 'LMN'.

For clinical purposes the cervical and thoracolumbar cord (areas A and C) may be considered as UMN-carrying areas. It can be seen from Fig. 42.2 that part of the LMN lies within the spinal cord; thus, lesions in certain areas of the cord will produce LMN signs in the limbs. Area B of the cord provides the LMN to the thoracic limbs, and area D the LMN to the pelvic limbs, bladder and perineum.

Lesions in the various areas will produce different combinations of neurological signs (Fig. 42.3).

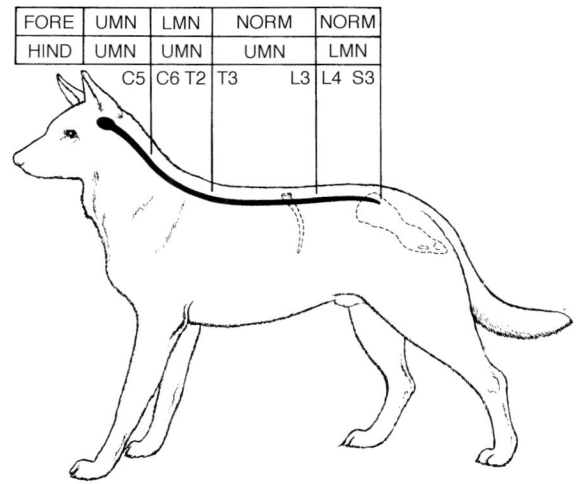

Figure 42.3 Spinal lesion localization areas (see text).

- A: C1–C5. Lesions in the cervical cord produce UMN signs in the thoracic or pelvic limbs, or both.
- B: C6–T2. Lesions of the brachial outflow segments produce LMN deficits in the thoracic limbs and UMN signs in the pelvic limbs. Asymmetrical lesions in this area may produce LMN signs in one thoracic limb only, with UMN signs in both the pelvic limbs and the other thoracic limb.
- C: T3–L3. Lesions in the thoracolumbar cord produce UMN signs in the pelvic limbs only, with normal thoracic limbs (although the Schiff–Sherrington sign may be present, where there is extensor rigidity of the thoracic limbs and possibly the neck).
- D: L4–S3. Lesions in the lumbosacral outflow segments produce LMN signs in the pelvic limbs, tail and perineum; the thoracic limbs are normal.

Variations in this pattern may occur. For example, in some Dobermanns with caudal cervical spondylomyelopathy, UMN signs in the pelvic limbs predominate even though the lesion is in the cervical cord. The possibility of a thoracolumbar lesion in such patients should not be overlooked.

The type of urinary incontinence also indicates the site of the lesion. The LMNs to the bladder are in the sacral segments. Lesions of these segments produce a LMN-type of incontinence with a flaccid, easily expressed bladder. Lesions cranial to the sacral segments produce a UMN-type of incontinence where the bladder is full and difficult to express.

Assessing the severity or extent of a spinal lesion

Assessing the severity of a lesion plays a major part in the diagnostic procedure. In certain patients, the severity of the lesion has as much bearing on the prognosis as the aetiology; if a poor prognosis is suggested, further investigations may be deemed unnecessary.

In general, LMN deficits have a worse prognosis than UMN deficits, because of destruction of the cell body in LMN spinal cord diseases. Patients with major LMN deficits have a poor prognosis for return to normal function, although associated UMN signs may resolve.

With UMN injuries, the rate of onset, and the duration and degree of the spinal cord damage all have a bearing on the clinical signs. The degree of dysfunction can be graded from mild ataxia, through paresis, to paralysis with loss of pain perception.

The severity of signs caused by spinal cord lesions is related to two anatomical features. These are the position in the spinal cord where the tracts lie that carry the respective function, and the size of the fibres transmitting that function. Superficial tracts are more susceptible to damage, and larger myelinated fibres are more easily damaged than small non-myelinated fibres.

Conscious proprioception loss is one of the earliest neurological deficits seen in mild spinal cord damage, because this function is normally transmitted by large myelinated fibres in superficial tracts. Deep pain sensation is transmitted throughout a large area of the cord in small, non-myelinated fibres (see Fig. 42.4). Thus, by inference, loss of this function indicates physiological or anatomical transection of the cord. The prognosis worsens with the increasing neurological deficit, reflecting an increased degree of spinal cord damage. Animals without pain sensation have a poor prognosis, especially if the situation has existed for longer than 48 h. Animals that have lost pain sensation following trauma carry a poor prognosis whatever the duration of the signs.

Peripheral neuromuscular system

Generalized disorders of the peripheral neuromuscular system may have their basis in the peripheral nerve, neuromuscular junction or muscle. Most diseases present with locomotor abnormalities although there are exceptions, for example, some sensory neuropathies may present with a history of self-mutilation.

Localization of neuromuscular lesions

Polyneuropathies

Most animals with polyneuropathy have weakness, ataxia, muscle atrophy and loss of reflexes. Progressive weakness with exercise is usually not a feature. Many patients are initially more severely affected in the pelvic limbs. Distal weakness may predominate, for example, cats with diabetic neuropathy walk with plantigrade hocks. Alterations of voice are also seen. Pain sensation and autonomic function are preserved in most neuropathies.

Neuromuscular junction disorders

Diseases of the neuromuscular junction tend to present with one of the following signs: exercise-induced collapse, stiffness or flaccid paralysis. One feature is that conscious proprioception is maintained. Thus, if the weight of the animal is supported, this function is intact. Regurgitation due to megaoesophagus may also be seen.

Myopathies

Muscle diseases also present with locomotor disturbances. Stiffness and a stilted gait, which worsens with exercise, are seen in many myopathies. Reflexes may be reduced. Some muscle diseases cause generalized weakness, for example, potassium-depletion myopathy in cats.

Monoparesis and monoplegia

Monoparesis and monoplegia are fairly common presentations in dogs (less so in cats). In traumatic neuropathies, for example brachial plexus root

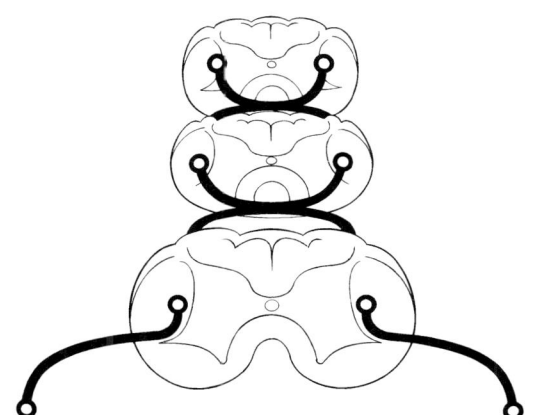

Figure 42.4 Fibres relaying deep pain sensation are small fibres that cross and recross extensively within the spinal cord of animals.

avulsion, there is an acute onset of LMN-type paralysis. Other causes such as brachial plexus tumours may present initially with lameness and only later do the more characteristic LMN signs develop.

DIAGNOSIS

Once the nature of the neurological problem and the location of the lesion have been established, a list of differential diagnoses can be made. Many factors should be considered when drawing up this list, including breed and age of the patient, history, presenting signs, progression, physical and neurological findings. Ancillary diagnostic aids are used to provide an aetiological diagnosis.

Diagnostic aids

Routine laboratory evaluations

Routine haematology and serum biochemistry screens are unlikely in most cases to provide definitive diagnostic information, but they nevertheless play an important role in the diagnostic process. Certain metabolic and systemic disorders may effect the nervous system, and the value of these tests is in identifying or ruling out such conditions. Also, they have an important role in evaluating the general health of the animal. In selected circumstances, the evaluation of blood parameters will be virtually diagnostic, for example, where creatine kinase (CK) concentrations are raised in myopathy or bile acid concentrations elevated in hepatic dysfunction.

Cerebrospinal fluid analysis

Cerebrospinal fluid (CSF) analysis is an important part of the investigation of most nervous system diseases. Cerebrospinal fluid is collected routinely from the cerebellomedullary cisterna (CMC), a straightforward procedure in the majority of dogs and cats. Fluid can also be collected from the lumbar spine. Although the technique is safe in experienced hands, practice on cadavers is recommended before attempting collection of CSF in clinical cases to allow the clinician to become familiar with the procedure. Cerebrospinal fluid collection is indicated in a number of situations:

- Where there is evidence, on the basis of the neurological examination, of a structural brain lesion (Note: CSF collection may be hazardous when increased intracranial pressure is suspected);
- In spinal cord diseases, where the diagnosis is not apparent by other means, particularly radiology. As the radiological investigation of spinal diseases often involves myelography, CSF should be collected before contrast medium is injected;
- In neurological diseases showing signs suggestive of multifocal involvement;
- Where signs of generalized peripheral polyneuropathy are present, as such signs may be due to nerve root diseases;
- In patients with epilepsy, where seizures are proving difficult to control with adequate anticonvulsant therapy or if other neurological signs indicate the presence of a structural lesion.

General anaesthesia is required for CSF collection in small animals. Patients should be intubated and ventilatory support must be available. The collection site must be clipped and prepared aseptically. Sterile needles are used for collection and the wearing of sterile surgical gloves is recommended. An assistant is required to hold the patient in the correct position.

The choice of collection site warrants some consideration. The two sites available are the CMC and the lumbar spine. Collection from the CMC is easier and is less likely to produce a sample contaminated with blood. However, as CSF flows in a cranial to caudal direction, abnormal CSF is more likely to be present caudal to a lesion (Thomson et al., 1990). Thus, lumbar CSF is more likely to be diagnostically useful. However, lumbar collection is more difficult and blood contamination occurs more frequently.

If raised intracranial pressure is present, lumbar collection is somewhat safer. This is not because brain herniation is any less likely, but the risk of direct damage to tissue which has already herniated is not a factor with lumbar collection.

Spinal needles are preferred for CSF collection but hypodermic needles may be used. The CSF is collected into sterile vials; plain vials without anticoagulant are generally used.

Collection from the cerebellomedullary cistern

Landmarks for CMC puncture are the edge of the wings of the atlas and the occipital protuberance. An imaginary line is drawn between the wings of the atlas. The site is in the midline of the patient, half way between the occipital protuberance and the line joining the wings of the atlas (Fig. 42.5).

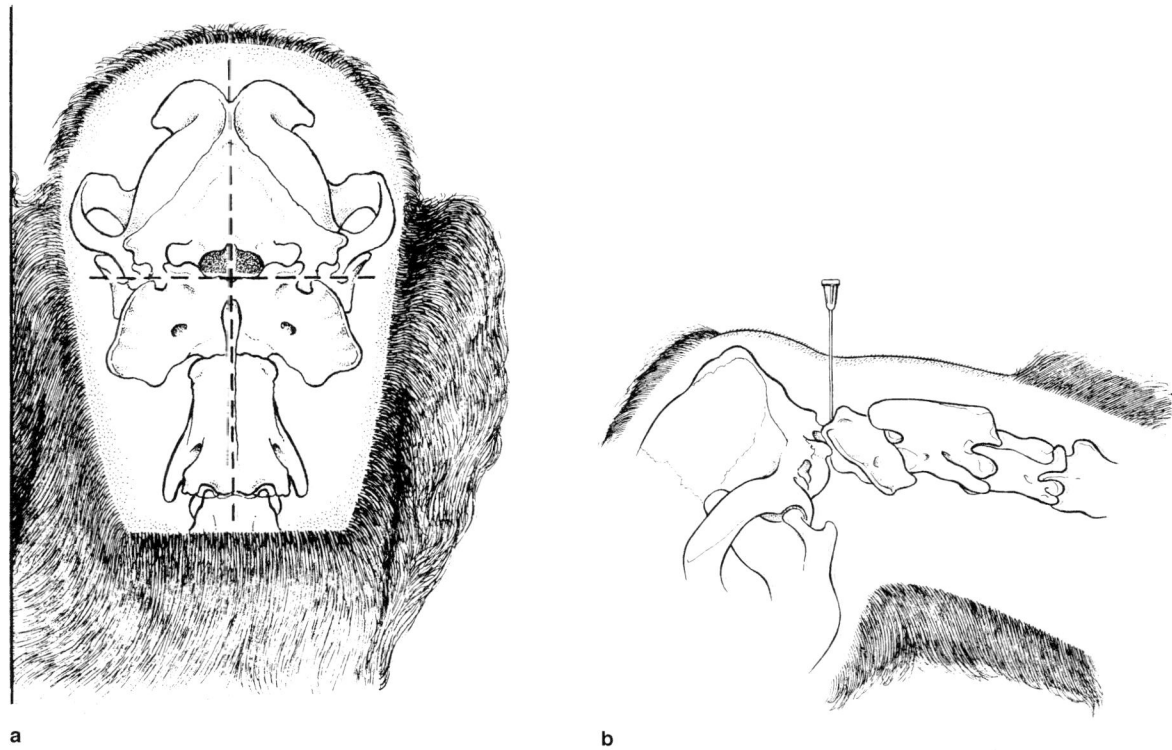

Figure 42.5a,b Anatomical landmarks for obtaining CSF by cisternal puncture.

Just behind the occipital protuberance, there is a slight depression in the musculature. This is not the site of needle penetration, but is cranial to it. Inserting the needle at this site usually leads to it striking the bone of the skull. The needle is inserted perpendicular to the skin in the midline.

There are a number of possible methods for advancing the needle.

(a) Remove the stilette once the tip of the needle is in muscle. The needle is than advanced until the dura mater is penetrated and CSF appears in the hub of the needle.
(b) Advance the needle with the stilette still in place in small increments, removing the stilette between each movement to check whether CSF is present in the needle. A slight 'pop' can sometimes be felt when the needle enters the subarachnoid space.

Because the neck is severely flexed, a kink-proof endotracheal tube should be used. Alternatively, the cuff is deflated to allow space around the tube for ventilation should the tube obstruct.

Collection from the lumbar spine

The site is between L5 and L6. The needle is inserted alongside the spinous process of L6 and directed cranially and ventrally through the ligamentum flavum into the vertebral canal. In the cat L6/7 can be used. The pelvic limbs are pulled cranially under the abdomen. The tip of the L6 spinous process is palpated. The needle is inserted alongside the caudal edge of the spinous process, slightly lateral to the midline. It is advanced in a cranioventral direction such that the point reaches the midline as it reaches the vertebral lamina. The stilette is removed intermittently to check progress. On penetrating the subarachnoid space, CSF will flow.

Collection of CSF from the lumbar site is more likely to fail than from the CMC. Contamination is also more frequent.

Sample handling and laboratory analysis

The routine analyses performed on CSF are gross examination, total and differential white cell (WBC) counts and total protein. White cell analysis must be performed on fresh CSF within 30 min of collection as the cells deteriorate rapidly. If this is not possible, the specimen should be preserved with an equal volume of 4% formalin solution (Evans, 1989). Normal CSF findings are given in Table 42.7.

Table 42.7 Normal CSF findings

Colour	Clear, colourless
Specific gravity	1.004–1.006
White cell count	< 5 mm^{-3}
Differential white cells	Mostly mononuclear cells (lymphocytes, monocytes, macrophages)
Total protein	
Cerebellomedullary cistern	10–30 mg dl^{-1}
Lumbar	10–45 mg dl^{-1}

Gross examination

Normal CSF is clear and colourless. Colour change and turbidity may be noted in some diseases. The most frequent colour changes are due to haemorrhage or to xanthochromia.

Cell counts

These are performed using a haemocytometer; cell numbers are too low to be accurately counted by automatic means. Undiluted CSF is used unless cell counts are particularly high. If this is so, the CSF will appear turbid.

Normal CSF is free of red blood cells. Normal white cell counts vary in different laboratories, but are generally less than 5 cells mm^{-3}. An increase in nucleated cells, usually white blood cells (WBC), is termed pleocytosis.

Cell counts and blood contamination

There are formulae for correcting CSF cell counts that take the peripheral blood WBC count into consideration. However, contaminating RBCs do not greatly alter markedly elevated WBC counts (Wilson and Stevens, 1977). It is probably adequate to remember that WBCs and RBCs are in a ratio of approximately 1:500 in blood, and to take this into account when viewing cell counts in blood-contaminated CSF.

Differential white cell counts and cytology

This is an important part of the examination of CSF, even in the face of a normal total WBC count. The WBCs must be concentrated either by centrifugation or sedimentation, mounted on a slide and stained (Mayhew and Beal, 1980). Most WBCs in CSF are mononuclear, i.e. lymphocytes, monocytes and occasional macrophages. Occasional neutrophils may be seen.

The differential WBC count is most useful in distinguishing acute and chronic inflammation, for example, granulomatous meningoencephalitis can be differentiated from non-infectious suppurative meningoencephalitis.

Bacteria may occasionally be seen in CSF. These may be pathogenic, but if present in the absence of a neutrophilic pleocytosis, they are most likely the result of contamination (see below). Bacterial meningoencephalomyelitis is very rare in the dog and cat.

Abnormal cells suggestive of neoplasia are rarely found in CSF. Large numbers of neoplastic lymphoid cells may be evident in cases of lymphoma which involve the meninges.

Protein content

Protein content of CSF can be estimated by a number of methods; use of a professional laboratory is advised. Normal CSF collected from the CMC has a protein concentration of less than 30 mg dl^{-1}; it may be up to 45 mg dl^{-1} at the lumbar site. Total protein may be increased in many diseases but is a non-specific finding. Increased protein in the absence of pleocytosis is usually indicative of non-inflammatory disorders. Electrophoresis provides information regarding the composition of the CSF protein.

Microbiology

Examination for the presence of bacteria may be performed microscopically, using a stained sample of CSF, and by culture. Care should be exercised when interpreting positive results in the absence of pleocytosis, as bacteria may be contaminants. Intracellular bacteria should always be viewed as being significant. It can be difficult to culture organisms from the CSF even in the face of fulminating infections, but attempts should be made to isolate pathogens and determine antibiotic sensitivity. Failure to obtain a positive result does not eliminate the possibility of central nervous system (CNS) infection being present. Blood cultures are useful in dogs with discospondylitis (Kornegay 1986a).

Serology

The evaluation of blood and CSF for viral antibodies has some application in canine neurology. It is most useful in attempting to confirm a diagnosis of viral infection of the central nervous system. A positive canine distemper virus (CDV) titre in the absence of other raised viral titres in the CSF is strongly indicative of CDV-related CNS disease.

Radiology

Radiology is the major diagnostic tool utilized in neurology, particularly for the identification of spinal and brain lesions. There are certain points regarding radiology that warrant emphasis. Survey radiography will provide a diagnosis in the majority of spinal disorders and has a role in other areas, for example, in evaluating the tympanic bullae in animals with signs of vestibular disease. Survey films are not particularly useful for evaluating intracranial lesions, other than those that involve the nasal cavity or the skull. Myelography is required for full evaluation of many spinal lesions. The indications for myelography are:

- Where the neurological examination indicates a spinal lesion but none is visible on survey radiographs;
- To determine the significance of multiple lesions identified on survey radiographs;
- To determine the presence of spinal cord compression;
- To assist in deciding the indications for surgery and type of procedure to be performed.

It is contraindicated if general anaesthesia or spinal puncture are unsafe, or where inflammatory disease of the CNS is present.

Other contrast techniques such as epidurography or discography may be useful in selected cases.

Computed tomography and magnetic resonance imaging

The diagnosis of brain lesions has been transformed by the use of central nervous system imaging. Although the availability of equipment is limited, its use is becoming more widespread in veterinary medicine.

Electrodiagnostic testing

The various electrodiagnostic procedures that are used in dogs are limited in their availability due to the expensive equipment required. The indications for performing the various techniques and interpretation of findings have been

Table 42.8 Important causes of neurological disease

	Forebrain	Brainstem	Cerebellum
Degenerative	Storage diseases	Storage diseases	Storage diseases Abiotrophies Hypomyelination Dysmyelination Neuroaxonal dystrophy Leukoencephalomalacia
Anomalous	Hydrocephalus	Hydrocephalus	Congenital malformations
Metabolic	Hepatic encephalopathy Hypoglycaemia Hyperglycaemia	Hepatic encephalopathy Hypoglycaemia Hyperglycaemia	
Neoplastic	Primary Secondary	Primary Secondary	Primary Secondary
Nutritional		Thiamine deficiency	
Inflammatory	Meningoencephalitis Infectious Non-infectious	Meningoencephalitis Infectious Non-infectious	Feline cerebellar hypoplasia
Idiopathic	Idiopathic epilepsy Narcolepsy Rage syndrome	Idiopathic peripheral vestibular disease Congenital vestibular disease Congenital deafness	
Traumatic	Cranial trauma	Cranial trauma	
Toxic	Various	Metronidazole	
Vascular	Various Feline ischaemic encephalopathy	Various Feline ischaemic encephalopathy	Various

Table 42.9 Storage diseases of dogs and cats

Disease	Enzyme deficient/Storage product	Breed/Age at onset	Clinical signs
Gangliosidosis GM₁ Type 1 (Norman Landing)	Beta-galactosidase	Beagle-cross (3 months); domestic cats (2–3 months)	Tremor; incoordination; spastic paraplegia; visual impairment
Type 2 (Derry's)	Beta-galactosidase	Siamese; Korat and domestic cats (2–3 months) Portuguese water dogs (5–6 months)	As with Type 1
Gangliosidosis GM₂ Type 1 (Tay–Sach's)	Hexosaminidase A	German short-haired pointer (6–9 months)	Ataxia; incoordination; visual impairment; dementia
Type 2 (Sandhoff's)	Hexosaminidase A and B	Domestic cats (2 months)	Same as with GM₁
Glucocerebrosidosis (Gaucher's)	Beta-glucosidase (Glucocerebroside)	Sydney silky dog (6–8 months)	Ataxia; incoordination; hypermetria
Sphingomyelinosis (Neimann–Pick)	Sphingomyelinase (Sphingomyelin)	Type C in Siamese and domestic cats (2–4 months) Poodles (2–4 months)	Ataxia; incoordination; hypermetria
(Six types of Nieman–Pick disease are recognized in human beings (A–F) based upon age of onset, degree of hepatosplenomegaly, extent of nervous system involvement and reduction in sphingomyelinase activity). With Type C in cats, sphingomyelinase activity is not dramatically decreased).			
Globoid cell leukodystrophy (Krabbe's)	Beta-galactosidase (galactocerebrosidase)	Cairn terrier; West Highland white terrier (2–5 months); beagle; blue tick hound (4 months); mixed-breed; poodle (2 year); basset hound (1–2 years); pomeranian (1.5 years); domestic cat (5–6 weeks)	Ataxia; incoordination; tremor; paraparesis; hypermetria; visual impairment
Metachromatic leukodystrophy	Arylsulphatase (sulphatide)	Domestic cat (2 weeks)	Progressive motor dysfunction; seizures; opisthotonos

Mucopolysaccharidosis I (Hurler's)	Alpha-L-iduronidase	Domestic cat (10 months)	Facial dysmorphia; corneal clouding; stunted growth; lameness; high incidence of meningioma in these cats
Mucopolysaccharidosis VI (Maroteaux–Lamy)	Arylsulphatase B (mucopolysaccharide)	Siamese and domestic cat (4–7 months)	As for Type I mucopolysaccharidosis; posterior paresis; skin nodules
Glycoproteinosis (Lafora's)	(Glycoprotein?)	Beagle, basset hound, poodle (5 months – 9 years)	Depression; seizures
Mannosidosis	Alpha-mannosidase (mannoside)	Domestic cat (7 months)	Ataxia; incoordination; tremor; aggression (calves)
Gycogenesis (Pompe's)	Alpha-glucosidase	Lapland dogs (1.5 years); domestic cats	Incoordination; exercise intolerance
Fucosidosis	Alpha-L-fucosidase	Springer spaniel dogs (2 years)	Incoordination; behavioural changes; dysphonia; dysphagia; seizures
Ceroid lipofuscinosis (Batten's)	Unknown	English setter (1 year); dachshund (3.5–7 years); cocker spaniel (1.5 years); chihuahua, Saluki (2 years); Australian cattle dogs; blue heeler; Siamese and domestic cats (2–7 years)	Personality change; visual impairment; ataxia; incoordination; jaw champing; seizures

reviewed elsewhere (see Further Reading for a list of specialist neurological textbooks). It is important to remember that none of these methods is a substitute for thorough neurological evaluation, and the information that they provide only enhances the clinical data. Electromyography and nerve conduction studies are most useful in peripheral neuropathies and some spinal diseases.

NEUROLOGICAL DISEASES

This section discusses commonly seen nervous system disorders in dogs and cats. This is not, however, intended to be a comprehensive review of all diseases of the nervous system in small animals. Specific infectious and metabolic disorders which are frequently associated with neurological signs are described in more detail elsewhere in this textbook. The disorders are listed in Table 42.8 under the areas of the nervous system which they may involve.

DISEASES OF THE BRAIN

Degenerative

Storage diseases are inborn errors of metabolism characterized by the absence of a vital enzyme necessary to break down an endogenous body substance. These substances then accumulate within the neurone or other cells within the nervous system and eventually cause cellular dysfunction. Because many of these diseases are inherited and congenital, clinical signs are usually seen in young animals of specific breeds. The numerous storage diseases of small animals are listed in Table 42.9.

Notable diseases from this list include globoid cell leukodystrophy because it may also involve peripheral nerves. Cats with mucopolysaccharidosis I (Hurler's syndrome) have an increased incidence of meningioma. An unclassified lysosomal storage disease exists in Abyssinian cats. Several unclassified leukodystrophies also exist in cats. Storage diseases can also involve the brainstem and cerebellum.

Cerebellar abiotrophies result from loss of a vital substance necessary for continued life of the neurone. These diseases are seen most notably in the Kerry blue terrier, Gordon setter, rough-coated collie, border collie, bull mastiff and rarely in samoyeds, Airedales, Finnish harriers, Labrador retrievers, golden retrievers, beagles, cocker spaniels, Cairn terriers and great Danes (deLahunta, 1980). In Gordon setters, a late onset cerebellar degeneration has been described (Steinberg *et al.*, 1981). Clinical signs are those of progressive cerebellar disease. Diagnosis is based on biopsy or necropsy. No treatment is effective.

Neuroaxonal dystrophy is a disease of rottweiler dogs (Chrisman, 1986); less frequently collies, Chihuahuas, and occasionally domestic cats may be affected. In rottweilers, neuroaxonal dystrophy is characterized by cerebellar signs (ataxia, hypermetria, loss of menace reflexes, head tremor) beginning at 1 to 2 years (ataxia) and progressing over the next 2 to 4 years (menace deficits, intention tremor). Conscious proprioception remains intact. The cell bodies in the grey matter are affected (showing axonal spheroids) throughout the nervous system except the cerebral cortex. The most severe lesions are in the spinocerebellar tracts and the Purkinje cells. Diagnosis is usually confirmed postmortem, however, ante-mortem biopsy of these areas may show pathological changes. No treatment is known.

Leukoencephalomyelopathy has been reported in two young rottweilers (Chrisman, 1986) with progressive ataxia and weakness. No cerebral signs were seen, even though pathologically the deep cerebellar white matter was abnormal (demyelination). Clinical signs suggested a pure spinal cord problem.

Anomalous

Hydrocephalus may be either acquired (usually due to obstruction of the ventricular system by neoplasia or inflammation) or congenital. Mentation changes and seizures are common. Hydrocephalus that involves the mesencephalic aqueduct or fourth ventricle can result in brain stem signs. Management can be difficult. If there is an underlying problem, such as inflammatory disease, this should be addressed. Surgical shunting of CSF into the peritoneal cavity is also described. Other anomalous conditions such as exencephaly, hydranencephaly, anencephaly and lissencephaly are uncommon and usually are congenital (Fig. 42.6).

Congenital malformations of the cerebellum are occasionally seen. Caudal vermian hypoplasia is described, with some dogs having associated ventricular dilation (Dandy Walker malformation) (Kornegay, 1986b). *Cerebellar hypoplasia*

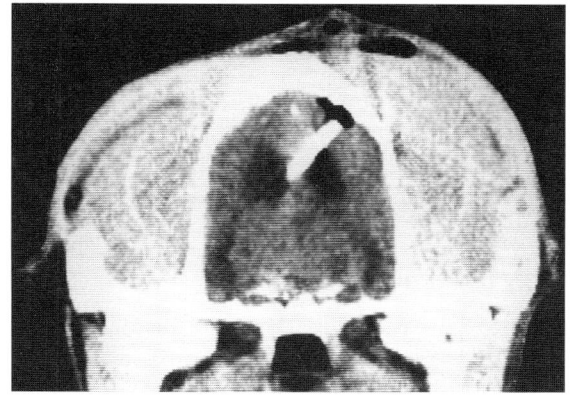

Figure 42.6 (a) Computed tomography (CT) of a boxer with seizures and mentation changes. Ventricular dilation is seen. (b) Postoperative CT showing decreased ventricular size following ventriculoperitoneal shunting.

has been recognized in chow chows, Irish setters and wire-haired fox terriers. The latter two breeds may have concurrent lissencephaly. Cerebellar aplasia has been reported in Siberian huskies.

Hypomyelination or dysmyelination of the CNS is seen in many breeds including the chow chow, springer spaniel, samoyed, Weimaraner, and Bernese mountain dog (Duncan, 1987). This disease is inherited in an X-linked manner in springer spaniels. Individual cases have been reported in a Dalmatian and a mixed breed dog. Clinical signs consist of tremor which may appear to be cerebellar in origin. This tremor usually worsens with excitement. Abnormal oligodendrocyte numbers or function is the suggested pathogenic mechanism. Tremor usually begins in these dogs within a few weeks of age. It is most commonly a generalized tremor, which helps distinguish it from the intention tremor seen with cerebellar disease which primarily involves the head. Diagnosis is based on clinical signs and signalment. Ante-mortem diagnosis requires brain biopsy. No treatment is helpful, however, oligodendrocyte transplant studies are ongoing. Spontaneous resolution of clinical signs occurs in chow chows and Weimaraners.

Metabolic

Numerous metabolic abnormalities may alter forebrain function. Liver disease (hepatic encephalopathy), renal disease (renal encephalopathy), pancreatic disease (pancreatic encephalopathy), glucose abnormalities (hyper- or hypoglycaemia), electrolyte abnormalities (sodium, potassium, chloride, calcium, magnesium), and acid–base abnormalities are examples. Metabolic disease can also result in depression of the sensorium, which may indicate brainstem (reticular activating system) disease.

Hepatic encephalopathy (HE) results when neurotoxins reach the brain, unmetabolized as they pass through an abnormally functioning liver. Suspected toxins include γ-aminobutyric acid, aromatic amino acids, mercaptans, ammonia and skatoles. Animals with HE are usually admitted for investigation of seizures, ptyalism and mentation changes. Clinical signs may be precipitated by feeding a high protein meal. Diagnosis is supported by clinical signs and abnormal liver function studies.

Hypoglycaemia can be associated with insulinoma, liver disease, hypoadrenocorticism, starvation, glycogen storage diseases, heavy work (hunting dog hypoglycaemia) and extrapancreatic neoplasia. Toy breed and neonates may become hypoglycaemic during times of stress. Because the central nervous system (CNS) requires a constant supply of glucose, clinical signs of hypoglycaemia relate to CNS dysfunction and include depression, seizures and tremors. A peripheral neuropathy has been occasionally seen in dogs with insulinoma (see Peripheral nerve disease).

Hyperglycaemia associated with diabetes mellitus more commonly results in clinical signs of peripheral nerve disease (see Peripheral Nerve Disease). In humans, hyperglycaemia can cause seizures (Brick et al., 1989). Dogs with diabetic ketoacidosis may have cerebral signs (depression), but whether these changes relate to the hyperglycaemia or other physiological or metabolic derangements is unknown.

Neoplastic

Neoplasia commonly involves the forebrain, particularly in older animals.

Primary tumours

Meningioma is the most common primary brain tumour in dogs and cats. Meningiomas arise from the arachnoid layer of the meninges and tend to occur in dolichocephalic breeds of dogs. Golden retrievers may be predisposed (Bagley *et al.*, 1993a).

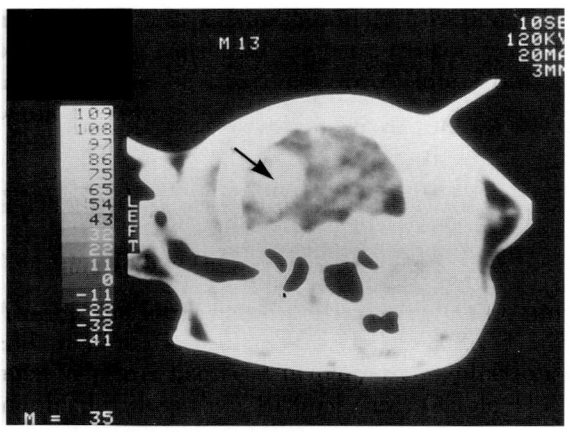

Figure 42.7 Contrast-enhanced computed tomographic image of a cat showing a broad based, extra-axial, contrast-enhancing mass (arrow) characteristic of a meningioma.

Meningiomas are usually histologically benign, but occasionally malignant. Solitary masses are seen in dogs. In cats, multiple masses may be seen. Computed tomography (CT) and magnetic resonance imaging (MRI) show a broad-based, extra-axial contrast enhancing mass in most animals (Turrel *et al.*, 1986) (Fig. 42.7). Cerebrospinal fluid may be normal, inflammatory, or contain increased protein without a concurrent pleocytosis (albuminocytological dissociation) (Carrillo *et al.*, 1986; Bailey and Higgins, 1986). Current treatment options include surgical resection and radiation therapy (Heidner *et al.*, 1991).

Gliomas arise from cells of the brain parenchyma. These include astrocytes, oligodendrogliocytes, ependymal cells, and choroid plexus cells. Brachycephalic dogs may be predisposed to development of these tumours. Choroid plexus tumours arise from areas where the choroid plexus is concentrated (the lateral, third and fourth ventricles). The CT and MRI appearance is varied, and enhancement following the administration of contrast material may not be evident (Turrel *et al.*, 1986) (Fig. 42.8). CSF changes will be similar to those mentioned with meningiomas. Treatment options include surgery, radiation, and chemotherapy (carmustine (BCNU), lomustine (CCNU)) (Dimski and Cook, 1990; Fulton, 1991).

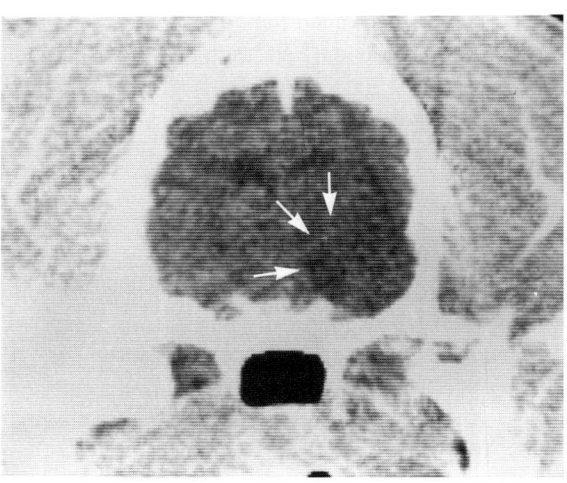

Figure 42.8 Contrast-enhanced computed tomography of a 5-year-old Mastiff with seizures. A hypodense, right to left mass effect with impingement on the right lateral ventricle is seen in the temporal lobe region (arrows). Histological diagnosis following biopsy was astrocytoma.

Pituitary tumours may result in signs of endocrine disease (e.g. hyperadrenocorticism, acromegaly) or signs primarily related to CNS dysfunction (Sarfaty *et al.*, 1988). Macroadenomas may enlarge dorsally from the sella and compress the diencephalon. Treatment options include radiation and surgery.

Other primary tumours involving the forebrain are uncommon and include lymphosarcoma, germ cell tumours, dermoid and epidermoid cysts and craniopharyngiomas.

Secondary tumours

Neoplasia can secondarily involve the brain either by metastasis or direct extension from an extraneural site. Numerous tumours metastasize to the brain including haemangiosarcoma, lymphosarcoma, mammary gland and other carcinomas. Tumours within the nasal cavity or frontal sinuses can extend directly into the brain (Fig. 42.9).

Clinical signs may be localized of multifocal. CT or MRI may show single or multiple masses. With diffuse meningeal tumours these studies may be normal. Occasionally, CSF will reveal neoplastic cells, most commonly with lymphosarcoma and carcinomatosis.

Both primary and metastatic neoplasia can involve the brainstem. Meningiomas (en plaque) can lie along the floor of the skull ventrally and result in brainstem compression. Choroid plexus tumours commonly involve the fourth ventricle (Fig. 42.10). Primary or secondary neoplasia involving the cerebellum is uncommon. Medulloblastoma is a primary brain tumour that may rarely involve the cerebellum in dogs.

Nutritional

Thiamine deficiency is the most common nutritional deficiency affecting the central nervous system. This deficiency results in lesions in the oculomotor and vestibular nuclei, the caudal colliculus and lateral geniculate nuclei. The earliest clinical sign is vestibular ataxia, progressing to seizures with ventral neck flexion and dilated, non-responsive pupils. Treatment consists of the administration of thiamine.

Inflammatory

Numerous inflammatory diseases can affect the brain. These include both infectious and non-infectious aetiologies. Again, clinical signs may be localized to one functional area or suggest multifocal levels of involvement.

Encephalitis and *meningitis* often exist concurrently in dogs and cats. Numerous infectious and non-infectious aetiological agents have been incriminated. The incidence of infectious agents causing meningitis varies with geographic location. Most meningitis syndromes (60%) in small animals do not have a definable infectious cause. A corticosteroid-responsive meningitis seen in young, large breed dogs is thought to occur as an idiopathic condition, however, extensive testing for infectious causes has not been performed. Eosinophilic encephalitis/meningitis of unknown aetiology occurs in dogs and cats. Usually, this disease entity responds to corticosteroid administration. Spinal cord vasculitis syndromes (beagle, German short-haired pointer and Bernese mountain dog), presenting with signs and CSF changes consistent with meningitis, have also been described.

Infectious diseases

Infectious agents causing brain disease include viruses (canine distemper, parvovirus, parainfluenza, herpes, adenovirus, feline infectious peritonitis, pseudorabies, rabies), bacteria, rickettsiae (Rocky Mountain spotted fever, ehrlichiosis), spirochaetes (Lyme disease, leptospirosis), fungae (blastomycosis, histoplasmosis, cryptococcosis, coccidioidomycosis, aspergillosis), protozoa (toxoplasmosis, neosporosis), and unclassified organisms (prothothecosis) (Meric, 1988).

Clinical signs may reflect multiple levels of neu-

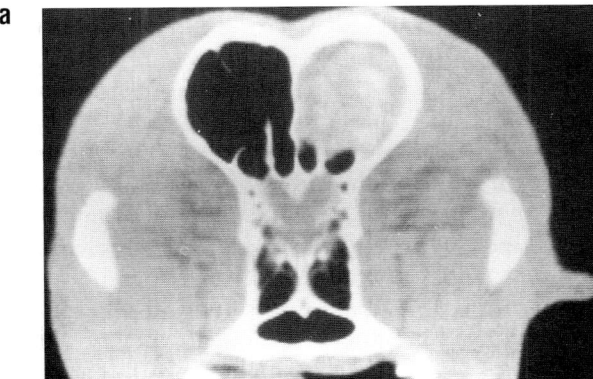
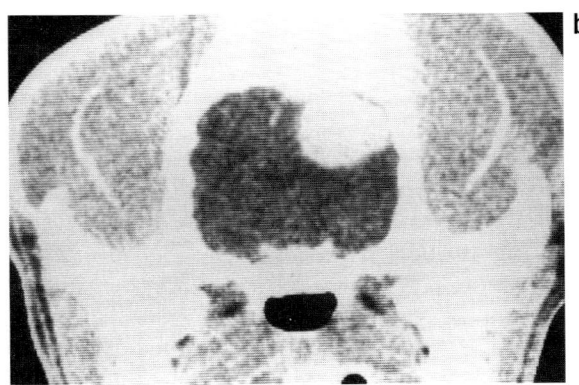

Figure 42.9 Contrast-enhanced computed tomography series of a 2-year-old Rottweiler with seizures, left menace deficit, left facial sensation deficit and left hemiparesis. A mass involving the right frontal sinus (a) extends caudally into the brain (b).

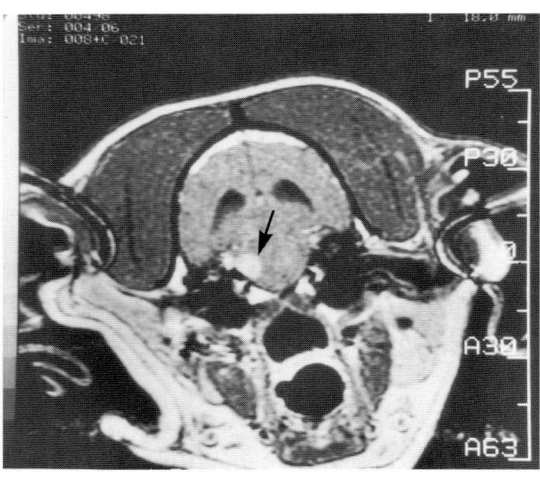

Figure 42.10 Contrast-enhanced T1 weighted magnetic resonance image showing a discrete, contrast-enhancing mass at the left cerebellopontinemedullary angle (arrow). (Intravenous gadolinium has been given, which accumulates in areas where there are alterations to the blood–brain barrier or increased vascularity, thus demonstrating lesions.) Histological diagnosis following biopsy was choroid plexus tumour. Reprinted from Bagley, R.S. (1996) *Veterinary Clinics of North America, Small Animal* **26**, 696.

rological involvement. Neck pain is often found in addition to other signs or as an isolated abnormality. Fundic examination is important and may provide evidence of a polysystemic problem. Imaging studies are helpful for defining structural lesions. Cerebrospinal fluid analysis is essential, however evidence of inflammation on CSF evaluation alone is not specific for meningitis as other CNS diseases (e.g. neoplasia) may result in a pleocytosis and increased CSF protein content.

Treatment is directed at a specific cause if found. Without a definable specific cause, the authors use trimethoprim-sulphadiazine, chloramphenicol, and corticosteroids in combination. If the animal is receiving phenobarbital, chloramphenicol must not be used as this drug will interfere (inhibit) the metabolism of the barbiturate and the animal may become comatose and possibly die.

Canine distemper is caused by a paramyxovirus. Clinical signs can occur in any age of dog, regardless of vaccination status. Most commonly, however, young dogs with inadequate protective immunity are affected. Any region of the nervous system can be involved. Clinical signs of a prior or concurrent systemic illness (respiratory, gastrointestinal) are not always found. Hyperkeratotic footpads in animals with distemper indicate that CNS involvement will occur.

Diagnosis is suggested by detecting inclusion bodies in cells of the conjunctival epithelium, blood or cerebrospinal fluid. Inclusion bodies found during histopathological examination of nervous tissue and elevated CSF antibody titre against distemper virus are also supportive of the diagnosis. Occasionally, however, dogs with CNS distemper do not have positive CSF distemper titres (Sorjonen *et al.*, 1989). No specific treatment is effective against the distemper virus. Corticosteroids, although seemingly contraindicated, may decrease inflammation and result in clinical improvement in some dogs.

Feline infectious peritonitis (FIP) is caused by a coronavirus infection in cats. This virus can involve various areas of the nervous system including the forebrain. Very young and very old cats are predisposed. Of the two forms of FIP that exist in the cat, the 'dry' form commonly affects the nervous system. This viral infection results in an immune complex vasculitis which is responsible for most of the pathological lesions and clinical signs. CSF analysis may show a pleocytosis, with either mononuclear cells or neutrophils as the predominant cell type. No specific treatment is effective. Immunosuppressive therapy may result in short-term improvement of clinical signs.

Toxoplasmosis (*Toxoplasma gondii*) most commonly affects the nervous system of cats. Dogs are infrequently affected. Clinical signs depend on the level of nervous system involvement and include both intracranial, spinal cord and lower motor neurone presentations.

Cerebrospinal fluid may show a pleocytosis, usually with increased numbers of mononuclear cells, and occasionally, eosinophils. Increasing IgG or a single positive IgM serum antibody titre is diagnostic of active infection (Lappin *et al.*, 1989). Treatment includes clindamycin (Greene *et al.*, 1985a) and trimethoprim-potentiated sulphonamide antibiotics.

Rabies is a dramatic, but uncommon cause of CNS disease. Unvaccinated animals and those exposed to wild animals are at greatest risk.

Parasites most commonly affect the forebrain during aberrant migration. Examples include *Toxocara* sp, heartworm and cuterebra larva. Treatment is directed at parasite removal. Anthelmintics are rarely effective when the CNS is involved.

Non-infectious diseases

Non-infectious diseases of the forebrain include *granulomatous meningoencephalitis (GME)* and *pug encephalitis*.

Granulomatous meningoencephalitis can occur as a disseminated disease, as a focal mass-lesion, or as a primary ocular disease. The cause is not known. Some animals initially thought to have this disease have been shown, upon further study, to have lymphoma. CSF usually shows a mononuclear pleocytosis. Occasionally the CSF will be normal or contain only increased protein. CT or MRI may show diffuse inflammatory changes or a mass lesion (Plummer *et al.*, 1992) (Fig. 42.11). Biopsy is needed for definitive diagnosis. Treatment options include immunosuppression (corticosteroids, azathioprine), surgery (if a focal mass is identified), or radiation therapy. Most dogs with GME die within 6 months to 1 year after diagnosis.

Pug encephalitis occurs in young pugs and is characterized histologically by forebrain inflammation and necrosis (Cordy and Holliday, 1989). This disease has been uniformly fatal and therapy (corticosteroids) has not altered the course of the disease.

Idiopathic meningitis is also known as aseptic or sterile meningitis (see under cervical spinal cord disease and multifocal diseases of the nervous system).

Generalized tremor syndrome ('white shaker dog') is described under multifocal diseases of the nervous system.

Many inflammatory diseases which can affect the forebrain can also affect the brainstem. Rocky Mountain spotted fever, for example, commonly involves the brainstem, particularly the vestibular system (Greene *et al.*, 1985b). Diagnosis is based on lack of mass lesion on imaging and a pleocytosis on CSF evaluation.

Parasites will occasionally migrate through the brainstem as described with forebrain disease.

Feline cerebellar hypoplasia is caused by *in utero* infection with the panleukopenia virus (parvovirus), which affects the external germinal layer of the cerebellum and prevents the formation of the granular layer. Some affected cats have a concurrent hydrocephalus and hydranencephaly.

The clinical signs are of diffuse cerebellar disease. The course is non-progressive. Diagnosis can be aided by history and clinical signs. Magnetic resonance imaging may help to define the nature of the lesion. No treatment is helpful.

Idiopathic

Idiopathic epilepsy is characterized by recurrent seizures without an underlying gross or microscopic cause. Seizures in animals with idiopathic epilepsy begin between 6 months and 4 years of age. Certain breeds of dogs, such as beagles, keeshounds and German shepherds, may be predisposed and a hereditary basis is proven in

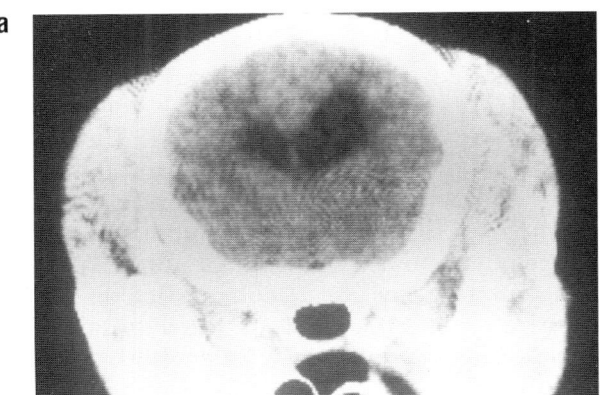 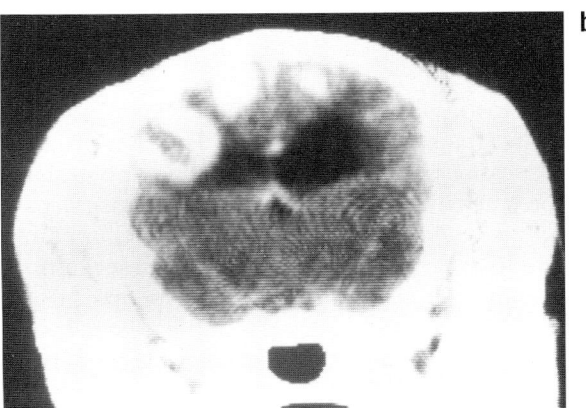

Figure 42.11 Non-contrast (a) and contrast-enhanced (b) CT showing multifocal contrast-enhancing lesions with ring pattern. Ring patterns are usually seen in inflammatory lesions, or neoplasms with fluid or necrotic centres. Diagnosis in this case was granulomatous meningoencephalitis.

some breeds and suspected in others. Seizures are typically of a grand mal type, where the animal becomes recumbent, there are paddling movements of the limbs, and urination, defecation and salivation. The episodes are usually followed by a period of depression – the post-ictal period. Diagnostic testing is normal but necessary to rule out other causes of seizures. Treatment initially consists of phenobarbitone (3 mg kg^{-1} p.o. bid). An assessment of efficacy of this treatment can be helped by determining serum concentrations of phenobarbitone. Trough serum phenobarbitone concentrations (collected just before the next dose) are used in combination with seizure control to determine treatment responses. The therapeutic range for serum phenobarbitone levels in most dogs is between 20 and 45 µg ml^{-1}. If this drug is ineffective and toxic serum levels are reached, additional anticonvulsants such as potassium bromide (20–60 mg kg^{-1} per day) can be used.

Narcolepsy (excessive daytime sleepiness) and *cataplexy* (periods of acute muscular hypotonia) usually occur without underlying structural brain disease. The actual anatomical or physiological abnormality may lie within the brainstem, however, clinical signs usually reflect a cerebral disturbance. Rarely, a structural brain abnormality is found. Disordered neurotransmitter metabolism or abnormalities of the reticular activating system are thought to be responsible, however, a true cause is not known.

Breeds of dogs predisposed to narcolepsy and cataplexy include the Dobermann pinscher, Labrador retriever, miniature poodle, dachshund, beagle and Saint Bernard. Clinical signs usually begin at a young age, however, dogs as old as 7 years have been diagnosed with this disease. Acute onset of REM sleep, usually occurring with stimulation such as eating, is characteristic of narcolepsy.

Physostigmine (0.025–0.1 mg kg^{-1} i.v.) potentiates the attacks for up to 45 min. The tricyclic antidepressant, imipramine, which potentiates serotonin may be helpful as therapy for narcolepsy.

Springer spaniel rage syndrome occurs in young to middle age Springer spaniels. These animals become aggressive usually toward people in the household. No pathological lesion has been found to explain this behaviour change. Treatment is with behaviour modification.

Idiopathic peripheral vestibular disease occurs in both dogs and cats. Older dogs and young to middle aged cats are most commonly affected. Clinical signs are of an acute peripheral vestibular disorder. The major differential diagnosis is otitis media/interna. Recurrence of the syndrome is possible.

Clinical signs usually improve dramatically in 1–2 weeks. The nystagmus usually resolves quickly whereas a mild head tilt may persist. No treatment has proved beneficial.

Congenital peripheral vestibular disease is seen in certain breeds including German shepherds, Dobermann pinschers, English cocker spaniels, and Siamese and Burmese cats. Bilateral congenital vestibular disease is seen in beagles and akitas. Clinical signs include a head tilt, nystagmus, ataxia and, in some, deafness. Animals with bilateral peripheral vestibular disease may not have a head tilt, but rather have wide head excursions. Also, bilaterally affected animals do not have either spontaneous or normal physiological nystagmus. Signs may persist throughout life or may improve spontaneously. There is no treatment.

Congenital deafness is found in a number of breeds including the Dalmatian, Australian heeler, English setter, Australian shepherd, Boston terrier, Old English sheepdog, and English bulldog (Holliday *et al.*, 1992; Strain *et al.*, 1992). White cats with blue irises may also be affected. Most studies have found degeneration or hypoplasia of the organ of Corti, spiral ganglion, and cochlear nuclei. One study has suggested that this may begin as a temporal lobe (auditory cortex) problem (Ferrara and Halnan, 1983). Diagnosis can be made subjectively by loss of Preyer's reflex (involuntary movement of the ears in response to a loud sound) or objectively by brainstem auditory evoked potential testing. No treatment is effective.

Trauma

Head trauma can result in forebrain signs due to haemorrhage, oedema, contusion, penetrating wounds, or depressed skull fractures. Treatment includes control of intracranial pressure and cerebral oedema. Aspects of treatment include maintenance of the airway, hyperventilation with oxygen, and possibly the use of corticosteroids and diuretics. Surgical decompression of compressive skull fractures or rarely, subdural haematoma (Hopkins and Wheeler, 1991), may be indicated.

Brainstem trauma usually carries a poorer prognosis than forebrain trauma alone. Brainstem function can be assessed by evaluation of cranial nerve function, particularly the oculovestibular response. Occasionally, dogs have brainstem signs with cranial cervical lesions, therefore, manipulation for the oculovestibular response should be made only after assessing for an unstable cervical fracture or luxation.

Toxic

Numerous *toxins* can affect the nervous system either primarily or secondarily. Examples of primary toxins include organophosphates, metaldehyde, lead, bromethalin and hexachlorophene.

Toxicity with metronidazole may result in central vestibular signs (Dow et al., 1989). Usually this is associated with high doses of the drug. Clinical signs suggest central vestibular disease. Discontinuation of the drug is imperative. Some dogs may die whereas others may recover completely.

Vascular

Vascular disease involving the forebrain is uncommon in animals compared to human beings (Joseph et al., 1988a). *Thrombosis, infarction and haemorrhage* can occur spontaneously, secondary to drug therapy (L-asparaginase, anticoagulants), with thrombocytopenia and other bleeding disorders, trauma, hypertension, atherosclerosis associated with hypothyroidism, and with infection (septic emboli). Clinical signs are usually acute in onset, and may be initially progressive as the vascular event results in secondary brain disease and oedema. Haemorrhage and infarction may be seen with CT and MRI.

Feline ischaemic encephalopathy is an ischaemic necrosis of the cerebral hemisphere of cats. The distribution of the infarction is usually in the area supplied by the middle cerebral artery. Vascular lesions, however, are infrequently found at necropsy. Clinical signs reflect a forebrain abnormality. Cerebrospinal fluid often contains mild elevations in protein. Computed tomography and MRI abnormalities have not been described. Prognosis for life is good after the first 48 h as this is a non-progressive disorder. Residual neurological deficits may persist.

Similar vascular diseases may involve the brainstem and, rarely, the cerebellum (Bagley et al., 1988).

DISEASES OF THE SPINAL CORD

There are numerous diseases that affect the spinal cord. Some affect selected spinal segments whereas others may occur anywhere along the spinal cord. This latter group will be discussed first. See Wheeler and Sharp (1994) for further details, particularly on surgical treatment.

Diseases which may affect any part of the spinal cord

Degenerative

Degenerative spinal cord disease is usually breed specific and occurs in younger animals, with the exception of degenerative myelopathy. Examples include Afghan myelomalacia, hereditary ataxia of smooth-haired fox terriers and Jack Russell terriers, and miniature poodle demyelination.

Intervertebral disc disease can occur in any area of the spinal cord caudal to C1–2. Dachshunds appear predisposed. Middle-aged dogs are most commonly affected. Dogs less than 1 year of age rarely have intervertebral disc disease (IVD). Geriatric dogs are occasionally affected. Clinical signs of IVD disease in cats are rare.

Two basic types of disc disease are seen. A Hansen type I intervertebral disc abnormality is seen in chondrodystrophic breeds of dog which have chondroid metaplasia of their discs beginning early in life. These discs usually extrude rather that protrude into the vertebral canal. The Hansen type II intervertebral disc abnormality is seen most commonly in older, larger non-chondrodystrophic dogs with fibroid metaplasia of the disc. These discs usually protrude rather than extrude into the vertebral canal.

Clinical signs of cervical IVD disease include neck pain and paresis. Root signature (holding one limb up or flexed) may occur. Neck pain may be the only clinical sign in some dogs. Diagnosis is made by myelography.

In the thoracolumbar area, the disc spaces between T11 and L2 are at high risk for extrusion. Accurate diagnosis requires myelography (Fig. 42.12). General guidelines have been established for therapy depending on the severity of clinical signs. Mildly affected animals (animals with pain alone or mild paresis) may be managed with cage confinement for at least two weeks. If after 2 weeks signs are not improved, diagnosis and surgery should be considered. If the animal worsens during this time, surgery should be considered sooner.

If improvement is noted, continuation of cage confinement is indicated for up to one to two weeks after the animal is clinically normal. Short-term oral corticosteroid administration may be used concurrently, but should never be used without cage confinement.

More severely affected animals (those who are unable to support weight) are considered surgical candidates for decompression of the spinal cord. Animals that retain deep pain sensation have an 80–90% chance of being able to walk at some time after surgery. When deep pain is absent, the prognosis for walking falls to 50%. If deep pain perception is absent for longer than 48 h, the prognosis for return to walking falls below 5% (although there are exceptions to these rules).

Signs of myelomalacia suggest irreversible damage to the spinal cord and surgery is not helpful. The debate as to whether surgery may stop myelomalacia and prevent extension is unresolved. The prognosis of return to walking of an animal with myelomalacia is nil. If myelomalacia ascends to involve the cervical spinal cord, death will ensue and euthanasia is the most sensible and humane course of action.

Corticosteroids (e.g. methylprednisolone) are useful if given within the first 8 h after a spinal trauma in human (Bracken *et al.*, 1990). Initial treatment is with methylprednisolone at 30 mg kg^{-1} i.v. A clinical study in humans suggests following this bolus dose with 5.4 mg kg^{-1} h^{-1} i.v. of methylprednisolone for the ensuing 23 h. Long-term treatment of patients with IVD disease with these drugs is not advantageous and can result in significant side effects, particularly gastrointestinal ulceration. Therefore, long-term corticosteroid therapy is not recommended. (Wheeler and Sharp, 1994).

Anomalous

Anomalies involving the spinal cord, vertebral column, or skin may result from abnormal development of the neural tube. Most often, these lesions occur in the caudal lumbar and sacral areas. Components of spinal dysraphism include spina bifida (defective fusion of the vertebral

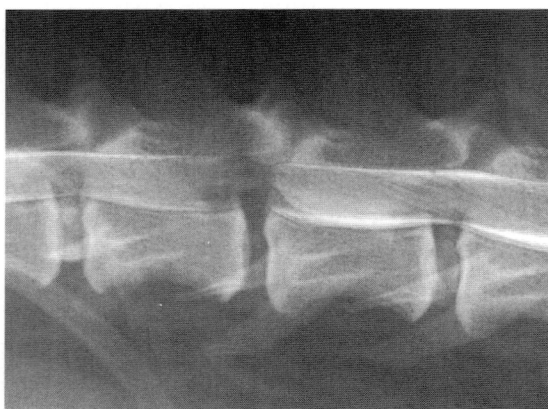

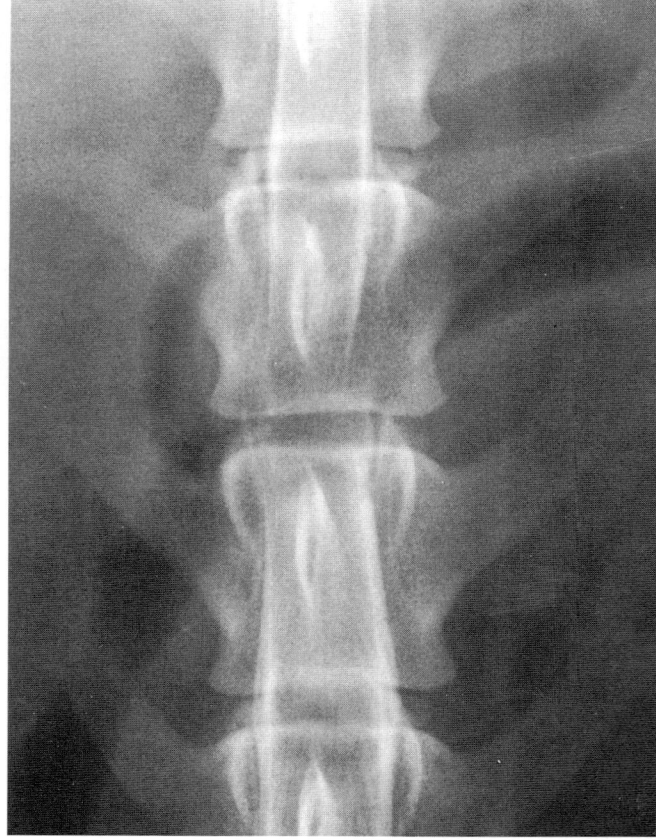

Figure 42.12 Lateral (a) and ventrodorsal (b) myelogram images of a dachshund dog with a lumbar disc extrusion.

arch), meningocele (protrusion of meninges through the defect), myelocele (protrusion of spinal cord through the defect) and meningomyelocele (protrusion of both meninges and spinal cord).

Defects are common in Manx cats and Weimaraner dogs. Rhodesian ridgeback dogs have a skin defect, a dermal sinus, that may communicate with the spinal cord. Intramedullary defects such as hydro- or syringomyelia may accompany these other more obvious defects. Surgical closure of the abnormality may be considered as a possible treatment in selected cases.

It is important to note that not all congenital vertebral anomalies result in spinal cord compression.

Neoplastic

Neoplasia of the spine is described anatomically as being extradural, intradural-extramedullary, and intramedullary. Extradural tumours are most common and include primary and secondary bone tumours (osteosarcoma, fibrosarcoma, chondrosarcoma), haemangiosarcoma, various carcinomas, multiple myeloma and other plasma cell tumours, lipomas, liposarcomas, and lymphosarcoma (especially in cats). Multiple cartilaginous exostoses are benign proliferations of cartilage and bone occurring in young, growing animals, with the thoracic and lumbar vertebrae most commonly affected. Some authors consider these benign tumours of the spine.

Intradural-extramedullary tumours include meningiomas and nerve sheath tumours (Fig. 42.13). Neuroepithelioma is an unusual intradural-extramedullary tumour that involves only the thoracolumbar area (deLahunta, 1983). The cell of origin of the tumour is unclear, and thoracic cord blastoma has been recently suggested as a more appropriate term. The German shepherd dog is commonly affected.

Intramedullary tumours include astrocytomas and ependymomas and, occasionally, intramedullary metastasis from haemangiosarcoma.

Clinical signs depend on the level of spinal cord involvement. Extradural and intradural extramedullary tumours usually result in pain, whereas intramedullary tumours are usually not painful (exceptions exist). The onset of clinical signs is often more chronic with extradural tumours, and acute with intramedullary tumours.

Diagnosis is made primarily with myelography. CT and MRI may also be helpful to localize and define the extent of the tumour. Treatment

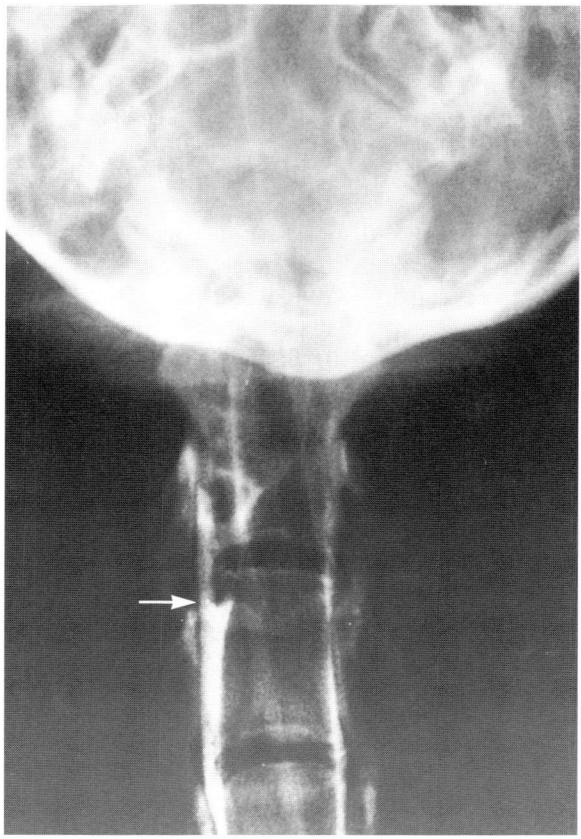

Figure 42.13 Intradural, extramedullary lesion identified with myelography (dorsoventral view) in a 9-year-old Yorkshire terrier with chronic neck pain. The classic 'golf-tee' appearance is seen (arrow). Surgical resection and biopsy revealed a nerve sheath tumour. Reprinted from Bagley, R.S. and Tucker, R.L. (1996) Progress in Veterinary Neurology **7**, 63.

options include surgical removal, radiation and possibly chemotherapy. Surgical removal is easiest with extradural tumours, however, intramedullary tumours have occasionally been successfully resected. Prognosis depends on tumour type.

Inflammatory

Infectious disease

Discospondylitis is infection in the intervertebral space and adjacent vertebral bodies. This can occur in any area of the spinal column, and can be in multiple sites. The most common organism cultured with this disease is *Staphylococcus intermedius; Brucella canis* and *Escherichia coli* are also found occasionally. Rarely, discospondylitis is caused by fungal infections such as aspergillosis.

Larger breeds of dogs are more commonly affected. Clinical signs include paresis and spinal pain. Paraspinal muscle atrophy may be severe.

Diagnosis is based on the typical radiographic findings of lytic vertebral end-plates on either side of the affected disc space(s) (Fig. 42.14) The causative organism may be isolated from blood and urine cultures. When routine bacterial cultures are negative, suspicion should be heightened for possible fungal disease. Rarely, curettage or disc space aspiration under fluoroscopy is needed to collect material for culture. *Brucella canis* titres in serum should also be evaluated. Radionuclide scanning may reveal lesions of bone inflammation/infection before changes are visible on survey radiographs.

The role of immunodeficiency in this disease is unclear. Many of these dogs have abnormal lymphocyte blastogenesis tests, but this may be a non-specific finding secondary to the underlying infection.

Treatment includes prolonged antibiotic administration. The choice of antibiotic depends on the sensitivity spectrum of the organism cultured. Before definitive culture results, or when cultures are negative but radiographic signs are suggestive of this disease, a cephalosporin should be used.

Non-infectious diseases

These are discussed in the section on multifocal diseases of the nervous system (p. 691).

Trauma

Trauma to the spinal column can occur as the result of falls or gunshot wounds, but most commonly is caused by road traffic accidents. Any age or breed can be affected. Clinical signs will depend on the level of spinal cord involvement.

Remember that the severity of injury is assessed from the neurological status, not the degree of displacement of vertebrae observed on radiographs. Radiographic evaluation provides only static information as to where the vertebrae lie presently; it does not give information as to how far the vertebrae were displaced at the time of the trauma. Animals that suffer a

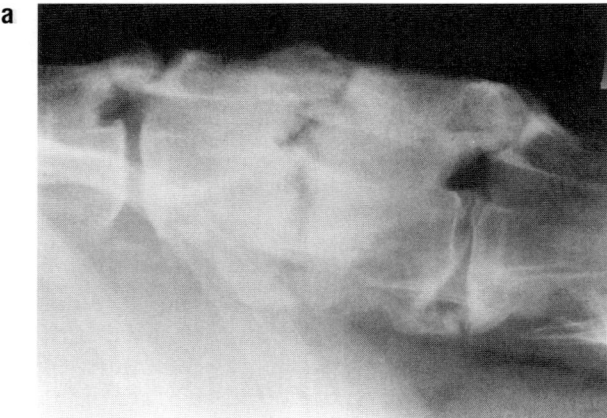
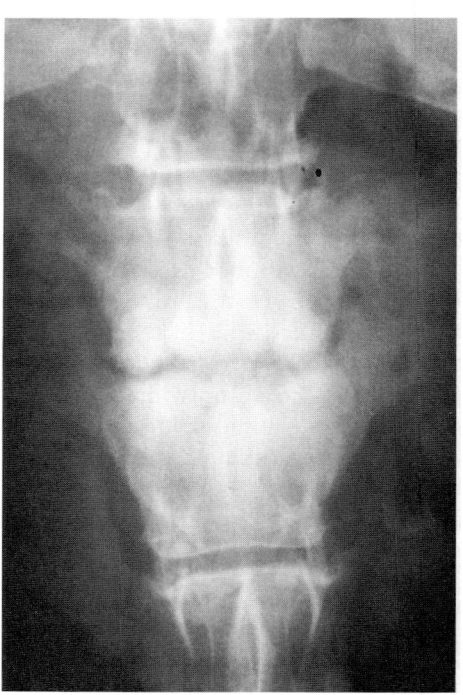

Figure 42.14 Survey lateral (a) and dorsoventral (b) radiographs of the thoracolumbar area of a 7-year-old German shepherd with back pain. Vertebral endplate lysis suggestive of discospondilitis is seen at L1–2. Blood cultures recovered a staphylococcal organism and neurological signs resolved following antibiotic therapy.

traumatic spinal injury should be assessed using a similar prognostic scale as for IVD disease. Absent deep pain sensation in an animal with known spinal trauma is a poor prognostic sign. If displacement of the vertebral canal is greater than 100% of the vertebral canal, the prognosis is similarly poor.

Vascular

Ischaemic myelopathy (fibrocartilaginous embolism) occurs secondary to vascular thrombosis and infarction of the spinal cord. Non-chondrodystrophic dogs are affected. Clinical signs of spinal cord dysfunction occur acutely. These dogs have no spinal pain, however, they may seem to be in pain initially (within the first 24 h) after onset. Spinal cord involvement is usually asymmetric and commonly involves an intumescence. Therefore, LMN signs in one or more limbs are common. The signs are not progressive after the first 24 h.

The infarction is thought to be due to embolization of fibrocartilaginous material of IVD origin. How this material enters the vascular system is unknown. Theories include disc extrusion into the vascular system, either directly or through neovascularization of the IVD due to degeneration. Others have suggested that the fibrocartilage may actually arise from within the vascular system.

Diagnosis is by exclusion of other possible causes of myelopathy. Myelography is often normal but, if performed during the acute phase of the disease, there may be evidence of cord swelling. Cerebrospinal fluid may be normal or there may be increased numbers of nucleated cells with an increased protein concentration.

There is no specific treatment for this condition. Prognosis depends on the severity of clinical signs. Loss of deep pain sensation is a poor prognostic sign for return to function. Similarly, LMN signs rarely improve.

Diseases localized to the cervical spine

Degenerative

Wobbler's syndrome encompasses a number of cervical vertebral abnormalities. These include vertebral malarticulation/malformation, disc extrusion, articular facet hypertrophy, and ligament hypertrophy. Older Doberman pinschers and young Great Danes are most commonly affected. Great Danes usually have dorsal articular facet hypertrophy whereas ventral compressive lesions are more common in Dobermanns.

Tetraparesis is frequently seen. Paraparesis may be more prominent in some dogs, with the thoracic limbs showing minimal neurological involvement. Spasticity of the forelimbs at gait may be noted. Neck pain is not always obvious, however, affected dogs tend to hold their heads downward in a flexed position. Atrophy of the supra- and infraspinatus muscle may be noted.

Myelography will reveal the compressed segments of the spinal cord. Both dynamic and static compressive lesions can be seen. Flexed and extended radiological views may be needed to reveal a dynamic compressive lesion. Commonly, this type of compression is worse when the neck is extended. Computed tomography may be helpful for detecting occult bony changes and spinal cord atrophy (Sharp *et al.*, 1992).

Medical and surgical treatments have been used for this disease. Numerous surgical techniques have been described suggesting that no one technique is adequate. A 75% success rate for either stopping the progression of the disease or improving clinical signs is given for dogs that can still walk. This percentage falls to 50% in dogs that are non-ambulatory.

Anomalous

Atlantoaxial subluxation most often occurs in young small breed dogs, particularly Yorkshire terriers, chihuahuas, pomeranians etc., where there is instability at the atlantoaxial joint due to an abnormality of the dens or its associated ligaments. Clinical signs are consistent with cervical spinal cord disease. Diagnosis is made by radiology. The most effective treatment is surgical stabilization (Thomas *et al.*, 1991).

Inflammatory

Meningitis frequently results in clinical signs suggestive of cervical spinal cord disease. This topic is discussed under multifocal diseases of the nervous system.

Diseases localized to the thoracolumbar spine

Degenerative

Degenerative myelopathy is a degenerative spinal cord disease. German shepherd dogs are commonly affected. The disease is usually chronic and progressive. Clinical signs resemble those of a T3–L3 spinal cord lesion, however, the actual histopathological lesions may be more severe in the caudal cervical area. UMN signs in the pelvic limbs are the rule with the exception that the patellar reflexes may be decreased (due to dorsal root involvement). Symmetrical paraparesis is common. Occasionally, asymmetry of clinical signs is noted. There is no spinal pain. As the disease progresses, the thoracic limbs and later the brain stem will become involved. Bladder and bowel function is maintained.

The cause of this disease is unknown. Speculation has centred on a disregulation of suppressor T-cell function as assessed by decreased lymphocyte blastogenesis in affected dogs.

Myelography is normal. Cerebrospinal fluid may be normal or have an increased protein concentration.

No curative treatment is known. One author has claimed success in stopping or slowing the progression of the disease using ε-aminocaproic acid (Clemmons, 1989). Other treatments, as yet unproven, include exercise and vitamin supplementation.

Diseases localized to the lumbosacral spine

Cauda equina syndrome is the name given to a variety of diseases that result in similar clinical signs of caudal spinal cord and nerve root compression. The most common cause is lumbosacral stenosis/compression. Rarely, however, tumour or inflammation (cauda equina neuritis) may occur.

Degenerative

Lumbosacral stenosis/compression can occur as a congenital stenosis of this region or be acquired due to malarticulation or malformation. Lumbosacral (LS) compression is most common in larger breeds of dogs. Occasionally, neoplasia or discospondilitis can result in LS compression. Compression of L7 and of the sacral nerve roots occurs as they traverse this disc space. Compression can result dorsally from the ligamentum flavum, or ventrally from the bulging annulus fibrosis. Clinical signs include LS pain, faecal and/or urinary incontinence, and LMN signs in the pelvic limbs (sciatic fields).

Diagnosis is based on myelography, epidurography, discography and CT or MRI studies. Cerebrospinal fluid analysis is usually not helpful. Electromyography and nerve conduction velocity studies of the pelvic limbs and tail may reveal spontaneous activity consistent with denervation or slowed conduction velocities, respectively (Sisson et al., 1992).

Treatment involves surgical decompression and/or stabilization of this area. Rest and analgesics are used when surgical decompression is not chosen. Antibiotics are indicated if an infectious process is present.

DISEASES OF THE PERIPHERAL NERVOUS SYSTEM, NEUROMUSCULAR JUNCTION AND MUSCLE

Degenerative/congenital

Degenerative peripheral neuropathies include hypertrophic neuropathy of the Tibetan mastiff, giant axonal neuropathy of German shepherds and progressive axonopathy of boxers. Globoid cell leukodystrophy may involve peripheral nerves (Vicini et al., 1988).

Degenerative muscle disorders are seen occasionally (see also Chapter 43). Breeds affected include the golden retriever, Irish terrier, English springer spaniel, labrador retriever, and Old English sheepdog. Affected animals may have increased serum creatine kinase (CK) concentrations and complex repetitive discharges may be evident on EMG. Muscle biopsy should be diagnostic. Currently there is no treatment.

An X-linked muscular dystrophy similar to Duchenne's disease and golden retriever myopathy has been described in cats (Gaschen et al., 1991).

Myotonia is a sustained muscle contraction which is initiated voluntarily or in response to external stimulation (percussion), and which is sustained involuntarily. Myotonia occurs as a congenital problem in various breeds including the chow chow. Rarely, myotonia results from toxicity. The excessive muscle contraction is thought to be due to an abnormal muscle cell membrane which supports persistent depolarization.

Motor neuronopathies are diseases which affect the cell bodies of the LMN. This leads to degeneration of the cell in the ventral horn of the spinal cord and occasionally the cranial nerve nuclei. Breeds of dogs affected include the Brittany spaniel, Swedish Lapland, rottweiler, German shorthaired pointer, and, experimentally, the offspring of Great Danes mated with bloodhounds or Saint Bernards.

Clinical signs are seen early in life in most dogs. The clinical course is chronic and progressive. No effective treatment is known.

Neuropathies have been seen that only involve the *sensory nerves*. Breeds affected include the dachshund, English pointer and Siberian husky. The English pointers begin self-mutilating their extremities at a young age. Anaesthesia of the pelvic limbs is seen. This self-mutilation may represent a paraesthesia or may be due to abnormal sensory impulses.

Metabolic

Diabetic neuropathy commonly affects the tibial nerve in cats resulting in a classic dropped hock appearance. Neuropathies have been reported in association with insulinomas (Shahar *et al.*, 1985; Braund *et al.*, 1987a), Other metabolic myopathies or neuropathies have been reported with hyperlipidaemia in cats (Jones *et al.*, 1986), and hyperadrenocorticism and hypothyroidism in dogs.

Polymyopathy of cats was initially described as an idiopathic acquired myopathy resulting in weakness. A *hypokalaemic myopathy* has since been described in cats also resulting in weakness (Dow *et al.*, 1987). Therefore, some of this original group of cats may have fallen into this latter category. Muscle weakness is a prominent clinical sign and may result in ventroflexion of the neck. Decreased serum potassium and increased serum CK concentrations with appropriate EMG, and muscle biopsy findings support this diagnosis. Increasing serum potassium via oral supplementation should improve clinical signs. Intravenous potassium administration should be performed with caution. Some of the original group of cats responded to corticosteroid treatment. In humans, horses, and less commonly in dogs, hyperkalaemia can result in muscle weakness. Other electrolyte disturbances including sodium, chloride, calcium and magnesium imbalances may also result in myopathic signs.

Neoplastic

Lymphoma commonly occurs extradurally in cats and can involve nerve roots. Rarely, only peripheral nerve involvement is seen (Presthus and Teige, 1986). Cranial nerves (V, VII) may be involved with haematogenous neoplasia (leukaemias) due to direct infiltration with the tumour cells (Carpenter *et al.*, 1987) (Fig. 42.15).

Nerve sheath tumours (Schwannoma, neurofibroma, neurofibrosarcoma) commonly involve the peripheral nerves of the thoracic limb in older dogs. These dogs present for lameness that in some animals may have been present for a year or more before presentation. Often dogs are initially diagnosed with arthritis or other orthopaedic diseases. Clinical clues include atrophy of selected thoracic limb muscles and pain on axillary palpation. In some instances, a discrete mass can be palpated in the axilla. Dogs with extreme pain may require general anaesthesia for adequate palpation.

Diagnosis often requires surgical exploration of the axilla. Electromyography and nerve conduction velocity studies may determine which peripheral nerves are involved.

Prognosis is poor when the tumour invades the vertebral canal. Local recurrence is common, and extensive resection and amputation is recommended. Preliminary unpublished observations by the authors using postoperative radiation therapy after tumour resection have been encouraging, but too few cases have been evaluated to make firm recommendations.

Paraneoplastic neuropathy is occasionally

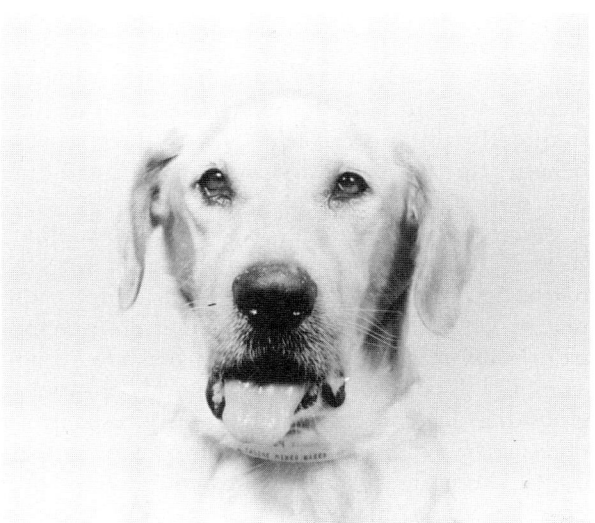

Figure 42.15 Dog presented with dropped jaw suggestive of bilateral trigeminal nerve paralysis. Lymphoma involving these and other cranial nerves was found at necropsy.

recognized in dogs (Braund et al., 1987a, b). The peripheral nervous system distant to the primary tumour is secondarily affected, often by unknown mechanisms. It is possible that the primary tumour results in metabolic alterations that affect the peripheral nerve, or that the nerve is destroyed by immune-mediated mechanisms. This sequel of systemic neoplasia is commonly overlooked as a cause of weakness in animals with cancer.

A recognized relationship between insulinoma and peripheral neuropathy has been reported (Shahar et al., 1985; Braund et al., 1987a, b). Whether the nerve damage is the result of insulin-induced hypoglycaemia or other factors is still unclear.

Inflammatory

Infectious

Botulism is due to the exotoxin of *Clostridium botulinum*. Many toxin types have been described, however, type C appears to cause the disease most readily in dogs. This exotoxin blocks the presynaptic release of acetylcholine from the neuromuscular junction.

Clinical signs include diffuse LMN disease. Cranial nerve involvement is common and can be used to differentiate botulism from tick or coonhound paralysis. Diagnosis is made by identifying the toxin in serum or vomitus. Electromyography and nerve conduction velocity studies may show decreased amplitude of the compound muscle action potential.

Treatment includes the administration of polyvalent antitoxin and supportive care. Other less frequently administered drugs with questionable benefit include neostigmine and guanidine hydrochloride.

Tetanus is due to a neurotoxin (tetanospasmin) secreted by the organism *Clostridium tetani*. This toxin binds to interneurones and inhibits the release of inhibitory neurotransmitter (glycine) from inhibitory interneurons (Renshaw cells). The organism gains access to the body through a wound. Dogs and cats are inherently resistant to this disease, with cats being more resistant than dogs. Therefore, although the wound on a dog may be undetectable, the wound on a cat is usually obvious.

Clinical signs include extensor rigidity, inability to open the mouth, salivation, prolapsed nictitating membranes, inability to urinate and seizures. Bradycardia (Panciera et al., 1988), megaoesophagus and hiatal hernia (Dieringer and Wolf, 1991) may be seen. Tetanus localized to one part of the body (e.g. one limb) is occasionally found (Malik et al., 1989).

Diagnosis is based on clinical signs. Culturing of a wound may reveal the organism. A serum test for antibodies is occasionally helpful (Baker et al., 1988). Treatment includes wound debridement and the administration of antitoxin (a single dose intravenously), penicillin and muscle relaxants (acepromazine or chlorpromazine), enteral or parental nutrition support, anticonvulsants if necessary, a quiet environment, and good supportive care.

Toxoplasma gondii and *Neospora caninum* are protozoal organisms that can affect any area of the nervous system resulting in encephalitis, myelitis, peripheral neuropathy or myositis. The disease is classically seen in young animals with hyperextended pelvic limb(s). Diagnosis is based on the presence of a single IgM titre or rising IgG titres to the organism (toxoplasmosis), or visualization of the protozoan in biopsy specimens (both). Clinical distinction between the two infections is not always possible, however serological testing and electron microscopic characteristics of the organisms may be helpful in identifying the causative agent.

Treatment for toxoplasmosis currently is clindamycin (Greene et al., 1985a). The same may be true for neosporosis, however, few cases with definitive treatment success have been reported.

Non-infectious

Myasthenia gravis literally means grave muscle weakness. There are two forms of this disease: a congenital form that is not associated with antibody production, and an acquired form that is associated with antibodies produced against acetylcholine receptors on the neuromuscular end-plates. The clinical consequence of either of these forms is neuromuscular junction dysfunction and muscle weakness after a short period of exercise.

The congenital form occurs in smooth-haired fox terriers, springer spaniels, samoyeds, Jack Russell terriers and Siamese cats.

The acquired form can occur idiopathically, or secondary to a variety of tumours (thymoma, cholangiosarcoma, osteosarcoma). In thymoma, the tumour either produces excess antibody similar to acetylcholine receptor antibody, or produces an antibody against an antigen in the tumour, which is similar to one found in muscle.

Diagnosis is based on clinical signs of exercise-induced weakness. Affected animals usually adopt a characteristic posture before collapsing (Fig. 42.16). Weakness of facial muscle may also be seen. Megaoesophagus may be the only clinical manifestation of disease in some dogs (Shelton et al., 1990). A positive response to edrophonium suggests a diagnosis of myasthenia gravis. Edrophonium is an anticholinesterase that potentiates acetylcholine at the neuromuscular junction. This drug when given intravenously can reverse the clinical weakness seen with myasthenia gravis for a short period of time.

Electromyography and nerve conduction velocity studies are normal. A decremental response may be seen during repeated stimulation of a peripheral nerve in some but not all cases. Single fibre EMG is a relatively new technique that may be an aid to diagnosis of this disease in the future (Hopkins et al., 1993).

Treatment depends on eliminating any underlying aetiology. With the congenital form of the disease, a long-acting anticholinesterase product (pyridostigmine) can be given to enhance the effect of acetylcholine at the neuromuscular junction. Additionally, immunosuppressive therapy with corticosteroids may be needed to control clinical signs in cases of acquired (immune-mediated) myasthenia gravis. Corticosteroids should not be given to patients with aspiration pneumonia secondary to megaoesophagus (see below).

Prognosis for some animals is good, with occasional spontaneous cures or remission. Complicating factors include severe weakness with respiratory embarrassment and aspiration pneumonia secondary to megaoesophagus.

Feline myasthenia gravis is similar to the canine disease. Abyssinian cats may be predisposed (Joseph et al., 1988b). Treatment responses may not be as dramatic, but spontaneous remission is still possible.

Coonhound paralysis or *polyradiculoneuritis* is a disease of dogs similar to Guillain–Barré disease in humans. A suspected antigen (raccoon saliva) results in an inflammatory response directed commonly toward the nerve root. Other antigens may also initiate this disease, as raccoon exposure in not a consistent factor in all animals. Clinical signs are consistent with LMN disease. Affected animals are often hyperaesthetic to minimal pressure. Treatment is supportive.

Brachial plexus neuritis is suspected to be an immune-mediated neuritis which preferentially affects the thoracic limbs. In one dog, horse meat in the diet was thought to be the inciting antigen. Treatment may be attempted with immunosuppression. Other inflammatory neuropathies such as *trigeminal neuritis* and *idiopathic polyneuropathy* occur without obvious cause.

Masticatory muscle myositis is a myopathy which preferentially affects the muscles of mastication. This is thought to arise as a result of an immune-mediated destruction of the type 2M fibres found selectively in these muscles (Gilmour et al., 1992). Clinical signs include muscle swelling and pain on opening the mouth and decreased ability to open the mouth. This disease can progress to atrophy and fibrosis of these muscles which significantly restricts jaw movement. Diagnosis is based on muscle biopsy. Creatine kinase elevations may be seen during the acute phase of the disease. Treatment consists of immunosuppressive doses of corticosteroids.

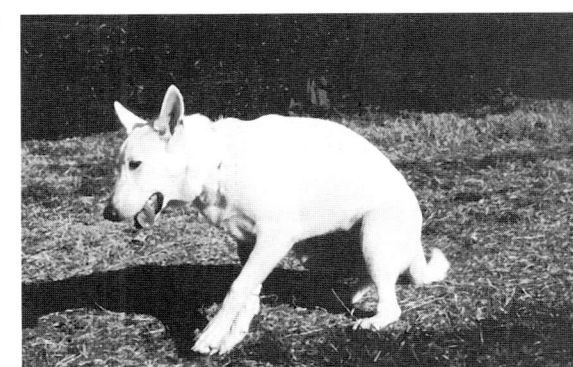
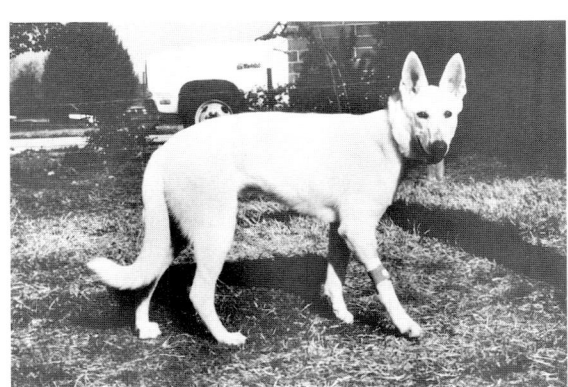

Figure 42.16 Dog showing episodic weakness and stilted gait (a). After edrophonium administration (b), the dog became normal. A subsequent diagnosis of myasthenia gravis was made.

Idiopathic

Laryngeal paralysis in most cases occurs without obvious cause. A tenuous association with hypothyroidism has been reported in a few cases. Laryngeal paralysis may also be a component of a diffuse peripheral neuropathy.

Idiopathic neuropathies include chronic relapsing polyneuritis, distal denervating disease and giant axonal neuropathy of German shepherds. Distal denervating disease causes generalized LMN dysfunction. Despite the profound neurological deficits, most of these dogs recover over a period of weeks.

Scotty cramp is characterized by paroxysms of muscular hypertonicity, usually precipitated by excitement or exercise although the underlying mechanism for these episodes is not known. It is believed to be inherited as a recessive trait. Treatment includes diazepam or promazine tranquillizers.

Familial myoclonus of Labrador retrievers is a disease characterized by marked, intermittent muscular hypertonicity in young dogs (Fox et al., 1984). Other breeds (e.g. Dalmatians) are occasionally affected. The cause is unknown. Treatment with diazepam is not helpful. Clonazepam, however, may provide some relief.

Dancing Dobermann syndrome is a disease characterized by alternating pelvic limb flexion when the animal is standing. A peripheral neuropathy of the pelvic limb nerves is suspected (Chrisman, 1990).

Dysautonomia is an idiopathic autonomic nervous system disease primarily seen in cats and occasionally dogs (Sharp et al., 1984; Wise and Lappin, 1991). Clinical signs reflect autonomic system dysfunction and include megacolon, dilated pupils, xerostomia (dry mouth), and keratoconjunctivitis sicca. No cause has been found and no effective treatment is available.

Trauma

Trauma can occur to a single nerve (e.g. misplaced injection into the sciatic nerve) or multiple nerves (e.g. brachial plexus avulsion). The severity of damage sustained by the nerves determines the prognosis. A neurapraxia (least severe injury) is an interruption in function and conduction in a nerve, usually associated with a lesion of the myelin without severe axonal involvement. Axonotmesis suggests separation and damage of axons, where neurotmesis (most severe injury) is complete severance of all structures of the nerve. The likelihood of regeneration is less with neurotmesis compared to neurapraxia.

Brachial plexus avulsion occurs as a result of a trauma (Wheeler et al., 1986). The roots of brachial plexus nerves are avulsed from the spinal cord. Clinical signs include LMN paresis/plegia in the affected thoracic limb. Ipsilateral loss of the cutaneous trunci reflex (due to damage to the lateral thoracic nerve that exits the spinal cord at C8–T1 area) and/or Horner's syndrome (sympathetic nerves exit the spinal cord at T1–3) may be associated signs. It is the nerve roots that are actually avulsed off the spinal cord. Treatment for primary avulsion is not useful. Tendon transpositions and arthrodesis of the carpus may be salvage options in selected patients. Nerve transpositions have been used in human beings, but have not been adequately evaluated in animals.

Toxic

Tick paralysis is due to infestation with ticks (in the USA) such as *Dermacentor* sp., *Amblyomma* sp. and *Ixodes* sp. These secrete a toxin that prevents release of acetylcholine from the neuromuscular junctions. Clinical signs are those of diffuse LMN disease. Diagnosis depends on clinical signs and the presence of ticks. One should be sure to look for ticks in hard to find places such as the ear canals. Treatment is tick removal, usually most easily accomplished by tick dipping.

Chronic *organophosphate toxicity* can result in weakness, primarily in cats (Jaggy and Oliver, 1990).

Vascular

Aortic thromboembolism occurs in cats most often as a consequence of cardiomyopathy (most frequently the hypertrophic form). Occasionally, these thrombi can lodge in vessels supplying a thoracic limb. Clinical signs include paraplegia, with firm, hard painful muscles in the affected limb(s) (Griffiths and Duncan, 1979). Absent femoral pulses, cold cyanotic extremities and absent bleeding when a toenail is cut are also found. Various treatments have been tried. Tissue plasminogen activator administration may be the most effective but carries the risk of significant mortality (50%) (Pion, 1988). Prognosis is usually poor for full long-term recovery because of the nature of the underlying heart disease.

MULTIFOCAL DISEASES OF THE NERVOUS SYSTEM

Multifocal diseases of the nervous system are those where more than one functional area is involved. Many of the inflammatory (infectious and non-infectious) diseases previously described may result in multifocal neurological signs (Meric, 1988).

Dogs with *generalized tremor syndrome* ('white shaker dog syndrome') present with diffuse, fine, whole body tremor. Dogs with white hair coats (e.g. Maltese terriers, West Highland white terriers) are more commonly affected, however, dogs with other coat colours are also affected (Farrow, 1986). Additional neurological abnormalities include nystagmus, menace response abnormalities, proprioceptive deficits and seizures. This syndrome is most often the result of a mild lymphocytic encephalitis. No aetiological agents have been identified to date.

Cerebrospinal fluid is usually abnormal and shows a mild lymphocytic pleocytosis. Protein concentration may be normal or mildly increased. Occasionally, CSF analysis is normal. Computed tomography has been reported in only a few cases. In one group of seven Maltese terriers with this disease, all four which were evaluated with CT had ventricular enlargement (Bagley *et al.*, 1993b). The significance of this finding is unknown, however, as there is a high incidence of ventricular enlargement in Maltese terriers without concurrent tremor.

Affected dogs generally respond to immunosuppressive doses of corticosteroid. Gradual tapering of the dose should be performed to prevent recurrence. Relapse is possible and corticosteroids may be required for the life of the animal to control clinical signs.

Aseptic meningitis occurs in certain breeds such as the beagle (beagle pain syndrome), Bernese mountain dog, and as a clinical entity in young, large breed dogs. Clinical signs usually resemble those of cervical spinal cord disease including neck pain and/or tetraparesis. Additional brain stem or forebrain signs may also result. Diagnosis is based on pleocytosis (neutrophilic, mononuclear or mixed) with or without elevated protein in the CSF. The numerous causes of meningitis should be excluded before a diagnosis of aseptic meningitis is made.

If an infectious cause is identified in a patient with inflammatory CNS disease, antibiotic therapy should be instigated. Trimethoprim potentiated sulphonamides and chloramphenicol achieve therapeutic concentrations in the CNS and spinal fluid. Corticosteroids are usually effective in improving clinical signs. Relapses can occur, especially if medication is withdrawn rapidly.

REFERENCES

Bagley, R.S., Anderson, W.I., deLahunta, A., Kallfelz, F.A. and Bowersox, T.S. (1988) Cerebellar infarction caused by arterial thrombosis in a dog. *Journal of the American Veterinary Medical Association* **192**, 785–787.

Bagley, R.S., Kornegay, J.N., Page, R.L. and Thrall, D.E. (1993a) Central nervous system neoplasia. In: *Textbook of Small Animal Surgery*, 2rd edn (Ed. D.H. Slatter), W.B. Saunders, Philadelphia, pp. 2137–2166.

Bagley, R.S., Kornegay, J.N., Wheeler, S.J., Plummer, S.B. and Cauzinille, L. (1993b) Generalized tremors in Maltese terriers: clinical findings in 7 cases (1984–1990). *Journal of the American Animal Hospital Association* **29**: 141–145.

Bailey, C.S. and Higgins, R.J. (1986) Characteristics of cisternal cerebrospinal fluid associated with primary brain tumours in the dog: a retrospective study. *Journal of the American Veterinary Medical Association* **188**, 414–421.

Baker, J.L., Waters, D.J. and deLahunta, A. (1988) Tetanus in two cats. *Journal of the American Animal Hospital Association* **24**, 159–164.

Bracken, M.B., Shepard, M.J., Collins, W.F. *et al.* (1990) A randomized, controlled trial of methylprednisolone or naloxone in the treatment of acute spinal cord injury. *New England Journal of Medicine* **322**, 1405–1411.

Braund, K.G. (1987) Degenerative and developmental diseases. In: *Veterinary Neurology* (Ed J.E. Oliver, Jr, B.F. Hoerlein and I.B. Mayhew). W.B. Saunders, Philadelphia, p. 186.

Braund, K.G., Steiss, J.E., Amling K.A. *et al.* (1987a) Insulinoma and subclinical peripheral neuropathy in two dogs. *Journal of Veterinary Internal Medicine* **1**, 86–90.

Braund, K.G., McGuire, J.A., Amling, K.A. and Henderson, R.A. (1987b) Peripheral neuropathy associated with malignant neoplasms in dogs. *Veterinary Pathology* **24**, 16–21.

Brick, J.F., Gutrecht, J.A. and Ringle, R.A. (1989) Reflex epilepsy and nonketotic hyperglycemia in the elderly. *Neurology* **39**, 394–399.

Carpenter, J.L., King Jr, N.W. and Abrams, K.L. (1987)

Bilateral trigeminal nerve paralysis and Horner's syndrome associated with myelomonocytic neoplasia in a dog. *Journal of the American Veterinary Medical Association* **191**, 1594–1596.

Carrillo, J.M., Sarfaty, D. and Greenlee, P. (1986) Intracranial neoplasm and associated inflammatory response from the central nervous system. *Journal of the American Animal Hospital Association* **22**, 367–373

Chrisman, C.L. (1986) Neuroaxonal dystrophy and leukoencephalomyelopathy of Rottweiler dogs. In: *Current Veterinary Therapy*, 9th edn (Ed. R.W. Kirk). W.B. Saunders, Philadelphia, pp. 805–806.

Chrisman, C.L. (1990) Dancing Doberman disease: clinical finding and prognosis. *Progress in Veterinary Neurology* **1**, 83–90.

Clemmons, R.M. (1989) Degenerative myelopathy. In: *Current Veterinary Therapy*, 10th edn (Ed. R.W. Kirk). W.B. Saunders, Philadelphia, pp. 830–833.

Cordy, D.R. and Holliday, T.A. (1989) A necrotizing meningoencephalitis of pug dogs. *Veterinary Pathology* **26**, 191–194.

deLahunta, A. (1980) Comparative cerebellar disease in domestic animals. *The Compendium on Continuing Education* **2**, 8–19.

deLahunta, A. (1983) Small animal spinal cord disease. In: *Veterinary Neuroanatomy and Clinical Neurology*, 2nd edn, W.B. Saunders, Philadelphia, p. 189.

Dieringer, T.M. and Wolf, A.M. (1991) Esophageal hiatal hernia and megaesophagus complicating tetanus in two dogs. *Journal of the Veterinary Medical Association* **199**, 87–89.

Dimski, D.S. and Cook, J.R. (1990) Carmustine-induced partial remission of an astrocytoma in a dog. *Journal of the American Animal Hospital Association* **26**, 179–182.

Dow, S.W., LeCouteur, R.A., Fettman, M.J. and Spurgeon, T.L. (1987) Potassium depletion in cats: hypokalemic polymyopathy. *Journal of the American Veterinary Medical Association* **191**, 1563–1568.

Dow, S.W., LeCouteur, R.A., Poss, M.L. and Beadleston, D. (1989) Central nervous system toxicosis associated with metronidazole treatment of dogs: five cases (1984–1987). *Journal of the American Veterinary Medical Association* **3**, 365–368.

Duncan I.D. (1987) Abnormalities of myelination of the central nervous system associated with congenital tremor. *Journal of Veterinary Internal Medicine* **1**, 10–23.

Evans, R.E. (1989) Haematology, biochemistry, cerebrospinal fluid analysis and other clinicopathological investigations. In: *Manual of Small Animal Neurology* (Ed. S.J. Wheeler). BSAVA Publications, Cheltenham, pp. 49–62.

Farrow, B.R.H. (1986) Generalized tremor syndrome. In: *Current Veterinary Therapy*, 9th edn (edn. R.W. Kirk). W.B. Saunders, Philadelphia, pp. 800–801.

Ferrara, M.L. and Halnan, C.R.E. (1983) Congenital structural brain defects in the deaf dalmatian. *Veterinary Record* **112**, 344–346.

Fox, J.G., Averill, D.F., Hallett, M. and Schunk, K. (1984) Familial reflex myoclonus in Labrador retrievers. *American Journal of Veterinary Research* **45**, 2367–2376.

Fulton, L. (1991) The use of lomustine in the treatment of brain masses. *Proceedings Ninth Annual Veterinary Medical Forum*, pp. 827–828.

Gaschen, F.P., Uhl, E.W., Senior, D.F., Pearle, L.K. and Hoffman, E.P. (1991) Muscular dystrophy and dystrophin deficiency in two kittens. *Proceedings Ninth Annual Veterinary Medical Forum*, p. 892.

Gilmour, M.A., Morgan, R.V. and Moore, F.M. (1992) Masticatory myopathy in the dog: a retrospective study of 18 cases. *Journal of the American Animal Hospital Association* **28**, 300–306.

Greene, C.E., Cook, J.R. Jr and Mahaffey, E.A. (1985a) Clindamycin for treatment of toxoplasma polymyositis in a dog. *Journal of the American Veterinary Medical Association* **187**, 631–634.

Greene, C.E., Burgdorfer, W., Cavagnolo, R., Philip, R.N. and Peacock, M.G. (1985b) Rocky Mountain spotted fever in dogs and its differentiation from canine ehrlichiosis. *Journal of the American Veterinary Medical Association* **186**, 465–472.

Griffiths, I.R. and Duncan, I.D. (1979) Ischaemic neuromyopathy in cats. *Veterinary Record* **104**, 518–522.

Heidner, G.L., Kornegay, J.N., Page, R.L., Dodge, R.K. and Thrall, D.E. (1991) Analysis of survival in a retrospective study of 86 dogs with brain tumours. *Journal of Veterinary Internal Medicine* **5**, 219–226.

Holliday, T.A., Nelson, H.J. Williams, D.C. and Willits, N. (1992) Unilateral and bilateral brainstem auditory-evoked response abnormalities in 900 dalmatian dogs. *Journal of Veterinary Internal Medicine* **6**, 166–174.

Hopkins, A.L. and Wheeler, S.J. (1991) Subdural hematoma in a dog. *Veterinary Surgery* **20**, 413–417.

Hopkins, A.L., Howard, J.F., Wheeler, S.J. and Kornegay, J.N. (1993) Stimulated single fiber electromyography in normal dogs. *Journal of Small Animal Practice* **34**, 271–276.

Jaggy, A. and Oliver, J.E. (1990) Chlorpyrifos toxicosis in two cats. *Journal of Veterinary Internal Medicine* **4**, 135–139.

Jones, B.R., Johnstone, A.C., Cahill, J.I. and Hancock, W.S. (1986) Peripheral neuropathy in cats with inherited primary hyperchylomicronaemia. *Veterinary Record* **119**, 268–272.

Joseph, R.J., Greenlee P.G., Carrillo, J.M., Kay W.J. (1988a) Canine cerebovascular disease: clinical and pathological findings in 17 cases. *Journal of American Animal Hospital Association* **24**, 569–576.

Joseph, R.J., Carrillo, J.M. and Lennon, V.A. (1988b) Myasthenia gravis in the cat. *Journal of Veterinary Internal Medicine* **2**, 75–79.

Kornegay, J.N. (1986a) Discospondylitis. In: *Current Veterinary Therapy* IX, W.B. Saunders, Philadelphia, pp. 810–814.

Kornegay, J.N. (1986b) Cerebellar vermian hypoplasia in dogs. *Veterinary Pathology* **23**, 374–379.

Lappin, M.R., Greene, C.E., Prestwood, A.K., Dawe, D.L. and Tarleton, R.L. (1989) Diagnosis of recent *Toxoplasma gondii* infection in cats by use of an enzyme-linked immunosorbent assay for immunoglobulin M. *American Journal of Veterinary Research* **50**, 1580–1585.

Malik, R., Church, D.B., Maddison, J.E. and Farrow, B.R. (1989) Three cases of local tetanus. *Journal of Small Animal Practice* **30**, 469–473.

Mayhew, I.G. and Beal, C.R. (1980) Techniques of analysis of cerebrospinal fluid. *Veterinary Clinics of North America, Small Animal Practice* **10**, 155–176.

Meric S.M. (1988) Review: canine meningitis: a changing emphasis. *Journal of Veterinary Internal Medicine* **2**, 26–35.

Panciera, D.L., Baldwin, C.J. and Keene, B.W. (1988) Electrocardiographic abnormalities associated with tetanus in two dogs. *Journal of the Veterinary Medical Association* **192**, 225–227.

Pion, P.D. (1988) Feline aortic thromboemboli and the potential utility of thrombolytic therapy with tissue plasminogen activator. *Veterinary Clinics of North America: Small Animal Practice* **18**, 79–86.

Plummer, S.B., Wheeler, S.J., Thrall, D.E. and Kornegay, J.N. (1992) Computed tomography of primary inflammatory brain disorders in dogs and cats. *Veterinary Radiology and Ultrasound*, **33**, 307–312.

Presthus, J. and Tege Jr J. (1986) Peripheral neuropathy associated with lymphosarcoma in a dog. *Journal of Small Animal Practice* **27**, 463–469.

Sarfaty, D., Carillo, J.M. and Peterson M.E. (1988) Neurologic, endocrinologic and pathologic findings associated with large pituitary tumours in dogs: eight cases (1976–1984). *Journal of the American Veterinary Medical Association* **143**, 854–856.

Shahar, R., Rousseaux, C. and Steiss, J. (1985) Peripheral polyneuropathy in a dog with functional islet B-cell tumour and widespread metastasis. *Journal of the American Veterinary Medical Association* **187**, 175–177.

Sharp, N.J.H., Nash, A.S. and Griffiths, I.R. (1984) Feline dysautonomia (the Key–Gaskell syndrome): a clinical and pathological study of forty cases. *Journal of Small Animal Practice* **25**, 599–615.

Sharp, N.J.H., Wheeler, S.J. and Cofone, M. (1992) Radiological evaluation of 'Wobbler' syndrome–caudal cervical spondylomyelopathy. *Journal of Small Animal Practice* **33**, 491–499.

Shelton, G.D., Willard, M.D., Cardinette, G.H. and Lindstrom, J. (1990) Acquired myasthenia gravis, selective involvement of esophageal, pharyngeal, and facial muscles. *Journal of Veterinary Internal Medicine* **4**, 281–284.

Sisson, A.F., LeCouteur, R.A., Ingram, J.T., Park, R.D. and Child, G. (1992) Diagnosis of cauda equina abnormalities by using electromyography, discography, and epidurography in dogs. *Journal of Veterinary Internal Medicine* **6**, 253–263.

Sorjonen, D.C., Cox, N.R. and Swango, L.J. (1989) Electrophoretic determination of albumin and gamma globulin concentrations in cerebrospinal fluid of dogs with encephalomyelitis attributable to canine distemper virus infection: 13 cases (1980–1987). *Journal of the American Veterinary Medical Association* **195**, 977–980.

Steinberg, H.S., Troncoso, J.C., Cork, L.C. and Price, D.L. (1981) Clinical features of inherited cerebellar degeneration in Gordon Setters. *Journal of the American Veterinary Association* **179**, 886–890.

Strain, G.M., Kearney, M.T., Gignac, I.J. *et al.* (1992) Brainstem auditory-evoked potential assessment of congenital deafness in Dalmatians: associations with phenotypic markers. *Journal of Veterinary Internal Medicine* **6**, 175–182.

Thomas, W.B., Sorjonen, D.C. and Simpson, S.T. (1991) Surgical management of atlantoaxial subluxation in 23 dogs. *Veterinary Surgery* **20**, 409–412.

Thomson, C.E., Kornegay, J.N. and Stevens, J.B. (1990) Analysis of cerebrospinal fluid from the cerebellomedullary and lumbar cisterns of dogs with focal neurologic disease: 145 cases (1985–1987). *Journal of the American Veterinary Medical Association* **196**, 1841–1844.

Turrel, J.M., Fike, J.R., LeCouteur, R.A. and Higgins, R.J. (1986) Computed tomographic characteristics of primary brain tumours in 50 dogs. *Journal of the American Veterinary Medical Association* **188**, 851–856.

Vicini, D.S., Wheaton, L.G., Zachary, J.F. and Parker, A.J. (1988) Peripheral nerve biopsy for diagnosis of globoid cell leukodystrophy in a dog. *Journal of the American Veterinary Medical Association* **192**, 1087–1090.

Wheeler, S.J., Wright, J.A. and Clayton Jones, D.G. (1986) The diagnosis of brachial plexus disorders in dogs: a review of twenty two cases. *Journal of Small Animal Practice* **27**, 147–152.

Wheeler, S.J. and Sharp, N.J.H. (1994) *Small Animal Spinal Disorders: Diagnosis and Surgery*, Mosby-Wolfe.

Wilson, J.B. and Stevens, J.B. (1977) Effects of blood contamination on cerebrospinal fluid analysis. *Journal of the American Veterinary Medical Association* **171**, 256–258.

Wise, L.A. and Lappin, M.R. (1991) A syndrome resembling feline dysautonomia (Key–Gaskell syndrome) in a dog. *Journal of the American Veterinary Medical Association* **198**, 2103–2106.

FURTHER READING

Braund, K.G. (1994) *Clinical Syndromes in Veterinary Neurology*, 2nd edn, Mosby-Wolfe.

deLahunta, A. (1983) *Veterinary Neuroanatomy and*

Clinical Neurology, 2nd edn. W.B. Saunders, Philadelphia.

Oliver, J.E., Hoerlein, B.F. and Mayhew, I.G. (1987) *Veterinary Neurology*. W.B. Saunders, Philadelphia.

Oliver, J.E. Jr and Lorenz, M.D. (1993) *Handbook of Veterinary Neurologic Diagnosis*, 2nd edn. W.B. Saunders, Philadelphia.

Wheeler, S.J. (1989) *Manual of Small Annual Neurology*. British Small Animal Veterinary Association Publications, Cheltenham, UK.

Wheeler, S.J. and Sharp, N.J.H. (1994) *Small Animal Spinal Disorders: Diagnosis and Surgery*. Mosby-Wolfe

43

Muscle Diseases of the Dog and Cat

R. E. McKerrell

Introduction	695	Non-inherited congenital muscle diseases of the dog	704
History taking	696	Acquired muscle diseases of the dog	704
Physical examination	696	Inherited/congenital muscle diseases of the cat	710
Investigative techniques	697	Acquired muscle diseases in the cat	712
Inherited muscle diseases of the dog	698		

INTRODUCTION

In 1958 Meier wrote in a review that 'although primary diseases of striated muscle have frequently been described in man, reference to spontaneous myopathies in animals especially the dog is rare.' By 1986 Duncan and Griffiths were able to include more than 20 canine myopathies in a chapter on neuromuscular disorders of the dog and cat, and there are now sufficient muscle conditions documented to warrant a separate chapter in this volume. The increase in the number of muscle diseases now recognized is attributable, at least in part, to advances in methods of investigation and the increasing adoption by veterinary specialists of techniques such as muscle biopsy and electromyography which are described below.

Anatomy and physiology

Muscle tissue is responsible for movement and may be divided into skeletal, smooth and cardiac. This chapter is concerned with diseases affecting skeletal or voluntary muscle although cardiac muscle is involved in some conditions. Smooth or involuntary muscle is rarely involved in myopathies in animals and will not be considered further.

Skeletal muscle is under voluntary control and is composed of striated muscle fibres. These fibres are multinucleate cells formed in development by the fusion of many myogenic precursors. A single muscle fibre may be from a few millimetres to 10 cm in length and have a diameter of 10–100 μm. In normal mature muscle the many nuclei are arranged beneath the outer cell membrane (sarcolemma) but in immature or regenerating muscle, and in some disease states, centrally placed nuclei may be present. Skeletal muscle is known as striated muscle since when examined using light microscopy the fibres are observed to have transverse striations. The muscle fibres are composed of myofibrils, which in turn are made up of myofilaments formed primarily of the proteins actin and myosin. It is as a result of the thin filaments of actin sliding between the thick myosin filaments that muscle contraction occurs.

It was realized early in the study of muscle that muscle fibres are not uniform. Initially two types were identified and these were referred to as red and white or fast and slow twitch fibres. It is now recognized that the situation is far more complex than this and many classification systems have been attempted on the basis of anatomical appearance, physiological behaviour, biochemical and histochemical features. However, for practical purposes a system based on staining using the myosin ATPase reaction provides a useful classification in humans and animals. Using this reaction two types of fibre can be identified. These are designated type 1 and type 2 fibres, and the type 2 fibres are then further subdivided on the basis of histochemical and biochemical characteristics.

The 'type' of a muscle fibre is determined by the motor neurone which innervates it. Each motor neurone provides innervation to many muscle fibres, and this ventral horn cell together with all the muscle fibres it supplies is known as a 'motor unit'. The fibres innervated by each ventral horn cell are not, as might be expected, grouped together within the normal muscle but are randomly distributed so that when stains showing the different fibre types are used, a random mosaic of fibres is seen.

Reaction of muscle to injury

A muscle fibre will atrophy if it is denervated. If reinnervation does not occur atrophy progresses and there is an increase in the connective tissue component, until eventually the muscle is completely replaced by fibrous tissue. When muscle fibres are damaged they can undergo repair providing some sarcolemmal tubes remain intact, but if the damage is very severe regeneration may not be possible. In this situation there is loss of muscle fibres and a proliferation of connective tissue resulting, once again, in the production of a fibrosed 'endstage' muscle.

HISTORY TAKING

The history is taken as described in Chapter 1 but in cases of suspected muscle disease the following points should be considered.

It is always important to ascertain when the onset of signs occurred. Since a number of muscle diseases are inherited or congenital it is useful to know whether any littermates are similarly affected and, if so, how many and of which sex. In adults it should be established whether the onset was sudden or insidious and whether the condition has deteriorated, remained stable or improved.

Vaccination status may be of importance since, for example, cases of toxoplasmosis are sometimes seen in association with canine distemper. Previous illnesses which seem irrelevant to the owner may also be of interest. An illustration of this is seen in acquired myasthenia gravis, signs of which may be preceded by a non-specific febrile episode.

Exercise tolerance should be investigated as part of the physical examination but in the artificial environment of the clinic it may be difficult to reproduce the abnormalities which characterize the problem at home. Careful history taking can elicit useful details from the owner regarding the willingness and ability of the dog to exercise and of factors which either improve or worsen the condition.

Questioning the owner about the patient's appetite also provides useful information. The owner may report that the dog eats well but fails to thrive or observe that although the dog appears to be hungry it has difficulty eating. This is particularly relevant as dysphagia is a feature of several muscle diseases. Cases of Labrador retriever myopathy and glycogen storage disease type II often lie down to eat. This observation may seem trivial but can provide another piece to fit into the clinical jigsaw.

It is important to ask whether the dog ever regurgitates or coughs since megaoesophagus is a common feature of muscle disease in the dog. It occurs due to the high proportion of striated muscle present throughout the length of the oesophagus in this species and can result in serious complications such as inhalation pneumonia.

Intermittent neurological signs such as collapse or fits may not be observed at the time of the clinical examination. By questioning the owner it may be possible to establish a history of central nervous system involvement, thus eliminating exclusively myopathic disorders from those, such as toxoplasmosis, which can affect both the nervous system and muscle.

In cases which collapse it is necessary to find out what else happens. Is the dog cyanosed? Is there loss of consciousness? Do any external factors govern whether and when the collapse occurs? The dog may resolutely refuse to collapse during the course of the investigation, so a detailed description from the owner is essential.

PHYSICAL EXAMINATION

Detailed clinical examination includes a full physical examination of the patient as outlined in Chapter 1, and since many muscle disorders present as abnormalities of gait, reduced exercise tolerance or possibly collapse, orthopaedic, metabolic and cardiac conditions must be ruled out.

A full neurological examination should be carried out in any case of suspected muscle disease, not only because some conditions affect both nervous tissue and muscle but also because many of the procedures highlight abnormalities pertinent to muscle disease. The so-called wheelbarrow test is a good way of showing up forelimb weakness, likewise postural tests such as hemiwalking, hopping and stepping can help to localize weakness in individual limbs.

The skeletal muscles themselves should be examined with particular care. Is there evidence of atrophy or hypertrophy? If so, is it localized or generalized? Are there discrete swellings within the muscle? Are the abnormalities symmetrical? The tone of the muscles should be assessed by passively manipulating the joints. Joints are lax in conditions where muscle tone is reduced. Conversely there will be reduction in joint movement where muscles are fibrosed or contractures have formed.

Palpation of the muscles may reveal them to be unusually swollen and firm and there may be evidence of muscle pain. In myotonia sharp percussion of the muscle belly produces a myotonic dimple. This is a simple but informative test which should be carried out on any case showing stiffness and hypertrophy.

Cases of muscle disease frequently show abnormalities of gait and/or exercise intolerance and must therefore be examined at exercise as well as at rest. Many dogs with myopathic disease have a stiff, stilted gait. This does not necessarily indicate stiffness of the joints or increased tone in the limbs, but is often noted in conditions characterized by weakness.

In cases with marked exercise intolerance a Camsilon test should be carried out as described below.

INVESTIGATIVE TECHNIQUES

Camsilon test

This is the diagnostic test for myasthenia gravis, a condition of the neuromuscular junction in which fatigue which improves after rest is the characteristic clinical feature. Camsilon (edrophonium chloride), is an ultrashort-acting anticholinesterase drug which effectively increases the amount of acetylcholine available at the neuromuscular junction. For the test a dose of 0.1–1.0 mg of Camsilon is given by slow or incremental intravenous injection. There is no precise dose per kilogram but a useful guide is to use 0.1 mg for a small breed of dog such as a Jack Russell terrier up to a total dose of 1 mg for a large breed such as a German shepherd. Since the available preparation is designed for use in humans it may be necessary to dilute the drug in saline to facilitate administration of low doses. Myasthenic patients show a dramatic improvement on administration of Camsilon which lasts for several minutes. Normal animals sometimes fasciculate and occasionally stop breathing. It is, therefore, advisable to have oxygen available although the ultra-short duration of this preparation means that the effect is short lived.

Serum enzymes

Serum creatine kinase (CK) is the most specific marker of muscle damage. Other enzymes are also raised in muscle disease but CK gives the best indication of the amount of muscle damage occurring at any particular time.

There are some potential pitfalls in the interpretation of CK levels which should be noted. CK can be raised after intramuscular injections, exercise and recumbency and there is a transient rise in CK after electromyography.

Since the CK is highest in myopathies where there is a large amount of muscle fibre destruction, the most dramatic elevations in CK are seen in myopathies characterized by massive necrosis, such as muscular dystrophy in the Golden retriever. It is equally important to stress that in low-grade, focal or chronic myopathies the amount of cell destruction occurring at any one time may be quite low and in these cases the CK may only be slightly raised or may indeed be normal. A normal CK level does not itself rule out the presence of myopathy.

Muscle biopsy

Muscle biopsy is a technique which can readily be performed in veterinary practice, using specially designed biopsy needles or open surgery. When selecting which muscle to biopsy it is important to choose a muscle which is involved in the disease process but to avoid areas where the disease is so far advanced that all the muscle has been replaced by fibrous tissue. If in doubt several biopsies should be taken from a range of different muscles. Orientation of the specimen is of great importance to the muscle pathologist due to the highly organized nature of muscle tissue. The rectangular specimen should be oriented so that the fibres run parallel to the long side. To avoid twisting or folding it should be pinned at resting length onto blocks of wax, or laid on a piece of card for a few minutes before fixation in a solution of, for example, 10% buffered formalin. Once the specimen has been fixed and embedded in paraffin it is stained. Specimens produced in this way are perfectly adequate for diagnosis of conditions such as toxoplasmosis or polymyositis. However, with the advent of frozen sections and histochemical staining it has become possible to reveal far more of the cellular detail of the muscle and to examine the proportions of each fibre type. In order to make the most of these techniques correct processing is essential. Samples for fibre typing are snap frozen in liquid nitrogen and must then remain at low temperatures throughout processing. For this reason, biopsies which require histochemical staining are generally taken at referral centres.

Electromyography

Electromyography (EMG) is used to examine the electrical activity within muscle by inserting needle electrodes into the muscle mass. The procedure requires specialist equipment comprising an oscilloscope, amplifiers, recording and reference electrodes.

Normal, relaxed, skeletal muscle is electrically silent but in some disease states so-called spontaneous activity is present. This can be recorded even when the patient is under general anaesthetic and is an indication of abnormality. Spontaneous activity takes the form of fibrillation potentials, positive sharp waves and bizarre high frequency discharges.

About a week after denervation fibrillation potentials are seen on the electromyogram. These are small biphasic potentials 20–300 µV in amplitude which are thought to arise from individual muscle fibres twitching when released from the control of the nerve. Positive sharp waves consist of an initial positive deflection followed by a slower negative potential. In the dog positive sharp waves have an amplitude similar to that of fibrillation potentials but are of longer duration. They often accompany fibrillation potentials in denervation. Both fibrillation potentials and positive sharp waves may also be present in myopathic disease.

Bizarre high frequency discharges are also known as complex repetitive discharges (CRDs). Myotonic discharges are a specific form of high frequency repetitive discharge which wax and wane in frequency and amplitude and give rise to a sound like a revving motor bike when played through the loudspeaker of the EMG machine. True myotonic discharges are diagnostic of myotonia. Whereas myotonic discharges wax and wane other forms of CRD may have an abrupt onset and ending. These 'pseudomyotonic' discharges are seen in a wide range of muscle diseases in the dog.

INHERITED MUSCLE DISEASES OF THE DOG (Table 43.1)

Canine muscular dystrophy

One of the most dramatic inherited muscle diseases to be described in the dog is a sex-linked, degenerative myopathy affecting golden retrievers which has been reported in the United States of America (Meier, 1958; Kornegay, 1984; Valentine et al., 1986). This condition has been studied closely and is now considered to be analogous to Duchenne muscular dystrophy of humans. The onset of clinical signs occurs by 6 to 8 weeks although examination of muscle from neonates has shown that pathological changes may be present from birth. Affected puppies are all males. They tire quickly and develop an abnormal shuffling gait, characterized by short stiff strides. They may show reduced ability to open

Table 43.1 Congenital muscle diseases of the dog

Inherited/familial	
Muscular dystrophy	Golden retriever
	Irish terrier
Labrador retriever myopathy	Labrador retriever
Myotonia	Chow Chow
	Staffordshire terrier
Mitochondrial myopathy	Clumber spaniel
	Sussex spaniel
	?Old English sheepdog
Myasthenia gravis	Jack Russell terrier
	Springer spaniel
	Smooth Haired Fox terrier
Glycogen storage disease type II	Lapland dog
Glycogen storage disease type III	German shepherd
Familial dermatomyositis	Collie
	Shetland sheepdog
Malignant hyperthermia	
Myopathy associated with 'falling cavaliers'	Cavalier King Charles spaniel
Central core myopathy	Great Dane
Hypotrophic myopathy	German shepherd dog
??Cramp	Norwich terriers
??Steroid responsive polymyositis	German pointer
Non-inherited	
'Swimmer' puppies	
Congenital quadriceps contracture	
Nutritional myopathy	
Congenital protozoal myositis	

the jaws and difficulty prehending and swallowing food. The condition progresses gradually and there is considerable variation in the severity of the clinical signs. Most skeletal muscles are atrophic but hypertrophy has been observed in some muscle groups and in the tongue. Gross hypertrophy of the tongue has been reported as early as 10 days of age resulting in inability to feed and respiratory difficulties (Meier, 1958). Affected dogs show no neurological deficits and spinal reflexes are normal. Cardiac involvement resulting in congestive heart failure has occurred.

An important diagnostic feature of canine muscular dystrophy is the massive elevation of serum CK. Values greater than 15 000 iu l^{-1} have been reported (reference range up to 300 iu l^{-1}) and clinically normal female carriers may also show an elevated CK. At electromyography positive sharp waves and bizarre high frequency discharges (pseudomyotonic) are recorded.

Histology of affected muscles shows fibre size variation, large rounded hyaline fibres, prominent necrosis, phagocytosis and mineralization together with some evidence of regeneration (Valentine et al., 1986). Many of the features of this condition are identical to those of the X-linked degenerative myopathy described in a litter of Irish terrier puppies (Wentink et al., 1972). Clinical signs included dysphagia, difficulty walking, lumbar kyphosis, hypertrophy of the base of the tongue, marked stiffness of skeletal muscles and dramatically elevated levels of serum CK. No further cases of Irish terrier myopathy have been reported but it seems certain that the condition is identical to the golden retriever myopathy and should therefore be classified as an example of canine muscular dystrophy. X-linked muscular dystrophy has also been observed in the samoyed, rottweiler and Belgian shepherd (Kornegay, 1992).

Breeding studies carried out on the golden retrievers suggest that the mode of inheritance is as an X-linked recessive trait. The clinical signs and muscle pathology observed in these dogs are very similar to those seen in the Duchenne form of muscular dystrophy of man, and the demonstration that the muscle protein 'dystrophin' is absent from muscles of affected animals (Cooper et al., 1988), confirmed that this example of canine muscular dystrophy is analogous to Duchenne muscular dystrophy.

The definition of the term muscular dystrophy gave rise to some confusion within the medical literature for many years and, in the veterinary field, the situation is further complicated by the fact that nutritional myodegeneration of farm animals has frequently been alluded to as 'muscular dystrophy' (Blood et al., 1983). It has been suggested that in humans the term 'muscular dystrophy' should be reserved for cases of 'progressive, genetically determined, primary degenerative myopathy' (Walton and Gardner-Medwin 1981) and it would seem desirable to adopt a similar definition in veterinary medicine.

Other cases of so-called muscular dystrophy have been reported in dogs (Innes, 1951; Whitney, 1958; Funkquist et al., 1980), but if the definition stated above is critically applied some of these examples do not fulfil the criteria.

Persistent atrial standstill has been described in the springer spaniel, in association with a facioscapulohumeral type of dystrophy (Bonagura and O'Grady, 1983), and three related English springer spaniels with a polysystemic disorder characterized by dyserythropoiesis, myopathy and cardiac disease have also been reported (Holland et al., 1991). A single litter of Old English sheepdog puppies showed a progressive disease which it was suggested might be a form of canine muscular dystrophy (Chrisman, 1982). In the Bouvier des Flandres a primary myopathy has been found to underly the swallowing difficulties described in 24 dogs (Peeters et al., 1991). The authors considered that this condition resembles oculopharyngeal muscular dystrophy of humans. The affected dogs showed no generalized weakness and no abnormalities were found in the muscles of the limbs suggesting that this is not the same condition as the degenerative polymyopathy previously described in four related Bouvier des Flandres dogs (Braund et al., 1990). The animals described in this report were all females. Two of the cases presented with generalized limb weakness and megaoesophagus, the other two were clinically normal.

Labrador retriever myopathy

This disease was first described in the United States (Kramer et al., 1976) and is widespread throughout the United Kingdom. The condition has been referred to as type 2 muscle fibre deficiency, generalized muscle weakness, myotonia, muscular dystrophy and Labrador retriever myopathy. The most common reason for presentation is apparent exercise intolerance with or without collapse. However some pups are presented as orthopaedic cases due to abnormalities of gait or as cases of lethargy. The age at which affected animals are presented also varies. Onset of signs usually occurs between 8 and 12 weeks of age although some dogs may appear to be normal until approximately 6 months (McKerrell and Braund, 1987). When exercised, the puppies move with a stiff, stilted gait and an arched back (Fig. 43.1). The head carriage is often low with the neck greatly flexed and many of the pups show abnormal joint posture such as overextended carpi, carpal valgus, overflexed hocks or 'cow hocks'. Exercise tolerance is reduced and as the puppies become tired the stride shortens and the head is lowered until the dog pitches forward onto its nose in a manner reminiscent of myasthenia gravis. However, in these cases there is no improvement following administration of Camsilon (see Camsilon test). There is no loss of consciousness during collapse and after a period of rest the puppy is usually able to resume exercise. Some older animals appear to regulate their exercise and rather than collapse merely sit down and obstinately refuse to move.

There is generalized atrophy of skeletal muscle which is often most noticeable over the temporal region and in the proximal forelimb. Muscle tone is reduced and postural testing reveals marked limb weakness. Affected puppies often cannot support the weight on the forelimbs in the wheelbarrow test and may be unable to perform hemiwalking or hopping and stepping tests. It is an interesting feature of these cases that the tail is always strong and wags normally! Neurological examination should be carried out since in all cases the patellar and triceps reflexes are reduced or absent. No other neurological abnormalities are present although megaoesophagus has developed in a few cases. Routine biochemical and haematological examination is of little use in diagnosis. CK levels may be slightly elevated but are more usually within the normal range. Electromyography can be an aid to confirming the diagnosis. Fibrillation potentials and positive sharp waves are generally present, particularly in younger animals whereas in older dogs bizarre high frequency discharges (pseudomyotonic) are commonly found throughout the skeletal muscles (Moore et al., 1987; McKerrell, 1989). The most reliable way of confirming the diagnosis is by muscle biopsy. The pathological changes present in the muscle are very variable including changes classically regarded as indicative of mild denervation but also those suggestive of myopathy (McKerrell and Braund, 1986). Myopathic changes include splitting of fibres, some necrosis and in some muscles, very large increases in the numbers of internal nuclei. Histochemistry reveals a deficiency of type 2 fibres in some muscles.

Although young puppies can be quite severely disabled the condition generally stabilizes by approximately one year of age. The dogs still have a reduced exercise tolerance and severe muscle atrophy but can often make good pets. Owners should be warned that exacerbations occasionally occur if affected animals are exposed to stress, particularly severe cold, and many dogs continue

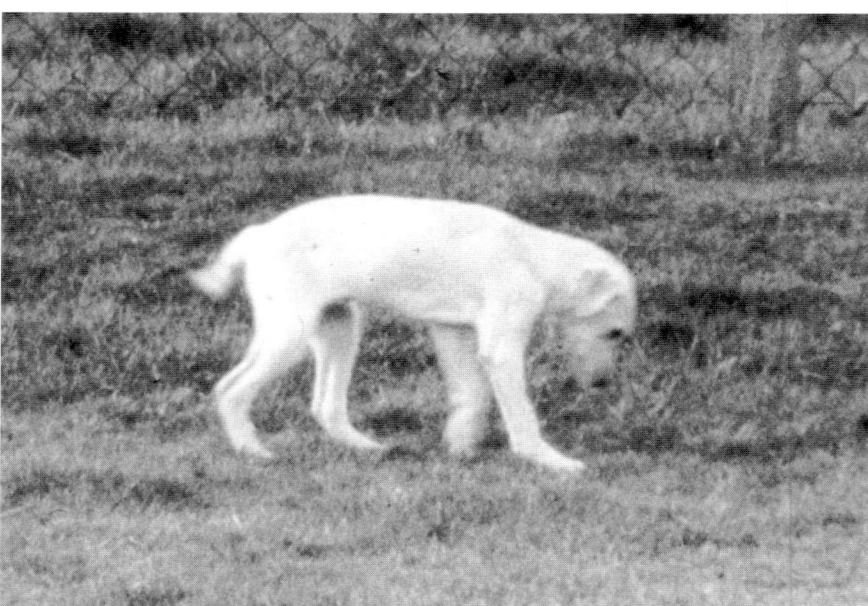

Figure 43.1 Labrador retriever myopathy in puppy showing abnormal posture with an arched back and low head carriage. From McKerrell and Braund (1987).

to suffer transient episodes of weakness when upset or excited. The condition is seen in Labrador retrievers of black and yellow coat colour and affects both sexes equally. In the UK the majority of cases have occurred in dogs from working strains although a few cases have been seen in show animals. Since the condition is inherited via an autosomal recessive trait (Kramer et al., 1981) both parents of an affected puppy are obligate carriers, although they will appear clinically normal. Furthermore, half of the litter are likely to be carriers of the affected gene. Thus the advice to breeders must be to avoid breeding from the parents or siblings of affected animals. There is no treatment for this condition although anecdotal evidence suggests that anabolic steroids may be of some use in preventing further muscle loss.

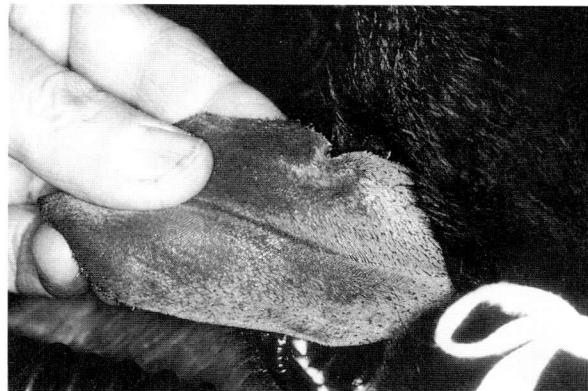

Figure 43.2 Canine myotonia in a 4-month-old chow chow. A myotonic dimple has been elicited by percussing the edge of the tongue in the anaesthetized patient. Photograph courtesy of Michael Herrtage.

■ Canine myotonia

Myotonia is characterized by the delayed relaxation of skeletal muscle following voluntary contraction or stimulation, and has been described in chow chows in Great Britain (Griffiths and Duncan, 1973), Australia (Farrow and Malik, 1981), New Zealand (Jones et al., 1978), Holland (Wentink et al., 1974) and the United States (Shores et al., 1986). Canine myotonia has also been seen in the Staffordshire terrier in the United States (Shires et al., 1983). Signs of myotonia are first seen when the puppies begin to walk. Affected dogs have difficulty in rising and stiffness of all four limbs which improves with exercise. The gait is waddling and the dog may 'bunny-hop'. In some cases the generalized muscle spasm is so severe that the dog falls over and remains in lateral recumbency for up to 30 s. The skeletal muscles are often greatly hypertrophied and percussion of these (or the tongue in the anaesthetized patient) results in the production of a myotonic dimple (Fig. 43.2). Characteristic myotonic discharges are recorded at electromyography. These high frequency discharges wax and wane in both frequency and amplitude, giving rise to the so-called 'dive bomber' sound when played through the amplifier. The pathological changes observed in the muscle are generally non-specific.

In both the chow chow and the Staffordshire terrier, the condition appears to be familial but the mode of inheritance has not been demonstrated. The chow was originally bred for meat and over the years a highly muscled appearance has been considered desirable in both breeds. It is interesting to speculate that this may have inadvertently resulted in selection for this disorder.

Treatment of canine myotonia has been attempted with some success using membrane stabilizers such as procainamide at a dose of 500 mg orally every 6 h (Farrow and Malik, 1981).

Occasional cases of myotonia-like conditions associated with myopathies have been reported in various other breeds, including the cavalier King Charles spaniel (Jones and Johnstone, 1982), Rhodesian ridgeback (Simpson and Braund, 1985), and Great Dane (Honhold and Smith, 1986). Myotonia is also seen in association with canine hyperadrenocorticism (Duncan et al., 1977), and transient myotonia occurred in dogs given oral doses of the herbicide 2,4-dichlorophenoxyacetic acid (Steiss et al., 1987).

The myopathies affecting the golden retriever, Irish terrier and Labrador retriever have been misleadingly referred to as myotonia or myotonic myopathies in the literature since in all cases bizarre high frequency discharges (pseudomyotonic) were recorded at electromyography. However, they do not show the classical signs of congenital myotonia and should not be confused with the well-recognized forms of the condition described above.

■ Mitochondrial myopathies

A condition has been described in the Clumber spaniel in which the primary abnormality was shown to be a defect in mitochondrial function (Herrtage and Houlton, 1979). These dogs were eager to exercise and appeared clinically normal when examined at rest. When exercised the gait was normal but exercise tolerance was dramatically reduced. After approximately 100 m affected puppies sank into sternal recumbency and refused to move. Excessive panting and tachycardia were observed and arterial blood samples confirmed that this was due to severe acidosis. After 10–15 min the dogs were able to rise but remained depressed for up to an hour after the collapse. The exercise-induced acidosis was found to be due to dramatic increases in both lactate and pyruvate. Light microscopic examination of muscle biopsies showed prominent lipid droplets in type 1 fibres, and at electron microscopy large lipid droplets were seen between the fibrils (Anderson, 1985). Although mitochondria were normal in appearance biochemical analysis of muscle showed that the defect lay in the mitochondria, which were unable to oxidize pyruvate due to a defect in the pyruvate dehydrogenase complex.

The condition was subsequently recognized in the Sussex spaniel, a breed closely related to the clumber (Houlton and Herrtage, 1980). Care should be taken when investigating such a case since exercise in an affected animal can result in sudden death, and is a possible explanation for the occasional anecdotal reports of 'heart attacks' in young dogs of these breeds.

Episodic weakness associated with exertional lactic acidosis and myopathy has also been described in two Old English sheepdog littermates. The condition was considered likely to be a mitochondrial myopathy but biochemical characterization of the defect was not carried out (Breitschwerdt et al., 1992).

A single case of a myopathy, in which bar-like inclusions were found in the mitochondria, was reported in a West Highland white terrier (Bradley et al., 1988).

Congenital myasthenia gravis

Congenital myasthenia gravis is an inherited disease seen in the Jack Russell terrier (Palmer and Goodyear, 1978), springer spaniel (Johnson et al., 1975) and the smooth haired fox terrier (Miller et al., 1983), and is inherited as an autosomal recessive trait (Wallace and Palmer, 1984). Puppies show signs of weakness from 6–8 weeks of age. They have difficulty standing or raising their heads and are often dysphagic. Diagnosis of this condition may be suspected from the clinical signs and is confirmed by the response to the Camsilon test (see p. 697). Treatment consists of the anticholinesterase pyridostigmine bromide at a dose of approximately 0.5–3.0 mg a day, and is best administered orally in the form of a syrup diluted in water.

Congenital myasthenia gravis is a condition of the neuromuscular junction but in contrast to acquired myasthenia gravis (qv), there are no circulating antibodies to acetylcholine receptors in this form of the disease. The condition appears to be due to a reduced number of acetylcholine receptors present in the postsynaptic membrane (Oda et al., 1984), and morphometric examination of the ultrastructure of the end-plate regions has demonstrated some alterations in the membrane folding pattern in affected animals (Wilkes et al., 1987).

A recessively inherited disorder of neuromuscular transmission has also been described in a Danish breed, the Gamel Dansk Honsehund (Trojaberg and Flagstad, 1982). Signs included weakness on exercise and electrophysiological responses similar to those seen in myasthenia gravis but there was no improvement on administration of edrophonium chloride. It is not clear whether the failure of neuromuscular transmission in this condition was pre- or postsynaptic but treatment with guanidine hydrochloride resulted in improved muscular function (Flagstad et al., 1986). Since guanidine is known to increase the number of quanta of acetylcholine released by a single nerve impulse, the response to guanidine may suggest the presence of a presynaptic defect in this breed.

Glycogen storage diseases

The glycogen storage diseases comprise a group of inherited disorders of carbohydrate metabolism which result in accumulation of glycogen and in which a predominant sign is muscle weakness. Two glycogen storage diseases analogous to those previously described in humans have been documented in the dog.

Glycogen storage disease type II (Pompe's disease)

A condition similar to glycogen storage disease type II (Pompe's disease) was described in four related Lapland dogs (Walvoort et al., 1984). Affected dogs showed no clinical signs in the first 6 months of life but gradually became weak and reluctant to exercise. Several of the dogs lay down to eat and were noticed to tire easily. Frequent vomiting and dysphagia were observed and megaoesophagus was found to be present. Electrocardiography revealed the presence of cardiac abnormalities and at electromyography bizarre high frequency discharges were recorded, particularly from the paraspinal and proximal limb muscles. Occasional fibrillation potentials and positive sharp waves were also present in some muscles. The prognosis of the disease is poor and death occurred by 18 months of age in all four cases.

Histology of various organs showed that cardiac and smooth muscle were among the tissues most severely affected. The altered cells contained accumulations of glycogen and an increase in acid phosphatase activity. In glycogen storage disease type II of man the enzyme deficiency is of acid maltase (alpha glucosidase deficiency) and it has been shown that in affected dogs the activity of this enzyme is greatly reduced.

Glycogen storage disease type III (Cori's disease)

Glycogen storage disease type III (Cori's) disease has been seen in German shepherd dogs where so far it has only been reported in females. Clinical signs are first observed at two months of age and include muscular weakness and apparent 'dizziness'. The dogs may appear undernourished and poorly grown and show signs of liver disease characterized by gross hepatomegaly and ascites (Rafiquzzaman et al., 1976). The defect in this disease is of the debranching enzyme, amylo-1, 6-glucosidase (Ceh et al., 1976). Histology reveals abnormally high levels of glycogen in hepatocytes, nerve cells and in the muscle fibres of skeletal, smooth and cardiac muscle. The disease is rare and the prognosis is poor with death occurring by 15 months of age.

Familial dermatomyositis

This condition is thought to be inherited as an autosomal dominant trait in collies and Shetland sheepdogs (Haupt et al., 1985a). Affected dogs develop lesions involving the skin of the head, feet and overlying joints. Severely affected animals may show generalized muscle atrophy, although weakness is not always obvious. Fibrillation potentials, positive sharp waves and bizarre high frequency discharges are present at electromyography. Muscle biopsies are characterized by the presence of atrophy, degeneration and regeneration of muscle fibres together with inflammatory cell infiltrates. There is no elevation of serum enzymes but high levels of circulating immune complexes have been found in affected dogs (Haupt et al., 1985b). Immunosuppressive doses of prednisolone and oral vitamin E have been used to treat the signs attributable to the myopathy.

Malignant hyperthermia

Malignant hyperthermia is a hypermetabolic disorder of skeletal muscle first described in humans (Denborough and Lovell, 1960), which has since been recognized in a number of species including the pig, dog, cat, horse and wild animals at capture. In humans and the pig, malignant hyperthermia has an inherited component and a colony of dogs with increased susceptibility to malignant hyperthermia has been described (O'Brien et al., 1983). This condition is further discussed in the section on acquired conditions.

Myopathy associated with 'falling cavaliers'

Episodic falling in the cavalier King Charles spaniel is characterized by intermittent collapse, often precipitated by exercise or excitement. In the two animals in which a post mortem was carried out, no abnormalities were found in any of the tissues examined (Herrtage and Palmer, 1983).

Ultrastructural changes have since been reported in the muscles of affected dogs including hydropic degeneration of mitochondria, dilatation of the sarcoplasmic reticulum and tubular proliferation in the vicinity of the triads (Wright et al., 1987). However, the authors acknowledged that such changes are non-specific and that the underlying cause of the disease remains obscure.

Central core myopathy

A myopathy has been reported in two Great Danes, in which the characteristic histological feature of the condition was the presence of central cores in many fibres (Newsholme and Gaskell, 1987; Targett et al., 1994). Both dogs were young adults which presented with signs of muscle weakness and exercise intolerance. In both cases clinical signs were progressive and severe, necessitating euthanasia at 15 and 18 months of age, respectively.

Hypotrophy of the pectineus muscle

A developmental myopathy of the pectineus muscle characterized by hypotrophy of type 2 fibres was described in a number of German shepherd dogs (Cardinet et al., 1969). The possibility that there could be an association between the muscle abnormality and the development of hip dysplasia was examined but failed to confirm any relationship between the conditions (Lust et al., 1972).

Cramp in Norwich terriers

For some years a condition has been recognized in Norwich terriers in which a 'spasm' of the hindquarters lasting approximately 5 min occurs during or after exercise. It has been suggested that dietary supplementation with selenium or seaweed may reduce its incidence (Furber, 1984), but the disease has not been documented in any detail. It is not clear if an inherited component is involved or whether it is an example of an acquired nutritional myopathy.

Polymyositis

A steroid-responsive polymyositis has been reported in two German pointer puppies (Presthus and Lindboe, 1988).

NON-INHERITED CONGENITAL MUSCLE DISEASES OF THE DOG (Table 43.1)

Swimmer puppies

'Swimmer puppies' are known to occur in several breeds. Affected puppies are unable to stand and the limbs are abducted. If allowed to remain in sternal recumbency, flattening of the sternum develops but if the limbs are bound together in an adducted position, or in flexion, the puppies recover (McKeown and Archibald, 1979).

Congenital contractures

Vaughan described congenital contracture of the quadriceps muscle in two 8-week-old Labrador retriever puppies and suggested that this might be a form of localized arthrogryposis (Vaughan, 1979).

Nutritional myopathies

Nutritional myopathies have been produced experimentally in puppies by feeding them diets known to be deficient in vitamin E and selenium (Van Vleet, 1975). Naturally occurring cases of congenital nutritional myopathy have also been reported in puppies (Manktelow, 1963; Kaspar and Lombard, 1963).

Congenital protozoal myositis

See acquired conditions.

ACQUIRED MUSCLE DISEASES OF THE DOG (Table 43.2)

Inflammatory

The inflammatory myositides are among the most common muscle diseases of the dog and may be

Table 43.2 Acquired muscle diseases of the dog

Inflammatory		
	Infectious	*Toxoplasma* myopathy
		Neospora myopathy
		Microfilaria
		Trichinella
		Leptospirosis
		Clostridia
	Immune mediated	Idiopathic myositis of masticatory muscles
		Polymyositis
		Myasthenia gravis
Endocrine		Hypothyroidism
		Hyperadrenocorticism
Metabolic		Hyperkalaemia (periodic paralysis)
		Hypokalaemia
		Malignant hyperthermia
		Exertional myopathy (Greyhound cramp)
Neoplasia		Rhabdomyoma
		Rhabdomyosarcoma
		Paraneoplastic myopathy
Miscellaneous/traumatic		Fibrotic myopathy of the semitendinosus
		Myositis ossificans
		Contractures –quadriceps –infraspinatus –gracilis
		Immobilization myopathy

subdivided into infectious and immune-mediated conditions. Leptospirosis and microfilariasis occasionally cause diffuse myositis in the dog and local clostridial myositis can develop either as a result of direct inoculation via a wound or as a consequence of osteomyelitis. In one report neuromuscular disease was associated with *Trichinella* infection (Lindberg *et al*., 1991), but it is the protozoal myopathies which are the most important muscle diseases of infectious origin in the dog and these are described below.

Toxoplasma myositis

Toxoplasma gondii is a coccidian parasite of the cat which can use almost any warm-blooded species as its intermediate host. *Toxoplasma* infection in the dog is often asymptomatic but can result in nervous signs with or without myositis. It has been suggested that for the organism to become clinically significant the animal must be immunosuppressed, hence it is often found in association with canine distemper virus. Since lesions may be present in brain, spinal cord, nerve roots, peripheral nerve or muscle, the clinical picture is very variable.

Puppies may acquire toxoplasma infection *in utero* in which case signs of protozoal myositis and/or radiculoneuritis become apparent soon after birth. A common feature of congenital toxoplasmosis is that the limbs, particularly the hindlimbs, are held so rigidly in extension that passive flexion is impossible.

Diagnosis of toxoplasma myositis is made from the muscle biopsy where an inflammatory response is seen together with evidence of the parasite. Serology can also be a useful aid to diagnosis, although the presence of the organism in many asymptomatic dogs means that serological evidence of infection must be interpreted with caution. In a case of flaccid posterior paralysis (McGlennon *et al*., 1990), examination of a centrifuged sample of cerebrospinal fluid proved a useful aid to diagnosis. In this case protozoal organisms were identified and the diagnosis of protozoal infection was confirmed following post-mortem examination.

Oral therapy using a combination of pyrimethamine (0.5–2.0 mg kg^{-1}) and sulphadiazine (60 mg kg^{-1}) or clindamycin (10–100 mg kg^{-1} in divided doses) are the treatments of choice for toxoplasmosis. McGlennon *et al*. (1990) described a dramatic response to a combination of oral trimethoprim, sulphadiazine and pyrimethamine in a 7-week-old puppy which was showing mild signs of flaccid hindlimb paresis, and was a littermate of a known case of protozoal myositis and encephalitis. This puppy improved rapidly after 48 h and appeared to make a complete recovery after receiving treatment for two weeks. However, in other cases treatment may have to be maintained for 6–8 weeks and in general the prognosis remains guarded. Corticosteroids must *not* be given in cases of toxoplasma myositis as exacerbation of the condition may occur.

Neospora myopathy

It has now been recognized that at least some cases of apparent toxoplasmosis in the dog are, in fact, due to infection with a serologically distinct parasite of similar appearance known as *Neospora caninum*. These organisms do not stain with sera raised against *Toxoplasma gondii* and differ in their ultrastructural appearance. *Neospora* has been found in dogs with encephalomyelitis and meningomyelitis and in a litter of young puppies which developed a rapidly ascending protozoal polyradiculoneuritis (Cummings *et al*., 1988). A case was described in a boxer puppy in which the predominant lesions were encephalomyelitis and myositis (Uggla *et al*., 1989), and Mayhew *et al*. (1991) described a 17-week-old bloodhound puppy in which progressive paralysis resulted in the pelvic limbs becoming fixed in extension (Fig. 43.3). It thus appears that this previously unrecognized sporozoan parasite produces a range of clinical syndromes identical to those associated with toxoplasmosis. Treatment is the same as for toxoplasma infection, namely a combination of sulphadiazine and pyrimethamine. Mayhew *et al*. (1991) described the successful treatment of an affected littermate of a case of *Neospora* encephalomyelitis and polyradiculoneuritis. Three puppies out of a subsequent litter from the same bitch also developed neurological signs which responded to antiprotozoal therapy.

To differentiate between *T. gondii* and *N. caninum* requires ultrastructural, serological and immunohistochemical analysis. It is, therefore, possible that a number of cases previously diagnosed as toxoplasmosis on the basis of light microscopy alone may in fact have been due to *Neospora*. Indeed, retrospective analysis of material from dogs in America collected over a period of 40 years did show that a number of cases previously diagnosed as toxoplasmosis were due to the newly identified organism (Dubey *et al*., 1988). The existence of this parasite may also explain the

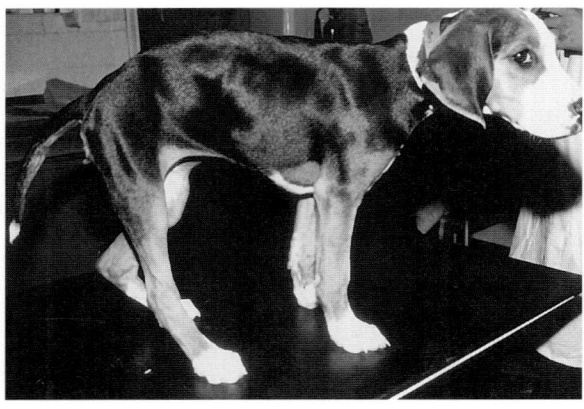 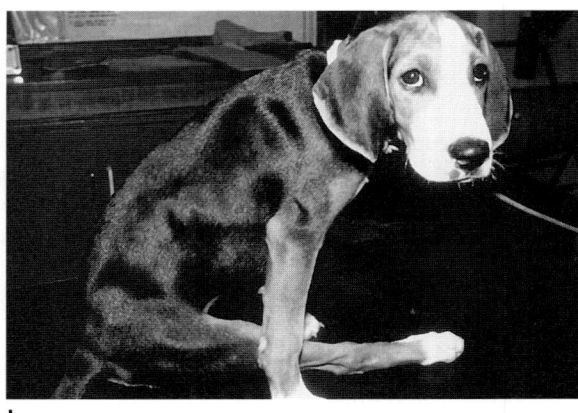

Figure 43.3 (a) and (b) A Hamilton stovare puppy with hindlimb extensor rigidity caused by *Neospora caninum* infection. Photographs courtesy of Michael Herrtage.

observation that many cases of protozoal disease were seronegative when tested for toxoplasmosis. The life cycle of *Neospora caninum* and the source of infection are still unknown.

Eosinophilic myositis/idiopathic myositis of the masticatory muscles

Eosinophilic myositis or idiopathic myositis of masticatory muscles is said to be one of the most frequently recognized canine muscle diseases, with a particularly high incidence in the German shepherd dog (McKeown and Archibald, 1979).

The clinical course may be acute or chronic and the condition may be unilateral or bilateral. In acute cases the muscles of mastication are swollen and painful and there is difficulty opening the mouth. The animal may be depressed and febrile, with enlarged tonsils and submaxillary lymph nodes. The acute phase lasts 2–3 weeks, during which time there is evidence of a peripheral neutrophilia and in some cases eosinophilia as well. Muscle biopsies show necrosis, haemorrhage, oedema and an inflammatory infiltrate, consisting primarily of mononuclear cells.

The chronic form of the condition may follow an acute episode or episodes, or may develop insidiously. Chronic cases are characterized by severe atrophy of the muscles of mastication. The condition may be unilateral but is often bilateral, resulting in limited ability to open the jaws. Biopsies from these cases show marked fibrosis of affected muscles. The aetiology of the condition is not fully understood but it seems likely that it is immune mediated. This is supported by the observation that treatment with glucocorticoids is generally of benefit in both acute and chronic cases and by the demonstration that affected dogs have circulating autoantibodies directed against type 2M fibres, a type of muscle fibre unique to the muscles of mastication (Shelton *et al.*, 1987).

Treatment consists of 0.5–1.5 mg kg^{-1} oral prednisolone twice daily until remission occurs. The dose is then gradually reduced and withdrawn if possible. In some cases alternate day therapy is necessary to prevent relapse.

Polymyositis

Polymyositis is a diffuse inflammatory disease which affects adult dogs of either sex and is said to be more common in large breeds. Presenting signs are variable and include weakness with fatigability, difficulty swallowing, lameness or stiffness and generalized muscle atrophy. Approximately one-third of cases have pain on palpation of skeletal muscles and megaoesophagus may be present.

Fibrillation potentials, positive sharp waves and increased insertional activity are present at electromyography. There is usually elevation of serum enzymes, but since only some may be raised CK, aspartate aminotransferase, aldolase and lactate dehydrogenase should all be evaluated. Diagnosis is confirmed by examination of muscle biopsies in which necrosis of muscle fibres and infiltration of muscle by plasma cells and lymphocytes are seen. The disease is likely to be immune mediated in most cases and treatment with corticosteroids often produces a rapid improvement (Kornegay *et al.*, 1980). Prednisolone is given at a dose of 0.25–1.5 mg kg^{-1} every 8 h. If there is no dramatic response the dose may be doubled until improvement occurs, maintained for 3 to 4 weeks and then reduced gradually.

It is of particular importance that corticosteroids should not be given to cases of toxoplasma myositis as this can produce exacerbation of the condition. Protozoal infection must, therefore, be ruled out before treatment with corticosteroids is initiated.

Idiopathic polymyositis is seen alone but has also been reported in association with other immune-mediated diseases such as systemic lupus erythematosus (Krum *et al.*, 1977), and polyarthritis (Bennett and Kelly, 1987). Steroid-responsive polymyositis was also reported in two 7-month-old German wire-haired pointer litter mates (Presthus and Lindboe, 1988).

Acquired myasthenia gravis

In acquired canine myasthenia gravis the neuromuscular junction is the site of immune-mediated destruction (Palmer, 1980; Lennon *et al.*, 1981). Most cases are seen in adult dogs of large breeds, although one acquired case was seen in a 7-week-old Jack Russell terrier-cross bitch (Palmer *et al.*, 1980). Signs are of severe muscular weakness, particularly of the forelimbs, and fatigue on exercise which improves with rest. Myasthenic dogs have a short choppy stride and a low head carriage which becomes more pronounced as the dog tires. If encouraged to exercise the stride becomes shorter and shorter until eventually the dog pitches forward onto its nose. Myasthenia gravis in the dog is frequently characterized by regurgitation due to megaoesophagus, and a number of cases have been seen in association with thymoma.

The condition is considered to be autoimmune in origin and circulating antibodies to acetylcholine receptors of the neuromuscular junction are detectable. Diagnosis is based on clinical signs and on the response to the Camsilon test (p. 697). Treatment consists of the oral administration of pyridostigmine bromide an anticholinesterase drug which effectively increases the availability of acetylcholine at the neuromuscular junction. The dose of pyridostigmine required varies according to the size of the dog, the severity of the signs and the response to treatment. The effective dose may therefore range from 7.5 mg orally once a day in a Jack Russell terrier to 60 mg two or three times a day in a German shepherd. Care should be taken when administering this drug since inadvertent overdose can result in a cholinergic crisis which if unrecognized may prove fatal. Since the condition is immune mediated, immunosuppressive levels of corticosteroids may be beneficial, and even curative in some cases, but it is important to note that glucocorticoids used in combination with anticholinesterase drugs may result in enhancement of muscle weakness.

The prognosis of myasthenia in the dog is variable. Some cases go into spontaneous remission and make a full recovery, but a proportion of dogs require continuous therapy. Complications such as inhalation pneumonia may arise in dogs which develop megaoesophagus. It is particularly important that these individuals should not be given corticosteroids until the pneumonia is controlled.

A focal form of myasthenia gravis has also been described in which megaoesophagus is the main feature although some of the dogs also showed weakness of laryngeal, pharyngeal and facial muscles (Shelton *et al.*, 1990). In a study of 152 dogs with idiopathic acquired megaoesophagus 40 had positive titres of antibody to acetylcholine receptors and in 48% of these cases decreasing titres correlated with improvement or remission of clinical signs.

■ Myopathies associated with endocrine disease

Myopathic changes have been found in dogs in association with endocrine disease. Muscle biopsies taken from dogs known to have primary hypothyroidism (see Chapter 39) have revealed an associated myopathy. The pathological changes included fibre size variation and reduction in diameter of type 2 fibres, although the electromyogram was normal and there were no clinical signs directly attributable to the myopathy (Braund *et al.*, 1981).

Cases of hyperadrenocorticism may also be associated with pathological changes in the muscle (Greene *et al.*, 1979; Braund *et al.*, 1980a). In these cases there is evidence of severe weakness and atrophy of skeletal muscle which improves as the underlying metabolic disease is treated. Some cases of canine Cushing's disease develop signs of myotonia and in these dramatic high frequency discharges are recorded at electromyography.

■ Metabolic myopathies

Hyperkalaemia and hypokalaemia

Muscle weakness is seen in animals in which alterations have occurred in potassium levels. Hypokalaemia is seen in association with vomiting, diarrhoea and urinary loss. Hyperkalaemia may be seen in hypoadrenocorticism, uncontrolled diabetes mellitus, renal failure and acidosis. One case has been described in which a dog suffered frequent short episodes of weakness associated with periods of exercise-induced hyperkalaemia (Jezyk, 1982).

Malignant hyperthermia

Malignant hyperthermia is a hypermetabolic disorder of skeletal muscle which has been reported in the dog and cat. It has been seen in a number of breeds and a colony of susceptible dogs has been described, suggesting a possible genetic component to the condition (O'Brien et al., 1983). In susceptible individuals episodes are usually initiated by the administration of certain halogenated anaesthetic agents such as halothane or by depolarizing muscle relaxants. The defect appears to lie in the sarcoplasmic reticulum. Calcium is released but the membrane fails to take it up again resulting in sustained contraction. Until an episode is precipitated the animal appears clinically normal although some susceptible dogs show hypertrophy of skeletal muscle and an increase in muscle tone. During an attack the limbs become rigid and trismus develops. The prolonged contraction of the muscles results in hyperthermia and acidosis, and if untreated may lead to respiratory and cardiac arrest. Stress or exercise may also be precipitating factors. In one case a greyhound developed malignant hyperthermia when it became excited on being reunited with its owner after an anaesthetic (Kirmayer et al., 1984). Exercise-induced hyperthermia was reported in a 2-year-old male English springer spaniel (Rand and O'Brien, 1987). In this case, moderate exercise resulted in hyperthermia (rectal temperature of 42.3°C), apparent cramping of hindlimb muscles and laboured respiration.

The treatment of choice for cases of malignant hyperthermia is to administer the muscle relaxant dantrolene at a dose of 5 mg kg^{-1} intravenously but the prognosis is guarded. Dantrolene did not prevent exercise-induced malignant hyperthermia in the case described above (Rand and O'Brien, 1987).

Exertional myopathy

Exertional myopathy is a syndrome most often seen in the racing greyhound and varies in both the severity of the clinical signs and the acuteness of the onset (Gannon, 1980). In hyperacute cases the dog becomes extremely distressed while exercising. There are signs of severe pain in the muscles, particularly of the back and hindquarters, and myoglobinuria develops. This may result in renal failure and death within 48 h. Acute cases also occur during the race but in these cases the muscle pain is more localized and myoglobinuria is only observed initially. In these cases mortality is less common and treatment may be successful. A third, subacute, form of the condition may be seen 24–72 hours after a race. In these cases there is no myoglobinuria and the muscle pain is confined to the longissimus thoracis. These cases are not fatal.

Predisposing factors for the condition include lack of physical fitness, a tendency to become overexcited and tense before racing, hot humid conditions and excessive racing of fit animals.

The pathogenesis of exertional myopathy is not fully understood and is dependent on a number of factors. It also differs between the acute and subacute forms of the syndrome.

When muscular exercise is undertaken hydrogen ions are produced and these must be buffered by the body. If an unfit animal is subjected to excessive fast work the production of hydrogen ions is too great for the intracellular buffers, osmotic pressure rises and water enters the cells. This produces local swelling which in turn results in local ischaemia and focal necrosis. The subacute form of the condition is associated with a relative potassium deficit rather than a failure of the ion pump and alkali reserve. This relative deficit may be seen in dogs which are raced too frequently. When the potassium level falls to a critical level there may be insufficient outflow of potassium ions, as the muscle contracts, to initiate local vasodilation, causing local hyperthermia and ischaemia. Thus it may be seen that although the mechanisms are different the end result in each case is focal necrosis of the muscle cell wall produced by local ischaemia. Once the cell wall has lysed myoglobin is released producing myoglobinuria. When large amounts of myoglobin are precipitated in the kidneys renal failure occurs.

Treatment of hyperacute and acute cases should be started as soon as possible if it is to be successful. Intravenous fluids must be given to prevent hypovolaemic shock and aid excretion of myoglobin through the kidneys. Any normal extracellular replacement fluid is suitable for this purpose. In addition 20 ml kg^{-1} of 4.2% bicarbonate solution should be administered in order to increase the buffering capacity of the extracellular fluid. Bicarbonate also aids the viability of the nephrons of the kidney as an alkaline environment reduces the precipitation of myoglobin protein.

Additional therapeutic measures include local cooling of affected muscles with cold packs in the early stages of the condition. Anabolic steroids, phenylbutazone and prophylactic antibiotics may also be useful.

The urine should be kept alkaline by the administration of oral sodium bicarbonate, at a dose of 100 mg kg^{-1} for ten days after the episode in order to protect the kidneys.

Treatment of the subacute form of the condition takes account of the fact that in these cases the underlying cause is the relative potassium deficit. The urine should be alkalinized to prevent myoglobin precipitation and phenylbutazone may be given to relieve muscle pain. Anabolic steroids are also of value.

Traumatic/miscellaneous muscle conditions

Fibrotic myopathy of the semitendinosus

This is a condition usually seen in the German shepherd dog between 2 and 7 years of age. A palpable band of fibrous connective tissue develops in the semitendinosus muscle extending from the tuber ischii to the tibia. Clinical signs include lameness and reduced extension of the limb. The cause of the condition is unknown although it has been suggested that it may be due to repeated trauma. Surgical excision results in improvement but the condition usually recurs (Moore et al., 1981). Similar fibrous bands have been described in the quadriceps and gracilis muscles.

Myositis ossificans

This term is used to refer to the formation of non-neoplastic bone in extraosseous sites often within skeletal muscles. It is a rare condition which can be localized or generalized and although uncommon, has been reported in the dog. Clinical signs include lameness, pain on palpation and swelling or enlargement of the affected muscles. Histology varies from mild interstitial fibrosis to the complete replacement of muscle by fibrous tissue and bone (Bone and McGavin, 1985). In localized lesions surgical removal of the ossified muscle generally results in recovery.

Contractures

In theory any muscle may undergo fibrosis and contracture following injury. In the dog, contractures are most commonly seen in the gracilis, infraspinatus and quadriceps muscles.

Quadriceps contracture together with stifle stiffness is seen in dogs with femoral fractures which have been treated by prolonged immobilization in extension. The limb is held in hyperextension, the muscles are atrophied and if examined histologically evidence of so-called immobilization myopathy (fibre size variation, focal necrosis, type 2 atrophy and fibrosis) is found (Braund et al., 1980b). Trauma appears to be the crucial factor influencing recovery since experimental studies suggest that the duration of the immobilization is not an important factor.

Infraspinatus contracture is often seen following trauma or with a history of sudden pain. The initial lameness improves but the dog is left with an abnormal gait and a prominent scapular spine. The underlying aetiology is unknown. It has been suggested that the suprascapular nerve is damaged where it crosses the scapular border, resulting in neurogenic atrophy and eventually fibrosis. Others suggest that the fibrosis follows acute rupture of muscle fibres. Treatment involves tenotomy or partial tenectomy of the tendon of insertion of infraspinatus together with separation of local adhesions and is said to give good results (Bennett, 1986; Vaughan, 1979).

Contractures are also seen in the gracilis. Most cases have been documented in German shepherd dogs, especially those which are particularly athletic. There is an alteration of gait and on examination the gracilis muscle is found to be taut, firm and narrow with thickening of the tenson of insertion. Tenotomy relieves the signs but the condition frequently recurs (Vaughan, 1969).

Neoplasia and muscle disease

Muscle tumours

Primary muscle tumours are rare and a third of striated muscle tumours are benign. Rhabdomyomas are congenital and affect the heart. Conversely, rhabdomyosarcoma is a malignant tumour which arises from muscle or non-muscle sites but is not seen in the heart. This tumour usually presents as a hard spherical mass palpable deep within the muscle of the limb, neck or head. It is locally invasive but also spreads via the lymphatics to the lymph nodes and via the blood to lungs, abdominal viscera and bones (see Chapter 50).

Paraneoplastic myopathy

Pathological changes consistent with both neuropathy and myopathy have been reported in dogs with tumours remote from the muscular or nervous system. The underlying mechanisms responsible for the pathology is not known but it is likely that it occurs more frequently than the few reported cases would suggest (Braund, 1986).

INHERITED/CONGENITAL MUSCLE DISEASES OF THE CAT (Table 43.3)

Hypokalaemic polymyopathy

Hypokalaemic polymyopathy has been widely reported in the cat and it has been suggested that there is an inherited predisposition to the condition in the Burmese (Blaxter *et al.*, 1986; Jones *et al.*, 1988). Hypokalaemia in Burmese kittens is characterized by episodes of transient weakness. Onset of signs occurs between 4 and 12 months and in between attacks there may be improvement. Affected cats show weakness of the limbs and persistent ventroflexion of the neck (Fig. 43.4) which is often accompanied by tremor or head nodding. They are reluctant to walk or jump, and the gait is stiff and stilted. Diagnosis is based on the demonstration of low serum potassium (less than 3.0 mmol l^{-1}). Histological examination of muscle biopsies reveals mild, diffuse necrosis, although CK levels may be very high (up to 97 000 iu l^{-1}). At electromyography there is increased insertional activity and the presence of positive sharp waves.

Table 43.3 Muscle diseases of the cat

Inherited/congenital	Hypokalaemic myopathy (Burmese) Hereditary myopathy (Devon Rex) Congenital myasthenia gravis Nemaline myopathy Muscular dystrophy Myotonia
Acquired	Ischaemic myopathy Acquired myasthenia gravis Nutritional myopathy Polymyopathy Hypokalaemic polymyopathy Myositis osssificans –? generalized – localized Fibrodysplasia ossificans Malignant hyperthermia Polymyositis

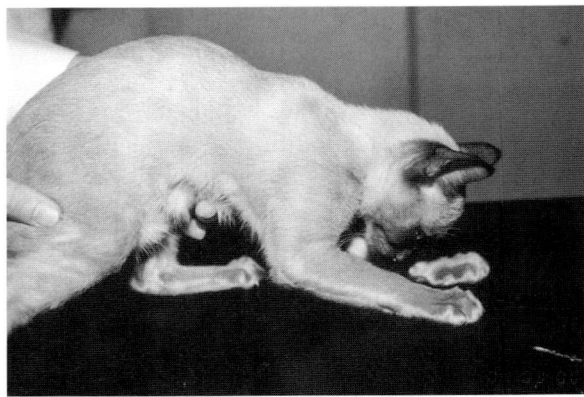

Figure 43.4 Hypokalaemic myopathy in a Burmese kitten. Note persistent ventroflexion of the neck. Photograph courtesy of Michael Herrtage.

Treatment consists of a high potassium diet, but in severe cases oral potassium supplementation (5–8 mmol potassium per day in divided doses) may be required. Restoration of normal levels of potassium generally results in considerable improvement in the clinical signs (Jones *et al.*, 1988) although full strength may take several weeks to return.

Hereditary myopathy of Devon rex cats

For many years an inherited condition characterized by muscle weakness has been recognized in Devon rex cats and has generally been referred to by breeders as 'spasticity'. The mode of inheritance was established as an autosomal recessive (Robinson, 1992), but although several cases were investigated no satisfactory aetiology was established.

A series of six cases has been described in which evidence is presented suggesting that so-called 'spasticity' in this breed should be regarded as an example of a hereditary myopathy (Malik *et al.*, 1993).

Clinical signs include ventroflexion of the head and neck, generalized appendicular weakness with protrusion of the scapulae and fatigability. Weakness is particularly apparent following exertion, stress or excitement and affected cats tire quickly with exercise, collapsing into sternal recumbency with the head resting beside or on top of the paws. Affected animals often have difficulty prehending and swallowing food and megaoesophagus is a common finding.

Furthermore, a number of cats have died suddenly due to laryngospasm following the accumulation of food in the pharynx or larynx, suggesting oropharyngeal weakness. There appears to be no positive response to the Camsilon test in this condition thus distinguishing it from feline myasthenia gravis (qv).

Routine haematology and biochemistry are normal. There is no elevation of CK and no evidence of hypokalaemia.

Muscle biopsies taken from five cases showed evidence of myopathic change (Malik et al., 1993). In mildly affected young animals the changes were subtle consisting of fibre size variation, occasional degenerating fibres, and an increase in the numbers of subsarcolemmal nuclei. In older animals and those in which clinical signs were more severe there was greater variation in fibre size, the presence of internal nuclei and evidence of fibre splitting. Necrotic and regenerating fibres were found and an increased amount of intrafascicular connective tissue was present. There was no alteration in fibre type proportions observed in the muscles examined using the ATPase reaction and immunofluorescence confirmed the presence of dystrophin. No abnormalities were found in either the peripheral or central nervous systems of the cases examined.

On electromyography sparse fibrillations and positive sharp waves were recorded from muscles of the proximal forelimb and neck. Conduction velocities of the tibial and ulnar nerves were normal.

Congenital myasthenia gravis

Two cases of myasthenia gravis have been reported in young cats and are considered to have been congenital (Indrieri et al., 1983; Joseph et al., 1988). See also acquired myasthenia gravis below.

Nemaline myopathy

An apparently inherited myopathy has been described in a group of related cats of unspecified breed. The clinical signs were seen between 6 and 18 months of age and included reluctance to move, depressed reflexes, jerky gait and muscle twitching. Histological findings consisted of fibre size variation, atrophy of both fibre types and the presence of so-called nemaline rods at electron microscopy (Cooper et al., 1986). Nemaline myopathy is a relatively rare human myopathy.

Nemaline rods have been induced experimentally, and are seen as non-specific findings in neuromyopathies in various species. This condition appears to be the first in which an accumulation of rods constitutes a dramatic feature of a naturally occurring disease of animals. Although affecting only a small number of cats it is, therefore, of comparative interest.

Muscular dystrophy

Two cases of a dystrophy-like myopathy were described in cats (Vos et al., 1986). Both presented with moderate locomotor disturbances such as inability to jump and 'kangaroo' gait. In each case there was evidence of a generalized myopathy involving skeletal muscles and also the diaphragm which became grossly hypertrophied. Histological features included the variation in fibre size, some necrosis and the presence of internal nuclei (Vos et al., 1986).

An apparently X-linked muscular dystrophy with deficiency of the muscle protein dystrophin has since been reported in two domestic shorthaired cats (Carpenter et al., 1989). These male siblings showed signs of progressive muscle stiffness and gait abnormalities, together with striking hypertrophy of most muscles. Weakness was not a feature but both cats tired easily. Histology of affected muscles revealed many necrotic fibres together with evidence of regeneration. Fibre splitting and variation in fibre size were also present. The demonstration that dystrophin was absent from the muscles of these two cats confirmed the diagnosis of a muscular dystrophy which is analogous to that documented in humans (Duchenne dystrophy) and the golden retriever (qv).

Myotonia

Myotonia has been widely reported in many species but only one case has been observed in the cat. Clinical signs first became apparent at a few months of age and the condition was therefore assumed to be congenital. The predominant sign was muscle stiffness which was most noticeable after rest but improved with exercise. If the cat was startled it fell to one side and the nictitating membranes would prolapse. Muscle hypertrophy was prominent and the diagnosis was confirmed by the presence of myotonic discharges on electromyography (Lievesley and Gruffydd-Jones, 1989).

ACQUIRED MUSCLE DISEASES IN THE CAT (Table 43.3)

Ischaemic myopathy

This condition is seen in association with cardiomyopathy (see Chapter 34) as a result of embolus formation. Emboli may travel to any part of the circulation but the most common site is the distal aorta where the so-called saddle thrombus extends into the iliac arteries resulting in loss of blood supply. The ischaemia results in a myopathy characterized by focal necrosis, phagocytosis and infiltration of the muscle by inflammatory cells.

Clinical signs include acute onset of pelvic limb pain, together with varying degrees of paresis. On examination the femoral pulse is weak or absent and the limbs are cold. The muscles may be firm and painful, particularly those beneath the stifle and there is loss of sensation from the distal limb. In some cases collateral circulation is re-established but there is evidence that this process may be inhibited due to the release of vasoactive substances from the thromboembolism itself. Although there may be some improvement in motor function after two to three weeks, the prognosis is very poor as the condition is likely to recur. If treatment is undertaken a prime consideration is the control of pain which may be very severe. Further treatment is aimed at the underlying disorder and should include aspirin (25 mg kg^{-1} every third day) to combat platelet aggregation together with low doses of acepromazine or cyproheptadine in order to prevent vasoconstriction (Robins et al. 1982; Flanders, 1986).

Acquired myasthenia gravis

Although rarer than myasthenia in the dog, a number of cases of feline myasthenia gravis have been reported (Dawson, 1970; Mason, 1976; Indrieri et al., 1983; Joseph et al., 1988; Cuddon, 1989). Myasthenic cats show an initial stiffnesss of gait and may appear to be lame. As they exercise they rapidly become weak and reluctant to stand. A common presenting sign in this species is trembling or muscle tremors, which are not a feature of myasthenia in other species. Dysphagia, salivation, changes in the voice, and facial weakness may also occur and two cases have been described in association with thymic masses (Scott-Moncrieff et al., 1990; O'Dair et al., 1991). Most recorded cases have been adult onset and are, therefore, likely to be acquired but two cases of probable congenital myasthenia have also been described (Indrieri et al., 1983; Joseph et al., 1988). Exotic cats seem to be over-represented; affected breeds include the Somali, Siamese and Abyssinian. In view of this it has been suggested that there may be some association with the major histocompatibility complex as in humans (Cuddon, 1992). It is interesting to speculate on the apparently low incidence of myasthenia gravis in the cat. It is possible that in some cases the unusual presenting sign of trembling may obscure the diagnosis. Another clue to the apparent rarity of the disease may be found in a case reported in Australia (Mason, 1976). The owners noticed that this 2-year-old DSH cat was unable to cross the road without a period of rest; a clinical feature which no doubt has considerable influence on the prognosis of the disease in the urban cat!

Treatment with pyridostigmine bromide orally at a dose of 2 mg kg^{-1} has been successful in conjunction with oral prednisolone at a dose of 1.5 mg kg^{-1} bid. Where possible a reducing dose of each drug should be given and in some cases it may be possible eventually to withdraw treatment altogether. Thymectomy may be indicated in those cases associated with thymic tumours.

Nutritional myopathy

Occasional cases of nutritional myopathy have been reported. One cat which had been fed entirely on boiled coley developed hot painful swellings in the limbs. Histologically there was severe muscle fibre degeneration and a diagnosis of vitamin E deficiency was made. Correction of the diet led to a complete recovery and the cat regained the use of its legs 14 days after the diet was changed (Dennis and Alexander, 1982). In another case of suspected nutritional myopathy a cat was fed only on raw mutton and milk and developed signs of acute myopathy. The cause was not established but selenium deficiency was suspected (Bradley and Fell, 1981).

Polymyopathy

In 1984 a polymyopathy unassociated with nutritional deficiency was diagnosed in 24 cats in the USA. The condition appeared to be acquired and to have no obvious age, sex or breed predilection. Diagnosis was based on appendicular weakness, low head carriage, elevated serum muscle enzymes, EMG abnormalities and histological evidence of myopathy in skeletal muscles. In a high proportion of cases there was evidence of low serum potassium (see hypokalaemia below). The aetiology of the disease is not known, indeed it is possible that several different conditions could be included in the cases reviewed (Schunk, 1984).

Hypokalaemic polymyopathy

Muscle weakness associated with hypokalaemia has been widely reported in the cat and hypokalaemic polymyopathy is currently thought to be one of the most common causes of generalized muscle weakness in this species (Dow and LeCouteur, 1989). Most cases are acquired (sporadic) and occur in adults, but a periodic muscle weakness related to low serum potassium has been reported in Burmese kittens (qv). A number of the cats described in the series of idiopathic polymopathy cases (Schunk, 1984) were noted to be hypokalaemic.

Total body potassium content depends on the balance between intake and loss. Therefore, for depletion to occur there must be reduced intake or increased loss of potassium via either the gastrointestinal tract or the kidneys. A retrospective study of a series of cats revealed a strong association between hypokalaemia and chronic renal disease. Hepatic disease was also significantly associated with the development of hypokalaemia (Dow et al., 1989). Hypokalaemia has also been reported in a case of primary hyperaldosteronism (Eger et al., 1983). The mechanism by which renal dysfunction produces potassium loss is not fully understood and may be peculiar to cats (Dow et al., 1989). If this loss occurs over several months there may be a severe depletion of total body potassium particularly if the diet is in any way deficient in potassium. It is also important to note that if hypokalaemic cats are treated with subcutaneous or intravenous fluids this can itself deplete the serum potassium to a level at which respiratory paralysis occurs (Dow and LeCouteur, 1989).

Severely affected cases of hypokalaemic polymyopathy show signs of generalized muscle weakness. They are reluctant to walk, have a stiff stilted gait, a low head carriage and there may be apparent muscle pain when handled. Diagnosis of hypokalaemic polymyopathy depends on demonstration of these signs together with a serum potassium concentration of less than 3.5 mmol l^{-1} and a good response to treatment with potassium. Serum CK is high indicating muscle damage and at electromyography, widespread abnormalities including positive sharp waves, fibrillation potentials and occasional bizarre high frequency discharges are found in most muscle groups. Histologically mild necrosis and macrophage infiltration may be seen in muscle biopsies but inflammatory changes are not a feature.

Although the onset of signs may be acute it has been suggested that a subclinical myopathy may exist for weeks to months without obvious signs and that hypokalaemic polymyopathy represents only the most dramatic manifestation of chronic potassium depletion (Dow and LeCouteur, 1989).

Oral treatment using potassium-containing elixirs is recommended for cases of hypokalaemia. Cats are given 5–8 mmol potassium l^{-1} day^{-1} in divided doses until serum concentrations return to normal. Most affected cats are then maintained on 2–4 mmol potassium l^{-1} day^{-1} although there is great individual variation in the doses required.

Some response to treatment is generally seen within 24 h although complete resolution of muscle weakness may take several weeks and the condition may recur if dietary supplementation is not continuous.

Myositis ossificans

A case of generalized myositis ossificans was diagnosed in a cat which had a history of stiffness, pain, progressive weakness and firm masses in the longissimus and limb muscles (Norris et al., 1980). However, it was later suggested that the condition was probably better described as fibrodysplasia ossificans since the process does not begin in muscle and is not inflammatory. Three further cases of fibrodysplasia ossificans were described and, in each, the clinical signs consisted of progressive stiffness and pain with radiographic evidence of soft tissue and bony densities in many muscles (Warren and Carpenter, 1984).

Localized myositis ossificans has also been reported in a cat. In this case lesions were restricted to the elbows and did not recur after surgical removal.

Malignant hyperthermia

Malignant hyperthermia occurs in many species but although a case has been described it appears to be rare in the cat (De Jong *et al.*, 1982.)

Polymyositis

Inflammatory muscle disease has not been widely reported in the cat. Although cats are the definitive hosts of *Toxoplasma gondii* infections are rarely clinically evident and when they are, muscle involvement is not a typical feature. No natural cases of *Neospora caninum* infection have been reported although experimental inoculation can produce a fatal disease in which polymyositis is present (Cuddon, 1992).

Three cases of inflammatory muscle disease associated with thymic tumours have been reported of which two showed evidence of myocardial involvement. Muscle wasting was extreme in two cases and those cats which had cardiac lesions were lethargic and dysphagic. Both these cats had difficulty swallowing, bouts of vomiting and tended to rest the head on the forepaws (Carpenter and Holzworth, 1982).

REFERENCES

Anderson, J.R. (1985) *Atlas of Skeletal Muscle Pathology*. MTP Press, Lancaster, p. 139.

Bennett, R.A. (1986) Contracture of the infraspinatus muscle in dogs: a review of 12 cases. *Journal of the American Animal Hospital Association* 22, 481–487.

Bennett, D. and Kelly, D.F. (1987) Immune-based non-erosive inflammatory joint disease of the dog. 2. Polyarthritis/polymyositis syndrome. *Journal of Small Animal Practice* 28, 891–908.

Blaxter, A.C., Lievesley, P., Gruffydd-Jones, T.J. and Wotton, P. (1986) Periodic muscle weakness in Burmese kittens. *Veterinary Record* 118, 619–620.

Blood, D.C., Radostits, O.M. and Henderson, J.A. (1983) *Veterinary Medicine*, 6th edn. Baillière Tindall, London, p. 1043.

Bonagura, J.D. and O'Grady, M. (1983) ECG of the month. *Journal of the American Veterinary Medical Association* 183, 658–659.

Bone, D.L. and McGavin, M.D. (1985) Myositis ossificans in the dog: a case report and review. *Journal of the American Animal Hospital Association* 21, 135–138.

Bradley, R. and Fell, B.F. (1981) Myopathies in animals. In: *Disorders of Voluntary Muscle*, 4th edn (Ed. J. Walton). Churchill Livingstone, Edinburgh, p. 859.

Bradley, R., McKerrell, R.E. and Barnard, E.A. (1988) Neuromuscular disease in animals. In: *Disorders of Voluntary Muscle*, 5th edn (Ed. J. Walton). Churchill Livingstone, Edinburgh, pp. 910–980.

Braund, K.G. (1986) *Clinical Syndromes in Veterinary Neurology*. Williams and Wilkins, Baltimore, p. 150.

Braund, K.G., Dillon, A.R., Mikeal, R.L. and August, J.R. (1980a) Subclinical myopathy associated with hyperadrenocorticism in the dog. *Veterinary Pathology* 17, 134–148.

Braund, K.G., Shires, P.K. and Mikeal, R.L. (1980b) Type I fiber atrophy in the vastus lateralis muscle in dogs with femoral fractures treated by hyperextension. *Veterinary Pathology* 17, 164–176.

Braund, K.G., Dillon, A.R., August, J.R. and Ganjam, V.K. (1981) Hypothyroid myopathy in two dogs. *Veterinary Pathology* 18, 589–598.

Braund, K.G., Steinberg, H.S., Mehta, J.R. and Amling, K.A. (1990) Investigating a degenerative polymyopathy in four related Bouvier des Flandres dogs. *Veterinary Medicine* 85, 558–570

Breitschwerdt, E.B., Kornegay, J.N., Wheeler, S.J., Stevens, J.B. and Baty, C.J. (1992) Episodic weakness associated with exertional lactic acidosis and myopathy in Old English Sheepdog littermates. *Journal of the American Veterinary Medical Association* 201, 731–736

Cardinet, G.H., Wallace, L.J., Fedde, M.R., Guffy, M.M. and Bardens, J.W. (1969) Developmental myopathy in the canine with type II muscle fiber hypotrophy. *Archives of Neurology* 21, 620–630

Carpenter, J.L. and Holzworth, J. (1982) Thymoma in 11 cats. *Journal of the American Veterinary Medical Association* 181, 248–251

Carpenter, J.L., Hoffman, E.P., Romanul, F.C.A., Kunkel, L.M., Rosales, R.K., Ma, N.S.F., Dasbach, J.J., Rae, J.F., Moore, F.M., McAfee, M.B. and Pearce, L.K. (1989) Feline muscular dystrophy with dystrophin deficiency. *American Journal of Pathology* 135, 909–919

Ceh, L., Hauge, J.G., Svenkerud, R. and Strande, A (1976) Glycogenosis type III in the dog. *Acta Veterinaria Scandinavica* 17, 210–222

Chrisman, C.L. (1982) Problems in small animal neurology. Lea and Febiger, Philadelphia, p 345

Cooper, B.J., de Lahunta, A., Gallagher, E.A. and Valentine, B.A. 1986 Nemaline myopathy of cats. *Muscle and Nerve* 9, 618–625

Cooper, B.J., Winand, N.J., Stedman, H., Valentine, B.A., Hoffman, E.P., Kunkel, L.M., Scott, M-O., Fischbeck, K.H., Kornegay, J.N., Avery, R.J., Schmickel, R.D. and Sylvester, J.E. (1988) The homologue of the Duchenne locus is defective in X-linked muscular dystrophy of dogs. *Nature* 334, 154–156

Cuddon, P.A. (1989) Acquired immune-mediated myasthenia gravis in a cat. *Journal of Small Animal Practice* 30, 511–516

Cuddon, P.A. (1992) Feline neuromuscular diseases. *Current Veterinary Therapy* **11**, 1024–1031

Cummings, J.F., deLahunta, A., Suter, M.M. and Jacobson, R.H. (1988) Canine protozoan polyradiculoneuritis. *Acta Neuropathologica* **76**, 46–54

Dawson, J.R.B. (1970) Myasthenia gravis in a cat. *Veterinary Record* **86**, 562–563

De Jong, R.H., Heavner, J.E. and Amory, D.W. (1982) Malignant hyperpyrexia in the cat. *Anaesthesiology* **41**, 608–609

Denborough, M.A. and Lovell, R.R.H. (1960) Anaesthetic deaths in a family. *Lancet* **2**, 45.

Dennis, J.M. and Alexander, R.W. (1982) Nutritional myopathy in a cat. *Veterinary Record* **111**, 195–196.

Dow, S.W. and LeCouteur, R.A. (1989) Hypokalaemic polymyopathy of cats. In: *Current Veterinary Therapy* X (Ed. R.W. Kirk). W.B. Saunders, Philadelphia, pp. 812–815.

Dow, S.W., Fettman, M.J., Curtis, C.R. and LeCouteur R.A. (1989) Hypokalaemia in cats: 186 cases (1984–1987). *Journal of the American Veterinary Medical Association* **194**, 1604–1608.

Dubey, J.P., Carpenter, J.L., Speer, C.A., Topper, M.J. and Uggla, A. (1988) *Journal of the American Veterinary Medical Association* **192**, 1269–1285.

Duncan, I.D. and Griffiths, I.R. (1986) Neuromuscular diseases. In: *Neurological Disorders* (Ed. J.N. Kornegay). Churchill Livingstone, New York, pp. 169–195.

Duncan, I.D., Griffiths, I.R. and Nash, A.S. (1977) Myotonia in canine Cushing's disease. *Veterinary Record* **100**, 30–31.

Eger, C.E., Robinson, W.F. and Huxtable, C.R.R. (1983) Primary aldosteronism (Conn's syndrome) in a cat: a case report and review of comparative aspects. *Journal of Small Animal Practice* **24**, 293.

Farrow, B.R.H. and Malik, R. (1981) Hereditary myotonia in the Chow Chow. *Journal of Small Animal Practice* **22**, 451–465.

Flagstad, A., Nielsen, P. and Trojaberg, W. (1986) Pharmacokinetics and pharmacodynamics of guanidine hydrochloride in an hereditary myasthenia gravis like disorder in dogs. *Journal of Veterinary Pharmacology and Therapeutics* **9**, 318–324.

Flanders, J.A. (1986) Feline aortic thromboembolism. *Compendium on Continuing Education for the Practising Veterinarian* **8**, 473–480.

Funkquist, B., Haraldsson, I. and Stahre, L. (1980) Primary progressive muscular dystrophy in the dog. *Veterinary Record* **106**, 341–346.

Furber, R.M., (1984) Cramp in Norwich terriers. *Veterinary Record* **115**, 46.

Gannon, J.R. (1980) Exertional rhabdomyolysis (myoglobinuria) in the racing greyhound. In: *Current Veterinary Therapy* VII (Ed. R.W. Kirk). W.B. Saunders, Philadelphia, pp. 783–787.

Greene, C.E., Lorenz, M.D., Munnell, J.F., Prasse, K.W., White, N.A. and Bowen, J.M. (1979) Myopathy associated with hyperadrenocorticism in the dog. *Journal of the American Veterinary Medical Association* **174**, 1310–1315.

Griffiths, I.R. and Duncan, I.D. (1973) Myotonia in the dog: a report of four cases. *Veterinary Record* **93**, 184–188.

Haupt, K.H., Prieur, D.J., Moore, M.P., Hargis, A.M., Hegreberg, G.A., Gavin, P.R. and Johnson, R.S. (1985a) Familial canine dermatomyositis: clinical, electrodiagnostic and genetic studies. *American Journal of Veterinary Research* **46**, 1861–1869.

Haupt, K.H., Prieur, D.J., Hargis, A.M., Cowell, R.L., McDonald, T.L., Werner, L.L. and Evermann, J.F. (1985b) Familial canine dermatomyositis: clinicopathologic, immunologic and serologic studies. *American Journal of Veterinary Research* **46**, 1870–1875.

Herrtage, M.E. and Houlton, J.E.F. (1979) Collapsing Clumber spaniels. *Veterinary Record* **105**, 334.

Herrtage, M.E. and Palmer, A.C. (1983) Episodic falling in the cavalier King Charles spaniel. *Veterinary Record* **112**, 458–459.

Holland, C.T., Canfield, P.J., Watson, A.D.J. and Allan, G.S. (1991) Dyserythropoiesis, polymyopathy and cardiac disease in three related English springer spaniels. *Journal of Veterinary Internal Medicine* **5**, 151–159.

Honhold, N. and Smith, D.A. (1986) Myotonia in the Great Dane. *Veterinary Record* **119**, 162.

Houlton, J.E.F. and Herrtage, M.E. (1980) Mitochondrial myopathy in the Sussex spaniel. *Veterinary Record* **106**, 206.

Indrieri, R.J., Creighton, S.R., Lambert, E.H. and Lennon, V.A. (1983) Myasthenia gravis in two cats. *Journal of the American Veterinary Medical Association* **182**, 57–60.

Innes, J.R.M. (1951) Myopathies in animals. *British Veterinary Journal* **107**, 131.

Jezyk, P.F. (1982) Hyperkalemic periodic paralysis in a dog. *Journal of the American Animal Hospital Association* **18**, 977–980.

Johnson, R.P., Watson, A.D.J., Smith, J. and Cooper, B.J. (1975) Myasthenia in springer spaniel littermates. *Journal of Small Animal Practice* **16**, 641–647.

Jones, B.R. and Johnstone, A.C. (1982) An unusual myopathy in a dog. *New Zealand Veterinary Journal* **30**, 119–121.

Jones, B.R., Anderson, L.J., Barnes, G.R.G., Johnstone, A.C. and Juby, W.D. (1978) Myotonia in related Chow Chow dogs. *New Zealand Veterinary Journal* **25**, 217–220.

Jones, B.R., Swinney, G.W. and Alley, M.R. (1988) Hypokalaemic myopathy in Burmese kittens. *New Zealand Veterinary Journal* **36**, 150–151.

Joseph, R.J., Carrillo, J.M. and Lennon, V.A. (1988) Myasthenia gravis in the cat. *Journal of Veterinary Internal Medicine* **2**, 75–79.

Kaspar, L.V. and Lombard, L.S. (1963) Nutritional myodegeneration in a litter of beagles. *Journal of the*

American Veterinary Medical Association **143**, 284–288.

Kirmayer, A.H., Klide, A.M. and Purvance, J.E. (1984) Malignant hyperthermia in a dog: case report and review of the syndrome. *Journal of the Veterinary Medical Association* **185**, 978–982.

Kornegay, J.N. (1984) Golden retriever myopathy. Proceedings of the XII Annual Scientific program of the American College of Veterinary Internal Medicine May 17–20 1984 Washington, DC, pp. 193–196.

Kornegay, J.N., Gorgaez, E.J., Dawe, D.L., Bowen, J.M., White, N.A. and DeBuysscher, E.V. (1980) Polymyositis in dogs. *Journal of the American Veterinary Medical Association* **176**, 431–437.

Kornegay, J.N. (1992) The X-linked muscular dystrophies. In: *Current Veterinary Therapy* XI (Ed. R.W. Kirk). W.B. Saunders, Philadelphia, pp. 1042–1047.

Kramer, J.W., Hegreberg, G.A., Bryan, G.M., Meyers, K. and Ott, R.L. (1976) A muscle disorder of Labrador retrievers characterised by deficiency of type II muscle fibres. *Journal of the American Veterinary Medical Association* **169**, 817–820.

Kramer, J.W., Hegreberg, G.A. and Hamilton, M.J. (1981) Inheritance of a neuromuscular disorder of Labrador retriever dogs. *Journal of the American Veterinary Medical Association* **179**, 380–381.

Krum, S.H., Cardinet, G.H., Anderson, B.C. and Holliday, T.A. (1977) Polymyositis and polyarthritis associated with systemic lupus erythematosis in a dog. *Journal of the American Veterinary Medical Association* **170**, 61–64.

Lennon, V.A., Lambert, E.H., Palmer, A.C., Cunningham, J.G. and Christie, T.R. (1981) Acquired and congenital myasthenia gravis in dogs – a study of 20 cases. In: *Myasthenia Gravis: Pathogenesis and Treatment* (Ed. E. Satoyoshi). University of Tokyo Press, Tokyo, pp. 41–54.

Lievesley, P. and Gruffydd-Jones, T.J. (1989) Episodic collapse and weakness in cats. *Veterinary Annual* **29**, 261–269.

Lindberg, R., Bornstein, S., Landerholm, A. and Zakrisson, G. (1991) Canine trichinosis with signs of neuromuscular disease. *Journal of Small Animal Practice* **32**, 194–197.

Lust, G., Craig, P.H., Ross, G.E. and Geary, J.C. (1972) Studies on pectineus muscles in canine hip dysplasia. *Cornell Veterinarian* **62**, 628–645.

Malik, R., Mepstead, K., Yang, F. and Harper, C. (1993) Hereditary myopathy of Devon rex cats. *Journal of Small Animal Practice* **34**, 539–546.

Manktelow, B.W. (1963) Myopathy of dogs resembling white muscle disease of sheep. *New Zealand Veterinary Journal* **11**, 52–55.

Mason, K.V. (1976) A case of myasthenia gravis in a cat. *Journal of Small Animal Practice* **17**, 467–472.

Mayhew, I.G., Smith, K.C., Dubey, J.P., Gatward, L.K. and McGlennon, N.J. (1991) Treatment of encephalomyelitis due to *Neospora caninum* in a litter of puppies. *Journal of Small Animal Practice* **32**, 609–612.

McGlennon, N.J., Jeffries, A.R. and Casas, C. (1990) Polyradiculoneuritis and polymyositis due to a toxoplasma-like protozoan: diagnosis and treatment. *Journal of Small Animal Practice* **31**, 102–104.

McKeown, D. and Archibald, J. (1979) The musculoskeletal system. In: *Canine Medicine*, 4th edn (Ed. E.J. Calcott). Veterinary Publications Inc., Santa Barbara, pp. 533–669.

McKerrell, R.E. (1989) Labrador retriever myopathy: clinical and pathological investigations. PhD thesis, University of Cambridge.

McKerrell, R.E. and Braund, K.G. (1986) Hereditary myopathy in Labrador retrievers: a morphologic study. *Veterinary Pathology* **23**, 411–417.

McKerrell, R.E. and Braund, K.G. (1987) Hereditary myopathy in Labrador retrievers: clinical variations. *Journal of Small Animal Practice* **28**, 479–489.

Meier, H. (1958) Myopathies in the dog. *Cornell Veterinarian* **48**, 313–330.

Miller, L.M., Lennon, V.A., Lambert, E.H., Reed, S.M., Hegreberg, G.A., Miller, J.B. and Ott, R.L. (1983) Congenital myasthenia gravis in 13 smooth Fox terriers. *Journal of the American Veterinary Medical Association* **182**, 694–697.

Moore, R.W., Rouse, G.P., Piermattei, D.L. and Ferguson, R.H. (1981) Fibrotic myopathy of the semitendinosus muscle in four dogs. *Veterinary Surgery* **10**, 169–174.

Moore, M.P., Reed, S.M., Hegreberg, G.A., Kramer, J.W., Alexander, J.E., Meyer, K.M. and Bryan, G.M. (1987) Electromyographic evaluation of adult Labrador retrievers with type II muscle fibre deficiency. *American Journal of Veterinary Research* **48**, 1332–1336.

Newsholme, S.J. and Gaskell, C.J. (1987) Myopathy with core-like structures in a dog. *Journal of Comparative Pathology* **97**, 597–600.

Norris, A.M., Pallett, L. and Wilcock, B. (1980) Generalized myositis ossificans in a cat. *Journal of the American Animal Hospital Association* **16**, 659–663.

O'Brien, P.J., Cribb, P.H., White, R.J., Olfert, E.D. and Steiss, J.E. (1983) Canine malignant hyperthermia: diagnosis of susceptibility in a breeding colony. *Canadian Veterinary Journal* **24**, 172–177.

Oda, K., Lambert, E., Lennon, V.A. and Palmer, A.C. (1984) Congenital canine myasthenia gravis: deficient junctional acetylcholine receptors. *Muscle and Nerve* **7**, 705–716.

O'Dair, H.A., Holt, P., Pearson, G.R. and Gruffydd-Jones, T.J. (1991) Acquired immune-mediated myasthenia gravis in a cat associated with a cystic thymus. *Journal of Small Animal Practice* **32**, 198–202.

Palmer, A.C. (1980) Myasthenia gravis. Symposium on Advances in Veterinary Neurology. *Veterinary Clinics of North America: Small Animal Practice* **10**, 213–221.

Palmer, A.C. and Goodyear, J.V. (1978) Congenital myasthenia in the Jack Russell terrier. *Veterinary Record* **103**, 433.

Palmer, A.C., Lennon, V.A., Beadle, C. and Goodyear, J.V. (1980) Autoimmune form of myasthenia gravis in a juvenile Yorkshire terrier × Jack Russell terrier hybrid contrasted with congenital (non-autoimmune) myasthenia gravis of the Jack Russell. *Journal of Small Animal Practice* **21**, 359–364.

Peeters, M.E., Venker-van Haagen, A.J., Goedegebuure, S.A. and Wolvekamp, W.Th.C. (1991) Dysphagia in Bouviers associated with muscular dystrophy; evaluation of 24 cases. *Veterinary Quarterly* **13**, 65–73.

Presthus, J. and Lindboe, C.F. (1988) Polymyositis in two German wire haired pointer littermates. *Journal of Small Animal Practice* **29**, 239–248.

Rafiquzzaman, M., Svenkerud, R., Strande, A. and Hauge, J.G. (1976) Glycogenosis in the dog. *Acta Veterinaria Scandinavica* **17**, 196–209.

Rand, J.S. and O'Brien, P.J. (1987) Exercise-induced malignant hyperthermia in an English springer spaniel. *Journal of the American Veterinary Medical Association* **190**, 1013–1014.

Robins, G.M., Wilkinson, G.T., Menrath, V.H., Atwell, R.B. and Riesz, G. (1982) Long term survival following embolectomy in two cats with aortic embolism. *Journal of Small Animal Practice* **23**, 165–174.

Robinson, R. (1992) Spasticity in the Devon rex cat. *Veterinary Record* **132**, 302.

Schunk, K.L. (1984) Feline polymyopathy. American College of Veterinary Internal Medicine Proceedings of the 2nd Annual forum, and 12th annual scientific program. Washington, pp. 197–200.

Scott-Moncrieff, J.C., Cook, J.R. and Lantz, G.C. (1990) Acquired myasthenia gravis in a cat with thymoma. *Journal of the American Veterinary Medical Association* **196**, 1291–1293.

Shelton, G.D., Cardinet, G.H. and Bandman, E. (1987) Canine masticatory muscle disorders: a study of 29 cases. *Muscle and Nerve* **10**, 753–766.

Shelton, G.D., Willard, M.D., Cardinet, G.H. and Lindstrom, J. (1990) Acquired myasthenia gravis. Selective involvement of esophageal, pharyngeal, and facial muscles. *Journal of Veterinary Internal Medicine* **4**, 281–284.

Shires, P.K., Nafe, L.A. and Hulse, D.A. (1983) Myotonia in a Staffordshire terrier. *Journal of the American Veterinary Medical Association* **183**, 229–232.

Shores, A., Redding, R.W., Braund, K.G. and Simpson, S.T. (1986) Myotonia congenita in a Chow Chow pup. *Journal of the American Veterinary Medical Association* **188**, 532–533.

Simpson, S.T. and Braund, K.G. (1985) Myotonic dystrophy-like disease in a dog. *Journal of the American Veterinary Medical Association* **186**, 495–498.

Steiss, J.E., Braund, K.G. and Clark, E.G. (1987) Neuromuscular effects of acute 2,4-dichlorophenoxyacetic acid (2,4-D) exposure in dogs. *Journal of the Neurological Sciences* **78**, 295–301.

Targett, M.P., Franklin, R.J.M., Olby, N.J., Dyce, J., Anderson, J.R. and Houlton, J.E.F.H. (1994) Central core myopathy in a great dane. *Journal of Small Animal Practice* **35**, 100–104.

Trojaberg, W. and Flagstad, A. (1982) A hereditary neuromuscular disorder in dogs. *Muscle and Nerve* **5**, 30–38.

Uggla, A., Dubey, J.P., Lundmark, G. and Olson, P. (1989) Encephalomyelitis and myositis in a boxer puppy due to a *Neospora*-like infection. *Veterinary Parasitology* **32**, 255–260.

Valentine, B.A., Cooper, B.J., Cummings, J.F. and deLahunta, A. (1986) Progressive muscular dystrophy in a golden retriever dog: light microscope and ultrastructural features at 4 and 8 months. *Acta Neuropathology* (Berlin) **71**, 301–310.

Van Vleet, J.F. (1975) Experimentally induced vitamin E–selenium deficiency in the growing dog. *Journal of the American Veterinary Medical Association* **166**, 769–774.

Vaughan, L.C. (1969) Gracilis muscle injury in greyhounds. *Journal of Small Animal Practice* **10**, 363–375.

Vaughan, L.C. (1979) Muscle and tendon injuries in dogs. *Journal of Small Animal Practice* **20**, 711–736.

Vos, J.H., Van der Linde-Sipman, J.S. and Goedegebuure, S.A. (1986) Dystrophy-like myopathy in a cat. *Journal of Comparative Pathology* **96**, 335–341.

Wallace, M.E. and Palmer, A.C. (1984) Recessive mode of inheritance in myasthenia gravis in the Jack Russell terrier. *Veterinary Record* **114**, 350.

Walton, J.N. and Gardner-Medwin, D. (1981) Muscular dystrophies and the myotonias. In: *Disorders of Voluntary Muscle*, 4th edn (Ed. J. Walton). Churchill Livingstone, Edinburgh, p. 482.

Walvoort, H.C., Van Nes, J.J., Stokhof, A.A. and Wolvekamp, W.T.C. (1984) Canine glycogen storage disease type II. A clinical study of four affected Lapland dogs. *Journal of the American Animal Hospital Association* **20**, 279–286.

Warren, H.B. and Carpenter, J.L. (1984) Fibrodysplasia ossificans in three cats. *Veterinary Pathology* **21**, 495–499.

Wentink, G.H., Hartman, W. and Koeman, J.P. (1974) Three cases of myotonia in a family of Chows. *Tijdschrift voor Diergeneeskunde* **99**, 729–731.

Wentink, G.H., Van der Linde-Sipman, J.S., Meijer, A.E.F.H., Kamphuisen, H.A.C., Van Vorstenbosch, C.J.A.H.V., Hartman, W. and Hendriks, H.J. (1972) Myopathy with a possible recessive X-linked inheritance in a litter of Irish terriers. *Veterinary Pathology* **9**, 328–349.

Whitney, J.C. (1958) Progressive muscular dystrophy in the dog. *Veterinary Record* **70**, 611–613.

Wilkes, M.K., McKerrell, R.E., Patterson, R.C. and Palmer, A.C. (1987) Ultrastructure of motor end-plates in canine congenital myasthenia gravis. *Journal of Comparative Pathology* **97**, 247–256.

Wright, J.A., Smyth, J.B.A., Brownlie, S.E. and Robins, M. (1987) A myopathy associated with muscle hypertonicity in the cavalier King Charles spaniel. *Journal of Comparative Pathology* **97**, 559–565.

44

Diseases of Bones and Joints

C. May

Structure and function of bones and joints	719	Bone diseases of cats	739
History	723	**JOINT DISEASES**	**740**
Physical examination	724	Joint diseases of dogs	741
Investigative techniques	725	Joint diseases of cats	755
BONE DISEASES	**727**		
Bone diseases of dogs	727		

STRUCTURE AND FUNCTION OF BONES AND JOINTS

Bones

Bones serve three major functions:

1. As lever arms for the action of muscles in movement and in resisting the force of gravity;
2. As protection and support for adjacent organs;
3. As a reservoir of minerals, particularly of calcium and phosphates, for metabolic homeostasis.

Bones may be classified as long bones (limb bones), flat bones (skull, scapula) and irregular bones (vertebrae, pelvis). Irregular bones may be simplistically regarded as a mixture of the bone types found in long bones and in flat bones.

Bone, like all connective tissues, consists of cells and fibrous elements (collagen) suspended in a matrix. It is mineralization of the matrix which most clearly distinguishes bone from all other connective tissues. Most mature bone can be classified as either cortical bone or cancellous bone. Cortical bone and cancellous bone differ primarily by the way in which the bone matrix is deposited. In cancellous bone, osteoblasts deposit the matrix in plate-like formation. The plate-like structures aggregate in stacks to form bony spicules typical of cancellous bone. The spicules associate loosely with one another and with bone marrow elements giving cancellous bone an elastic structure which is shock-absorptive but which lacks strength. Conversely, cortical bone is formed from a strong and relatively rigid system of bone cylinders referred to as Haversian systems or osteones. Each osteone consists of concentric cylinders of bone matrix surrounding a central blood vessel. The collagen fibres in each cylinder are arranged in helical fashion and the direction of the helix in adjacent cylinders is reversed so that adjacent sets of collagen fibres lie approximately at right angles to one another. It is this organization of the collagen fibres that lends great strength to cortical bone.

There are primarily three cell types in bone, osteoblasts, osteoclasts and osteocytes. Osteoblasts are round cells with an abundant endoplasmic reticulum signifying their role in the synthesis and secretion of bone matrix. As a result of their own activity, they become entombed within the matrix but continue to communicate with neighbouring cells via small cytoplasmic processes. The cytoplasmic processes extend along channels, called canaliculi, that ramify through the mineralized matrix. Once entombed, the cells cease their secretory function and lose their abundant endoplasmic reticulum. They are henceforth known as osteocytes. The precise function of osteocytes is at present unclear although they may contribute to a cellular pump mechanism for transporting labile calcium out of bone and into the extracellular fluid (Capen and Weisbrode, 1982). The third type of bone cell is the osteoclast. Osteoclasts are large multinucleate cells located on the surface of mineralized matrix.

DISEASES OF BONES AND JOINTS

They are responsible for the bone resorption which occurs during remodelling, as a normal part of calcium and phosphate homeostasis and in pathological processes characterized by excessive bone resorption.

Much of the external surface of bones is surrounded by a fibrous capsule called the periosteum. A second fibrous membrane, the endosteum, separates diaphyseal cortical bone from its marrow cavity.

Bone tissue is unique in having an inorganic mineral component deposited within its organic matrix. The mineral content of the bone matrix consists of small crystals of hydroxyapatite, with many impurities. The bone matrix is continually resorbed by osteoclasts whereas osteoblasts simultaneously deposit new bone matrix. This constant state of flux is known as remodelling. Remodelling contributes not only to the growth and development of bone but also to the repair of damaged bone and to the homeostasis of normal mature bone. The turnover of normal bone by the remodelling process ensures that it does not fatigue and fracture along lines of mechanical stress. Bone turnover is primarily governed by three hormones. Parathyroid, vitamin D and calcitonin (Figs 44.1 and 44.2). The function of these hormones is to maintain serum calcium levels in the normal range of 2.3–2.8 mmol l^{-1}. Parathyroid hormone (PTH) and vitamin D function together to elevate serum calcium levels whereas calcitonin functions to depress serum calcium levels. It is the balance between these hormones that maintains serum calcium homeostasis. PTH increases circulating calcium by its actions in the kidneys, in the small intestine and in bone. In the kidneys, PTH increases active uptake of calcium whilst depressing active phosphate absorption, resulting in increased phosphate excretion in the urine (phosphaturic effect). In the small intestine, PTH increases absorption of calcium from the diet by an energy dependent mechanism. In bone, PTH increases the rate of bone resorption over the rate of bone deposition causing a net movement of mineral from the bone reservoir into the serum. Vitamin D$_3$ is a hormone produced in the skin under the influence of ultraviolet radiation or

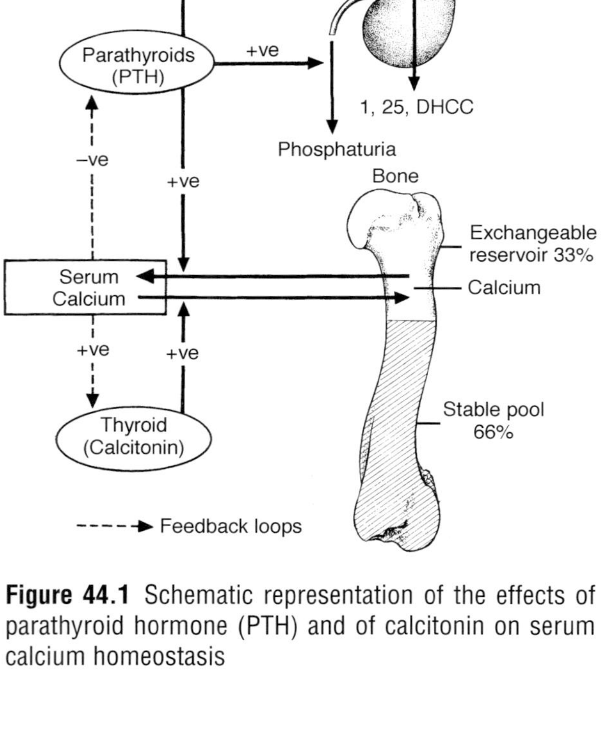

Figure 44.1 Schematic representation of the effects of parathyroid hormone (PTH) and of calcitonin on serum calcium homeostasis

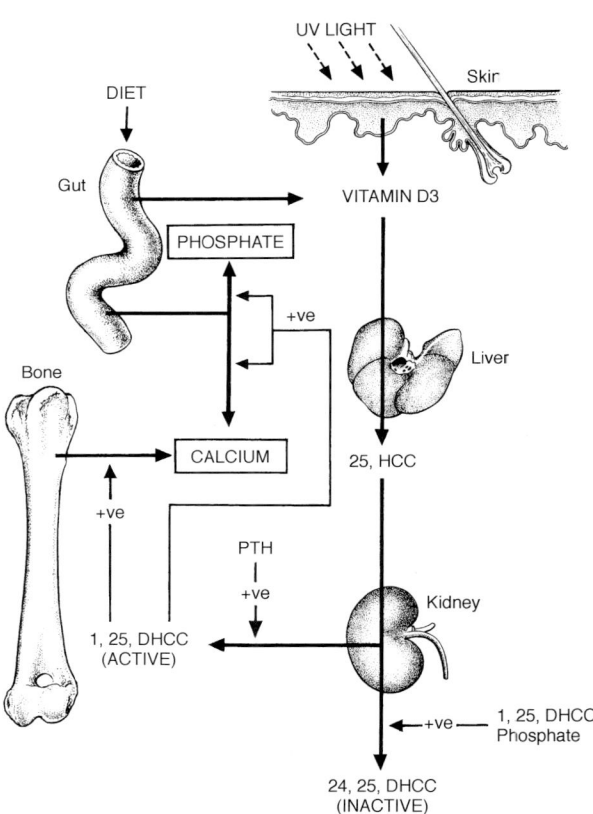

Figure 44.2 Schematic representation of vitamin D metabolism and the effects of vitamin D on serum calcium homeostasis. HCC = hydroxycholecalciferol, DHCC = dihydroxycholecalciferol, PTH = parathyroid hormone

absorbed from the diet in the small intestine. Dogs have a daily dietary requirement for vitamin D of 450 iu kg^{-1} (Hazewinkel, 1989). Vitamin D_3 is processed in the liver and in the kidney to form its functional metabolite 1,25-dihydroxycholecalciferol (1,25-DHCC) or its inactive form 24,25-dihydroxycholecalciferol (24,25-DHCC). 1,25-DHCC interacts with PTH in the kidneys, small intestine and bone to cause a net increase in serum calcium levels. Calcitonin is a thyroid peptide hormone which acts directly on osteoclasts to decrease the rate of bone resorption in relation to the rate of bone deposition. The net effect of this is to depress serum calcium levels. All these hormonal systems are controlled by feedback loops which maintain both serum calcium and serum phosphate homeostasis (Capen and Weisbrode, 1982).

Bone growth

Endochondral ossification is the development of bone by the production of a cartilage model which is subsequently calcified, ossified and remodelled (Olsson, 1982). It is an important method of bone production, responsible for the gain in length of long bones (Fig. 44.3). Briefly, chondrocytes from the reserve zone of the growth plate sporadically undergo mitosis to form proliferating columns of flattened cells which secrete cartilage matrix. The proliferation of cells and secretion of matrix are responsible for the gain in bone length. In the zone of degeneration, the chondrocytes begin to accumulate calcium within their mitochondria and their glycogen stores become gradually depleted (zone of maturation). Once the chondrocyte glycogen stores are exhausted, calcium is released from the cells and the surrounding matrix becomes calcified. Vascularization of the calcified matrix marks the beginning of the metaphysis where remodelling into mature bone occurs.

Membranous ossification is bone growth under a fibrous membrane, usually the periosteum, which occurs without a cartilaginous precursor. Membranous ossification is responsible for the development of flat bones and for the increase in diameter of long bones.

Joints

Joints are formed when two or more bones are united by fibrous, elastic or cartilaginous tissue, or by a combination of these tissues (Evans and Christensen, 1979). Joints are most often classified according to the type of motion they allow (Table 44.1). For the purposes of this chapter the synovial joints are of most importance and these can be further classified (Table 44.2). Not all synovial joints conform exactly to this classification and some synovial joints may fit into more than one category. Synovial joints perform two major functions.

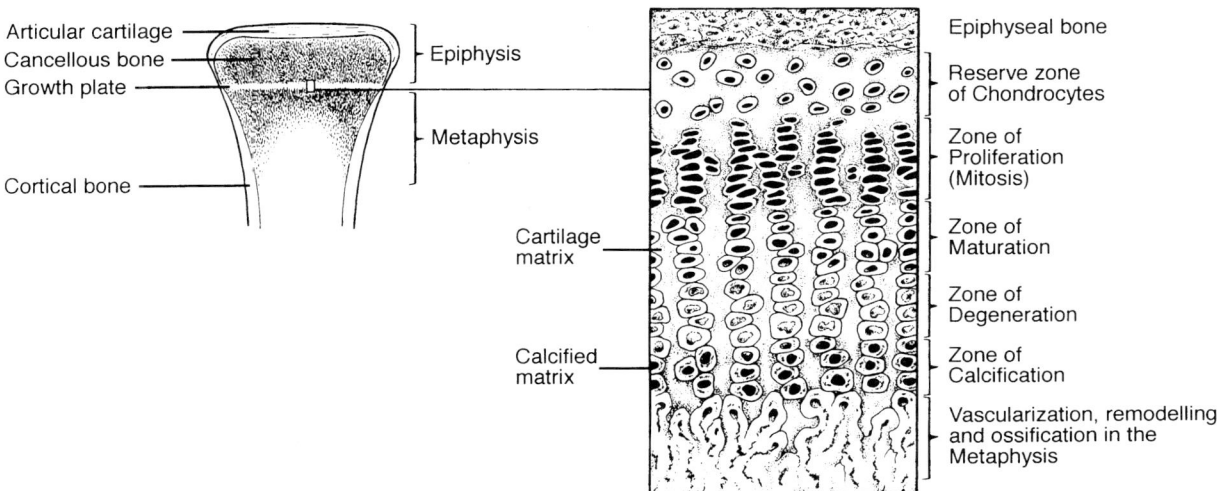

Figure 44.3 Schematic representation of endochondral ossification in the growth plate of a long bone

1. They facilitate almost frictionless mobility.
2. They provide stability to prevent abnormal movements and slipping when loaded.

Figure 44.4 is a schematic representation of a synovial joint. The adjacent ends of the bones are covered with a specialized connective tissue, hyaline cartilage, which provides an ultra-low friction weight-bearing and gliding surface. The hyaline cartilage is tightly adherent to an underlying plate of dense cortical bone known as the articular end plate and beneath this lies the shock-absorptive

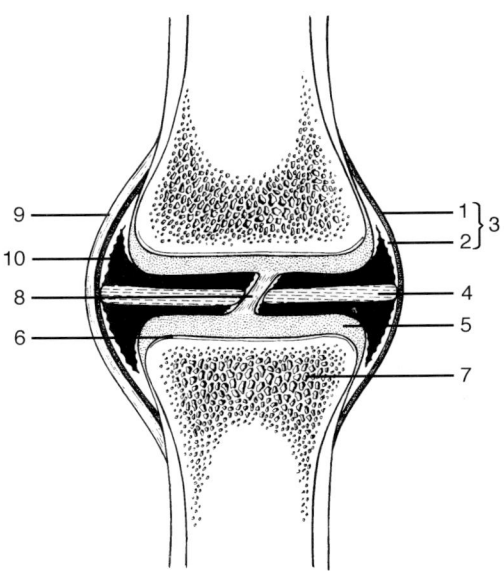

Figure 44.4 Schematic representation of a synovial joint. The fibrous joint capsule (1) and the synovial membrane (2) together make up the articular capsule (3). In some joints, menisci (4) are interposed between the joint surfaces. Articular cartilage (5) is supported on a plate of dense bone, the epiphyseal plate (6), which is in turn seated on cancellous bone (7). Ligaments may traverse the joint (8) or occur as part of the joint capsule (9). The joint cavity (10) contains synovial fluid.

Table 44.1 Classification of joints according to the degree of movement between the opposing bones in the joint

Type of joint	Mobility	Examples
Synarthroses	Immovable	Suture lines of the skull, syndesmoses (e.g. hyoid-petrous temporal bone), gomphoses (tooth/bone)
Amphiarthroses	Partially movable	Intervertebral discs, sternebrae, pelvic and mandibular symphyses
Diarthroses	Freely movable	All synovial joints

Table 44.2 Classification of diarthroses according to the anatomy of the articulating surfaces

Type of diarthrosis	Examples	Major features
Enarthrosis (Ball and socket)	Hip, Shoulder	Permit flexion, extension abduction, adduction and rotation
Ellipsoidal	Radial–carpal	Similar to enarthrosis, but the joint surfaces are ellipsoidal rather than spheroidal
Sellar joint (Saddle shaped)	Interphalangeal	Opposing surfaces of the joint are convex in one direction and concave in another (usually at right angles to each other)
Condylarthrosis (Condylar)	Stifle	One joint surface has rounded prominences which fit into depressions in the adjacent surface. Functionally, condylar joints often resemble hinge joints
Ginglymus (Hinge)	Elbow	Permit flexion, extension and limited rotation
Trochoid (Pivot)	Atlanto-axial	Primarily permit rotation
Arthrodial (Plane joint)	Intercarpal, Intertarsal	Flat surfaced joints. Permit a slight gliding action

cancellous bone. The entire joint is surrounded by a specialized structure called the articular capsule. The articular capsule consists of an outer fibrous layer called the joint capsule and an inner layer, the synovial membrane. The tissue space within the articular capsule is the joint cavity and this contains a very small amount of viscous synovial fluid. Synovial fluid is essentially a transudate of blood to which the large glycoprotein molecule, hyaluronate, is added by synoviocytes. Contrary to popular belief, hyaluronate is not of major importance in lubricating weight-bearing cartilage surfaces of the joint. When working under load, these surfaces are primarily lubricated by water displaced from the loaded cartilage; so-called hydrostatic lubrication. Hyaluronate serves mainly as a boundary lubricant, by binding to the surfaces of intra-articular structures and preventing them from making contact with one another. Boundary lubrication is important at the initiation of movement, in joints working under light compressive loads, and in reducing friction developed by synovial membrane–cartilage, synovial membrane–bone and synovial membrane–synovial membrane contact. In this respect it is worth noting that even unlubricated cartilage on cartilage movement is low friction and most friction in the joint arises from the relatively large area of synovial membrane–synovial membrane contact. This is exacerbated in disease states in which the efficiency of boundary lubrication is reduced due to changes in the synovial fluid (Le Gros Clark, 1975).

In addition to its role in the formation of synovial fluid, the synovial membrane lining layer contains macrophage-like cells responsible for the phagocytosis of intra-articular debris. The supporting layer of the synovial membrane is highly vascular and contains loose nerve endings, as does the fibrous joint capsule. The nerve endings in the articular capsule contribute to proprioceptive responses that facilitate complex joint movements and provide deep pain responses that protect the joints.

Joint stability is provided by a combination of bone congruency, support from the articular ligaments and capsule, and support from the muscles and tendons surrounding the joint. In most joints, the joint capsule, its associated ligaments and the surrounding muscles and tendons are the prime effectors in maintaining articular integrity. In the stifle and temporomandibular joints of dogs and cats, joint congruency is improved by fibrocartilaginous discoid structures, called menisci, interposed between the articular surfaces. The joint capsule and ligaments consist of dense connective tissue. Most ligaments form as thick bands of parallel collagen fibres within the joint capsule, but some, like the cruciate ligaments of the stifle and the round ligament of the femoral head, are not incorporated into the joint capsule but freely traverse the joint cavity. The tautness of ligaments varies enormously from site to site and is often dependent on the position in which the joint is placed.

In summary, the bones and joints form a rigid structure of support and protection for the soft tissues of the body whilst allowing sufficient movement for locomotion and prehension. In addition, bone serves as an important homeostatic reservoir for calcium and phosphate metabolism.

HISTORY

An accurate history is essential to satisfactory diagnosis of orthopaedic cases. Even the signalment and pedigree history can yield useful information as many bone and joint diseases have well documented age, breed or sex predilections. The primary complaint, including the limb (or limbs) involved, should be noted. The remaining history may usefully be considered in three sections; background history, orthopaedic history and disease specific history.

Background history

The background history is frequently of great help, not only in reaching a diagnosis, but also in formulating a prognosis and treatment plan. Previous illnesses and vaccination status are relevant, whether these are directly related to the locomotor system or not. The relevance of previous orthopaedic disease is obvious but the general health of the animal is also important as some systemic diseases present with skeletal signs and certain bone and joint diseases have systemic manifestations. The prognosis for many skeletal diseases varies with the required function of the animal and it is important to establish whether the animal is kept as a pet, for show purposes or for some form of work. Diet is a pivotal factor in many skeletal disorders. The number of feeds given daily, the amount given in each feed, the constituents of the feed, any dietary supplements that are given and any tit-bits that are fed should all be recorded. Information on the temperament of the patient is frequently useful. Some animals undergo a temperament change associated with persistent pain whereas other, more stoic, animals show no outward signs of distress even in the face of lesions which are presumably quite painful.

Orthopaedic history

Previous history of orthopaedic disease, no matter how ancient, should always be considered pertinent to a current orthopaedic problem. Good examples of this lie in the onset of osteoarthritis in old-age secondary to hip dysplasia, patellar luxation, osteochondrosis or other joint disease in youth and in the predilection of osteosarcoma at old fracture sites.

The onset of disease should be defined by its duration, whether there was a gradual or acute onset of clinical signs and whether or not there has been any progressive change in the lameness. When there is an acute onset of disease, it should be established whether this was associated with particular trauma, whether it occurred during normal exercise or whether the event leading to lameness was unnoticed. In some skeletal diseases the lameness may be intermittent or migratory, and in many joint diseases the lameness worsens following periods of rest or vigorous exercise. Severe and prolonged stiffness after rest, associated with inflammatory joint disease, should be differentiated from short-lived stiffness after rest (articular gelling) which is most commonly encountered in association with degenerative joint diseases. Stiffness after rest may also occur with certain muscle disorders.

When dealing with a chronic disease it is extremely important to note the nature of any previous treatments and the response, if any, to those treatments. Specific points of history are sometimes useful in reaching a definitive diagnosis from a list of differential diagnoses. Examples of such points include known exposure to sheep ticks in cases of suspected Lyme disease, a high liver diet in hypervitaminosis A of cats and recent gastrointestinal disease in some cases of polyarthritis.

PHYSICAL EXAMINATION

More than one clinical disorder may co-exist and contribute to the lameness in any one animal and musculoskeletal abnormalities may be only one aspect of a multisystemic disease. All orthopaedic examinations should therefore be precluded by a thorough general examination and, in some cases, the orthopaedic examination should be supplemented by a neurological examination. Comparison of an affected limb with the contralateral limb is of recurring benefit in all evaluations of animals with musculoskeletal disorders affecting locomotion.

An orthopaedic examination begins with observation, paying particular attention to the animal's general body condition, conformation, limb positions, musculoskeletal symmetry and any outward signs of injury, such as puncture wounds, lacerations or contusions. Muscle atrophy is commonly seen in chronic lameness cases, but severe, rapidly progressing or highly localized muscle wastage may be indicative of neuromuscular disease rather than skeletal disease. Abnormal postures may be adopted to compensate for painful lesions; dogs with elbow arthritis will frequently stand with the elbows adducted, but will circumduct the elbows during the swinging leg phase of the gait. Weight transfer from the affected limb to the contralateral limb may cause excessive splaying of the toes on the unaffected side. Similarly dogs with bilateral hindlimb or forelimb pain may compensate by shifting their weight forwards or backwards. Dogs and cats with stifle or hock pain usually stand with a very straight hindlimb conformation; this is often more accentuated with disease of the hock than with disease of the stifle. If there is bilateral hock or stifle pain, especially in large breeds of dog, the animal will often continually shift weight from one limb to the other.

All lame animals should be observed in locomotion. Cats should be observed in free moving exercise in a secure consulting area. Dogs of all sizes should be observed whilst leash-exercised at the walk and trot. It is sometimes helpful to observe an animal through a prolonged period of exercise to appreciate exercise-related changes in the lameness. In addition to noting which limb, or limbs, the animal is lame on, the object of observing the animal in motion is to identify and note specific abnormalities of gait such as shortened stride length, limited voluntary movement of joints through their range of motion, abnormal limb movements during the swinging leg phase or supporting leg phase of the stride, whether abnormalities of gait are consistent in every stride, whether there is any progressive change in limb usage with exercise and whether a painful lesion is present to such an extent that the dog or cat resents exercise.

After observing the animal both standing and in locomotion, individual attention should be paid to observation, manipulation and palpation of the spine and all the bones and joints of the limbs even in animals lame in only one leg. It is often helpful to reserve examination of an obviously affected limb until last. In this way one can familiarize oneself with the normal limbs of the animal and gauge the response of the animal to being handled in an unfamiliar environment. Reactions to manipulation of the abnormal limb are then more readily placed in context.

Careful palpation of the limbs will reveal subtle changes in muscle symmetry, joint size and bone contour not readily detectable by observation alone. Every bone and every joint must be palpated for signs of heat, pain, swelling and crepitus. The nature of a detectable swelling should be characterized as fluid, soft tissue or bone. Each joint should be manipulated through its normal range of movement and any reduced range of movement noted. Joints should also be manipulated for abnormal movements resulting in luxations or subluxations. Good examples of such manipulations include the cranial drawer sign detectable in the subluxating stifle joint of animals with rupture of the cranial cruciate ligament, displacement of the patella in dogs and cats with patellar luxation and hyperextension of the carpus or hock in luxations and subluxations of the carpal joints or tarsal joints. The ease with which luxated or subluxated joints can be reduced should also be noted.

It is often necessary to sedate or anaesthetize orthopaedic patients for further examinations, such as radiology or arthrocentesis and this is a good opportunity to perform a second orthopaedic examination with the patient fully relaxed. Useful information is frequently forthcoming from such an examination; for example, large breeds of dog with rupture of the cranial cruciate ligament often have a palpable drawer sign when anaesthetized even if no such sign is palpable with the animal fully conscious. Examination under sedation should always be additional to, and never a substitute for, examination of the fully conscious patient.

It is rarely possible to establish a definitive diagnosis of bone and joint disorders from the history and clinical examination alone. A list of differential diagnoses should be considered at the end of the clinical examination and procedures devised to investigate the clinical findings further.

INVESTIGATIVE TECHNIQUES

Diagnostic imaging

Radiography is indicated in the investigation of virtually all orthopaedic problems in the dog and cat. Good quality radiographs are essential for adequate interpretation of bone and joint disorders. At least two views should be taken of any one region under investigation and these should ideally be perpendicular to one another. In areas where the anatomical configuration is complex, such as the elbow joint, there may be benefit in taking oblique views in addition to the standard views. Further information may be gained by radiographing joints in varying degrees of flexion or extension. With ligament injuries it is often useful to take stressed radiographs to demonstrate possible subluxation of a joint. Contrast studies of use in the radiographic evaluation of orthopaedic patients include myelography (Widmer and Blevins, 1991) and contrast arthrography (Suter and Carb, 1969; Muhumuza et al., 1988; van Bree, 1990). Orthopaedic radiographs should always be viewed under bright light conditions as well as on a normal viewer.

In some cases, additional survey radiographs should be considered. Trauma patients and those with bone tumours warrant radiographic investigation of the thorax and abdomen. Certain orthopaedic diseases may present with one clinically apparent lesion while other, clinically silent, lesions exist elsewhere. For example, osteochondrosis may present as a single limb lameness, but bilaterally symmetrical lesions can often be demonstrated radiographically and some dogs presenting with unilateral cranial cruciate ligament rupture have subclinical cruciate disease in the contralateral limb. In such cases radiographic surveys of several bones or joints may be indicated to fully evaluate the patient.

Some other diagnostic imaging techniques are helpful in evaluating small animal bone and joint disorders but are not in common use at the present time. Ultrasonography may be used to assess joint effusions and other abnormalities of articular soft tissues (Koski et al., 1990). Bone scintigraphy is a useful method of imaging bone lesions that are not readily appreciated on conventional radiographs (Lamb, 1987; Berg et al., 1990). The technique evaluates the degree of localization of an intravenously administered radioisotope into bone. The uptake of radioisotope is dependent on the local blood supply and metabolic activity of the bone, so scintigraphy provides a functional assessment which complements the structural assessment of conventional radiography. Nuclear magnetic resonance imaging has the potential to produce excellent bone and joint images but the cost may be prohibitive (Stoller and Genant, 1989, Parchman et al., 1989).

■ Arthrocentesis

Arthrocentesis is a simple procedure easily performed in sedated animals and it is often convenient to aspirate synovial fluid at the time of sedation for radiographic investigation (for details of arthrocentesis technique, see Lipowitz, 1985). Synovial fluid analysis is a valuable diagnostic screening test for the investigation of all forms of articular disease (Freemont et al., 1991). Specific indications include investigation of articular effusions, polyarthritis or polyarthralgia, joint stiffness or pain, and migratory arthropathies. There are no absolute contraindications, but asepsis should be maintained at all times and arthrocentesis through damaged or infected skin is to be avoided. The yield of synovial fluid may be small, particularly in cats and toy breeds of dog, and in some cases it is not possible to aspirate fluid even from joints with a significant effusion. Aspirated fluid is transferred to a sterile container or to a sterile container with EDTA as an anticoagulant.

Normal synovial fluid is a clear, viscous, colourless or straw-coloured fluid which does not clot on exposure to air. Synovial fluid from diseased joints is thin, increased in volume and may be turbid. Routine synovial fluid analyses include gross assessment of volume, viscosity, clarity and colour; cytological examination; aerobic and anaerobic culture; assessment of hyaluronate polymerization (mucin clot test); estimation of synovial fluid protein and glucose (and estimation of plasma parameters in parallel) and examination for crystals (Table 44.3). Many other parameters can be assayed in synovial fluid, including proteoglycan components, rheumatoid factor, antinuclear antibodies, immune complexes, immunoglobulins and complement. These parameters are of uncertain diagnostic significance in canine and feline joint diseases.

■ Biopsy

Biopsy of bone or synovial membrane may be necessary to establish a definitive diagnosis. Bone biopsy is most frequently indicated in the investigation of aggressive destructive or proliferative bone lesions. Bone biopsy material can be submitted for aerobic and anaerobic culture, or cut into several thin sections and fixed in buffered formalin for histopathological examination. Biopsies may be obtained as open incisional biopsies, open or closed trephine biopsies or by a closed bone marrow needle biopsy technique (Powers et al., 1988). Some aggressive bone lesions are accompa-

Table 44.3 Synovial fluid analysis in dogs and cats

	Joint status			
	Normal	OA[a]	IJD	BIA
Cytology[b]				
Total cell count ($\times 10^{-9}$ l^{-1})	0–2	1–5	2–>100	20–>200
Mononuclear cells (%)	>95	>90	5–90	<10
PMN (%)	<5	<10	10–95	>90
Biochemistry[c]				
Protein (g dl^{-1})	1–2.5	2–3	2–>5	often >5
Glucose (cf. serum)	equivalent	± reduced	+ reduced	+++ reduced
Mucin clot	good	fair to good	fair to poor	poor

[a]OA, osteoarthritis; IJD, immune-mediated joint disease; BIA, bacterial infective arthritis.
[b]The cytological values quoted are guidelines only; there is considerable overlap in the range of values seen in different disease categories.
[c]In addition to the these tests, synovial fluid should be grossly assessed for appearance (quantity, colour, turbidity and viscosity) and may be submitted for microbiological culture and/or various other assessments (e.g. rheumatoid factor, antinuclear antibodies, crystals).

nied by large amounts of reactive new bone and it is important to ensure that the biopsy material does not consist solely of reactive bone. The diagnostic accuracy of biopsies varies between 66% and 94% (Wykes et al., 1985; Powers et al., 1988). Multiple core biopsies from a single lesion and biopsy of the radiological centre of the lesion rather than the transitional zone both increase the likelihood of an accurate histological diagnosis (Wykes et al., 1985). Complications following bone biopsy include haematoma formation, infection, wound breakdown, local seeding of tumours and pathological fracture (Simon, 1982).

Synovial membrane biopsies can be obtained arthroscopically (May and Bennett, 1991) or at arthrotomy. Although these measures are invasive, it is sometimes necessary to explore joints surgically to establish the definitive diagnosis. Aerobic and anaerobic bacteriological culture of synovial membrane may be more successful than culture of synovial fluid in the investigation of suspected infectious arthropathies (Bennett and Taylor, 1988a). However, success with culture from synovial fluid is dramatically improved if the sample is transferred to blood culture medium before transport to the laboratory. Histological examination of formalin-fixed synovial membrane biopsies is a useful adjunct in the diagnosis of certain arthropathies, particularly the 'immune-mediated' joint diseases.

Haematological, biochemical and serological analyses

Haematological and biochemical profiles may be indicated as part of the preoperative investigation of potential orthopaedic surgical candidates or in the investigation of orthopaedic and rheumatological disorders that present as part of a multisystemic illness. In some instances specific serological tests are indicated, particularly in the investigation of certain rheumatological disorders. Rheumatoid factor, antinuclear antibodies and antibodies to *Borrelia burgdorferi* are some of the more common serological parameters measured in the investigation of joint diseases. It is important to remember that serological parameters merely lend support to a clinical diagnosis and it is the responsibility of the clinician to understand the relevance of any serological tests he or she may request. No single serological parameter is diagnostic for a specific joint disease and laboratory findings should always be considered in association with the history, clinical and radiographic findings.

Bone Diseases

Bone disorders may be classified on an aetiological basis (Table 44.4). The term 'metabolic bone disease' is often used to describe bone diseases with hormonal, nutritional or unknown aetiologies characterized by changes in the rate of production or resorption of bone. This usage is confusing and is best avoided (Watson, 1990). Only diseases of bone associated with constitutional metabolic derangement should be referred to as 'metabolic' bone diseases. Some bone diseases fall into more than one category of classification. For example, the idiopathic bone disease, metaphyseal osteopathy, has an inflammatory component and nutritional secondary hyperparathyroidism has a nutritional aetiology, but is mediated via increased secretion of parathormone by the parathyroid glands.

BONE DISEASES OF DOGS

Constitutional bone disease

Constitutional abnormalities of bone may arise as rare, sporadic events resulting either from new mutations or from the expression of rare recessive traits. Such anomalies are often rapidly removed from the genetic pool. However, some inherited bone anomalies have been positively selected by breeders because they are perceived as desirable. A complex system of classification of constitutional bone anomalies, originally designed for human disorders, has been adapted for use in dogs and cats (Rimoin, 1978; Jezyk, 1985). The system of classification is too extensive to cover here, but certain disease categories are of particular relevance in dogs.

Table 44.4 Classification of bone disease in dogs and cats

Constitutional bone disease
  Osteochondrodysplasias
    Achondroplasia
    Hypochondroplasia
    Chondrodysplasia punctata
    Dyschondrosteosis
    Arthro-ophthalmopathy
    Multiple cartilaginous exostoses
  Dysostoses
    Vertebral segment defects
    Apodia
    Amelia/hemimelia
    Ectrodactyly
    Polydactyly
    Syndactyly
  Chromosomal aberrations
    Mucopolysaccharidoses (rare in dogs)
  Congenital hormonal deficiencies
    Panhypopituitarism
    Growth hormone deficiency
    Hypothyroidism
Traumatic bone disease
  Fractures
  Contusion
Nutritional bone disease
  Nutritional secondary hyperparathyroidism
  Rickets
  Overnutrition
  Hypervitaminosis A (cats)
  Hypovitaminoses
Hormonal bone disease
  Hyperparathyroidism
    Secondary hyperparathyroidism
      Nutritional (qv)
      Renal
    Primary Hyperparathyroidism
      Parathyroid adenoma
      Parathyroid adenocarcinoma (rare)
  Hyperadrenocorticism
  Hyperthyroidism
  Acromegaly
Inflammatory bone disease
  Osteomyelitis
    Bacterial
    Mycotic
    ?Viral
    Metallosis
Bone neoplasia
  Primary benign bone tumours
    Osteoma
    Chondroma
    Multilobular osteoma/chondroma of the skull
  Primary malignant bone tumours
    Osteosarcoma
    Parosteal osteosarcoma (cats)
    Chondrosarcoma
    Fibrosarcoma
    Haemangiosarcoma
    Liposarcoma
    Osteoclastoma
    Primary lymphosarcoma
    Plasma cell myeloma
  Non-osseous tumours invading bone
    From adjacent soft tissues
      Squamous cell carcinoma
      Acanthomatous epulis
      Melanoma
      Fibrosarcoma
      Prostatic carcinoma
      Synovial sarcoma
      Malignant histiocytosis
    By metastasis
      Mammary carcinoma
      Prostatic carcinoma
      Bronchial carcinoma (cats)
Idiopathic bone disease
  Metaphyseal osteopathy
    Cranio-mandibular osteopathy
    Panosteitis
Miscellaneous bone disease
  Hypertrophic pulmonary osteopathy
  Retained cartilaginous cores

Osteochondrodysplasias

Osteochondrodysplasias are abnormalities of cartilage growth and/or bone growth.

Achondroplasia

Achondroplasia is a characteristic of several breeds of dog, including Bulldogs, Boston terriers, Pekingese, Lhasa Apsos and shih tzus. Achondroplasia presents at birth with shortened limbs, flared metaphyses, shortened maxilla and a depressed nasal bridge.

Hypochondroplasia

Hypochondroplasia presents with limb shortening and metaphyseal flaring but no skull abnormalities. This defect has also been selected for in several breeds of which basset hounds, dachshunds and Scottish terriers are typical.

Chondrodysplasia punctata

Osteochondrodysplasias presenting with stippling of the epiphyses (chondrodysplasia punctata) have been reported in Beagles (Rasmussen, 1971) and miniature poodles (Cotchin and Dyce, 1956).

Dyschondrosteosis

A syndrome of Alaskan malamutes characterized by chondrodysplastic dwarfism and inherited as an autosomal recessive trait bears similarities to dyschondrosteosis of humans (Fletch *et al.*, 1973). However, the inherited dyschondrosteosis of Alaskan malamutes is associated with defective zinc metabolism and responds to zinc supplementation at four times the normal dietary requirement (normal = 0.22 mg kg^{-1} daily (juveniles), 0.11 mg kg^{-1} daily (adults)) (Brown *et al.*, 1978). Inherited chondrodysplastic dwarfism has also been reported in Norwegian elkhounds (Bingel and Sande, 1982), English pointers (Whitbread *et al.*, 1983) and Scottish deerhounds (Breur *et al.*, 1989).

Artho-ophthalmopathy

Syndromes of dwarfism, limb deformity and ophthalmopathy, similar to arthro-ophthalmopathy of humans, have been described in Labrador retrievers (Carrig *et al.*, 1988) and samoyeds (Meyers *et al.*, 1983).

Multiple enchondromatosis

An osteochondrodysplasia of bull terriers has been described which radiographically resembles nutritional secondary hyperparathyroidism, but with pathological features suggestive of failed chondrocyte maturation (Watson *et al.*, 1991).

Multiple cartilaginous exostoses (MCE)

MCE arise from disorganized development of cartilaginous or fibrous elements of the skeleton. Affected dogs are often immature and present with palpable, painless, discrete, partially ossified protuberances from bone cortices. Neuromuscular dysfunction occurs only rarely as a result of the developing mass impinging on neighbouring soft tissues. MCE probably arise as a consequence of displacement of developing chondrocytes from the physis into the neighbouring metaphysis. MCE may be diagnosed radiographically as a non-aggressive partially mineralized exostosis. The diagnosis can be confirmed by biopsy. MCE is often an incidental finding without need of treatment, although malignant transformation has been documented (Owen and Bostock, 1971). If required, treatment is by complete surgical resection.

Dysostoses

Dysostoses are malformations or a congenital absence of individual bones. They include vertebral segment defects (e.g. hemivertebra), apodia (absence of a limb), amelia and hemimelia (absences of parts of a limb), ectrodactyly ('lobster claw syndrome'), polydactyly (extra digits) and syndactyly (fusion of bone and/or soft tissue between two or more digits).

Chromosomal aberrations

Chromosomal aberrations are extremely rare in dogs, but more commonly recognized in cats as mucopolysaccharidoses (MPS) (qv cats). Sporadic examples of MPS have been documented in dogs (Jezyk, 1985).

Congenital hormonal deficiencies

Some congenital hormonal deficiencies present with dwarfing syndromes. Panhypopituitarism or growth hormone deficiency dwarfing has been documented in German shepherd dogs (Andresen and Willeberg, 1976). Dwarfism and cretinism associated with congenital hypothyroidism has been reported in boxers (Jezyk, 1985; Saunders and Jezyk, 1991).

Traumatic bone disease

Clinically, most involvement with bone trauma takes the form of fracture repair. The reader is referred to the many suitable surgical textbooks for full discussion of the topic (see Further Reading).

Nutritional bone disease

Nutritional secondary hyperparathyroidism

Excessive secretion of parathyroid hormone (PTH) in nutritional secondary hyperparathyroidism is a response to dietary deficiency of calcium. The deficiency may be exacerbated by high levels of dietary phosphates. Persistently depleted serum calcium levels lead to chronic and excessive secretion of PTH which maintains serum calcium levels within the normal range, but at the expense of bone mineralization (see Structure and Function of Bones).

Nutritional secondary hyperparathyroidism is seen most commonly in immature, rapidly growing breeds of dog, fed on a predominantly meat diet. It is occasionally seen in breeding bitches maintained on an inappropriate diet for prolonged periods. Affected dogs present with bone pain and lameness which may be mild to severe. Pathological fractures may occur in the limbs or vertebrae following minimal trauma. Vertebral fractures may result in neurological abnormalities. Some affected dogs are unable, or unwilling, to stand. Resorption of bone from the mandible may result in the loss of teeth and increased pliability of the jaw, but this is most commonly reported in adult dogs with renal secondary hyperparathyroidism.

Serum calcium and phosphate evaluations are of limited diagnostic value as they remain within the normal range in many animals with nutritional secondary hyperparathyroidism. Serum alkaline phosphatase levels may be elevated, but this is a non-specific finding associated with increased bone turnover. A radiological skeletal survey demonstrates poor mineralization of the bones, which have an opacity similar to that of surrounding soft tissues ('ghost bones'). The cortices are thinned and they may appear lamellated. Pathological fractures may be seen. The area of primary calcification adjacent to the physis may be seen as a relatively well mineralized band (Riser, 1964) (Fig. 44.5). A history of dietary calcium insufficiency (particularly in a dog of susceptible size and age), the characteristic radiological findings and raised serum alkaline phosphatase levels are sufficient to establish a diagnosis of nutritional secondary hyperparathyroidism.

DISEASES OF BONES AND JOINTS

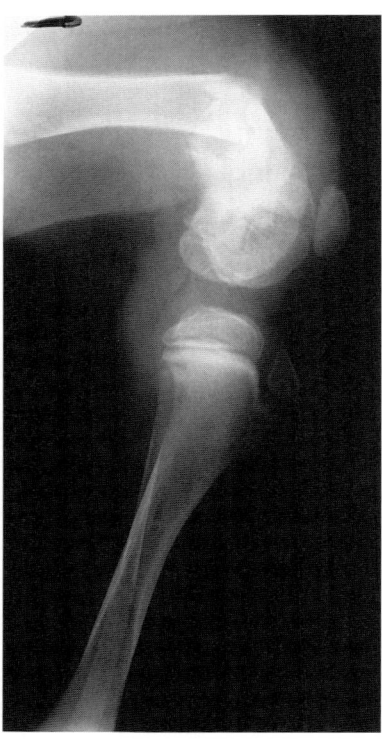

Figure 44.5 Medial-lateral radiograph of the stifle joint of a dog with nutritional secondary hyperparathyroidism. There is cortical thinning and lamellation consistent with osteopenia. There is a pathological fracture of the distal femoral diaphysis.

Rickets

Rickets is a juvenile form of osteomalacia most frequently associated with dietary deficiency of calcium, phosphate and vitamin D. The condition is now extremely rare. Diagnosis of rickets centres on a history of dietary insufficiency and characteristic radiographic changes which include widening of the physeal zone of cartilage due to delayed endochondral ossification and flaring of the metaphyses (Fig. 44.6). Rickets is managed by providing a normal balanced diet (see nutritional secondary hyperparathyroidism). Vitamin D supplements should only be given together with adequate feeding of calcium and phosphates. Rickets-like syndromes are sometimes seen in constitutional osteochondrodysplasias.

Overnutrition and bone disease

Feeding of high calorie diets and excesses of protein and calcium to growing dogs are associated with increased risk of a variety of bone disorders

Nutritional secondary hyperparathyroidism is managed by providing a normal balanced diet containing calcium and phosphate at approximately 1% of the dry matter weight of the diet, in a calcium/phosphate ratio of 1:1 to 1.2:1. Most commercially available diets are adequate for this purpose. During the recovery phase of the disease, additional calcium may be provided to increase the dietary calcium/phosphate ratio to 2:1. Vitamin D supplementation is usually unnecessary and may be harmful. The prognosis is limited by secondary injuries resulting from pathological fractures. Most uncomplicated cases have a good prognosis, but require skilled nursing care to avoid further fracture injury and decubitus ulcer formation. Many dogs show clinical improvement within one week of dietary correction, but they should be confined for at least one month as complete recovery may take several weeks.

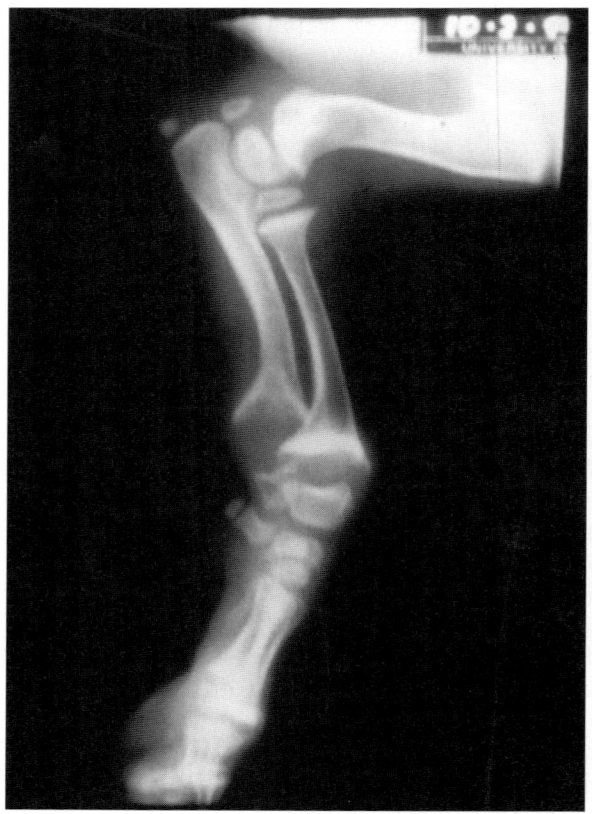

Figure 44.6 Medial-lateral radiograph of the forelimb of a puppy with rickets. There is a wide band of growth plate cartilage and flaring of the metaphyses.

including panosteitis, metaphyseal osteopathy and osteochondroses causing retarded physeal growth (Hedhammer *et al.*, 1974; Hazewinkel *et al.*, 1985; Hazewinkel, 1989). Hypervitaminosis A is rare in dogs and most commonly causes skeletal disease in cats (see below).

Hypovitaminoses

Skeletal diseases associated with hypovitaminoses are extremely rare in both dogs and cats. Apart from the aforementioned association with rickets, hypovitaminosis D may cause osteoporosis. Hypovitaminosis A has been associated with lameness and bone deformity (Bennett, 1976). Neither dogs nor cats have a dietary requirement for vitamin C and there is no conclusive evidence of skeletal disease associated with vitamin C deficiency in either species.

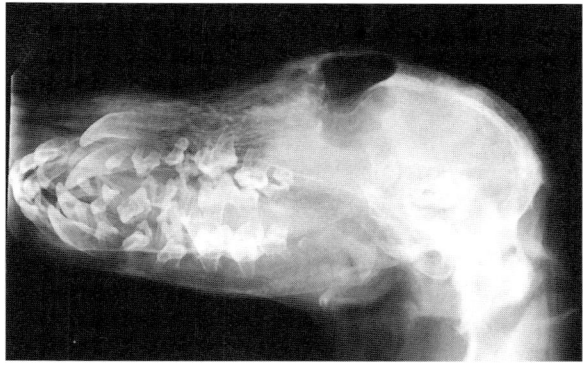

Figure 44.7 Lateral radiograph of the skull of a 5-month-old Afghan hound with renal secondary hyperparathyroidism. Note the mottled appearance of the bone particularly over the cranium and the reduced density of the bone of the mandible when compared to the teeth.

■ Hormonal bone disease

Hyperparathyroidism

Three forms of hyperparathyroidism are recognized:

1. Nutritional secondary hyperparathyroidism (see Nutritional bone disorders);
2. Renal secondary hyperparathyroidism;
3. Primary hyperparathyroidism.

Renal secondary hyperparathyroidism

Renal secondary hyperparathyroidism occurs as a result of reduced glomerular filtration in progressive renal disease leading to retention of phosphate. Persistent elevation of serum phosphate has a chronic depressive effect on serum calcium levels resulting in parathyroid stimulation. Impaired renal metabolism of vitamin D in chronic renal disease may lead to reduced production of 1,25-dihydroxycholecalciferol and diminished intestinal absorption of dietary calcium which exacerbates the effects of excessive PTH secretion. Most commonly, renal secondary hyperparathyroidism is seen in aged dogs with chronic renal insufficiency, but it may also be seen in young dogs with congenital renal abnormalities.

Bone resorption in renal secondary hyperparathyroidism is often seen first in the cancellous bones of the head. Resorption of bone from the maxilla gives rise to 'rubber jaw' in which the mandibles become pliable but painful to manipulate. Pathological fractures may occur. The predominant clinical signs are usually associated with chronic renal failure rather than bone disease.

Serum evaluations of calcium and phosphate must be interpreted with care. Most dogs with chronic renal failure have normal or elevated serum phosphate concentrations. Only rarely are serum calcium concentrations depressed and in some cases there may even be hypercalcaemia.

A diagnosis of renal secondary hyperparathyroidism is confirmed by the characteristic radiological changes and confirmation of chronic renal failure. The radiological interpretation of bone changes is essentially similar to that described for nutritional secondary hyperparathyroidism. Mandibular involvement manifests radiologically with reduced mineral opacity surrounding the tooth roots. The skull may have a 'moth-eaten' appearance (Fig. 44.7).

Management of dogs with renal secondary hyperparathyroidism should be directed at management of the underlying renal disease (see Chapter 41). The prognosis is generally poor because of the progressive renal disease.

Primary hyperparathyroidism

Primary hyperparathyroidism is rare. Excessive PTH secretion in primary hyperparathyroidism is most commonly attributable to a chief cell adenoma in the parathyroid glands or, occasionally, in cranial mediastinal ectopic parathyroid tissue. Parathyroid carcinomas are extremely rare. The clinical and radiological skeletal abnormalities are similar to those seen in renal secondary hyperparathyroidism. Dogs with primary hyperparathyroidism usually have a consistent and substantial elevation in serum calcium levels (3.5 mmol l^{-1} or above) and serum phosphate levels are usually low, or in the low normal range. Since primary hyperparathyroidism is relatively rare other more common differential diagnoses of hypercalcaemia should be considered (see Chapter 39). Treatment of primary hyperparathyroidism is by surgical excision of the neoplasm. Care must be taken to ensure that residual normal parathyroid tissue is left intact. Reflex hypocalcaemia may occur during the postoperative phase due to negative feedback suppression of normal parathyroid tissue.

Other hormonal bone diseases

Secondary osteoporosis may occur in hyperadrenocorticism, hyperthyroidism and acromegaly. The skeletal disorder is usually of minor importance when compared to the other clinical manifestations of these syndromes.

■ Inflammatory bone disease

Bacterial osteomyelitis

Bacterial osteomyelitis usually presents with an obvious lameness and a localized painful and swollen bone lesion. The disease may or may not be accompanied by systemic signs of infection, including local lymphadenopathy, pyrexia, depression and inappetence. In chronic cases there may be weight loss and discharging sinus tracts may develop. Joint infection may occur in association with infection of a neighbouring bone and it may be difficult to determine whether infective arthritis or osteomyelitis was the primary event. It is rare for bacterial osteomyelitis to spread from one bone to another across a joint.

Staphylococcus aureus is the most frequently isolated bacterium from bone infections of dogs (Caywood *et al.*, 1978) but many other bacteria have been associated with bacterial osteomyelitis. Mixed infections may occur, and in some cases both aerobic and anaerobic bacteria are present simultaneously.

Bacterial invasion of bone may occur by any of three routes:

1. Haematogenous spread;
2. Invasion from local soft tissue infection;
3. By direct penetration (usually iatrogenic or as a result of an open fracture).

Bone inflammation resulting from bacterial infection is characterized by leucocytic infiltration, phagocytosis of the infecting organisms and the release of proteolytic enzymes which cause further local tissue injury. If the infection is not controlled by this inflammatory response, bacteria persist and the suppurative lesion expands within the affected bone. Localized ischaemia may be a contributory factor in the establishment of some cases of bacterial osteomyelitis. In other cases ischaemia occurs as a secondary event due to intraosseous vascular thrombosis. Severe localized ischaemia may lead to bone death and sequestrum formation. Draining sinuses develop in chronic lesions.

Haematological and serum biochemical analyses are often of little help in confirming a suspected diagnosis of bacterial osteomyelitis. Often there is no significant change in the leucogram. Some animals have a neutrophilia and a left shift, but this is usually mild.

Radiologically, bacterial osteomyelitis usually has an aggressive pattern of bone destruction and/or new bone production (Fig. 44.8).

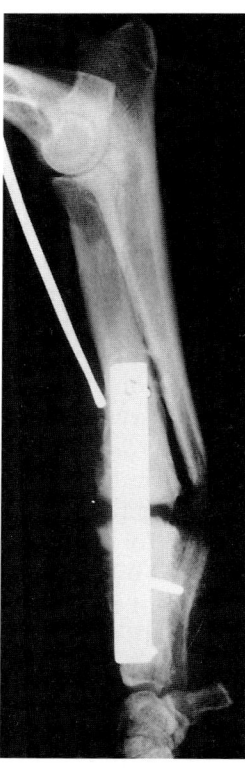

Figure 44.8 Medial-lateral radiograph of the antebrachium of a dog with osteomyelitis following internal fixation of a fracture of the distal radius and ulna. There is bone lysis around the proximal part of the implant and extensive periosteal new bone proliferation. The probe is inserted in a sinus communicating from the infected site to the skin surface.

Periosteal new bone production may be extensive. In early infections, less than 14 days old, bone changes may not be evident on radiographs, but soft tissue swelling may be appreciated within the first 24 hours (Boland, 1972; Walker et al., 1975). Radiographs should be carefully scrutinized for sequestra. The aggressive radiological picture of acute osteomyelitis may be difficult to differentiate from that of malignant bone tumours.

In all cases, a biopsy taken directly and aseptically from the infected bone at the time of surgery, should be submitted for aerobic and anaerobic bacteriological culture and antimicrobial sensitivity testing. Swabs from draining sinus tracts are less satisfactory because the tracts are commonly invaded by secondary bacteria. If there is any uncertainty about the diagnosis, a further biopsy should be formalin fixed and submitted for histopathological examination.

Treatment of osteomyelitis often depends on a combination of surgical and medical therapies. Sequestra are surgically removed, as are any surgical implants which may act as a continuing focus for infection. Dead bone is removed by curettage to leave only healthy, vascularized bone. It is important in all cases to establish drainage and if necessary holes are drilled through the cortex to allow drainage from the medullary cavity. Drainage tubes may be inserted or drainage may be maintained by open-wound management (Daly, 1985). A soft, padded dressing is used to protect the surgical drains, which are usually left in place for 4 to 7 days. Antibiotic therapy is based on the results of antimicrobial sensitivity testing. While awaiting laboratory results antibiotic therapy should be instigated using a broad-spectrum bactericidal agent, effective against the commonly isolated Gram-positive cocci. Suitable antibiotics for use during this interim period include clavulanate-potentiated amoxycillin and cephalosporin derivatives. Metronidazole may be included for its action against anaerobes. High doses of antibiotics may be necessary to facilitate penetration of areas with poor blood perfusion. Resolution of the disease may be a prolonged process and some cases, particularly cases of chronic osteomyelitis, either persist or are prone to relapse. Even with a good clinical response, the administration of systemic antibiotics should continue for a minimum of 6–8 weeks, or for two weeks after the complete resolution of clinical signs. Surgical implantation of gentamycin impregnated polymethylmethacrylate beads may be helpful in selected cases with multiple antibiotic resistant infections (Brown and Bennett, 1989).

Nursing adjuncts to therapy include regular attention to dressings and drains, cage rest and even immobilization of the affected limb during the initial stages of treatment. Prolonged exercise restriction is inadvisable as this may support the formation of adhesions.

Polyostotic bone infection, probably resulting from the haematogenous spread of bacteria, is occasionally seen in young dogs (Dunn et al., 1992). The term metaphyseal osteomyelitis has been used to describe this condition which is characterized by generalized stiffness and multiple bone pain in immature dogs. Radiographically, the lesions present as diffuse areas of bone lysis with associated periosteal new bone proliferation in the metaphyses of many long bones. Metaphyseal osteomyelitis is an important differential diagnosis for metaphyseal osteopathy. Treatment is by prolonged antibiotic administration.

Mycotic osteomyelitis

Fungal infections of bone documented in dogs and cats include aspergillosis (Sharp et al., 1991), blastomycosis (Roberts, 1979), coccidioidomycosis (Brodey et al., 1970), cryptococcosis (Brearley and Jeffrey, 1992; Small, 1969), nocardiosis (Small, 1969) and histoplasmosis (Small, 1969) among others. With the exception of aspergillosis all are rare, most have a restricted geographical distribution and some have never been diagnosed in the UK. Aspergillosis usually causes bone infection as an extension of mycotic rhinitis or sinusitis. Treatment hinges on the administration of antifungal agents (Sharp et al., 1991).

Metallosis

Sterile, non-suppurative bone inflammation can be associated with corrosion of metal implants. Metallosis predisposes to secondary bacterial infection and should be treated by implant removal.

Bone neoplasia

Neoplasms of bone can be considered in three groups:

1. Primary benign bone tumours;
2. Primary malignant bone tumours;
3. Non-osseous tumours invading bone.

Primary benign bone tumours

Primary benign bone tumours include osteoma, chondroma, multilobular osteoma and chondroma of the skull, and multiple cartilagenous exostoses (see constitutional bone disease).

Primary benign tumours of bone are uncommon in dogs and they are often of little clinical significance, except as differential diagnoses for more aggressive bone lesions. Some may occasionally undergo malignant transformation. If treated, they have a good prognosis following complete excision.

Primary malignant bone tumours

Primary malignant bone tumours include osteosarcoma, chondrosarcoma, fibrosarcoma, haemangiosarcoma, liposarcoma, osteoclastoma (giant cell tumour), primary lymphosarcoma and plasma cell myeloma.

Osteosarcoma is by far the most common primary malignant bone tumour of dogs. Chondrosarcoma accounts for approximately 10% of all canine bone sarcomas and haemangiosarcoma and fibrosarcoma between them account for approximately 7% of primary bone tumours in dogs (Goldschmidt and Thrall, 1985). The others are rare.

Primary malignant bone tumours of the appendicular skeleton most commonly present with pain, bone swelling and lameness, which is usually gradual in onset but may have an acute presentation. Most osteosarcomas and haemangiosarcomas are appendicular but chondrosarcomas are predominantly found in the axial skeleton, especially the ribs and nasal cavity (Goldschmidt and Thrall, 1985). Rib-based chondrosarcomas may cause relatively few clinical problems, but intranasal chondrosarcomas often present with sneezing, nasal obstruction, discharge and epistaxis. Approximately 60% of fibrosarcomas are associated with the bones of the skull and mandible and 30% with the bones of the axial skeleton.

All primary malignant bone tumours are locally invasive, but not all metastasize readily and this is important with regard to their prognosis. Most osteosarcomas and haemangiosarcomas, particularly those of the appendicular skeleton, metastasize readily to the lungs and other organs. Metastasis of chondrosarcomas and fibrosarcomas is uncommon. Only 10% of chondrosarcomas metastasize and fibrosarcomas will usually only do so if they are anaplastic.

Radiography of a suspected primary malignant bone tumour demonstrates cortical bone destruction, poor margins between normal and abnormal tissues and active periosteal bone proliferation (Fig. 44.9). These are features of an aggressive bone lesion and differential diagnoses include infection, trauma, metaphyseal osteopathy and hypertrophic pulmonary osteopathy. A definitive diagnosis can only be achieved by bone biopsy. Thoracic and abdominal survey radiographs should be taken to check for metastases in all cases with suspected primary malignant bone tumours. Skeletal survey radiographs may reveal further clinically undetectable bone neoplasms in approximately 7% of dogs with confirmed primary malignant bone sarcomas (LaRue et al., 1986). Bone scintigraphy may also be helpful in a search for occult metastases (Berg et al., 1990).

The treatment options available for primary malignant bone tumours vary with the type of tumour, site of tumour and stage of the disease, paying particular regard to the presence of metastases. Treatment options include palliative support (analgesia), radical excision, amputation,

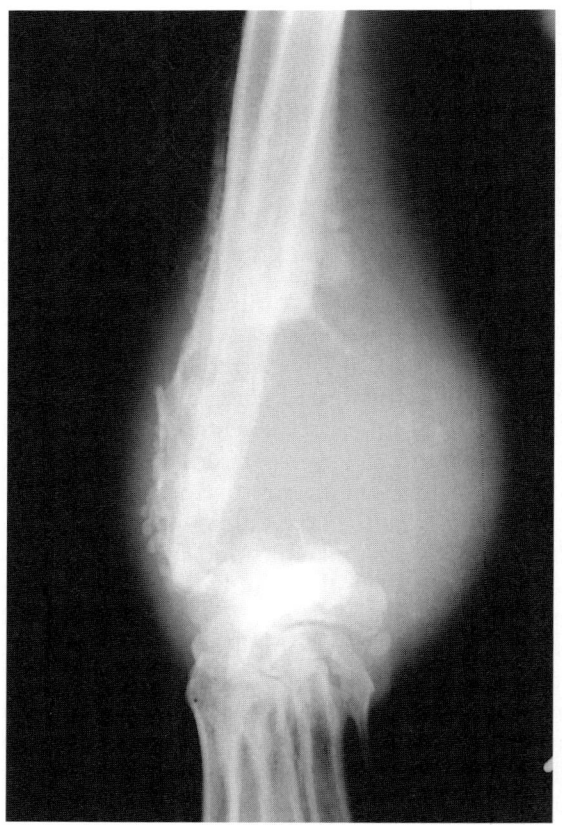

Figure 44.9 Cranial-caudal radiograph of the antebrachium and carpus of a dog with a primary malignant bone tumour. In addition to soft tissue swelling there is extensive lysis of bone and aggressive periosteal new bone production in the radius and ulna.

amputation and adjunctive therapy (e.g. chemotherapy) (Shapiro et al., 1988) or limb salvage surgery and adjunctive therapy (LaRue et al., 1989). Chemotherapy combined with surgery has the potential to double the median life expectancy of dogs with appendicular osteosarcoma. However, the most commonly used chemotherapeutic agent, cisplatin, has a number of potentially serious side effects, including severe nephrotoxicity. Chemotherapy for osteosarcoma should only be used by suitably experienced veterinary surgeons with adequate facilities for the specialist care required during its administration.

Non-osseous tumours invading bone

Invasion of bone by non-osseous tumours may occur by direct extension from adjacent soft tissues or by metastasis.

Tumours which may locally invade bone include melanoma, squamous cell carcinoma, acanthomatous epulis, oral fibrosarcoma, synovial sarcoma and intrapelvic tumours, particularly prostatic carcinoma. In some cases, radical excision may be feasible, particularly with oral tumours. However, the prognosis is usually poor.

Skeletal metastasis only occurs in approximately 17% of all metastasizing tumours in dogs and usually warrants a poor prognosis (Goedegebuure, 1979). Tumours metastasizing to bone are most often carcinomas, particularly mammary carcinoma, primary lung carcinoma and prostatic carcinoma (Brodey et al., 1966). Some connective tissue tumours, for example haemangiosarcoma, fibrosarcoma and lymphosarcoma, may metastasize to bone. Most bone metastases occur by the haematogenous route and consequently have a polyostotic distribution. Radiographically they present as aggressive bone lesions which cannot reliably be differentiated from primary bone tumours.

Some tumours, such as malignant melanoma, lymphosarcoma and malignant histiocytoma may invade bone both by localized spread and by metastasis.

Idiopathic bone disease

Metaphyseal osteopathy

Metaphyseal osteopathy is a disease with many synonyms, the most common of which is hypertrophic osteodystrophy. Grondalen (1976) coined the term metaphyseal osteopathy in a seminal paper on the disease.

Metaphyseal osteopathy is a relapsing disease which most frequently presents in large breeds of dog at the age of 3–4 months (range 2–8 months). Respiratory or gastrointestinal illness may precede the onset of skeletal disease. Clinical signs vary from mild lameness to severe systemic illness, pyrexia, depression, inappetence, weight loss and inability or unwillingness to stand. In mild cases, pain can be elicited by digital pressure on the metaphyses. In severe cases, the long bone metaphyses are visibly swollen, hot and painful on palpation. The long bones distal to the stifle and elbow are usually most severely affected. Active periods of disease may last several days. Relapses occur in some, but not all, cases at intervals of 1 to 6 weeks. A small number of affected dogs may die naturally and others suffering severe and repeated bouts of illness may be euthanatized at the request of their owners.

Histologically the lesions of metaphyseal osteopathy are characterized by a band of trabecular disruption, necrosis, haemorrhage and inflammatory cell infiltrate in the metaphyseal bone. The lesion usually lies parallel to the physis at the level of endochondral cartilage vascularization. The calcified cartilage between the disrupted layer and the physis also contains haemorrhage and an inflammatory infiltrate. Disruption of the metaphyseal blood supply may lead to irregular widening of the physis. There is often extensive osteoclastic resorption of adjacent metaphyseal bone trabeculae. Subperiosteal haemorrhage and periosteal reactive new bone formation are inconsistent features.

The aetiology of metaphyseal osteopathy is unknown. However, the occurrence of respiratory or gastroenteric illness before the onset of skeletal disease, coupled with the presence of an intraosseous inflammatory infiltrate during the disease, is consistent with an infectious aetiology and it has been suggested that metaphyseal osteopathy may be a viral osteomyelitis. This hypothesis is supported by the demonstration of metaphyseal lesions in both naturally occurring and experimental canine distemper virus (CDV) infection (Boyce et al., 1983) and by the demonstration of CDV-infected bone cells in the metaphyses of dogs (Mee et al., 1992, 1993).

Haematological and serum biochemical parameters are often unremarkable in metaphyseal osteopathy. The diagnosis is usually confirmed radiologically by the recognition of irregular, radiolucent lines, parallel to the physis, in the metaphyses of long bones (Fig. 44.10). In cases with hypertrophic bone proliferation, a cuff of

736 | DISEASES OF BONES AND JOINTS

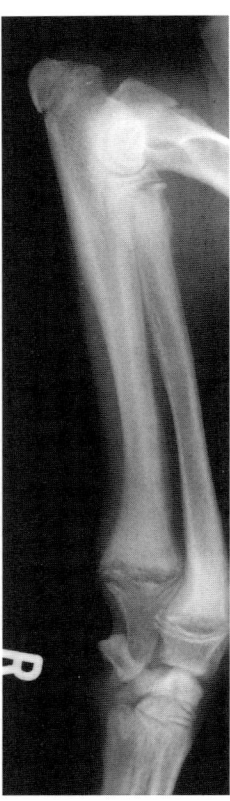

Figure 44.10 Medial-lateral radiograph of the radius and ulna of a dog with metaphyseal osteopathy. Irregular areas of bone sclerosis and lysis are seen parallel to the growth plates in the distal metaphyses of the radius and ulna.

periosteal new bone is seen developing around the metaphysis (Riser, 1964).

Only palliative treatment is given. Nonsteroidal anti-inflammatory drugs or corticosteroids used at anti-inflammatory doses can be administered during the acute phase of the disease. Overnutrition is associated with an increased risk of developing metaphyseal osteopathy and normalization of the diet should form part of the treatment regime. Adjunctive therapy includes fluid replacement, appetite stimulation or feeding through a gastrostomy tube and careful avoidance of decubitus ulcer formation in recumbent patients.

The prognosis is dependent on the severity of the illness and the frequency of relapse, but it is generally good as relapse is uncommon and almost all affected dogs become asymptomatic when they mature. Metaphyseal osteopathy may be complicated by limb deformity as a result of either physeal bridging by hypertrophic new bone or retarded growth associated with impaired vascularization of the developing endochondral cartilage.

Craniomandibular osteopathy (CMO)

Like metaphyseal osteopathy, CMO is a relapsing disease with onset usually between 2 and 4 months of age. West Highland white terriers, Cairn terriers and Scottish terriers present most commonly with CMO although it has also been reported in Labrador retrievers, Great Danes, boxers and Dobermanns (Watson, 1990). The most common presenting sign is jaw-pain accompanied by inability to open the mouth and intermittent fever. Acute episodes last for several days and relapses occur at intervals ranging from days to weeks.

The mandibles and tympanic bullae are the most commonly affected bones although other bones of the calvarium and, rarely, limb bones may also be affected. The pathological changes are characterized by osteoclastic resorption of bone with an associated inflammatory infiltrate. Lamellar bone and bone marrow spaces are replaced by coarse bone and fibrous stroma. There is periosteal bone proliferation. The aetiology of CMO is unknown (Riser, 1966).

CMO should be suspected in young dogs with jaw pain and fever, particularly if the dog is of the Scottish terrier type. Heat and swelling may be palpated in the mandibles and the diagnosis can be confirmed by the radiographic demonstration of proliferative new bone on the mandibles (Fig. 44.11). Although both mandibles are usually affected, CMO may be seen localized to one mandible.

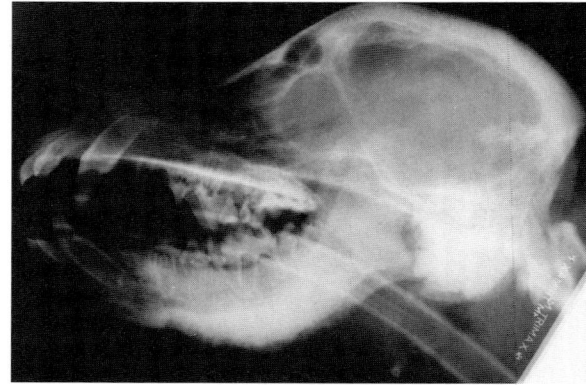

Figure 44.11 Lateral radiograph of the skull of a West Highland white terrier with craniomandibular osteopathy. There is irregular new bone production in the area of the tympanic bullae and along the ventral aspect of the mandibles.

Treatment is palliative. Non-steroidal anti-inflammatory drugs or corticosteroids are used to control the painful episodes and relapses usually cease when the dog reaches approximately one year of age. There is often some residual impairment of jaw function, but this does not usually interfere with normal mastication. The proliferative new bone eventually remodels, but there is often residual thickening of the jaw. Uncommonly, dogs with uncontrollable pain, frequent relapses or severely impaired jaw function may be euthanatized.

Panosteitis

Panosteitis is a self-limiting, recurrent disease of the diaphyses and metaphyses of long bones of dogs. Immature, large breeds of dog, particularly German shepherd dogs, are most commonly affected, but panosteitis has been reported in breeds of all sizes and in adult dogs (Lenehan et al., 1985). Affected dogs present with acute onset lameness in one or more limbs, sometimes accompanied by pyrexia, lethargy and inappetence. There is no history of trauma and the severity of lameness does not fluctuate with exercise or rest. There may be spontaneous recovery after a few days and relapses occur at periods ranging from days to weeks. The lameness may shift from limb to limb during episodes and from one episode to the next. The severity and frequency of attacks reduce with age and most dogs are free of disease by one to two years of age. Clinical examination is usually unremarkable except that pain can be elicited by firm palpation of affected long bones.

The aetiology of panosteitis is unknown. Pathologically, there is episodic degeneration of medullary adipose tissue followed by stromal proliferation and endosteal and subperiosteal intramembranous bone proliferation.

The diagnosis of panosteitis is usually confirmed radiographically. A patchy increase in medullary opacity, with or without well-defined borders, is the most common radiographic sign (Fig. 44.12). In some cases the endosteal new bone may be seen as cortical bone thickening and there may also be some periosteal new bone formation. In early cases there may be increased radiolucency of the medulla. Occasionally, no radiographic abnormalities will be seen. In such cases it is sometimes helpful to re-radiograph after a period of two weeks.

No specific treatment is necessary. Symptomatic control of painful episodes can be achieved with non-steroidal anti-inflammatory drugs. The prognosis is good.

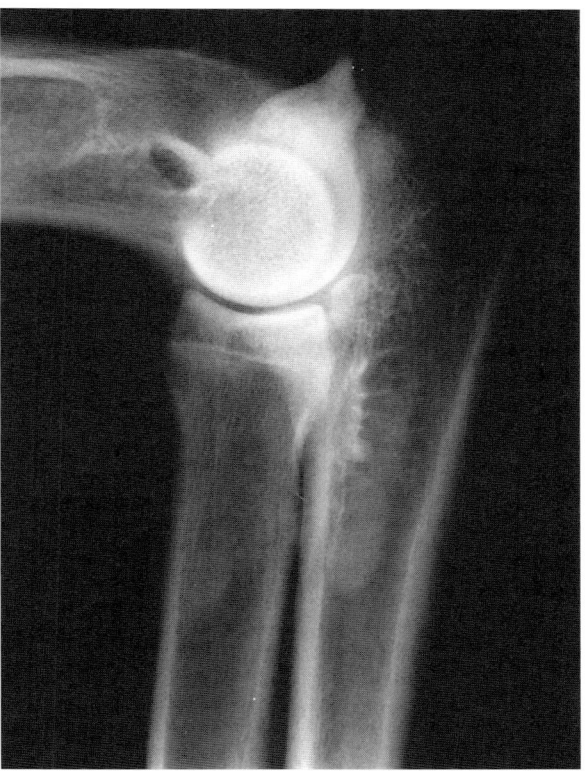

Figure 44.12 Medial-lateral radiograph of the elbow joint of an immature German shepherd dog with panosteitis. Patchy radiodensities are seen within the medullae of the proximal radius and ulna.

Miscellaneous bone diseases

Hypertrophic pulmonary osteopathy

Hypertrophic pulmonary osteopathy (HPO) typically presents as warm, painful swelling of the extremities of all four limbs. The swelling is associated with characteristic periosteal new bone formation along the diaphyses and metaphyses of many long bones (Brodey, 1971). Radiographically there is a varied appearance to the new bone which may be spiculated, smooth, lamellar or irregular (Fig. 44.13). Demonstration of extensive periosteal new bone along the long bones of all four limbs is usually sufficient to justify a diagnosis of HPO.

HPO occurs secondary to chronic thoracic or abdominal pathology. Most commonly the inciting factor is pulmonary neoplasia. Primary lung tumours and pulmonary metastases of primary bone tumours seem to give rise to HPO more commonly than other tumour types. HPO has

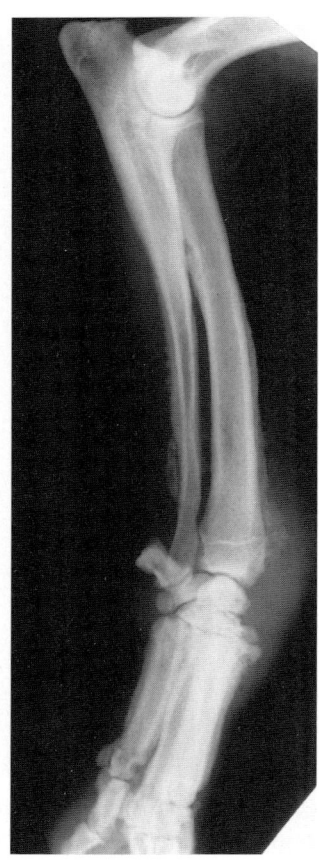

Figure 44.13 Medial-lateral survey radiograph of the distal forelimb of a dog with hypertrophic pulmonary osteopathy. There is soft tissue swelling and irregular new bone formation along the diaphyses of the long bones. Similar changes were seen on survey radiographs of all four limbs.

changes eventually remodel, but this is a slow process and radiographically identifiable bone changes persist long after the symptoms of HPO have resolved (Brockus and Hathcock, 1988).

Retained cartilaginous cores

Retained cores of endochondral cartilage may be identified on radiographs of young, large breed dogs. The distal ulnar, distal tibia and distal femur are common sites of retention of endochondral cartilage. The cartilage core is retained as a result of delayed ossification of the hypertrophied cartilage cells emanating from the physis. This may be regarded as a form of osteochondrosis. Retained cartilage cores are sometimes asymptomatic, but in some dogs the retarded growth resulting from delayed endochondral ossification can lead to bone deformities requiring surgical correction (Fig. 44.14).

also been reported as a sequel to pulmonary abscessation, chronic bronchopneumonia, pulmonary tuberculosis, rib tumours, abdominal neoplasms, bacterial endocarditis, *Dirofilaria immitis* infection *Spirocerca lupi* infection and blastomycosis (Susanek, 1982; Brockus and Hathcock, 1988). The most common abdominal disease giving rise to HPO is neoplasia of the bladder both with and without pulmonary metastases.

The pathogenesis of HPO remains unclear, but is thought to relate to an increase in peripheral blood supply to the affected bones. The vascular change is mediated by afferent impulses arising in the thorax and transmitted along the vagus nerve. The precise nature of the afferent stimulus and the efferent pathway have yet to be determined.

Treatment of HPO is dependent on treatment of the primary lesion. Successful removal of the inciting cause usually results in resolution of the clinical signs of HPO within weeks. The bony

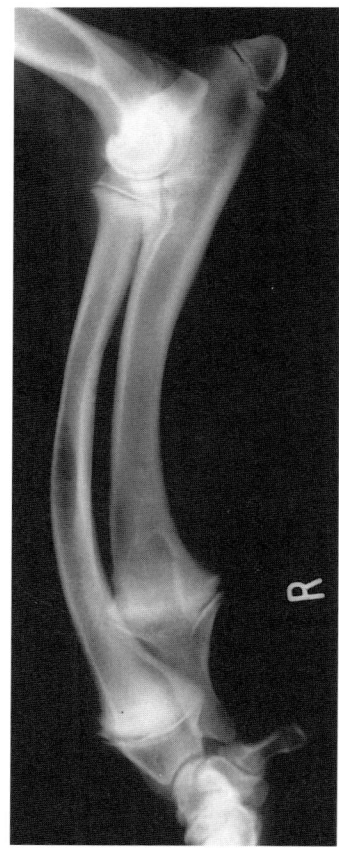

Figure 44.14 Medial-lateral radiograph of the radius and ulna of a great Dane with radius curvus syndrome secondary to retardation of ulnar growth relative to radial growth. A retained cartilaginous core is seen as a well demarcated area of soft tissue opacity in the distal ulnar metaphysis.

Bone cysts

Bone cysts are rare in small animals and are often asymptomatic. They are identified on radiographs as well defined, radiolucent monostotic or polyostotic lesions (Huff and Brodey, 1964). The very sharp boundary between the cyst and normal bone is helpful in differentiating bone cysts from neoplasms. A bone biopsy may be necessary to establish a definitive diagnosis in some cases. Treatment is by curettage. The resulting defect may be packed with cancellous bone.

BONE DISEASES OF CATS

Cats suffer many of the bone diseases suffered by dogs and their classification, diagnosis and management is essentially similar (Table 44.4). The following bone conditions are worthy of particular consideration in feline medicine.

Mucopolysaccharidosis

The mucopolysaccharidoses fall into the class of true metabolic bone diseases, resulting from inherited chromosomal abnormalities which give rise to a congenital enzyme deficiency. In humans, the mucopolysaccharidoses have been classified into several groups and this classification has been adapted for use in animals (Jezyk, 1985). Mucopolysaccharidosis is seen uncommonly, but two types have been recognized in cats. Mucopolysaccharidosis I occurs in domestic short-haired cats. Affected kittens have a large, broad head, small ears and wide-spaced eyes with corneal clouding and mitral insufficiency in some cases. Skeletal lesions include fusion of cervical vertebrae, pectus excavatum and joint abnormalities including hip subluxation. Mucopolysaccharidosis VI has been recorded in Siamese cats (Cowell et al., 1976; Konde et al., 1987). Affected animals are dwarfed and may suffer multiple skeletal, neurological and retinal deficits. Affected joints show radiographic changes reminiscent of hypervitaminosis A (see below). Some cats with mucopolysaccharidosis lead acceptable lives as pets, but there is no specific treatment available.

Hypervitaminosis A

Hypervitaminosis A usually presents in cats fed a diet consisting entirely or predominantly of liver which is a rich source of vitamin A. Affected cats present with lameness, discomfort and neck stiffness (Seawright et al., 1967). There may be associated lethargy and the cat may appear unkempt as a result of unwillingness to groom. Gingival oedema, hyperaemia and abdominal distension have also been reported. In young animals there may be retarded bone growth and deformity.

Pathologically, there is extensive formation of bone exostoses. These are most commonly recognized radiographically in the cervical spine, but they also affect other vertebrae and some appendicular joints (Fig. 44.15a and b). The exostoses are often so extensive they fuse several adjacent vertebrae.

Hypervitaminosis A is diagnosed by the radiographic demonstration of extensive bridging

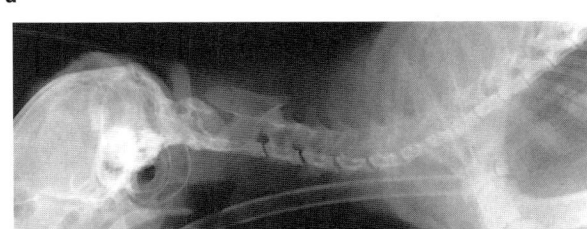
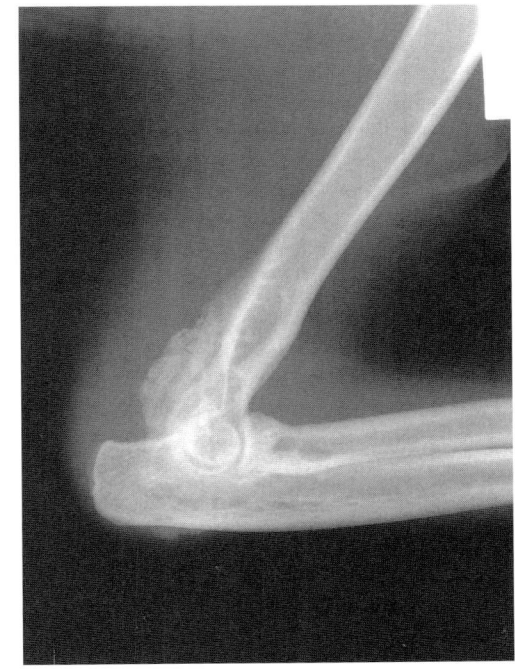

Figure 44.15 Radiographs of a cat with hypervitaminosis A. (a) Fusion of cervical vertebrae and ventral spondylosis. (b) Periarticular soft tissue swelling and osteophyte production in the elbow.

spinal or articular exostoses in cats with a history of excessive vitamin A supplementation or a predominantly liver diet. If necessary, plasma vitamin A (retinol) levels may be measured (normal = 12–100 µg dl^{-1}).

Treatment relies on dietary correction and most mature cats will show significant clinical improvement as a result. Immature cats suffer permanently retarded long bone growth. Some cats are difficult to wean off their liver diet.

Bone neoplasia

Primary bone tumours are uncommon in cats and their biological behaviour sometimes differs from that seen in dogs. The most common primary bone tumour of cats is osteosarcoma. Most osteosarcomas of cats occur in the appendicular skeleton, but some arise from the bones of the skull, pelvis or vertebrae. The main presenting clinical sign is usually painful lameness and bone swelling. Radiographically, osteosarcoma appears as an aggressive, usually lytic, bone lesion in cats. The diagnosis is confirmed by bone biopsy. Metastasis of osteosarcoma occurs less commonly in cats than in dogs and mean survival following radical surgical excision or amputation may be in excess of four years (Bitetto et al., 1987).

Parosteal osteosarcoma of cats is a slow-growing tumour that arises from the outer bone cortex. Metastasis is rare and most cats present with bony swelling and/or lameness. The most common sites for parosteal osteosarcoma are the humerus, femur, mandible and frontal bones. Complete excision is usually curative.

Osteochondromas may present in cats as solitary masses or as multiple cartilaginous exostoses. Clinical signs are usually only associated with displacement of adjacent structures by the enlarging mass, but the condition is important as a differential diagnosis of aggressive bone tumours.

Soft tissue tumours may invade bone or metastasize to bone in cats as in dogs. In particular, primary bronchial carcinoma of cats may metastasize to the digits. Some affected cats present with painful lameness and multiple digital swelling before there are signs of respiratory disease (May and Newsholme, 1989) (Fig. 44.16).

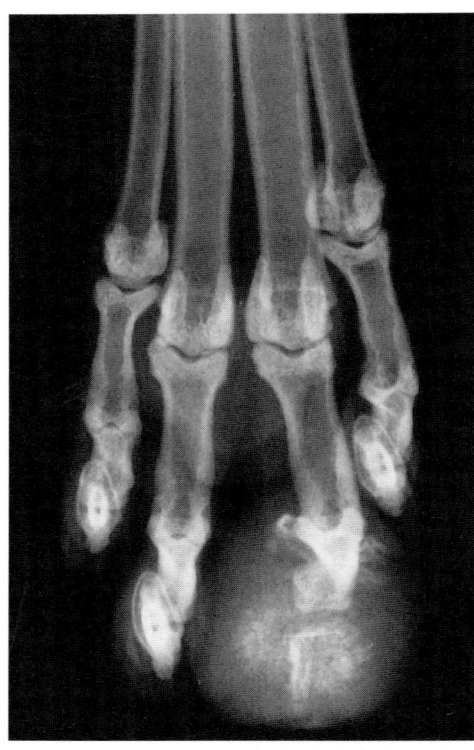

Figure 44.16 Dorsal-palmar radiograph of the digits of a cat with metastasis of primary bronchial carcinoma to digit IV. There is loss of the claw, soft tissue swelling, aggressive new bone production and bone lysis.

Joint Diseases

Joint diseases can be classified on the basis of the predominant type of intra-articular pathology (Table 44.5). However, it should be remembered that few cases present with pure pathology of one type or another. Joint diseases of all types are often accompanied by a degree of secondary degenerative change (secondary osteoarthritis). Conversely, 'degenerative' joint diseases may have an inflammatory component. A full discussion of all joint disease is beyond the scope of this chapter and the reader is referred to specialist texts listed at the end of this chapter for more detailed information (see Further Reading).

Table 44.5 Classification of synovial joint disease in dogs and cats

Traumatic joint disease
  Sprain
  Contusion
  Articular fracture
  Cartilage trauma
  Meniscal trauma

Degenerative joint disease
  Constitutional
    Mucopolysaccharidoses (Types I and VI in cats. Rare in dogs)
  Dietary
    Hypervitaminosis A (cats)
  Neuropathic
    ?Chronic diabetes mellitus (cats)
  Osteoarthritis
    Primary
    Secondary
      Trauma
      Luxation/subluxation
      Developmental disorders
      Inflammatory joint disease

Inflammatory joint disease
  Infectious
    Bacterial (suppurative)
      Spirochaetal (Lyme disease)
    Fungal
    Protozoal
    Mycoplasmal
    Viral
  'Immune mediated'
    Erosive
      Rheumatoid-like arthritis
      Polyarthritis of greyhounds
      Feline progressive polyarthritis
    Non-erosive
      Idiopathic polyarthritis
      Reactive arthritis
      Malignancy-associated arthritis
      Enteropathic arthritis
      Drug-associated arthritis
      Systemic lupus erythematosus
      Polyarthritis of Japanese Akitas
      Shar Pei fever
      Feline progressive polyarthritis
      Crystal arthropathies

Joint neoplasia
  Primary
    Synovial sarcoma
  Secondary
    Osteosarcoma
    Malignant histiocytosis (dogs)
    Lymphosarcoma (cats)

JOINT DISEASES OF DOGS

Traumatic joint disease

Repetitive trauma may contribute to the gradual progression of many joint diseases, but the term traumatic joint disease refers to an acute episode of arthritis induced by physical insult. *Sprain* refers to injury of ligaments and should be differentiated from *strain* which refers to injuries of the muscle–tendon unit. Sprain and strain injuries can be classified on the basis of the severity of the injury, which may range from minimal tearing and associated haemorrhage and contusion, through to complete rupture. Acute synovitis invariably complicates traumatic arthritis and there may be areas of haemorrhage, haemosiderin deposition and an infiltrate of acute inflammatory cells into the synovial membrane and associated joint capsule and ligaments. These changes may be reflected in synovial fluid analysis (Table 44.3). Traumatic arthritis can usually be diagnosed after physical and radiological examination of a patient with a recent history of trauma. Radiological findings may range from minimal joint effusion through to obvious articular fractures. Treatment and prognosis is governed by the particular problems of individual cases. Mild cases may only require rest, others may require analgesia, external support dressings or even surgical repair of ligament ruptures and fractures. Severe or repeated episodes of traumatic joint disease may give rise to secondary osteoarthritis.

Degenerative joint disease

Constitutional joint disease (mucopolysaccharidosis) and dietary joint disease (hypervitaminosis A) are covered under bone disorders. Neuropathic arthritis is dealt with under joint diseases of cats.

Osteoarthritis

Osteoarthritis (OA) may be defined as an inherently non-inflammatory disorder of movable joints characterized by deterioration and abrasion of articular cartilage and by the formation of new bone at the joint surfaces and margins (Hough, 1993). It is not a distinct disease, but more a pattern of reaction to joint injury. Secondary OA is a term used to describe OA developing as a result of other recognizable joint disease, particularly when this leads to chronic joint incongruity and instability (e.g. rupture of the cranial cruciate ligament, osteochondrosis, hip dysplasia). Primary, or idiopathic, OA may result from changes arising in the metabolism of the articular cartilage itself. Primary OA is usually diagnosed when there is no readily recognizable predisposing disease. In mild to moderate cases of secondary OA, the underlying disease process is usually recognizable, but in advanced cases it may be difficult to differentiate primary from secondary disease (Olsson, 1971). Heritability is a factor in the development of some forms of OA, notably OA secondary to hip dysplasia (Leighton et al., 1977) and elbow arthrosis presumed to be secondary to osteochondrosis (Guthrie and Pidduck, 1990; Grondalen and Lingaas, 1991).

The main presenting clinical sign of OA is lameness, which may be subtle or pronounced to the extent of non-weightbearing. Short-lived stiffness after rest (articular gelling) is common in OA and the lameness may be exacerbated by exercise. Physical examination may reveal pain on palpation and resentment of forced extension or flexion. There may be reduced range of joint movement. Joint enlargement is frequently encountered in OA as a result of moderate effusion in acute cases and osteophyte formation and thickening of the joint capsule in chronic cases. Crepitus may be detected by palpation. A diagnosis of OA can be confirmed in dogs with appropriate clinical signs, radiological findings (Fig. 44.17) and synovial fluid analysis (Table 44.3). Morgan (1981) listed the following characteristic radiological features of OA:

1. Periarticular osteophyte formation
2. Subchondral bone sclerosis
3. Attrition of subchondral bone
4. Subluxation
5. Remodelling of bones adjacent to the joint
6. Intra-articular or periarticular soft tissue calcification
7. Subchondral bone cysts
8. Joint space narrowing

Periarticular and intra-articular soft tissue swelling is also commonly recognized radiologically in osteoarthritic joints. In chronic cases, atrophy of the muscles surrounding the affected joint may also be appreciated on radiographs. Subchondral bone cysts are rare in small animals. Joint space narrowing may be difficult to evaluate on non-weightbearing radiographs, particularly when these are obtained with the animal sedated or anaesthetized and positioned using ties and sandbags.

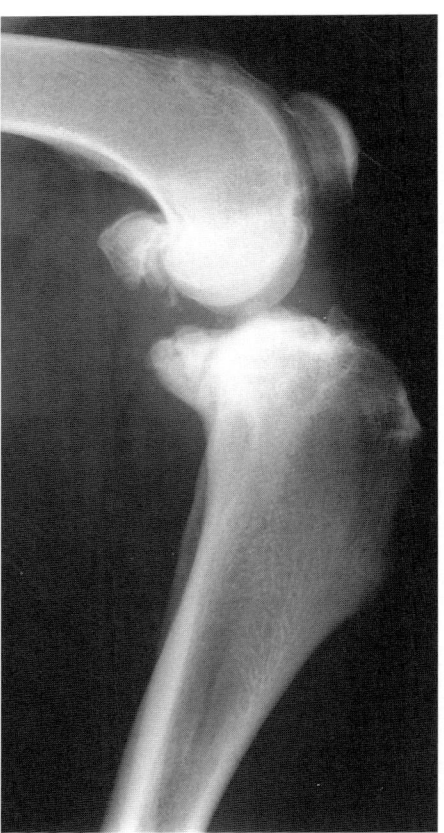

Figure 44.17 Medial-lateral radiograph of an advanced case of stifle osteoarthritis in a dog. There is periarticular soft tissue swelling, periarticular osteophyte formation, remodelled bone and subchondral bone sclerosis.

Treatment of secondary OA should first and foremost be directed at early correction of the inciting cause. It is therefore imperative that all dogs presenting with OA are fully evaluated for underlying joint diseases. Many of these diseases are amenable to surgical therapy and they have received considerable attention in the surgical literature. Relatively little attention has concentrated on the management of patients with established OA. This is surprising when the ever-increasing age of the pet population and the high prevalence of OA within that population is considered. Furthermore, there is now a bewildering range of pharmaceutical preparations available for the treatment of OA and some animals are prescribed these drugs inappropriately. Once initiated, the general clinical signs, symptoms, radiological findings and progression of disease are similar for both primary and secondary OA. They are amenable to similar methods of management.

The many different aetiologies of OA are thought to converge in a 'final common pathway' of pathology characterized by damage to the proteoglycan matrix, chondrocyte injury and disturbance of normal chondrocyte functions. Enzymes produced by the chondrocytes, and perhaps the synovial membrane, lead to increased breakdown of the cartilage proteoglycans matrix (Pelletier et al., 1983a, b; Martel-Pelletier et al., 1984). Somewhat paradoxically, the increased net loss of cartilage matrix is accompanied by chondrocyte proliferation and an increase in the synthesis of matrix by the chondrocytes. Chondrocyte proliferation may result in local aggregations of chondrocytes appearing at sites of cartilage damage. Breakdown products from the cartilage (so-called 'wear particles') may be phagocytosed by synovial membrane macrophages and this is thought to be one factor that initiates a chronic inflammatory synovitis in some OA joints.

Treatment of OA is palliative and it is important that owners of pets with OA fully understand that there is currently no cure. Therapeutic intervention is largely for relief of pain, to combat inflammation and, wherever possible, to minimize progression of the disease. The management of OA patients can be considered in three stages.

1. Goal planning/lifestyle adjustment
2. Pharmacological support
3. Surgical treatment

Goal planning/lifestyle adjustment

Goal planning is important as the aims of treatment vary with individual patients and a blanket approach to the management of OA is too inflexible. Continual dosing with anti-inflammatory drugs is no substitute for good management of the lifestyle of dogs with OA and it is unfortunate that lifestyle adjustment is sometimes overlooked by clinicians treating OA patients. Most of the drugs currently prescribed for OA do not beneficially alter the progression of the disease and many drugs may actually hasten the demise of the affected joints (Lees et al., 1991; Clark, 1991). Moreover, for many OA patients the discomfort suffered is often both intermittent and transient, rather than crippling and unrelenting. These factors mitigate against a heavy reliance on drug therapy or major surgical therapies and in favour of good lifestyle management in many cases.

It is important before embarking on any course of treatment for OA to establish therapeutic goals that are acceptable to the patient, the client and the clinician. The goals may vary depending on many factors including the major problem (stiffness after rest, pain, exercise intolerance), the type of dog (gundog, working dog, show dog, pet), the requirements of the owner, financial restraints, age of dog, size of dog and intercurrent disease or drug therapy that may interfere with the use of anti-inflammatory drugs. If adjustment of a dog's lifestyle is to be made successfully, it is imperative that OA and its management are fully discussed with the owner during a goal planning session and that the agreed goals and necessary lifestyle adjustments are recorded both for the clinician and the client.

No dog with clinical OA should be overweight. Weight reduction is perhaps the single most important factor that will benefit many dogs with OA. Continual use of an osteoarthritic joint in a manner which is painful is thought to accelerate the rate of cartilage degradation (Clark, 1991). The dog's exercise should therefore be restricted to avoid exercise-induced pain or discomfort. That is not to say that dogs with OA should not be exercised. Regular, controlled exercise helps to maintain muscle tone and ligament strength, both of which are beneficial to the joints. Rest may be imposed, with or without anti-inflammatory therapy, during periods of acute pain associated with OA. At other times a regime of moderate exercise is advisable. In this context, moderate exercise may be defined as exercise within the capability of the patient that does not induce pain, lameness or excessive articular gelling during or following the exercise period. The definition of moderate requires that the level of acceptable exercise is established for each patient and is maintained under constant review. Most OA patients cope best with several short exercise periods each day rather than with one or two extended periods of exercise. Every effort should be made to maintain an exercise routine that does not vary significantly from day to day. As the disease progresses it will usually be necessary to gradually to reduce the permissible level of daily exercise whilst taking care to maintain body weight at an optimum. Non-weightbearing exercise, such as swimming, may be helpful in some cases, provided it is performed frequently and regularly.

Pharmacological support

Synovial membranes and periarticular soft tissues are often inflamed in OA. The inflammation may be an important source of pain and a target for symptomatic relief by the administration of either non-steroidal anti-inflammatory drugs (NSAIDS) or steroids. However, it is important to remember that many anti-inflammatory drugs have systemic side effects and some drugs may hasten the progress of joint disease. Both NSAIDS and corticosteroids cause depletion of articular cartilage proteoglycans in normal joints and it has been suggested that these drugs may hasten cartilage degradation in osteoarthritic joints (Behrens et al., 1975; Willhelmi and Maier, 1983; Trotter et al., 1991). However, the use of corticosteroids in the management of OA remains controversial as there is mounting evidence that, in inflamed OA joints, low doses of corticosteroid actually reduce the severity of cartilage degradation and reduce osteophyte formation; a so-called 'chondroprotective' effect (Colombo et al., 1983; Williams and Brandt, 1985; Moskowitz and Goldberg, 1987; Pelletier and Martel-Pelletier, 1989).

The systemic side effects of NSAIDS are mainly gastrointestinal irritation (diarrhoea and/or vomiting) with associated gastric hyperaemia and ulceration in some cases. Gastric mucosal damage by NSAIDS has a multifactorial basis, but local impairment of the cyclo-oxygenase pathway is thought to be an important mechanism. This leads to local suppression of prostaglandin production, giving rise to gastric mucosal ischaemia, increased membrane permeability, mast cell degranulation and increased secretion of pepsin and gastric acid (Hazleman, 1986). Acidic drugs may also have a direct irritant effect on the gastric mucosa. Gastrointestinal side effects in animals on NSAID therapy may be exacerbated by the simultaneous administration of other anti-inflammatory drugs, particularly corticosteroids. Gastrointestinal side effects are treated by complete withdrawal of anti-inflammatory drugs and supportive care including the administration of anti-ulcerogenic drugs, intravenous fluids and whole blood if necessary. Some NSAIDS cause a reduction in the glomerular filtration rate and they may significantly impair the renal function of dogs in compensated chronic renal failure. Reduced excretion of anti-inflammatory drugs in dogs with clinical or subclinical renal or hepatic disease may necessitate lowering the administered dose to achieve satisfactory, non-toxic, serum drug levels. In many cases anti-inflammatory therapy can be reserved for short-term treatment of acute, painful episodes. Prolonged usage of anti-inflammatory drugs should be avoided if at all possible and NSAID therapy should be withdrawn immediately if side effects are recognized. In many cases, it is possible to control the symptoms of OA with doses of NSAIDS below the minimum recommended by drug manufacturers. After a short period of dosing at the normal levels, it is always advisable to try reducing the dose of administered NSAID to the lowest effective level.

There are several excellent reviews of anti-inflammatory therapy in dogs and cats (Clark, 1991; Lees et al., 1991; McKellar et al., 1991a). Some of the anti-inflammatory drugs used in dogs are summarized in Table 44.6. Aspirin and phenylbutazone are still in common use for the management of OA in dogs, as is a combination of cincophen and prednisolone (McKellar et al., 1991b). In human medicine, many new NSAIDS are now becoming available. However, few are licensed for use in the dog and there is wide interspecies variation in the efficacy and toxicity of NSAIDS, making direct extrapolation from human drug data sheets dangerous. Moreover, no study has suggested that any of the new agents is more effective than aspirin (Clark, 1991).

Ibuprofen is a propionic acid derivative which is available for use in man without prescription and some owners may therefore administer ibuprofen to their animals. Ibuprofen carries a high risk of gastrointestinal side effects in dogs and has no therapeutic advantages over other NSAIDS (Scherkl and Frey, 1987). Its use in the dog should be discouraged.

Ketoprofen is a propionic acid derivative licensed for short term use in dogs and cats. Ketoprofen may inhibit both the cyclo-oxygenase pathway leading to prostaglandin production and the lipoxygenase pathway leading to leucotriene production. It is an extremely potent anti-inflammatory drug.

Carprofen is a carbazole acetic acid derivative that is licensed for use in dogs. At doses of 0.7 mg kg^{-1} daily, carprofen produces little cyclo-oxygenase pathway inhibition (McKellar et al., 1990). However, at this low dose carprofen may be effective only as an analgesic, not as an anti-inflammatory drug. At anti-inflammatory doses (>4 mg kg^{-1} daily), carprofen has been shown to inhibit prostaglandin production (Baruth et al., 1986; Enthoven et al., 1987). Nevertheless, the dog gastrointestinal tract seems particularly resistant to carprofen-induced ulceration and clinical trials in humans suggest that carprofen does have a moderately low incidence of gastrointestinal side effects (Coutinho et al., 1975; Rainsford, 1988). It is possible that carprofen is a highly specific inhibitor of prostaglandin synthetase with a high potency at sites of inflammation but causing relatively little inhibition of the intestinal cyclo-oxygenase pathway. This may explain the appar-

Table 44.6 Anti-inflammatory drugs used in the management of canine osteoarthritis

Drug	Dose
Aspirin	20–25 mg kg^{-1} tid p.o. (anti-inflammatory dose) 10–15 mg kg^{-1} tid p.o. (analgesic dose)
Phenylbutazone	15 mg kg^{-1} tid p.o. (loading dose for up to 48 h); maximum 800 mg daily. Reduce to lowest effective dose for maintenance (may be given on alternate days)
Cincophen/Prednisolone	Cincophen 12.5 mg kg^{-1}; prednisolone 0.125 mg kg^{-1} bid p.o.
Flunixin meglumine	1 mg kg^{-1} daily for a maximum of 3 days i.m. or p.o.
Carprofen	2 mg kg^{-1} bid p.o. Reduce to lowest effective dose for maintenance
Ketoprofen	2 mg kg^{-1} s.c., i.m or i.v daily for a maximum of 3 days or 1 mg kg^{-1} p.o. daily for a maximum of 5 days
Meloxicam	0.2 mg kg^{-1} daily p.o.; after 7–21 days reduce to 0.1 mg kg^{-1} daily, or lowest effective dose for maintenance
Piroxicam	0.3 mg kg^{-1} every 48 h p.o.
Mefenamic acid	20–30 mg kg^{-1} bid p.o. (loading dose for up to 2 weeks); 5 mg kg^{-1} bid p.o. (maintenance)
Sodium hyaluronate	0.3–0.5 ml intra-articular
Pentosan polysulphate	3 mg kg^{-1} s.c. Five doses administered at intervals of 5–7 days
Prednisolone	1–2 mg kg^{-1} daily p.o. initially in divided doses (anti-inflammatory). Reduce to minimum effective dose. May be given on alternate days

bid = twice daily; tid = three times daily; p.o. = per os; i.m. = intramuscular; s.c. = subcutaneous.

ent safety of the drug. Pharmacological safety evaluations have also shown no significant adverse effects of carprofen on the renal system (Baruth *et al.*, 1986).

Meloxicam is the only member of the oxicam group of NSAIDS licensed for use in dogs. Another oxicam, piroxicam, has been used empirically in dogs (Thomas, 1987; Galbraith and McKellar, 1991; McKellar *et al.*, 1991a). Meloxicam is an extremely potent NSAID with a greater therapeutic ratio than aspirin in dogs. Available evidence indicates that it does not hasten cartilage degeneration in osteoarthritic joints in dogs.

Flunixin meglumine is licensed for use in dogs in the UK in both parenteral and oral form and it is effective in the control of musculoskeletal pain and inflammation. Administration of flunixin for more than three successive days is not recommended by the manufacturers and this period should not be exceeded.

Other non-steroidal drugs which may be used for the treatment of OA include hyaluronic acid derivatives, polysulphated glycosaminoglycans (PSGAG) derivatives, orgotein and dimethylsulphoxide. Only one of these (pentosan polysulphate, a PSGAG) is licensed for use in dogs. The role of PSGAGs in the management of OA has not been fully evaluated, but they have several effects which may be beneficial. The most important of these are anti-inflammatory activity and evidence that PSGAGs are chondroprotective in dogs (Altman *et al.*, 1989). Chondroprotection is a property of drugs which arrest or moderate the degradative processes in articular cartilage while simultaneously supporting anabolic pathways essential for its repair (Ghosh, 1988).

Glucocorticoids are powerful inhibitors of inflammation. However, their usefulness in the long-term management of OA is limited because they have serious systemic side effects and because the effect of glucocorticoids on OA cartilage awaits further clarification (Ghosh, 1988; Pelletier and Martel-Pelletier, 1989). At present it is advisable to reserve glucocorticoid therapy for short-term control of acute episodes of synovitis in OA or for the control of inflammation associated with severe, end-stage OA. Glucocorticoids should only be used in OA at their lowest effective dose and in many cases it is possible to maintain adequate quality of life by dosing on an every other day basis.

Surgical treatment

Most surgical management in OA of dogs and cats is aimed at removing the primary cause. Such procedures include replacement of a torn cranial cruciate ligament, stabilization of a luxating patella, triple pelvic and/or intertrochanteric osteotomy to improve the biomechanics of hip joint function and removal of cartilage flaps from joints with osteochondrosis dissecans. Surgical treatment of OA itself may include subtotal synovectomy as a palliative measure, but this is rarely performed in dogs and cats. Most surgical procedures that aim to manage OA directly are salvage procedures which include excision arthroplasties and arthrodeses. Joint replacement arthroplasties are used with ever-increasing frequency in the management of serious joint disease in people and this technology is now becoming more readily available in veterinary medicine. The most common joint arthroplasty procedure at the moment is the total hip replacement (THR). The main indication for THR in humans is as a salvage procedure for end-stage joint disease. However, some veterinary surgeons now use THR as a primary management technique in young dogs with severe hip subluxation as a result of hip dysplasia, long before the dogs have serious OA.

■ Inflammatory joint disease

Inflammatory joint disease is characterized by synovitis with or without accompanying systemic illness. Inflammatory joint diseases of humans have infectious, crystal-induced, drug-induced and idiopathic aetiologies. Crystal arthropathies are rare in dogs and cats and most cases of inflammatory joint disease have either infectious or idiopathic aetiologies.

Infectious arthropathies

Arthritis may be caused by many infectious agents, including bacteria, viruses, fungi, mycoplasma and rickettsia. Rickettsial arthritides are unimportant in the UK but in some areas of the USA they are increasingly associated with non-erosive inflammatory polyarthritis (Cowell *et al.*, 1988; Pedersen *et al.*, 1989).

Bacterial infective arthritis (suppurative arthritis)

Bacterial infective arthritis (BIA) is seen in all ages of dog. It is most common in large breeds and in males. Affected animals usually present with acute onset lameness in a single limb which is associated with pathology in a single joint. Simultaneous infection in more than one joint is occasionally seen and in some cases the onset of disease is insidious. Affected joints show signs of inflammation, including heat, pain, swelling, disuse and, in some cases, crepitus. There may be local limb oedema and lymphadenopathy. Pyrexia, depression, lethargy and inappetence may be seen, but in most cases there are no signs of systemic illness (Bennett and Taylor, 1988a).

Bacterial infective arthritis is caused by many different organisms but most cases are associated with either staphylococci or β-haemolytic streptococci. The type of pathology evident in the joint is dependent on the infecting organism. Staphylococci and some coliforms tend to cause rapid joint destruction, whereas infections by streptococci and *erysipelas* tend to be less aggressive (Pedersen *et al.*, 1989). Bacteria gain access to the joint by any one of several routes:

1. Penetrating wounds (including surgical incisions and intra-articular injections);
2. Extension from neighbouring osteomyelitis or soft tissue infection;
3. Haematogenous spread from a distant site of infection (e.g. bacterial endocarditis, urogenital tract infection, umbilical infection);
4. Tracking foreign bodies.

Involvement of more than one joint is most common when joint penetration is by haematogenous spread, particularly in cases of bacterial endocarditis and umbilical infection. It is important to differentiate BIA from traumatic joint disease and this is particularly difficult in the early stages of disease when radiographic evidence of BIA may be minimal (Bennett and Taylor, 1988a). Synovial fluid analysis is helpful in such cases (Table 44.3). The earliest radiographic changes in BIA are periarticular and intra-articular soft tissue swelling. Later changes include periarticular periosteal bone proliferation, calcification of periarticular soft tissues, decreased joint space, subchondral bone erosion, subchondral sclerosis and regional osteoporosis (Fig. 44.18).

A presumptive diagnosis of BIA can often be made on the basis of clinical and radiological findings and the cytological features of aspirated synovial fluid. Haematology profiles may reflect systemic infection in some cases, but often there

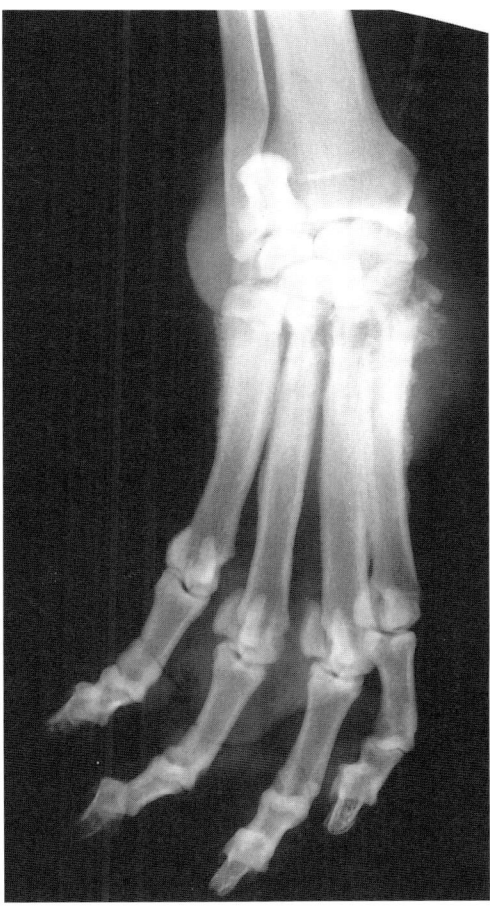

Figure 44.18 Cranial-caudal radiograph of the carpal joint of a dog with bacterial infective arthritis. There is marked soft tissue swelling and aggressive periarticular new bone proliferation. Erosion of bone is seen in the distal row of carpal bones and the proximal epiphyses of metacarpals II–IV.

are no significant haematological changes. Definitive diagnosis requires isolation and identification of the causative organism. Attempts to culture the organism should be made from synovial fluid, synovial membrane, blood or urine before any antibiotic therapy is initiated. Culture is often most successful from synovial membrane biopsy (Bennett and Taylor, 1988a), although pre-incubating synovial fluid in blood culture medium increases the chances of success (Abercromby, 1994). If needed, synovial membrane biopsies can sometimes be obtained at surgery to implant intra-articular drains. Antibiotic sensitivities should be obtained.

Treatment is by prolonged antibiotic therapy given systemically and/or locally. Most antibiotics will penetrate the inflamed joint and systemic administration of antibiotics is usually effective. A broad-spectrum, bactericidal antibiotic should be given initially and should only be changed if specifically indicated by bacteriological culture and sensitivity results. Cephalosporin derivatives or clavulanate potentiated amoxycillin are suitable in many cases. Surgical drainage and lavage may be used to supplement systemic antibiotic therapy in cases with particularly severe and rapidly progressive joint disease. Drainage may be by needle aspiration or, more commonly, by the use of surgical drains which are left in place for three to five days. Adjunctive treatment includes protecting the joint by bandaging, analgesia, daily flushing of the drains with sterile saline and good nursing care. Most cases require an Elizabethan collar to prevent interference with the drains. The technique of distension irrigation is beneficial in some cases, particularly when there is excessive suppuration. Distension irrigation is performed by infusing fluid into the joint whilst preventing outflow through the drains. The joint is left in distension for a few minutes before releasing the outflow. This technique requires good patient co-operation as it produces some discomfort, but it is a valuable way of clearing inflammatory debris and limiting the formation of adhesions. Antibiotic impregnated polymethylmethacrylate beads may also be useful in the management of joint infections, particularly when the causative agent shows multiple antibiotic resistance (Brown and Bennett, 1989). Antibiotic treatment should be continued for a minimum of two weeks after the signs of infection have subsided. Rest is important during the initial phases of treatment, but gentle exercise and passive motion help to limit adhesions during the recovery phase. In a small number of cases, BIA may be superseded by sterile inflammation associated with persistence of bacterial antigens and/or immune complexes. Such cases respond to anti-inflammatory therapy with corticosteroids, but it is essential that the joint is sterile before these are administered (Bennett and Taylor, 1988a).

Osteoarthritis is an almost inevitable sequel to joint infection and in some cases it progresses rapidly. Consequently, the prognosis for return of normal joint function is poor. Cases of bacterial endocarditis carry a particularly poor prognosis and they may be complicated by an immune-mediated arthropathy. Many cases of bacterial endocarditis succumb to severe systemic illness which shows a poor response to therapy (Bennett and Taylor, 1988b).

Discospondylitis

Bacteria may lodge in the intervertebral disc spaces and give rise to discospondylitis. Most cases are reported in young, large breeds of dog presenting with spinal pain and stiffness or hindlimb lameness (Denny et al., 1982). Neurological deficits occur in some cases. Pain can often be localized to the affected area of the spine and some cases show signs of systemic illness. Staphylococci and coliforms are the most common organisms isolated from discospondylitis lesions. Initial infection is presumably by the haematogenous route and local trauma may play a role in predisposing individual disc spaces to bacterial lodgement. Urinary tract infections have been implicated in the pathogenesis of discospondylitis, but this finding is controversial and some authors suggest that the co-existence of urinary tract infection is coincidental in affected dogs (Turnwald et al., 1986).

The earliest radiographic finding in discospondylitis is widening of the affected intervertebral disc space. Later there is destruction of the vertebral body endplates on either side of the disc space. The resulting irregular lytic area is surrounded by sclerotic bone and periosteal new bone proliferation (Fig. 44.19). If necessary, the diagnosis can be confirmed by bacterial culture of material curetted from the affected disc space. Antibiotic sensitivities should be obtained.

If diagnosed promptly, most cases respond to systemic antibiotic therapy for 6–8 weeks, rest and supportive anti-inflammatory therapy (Gilmore, 1987). Other cases require curettage and debridement of the affected area to remove necrotic tissue in addition to systemic antibiotic therapy. Emergency spinal decompressive surgery is indicated in those animals with neurological deficits associated with compression of the spinal cord by the expansile lesion. Spinal decompression may be combined with vertebral body fusion to increase vertebral stability (McKee et al., 1990). Prognosis is dependent on the severity of presenting signs. Dogs with mild disease, treated promptly, have a good prognosis, but those with severe neurological deficits warrant a poor prognosis.

Lyme disease

Lyme disease is a multisystemic inflammatory disorder caused by infection with the tick-borne spirochaete *Borrelia burgdorferi* (Steere, 1989; Appel, 1990). *Ixodes ricinus* is probably the main vector of *B. burgdorferi* in the UK.

Many different syndromes have been associated with *B. burgdorferi* infection, including dermatological, neurological, cardiological and rheumatological diseases. There is no conclusive evidence that significant dermatological disease occurs in dogs with Lyme disease and there is little definitive work on cardiological or neurological manifestations of the disease in small animals. Most dogs with Lyme disease have lameness associated with inflammatory synovitis which is commonly monoarticular or pauciarticular. True polyarthritis is rare (Kornblatt et al., 1985; May et al., 1990). Joint signs normally commence some weeks or months after exposure to *Ixodes ricinus* and they may be accompanied by mild signs of systemic illness, including pyrexia and low-grade, localized, lymphadenopathy. The lameness often spontaneously resolves after a few days, but repeated relapses may occur. Some dogs have a history of non-specific pyrexic illness soon after tick-exposure.

The synovitis in Lyme disease is associated with the presence of *B. burgdorferi* in joint tissues, but the degree of inflammation is out of proportion to the number of organisms present and it is thought that host immune-responses also contribute to the pathogenesis of disease. *B. burgdorferi* can persist for months or years in its host and untreated individuals may develop chronic disease which could be confused with the idiopathic inflammatory joint disorders. A small number of dogs with Lyme disease may develop an aggressive joint disease similar to rheumatoid arthritis.

A diagnosis of Lyme disease is difficult to con-

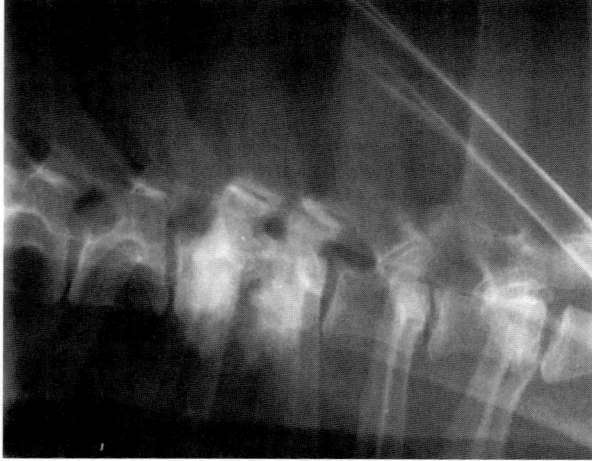

Figure 44.19 Lateral radiograph of a dog with advanced discospondylitis. There is collapse of the disc space, destruction of the adjacent vertebral body endplates and aggressive new bone proliferation.

firm. Most affected dogs have non-erosive inflammatory joint disease and the only visible radiographic changes include moderate periarticular and intra-articular soft tissue swelling. Synovial fluid analysis is similar to that of the non-infective inflammatory arthritides. The following criteria have been suggested for the diagnosis of Lyme disease in dogs (Bennett et al., 1992):

1. A history of potential exposure to *B. burgdorferi*;
2. Seasonal incidence; most cases of Lyme disease in the USA are associated with times of peak activity of ixodid nymph (spring) or adult (autumn) stages;
3. Appropriate clinical signs; these include fever, malaise, lethargy, inappetence, lymphadenopathy, lameness, myocarditis (heart block), neurological signs and possibly glomerulonephritis;
4. Laboratory and radiological support for the diagnosis; for example, in the case of arthropathy, there may be an associated articular effusion and aspirated synovial fluid will be characteristic of an inflammatory arthropathy;
5. A positive serological test for *B. burgdorferi*; some asymptomatic animals may be positive for anti-*Borrelia* antibodies (May et al., 1991);
6. Response to antibiotic therapy;
7. Identification of *B. burgdorferi* in blood, urine, synovial fluid, CSF or tissues;
8. Culture of *B. burgdorferi* from blood, urine, synovial fluid, CSF, or tissues;
9. Exclusion of other possible causes of similar clinical signs; for example, canine rheumatoid arthritis and systemic lupus erythematosus should be considered and excluded as differential diagnoses for Lyme disease.

A diagnosis of Lyme disease in dogs should satisfy criteria 1, 3, 4, 5 and 9. Criterion 6 should be subsequently satisfied in most cases. Ideally, criteria 7 and 8 should also be satisfied, but this may be impractical as *B. burgdorferi* is often present in low numbers in Lyme disease patients and the organism is notoriously difficult to culture.

Most cases of Lyme arthritis in dogs respond to antibiotic therapy, particularly if they are diagnosed and treated promptly. A response to antibiotics should be seen within seven days of the start of treatment, but it is advisable to continue antibiotic therapy for at least two weeks after complete clinical recovery. Oxytetracycline is commonly recommended for the treatment of *B. burgdorferi* infections on the basis of *in vitro* sensitivity results. However, *B. burgdorferi* is capable of evading immune responses and it may be more advisable to use a bactericidal antibiotic. Ampicillin is effective *in vivo*.

Other infective arthritides

Canine tuberculosis is now exceedingly rare in the UK but is important because affected animals are an obvious public health risk. Arthritis is a feature of some *Mycobacterium tuberculosis* infections.

Mycoplasma species have occasionally been isolated from the joints of dogs with inflammatory arthropathies, but their significance remains unclear (Bennett, 1990).

No cases of fungal arthritis in the dog have yet been reported in the UK. Outside the UK fungal arthritis is uncommon and has a restricted geographical distribution. Most often fungal arthritis is an extension of fungal osteomyelitis, but primary fungal synovitis may occur in some cases. The organisms most frequently implicated in fungal arthritis are *Coccidioides* sp., *Blastomyces* sp. and *Cryptococcus* sp. Multiple discospondylitis is one presenting feature in dogs with extranasal forms of aspergillosis (Neer, 1988). The German shepherd dog is over-represented for this condition, possibly as a consequence of defective IgA production (Day and Penhale, 1988). Common clinical features include weight loss, anorexia, fever, depression, back pain, weakness, paresis or paralysis. Infection is often due to *Aspergillus terreus* and it is important to note that serodiagnostic tests for *A. fumigatus* (the most common nasal form of aspergillosis) will be negative in affected dogs.

Leishmania donovani is a protozoan parasite which may cause shifting lameness or polyarthritis and systemic illness in dogs (Yamaguchi et al., 1983; May, 1989). Leishmaniasis is endemic in certain countries including the Mediterranean basin and South America. The disease has a long latent period and some dogs imported into the UK may remain asymptomatic throughout their quarantine period. Leishmaniasis is important as a potentially serious zoonosis.

Specific viral infections of joints are unknown in dogs but arthralgia is a complicating feature of some systemic viral infections. Some dogs suffer a transient inflammatory polyarthritis as a sequel to vaccination, particularly with live virus vaccines, but it is not known which component of the vaccine is the phlogistic agent (Pedersen et al., 1989). The inflammation of canine rheumatoid arthritis has been associated with a persistent immune response to canine distemper viral antigens (Bell et al., 1991).

Immune-mediated

The term 'immune-mediated' joint disease (IJD) encompasses several inflammatory syndromes characterized by chronic synovial inflammation (Table 44.5). Excessive or persistent immune-responses and/or autoimmunity contribute to the pathogenesis of these syndromes. The pathology of canine IJD may be explained by chronic immune responses to a persistent intra-articular antigen or antigens. Some IJD syndromes are associated with known causes, such as adverse drug reactions, but most cases are idiopathic. It is a common hypothesis that some of the IJD syndromes with hitherto unknown aetiologies are associated with persistent microbial infection (Zvaifler, 1989). Furthermore, it is clear in humans that genetically determined factors, particularly major histocompatibility complex (MHC) antigens, predispose individuals to particular types of IJD (Arnett, 1989). Little is known about canine MHC in this regard, but it is possible that canine IJD results from exposure of a genetically susceptible individual to an infectious agent or agents which may be ubiquitous in the canine population. The precise clinical presentation may vary, not with the aetiology, but with the particular genetic susceptibility of the individual. Thus, it is wrong to presume that the clusters of clinical signs recognized as IJD with differing prognoses are in fact different disease entities. Canine idiopathic IJD should only be regarded as syndromes until their aetiologies become clear. Diagnostic criteria based on clinical and paraclinical findings help to standardize the diagnosis of these syndromes.

Canine rheumatoid arthritis

Canine rheumatoid arthritis (CRA) typically presents with lameness and joint stiffness which is often worse after prolonged periods of inactivity. CRA affects both sexes and many breeds of dog, particularly in middle age (Bennett, 1987a). Affected dogs are usually lame and often reluctant to move. They may show signs of systemic illness including pyrexia, inappetence, respiratory disease, gastrointestinal disorders and conjunctivitis (Halliwell et al., 1972; Schiefer et al., 1974; Bennett, 1987a). The lameness is always progressive, sometimes with periods of remission interspersed with relapses. In some cases there is marked muscle atrophy, but the most prominent changes are always seen in the joints. Several joints may be diseased at any one time and the joint disease frequently has a bilaterally symmetrical distribution. Any joint may be involved in CRA but the joints of the distal limb are most commonly affected. The affected joints show signs typical of inflammation including heat, soft tissue swelling and pain. Instability may result from ligament rupture secondary to the inflammation and there may be crepitus. In chronic cases there is often severe joint deformity associated with the loss of periarticular soft tissue support and erosion of cartilage and subchondral bone. Granulation tissue (pannus) develops in some cases within the joint and invades both over and under the articular cartilage. The development of pannus is associated with particularly severe erosive disease (Bennett, 1987b).

The commonly used criteria for diagnosing CRA are derived from criteria designed for the diagnosis of rheumatoid arthritis in humans (Ropes et al., 1959; Bennett, 1987a):

1. Stiffness after rest;
2. Pain or tenderness in at least one joint;
3. Soft tissue swelling or effusion in at least one joint;
4. Swelling of at least one other joint within 3 months;
5. Symmetrical joint swelling;
6. Subcutaneous nodules over bony prominences, extensor surfaces or in juxta-articular regions;
7. Destructive radiographic changes typical of rheumatoid arthritis;
8. Positive laboratory test for serum rheumatoid factor;
9. Appropriate cytological abnormalities in synovial fluid and poor mucin precipitate from synovial fluid;
10. Characteristic histopathological changes in the synovial membrane with three or more of the following: marked villous hypertrophy, proliferation of superficial synovial cells, marked infiltration of chronic inflammatory cells (lymphocytes and plasma cells predominating) with a tendency to form 'lymphoid nodules', deposition of fibrin and foci of cell necrosis;
11. Characteristic histopathological changes in subcutaneous nodules showing granulomatous foci with central zones of cell necrosis surrounded by proliferated fixed cells, peripheral fibrosis and a chronic inflammatory cell infiltration, predominantly perivascular.

Classical CRA is diagnosed when seven criteria are satisfied and *definite* CRA when five are satisfied. The joint signs in criteria 1–5 must be present for at least six weeks. At least two of criteria 7, 8 and 10 must be satisfied. *Possible* and *probable* RA are also diagnosed in humans, but these diagnoses are not extrapolated for CRA.

The most prominent radiographic features in the joints of affected dogs are symmetrical deformity and the presence of subchondral bone erosions or loss of mineralization in the epiphyses (Fig. 44.20a and b). The erosions may be well demarcated, or poorly defined. Joint space may increase during the early stages of the disease due to effusion or synovial proliferation, but during the later stages there is joint space narrowing as a result of cartilage destruction (Newton et al., 1976; Pedersen et al., 1976a). In addition to the destructive changes there may be radiological evidence of bone proliferation, including subchondral bone sclerosis and periarticular periosteal new bone formation. In early CRA, the only joint abnormality recognized radiographically may be soft tissue swelling (Biery and Newton, 1975), and it is possible for dogs to satisfy sufficient criteria to justify a diagnosis of classical or definite CRA without evidence of erosive joint disease.

The synovial fluid abnormalities in CRA are common to all forms of inflammatory joint disease (Table 44.3).

Serum rheumatoid factor (RF) levels are a useful adjunct to the diagnosis of CRA. However, only 40–75% of dogs with CRA test positive for RF by the Rose–Waaler method (Bennett, 1980, 1987a). A titre of greater than 1:16 is usually considered positive but variation may occur between laboratories. Recently, a more sensitive enzyme-linked immunosorbent assay (ELISA) has been developed for measuring canine RF (Carter et al., 1989). As in humans, RF levels alone are not specific for CRA and raised levels may occur in a variety of arthritides (Carter et al., 1989).

The prognosis in CRA is poor. The disease is inevitably progressive and the resulting disability often necessitates eventual euthanasia. However, extended periods of remission can be achieved and dogs with CRA lead quite acceptable lives as pets for many years.

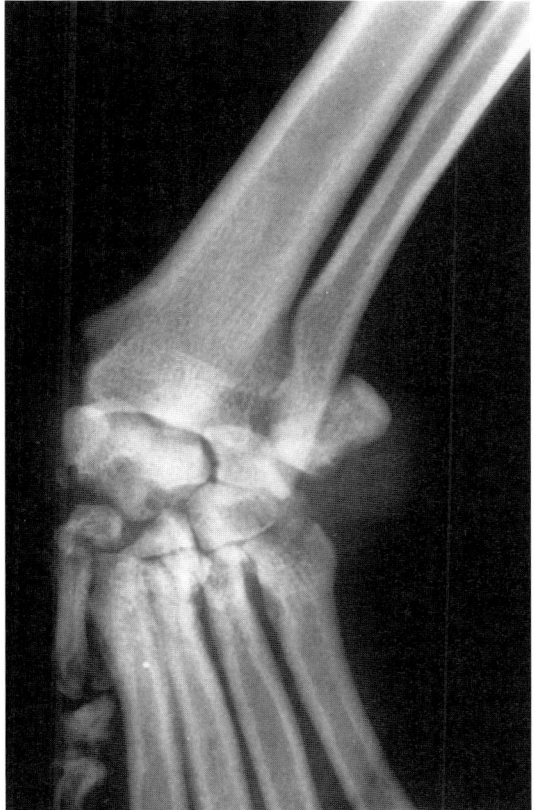 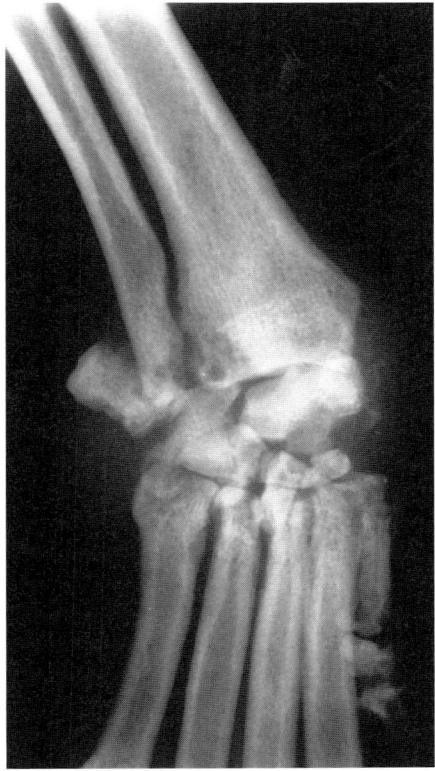

Figure 44.20 Cranial-caudal radiographs of the left (a) and right (b) carpal joints of a dog with rheumatoid arthritis. Both joints show soft tissue swelling, subluxation, subchondral bone erosion and periarticular new bone proliferation. The changes are very symmetrical.

Non-steroidal anti-inflammatory drugs are the mainstay of treatment in humans with rheumatoid arthritis, but they are not commonly used to control CRA. Prednisolone is the most commonly used drug in the treatment of CRA, either on its own or in combination with other therapies (Table 44.7). Once remission is achieved, the dose is gradually reduced to the minimum level which adequately controls the arthritis without giving rise to excessive corticosteroid side effects. Every-other-day dosing can be achieved in many cases. When combination therapies with cytotoxic drugs are used, it is important to monitor peripheral blood cell counts for evidence of bone marrow suppression and to monitor for other side effects (Table 44.7). Sterile haemorrhagic cystitis commonly occurs when cyclophosphamide is used for more than three to four consecutive months. This complication is potentially serious and is best avoided. Azathioprine is the preferred drug to combine with prednisolone if prolonged cytotoxic therapy is necessary.

Prednisolone therapy may also be supplemented with the administration of gold salts in either injectable (sodium aurothiomalate) or oral (auranofin) form (Table 44.7). Patients receiving crysotherapy should be regularly monitored for serious side effects which include bone marrow suppression, renal impairment, pulmonary fibrosis, dermatoses and corneal ulceration. Orally administered gold salts are supposedly safer than parenteral forms, although there are few objective data available in dogs (Serra and White, 1989). Many dogs develop an osmotic diarrhoea with oral gold therapy. This may be difficult to control and some owners consequently request withdrawal of the drug.

With the possible exception of gold salts, there is no current evidence that the above-mentioned drugs will favourably modify the progression of CRA in any way and all are given for symptomatic relief only. Bearing in mind the toxicity of these agents, one should always aim to administer the minimum dose that is required for adequate control of the disease and complete withdrawal of the drugs should be attempted periodically during extended periods of remission. It is also important to note that, prednisolone aside, none of these drugs are licensed for use in dogs. Many other drugs are available for the management of chronic inflammatory joint diseases, but few have been sufficiently evaluated to recommend their routine use in dogs.

In selected cases, surgical procedures may be indicated for the relief of pain or disability in individual joints. These procedures may include synovectomy, ligament repair, arthrodesis and joint replacement therapy.

Table 44.7 Drug therapies in immune-mediated joint disease of dogs and cats

Drug	Notes
Prednisolone	Initially 2–4 mg kg^{-1} p.o. daily (immunosuppressive dose). After 2–4 weeks, gradually reduce the dose over 2–3 months. Aim for complete withdrawal or every other day treatment.
Cyclophosphamide	50 mg m^{-2} p.o. given on four consecutive days each week. Combine with prednisolone (initial dose 1–2 mg kg^{-1} daily). Monitor for myelosuppression[a] every 7–14 days. High risk of haemorrhagic cystitis after 3–4 months.
Azathioprine	2 mg kg^{-1} p.o. on alternate days with prednisolone (1–2 mg kg^{-1}). Monitor for myelosuppression.[a] High risk of toxicity in cats.
Sodium aurothiolomate	0.5–1 mg kg^{-1} i.m. weekly for 6 weeks in combination with prednisolone (2–4 mg kg^{-1} p.o. initially). Monitor for myelosuppression,[a] renal failure, dermatitis, pulmonary fibrosis, corneal ulceration. Can repeat course after 2–3 months. Poorly evaluated in cats.
Auranofin	0.05–2.0 mg kg^{-1} p.o. twice daily (max. 9 mg day^{-1}) in combination with prednisolone (2–4 mg kg^{-1} p.o. initially). May use continuously. Monitor for osmotic diarrhoea and for same side effects as aurothiolamate. Not evaluated in cats.

[a] Myelosuppression may occur weeks or months after initiation of therapy. Reduce dose by 25% if WBC count falls below 6×10^9 l^{-1} or platelet count falls below 125×10^9 l^{-1}. Discontinue therapy for at least 2 weeks if WBC count falls below 4×10^9 l^{-1} or platelet count falls below 100×10^9 l^{-1}. Reinstate therapy at 50% of original dose.
p.o. = per os; i.m. = intra-muscular; WBC = white blood cell.

Canine systemic lupus erythematosus

In humans, systemic lupus erythematosus (SLE) is an idiopathic, multisystemic inflammatory disorder characterized by the presence of multiple autoantibodies that participate in immunologically mediated tissue injury (Rothfield, 1989). Autoantibodies against nuclear antigens (antinuclear antibodies, ANA) are a consistent finding in patients with SLE (Friou, 1967).

Canine SLE is also a multisystemic disease but its diagnosis is controversial. Some workers diagnose canine SLE on the basis of multisystemic involvement, even if the patient is seronegative for ANA (Werner and Halliwell, 1984). Others insist that canine SLE should only be diagnosed if circulating ANA are present (Bennett, 1987c).

SLE in dogs presents with a bewildering range of clinical signs and symptoms dependent on the organ systems involved. It has been associated with non-erosive polyarthritis, autoimmune haemolytic anaemia (AIHA), thrombocytopenia, leucopenia, glomerulonephritis, mucocutaneous ulceration, skin lesions (alopecia, erythema, crusting), polymyositis, neurological disorders (behavioural changes, seizures, ataxia), gastrointestinal disease (vomiting, diarrhoea, abdominal pain), polydypsia, tachypnoea, pyrexia, lethargy and inappetence. Pyrexia, polyarthritis, proteinuria and blood dyscrasias are the most common clinicopathological findings.

Criteria have been developed to simplify the diagnosis of SLE in dogs. Several different sets of criteria have been reported in the literature, but all aim to demonstrate multisystem involvement and an autoimmune response (Werner and Halliwell, 1984; Bennett, 1987c). Bennett (1987c) recommends the following criteria.

1. Evidence of involvement of more than one body system. It is unlikely that any one patient will show evidence of involvement of more than two or three organ systems at any one time.
2. Serum ANA detectable at a significantly high titre. A titre of greater than 1:16 is usually considered positive, but there may be variation between individual laboratories.
3. Immunopathological features consistent with the clinical findings. For example, if AIHA, thrombocytopenia or leucopenia are present, antibodies should be shown against red blood cells, platelets or white blood cells, respectively.

Criteria 1 and 2 must always be satisfied (*probable* canine SLE). If all three are satisfied, *definite* canine SLE may be diagnosed.

Joint abnormalities may not be identified radiographically in all cases. Joint abnormalities which are demonstrable radiographically include soft tissue swelling associated with synovial membrane proliferation or synovial fluid effusion and, uncommonly, periarticular bone proliferation. Destructive change in the joints is not a feature of SLE.

Haematology and serum biochemistry profiles are helpful in determining which organ systems are involved in SLE, but further assays are needed to confirm the diagnosis. Blood from dogs with suspected SLE should be tested for autoagglutination of erythrocytes. Those not showing autoagglutination should undergo a test for immunoglobulins attached to erythrocytes (Coombs' test) at 37°C and 4°C (Bennett, 1980). Bennett (1987c) found five of 13 dogs with SLE had anaemia; all five were either Coombs' positive or showed autoagglutination. Similarly, Werner and Halliwell (1984) maintain that the anaemia associated with SLE in dogs should always be Coombs' positive. Conversely, in humans, although mild anaemia is common in SLE patients, less than 5% suffer haemolytic, Coombs' positive anaemia (Huskisson and Hart, 1987). Antinuclear antibodies in dog serum may be assayed by any of several methods, but some commonly used tests are unreliable and may give rise to false negative or false positive results. An indirect immunofluorescence assay, using rat liver as a substrate and a fluorescein-conjugated anti-dog IgG reagent, is reported to be the most reliable method (Bennett and Kirkham, 1987). The LE cell test is a measure of polymorphonuclear phagocyte engulfment of nuclear material coated with antinuclear antibodies. The LE phenomenon, performed *in vitro*, may also be used as an assay of ANA in the diagnosis of SLE. Some dogs with SLE may be seropositive for RF at low titres (Bennett, 1987c).

The prognosis for SLE is guarded; there is no cure and most animals require lifelong therapy. Treatment is with immunosuppressive therapy using prednisolone alone or in combination with cyclophosphamide or azathioprine (Table 44.7 and see canine rheumatoid arthritis).

Canine idiopathic polyarthritis

Canine idiopathic polyarthritis (CIP) is a descriptive term for cases of IJD of dogs that cannot be classified into more clearly defined groups (Pedersen *et al.*, 1976b; Bennett, 1987d). Affected animals are usually young adults presenting with pyrexia, lethargy and inappetence as well as lameness due to inflammation in multiple joints. Additional body systems may be involved, giving a variety of clinical signs, including lymphadenopathy, splenomegaly, oral haemorrhages, retinal haemorrhage and hyperreflexia, polydipsia, proteinuria, neurological disease and muscle atrophy. Dogs with CIP are seronegative for ANA and RF.

Synovitis in dogs with CIP is thought to arise, in part, from the chronic perivascular deposition of immune-complexes in the synovial membrane supporting layer. The antigen–antibody complexes activate complement components which act as inflammatory mediators. Immune-complex formation is a normal part of the immune-response to non-self ('foreign') antigens. However, in some cases, immune-complexes may be formed persistently and at levels which cannot adequately be cleared. The immune-complexes localize to certain tissues, including the joints, either because they are formed locally, or because they are carried to the tissues via the circulation after forming elsewhere in the body.

The underlying pathology remains obscure in approximately 50% of CIP cases (Bennett, 1987d). However, some cases are not truly idiopathic. Episodes of polyarthritis are often associated with a recent history of other illness, commonly gastroenteritis, but occasionally urogenital infection, respiratory tract infection, skin infection or abscessation. In humans, polyarthritis associated with infection occurs commonly in males who carry a particular MHC antigen (called HLA-B27). Individuals with this genotype, who are exposed to certain infections are at greater risk of developing polyarthritis as a complication (Calin and Fries, 1976). Certain gastroenteric and urogenital infections are particularly important in the aetiology of this form of arthritis, notably those caused by *Chlamydia* spp., *Salmonella* spp., *Yersinia* spp., *Shigella* spp., *Campylobacter* spp. and *Ureaplasma* spp. (Ford, 1989). No microbes have been definitively associated with canine or feline idiopathic polyarthritides, but it is possible that CIP of dogs (and cats), associated with infection elsewhere in the body, has a similar pathogenesis to human HLA-B27-associated disease.

Inflammatory synovitis associated with infection and HLA-B27 is called reactive arthritis or, if there is a triad of clinical signs which includes urethritis, conjunctivitis and polyarthritis, the term Reiter's syndrome may be substituted for reactive arthritis (Huskisson and Hart, 1987). Reiter's syndrome has been used in the veterinary literature to describe periosteal proliferative polyarthritis of cats, but this usage may be incorrect and should be discouraged.

Polyarthritis may also be seen as a complication of neoplasia and it is probable that in these cases the tumour acts as a chronic source of self-antigens which are so altered as to break tolerance and result in persistent immune-complex formation. Rarely, polyarthritis may accompany chronic bowel disease, such as histiocytic colitis. Very little is known about this syndrome, but it may be an analogue of enteropathic arthritis in humans (Huskisson and Hart, 1987).

Radiographically, the joints of dogs with CIP show changes similar to those seen in SLE. There is early joint effusion and an increased joint space may be apparent. Later, secondary degenerative changes and periarticular bone proliferation are seen. In some cases there is calcification of periarticular soft tissues. Subchondral bone erosions, as seen in canine rheumatoid arthritis, are not a feature of CIP.

Most laboratory tests are directed towards excluding diagnoses of canine rheumatoid arthritis and systemic lupus erythematosus. Synovial fluid analyses are consistent with all forms of immune mediated joint disease (Table 44.3).

Treatment of CIP is aimed at the inciting pathology if this can be recognized. If the primary pathology is successfully treated, the polyarthritis will often resolve. It is sometimes necessary to supplement treatment of the primary disease with immunosuppressive doses of prednisolone (Table 44.7) to control the synovitis. Prednisolone is the mainstay of treatment in those cases in which no underlying pathology can be recognized.

Many dogs with CIP respond well to prednisolone therapy and in some cases the drug can eventually be completely withdrawn. Some dogs require lifelong therapy; in these cases the drug should be given at the minimal effective dose (usually every other day). A small number of cases require combination therapy with prednisolone and cyclophosphamide or azathioprine (Table 44.7 and see canine rheumatoid arthritis). Canine idiopathic polyarthritis is usually more readily controlled than either canine rheumatoid arthritis (CRA) or systemic lupus erythematosus (SLE). If a case of CIP is difficult to control with just prednisolone, the diagnosis should be reviewed; CRA, SLE, bacterial endocarditis, underlying infections, malignancy, gastrointestinal disease, Lyme disease and infectious arthritides (bacterial, fungal, viral, mycoplasmal, rickettsial and protozoal) should all be considered as differential diagnoses.

Other polyarthritis syndromes of dogs

A syndrome of dogs, particularly the spaniel breeds, has been described that is characterized by non-infective inflammatory polyarthritis (non-erosive) and polymyositis (Bennett and Kelly, 1987). All the cases were seronegative for ANA and RF. Similarly, a syndrome in which polyarthritis is associated with clinical signs of meningitis has been described (Bennett, 1984). Some breed-related inflammatory arthropathy syndromes have been reported, including an erosive inflammatory arthropathy of greyhounds (Woodard *et al.*, 1991) and an inflammatory arthropathy of Japanese Akitas (Dougherty *et al.*, 1991). Inflammatory synovitis is one component of a fever syndrome recognized in Chinese sharpei dogs (May *et al.*, 1992). Drug idiosyncrasies may give rise to polyarthritis and systemic illness as a result of hypersensitivity reactions. Such reactions are most commonly associated with antibiotics (e.g., sulphonamides, erythromycin, lincomycin, cephalosporins, penicillin derivatives). The polyarthritis usually responds to withdrawal of the causative drug.

Joint neoplasia

Primary joint neoplasia

Synovial cell sarcoma is rarely diagnosed, but it is probably the most common joint tumour in dogs. The tumour usually affects the stifle or elbow (McGlennon *et al.*, 1988). There is great variation in the tendency to develop metastases and most metastatic disease occurs in local lymph nodes or lungs. Lameness is an early presenting feature and may precede significant radiological changes. Eventually, lysis of bone occurs on either side of the joint and there is periarticular soft tissue swelling. The diagnosis can be confirmed by histopathological examination of a synovial membrane biopsy.

Amputation is the usual treatment for synovial sarcoma but chemotherapeutic management with doxorubicin has been described (Tilmant *et al.*, 1986).

Secondary joint neoplasia

Tumours may secondarily invade joints either by local extension or by metastasis. Osteosarcoma may extend into joints from neighbouring bone, but rarely completely traverses a joint. Metastasis to joints is rare but has been documented in lymphosarcoma of cats. Malignant histiocytosis of Bernese mountain dogs may affect joints, either as a primary entity, or by extension from neighbouring tissues.

JOINT DISEASES OF CATS

The classification of joint disease in cats is based on the same principles as the classification of joint disease in dogs. The principles of diagnosis and management of traumatic joint disease are precisely similar to the dog. Some diseases may present as joint disease, but the primary pathology affects bone. These include the mucopolysaccharidoses and hypervitaminosis A, both of which are discussed in the section on bone disorders. Joint tumours are rarely diagnosed in cats. Synovial sarcoma is the most common primary joint tumour of cats. It should be treated by radical excision or amputation.

Like dogs, cats suffer both degenerative and inflammatory joint diseases. The following discussion supplements the section on joint disease of dogs by covering aspects of feline joint disease which differ significantly from their canine counterparts. It cannot be overemphasized that synovial fluid analysis is a powerful tool in the investigation of arthropathies. Interpretation of synovial fluid analysis in cats is similar to that in dogs (Table 44.3).

Degenerative joint disease

Osteoarthritis

Most osteoarthritis (OA) in cats is 'secondary' OA. Joint diseases giving rise to secondary OA in cats include rupture of the cranial cruciate ligament (Scavelli and Schrader, 1987), hip dysplasia (Holt, 1978) and patellar luxations (Houlton and Meynink, 1989). These joint diseases are all diagnosed less commonly in cats than in dogs and it is possible that there are several explanations for this. First, there is far less inbreeding in cats and it is therefore unlikely that genetic predispositions to disease are selected for as they are in dogs. Secondly, loading of the joint is a significant contributory factor in many joint diseases and this may be related to both size and activity. Finally, cats tolerate joint disease far better than dogs and this may also be related to their small size and sedentary lifestyle. For example, hip dysplasia of cats is often only recognized as an incidental finding on pelvic radiographs and is usually of no clinical significance. Rupture of the cranial cruciate ligament in cats is almost always amenable to conservative management, with clinical signs resolving in three to five weeks. Secondary OA and remodelling of the affected stifle invariably occurs, but this does not usually affect the gait or lifestyle of the cat. Only cats that do not respond to conservative therapy need surgical replacement of the cranial cruciate ligament.

It is also uncommon for established OA to present as a clinical problem in cats and this is fortuitous as there are many toxicity problems associated with anti-inflammatory therapy in this species. However, some cats with advanced OA may present with lameness that has an insidious onset and is gradually progressive. Stiffness after rest may be a feature.

Obviously it is difficult to make significant adjustments to a cat's lifestyle as part of the management of OA, but in some cases there may be benefit in a weight reduction programme. Enforced rest may be of help during acute, painful episodes associated with OA.

Some drugs that may be used in the management of OA in cats are listed in Table 44.8. Extreme caution should always be exercised when using NSAIDs in cats; the stated dose must not be exceeded and NSAIDs should not be administered for periods of more than a few days.

Corticosteroids have the advantage of relative safety for treating OA in cats; the obvious disadvantages are the systemic side effects and possible deleterious effects of cartilage degradation. Nevertheless, significant clinical improvement can be achieved with low steroid doses. Prolonged administration of corticosteroids is not recommended.

The polysulphated glycosaminoglycan group of drugs that show promise in the management of canine and equine OA have not been evaluated in cats and cannot yet be recommended for use in this species. Sodium hyaluronate may be given to cats by intra-articular injection at a dose of 0.1 ml per joint.

Surgical salvage procedures are rarely called for in cats with OA, but they may include excision arthroplasty, replacement arthroplasty, arthrodesis or amputation.

Neuropathic arthritis (Charcot joints)

Neuropathic arthritis is a progressive degenerative joint disease which develops as a result of continued weight bearing in the face of sensory nerve loss (Ellman, 1989). The classical clinical presentation is sudden onset, effusive swelling, crepitus and luxations or subluxations in joints of the feet of patients with peripheral neuropathy secondary to diabetes mellitus. Most patients experience relatively less pain than expected for their clinical signs and this allows continued use of the joint, resulting in further damage. The author is aware of a syndrome of carpal joint collapse in cats with chronic diabetes mellitus. The carpal luxation is often bilateral and is associated with relatively little pain. Clinically, this syndrome resembles diabetes mellitus-associated Charcot joint disease, but it is not known for certain that the disease in cats is a true neuropathic arthritis.

Inflammatory joint disease

Bacterial infective arthritis

Bacterial infective arthritis (BIA) of cats most commonly occurs as a result of a penetrating bite wound and presents as acute onset lameness with

Table 44.8 Anti-inflammatory drugs used in the management of feline osteoarthritis

Drug	Dose
Aspirin	15 mg kg^{-1} eod p.o. Avoid prolonged dosing. Paediatric suspension useful for administering small doses
Ketoprofen	2 mg kg^{-1} s.c. daily for a maximum of 3 days *or* 1 mg kg^{-1} p.o. daily for a maximum of 5 days
Phenylbutazone	Maximum of 5–8 mg kg^{-1} bid p.o. (alternate weeks). Avoid prolonged dosing
Sodium hyaluronate	0.1 ml intra-articular
Prednisolone	1–2 mg kg^{-1} daily p.o. initially in divided doses (anti-inflammatory). Reduce to minimum effective dose. May be given on alternate days.

bid = twice daily; eod = every other day; p.o. = per os.

Note: All non-steroidal anti-inflammatory drugs (NSAIDs) should be used with extreme caution in cats. Data for NSAIDs use in other species should never be extrapolated for use in cats.

pain and swelling in a single joint. Management is as for BIA in dogs. Gentamycin-impregnated polymethylmethacrylate beads (Brown and Bennett, 1989) have not been evaluated in cats.

Discospondylitis is rarely documented in cats (Malik et al., 1990).

Lyme disease

Although cats are undoubtedly exposed to *Borrelia burgdorferi*, the available evidence suggests that they do not suffer clinical Lyme disease to the same extent as dogs (Magnarelli et al., 1990).

Viral arthritis

A transient, self-limiting polyarthritis and fever has been documented in cats, particularly kittens, with certain strains of calicivirus acquired by either natural infection or by vaccination (Bennett et al., 1989). In many cases resolution occurs within one week and no specific treatment is necessary. Corticosteroids may be given in cases in which the arthritis persists.

Other infective arthritides

Fungal and mycoplasmal arthritides have both been documented in cats, but they are rare (Pedersen et al., 1989). Mycoplasmal arthritis has only been recorded in debilitated or immunosuppressed cats. Synovial fluid cytology from affected joints reflects synovial inflammation, with many neutrophils which do not show the toxic changes that occur in cases of bacterial infective arthritis (Moise et al., 1983). Mycoplasmal arthritis may be treated with erythromycin or gentamycin, but possible causes of underlying debility should be carefully investigated with particular regard to the feline lymphotropic viruses.

'Immune-mediated' inflammatory joint disease

Immune-mediated inflammatory joint disease is rare in cats, but all the idiopathic inflammatory polyarthritis syndromes seen in dogs (rheumatoid arthritis, systemic lupus erythematosus, canine idiopathic polyarthritis) have their counterparts in cats (Bennett and Nash, 1988). The clinical, radiological and laboratory findings are similar in the feline and canine diseases.

Periosteal proliferative polyarthritis

Periosteal proliferative polyarthritis (PPP) is a form of idiopathic inflammatory arthritis rare in dogs, but recognized relatively commonly in cats (Pedersen et al., 1980). Periosteal proliferative polyarthritis has a marked male sex predisposition. The clinical presentation of PPP is similar to other forms of immune-mediated polyarthritis as are the laboratory features and synovial fluid analyses. Some cats with PPP have conjunctivitis, but this feature is occasionally seen in many other polyarthritis syndromes.

The distinguishing feature of PPP is the marked periosteal new bone that develops around affected joints and may lead to ankylosis. The joints of affected cats are often markedly swollen by the new bone which is readily demonstrated radiographically (Fig. 44.21). Some cases are characterized by erosions of cartilage and subchondral bone with joint instability leading to subluxation or luxation rather than by marked periosteal new bone proliferation.

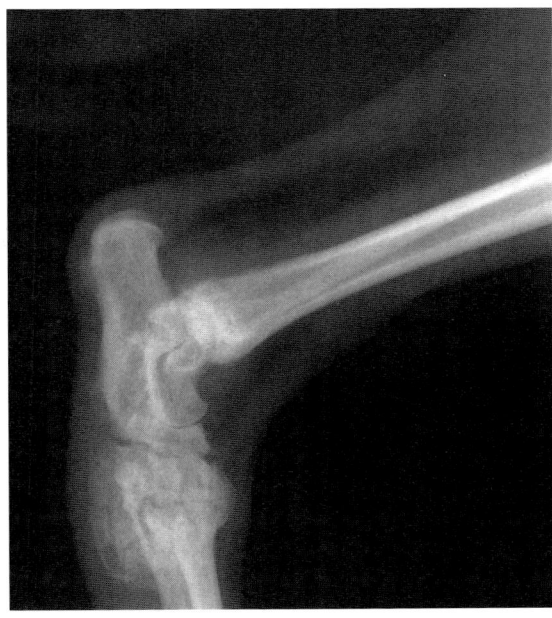

Figure 44.21 Medial-lateral radiograph of the hock joint of a cat with periosteal proliferative polyarthritis. There is soft tissue swelling, but the most prominent feature is the periarticular bone proliferation. Symmetrical changes were seen on a radiograph of the opposite hock joint.

Suggestions that PPP is associated with feline leukaemia virus and feline syncytium forming virus infection have not been substantiated (Pedersen *et al.*, 1980; Bennett and Nash, 1988). It is possible that these viruses are opportunist invaders of the diseased joint.

Treatment of immune-mediated inflammatory joint diseases in cats is similar to that in dogs (Table 44.7). Prednisolone is the mainstay of therapy and should be administered initially at immunosuppressive doses. The dose is gradually reduced over a period of 2–3 months, aiming for the minimum possible dose that controls the joint disease. In refractory cases, cyclophosphamide is the preferred drug in combination with prednisolone (Table 44.7). The constraints that apply for the use of these drugs in dogs also apply in cats. Only the minimum effective dose should be used and gradual withdrawal of combination drug therapy should be attempted if remission is sustained for more than one month. Low dose prednisolone therapy will often be effective in maintaining remission gained in this way and, in some cases, all drug therapy can eventually be withdrawn. It is important to understand that these diseases are not curable. Relapses are likely to occur and these require repeated therapeutic intervention. Some cases need permanent drug therapy. The ultimate prognosis is guarded to poor. Rheumatoid arthritis and PPP may eventually produce such severe joint deformity that euthanasia is indicated on humane grounds.

REFERENCES

Abercromby, R. (1994) Infective arthritis. In: *Manual of Small Animal Arthrology* (Eds Houlton, J.E.F. and Collinson, R.W.). BSAVA, Cheltenham, England.

Altman, R.D., Dean, D.D., Muniz, O.E. and Howell, D.S. (1989). Prophylactic treatment of canine osteoarthritis with glycosaminoglycan polysulfuric acid ester. *Arthritis and Rheumatism* **32**, 759–766.

Andresen, E. and Willeberg, P. (1976) Pituitary dwarfism in German shepherd dogs: additional evidence of simple autosomal recessive inheritance. *Nordisk Veterinaer Medicin* **28**, 481–486.

Appel, M. (1990) Lyme disease in dogs and cats. *Compendium of Continuing Education for the Practising Veterinarian* **12**, 617–627.

Arnett, F.C. (1989) Immunogenetics and rheumatic diseases. In: *Arthritis and Allied Conditions*, 11th edn (Ed. D.J. McCarty). Lea and Febiger, Philadelphia. pp. 453–464.

Baruth, H., Berger, L., Bradshaw, D., Costin, C.H., Coffey, J.W., Gupta, N., Konikoff, J., Roberts, N.A. and Wyler-Plaut, R.S. (1986) Carprofen. In: *Anti-inflammatory and Anti-rheumatic Drugs*, Vol. II, *Newer anti-inflammatory drugs* (Ed. K.D. Rainsford). CRC Press, Boca Raton, Florida.

Behrens, F., Shepard, N. and Mitchell, N. (1975) Alterations of rabbit articular cartilage by intra-articular injections of glucocorticoids. *Journal of Bone and Joint Surgery* **57A**, 70–76.

Bell, S.C., Carter, S.D. and Bennett, D. (1991) Canine distemper viral antigens and antibodies in dogs with rheumatoid arthritis. *Research in Veterinary Science* **50**, 64–68.

Bennett, D. (1976) Nutrition and bone disease in the dog and cat. *Veterinary Record* **98**, 313.

Bennett, D. (1980) The naturally occurring inflammatory arthropathies of the dog. PhD Thesis, University of Glasgow.

Bennett, D. (1984) Joint disease. In: *Canine Medicine and Therapeutics* (Eds E.A. Chandler, J.B. Sutton and D.J. Thompson). Blackwell Scientific Publications, Oxford, pp. 167–205.

Bennett, D. (1987a) Immune based erosive inflammatory joint disease of the dog. Canine rheumatoid arthritis 1: Clinical, radiological and laboratory investigations. *Journal of Small Animal Practice* **28**, 779–798.

Bennett, D. (1987b) Immune based erosive inflammatory joint disease of the dog. Canine rheumatoid arthritis 2: Pathological investigations. *Journal of Small Animal Practice* **28**, 799–820.

Bennett, D. (1987c) Immune based non-erosive inflammatory joint disease of the dog 1: Canine systemic lupus erythematosus. *Journal of Small Animal Practice* **28**, 871–890.

Bennett, D. (1987d) Immune based non-erosive inflammatory joint disease of the dog 3: Canine idiopathic polyarthritis. *Journal of Small Animal Practice* **28**, 909–928.

Bennett, D. (1990) Joints and joint diseases. In: *Canine Orthopaedics* (Ed. W.G. Whittick). Lea and Febiger, Philadelphia, pp. 761–856.

Bennett, D. and Kelly, D.F. (1987) Immune based non-erosive inflammatory joint disease of the dog 2: Polyarthritis/polymyositis syndrome. *Journal of Small Animal Practice* **28**, 891–908.

Bennett, D. and Kirkham, D. (1987) The laboratory identification of serum antinuclear antibody in the dog. *Journal of Comparative Pathology* **97**, 523–539.

Bennett, D. and Nash, A.S. (1988) Feline immune-based polyarthritis: a study of 31 cases. *Journal of Small Animal Practice* **29**, 501–524.

Bennett, D. and Taylor, D.J. (1988a) Bacterial infective arthritis in the dog. *Journal of Small Animal Practice* **29**, 207–230.

Bennett, D. and Taylor, D.J. (1988b) Bacterial endocarditis and inflammatory joint disease in the dog. *Journal of Small Animal Practice* **29**, 347–366.

Bennett, D., Gaskell, R.M., Mills, A., Knowles, J.O., Carter, S.D. and McCardle, F. (1989) Detection of feline calicivirus antigens in the joints of infected cats. *Veterinary Record* 124, 329–332.

Bennett, D., May, C. and Carter, S.D. (1992) Lyme disease in dogs and cats. In: *The Veterinary Annual* 32 (Eds C.S.G. Grunsell, M.-E. Raw and F.W.G. Hill), Wright, London, pp. 154–156.

Berg, J., Lamb, C.R. and O'Callaghan, M.W. (1990). Bone scintigraphy in the initial evaluation of dogs with primary bone tumours. *Journal of the American Veterinary Medical Association* 196, 917–920.

Biery, D.N. and Newton, C.D. (1975) Radiographic appearance of rheumatoid arthritis in the dog. *Journal of the American Animal Hospitals Association* 11, 607–612.

Bingel, S.A. and Sande, R.D. (1982) Chondrodysplasia in the Norwegian Elkhound. *American Journal of Pathology* 107, 219–229.

Bitetto, W.V., Patnaik, A.K., Schrader, S.C. and Mooney, S.C. (1987) Osteosarcoma in cats, 22 cases (1974–1984). *Journal of the American Veterinary Medical Association* 190, 91–93.

Boland, A.L. Jr. (1972) Acute hematogenous osteomyelitis. *Orthopaedic Clinics of North America* 3, 225–239.

Boyce, R.W., Axthelm, M.K., Krakowka, S. and Weisbrode, S.E. (1983) Metaphyseal bone lesions associated with canine distemper virus infection. In: *Proceedings of the 24th Annual Meeting of the American College of Veterinary Pathologists*, San Antonio, Texas, p. 126.

Brearley, M.J. and Jeffery, N. (1992) Cryptococcal osteomyelitis in a dog. *Journal of Small Animal Practice* 33, 601.

Breur, G.J., Zerbe, C.A., Slocombe, R.F., Padgett, G.A. and Braden, T.D. (1989) Clinical, radiographic, pathologic and genetic features of osteochondrodysplasia in Scottish deerhounds. *Journal of the American Veterinary Medical Association* 195, 606–612.

Brockus, C.W. and Hathcock, J.T. (1988) Hypertrophic osteopathy associated with blastomycosis in a dog. *Veterinary Radiology* 29, 184–190.

Brodey, R.S. (1971) Hypertrophic osteoarthropathy in the dog: a clinicopathological survey of 60 cases. *Journal of the American Veterinary Medical Association* 159, 1242–1246.

Brodey, R.S., Reid, C.F. and Sauer, R.M. (1966) Metastatic bone neoplasms in the dog. *Journal of the American Veterinary Medical Association* 148, 29–43.

Brodey, R.S., Roszel, J.F. and Rhodes, W.H. (1970) Disseminated coccidioidomycosis in a dog. *Journal of the American Veterinary Medical Association* 157, 926–933.

Brown, A. and Bennett, D. (1989) The use of gentamycin impregnated methylmethacrylate beads for the treatment of bacterial infective arthritis. *Veterinary Record* 123, 625–626.

Brown, R.G., Hoag, G.N., Smart, M.E. and Mitchell, L.H. (1978) Alaskan Malamute chondrodysplasia V. Decreases in gut zinc absorption. *Growth* 42, 1–6.

Calin, A. and Fries, J.F. (1976) An 'experimental' epidemic of Reiter's syndrome revisited: follow-up evidence on genetic and environmental factors. *Annals of Internal Medicine* 84, 564–566.

Capen, C.C. and Weisbrode, S.E. (1982) Hormonal control of mineral metabolism and bone cell activity. In: *Bone in Clinical Orthopaedics: a Study in Comparative Osteology* (Ed. G. Sumner-Smith). W.B. Saunders, Philadelphia, pp. 197–252.

Carrig, C.B., Sponenberg, D.P., Schmidt, G.M. and Tvedten, H.W. (1988) Inheritance of associated ocular and skeletal dysplasia in Labrador retrievers. *Journal of the American Veterinary Medical Association* 193, 1269–1272.

Carter, S.D., Bell, S.C., Bari, A.S.M. and Bennett, D. (1989) Immune complexes and rheumatoid factors in canine arthritides. *Annals of the Rheumatic Diseases* 48, 986–991.

Caywood, D.D., Wallace, L.J. and Braden, T.D. (1978) Osteomyelitis in the dog. A review of 67 cases. *Journal of the American Veterinary Medical Association* 172, 943–946.

Clark, D.M. (1991) Current concepts in the treatment of degenerative joint disease. *Compendium of Continuing Education for the Practising Veterinarian* 13, 1439–1446.

Colombo, C., Butler, M., Hickman, L., Selwyn, M., Chart, J. and Steinetz, B. (1983) A new model of osteoarthritis in rabbits. II. Evaluation of anti-osteoarthritic effects of selected anti-rheumatic drugs administered systemically. *Arthritis and Rheumatism* 26, 1132–1139.

Cotchin, E. and Dyce, K.M. (1956) A case of epiphyseal dysplasia in a dog. *Veterinary Record* 68, 427–428.

Coutinho, C.B., Cherpiko, J.A., Crews, T., Min, B.H. and Levy, A.C. (1975) The usefulness of drug blood level studies during toxicological safety evaluation. *Toxicology and Applied Pharmacology* 33, 163–177.

Cowell, K.R., Jezyk, P.F. and Haskins, M.E. (1976) Mucopolysaccharidosis in a cat. *Journal of the American Veterinary Medical Association* 169, 334–339.

Cowell, R.L., Tyler, R.D., Clinkenbeard, K.D. and Meinkoth, J.H. (1988) Ehrlichiosis and polyarthritis in three dogs. *Journal of the American Veterinary Medical Association* 192, 1093–1095.

Daly, W.R. (1985) Orthopaedic infections. In: *Textbook of Small Animal Surgery* (Ed. D.H. Slatter). W.B. Saunders, Philadelphia, pp. 2020–2034.

Day, M.J. and Penhale, W.J. (1988) Humeral immunity in disseminated *Aspergillus terreus* infection in the dog. *Veterinary Microbiology* 16, 283.

Denny, H.R., Gibbs, C. and Holt, P.E. (1982) The diagnosis and treatment of cauda equina lesions in the dog. *Journal of Small Animal Practice* 23, 425–443.

Dougherty, S.A., Center, S.A., Shaw, E.E. and Erb,

H.A. (1991) Juvenile-onset polyarthritis syndrome in Akitas. *Journal of the American Veterinary Medical Association* **198**, 849–856.

Dunn, J.K., Dennis, R. and Houlton, J.E.F. (1992) Successful treatment of two cases of metaphyseal osteomyelitis in the dog. *Journal of Small Animal Practice* **33**, 85–89.

Ellman, M.H. (1989) Neuropathic joint disease (Charcot joints). In: *Arthritis and Allied Conditions*, 11th edn (Ed. D.J. McCarty). Lea and Febiger, Philadelphia, pp. 1255–1272.

Enthoven, D., Coffey, J.W. and Wyler-Plaut, R.S. (1987) Carprofen. In: *Nonsteroidal Anti-inflammatory Drugs. Mechanisms and Clinical Use* (Eds A.J. Lewis and D.E. Furst). Marcel Dekker, New York.

Evans, H.E. and Christensen, G.C. (1979) Arthrology. *Miller's Anatomy of the Dog*. 2nd edn. WB Saunders, Philadelphia, pp. 95–130.

Fletch, S.M., Smart, M.E. and Pennock, P.W. (1973) Clinical and pathological features of chondrodysplasia (dwarfism) in the Alaskan malamute. *Journal of the American Veterinary Medical Association* **162**, 357–361.

Ford, D.R. (1989) Reiter's syndrome. Reactive arthritis. In: *Arthritis and Allied Conditions*, 11th edn (Ed. D.J. McCarty). Lea and Febiger, Philadelphia, pp. 944–953.

Freemont, A.J., Denton, J., Chuck, A., Holt, P.J.L. and Davies, M. (1991) Diagnostic value of synovial fluid microscopy: a reassessment and rationalisation. *Annals of the Rheumatic Diseases* **50**, 101–107.

Friou (1967) Antinuclear antibodies: diagnostic significance and methods. *Arthritis and Rheumatism* **10**, 151–159.

Galbraith, E.A. and McKellar, Q.A. (1991) Pharmacokinetics and pharmacodynamics of piroxicam in the dog. *Veterinary Record* **128**, 561–565.

Ghosh, P. (1988) Anti-rheumatic drugs and cartilage. *Clinical Rheumatology International Practice and Research* **2**, 309–331.

Gilmore, D.R. (1987) Lumbosacral diskospondylitis in 21 dogs. *Journal of the American Animal Hospitals Association* **23**, 57–61.

Goedegebuure, S.A. (1979) Secondary bone tumours in the dog. *Veterinary Pathology* **16**, 520–526.

Goldschmidt, M.H. and Thrall, D.E. (1985) Malignant bone tumours in the dog. In: *Textbook of Small Animal Orthopaedics* (Eds C.D. Newton and D. Nunamaker). Lippincott, Philadelphia, pp. 887–898.

Grondalen, J. (1976) Metaphyseal osteopathy (hypertrophic osteodystrophy) in growing dogs. A clinical study. *Journal of Small Animal Practice* **17**, 721–735.

Grondalen, J. and Lingaas, F. (1991) Arthrosis in the elbow joint of young rapidly growing dogs. A genetic investigation. *Journal of Small Animal Practice* **32**, 460–464.

Guthrie, S. and Pidduck, H.G. (1990) Heritability of elbow osteochondrosis within a closed population of dogs. *Journal of Small Animal Practice* **31**, 93–96.

Halliwell, R.E.W., Lavelle, R.B. and Butt, K.M. (1972) Canine rheumatoid arthritis – a review and a case report. *Journal of Small Animal Practice* **13**, 239–243.

Hazewinkel, H.A.W. (1989) Nutrition in relation to skeletal growth deformities. *Journal of Small Animal Practice* **30**, 625–630.

Hazewinkel, H.A.W., Goedegebuure, S.A., Poulos, P.W. and Wolvekamp, W.Th.C. (1985) Influences of chronic calcium excess on the skeletal development of growing Great Danes. *Journal of the American Animal Hospitals Association* **21**, 377–391.

Hazleman, B.L. (1986) Drug-induced syndromes and drug toxicity. In: *Therapeutics in Rheumatology* (Eds J.M.H. Moll, H.A. Bird and A. Rushton). Chapman & Hall, London.

Hedhammer, A., Wu, F., Rrook, L., Schrijver, H.F., De Lahunta, A., Whalen, J.P., Rallfelz, F., Nunez, E.A., Hintz, H.F., Sheffy, B.E. and Ryan, A.D. (1974) Overnutrition and skeletal disease. An experimental study in growing Great Dane dogs. *Cornell Veterinarian Supplement* **5**, 11–16.

Holt, P.E. (1978) Hip dysplasia in a cat. *Journal of Small Animal Practice* **19**, 273–276.

Hough, A.J. (1993) Pathology of osteoarthritis. In: *Arthritis and Allied Conditions*, 12th edn (Ed. D.J. McCarty). Lea and Febiger, Philadelphia, pp. 1571–1594.

Houlton, J.E.F. and Meynink, S.E. (1989) Medial patellar luxation in the cat. *Journal of Small Animal Practice* **30**, 349–352.

Huff, R.W. and Brodey, R.S. (1964) Multiple bone cysts in a dog – a case report. *Journal of the American Veterinary Radiology Society* **5**, 40–45.

Huskisson, E.C. and Hart, F.D. (1987) *Joint disease: All the arthropathies*, 4th edn. IOP Publishing, Bristol.

Jezyk, P.F. (1985) Constitutional disorders of the skeleton in dogs and cats. In: *Textbook of Small Animal Orthopaedics* (Eds C.D. Newton and D. Nunamaker). Lippincott, Philadelphia, pp. 637–654.

Konde, L.J., Thrall, M.A., Gasper, P., Dial, S.M., McBiles, K., Colgan, S. and Haskins, M. (1987) Radiographically visualized skeletal changes associated with mucopolysaccharidosis VI in cats. *Veterinary Radiology* **28**, 223–228.

Kornblatt, A.N., Urband, P.H. and Steere, A.C. (1985) Arthritis caused by *Borrelia burgdorferi* in dogs. *Journal of the American Veterinary Medical Association* **191**, 1089–1094.

Koski, J.M., Antilla, P., Hamalainen, M. and Isomaki, H. (1990) Hip joint ultrasonography: correlation with intra-articular effusion and synovitis. *British Journal of Rheumatology* **29**, 189–192.

Lamb, C.R. (1987) Bone scintigraphy in small animals. *Journal of the American Veterinary Medical Association* **191**, 1616–1622.

LaRue, S.M., Withrow, S.J. and Wrigley, R.H. (1986) Radiographic bone surveys in the evaluation of primary bone tumors in dogs. *Journal of the American*

Veterinary Medical Association **188**, 514–516.

LaRue, S.M., Withrow, S.J., Powers, B.E., Wrigley, R.H., Gilette, E.L., Schwarz, P.D., Straw, R.C. and Richter, S.L. (1989) Limb-sparing treatment for osteosarcoma in dogs. *Journal of the American Veterinary Medical Association* **195**, 1734–1744.

Le Gros Clark, W.E. (1975) The tissues of the joints. In: *The Tissues of the Body*, 6th edn. Oxford University Press, Oxford, pp. 165–185.

Lees, P., May, S.A. and McRellar, Q.A. (1991) Pharmacology and therapeutics of non-steroidal anti-inflammatory drugs in the dog and cat: 1 general pharmacology. *Journal of Small Animal Practice* **32**, 183–193.

Leighton, E.A., Linn, J.M., Wilham, R.L. and Castleberry, M.W. (1977) A genetic study of canine hip dysplasia. *American Journal of Veterinary Research* **38**, 241–244.

Lenehan, T.M., van Sickle, D.C. and Biery, D.N. (1985) Canine panosteitis. In: *Textbook of Small Animal Orthopaedics* (Eds C.D. Newton and D. Nunamaker) Lippincott, Philadelphia, pp. 591–596.

Lipowitz, A.J. (1985) Synovial fluid. In: *Textbook of Small Animal Orthopaedics* (Eds C.D. Newton and D. Nunamaker) Lippincott, Philadelphia, pp. 1015–1028.

Magnarelli, L.A., Anderson, J.F., Levine, H.R. and Levy, S.A. (1990) Tick parasitism and antibodies to *Borrelia burgdorferi* in cats. *Journal of the American Veterinary Medical Association* **197**, 63–66.

Malik, R., Latter, M. and Love, D.N. (1990) Bacterial discospondylitis in a cat. *Journal of Small Animal Practice* **31**, 404–406.

Martel–Pelletier, J., Pelletier, J-P., Cloutier, J-M., Howell, D.S., Ghandur-Mnaymneh, L. and Woessner, J.F. Jr. (1984) Neutral proteases capable of proteoglycan digesting activity in osteoarthritic and normal human cartilage. *Arthritis and Rheumatism* **27**, 305–312.

May, C. (1989) Leishmaniasis associated with polyarthritis in a dog. *Proceedings of the World Small Animal Veterinary Association. Annual Congress*, Harrogate, England, p. 254.

May, C. and Bennett, D. (1991) Canine arthroscopy. In: *A Colour Atlas of Small Animal Endoscopy* (Eds M.J. Brearley, J.E. Cooper and M. Sullivan), Wolfe Publishing, Aylesbury, pp. 93–96.

May, C. and Newsholme, S.J. (1989) Metastasis of feline pulmonary carcinoma presenting as multiple digital swelling. *Journal of Small Animal Practice* **30**, 302–310.

May, C., Bennett, D. and Carter, S.D. (1990) Lyme disease in the dog. *Veterinary Record* **126**, 293.

May, C., Bennett, D. and Carter, S.D. (1991) Serodiagnosis of Lyme disease in UK dogs. *Journal of Small Animal Practice* **32**, 170–174.

May, C., Hammill, J. and Bennett, D. (1992) Chinese shar pei fever syndrome: a preliminary report. *Veterinary Record* **131**, 586–587.

McGlennon, N.J., Houlton, J.E.F. and Gorman, N.T. (1988) Synovial sarcoma in the dog – a review. *Journal of Small Animal Practice* **29**, 139–152.

McKee, W.M., Mitten, R.W. and Labuc, R.H. (1990) Surgical treatment of lumbosacral discospondylitis by a distraction-fusion technique. *Journal of Small Animal Practice* **31**, 15–20.

McKellar, Q.A., Pearson, T., Bogan, J.A., Galbraith, E.A., Lees, P., Ludwig, B. and Tiberghien, M.P. (1990) Pharmacokinetics, tolerance and serum thromboxane inhibition of carprofen in the dog. *Journal of Small Animal Practice* **31**, 443–448.

McKellar, Q.A., May, S.A. and Lees, P. (1991a) Pharmacology and therapeutics of non-steroidal anti-inflammatory therapy in the dog and cat: 2 Individual agents. *Journal of Small Animal Practice* **32**, 225–235.

McKellar, Q.A., Pearson, T., Galbraith, E.A., Boyle, J. and Bell, G. (1991b) Pharmacokinetics and clinical efficacy of a cincophen and prednisolone combination in the dog. *Journal of Small Animal Practice* **32**, 53–58.

Mee, A.P., Webber, D.M., May, C., Bennett, D., Sharpe, P.T. and Anderson, D.C. (1992) Detection of canine distemper virus in bone cells in the metaphyses of distemper-infected dogs. *Journal of Bone and Mineral Research* **7**, 829–833.

Mee, A.P., Gordon, M.T., May, C., Bennett, D., Anderson, D.C. and Sharpe, P.T. (1993) Canine distemper viral transcripts detected in the bone cells of a dog with metaphyseal osteopathy. *Bone* **14**, 59–67.

Meyers, V.N., Jezyk, P.F., Aguirre, G.D. and Patterson, D.F. (1983) Short limbed dwarfism and ocular defects in the Samoyed dog. *Journal of the American Veterinary Medical Association* **183**, 975–979.

Moise, N.S., Crissman, J.W., Fairbrother, J.F. and Baldwin, C. (1983) *Mycoplasma gatae* arthritis and tenosynovitis in cats: case report and experimental reproduction of the disease. *American Journal of Veterinary Research* **44**, 16–21.

Morgan, J.P. (1981) Radiographic evaluation of extremital disease. In: *Radiology of Skeletal Disease – Principles of Diagnosis in the Dog*. Iowa State University Press, Iowa, pp. 20–46.

Moskowitz, R.W. and Goldberg, V.M. (1987) Osteophyte evolution: studies in an experimental partial meniscectomy model. *Journal of Rheumatology* (suppl) **14**, 116–118.

Muhumuza, L., Morgan, J.P., Miyabayashi, T. and Atilola, A.O. (1988) Positive contrast arthrography. A study of the humeral joints in normal beagle dogs. *Veterinary Radiology* **29**, 157–161.

Neer, T.M. (1988) Disseminated aspergillosis. *Compendium of Continuing Education for the Practising Veterinarian* **10**, 465.

Newton, C.D., Lipowitz, A.J., Halliwell, R.E.W., Allen, H.I., Biery, D.N. and Schumacher, H.R.

(1976) Rheumatoid arthritis in dogs. *Journal of the American Veterinary Medical Association* **168**, 113–121.

Olsson, S.-E. (1971) Degenerative joint disease (osteoarthrosis): a review with special reference to the dog. *Journal of Small Animal Practice* **12**, 333–342.

Olsson, S.-E. (1982) Morphology and physiology of the growth cartilage under normal and pathologic conditions. In: *Bone in Clinical Orthopaedics: A Study in Comparative Osteology* (Ed. G. Sumner-Smith). W.B. Saunders, Philadelphia, pp. 159–196.

Owen, L.N. and Bostock, D.E. (1971) Multiple cartilaginous exostoses with development of metastasizing osteosarcoma in a Shetland sheepdog. *Journal of Small Animal Practice* **12**, 507–512.

Parchman, M.B., Flanders, J.A., Erb, H.N., Wallace, R. and Rallfelz, F.A. (1989) Nuclear medical bone imaging and targeted radiography for evaluation of skeletal neoplasms in 23 dogs. *Veterinary Surgery* **18**, 454–458.

Pedersen, N.C., Pool, R.C., Castles, J.J. and Weisner (1976a) Non-infectious canine arthritis. Rheumatoid arthritis. *Journal of the American Veterinary Medical Association* **169**, 304–310.

Pedersen, N.C., Weisner, K., Castles, J.J., Ling, G.V. and Weisner, G. (1976b) Non-infectious canine arthritis. The inflammatory non-erosive arthritides. *Journal of the American Veterinary Medical Association* **169**, 304–310.

Pedersen, N.C., Pool, R.R. and O'Brien, T. (1980) Feline chronic progressive polyarthritis. *American Journal of Veterinary Research* **41**, 522–535.

Pedersen, N.C., Wind, A., Morgan, J.P. and Pool, R.R. (1989) Joint diseases of dogs and cats. In: *Textbook of Veterinary Internal Medicine*, 3rd edn (Ed. S.J. Ettinger). W.B. Saunders, Philadelphia, pp. 2329–2377.

Pelletier, J.-P. and Martel-Pelletier, J. (1989) Protective effects of corticosteroids on cartilage lesions and osteophyte formation in the Pond-Nuki dog model of osteoarthritis. *Arthritis and Rheumatism* **32**, 181–193.

Pelletier, J.-P., Martel-Pelletier, J., Howell, D.S., Ghandur-Mnaymneh, L., Enis, J.E. and Woessner, J.F. Jr. (1983a) Collagenase and collagenolytic activity in human osteoarthritic cartilage. *Arthritis and Rheumatism* **26**, 63–68.

Pelletier, J.-P., Martel-Pelletier, J., Altman, R.D., Ghandur-Mnaymneh, L., Enis, J.E., Howell, D.S. and Woessner, J.F. Jr. (1983b) Collagenolytic activity and collagen matrix breakdown of the articular cartilage in the Pond-Nuki dog model of osteoarthritis. *Arthritis and Rheumatism* **26**, 866–874.

Powers, B.E., LaRue, S.M., Withrow, S.J., Straw, R.C. and Richter, S.L. (1988). Jamshidi needle biopsy for diagnosis of bone lesions in small animals. *Journal of the American Veterinary Medical Association* **193**, 205–210.

Rainsford, K.D. (1988) Novel non-steroidal anti-inflammatory drugs. *Clinical Rheumatology International Practice and Research* **2**, 485–512.

Rasmussen, P.G. (1971) Multiple epiphyseal dysplasia in a litter of beagle puppies. *Journal of Small Animal Practice* **12**, 91–97.

Rimoin, D.L. (1978) International nomenclature of constitutional diseases of bone. Revision, May 1977. *Birth Defects* **14**, 39–45.

Riser, W.H. (1964) Radiographic differential diagnosis of skeletal diseases in young dogs. *Journal of the American Veterinary Radiology Society* **5**, 15–27.

Riser, W.H. (1966) Hypertrophic osteopathy of the mandibles and cranium in West Highland terriers. *Journal of the American Veterinary Medical Association* **148**, 1543–1547.

Roberts, R.E. (1979) Osteomyelitis associated with disseminated blastomycosis in dogs: some radiographic observations. *Journal of the American Veterinary Radiology Society* **20**, 21–24.

Ropes, M.W., Bennett, G.A. and Cobb, S. (1959) 1958 revision of the diagnostic criteria for rheumatoid arthritis. *Arthritis and Rheumatism* **2**, 16–20.

Rothfield, N.F. (1989) Systemic lupus erythematosus: clinical aspects and treatment. In: *Arthritis and Allied Conditions*, 11th edn (Ed. D.J. McCarty). Lea and Febiger, Philadelphia.

Saunders, H.M. and Jezyk, P.K. (1991) The radiographic appearance of canine congenital hypothyroidism: skeletal changes with delayed treatment. *Veterinary Radiology* **32**, 171–177.

Scavelli, T.D. and Schrader, S.C. (1987) Non-surgical management of rupture of the cranial cruciate ligament in 18 cats. *Journal of the American Animal Hospitals Association* **23**, 337–340.

Scherkl, R. and Frey, H.-H. (1987) Pharmacokinetics of ibuprofen in the dog. *Journal of Veterinary Pharmacology and Therpeutics* **10**, 261–265.

Schiefer, B., Hurov, L. and Seer, G. (1974) Pulmonary emphysema and fibrosis associated with polyarthritis in a dog. *Journal of the American Veterinary Medical Association* **164**, 408–413.

Seawright, A., English, P. and Gartner, R.J.W. (1967) Hypervitaminosis A and deforming cervical spondylosis of the cat. *Journal of Comparative Pathology* **77**, 29–35.

Serra, D.A. and White, S.D. (1989) Oral chrysotherapy with auranofin in dogs. *Journal of the American Veterinary Medical Association* **194**, 1327–1330.

Shapiro, W., Fossum, T.W., Ritchell, B.E., Couto, C.G. and Theilen, G.H. (1988) Use of cisplatin for treatment of appendicular osteosarcoma in dogs. *Journal of the American Veterinary Medical Association* **192**, 507–511.

Sharp, N.J., Harvey, C.E. and O'Brien, J.A. (1991) Treatment of canine nasal aspergillosis/penicillosis with fluconazole (UR-49,858). *Journal of Small Animal Practice* **32**, 513–516.

Simon, M.A. (1982) Biopsy of musculoskeletal

tumours. *Journal of Bone and Joint Surgery* (American issue) **64-A**, 1253–1257.

Small, E. (1969) Systemic mycoses. *Journal of the American Veterinary Medical Association* **155**, 2002–2004.

Steere, A.C. (1989) Lyme disease. *New England Journal of Medicine* **321**, 586–589.

Stoller, D.W. and Genant, M.D. (1989) Magnetic resonance imaging of the joints. In: *Arthritis and Allied Conditions* (Ed. D.J. McCarty). Lea and Febiger, Philadelphia, pp. 91–131.

Susanek, S.J. (1982) Hypertrophic osteopathy. *Compendium on Continuing Education for the Practising Veterinarian* **4**, 689–693.

Suter, P.F. and Carb, A.V. (1969) Shoulder arthrography in dogs: radiographic anatomy and clinical application. *Journal of Small Animal Practice* **10**, 407–413.

Thomas, N.W. (1987) Piroxicam-associated gastric ulceration in the dog. *Compendium on Continuing Education for the Practising Veterinarian* **9**, 1004–1006.

Tilmant, L.L., Gorman, N.T., Ackerman, N., Calderwood Mays, M.B. and Parker, R. (1986) Chemotherapy of synovial sarcoma in a dog. *Journal of the American Veterinary Medical Association* **188**, 530–532.

Trotter, G.W., McIlwraith, C.W., Yovich, J.V., Norrdin, R.W., Wrigley, R.H. and Lamar, C.H. (1991) Effects of intra-articular administration of methylprednisolone acetate on normal equine articular cartilage. *American Journal of Veterinary Research* **52**, 83–87.

Turnwald, G.H., Shires, P.R., Turk, M.A.M., Cox, H.U., Pechman, R.D., Reaney, M.T., Hugh-Jones, M.E., Balsamo, G.A. and Helouin, C.M. (1986) Diskospondylitis in a kennel of dogs. Clinicopathological findings. *Journal of the American Veterinary Medical Association* **188**, 178–183.

van Bree, H. (1990) Evaluation of the prognostic value of positive-contrast shoulder arthrography for bilateral osteochondrosis lesions in dogs. *American Journal of Veterinary Research* **51**, 1121–1125.

Walker, M.A., Lewis, R.E., Kneller, S.R., Thrall, D.E. and Losonsky, J.M. (1975) Radiographic signs of bone infection in small animals. *Journal of the American Veterinary Medical Association* **166**, 908–910.

Watson, A.D.J. (1990) Diseases of muscle and bone. In: *Canine Orthopaedics*, 2nd edn (Ed. W.G. Whittick). Lea and Febiger, Philadelphia, pp. 657–692.

Watson, A.D.J., Miller, A.S.C., Allan, G.S., Davis, P.E. and Howlett, C.R. (1991) Osteochondrodysplasia in bull terrier littermates. *Journal of Small Animal Practice* **32**, 312–317.

Werner, L.L. and Halliwell, R.E.W. (1984) Diseases associated with autoimmunity. In: *Canine Medicine and Therapeutics* (Eds E.A. Chandler, J.B. Sutton and D.J. Thompson). Blackwell Scientific, Oxford, pp. 270–296.

Whitbread, T.J., Gill, J.J.B. and Lewis, D.G. (1983) An inherited enchondrodystrophy in the English Pointer dog. A new disease. *Journal of Small Animal Practice* **24**, 399–411.

Widmer, W.R. and Blevins, W.E. (1991) Veterinary myelography: a review of contrast media, adverse effects and technique. *Journal of the American Animal Hospitals Association* **27**, 163–177.

Willhelmi, G. and Maier, R. (1983) Experimental studies on the effects of drugs on cartilage. In: *Articular Cartilage and Osteoarthrosis*. Hansuber Publishers, Bern, Switzerland, pp. 67–78.

Williams, J.M. and Brandt, K.D. (1985) Triamcinolone hexacetonide protects against fibrillation and osteophyte formation following chemically induced articular cartilage damage. *Arthritis and Rheumatism* **28**, 1267–1274.

Woodard, J.C., Riser, W.H., Bloomberg, M.S., Gaskin, J.M. and Goring, R.L. (1991) Erosive polyarthritis in two greyhounds. *Journal of the American Veterinary Medical Association* **198**, 873–876.

Wykes, P.M., Withrow, S.J. and Powers, B.E. (1985) Closed biopsy for the diagnosis of long bone tumors: accuracy and results. *Journal of the American Animal Hospitals Association* **21**, 489–494.

Yamaguchi, R.A., French, T.W., Simpson, C.F. and Harvey, J.W. (1983) *Leishmania donovani* in the synovial fluid of a dog with visceral leishmaniasis. *Journal of the American Animal Hospitals Association* **19**, 723–726.

Zvaifler, N.J. (1989) Etiology and pathogenesis of rheumatoid arthritis. In: *Arthritis and Allied Conditions*, 11th edn (Ed. D.J. McCarty). Lea and Febiger, Philadelphia, pp. 659–673.

FURTHER READING

Bennett, D. and May, C. (1995) Joint diseases in dogs and cats. In: *Textbook of Veterinary Internal Medicine* (Eds S.J. Ettinger and E.C. Feldman). WB Saunders, Philadelphia.

Brinker, W.O., Piermattei, D.L. and Flo, G.L. (1990) *Handbook of Small Animal Orthopaedics and Fracture Treatment*, 2nd edn. WB Saunders, Philadelphia.

Houlton, J.E.F. and Collinson, R.W. (Eds) (1994) *Manual of Small Animal Arthrology*. BSAVA, Cheltenham, England.

Johnson, K.A., Watson, A.D.J. and Page, R.L. Skeletal diseases. In: *Textbook of Veterinary Internal Medicine* (Eds S.J. Ettinger and E.C. Feldman). WB Saunders, Philadelphia.

Newton, C.D. and Nunamaker, D. (Eds) (1985) *Textbook of Small Animal Orthopaedics*, Lippincott, Philadelphia.

Slatter, D.H. (Ed.) (1993) *Textbook of Small Animal Surgery* (2nd edn). WB Saunders, Philadelphia.

Whittick, W.G. (Ed.) (1990) *Canine Orthopaedics*, 2nd edn. Lea and Febiger, Philadelphia.

45

Diseases of Blood and Blood-forming Organs

J. D. Littlewood

Introduction	765
Clinical history	771
Physical examination	771
Investigative techniques	772
Laboratory investigations	775
SPECIFIC CONDITIONS IN THE DOG	**784**
Anaemias	784
Leucocyte abnormalities	790
Bone marrow neoplasia	790
Disorders of haemostasis	796
SPECIFIC CONDITIONS IN THE CAT	**805**
Anaemias	805
Leucocyte abnormalities	807
Bone marrow neoplasia	807
Disorders of haemostasis	809
Blood transfusion in the dog and cat	811

INTRODUCTION

Blood consists of cellular elements derived from the bone marrow and plasma which contains various proteins and electrolytes as well as nutrients and metabolites. This chapter considers disorders which affect the cellular components of the blood, the bone marrow and those plasma proteins which are involved in haemostasis.

Normal haematopoiesis

In the fetus, haematopoiesis takes place initially in the yolksac, and later in the liver and spleen. The bone marrow becomes the principal site of haematopoiesis during the last third of pregnancy and remains as the major site in the healthy animal. All blood cells are derived from pluripotential (or totipotent) haematopoietic stem cells (HSC). These cells, present in only small numbers, are capable of self-proliferation and the generation of both lymphoid and non-lymphoid progenitor cells (Fig. 45.1). *In vitro* studies of bone marrow-derived cultures have identified partially committed progenitor cells known as colony forming units (CFU), which are further classified according to the cell lineage(s) to which they give rise. The non-lymphoid, multipotent stem cell (termed CFU-GEMM) produces erythroid progenitors, granulocyte-macrophage progenitors (CFU-GM) (from which granulocyte (CFU-G) and macrophage/monocyte (CFU-M) progenitors are derived), eosinophil (CFU-Eo) progenitors, basophil progenitors (CFU-Bas) and megakaryocyte progenitors (CFU-Meg). These committed stem cells are capable of both regeneration and differentiation under the influence of various growth factors produced by activated lymphocytes and macrophages, including interleukins, colony stimulating factors (e.g. granulocyte/macrophage colony stimulating factor (GM-CSF) and granulocyte colony stimulating factor (G-CSF)), erythropoietin and thrombopoietin. The erythroid precursors form blast forming units (BFU-E) whose progeny are CFU-E. CFU cells of all lineages give rise to blast cells which further differentiate through various immature stages to produce the mature blood cells released into the circulation.

Haematopoiesis takes place in the marrow, but outside the vascular channels, in a stroma of fibroblasts, fat-cells, endothelial cells and macrophages. This microenvironment is vital to the maintenance of the stem cell population and to normal proliferation and differentiation of precursor cells.

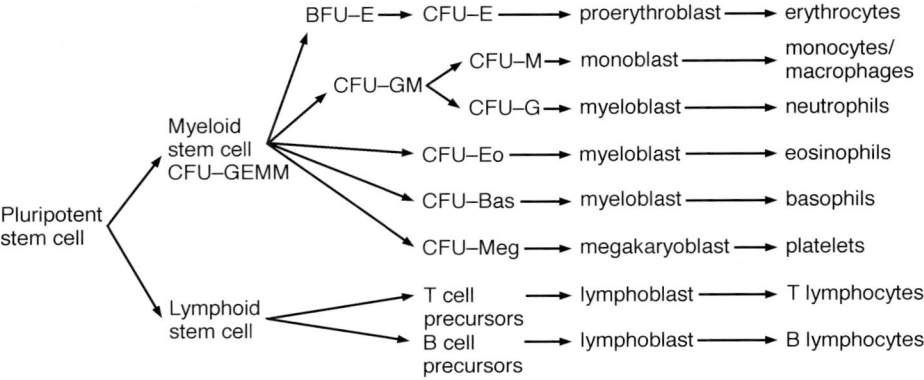

Figure 45.1 Simplified schematic representation of haematopoiesis

Erythrocytes

Erythropoiesis

The proerythroblast is the earliest cell of the red cell series which can be recognized. Division is followed by maturation through three stages of normoblast, at which stage the nucleus is extruded to form a reticulocyte. This process takes about five days. After a further 2–3 days reticulocytes are released into the circulation where it takes 24 h to become fully functional red cells. Under normal circumstances the rate of production of red cells is sufficient to compensate for the removal of erythrocytes at the end of their life span by the monocyte–phagocyte system (MPS). Erythropoietin is the main humoral mediator influencing the production of red cells and their release into the circulation. Erythropoietin is produced by the kidney with a small contribution from the liver and its rate of synthesis is enhanced by reduced tissue oxygen tension. This results in increased production of committed stem cells, accelerated differentiation and earlier release of reticulocytes and even late normoblasts into the circulation. Maturation can be reduced from five to seven days down to three to four days. Erythropoietin has also been shown to influence the proliferation of fibroblasts in the marrow stroma (Giger, 1992).

Erythrocyte function

Erythrocytes are biconcave spheres with a flexible cell membrane, containing haemoglobin, and their function is to deliver oxygen to peripheral tissues. Canine red cells are 7 µm in diameter and have a circulating lifespan of 100–120 days. Feline erythrocytes are smaller, mean 5.7 µm diameter, with a less obvious area of central pallor. They have a shorter lifespan ranging between 50 and 80 days. Normal cats may have refractile Heinz bodies (denatured haemoglobin) in up to 10% of erythrocytes and Howell–Jolly bodies (nuclear chromatin remnants) in about 1% of cells.

Erythrocyte antigens

Eight different red cell antigens have been described in the dog, designated DEA (dog erythrocyte antigen) 1 to 8, with two subtypes DEA1.1 and DEA1.2 occurring (Dodds, 1985). The population incidence is shown in Table 45.1. More recently a third subtype of the DEA1 group has been recognized which can induce an immune response to the other subtypes (Symons and Bell, 1991). Naturally occurring isoantibodies have been identified in about 15% of dogs against blood groups DEA3, 4, 5 and 7; 40–50% of dogs are positive for DEA1 and DEA7 which are generally regarded as the two most important blood group antigens in terms of incompatible blood transfusion reactions. DEA1 antigens are the most potent stimulators of isoantibody production. Fortunately, dogs have no naturally occurring isoantibodies against the DEA1 blood group antigens, therefore acute transfusion reactions are rare following a first blood transfusion. Acute transfusion reactions characterized by rapid destruction of transfused red cells will occur, however, if a DEA1-negative dog, transfused with DEA1-positive blood, is subsequently transfused with the same mismatched blood. DEA7 (also referred to as Tr antigen) is not a true erythrocyte antigen and is adsorbed onto the erythrocytes from plasma (Smith, 1991). Dogs which are DEA7

Table 45.1 Population incidence of canine blood groups in dogs in the United States

Blood group	Incidence (%)
DEA1.1	40
DEA1.2	20
DEA 3	5
DEA 4	98
DEA 5	25
DEA 6	98
DEA 7	45
DEA 8	40

After Dodds (1985).

negative acquire anti-DEA7 antibodies following exposure to certain environmental antigens present on common bacteria. Naturally occurring anti-DEA7 antibodies may be of significance in animals receiving blood transfusions and may cause delayed destruction of transfused red blood cells (10–14 days post-transfusion).

Three feline blood groups are recognized: A, B and AB. The incidence of type A varies from 73% to 99% of the feline population in surveys from different countries and different geographical locations (Giger et al., 1989). The incidence of type B blood in purebred cats may be markedly higher than the general cat population (Giger, 1990; Giger et al., 1991a). Cats with type B blood invariably have naturally occurring isoantibodies against type A cells and 30–35% of cats with blood group A have low titres of anti-B isoantibodies (Auer and Bell, 1986).

Leucocytes

Granulocyte production and function

The granulocytic cells of the marrow can be divided into three distinct cell pools. The mitotic pool is those cells capable of division, i.e. the myeloblasts, promyelocytes and myelocytes. The maturing pool consists of metamyelocytes and band cells. Passage from myeloblast to mature granulocyte takes about seven days. Mature cells remain in the marrow storage pool for a further three to five days before release into the circulation.

Neutrophils

In the circulation about half the neutrophils are freely circulating and the rest constitute the marginated or marginal pool, adherent to the walls of small vessels. From here they enter the tissue pool, attracted by numerous chemotactic factors to sites of inflammation, where their principal function is the production of bactericidal molecules (e.g. lysozyme, lactoferrin, esterases, elastases and collagenases) and phagocytosis of bacteria. The length of time spent in the peripheral circulation is approximately 8–12 h.

Eosinophils

There is minimal storage of eosinophils in the marrow and the time spent in the circulation is only minutes to hours. The eosinophil is attracted to sites of antigen–antibody complex formation or deposition. The primary functions of eosinophils are twofold: they kill parasites and modulate immune reactions, particularly hypersensitivity reactions. This is achieved by an array of biologically active molecules derived from the cytoplasmic granules, including major basic protein, peroxidase, histaminase to inactivate histamine released by basophils and mast cells, and other enzymes. As well as the beneficial effects of these substances in the host defences against parasitism, release of eosinophil granule contents also results in tissue damage. Eosinophils may persist in the tissues for several days after which they are phagocytosed by macrophages.

Basophils

Bone marrow storage is minimal. Basophils, like tissue mast cells, are involved in IgE-mediated and other immune-mediated inflammatory reactions, releasing various mediators from granules including histamine, heparin and eosinophil chemotactic factor.

Monocyte production and function

Monocytes are derived from a common stem cell to granulocytes but there is no marrow storage pool; rather they are produced and released on demand. Monocytes and their precursors are therefore only present in small numbers in normal marrow. Monocyte production takes about 15 h. In the circulation there is both a freely circulating and marginal pool. After approximately 24 h the monocyte migrates into the tissues where it becomes a macrophage, performing a number of functions. The macrophages of the spleen, lymph nodes, bone marrow, Kupffer cells of the liver, pleural and peritoneal macrophages, tissue histiocytes and Langerhans cells of the skin are all monocyte-derived. Their primary function is the phagocytosis of particulate debris. Since they carry both immunoglobulin (Fc component of

IgG) and complement receptors they can phagocytose appropriately coated (opsonized) organisms and antigens. They also play a vital role in processing antigens to render them more immunogenic for presentation to lymphocytes. Various substances important in the immune response are produced by activated monocytes/macrophages including interferon, interleukins, lymphokines, complement components and proteolytic enzymes. Tissue macrophages are involved in iron metabolism. After red cell breakdown, iron from degraded haemoglobin is stored in macrophages as haemosiderin or ferritin and subsequently released for reutilization in the marrow for red cell production.

Lymphocyte production and function

Lymphoid precursors are derived from pluripotent stem cells. The committed stem cell or lymphoblast produces prolymphocytes which progress to mature lymphocytes. The lymphoid system comprises the bone marrow, thymus, spleen, lymph nodes, gut-associated lymphoid tissue (GALT), bronchial-associated lymphoid tissue (BALT) and blood. Although continued lymphopoiesis is dependent on the stem cells in the marrow, the majority of lymphocytes in the adult are derived from peripheral lymphoid tissues. Lymphocytes processed in the thymus are termed T-lymphocytes and bone marrow processed cells are known as B-lymphocytes. B-lymphocytes are involved in humoral immunity. After antigenic stimulation B cells transform into antibody-producing plasma cells. Several subsets of T-lymphocyte are variously involved in cell-mediated immunity, by modulating the activity of other cells (T-helper and T-suppressor cells) and by killing infected and tumour cells (cytotoxic T-cells).

Lymphocytes in the blood represent only about 5% of the total body lymphocyte population. There is constant recirculation of lymphocytes through the peripheral tissue from which they derived, via the lymphatics, thoracic duct, into the circulation and back out into the peripheral lymphoid tissues. This recirculation allows constant immune surveillance, antigen exposure and recognition, and subsequent mobilization of sensitized lymphocytes. The majority of circulating lymphocytes in the blood are T-cells. Occasionally large transformed lymphocytes and plasma cells may be seen on a blood film especially after an antigenic challenge such as vaccination.

Platelets

Platelets, also known as thrombocytes, are produced in the bone marrow by budding off and shedding from the cytoplasm of megakaryocytes. Megakaryocytes are large mutinucleate cells whose cytoplasmic arms extend into the venous sinuses. The production of megakaryocytes from progenitor cells and platelets from megakaryocytes is influenced by the humoral factor thrombopoietin as well as other colony stimulating factors, the whole process taking about three days. Circulating platelets are oval in shape, approximately 3 µm in diameter, with granular cytoplasm. Immature platelets are larger and known as shift platelets. At any one time up to 30% of the platelet population may be sequestered in the spleen. The lifespan of the circulating platelet is 6–10 days.

Platelet function: primary haemostasis

Platelets interact with endothelial cells to ensure normal vascular integrity. The role of platelets in haemostasis is summarized in Fig. 45.2. When a vessel is injured platelets adhere to collagen in the subendothelium via membrane glycoprotein receptors. The receptor GP Ib which binds von Willebrand factor (vWF) is important in platelet adhesion. Shape change and release reactions follow adhesion with secretion of substances from granules which potentiate platelet aggregation and contraction of the platelet plug. The receptor GP IIb–IIIa, which binds ADP and fibrinogen, is important in platelet–platelet interactions. Primary platelet aggregation is followed by further release reactions which potentiate aggregation and result in further recruitment of platelets into the aggregate, forming the primary haemostatic plug. Prostaglandin synthesis results in the production of thromboxane A_2 by the platelet which counteracts the effects of prostacyclin (PGI_2) produced by endothelial cells. Prostacyclin is an inhibitor of platelet aggregation and a vasodilator. The responsiveness of platelets is regulated by these prostaglandins via effects on cyclic AMP concentration in platelets. Stabilization of the platelet plug is achieved by the deposition of fibrin, the end-product of the coagulation cascade (secondary haemostasis). Membrane receptors on the surface of activated platelets provide binding sites for many of the coagulation proteins and the phospholipid, termed platelet factor 3, which is required for several steps in the coagulation pathway. This has the effect of localizing clot formation to the site of vascular injury.

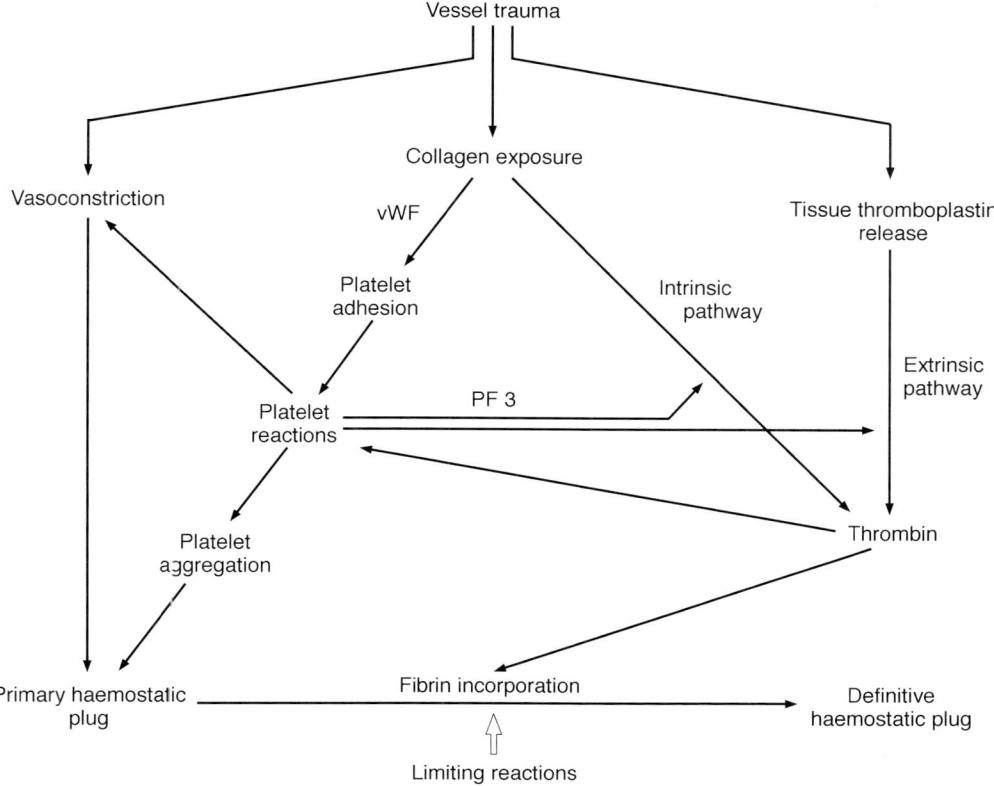

Figure 45.2 Simplified scheme of the mechanisms involved in haemostasis. vWF, von Willebrand factor; PF3, platelet factor 3 phospholipid. Reproduced from Littlewood (1986).

Plasma proteins involved in haemostasis

Von Willebrand factor

This is a highly glycosylated, multimeric protein of high molecular weight which is derived from vascular endothelial cells. Although it is also present in megakaryocytes and platelets of other species there is little, if any, vWF in canine platelets (Meyers *et al.*, 1987; Parker *et al.*, 1991). In plasma, vWF circulates non-covalently bonded with the antihaemophilic coagulation factor, factor VIII (F.VIII). However, it is a completely distinct protein, coded for by an autosomal gene, with a different role in haemostasis from F.VIII. The close association has led to confusion regarding terminology and vWF was originally known as factor VIII-related antigen. This name is now outmoded.

vWF has a pivotal role in platelet adhesion to collagen. The protein is released from endothelial stores by the action of vasopressin, after exercise and stress. These and other hormonal influences may cause great variability in circulating vWF concentrations in people and the same is likely to be the case in dogs.

Coagulation proteins: secondary haemostasis

The coagulation proteins or factors are designated by Roman numerals. The majority are serine proteases which are sequentially activated. Classically, the coagulation cascade is divided into intrinsic and extrinsic pathways with a final common pathway (Fig. 45.3) although there is extensive interaction *in vivo*. Factors II, VII, IX and X are synthesized in the liver and are vitamin K dependent. Factors V and VIII are essential cofactors, also liver derived, and are activated by the action of thrombin. The intrinsic pathway is initiated by the activation of F.XII after surface (subendothelial) contact or exposure. F.XIIa also plays an important role in inflammation by the release of kinins and kallikrein production and in the activation of complement, as well as triggering fibrinolysis by conversion of plasminogen to plasmin. The extrinsic pathway comprises F.VII and tissue factor (thromboplastin), a lipoprotein complex derived from the membranes of many cells

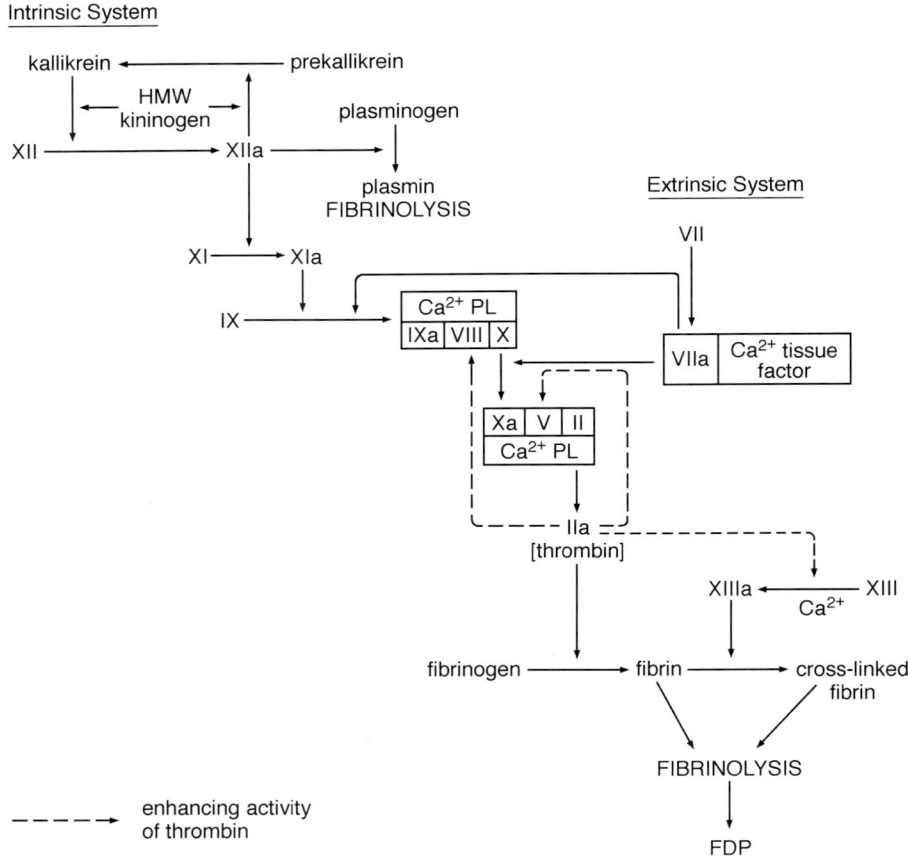

Figure 45.3 A simplified scheme of the coagulation cascade, omitting feedback and inhibition interactions. HMW, high molecular weight; FDP, fibrin/fibrinogen degradation products; PL, phospholipids. Reproduced from Littlewood (1986).

including monocytes and macrophages. The common pathway consists of conversion of prothrombin into thrombin by F.Xa and finally the production of insoluble fibrin from fibrinogen. This polymerizes to form a clot under the influence of F.XIIIa. Thrombin activates many of the enzymes and thus feedback amplification occurs. Calcium ions and phospholipid (PF3) are essential for many of the enzyme reactions. Fibrin polymer is deposited in a meshwork to form a definitive platelet plug, preventing further loss of blood.

Limiting reactions: tertiary haemostasis

Localization of these reactions to the surface of activated platelets limits the extent of clot and thrombus formation. The antithrombotic effects of prostacyclin derived from endothelial cells has already been mentioned. Thrombin, in addition to activating cofactors and other enzymes, also inactivates molecules by further enzymatic cleavage. Protein C and protein S are vitamin K-dependent factors which inactivate cofactors V and VIII. This action is enhanced by thrombomodulin, an endothelial cell surface receptor which binds thrombin. The major physiological inhibitor of coagulation is antithrombin III (AT III). This, in association with heparin, inactivates thrombin and serine proteases. Various other natural inhibitors have been identified. In addition to these localized limiting reactions any activated factors reaching the circulation are removed by the liver.

Fibrinolysis

The fibrin clot is broken down by the action of plasmin. Plasmin is derived from plasminogen which is activated by a number of molecules, the most important of which is tissue plasminogen activator (tPA), which is produced by endothelial cells. Urokinase, F.XIIa and kallikrein also activate plasminogen. The action of tPA is regulated by several inhibitors. The breakdown products of fibrin and fibrinogen, resulting from the action of plasmin, are known as fibrin(ogen) split or degradation products (FSP, FDP). These possess anticoagulant properties, interfering with the polymerization of fibrin and also platelet function. Circulating plasmin is inactivated by α_2-antiplasmin and α_2-macroglobulin. Healing of damaged vessels is completed by fibroblastic and endothelial repair, under the stimulus of platelet derived growth factors.

In summary, the normal haemostatic system is a complex, well-regulated balance between the vascular responses, platelets, coagulation proteins, fibrinolytic mechanisms and natural inhibitors. These mechanisms serve to limit haemorrhage, prevent excessive thrombosis, stimulate local repair and thus maintain homeostasis.

CLINICAL HISTORY

The history of animals with haematological abnormalities is often non-specific and, particularly in cats whose owners may not notice compensatory changes in lifestyle, inapparent until the disease process is quite advanced. Although there are conditions with a rapid rate of onset and acute signs, many dogs and cats with red or white blood cell abnormalities follow a chronic course, sometimes with repeated episodes of illness. Bleeding disorders, however, generally progress more rapidly, although repeated episodes of bleeding may be encountered in inherited disorders and a more prolonged course may be seen with some low-grade acquired disorders of haemostasis.

Lethargy and/or generalized weakness are common features of most haematological disorders. Anorexia is also frequently encountered, together with weight loss, the severity of which is dependent on the duration of the condition. Some animals with anaemia may show cold sensitivity. Exercise intolerance is common, with dyspnoea and even collapse resulting from any exertion. Owners may have noticed pallor of the mucous membranes and, in the case of bleeding disorders, the presence of petechial or ecchymotic haemorrhages affecting the mucosae and skin. Occasionally ocular haemorrhage may be the presenting complaint.

Owners should be questioned about external blood loss, such as epistaxis, haemoptysis, haematemesis, melaena and haematuria. The presence of large swellings and shifting lameness may indicate the presence of soft tissue haematomas and haemarthroses, respectively. In some bleeding disorders haemorrhage may be spontaneous; in others it may only be apparent after trauma. A history of uneventful surgery or dental extractions in the past suggests an acquired rather than an inherited disorder of haemostasis. Details of previous bleeding episodes, age of onset, frequency and type of bleeding should be documented. The incidence of any similar problems in related animals would indicate an inherited condition.

Many haematological disorders are associated with underlying systemic disease. There may be a history of recurrent infections and fever in immunocompromised animals, e.g. animals with myelo- or lymphoproliferative disease or which are neutropenic. Polydipsia and polyuria may indicate the presence of renal or hepatic disease, both of which are commonly associated with anaemia. Diarrhoea and vomiting may be features of several conditions which result in haematological abnormalities.

The owner should be questioned about the diet of the animal. In some cases of anaemia, for example, pica may be a feature. A detailed history of drug administration, particularly antibiotics, hormones and anti-inflammatory preparations, both prescribed and owner initiated, is essential. Possible exposure to toxins should also be considered.

PHYSICAL EXAMINATION

Animals with haematological disorders are commonly rather quiet and may be depressed. Pyrexia is not uncommon in animals with bone marrow neoplasia or aplasia and other causes of immunosuppression, e.g. FeLV or FIV infections in cats. Fever spikes may accompany acute haemolytic episodes.

Pallor of mucous membranes is characteristic of many haematological conditions, although some animals with a slowly progressive anaemia may show little pallor until the disease is advanced. However, it should be remembered that anaemia is not the only cause of pale mucosae; peripheral vasoconstriction, for example in dogs with severe congestive heart failure, may also result in mucosal pallor. An assessment of capillary refill time may be helpful in distinguishing pallor due to decreased perfusion and anaemia. When a bleeding disorder is suspected all mucosal surfaces should be examined for the presence of petechial haemorrhages which are characteristic of vascular or, more usually, platelet disorders. Cases of oxidant poisoning (e.g. paracetamol toxicity) may show cyanosis of the mucosae. Polycythaemic animals may show injection and hyperaemia of the mucous membranes which are difficult to blanche. Oropharyngeal inflammation and ulceration are common in immunosuppressed FeLV and/or FIV-infected cats and may be associated with haematological abnormalities. Tachycardia, a frequent finding in anaemic animals, is a compensatory mechanism to maintain oxygen delivery to the tissues, although at rest it is worth noting that the heart rate may be normal especially in animals with slowly progressive, chronic anaemias. Peripheral pulse pressure is variable; it is often increased in chronically anaemic animals and is typically weak and easily compressed in animals following acute blood loss. Haemic murmurs are commonly audible in anaemic dogs but the tachycardia in cats often makes it difficult to detect any heart murmur. The murmur is due to increased ejection velocity and decreased blood viscosity, is heard during mid-systole and is usually graded I to III out of VI. Anaemia may exacerbate pre-existing heart disease. Tachypnoea at rest progressing to dyspnoea on exertion is common, particularly in anaemic cats. Bleeding into the thoracic cavity is accompanied by respiratory distress and heart and lung sounds may be reduced in amplitude.

Haematological abnormalities are common in animals with superficial lymphadenopathy, especially cases of multicentric lymphoma with bone marrow involvement or immunocompromised animals with generalized reactive lymph node enlargement. Hepatosplenomegaly is similarly a feature of many cases of lymphoproliferative and myeloproliferative diseases and immune-mediated anaemia. Abdominal palpation may indicate the presence of pain in some instances, e.g. hepatic disease, especially necrosis, ruptured splenic masses or other causes of intra-abdominal bleeding. Rectal examination is indicated in male dogs, since prostatic carcinoma may be a cause of disseminated intravascular coagulation (DIC).

Examination of the skin may show ecchymotic haemorrhages in cases of platelet disorders. In cats with immunosuppressive viral infections signs of chronic abscessation may be present. Coagulopathies frequently result in the presence of swellings due to haematomas; bleeding may occur subcutaneously, between fascial planes or into muscles. Joint swelling may also be encountered.

Animals with neoplastic disease involving bone marrow may occasionally show pain on deep palpation of the bones.

Ocular examination may reveal haemorrhage into the anterior chamber in bleeding disorders. Ophthalmic examination of the fundus can be helpful, marked pallor being evident in anaemic cases, retinal haemorrhages in bleeding disorders, tortuous vessels in polycythaemia and inflammatory infiltrates in some infectious diseases of cats, e.g. FeLV, FIP and toxoplasmosis. Uveitis may accompany the latter conditions.

In summary, a full and thorough clinical examination is indicated in all animals with suspected haematological disorders, both cellular and haemostatic. The detailed investigation of the animal with pallor of the mucous membranes or suspected bleeding disorders is described in Chapters 14 and 21, respectively.

INVESTIGATIVE TECHNIQUES

Blood sampling

Examination of blood samples is mandatory in all cases of suspected haematological disorders. It should be remembered that the peripheral blood picture is a dynamic and constantly changing state and a blood sample provides only a window on events. Although a single blood sample may yield much valuable information, repeated samples are necessary to document changes in blood cell kinetics and are essential for monitoring the progession of haematological disorders.

Venepuncture technique

The usual sites for blood sampling in dogs and cats are the cephalic or jugular veins, although other superficial veins may be used (Patteson and Williams, 1988). The jugular vein has advantages, allowing for more rapid sampling with a larger needle and the removal of larger volumes of blood. The secret to successful jugular venepuncture is effective restraint and correct positioning of the patient, combined with adequate clipping of the neck to give optimum visibility of the vein. In order to avoid artefacts due to lipaemia the patient should, in preference, be fasted before sampling.

Blood samples from different sites may show differences in cell counts, particularly platelet counts, and any difficulty or delay in obtaining the sample will dramatically reduce the platelet count. Similarly, sampling difficulties have a seriously detrimental effect on the results of clotting assays, due to triggering of the coagulation cascade. Interruption of blood flow through a vessel will affect the balance between marginated and circulating pools of cells so compression of the vein during collection should be minimal. Samples collected into vacuum tubes are prone to haemolysis which will affect the red cell parameters and influence the results of clotting assays. Needles should be removed from syringes for transfer of blood into tubes, again to prevent haemolysis. Haemolysis, artefactual changes in cell morphology and platelet clumping occur in blood samples which have 'aged' or have been exposed to high environmental temperature. Rapid delivery to the laboratory is desirable, therefore; if there is to be an unavoidable delay, air-dried smears should be prepared and the sample refrigerated at 4°C before submission to the laboratory.

Anticoagulants

Routine haematology

The usual anticoagulant for haematological investigation is ethylenediaminetetra-acetate (EDTA). The correct amount of blood should be added to the tube, since excessive anticoagulant reduces the packed cell volume (PCV) and derived red cell indices. Gentle mixing of blood with anticoagulant also reduces the risk of haemolysis.

Clotting assays

The anticoagulant of choice for assessment of all clotting factors is 3.8% sodium citrate in the proportions of nine parts blood to one part anticoagulant. It is vital that the correct ratio is maintained as excess anticoagulant will have a profound effect on clotting times (Johnstone, 1993). Some sample tubes contain solid anticoagulant and adequate mixing (>20 inversions of the tube) is required to prevent clotting. When submitting samples to a laboratory it is often helpful to sample a normal animal at the same time as the patient to act as a control for sample handling. Delivery to the laboratory within hours of sampling is desirable, but there is evidence that next day delivery results in no significant deterioration (Mansell and Parry, 1989; Johnstone et al., 1991). Clotting times and factor levels are well preserved in samples kept as plasma for up to 24 h at either 4°C or 22°C (Johnstone et al., 1991). If there is to be a delay of more than 24 h the plasma should be separated and frozen for subsequent transport to the laboratory in the frozen state. Whole blood samples kept at 22°C for up to 48 h give reliable results for von Willebrand factor antigen (Johnstone et al., 1991). However in whole blood, factor VIII concentrations fall unless the sample is refrigerated and this is unsuitable for von Willebrand factor measurement. Patients should be sampled before commencement of any therapy as this may affect results and render interpretation difficult, if not impossible.

Bone marrow aspiration and biopsy

The indications for bone marrow biopsy are outlined in Table 45.2. Biopsy should be undertaken initially prior to therapy since administration of chemotherapeutic agents may dramatically affect the relative cell populations and their maturation, and corticosteroids have an adverse effect on the morphological features of lymphoid and reticuloendothelial cells. Aspirates of marrow can be obtained for cytological examination using a Klima biopsy needle (14–18 guage). Core biopsies taken with a Jamshidi biopsy needle have the advantage of preserving the architecture of the marrow, and are particularly helpful when 'dry' taps are obtained following repeated attempts to aspirate marrow, a common finding in myelophthisic disorders.

The usual site for aspiration or biopsy is the iliac crest (Fig. 45.4). In small dogs and cats marrow may be aspirated from the wing of the ilium using a transverse approach, or from the shaft of the femur via the trochanteric fossa. In obese animals the author has had success in obtaining samples from the ischium. An alternative site is the craniolateral aspect of the humerus in its proximal

Table 45.2 Indications for bone marrow aspiration and biopsy

Non-regenerative anaemia
Anaemia with an inappropriate erythroid marrow response
Abnormal cells in peripheral blood
Persistent leucopenia
Persistent leucocytosis
Thrombocytopenia
Lymphosarcoma (to assist staging of the disease)
Pyrexia of unknown origin
Hypergammaglobulinaemia
Unexplained hypercalcaemia
Focal lytic bone lesions (vertebral bodies, pelvis and long bones)
Periodic monitoring of cases to assess progression and/or response to therapy

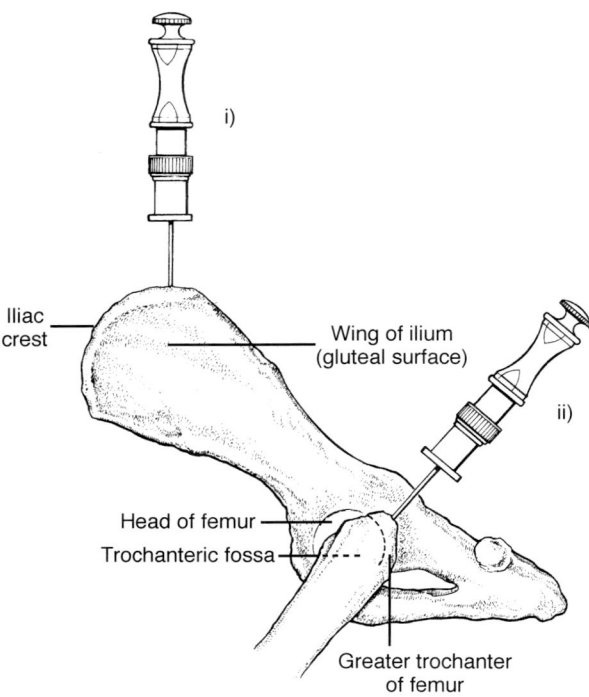

Figure 45.4 Diagram of sampling sites for bone marrow aspiration or core biopsy.

third. Samples can be obtained under sedation and local analgesia, with infiltration of local anaesthetic down to the periosteum. The needle is introduced with a rotating action through the cortex until it is firmly seated. The marrow is aspirated with a 10 ml syringe and immediately expressed onto clean glass slides, tilted at an angle to allow excess blood to drain away leaving marrow flecks which are spread with another slide. Anticoagulant (3% EDTA) can be introduced into the syringe nozzle to prevent clotting. Smears should be rapidly air dried and submitted, together with a blood sample for full haematological examination taken at the same time, to a laboratory with experience of marrow examination. Significant haemorrhage after biopsy is extremely unusual. For a more detailed description and illustrations of bone marrow aspiration and biopsy techniques see Dunn (1990) and Relford (1991).

Assessment of haemostatic function

Bleeding time

The bleeding time gives an assessment of primary haemostasis. It is particularly useful where platelet counts are normal and a defect of platelet adhesion or function is suspected.

Buccal mucosal bleeding time

A standardized injury is made on the inner aspect of the upper lip, rostral to a strip of gauze bandage which holds the lip up, using a bleeding time device (Simplate II, Organon Teknika, General Diagnostics, Cambridge, UK; Surgicutt, Ortho Diagnostic Systems, High Wycombe, UK). Blood is blotted every 30 s, taking care not to touch the wound itself. The technique is illustrated in Fig. 45.5. The bleeding time in normal dogs is 1.7–4.2 min, mean 2.6 min (Jergens et al., 1987). In this study, times were not significantly affected by sedation or anaesthesia. The technique is equally appropriate to cats, with the bleeding time of normal cats being similar to that of dogs.

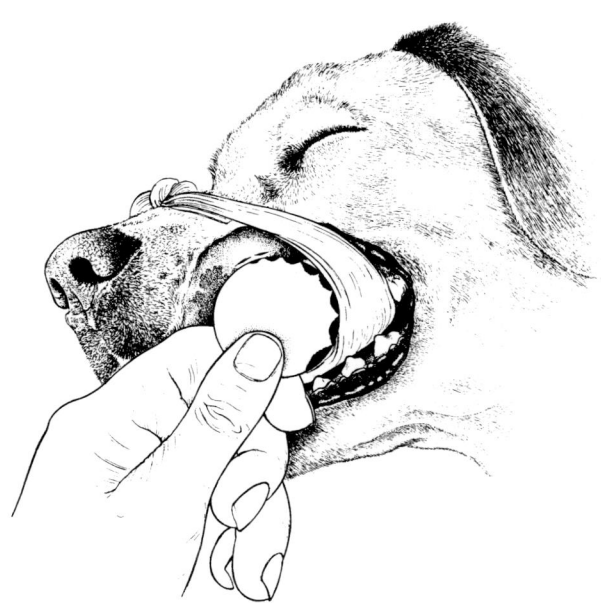

Figure 45.5 Technique for determination of the buccal mucosal bleeding time in the dog. Reproduced from Jergens et al. (1987).

Cuticle bleeding time

This technique is described in the literature as an experimental model of bleeding in haemophilic dogs to assess the haemostatic efficacy of potential procoagulant therapies (Giles et al., 1982). However, the test should be sensitive to disorders of both primary and secondary haemostasis and may be useful as a presurgical screen of haemostatic function. The technique involves cutting a toenail into the quick with guillotine nail clippers and the time taken for blood to stop dripping is noted.

Since the injury itself is painful and cautery is required to stop bleeding if there is a haemostatic defect, the technique can only be recommended for use in anaesthetized animals. Although the technique sounds deceptively easy and potentially useful, there can be difficulties in deciding when the end point is reached and some animals with severe secondary haemostatic defects may have apparently normal cuticle bleeding times (Giles et al., 1982, Pijnappels et al., 1986)

Other investigative techniques

Other procedures which may be indicated in the investigation of patients with haematological abnormalities include radiography. Survey chest and abdominal radiographs are indicated in the work-up of animals with suspected lymphosarcoma and cases which present with a history of pyrexia of unknown origin (see Chapter 4). Screening radiographs of the thorax and abdomen are indicated in most anaemic animals particularly those where intrathoracic or intra-abdominal haemorrhage is suspected. Abdominal films should be taken in animals with hepatic or splenic enlargement, or which have other abdominal masses and/or abdominal pain. If a gut lesion resulting in chronic blood loss is suspected as a cause of anaemia then barium contrast studies may be indicated.

Survey radiographs of the skeletal system are indicated in animals with hypergammaglobulinaemia, looking for the lytic lesions of plasma cell (multiple) myeloma. Animals with myeloproliferative disease, notably myelosclerosis, may show radiographic changes of osteosclerosis in the medullary cavity of long bones.

Lymph node aspiration may give useful additional information in animals with peripheral lymphadenopathy, allowing differentiation between neoplastic and reactive node enlargement. (See Chapter 20).

LABORATORY INVESTIGATIONS

Routine haematology

Normal reference ranges for haematological parameters of adult dogs and cats are shown in Table 45.3. The values for young and aged animals may fall outside these ranges, e.g. animals less than 3 months of age tend to have lower red cell counts and packed cell volumes. Blood smears are usually stained with Romanowsky stains (e.g. Wright or Giemsa stains) for examination of cell type and morphology.

Red cell parameters

Feline erythrocytes are smaller than those of dogs and the total red cell mass is less in cats. Inadequate filling of sample tubes resulting in an excessive anticoagulant concentration will artefactually reduce the PCV and derived red cell indices. PCV should be interpreted in association with the total plasma protein concentration.

Table 45.3 Normal reference ranges for haematological parameters in adult animals[a]

Parameter	Dog	Cat	Units
Haemoglobin (Hb)	12–18	9–15	g dl^{-1}
Red blood cells (Rbc)	5.5–8.5	5.5–10	$\times 10^{12}$ l^{-1}
Packed cell volume (PCV)	0.37–0.55	0.27–0.45	l l^{-1}
Mean cell haemoglobin (MCH)	19.5–24.5	12–17	pg
Mean cell volume (MCV)	62–77	40–55	fl
Mean cell haemoglobin concentration (MCHC)	32–36	32–35	g dl^{-1}
White blood cells (WBC)	6–18	5–20	$\times 10^9$ l^{-1}
Band neutrophils	0–0.5	0–0.3	$\times 10^9$ l^{-1}
Neutrophils	4.0–12.0	2.5–13.0	$\times 10^9$ l^{-1}
Lymphocytes	1.0–4.8	1.5–7.0	$\times 10^9$ l^{-1}
Eosinophils	0.2–1.2	0.1–2.0	$\times 10^9$ l^{-1}
Basophils	0	0	$\times 10^9$ l^{-1}
Monocytes	0.1–1.8	0–0.8	$\times 10^9$ l^{-1}

[a] Normal referance range at the Peter E. Burrell Laboratories, Animal Health Trust, Newmarket.

Red cell morphology

A list of definitions of terms applied to describe the appearance of red cells and red cell inclusions is given in Table 45.4. Care must be exercised when interpreting several of these findings in cats, since crenation is commonly observed. Feline erythrocytes are normally more spherical in appearance compared to dogs and both Howell–Jolly bodies and Heinz bodies may be seen in normal, healthy cats. Increased numbers of Howell–Jolly bodies may be seen in markedly responsive anaemias, regardless of cause. Heinz bodies disrupt the erythrocyte membrane, making the cell more prone to haemolysis or phagocytosis. They may be single or multiple and are better demonstrated by new methylene blue stains.

Reticulocyte counts

The normal rate of replacement of effete red cells means that approximately 1% of circulating erythrocytes are reticulocytes which appear as polychromatophilic, macrocytic red cells on Romanowsky-stained smears. They can be better demonstrated with a supravital stain such as new methylene blue. Cats have two populations of reticulocytes: coarse (aggregate) and fine (punctate) reticulocytes. The number of coarse reticulocytes corresponds well to the degree of current marrow activity. Feline reticulocytes have a relatively longer maturation period (up to 3 days compared to the 24 h of canine reticulocytes) and pass through a phase of fine, punctate reticulation before becoming fully mature erythrocytes. Simply counting the percentage of fine reticulocytes may provide an erroneously false (high) estimate of the degree of erythroid activity.

An increase in the reticulocyte count is an indication of increased marrow activity in response to erythrocyte loss. Adequacy of this reticulocyte response is a useful tool in assessing the state of the bone marrow. To gain a true indication of marrow activity the reticulocyte count must be considered in the light of the reduction in red cell count and prolonged maturation of younger reticulocytes. Various correction factors can be calculated as follows.

1. The absolute reticulocyte count corrects for variation in red cell number, i.e. the degree of anaemia, and is calculated as follows:

   Absolute reticulocyte count ($\times 10^9$ l^{-1}) = observed % reticulocytes $\times$ RBC count ($\times 10^{12}$ l^{-1}) $\times$ 10

   An absolute reticulocyte count >60 $\times 10^9$ l^{-1} in the dog (an aggregate reticulocyte count >50 $\times 10^9$ l^{-1} in the cat) is evidence of a responsive anaemia.

2. The corrected reticulocyte count can be defined as follows:

Table 45.4 Glossary of terms used to describe red blood cell morphology and cellular inclusions

Term	Definition	Significance
Anisocytosis	Variable cell size	Common in responsive anaemias
Poikilocytosis	Abnormal shape	Depends on category
Acanthocyte	Surface projections	Increased in liver disease and splenic tumours
Crenation	Artefactual spurs	Old sample, excess EDTA common in cats
Spherocyte	Small, round cells	Partially phagocytosed cells seen in immune-mediated haemolysis
Schistocyte	Fragmented cells	Feature of damage in microcirculation, e.g. DIC
Leptocyte	Thin, flat cells	Feature of anaemia of chronic disease, portosystemic shunts
Target cell	Leptocyte with dark-staining centre	
Howell–Jolly bodies	Nuclear remnants, appear as basophilic spheres	Rare in dogs, present in up to 1% of cat cells
Heinz bodies	Small, irregular, refractile areas of denatured haemoglobin	Oxidant or drug damage, present in up to 10% of cells in normal cats

Corrected % reticulocyte count = observed % count × observed PCV/mean species PCV (0.45 l l⁻¹ for dogs and 0.37 l l⁻¹ for cats).

Values greater than 1% are indicative of active erythropoiesis in the dog and cat.

3. A further adjustment must be made for the longer maturation time of reticulocytes due to earlier release from the marrow in anaemic states (see Table 45.5 for different maturation times). The reticulocyte production index (RPI) is calculated as follows:

RPI = corrected % reticulocyte count/maturation time

In normal healthy dogs the RPI is 1–1.5% and 0.5% for cats. Values less than 1.0 indicate non-regenerative anaemia; values greater than 2.0 indicate accelerated erythropoiesis.

Table 45.5 Lifespan of reticulocytes

PCV (l l⁻¹)	Maturation time (days)
Dogs	
0.45	1
0.35	1.5
0.25	2
0.15	2.5
Cats	
0.32	1
0.24	1.5
0.16	2
0.10	2.5

Erythropoietin assay

Immunoassays for human erythropoietin have been shown to be valid for the measurement of canine serum erythropoietin (Giger, 1992; King et al., 1992; Cook and Lothrop, 1994; Suzuki and Kubo, 1996) and commercial kits are readily available (Giger, 1992; Suzuki and Kubo, 1996). Evaluation of erythropoietin concentrations may aid in the investigation of anaemic animals and those with polycythaemia (Cook and Lothrop, 1994). A low or normal serum erythropoietin value in a polycythaemic cat was found to be consistent with primary polycythaemia, but did not rule out secondary polycythaemia, whereas elevated erythropoietin concentrations were consistent with secondary polycythaemia (Hasler and Giger, 1996).

Red cell responses to disease

Anaemia

Anaemia is defined as a reduction in the circulating red cell mass, reflected by haemoglobin, packed cell volume and red cell counts below the normal reference range. The haemoglobin concentration is the most sensitive indicator of anaemia. Anaemias can be classified according to erythrocyte morphology (Table 45.6), but an aetiopathological classification according to the

Table 45.6 Morphological classification of anaemia

Morphology	Aetiology
Macrocytic, hypochromic	Haemorrhage, haemolysis
Macrocytic, normochromic	Maturation defects, myeloproliferative disease, FeLV infection, folate/B$_{12}$ deficiency
Normocytic, normochromic	Recent haemorrhage, marrow aplasia/hypoplasia, anaemia of chronic disease
Microcytic, hypochromic	Iron deficiency due to chronic blood loss, chronic lead poisoning, occasionally portosystemic shunts in dogs

bone marrow response may be more helpful (Table 45.7). Regenerative anaemias are the result of either blood loss or increased red cell destruction. The features of a regenerative or responsive marrow are a reticulocytosis with an RPI >2, polychromasia, anisocytosis, increased mean cell volume (MCV) and, in severe anaemias, the appearance of significant numbers of nucleated red blood cells in the circulation. A marked normoblastosis without a corresponding reticulocytosis represents an inappropriate red cell response (see Table 45.7 for diseases associated with an inappropriate red cell response).

Non-regenerative anaemias caused by primary conditions affecting the bone marrow and production of all the cellular elements of blood are covered in detail later. Non-regenerative anaemia is also a common secondary feature of numerous systemic diseases. Mild to moderate anaemia commonly accompanies chronic inflammatory disease, due to interference with iron metabolism; increased bone marrow stores of haemosiderin are present, but these stores are not mobilized and incorporated into haemoglobin. Anaemia may also be associated with various neoplastic conditions, possible mechanisms including haemorrhage, haemolysis and DIC. Renal disease may result in anaemia because of shortened red cell lifespan, haemorrhage associated with uraemic ulceration of the gastrointestinal tract, haemolysis

Table 45.7 Classification of anaemia according to marrow response

Regenerative anaemias	Haemorrhage
	Haemolysis
Non-regenerative anaemias	Erythroid hypoplasia/aplasia
	Aplastic anaemia/pancytopenia
	Myeloproliferative disease
	Myelodysplasia
	Myelofibrosis
	Lymphoproliferative disease
	Chronic inflammatory disease
	Renal disease
	Chronic liver disease
	Hypothyroidism, hypoadrenocorticism
Inappropriate marrow response	Myeloproliferative disease (erythraemic myelosis, erythroleukaemia)
	Myelodysplasia
	Lead poisoning

associated with uraemic vasculitis, toxic effects on the bone marrow and reduced or absent erythropoietin production, as well as the anaemia associated with the chronic disease state. The anaemia associated with hepatic disease similarly may occur due to chronic inflammation and the effect of toxins, with additional contributions from microangiopathic damage due to disrupted sinusoids and a bleeding tendency (see later). The mild anaemia which may be a feature of hypothyroidism is physiological and is associated with reduced metabolic rate. Mild anaemia is common in hypoadrenocorticism, but is often masked by haemoconcentration due to dehydration.

Polycythaemia

Polycythaemia is characterized by an increase in erythrocyte numbers above normal and may be relative or absolute. Relative polycythaemia is usually the result of dehydration (i.e. haemoconcentration) or possibly splenic contraction. Absolute polycythaemia may be primary or secondary. Primary polycythaemia (polycythaemia vera) is a chronic myeloproliferative condition and is covered later. Secondary polycythaemia may occur as a physiological response to hypoxia resulting in an *appropriate* increase in erythropoietin production. It is a feature of congenital cardiac anomalies such as tetralogy of Fallot which are characterized by the right to left shunting of blood. Secondary polycythaemia, in association with *inappropriate* erythropoietin production, most commonly occurs with renal tumours (Crow et al., 1995) and other renal diseases.

White cell parameters

Differential white cell counts should always be interpreted on the basis of absolute values rather than relative percentages. The morphological features which allow discrimination between leucocytes and the species differences are well covered elsewhere (see Further Reading). Romanowsky stains permit differentiation of normal, mature leucocytes, but it may be difficult to discriminate between morphologically abnormal cells and poorly differentiated neoplastic myeloid and lymphoid cell lines without the use of cytochemical stains (Jain, 1986, 1989).

Normal reference ranges for leucocytes are given in Table 45.3. It must be remembered that a single blood sample provides only one picture of the transient journey of white cells from bone marrow to tissue and repeated counts are necessary to gain a fuller understanding of the reasons for an abnormal white cell count. Serial counts are also helpful in monitoring the progress of a disease process and its response to therapy.

Leucocyte responses

Physiological leucocytosis

Physiological leucocytosis occurs with excitement, fear and exercise. The release of catecholamines increases blood flow and mobilizes marginated neutrophils resulting in a mild neutrophilia. Physiological leucocytosis, particularly a lymphocytosis, is a common occurrence in cats.

Physiological leucopenia
Samples taken from sedated or anaesthetized animals may show a physiological leucopenia due to increased margination of neutrophils.

Stress leucocytosis
Corticosteroids have several effects on the release and distribution of neutrophils resulting in a neutrophilia, including reduced egress of cells into tissues, a shift from the marginated to circulating pool, and increased release from the marrow storage pool. There may be nuclear hypersegmentation associated with prolongation of the circulation time of neutrophils. Eosinopenia and lymphopenia are usually present as a result of the lytic effect of corticosteroids on these cells and/or a shift of cells into the marginated pool. There may also be an accompanying monocytosis. This typical picture of a neutrophilic leucocytosis with eosinopenia and lymphopenia is commonly referred to as the *stress leucogram*. It may be seen after trauma, pain, surgery and many chronic non-inflammatory conditions, and is a hallmark of spontaneous or iatrogenic hyperadrenocorticism (Cushing's disease).

Leucocyte responses in inflammation

Peracute inflammation
Early in the response to severe tissue damage neutrophils move from the circulating to marginated pool and pass into the tissues in reponse to chemotactic factors. This results in a leucopenia, due to neutropenia. In most cases this phase is transient and the response progresses to that more typical of acute inflammation. However, in the face of overwhelming infection such as endotoxaemia this leucopenia (neutropenia) may persist accompanied by a *degenerative left shift*, i.e. the number of band neutrophils released into the circulation is out of proportion to the number of mature segmented neutrophils (the number of band cells usually exceeds the number of mature neutrophils by at least 10%). This picture carries a more guarded prognosis.

Acute inflammation
Neutrophils continue to pass into the tissues and at the same time cells are released from the marrow storage pool. The mobilization of neutrophils causes increased marrow production of granulocytes. In the peripheral blood acute inflammation is characterized by a neutrophilia and the presence of immature band neutrophils, a left shift. This leucocytosis (neutrophilia) and *regenerative left shift* is the appropriate response to an inflammatory reaction. It also accompanies acute haemorrhage and haemolysis.

Chronic inflammation
In the face of ongoing, unresolved inflammation there are several possible sequelae. If the reaction becomes stabilized and the tissue demand for neutrophils is balanced by expanded marrow production, the total white cell count may be at the upper limits of normal or a mild neutrophilia is seen with a variable left shift and monocytosis. If the marrow response becomes exhausted by tissue demands then a low normal neutrophil count or a neutropenia may be seen, with a degenerative left shift. A more guarded prognosis is warranted in such cases

Leukaemoid response
A severe localized infection such as closed pyometra or pyothorax may result in a profound leucocytosis with an extreme left shift with bands, myelocytes and occasionally myeloblasts present in the circulation. Total white cell counts may be in the region of $50–80 \times 10^9$ l^{-1} or more. Leukaemoid reactions may be difficult to distinguish from chronic granulocytic (myeloid) leukaemia.

Morphological changes
Toxic changes, refelecting abnormal maturation, may be seen in neutrophils in association with severe toxaemic states. Changes include purple–black cytoplasmic granules, diffuse cytoplasmic basophilia, cytoplasmic vacuolation, pale blue, angular cytoplasmic inclusions (Dohle bodies) and giant neutrophils with bizarre nuclei. Toxic changes are commonly encountered in feline neutrophils.

Neutropenia
In addition to the situations described above neutropenia may result from the use of cytotoxic drugs and is a common feature of myeloproliferative disease (see later). Whatever the cause, neutropenia always carries a guarded prognosis for the patient since affected animals are more likely to succumb to infection.

Lymphocyte responses

Lymphocytosis
A physiological lymphocytosis may be part of the leucocytosis seen in response to fear and excitement, especially in the cat. Lymphocytosis can be seen after vaccination and in response to

prolonged immunogenic challenge. Large reactive lymhocytes may be seen in the circulation in such circumstances. Lymphocytosis is occasionally seen in dogs with hypoadrenocorticism. Lymphoproliferative disorders are covered elsewhere.

Lymphopenia
The commonest cause of lymphopenia is stress or exogenous corticosteroid administration. Other causes include the acute phase of viral infections, chylothorax due to ruptured thoracic duct, lymphangiectasia and immunosuppressive drug therapy.

Eosinophil responses

Eosinophilia
Eosinophils are primarily involved in hypersensitivity reactions and parasitic infections. In such cases eosinophilia is sometimes accompanied by a basophilia. An increase in the number of circulating eosinophils may accompany a number of conditions characterized by tissue infiltration with eosinophils, such as eosinophilic gastroenteritis, myositis, panosteitis and pulmonary eosinophilic infiltration in dogs, and hypereosinophilic syndrome and eosinophilic granuloma complex in cats. Occasionally eosinophilia, in association with a lymphocytosis, is seen in dogs with hypoadrenocorticism. Eosinophilic leukaemia is rare in dogs and cats.

Eosinopenia
Endogenous or exogenous glucocorticoids are the commonest cause of eosinopenia. Acute infection and inflammation may also reduce the eosinophil count, possibly as a result of 'stress'.

Monocytosis
Monocytosis is a feature of the chronic inflammatory response and may be associated with a neutrophilia with or without a left shift. Chronic inflammatory conditions, especially those involving a significant degree of tissue necrosis, or pyogranulomatous disorders (e.g. mycotic infections), frequently result in an increase in the number of circulating monocytes. Monocytosis may also be a feature of the 'stress leucogram'. Leukaemic causes are covered later.

Basophilia
Basophilia rarely occurs in the absence of an eosinophilia, hence many of the allergic and parasitic causes of eosinophilia may also give rise to a basophilia (one of the more common causes being canine heartworm disease). Increased numbers of circulating basophils may also occur with hyperlipoproteinaemia and some of the less common myeloproliferative disorders such as polycythaemia vera and essential thrombocythaemia. Basophilic leukaemia is rare.

Bone marrow examination
Bone marrow smears are usually stained with a Romanowsky stain, e.g. May–Grunwald Giemsa. Detailed descriptions and illustrations of marrow cytology can be found elsewhere (see Further Reading). An assessment of cellularity is made and cell lines identified. Cell morphology should be examined for evidence of normal differentiation and maturation. The normal myeloid to erythroid ratio varies from 1:1 to 2:1. Smears can also be stained with Prussian blue to demonstrate marrow iron (haemosiderin) stores. Cytochemical stains may be required to differentiate the cell lines involved in acute myeloproliferative or lymphoproliferative conditions (Jain, 1989). Immunofluorescent staining of marrow aspirates may be helpful in the investigation of suspected immune-mediated conditions. Core biopsies require histological processing and staining as appropriate.

Descriptions of bone marrow abnormalities relating to specific conditions are covered briefly in the appropriate sections.

Laboratory assessment of haemostasis

Platelets

Platelet count
Normal platelet counts are shown in Table 45.3. Most commercial laboratories use automated platelet counters, with the thresholds adjusted for the particular species under investigation. Since feline platelets are not much smaller than erythrocytes, platelet counts must be performed manually in this species or an automated count can be performed using platelet-rich plasma. Some machines also give a profile of the frequency distribution of platelet size, which is helpful in detecting increased numbers of large shift platelets, evidence of platelet clumping and other divergencies from normal profiles. Thrombocytosis is a common finding following acute haemorrhage. Macrothrombocytosis is indicative of active thrombopoiesis and is especially marked with chronic blood loss. Macrothrombocytes have also been reported as a normal finding in healthy cavalier King Charles spaniels (Eksell et al., 1994). Microthrombocytosis has been found to be a spe-

cific indicator of immune-mediated thrombocytopenia which is present at the onset of the condition (Northern and Tvetden, 1992). Mega- or macrothrombocytosis has been shown to be a good predictor of adequate bone marrow response (Sullivan et al., 1995). Manual platelet counts using haemocytometer chambers are notoriously inaccurate, even in the hands of experienced technicians. However, a reasonable estimate of the platelet count can be made by examination of the feathered edge region of a stained blood smear. One platelet per oil immersion field is roughly equivalent to a count of $15 \times 10^9 \text{ l}^{-1}$. An assessment of morphology can also be made on examination of the smear, elongated platelets indicating activation.

Although counts below the reference ranges constitute a thrombocytopenia, haemorrhage is not likely to ensue until the count falls below $50 \times 10^9 \text{ l}^{-1}$. Counts above this, but below normal, in bleeding patients are usually the result of, rather than the cause of, the haemorrhage.

The presence of large numbers of macrothrombocytes should be taken into consideration when interpreting platelet counts in cavalier King Charles spaniels (erroneously low counts may occur with automated counters since large platelets are counted as red cells). In one study involving 102 cavalier King Charles spaniels with no history of abnormal bleeding, 31% had platelet counts below $100 \times 10^9 \text{ l}^{-1}$ and males had significantly lower counts than females (Eksell et al., 1994). Platelets should therefore be counted manually in this breed to gain a more accurate assessment of true platelet numbers.

Clot retraction

Blood collected into a glass tube is allowed to clot and left for two hours, after which time the clot should have retracted to approximately 50% of its original volume. This retraction is a function of platelet contractile fibres and the test is thus a crude assessment of platelet numbers and function.

Platelet function tests

Tests of platelet function require fresh blood samples and, for aggregometry, specialized equipment which largely limits their availability to research establishments. Aggregometry is the story of the response of platelets to agonists such as ADP, collagen and arachidonic acid. Platelet adhesion can be assessed by measuring the retention of platelets on a glass bead column (Weiss, 1975). These assays are not routinely available for investigation of clinical cases.

Von Willebrand factor assays

Laurell rocket immunoelectrophoresis is the classic method of assessment of vWF antigen (vWF:Ag). Specific rabbit anti-canine vWF:Ag antibody can be prepared, but cross-reactivity with human reagent occurs. Enzyme-linked immunosorbent assays (ELISA) are also available. These assays give a measure of protein concentration rather than biological activity. Botrocetin cofactor assays correlate better with function. A more detailed review of assays is given by Littlewood (1991). The normal range for vWF:Ag is 60–150% of pooled normal canine plasma, alternatively expressed as 0.6–1.5 units ml^{-1}. Individual animals may show considerable variation in vWF concentrations in repeated blood samples over time (Moser et al., 1996a) although this is only likely to be of clinical relevance in the mid-range values of 0.3–0.75 units ml^{-1}, where some dogs, on repeat sampling, had concentrations in the high vWF range. This study highlighted the difficulty of attempting to assess genotype from a single vWF measurement.

Coagulation assays

Whole blood clotting time (WBCT)

The WBCT is a simple test to perform, giving a crude measure of the intrinsic pathway of coagulation. Immediately after venepuncture and sampling, 1 ml of blood is introduced into each of two clean glass tubes; the tubes are tilted every 30 s and the time taken to clot formation is noted. The WBCT of normal dogs, performed at room temperature, is 6.1 min (SD 0.2 min), and that of cats is also 6.1 (SD 0.3 min) (Osbaldiston et al., 1970). Since no exogenous phospholipid is added, this test is also prolonged in severe thrombocytopenia. The activated clotting time (ACT) is the same test in principle, but special tubes containing an activator accelerate the normal clotting time to about 2 min.

Screening assays

Clotting assays are performed with platelet-poor plasma using citrate as anticoagulant. Plasma from the patient is compared to a standard which is pooled plasma from at least ten animals of the same species. The end point of coagulation or clotting assays is the formation of a fibrin clot. These tests are performed at 37°C and the clot detected by manual or automated techniques. Test and control clotting times are performed simultaneously, in duplicate. Normal ranges vary according to the reagents and assay conditions used in each laboratory. Clotting times which are >30% longer than control times can be considered abnormal. The screening tests are relatively insensitive and abnormal times only become evident when individual factors are reduced to about one third of their normal concentration.

Prothrombin time (PT)
A source of tissue factor, most commonly rabbit brain thromboplastin, is added to plasma, which is then recalcified and the time to clot formation noted. Normal values vary according to the reagents used, but are commonly of the order of 10 s in both dog and cat. The test is a measure of the extrinsic and common pathways.

Activated partial thromboplastin time (APTT)
Plasma is incubated with an activator, usually kaolin or ellagic acid and phospholipid added prior to recalcification. Normal ranges are very dependent on reagents and assay conditions and may vary from day to day. In the author's laboratory the APTT of pooled normal canine plasma is 15–17 s and that of pooled normal feline plasma is 14–16 s. The APTT is a measure of the intrinsic and common pathways.

Specific factor assays
Abnormalities detected in screening tests are further characterized by correction assays and performance of specific factor assays, using plasma (usually human) which is deficient in a single factor as the substrate. To this, dilutions of test and standard plasma are added and the appropriate clotting assay (PT or APTT) performed. The concentration of the factor in the test sample is calculated by comparison with the clotting times of the standard (of the same species). Pooled normal plasma is considered to contain 100% of each factor, alternatively expressed as 1 unit ml^{-1}.

Fibrinogen (Factor I)
Heat precipitation is an adequate method of assessing normal or elevated fibrinogen concentrations. The thrombin time (TT) gives a more accurate measurement of low concentrations of fibrinogen as occur in consumptive coagulopathies or abnormalities of fibrin formation. The TT is affected by the presence of heparin and fibrin degradation products. The batroxobin (Reptilase) time similarly converts fibrinogen into fibrin, but is unaffected by circulating heparin.

Fibrin degradation products (FDPs)
There is sufficient immunological cross-reactivity between canine and human FDPs to enable the commercially available antibody-coated latex bead agglutination tests for the estimation of FDPs in serum (ThromboWellcotest) to be clinically useful. Blood must be collected into special tubes which contain thrombin to promote clot formation and an inhibitor of fibrinolysis to prevent further degradation of fibrin(ogen) in the sample. Failure of blood to clot in the tube is indicative of hypofibrinogenaemia which may be a feature of disseminated intravascular coagulation (DIC). Agglutination of latex beads at sample dilutions of >1:25 indicates the presence of ongoing fibrinolysis.

The delayed formation of a clot or the production of a loose clot in the TT or batroxobin time tests indicates the presence of FDPs since they interfere with fibrin polymerization.

Other haemostatic factors
Assays for inhibitors such as antithrombin III are performed in certain specialist laboratories. Conditions associated with decreased AT III concentrations are covered on p. 804.

Other laboratory tests

Immunological tests

Direct antiglobulin Coombs' test
This test identifies the presence of IgG, IgM or complement fraction C3 attached to the surface of erythrocytes by a rabbit antiserum (a polyvalent antiserum is usually used) (Fig. 45.6). The rabbit antiserum must be species-specific. As well as detecting autoantibodies, false positive results may occur due to the presence of antibodies attached to parasites, e.g. *Haemobartonella* or drugs on the surface of cells, to non-specific immunoglobulin adsorption on red cells, in some neoplastic conditions, after whole blood transfusion, and if the Coombs' antiserum was inadequately adsorbed with normal erythrocytes during preparation. False negative results may occur with antisera of incorrect strength or specificity, if there are too few antibodies on the red cells, if the antiserum is too strong (prozone effect), when the disease is in remission or following the administration of corticosteroids.

Antiplatelet antibody test
The platelet factor 3 test (PF3) for detection of immune-mediated damage to platelet membranes by a clotting method has largely fallen from favour. Direct immunofluorescent staining tests

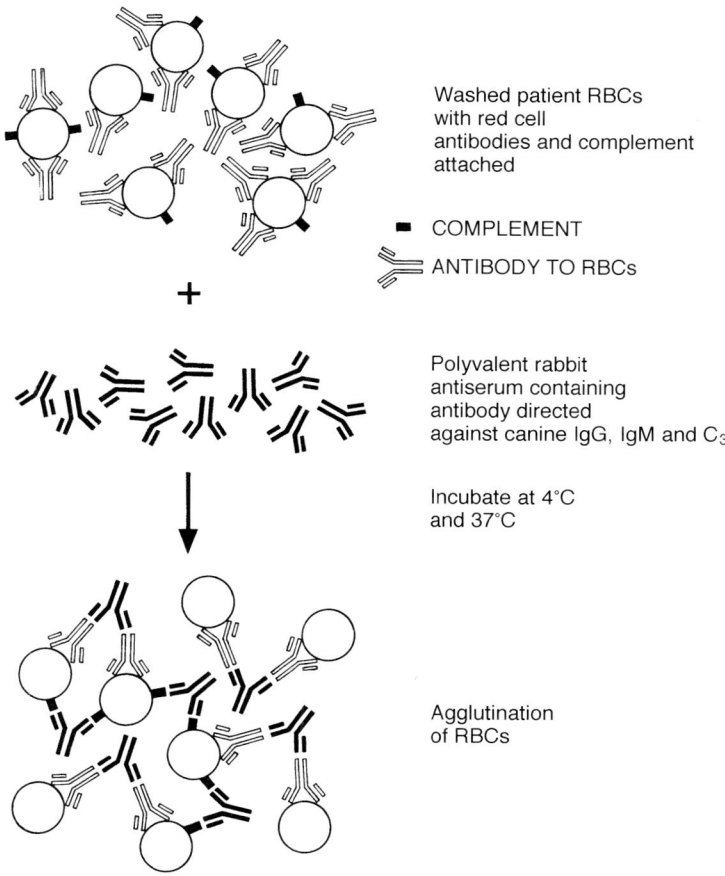

Figure 45.6 Schematic representation of the direct antiglobulin (Coombs') test.

will demonstrate the presence of antibodies on the surface of platelets, but severe thrombocytopenia may result in false negative results. More recently, an indirect fluorescent antibody test to detect anti-platelet antibodies in patient plasma has been described (Kristensen et al., 1994a). Positive staining of megakaryocytes in bone marrow aspirates is an alternative method of identifying autoantibodies (Jain, 1993). ELISA tests for anti-platelet antibody detection are used in human medicine, but have yet to become widely available in the veterinary field. A study comparing an ELISA test for detection of platelet-bound antibodies, a direct test, with an ELISA for detection of anti-platelet antibodies in plasma, an indirect test, found that the direct test was more sensitive in confirming a diagnosis of idiopathic thrombocytopenia, but was not specific since it also detected other causes of immune-mediated thrombocytopenia (Lewis et al., 1995).

Others

In cases where systemic lupus erythematosus is suspected then an antinuclear antibody test should be requested. Occasionally other immunological screening tests may be indicated, e.g. anti-neutrophil antibody or rheumatoid factor.

Biochemistry

A measure of the total plasma protein (TPP) concentration is almost essential for the interpretation of PCV. A low PCV in association with a decreased TPP concentration is suggestive of blood loss; dehydration may result in an increase in PCV and TPP concentration. Serum protein electrophoresis will identify hypergammaglobulinaemias and monoclonal gammopathies.

A full biochemical screen is advocated, especially in cases of non-regenerative anaemia, to rule out the presence of systemic disease. Particular attention should be paid for evidence of renal failure, hepatic disease, and the presence of hypercalcaemia, a paraneoplastic condition which may be seen in association with haematological malignancies such as lymphoma and plasma cell myeloma.

Tests to detect abnormalities in iron metabolism such as serum iron, total iron binding capacity, percentage saturation of transferrin and serum ferritin may be helpful in the investigation of anaemia, particularly non-regenerative anaemias. For example serum ferritin assays may differentiate between true iron-deficiency anaemia due to chronic blood loss and anaemia of chronic disease both of which may result in low concentrations of serum iron. The interpretation of these tests is described in more detail in Chapter 14.

Urinalysis

Urine may be examined for evidence of renal failure (fixed range specific gravity, abnormal urine:plasma urea/creatinine ratios, increased fractional excretion of sodium), proteinuria which may indicate immune complex glomerular damage, or paraproteinuria (Bence–Jones proteins) which may be seen in some cases of plasma cell myeloma.

Tests for viral infection

Tests for feline leukaemia virus (FeLV) and feline immunodeficiency virus (FIV) status are indicated in all cats with haematological disorders.

SPECIFIC CONDITIONS IN THE DOG

ANAEMIAS

Responsive anaemias

Acute haemorrhage

Acute haemorrhage following trauma or during surgery is usually obvious. Haemorrhage due to defects of haemostasis or from visceral masses, particularly splenic tumours, and acute gastrointestinal ulceration may not be immediately apparent. Dogs may be presented in various stages of hypovolaemic shock, depending upon the rate of blood loss and degree of owner observation. Thorough clinical examination, followed by appropriate radiographic examination should point the clinician towards a diagnosis of haemorrhage and the underlying cause.

During and immediately after acute haemorrhage, red cell parameters and plasma proteins may be normal, since whole blood is lost and splenic contraction helps to offset erythrocyte loss. It may be 12 h or more before fluid shifts attempt to restore circulating volume and haematological evidence of anaemia, i.e. decreased PCV, total red cell count, haemoglobin concentration (with reduced plasma protein concentration), become apparent in blood samples. At this stage the anaemia is normocytic and normochromic.

After two to three days there is evidence of a marrow response and the anaemia typically becomes macrocytic and hypochromic. A leucocytosis due to a neutrophilia is commonly seen and reflects a general bone marrow response. Thrombocytosis and shift platelets are produced in response to blood loss. When haemorrhage occurs into a body cavity erythrocytes may be resorbed into the circulation. This results in membrane damage, and poikilocytes and acanthocytes may be seen on peripheral blood smears.

The management of haemorrhagic anaemia depends on the specific cause of blood loss. Obviously, efforts must be made to arrest the haemorrhage and correct the underlying abnormality where appropriate. Initial therapy should be directed towards reversal of hypovolaemic shock by restoration of circulating volume, using plasma expanders and fluid therapy. Whole blood and/or plasma may be indicated, particularly in the management of haemorrhage due to haemostatic defects. The decision to transfuse whole blood or red cells should be based on the patient's clinical requirement for oxygen-carrying capacity. As a rule of thumb, in cases of acute blood loss, red cell replacement is not usually indicated in the dog unless the PCV falls below $0.20\ l\ l^{-1}$ (after correction of hypovolaemia) and there is evidence of continued blood loss (see section on blood transfusion p. 810). If blood is not readily available, hypertonic saline may be administered to animals which have lost more than 40% of their total blood volume in an attempt to rapidly increase and maintain plasma volume in the short term.

Haemolytic anaemias

Most cases of haemolytic anaemia in the dog have an immune-mediated pathogenesis. The presence of antibodies and/or complement components on the surface of erythrocytes may lead to intravascular haemolysis or removal of cells by the reticulo-endothelial system (extravascular haemolysis). Extravascular red cell destruction takes place principally in the spleen, since splenic macrophages possess receptors for the Fc portion of the IgG molecule and also for C3.

Autoimmune haemolytic anaemia (AIHA)

Pathophysiology

AIHA is one of the more common causes of anaemia in the dog (Halliwell and Gorman, 1989). It may be primary or idiopathic, where there is no apparent underlying cause, i.e. it may occur as a true autoimmune disease, or it may be secondary to or occur in association with another disease process. AIHA may be a feature of other immune-mediated conditions such as immune-mediated thrombocytopenia and systemic lupus erythematosus. Secondary AIHA has also been described in association with neoplasia, particularly myeloproliferative disease and lymphoproliferative disease; infections (including severe bacterial infections and red cell parasites) and, in some cases, may be drug-induced (Slappendel, 1979; Halliwell and Gorman, 1989). The antibodies in drug-associated AIHA may arise due to membrane binding of the drug (hapten), or by alteration of surface antigens initiating an immune response against the host's red cells. A number of drugs have been implicated including sulphonamides, penicillin, cephalosporins, dipyrone, quinidine, phenylbutazone and chlorpromazine, although there is a paucity of case reports in the literature. However, an association with potentiated sulphonamide (trimethoprim-sulphadiazine) administration and secondary AIHA has been recognized in a number of cases (Werner and Bright, 1983), particularly in Dobermanns in which it may cause a lupus-like syndrome (Giger et al., 1985a). In these cases the immune-mediated response has been attributed to the sulphadiazine and withdrawal of the drug usually results in rapid resolution of signs.

Recent vaccination has been implicated, anecdotally, for some time as a trigger for immune-mediated disease and recently the first clinical evidence for a temporal relationship between vaccination and development of AIHA has been published (Duval and Giger, 1996). About 26% of the dogs studied with idiopathic AIHA had been vaccinated within the previous month, whereas no increased frequency of presentation after vaccination was seen in the control group. Combination vaccines had been administered in all cases, from various manufacturers.

AIHA can be further classified according to the nature of the autoantibodies present.

1. In saline agglutinins: cross-linking IgM or IgG antibodies which cause agglutination of red cells *in vitro* which is not disrupted by addition of a drop of normal saline. This autoagglutination precludes the need to perform a Coombs' test.
2. Intravascular haemolysins: usually IgM antibodies which fix complement and result in acute and severe intravascular haemolysis *in vivo*.
3. Incomplete antibodies: IgG class antibody, not cross-linking, which result in removal of erythrocytes from the circulation and their extravascular destruction.
4. Cold haemagglutinins: IgM antibodies active at temperatures below normal body temperature which cause agglutination of erythrocytes *in vitro* on glass slides cooled to 4°C and *in vivo* result in erythrocyte clumping and microthrombi formation in the cooler peripheral extremities.
5. Cold haemolysins: rare IgG class, non-agglutinating antibodies which result in intravascular haemolysis in cold weather.

In a series of 14 dogs, IgG autoantibody alone was most frequently identified (57%) with both IgG and IgM autoantibodies recognized in a further 21% and IgM autoantibody alone in 14% (Day, 1996).

Studies to identify the antigens on the erythrocyte surface in canine AIHA by immunoprecipitation have shown at least three patterns of autoantigen, some of which may be equivalent to the human Rhesus complex (Barker et al., 1991). The varied patterns of antigen identified may reflect the differences in aetiology of AIHA.

History and clinical findings

The clinical presentation and course of canine AIHA is quite variable (Halliwell and Gorman, 1989). The condition may affect any age of dog, but is more common in young adults and juveniles. As in humans, the condition is more common in females and episodes of disease may be related to recent oestrus. A number of breeds appear to be over-represented including poodles, old English sheepdogs, cocker spaniels and Dobermann pinschers.

The onset of anaemia and severity of associated symptoms is more acute in those cases with autoagglutinating and intravascular haemolytic antibodies. These dogs may have a sudden onset of lethargy, depression, pyrexia and marked pallor of the mucous membranes in association with haemoglobinaemia and haemoglobinuria (Fig. 45.7). Affected animals become rapidly icteric due to the high circulating levels of unconjugated bilirubin (Fig. 45.8). Hypoxic damage to the liver frequently results in elevation of liver enzymes. Haemoglobinuria may cause renal tubular damage. The presence of large amounts of damaged erythrocyte membrane may lead to complications of thrombotic disease including pulmonary embolism and disseminated intravascular coagulation.

More often AIHA follows a more protracted course, since the majority of cases are due to the formation of warm incomplete antibodies which result in the opsonization and extravascular destruction of red blood cells. In these cases

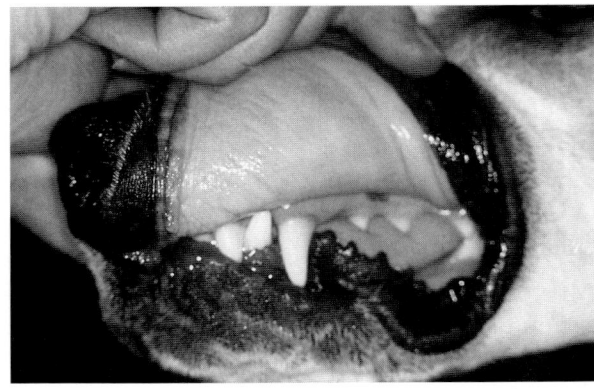

Figure 45.8 Icteric oral mucous membranes in a 1-year-old German short-haired pointer with acute autoimmune haemolytic anaemia. Courtesy of J.K. Dunn. See colour plate.

splenomegaly is a common finding; hepatomegaly and generalized peripheral lymphadenopathy may also occur.

Dogs with cold-acting antibodies show somewhat different signs. Cold agglutinin disease is characterized by ischaemic necrosis of the ear tips, tail and feet. Cold non-agglutinating AIHA is a rare condition and affected animals experience recurrent episodes of anaemia and haemoglobinuria in association with cold weather (Halliwell and Gorman, 1989).

Diagnosis

Haematological examination usually reveals a markedly regenerative anaemia. A reticulocyte production index greater than 3 is highly suggestive of a diagnosis of AIHA, and in some cases the RPI may be as high as 8. The reticulocytosis is usually an accompanied by a neutrophilic leucocytosis. The presence of spherocytes, red cells which have been partially phagocytosed by reticuloendothelial macrophages during passage through the liver and/or spleen, is highly suggestive of AIHA, although an absence of spherocytes does not rule out such a diagnosis. Occasionally the autoantibodies may also be directed against erythrocyte precursors in the marrow so that the resultant anaemia appears non-regenerative (Weiss, 1986). In such cases bone marrow examination is mandatory to rule out other causes of erythroid hypoplasia or aplasia. Bone marrow cytology in AIHA typically reveals marked erythroid hyperplasia, often with concurrent myeloid hyperplasia and an increased number of plasma cells. Erythrophagocytosis and/or erythrocyte rosettes around macrophages are also highly suggestive of immune-mediated erythrocyte destruction.

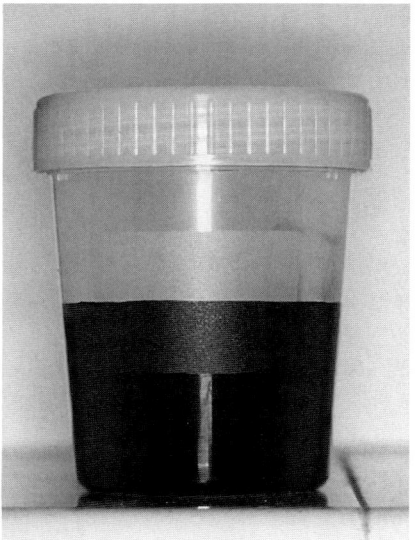

Figure 45.7 Haemoglobinuria resulting from acute intravascular haemolysis. Courtesy of J.K. Dunn. See colour plate.

The presence of non-agglutinating antibodies is confirmed by a positive direct antiglobulin (Coombs') test, which should be performed at 37°C and 4°C. Most cases have high titres against IgG and C3. Titres below 1:16 should be interpreted with caution, particularly in the absence of other evidence of haemolysis, and low titres of cold agglutinins may be present in healthy dogs (Slappendel, 1979) and cats (Dunn et al., 1984a). Other tests for autoantibodies have been described including the papain test (Jones and Darke, 1975), and enzyme-linked direct antiglobulin tests (Jones, 1986; Jones et al., 1987) and an ELISA test (Porter et al., 1989). Factors influencing the canine antiglobulin test have also been studied (Jones et al., 1990).

Another test which may be useful, which does not require the use of sophisticated reagents, is an assessment of osmotic fragility of red cells. A few drops of patient blood is mixed with the same volume of 0.54% saline (made by diluting three volumes of normal saline with two volumes of water). The presence of haemolysis indicates increased fragility of erythrocytes. Decreased osmotic resistance can be present in 85% of dogs with AIHA (Slappendel, 1986).

Management

Immunosuppressive doses of corticosteroids are recommended for therapy, prednisolone being the drug of choice at doses of 2–4 mg kg^{-1} daily in two divided doses. If an adequate response is not seen within five to seven days then other immunomodulating drugs should be introduced. Cyclophosphamide is the usual choice, at doses of 50 mg m^{-2} *per os* given on alternate days. Haemoglobin concentration and PCV should be monitored regularly and therapy gradually withdrawn over a period of not less than three months. Some cases require no further treatment whereas others need permanent therapy to prevent relapses. The undesirable side effects of cyclophosphamide on the bladder render it unsuitable for long-term management and azathioprine is a suitable alternative, at doses of 1–2 mg kg^{-1} every other day alternating with prednisolone at the lowest possible dose. Azathioprine, like cyclophosphamide, may have bone marrow suppressive effects, therefore regular haematological assessments are advised, e.g. every 2–3 weeks initially (see Chapter 50).

Blood transfusion may be essential in cases of severe anaemia, but may be followed by acute haemolysis and is not without risk. It is best to perform a cross-match with potential donors beforehand and transfuse with blood which shows the least degree of incompatability. Cases with repeated life-threatening relapses and those requiring unacceptably high levels of corticosteroid to maintain a normal PCV may benefit from splenectomy, since this removes the major organ responsible for red cell removal and a site of autoantibody production. In the case of secondary AIHA appropriate therapy should be directed towards management of the intercurrent disease. Ovariohysterectomy is indicated in bitches which suffer oestrus-related relapses.

The prognosis for complete recovery from AIHA is guarded, with a poor outcome in acute cases with thrombotic complications. Persistent autoagglutination has been found to be a negative prognostic indicator (Duval and Giger, 1996), but no correlation has been noted between haematological and immunological parameters at presentation and the subsequent response to therapy or long-term clinical behaviour (Day, 1996). Repeated relapses may occur in cases which respond well to treatment in the first instance.

Isoimmune haemolytic anaemia

Haemolytic anaemia may develop in the first 48 h of life in pups born to bitches with circulating isoantibodies to erythrocyte antigens on their red cells, after ingestion of colostrum. Sensitization of the bitch may occur due to previous mismatched blood transfusion or if leakage of mismatched fetal erythrocytes has occurred during previous pregnancies. Replacement transfusion therapy may be necessary in such cases and steps should be taken to prevent the further ingestion of colostrum.

Red cell parasites

Babesiosis

Three species of *Babesia* are known to affect dogs (Hribernik and Barr, 1989), the commonest of which is *B. canis*. The disease occurs worldwide, although is more commonly reported in tropical and subtropical regions of the world. In the UK infection occasionally occurs in quarantined animals. Babesiosis is a tick-transmitted, intraerthrocytic protozoal disease which may be subclinical, peracute, acute or chronic. Typical clinical findings include anorexia, lethargy, weakness, pyrexia, pallor of mucous membranes, generalized lymphadenopathy, splenomegaly, emaciation and icterus (Abdullahi et al., 1990). Chronic cases show weight loss and intermittent fever; terminally hepatic and renal failure become evident. The parasite causes anaemia by direct damage to red cells and by stimulating an immune response, both of which lead to haemolysis. Diagnosis is by identification of organisms in peripheral blood smears or by an indirect immunofluorescent antibody test. Therapy consists of antibabesial drugs such as imidocarb dipropionate (a single intramuscular dose of 5 mg kg^{-1}), appropriate supportive measures such as blood transfusion, fluid therapy and tick control.

Haemobartonellosis

Haemobartonella canis is a tick-transmitted rickettsial organism found on the surface of erythrocytes. Splenectomy or intercurrent infection or illness is generally required for *H. canis* to cause disease. Red cell destruction may be a direct result of parasite damage or secondary to antibody production. The parasite is identified in Giemsa-stained blood smears as blue coccoid or rod-like organisms across the surface of erythrocytes. Any underlying disease should be appropriately managed. If clinical disease occurs in splenectomized animals then treatment with oral tetracyclines is indicated.

Oxidant poisoning

Oxidant chemicals result in the formation of Heinz bodies in erythrocytes which lead to disruption of the cell membrane making it more susceptible to haemolysis and phagocytosis. Heinz body haemolytic anaemia has been reported in the dog in association with ingestion of large quantities of onions and after administration of paracetomol in doses exceeding 150 mg kg^{-1} (Oehme, 1986). Vitamin K-induced Heinz body formation and subsequent haemolytic anaemia has been described, vitamin K$_3$ being of greater risk than vitamin K$_1$ (Fernandez *et al.*, 1984). Treatment consists of appropriate supportive therapy. For paracetomol toxicity *N*-acetylcysteine may be given orally or intravenously at an initial loading dose of 140–280 mg kg^{-1} then 70 mg kg^{-1} every 4 h for three to five treatments (Oehme, 1986).

Fragmentation/microangiopathic anaemia

Red cells passing through abnormal microvasculature as occurs with disseminated intravascular coagulation (DIC) and large vascular neoplasms such as splenic haemangiosarcoma are subject to mechanical damage which may result in intravascular haemolysis and the formation of fragmented erythrocytes (schistocytes) which are then phagocytosed in the spleen and liver. DIC is discussed in the section on bleeding disorders, p. 801.

Metabolic defects causing haemolytic anaemia

Rare inherited defects of erythrocyte metabolism may cause intrinsic haemolytic anaemia. Red cell pyruvate kinase deficiency causing anaemia has been described in the beagle and basenji, which may lead to myelofibrosis and osteosclerosis (Prasse *et al.*, 1975; Searcy *et al.*, 1979; Giger *et al.*, 1991b). More recently the defect has been recognized in the West Highland white terrier (Chapman and Giger, 1990). This autosomal recessive condition can be controlled by metabolic screening to identify affected and heterozygote animals. Red cell phosphofructokinase deficiency has been reported in springer spaniels with an associated haemolytic anaemia (Giger *et al.*, 1985b; Harvey and Smith, 1994).

■ Non-responsive anaemias

Primary failure of erythropoiesis

Pure red cell aplasia

Erythroid hypoplasia in the presence of normal white cell and platelet counts implies selective damage to red cell precursors. Infection with viruses which replicate in haematopoietic cells may result in such a picture. Parvovirus infection has been reported as a cause of pure red cell aplasia. However, many cases of pure red cell aplasia are likely to be immune-mediated (Weiss, 1986). Some cases show a positive direct Coombs' test and antibodies directed towards erythroid precursors have been identified (Weiss, 1986). Response to immunosuppressive therapy (as for AIHA) provides supportive evidence for an immune-mediated aetiology. Bone marrow aspirates show an increased myeloid to erythroid ratio, with a relative absence of erythroid precursors or a maturation arrest involving the erythroid cell lines and normal granulocyte maturation. Increased numbers of plasma cells and erythrophagocytosis are indicative of immune-mediated mechanisms. Other therapeutic measures include whole blood or packed red cell transfusions and the administration of androgens to stimulate erythropoiesis (e.g. nandrolone decanoate 1–2 mg kg^{-1} intramuscularly weekly for 3 weeks then every 3 weeks).

Marrow hypoplasia/aplasia

Generalized suppression of the bone marrow is reflected in the blood as pancytopenia. Reduction in numbers of all marrow-derived cells as a result of damage to stem cells and/or the microenvironment of the marrow stroma may be a sequel to a number of agents. Infectious causes include canine distemper virus, canine parvovirus and the intracellular rickettsial organism *Ehrlichia canis*. Ehrlichiosis is seen in the UK only in dogs imported from tropical regions. The intermediate host for *E. canis* is the brown dog tick, *Rhipicephalus sanguineus*. Pancytopenia is a feature of the chronic form of the disease and hyperglobulinaemia and proteinuria may accompany the bone marrow suppression. A buffy coat smear may be examined for the presence of inclusions in white blood cells and the diagnosis is confirmed by indirect fluorescent antibody test (Breitschwerdt, 1988). Hyperoestrogenism and bone marrow suppression may occur with functional Sertoli cell tumours. Drugs and ionizing radiation employed in cancer chemotherapy have a dose-related suppressive effect on the bone marrow. Other drugs which have been implicated in marrow hypoplasia include phenylbutazone (Fredrikson and Grøndalen, 1988) and oestrogen compounds (Weiss and Klausner, 1990). Aplastic anaemia has also been associated with the administration of potentiated sulphonamides (Weiss and Adams, 1987; Fox et al., 1993). Since relatively few animals develop problems when given these drugs, the bone marrow suppression probably represents an idiosyncratic response to the drug by an individual animal. An immune-mediated pathogenesis has been implicated in some cases of aplastic anaemia in humans.

Clinical signs in aplastic anaemia reflect the severity of anaemia, leucopenia and thrombocytopenia. Affected animals are susceptible to infection, prone to haemorrhage and show the typical signs associated with severe non-responsive anaemia. The diagnosis is confirmed and differentiated from neoplastic (myelophthisic) causes of pancytopenia by bone marrow examination. Core biopsies are useful to confirm that a marrow aspirate is genuinely hypocellular and will also show whether there is any significant reticulin or collagen fibre deposition within the medullary cavity. Myelofibrosis may be a sequel to prolonged bone marrow suppression. The prognosis for recovery is poor, although a few cases will respond to prolonged (up to 3 months) supportive therapy consisting of repeated blood transfusions and administration of bone marrow stimulants, e.g. anabolic steroids. If an immune-mediated pathogenesis is suspected then immunosuppressive therapy, e.g. prednisolone may be employed.

Myelophthisis

This results from infiltration of bone marrow by fibrous tissue (myelofibrosis) or neoplastic cells. Primary bone marrow neoplasia is covered more fully later (page 790). Occasionally metastatic spread from a distant neoplasm may invade bone marrow. Myelophthisic anaemia is usually non-responsive, severe and may be accompanied by leucopenia and variable platelet numbers.

Primary myelofibrosis is regarded as a chronic myeloproliferative disorder (see later) involving the proliferation of fibroblasts. Secondary myelofibrosis is more common and represents the end stage of other conditions causing prolonged damage to the marrow stroma, e.g it may occur as a sequel to marrow necrosis. Repeated attempts to obtain bone marrow aspirates are generally unsuccessful ('dry tap') and histopathological examination of core biopsies is required to confirm a diagnosis. The prognosis depends on the severity of myelofibrosis and the degree of marrow suppression, but is at best guarded. However, some cases can be reversed with conventional immunosuppressive therapy, anabolic steroids and blood transfusions, presumably when the underlying condition has an immune-mediated pathogenesis.

Secondary failure of erythropoiesis

Anaemia of chronic disease

The most common cause of mild to moderate non-regenerative anaemia at least in the dog is that associated with chronic disease. This includes anaemia associated with inflammatory disease (Feldman et al., 1981; Stone and Freden, 1990), neoplasia, renal disease (King et al., 1992) and other systemic disorders (see page 778). Anaemia of chronic disease is characterized by low serum iron, low or low normal total iron binding capacity, increased serum ferritin, and increased bone marrow stores of haemosiderin. Characterization of the nature and extent of the underlying disease followed by successful treatment may result in resolution of the anaemia.

Erythrocyte maturation defects

Maturation defects are rare causes of non-regenerative anaemia in the dog. Bone marrow aspirates are often hypercellular, but maturation arrest is present, i.e. red cell maturation and morphology is abnormal so that erythrocytes are not released into the circulation.

Iron deficiency anaemia

Chronic blood loss occurs most commonly via the gastrointestinal tract as a result of bleeding ulcers and neoplasms; less frequently it is the result of urinary tract haemorrhage. Heavy parasitic burdens, such as hookworm infestation, flea infestations and sometimes lice or ticks, may also cause chronic blood loss. In such situations the iron stores are gradually depleted, serum iron decreases, and the anaemia becomes less responsive with the production of microcytic and hypochromic red cells. A leucocytosis and marked thrombocytosis may also be present. In dogs there is usually no significant change in total iron binding capacity (Smith, 1989). The concentration of serum ferritin, a more accurate indicator of total body iron reserves than serum iron, is reduced (Stone and Freden, 1990). Bone marrow examination reveals erythroid hyperplasia but greatly reduced or absent iron stores.

Successful therapy depends on identification and correction of the underlying reason for the blood loss. Iron supplementation may take the form of intramuscular injections of iron dextrans or oral ferrous sulphate or ferrous gluconate (200 mg tid), but absorption from the gut may be poor.

Megaloblastic anaemia

Defects in nuclear maturation result in large erythroid precursors (megaloblasts) in the marrow and macrocytic, normochromic cells may be present in the peripheral blood. True folate/vitamin B_{12} deficiency is rare in the dog, but drugs which interfere with folate mebabolism such as trimethoprim and methotrexate may cause megaloblastosis. Prolonged anticonvulsant therapy has also been implicated as a cause, as has chronic small intestinal disease and prolonged anorexia. The effect on nuclear maturation may also be reflected by an accompanying leucopenia and thrombocytopenia.

LEUCOCYTE ABNORMALITIES

Canine granulocytopathy syndrome

An abnormality of neutrophil function has been described in Irish setters initially thought to be a defect of bacterial activity (Renshaw and Davis, 1979), but subsequently recognized as defective chemotaxis and adhesion (Giger et al., 1987). More recent studies have confirmed that the condition is similar to leucocyte adhesion deficiency in humans (Troward-Wigh et al., 1992). The condition is inherited as an autosomal recessive trait. Affected animals suffer from repeated infections, particularly of the skin, and have a shortened life expectancy. The neutrophil counts are usually very high, of the order of $100–200 \times 10^9 \, l^{-1}$. Permanent antibiotic therapy is necessary to maintain affected dogs. A diagnostic test is available to identify affected animals (Kennel Club and BSAVA Scientific Committee, 1997).

Pelger–Hüet anomaly

Pelger–Hüet anomaly is a rare condition characterized by failure of nuclear segmentation in granulocytes, giving an appearance of a persistent left shift. It has been described in foxhounds. The inheritance is autosomal dominant. The morphological defect is not accompanied by functional impairment (Latimer et al., 1989) and affected animals are clinically normal.

Cyclic haematopoiesis

Originally termed cyclic neutropenia, this autosomal recessive condition occurs in grey collies (Jones and Lange, 1983). All bone marrow elements are affected with cyclical rises and falls of cell counts. The periodicity is the same in any individual, but different cell lines are low at different times, reflecting the differing maturation times. Neutropenia and impaired bactericidal activity of neutrophils results in recurrent episodes of infection. Bleeding due to cyclical thrombocytopenia is also encountered. The condition is usually fatal, affected animals rarely reaching middle age. With careful management and supportive therapy dogs can be maintained successfully for some time. Lithium carbonate therapy has been found to be effective in restoring normal cell counts, but the condition relapses on withdrawal of treatment.

BONE MARROW NEOPLASIA

Myeloproliferative disease

The term myeloproliferative disease (MPD) can be applied to all non-lymphoid dysplastic and neoplastic conditions arising from the haematopoietic stem cell or its progeny (Evans and Gorman, 1987). This concept of a single disease process is helpful since involvement of more than one cell line is common, as is transition from one form of disease to another. These conditions are not static and can evolve over a period of months or years. The classification of MPD depends on the cell lines involved, the degree of maturation occurring and whether abnormal cells are restricted to the bone marrow or seen in peripheral blood. The pathological classification of MPD is shown in Table 45.8. The term *leukaemia* implies the presence of increased numbers of neoplastic cells in the circulation. If the bone marrow is dominated by a population of abnormal cells, but these neoplastic cells are not released into the circulation, the term *aleukaemic leukaemia* or *smouldering leukaemia* may be used. In the latter case cell counts may be depressed (e.g. selective cytopenia or even pancytopenia) and morphological abnormalities, reflecting abnormal differentiation and maturation of the cell line(s) involved, are often present.

Myelodysplasia is the term applied to bone marrow abnormalities which are not overtly neoplastic and which may account for a number of changes seen in the peripheral blood, e.g. a maturation arrest or abnormal maturation of bone marrow precursors may result in cytopenia of one or more cell lines and abnormalities of cellular morphology and function. Clinical and haematological signs may be subtle initially, but over a variable period of time these myelodysplastic syndromes often progress into overt leukaemias, hence the term *preleukaemia*.

The degree of differentiation of the major cell lines involved is indicated by the classification of the condition as *acute* or *chronic*. In acute MPD, differentiation is disrupted at an early stage of cellular development, maturation is incomplete, and the bone marrow, and often the peripheral blood, are dominated by a population of blast cells. In chronic MPD, cellular differentiation and maturation progress to completion and there is clonal expansion of relatively normal appearing cells, which commonly results in crowding out of other cell lines. The clinical presentation may be very similar in both acute and chronic MPD, but disease progression is more rapid with acute MPD. The prognosis differs between the two forms of the disease; acute MPD tends to respond poorly to chemotherapy and the consequences of the severe haematological disturbances are usually serious.

A classification scheme for myeloid leukaemias and myelodysplastic syndromes, based on the human FAB system, has been described for use in dogs and cats (Jain et al., 1991).

Acute myeloproliferative disease

In acute MPD blast cells predominate in the bone marrow and may also be present in the peripheral blood, and involvement of spleen, liver and lymph nodes in the neoplastic process is common. The forms most commonly encountered in the dog are *acute myeloid (granulocytic) leukaemia*, *acute monocytic* and *acute myelomonocytic leukaemia*. In addition sporadic cases of *megakaryoblastic leukaemia* have been reported (Shull et al., 1986; Bolton et al., 1989; Messick et al., 1990).

Clinical signs
Weakness, lethargy, fever, and bleeding tendencies are common presenting signs in acute MPD (Gorman and Evans, 1987). Anaemia may also be present, which in most cases is non-regenerative. Coombs'-positive anaemias, both regenerative and non-regenerative, have also been reported in association with acute MPD. The bleeding may be the result of reduced bone marrow production of platelets, secondary immune-mediated thrombocytopenia, thrombocytopathy, coagulopathy or disseminated intravascular coagulation. Hepatosplenomegaly is a fairly consistent finding and may be due to extramedullary haematopoiesis or, more usually, infiltration by neoplastic cells. Lymphadenopathy, if present, is usually mild.

Diagnosis
The peripheral blood picture can be quite variable, but circulating blasts are common in acute MPD. The diagnosis is confirmed by cytological examination of bone marrow aspirates. If the marrow is heavily infiltrated it may be necessary to obtain core biopsies for histological examination.

Table 45.8 Pathological classification of myeloproliferative disease

Acute myeloproliferative diseases
Acute granulocytic/myeloid leukaemia
Acute monocytic leukaemia
Acute myelomonocytic leukaemia
Erythroleukaemia/erythraemic myelosis complex
Megakaryoblastic leukaemia
Eosinophilic leukaemia
Basophilic leukaemia

Chronic myeloproliferative diseases
Chronic granulocytic/myeloid leukaemia
Polycythaemia vera/primary polycythaemia
Primary (essential) thrombocythaemia
Myelofibrosis
Myelodysplastic syndromes

Identification of cell lines and differentiation from lymphoid precursors may require the use of cytochemical stains.

Management
Treatment of acute MPD in the dog is generally unsatisfactory. The rapid proliferation of malignant cells results in the development of haematological crises which are difficult to manage, and it is virtually impossible successfully to suppress the proliferation of neoplastic cells with chemotherapeutic agents without also damaging remaining normal marrow elements. The prognosis is, therefore, grave.

Chronic myeloproliferative disease
Chronic granulocytic leukaemia (CGL)
CGL is characterized by the production of large numbers of relatively well-differentiated neutrophils, which may or may not be released from the marrow into the peripheral circulation, depending on the degree of maturation reached.

Clinical signs
As with acute MPD, lethargy, weakness, febrile episodes, inappetance and anaemia are common presenting signs. Bleeding tendencies may also be seen. The onset of clinical signs in CGL may be sudden or there may be a more prolonged course, with a history of recurrent episodes of unexplained fever. Hepatosplenomegaly may be present. The anaemia is commonly non-regenerative, but regenerative immune-mediated anaemia may occasionally be present.

Diagnosis
Peripheral blood samples may show a marked neutrophilic leucocytosis with a disorderly left shift due to the presence of large numbers of mature and immature neutrophils and/or neutrophils with abnormal morphology. The total white blood cell count and neutrophil count may fluctuate during the course of the disease and at some stages of the disease the cell counts may be within normal limits or only marginally increased and not diagnostic for leukaemia. Bone marrow examination may reveal the presence of large numbers of myeloid cells with a preponderance of younger granulocyte precursors. In some cases maturation is more orderly making it difficult to differentiate CGL from the marked granulocytic hyperplasia of a reactive marrow. In such cases the presence of other findings such as splenomegaly and/or the absence of an identifiable inflammatory focus is helpful in reaching a diagnosis of CGL.

Management
The aim of treatment is to reduce the number of neutrophils produced, using the drug busulphan (Myeleran, Wellcome) which is specific for the granulocyte series, usually in combination with prednisolone. Busulphan is given at an initial dose of 2–6 mg m^{-2} *per os* until the leucocytosis or other haematological abnormalities have resolved and cell counts have returned to their normal reference values. The drug may then be used at a lower maintenance dose (2 mg m^{-2}). Regular examination of peripheral blood is required to detect signs of drug-induced bone marrow suppression and to identify relapses.

With careful monitoring and appropriate adjustment to therapy it is possible to maintain dogs with CGL for extended periods. Ultimately, however, most cases progress to an acute blast cell crisis which carries a grave prognosis.

Polycythaemia vera
This condition is characterized by an increased red cell mass and the clinical signs relate to the resultant hyperviscosity syndrome.

Clinical signs
Visual defects and neurological disturbances (ataxia, occasionally seizures) are common findings. Lameness and bleeding diatheses may occur. Mucosal erythema is evident (Fig. 45.9) and fundoscopic examination of the eye reveals distended, tortuous retinal vessels (Fig. 45.10), sometimes with haemorrhage and/or retinal detachment. Unlike the disease in humans, splenomegaly is not a feature.

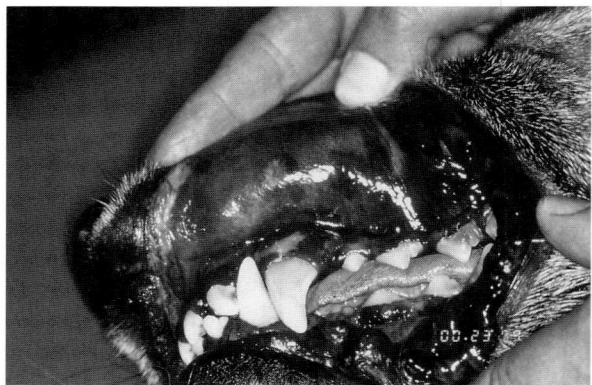

Figure 45.9 Marked congestion of the buccal mucosa in a German shepherd dog with polycythaemia secondary to bilateral renal lymphoma. Courtesy of J.K. Dunn. See colour plate.

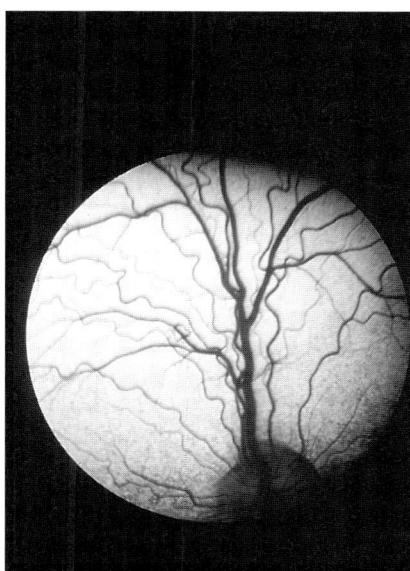

Figure 45.10 Distended and tortuous retinal blood vessels of a dog with polycythaemia vera. Courtesy of Mosby Year Book Europe Ltd. See colour plate.

Diagnosis

The PCV is usually in the range 0.65–0.80 l l^{-1}, with corresponding elevations of haemoglobin concentration and total red cell count. White cell counts and platelets are often within normal ranges. Bone marrow examination generally reveals both erythroid and myeloid hyperplasia and there may be an absence of stainable iron (J.K. Dunn, personal communication). The diagnosis is confirmed on the basis of low or undetectable serum erythropoietin levels, in contrast to cases of secondary polycythaemia where erythropoietin levels are either within normal limits or increased.

Management

Dogs with polycythaemia vera can be successfully managed for extended periods by periodic phlebotomy, and this is the treatment of choice in an emergency precipitated by hyperviscosity. Initially sufficient blood should be removed to reduce the PCV by one sixth, and the volume lost replaced with plasma expanders and crystalloid solutions. If facilities are available the red cells may be spun off and the plasma reinfused into the patient. Subsequently 20 ml kg^{-1} of blood can be removed on a regular basis to maintain the red cell mass within normal limits. After initial phlebotomy the antineoplastic drug hydroxyurea may be used for long-term maintenance. The initial dose rate is 30 mg kg^{-1} orally daily for 10 days, reducing to a maintenance dose of 15 mg kg^{-1} daily. Myelosuppression is a potential side effect and regular monitoring of haematological parameters and appropriate dosage adjustment is required. Other side effects may include anorexia and gastrointestinal disturbances (Peterson and Randolph, 1982).

Myelofibrosis

Myelofibrosis may be a true primary neoplastic condition of the bone marrow or may be an end stage of other forms of MPD. The mechanism is probably due to the production of growth factors by megakaryocytes which stimulate polyclonal fibroblast proliferation and explains why cases of megakaryoblastic leukaemia and to a lesser extent essential thrombocythaemia, are associated with reticulin fibrosis of the bone marrow (Valli and Parry, 1993). Myelofibrosis may also occur as a sequel to marrow damage, for example toxic or immune-mediated damage (resulting in inflammation or necrosis of the marrow) or metastatic disease. In the majority of cases an underlying cause is not identified so the myelofibrosis is described as idiopathic. The haematopoietic tissue is replaced by fibrous tissue and in some cases osteosclerosis develops (Dunn et al., 1986). Haematological findings usually include a non-responsive anaemia and initially relatively normal white cell and platelet counts progressing to leucopenia and thrombocytopenia. Misshapen red cells and giant platelets may be seen in blood smears. Attempts to aspirate bone marrow usually result in 'dry' taps and histopathological examination of a core biopsy is necessary to confirm the diagnosis. The prognosis is guarded. Some cases of myelofibrosis, providing they are given adequate supportive therapy in the form of blood transfusions and anabolic steroids, appear to respond to immunosuppressive therapy suggesting an underlying immune-mediated mechanism for the marrow damage.

Myelodysplasia

The history and clinical signs in myelodysplasia are often vague and variable, but episodes of pyrexia with accompanying lethargy and inappetence are commonly encountered. Various haematological abnormalities may be evident including non-regenerative anaemia, unexplained neutropenia, thrombocytopenia, circulating nucleated erythrocytes and abnormal platelet morphology. A diagnosis of myelodysplasia is based on bone marrow examination. The abnormalities of bone marrow cytology are non-neoplastic and may be subtle. The condition may ultimately progress to an overtly neoplastic state.

However, affected dogs may remain relatively well for extended periods of time, often without therapy. Anabolic steroids may be employed to stimulate erythropoiesis and antibiotic cover may be required during pyrexic episodes. If problems such as thrombocytopenia are present then therapy with prednisolone should be considered.

Basophilic leukaemia is rarely encountered in the dog (Mahaffey et al., 1987). *Essential thrombocythaemia* is a rare condition associated with platelet counts often exceeding 1000×10^9 l^{-1}. In humans the disease is characterized clinically by a haemorrhagic syndrome and thromboembolic disease. In dogs signs of bleeding appear to be less common (Evans et al., 1982). Essential thrombocythaemia can be regarded as a chronic form of megakaryocytic or megakaryoblastic leukaemia. Successful management of a case of essential thrombocythaemia in a dog with vincristine, cytosine arabinoside, cyclophosphamide and prednisolone has been documented (Simpson et al., 1990).

Lymphoproliferative disease

(See Chapter 50)
Lymphoid neoplasia can be classified on an anatomical basis (Holmberg, 1985), which is useful from a clinical standpoint. The advent of specific markers for surface antigens on canine lymphocytes is likely to clarify the cell types involved and assist in the classification and prognosis of these conditions.

Multicentric malignant lymphoma (lymphosarcoma)

Lymphoid infiltration of the bone marrow occurs in about 10–15% of animals with the multicentric form of malignant lymphoma (Raskin and Krehbiel, 1989; Dobson and Gorman, 1993). Abnormal lymphocytes may not always be found in the circulation and, if present, are few in number until the terminal stages of the disease.

Clinical signs

Dogs with multicentric malignant lymphoma may present with a history of lethargy, anorexia and weight loss although these signs are very variable. On clinical examination there is marked symmetrical enlargement of peripheral lymph nodes and hepatosplenomegaly. When there is bone marrow involvement a mild to moderate degree of anaemia is usually present with accompanying pallor of mucous membranes. The anaemia may be that of chronic disease and/or may be haemorrhagic, immune-mediated, microangiopathic and dyserythropoietic in origin. Animals with multicentric malignant lymphoma with bone marrow involvement generally have less severe clinical signs than those with true lymphoblastic leukaemia (Morris et al., 1993). Thrombocytopenia may result in a bleeding tendency and occasionally signs related to hyperviscosity may occur in association with immunoglobulin-producing B cell tumours. Hypercalcaemia may also occur as a paraneoplastic syndrome.

Diagnosis

Most cases have a mild to moderate non-regenerative anaemia, but some dogs may have a regenerative anaemia due to concurrent Coombs' positive haemolytic anaemia. White cell and platelet counts may be normal or moderately reduced. Radiography may reveal enlargement of the intrathoracic, retroperitoneal and sublumbar lymph nodes. Lymph node aspirate and/or biopsy is necessary to confirm the diagnosis of lymphoma. Infiltration by a monomorphic population of lymphoid cells is seen, with loss of normal lymph node architecture. Confirmation of bone marrow involvement requires bone marrow aspiration and/or histological examination of a core biopsy. Initially, bone marrow infiltration may be patchy and may be missed in marrow aspirates.

Management

Cases of multicentric lymphoma with or without bone marrow involvement are usually treated by combination chemotherapy. A number of therapeutic protocols have been described for the management of canine malignant lymphoma, vincristine, cyclophosphamide and prednisolone being the most commonly used drugs. Cytosine arabinoside and adriamycin may also be useful (see Chapter 50). Animals with signs relating to paraneoplastic syndromes may require appropriate therapy as a matter of urgency (see Chapter 50).

The prognosis is generally regarded as being less favourable for those cases of multicentric malignant lymphoma with bone marrow involvement, however extended periods of remission in response to chemotherapy have been reported (Dobson and Gorman, 1994).

Lymphocytic/lymphoid leukaemias

Lymphocytic leukaemia represents only about 1% of lymphoid neoplasms in the dog. The proliferation of leukaemic cells occurs primarily in the bone marrow with secondary infiltration occurring in the liver, spleen and lymph nodes. On a clinical basis it may be difficult to differentiate the lymphoid leukaemias, particularly acute lymphoblastic leukaemia (see below), from cases of multicentric lymphoma with terminal bone marrow involvement.

Acute lymphoblastic leukaemia (ALL)
The bone marrow and lymphatic organs are infiltrated by immature, poorly differentiated lymphocytes (lymphoblasts).

Clinical signs
The most common presenting signs are lethargy, anorexia, vomiting and diarrhoea. The onset of signs and progression of the disease is usually rapid and affected dogs are systemically ill. Many abnormalities may be found on clinical examination including mucosal pallor, petechial and ecchymotic haemorrhages, hepatosplenomegaly, moderate lymph node enlargement, bone and joint pain, neurological deficits and ocular changes. Affected dogs have defective humoral and cellular immune responses and are susceptible to infection.

Diagnosis
Blood samples often show a severe anaemia and thrombocytopenia (Morris et al., 1993). The total white cell count may be normal, increased or low, with variable numbers of abnormal immature lymphocytes in the peripheral blood. Bone marrow examination reveals diffuse infiltration with lymphoblasts and suppression of erythroid, myeloid and megakaryocyte elements. Cytochemical stains may be needed to differentiate ALL from other acute leukaemias.

Management
The response to antineoplastic therapy in dogs with ALL is poor due to rapid disease progression and death resulting from major haemorrhage or infection ensues. Improved survival times may be secured in a minority of cases with combination chemotherapy (Leifer and Matus, 1985). Bone marrow transplantation after total body irradiation may offer more extended remission, but intensive supportive therapy is needed and in most cases this approach is not a practical proposition.

Chronic lymphocytic leukaemia (CLL)
This form of leukaemia is characterized by the abnormal proliferation of small lymphocytes. In CLL the bone marrow is primarily involved from the outset and lymph node enlargement is usually less marked.

Clinical signs
CLL may be diagnosed incidentally following haematological examination to investigate a non-specific problem such as weight loss or inappetence. There may be a long history of vague signs such as lethargy, reduced appetite, intermittent vomiting and diarrhoea, fever, polydipsia and polyuria. Mild to moderate lymphadenopathy is common and hepatosplenomegaly (splenomegaly may be particularly pronounced) and mucosal pallor are frequently present. Signs referrable to hyperviscosity may occasionally be evident.

Diagnosis
Haematological examination generally reveals a non-regenerative anaemia (possibly regenerative if secondary haemolytic disease is present). Platelet counts are usually low normal or slightly reduced and total white cell counts are classically markedly increased due to lymphocytosis. Absolute lymphocyte counts are in the range $5–100 \times 10^9 \, l^{-1}$. Circulating lymphocytes are well differentiated, i.e. they have the appearance of small, mature lymphocytes. The bone marrow is progressively replaced by neoplastic lymphocytes and aspiration may be difficult in advanced cases. Most dogs with CLL show normal serum globulin values, but more than 50% show a monoclonal peak on electrophoresis (Leifer and Matus, 1986). In most cases this was IgM and about half were positive for Bence–Jones proteins in the urine.

Management
The prognosis for CLL is generally better than for ALL, but the course of the disease may be extremely variable. Some may remain quite well without treatment for some time. If anaemia and systemic signs are present then treatment is advisable. Both cyclophosphamide and chlorambucil ($0.2 \, mg \, kg^{-1}$ orally once daily for a week reducing to $0.1 \, mg \, kg^{-1}$) have been used in combination with prednisolone, chlorambucil having less serious side effects. Pulse therapy may be better than continuous maintenance therapy. A more rapid remission can be induced initially with vincristine used in conjunction with the above. Appropriate supportive therapy may be required in cases with paraneoplastic complications such as anaemia or hypercalcemia. Frequent haematological monitoring of patients is necessary.

Multiple myeloma

This is a neoplasm of plasma cells proliferating in the bone marrow associated with either an IgG or

IgA monoclonal gammopathy. Multiple myeloma comprised 8% of canine haematopoietic tumours in one survey (Matus and Leifer, 1985).

Clinical signs

These are often vague and ill defined. The onset of multiple myeloma tends to be insidious and the tumour burden may be large at presentation. The major signs tend to relate to the monoclonal gammopathy. Platelet function is affected by the hyperglobulinaemia and animals may present with a bleeding tendency. Immune competence is affected and may lead to recurrent infections. Hyperviscosity is more common with IgA-producing tumours, because of the tendency for the immunoglobulin molecules to polymerize, and may result in severe neurological disturbances and ocular pathology.

Tumour proliferation in the bone marrow is associated with osteoclast activation and the development of multiple, discrete, punched-out lytic lesions in bones or more diffuse osteoporosis. This is associated with pain, weakness and a predisposition to pathological fractures. If these involve vertebrae, paralysis may ensue.

A mild to moderate non-regenerative anaemia is common; occasionally the anaemia is Coombs' positive. Mild leucopenia is also not an uncommon feature. Platelet counts usually remain normal until there is extensive infiltration of the bone marrow. Hypercalcaemia may be present which can result in nephropathy and ultimately irreversible renal failure. Light chain proteinuria (Bence–Jones proteins) is present in about a third of cases and may result in renal damage and renal failure.

The presence of these paraneoplastic syndromes significantly affects the morbidity and prognosis of patients with multiple myeloma (Hammer and Couto, 1994).

Diagnosis

At least two of the following criteria should be present (MacEwen and Hurvitz, 1977): monoclonal gammopathy; Bence–Jones proteinuria; osteolytic or osteoporotic lesions on radiographs; clusters or sheets of plasmacytoid cells in bone marrow aspirates or biopsies.

Management

The alkylating agent melphalan and prednisolone are the drugs of choice for treatment of multiple myeloma. After induction of remission there appears to be no difference between continuous maintenance therapy and intermittent pulse dosing on the incidence of relapse (Matus and Leifer, 1985). Prolonged survival times can be achieved, depending on the severity of other systemic signs. Other therapeutic measures required depend on these associated complications, and aggressive supportive therapy may be indicated (Hammer and Couto, 1994). In the case of hyperviscosity syndromes, phlebotomy followed by centrifugation of blood, separation of plasma and reinfusion of packed cells in normal saline is a simpler option than plasmapheresis.

DISORDERS OF HAEMOSTASIS

Platelet abnormalities

Thrombocytopenia

Thrombocytopenia is the commonest cause of haemostatic defects in the dog. Reduced platelet numbers may be the result of defective platelet production, accelerated destruction or loss from the circulation (see Table 45.9). Of these immune-mediated thrombocytopenia is the most common cause.

Immune-mediated thrombocytopenia (IMTP)

Pathophysiology

As for autoimmune haemolytic anaemia, IMTP may be primary (idiopathic) or secondary in nature. Canine idiopathic IMTP is analogous to human chronic idiopathic thrombocytopenia purpura (Lewis and Meyers, 1996). Secondary IMTP may be seen in association with other autoimmune diseases, drug administraton, viral or rickettsial infections (see Ehrlichiosis above) and lymphoproliferative or myeloproliferative diseases. Drugs may become attached to the surface of platelets, acting as haptens, or may expose or alter surface antigens causing autoantibody production, or drug–antibody complexes may be adsorbed onto the platelet surface (innocent bystander mechanism). Drugs implicated include sulphonamides, chlorothiazides, arsenicals, digitoxin and quinidine (Feldman, 1989). Of these, sulphonamides appear to be the most commonly implicated (Weiss and Adams, 1987; McEwan, 1992; Littlewood, unpublished observations). Whatever the initiating cause, the presence of immunoglobulins on platelets leads to their removal from the circulation and destruction, primarily in the spleen. There is evidence that these antibodies may also cause platelet dysfunction in many patients (Kristensen et al., 1994).

Table 45.9 Pathogenesis of thrombocytopenia

Defective platelet production
  Drug-induced marrow hypoplasia
  Chemical/toxic marrow suppression
  Idiopathic marrow aplasia/pancytopenia
  Chronic infections, particularly viral and rickettsial
  Myelophthisis
  Antibodies directed against megakaryocytes
  Cyclic thrombocytopenia
  Other rare genetic defects of bone marrow
  Radiation exposure

Accelerated platelet removal
  Immune-mediated destruction
  Consumption in microangiopathic conditions (DIC, vasculitis)
  Acute infections

Platelet sequestration or loss
  Splenomegaly
  Vascular pooling
  Acute ongoing haemorrhage

History and clinical findings

Idiopathic IMTP is more common in young adult dogs. Females are affected slightly more frequently than males and certain breeds appear to be predisposed. Analysis of positive antiplatelet antibody tests at the University of Cambridge revealed over-representation of spaniel breeds and Dobermann pinschers (unpublished data). The onset of disease may be acute or more insidious in chronic cases. The typical clinical signs in IMTP are petechial and ecchymotic haemorrhages on the skin and mucosal surfaces (Figs 45.11 and 45.12). Melaena, haematuria, epistaxis and scleral and intraocular haemorrhages (Fig. 45.12) may be observed. Dogs with primary IMTP may appear generally healthy in other respects, although a precipitous fall in platelet numbers may result in fatal gastrointestinal haemorrhage or bleeding involving the central nervous system. Systemic signs in secondary IMTP depend on the nature of the underlying primary disease process.

Diagnosis

Clinical signs are associated with platelet counts of the order of $50 \times 10^9 \, l^{-1}$ and below. Young shift platelets may be present in blood smears. Direct immunofluorescent staining of a peripheral blood smear (blood collected into EDTA) may demonstrate the presence of autoantibodies on platelets, but false negative results do occur. An indirect fluorescent antibody test to detect antiplatelet antibodies in patient plasma has also been described (Kristensen et al., 1994a) but this test has been shown to be less sensitive for the diagnosis of IMTP than direct detection of platelet-bound antibodies (Lewis et al., 1995). Bone marrow examination is indicated to rule out causes of inadequate platelet production. Findings in IMTP include increased numbers of actively budding megakaryocytes and increased numbers of plasma cells. Immunofluorescent staining of bone marrow megakaryocytes may be positive when negative results are obtained in peripheral blood samples due to inadequate platelet numbers (Jain, 1993).

Management

Treatment of underlying disease should be initiated as appropriate. For management of IMTP prednisolone is the drug of first choice at doses of $2\text{--}4 \, mg \, kg^{-1} \, day^{-1}$ divided bid. Steroids usually have a rapid effect since they interfere with phagocytic removal of antibody-coated platelets as well as being immunosuppressive. If a rise in

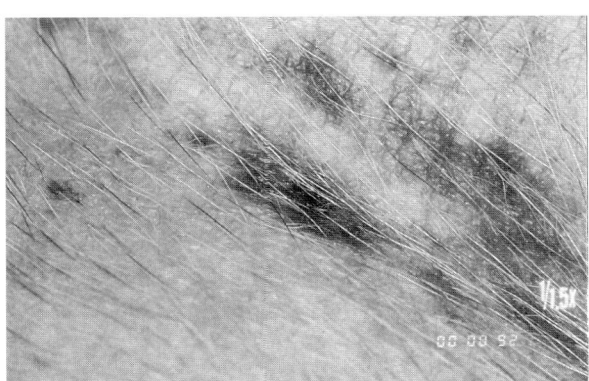
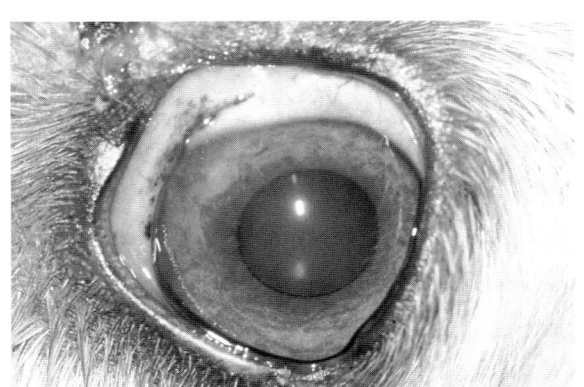

Figure 45.11 Clinical signs of thrombocytopenic purpura. (a) Petechial and ecchymotic haemorrhages on the skin of the ventral abdomen; (b) small petechial conjunctival haemorrhages. Courtesy of J.K. Dunn. See colour plate.

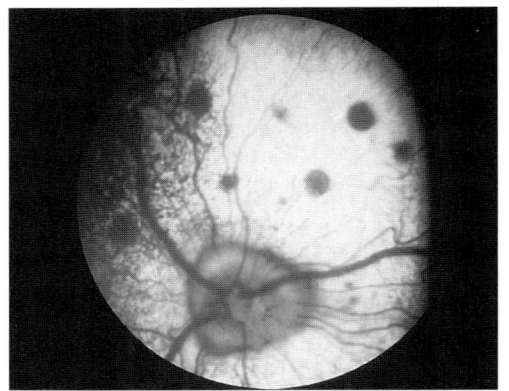

Figure 45.12 Clinical signs of thrombocytopenic purpura. (a) Extensive scleral haemorrhage. Courtesy of J.K. Dunn. (b) Retinal haemorrhages. Courtesy of the *Journal of Small Animal Practice*. See colour plate.

platelet count is not observed within two to three days then addition of further drugs to the treatment regime is indicated. Vincristine is helpful since it encourages shedding of platelets from megakaryocytes and is immunosuppressive. A dose of 0.25–0.5 mg m^{-2} should be given intravenously and may be repeated once or twice at weekly intervals. Cases which are refractory to this combination may require cyclophosphamide or azathioprine using the same doses as for AIHA. Once the platelet count exceeds 100×10^9 l^{-1} the dosage of drugs can be gradually tapered over a period of weeks to months. The minimum treatment period is usually around 3 months.

Cases of acute thrombocytopenia associated with potentially serious haemorrhage benefit from platelet-rich plasma transfusions. In a series of cases reported by Jans *et al.* (1990), dogs which received platelet-rich plasma had a better long-term prognosis and it may be that transfusion has some modulating effect on future autoantibody production. The initial prognosis in IMTP must be guarded since fatal haemorrhage can occasionally occur. Although many cases respond well to treatment and suffer no further episodes, a significant number have repeated relapses and may require permanent therapy to maintain the platelet count above $75–80 \times 10^9$ l^{-1}. Alternate day prednisolone and azathioprine, using the lowest possible maintenance doses, should be used in such cases. Splenectomy may be helpful in the management of these cases of chronic refractory IMTP.

Drug-induced bone marrow suppression

A number of drugs cause bone marrow suppression in a predictable and dose-related way including cytotoxic drugs, oestrogens, heparin, phenylbutazone and gold compounds whereas others, including sulphonamides, primidone and phenobarbital may occasionally cause marrow suppression (Feldman, 1989). Although all cell lines in the marrow may be affected, the effect on megakaryocytes and thus circulating platelet numbers is generally the earliest sign. Of these drugs it is oestrogen compounds which have been most commonly associated with clinical cases. In some animals irreversible bone marrow suppression may be seen after the use of oestrogenic drugs at normal recommended dose rates on a single occasion and this probably represents an individual idiosyncratic response (Teske, 1986).

History and clinical findings

A history of a recent illness or other problem requiring the administration of one of the above drugs is sought, for example misalliance and urinary incontinence are common reasons for the use of oestrogens. It should be noted that endogenous hyperoestrogenism may occur in association with functional Sertoli cell tumours. Generalized bone marrow suppression may result in anaemia, neutropenia and thrombocytopenia, i.e. true pancytopenia. Affected animals may present with a history of intermittent pyrexia, have a tendency to bleed, and are susceptible to recurrent infections. Bone marrow aspirates are hypocellular and histopathological examination of a trephine core biopsy may show evidence of myelofibrosis.

Diagnosis

A presumptive diagnosis is made on the basis of the clinical signs and typical haematological and bone marrow findings with a history of having received a potentially marrow suppressive drug before the onset of clinical signs.

Management
The offending drug should be withdrawn and supportive therapy initiated (transfusion, anabolic steroids, antibiotic cover). The prognosis for recovery is guarded although some dogs may show return of marrow function. As a guide the author gives monthly whole blood transfusions for a period of three months before considering the prognosis hopeless.

Myeloproliferative and lymphoproliferative disease
Thrombocytopenia and occasionally thrombocytosis may be features of myeloproliferative (Degen et al., 1989) and lymphoproliferative disease (Morris et al., 1993), and can be associated with a bleeding tendency.

Isoimmune thrombocytopenia
Rarely dogs may become sensitized to platelet antigens after blood transfusion resulting in thrombocytopenia. Similarly, haemorrhagic disease of the newborn may occur by colostral transfer of maternal antibodies directed against platelets in the pups.

Abnormalities of platelet function

von Willebrand's disease (vWD)
Pathophysiology
Canine vWD is the commonest inherited disorder of haemostasis. The condition is characterized by the presence of reduced concentrations and/or an abnormal molecular structure of vWF, the plasma protein essential for normal platelet adhesion *in vivo*. In most dogs the inheritance is autosomal dominant with incomplete penetrance or partial expression (Type 1). Recent studies in Doberman pinschers suggest that vWF deficiency is due to a single gene defect, with dogs with low plasma vWF concentrations (<0.3 units ml^{-1}) probably being homozygous for the defect (Moser et al., 1996b). The authors considered that dogs with mid-range values (0.3–0.75 units ml^{-1}) may be heterozygotes, although it may be difficult to distinguish heterozygotes from normal dogs. In the Scottish terrier and Chesapeake Bay retriever the condition is autosomal recessive (Type III) and Type II disease has been described in German short-haired pointers (Johnson et al., 1987) and German wire-haired pointers (Brooks et al., 1996). Subnormal concentrations of vWF have been identified in 54 breeds of dog in the USA (Dodds, 1989) and 16 in the UK (Littlewood, 1991), although the number of asymptomatic carriers of the trait exceeds the number of clinical bleeders. Some breeds, including Doberman pinschers, German shepherd dogs and labrador retrievers, have a high prevalence of the trait. vWD is also a significant problem in Dobermann dogs in Australia (Stokol et al., 1995a).

History and clinical findings
The bleeding tendency and severity of bleeding in animals with vWD is variable and the bleeding tendency of affected individuals may vary, often decreasing with advancing age. Intercurrent disease tends to exacerbate the risk and severity of bleeding. Clinical manifestations may include easy bruising, prolonged oozing of blood after minor injuries and surgery, excessive bleeding during oestrus and post-partum. Mild vWD may exacerbate the bleeding tendency associated with other conditions, such as IMTP (Littlewood et al., 1987; Woods et al., 1995).

Although some authors have proposed an association between hypothyroidism and canine vWD, citing it as a cause of 'acquired vWD' there is a paucity of data to substantiate this, with a notable lack of confirmation of the hypothyroid state by dynamic thyroid testing or measurement of endogenous thyroid stimulating hormone, the diagnosis often being erroneously assumed on the basis of a single total thyroxine (TT4) measurement. In fact, investigations in dogs with naturally occurring hypothyroidism revealed concentrations of vWF antigen within reference limits and a significant reduction after treatment with thyroid supplementation (Panciera and Johnson, 1994). This finding was confirmed in a study of experimentally induced hypothyroidism which also showed no significant changes in buccal mucosal bleeding times of dogs after induction of hypothyroidism (Panciera and Johnson, 1996). These data refute a causal association between hypothyroidism and vWD.

Diagnosis
Platelet counts and coagulation screening tests are normal in vWD. The buccal mucosal bleeding time (BMBT) is prolonged. The diagnosis is confirmed by demonstration of low vWF concentrations.

Management
Bleeding episodes should be treated by the administration of plasma or cryoprecipitate infusion. Shortening of the BMBT after administration of the synthetic vasopressin analogue, desmopressin (DDAVP) at doses of 1 µg kg^{-1} subcutaneously, has been demonstrated in affected

dogs (Kraus et al., 1989; Meyers et al., 1990). This drug has been used successfully to manage surgical haemorrhage in an affected Dobermann undergoing spinal surgery (Kraus et al., 1988). With correct management vWD is a disease of low mortality in most cases. Affected animals should not be used for breeding and screening of potential breeding stock is advisable to identify asymptomatic carriers of the trait. Genomic DNA studies of Dobermanns have shown a polymorphic DNA marker within the vWF gene which may correlate with disease status (Holmes et al., 1996). This test may help to clarify the status of animals intended for breeding and help to reduce the incidence of the disease in the breed.

Inherited thrombopathia

An autosomally inherited thrombasthenic thrombopathia has been described in otterhounds in the USA. Platelets from affected dogs fail to aggregate in response to physiological stimuli and do not support clot retraction (Catalfamo and Dodds, 1988). Giant platelets with abnormal morphology may be seen in the circulation.

A severe platelet dysfunction and clinical bleeding has been seen in basset hounds in North America, attributable to aberrant cyclic AMP metabolism. Platelets from thrombopathic animals fail to aggregate to all physiological stimuli except thrombin, but do support normal clot retraction. No definite conclusions have yet been reached concerning the mode of inheritance (Catalfamo and Dodds, 1988). A similar defect has been described in a family of spitz dogs (Boudreaux et al., 1994).

Acquired defects of platelet function

Various drugs are known to affect platelet function (Feldman, 1989), particularly the nonsteroidal anti-inflammatory drugs such as aspirin and phenylbutazone, which interfere with prostaglandin synthesis. A state of platelet refractoriness can be induced by heparin preparations and dextrans (Evans and Gordon, 1974).

The platelet dysfunction resulting from these drugs is unlikely to result in spontaneous bleeding in normal animals, but may aggravate a bleeding tendency in animals with inherited disorders of haemostasis or in dogs undergoing surgery.

Platelet function defects have also been demonstrated in the acute stage of canine ehrlichiosis and may, in addition to the thrombocytopenia which is the predominant haematological abnormality found in affected dogs, contribute to the bleeding tendency commonly observed in this disease (Harrus et al., 1996).

Platelet dysplasia

Abnormalities of platelet structure and function are commonly encountered in myeloproliferative disease (Cain et al., 1986) and other forms of neoplasia (Helfand, 1988).

Coagulopathies

Acquired coagulation defects

Vitamin K antagonism

Anticoagulant rodenticides interfere with vitamin K metabolism in the liver, blocking the conversion of inactive vitamin K epoxide to the active vitamin K_1 which is required for conversion of precursor proteins into active clotting factors (Fig. 45.13). This results in depletion of clotting factors II, VII, IX and X. The widespread use of coumarin and inandione compounds to control rats in both rural and urban situations provides opportunities for accidental ingestion by dogs. In most cases of poisoning in dogs there is a known possible exposure to rodenticides.

Clinical signs

Clinical signs of poisoning may appear within one to three days of ingestion of second generation compounds (bromadiolone, brodifacoum, flocoumafen) and four to five days after exposure to first generation compounds (warfarin, dicoumarol, diphacinone, chlorphacinone). Haemorrhage may occur in a large number of sites, both externally and particularly into body cavities (Fig. 45.14). Affected animals show depression, weakness and pallor, depending on the severity of haemorrhage. Intrathoracic haemorrhage is the most common cause of acute death, and animals with clinical or radiographic evidence of pleural fluid accumulation require emergency treatment.

Diagnosis

A history of exposure is most helpful in making a definitive diagnosis. Screening coagulation assays are imperative to confirm the suspicion and rule out other causes of bleeding. Factors in both the intrinsic and extrinsic pathways become depleted. Since factor VII has a shorter half life than other factors, the prothrombin time (PT) is prolonged initially but later the activated partial thromboplastin time (APTT) also increases. The platelet count may decrease slightly due to acute blood loss.

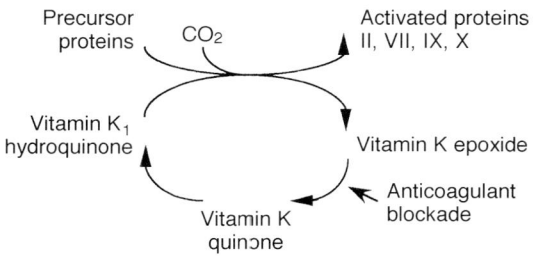

Figure 45.13 The role of vitamin K in the activation of clotting factors

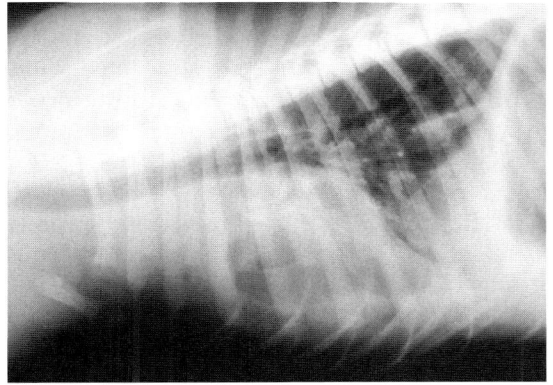

Figure 45.14 Lateral thoracic radiograph of a dog with pleural haemorrhage due to vitamin K antagonism.

Therapy

The specific antidote in vitamin K antagonism is the active form, vitamin K_1 (Konakion, Roche). Doses of 0.5–2.5 mg kg^{-1} daily in divided doses for a week are usually adequate for warfarin poisoning. However, the half-life of diphacinone and the second generation rodenticides such as bromadiolone is far longer than that of warfarin (Mount et al., 1986) and inadequate dosing and premature cessation of therapy may be responsible for relapses of clinical signs and life-threatening haemorrhage. When it is known that a long-acting anticoagulant has been ingested doses of 5 mg kg^{-1} two to three times daily for at least three weeks are recommended. Prolonged therapy may be necessary in some cases (Hall, 1990). Since anaphylaxis may occur in association with the intravenous administration of vitamin K_1, some authors advise against this route. However, both intramuscular and subcutaneous injections may precipitate haematoma formation and these routes should be avoided. Oral absorption is good, and this author prefers an initial intravenous loading dose (1–5 mg kg^{-1}) followed by oral dosing.

The PT promptly returns to normal with appropriate therapy, but if therapy is withdrawn too soon it will become prolonged again. The PT should be checked 48 h after cessation of therapy and if significantly prolonged (30% longer than control) therapy should be reinstituted for a further two to three weeks.

In animals suffering from respiratory distress and/or hypovolaemic shock, plasma or whole blood transfusion is indicated to supply clotting factors and expand the plasma volume. Exercise restriction (cage confinement if possible) is essential. Thoracocentesis should be attempted after therapy has been initiated only in animals which are severely dyspnoeic.

With proper management of life-threatening bleeding episodes and adequate duration of vitamin K therapy the outcome in most cases is favourable.

Hepatic disease

Many of the clotting factors as well as inhibitors of coagulation are synthesized in the liver and, moreover, active clotting factors in the circulation are cleared by the liver. In addition, there may be qualitative and quantitative alterations in platelets in liver diseases. Animals with acute, diffuse liver disease, in particular acute hepatic necrosis or diffuse tumour infiltration, may present with a bleeding diathesis. Chronic liver conditions such as portosystemic shunts often result in increased clotting times but are rarely associated with signs of spontaneous haemorrhage.

History and clinical signs indicative of liver involvement will be evident. Laboratory tests of coagulation reveal elevation of both PT and APTT tests. Increased plasma concentrations of alkaline phosphatase and alanine aminotransferase confirm the presence of liver damage; increased bile salt concentrations indicate hepatic dysfunction. Treatment is primarily supportive and the prognosis depends on the nature and severity of the hepatic pathology.

Disseminated intravascular coagulation (DIC)

DIC or disseminated intravascular thrombosis (DIT) is a disorder of both primary and secondary haemostasis. It is also known as consumption coagulopathy. Generalized or diffuse activation of haemostasis occurs, triggered by several mechanisms including release of tissue substances into the blood, exposure of damaged endothelium and procoagulant factors produced by various neoplasms. This results in the formation of thrombi in the microvasculature and the consumption of both platelets and clotting factors, and in the triggering of fibrinolysis and the production of fibrin degradation products (FDPs), which are themselves anticoagulants, interfering with the action of thrombin on fibrinogen. Inhibitors such as antithrombin III (AT III) are utilized and also depleted. The net result of these events is a tendency to bleed.

DIC is always a secondary complication of an underlying disease process and may occur in association with a number of conditions (Table 45.10).

Table 45.10 Diseases associated with DIC

Tissue damage:	trauma
	shock
	heat stroke
	vasculitis
	obstetrical complications
	haemolysis
Infections:	infectious canine hepatitis
	leptospirosis
	peritonitis
	endotoxaemia
	septicaemia
	angiostrongylasis
Neoplasia:	carcinoma
	haemangiosarcoma
	lymphoma/lymphoid leukaemias
	myeloproliferative disease

Clinical signs

The onset of DIC may be insidious or abrupt and the condition may be acute or chronic, depending on the extent of microvascular thrombosis and consumption of platelets and clotting factors. The bleeding manifestations seen include prolonged bleeding after venepuncture, prolonged bleeding from minor wounds or after minor surgery, epistaxis and bleeding from other body orifices. Other specific clinical signs will depend upon the underlying disease present.

Diagnosis

Platelet numbers are reduced and clotting times (WBCT, ACT, PT, APTT) are prolonged. Poor clot formation due to FDPs interfering with fibrin polymerization is evident in clotting assays. AT III concentrations are reduced. Fibrinogen may be markedly reduced, but may remain in the normal range if the primary disease process is inflammatory and thus is likely to result in elevation of fibrinogen concentrations. Elevation of FDPs is usually, although not always, detected.

Management

Successful management of cases of DIC depends on the nature of the primary disease process and how amenable this is to therapy. Treatment should consist of aggressive fluid therapy to re-establish tissue perfusion. Plasma transfusion provides a source of clotting factors and the thrombin antagonist AT III. Heparin complexes with and potentiates the actions of AT III. The aim of heparin therapy is to prevent further coagulation. (Heparin can be given subcutaneously or intravenously.) Mini-dose heparin therapy (5–10 units heparin kg^{-1} s.c. tid) in combination with blood or plasma transfusions, has been advocated (Couto, 1992a). Doses of this magnitude do not prolong the ACT or APTT in normal dogs (this requires doses in excess of 150–250 units kg^{-1}) so any increase in these times during therapy is indicative of a deterioration in haemostatic function and worsening of the DIC. Higher doses of heparin varying from 300 to 1000 units kg^{-1} tid can be given either subcutaneously or intravenously in cases of acute DIC but the ACT or APTT should be monitored once or twice daily during therapy, the aim being to prolong these clotting times by no more than 2–2.5 times the normal baseline values. Heparin therapy must be tapered off slowly to avoid a rebound hypercoagulable state. Successful treatment should result in fibrinogen concentrations returning to normal. The use of drugs to inhibit platelet function (e.g. aspirin) have not been fully evaluated in veterinary patients as a treatment for DIC.

Inherited coagulopathies

Factor VIII deficiency (haemophilia A, or 'classic' haemophilia)

Factor VIII (F.VIII) deficiency is a sex-linked inherited defect in the dog, as in other species; affected animals are males and females may be asymptomatic carriers, although homozygous affected females may occur. It is the commonest of the severe inherited bleeding disorders and has been described in many breeds of dogs including mongrels. The bleeding tendency may be severe, moderate or mild, depending on the severity of the F.VIII deficiency. Animals with less than 1% of normal F.VIII concentrations suffer from spontaneous, life-threatening bleeding episodes, which are usually apparent from a young age. It is unusual for severely affected animals to reach maturity. For this reason the defect is usually self-limiting and not passed to subsequent generations if female relatives (dam and siblings) are prevented from future breeding. Most of the cases of severe F.VIII deficiency represent new genetic mutations. However, in the German shepherd breed, a moderate form of the disease occurs (F.VIII 2–10% of pooled normal plasma) and affected males living a relatively sedate lifestyle may survive to maturity and breed. This has led to the production of new generations of carrier bitches and perpetuation of the defect, which has become disseminated throughout the world (Fogh, 1988; Littlewood, 1988; Parry et al., 1988).

Clinical signs

A history of excessive bleeding when deciduous teeth are lost, shifting lameness, and unexplained joint and soft tissue swellings are common (Fig. 45.15). Neurological abnormalities may be the presenting clinical sign (Stokol et al., 1995a). Trauma or surgery may precipitate severe haemorrhage in moderately affected animals, but minor surgery with good surgical haemostasis may proceed uneventfully.

Diagnosis

F.VIII is an essential cofactor in the intrinsic pathway and deficiencies result in prolongation of the APTT. The diagnosis is confirmed by a specific F.VIII assay.

Management

Bleeding episodes are treated by factor replacement, either by plasma or cryoprecipitate infusions. Whole blood is not usually effective in raising F.VIII concentration to haemostatic levels. Heterologous F.VIII concentrates, particularly porcine F.VIII (Hyate C, Speywood Laboratories, Porton Products) have been used successfully in the management of bleeding episodes, but repeated use is accompanied by the risk of anaphylaxis due to antibody formation. The production of anti-F.VIII antibodies renders patients resistant to further treatment.

Severe F.VIII deficiency is not really consistent with life as a pet dog, although moderately affected animals may survive for some time. However, many owners request euthanasia after diagnosis because of the incurable and serious nature of the condition. The problem of detecting affected males and carrier females and removing them from breeding programmes in the German

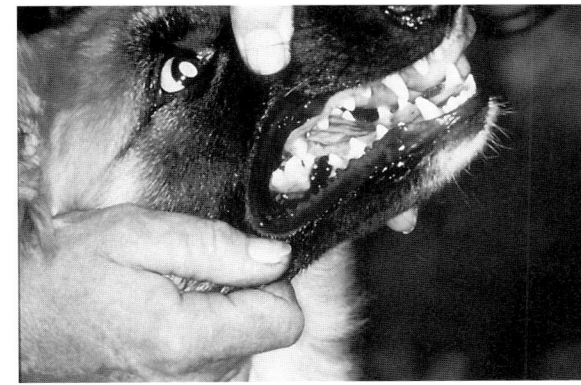

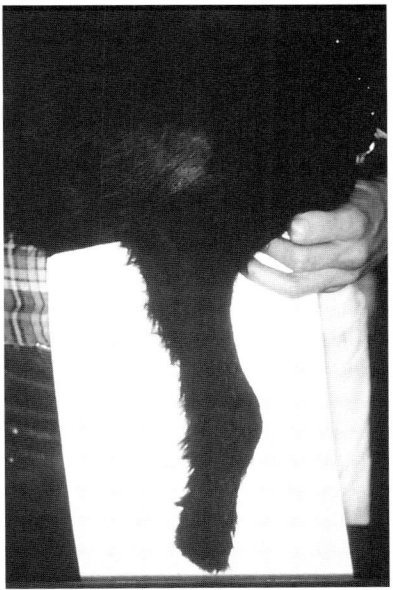

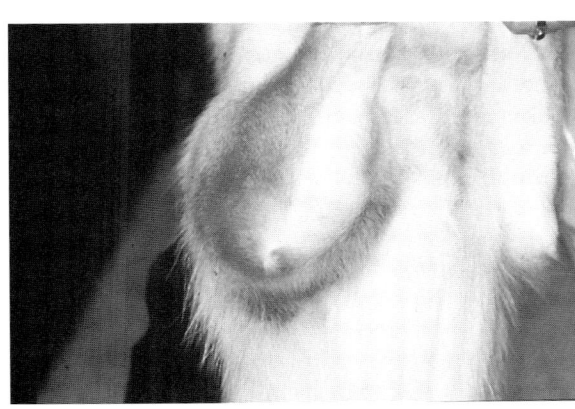

Figure 45.15 Bleeding manifestations of Factor VIII deficiency (haemophilia A). (a) Excessive bleeding after loss of deciduous teeth; (b) carpal haemarthrosis (photograph courtesy of Dr R.A.S. White); (c) haematoma in the soft tissues around the elbow. See colour plate.

shepherd breed remains. Screening of animals is practised in the UK and Australia, with restrictions on registration imposed by the Kennel Club to try and control the problem.

Factor IX deficiency (haemophilia B, Christmas disease)

Like F.VIII deficiency, factor IX (F.IX) deficiency is a sex-linked inherited condition, which is clinically identical to F.VIII deficiency, since both factors are active at the same point in the coagulation cascade. As with F.VIII deficiency, prolongation of the APTT is seen. F.IX deficiency is less common than F.VIII deficiency. It has been reported in 11 breeds in the USA (Verlander et al., 1984) and a moderate form of the disease has been described in a spaniel cross in the UK (Littlewood et al., 1986). This latter dog suffered from only occasional bleeding episodes in association with trauma and dental extractions which were successfully managed by plasma transfusion and the dog was maintained as a pet until old age. More recently factor IX deficiency has also been reported in a family of German shepherd dogs (Feldman et al., 1995).

Factor X deficiency

Factor X (F.X) deficiency has been reported in cocker spaniels in the USA (Dodds, 1973) and in a Jack Russell terrier (Cook et al., 1993). The pattern of inheritance is autosomal dominant, with variable severity of clinical bleeding. Severely affected pups die young at only a few weeks of age, those that survive to adulthood being mildly to moderately affected. Since F.X is in the common pathway, both PT and APTT clotting times are prolonged. Bleeding episodes are managed by plasma transfusion.

Factor XI deficiency

This severe and often lethal bleeding disorder has been reported in springer spaniels, Pyrenean mountain dogs and Kerry blue terriers (Dodds and Kull, 1971; Dodds, 1977; Knowler et al., 1994). It has an autosomal dominant pattern of inheritance. The APTT is prolonged in screening tests.

Factor VII deficiency

This condition has been identified in several colonies of beagles and has also been described in the Alaskan malamute (Spurling, 1980). The bleeding tendency is usually mild. Inheritance is autosomal dominant, with heterozygotes being asymptomatic. Coagulation screening tests reveal a prolonged PT but normal APTT.

Other inherited defects

There are occasional reports of other rare inherited disorders including hypofibrinogenaemia, dysfibrinogenaemia and hypoprothrombinaemia (Fogh and Fogh, 1988).

Thrombotic disorders

Hypercoagulable states are uncommon in canine patients, but embolic complications may arise secondary to other disease processes, e.g. hyperadrenocorticism. Acquired antithrombin III (AT III) deficiency has been identified as the causative mechanism in a number of thrombotic disorders in dogs. Glomerulonephropathy leads to urinary loss of a number of important proteins including AT III, and dogs with concentrations of less than 50% have a high risk of thrombotic complications (Green, 1988).

AT III becomes depleted in patients suffering from DIC and AT III measurement has been found to be helpful prognostically in this condition. AT III concentrations are also reduced in liver disease, but the corresponding reduction in synthesis of clotting factors tends to balance any tendency to develop a thrombotic tendency.

A case has been described in which a lupus-type anticoagulant was identified in a dog suffering from haemolytic anaemia and fatal pulmonary thromboembolism (Stone et al., 1994). Antiphospholipid antibodies occur in a number of human patients with systemic lupus erythematosus and a number of other diseases, but this is the first documented case in a dog. Although coagulation tests show abnormal prolongation of tests of the intrinsic pathway (WBCT, ACT, APTT) patients with antiphospholipid antibodies are at risk from thrombotic complications rather than bleeding, as in the dog described above.

SPECIFIC CONDITIONS IN THE CAT

ANAEMIAS

Responsive anaemias

Haemorrhage

Acute blood loss in the cat most commonly occurs as a result of trauma, but may also be due to internal haemorrhage and coagulopathies. The earlier comments concerning the interpretation of red cell parameters immediately after haemorrhage apply. In addition to the normal features of a marrow response, cats with regenerative anaemias frequently have increased numbers of red cells containing Howell–Jolly bodies. It should be noted that there are two populations of reticulocytes in cats; the number of coarse or aggregate reticulocytes correlates more closely with the marrow response than does the number of fine or punctate reticulocytes (see page 776). The same therapeutic considerations apply as for dogs.

Haemolytic anaemias

Autoimmune haemolytic anaemia

AIHA is much less frequently encountered in the cat than the dog. Most cases are secondary to other diseases, with feline leukaemia virus (FeLV) infection being commonly implicated (Dunn et al., 1984a). In 43 cats with AIHA more than half had FeLV infection and a further 25% were suffering from myeloproliferative disease. Six had haemobartonellosis, three were cases of lymphoma and one cat was diagnosed as suffering from systemic lupus erythematosus. Only one cat had primary idiopathic AIHA (Gorman and Evans, 1987). A case of cold agglutinin disease has been described in a cat in association with trauma and exposure to lead (Godfrey and Andersen, 1994).

Clinical signs are similar to those seen in the dog, but the onset is usually more insidious and the course more chronic. A positive Coombs' test, using species-specific antisera, in combination with the typical clinical and laboratory signs, is supportive of the diagnosis of AIHA in the cat. However, positive Coombs' tests must be interpreted with caution since normal cats may show a positive test (especially low titres of cold agglutinins), as may cats infected with FeLV and those suffering from feline infectious anaemia (Dunn et al., 1984a).

If other causes of haemolytic disease have been ruled out, treatment with immunosuppressive doses of prednisolone (2 mg kg^{-1} twice daily) may be instituted. Once a satisfactory response has been achieved this dose can be gradually reduced over a 2–3 month period until, in some cases, therapy is discontinued. Too few cases have been documented to permit generalizations concerning the prognosis in primary AIHA. The nature of the underlying disease is the determining factor in the outcome of secondary AIHA.

Feline infectious anaemia

Infection with the parasite *Haemobartonella felis* is a significant cause of anaemia in cats. The course of the illness may be acute and severe or more chronic, with cyclical episodes of parasitaemia. Lethargy, anorexia, depression and marked pallor of mucous membranes are common presenting signs. In acute cases icterus and splenomegaly may be present. Chronic cases may show only weight loss and pallor.

After acute haemolysis a regenerative anaemia is seen. This anaemia may be Coombs' positive and is frequently accompanied by a reactive neutrophilia and increased bilirubin levels. Large histiocytic-type cells containing phagocytosed red cells may occasionally be noted on a peripheral blood film. The diagnosis is confirmed by identification of the parasite on red cells. The organism is demonstrated better by acridine orange than Romanowsky stains. In chronic cases, examination of blood smears may need to be repeated on several consecutive days to detect parasitized red cells.

Affected cats should be treated with oral tetracyclines at a dose rate of 20 mg kg^{-1} three times daily for three weeks. Blood transfusion may be necessary in some cases.

It should be remembered that it is common to find *H. felis* in the blood of cats with concurrent illness, particularly FeLV infection, and the presence of organisms in a cat without evidence of a marrow response should alert the clinician to look for other underlying problems.

FeLV-associated haemolytic anaemia

Haemolytic anaemia in FeLV-infected cats may be immune-mediated or a direct effect of viral effects in red cells (Cotter, 1979). Experimentally, haemolytic anaemia has been shown to be associated with subgroup A virus (Jarrett, 1991). Affected cats may recover from a transient haemolytic episode, or suffer from a persistent anaemia with recurrent haemolytic episodes. In a few the haemolysis is persistent and fatal. Only occasionally does an acute haemolytic episode result in death.

Although in many cats the haemolysis is not life threatening, the long-term prognosis is guarded to poor. Supportive therapy may be given until other FeLV-related illness supervenes which might necessitate euthanasia.

Oxidant poisoning

Paracetamol poisoning is common in cats due to owner administration of this widely available analgesic (Evans, 1985; Oehme, 1986). Cats are unable to metabolize and excrete this phenolic drug efficiently and are poisoned by as little as 50–60 mg kg^{-1}.

Clinical signs

Signs of toxicity develop within hours of dosing. Anorexia, salivation and vomiting are followed by depression. Methaemoglobinaemia develops rapidly and red cells undergo intravascular haemolysis. Brown discoloration of the mucous membranes becomes apparent and dark, chocolate-coloured urine is characteristic. Facial oedema and swelling of the paws is also common. When the methaemoglobin concentration exceeds 50% the cat may die during exertion or handling, due to anoxia. The duration of clinical signs depends on the dose of paracetamol received and death due to methaemoglobinaemia occurs 18–36 hours after ingestion.

Management

If less than 6 h has passed since ingestion than gastric emptying by the use of emetics and gastric lavage should be attempted followed by oral administration of activated charcoal (2 g kg^{-1}).

The drug N-acetylcysteine can be used to conjugate the reactive paracetamol metabolite. Treatment should be initiated immediately if high doses of paracetamol are known to have been given or as soon as clinical signs are apparent. A loading dose of 140 mg kg^{-1} is given intravenously or orally, followed by 70 mg kg^{-1} every 4 h. Treatment has been shown to be effective in cats receiving two or three times the lethal dose, but persistent and conscientious therapy is required. Additional supportive therapy such as blood transfusion to replace haemolysed red cells and fluid therapy may be helpful. With appropriate treatment cats may appear normal within 48 h of initial therapy.

Methylene blue toxicity has been encountered in cats. Marked Heinz body formation is accompanied by severe haemolysis, followed by a bone marrow response in those cats which survive the acute event. Other drugs which have been implicated in cases of haemolytic anaemia include phenylhydrazine and the phenothiazines. Treatment consists of withdrawal of the drug and institution of supportive therapy.

Fragmentation haemolytic anaemia

This may be a feature of DIC in the cat, in the same way as it is in the dog.

Congenital haemolytic anaemias

Isoimmune haemolytic anaemia (neonatal isoerythrolysis) is a problem in breeds of cats which have a high incidence of type B blood. Abyssinian, Birman, British shorthair, Devon Rex, Himalayan, Persian and Somali cats in the USA have been found to have a high proportion of type B blood (Giger, 1990). Maternal–fetal incompatability occurs when a queen with type B blood is mated with a type A (rarely type AB) sire, since type A is dominant. Anti-A isoantibodies in the colostrum are strongly agglutinating, resulting in extravascular haemolysis in the type A kittens. Tail tip necrosis in Birman kittens due to cold-acting isoagglutinins has been reported (Bridle and Littlewood, 1998).

Congenital erythropoietic porphyria has been reported in the cat (Watson, 1990). Abnormal haemoglobin synthesis results in a haemolytic anaemia. Other signs include accumulation of pinkish-brown pigment in teeth, bones and other tissues. The condition is inherited in an autosomal dominant fashion.

Spontaneous Heinz body haemolytic anaemia has been described in Siamese kittens (T/F).

■ Non-responsive anaemias

Primary failure of erythropoeisis

Anaemia due to reduced red cell production is very common in the cat and the majority of cases are associated with FeLV infection.

Pure red cell aplasia

Erythroid hypoplasia is a characteristic of infection with FeLV subgroup C experimentally. Clinical cases of FeLV-induced pure red cell aplasia, with no involvement of other cell lines, may be encountered. Occasionally, cases of red cell aplasia may be secondary to drugs or toxins or may be idiopathic. In all cases the prognosis is poor.

Marrow hypoplasia/aplasia

Non-regenerative anaemia may be accompanied by a reduction in granulocyte and/or platelet production. In a large proportion of these cases the cats are FeLV positive. Other causes of marrow hypoplasia/aplasia include chronic feline infectious enteritis, feline immunodeficiency virus (FIV) infection (Shelton et al., 1990; Fleming et al., 1991), drugs (e.g. chloramphenicol) and toxins. Affected animals may present with pyrexia or overwhelming infection before the anaemia is well developed.

Bone marrow examination reveals a hypocellular marrow with depletion of all cell series. In FeLV-associated marrow hypoplasia or pancytopenia the marrow may be normo- to hypocellular and maturation arrest or megaloblastoid changes are common in the erythroid series. Regardless of the cause of the marrow suppression the prognosis is invariably poor.

Secondary failure of erythropoiesis

Anaemia of chronic disease

Anaemia in association with chronic disease is common in the cat. Underlying conditions include chronic renal failure, feline infectious peritonitis and FIV-associated disease. The anaemia is mild to moderate and normocytic, normochromic in nature. The white cell count depends on the associated disease. Management of the inciting cause is the important consideration, but administration of bone marrow stimulants may be of some benefit.

Erythrocyte maturation defects

Iron deficiency anaemia

Chronic blood loss in the cat is ultimately associated with a microcytic, hypochromic, non-regenerative anaemia, once iron stores are depleted. Gastrointestinal and urinary tract lesions may be the site of blood loss, but heavy flea burdens may also result in this type of anaemia, particularly in kittens whose iron intake and reserves are marginal. Coccidiosis in kittens may also cause anaemia which may become hypochromic in nature. Bone marrow samples should be assessed for iron stores although, compared to dogs, cats have relatively sparse iron stores in the marrow in normal circumstances (Evans, 1985). Treatment is directed at preventing further blood loss and supportive therapy (blood transfusion, iron supplements).

Macrocytic non-responsive anaemia

Macrocytic or megaloblastic anaemia with no reticulocytosis, sometimes with nucleated red blood cells in the circulation, is indicative of dyserythropoiesis and is most often associated with FeLV infection (Cotter, 1979; Hirsch and Dunn, 1983; Dunn et al., 1984b). Dyserythropoietic anaemia may be a feature of acute myeloid leukaemia and myelodysplasia (sometimes referred to as preleukaemic myeloproliferative disease). Cats with megaloblastic anaemia usually have normal Vitamin B_{12} and folate levels (Dunn et al., 1984b). The white cell count may be normal or increased and the platelet count is usually normal, although large, bizarre platelets may be present. Bone marrow examination confirms abnormal megaloblastic red cell precursors or arrested red cell maturation. The myeloid to erythroid ratio is increased. Increased numbers of immature myeloid precursors may be present in preleukaemic cases. The long-term prognosis is poor.

LEUCOCYTE ABNORMALITIES

The leucocyte responses in physiological situations and to pathological states are covered elsewhere. Rare inherited abnormalities of granulocytes may be encountered in the cat, and it is worth noting that abnormal vacuolation of leucocytes is a feature of a number of metabolic storage diseases, but presenting signs in these conditions are not usually referrable to the haematopoietic system. Abnormal (neoplastic) proliferation of leucocytes is not uncommon in the cat.

BONE MARROW NEOPLASIA

Haematopoietic neoplasia is common in the cat accounting for almost a third of all neoplasms in this species. Between 80 and 90% of these neoplasms are cases of malignant lymphoma (lymphosarcoma) (Hardy, 1981). The rest constitute the myeloproliferative diseases and true lymphoid leukaemias. There is a strong association with FeLV infection in all haematopoietic (myeloid and lymphoid) neoplasms in the cat.

Myeloproliferative disease (MPD)

Although many cases of feline MPD may be negative for FeLV using the commonly used tests which detect circulating viral antigen, involvement of FeLV has been demonstrated by immunofluorescent or nucleic acid hybridization techniques in feline MPD (Tzavaras et al., 1990). A classification system for myeloid leukaemias and myelodysplastic syndromes in dogs and cats, based on the FAB criteria used in humans, has been described by Jain et al. (1991). The most commonly encountered forms of MPD in the cat are the *acute myeloid leukaemias* (AML) and *myelodysplasia* (MDS) (Blue et al., 1988). Acute myeloblastic leukaemia, erythroleukaemia and erythremic myelosis appear to be the most common forms of acute myeloid leukaemia reported in cats (Blue et al., 1988; Jain et al., 1991). Cases of monoblastic leukaemia, myelomonocytic leukaemia and megakaryocytic myelosis (megakaryoblastic leukaemia) occur sporadically. Chronic myeloproliferative disorders such as polycythaemia vera (Khanna and Bienzele, 1994; Evans and Caylor, 1995), essential thrombocythaemia and chronic granulocytic leukaemia are rare. Primary erythrocytosis rather than polycythaemia vera has been reported in a series of cats, because features often associated with the latter were either uncommon or absent (Watson et al., 1994).

Various clinical signs may be seen in feline MPD but inappetence and weight loss are consistent features, present in all cases in a series described by Gorman and Evans (1987). Recurrent infections and intermittent or persistent pyrexia were also common findings. Moderate lymphadenopathy and splenomegaly were evident on physical examination in some cases. Anaemia was present in all 17 cats, ten of which showed a positive Coombs' test.

Peripheral white blood cell parameters are variable. Pronounced leucocytosis is not a consistent feature of AML in the cat although in some cases the total WBC count may exceed 200×10^9 l^{-1}; in one study almost 50% of cats with AML were neutropenic and many were also thrombocytopenic (Blue et al., 1988). Circulating blast cells are present in most cases of AML and the bone marrow examination reveals a high percentage of blast cells (by definition at least 30% of all nucleated cells counted in the marrow are myeloblasts in cases of myeloblastic leukaemia). In some cases, circulating myeloblasts are accompanied by a significant number of proerythroblasts, the so-called leucoerythroblastic reaction that is typical of erythroleukaemia. Cytochemistry may be helpful in identifying the cell line involved in cases of AML where the blast cells are poorly differentiated (Jain et al., 1991). In some cases of myeloblastic leukaemia bone marrow cytology may show evidence of cellular differentiation and a degree of normal maturation of the granulocytic series making differentiation from a highly reactive marrow difficult unless there is supportive clinical evidence of leukaemic infiltration of other organs (both of these disease states may result in a neutrophilia with a pronounced left shift).

Erythroid maturation is frequently abnormal in cats with myelodysplasia resulting in the appearance of macrocytic and/or increased numbers of nucleated blood cells in the circulation (see maturation defect anaemias). The anaemia is typically non-regenerative and may be accompanied by neutropenia and thrombocytopenia. Large bizarre platelets may be present in the peripheral blood. Circulating myeloblasts are rarely seen and although myeloblasts are present in increased numbers in the marrow they constitute less than 30% of all nucleated cells counted (Jain et al., 1991). Myelofibrosis may be a sequel to both myelodysplasia and acute myeloid leukaemia in the cat (Blue, 1988).

Cases of AML usually respond poorly to combination chemotherapy with survival times rarely exceeding 2–10 weeks (Couto, 1992b). Cats with polcythaemia vera (Evans and Caylor, 1995) and primary erythrocytosis (Watson et al., 1994) have been managed successfully with hydroxyurea. The decision to treat cats with myelodysplastic syndromes is based on the nature and severity of the haematological abnormalities and the presence or absence of associated clinical signs. Although the long-term prognosis is usually poor, supportive therapy may improve the quality and duration of life. Anabolic steroids may be used to stimulate erythropoiesis, using either 10 mg nandrolone decanoate (Deca Durabolin, Organon) intramuscularly once weekly for six weeks, or up to 50 mg oxymethalone (Anapolon, Syntex) daily by mouth. Prednisolone at doses of 2–4 mg kg^{-1} daily may prolong the lifespan of red cells and platelets and improve the appetite and general well-being of patients. Low doses of cytosine arabinoside have been given to cats with MDS with varying degrees of success in an attempt to induce cellular differentiation (5–10 mg m^{-2} s.c. bid for

2–3 weeks then on alternative days; Couto, 1992b). Ultimately about 30% of cats with MDS progress to AML or, less frequently, acute lymphoblastic leukaemia (ALL) (Couto, 1992b).

Lymphoproliferative disease

The role of FeLV infection in the development of lymphoid neoplasia in the cat is well recognized. As in the dog, there may be bone marrow involvement in cases of *multicentric lymphoma*. In such cases anaemia is common, though not always present, with variable circulating lymphocyte counts. The diagnosis is confirmed by identification of abnormal lymphocytes in bone marrow and lymph node aspirates or histological examination of biopsies. Survival times for cats with lymphoma are shorter than those reported for dogs. Combination chemotherapy may result in survival times of between six and nine months with only 20% of cats surviving longer than one year (Couto, 1992c).

Lymphoid leukaemia

Acute lymphoblastic leukaemia (ALL)

Lymphoid leukaemia in the cat is usually lymphoblastic and has a rapid clinical course. Large numbers of neoplastic lymphoblasts are found in the circulation and infiltrating the bone marrow. There is usually a profound anaemia. The prognosis for ALL is poor although slightly better than AML, survival times in response to chemotherapy varying between one and seven months (Couto, 1992b).

Chronic lymphocytic leukaemia (CLL)

CLL is a more slowly progressive condition characterized by the proliferation of a monomorphic population of small, well-differentiated lymphocytes in the bone marrow. Large numbers of these cells are present in the circulation and the total white cell count in some cases may be as high as 200×10^9 l^{-1}. Progression to a blast cell crisis may result in death. Compared to the dog, reports of CLL and long-term survival in cats are scarce, but one cat treated with chorambucil and prednisolone survived for five years (Couto, 1992b).

Multiple myeloma

Occasional cases of multiple myeloma may be encountered in the cat. Clinical and laboratory findings are as for the dog.

DISORDERS OF HAEMOSTASIS

Platelet abnormalities

Thrombocytopenia

Primary immune-mediated thrombocytopenia is much less frequently encountered in the cat than in the dog and only three cases have been reported (Halliwell and Gorman, 1989). The thrombocytopenia which is seen in association with a number of viral infections in the cat may well have an immune-mediated component.

As in the dog, failure of platelet production may be a feature of conditions involving the bone marrow, including neoplasia, with abnormalities in other cell lines also present. Thrombocytopenia may be a feature of FeLV-related myelodysplasia (see above). Bone marrow examination is indicated in such cases.

Abnormalities of platelet function

Chediak–Higashi syndrome

This autosomally recessive condition has been reported in a line of blue-smoke Persian cats with yellow eyes. There is abnormal granulation of platelets and granulocytes (Menard *et al.*, 1990). Clinical signs of a bleeding tendency due to defective platelet function and recurrent infections may be seen.

von Willebrand's disease

Feline vWD has been reported in a Himalayan cat (French *et al.*, 1987).

Coagulopathies

Acquired coagulation defects

Vitamin K antagonism

Although not common, coumarin toxicity may be encountered in the cat. It is usually the result of ingesting poisoned rodents rather than direct ingestion of bait. The clinical signs may include pulmonary haemorrhage and bleeding from other sites. The diagnosis, principles of management and monitoring of cases is as for dogs. The dose of vitamin K recommended for cats is 1–2 mg kg^{-1} daily, with an initial double loading dose or two doses given on the first day.

Disseminated intravascular coagulation

DIC has not been widely reported in the cat. It has been recognized as a complication of severe infections such as panleucopenia, FeLV-induced panleucopenia syndrome and feline infectious peritonitis. DIC should be suspected in a cat which develops abnormal bleeding with features of both platelet and coagulation factor abnormalities in association with a pre-existing condition.

Similar laboratory features are encountered to DIC in the dog. The latex agglutination test appears to give satisfactory results for identification of FDPs in the cat. Therapeutic considerations are as for the dog and the prognosis is dependent on early identification of the problem and successful management of the underlying precipitating cause.

Inherited coagulopathies

Factor VIII deficiency (haemophilia A)
F.VIII deficiency has been reported in a number of breeds of cats. The pattern of inheritance is the same as for the dog. Both severe and moderate forms may be encountered. In general, haemophilic cats would appear to be less likely to suffer from serious spontaneous haemorrhage than haemophilic dogs, possibly reflecting the different lifestyle of the two species. However, trauma and elective surgery may be accompanied by severe and fatal haemorrhage (Cotter et al., 1978; Littlewood, 1986). The author has also encountered moderate haemophilia in a cat which had survived castration, but bled excessively after removal of a lump which proved to be a resolving haematoma on histological examination.

Factor IX deficiency (haemophilia B)
This condition has been recognized in the British short-haired cat (Dodds, 1984) and in the Siamese (W.J. Dodds, personal communication). A combined defect of F.IX and F.XII has been reported in a litter of Siamese-cross domestic short haired (DSH) kittens (Dillon and Boudreaux, 1988).

Factor XII (Hageman factor) deficiency
Deficiency of F.XII is not associated with a symptomatic bleeding tendency, although it results in a dramatic prolongation of the APTT. The defect has been recognized in a number of cats and the inheritance has been shown to be autosomal recessive (Kier et al., 1980). A combined defect of F.VIII and F.XII deficiency has been encountered in one family of cats (Littlewood and Evans, 1990) where the importance of the condition as a laboratory abnormality confusing the identification of haemophilic kittens was illustrated.

Devon Rex coagulopathy
A coagulopathy of complex nature has been recognized in this breed for some time (Evans, 1985). A vitamin K-dependent multifactorial coagulopathy was described in several related Devon Rex cats in Australia (Maddison et al., 1990). Laboratory investigations revealed two- to threefold prolongation of PT and APTT. Factors II, IX and X were reduced to less than 20% of normal and F.VII to less than 50%. Oral vitamin K (5 mg daily) corrected the coagulation factor abnormalities and bleeding tendency. Cats of both genders were affected, but the pattern of inheritance was not elucidated. A case of Devon Rex coagulopathy has been confirmed in the UK (Littlewood et al., 1995).

Thrombotic disorders

Aortic thromboembolism
Feline aortic thromboembolism is a common clinical condition which in most cases arises secondary to cardiomyopathy (see Chapter 34). Stasis of blood gives rise to thrombus formation in the auricular appendage of the left atrium with subsequent embolic shedding. The bifurcation of the terminal aorta is the usual site for emboli to lodge, resulting in clinical signs of hind limb paresis, pain and ischaemic myopathy. Experimental studies have shown that the clinical syndrome is associated with the thrombus and vasoactive substances arising from its presence rather than simple obstruction to blood flow at this point; hence the poor results associated with surgical removal of the thrombus.

Alternative approaches to management of this distressing syndrome include the use of inflammatory and vasoactive inhibitors such as the serotonin antagonist cyproheptadine (Olmstead and Butler, 1977). Encouraging results have been obtained by the use of aspirin at a dose of 25 mg kg^{-1} every three days (Fox, 1983), with approximately 50% of treated cats regaining hind limb function within six weeks. Aspirin may also be used prophylactically in cats which have suffered a previous thrombotic episode, although there is still a high rate of re-thrombosis (Greene, 1985). The anticoagulant drug warfarin has been used with success to prevent recurrence (Harpster, 1986). More recently, reperfusion has been achieved by using genetically engineered tissue plasminogen activator (tPA), with a rapid return of function and a favourable outcome in 50% of cases, but a high incidence of complications (including death) associated with thrombolysis and hyperkalaemia was recorded in the rest (Pion, 1989).

BLOOD TRANSFUSION IN THE DOG AND CAT

A number of conditions may require the use of whole blood or blood component transfusions. The use of transfusion therapy in a large number of cases has been reviewed by Stone et al. (1992) and Callan et al. (1996). This topic is covered more fully elsewhere (Pilcher and Turnwald, 1985; Turnwald and Pilcher, 1985; Cotter, 1991) and general principles only will be considered here.

Where possible, the clinician should select the most appropriate product to treat the needs of the individual patient. The options include whole blood, packed red cells, fresh or fresh-frozen whole plasma, platelet-rich plasma and cryoprecipitate. Further fractionation of plasma is possible, but rarely (if ever) used in veterinary medicine.

Donor considerations

Blood groups

Of the eight canine erythrocyte antigens recognized DEA 1 antigens (DEA 1.1 and 1.2) and DEA 7 are the most immunogenic. The ideal donor should be negative for these blood groups. Although pre-existing isoantibodies are not a significant problem in canine transfusion medicine and do not cause acute transfusion reactions (unlike the cat), anti-DEA 7 isoantibodies may be responsible for a delayed incompatability reaction resulting in reduced lifespan of the transfused red cells. Anti-DEA 1 isoantibodies are not present in dogs which have never been transfused previously, but an immune response will occur within seven to ten days of administration of incompatible blood to a dog. Subsequent incompatible transfusions will elicit a rapid and severe reaction (Gelens et al., 1992).

The incidence of type B cats is less than 1% of the DSH cat population, but may be up to 50% in some pure breeds (Giger, 1990). Since up to 35% of type A and all of type B cats carry naturally occurring isoantibodies to foreign blood group antigens, the potential exists for a transfusion reaction with the first transfusion of incompatible blood to feline patients (Auer and Bell, 1986; Giger and Akol, 1990; Giger and Bucheler, 1991).

Management of donors

Animals maintained as blood donors should be adult animals in good health and free of infections which may be transmitted in blood (red cell parasites, toxoplasma, FeLV, FIV, FIP). Donor dogs preferably should be at least 25–30 kg to allow removal of large quantites of blood. Regular monitoring of body weight and haematological parameters should be performed, in addition to clinical examination. Donor animals may be used as frequently as every three to four weeks, providing they are on a high plane of nutrition. Approximately 15% of blood volume may be safely removed (this equates to approximately 13.5 ml kg^{-1} for dogs and 10.5 ml kg^{-1} for cats).

Storage and delivery

Commercially available blood bags containing citrate–phosphate–dextrose–adenine (CPD-A) are appropriate for collecting and storing canine blood. For feline blood an appropriate volume of anticoagulant can be taken from a bag into a syringe to allow collection of small volumes of blood (7 ml anticoagulant per 50 ml blood). Red cell viability is maintained for up to a month. Beyond this the fall in pH and lactate production due to glucose metabolism results in increased rigidity of erythrocytes, and reduced concentrations of 2,3-diphosphoglycerate in red cells results in decreased oxygen release to tissues. Heparin can be used in the ratio of 625 units heparin per 50 ml blood, but this anticoagulant has no preservative properties and blood must be used within 24–48 h.

Blood collection packs with satellite or transfer bags allows separation of plasma by squeeze devices after centrifugation. Slow thawing of frozen plasma at 4°C and centrifugation provides cryoprecipitate, which increases the concentration of vWF and F.VIII compared to whole plasma. The details for producing component products have been described by Authement et al. (1987).

Whole blood, packed cells and platelet-rich plasma (PRP) should be stored at 4°C. Platelets (in PRP or whole blood) should be used within 8–12 h of collection. Plasma and plasma products can be frozen and stored for up to three months at −20°C or one year at −70°C without a significant decrease in concentration of clotting factors.

Patient considerations

Crossmatch

Major and minor crossmatching is a simple and essential prerequisite to successful transfusion.

Table 45.11 Method for crossmatching blood for transfusion

1. Take blood from patient and donor(s), in EDTA or ACD
   Spin and separate plasma
   Wash cells 3 times in warm isotonic saline
   Make a 3% cell suspension
2. Label three tubes for each donor: Major, Minor, Control
   Add cells and plasma (serum) as follows:
   Major: 2 drops donor cells added to 2 drops patient plasma
   Minor: 2 drops patient cells added to 2 drops donor plasma
   Control: 2 drops patient cells added to 2 drops patient plasma
3. Incubate 30 min at 37°C (or room temperature)
   Spin gently, 280 *g*, for 1 min
   Look for haemolysis
   Tap to look for agglutination
   Microscopic examination for agglutination

The major crossmatch detects recipient antibodies to donor cell, and the minor crossmatch detects antibodies in donor plasma to recipient cells. The method is outlined in Table 45.11.

Administration

The amount of blood required can be calculated from the following equation:

$$\text{Volume (ml)} = \frac{\text{Desired rise in PCV} \times \text{patient blood volume} \times 100}{\text{PCV of donated blood}}$$

The blood volume of dogs is about 90 ml kg^{-1} and that of cats is 70 ml kg^{-1}. An alternative rule of thumb is that 2.2 ml of blood per kg bodyweight raises the PCV by 0.01 l l^{-1} when the PCV of the transfused blood is 0.40 l l^{-1}.

Plasma administered for management of coagulopathies or hypoproteinaemia should be given at doses of 6–10 ml kg^{-1} and repeated two or three times daily as required.

All blood products should be warmed to 37°C before administration and given through a giving set which includes a blood filter. Filters for use with syringes can be obtained for feline transfusions (Monoject-type filter needles, Sherwood Medical, Crawley, Surrey, UK). The rate of infusion of blood products should not exceed 1 ml kg^{-1} in normovolaemic patients although in acute blood loss rates of 10–20 ml kg^{-1} may be given safely.

■ Complications

Potential complications include acute (Giger *et al.*, 1995) and delayed haemolytic reactions and reactions to leucocytes, platelets and plasma proteins. To minimize the risks of these reactions an antihistamine, e.g. diphenhydramine (Piriton) may be administered intravenously before transfusion. Glucocorticoids are indicated if such reactions occur. Non-immunological reactions which may occur include septic complications due to administration of contaminated blood, circulatory overload, thrombosis and hypothermia. Dogs receiving multiple transfusions may occasionally become hypocalcaemic (excessive volumes of citrate, if administered quickly, may chelate ionized calcium) or suffer iron overload. There is also the potential for disease transmission.

■ REFERENCES

Abdullahi, S.U., Mohammed, A.A., Trimnell, A.R., Sannusi, A. and Alafiatayo, R. (1990) Clinical and haematological findings in 70 naturally occurring cases of canine babesiosis. *Journal of Small Animal Practice* **31**, 145–147.

Auer, L.A. and Bell, K. (1986) Feline blood transfusion reactions. In: *Current Veterinary Therapy IX* (Ed. R.W. Kirk). W.B. Saunders, Philadelphia, pp. 515–521.

Authement, J.M., Wolfsheimer, K.J. and Catchings, S. (1987) Canine blood component therapy: product preparation, storage and administration. *Journal of the American Animal Hospitals Association* **23**, 483–493.

Barker, R.N., Gruffydd-Jones, T.J., Stokes, C.R. and Elson, C.J. (1991) Identification of autoantigens in canine autoimmune haemolytic anaemia. *Clinical and Experimental Immunology* **85**, 33–40.

Blue, J.T. (1988) Myelofibrosis in cats with myelodysplastic syndrome and acute myelogenous leukemia. *Veterinary Pathology* **25**, 154–160.

Blue, J.T., French, T.W. and Kranz, J.S. (1988) Non-lymphoid hematopoietic neoplasia in cats: a retrospective study of 60 cases. *Cornell Veterinarian* **78**, 21–42.

Bolton, B., Buergelt, C.D., Harvey, J.W., Meyer, D.J. and Kaplan-Stein, D. (1989) Megakaryoblastic leukemia in a dog. *Veterinary Clinical Pathology* **18**, 69–72.

Boudreaux, M.K., Crager, C., Dillon, A.R., Stanz, K. and Toivio-Kinnucan, M. (1994) Identification of an intrinsic platelet function defect in spitz dogs. *Journal of Veterinary Internal Medicine* **8**, 93–98.

Breitschwerdt, E.B. (1988) Infectious thrombocytopenia in dogs. *Compendium of Continuing Education for the Practicing Veterinarian* **10**, 1177–1190.

Bridle, K.H. and Littlewood, J.D. (1998) Tail tip necrosis in two litters of Birman kittens. *Journal of Small Animal Practice* **32**, 88–89.

Brooks, M., Raymond, S. and Catalfamo, J. (1996) Severe, recessive von Willebrand's disease in German wirehaired pointers. *Journal of the American Veterinary Medical Association* **209**, 926–929.

Cain, G.R., Feldman, B.F., Kawakami, T.G. and Jain, N.C. (1986) Platelet dysplasia associated with megakaryoblastic leukemia in a dog. *Journal of the American Veterinary Medical Association* **188**, 529–530.

Cain, G.R., Kawakami, T.G. and Jain, N.C. (1985) Radiation-induced megakaryoblastic leukaemia in a dog. *Veterinary Pathology* **22**, 641–643.

Callan, M.B., Oakley, D.A., Shofer, F.S. and Giger, U. (1996) Canine red blood cell transfusion practice. *Journal of the American Animal Hospital Association* **32**, 303–311.

Catalfamo, J.L. and Dodds, W.J. (1988) Hereditary and acquired thrombopathias. *Veterinary Clinics of North America Small Animal Practice* **18**, 185–193.

Chapman, B.L. and Giger, U. (1990) Inherited erythrocyte pyruvate kinase deficiency in the West Highland white terrier. *Journal of Small Animal Practice* **31**, 610–616.

Cook, A.K., Werner, L.L., O'Neill, S.L., Brooks, M. and Feldman, B.F. (1993) Factor X deficiency in a Jack Russell terrier. *Veterinary Clinical Pathology* **22**, 68–71.

Cook, S.M. and Lothrop, C.D. (1994) Serum erythropoietin concentrations measured by radioimmunoassay in normal, polycythemic and anemic dogs and cats. *Journal of Veterinary Internal Medicine* **8**, 18–25.

Cotter, S.M. (1979) Anemia associated with feline leukemia virus infection. *Journal of the American Veterinary Medical Association* **175**, 1191–1194.

Cotter, S.M. (1991) Clinical transfusion medicine. *Advances in Veterinary Science and Comparative Medicine* **36**, 188–224.

Cotter, S.M., Brenner, R.M. and Dodds, W.J. (1978) Hemophilia A in three unrelated cats. *Journal of the American Veterinary Medical Association* **172**, 166–168.

Couto, C.G. (1992a) Disorders of hemostasis. In: *Essentials of Small Animal Internal Medicine* (Eds R.W. Nelson and C.G. Couto). Mosby Year Book, St Louis, pp. 926–940.

Couto, C.G. (1992b) Leukaemias. In: *Essentials of Small Animal Internal Medicine* (Eds R.W. Nelson and C.G. Couto). Mosby Year Book, St Louis, pp. 871–878.

Couto, C.G. (1992c) Lymphoma in the dog and cat. In: *Essentials of Small Animal Internal Medicine* (Eds R.W. Nelson and C.G. Couto). Mosby Year Book, St Louis, pp. 861–870.

Crow, S.E., Allen, D.P., Murphy, C.J. and Culbertson, R. (1995) Concurrent renal adenocarcinoma and polycythemia in a dog. *Journal of the American Animal Hospital Association* **31**, 29–33.

Day, M.J. (1996) Serial monitoring of clinical, haematological and immunological parameters in canine autoimmune haemolytic anaemia. *Journal of Small Animal Practice* **37**, 523–534.

Degen, M.A., Feldman, B.F., Tuernel, J.M., Goding, B., Kitchell, B., and Mandell, C.P. (1989) Thrombocytosis associated with a myeloproliferative disorder in a dog. *Journal of the American Veterinary Medical Association* **194**, 1457–1459.

Dillon, A.R. and Boudreaux, M.K. (1988) Combined factors IX and XII deficencies in a family of cats. *Journal of the American Veterinary Medical Association* **193**, 833–834.

Dobson, J.M. and Gorman, N.T. (1993) Canine multicentric lymphoma 1: clinico-pathological presentation of the disease. *Journal of Small Animal Practice* **34**, 594–598.

Dobson, J.M. and Gorman, N.T. (1994) Canine multicentric lymphoma 2: comparison of response to two chemotherapuetic protocols. *Journal of Small Animal Practice* **35**, 9–15.

Dodds, W.J. (1973) Canine factor X (Stuart–Power factor) deficiency. *Journal of Clinical Laboratory Medicine* **82**, 560–566.

Dodds, W.J. (1977) Inherited hemorrhagic defects. In: *Current Veterinary Therapy* VI (Ed. R.W. Kirk). W.B. Saunders, Philadelphia, pp. 438–445.

Dodds, W.J. (1984) Hemophilia in cats. *Cat World (USA)* November issue, p. EE13.

Dodds, W.J. (1985) Canine and feline blood groups. In: *Textbook of Small Animal Surgery*, 1st edn (Ed. D.H. Slatter), W.B. Saunders, Philadelphia, pp. 1195–1198.

Dodds, W.J. (1989) Acquired von Willebrand's disease, In: *Proceedings of the American Animal Hospital Association* 56th Annual Meeting, pp. 614–619.

Dodds, W.J. and Kull, J.E. (1971) Canine factor XI (plasma thromboplastin antecedent) deficiency. *Journal of Clinical Laboratory Medicine* **78**, 746–752.

Dunn, J.K. (1990) Bone marrow aspiration and biopsy in the dog and cat. *In Practice* **12**, 200–206.

Dunn, J.K., Seary, G.P. and Hirsch, V.M. (1984a) The diagnostic significance of a positive direct antiglobulin test in anaemic cats. *Canadian Journal of Comparative Medicine* **48**, 349–353.

Dunn, J.K., Hirsch, V.M. and Searcy, G.P. (1984b) Serum folate and vitamin B_{12} levels in anemic cats. *Journal of the American Animal Hospital Association* **20**, 999–1002.

Dunn, J.K., Doige, C.E., Searcy, G.P. and Tamke, P. (1986) Myelofibrosis–osteosclerosis syndrome associated with erythroid hypoplasia in a dog. *Journal of Small Animal Practice* **27**, 799–806.

Duval, D. and Giger, U. (1996) Vaccine-associated immune-mediated hemolytic anemia in the dog. *Journal of Veterinary Internal Medicine* **10**, 290–295.

Eksell, P., Häggström, J., Kvart, C. and Karlsson, A. (1994) Thrombocytopenia in the cavalier King Charles spaniel. *Journal of Small Animal Practice* **35**, 153–155.

Evans, L.M. and Caylor, K.B. (1995) Polycythemia vera in a cat and management with hydroxyurea. *Journal of the American Animal Hospital Association* **31**, 434–438.

Evans, R.J. (1985) The blood and haematopoietic system. In: *Feline Medicine and Therapeutics* (Eds E.A. Chandler, C.J. Gaskell and A.D.R. Hilbery). Blackwell Scientific Publications, Oxford, pp. 110–132.

Evans, R.J. and Gordon, J.L. (1974) Mechanism of the antithrombotic action of dextran. *New England Journal of Medicine* **290**, 748.

Evans, R.J. and Gorman, N.T. (1987) Myeloproliferative disease in the dog and cat: definition, aetiology and classification. *Veterinary Record* **121**, 437–443.

Evans, R.J., Jones, D.R.E. and Gryffydd-Jones, T.J. (1982) Essential thrombocythaemia in the dog and cat. *Journal of Small Animal Practice* **23**, 457–467.

Feldman, B.F. (1989) Disorders of platelets. In: *Current Veterinary Therapy* X (Ed. R.W. Kirk). W.B. Saunders, Philadelphia, pp. 457–464.

Feldman, B.F., Kaneko, J.J. and Farver, T.B. (1981) Anemia of inflammatory disease in the dog: clinical characterization. *American Journal of Veterinary Research* **42**, 1109–1113.

Feldman, D.G., Brooks, M.B. and Dodds, W.J. (1995) Hemophilia B (factor IX deficiency) in a family of German shepherd dogs. *Journal of the American Veterinary Medical Association* **206**, 1901–1905.

Fernandez, F.R., Davies, A.P., Teachout, D.J., Krake, A., Christopher, M.M. and Perman, V. (1984) Vitamin K-induced Heinz body formation in dogs. *Journal of the American Animal Hospital Association* **20**, 711–720.

Fleming, E.J., McCaw, D.L., Smith, J.A., Buening, G.M. and Johnson, C. (1991). Clinical, hematologic and survival data from cats infected with feline immunodeficiency virus: 42 cases (1983–1988). *Journal of the American Veterinary Medical Association* **199**, 913–916.

Fogh, J.M. (1988) A study of hemophilia A in German shepherd dogs in Denmark. *Veterinary Clinics of North America Small Animal Practice* **18**, 245–254.

Fogh, J.M. and Fogh, I.T. (1988) Inherited coagulation disorders. *Veterinary Clinics of North America Small Animal Practice* **18**, 231–244.

Fox, L.E., Ford, S., Alleman, A.R., Homer, B.L. and Harvey, J.W. (1993) Aplastic anemia associated with prolonged high-dose trimethoprim-sulfadiazine administration in two dogs. *Veterinary Clinical Pathology* **22**, 89–92.

Fox, P.R. (1983) Feline myocardial diseases. In: *Current Veterinary Therapy VIII* (Ed. R.W. Kirk). W.B. Saunders, Philadelphia, pp. 337–348.

Fredrikson, B and Grøndalen, J. (1988) Phenylbutazone intolerance: a cause of bone marrow depression in the dog. *Norsk Veterinær Tidsskrift* **100**, 793–798.

French, T.W., Fox, L.E., Randolph, J.F. and Dodds, W.J. (1987) A bleeding disorder (von Willebrand's disease) in a Himalayan cat. *Journal of the American Veterinary Medical Association* **190**, 437–439.

Gelens, C.J., Giger, U., Callan, M.B. and Oakley, D.A. (1992) Canine blood type frequencies and an acute hemolytic transfusion reaction. *Journal of Veterinary Internal Medicine* **6**, 141.

Giger, U. (1990) Frequency of feline A and B blood types in purebred cats and their clinical significance. *Veterinary Clinical Pathology* **19**, 7.

Giger, U. (1992) Erythropoietin and its clinical use. *Compendium of Continuing Education for the Practicing Veterinarian* **14**, 25–34.

Giger, U. and Akol, K.G. (1990) Acute haemolytic transfusion reaction in an Abyssinian cat with blood type B. *Journal of Veterinary Internal Medicine* **4**, 315–316.

Giger, U. and Bucheler, J. (1991) Transfusion of type A and type B blood to cats. *Journal of the American Veterinary Medical Association* **198**, 411–418.

Giger, U., Werner, L.L., Millichamp, N.J. and Gorman, N.T. (1985a) Sulfadiazine-induced allergy in six dobermann pinschers. *Journal of the American Veterinary Medical Association* **186**, 479–484.

Giger, U., Harvey, J.W., Yamaguchi, R.A., McNulty, P.K., Chiapella, A. and Beutler, E. (1985b) Inherited phosphofructokinase deficiency in dogs with hyperventilation-induced haemolysis: increased *in vitro* and *in vivo* alkaline fragility of erythrocytes. *Blood* **65**, 345–351.

Giger, U., Boxer, L.A., Simpson, P.J., Lucchesi, B.R. and Todd, R.F. (1987) Deficiency of leukocyte surface glycoproteins Mo1, LFA-1 and Leu M5 in a dog with recurrent infections: an animal model. *Blood* **69**, 1622–1630.

Giger, U., Kilrain, C.G., Filippich, L.J. and Bell, K. (1989) Frequencies of feline blood groups in the United States. *Journal of the American Veterinary Medical Association* **195**, 1230–1232.

Giger, U., Bucheler, J. and Patterson, D.F. (1991a) Frequency and inheritance of A and B blood types in feline breeds of the United States. *Journal of Heredity* 82, 150–20.

Giger, U., Wang, P. and Mason, G.D. (1991b) Inherited erythrocyte pyruvate kinase deficiency in a Beagle dog. *Veterinary Clinical Pathology* 20, 83–86.

Giger, U., Gelens, C.J., Callan, M.B. and Oakley, D.A. (1995) An acute hemolytic transfusion reaction caused by dog erythrocyte antigen 1.1 incompatibility in a previously sensitized dog. *Journal of the American Veterinary Medical Association* 206, 1135–1362.

Giles, A.R., Tinlin, S. and Greenwood, R. (1982) A canine model of hemophilic (factor VIII:C deficiency) bleeding. *Blood* 60, 727–730.

Godfrey, D.R. and Andersen, R.M. (1994) Cold agglutinin disease in a cat. *Journal of Small Animal Practice* 35, 267–270.

Gorman, N.T. and Evans, R.J. (1987) Myeloproliferative disease in the dog and cat: clinical presentations, diagnosis and treatment. *Veterinary Record* 121, 490–496.

Green, R.A. (1988) Pathophysiology of antithrombin III deficiency. *Veterinary Clinics of North America Small Animal Practice* 18, 95–104.

Greene, C.E. (1985) Effects of aspirin and propranolol on feline platelet aggregation. *American Journal of Veterinary Research* 46, 1820–1823.

Hall, E.J. (1990) Prolonged coagulopathy associated with brodifacoum poisoning in two dogs. *Journal of Small Animal Practice* 31, 574–579.

Halliwell, R.E.W. and Gorman, N.T. (1989) Autoimmune blood diseases. In: *Veterinary Clinical Immunology* (Eds R.E.W. Halliwell and N.T. Gorman). W.B. Saunders, Philadelphia, pp. 308–336.

Hammer, A.S. and Couto, C.G. (1994) Complications of multiple myeloma. *Journal of the American Animal Hospital Association* 30, 9–14.

Hardy, W.D. (1981) Hematopoietic tumours of cats. *Journal of the American Animal Hospital Association* 17, 921–940.

Harpster, N.K. (1986) Feline myocardial diseases. In: *Current Veterinary Therapy IX* (Ed. R.W. Kirk). W.B. Saunders, Philadelphia, pp. 380–398.

Harrus, S., Waner, T., Eldor, A., Zwang, E. and Bark, H. (1996) Platelet dysfunction associated with experimental acute canine ehrlichiosis. *Veterinary Record* 139, 290–293.

Harvey, J.W. and Smith, J.E. (1994) Haematology and clinical chemistry of English springer spaniel dogs with phosphofructokinase deficiency. *Comparative Haematology International* 4, 70–75.

Hasler, A.H. and Giger, U. (1996) Serum erythropoietin values in polycythemic cats. *Journal of the American Animal Hospital Association* 32, 294–301.

Helfand, S.C. (1988) Platelets and neoplasia. *Veterinary Clinics of North America Small Animal Practice* 18, 131–156.

Hirsch, V.M. and Dunn, J.K. (1983) Megaloblastic anaemia in the cat. *Journal of the American Animal Hospital Association* 19, 873–880.

Holmberg, C.SA. (1985) Classification of hematopoietic system neoplasia in the dog. *Veterinary Clinics of North America Small Animal Practice* 15, 697–708.

Holmes, N.G., Shaw, S.C., Dickens, H.F., Coombes, L.M., Ryder, E.J., Littlewood, J.D. and Binns, M.M. (1996) Von Willebrand's disease in UK dobermanns: possible correlation of a polymorphic DNA marker with disease status. *Journal of Small Animal Practice* 37, 307–308.

Hribernik, T.N. and Barr, W.C. (1989) Parasitic blood diseases of dogs and cats. In: *Current Veterinary Therapy X, Small Animal Practice* (Ed. R.W. Kirk). W.B. Saunders, Philadelphia, pp. 419–424.

Jain, N.C. (1986) Cytochemistry of normal and leukaemic leukocytes. In: *Schalm's Veterinary Haematology*, 4th edn. Lea and Febiger, Philadelphia, pp. 909–939.

Jain, N.C. (1989) Cytochemistry of canine and feline leukocytes and leukemias. In: *Current Veterinary Therapy X, Small Animal Practice* (Ed. R.W. Kirk). W.B.Saunders, Philadelphia, pp. 465–468.

Jain, N.C. (1993) Immunohematology. In: *Essentials of Veterinary Hematology*. Lea and Febiger, Philadelphia, pp. 381–407.

Jain, N.C., Blue, J.T., Grindem, C.B., Harvey, J.W., Kociba, G.J., Krehbiel, J.D., Latimer, K.S., Raskin, R.E., Thrall, M.A. and Zinkl, J.G. (1991) A report of the animal leukaemia study group: proposed criteria for classification of acute myeloid leukaemia in dogs and cats. *Veterinary Clinical Pathology* 20, 63–82.

Jans, H.E., Armstrong, J. and Price, G.S. (1990) Therapy of immune mediated thrombocytopenia: a retrospective study of 15 dogs. *Journal of Veterinary Internal Medicine* 4, 4–7.

Jarrett, O. (1991) Overview of feline leukaemia virus research. *Journal of the American Veterinary Medical Association* 199, 1279–1281.

Jergens, A.E., Turrentine, M.A., Kraus, K.H. and Johnson, G.S. (1987) Buccal mucosal bleeding time of healthy dogs and of dogs in various pathological states, including thrombocytopenia, uremia and von Willebrand's disease. *American Journal of Veterinary Research* 48, 1337–1342.

Johnson, G.S., Turrentine, M.A. and Dodds, W.J. (1987) Type II von Willebrand's disease in German shorthair pointers. *Veterinary Clinical Pathology* 16, 7.

Johnstone, I.B. (1993) The importance of accurate citrate to blood ratios in the collection of canine blood for hemostatic testing. *Canadian Veterinary Journal* 34, 627–629.

Johnstone, I.B., Keen, J., Halbert, A. and Crane, S. (1991) Stability of factor VIII and von Willebrand factor in canine blood samples during storage. *Canadian Veterinary Journal* 32, 173–175.

Jones, D.R.E. (1986) Use of an enzyme indirect antiglobulin test for the diagnosis of autoimmune haemolytic anaemia in the dog. *Research in Veterinary Science* 41, 187–190.

Jones, D.R.E. and Darke, P.G.G. (1975) Use of papain for the detection of incomplete erythrocyte autoantibodies in autoimmune haemolytic anaemia of the dog and cat. *Journal of Small Animal Practice* **16**, 273–279.

Jones, D.R.E., Stokes, C.R., Gruffydd-Jones, T.J. and Bourne, F.J. (1987) An enzyme-linked antiglobulin test for the detection of erythrocyte-bound autoantibodies in canine autoimmune haemolytic anaemia. *Veterinary Immunology and Immunopathology* **16**, 11–21.

Jones, D.R.E., Gruffydd-Jones, T.J., Stokes, C.R. and Bourne, F.J. (1990) Investigation into factors influencing performance of the canine antiglobulin test. *Research in Veterinary Science* **48**, 53–58.

Jones, J.B. and Lange, R.D. (1983) Cyclic hematopoiesis: animal models. *Experimental Hematology* **11**, 571–580.

Kennel Club and British Small Animal Veterinary Association Scientific Committee (1997). Canine granulocytopathy syndrome in Irish setters. *Journal of Small Animal Practice* **38**, 591.

Khanna, C. and Bienzele, D. (1994) Polycythemia vera in a cat: bone marrow culture in erythropoietin-deficient medium. *Journal of the American Animal Hospital Association* **30**, 45–49.

Kier, A.B., Bresnaham, J.F., White, F.J. and Wagner, J.E. (1980) The inheritance pattern of factor XII deficiency in domestic cats. *Canadian Journal of Comparative Medicine* **44**, 309–314.

King, L.G., Giger, U., Diserens, D. and Nagode, L.A. (1992) Anemia of chronic renal failure in dogs. *Journal of Veterinary Internal Medicine* **6**, 264–270.

Knowler, C., Giger, U., Dodds, W.J. and Brooks, M. (1994) Factor XI deficiency in Kerry blue terriers. *Journal of the American Veterinary Medical Association* **205**, 1557–1561.

Kraus, K.H., Turrentine, M.A. and Johnson, G.S. (1988) Use of DDAVP for management of surgical hemorrhage from a dobermann pinscher with von Willebrand's disease. *Veterinary Clinics of North America Small Animal Practice* **18**, 276.

Kraus, K.H., Turrentine, M.A., Jergens, A.E. and Johnson, G.S. (1989) Effect of desmopressin acetate on bleeding times and plasma von Willebrand factor in Dobermann Pinscher dogs with von Willebrand's disease. *Veterinary Surgery* **187**, 103–109.

Kristensen, A.T., Weiss, D.J., Klausner, J.S. and Christie, D.J. (1994a) Detection of antiplatelet antibody with a platelet immunofluorescence assay. *Journal of Veterinary Internal Medicine* **8**, 36–39.

Kristensen, A.T., Weiss, D.J. and Klausner, J.S. (1994b) Platelet dysfunction associated with immune-mediated thrombocytopenia purpura. *Journal of Veterinary Internal Medicine* **8**, 323–327.

Latimer, K.S., Kircher, I.M., Lindl, P.A., Dawe, D.L. and Brown, J. (1989) Leukocyte function in Pelger–Huët anomaly of dogs. *Journal of Leukocyte Biology* **45**, 301–310.

Leifer, C.M. and Matus, R.E. (1985) Lymphoid leukemia in the dog: acute lymphoblastic leukemia and chronic lymphocytic leukemia. *Veterinary Clinics of North America Small Animal Practice* **15**, 723–740.

Leifer, C.M. and Matus, R.E. (1986) Chronic lymphocytic leukemia in the dog: 22 cases (1974–1984). *Journal of the American Veterinary Medical Association* **189**, 214–217.

Lewis, D.C. and Meyers, K.M. (1996) Canine idiopathic thrombocytopenic purpura. *Journal of Veterinary Internal Medicine* **10**, 207–218.

Lewis, D.C., Meyers, K.M., Callan, B., Bucheler, J. and Giger, U. (1995) Detection of platelet-bindable antibodies for diagnosis of idiopathic thrombocytopenic purpura in dogs. *Journal of the American Veterinary Medical Association* **206**, 47–52.

Littlewood, J.D. (1986) Haemophilia A (factor VIII deficiency) in the cat. *Journal of Small Animal Practice* **27**, 541–546.

Littlewood, J.D. (1988) Haemophilia A (factor VIII deficiency) in German shepherd dogs. *Journal of Small Animal Practice* **29**, 117–128.

Littlewood, J.D. (1991) Von Willebrand's disease in the dog. In: *Veterinary Annual*, 31st edn (Eds C.S.G. Grunsell and M.E. Raw). Blackwell Scientific Publications, Oxford, pp. 163–172.

Littlewood, J.D. and Evans, R.J. (1990) A combined deficiency of factor VIII and contact activation defect in a family of cats. *British Veterinary Journal* **146**, 30–35.

Littlewood, J.D., Matic, S.M. and Smith, N. (1986) Factor IX deficiency (Haemophilia B, Christmas disease) in a cross-bred dog. *Veterinary Record* **118**, 400–401.

Littlewood, J.D., Herrtage, M.E., Gorman, N.T. and McGlennon, N.J. (1987) von Willebrand's disease in dogs in the United Kingdom. *Veterinary Record* **121**, 463–468.

Littlewood, J.D., Shaw, S.C. and Coombes, L.M. (1995) Vitamin K-dependent coagulopathy in a British Devon rex cat. *Journal of Small Animal Practice* **36**, 115–118.

MacEwen, E.G. and Hurvitz, A.I. (1977) Diagnosis and management of monoclonal gammopathies. *Veterinary Clinics of North America* **7**, 119–131.

Maddison, J.E., Watson, A.D.J., Eade, I.G. and Exner, T. (1990) Vitamin K-dependent multifactor coagulopathy in Devon rex cats. *Journal of the American Veterinary Medical Association* **197**, 1495–1497.

Mahaffey, E.A., Brown, T.P., Duncan, J.R., Latimer, K.S. and Brown, S.A. (1987) Basophilic leukaemia in a dog. *Journal of Comparative Pathology* **97**, 393–399.

Mansell, P.D. and Parry, B.W. (1989) Stability of canine factor VIII:C coagulant activity in vitro. *Canadian Journal of Veterinary Research* **53**, 264–267.

Matus, R.E. and Leifer, C.M (1985) Immunoglobulin-producing tumors. *Veterinary Clinics of North America Small Animal Practice* **15**, 741–754.

McEwan, N.A. (1992) Presumptive trimethoprim-sulphamethoxazole associated thrombocytopenia and anaemia in a dog. *Journal of Small Animal Practice* **33**, 27–29.

Menard, M., Meyers, K.M. and Prieur, D.J. (1990) Absence of dense granule precursors in megakaryocytes from cats with Chediak–Higashi syndrome. *Veterinary Clinical Pathology* **19**, 6–7.

Messick, J., Carothers, M. and Wellman, M. (1990) Identification and characterization of megakaryoblasts in acute megakaryoblastic leukemia in a dog. *Veterinary Pathology* **27**, 212–214.

Meyers, K.M., Wardrop, K.J., Helmick, C.M. and White, F.P. (1987) Presence of VWF in vascular endothelium but not platelets from control dogs and VIIIR:Ag deficient dogs. *Thrombosis and Haemostasis* **58**, 460, Abstract 1702.

Meyers, K.M., Wardrop, K.J., Dodds, W.J. and Brassard, J. (1990) Effect of exercise, DDAVP and epinephrine on the factor VIII:C/von Willebrand factor complex in normal dogs and von Willebrand factor deficient Doberman pinscher dogs. *Thrombosis Research* **57**, 97–98.

Morris, J.S., Dunn, J.K. and Dobson, J.M. (1993) Canine lymphoid leukaemia and lymphoma with bone marrow involvement: a review of 24 cases. *Journal of Small Animal Practice* **34**, 72–79.

Moore, A.H., Day, M.J. and Graham, M.W.A. (1993) Congenital pure red blood cell aplasia (Diamond–Blackfan anaemia) in a dog. *Veterinary Record* **132**, 414–415.

Moser, J.M., Meyers, K.M., Meinkoth, J.H. and Brassard, J.A. (1996a) Temporal variation and factors affecting measurement of canine von Willebrand factor. *American Journal of Veterinary Research* **57**, 1288–1293.

Moser, J.M., Meyers, K.M. and Russon, R.H. (1996b) Inheritance of von Willebrand factor deficiency in dobermann pinschers. *Journal of the American Veterinary Medical Association* **209**, 1103–1106.

Mount, M.E., Woody, B.J. and Murphy, M.J. (1986) The anticoagulant rodenticides. In: *Current Veterinary Therapy IX* (Ed. R.W. Kirk). W.B. Saunders, Philadelphia, pp. 156–165.

Northern, F. and Tvedten, H.W. (1992) Diagnosis of microthrombocytosis and immune-mediated thrombocytopenia in dogs with thrombocytopenia: 68 cases (1987–1989). *Journal of the American Veterinary Medical Association* **200**, 368–372.

Oehme, F.W. (1986) Aspirin and acetaminophen. In: *Current Veterinary Therapy IX* (Ed. R.W. Kirk). W.B. Saunders, Philadelphia, pp. 188–190.

Olmstead, M.L. and Butler, H.C. (1977) Five-hydroxytryptamine antagonists and feline aortic embolism. *Journal of Small Animal Practice* **18**, 247–259.

Osbaldiston, G.W., Stowe, E.C. and Griffith, P.R. (1970) Blood coagulation: comparative studies in dogs, cats, horses and cattle. *British Veterinary Journal* **126**, 512–521.

Panciera, D.L. and Johnson, G.S. (1994) Plasma von Willebrand factor antigen concentration in dogs with hypothyroidism. *Journal of the American Veterinary Medical Association* **205**, 1550–1553.

Panciera, D.L. and Johnson, G.S. (1996) Plasma von Willebrand factor antigen concentration and buccal mucosal bleeding time in dogs with experimental hypothyroidism. *Journal of Veterinary Internal Medicine* **10**, 60–64.

Parker, M.T., Turrentine, M.A. and Johnson, G.S. (1991) Von Willebrand factor in lysates of washed platelets from normal dogs and dogs with von Willebrand's disease. *American Journal of Veterinary Research* **52**, 119–125.

Parry, B.W., Howard, M.A., Mansell, P.D. and Holloway, S.A. (1988) Haemophilia A in German shepherd dogs in Australia. *Australian Veterinary Journal* **65**, 276–279.

Patteson, M and Williams, P. (1988) Blood sampling in the dog and cat. *In Practice* **10**, 105–111.

Peterson, M.E. and Randolph, J.F. (1982) Diagnosis of canine primary polycythemia and management with hydroxyurea. *Journal of the American Veterinary Medical Association* **180**, 415–418.

Pilcher, M.E. and Turnwald, G.H. (1985) Blood transfusion in the dog and cat. Part I. Physiology, collection, storage and indications for whole blood therapy. *Compendium of Continuing Education for the Practicing Veterinarian* **7**, 64–71.

Pijnappels, M.I.M., Briet, E., van der Zweet, G.Th., Huisden, R., van Tilburg, N.H. and Eulderink, F. (1986) Evaluation of the cuticle bleeding time in canine haemophilia A. *Thrombosis and Haemostasis* **55**, 70–73.

Pion, P.D. (1989) Aortic thromboemboli and thrombolytic therapy. *Veterinary Clinics of North America Small Animal Practice* **18**, 79–86.

Porter, R.E., Weiser, M.G. and Callahan, G.N. (1989) Development of an enzyme-linked immunosorbent assay to detect IgG, IgM and complement (C_3) on canine erythrocytes. *American Journal of Veterinary Research* **50**, 1365–1369.

Prasse, K.W., Crouser, D., Beutler, E., Walker, M. and Schall, W.D. (1975) Pyruvate kinase deficiency anemia with terminal myelofibrosis and osteosclerosis in a beagle. *Journal of the American Veterinary Medical Association* **166**, 1170–1175.

Raskin, R.E. and Krehbiel, J.D. (1989) Prevalence of leukemic blood and bone marrow in dogs with multicentric lymphoma. *Journal of the American Veterinary Medical Association* **194**, 1427–1429.

Relford, R.L. (1991) The steps in performing a bone marrow aspiration and core biopsy. *Veterinary Medicine* **6**, 670–688.

Renshaw, H.W. and Davis, W.C. (1979) Canine granulocytopathy syndrome: an inherited disorder of leukocyte function. *American Journal of Pathology* **95**, 731–744.

Searcy, G.P., Tasker, J.B. and Miller, D.R. (1979) Animal model of human disease: pyruvate kinase deficiency. *American Journal of Pathology* **94**, 689–692.

Shelton, G.H., Linenberger, M.L., Grant, C.K. and Abkowitz, J.L. (1990) Hematologic manifestations of feline immunodeficiency virus infection. *Blood* 76, 1104–1109.

Shull, R.M., DeNovo, R.C. and McCracken, M.D. (1986) Megakaryoblastic leukemia in a dog. *Veterinary Pathology* 23, 533–536.

Simpson, J.W., Else, R.W. and Honeyman, P. (1990) Successful treatment of suspected essential thrombocythaemia in the dog. *Journal of Small Animal Practice* 31, 345–348.

Slappendel, R.J. (1979) The diagnostic significance of the direct antiglobulin test (DAT) in anaemic dogs. *Veterinary Immunology and Immunopathology* 1, 49–59.

Slappendel, R.J. (1986) Interpretation of tests for immune-mediated blood diseases. In: *Current Veterinary Therapy IX* (Ed. R.W. Kirk). W.B. Saunders, Philadelphia, pp. 498–505.

Smith, J.E. (1989) Iron metabolism and its diseases. In: *Clinical Biochemistry of Domestic Animals*, 4th edn (Ed. J.J. Kaneko). Academic Press, San Diego, pp. 256–273.

Smith, J.E. (1991) Erythrocytes. *Advances in Veterinary Science and Comparative Medicine* 36, 9–55.

Spurling, N.W. (1980) Hereditary disorders of haemostasis in dogs: a critical review of the literature. *Veterinary Bulletin* 50, 151–173.

Stokol, T., Parry, B.W. and Mansell, P.D. (1995a) von Willebrand's disease in dobermann dogs in Australia. *Australian Veterinary Journal* 72, 257–262.

Stokol, T., Parry, B.W., Mansell, P.D. and Richardson, J.L. (1995b) Hematorrhachis associated with hemophilia A in three German shepherd dogs. *Journal of the American Animal Hospital Association* 239.

Stone, M.S. and Freden, G.O. (1990) Differentiation of anemia of inflammatory disease from anemia of iron deficiency. *Compendium of Continuing Education for the Practicing Veterinarian* 12, 963–966.

Stone, E., Badner, D. and Cotter, S.M. (1992) Trends in transfusion medicine in dogs at a veterinary school: 315 cases (1986–1989). *Journal of the American Veterinary Medical Association* 200, 1000–1004.

Stone, M.S., Johnstone, I.B., Brooks, M., Bollinger, T.K. and Cotter, S.M. (1994) Lupus-type 'anticoagulant' in a dog with hemolysis and thrombosis. *Journal of Veterinary Internal Medicine* 8, 57–61.

Sullivan, P.S., Manning, K.L. and McDonald, T.P. (1995) Association of mean platelet volume and bone marrow megakaryocytopoiesis in thrombocytopenic dogs: 60 dogs (1984–1993). *Journal of the American Veterinary Medical Association* 206, 332–334.

Suzuki, K. and Kubo, A. (1996) Validation and application of an enzyme-linked immunoassay for human erythropoietin to canine serum. *Research in Veterinary Science* 61, 13–16.

Symons, M. and Bell, K. (1991) Expansion of the canine A blood group system. *Animal Genetics* 22, 227–235.

Teske, E. (1986) Estrogen-induced bone marrow toxicity. In: *Current Veterinary Therapy IX* (Ed. R.W. Kirk). W.B. Saunders, Philadelphia, pp. 495–498.

Troward-Wigh, G., Hakansson, L., Johannisson, A., Norrgren, L. and Hard-af-Segersted, C. (1992) Leucocyte adhesion protein deficiency in Irish setter dogs. *Veterinary Immunology and Immunopathology* 32, 261–280.

Turnwald, G.H. and Pilcher, M.E. (1985) Blood transfusion in the dog and cat. Part II. Administration, adverse effects and component therapy. *Compendium of Continuing Education for the Practicing Veterinarian* 7, 115–125.

Tzavaras, T., Stewart, M., McDougall, A., Fulton, R., Testa, N., Onions, D.E. and Neil, J.C. (1990) Molecular cloning and characterization of a defective recombinant feline leukaemia virus associated with myeloid leukaemia. *Journal of General Virology* 71, 343–354.

Valli, V.E.O. and Parry, B.W. (1993) The haemopoietic system. In: *Pathology of Domestic Animals*, 4th edn (Eds K.V.F. Jubb, P.C. Kennedy and N. Palmer). Academic Press, San Diego, pp. 101–265.

Verlander, J.W., Gorman, N.T. and Dodds, W.J. (1984) Factor IX deficiency (hemophilia B) in a litter of labrador retrievers. *Journal of the American Veterinary Medical Association* 185, 83–84.

Watson, A.D.J. (1990) Feline precursor porphyria, characterised by persistent delta aminolevulinic aciduria. *Journal of Small Animal Practice* 31, 393–397.

Watson, A.D.J., Moore, A.S. and Helfand, S.C. (1994) Primary erythrocytosis in the cat: treatment with hydroxyurea. *Journal of Small Animal Practice* 35, 320–325.

Weiss, D.J. (1986) Antibody-mediated suppression of erythropoiesis in dogs with red blood cell aplasia. *American Journal of Veterinary Research* 47, 2647–2648.

Weiss, D.J. and Adams, L.J. (1987) Aplastic anemia associated with trimethoprim-sulfadiazine and fenbendazole administration in a dog. *Journal of the American Veterinary Medical Association* 191, 1119–1120.

Weiss, D.J. and Klausner, J.S. (1990) Drug-associated aplastic anemia in dogs: eight cases (1984–1988) *Journal of the American Veterinary Medical Association* 196, 472–475.

Weiss, H.J. (1975) Platelet physiology and abnormalities of platelet function. *New England Journal of Medicine* 293, 580–588.

Werner, L.L. and Bright, J.M. (1983) Drug-induced immune hypersensitivity disorders in two dogs treated with trimethoprim-sulphadiazine: case reports and drug challenge studies. *Journal of the American Animal Hospital Association* 19, 783–790.

Woods, J.P., Johnstone, I.B., Bienzle, D., Balson, G. and Gartley, C.J. (1995) Concurrent lymphangioma, immune-mediated thrombocytopenia and von Willebrand's disease in a dog. *Journal of the American Animal Hospital Association* 31, 70–76.

FURTHER READING

Brown. N.O. (1985) Guest editor. Canine hematopoietic tumors. *Veterinary Clinics of North America* **15** (4).

Carr, A.P. and Johnson, G.S. (1994) A review of hemostatic abnormalities in dogs and cats. *Journal of the American Animal Hospital Association* **30**, 475–482.

Davenport, D.J. and Carakostas, M.C. (1982) Platelet disorders in the dog and cat. Part 1: Physiology and pathogenesis. *Compendium on Continuing Education for the Practicing Veterinarian* **4**, 762–772.

Feldman, B.F. (1988) Guest editor. Hemostasis. *Veterinary Clinics of North America Small Animal Practice* **18** (1).

Fineman, L.S. (1996) Diagnosing and treating canine idiopathic thrombocytopenic purpura. *Veterinary Medicine*, September issue 829–840.

Halliwell, R.E.W. and Gorman, N.T. (1989) Diseases associated with immunodeficiency. In: *Veterinary Clinical Immunology* (Eds R.E.W. Halliwell and N.T. Gorman). W.B. Saunders, Philadelphia, pp. 449–466.

Harvey, J.W. (1984) Canine bone marrow: normal haematopoiesis, biopsy techniques and cell identification and evaluation. *Compendium of Continuing Education for the Practicing Veterinarian* **6**, 909–927.

Hawkey, C.M. and Dennett, T.B. (1989) *A Colour Atlas of Comparative Veterinary Haematology*. Wolfe Medical Publications, London.

Honeckman, A.L., Knapp, D.W. and Reagan, W.J. (1996) Diagnosis of canine immune-mediated haematologic disease. *Compendium on Continuing Education for the Practicing Veterinarian* **18**, 113–127.

Jain, N.C. (1986) *Schalm's Veterinary Haematology*, 4th edn. Lea and Febiger, Philadelphia.

Jain, N.C. (1993) *Essentials of Veterinary Haematology*. Lea and Febiger, Philadelphia.

Jain, N.M. and Zinkl, J.G. (1981) Guest editors. Clinical Hematology. *Veterinary Clinics of North America* **11** (2).

Lewis, D.C. and Meyers, K.M. (1996) Canine idiopathic thrombocytopenic purpura. *Journal of Veterinary Internal Medicine* **10**, 207–218.

Lewis, H.B. and Rebar, A.H. (1979) *Bone Marrow Evaluation in Veterinary Practice*. Ralston Purina Co., St Louis.

Littlewood, J.D. (1986) A practical approach to bleeding disorders in the dog. *Journal of Small Animal Practice* **27**, 397–409.

Littlewood, J.D. (1989) Inherited bleeding disorders of dogs and cats. *Journal of Small Animal Practice* **30**, 140–143.

Littlewood, J.D. (1992) Differential diagnosis of haemorrhagic disorders in dogs. *In Practice* **14**, 172–180.

Mackey, L. (1977) Haematology of the cat. In: *Comparative Clinical Haematology* (Eds R.K. Archer and L.B. Jeffcot). Blackwell Scientific Publications, Oxford, pp. 441–482.

Morris, J.S. and Dunn, J.K. (1992) Haematology. *In Practice* **14**, 67–72.

Parry, B.W. (1989) Guest editor. Clinical Pathology: Part I. *Veterinary Clinics of North America* **19** (4).

Perman, V., Alsaker, R.D. and Riis, R.C. (1979) *Cytology of the Dog and Cat*. American Animal Hospital Association publication, Indiana.

Raskin, R.E. and Krehbiel, J.D. (1988) Histopathology of canine bone marrow in malignant lymphoproliferative disorders. *Veterinary Pathology* **25**, 83–88.

Rebar, A.H. (1987) *Handbook of Veterinary Cytology*. Ralston Purina Company, St Louis, Missouri.

Rich, L.J. (1974) *The Morphology of Canine and Feline Blood Cells*. Ralston Purina Company, St Louis, Missouri.

Slappendel, R.J. (1989) Disseminated Intravascular Coagulation. In: *Current Veterinary Therapy* X (Ed. R.W. Kirk). W.B. Saunders, Philadelphia, pp. 451–457.

Smith, C.A., Andrews, C.M., Collard, J.K., Hall, D.E. and Walker, A.K. (1994) *Color Atlas of Comparative Diagnostic and Experimental Hematology*. Wolfe Publishing, Mosby Year Book, London.

Squires, R. (1993) Differential diagnosis of anaemia in dogs. *In Practice* **15**, 29–36.

Squires, R. (1993) Management of anaemia in dogs. *In Practice* **15**, 92–94.

Thomas, J.S. (1996) Von Willebrand's disease in the dog and cat. *Veterinary Clinics of North America: Small Animal Practice* **26**, 1089–1110.

Young, K.M. (1985) Myeloproliferative disorders. *Veterinary Clinics of North America* **15**, 769–781.

46

Diseases of the Eye

S. M. Petersen-Jones

Introduction	820	Conditions of the fundus	847
History taking	820	Conditions of the optic nerve and optic disc	854
Physical examination	821	Neuro-ophthalmology	855
Ophthalmological examination	821		
OCULAR CONDITIONS OF THE DOG	**823**	**OCULAR CONDITIONS OF THE CAT**	**858**
Conditions of the orbit and globe	823	Conditions of the globe and orbit	858
Conditions of the eyelids	825	Conditions of the eyelids	858
Conditions of the lacrimal and nasolacrimal systems	828	Conditions of the third eyelid	859
		Conditions of the conjunctiva	859
Conditions of the third eyelid	829	Conditions involving the tear film	860
Conditions of the conjunctiva	830	Conditions of the cornea	860
Conditions of the cornea and sclera	831	Conditions of the anterior uvea	861
Conditions of the anterior uvea	836	Glaucoma	863
Glaucoma	839	Conditions of the lens	863
Conditions of the lens	842	Conditions of the posterior segment	863
Conditions of the vitreous	846	Neuro-ophthalmology	865

INTRODUCTION

The eye is a unique organ which by its very function, can be observed in great detail often allowing direct visualization of pathological change and rapid diagnosis. Its response to disease can be deleterious to function, therefore early diagnosis and appropriate medication to modify this response is required. This chapter starts with a brief description of the examination of the eye, then using an anatomical approach considers the ocular diseases of the dog and then finally covers those conditions of the cat which are unique to this species or differ from those described in the dog.

HISTORY TAKING

A full clinical history is an essential part of any ophthalmic examination. The signalment can be very useful: many ocular conditions, particularly in the dog, are breed related and some develop at characteristic ages. The order in which clinical signs develop can also be useful and should be ascertained by careful questioning, as should the speed of onset, rate of progression and details of any treatment already administered. Ocular disorders can result from systemic disease, therefore the animal's general health and medical history should be determined.

PHYSICAL EXAMINATION

A full clinical examination is an important part of the investigation of ocular disease.

OPHTHALMOLOGICAL EXAMINATION (Mould, 1993; Cottrell and Petersen-Jones, 1993)

Equipment

A few basic facilities and pieces of equipment are required to perform a thorough ophthalmic examination.

Examination room

A well lit room, which can be darkened, is essential.

Focal illumination

A bright focal light source is required. A pen-torch or transilluminator (e.g. a Finnoff transilluminator) can be used.

Magnification

Magnification is helpful, and sometimes essential. The direct ophthalmoscope provides some magnification (positive dioptre lenses are selected) or loupes may be used. The slit-lamp biomicroscope is the most useful instrument for detailed examination of the eye and offers great benefits in detecting and localizing lesions.

Direct ophthalmoscopy

The direct ophthalmoscope may be used for distant or close ophthalmoscopy. *Distant direct ophthalmoscopy* is useful for visualizing opacities within the transparent structures of the eye and for comparing pupil size. The examiner observes the eye from arm's length through the direct ophthalmoscope with a zero lens selected. Opacities appear as dark shadows against the reflection from the tapetum. When performing *close direct ophthalmoscopy* the instrument should be held at 2–3 cm from the cornea. Table 46.1 shows the power of lens used to examine the various parts of the eye.

Table 46.1 Power of direct ophthalmoscope lens required for examination of various areas of the eye

Structure	Power of lens in dioptres (for emmetropic examiner)
Cornea	+20 – +40
Anterior surface of lens	+12
Posterior surface of lens	+8
Vitreous	+8 – 0
Fundus	0
Depths of colobomas of the fundus	0 – several minus dioptres (depending on depth)

Indirect ophthalmoscopy

The examiner stands at arm's length from the patient and looks along a beam of light with a condensing lens (15–30 dioptre) positioned at 4–8 cm from the animal's cornea. An inverted and reversed aerial image of a relatively wide area of the fundus is formed.

Table 46.2 compares direct and indirect ophthalmoscopy.

Other examination equipment and materials

- Schirmer tear test strips
- Fluorescein dye (impregnated paper strips or single dose bottles)
- Local anaesthetic drops, e.g. proxymetacaine (Ophthaine, Squibb)
- Mydriatic drops, e.g. tropicamide (Mydriacyl, Alcon)

Table 46.2 Comparison of fundoscopy by direct and indirect ophthalmoscopy

Feature	Direct ophthalmoscope	Indirect ophthalmoscope
Position of image	Direct visualization of fundus	Aerial image
Field of view	9–10°	40° (with 20 dioptre lens)
Magnification of image	15–17 times	2–4 times
Image orientation	Real and erect	Inverted and reversed
Stereopsis?	No	Yes with most commercial types
Visualization through opacities	Can be poor	Good
Visualization of peripheral fundus	Can be difficult	Good

- Nasolacrimal cannulae
- Tonometer
- Gonioscopy lens

Procedure for an ophthalmic examination

A thorough systematic approach should be used. Certain tests must, by necessity, be performed before others; for example, a Schirmer tear test must be performed before any eye drops are administered, and the pupillary light responses examined before the administration of a mydriatic.

Initial examination under normal lighting conditions

The unrestrained animal is observed from a distance, looking for any asymmetry of the head and eyes, ocular discharges and eye and lid movements and positions. Gentle restraint is then employed and the adnexa, eyelids and ocular surface are examined more closely. The eyelid margins are carefully examined and each eyelid retracted in turn to expose the conjunctival sacs. A healthy cornea and coating tear film should result in an even reflection of light. The external surface of the third eyelid is examined by pressing on the globe through the upper eyelid thus protruding the third eyelid; this additionally allows an assessment of the degree to which the globes can be repelled into the orbits. Vision testing may be performed at this stage: the menace response and the ability to follow cotton wool balls are useful for assessing vision in puppies and cats; in addition obstacle courses, coupled with unilateral blindfolding, can be used in most dogs.

Detailed examination in a darkened room

A focal light source is used to examine the eyes in more detail. Examination of adnexa, lids and ocular surface is repeated, again comparing the two sides. When reduced tear production is suspected a *Schirmer tear test* should be performed before further manipulation. A standard strip of filter paper is bent at 90° 5 mm from one end. The short end is hooked between lower lid and cornea for one minute and the length of paper which becomes wet is measured. A normal result is in the region of 15–25 mm min^{-1}.

The *pupillary light responses* (PLRs) are checked. A swinging flash light test can be used: the light is initially shone into one eye and the direct PLR noted; it is quickly swung across to illuminate the other eye, the pupil of which should already be constricted (consensual response), and should remain so. When initially examined the PLR of nervous animals is often poor but will improve in a few minutes.

Fluorescein dye is used to stain corneal ulcers. Excess dye should always be flushed from the ocular surface with sterile saline, to prevent false positives. The appearance of dye at the external nares indicates that tear drainage is occurring.

The eye is *viewed obliquely*, as well as from directly in front, looking both along the beam of light and across it. This aids in the localization of lesions.

A *mydriatic* such as tropicamide is used to allow a full ophthalmic examination.

Examination of the fundus is performed using an ophthalmoscope as described above.

Laboratory examination

A number of samples for laboratory tests may be required to investigate ocular disease:

- Swabs for bacterial, chlamydial or viral culture
- Scrapes for surface cytology
- Biopsies
- Blood for haematology, biochemistry and serology

Further investigations

Tonometry: assessment of intraocular pressure (IOP)

The simplest and cheapest tonometer is the Schiøtz tonometer which uses a corneal indentation method for measuring IOP. Conversion tables for the dog are available (Peiffer *et al.*, 1977), although it has been suggested that conversion tables used for humans may be more accurate (Miller and Pickett, 1992). Most veterinary ophthalmologists favour applanation tonometers such as the Tonopen (Carelton Optical Equipment Co. Ltd, London).

Digital assessment of IOP can detect gross alterations and is of limited value in the diagnosis and management of glaucoma.

Gonioscopy

Examination of the iridocorneal drainage angle using a diagnostic contact lens (goniolens) is important in the investigation of glaucoma. The drainage angle is the opening into the ciliary cleft at the iris base via which aqueous drains from the eye (Bedford, 1977 gives a description of the normal canine drainage angle). The Barkan Lo-vac lens (Medical Workshop, Holland) is relatively easy to use in dogs and cats.

Imaging

- *Radiography* may be useful in the investigation of orbital disease where there is bony involvement.
- *Ultrasonography* of the globe can detect intraocular lesions where opacity prevents direct visualization and is also useful for investigating orbital disease (Cottrill *et al.*, 1989; Dziezyc *et al.*, 1987).
- *Computerized axial tomography* and *magnetic resonance imaging* are newer methods which offer greatly superior imaging of the globe and retrobulbar area.

Electrophysiology

Electroretinography (measuring retinal electrical responses) can be used to detect generalized retinal disease before ophthalmoscopic signs are present, or if other lesions prevent funduscopy (Acland, 1988).

Ocular Conditions of the Dog

CONDITIONS OF THE ORBIT AND GLOBE

Microphthalmos

Microphthalmos (a congenitally small eye) varies in severity from cases where only a small amount of rudimentary ocular tissue is present, to cases with an abnormally small but functional eye.

Microphthalmos accompanied by cataract (often non-progressive), persistent pupillary membranes (Fig. 46.1) and sometimes retinal dysplasia is seen in a number of breeds of dog, although inheritance has not been proven in many instances:

- Cavalier King Charles spaniel (Narfström and Dubielzig, 1984)
- Dobermann (Peiffer and Fischer, 1983; Lewis *et al.*, 1986)
- English cocker spaniel (Olesen *et al.*, 1974; Strande *et al.*, 1988)
- Lancashire heeler (Barnett, 1988)
- Miniature schnauzer (Gelatt *et al.*, 1983)
- Old English sheepdog (Barnett, 1985)
- West Highland white terrier (Narfström, 1981)

Environmental and genetic factors have been implicated in this condition.

Colour dilute animals such as Harlequin great Danes and merle collies may suffer from multiple congenital abnormalities including microphthalmos with multiple ocular defects and deafness (Gwin *et al.*, 1981).

Phthisis bulbi

Destruction of the ciliary body due to severe intraocular disease results in an eye with a low intraocular pressure which slowly shrinks down in size i.e. becomes phthisical (Fig. 46.2).

Buphthalmos

A chronically enlarged glaucomatous globe (Fig. 46.2).

Exophthalmos

The abnormal anterior displacement of the globe as a result of an orbital space-occupying lesion.

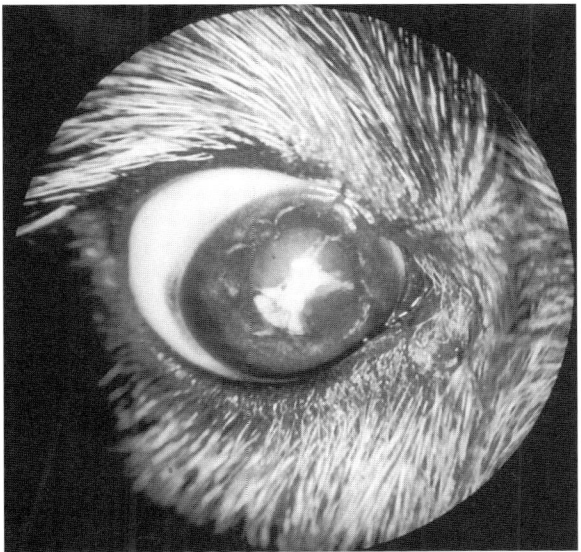

Figure 46.1 Microphthalmos, congenital cataracts and persistent pupillary membranes in an English cocker spaniel puppy.

824 DISEASES OF THE EYE

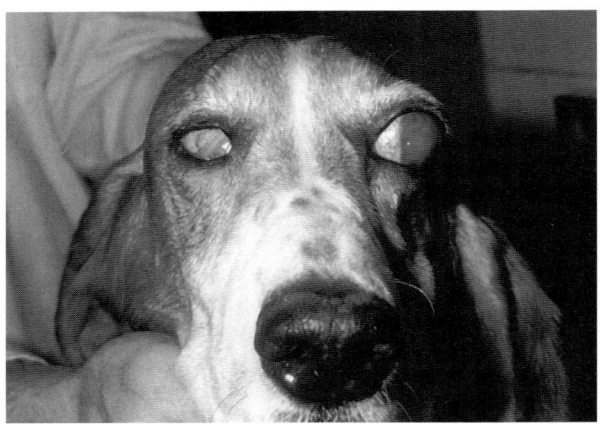

Figure 46.2 Bassett hound with phthisis bulbi of the right eye and buphthalmos of the left eye. The changes are both due to chronic glaucoma.

The site of the mass affects the direction of displacement; for example, a mass ventrally positioned within the orbit will cause an anterior and dorsal deviation of the globe. Exophthalmos may be accompanied by protrusion of the third eyelid (Fig. 46.3), conjunctivitis or chemosis, ocular discharge, and exposure keratitis, if the lids are unable to close completely.

The causes of exophthalmos are considered in Table 46.3.

■ Enophthalmos

Enophthalmos is an abnormally deep-set globe. It occurs commonly in some breeds (e.g. Dobermann, rough collie) and results in accumulation of mucus in the deep medial canthal pocket. Acquired enophthalmos may result from:

Table 46.3 Causes of exophthalmos

Cause of exophthalmos	Typical presentation	Aids in diagnosis	Treatment
Retrobulbar abscess/cellulitis (most common)	Unilateral, rapid onset, painful, pain on opening mouth, may have a discharge of pus. May result from penetrating wounds in the mouth or pharynx	Clinical signs, haematology, ultrasonography	Surgical drainage via blunt dissection through the oral mucosa behind the last upper molar tooth. Provide antibiotics (following culture and sensitivity testing)
Retrobulbar tumour (most common)	Usually unilateral, slow onset of signs not usually painful. May be primary or secondary tumours (Fig. 46.3) or extension from adjacent structures (e.g. sinuses, nasal chambers, cranial and oral cavities)	Clinical signs, haematology, ultrasonography, radiography. Fine needle aspiration can be used with care, ideally with ultrasonographic guidance	Complete excision unlikely to be possible. Chemotherapy, radiotherapy
Masticatory myositis	Bilateral, acute onset, painful, particularly on opening mouth. German shepherd dogs, weimeraner	Clinical signs, breed, swelling of masticatory muscles, muscle biopsy	Corticosteroids
Zygomatic mucocoele	Unilateral, gradual onset, painless	Clinical signs, dorsal deviation of globe, ultrasonography, sialography	Extirpation of gland
Temperomandibular osteopathy	Young West Highland white or Scottish terriers, or occasionally other breeds. Exophthalmos is a rare complication	Clinical signs, radiography	Symptomatic therapy
Arteriovenous shunts	Congenital, unilateral, rare. Pulsatile, palpable bruit	Clinical signs. Venography or arteriography	Ligation difficult

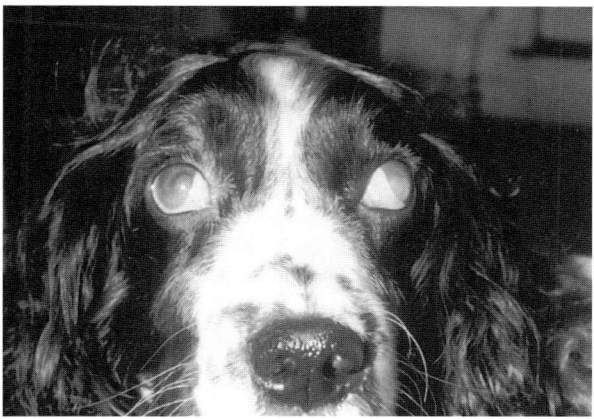

Figure 46.3 Bilateral exophthalmos in a young English springer spaniel with lymphoma. Both third eyelids are protruded due to the orbital swelling. There is also anterior uveal involvement.

- Retraction of a painful eye
- Horner's syndrome
- Loss of orbital tissue – dehydration, cachexia, masticatory muscle atrophy, neoplastic destruction
- Tissue contracture, e.g. contracture of extraocular muscles following myositis

Traumatic proptosis and prolapse of the globe

Proptosis is an anterior displacement of the globe whereas prolapse is the dislocation of the globe beyond the plane of the eyelids which occurs relatively easily in brachycephalic breeds. Accompanying intraocular and optic nerve damage may be present and tearing of the extraocular muscles (especially the medial rectus) can, in the long-term, result in a squint. Prompt treatment is required. The cornea should be kept moistened until the globe can be replaced and a temporary tarsorraphy performed. Sutures are removed once the swelling has resolved.

Other trauma to the globe

Blunt trauma to the globe can cause severe injury such as rupture of the globe or luxation of the lens, hyphaema and retinal detachment.

CONDITIONS OF THE EYELIDS

Ophthalmia neonatorum

Infections sometimes develop in the conjunctival sac before the eyelids open. The fused eyelids appear swollen and a small amount of purulent discharge may escape from the medial canthus. Corneal penetration can develop if the condition is not treated promptly by opening the lids along their line of fusion using fine, blunt-ended scissors. Material should be collected for culture and the conjunctival sac irrigated thoroughly. Antibiotic ointment should be applied frequently until the infection has resolved and tear production has become established.

Macropalpebral fissure

Breeds such as bloodhounds, Saint Bernards and clumber spaniels have an overlong palpebral fissure associated with a 'diamond eye'. Brachycephalic breeds often have a macropalpebral fissure and an inadequate blink resulting in an exposure keratitis. Surgical shortening of the eyelids may be required.

Abnormalities of eyelid position

Entropion

Inturning of the eyelids is common in dogs and is probably inherited in some breeds (Gelatt, 1991). Eyelid hair contacts the cornea causing discomfort, increased lacrimation, blepharospasm and even keratitis or ulceration. The age of onset differs between breeds. Some, such as the shar pei can develop entropion shortly after the lids open. A temporary eversion of the eyelids using 'tacking sutures' may be sufficient treatment in such cases (Johnson et al., 1988). Some breeds, such as retrievers and the chow chow develop entropion at a slightly later age. Permanent surgical eversion of the affected portion of the lid is often required in these cases (Gelatt, 1991).

Upper eyelid entropion/trichiasis, in which the eyelid turns in and hairs on its outer surface are directed onto the cornea, often coupled with lower eyelid ectropion occurs in older English cocker spaniels. The drooping and inturned upper eyelid may cause ulcerative keratitis and also obscure vision (Fig. 46.4). A procedure to evert the lid and create a band of hairless skin adjacent

DISEASES OF THE EYE

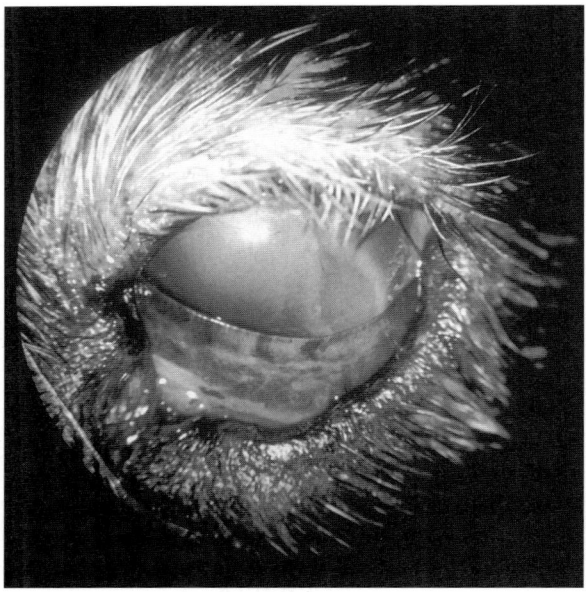

Figure 46.4 Upper eyelid entropion/trichiasis in a middle-aged English cocker spaniel. The trichiasis has resulted in a superficial ulcerative keratitis.

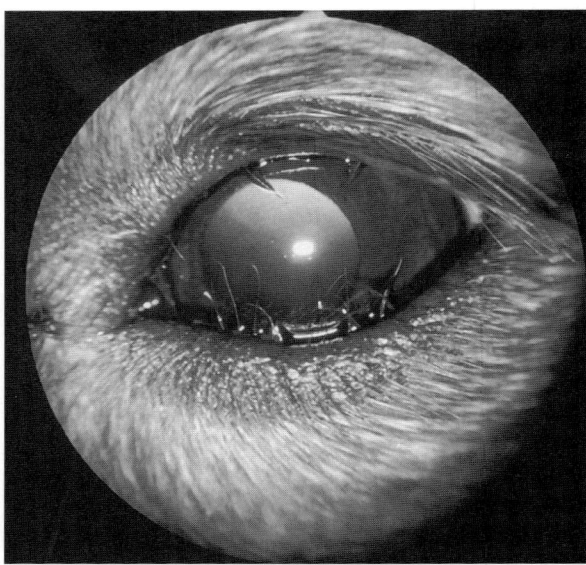

Figure 46.5 Distichiasis in a Shetland sheepdog.

to the eyelid margin is the most effective treatment (Stades, 1987).

Ectropion

An outward turning of the lower eyelid (ectropion) is a common breed related problem. Ectropion tends to worsen with fatigue. Only rarely is surgical intervention necessary.

Dogs with a 'diamond eye' conformation can suffer from entropion in addition to ectropion. This is associated with macropalpebral fissure and a weak lateral canthal ligament. When entropion or excessive ectropion is present, surgical correction is indicated (Wyman, 1971).

■ Conditions involving cilia

Distichiasis (Fig. 46.5 and 46.6)

Distichia are cilia which emerge along the eyelid margin and are common in certain breeds. The cilia emerge at a young age and in many cases do not cause significant clinical signs. When distichia cause problems such as irritation or corneal ulceration, surgery to destroy or remove the offending follicles is indicated. This may be performed by electrolysis, cryosurgery or surgical excision (see Gelatt, 1991, for a review).

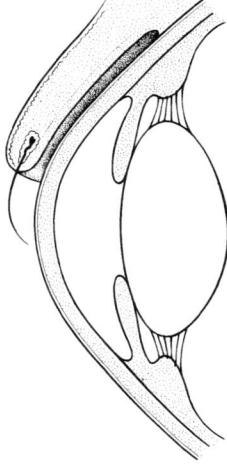

Figure 46.6 Diagram of a cross section of an eyelid demonstrating the presence of a distichium.

Ectopic cilia (Fig. 46.7)

An ectopic cilium emerges through the palpebral conjunctiva often midway along the upper eyelid. It is less common than distichiasis and usually unilateral. The offending hair(s) usually emerges in the young adult and may be difficult to see. They do cause irritation and often a superficial keratitis and ulceration. Surgical excision of the follicle is required.

Infections and inflammation of the eyelids

Inflammation of the eyelids (blepharitis) occurs commonly in the dog. It may be associated with more widespread dermatitis or accompany ocular surface disease. The various aetiologies of blepharitis are listed in Table 46.4. Many of these conditions are covered in Chapter 47.

Eyelid injuries

Traumatic eyelid injuries are common. Reconstructive surgery should be performed promptly, paying particular attention to restoring a normal lid–cornea relationship. Cicatrix formation can result in ectropion or trichiasis.

Eyelid neoplasia

Eyelid neoplasia is common in older dogs. Benign sebaceous adenomas arising from the meibomian

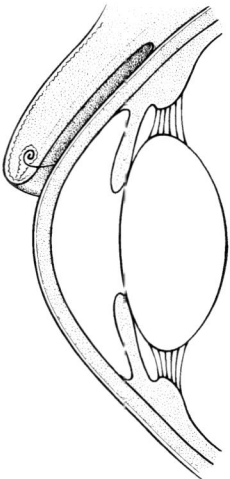

Figure 46.7 Diagram of a cross section of an eyelid demonstrating the presence of an ectopic cilium.

Trichiasis

This is a condition whereby facial hair contacts the ocular surface. The nasal folds of some brachycephalic breeds may contact the cornea causing a superficial pigmentary keratitis. Surgical resection of the nasal folds may be required (Carter, 1973).

Table 46.4 Causes of blepharitis

Aetiology	Diagnosis
Parasitic • *Sarcoptes* • *Demodex*	• Skin scrapings
Bacterial infection • blepharitis • external stye • meibomianitis and chalazion	• Swabs for bacteriology • drain abscess or chalazion or express meibomian secretion for culture (staphylococcal spp. often isolated)
Fungal infection (ringworm)	• Woods lamp examination • Skin scrape • Fungal culture
Immune-mediated • pemphigus • uveodermatological syndrome – eyelid poliosis and vitiligo	• Biopsy – histopathology and immunopathology • Clinical signs
Allergic • food • contact • drugs • atopy	• Clinical signs • Hypoallergenic diets • Intradermal skin testing
Postparotid duct transposition (occurs with overflow of saliva)	• Swab for bacteriology
Secondary to ocular irritation (due to self-inflicted trauma)	• Demonstrate primary source of irritation
Seborrhoeic	• Clinical signs
Endocrine related • Hyperadrenocorticism • Hypothyroidism	• Clinical signs • Endocrine assessment

gland are the most common. Other neoplasms include squamous papilloma, melanoma, sebaceous adenocarcinoma, histiocytoma, mastocytoma, basal cell carcinoma and squamous cell carcinoma (Roberts et al., 1986). Complete surgical excision is the treatment of choice.

CONDITIONS OF THE LACRIMAL AND NASOLACRIMAL SYSTEMS

The tear film, consisting of lipid, aqueous and mucus layers, coats the corneal and conjunctival surfaces and is extremely important in maintaining a healthy and functional ocular surface. Drainage of tears to the nasal chambers occurs via the nasolacrimal system (Fig. 46.8).

Keratoconjunctivitis sicca (KCS)

KCS primarily results from a deficiency of the aqueous phase of the tear film. It can occur congenitally or, more commonly, as an acquired problem. The commonest cause is a probable immune-mediated destruction of the lacrimal and nictitans glands. Drug toxicity (for example sulphonamides), systemic disease (for example distemper), trauma and denervation of the tear-producing glands are other possible causes. The West Highland white terrier has a strong breed predilection for KCS with approximately 35% of cases in the UK occurring in this breed (Sansom and Barnett, 1985). Other breeds commonly

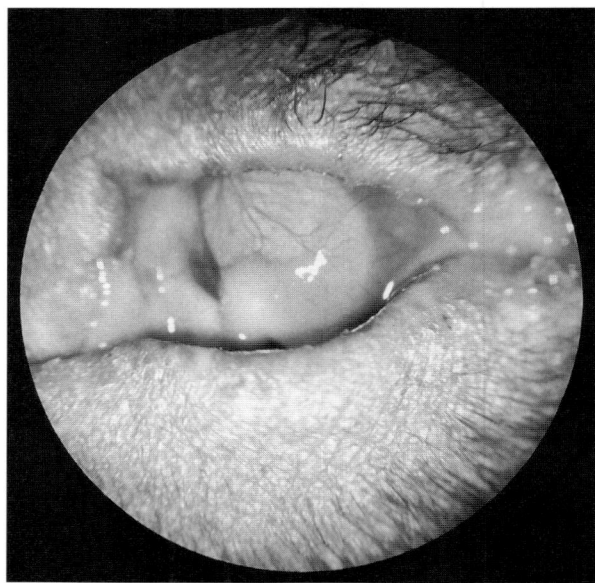

Figure 46.9 Keratoconjunctivitis sicca in a 6-year-old Irish water spaniel. Note the typical tenaceous mucopurulent ocular discharge and the resulting superficial keratitis. See colour plate.

affected include the English cocker spaniel, cavalier King Charles spaniel, English bulldog, Lhasa apso and shih tzu.

Clinical signs

KCS is usually a chronic condition with an insidious onset. Initially it may present as a recurrent conjunctivitis, but typically more severe ocular surface pathology develops. Tenacious mucopurulent material accumulates within the conjunctival fornices and adheres to the corneal surface (Fig. 46.9). Conjunctival hyperaemia, thickening and pigmentation are features; the cornea lacks lustre and develops a pigmentary superficial keratitis. Corneal ulceration occasionally occurs and may be complicated by secondary bacterial infection.

Acute onset of KCS is less common, but often results in corneal ulceration and even perforation.

Diagnosis

Diagnosis is based on history, clinical signs, visual assessment of the tear film and measurement of aqueous tear production using the Schirmer tear test (STT). Dogs with clinical signs of KCS usually have STT levels below 10 mm min^{-1}. It is not uncommon for more severely affected eyes to have STT levels of 0 mm min^{-1}.

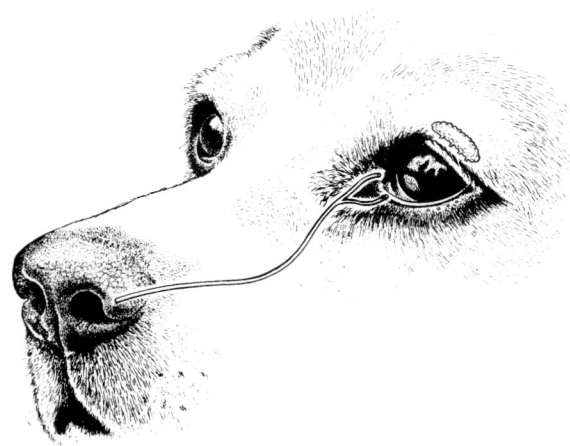

Figure 46.8 Diagram showing tear production and drainage.

Treatment

- *Nursing* – regular cleaning of the eye with sterile water or saline.
- *Treatment of surface pathology* – corneal ulceration often requires surgical management (for example third eyelid flap, or if deep, conjunctival flaps or grafts). Topical antibiotics are applied if a secondary bacterial infection develops. Superficial keratitis may be treated by topical cyclosporin, or if non-ulcerative topical corticosteroids.
- *Tear replacement* – many different artificial tear replacement preparations are available. These need to be applied four to six times daily or sometimes more frequently.
- *Stimulation of lacrimation* – cyclosporin has a lacrimogenic effect (Kaswan and Salisbury, 1990). Animals with denervation of the lacrimal gland may respond well to oral administration of pilocarpine (1–4 drops of 1% pilocarpine 12 hourly).
- *Treatment of immune-mediated dacryoadenitis* – cyclosporin, applied twice daily, has become widely used to treat KCS (Kaswan and Salisbury, 1990). Topical corticosteroids have also been used to suppress active dacryoadenitis.
- *Surgical treatment* – transposition of the parotid duct can be very effective at controlling the condition when medical therapy has failed to do so. Complications include salivary epiphora (especially at meal times) resulting in blepharitis, and corneal crystallization causing irritation.

Abnormalities of the tear drainage system

Tear overflow

A tear overflow may result from inadequate tear drainage and/or increased lacrimation (due to pain or irritation). Fluorescein passage tests assess overall tear drainage. The dye is placed in the conjunctival sac and should appear at the ipsilateral naris within 3–4 min. Tears may drain to the caudal nasal chambers in brachycephalic breeds giving a negative result. The patency of the nasolacrimal system is further investigated by cannulation and flushing.

Inadequate passage of tears into the nasolacrimal system

Epiphora is common in breeds such as miniature and toy poodles and bichon frisé. The resultant tear staining (particularly noticeable in white coated dogs) is a cosmetic problem. There are a number of factors involved:

- hairs on the caruncle act as a wick to draw tears on to the face
- impaired drainage through the lower punctum due to a prominent globe with tight apposition to the lower lid or medial lower eyelid entropion
- a shallow medial canthal tear lake (tears squeezed on to the face during blinking)

Congenital abnormalities of the nasolacrimal system

- *Imperforate lower punctum* – epiphora is often not noticed until the animal is several months of age. Cannulation and flushing via the upper punctum causes conjunctiva over the lower canaliculus to bulge. A lower punctal opening may be created surgically.
- *Micropunctum* – an abnormally small lower punctum is said to impede tear drainage.
- *Agenesis of other components of the nasolacrimal system* – occasionally more extensive agenesis of parts of the nasolacrimal system occurs.
- *Acquired obstructions of the nasolacrimal system*. This may result from foreign bodies, inflammation or neoplasia.

Dacryocystitis

This is uncommon and is usually due to a nasolacrimal foreign body. There is a profuse, mucopurulent discharge and further discharge can be expressed by pressing on the medial canthal region. The system should be gently irrigated after collecting fresh discharge for culture. Care must be taken not to flush any foreign bodies further along the system. Surgically opening the canaliculi may facilitate foreign body removal.

CONDITIONS OF THE THIRD EYELID

The third eyelid (membrana nictitans) plays an important role in corneal protection and distribution of tears. It should therefore be preserved whenever possible.

Scrolling of the third eyelid (Fig. 46.10)

Scrolling of the T-shaped cartilage skeleton usually results in eversion of the leading edge of the third eyelid. Correction is by excision of the

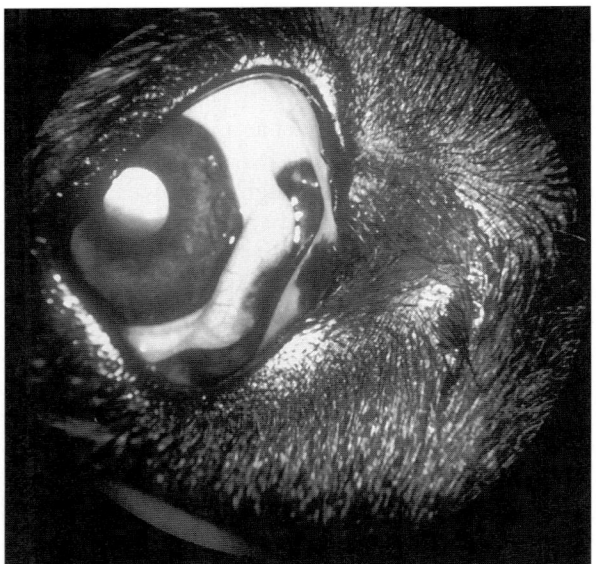

Figure 46.10 Scrolling of the third eyelid in a great Dane.

scrolled portion of cartilage via an incision through the bulbar conjunctival surface (Gelatt, 1972).

Prolapse of the nictitans gland (Fig. 46.11)

The prolapsed gland appears as a pink swelling in the medial canthal region (cherry eye). As the gland contributes significantly to the precorneal tear film it should be preserved. Suturing the prolapsed gland to the orbital rim is an effective treatment (Kaswan and Martin, 1985).

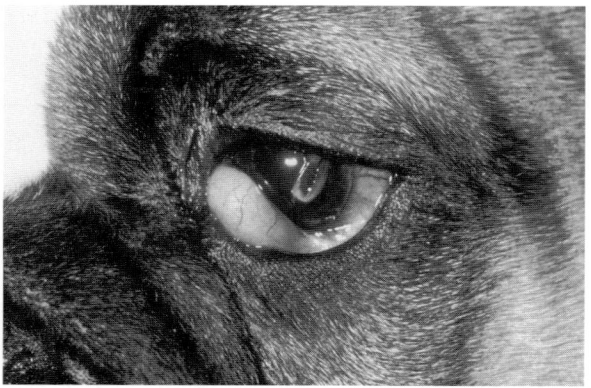

Figure 46.11 Prolapse of the nictitans gland (cherry eye) in a young bulldog.

Inflammations of the third eyelid

Plasma cell infiltration (plasma cell conjunctivitis) of the free border of the third eyelid resulting in depigmentation and pink/purple thickening occurs in some breeds, notably the German shepherd dog. It may accompany chronic superficial keratitis (pannus). Topical cyclosporin or corticosteroids can help control the condition.

Foreign bodies

Foreign bodies sometimes lodge between the third eyelid and the globe. This area should always be examined if the presence of a foreign body is suspected.

Neoplasia of the third eyelid

Neoplasia of the third eyelid is uncommon. Reported tumours include adenomas, adenocarcinomas and squamous cell carcinomas.

Protrusion of the third eyelid (Fig. 46.3)

Protrusion of the third eyelid is a common sign which may result from a number of causes (Table 46.5).

CONDITIONS OF THE CONJUNCTIVA

The conjunctiva lines the inner surface of the eyelids and is reflected at the fornix to overlay the globe as the bulbar conjunctiva. Goblet cells within the conjunctiva (of greatest density within the fornix) produce mucus which is an important constituent of the tear film. The normal canine conjunctival sac often harbours low numbers of bacteria such as staphylococci and diphtheroids.

Conjunctivitis

Conjunctivitis occurs commonly. It must be differentiated from other causes of a 'red eye'. Hyperaemia, irritation and discharge (serous to mucopurulent) are signs of conjunctival inflammation. There are many factors which predispose towards conjunctivitis (Table 46.6). Bacterial conjunctivitis usually resolves quickly if no predis-

Table 46.5 Causes of protrusion of the third eyelid in dogs

Causes of third eyelid protrusion	Accompanying signs
Reduced globe size	May be due to microphthalmos or phthisis bulbi
Enophthalmos	May be due to reduced orbital contents, e.g. cachexia, dehydration, masseter and temporal muscle atrophy
Active globe retraction	Painful ocular lesion – other signs of pain will be present
Orbital space occupying lesion (Fig. 46.3)	Prominent globe
Horner's syndrome	Miosis, ptosis and possibly conjunctival hyperaemia will also be present

Table 46.6 Canine conjunctivitis

Aetiology	Influencing factors
Irritation	• Poor lid conformation leading to conjunctival exposure • Lesions on eyelid margin • Abnormal cilia abrading conjunctiva • Foreign bodies in conjunctival sac
Trauma	• May see conjunctival wound
Tear film abnormalities	• Recurrent conjunctivitis may be first sign of keratoconjunctivitis sicca
Infection	• Predisposing factors may allow bacteria to cause an infection • viral infection (distemper)
Allergy/autoimmune conditions	• May occur in atopic dogs • Contact allergy (e.g. drugs) • Hypersensitivity to metabolites from microbes may play a role in bacterial conjunctivitis

posing factors are present. If the signs do not resolve the diagnosis should be reconsidered. Swabs for bacteriology and scrapes for cytology may aid in the investigation of such cases.

Follicular conjunctivitis

Lymphoid follicle proliferation can be caused by non-specific conjunctival irritation. The follicles appear as multiple, semi-spherical, raised, pink lesions. They may themselves cause mild irritation, in which case mechanical debridement and topical corticosteroids can be utilized as treatment.

Conjunctival foreign bodies

Foreign bodies, such as grass seeds, may penetrate through the conjunctival sac resulting in either acute cellulitis or a chronic discharging sinus characterized by profuse mucopurulent discharge. Careful examination of the conjunctival sac under general anaesthesia and exploration of any sinuses is required.

CONDITIONS OF THE CORNEA AND SCLERA

Congenital conditions

Corneal opacity

The corneas of young puppies normally have a diffuse opacity which usually clears a few weeks after birth. Abnormal causes of opacity include persistent pupillary membranes attaching to the posterior corneal surface; these cause an area of corneal fibroplasia and a permanent focal opacity.

Dermoids (Fig. 46.12)

Dermoids are abnormally positioned pieces of skin-like tissue which may be present on the lids,

832 DISEASES OF THE EYE

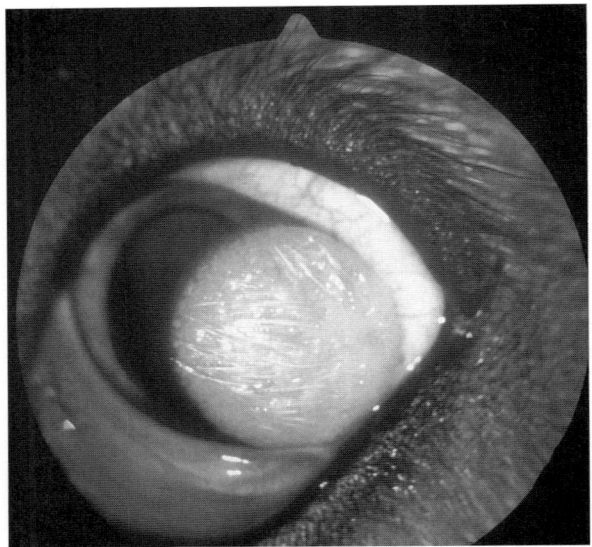

Figure 46.12 Non-pigmented dermoid in a young Bassett hound. The dermoid is affecting the lateral cornea. Hairs can be seen on its surface. A keratectomy can be used to remove it.

conjunctiva or cornea, usually laterally. Surgical removal is required.

Acquired conditions

Keratitis

Corneal inflammation may be superficial, or deep, ulcerative or non-ulcerative. Inflammation results in discomfort, opacity (oedema, scarring or pigmentation) and vascularization. Corneal vascularization may occur at varying depths within the cornea (Table 46.7). Keratitis results from infection, trauma, irritation, chemical burns, tear film abnormalities (as previously described), immune-mediated problems, or systemic disease.

Ulcerative keratitis (Fig. 46.13)

A corneal ulcer is a full thickness loss of corneal epithelium, which may be accompanied by a loss of stroma. It results in discomfort or pain, exhibited as blepharospasm and increased lacrimation. There are many causes of corneal ulceration (Table 46.8).

Table 46.7 Differences between superficial and deep corneal vascularization

	Superficial vascularization	Deep vascularization
Origin of vessels	Conjunctival vessels	Vessels within deeper layers of sclera
Are they seen crossing the limbus?	Yes	No. Obscured by scleral shelf
Appearance	Branching within superficial layers of cornea	Deep straight vessels appearing at limbus – 'paint brush like'

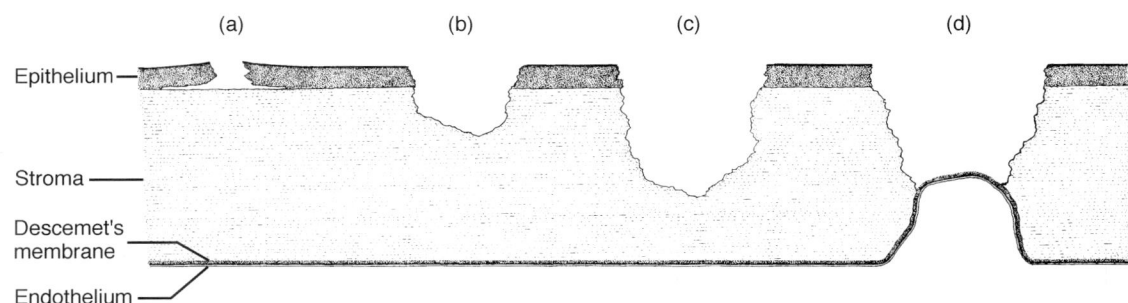

Figure 46.13 Diagram of a corneal section showing various depths of ulceration. (a) A superficial indolent type ulcer with underrunning of the surrounding epithelium. (b) An ulcer extending to mid-stroma: this type of ulcer may deepen rapidly and surgical intervention may be required. (c) A deep ulcer: surgery to support the weakened cornea while it heals may be required. (d) A descemetocele: corneal penetration is imminent.

Table 46.8 Aetiology of corneal ulceration

Aetiology	Examples
Adnexal and eyelid lesions	• Entropion • Eyelid deformities • Eyelid neoplasia • Trichiasis, distichiasis, ectopic cilia • Inadequate blink due to lagophthalmos or neurological damage (e.g. trigeminal denervation or facial paralysis).
Abnormal tear film	• Keratoconjunctivitis sicca
Irritants and chemicals	• Heat/smoke • Alkalis – deepening ulcers • Acids – coagulation of protein (lesions do not deepen)
Trauma	• Sharp trauma • Foreign bodies
Infection	• Bacteria may secondarily infect ulcers
Immune-mediated	• Unusual cause of ulcers but involved in some types of keratitis
Dystrophies and degenerations	• May cause specific types of ulcer

Superficial corneal ulceration heals very rapidly if simple and uncomplicated. Bacterial infection can lead to deepening of the ulcer. If an ulcer does not heal rapidly a predisposing factor should be searched for. Indolent or refractory type ulcers are epithelial defects which show little tendency to heal. The surrounding epithelium is often non-adherent for quite a distance from the actual ulcer. Fluorescein may underrun this loose epithelium. Some indolent ulcers are due to corneal epithelial basement dystrophy (see below). Treatment consists of removal of the surrounding loose epithelium followed by a grid or punctate keratotomy (Champagne and Munger, 1992) in which shallow abrasions or puncture wounds into the exposed stroma are made using a hypodermic needle (Fig. 46.14).

Deeper corneal ulceration (Fig. 46.15) or ulcers which are deepening may be complicated by corneal liquefaction due to the release of proteases from bacteria (especially *Pseudomonas aeruginosa*), neutrophils or damaged corneal cells. Such ulcers must be treated aggressively. Deeper ulcers, including descemetoceles (ulcers down to

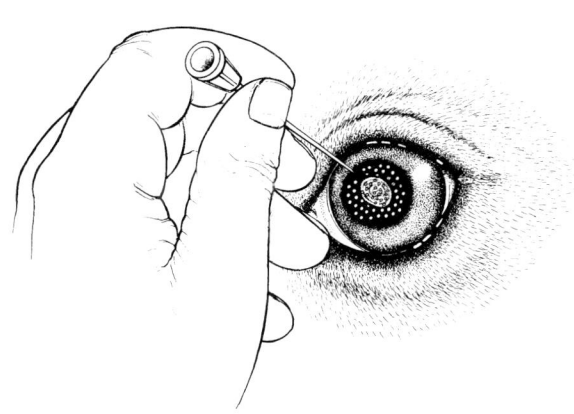

Figure 46.14 Diagram showing punctate keratotomy for the treatment of indolent-type ulcers.

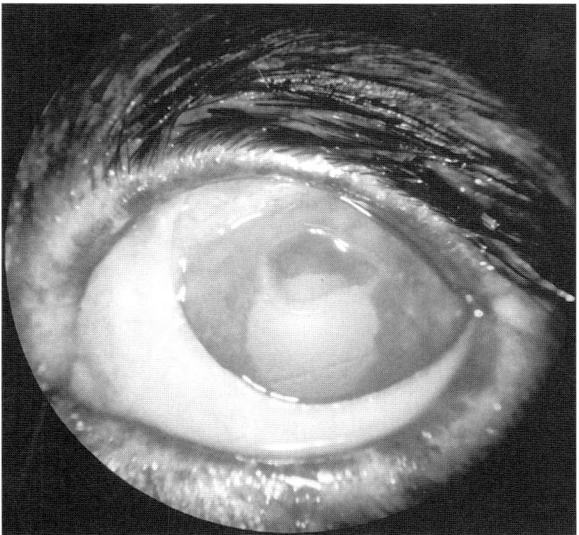

Figure 46.15 An ulcer extending to mid-stroma in an elderly English springer spaniel.

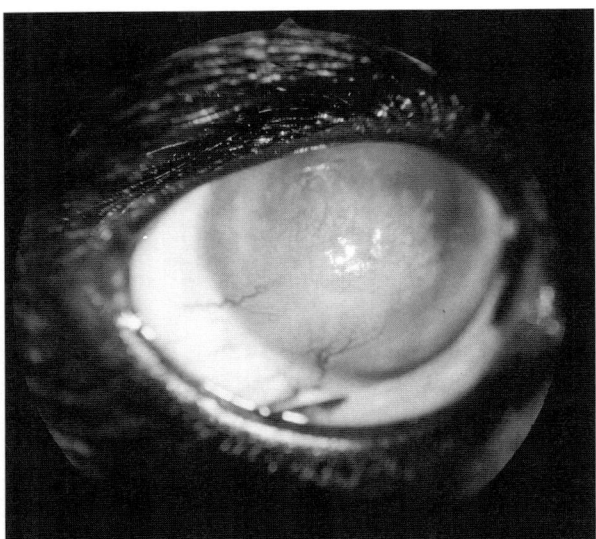

Figure 46.16 Chronic superficial keratitis (pannus) in a cross-bred dog. See colour plate.

Descemet's membrane) require some form of surgical treatment in addition to medical therapy. Conjunctival flaps of various types are easily performed and effective in providing support and blood supply to help heal the ulcer (Håkanson et al., 1988). Medical therapy includes the selection of an appropriate topical antibiotic. A swab and smear of material from the ulcer edge should be collected for Gram-staining (to allow rapid identification of bacterial involvement) and culture. Anticollagenases such as EDTA have been suggested for the treatment of melting ulcers. Corticosteroids should be avoided when the cornea is ulcerated. However, once the ulcer has fully healed they may be useful to reduce corneal scarring and vascularization.

Non-ulcerative keratitis

Chronic superficial keratitis (pannus) is a bilateral progressive, inflammatory condition which can result in blindness (Fig. 46.16). It occurs most commonly in German shepherd dogs, although border collies and greyhounds may also be affected. The condition starts at the lateral or ventrolateral limbal region leading to inflammatory cell infiltration of the adjacent cornea, superficial corneal vascularization and usually pigmentation. Treatment with cyclosporin or potent topical corticosteroids will reverse many of the changes. Affected dogs should be regularly checked to ensure that treatment is effectively controlling the condition. If extensive corneal pigmentation has developed, a keratectomy may be required to restore sight. Exposure to ultraviolet light should be reduced because it is a predisposing factor for the condition.

Pigmentary keratitis is often a feature of chronic superficial corneal disease. Dogs with prominent eyes, lagophthalmos, distichiasis, trichiasis or keratoconjunctivitis sicca may develop corneal pigmentation. Corticosteroids or cyclosporin should be used to suppress active, non-ulcerative keratitis, and the predisposing factors treated.

Neurotrophic keratitis – corneal denervation results in a superficial keratitis affecting the portion of the cornea exposed within the palpebral fissure.

Exposure keratitis occurs when an inability to close the eyelids results in poor spreading of the tear film and a superficial keratitis. The third eyelid can adequately spread the tear film in most dogs with an inability to blink due to facial nerve paralysis, except those with prominent eyes.

Deep keratitis may result from intraocular disease such as uveitis and glaucoma. This is manifested by corneal oedema and vascularization.

Corneal oedema

An oedematous cornea has a bluish/white appearance. There are several causes of corneal oedema (Table 46.9).

Corneal trauma

Full thickness lacerations may require suturing. If iris prolapse occurs the iris should be carefully cleaned and replaced, the corneal wound sutured and the anterior chamber reformed.

Corneal foreign bodies should be removed. Superficial foreign bodies can often be removed by cilia forceps or a hypodermic needle. Care must be taken not to push them deeper into the cornea. Deeper and penetrating foreign bodies can be more difficult to remove and referral should be considered.

Corneal dystrophy

Epithelial basement membrane dystrophy

This condition is due to abnormal attachment of the epithelium to the basement membrane and results in bilateral recurrent epithelial erosion or indolent ulcers as already discussed. It occurs particularly in boxers and corgis.

Table 46.9 Aetiology of corneal oedema

Aetiology	Mechanism
Corneal ulceration	• Allows fluid from tear film access to stroma
Canine adenovirus 1 infection	• Antigen/antibody deposition in endothelial cells causes 'blue eye', e.g. infection with CAV1 (or historically use of live CAV1 vaccine) can cause it
Anterior uveitis	• Endothelial cells may be affected by inflammation or toxic by-products
Glaucoma	• Increased intraocular pressure can force fluid into cornea and damage endothelial cells
Anterior lens luxation	• A patch of oedema results from contact between luxated lens and endothelium • Oedema may also result from secondary glaucoma
Iatrogenic	• Inexperienced intraocular surgeons may damage endothelial cells
Trauma	• If damages endothelial cells
Endothelial dystrophy	• A gradual loss of endothelial cells occurs resulting in progressive oedema. Epithelial bullae may form and rupture causing superficial ulceration

Crystalline stromal dystrophy (Fig. 46.17)

Lipid is deposited in the central superficial corneal stroma resulting in a white/grey circular or ring-shaped opacity. The epithelium is intact and the lesions are not usually clinically significant (cf. lipid keratopathy). Typically both eyes are affected although the lesions may not be bilaterally symmetrical. This condition is seen in the rough collie, Shetland sheepdog, cavalier King Charles spaniel, German shepherd dog and several other breeds (Crispin and Barnett, 1983). The Siberian husky suffers from a second form of crystalline stromal dystrophy in which lipid deposits may be more extensive and involve the full thickness of the corneal stroma (MacMillan et al., 1979).

Corneal endothelial dystrophy

This condition results in a progressive loss of endothelial cells and progressive corneal oedema (Gwin et al., 1982). It has been described in Boston terriers and chihuahuas although other breeds, notably the English springer spaniel, may also be affected. Medication is ineffective in preventing progression of the lesions.

Other corneal lipid depositions

Lipid keratopathy

Lipid deposition may follow corneal trauma or injury, or may be secondary to other ocular disease, or circulating lipid abnormalities (Crispin, 1987). The lesions are vascularized.

Calcareous (calcific) corneal degeneration

Calcium and lipid deposition in the central superficial cornea, sometimes accompanied by ulceration, is occasionally encountered in elderly dogs. Hypercalcaemia and uraemia are reported to be predisposing factors (Whitley, 1991).

Corneal inclusion cysts

These are white, raised, non-ulcerated lesions which consist of an epithelial-lined cavity filled with amorphous white material. Excision is curative.

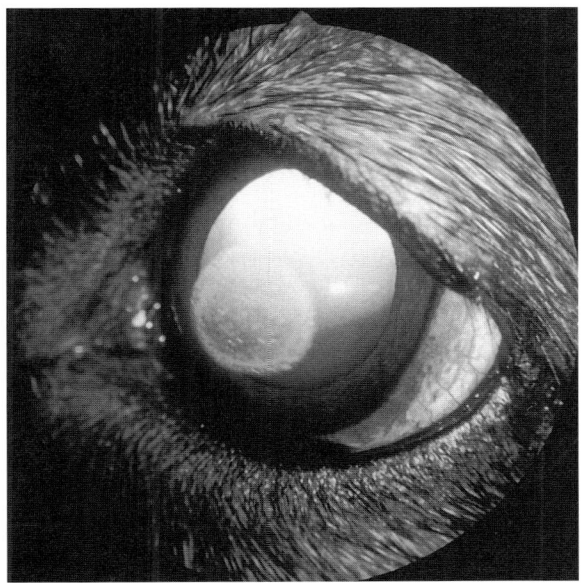

Figure 46.17 Crystalline stromal dystrophy in a German shepherd dog.

Episcleritis and scleritis

Episcleritis is divided into nodular and diffuse forms. There is often corneal involvement. The lesions are usually responsive to corticosteroids although surgical excision may be required. Inflammation involving the sclera may also affect the adjacent uveal tract.

Neoplasia of cornea and sclera

Limbal melanomas are the commonest form of corneal or scleral neoplasm. German shepherd dogs are most commonly affected. Limbal melanomas usually occur in older dogs and are only slowly progressive. Younger dogs are sometimes affected by a more invasive form of limbal melanoma (Martin, 1981). They appear as pigmented, smooth, raised lesions which arise at the limbus and encroach into the adjacent cornea and sclera. Surgical excision is feasible if performed early.

Other corneal and scleral tumours are uncommon.

CONDITIONS OF THE ANTERIOR UVEA

Congenital conditions

Mesodermal dysgenesis

Occasionally a lack of differentiation of the anterior chamber occurs resulting in congenital blindness. This has been reported in the Dobermann (Peiffer and Fischer, 1983; Lewis *et al.*, 1986).

Persistent pupillary membranes (Fig. 46.1)

These abnormal remnants of embryonal blood vessels originate from the anterior surface of the iris and may insert on the iris, anterior lens capsule or cornea. They are inherited in the basenji (Barnett and Knight, 1969).

Other congenital conditions of the iris

These include iris coloboma (a portion of the iris is absent), iris hypoplasia and heterochromia irides (in which there is a congenital difference in iris colour, either between the two irides or within one iris).

Acquired conditions

Uveitis (Fig. 46.18)

Inflammation may involve the anterior (iris and ciliary body) and/or posterior (choroid) uveal

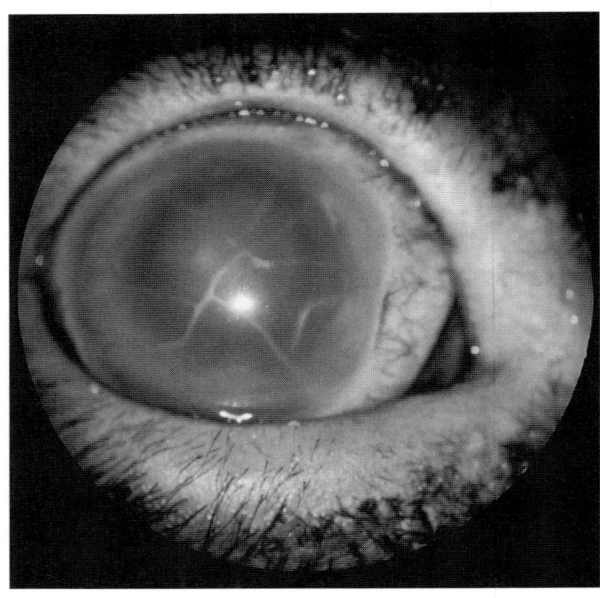

Figure 46.18 A St Bernard suffering from the uveodermatological syndrome. There is some loss of pigmentation in the eyelids. Uncontrolled uveitis has resulted in a secondary glaucoma with globe enlargement, splits in Descemet's membrane (corneal striae) and episcleral and conjunctival congestion. See colour plate.

tract. Adjacent structures such as cornea, sclera, lens and retina may also be involved. Uveitis is a serious, sight-threatening condition.

Table 46.10 indicates some aetiologies of uveitis in dogs. The signs and sequelae of anterior uveitis are listed in Tables 46.11 and 46.12.

Treatment of anterior uveitis

Therapy in most cases is symptomatic. If the aetiology has been identified it should be specifically treated, whenever possible.

Anti-inflammatory drugs to suppress sight-threatening intraocular inflammation are of prime importance. Corticosteroids are useful topically and systemically. Topical corticosteroids which can adequately penetrate an intact cornea should be used (for example prednisolone acetate). Subconjunctival corticosteroids may be used to achieve high drug levels within the eye although there is significant and rapid systemic absorption from this site (Regnier and Toutain, 1991). Topical and subconjunctival steroids should be avoided if the cornea is ulcerated and systemic steroids may be contraindicated if bacteraemia or systemic mycoses (rare in UK) are suspected. Oral prednisolone at an initial dose rate of 1–2 mg kg^{-1} day^{-1} is suggested.

Table 46.10 Aetiology of canine anterior uveitis

Aetiology	Features
Trauma	• Blunt • Sharp
Iatrogenic	• Any intraocular surgery
Infection	
• Bacterial	• Septicaemia/bacteraemia. *Leptospira* spp., *Brucella canis*, *Borrelia burgdorferi*
• Viral	• Distemper virus. Canine adenovirus I.
• Rickettsial	• Not seen in UK
• Protozoal	• *Toxoplasma gondii*, *Leishmania donovani* (imported dogs)
• Fungal	• Not common in UK (common in some parts of the world)
• Algal	• Not seen in UK (common in some parts of the world)
• Parasitic	• Ocular larval migrans. Ophthalmomyiasis interna posterior (rare)
Toxic	• Circulating toxins (e.g. pyometra)
Immune-mediated	• Uveodermatological syndrome • Lens induced • Many idiopathic cases probably fall into this catagory
Neoplasia	• Primary or secondary
Idiopathic	• Some have immunological causes

Table 46.11 Signs of canine anterior uveitis

Sign	Features
Pain	• Variable (mild to severe)
'Red eye'	• Ciliary flush • Congestion of conjunctival and episcleral blood vessels
'Cloudy eye'	• May have corneal oedema (and deep vascularization) • Inflammatory material in aqueous. Varies from protein to white blood cells • Deposition of inflammatory material ventrally in anterior chamber (hypopyon) • Lens changes (cataract)
Iris changes	• Pigmentary changes (usually increased pigmentation) • Hyperaemia and neovascularization (visible if iris is light coloured) • Iris swelling • Pupillary constriction

Table 46.12 Possible sequelae to uveitis

Part of eye	Lesion
Globe	• Phthisis bulbi • Secondary glaucoma
Cornea	• Permanent oedema/opacity
Iris	• Adhesions to anterior lens capsule (synechiae) • Pigmentary changes
Lens	• Adhesions to iris • Iris rests (pigment deposits) • Cataract formation
Posterior segment	• Vitreal changes • Retinal detachments • Retinal degeneration

Non-steroidal anti-inflammatory drugs can be useful. Systemic aspirin or flunixin meglumine have been used. Care should be taken because gastrointestinal ulceration, renal damage (particularly associated with anaesthesia and hypovolaemia) and prolonged clotting times can occur.

Immunosuppressive drugs such as azathioprine may be required to control uveitis in dogs with the uveodermatological syndrome (Wilkie, 1990).

Cycloplegic/mydriatics reduce anterior uveal muscle spasm reducing discomfort and dilating the pupil. The aim is to keep the pupil moderately dilated to reduce the area of iris to lens contact and thus decrease the chances of posterior synechiae formation (and hence the associated risk of pupil block and iris bombé, see Fig. 46.22). Atropine (1% ophthalmic drops) is applied to effect (maximum of four times daily as there is a risk of systemic effects in smaller patients).

Antibiotics Intraocular bacterial infections are rare, they are difficult to treat and may require surgical drainage and intraocular injection of antibiotics.

Iris cysts (Fig. 46.19)

Iris cysts may be congenital but most appear in older dogs. They arise from the posterior epithelium of the iris and pass into the anterior chamber as pigmented hollow spheres that can be transilluminated by a bright light. They are of no clinical significance.

Anterior uveal neoplasia

Neoplasia may present as a mass involving the anterior uvea, in which case the diagnosis is relatively easy. However, sometimes uveitis or glaucoma may be the presenting sign. Ultrasonography may help in the detection of intraocular masses in such cases.

Tumours may be primary or secondary. Melanomas are the commonest primary tumours, others include ciliary body adenomas, adenocarcinomas, and medulloepitheliomas. Enucleation is the treatment of choice for primary tumours, following thoracic radiography and possibly ultrasonography of the abdomen to check for metastasis. Some adenomas, if recognized early may be excisable. Lymphoma is the commonest secondary tumour. It may result in a panuveitis, conjunctival infiltration, exophthalmos, interstitial keratitis, hyphaema, retinal haemorrhages and secondary glaucoma. Other secondary tumours include melanomas, haemangiosarcomas and adenocarcinomas.

Hyphaema

Blood in the anterior chamber may result from a number of conditions (Table 46.13). Ultrasonographic examination of eyes with hyphaema is useful for detecting other intraocular changes. Investigation of possible systemic disorders should also be undertaken. Simple hyphaema can

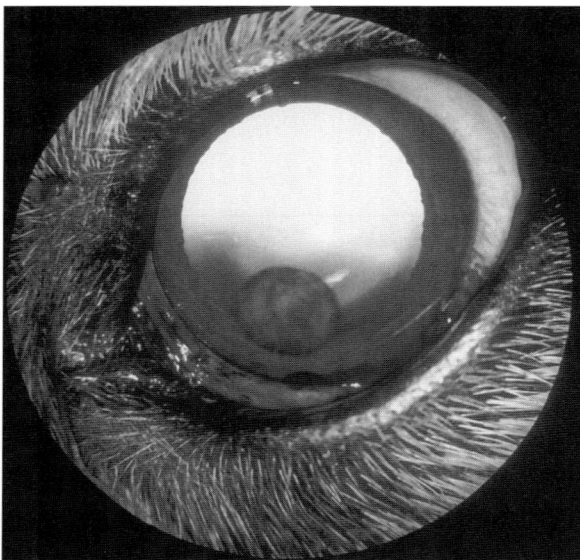

Figure 46.19 An iris cyst is present in the ventral anterior chamber of this dog's eye.

Table 46.13 Causes of hyphaema

Aetiology	Features
Trauma	• Blunt or penetrating
Anomalous vessels	• Persistent hyaloid vessels • Associated with collie eye anomaly
Retinal detachment	• Tearing of blood vessels may occur leading to vitreal haemorrhage, the blood may reach the aqueous
Accompanying uveitis	• Also inflammatory cells as well as erythrocytes
Neoplasia	• Especially malignant lymphoma
Generalized clotting disorders	• Toxicity (warfarin, dicoumarin, non-steroidal anti-inflammatory drugs) • Inherited clotting defect • Thrombocytopenia
Other systemic disorders	• Systemic hypertension • Hyperviscosity syndrome

clear very quickly, but there is a risk of secondary glaucoma. Most authors advocate treating as for a uveitis but avoiding non-steroidal anti-inflammatory drugs.

GLAUCOMA

Aqueous is the fluid which fills the anterior and posterior chambers of the eye (Fig. 46.20). Its production (by the ciliary body) is normally matched by drainage (predominantly via the iridocorneal drainage apparatus), thus maintaining a constant intraocular pressure (IOP). The normal IOP of the dog is approximately 15–25 mmHg.

Glaucoma (a raised IOP) is classified into primary and secondary forms (Table 46.14). It is important that the aetiology is identified so that appropriate treatment can be undertaken. Glaucoma always results from interference with aqueous passage within the eye, or out of the eye via the iridocorneal drainage apparatus. Gonioscopy, to examine the opening into the iridocorneal drainage pathway, is very important. Referral to a veterinary ophthalmologist should always be considered because an acute rise in IOP can rapidly cause irreversible blindness.

Clinical signs of glaucoma (Table 46.15 and Fig. 46.21)

Globe enlargement is not the presenting sign in most cases of canine glaucoma, with the exception of open angle glaucomas and some forms of secondary glaucoma. The presenting signs in most instances are pain, loss of function, a red eye and some degree of corneal oedema.

Primary glaucoma

Narrow (closed) angle glaucoma

In this form of glaucoma abnormal formation of the opening into the ciliary cleft predisposes affected individuals to glaucoma. The opening may be abnormally narrow and may be partly

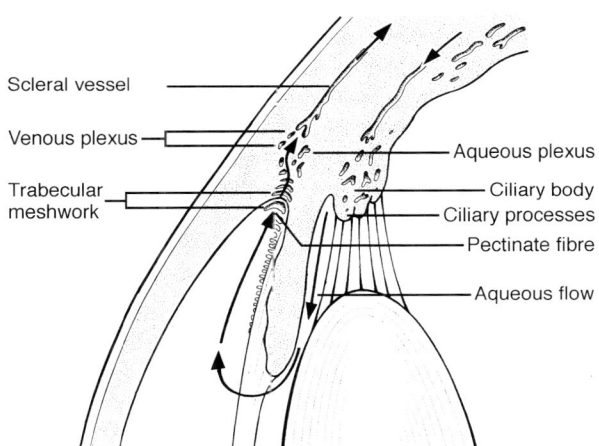

Figure 46.20 Diagram showing the sites of aqueous production and drainage.

Table 46.14 Classification of glaucoma

Category	Examples
Primary	• Narrow angle • Open angle • Congenital (abnormal anterior segment differentiation)
Secondary	• Uveitis • Lens luxation • Neoplasia • Ocular melanocytosis • Trauma

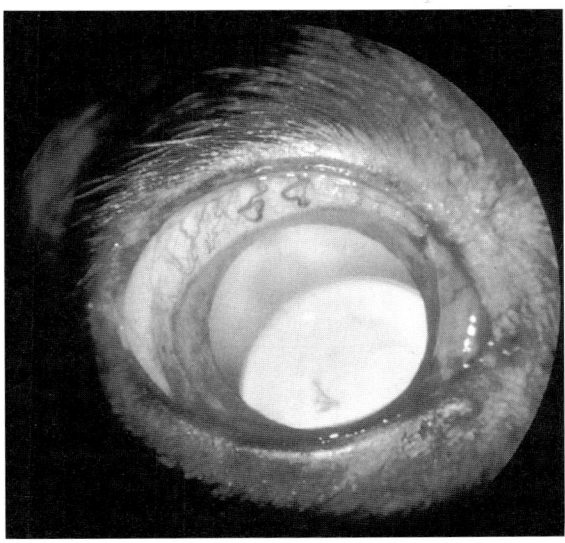

Figure 46.21 An English cocker spaniel with narrow angle glaucoma. The globe is enlarged, the pupil dilated and lens subluxated; an aphakic crescent can be seen between the equator of the lens and the pupil edge.

Table 46.15 Signs resulting from glaucoma

Sign	Features
Acute changes	
Pain	• Variable severity, depending on acuteness and magnitude of rise in IOP
Loss of vision	• Large increases in IOP cause acute vision loss (may not be apparent if unilateral)
Redness	• Ciliary flush, episcleral and conjunctival congestion and oedema may be present
Corneal changes	• Corneal oedema results from high IOP • Corneal vascularization develops in first few days
Anterior chamber and anterior uvea	• May see luxated lens • May see evidence of uveitis • Pupil often dilated (unless synechiae or iris bombé present) and non-responsive
Lens	• May be primarily luxated
Posterior segment	• May see retinal oedema, vitreous inflammatory material (from retina and disc)
Chronic changes which develop in addition to the acute changes	
Globe enlargement	• Degree depends on duration and elevation of IOP and elasticity of sclera
Descemet's membrane splits	• Appear as 'tram lines' as cornea stretches
Scleral staphyloma	• Sclera is weakened by stretching and intraocular contents bulge through weakened wall
Iris atrophy	• Occurs with chronicity
Lens subluxation	• Lens zonules torn as globe enlarges, gap between pupil edge and lens equator is known as an aphakic crescent
Posterior segment	• Cupping of optic disc, retinal atrophy

obscured by sheets of dysplastic pectinate material (goniodysgenesis). Although the abnormality is present from an early age, glaucoma does not occur until later in life. Some breeds such as the Welsh springer spaniel and great Dane typically develop glaucoma in the first few years of life (Cottrell and Barnett, 1988; Mason and Barnett, 1994), but most breeds develop glaucoma in middle or old age. The breeds of dog suffering from this condition in the UK are listed in Table 46.16.

Clinical signs

There may be a history of periods of discomfort, a 'red eye' and possibly corneal oedema. These are presumably due to short episodes of increased IOP. Most cases, however, present with a sudden, large increase in IOP. The affected eye can be very painful causing depression. There is marked episcleral and conjunctival congestion and corneal oedema. The pupil is usually moderately to

Table 46.16 Breeds of dog suffering from narrow-angle glaucoma

American cocker spaniel		listed on BVA/KC/ISDS eye scheme in UK
Basset hound		
English cocker spaniel		
Siberian husky		
Welsh springer spaniel		
Great Dane		Mason and Barnett (1994)
Other breeds:	miniature poodle	also seen in other breeds in UK (Bedford, 1980)
	English springer spaniel	
	golden retriever	
	flat coat retriever	

widely dilated and non-responsive. There may be slight aqueous flare and the fundus may have areas of oedema. Although in affected dogs both eyes have drainage angle abnormalities, one is usually affected before the other. Visualization of the opening into the drainage apparatus of the affected eye may be difficult, so the second eye (if unaffected) should be examined by gonioscopy (Bedford, 1982a).

Treatment
This is an ocular emergency. Osmotic diuretics should be used to lower the IOP before extensive retinal necrosis and optic nerve head damage occurs. Medical therapy is not usually effective and surgical procedures should be considered if the eye is still visual. Prompt referral to a veterinary ophthalmologist is recommended. The onset of glaucoma in the second eye may be delayed by the use of medication to reduce IOP (for example carbonic anhydrase inhibitors).

Open angle
This is uncommon in dogs. The opening into the ciliary cleft, through which aqueous drainage occurs, is initially open. The resistance to outflow is further along the drainage pathway.

The onset of clinical signs is insidious. Globe enlargement and lens subluxation result. Acute rises in IOP may occur resulting in episcleral and conjunctival congestion, corneal oedema and discomfort. The breeds affected in the UK include the Norwegian elkhound, Keeshond, miniature poodle (Bedford, 1980) and the German shepherd dog (personal observations).

Treatment
Medical therapy consisting of carbonic anhydrase inhibitors, miotics and possibly adrenergic agents and beta adrenergic blockers (Table 46.17) can slow down the progression of the disease. However, surgical intervention (Table 46.18) may eventually be required.

Secondary glaucoma

Secondary to uveitis
Glaucoma may occur secondarily to anterior uveitis, either due to extensive posterior synechiae (iris to lens adhesions) preventing the passage of aqueous passage through the pupil and resulting in iris bombé (anterior bulging of iris, Fig. 46.22), or direct blockage of the drainage pathways.

Table 46.17 Medication for the treatment of glaucoma

Class	Action	Example, route, dose	Contraindication and side effects
Osmotic diuretics	Emergency reduction in IOP (by osmosis)	• mannitol i.v. 1–1.5 g kg^{-1} • glycerin orally	Exacerbates pulmonary oedema (cardiovascular overload). Care with methoxyflurane. Cerebral dehydration.
Carbonic anhydrase inhibitors	Reduce aqueous production	• dichlorphenamide orally 2–10 mg kg^{-1} 2 to 3 times daily. • acetazolamide i.v. or orally 10 mg kg^{-1} 2 to 3 times daily. • dorzolamide topically 3 times daily.	Diuresis, GI tract disturbances, metabolic acidosis (increased respiration), potassium depletion. Dichlorphenamide has less side effects. Dorzolamide avoids systemic side effects.
Miotics	Constrict pupil, increase aqueous outflow.	• 1% or 2% pilocarpine topically 2 to 4 times daily.	Do not use if uveitis is present. Transient stinging.
Adrenergics	α and β actions. Increase outflow and decrease production.	• Adrenaline 1% drops 2 to 3 times daily. • Dipivefrine 0.1% drops twice daily.	Local irritation
β adrenergic blockers	Reduce aqueous production	• Timolol maleate 0.5% drops 2 to 3 times daily. • Betaxolol HCl 0.5% drops twice daily.	May cause bradycardia. Risk if concurrent cardiac disease?

Table 46.18 Surgical control of glaucoma

Method	Technique	Comments
Damage ciliary body to reduce aqueous production	• Diathermy • Cryosurgery • Laser • Intravitreal gentamicin (25 mg) and dexamethasone injection (1 mg)	• Marked inflammation • Post freezing rise in IOP and risk of retinal detachment • Causes some inflammatory reaction • Also destroys retina (not for visual eyes)
Filtration procedures – create alternative aqueous drainage pathway	Many procedures described. The best results are from the use of a drainage tube and plate. See Gelatt (1992) for a review.	Specialist procedure (Bedford 1989)
Enucleation	Transpalpebral or subconjunctival	To treat painful blind eyes

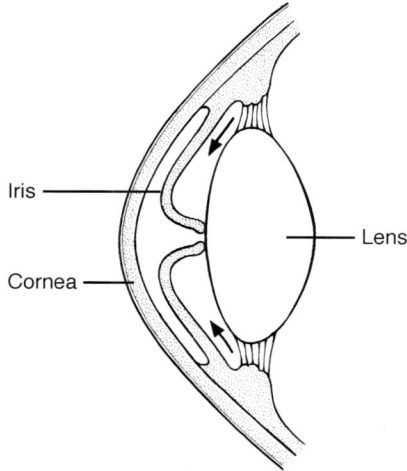

Figure 46.22 Diagram of a cross section of an eye with iris bombé which has resulted from posterior synechiae formation preventing aqueous drainage from the posterior chamber through the pupil into the anterior chamber.

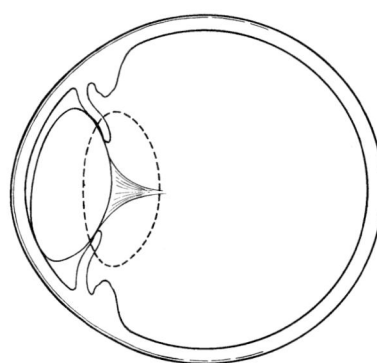

Figure 46.23 Diagram of pupil block resulting from an anteriorly luxated lens.

Treatment

Uveitis should be treated aggressively. If an iris bombé is starting to develop, mannitol (used with care, in case it crosses the blood:aqueous barrier) and carbonic anhydrase inhibitors can be administered to lower the IOP. Mydriatics can help break down the synechiae. Miotics should be avoided. Surgical iridectomies have a poor success rate. The prognosis is very guarded.

Secondary to lens luxation

Primary anterior lens luxation can result in 'pupil block' and secondary glaucoma (Figs 46.23 and 46.26). See under the conditions of the lens.

Secondary to neoplasia

Uveal neoplasia may interfere with aqueous drainage.

Secondary to intraocular pigment deposition (Fig. 46.24)

Ocular melanocytosis in cairn terriers results in secondary glaucoma (Petersen-Jones, 1990a). Uveal pigment is liberated into the aqueous and becomes deposited ventrally in the anterior chamber, eventually occluding the drainage angle. Raised scleral and episcleral pigment patches are also present. The resultant glaucoma has an insidious onset and is generally intractable.

CONDITIONS OF THE LENS

The lens is a transparent, biconvex structure (Fig. 46.25). It is positioned in the patella fossa of the anterior face of the vitreous. The vitreous is firmly attached to the posterior capsule of the lens. Zonular fibres run from the lens equator to the ciliary body thus holding the lens in position and allowing accommodation (which is limited in the dog). New lens fibres are produced throughout life.

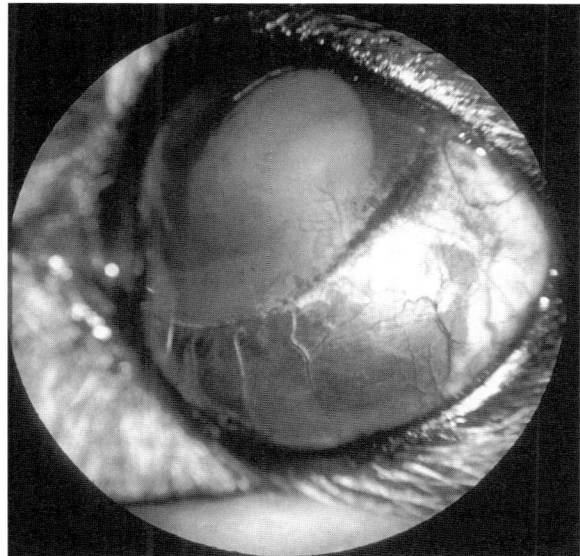

Figure 46.24 Glaucoma secondary to pigment deposition in a Cairn terrier. A large pigment patch is visible on the ventral sclera and a line of pigment is deposited ventrally in the anterior chamber and can be seen through the cornea.

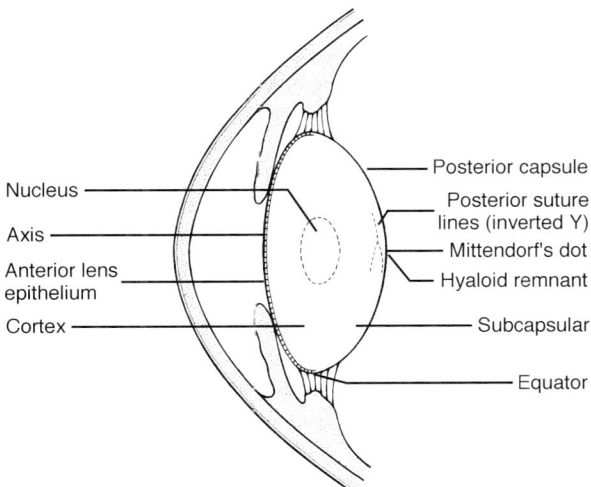

Figure 46.25 Diagram of a cross section of the eye showing the features of the lens.

Primary lens luxation (Curtis, 1990, Fig. 46.26)

This is an inherited condition which affects the terrier breeds (Jack Russell terrier, Tibetan terrier, Sealyham terrier, miniature bull terrier) and the border collie. It is occasionally seen in other breeds and cross breeds. Affected dogs are typically three to six years of age. Gradual zonular breakdown allows the lens to move relative to the rest of the globe under the effects of inertia. Lens instability and iridodonesis ('iris wobble') are early signs, best detected when closely viewing the anterior chamber from an oblique angle, just after an eye movement. Zonular breakdown allows strands of vitreous to pass anteriorly to appear through the pupil as faint wisps of slightly translucent material. Eventually the lens luxates fully. Most lenses luxate anteriorly through the pupil and will often cause a 'pupil block' and secondary glaucoma. In addition to the signs of glaucoma an area of corneal oedema just ventral to the centre of the cornea develops, due to contact with the lens. Sometimes the anteriorly luxated lens moves posteriorly through the pupil into the vitreous, and the IOP returns to normal, but the patch of corneal oedema remains.

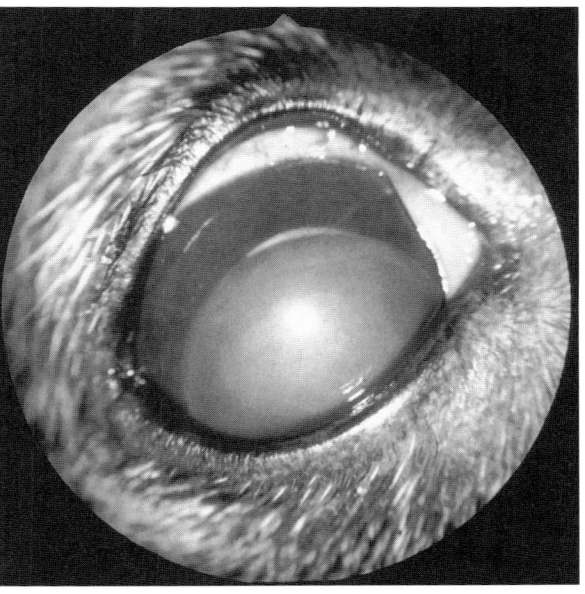

Figure 46.26 An anteriorly luxated lens in a Tibetan terrier. Aqueous drainage past the lens was still occurring in this eye, therefore a secondary glaucoma had not developed.

Treatment

Anteriorly luxated lenses should be surgically removed. Osmotic diuretics are used preoperatively to reduce the IOP. Referral to a veterinary ophthalmologist equipped for intraocular surgery is recommended. The lens of the second eye will also luxate at some stage and owners should be warned of this.

■ Secondary lens luxation

This may occur secondary to glaucoma, cataract formation, trauma or associated with uveitis.

■ Cataract

A cataract is an opacity of the lens or its capsule. Cataracts may be classified by their stage of development:

- Incipient – very early lens changes.
- Immature – the entire lens is not yet involved and a fundus reflex can still be seen. The fundus may still be visible by indirect ophthalmoscopy.
- Mature – the lens is totally opaque. It may take up fluid and swell (intumescence).
- Hypermature – liquefaction of cataractous material occurs. This leaks out through the capsule causing a low-grade uveitis and sometimes a secondary glaucoma. The lens shrinks in size and the capsule becomes wrinkled. Significant clearing of the visual axis sometimes occurs and sight may be restored. A dense remnant of cataractous material is sometimes left ventrally within a relatively clear lens capsule. This is known as a morgagnian cataract. Retinal detachment may be associated with hypermature cataracts.

There are several causes of cataract as listed in Table 46.19.

Congenital cataract (Fig. 46.1)

These are often associated with microphthalmos and other ocular abnormalities (Tables 46.20 and 46.21). They are often non-progressive. If the opacity is mainly axial use of a mydriatic may help the animal 'see around' the opacities.

Hereditary cataracts

Several breeds of dog are reported to suffer from inherited cataracts. These follow a characteristic pattern in most instances. Before condemning a dog as having hereditary cataracts it is important to ascertain that it follows the characteristics for that particular breed. Tables 46.20 and 46.21 show details of the cataracts known, or thought to be inherited in the UK. The BVA/KC/ISDS eye examination scheme literature lists breeds with known inherited cataracts in the UK (BVA/KC/ISDS, 1994).

Table 46.19 Aetiology of cataracts

Category	Examples
Congenital	• Inherited • *in utero* insult
Inherited	• Age of onset, rate of progression and appearance of cataract, depends on breed (see Tables 46.20 and 46.21)
Secondary to other ocular disease	• Glaucoma • Uveitis • Generalized progressive retinal atrophy • Chronic lens luxation • Persistent hyperplastic primary vitreous
Trauma	• Penetrating wounds which damage the lens capsule • Blunt trauma
Metabolic	• Diabetes mellitus • Hypoparathyroidism
Toxic or dietary	• Orphaned puppies fed inappropriate milk substitutes • Various drugs and toxins are reported to be cataractogenic

Table 46.20 Inherited cataracts in dogs as recoded on the BVA/KC/ISDS eye examination scheme literature (BVA/KC/ISDS, 1996)

Type of cataract	Breeds affected	Features	Mode of inheritance	Reference
Congenital with microphthalmos and rotatory nystagmus	Miniature schnauzer	Mainly nuclear sometimes cortical, rarely progressive. Some have posterior lenticonus and microphakia.	Autosomal recessive	Gelatt et al. (1983); Barnett (1985)
Early-onset and progressive	Boston terrier	Bilateral, spreads from nucleus and suture lines, leads to total cataract. Starts 8–10 wks	Autosomal recessive	Barnett (1978)
	Cavalier King Charles spaniel	Progressive, bilateral and symmetrical. Becomes total in young adult	Unknown	Barnett (1985)
	German shepherd dog	Bilateral, slowly progressive. Starts as vacuoles at suture lines at 8 wks	Autosomal recessive	Barnett (1986)
	Miniature schnauzer	Similar to Boston terrier (early-onset form)	Autosomal recessive	Barnett (1978)
	Old English sheepdog	Bilateral, asymmetrical, progressive. Starts at 7 months–2 years	Unknown	Barnett (1978)
	Staffordshire bull terrier	Similar to Boston terrier	Autosomal recessive	Barnett (1978)
	Standard poodle	Bilateral, symmetrical, progressive, cortical. Starts from 5 months	Autosomal recessive	Rubin and Flowers (1972); Barnett and Startup (1985)
	Welsh springer spaniel	Bilateral, symmetrical, progressive, cortical vacuolation. Starts from 8 wks	Autosomal recessive	Barnett (1980)
Posterior, polar cataracts – affect confluence of suture lines. Inverted Y-shaped, triangular or pyramidal	Chesapeake Bay retriever	Posterior polar cataract, may involve suture lines and equatorial area of lens as well. May progress.	? Dominant with incomplete penetrance	Gelatt et al. (1979)
	Golden retriever	Typical posterior polar subcapsular cataract at confluence of suture lines. A second progressive form exists which is believed to be due to same gene	? Dominant with incomplete penetrance	Curtis and Barnett (1989)
	Labrador retriever	Similar to golden retriever	? Dominant with incomplete penetrance	Curtis and Barnett (1989)
	Large Munsterlander	Similar to golden retriever	Unknown	Barnett (1985)
	Siberian Husky	Inverted Y shape	? Autosomal recessive	Peiffer (1982)
Other forms of cataract	American cocker spaniel	Onset 2 months–6 years. Variable appearance non-symmetrical, stationary or progressive.	Autosomal recessive	Yakely (1978)
	Boston terrier (2nd form)	Onset from 3–10 years. Subcapsular, anterior radial wedges (spokes) from equator	Unknown	Curtis (1984)
	Norwegian buhund	Onset from 3–4 months. Posterior polar cataract with extensions around the suture lines. Anterior cortex may be involved.	Unknown	Barnett (1988)

Metabolic cataracts

Diabetes mellitus is a common cause of cataracts. The resulting cataracts usually develop rapidly and progress to maturity. Hypocalcaemia such as that resulting from hypoparathyroidism can result in the formation of multiple small, linear or punctate opacities in the anterior and posterior subcapsular cortical region of the lens (Kornegay et al., 1980). These do not affect vision.

Treatment of cataracts

The only treatment for cataracts is surgical removal, employed once the cataracts significantly impair vision. Using newer techniques

Table 46.21 Breed-related cataracts which may be inherited (most are 'under investigation' in the BVA/KC/ISDS eye scheme – BVA/KC/ISDS, 1996)

Type of cataracts	Breeds	References
Congenital associated with multiple ocular abnormalities, e.g. microphthalmos, persistent pupillary membrane, abnormal lens shape, retinal dysplasia	Cavalier King Charles spaniel Dobermann English cocker spaniel Golden retriever Old English sheepdog Rottweiler Rough collie Standard poodle West Highland white terrier	Narfström and Dubielzig (1984) Lewis *et al.* (1986) Olesen *et al.* (1974) Gelatt (1972); Barnett and Grimes (1975) – quoted by Barnett (1978) Barrie *et al.* (1979); Barnett (1985) BVA/KC/ISDS (1994) BVA/KC/ISDS (1994) Barnett and Startup (1985) Barnett (1985)
Congenital	Golden retriever Old English sheepdog West Highland white terrier	Gelatt (1972) Koch (1972) Narfström (1981)
Early developing	Belgian shepherd dog Bichon frisé French bulldog Border collie Griffon Bruxellois Field spaniel Lancashire heeler Leonberger Tibetan terrier	BVA/KC/ISDS (1994) BVA/KC/ISDS (1994) BVA/KC/ISDS (1994) BVA/KC/ISDS (1994) BVA/KC/ISDS (1994) BVA/KC/ISDS (1994) BVA/KC/ISDS (1994) BVA/KC/ISDS (1994) BVA/KC/ISDS (1994)
Late onset	Yorkshire terrier Border terrier	BVA/KC/ISDS (1994) BVA/KC/ISDS (1994)

removal of immature cataracts is successful, indeed at this stage there are fewer complications than associated with removal of mature or hypermature cataracts. This is a skilled procedure best left to veterinary ophthalmologists (Petersen-Jones, 1990b; Nasisse *et al.*, 1991).

Nuclear sclerosis

The continual production of lens fibres results in progressive compression and loss of hydration of the nuclear area. This causes a change in refractive index and an apparent greying of the lens nucleus in all older dogs. There is no noticeable effect on vision, but this appearance is often mistaken for cataract formation.

CONDITIONS OF THE VITREOUS

The vitreous is a clear gel-like substance within which a few faint membranes can normally be seen. It fills the cavity posterior to the lens. The development of the vitreous is divided into three phases. The primary vitreous is the hyaloid vascular system which supplies the developing lens. This resolves and the secondary or adult vitreous is formed. The lens zonules are considered to be the tertiary vitreous.

Persistent hyperplastic primary vitreous/persistent hyperplastic tunica vasculosa lentis

This is the persistence into adult life, coupled with proliferation, of the vascular supply to the developing lens. Typically a fibrovascular plaque is present on the posterior lens surface. The lens capsule is involved and the lens itself may be abnormally shaped and cataractous. The presence of blood vessels within the plaque on the posterior lens capsule help distinguish this from an uncomplicated cataract. Persistent hyaloid vasculature may also be present. Intravitreal or intralenticular haemorrhage can also occur. The condition is congenital and variable in its severity with the more severely affected eyes being blind.

It occurs sporadically, but has been shown to be inherited in the Staffordshire bull terrier in the UK (Leon et al., 1986) and the Dobermann in the Netherlands (Stades, 1983).

Persistent hyaloid artery

The hyaloid artery, which originates on or adjacent to the optic disc and reaches to the posterior surface of the lens, occasionally persists into adult life. On close examination it is often possible to see a small remnant of hyaloid artery attached to the posterior surface of the lens.

Vitreal haemorrhage

This may result from anomalous vessels, trauma or retinal disease such as detachments and hypertensive retinopathy. Blood within the vitreous can be slow to clear.

Syneresis

Vitreal degeneration leading to liquefaction is known as syneresis. It can result from posterior segment disease and may itself predispose to retinal detachments.

Asteroid hyalosis

This is a degenerative, often age-related, condition in which numerous small spherical bodies become suspended in the vitreous and can be seen moving slightly under the effects of inertia. They are of no clinical significance.

Synchisis scintillans

This condition is characterized by vitreous liquefaction and the formation of crystalline deposits. Unlike asteroid hyalosis these structures gravitate ventrally, to be resuspended with eye movements. This is a rare condition. It may result from retinal disease or vitreal haemorrhage.

CONDITIONS OF THE FUNDUS

Appearance of the fundus (Figs 46.27 and 46.28)

It is important to be able to recognize the wide range in normal appearances of the canine fundus.

Tapetal fundus

This is a reflective, brightly coloured, roughly triangular area positioned at and above the axial part

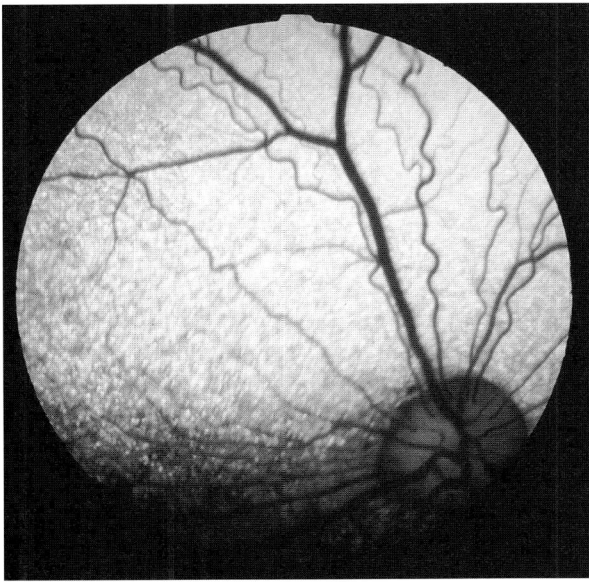

Figure 46.27 Normal fundus in an English springer spaniel. See colour plate.

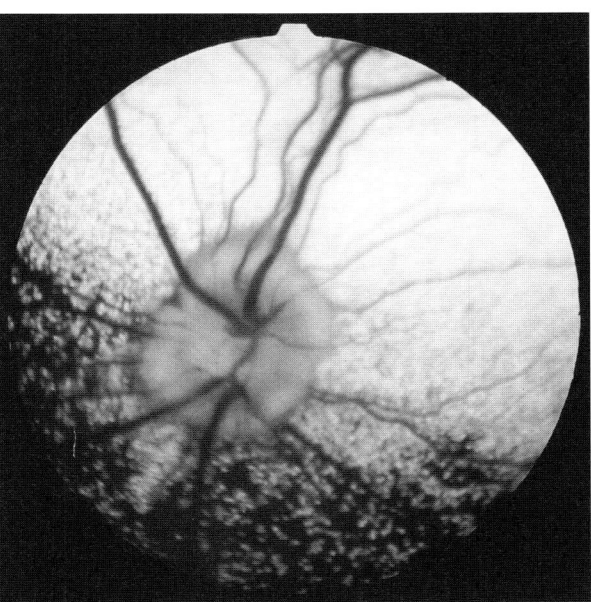

Figure 46.28 Normal fundus in a golden retriever. The retinal nerve fibres gain a myelin sheath just adjacent to the site that they join to form the optic nerve. This gives the optic disc an irregular, swollen appearance (pseudopapilloedema). See colour plate.

of the fundus. Its colour is variable, typically from yellow to blues and greens. Sometimes it is reduced in size or even absent.

Non-tapetal fundus

This is the area of the fundus not occupied by the optic disc or tapetum. Typically it is a non-reflective dark brown–grey colour. Dogs with a light coat colour may have a less heavily pigmented non-tapetal fundus. Merles often lack non-tapetal pigmentation allowing choroidal vessels and sclera to be visualized.

Optic disc

The optic disc is situated near the visual axis, close to the ventral tapetal/non-tapetal junction. The extent of myelination of nerve fibres at and adjacent to the disc is variable. Myelination of nerve fibres just prior to the area of the lamina cribrosa gives the disc an irregular ('fluffy'), slightly elevated appearance (pseudopapilloedema, Fig. 46.28), not to be confused with a pathological swelling of the disc.

Retinal vasculature

Arterioles and venules can be identified. The arterioles are smaller and radiate out from the disc periphery. There are three or four larger venules which form a complete or partial venous circle on the disc.

Congenital and developmental conditions of the fundus

Collie eye anomaly (Fig. 46.29)

This is an inherited (autosomal recessive), congenital condition primarily affecting collie breeds. It is bilateral, although not necessarily symmetrical. There is a high incidence in the Shetland sheepdog and the rough collie.

The condition is essentially non-progressive and does not seriously affect vision except in a small percentage of cases in which retinal detachment or intraocular haemorrhage occur.

Choroidal hypoplasia is the primary diagnostic lesion. The area adjacent and lateral to the disc is affected. There is an absence of pigment in the hypoplastic area allowing visualization of choroidal blood vessels (which may be abnormally shaped) and often sclera. This lesion is readily identified in puppies of about 6–8 weeks of age as a pale patch lateral to the disc, highlighted

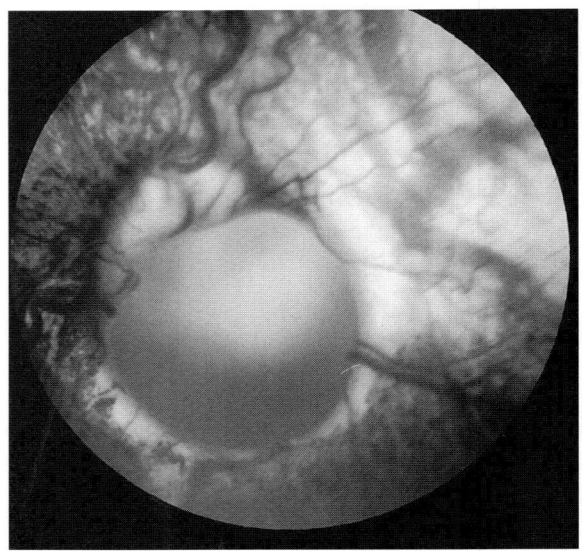

Figure 46.29 Collie eye anomaly in a rough collie (left eye). A deep coloboma involving the majority of the optic disc is present. An area of choroidal hypoplasia, in which abnormal choroidal vessels are present and the underlying sclera is showing through, is present lateral to the disc.

against the bluish colour of the developing fundus. Pigmentation which develops after this age may obscure the lesions of choroidal hypoplasia in a significant number of cases (Bjerkås, 1991). Dogs so affected are called 'go-normals' which is a rather misleading term because although the lesions are no longer ophthalmoscopically visible the animal is still genotypically affected. Diagnosis is also complicated by the blue merle fundus in which a general lack of pigmentation makes recognition of milder lesions difficult.

Colobomas of the disc or adjacent area are also features of collie eye anomaly having an incidence of about 30% (Bedford, 1982b).

Retinal detachments and *intraocular haemorrhage* affect a small percentage of cases.

Control

All puppies should be screened at 6–8 weeks of age. Test matings are required to distinguish the phenotypically normal carriers (heterozygotes) from the genotypically normal animal.

Retinal dysplasia (Fig. 46.30)

This is a group of congenital conditions characterized by abnormal retinal differentiation. Retinal dysplasia is inherited in certain breeds or may result from insults *in utero*.

CONDITIONS OF THE FUNDUS | 849

Hereditary retinal dysplasia (Table 46.22 lists affected breeds)

Two main forms are described:

1. *Total retinal dysplasia* in which there is retinal non-attachment and congenital blindness. Other ocular and sometimes skeletal or systemic defects may be present.
2. *Multifocal retinal dysplasia* varies in severity from just a few retinal folds or rosettes to larger areas of retinal degeneration or even retinal detachment. The folds or rosettes appear as vermiform streaks often situated in the tapetal fundus dorsal to the disc. In the tapetal fundus streaks appear darker than the surrounding fundus and are often surrounded by a narrow hyperreflective zone. When present in the non-tapetal fundus the streaks are a lighter grey than the normal non-tapetal fundus.

English springer spaniels with retinal dysplasia differ, often having larger areas of dysplastic retina. These lesions are characterized by tapetal hyperreflectivity coupled with pigment hypertrophy (appearing similar to postinflammatory lesions) and are situated among the dorsal retinal

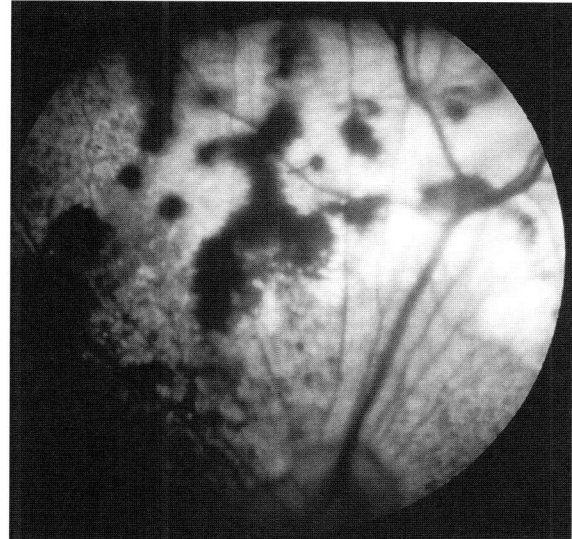

Figure 46.30 Multifocal retinal dysplasia in an English springer spaniel. The lesions are among the retinal vessels dorsal to the disc in the tapetal fundus. They have pigmented centres (due to hypertrophy of retinal pigment epithelium) with surrounding zones of tapetal hyperreflectivity (due to retinal thinning). The lesions are similar in appearance to postinflammatory lesions.

Table 46.22 Inherited or breed related retinal dysplasia in dogs

Breed	Features	Inheritance	References
American cocker spaniel	Multifocal	Recessive	MacMillan and Lipton (1978)
Beagle	Multifocal	?	Heywood and Wells (1970)
Bedlington terrier	Total + microphthalmos and cataracts	Recessive	Rubin (1968)
Cavalier King Charles spaniel	Multifocal	?	Curtis et al. (1991)
English springer spaniel	Multifocal – sometimes retinal detachments occur	Recessive	Lavach et al. (1978); Schmidt et al. (1979); O' Toole et al. (1983)
Field spaniel	Multifocal	?	BVA/KC/ISDS (1995)
German shepherd dog	Multifocal	?	BVA/KC/ISDS (1995)
Golden retriever	Multifocal	?	Curtis et al. (1991)
Hungarian puli	Multifocal	?	Curtis et al. (1991)
Labrador retriever	Multifocal or total + other ocular abnormalities and skeletal abnormalities	? Recessive effects on skeleton and incomplete dominant effects on eye	Carrig et al. (1977, 1988); Nelson and MacMillan (1983); Blair et al. (1985a, b)
	Total and cardiac defects	Recessive	Barnett and others (1970)
	Multifocal	?	BVA/KC/ISDS (1995)
Norwegian elkhound	Multifocal	?	BVA/KC/ISDS (1995)
Rottweiler	Multifocal	?	Bedford (1982c)
Rough collie	Multifocal	?	Curtis et al. (1991)
Sealyham terrier	Total + microphthalmos and cataracts	Recessive	Ashton et al. (1968)
Sussex spaniel	Multifocal	?	BVA/KC/ISDS (1995)
Yorkshire terrier	Total	?	Stades (1978)

vasculature (Fig. 46.30). Retinal detachment may develop in severe cases. An incidence of 16% was recorded in field trial of English springer spaniels in the UK (Bedford, 1984a).

Control
Puppies can be screened for hereditary retinal dysplasia from about 6–8 weeks of age.

Inherited retinal dystrophies and degenerations

Generalized progressive retinal atrophy

Generalized progressive retinal atrophy (gPRA) describes a number of different, inherited conditions with similar ophthalmoscopic signs, but differing ages of onset. With exception of an X-linked form in the Siberian husky (Acland et al., 1994), the inheritance of all other forms in the dog which have been investigated is autosomal recessive.

Clinical signs (Fig. 46.31)
Loss of night vision occurs initially and then day vision gradually deteriorates eventually resulting in total blindness. Ophthalmoscopically progressive tapetal hyperreflectivity (due to retinal thinning) develops over the entire tapetal area. In some forms a prominent band of hyperreflectivity may develop dorsal to the tapetal/non-tapetal junction. There is also a gradual attenuation of superficial retinal vasculature and the non-tapetal fundus develops a patchy distribution of pigment described as 'pavementing'. Atrophy of the optic disc occurs, the affected disc appearing dull and grey. Secondary cataract formation is very common. The pupillary light reflex is often reduced, although not reliably so.

Types of generalized PRA
Generalized PRA may be divided into early-onset and later-onset forms (see Millichamp, 1990; Curtis et al., 1991; Clements et al., 1996 for reviews).

The early-onset forms are rare in the pet population, but laboratory colonies of affected dogs have been established and extensively studied. This has led to the identification of a mutation in the gene for cyclic GMP phosphodiesterase β (a transduction cascade protein) as causal for the rod–cone dysplasia type 1 form of gPRA in Irish setters (Clements et al., 1993; Suber et al., 1993).

The later-onset forms are commoner. Miniature and toy poodles, English cocker spaniels and to a lesser extent Labrador retrievers are commonly affected in the UK. Night blindness occurs at 3–5 years of age in most cases. However, there is considerable variation in the age of onset and rate of progression of the condition within the same breed. Electroretinographic changes are present well before clinical signs are obvious (Aguirre et al., 1982).

Table 46.23 shows the breeds of dog suffering from gPRA on the BVA/KC eye scheme.

Control
Carriers (heterozygotes) can only be detected by pedigree analysis or test mating. Dogs affected with late onset forms can be identified by electro-retinography before they are bred from. The diagnosis in early-onset forms is usually possible well before animals are at breeding age and in rod–cone dysplasia type 1 in the Irish setter a DNA-based diagnostic test has been developed (Clements et al., 1993).

Retinal pigment epithelial dystrophy (central progressive retinal atrophy)

Retinal pigment epithelial dystrophy (RPED) encompasses a group of conditions which occur in a number of breeds (Table 46.24).

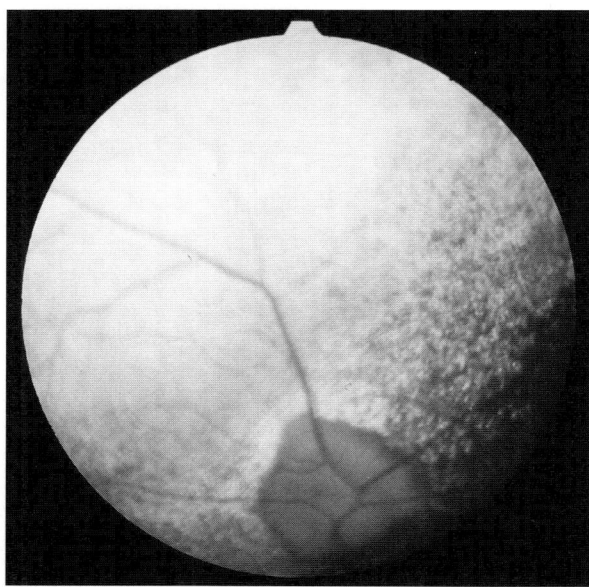

Figure 46.31 Generalized progressive retinal atrophy in a miniature poodle. There is marked retinal thinning manifested by tapetal hyperreflectivity and also attenuation of retinal blood vessels. See colour plate.

Table 46.23 Canine generalized progressive retinal atrophy: breeds on UK BVA/KC/ISDS eye scheme (BVA/KC/ISDS, 1995)

Breed	Age from which ophthalmoscopic diagnosis can be made
American cocker spaniel	3–5 years
Cairn terrier	5–7 months
Cardigan Welsh corgi	3–4 months
Chesapeake Bay retriever	3–5 years
English cocker spaniel	3–8 years
English springer spaniel	1–2 years
Irish setter	3–4 months
Labrador retriever	2–5 years
Miniature long-haired dachshund	5–7 months
Miniature schnauzer	1–3 years
Miniature and toy poodle	3–5 years
Norwegian elkhound	6–24 months
Rough collie	3–4 months
Tibetan spaniel	1–2 years
Tibetan terrier	1–2 years

Note that PRA-like disease is seen in many other breeds (see Rubin, 1989)

Table 46.24 Canine retinal pigment epithelial dystrophy: breeds on UK BVA/KC/ISDS eye scheme (BVA/KC/ISDS, 1995)

Border collie
Briard
Cardigan Welsh corgi
English cocker spaniel
English springer spaniel
Golden retriever
Labrador retriever
Rough and smooth collie
Shetland sheepdog

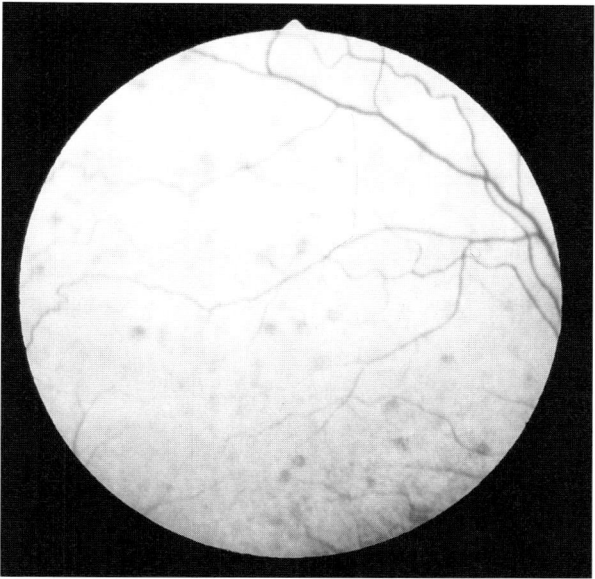

Figure 46.32 Pigmentary retinopathy in a Staffordshire bull terrier. This has the appearance of retinal pigment epithelial dystrophy, which has been seen in some dogs of this breed. Numerous light brown pigment spots can be seen across the tapetal fundus. See colour plate.

Clinical signs (Fig. 46.32)

Light brown pigment foci (lipofuscin) develop across the tapetal fundus (Bedford, 1984b). The pigment patches migrate and may coalesce during the course of the disease and retinal thinning, demonstrated by tapetal hyperreflectivity, may occur. There is sparing of the non-tapetal fundus. Affected dogs are described as having reduced central vision. Peripheral vision is preserved and moving objects more readily seen than stationary ones. Affected dogs have poorer vision in bright sunlight, but do not necessarily go totally blind.

Aetiology of RPED

The precise aetiologies of this group of conditions is unknown and although simple modes of inheritance have in the past been suggested it is now thought that environmental factors may play a role in the aetiopathogenesis (Millichamp, 1990).

Inflammation of the fundus

Inflammation affecting the fundus usually involves both choroid and retina (chorioretinitis or posterior uveitis). Anterior uveitis may accompany posterior uveitis.

Appearance

Active inflammation causes oedema and inflammatory cell infiltration, sometimes as perivascular cuffing. Lesions in the tapetal fundus appear grey and dull, in the non-tapetal fundus they are grey or white. Retinal oedema and exudative retinal detachments and retinal or subretinal haemorrhage may develop.

Postinflammatory lesions within the tapetal fundus typically appear as distinct hyperreflective areas coupled with pigment proliferation. The tapetal colour may be changed or in severe cases the tapetum may be destroyed.

Lesions within the non-tapetal fundus show depigmentation and pigment migration. Optic disc atrophy may also occur.

Aetiology

There are many possible causes of posterior uveitis (Table 46.25).

Treatment

Measures should be taken to identify and treat the cause. This is especially important when mycotic or algal infections are suspected because anti-inflammatory medication would be contraindicated in active infections.

Most cases are treated symptomatically using systemic corticosteroids such as prednisolone.

Table 46.25 Posterior uveitis in dogs

Category		Features	References
Viral	Distemper	Irregular focal areas of retinochoroiditis, with proliferation of retinal pigment epithelium. Sometimes get optic neuritis.	Jubb et al. (1957)
	Infectious rhinotonsillitis	Similar lesions to distemper.	Fontaine (1961)
Bacterial	Brucella canis	Zoonosis. Endophthalmitis, optic neuritis, retinitis.	Gwinn et al. (1980)
	Borrelia burgdorferi	Not proven to cause canine posterior uveitis.	–
	Bacteraemia or septicaemia	Experimentally causes multifocal choroiditis with exudative retinal detachment.	Meyers et al. (1982)
Rickettsial	Ehrlichosis Rocky mountain fever	Specific to certain geographical locations not seen in UK. Cause a generalized disease as well as ocular changes.	See Curtis et al. (1991) for a review.
Mycotic	Blastomycosis, Histoplasmosis, Cryptococcosis, Coccidioidomycosis, Geotrichosis	Specific to certain geographical locations rarely seen in UK. Cause a generalized disease as well as ocular changes.	See Curtis et al. (1991) for a review.
Algal	Prototheocosis	Specific to certain geographical locations not seen in UK. Cause a generalized disease as well as ocular changes.	See Curtis et al. (1991) for a review.
Protozoan	Toxoplasmosis	Retinochoriditis, optic neuritis in some. Animal may be immunodeficient. May also cause pneumonia, hepatitis, encephalitis.	Piper et al. (1970)
	Leishmaniasis	Occurs in Mediterranean countries. Keratouveitis and endophthalmitis.	See Curtis et al. (1991) for a review.
Parasitic	Toxocara (intraocular larval migrans)	Reported to cause slightly elevated nodules – translucent in tapetal fundus and grey in non-tapetal fundus.	See Curtis et al. (1991) for a review.
	Ophthalmomyiasis	Migrating fly larvae – cause subretinal tracks, retinal haemorrhage.	See Curtis et al. (1991) for a review.
Toxic	Toxic drugs and bacterial toxins	May be associated with retinopathies	See Curtis et al. (1991) for a review.
Immune mediated	Uveodermatological syndrome	Panuveitis as well as skin changes.	Kern et al. (1985)
	Immune-mediated vasculitis	Retinitis as well as systemic signs.	Randell and Hurvitz (1983)
Neoplastic and proliferative	Granulomatous meningoencephalitis	Chorioretinitis, retinal detachments, optic neuritis. Neurological signs.	See Curtis et al. (1991) for a review.
	Hyperviscosity syndrome (e.g. with monoclonal gammopathy due to multiple myeloma)	Retinal vascular dilatation, retinal haemorrhage, retinal detachment, papilloedema.	See Curtis et al. (1991) for a review.
Hypertension	Hypertensive retinopathy	Serous retinal detachment and haemorrhage. Systemic signs may be present.	Spangler et al. (1977)
Idiopathic	May have immune-mediated basis	Cause may be difficult to identify	

Sudden acquired retinal degeneration (SARD)

This is a condition of unknown aetiology affecting adult dogs and resulting in a rapid and permanent loss of vision over a period of a few days. Ophthalmoscopically, apart from dilated non-responsive pupils, no significant abnormalities are seen initially. The electroretinogram is extinguished, allowing differentiation from central causes of sudden-onset blindness. Some owners report an accompanying polyuria, polydipsia and polyphagia. Raised serum alkaline phosphatase, aminotransferase, cholesterol and bilirubin have been noted. After several weeks retinal thinning becomes ophthalmoscopically apparent. See Millichamp (1990) for a review.

Retinal vascular abnormalities

Hyperviscosity syndrome

Macroglobulinaemia, for example, due to myelomas, results in sludging of blood in dilated retinal vasculature, and retinal haemorrhages.

Anaemia

Severe anaemia can result in light-coloured retinal vasculature, the smaller vessels of which are less readily seen.

Clotting disorders

These can result in retinal haemorrhages.

Hypertension

Extremely engorged and enlarged retinal venules can be present in puppies with severe congenital cardiac abnormalities.

Hypertension (idiopathic, or secondary to hypothyroidism or chronic renal failure) can cause retinal haemorrhages, oedema and detachments (Spangler et al., 1977).

Retinal detachments

Retinal detachment is quite common. The extent of detachment varies from small areas to complete detachment. The detached retina usually remains attached around the optic disc, although it may become torn (disinserted) from the ora ciliaris retinae (anterior continuation of the neuroretina). Focal, flat detachments appear as 'fuzzy' areas of retina which are at a slightly dif-

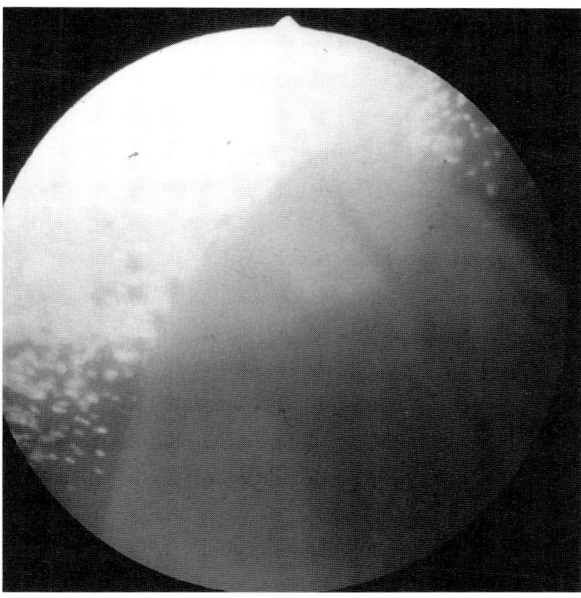

Figure 46.33 Retinal detachment with disinsertion at the ora ciliaris retinae. The retina appears as folds of grey membrane with surface blood vessels hanging ventrally from the optic disc. As there is no retina overlying the tapetum this structure appears very reflective.

ferent plane of focus when examined by direct ophthalmoscopy.

When larger areas are detached the affected retina may be seen ballooning forward in the vitreous as a grey membrane with surface blood vessels. Retinal tears (rhegmatogenous detachments) allow liquefied vitreous to pass between the neuroretina and retinal pigment epithelium making re-attachment very unlikely. If the detached retina tears at the ora ciliaris retinae it may hang ventrally within the vitreous obscuring the optic disc and revealing the very reflective tapetum (Fig. 46.33).

There are many possible causes of retinal detachment (Table 46.26).

Non-rhegmatogenous bullous detachments may re-attach with restoration of vision. Systemic corticosteroids are usually given to treat these detachments.

Surgical treatment for retinal detachment is in its infancy in veterinary ophthalmology (Dziezyc et al., 1986).

Neoplasia

Primary neoplasia affecting the ocular fundus is very rare. Secondary neoplasms occur more commonly. Lymphoma is one of the commoner types.

Table 46.26 Causes of retinal detachment in the dog

Category	Causes
Secondary to developmental abnormalities	• Collie eye anomaly • Retinal dysplasia
Secondary to other ocular disease	• Advanced retinal degeneration • Posterior uveitis (exudative detachment) • Neoplasia (solid or exudative detachments) • Associated with hypermature cataracts
Secondary to systemic disease	• Hypertension (serous detachment) • Hyperviscosity syndrome
Traction band detachment	• Following intraocular surgery and contraction of a fibrin band inserting on the retina
Traumatic	• Particularly blunt trauma
Idiopathic	?

CONDITIONS OF THE OPTIC NERVE AND OPTIC DISC

Coloboma

Colobomas of the optic disc are most commonly seen as part of collie eye anomaly. Large colobomas may be associated with visual impairment.

Optic nerve hypoplasia

This may occur unilaterally or bilaterally. The affected eye is usually blind and has no direct or consensual pupillary light responses. Ophthalmoscopy reveals an abnormally small, and often dark, optic disc. There is some evidence to suggest that the condition may be inherited in miniature and toy poodles (Kern and Riis, 1981; Barnett, 1988).

Optic neuritis

Inflammation of the optic nerve head results in visual impairment or blindness with a reduced or absent pupillary light response. The affected disc is swollen and hyperaemic with haemorrhages on or adjacent to it and there may be oedema and slight elevation of the peripapillary retina. When the retrobulbar portion of the optic nerve is affected the fundus appears normal. Retrobulbar optic neuritis and other central causes of sudden-onset blindness may be distinguished from SARD because the electroretinogram is preserved (it is extinguished in SARD).

Canine distemper, toxoplasmosis, and granulomatous meningoencephalitis have all been recorded as causes of optic neuritis. However, in many cases the aetiology remains obscure. Treatment consists of high levels of systemic corticosteroids. Recurrence can occur and optic atrophy may result.

Papilloedema

This is a pathological swelling of the optic disc (not to be confused with pseudopapilloedema). It may be associated with the presence of brain tumours, particularly those in the region of the optic chiasma (Palmer et al., 1974).

Neoplasia of the optic nerve

Primary tumours of the optic nerve are uncommon. Meningiomas compressing the optic nerve are occasionally encountered. Papilloedema and blindness may result.

Optic atrophy

Optic atrophy may occur as a result of optic neuritis, trauma, advanced generalized PRA or widespread retinal degenerations and lesions involving the optic nerve. The affected disc is smaller than usual due to loss of myelinated fibres and appears dull and flat or depressed with a pigmented border.

NEURO-OPHTHALMOLOGY

Central blindness

Figure 46.34 shows the central visual pathways. It should be noted that in domestic animals more than 50% of axons in the optic nerve cross in the chiasm to the contralateral optic tract. Additionally a similar percentage of fibres concerned with pupillary response cross back to the Edinger–Westphal nucleus on the original side. This has the following consequences: first, when a bright light is shone into one eye the pupil of that eye will constrict slightly more than that of the contralateral eye; secondly, lesions of one optic tract will predominantly affect vision from the contralateral eye.

Lesions affecting the central visual pathways can cause blindness with no funduscopically detectable lesions. However, lesions of the optic nerves or tracts (i.e. involving the central projection of the axons of the retinal ganglion cells) result in retrograde axonal degeneration which eventually progresses to optic disc atrophy. It is possible to localize the site of lesions causing central blindness using simple examination techniques, having first performed an ophthalmoscopic examination and electroretinography to rule out ocular causes of blindness. Table 46.27 shows the effect of lesions at various sites of the central visual pathways on vision and pupillary responses. Abnormalities of the central visual pathways may result from congenital hypoplasia, trauma, infective causes (for example distemper, bacterial abscessation), neoplastic and proliferative conditions.

Anisocoria

Anisocoria, a difference in size between the two pupils, may result from intraocular disease or neuro-ophthalmological disorders.

The pupillary constrictor muscles are innervated by parasympathetic nerve fibres originating in the Edinger–Westphal nucleus within the oculomotor nucleus and conveyed via the oculomotor nerve. These fibres synapse in the ciliary ganglion and continue via the short ciliary nerves.

Lesions of the parasympathetic nerve supply to the iris

Afferent arm lesions
The effect of optic nerve or optic tract lesions on the pupillary responses is described in Table 46.27.

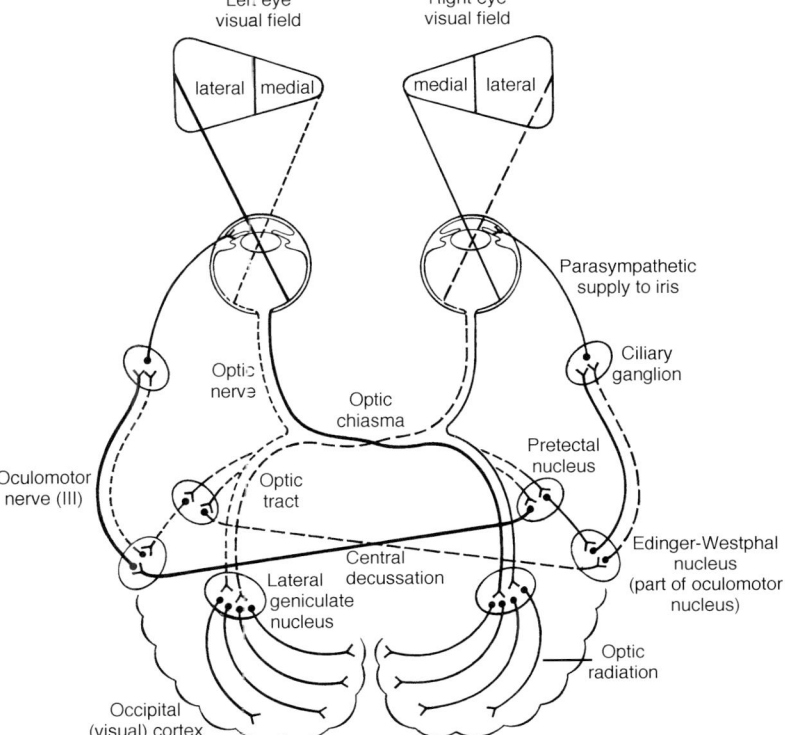

Figure 46.34 Diagram of the central visual pathways.

Table 46.27 Effect on vision and pupillary responses of lesions of the central visual pathways

Region of central visual pathway	Vision testing results	Pupillary response testing
Optic nerve	Vision of ipsilateral eye affected	No direct or consensual pupillary light response from eye on affected side. Pupil of ipsilateral eye will contract when contralateral eye is illuminated
Optic tract	Vision to opposite side of body affected. More severe deficit in the vision of eye contralateral to the lesion	Anisocoria, pupil of the eye contralateral to the lesion is always more dilated in the light 'static anisocoria'. However, pupil dilates normally in the dark
Lateral geniculate body, optic radiation, optic cortex	Vision to opposite side of body affected. More severe deficit in the vision of eye contralateral to the lesion	No effect on pupillary responses. (Fibres for pupillary response diverge from central visual pathway prior to lateral geniculate nucleus)

Efferent arm lesions

Complete lesions of the parasympathetic nerve supply to the iris results in a fully dilated non-responsive pupil. If the lesion affects the oculomotor nerve strabismus and upper eyelid ptosis will also be present.

Lesions of the sympathetic nerve supply to the iris

The sympathetic nervous system innervates the pupillary dilator muscle. Denervation of the sympathetic nerve supply to the head is quite a common finding and gives rise to *Horner's syndrome* (see Fig. 46.44). The signs of which are:

- miosis
- ptosis
- protrusion of the third eyelid
- enophthalmos
- (conjunctival hyperaemia may also be apparent)

Fig. 46.35 shows the route of the sympathetic nerve supply to the eye. Other clinical signs and pharmacological differentiation (Table 46.28) can

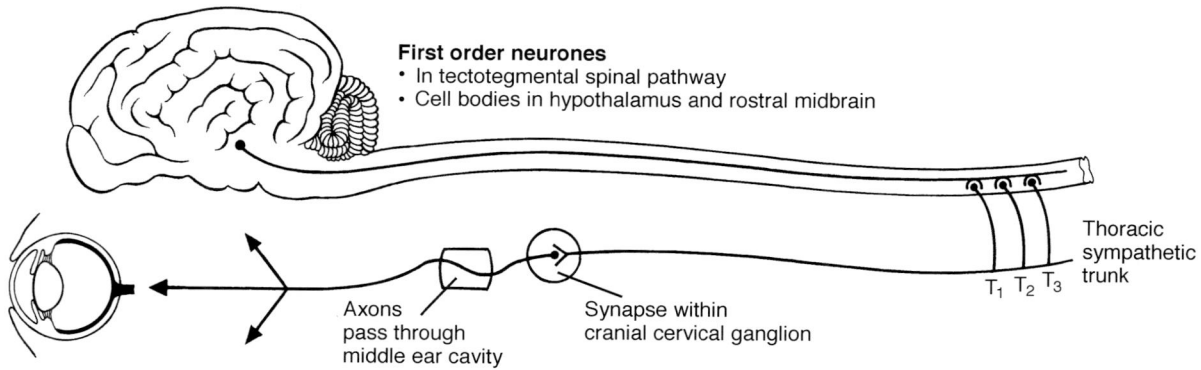

First order neurones
- In tectotegmental spinal pathway
- Cell bodies in hypothalamus and rostral midbrain

Thoracic sympathetic trunk T_1 T_2 T_3

Axons pass through middle ear cavity

Synapse within cranial cervical ganglion

Sympathetic nerves innervate:
- Pupillary dilator muscle
- Smooth muscle in orbit and in upper, lower and third eyelids

Actions:
- Slight pupillary dilation
- Eyeball protrusion
- Widen palpebral fissure
- Third eyelid retraction

Second order neurones (preganglionic neurones)
- Cell bodies in intermediate grey column $T_1 - T_3$
- Leave cord in $T_1 - T_3$ ventral roots and join vago-sympathetic trunk via rami communicantes
- Synapse in cranial cervical ganglion

Third order neurones (postganglionic neurones)
- Cell bodies in cranial cervical ganglion join trigeminal (V) nerve at trigeminal ganglion, provide sympathetic supply to structures of the head
- Sympathetic axons to the eye are conveyed via the ophthalmic branch of the trigeminal nerve

Figure 46.35 Sympathetic nerve supply to the eye.

Table 46.28 Localization of the lesion causing Horner's syndrome

Order of sympathetic neurone	Causes of lesions	Additional lesions	Results of pharmacological differentiation[a]
First	• Severe cervical spinal cord lesions	• Quadraplegic, paraplegic	Pupil very slow to dilate (may not dilate fully)
Second	• Brachial plexus avulsions or tumours • Injury to soft tissues of neck	• Lame on affected leg, pain on palpation • Injury to soft tissues visible	Pupil may take 45–60 min to dilate.
Third	• Middle ear disease or surgery • Skull fractures • Retrobulbar contusions	• Accompanying otitis externa, vestibular signs • Other neurological signs • Signs of injury	Pupil dilates in about 20–30 min

[a] Pharmacological differentiation is performed by applying 10% phenylephrine to both eyes (Bistner et al., 1970). The time taken for the pupil of the affected eye to dilate (and the other ocular signs of Horner's syndrome to resolve) is compared with the time taken for the normal pupil to dilate (normal pupil takes 60–90 min to dilate or may not dilate fully).

help to localize lesions responsible for Horner's syndrome. An apparently idiopathic Horner's syndrome occurs in golden retrievers (Boydell, 1995). After time partial or complete resolution may occur. Other possible causes of neuropathies such as hypothyroidism should be considered.

Eye position and movement

Strabismus

The action and nerve supply to the extraocular muscles is shown in Fig. 46.36. Strabismus (a squint) may be congenital or acquired. Acquired strabismus can result from lesions affecting the nerve supply to the extraocular muscles.

Nystagmus

Nystagmus is an involuntary rhythmical eye movement with a slow and fast phase. It is described as occurring in the direction of the fast phase. Normal nystagmus may be evoked by rotating an animal's head, both eyes should move in unison.

The features of abnormal nystagmus are shown in Table 46.29.

Disorders of blink

Blinking may be induced by corneal or periocular sensation, visual menacing actions, sudden bright lights or sudden loud noises. The corneal or palpebral reflex is often utilized to assess sensa-

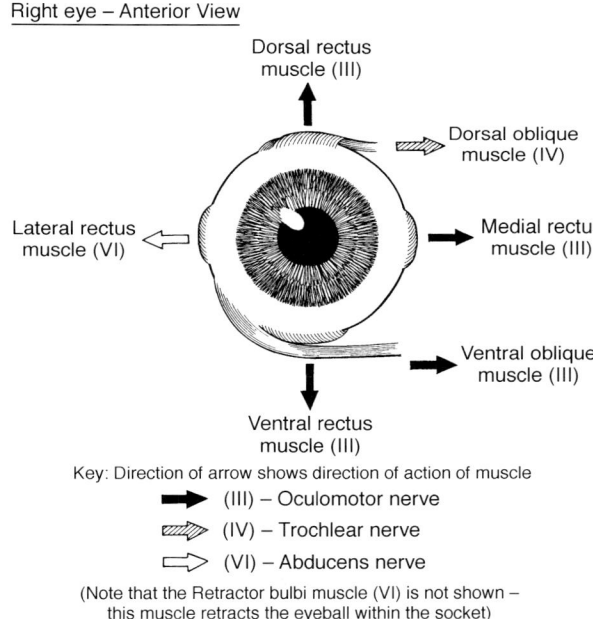

Figure 46.36 Diagram of the extraocular muscles and their actions and innervations.

tion (trigeminal nerve) and the motor innervation to the orbicularis oculi muscle (facial nerve).

Sensory deficits

Lesions affecting the ophthalmic branch of the trigeminal nerve result in a lack of corneal sensation, reduced blink rate and decreased lacrimation. This results in a neurotrophic keratitis involving the cornea exposed within the palpebral fissure.

Table 46.29 Features of abnormal nystagmus

Category of disease	Features of nystagmus
Congenital	Fine oscillatory nystagmus not associated with ocular disease 'Wandering' or 'searching' nystagmus associated with microphthalmos and multiple ocular abnormalities or congenital or very early-onset blindness
Peripheral vestibular disease	Horizontal nystagmus with fast phase away from the side of the lesion (plus other signs of vestibular disease)
Central vestibular disease	Vertical nystagmus, positional nystagmus (direction of nystagmus alters if head position is altered)
Cerebellar disease	Described as a form of intention tremor of the extraocular muscles

Motor deficits

The facial nerve innervates the muscles of facial expression and within its initial portion conveys parasympathetic fibres to innervate the lacrimal and nictitans glands. Idiopathic facial palsy is quite common (the parasympathetic nerves concerned with lacrimation are usually spared). The outer lids do not close when attempting to blink but the eye is retracted and the third eyelid passes across the corneal surface. This spreads the tear film and keeps the ocular surface healthy, except in breeds with prominent globes in which the third eyelid can not sweep across the entire corneal surface. The possibility of underlying causes of neuropathies such as hypothyroidism should be considered.

Ocular Conditions of the Cat

This section will only mention the conditions which are unique to the cat or differ markedly from those already described in the dog.

CONDITIONS OF THE GLOBE AND ORBIT

Congenital conditions

Multiple ocular defects are rare in cats but may result if the queen is dosed with griseofulvin in the first half of gestation (Scott *et al.*, 1975).

Acquired conditions

Lymphosarcoma is one of the commoner orbital tumours of the cat.

CONDITIONS OF THE EYELIDS

Coloboma

Eyelid colobomas occur sporadically in cats. The upper lateral portion of the eyelid is most commonly affected, usually bilaterally. There is a range of severity from an abnormally thin portion of lid, to a large defect where the majority of the lid is absent. Inadequate eyelid closure and an exposure keratitis results. Facial hair may be directed on to the cornea (trichiasis) thus exacerbating the situation.

Surgical reconstruction of the eyelid is required to prevent progression of the corneal pathology (Dziezyc and Millichamp, 1989).

Entropion

Entropion secondary to painful ocular surface lesions is occasionally encountered (Fig. 46.37). Surgical correction is usually required.

Ectropion

Cicatrical ectropion can result from periocular injuries. Surgical correction is performed if conjunctivitis or keratitis results.

Other eyelid tumours include basal cell carcinoma and fibrosarcoma.

CONDITIONS OF THE THIRD EYELID

Protrusion of the third eyelid is a common occurrence in the cat. The causes are listed in Table 46.30.

CONDITIONS OF THE CONJUNCTIVA

Infectious conjunctivitis is common in cats. Feline herpesvirus and *Chlamydia psittaci* are both important causes of ocular surface disease in the cat.

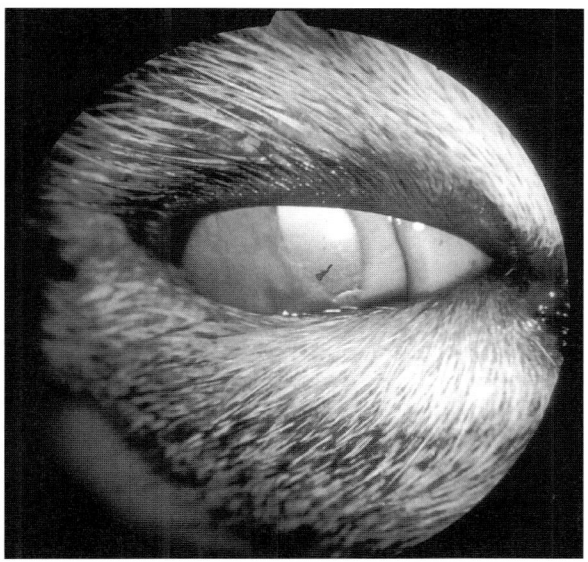

Figure 46.37 Lower eyelid entropion in a domestic cat.

Feline herpesvirus conjunctivitis (see Nasisse, 1990 for a review)

Feline herpesvirus can cause a severe conjunctivitis coupled with upper respiratory disease. Kittens and young adults are typically affected. Latent infections can develop leading to recurrence of clinical disease later in life, especially in immunocompromised or stressed animals. Infection in younger cats typically causes bilateral conjunctival hyperaemia and a serous to mucopurulent discharge. Corneal involvement is also possible and concurrent infection with other organisms may occur. Many affected kittens make a good recovery, but severe inflammation can cause extensive conjunctival adhesions (symblepharon). Resulting lesions include: conjunctiva being drawn on to the corneal surface; obliteration of the conjunctival fornices (often preventing normal tear drainage); and adherence of the third

Distortion due to symblepharon

Extensive conjunctival adhesions (symblepharon) resulting from a severe conjunctivitis may distort the eyelid margins.

Neoplasia

Squamous cell carcinoma is the commonest eyelid neoplasm of the cat. It most commonly affects white cats and exposure to sunlight is a contributory factor. The tumour appears as a slightly raised or depressed ulcerative lesion, the margins of which can be difficult to identify. Treatment may be by surgical excision, cryotherapy or radiotherapy (see Nasisse, 1991 for a review).

Table 46.30 Causes of protrusion of the third eyelid in cats

Causes of third eyelid protrusion	Accompanying signs
Reduced globe size	May be due to microphthalmos or phthisis bulbi
'Haws' syndrome	Cats with mild diarrhoea may present with bilateral third eyelid protrusion (viral aetiology suggested)
Enophthalmos	May be due to reduced orbital contents, e.g. cachexia, dehydration, masseter and temporal muscle atrophy
Active globe retraction	Painful ocular lesion – other signs of pain will be present
Orbital space occupying lesion	Prominent globe
Horner's syndrome	Miosis, ptosis and possibly conjunctival hyperaemia will also be present

eyelid to the palpebral conjunctiva. Surgery to free adhesions holds a poor prognosis because they tend to reform postoperatively.

Diagnosis
Feline herpesvirus may be isolated from conjunctival and pharyngeal swabs collected into an appropriate transport media (for example viral and chlamydial transport media). Recently a polymerase chain reaction-based test has been developed to detect the presence of viral material.

Treatment
Good nursing is important and antiviral medication, such as trifluorothymidine may be given. Corticosteroids should be avoided (Nasisse, 1990). Vaccination of at-risk cats should be undertaken to prevent them from being affected.

Chlamydia psittaci infection

This is a common cause of feline conjunctivitis. Young kittens are at risk when maternally derived antibody levels decrease, although cats of all ages may be affected. Typically the condition starts unilaterally with involvement of the second eye a few days later. Chemosis and serous discharge are present. Some animals may develop a chronic conjunctivitis and conjunctival follicles (Hoover *et al.*, 1978).

Diagnosis
Swabs collected into viral and chlamydial transport media should be sent to an appropriate laboratory for culture. Intracytoplasmic inclusion bodies may be seen on conjunctival scrapings stained with Giemsa or by fluorescent antibody technique. Paired serum samples show a rising titre.

Treatment
Chlamydia psittaci is sensitive to tetracyclines. Doxycycline, at a dose rate of 5 mg kg^{-1} day^{-1} orally, is useful. Tetracycline ointment should be applied topically (Nasisse, 1991). A vaccine is available, but should only be used on healthy cats.

Other causes of feline conjunctivitis

Mycoplasma spp. may also be involved in conjunctival infections. They are sensitive to most topical antibiotics. Reovirus, bacteria and calicivirus are also potential conjunctival pathogens although not necessarily as primary agents.

CONDITIONS INVOLVING THE TEAR FILM

Epiphora

Tear overflow is common in brachycephalic breeds such as Persians. Congenital abnormalities of the nasolacrimal system also occur resulting in epiphora. Symblepharon formation may also impair normal tear drainage.

Keratoconjunctivitis sicca

Keratoconjunctivitis sicca is uncommon in cats.

CONDITIONS OF THE CORNEA

Dermoids

Epibulbar dermoids have been reported as an inherited condition in the Birman breed (Hendy-Ibbs, 1985).

Feline herpesvirus keratitis

Feline herpesvirus may cause dendritic (branching) corneal ulcers or erosions which are best demonstrated by staining with rose bengal (Nasisse *et al.*, 1989a). They most commonly occur in adults, probably as a result of latent infections. Treatment using antiviral drugs such as idoxuridine or trifluorothymidine can be effective (Nasisse, 1991). Acyclovir is favoured by some clinicians although studies *in vitro* failed to demonstrate its efficacy (Nasisse *et al.*, 1989b). Stromal keratitis may also occur. Corneal oedema, vascularization and cellular infiltration are features and significant corneal scarring can result. The possibility of affected animals being immunocompromised should always be considered.

Corneal dystrophy

An apparent corneal endothelial dystrophy resulting in progressive corneal oedema has been reported in young cats (Crispin, 1982).

Corneal sequestrum (corneal nigrum, corneal necrosis, black body)

This condition is characterized by a brown to black-coloured corneal lesion (Fig. 46.38). The

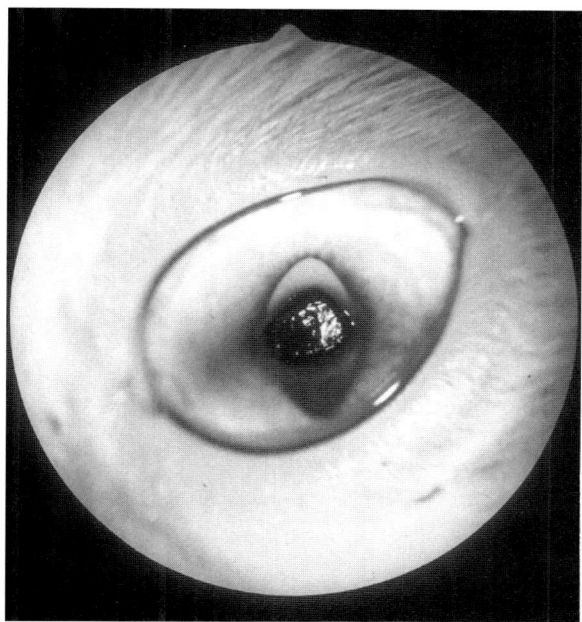

Figure 46.38 A corneal sequestrum in a domestic cat. This condition has a very characteristic appearance.

aetiology is unknown but it can occur secondarily to chronic corneal disease. A brown staining of the anterior stroma, usually of the central cornea, is initially observed. The affected area often becomes black and eventually a dense black plaque sloughs from the surface. Corneal vascularization accompanies many lesions. Occasionally the lesions extend deeply into the stroma. There is a variable degree of discomfort, with some lesions appearing to cause very little irritation at all. Colourpoints are reported to be most commonly affected (Startup, 1988). Some cases are associated with feline herpes virus infections.

Treatment
Lesions often slough on their own. Alternatively, if they are causing discomfort they may be removed by keratectomy. Recurrence is common. Conjunctival pedicle flaps may be used if the lesions are deep and may prevent recurrence.

Eosinophilic keratoconjunctivitis

This condition is manifest as a proliferative white to pink-coloured lesion affecting areas of the cornea and conjunctiva often with a whitish exudate adherent to the surface ('cottage cheese-like'). Scrapings from the lesions reveal eosinophils or eosinophilic material, in addition to lymphocytes and plasma cells (Paulsen *et al.*, 1987).

Treatment
Topical corticosteroids will control the condition. Megoestrol acetate therapy results in rapid resolution of the lesions, but its use may not be desirable because of the possibility of systemic side effects.

CONDITIONS OF THE ANTERIOR UVEA

Persistent pupillary membranes and *iris cysts* are occasionally encountered in cats.

Anterior uveitis

Anterior uveitis is important because it is relatively common and may be a presenting sign of systemic disease.

Clinical signs (Fig. 46.39)
Chronic uveitis is commoner in cats than acute uveitis and is not usually associated with obvious pain. There are other differences in the signs of feline anterior uveitis compared to canine anterior uveitis (Table 46.31).

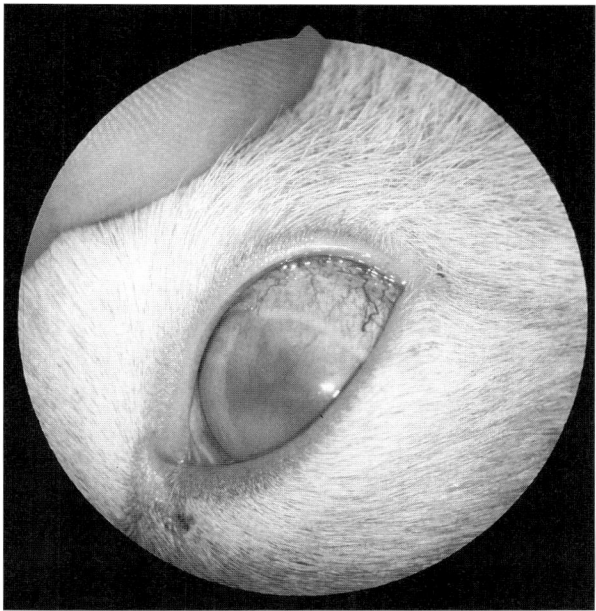

Figure 46.39 Anterior uveitis in a cat following a penetrating corneal wound. There is marked conjunctival and episceral blood vessel congestion and a large mass of inflammatory material can be seen ventrally in the anterior chamber. See colour plate.

Table 46.31 Signs of feline anterior uveitis

Signs	Features
Pain	• Variable, often mild unless resulting from corneal penetration or with secondary glaucoma
'Red eye'	• Ciliary flush • Congestion of conjunctival and episcleral blood vessels
Loss of transparency	• May have corneal oedema, although this is less common in the cat • Inflammatory material in aqueous. Varies from protein to white blood cells or red blood cells • Deposited inflammatory material ventrally in anterior chamber (hypopyon) • Keratic precipitates. These are inflammatory deposits on the corneal endothelium. They may be small punctate spots or large clumps. The ventral cornea is affected • Lens changes (cataract) • Iris rests. These are deposits of posterior iris pigment on the anterior lens capsule
Iris changes	• 'Rubeosis iridis' due to hyperaemia and neovascularization, is a common feature. New blood vessels may also grow from the iris onto adjacent structures • Iris nodules are often seen (these are 'nests' of inflammatory cells) • Iris swelling • Pupillary constriction – this occurs in acute inflammation but less so in chronic uveitis

The sequelae to anterior uveitis include phthisis bulbi, iris atrophy which is recognizable as a darker, thinner translucent iris, cataracts and glaucoma.

Aetiology
Table 46.32 lists the causes of uveitis in the cat.

Diagnosis
Serological testing for the infectious causes of uveitis should always be performed.

Treatment
As with the dog, symptomatic therapy using topical and possibly systemic corticosteroids and

Table 46.32 Aetiology and diagnosis of feline uveitis

Aetiology	Features	Diagnosis
Feline leukaemia virus	Lymphosarcoma is a common uveal neoplasm. FeLV has been associated with uveitis. Severe anaemia caused by FeLV may cause a retinopathy. Brightman *et al.* (1991) suggest it is not a major cause of ocular disease	Other clinical signs, serology
Feline infectious peritonitis virus	Can cause anterior and posterior uveitis. May see a vasculitis and perivascular cuffing, retinal haemorrhage or detachment and optic neuritis	Other clincial signs, lymphopenia, raised plasma proteins, serology (interpret with care, Addie, 1989)
Feline immunodeficiency virus	Associated with anterior uveitis, inflammation of the pars plana (pars planitis) (English *et al.*, 1990) and posterior uveitis	Serology
Toxoplasma gondii infection	Can cause an anterior uveitis but typically associated with a chorioretinitis with localized inflammation and possible retinal detachment	Serology (rising IgM titres considered to indicate active infection)
Others	Systemic fungal or algal infections – rare in UK Septicaemia, bacteriaemia, trauma etc.	Fungal and algal uveitis may be diagnosed by serology (not always reliable) or isolation from aspirates
Idiopathic	Davidson *et al.* (1991) found that despite full investigations the aetiology remained obscure in 70% of cases with uveitis. (Some of these cats may have had FIV.) Immune-mediated cases are difficult to prove	

mydriatic/cycloplegics is utilized. Atropine ointment is better tolerated than drops, as cats find the bitter taste of atropine particularly unpleasant.

Neoplasia of the anterior uvea

Lymphosarcoma is the commonest ocular neoplasm. Primary neoplasms include melanomas (pigmented or non-pigmented, diffuse or nodular), adenomas and adenocarcinomas of the ciliary body. Most of the primary tumours of the uveal tract are malignant, therefore early enucleation should be considered and the prognosis is guarded. Enucleation with curative intent is not indicated for secondary tumours or where metastatic spread has already occurred. Chronically damaged feline globes are at risk of sarcoma development (Peiffer et al., 1988), therefore enucleation of blind and severely damaged globes should be considered.

Hyphaema

Hypertension can result in hyphaema and is often associated with posterior segment haemorrhage.

GLAUCOMA

This most commonly occurs secondary to anterior uveitis or anterior uveal neoplasia. Anterior lens luxation occurs occasionally in cats, but does not invariably cause a secondary glaucoma. Glaucoma in the cat appears to cause remarkably little pain and affected individuals are often only presented once buphthalmos (and often marked vision loss) has developed. Corneal changes due to glaucoma in the cat are less severe than those seen in the dog. Apart from these differences the clinical signs are similar to those described for the dog.

CONDITIONS OF THE LENS

Cataract

Most cataracts develop secondary to penetrating wounds, blunt trauma or anterior uveitis.

Lens luxation

Lens luxation or subluxation results from trauma, glaucoma, or uveitis (particularly that associated with FIV infection) or cataract formation. Primary lens luxation is not recognized in the cat, but apparently spontaneous luxations occur in older cats. Removal of anteriorly luxated lenses is advisable.

CONDITIONS OF THE POSTERIOR SEGMENT

The normal fundus (Fig. 46.40)

The tapetum is typically a yellow–green colour but may be orange, red or occasionally blue. It occupies a similar position to that of the dog. The optic disc is round, flat and grey–white in colour. It is usually positioned just above the tapetal/non-tapetal junction. There may be a thin rim of pigment or hyperreflectivity around the disc. Retinal arteries and veins leave the edge of the disc usually in three main groups, with additional vessels in between. The non-tapetal fundus is normally dark grey–brown with retinal vessels visible on its surface. White or cream cats and Siamese cats may have a lack of pigment in the non-tapetal fundus exposing the choroid and its closely aligned, roughly parallel vessels. This gives a striped (tigroid) appearance. Sometimes choroidal vessels may be exposed in the tapetum as red streaks or the tapetum may be absent and choroidal vessels visible over the entire fundus.

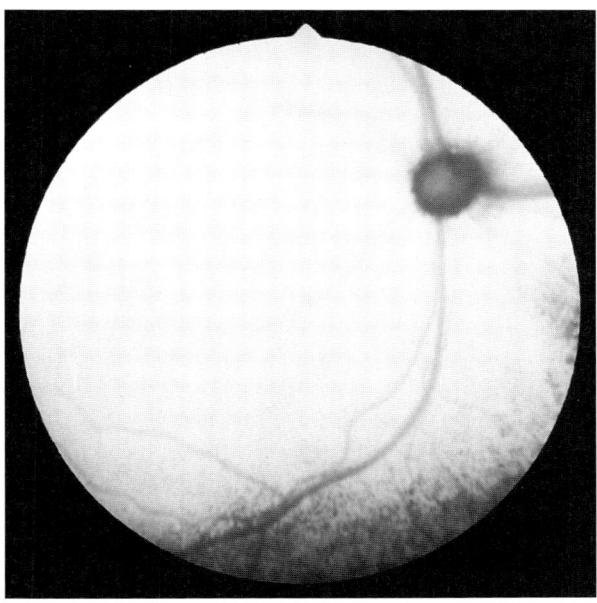

Figure 46.40 Normal feline fundus. Note the small and dark optic disc in comparison with that of the dog. See colour plate.

Congenital conditions

Retinal dysplasia

In utero infection with panleucopenia virus (Percy *et al.*, 1975) and feline leukaemia virus (Albert *et al.*, 1977) can cause retinal dysplasia. There may be large focal or multifocal areas of retinal degeneration across the tapetal and non-tapetal fundus. Lesions in the tapetal area appear as sharply demarcated areas of increased reflectivity and colour change whereas in the non-tapetal area, foci of pigmentary change are seen. Panleucopenia virus can also cause cerebellar hypoplasia.

Acquired conditions

Retinal haemorrhage (Fig. 46.41)

This may be caused by trauma, posterior uveitis, hypertension, coagulopathies, or severe anaemia. Retinal detachment may also be present. A full clinical and laboratory work up of all cats with retinal haemorrhage should be performed.

Retinal detachments

These are often associated with systemic disease and frequently occur bilaterally. The causes are similar to those of retinal haemorrhage.

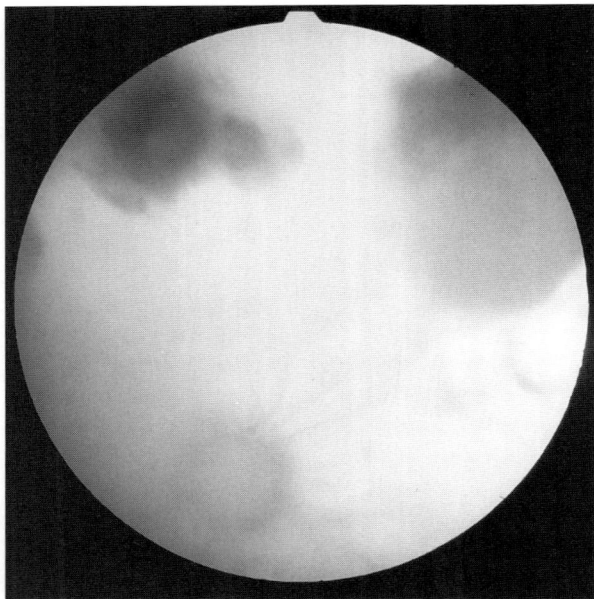

Figure 46.41 Large retinal and preretinal haemorrhages and partial retinal detachment in a cat with hypertension. See colour plate.

Hypertensive retinopathy (Fig. 46.41)

This condition is probably under diagnosed, and would appear to be relatively common in older cats. Hypertension results in retinal vascular tortuosity, vitreal and retinal haemorrhage and retinal detachment (Morgan, 1986). Hyphaema is occasionally seen. Causes include hyperthyroidism and chronic renal failure. The retinal changes may be irreversible by the time the diagnosis is made.

Diabetic retinopathy

An apparent diabetic retinopathy is reported (Herrtage *et al.*, 1985) which was manifest as retinal haemorrhage and detachment. The possibility of hypertension in cats with this presentation should always be considered.

Retinal and choroidal inflammation (posterior uveitis)

The ophthalmoscopic signs of posterior uveitis in the cat are broadly similar to those that may be encountered in the dog, although the aetiologies are different (Table 46.32). Treatment consists of identification and treatment of the cause, if possible, and symptomatic therapy consisting of systemic corticosteroids.

Nutritional retinal degeneration (Fig. 46.42)

Cats fed on a low taurine diet (e.g. some commercial dog foods or inappropriate home-made diets) are at risk of developing feline central retinal degeneration (Barnett and Burger, 1980). The initial lesions are oval areas of tapetal hyperreflectivity in the area centralis (dorsolateral to the optic nerve head). As the condition progresses a second lesion dorsomedial to the optic disc appears. The two areas eventually join to form a hyperreflective band. Degeneration of the entire tapetal retina may eventually occur. Provision of adequate dietary taurine will prevent progression of the condition.

Inherited retinal degeneration (Fig. 46.43)

Generalized progressive retinal atrophy (gPRA) is less common in the cat than dog. The affected breeds are shown in Table 46.33. Ophthalmoscopic signs are similar to those in the dog, except that secondary cataract formation is much less common. Typically the degeneration is advanced at the time of presentation, probably because cats cope with failing vision extremely well.

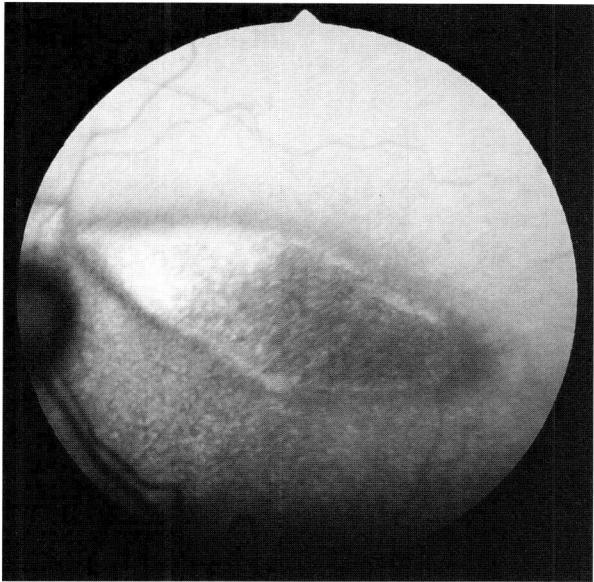

Figure 46.42 Feline central retinal degeneration due to dietary taurine deficiency. A large lozenge-shaped area of retinal thinning is seen dorsolateral to the optic disc encompassing the area centralis (area of greatest cone density). See colour plate.

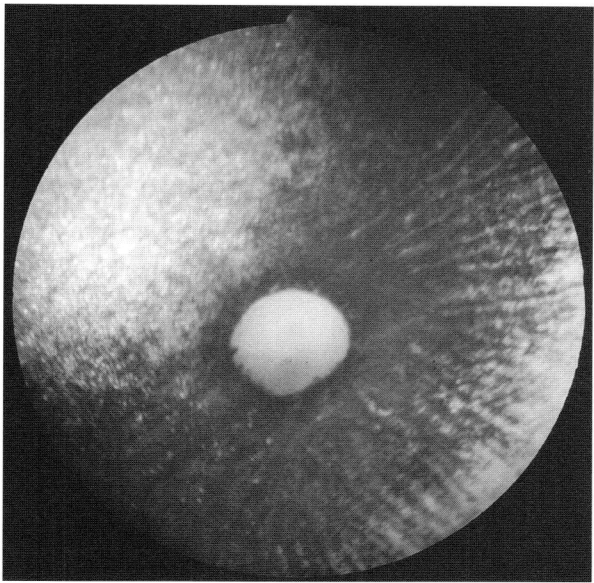

Figure 46.43 The fundus of one member of a litter of kittens with a generalized retinal atrophy of unknown aetiology. The optic disc has a small coloboma ventrally. No superficial retinal blood vessels are visible. See colour plate.

Table 46.33 Generalized progressive retinal atrophy in the cat

Breed	Features	Inheritance	References
Abyssinian	Onset 8–12 weeks, occasionally seen in UK Onset 1.5–2 years common in Scandinavia	Autosomal dominant Autosomal recessive	See Nasisse (1991) for a review
Siamese	Older cats affected, seen in UK	?	
Persian	Kittens affected, reported in USA	Autosomal recessive	

NEURO-OPHTHALMOLOGY

The general principles of neuro-ophthalmology described for the dog also apply to the cat.

Central blindness

The principles illustrated in Table 46.27 which allow localization of lesions of the central visual pathways also apply to the cat.

Tumours such as lymphosarcoma are among the commoner causes of lesions of the central visual pathways.

Ischaemic encephalopathy is recorded in the cat and may result in central blindness in addition to other neurological signs (DeLahunta, 1983).

Central blindness (sometimes temporary) may occasionally occur following general anaesthesia, presumably the affected cats have suffered a period of anoxia resulting in cerebral damage.

Pupillary abnormalities

Horner's syndrome (Fig. 46.44) is a relatively common condition in cats. Cats suffering from feline dysautonomia have dilated, poorly responsive pupils.

Eye position and movement

The Siamese cat has abnormal central projection of the fibres of the central visual pathways. This

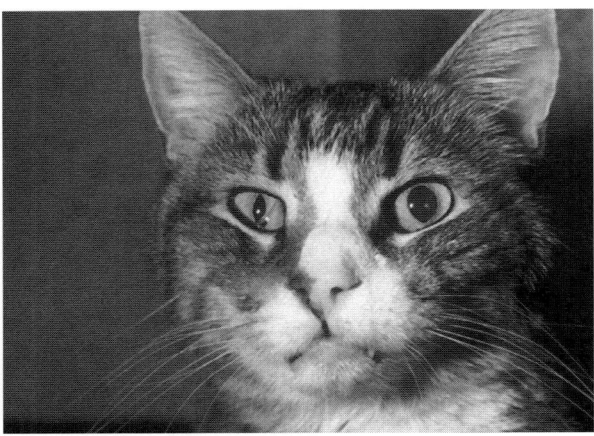

Figure 46.44 Horner's syndrome in a cat. The right eye has third eyelid protrusion, a miotic pupil and a narrowed palpebral fissure.

abnormality has no noticeable effect on vision but may result in a convergent strabismus or a congenital fine, oscillatory nystagmus.

As with puppies, kittens with severe visual defects may exhibit a 'wandering' or 'searching' nystagmus.

REFERENCES

Acland, G.M. (1988) Diagnosis and differentiation of retinal disease in small animals by electroretinography. *Seminars in Veterinary Medicine and Surgery (Small Animal)* **3**, 15–27.

Acland, G.M., Blanton, S.H., Hershfield, B. and Aguirre, G.D. (1994) XLPRA: A canine retinal degeneration inherited as an X-linked trait. *American Journal of Medical Genetics* **52**, 27–33.

Addie, D.D. (1989) Interpretation of feline coronavirus serology. *In Practice* **11**, 232–235.

Aguirre, G., Alligood, J., O'Brien, P. and Buyukmihci, N. (1982) Pathogenesis of progressive rod-cone degeneration in miniature poodles. *Investigative Ophthalmology and Visual Science* **23**, 610–630.

Albert, D.M., Lahav, M., Colby, E.D., Shadduck, J.A. and Sang, D.N. (1977) Retinal neoplasia and dysplasia. I. Induction by feline leukaemia virus. *Investigative Ophthalmology and Visual Science* **16**, 325–337.

Ashton, N., Barnett, K.C. and Sachs, D.D. (1968) Retinal dysplasia in the Sealyham terrier. *Journal of Pathology and Bacteriology* **96**, 269–272.

Barnett, K.C. (1978) Hereditary cataract in the dog. *Journal of Small Animal Practice* **19**, 109–120.

Barnett, K.C. (1980) Hereditary cataract in the Welsh springer spaniel. *Journal of Small Animal Practice* **21**, 621–625.

Barnett, K.C. (1985) The diagnosis and differential diagnosis of cataract in the dog. *Journal of Small Animal Practice* **26**, 305–316.

Barnett, K.C. (1986) Hereditary cataract in the German shepherd dog. *Journal of Small Animal Practice* **27**, 387–395.

Barnett, K.C. (1988) Inherited eye disease in the dog and cat. *Journal of Small Animal Practice* **29**, 462–475.

Barnett, K.C. and Burger, I.H. (1980) Taurine deficiency retinopathy in the cat. *Journal of Small Animal Practice* **21**, 521–534.

Barnett, K.C. and Knight, G.C. (1969) Persistent pupillary membranes and associated defects in the Basenji. *Veterinary Record* **85**, 242–248.

Barnett, K.C. and Startup, F.G. (1985) Hereditary cataract in the standard poodle. *Veterinary Record* **117**, 15–16.

Barnett, K.C., Bjorck, G.R. and Kock, E. (1970) Hereditary retinal dysplasia in the Labrador retriever in England and Sweden. *Journal of Small Animal Practice* **10**, 755–759.

Barrie, K.P., Peiffer, R.L., Gelatt, K.N. and Williams, L.W. (1979) Posterior lenticonus, microphthalmia, congenital cataracts, and retinal folds in an old English sheepdog. *Journal of the American Animal Hospital Association* **15**, 715–717.

Bedford, P.G.C. (1977) Gonioscopy in the dog. *Journal of Small Animal Practice* **18**, 615–629.

Bedford, P.G.C. (1980) The aetiology of canine glaucoma. *Veterinary Record* **107**, 76–82.

Bedford, P.G.C. (1982a) Gonioscopy in the assessment of the canine glaucoma patient. *Veterinary Annual* **22**, 319–326.

Bedford, P.G.C. (1982b) Collie eye anomaly in the United Kingdom. *Veterinary Record* **111**, 263–270.

Bedford, P.G.C. (1982c) Multifocal retinal dysplasia in the rottweiler. *Veterinary Record* **111**, 304–305.

Bedford, P.G.C. (1984a) Retinal dysplasia in the dog. *Veterinary Annual* **24**, 325–328.

Bedford, P.G.C. (1984b) Retinal pigment epithelial dystrophy (CPRA): a study of the disease in the briard. *Journal of Small Animal Practice* **25**, 129–138.

Bedford, P.G.C. (1989) A clinical evaluation of a one-piece drainage system in the treatment of canine glaucoma. *Journal of Small Animal Practice* **30**, 68–75.

Bistner, S., Rubin, L., Cox, T.A. and Condon, W.E. (1970) Pharmacological diagnosis of Horner's syndrome in the dog. *Journal of the American Veterinary Medical Association* **157**, 1220–1224.

Bjerkås, E. (1991) Collie eye anomaly in the rough collie in Norway. *Journal of Small Animal Practice* **32**, 89–92.

Blair, N.P., Dodge, J.T. and Schmidt, G.M. (1985a) Rhegmatogenous retinal detachments in Labrador retrievers. I. Development of retinal tears and detachment. *Archives of Ophthalmology* **103**, 842–847.

Blair, N.P., Dodge, J.T. and Schmidt, G.M. (1985b) Rhegmatogenous retinal detachments in Labrador retrievers. II. Proliferative vitreoretinopathy. *Archives of Ophthalmology* **103**, 848–854.

Boydell, P. (1995) Idiopathic Horner's syndrome in the golden retriever. *Journal of Small Animal Practice* **36**, 382–384.

Brightman, A.H., Ogilvie, G.K. and Tompkins, M. (1991) Ocular disease in FeLV-positive cats: 11 cases (1981–1986). *Journal of the American Veterinary Medical Association* **198**, 1049–1051.

BVA/KC/ISDS (1995) Hereditary eye disease and the BVA/KC/ISDS. *In Practice* **17**(6), 254–264.

Carrig, C.B., MacMillan, A.D., Brundage, S., Pool, R.R. and Morgan, J.P. (1977) Retinal dysplasia associated with skeletal abnormalities in Labrador retrievers. *Journal of the American Veterinary Medical Association* **170**, 49–57.

Carrig, C.B., Sponenberg, D.P., Schmidt, G.M. and Tvedten, H.W. (1988) Inheritance of associated ocular and skeletal dysplasia in Labrador retrievers. *Journal of the American Veterinary Medical Association* **193**, 1269–1272.

Carter, J.D. (1973) Surgery of congenital eyelid defects. *Veterinary Clinics of North America: Small Animal Practice* **3**, 423–432.

Champagne, E.S. and Munger, R.J. (1992) Multiple punctate keratotomy for the treatment of recurrent epithelial erosions in dogs. *Journal of the American Animal Hospital Association* **28**, 213–216.

Clements, P.J.M., Gregory, C.Y., Petersen-Jones, S.M., Sargan, D.R. and Bhattacharya, S.S. (1993) Confirmation of the rod cGMP phophodiesterase β-subunit (PDEβ) nonsense mutation in affected rcd-1 Irish setters in the UK and development of a diagnostic test. *Current Eye Research* **12**, 861–866.

Clements, P.J.M., Sargan, D.R., Gould, D.J. and Petersen-Jones, S.M. (1996) Recent advances in understanding the spectrum of canine generalised progressive retinal atrophy. *Journal of Small Animal Practice* **37**, 155–162.

Cottrell, B.D. and Barnett, K.C. (1988) Primary glaucoma in the Welsh springer spaniel. *Journal of Small Animal Practice* **29**, 185–199.

Cottrell, B.D. and Petersen-Jones, S.M. (1993) Special examination techniques. In: *Manual of Small Animal Ophthalmology* (Eds S.M. Petersen-Jones and S.M. Crispin). BSAVA Publications, Cheltenham, pp. 27–35.

Cottrill, N.B., Banks, W.J. and Pechman, R.D. (1989) Ultrasonographic and biometric evaluation of the eye and orbit in dogs. *American Journal of Veterinary Research* **50**, 898–903.

Crispin, S.M. (1982) Corneal dystrophies in small animals. *Veterinary Annual* **22**, 298–310.

Crispin, S.M. (1987) Lipid keratopathy in the dog. *Veterinary Annual* **27**, 196–208.

Crispin, S.M. and Barnett, K.C. (1983) Dystrophy, degeneration and infiltration of the canine cornea. *Journal of Small Animal Practice* **24**, 63–68.

Curtis, R. (1984) Late-onset cataract in the Boston terrier. *Veterinary Record* **115**, 577–578.

Curtis, R. (1990) Lens luxation in the dog and cat. *Veterinary Clinics of North America: Small Animal Practice* **20**, 755–773.

Curtis, R. and Barnett, K.C. (1989) A survey of cataracts in golden and Labrador retrievers. *Journal of Small Animal Practice* **30**, 277–286.

Curtis, R., Barnett, K.C. and Leon, A. (1991) Diseases of the canine posterior segment. In: *Veterinary Ophthalmology*, 2nd edn (Ed. K.N. Gelatt). Lea and Febiger, Philadelphia, pp. 461–525.

Davidson, M.G., Nasisse, M.P., English, R.V., Wilcock, B.P. and Jamieson, V.E. (1991) Feline anterior uveitis: a study of 53 cases. *Journal of the American Animal Hospital Association* **27**, 77–83.

DeLahunta, A. (1983) Visual system – special somatic afferent system. In: *Veterinary Neuroanatomy and Clinical Neurology*. W.B. Saunders, Philadelphia, pp. 279–303.

Dziezyc, J. and Millichamp, N.J. (1989) Surgical correction of eyelid agenesis in a cat. *Journal of the American Animal Hospital Association* **25**, 513–516.

Dziezyc, J., Wolf, E.D. and Barrie, K.P. (1986) Surgical repair of rhegmatogenous retinal detachments in dogs. *Journal of the American Veterinary Medical Association* **189**, 902–904.

Dziezyc, J., Hager, D.A. and Millichamp, N.J. (1987) Two-dimension real-time ultrasonography in the diagnosis of ocular lesions in dogs. *Journal of the American Animal Hospital Association* **23**, 501–508.

English, R.V., Davidson, M.G., Nasisse, M.P., Jamieson, V.E. & Lappin, M.R. (1990) Intraocular disease associated with feline immunodeficiency virus infection in cats. *Journal of the American Veterinary Medical Association* **196**, 1116–1119.

Fontaine, M. (1961) Contagious rhino-tonsillitis (CRT): a new virus unrelated to other infectious diseases in the dog. *Journal of Small Animal Practice* **2**, 71–96.

Gelatt, K.N. (1972) Surgical correction of everted nictitating membrane in the dog. *Veterinary Medicine/Small Animal Clinician* **67**, 291–292.

Gelatt, K.N. (1991) The canine eyelids. In: *Veterinary Ophthalmology*, 2nd edn (Ed. K.N. Gelatt). Lea and Febiger, Philadelphia, pp. 256–275.

Gelatt, K.N. (1992) Issues in ophthalmic therapy: the development of anterior chamber shunts for the clinical management of the canine glaucomas. *Progress in Veterinary and Comparative Ophthalmology* **2**, 59–64.

Gelatt, K.N., Whitley, D., Lavach, J.D., Barrie, K.P. and Williams, L.W. (1979) Cataracts in Chesapeake Bay retrievers. *Journal of the American Veterinary Medical Association* **175**, 1176–1178.

Gelatt, K.N., Samuelsen, D.A., Barrie, K.P., Das, N.D., Wolf, E.D., Bauer, J.E. and Andersen, T.L. (1983) Biometry and clinical characteristics of congenital cataracts in the miniature schnauzer. *Journal of the American Veterinary Medical Association* **183**, 99–102.

Gwin, R.M., Kolwalski, J.J., Wyman, M. and Winston,

S. (1980) Ocular lesions associated with *Brucella canis* infection in a dog. *Journal of the American Animal Hospital Association* **16**, 607–610.

Gwin, R.M., Wyman, M., Lim, D.J., Ketring, K. and Werling, K. (1981) Multiple ocular defects associated with partial albinism and deafness in the dog. *Journal of the American Animal Hospital Association* **17**, 401–408.

Gwin, R.M., Polack, F.M., Warren, J.K., Samuelson, D.A. and Gelatt, K.N. (1982) Primary canine corneal endothelial cell dystrophy: specular microscopic evaluation, diagnosis and therapy. *Journal of the American Animal Hospital Association* **18**, 471–479.

Håkanson, N., Lorimer, D. and Meredith, R.E. (1988) Further comments on conjunctival pedicle grafting in the treatment of corneal ulcers in the dog and cat. *Journal of the American Animal Hospital Association* **24**, 602–605.

Hendy-Ibbs, P.M. (1985) Familial feline epibulbar dermoids. *Veterinary Record* **116**, 13–14.

Herrtage, M.E., Barnett, K.C. and MacDougal, D.F. (1985) Diabetic retinopathy in a cat with megestrol acetate-induced diabetes. *Journal of Small Animal Practice* **26**, 595–601.

Heywood, R. and Wells, G.A.H. (1970) A retinal dysplasia in the beagle dog. *Veterinary Record* **87**, 178–180.

Hoover, E.A., Kahn, D.E. and Langloss, J.M. (1978) Experimentally induced feline chlamydial infection (feline pneumonitis). *American Journal of Veterinary Research* **39**, 541–547.

Johnson, B.W., Gerding, P.A., McLaughlan, S.A., Helper, L.C., Szajerski, M.E. and Cormany, K.A. (1988) Nonsurgical correction of entropion in shar pei puppies. *Veterinary Medicine/Small Animal Clinician* **83**, 482–483.

Jubb K.V., Saunders, L.Z. and Coates, H.V. (1957) The intraocular lesions of canine distemper. *Journal of Comparative Pathology* **67**, 21–29.

Kaswan, R.L. and Martin, C.L. (1985) Surgical correction of third eyelid prolapse in dogs. *Journal of the American Veterinary Medical Association* **186**, 83.

Kaswan, R.L. and Salisbury M.A. (1990) A new perspective on canine keratoconjunctivitis sicca: treatment with ophthalmic cyclosporin. *Veterinary Clinics of North America: Small Animal Practice* **20**, 583–613.

Kern, T.J. and Riis, R.C. (1981) Optic nerve hypoplasia in three miniature poodles. *Journal of the American Veterinary Medical Association* **178**, 49–54.

Kern, T.J., Walton, D.K., Riis, R.C., Manning, T.O., Laratta, L.J. and Dziezyc, J. (1985) Uveitis associated with poliosis and vitiligo in six dogs. *Journal of the American Veterinary Medical Association* **187**, 408–414.

Koch, S.A. (1972) Cataracts in interrelated old English sheepdogs. *Journal of the American Veterinary Medical Association* **160**, 299–301.

Kornegay, J.N., Greene, C.E., Martin, C., Gorgacz, E.J. and Melcon, D.K. (1980) Idiopathic hypocalcaemia in four dogs. *Journal of the American Animal Hospital Association* **16**, 723–734.

Lavach, J.D., Murphy, J.M. and Severin, G.A. (1978) Retinal dysplasia in the English springer spaniel. *Journal of the American Animal Hospital Association* **14**, 192–199.

Leon, A., Curtis, R. and Barnett, K.C. (1986) Hereditary persistent hyperplastic primary vitreous in the Staffordshire bull terrier. *Journal of the American Animal Hospital Association* **22**, 765–774.

Lewis, D.G., Kelly, D.F. and Sansom, J. (1986) Congenital microphthalmia and other developmental ocular abnormalities in the dobermann. *Journal of Small Animal Practice* **27**, 559–566.

MacMillan, A.D. and Lipton, D.E. (1978) Heritability of multifocal retinal dysplasia in American cocker spaniels. *Journal of the American Veterinary Medical Association* **172**, 568–572.

MacMillan, A.D., Waring, G.O., Spangler, W.L. and Roth, A.M. (1979) Crystalline corneal opacities in the Siberian husky. *Journal of the American Veterinary Medical Association* **175**, 829–832.

Martin, C.L. (1981) Canine epibulbar melanomas and their management. *Journal of the American Animal Hospital Association* **17**, 83–90.

Mason, I. K. and Barnett, K.C. (1994) Primary glaucoma in the great Dane. *BSAVA Paper Synopsis*. 185.

Meyers, S.M., Vasil, M.L. and Yamamoto. L. (1982) Pathologic mechanisms of multifocal choroiditis with retinal detachment after carotid injection of *Streptococcus mutans* and other bacteria in dogs. *Investigative Ophthalmology and Visual Science* **22**, 165–173.

Miller, P.E. and Pickett, J.P. (1992) Comparison of the human and canine Schiøtz tonometry conversion tables in clinically normal dogs. *Journal of the American Veterinary Medical Association* **201**, 1021–1025.

Millichamp, N.J. (1990) Retinal degeneration in the dog and cat. *Veterinary Clinics of North America: Small Animal Practice* **20**, 799–835.

Morgan, R.V. (1986) Systemic hypertension in four cats: ocular and medical findings. *Journal of the American Animal Hospital Association* **22**, 615–621.

Mould, J.R.B. (1993) Approach to an ophthalmic examination. In: *Manual of Small Animal Ophthalmology* (Eds S.M. Petersen-Jones and S.M. Crispin). BSAVA Publications, Cheltenham, pp. 11–25.

Narfström, K. (1981) Cataract in the West Highland white terrier. *Journal of Small Animal Practice* **22**, 467–471.

Narfström, K. and Dubielzig, R. (1984) Posterior lenticonus, cataracts and microphthalmia: congenital ocular defects in the Cavalier King Charles spaniel. *Journal of Small Animal Practice* **25**, 669–677.

Nasisse, M.P. (1990) Feline herpesvirus ocular disease. *Veterinary Clinics of North America: Small Animal Practice* **20**, 667–680.

Nasisse, M.P. (1991) Feline ophthalmology. In:

Veterinary Ophthalmology, 2nd edn (Ed. K.N. Gelatt). Lea and Febiger, Philadelphia, pp. 529–575.

Nasisse, M.P., Guy, J.S., Davidson, M.G., Sussman, W.A. and Fairley, N.M. (1989a) Experimental ocular herpesvirus infection in the cat: sites of virus replication, clinical features and effects of corticosteroid administration. *Investigative Ophthalmology and Visual Science* **30**, 1758–1768.

Nasisse, M.P., Guy, J.S., Davidson, M.G., Sussman, W.A. and De Clercq, E. (1989b) In vitro susceptibility of feline herpesvirus-1 to vidarabine, idouridine, acyclovir, or bromovinyldeoxyuridine. *American Journal of Veterinary Research* **50**, 158–160.

Nasisse, M.P., Davidson, M.G., Jamieson, V.E., English, R.V. and Olivero, D.K. (1991) Phaco-emulsification and intraocular lens implantation: a study of technique in 182 dogs. *Progress in Veterinary and Comparative Ophthalmology* **1**, 225–232.

Nelson, D.L. and MacMillan, A.D. (1983) Multifocal retinal dysplasia in field Labrador retrievers. *Journal of the American Animal Hospital Association* **19**, 388–392.

Olesen, H.P., Jensen, O.A. and Norn, M.S. (1974) Congenital hereditary cataract in Cocker Spaniels. *Journal of Small Animal Practice* **15**, 741–750.

O'Toole, D., Young, S., Severin, G.A. and Neuman, S. (1983) Retinal dysplasia of English springer spaniel dogs: light microscopy of the postnatal lesions. *Veterinary Pathology* **20**, 298–311.

Palmer, A.C., Malinowski, W. and Barnett, K.C. (1974) Clinical signs including papilloedema associated with brain tumours in twenty-one dogs. *Journal of Small Animal Practice* **15**, 359–386.

Paulsen, M.E., Lavach, J.D., Severin, G.A. and Eichenbaum, J.D. (1987) Feline eosinophilic keratitis: a review of 15 clinical cases. *Journal of the American Animal Hospital Association* **23**, 63–69.

Peiffer, R.L. (1982) Inherited ocular disease of the dog and cat. *Compendium on Continuing Education for the Practicing Veterinarian* **4**, 152–168.

Peiffer, R.L. and Fischer, C.A. (1983) Microphthalmia, retinal dysplasia and anterior segment dysgenesis in a litter of doberman pinschers. *Journal of the American Veterinary Medical Association* **183**, 875–878.

Peiffer, R.L., Gelatt, K.N., Jessen, C.R., Gum, G.G., Gwin, R.M. and Davis, J.D. (1977) Calibration of the Schiøtz tonometer for the normal canine eye. *American Journal of Veterinary Research* **38**, 1881–1889.

Peiffer, R.L., Monticello, T. and Bouldin, T.W. (1988) Primary ocular sarcomas in the cat. *Journal of Small Animal Practice* **29**, 105–116.

Percy, D.H., Scott, F.W. and Albert, D.M. (1975) Retinal dysplasia due to feline panleucopenia virus infection. *Journal of the American Veterinary Medical Association* **167**, 935–937.

Petersen-Jones, S.M. (1990a) Abnormal pigment deposition associated with glaucoma in the cairn terrier. *Journal of Small Animal Practice* **32**, 19–22.

Petersen-Jones, S.M. (1990b) Intraocular lenses for dogs. *Veterinary Practice* **22** (14), 1–5.

Piper, R.C., Cole, C.R. and Shadduck, J.A. (1970) Natural and experimental ocular toxoplasmosis in animals. *American Journal of Ophthalmology* **69**, 662–668.

Randell, M.G. and Hurvitz, A.I. (1983) Immune-mediated vasculitis in five dogs. *Journal of the American Veterinary Medical Association* **183**, 207–211.

Regnier, A. and Toutain, P.L. (1991) Ocular pharmacology and therapeutic modalities. In: *Veterinary Ophthalmology*, 2nd edn (Ed. K.N. Gelatt). Lea and Febiger, Philadelphia, pp. 162–194.

Roberts, S.M., Severin, G.A. and Lavach, J.D. (1986) Prevalence and treatment of palpebral neoplasms in the dog: 200 cases (1975–1983). *Journal of the American Veterinary Medical Association* **189**, 1355–1359.

Rubin, L.F. (1968) Heredity of retinal dysplasia in Bedlington terriers. *Journal of the American Veterinary Medical Association* **152**, 260–262.

Rubin, L.F. (1989) *Inherited Eye Disease in Purebred Dogs*. Williams and Wilkins, Baltimore.

Rubin, L.F. and Flowers, R.D. (1972) Inherited cataract in a family of standard poodles. *Journal of the American Veterinary Medical Association* **161**, 207–208.

Sansom, J. and Barnett, K.C. (1985) Keratoconjunctivitis sicca in the dog: a review of two hundred cases. *Journal of Small Animal Practice* **26**, 121–131.

Schmidt, G.M., Ellersieck, M.R., Wheeler, C.A., Blanchard, G.L. and Keller, W.F. (1979) Inheritance of retinal dysplasia in the English springer spaniel. *Journal of the American Veterinary Medical Association* **174**, 1089–1090.

Scott, F.W., de Lahunta, A., Schultz, R.D., Bistner, S.I. and Riis, R.C. (1975) Teratogenesis in cats associated with griseofulvin therapy. *Teratology* **11**, 79–86.

Spangler, W.L., Gribble, D.H. and Weisser, M.G. (1977) Canine hypertension: a review. *Journal of the American Veterinary Medical Association* **170**, 995–998.

Stades, F.C. (1978) Hereditary retinal dysplasia (RD) in a family of Yorkshire terriers. *Tijdschrift voor Diergeneeskunde* **103**, 1087–1090.

Stades, F.C. (1983) Persistent hyperplastic tunica vasculosa lentis and persistent hyperplastic primary vitreous in doberman pinschers: genetic aspects. *Journal of the American Animal Hospital Association* **19**, 957–964.

Stades, F.C. (1987) A new method for correction of upper eyelid trichiasis-entropion: operation method. *Journal of the American Animal Hospital Association* **23**, 603–606.

Startup, F.G. (1988) Corneal necrosis and sequestration in the cat: a review and record of 100 cases. *Journal of Small Animal Practice* **29**, 476–486.

Strande, A., Nicolaissen, B. and Bjerkås, I. (1988) Persistent pupillary membrane and congenital cataract in a litter of English cocker spaniels. *Journal of Small Animal Practice* **29**, 257–260.

Suber, M.L., Pittler, S.J., Qin, N., Wright, G.C., Holcombe, V., Lee, R.H., Craft, C.M., Lolley, R.N., Baehr, W. and Hurwitz, R.L. (1993) Irish setter dogs affected with rod–cone dysplasia contain a nonsense mutation in the rod cGMP phosphodiesterase β-subunit gene. *Proceedings of the National Academy of Sciences of the USA* **90**, 3968–3972.

Whitley, R.D. (1991) Canine cornea. *Veterinary Ophthalmology*, 2nd edn (Ed. K.N. Gelatt). Lea and Febiger, Philadelphia, p. 339.

Wilkie, D.A. (1990) Control of ocular inflammation. *Veterinary Clinics of North America: Small Animal Practice* **20**, 693–713.

Wyman, M. (1971) Lateral canthoplasty. *Journal of the American Animal Hospital Association* **7**, 196–201.

Yakely, W.L. (1978) A study of heritability of cataracts in the American cocker spaniel. *Journal of the American Veterinary Medical Association* **172**, 814–817.

47

Skin Diseases of the Dog and Cat

S. E. Shaw and S. E. Kelly

DISEASES OF THE SKIN	**871**	Skin diseases associated with keratinization	
Introduction	871	disorders	901
History taking	873	Genetic/congenital dermatoses	902
Physical examination	875		
Diagnostic procedures	876	**SKIN DISEASES OF THE CAT**	**903**
		Allergic skin disease	903
SKIN DISEASES OF THE DOG	**880**	Eosinophilic granuloma complex	905
Allergic skin disease	880	Psychogenic alopecia	906
Infectious skin disease	883	Infectious skin disease	907
Protozoal skin disease	888	Parasitic skin disease	911
Parasitic skin disease	889	Endocrine dermatoses	912
Neoplastic skin diseases	891	Neoplastic skin disease	913
Endocrine dermatoses	893	Immune-mediated diseases	914
Immune-mediated skin diseases	897	Congenital and genetic dermatoses	915

DISEASES OF THE SKIN

INTRODUCTION

It has often been stated that the skin is the body system most often involved in requests for veterinary attention. Estimates vary but 20% or more of all cases seen in an average small animal practice involve dermatology.

In dealing with dermatological cases, the clinician is in the unusual situation of having the whole organ system available for visual inspection. Clinical signs can be related to the part or parts of skin affected. Recognition that deeper rather than superficial areas of the skin are involved may result in different treatment recommendations and prognoses. Consequently it is useful to understand the normal structure of the skin and its appendages.

The skin is made up of three components:

- Epidermal structures;
- Dermis;
- Hypodermis and panniculus.

Epidermal structures

Surface epidermis

The epidermis consists of layered sheets of cells supported by a system of fibres and fibrils adjacent to the basement membrane zone and anchored to the dermis by hair follicles. In small animals, the epidermis is relatively thin: 1–3 cells in thickness or 0.1–0.5 mm (Fakhri and Lovell, 1979; Lloyd and Garthwaite, 1982). It consists primarily of keratinocytes developing in orderly sequence from the basal layer but also contains cells which are not of epidermal origin. These include the melanocyte and the Langherhans cell. It has been suggested that there is interaction between all three cell types in the maintenance of cutaneous integrity. Melanocytes are not only responsible for the distinctive marking of normal skin but have an integral role in protecting against ultraviolet radiation damage. The Langerhans cells are immigrants from bone marrow and are immunologically active; they phagocytose and process antigen for presentation to lymphocytes and produce numerous cytokines. There is concerted action of Langerhans cells, epidermotropic T lymphocytes, keratinocytes and local lymph nodes in maintaining cutaneous immunosurveillance. Together they are referred to as skin-associated lymphoid tissue or SALT (Breathnach, 1986; Yager, 1993).

The keratinocytes of the epidermis represent a dynamic cell renewal system which in the normal state, ensures physical protection of underlying structures by production of the complex fibrous protein, keratin. Estimates of epidermal turnover time vary but in the normal dog it is approximately 22 days. This may be decreased dramatically in primary hyperproliferative disorders of the epidermis such as idiopathic seborrhoea in Cocker spaniels where the cell renewal time may be as rapid as 8 days (Kwochka and Rademakers, 1989). Inflammatory mediators such as arachidonic acid and leucotrienes have also been incriminated in producing a secondary hyperproliferative epidermis in dogs (Campbell, 1990). The complex sequence involved in producing an adherent layer of flattened keratin scales (stratum corneum) from the basal layer of mitotically active keratinocytes is illustrated in Fig. 47.1.

The pilosebaceous unit

Hair and hair follicles

The basal layer of the epidermis is contiguous with that of the hair follicles. Hair shafts are formed by keratinocytes based in the hair matrix. Cells in this area have the most actively renewing population in the body (Kwochka, 1990). The process of epidermopoiesis is otherwise similar to that in the surface epidermis. The colour of hair is derived from follicular melanocytes also using a process similar to that in the surface epidermis. The dendritic processes of melanocytes primarily in the basal layer extend to transfer melanin to differentiating keratinocytes in the spinous layer.

Ducts of both sebaceous and sweat glands open into the top third of the hair follicle or infundibulum. This anatomical association is important clinically because the follicular epithelium represents the only barrier between 'foreign' lipids and protein (follicular keratin, sebum and sweat) and the dermis. Release of these products into the dermis if follicular rupture occurs, results in a severe inflammatory response.

The growth of hair is a poorly understood but complex process. Continuous hair growth does not occur but a cyclical progression from anagen to telogen is recognized and illustrated in Fig. 47.2. Hairs are normally shed in a mosaic fashion as adjacent follicles are in different phases of the cycle. As the anagen hair displaces the poorly anchored telogen shaft, shedding will be inevitable. Alterations in photoperiod, hormonal activity and nutritional status may shorten the anagen period to produce excessive shedding and in some cases, alopecia.

Sebaceous and sweat glands

Sebum acts as a lubricant to maintain the quality of the hair coat and diffuses through the stratum corneum to provide a physical and chemical barrier. Sebaceous and stratum corneum lipids may act as both nutrients for and inhibitors of microbial growth. Unsaturated fatty acids such as linoleic, oleic and lauric acids are generally inhibitory and saturated fatty acids inhibit dermatophytes *in vitro* (Hay, 1992). More recently, sphingosines present in the stratum corneum have been found to have profound antimicrobial activities both *in vivo* and *in vitro* (Bibel et al., 1992).

Both sweat and sebaceous glands discharge their products into the hair follicle, although sweat glands in the footpad discharge directly on to the skin surface. Sweat gland activity in dogs and cats is regulated by sympathetic adrenergic and cholinergic nerves. Sweat contains IgA and is therefore also important in skin immunity. The

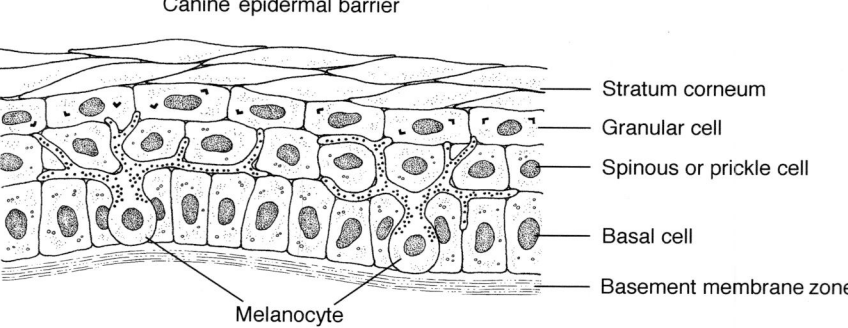

Figure 47.1 Schematic diagram showing the layers of the epidermis.

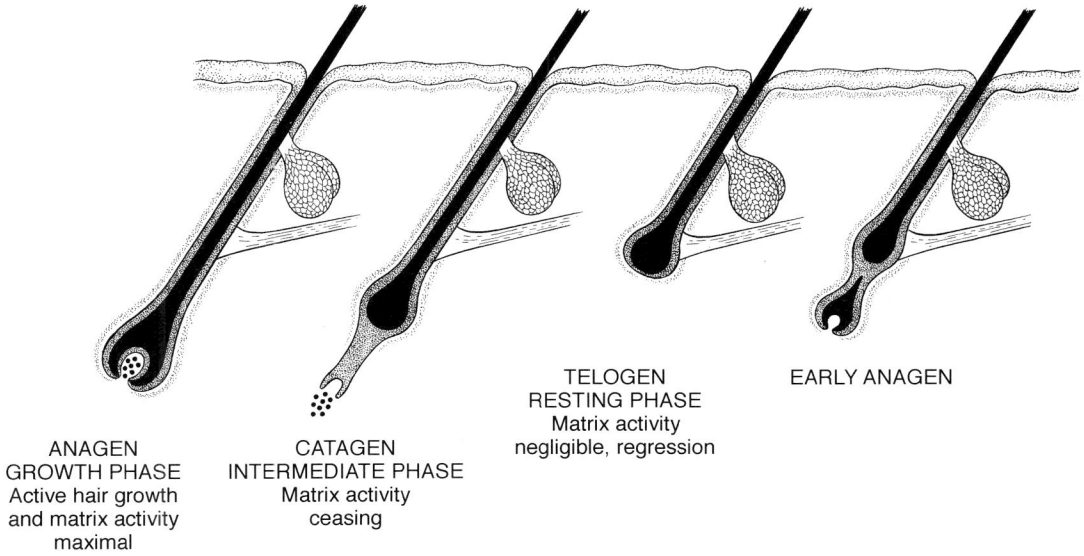

Figure 47.2 Schematic diagram of a simple hair follicle during the hair cycle.

traditional concepts of apocrine (follicular) and eccrine (footpad) secretion has been challenged; Jenkinson (1989) has presented evidence which suggests that both cell death and secretion are important processes in sweat formation. Accordingly, he proposed that sweat glands associated with follicles are termed 'epitrichial' and those on the footpads 'atrichial'.

Dermis

The dermis is a tough but pliable combination of collagen and elastin fibres surrounded by proteoglycan ground substance. It provides both the vascular and nerve supply to the epidermis. These include specialized receptors for the senses of touch, pain and pressure which are vital for survival. The sensation of pruritus is initiated in small non-myelinated nerve endings situated in the upper dermis, making it a very superficial sensation. The dermis also contains a diffuse population of mast cells, histiocytes and lymphocytes which are often involved in skin disease.

Hypodermis

The hypodermis is composed of adipose connective tissue, the panniculus muscle and an extensive blood supply. These structures give animal skin elasticity, an ability to express adaptive behaviour (piloerection), insulation and a deep anchor for the epidermis. It is also the site for a group of skin diseases which are inherently difficult to treat.

HISTORY TAKING

A general medical history combined with specific questions oriented to the skin problem is required (Table 47.1).

Certain breeds are predisposed to skin disease (Muller et al., 1989a). However, it is important to relate this information to differences in geographical influences and in some cases, to the narrow gene pools that have been investigated. Universally, West Highland white terriers have an increased risk for atopy, the Rhodesian ridgeback for dermoid sinus formation, the English bull terrier for furunculosis, and the boxer for mast cell neoplasia. Long-haired cats, particularly Persians in the UK, are predisposed to dermatophytosis.

The age of a dog or cat presented with skin disease can help in narrowing the diagnostic possibilities. In the group less than 6 months of age congenital and infectious causes are of primary concern. Dermatophytosis and demodicosis are more commonly seen than the congenital diseases such as ichthyosis and hypotrichosis. In general,

Table 47.1 Historical database for dogs and cats with skin disease

- Breed, age and gender
- Age of onset and duration of the problem
- Location of initial lesion/s and description of change in character and distribution
- Seasonal variation, i.e. lesions only during certain months of the year or present all the year round
- Determination of the degree of pruritus
  1. Scratching: mild (scratches occasionally) to severe (still scratching in stressful situations or at night)
  2. Overgrooming or licking excessively
- In contact pets or humans affected
- Environment
  1. Bedding and housing
  2. Access to sylvatic reservoirs of infectious disease: foxes, hedgehogs, voles
- Nutrition
  Determine that the nutritional profile is appropriate for age, growth, special work, activity and reproduction
- Determine the presence of systemic signs: polyuria, polydipsia, lethargy, abdominal enlargement, abnormal oestrus cycles, lack of libido
- Determine the stage of reproductive cycle
- Response to prior treatment

hypersensitivity disorders are seen in the 1–5-year age group and are uncommon over the age of 7. However, 34% of dogs with atopy in a Californian survey showed clinical signs by 9 months of age (Griffin, 1993a). Food allergy is also reported to occur before the age of 6 months. In dogs and cats over the age of 8 years, the prevalence of neoplasia and endocrine-mediated skin disease increases.

Gender predisposition to disease is important and collecting a full reproductive history is required. A cryptorchid male dog may appear to have been castrated and yet have a funtional tumour in a retained testis.

A useful piece of history is seasonality of clinical signs.

Flea allergy dermatitis may be worse in summer and certain plants cause contact dermatitis and atopic disease when they are flowering. However, allergic signs associated with house dust mite or food are non-seasonal.

Nutritional information is essential. Not only does this determine the possible basis for food allergy but imbalances in nutritional components may lead to specific dermatological syndromes. Generic dry foods may be deficient in fatty acids, high in dietary fibre and low in available zinc (Sousa et al., 1988). Feeding of excessive calcium in rapidly growing dogs on a high fibre diet may decrease the bioavailability of zinc, leading to relative zinc deficiency (Van den Broek and Thoday, 1986).

Dermatological diseases may reflect internal disorders. Vomiting and diarrhoea may be associated with food hypersensitivity dermatitis. Alopecia seen in conjunction with polyuria and polydipsia, changes in appetite, exercise intolerance or sexual activity often indicate an underlying endocrine cause.

Response to previous therapy may provide a useful diagnostic marker. Table 47.2 indicates the expected response of some common pruritic

Table 47.2 Glucocorticoid responsiveness of common pruritic skin diseases

Responsive	Partially or poorly responsive
Flea allergy dermatitis	Sarcoptic mange
Atopy	Superficial staphylococcal folliculitus
Contact allergy	Atopy with secondary pyoderma
	Demodicosis with secondary pyoderma
Pyotraumatic dermatitis	

dermatoses to glucocorticoids. Skin disease in which bacterial infection (*Staphylococcus intermedius*) plays a role may be markedly pruritic but only partially or poorly responsive to glucocorticoids. The pruritus associated with uncomplicated atopy is frequently very sensitive to these drugs. However, sarcoptic mange which has a similar distribution to atopy is only partially responsive. Complete clinical response to a previous course of antibiotics suitable for *S. intermedius* implicates this organism as the major pathogenetic factor but a partial response may indicate pyoderma secondary to an underlying disease such as allergy or demodicosis.

PHYSICAL EXAMINATION

A full general physical examination should be performed before concentrating on the skin since the skin often reflects signs of internal disease.

When examining the skin and hair coat, good, preferably natural, lighting is essential and a source of magnification useful. The entire skin surface should be examined by sight and palpation. If skin lesions are obscured by hair a 'window' should be clipped allowing the clinician to examine areas which are likely to be less altered by self-trauma and secondary change. Particular attention should be paid to those areas that are less obviously visible: the periocular region, lips, gingiva, ear canals and pinnal margins, the footpads and interdigital spaces, and the perineum including external genitalia and anal sacs. Evidence of parasites particularly fleas and flea faeces can be collected as part of the physical examination using coat brushing or combing.

Skin lesions are commonly described as primary or secondary lesions. Primary lesions are produced directly by the underlying disease process. Searching for them and interpreting their significance narrows the diagnostic possibilities. They are frequently masked by secondary lesions produced by self trauma and grooming.

Interpreting the various patterns of primary and secondary lesions in an individual case is often difficult. This is particularly the case in inflammatory skin disease. However, even though an aetiological diagnosis is rarely made based on lesion recognition alone, it may narrow the diagnostic possibilities to certain pathophysiological groups as illustrated in Table 47.3. This information aids planning of laboratory tests and appropriate interim therapy. It is important to determine the predominant lesion as several may be present simultaneously.

Certain diseases tend to affect specific areas of the skin. An uncomplicated case of flea allergy dermatitis has the classical dorsal tail head and gluteal distribution. However, the distribution pattern may be misleading in chronic disease. A chronic flea allergy case may have a more generalized distribution of lesions which provides fewer clues regarding the aetiology. The initial distribution pattern should be elicted by history and changes correlated with the pattern at presentation.

Table 47.3 Association of some skin lesions with diagnostic category

Primary lesion	Secondary lesion	Diagnosis
Papules Macules Wheals	Excoriations, erosions, lichenification and hyperpigmentation	Inflammatory Parasitic Allergic
Vesicles Bullae	Erosions, crusts and ulcers	Immune-mediated Autoimmune
Pustules	Epidermal collarettes	Inflammatory bacterial (immune-mediated)
Nodules	Ulcers	Neoplastic Inflammatory (infectious or sterile)
	Hyperpigmentation, scales	Endocrine
Scales	Scales	Keratinization defects: secondary or primary

DIAGNOSTIC PROCEDURES

Skin scrapings and coat brushings

These are some of the most cost effective and easy tests to perform in veterinary dermatology and should be routine in almost all cases (other than the most simple). All lesions associated with scale formation should be scraped. This also applies to all lesions of the face and feet, particularly in animals less than 9 months of age. Skin scrapings and coat brushings are primarily used in the diagnosis of parasitic disease. The method and site of scraping depends on the suspected aetiology. For sarcoptic mange the elbows, ear margins and any areas with a papular eruption are the sites of choice. Scabies mites can be difficult to find in some cases and failure to recover the parasite does not exclude the diagnosis; trial therapy is warranted whenever scabies is suspected but not proven by scrapings. Identification of one mite or egg supports the diagnosis. Demodectic mites reside in hair follicles and squeezing a fold of skin will aid in extruding them to the surface. Scraping should be continued to a depth where capillary ooze occurs. Demodectic mites are more easily found and in greater numbers than *Sarcoptes scabiei*. The site of scraping depends on lesion location.

Skin scrapings are performed using a scalpel blade moistened with mineral oil. The area to be scraped can be gently clipped of hair and also moistened with mineral oil to facilitate adherence of material to the blade. The material is dispersed on a microscope slide for examination. Although mineral oil is preferred by many, 6% potassium hydroxide may be used as an alternative (Baker and Thomsett, 1990). Ectoparasites can normally be observed using the scanning (×4) objective.

Suitable material for the diagnosis of superficially dwelling mites (*Cheyletiella*, *Otodectes*), small ticks and lice may be obtained by applying clear adhesive tape to the same skin surface several times. The tape is applied to a slide for examination. The same technique may be used for identification of the yeast, *Malassezia pachydermatis*, but the tape is stained with a routine cytological stain (Diff Quik) and examined directly under high-power or oil immersion.

Microscopic examination of hair shafts

This diagnostic test can be useful in two ways. Plucked hairs may be mounted on a microscope slide with adhesive tape and examined (trichogram). Where a history of self-trauma is difficult to elicit, microscopic examination may reveal broken and frayed proximal hair shafts indicative of excessive licking or biting. Examination of the distal end of the hair shaft can be used to evaluate the stage of the hair cycle.

Hairs and skin scrapings can also be examined for the presence of fungal elements. Estimations of the diagnostic value vary as the technique requires practice and experience in interpretation. Hairs and skin scales should be collected from the lesions using forceps. The collected specimen is placed on a slide and cleared of keratin. Various clearing agents have been recommended. Potassium hydroxide (20%) can be added to the sample and gently heated to decrease preparation time. At room temperature 20–30 min are required for clearing. More rapid digestion can be obtained with a mixture of potassium hydroxide and dimethylsulphoxide (DMSO) or by using a combination of chloral hydrate, liquid phenol and lactic acid (chlorphenolac). Some authors recommend mineral oil (Muller *et al.*, 1989a).

Hair and scales are examined for the presence of yeasts, conidia and hyphae. Most species of dermatophyte in animals produce ectothrix invasion of hair shafts. Fungal hyphae may be present within the hair shaft but their arthroconidia tend to encircle the surface of the hair in chains or as a sheath. They are relatively symmetrical and refractile resembling 'beads of mercury' on microscopy. A ×40 objective is usually required for identification. The technique is prone to artefact in inexperienced hands. Cotton fibres can be mistaken for hyphae and melanin granules for arthroconidia.

Wood's lamp examination

The use of a Wood's lamp may be helpful but has several limitations. Of the dermatophytes affecting small animals *Microsporum canis* is the only common species in dogs and cats which exhibits fluorescence. Although reports vary, only 30–40% of cases identified by culture will fluoresce. False positive fluorescence is a common problem. Normal scale, topical medications, dyes and soaps fluoresce usually without the classic 'apple green' colour. Only fluorescence of the correct hue seen on short broken hairs should be considered as positive. If positive, this technique can aid in identifying those hairs best suited for direct microscopic examination and culture but absence of fluorescence does not exclude the diagnosis.

Cytological examination

Material for cytological examination can be collected by fine needle aspiration or impression smears.

Impression smears are made by applying a microscope slide directly onto the surface of a lesion or the cut edge of a biopsy specimen. More practically a cotton swab may be used to collect material from the skin or external ear canal which is then rolled onto a slide. This is a useful technique for demonstrating cutaneous yeast infections and for evaluation of the cellular and microbiological components of otitis externa. For impression smears to be diagnostic, cells from the lesion must be easily exfoliated and the amount of superficial debris minimal. Fine needle aspiration may be used to collect material from pustules, bullae and nodules. Aspiration of intact pustular lesions is a rapid test for bacterial skin disease. Neutrophils are degenerate and intracellular bacteria should be present. An idea of the type of bacteria present will aid the empirical choice of antibiotics. Identification of acantholytic keratinocytes within a pustular or bullous lesion is suggestive of an immune-mediated process, particularly the pemphigus group of skin diseases.

Aspiration or impression smears are stained with a routine cytological stain such as Diff Quik for cellular cytology or with Gram stain for microbiological examination.

Bacterial culture and sensitivity

To obtain reliable results, material should be carefully selected as superficial erosions and ulcers are nearly always secondarily contaminated with coagulase-positive staphyloccoci. Intact pustules are the lesions of choice from which to obtain meaningful results. The pustule should be opened using a sterile 26 gauge needle and the contents swabbed. Bacterial culture from a skin biopsy is particularly useful when a deep pyoderma or pyogranulomatous infection is present. Transport media is recommended should there be any delay in transit to a laboratory.

The results of culture and sensitivity should be considered in the light of other diagnostic information. The *in vitro* sensitivity of an antibiotic may not correlate with its *in vitro* action for a number of reasons. An antibiotic may not penetrate the skin or a walled off lesion in an adequate antibacterial concentration even though it achieves an effective blood concentration.

Fungal culture

Broken or fragile hairs and hairs that fluoresce under Wood's lamp are the best specimens to choose for culture. If in doubt, the animal should be brushed with a sterile toothbrush or Denman brush to give a representative sample. This is particularly important in asymptomatic carrier cats. Samples should be placed in a dry airtight container for transport. As for bacterial skin disease, culture from a skin biopsy is recommended if an intermediate or deep fungal infection is suspected, in cases of nail bed infection and when a dermatophyte may be the cause of granuloma formation (kerion or pseudomycetoma).

The media available for isolation of fungi are essentially based on Sabouraud's dextrose agar with or without antibiotics to inhibit the growth of bacteria and saprophytic fungi. Neutral Sabouraud's dextrose agar and Mycobiotic media (chloramphenicol and cycloheximide added) allow identification of fungi by colony characteristics and pigmentation but do not selectively identify dermatophytes. Incubation for 1–3 weeks is required. Dermatophyte test medium (DTM) which consists of Sabourauds's dextrose agar, gentamycin, cycloheximide, chlortetracycline and phenol red provides an environment conducive to the differential growth of dermatophytes. The phenol red indicator is the basis for its selective qualities. Dermatophytes will use protein in the medium initially and the alkaline metabolites produced will turn the indicator dark red. Conversely saprophytic fungi will first use the dextrose substrate producing acid end products. In this case, DTM will remain yellow or amber. Evaluation of the colour change should be made daily for 10 days. Many dermatophytes take 7–10 days to appear but in heavily infected specimens a colour change under the colony may be detected in 72 h. Care should be taken when results are interpreted after two weeks incubation, since after exhausting the carbohydrate source, saprophytic fungi will digest protein and also turn the medium red.

Hairs or scale should be placed into the media using sterile forceps. Alternatively, the media may be inoculated directly from brush specimens. The optimal incubation temperature for all media is 30°C. If DTM is left at room temperature, fungal growth will be retarded and this should be taken into account when evaluating the rate of colour change. Specific identification of fungi should be made from colonies growing on neutral Sabouraud's or Mycobiotic media. DTM may alter the colony characteristics and mask pigmentation. The simplest technique for collecting material from a fungal colony is to use clear adhesive tape held with forceps so that the adhesive side gently brushes the colony surface. The tape is then placed on a slide with several drops of lactophenol cotton blue and examined under the microscope for conidial and hyphal characteristics.

Skin biopsies

Information obtained from a skin biopsy depends on three factors: the choice of the lesion biopsied, the method by which the biopsy is taken and the pathologist or microbiologist who interprets the biopsy. A skin biopsy is highly recommended in the following dermatological conditions: suspected neoplasia, persistent ulceration, cases that in the experience of the clinician are unusual or appear serious, skin diseases that do not respond to rational therapy and in any skin disease where the tentative diagnosis involves expensive treatment or is life threatening.

If there are multiple lesions, the most developed primary lesion is the choice for biopsy. Multiple biopsies should always be taken in order to provide a representative histopathological picture. If the lesion is small, total excision is preferred. Where lesions are more widespread, either punch or incisional scalpel biopsies can be taken. The biopsies should be full thickness and include the subcutis and some panniculus.

Punch biopsies are usually taken under sedation and local anaesthesia but biopsies of the face and feet may require the restraint of general anaesthesia. When using local anaesthesia, care must be taken to block the area without interfering with the lesions to be biopsied. Between 1 and 2 ml of lignocaine is injected adjacent to and underneath the lesion. Volumes larger than this are unnecessary and increase the risk of systemic absorption and toxicity if multiple biopsies are taken or when small dogs and cats are being biopsied. The area to be biopsied should be gently clipped and swabbed with 70% alcohol. Surgical scrub preparation is not recommended as epidermal pathology may be altered or obscured.

Correct handling of the specimen maximizes the chance of informative histopathological interpretation. Thin skin biopsies such as those taken from the ventral abdomen should be pinned on cardboard before fixing to prevent 'curling' artefact. Avoid handling the specimen with forceps except on the very periphery to minimize 'crush' artefact.

Before fixation, the biopsy specimens may be divided depending on the tentative diagnosis. If deep bacterial or fungal disease is suspected, samples are placed on a sterile gauze swab in an autoclaved container to which saline has been added. If autoimmune disease is suspected, some laboratories require samples submitted in Michel's fixative. However, recent developments in immunostaining techniques allow the use of formalin-fixed specimens. For routine histopathology, 10% buffered formalin is a satisfactory fixative.

Histopathology should be interpreted by a veterinary pathologist with an interest in cutaneous pathology. In order to obtain as much information as possible from histopathological interpretation, a full clinical history and summary of physical findings should accompany the biopsy. The sites from which the biopsies were taken and the distribution of the lesions should be identified. A tentative diagnosis might indicate to the pathologist that special stains would aid the definitive diagnosis. This is particularly the case where fungal or mycobacterial skin diseases are suspected.

Immunological testing

Immunostaining

Immunostaining technology has improved greatly in recent years. These techniques aim to identify the presence of immunoglobulin (IgG, IgA, IgM) and/or complement in intercellular or basement membrane locations of the skin and are used in the diagnosis of autoimmune and immune-mediated skin diseases. Immunofluorescent techniques using Michel's fixed specimens have largely been replaced by peroxidase labelling of formalin fixed tissue. This has increased the sensitivity of testing (Haines et al., 1986; Moore et al., 1987) and its practicality. Unlike immunofluorescence, peroxidase staining is permanent and the sections may be counterstained with routine stains. Since formalin is used as the fixative, sections may first be evaluated for histopathology and if compatible with autoimmune skin disease further sections from the same sample may be immunostained.

Both false positive and false negative results do occur, however. Poor lesion choice or concurrent glucocorticoid use may result in a negative immunostaining result and this should not be used to discount the diagnosis of autoimmune skin disease based on compatible clinical signs, histopathology and response to appropriate therapy. In addition, positive peroxidase staining may occur in skin diseases other than those with an autoimmune pathogenesis. Diffusion of immunoglobulins through the basement membrane zone into the epidermis may occur secondary to any inflammatory response increasing permeability. Consequently, care must be taken in interpreting the histopathological pattern before proceeding to immunostaining.

Antinuclear antibody (ANA) testing

A positive ANA test is primarily used as supporting evidence to identify systemic lupus erythematosus. ANA antibodies are directed towards multiple nuclear antigens exposed during cellular damage. Methods for testing for ANA are not standardized and results may be variable with respect to antibody titre and pattern of fluorescence. There is debate in the veterinary literature as to the diagnostic significance of either of these factors. In addition, positive results may be obtained in other diseases, after therapy with certain drugs, and in some normal individuals.

Allergy testing

Intradermal skin testing

Intradermal skin testing is used to support the diagnosis of atopic and flea allergy dermatitis. In both cases, the basis of the test is the cross-linking of mast cell-bound IgE and the injected allergen. Subsequent mast cell degranulation releases inflammatory mediators including histamine which results in a wheal and flare reaction. This is evaluated at 20 min for an immediate reaction, and at 12 and 24–48 h for intermediate and delayed reactions. Choice of allergens is important and when considering pollens, the geographical distribution of plant species must be considered. Extracts of moulds and other potential indoor allergens such as house dust, house dust mite, epidermals, wool and cotton may be added to the test range. In Europe, house dust mites account for approximately 80% of positive reactions in atopic dogs (Carlotti and Costargent, 1994).

Standardization of extracts is currently poor in veterinary medicine. Two methods are commonly used: protein nitrogen units (PNU) and weight by volume (w/v) assessment. Both have disadvantages. The protein as measured by PNU (0.00001 mg of protein nitrogen) may include non-allergic components and thus may not correlate with degree of biological activity. Weight by volume estimation uses the ratio of crude dry pollen to the volume of extracting fluid which may vary with the time of year.

In most reports in the literature, testing without the use of tranquillizers has been recommended. However, more recently, physical restraint alone has been associated with increased levels of endogenous cortisol in skin-tested dogs making interference with test results a possibility. A sedative with no antihistaminic or immunosuppressive effects should be used. Phenothiazine tranquillizers have been traditionally avoided for their antihistaminic properties. A combination of zylazine or metatomidine provide useful sedation, analgesia and minimal interference with skin test results.

Before intradermal testing, the animal must have been withdrawn from glucocorticoids, immunosuppressants, antihistamines and tranquillizers. The duration of therapy, type of drug, dose and frequency of administration will determine the interval between withdrawal and skin testing but it may vary from 14 days for antihistamines to 8 weeks for long-acting glucocorticoids. If there is doubt about an animal still being affected, the reaction to a positive and negative control injection can be evaluated. If the histamine reaction is weak, full skin testing should be delayed for at least 2 weeks.

The skin test is performed on the lateral part of the thorax. After gentle clipping, the area may be prepared by cleaning with alcohol and injection sites are marked with a permanent felt-tipped pen. The recommended volume of allergen to inject intradermally varies between 0.02 ml, 0.05 ml and 0.1 ml depending on the author. A 25–26 gauge needle should be used and test sites should be 2 cm apart. The tests are read after 15–20 min.

Interpretation of intradermal reactions is not standardized. Using 0.05 ml as the injected volume, a positive reaction is one where the diameter of the wheal exceeds the negative control by 3 mm or more (Fig. 47.3). Reactions may be graded on a scale of 0 (the test reaction has the same diameter as the negative control) to 4 (the test reaction is equal to the size of the positive control). Increased steepness of the wall, turgidity and flare are factors that influence the grade of the reaction. Use of a tangential light source in a dimmed room may facilitate interpretation of wheal size.

False negative intradermal reactions may be caused by improper injection techniques, for example, as subcutaneous injection of allergen or injection of air instead of allergen, the influence of anti-inflammatory and immunosuppressive agents, and the use of outdated, impotent or improperly prepared test allergens. The dilution effect of mixed allergens for intradermal testing may result in false-negative reactions and a contaminated or irritant negative control may result in a larger wheal for comparison. Other possible causes of false-negative reactions include the wrong selection of allergens, so that the offending allergen is omitted from the test, or low allergen-specific IgE levels.

In vitro diagnostic tests (RAST and ELISA)

There are two tests available commercially for the determination of circulating IgE antibodies in canine serum. The RAST (radioallergosorbent test) has widespread use in human medicine and detects IgE using an isotope-labelled anti-IgE. The ELISA (enzyme-linked immunosorbent assay) uses horseradish peroxidase conjugated with anti-canine IgE for detection of allergen-specific IgE. The majority of commercial laboratories in Europe currently use ELISA technology.

The advantages of using these tests is that there is minimum discomfort and risk to the patient, they are less time consuming and are easier to interpret. They may also be used in animals with extensive cutaneous inflammation where intradermal skin testing would be difficult. Limited studies suggest that recent glucocorticoid therapy does not affect serological test results in dogs (Miller *et al.*, 1992).

An important concern in serological allergy testing is the high prevalence of positive reactions to certain allergens, especially house dust mites, in dogs which do not show signs of atopic disease (Bond *et al.*, 1994; Scott *et al.*, 1995). Serological (and intradermal) tests cannot be used to discriminate between atopic and non-atopic dogs. However, dogs can be successfully hyposensitized using vaccines based on the results of serological tests. For these reasons, the use of allergy tests should not be considered until other differential diagnoses have been carefully excluded.

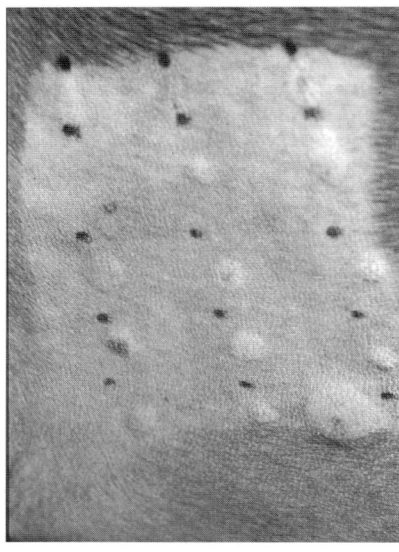

Figure 47.3 An intradermal skin test in a boxer, showing a number of positive reactions. The negative control is top left and the positive control is bottom right. Photograph courtesy of Michael Herrtage. See colour plate.

SKIN DISEASES OF THE DOG

ALLERGIC SKIN DISEASE

Immune-mediated reactions involving hypersensitivity are an important aetiology of canine skin disease.

Atopy

Atopic skin disease is associated with hypersensitivity reactions to environmental allergens. Although the mechanisms of the immune process are not fully understood antibody-mediated immediate and delayed hypersensitivity are

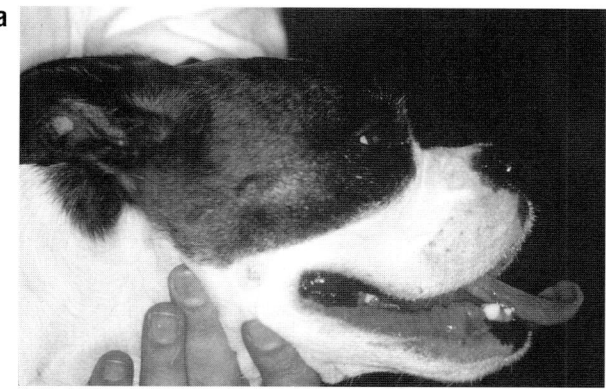 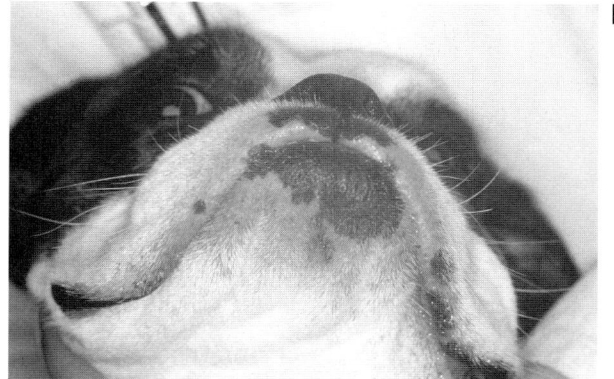

Figure 47.4 (a and b) Alopecia and erythema around the lips, muzzle, eyes and ears in a boxer with atopy. Photographs courtesy of Michael Herrtage. See colour plate.

involved. Sensitization may involve percutaneous transport of allergens and the tendency to develop atopy appears to have an hereditary component.

Onset of signs occurs most commonly from 1 to 3 years and is rare before 6 months and after 6 years of age. The major sign of atopy is pruritus which may occur anywhere but most commonly affects the face (muzzle, eyes, ears), feet and axilla (Fig. 47.4). Pruritus may be seasonal initially. Clinical signs are associated with self-trauma and development of secondary bacterial and *Malassezia* infections and include alopecia, erythema, excoriation, hyperpigmentation, seborrhoea and lichenification depending on the chronicity of disease.

Although firm diagnostic criteria have not been agreed, the diagnosis is based on history, clinical signs and exclusion of other diseases. Positive intradermal or serological test results should be considered to be supportive but not conclusive.

Flea allergy dermatitis

Infestation of dogs with the cat flea, *Ctenocephalides felis*, may result in hypersensitivity to flea saliva mediated by type I and/or type IV hypersensitivity reactions. A primary eruption with papules may be seen particularly on the caudal dorsum. Pruritus is a prominent feature of disease and secondary changes associated with self-trauma are common (Fig. 47.5).

The disease occurs in summer in regions with cold winters but may be non-seasonal where environmental contamination of fleas is heavy and in warm, moist, temperate climates. Demonstration of fleas, or flea faeces from coat brushings and intradermal skin testing with flea antigen can be used to support the diagnosis as can a response to an effective flea control programme.

Food allergy/intolerance

The prevalence of food allergies is subject to controversy as is the exact pathogenic mechanism which may involve immediate and delayed hypersensitivity reactions as well as complement fixation (Halliwell, 1987; White, 1992). Clinical signs are variable, non-seasonal and may occur at any age. A primary eruption may be evident although pruritus especially of the face, ears and ventrum is the major sign of disease. Gastrointestinal signs such as vomiting or diarrhoea occur occasionally.

Diagnosis is by amelioration of signs following an elimination diet and can only be confirmed by return of pruritus after rechallenge with the original diet. The recommended duration for feeding an elimination diet varies with author and ranges from 3 to 8 weeks (White, 1992; Rosser, 1993a,c).

Contact allergy

Contact allergies are thought to be uncommon and represent about 1% of all canine dermatological cases seen in practice. The pathogenesis involves T lymphocyte-mediated delayed hypersensitivity involving allergens (haptens) which bind to a carrier protein and become antigenic. The distribution of signs depends on the source of the allergen and generally affects thinly haired areas of skin. Potential contact allergens include topical medications and shampoos, material on the ground and floor, objects in contact with the

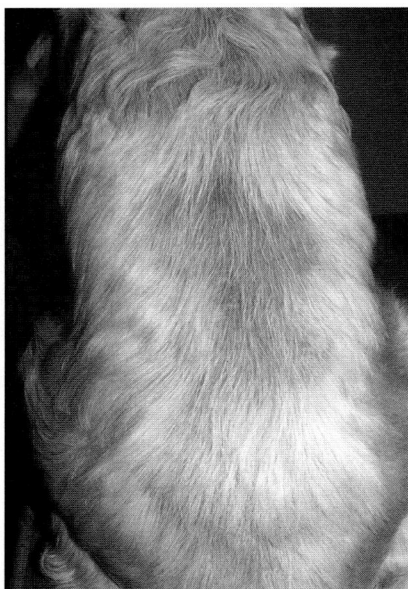

Figure 47.5 Alopecia and hyperpigmentation of the skin on the dorsum of a golden retriever with flea allergy dermatitis. Photograph courtesy of Michael Herrtage. See colour plate.

mouth (e.g. bowls, toys) and collars and clothing placed on the dog. Primary lesions (papules, macules) occur but are modified by self-trauma associated with pruritus. Diagnosis is based on history, improvement of signs on eliminating a putative allergen, and patch testing.

Therapy of canine allergic skin disease

The prime objective for the treatment of allergic skin disease should be identification and removal of substances to which the dog is allergic. This is rarely practical and other means may be used to reduce the degree of pruritus and self-trauma.

Glucocorticoids

These drugs are inexpensive and very effective for short periods of time. Use for extended periods of time is undesirable due to the potential for side effects associated with the numerous metabolic effects of glucocorticoids which mimic those of spontaneous hyperadrenocorticism. Glucocorticoids also cause immunosuppression and suppression of the adrenocortical pituitary axis. Oral prednisolone ($1\ mg\ kg^{-1}$) or methylprednisolone ($0.8\ mg\ kg^{-1}$) daily for 7 days is recommended for induction of an anti-inflammatory effect followed by alternate day dosing. Combination with antihistamines and essential fatty acid supplements may allow a significant decrease in the effective glucocorticoid dose.

Antihistamines

These may be used alone or in combination with glucocorticoids to control pruritus. The individual response to antihistamines is variable and the effect should be evaluated after a 2 week therapeutic trial. Many of the drugs have a sedative effect and their cost may be prohibitive. Available antihistamines and their dose rates are listed in Table 47.4. Many dose rates are extrapolated from those used in humans and most of these drugs are not licensed for animal use.

Table 47.4 Antihistamines used to treat allergic skin diseases in dogs

Drug	Dose
Hydroxyzine	$2.2\ mg\ kg^{-1}$ tid
Diphenhydramine	$2.2\ mg\ kg^{-1}$ tid
Clemastine	$0.05\ mg\ kg^{-1}$ bid
Chlorpheniramine	$0.5\ mg\ kg^{-1}$ bid or tid
Promethazine	$0.2–1\ mg\ kg^{-1}$ bid or tid
Terfenadine	10–30 mg bid (human dose)
Trimeprazine	$0.3–0.5\ mg\ kg^{-1}$ bid
Cyproheptadine	$0.3–2\ mg\ kg^{-1}$ bid
Amitryptyline	$1\ mg\ kg^{-1}$ bid

Essential fatty acids

Supplementation with essential fatty acids (EFA) especially γ-linolenic (GLA) and eicosapentaenoic acid (EPA) provides beneficial anti-inflammatory/antipruritic effects in certain dogs with allergic skin disease. The success rate varies with the author, dose rate and the source of EFA. Using evening primrose oil as a source of GLA, Scarff and Lloyd (1992) showed marked decrease in the degree of pruritus in atopic dogs whereas results from other studies have been less convincing (Scott and Buerger, 1988; Lloyd and Mason, 1993). Several authors have suggested that dose rates of 3–4 times those recommended by the manufacturers may be necessary to achieve the desired effect (Scott and Miller, 1990; Lloyd and Mason, 1993).

Essential fatty acids may have a synergistic effect with the antihistamines, clemastine and chlorpheniramine. A reduction of up to 50% in alternate day prednisolone dose rates has been achieved when concurrent essential fatty acid supplementation has been used (Miller, 1989a; Bond and Lloyd, 1993).

Hyposensitization (immunotherapy)

Hyposensitization involves the administration of allergens to atopic individuals to reduce the clinical response following exposure to natural allergens. The exact mechanism by which this procedure is effective is subject to controversy. It is currently the best alternative to glucocorticoids for treating atopic dogs. The success of hyposensitization depends on the accuracy and quality of the allergy test (intradermal or serological tests) which allows appropriate selection of allergens. Although the principle of subcutaneous injection of increasing concentrations of allergens is common, a number of protocols exist. Variables which affect the success rate such as the optimum dose and frequency of injections have not been determined. Finally, success is dependent on control of 'flare' factors which accentuate the sensation of pruritus (for example fleas or bacterial infection).

Hyposensitization may significantly reduce pruritus in up to 50–80% of atopic dogs (Angarano and MacDonald, 1992). In one placebo-controlled study, 59% showed a favourable response to active treatment and 21% responded favourably to placebo therapy (Willemse *et al.*, 1984). Hyposensitization may reduce the need for other treatment even if not effective alone. In one recent study, 21.5% of 277 dogs were reported to respond such that hyposensitization plus topical therapy was able to control the clinical signs, and 40% of dogs required additional systemic therapy (Nuttal, 1996). However, response to therapy may be slow.

Serious side effects such as anaphylaxis are rare but minor exacerbation of pruritus may occur during the first 1–2 months of treatment. Concurrent treatment with antihistamines and essential fatty acids is recommended. Although controversial, alternate day prednisolone may be used with immunotherapy although some authors prefer to avoid glucocorticoids during the first 1–2 months (Griffin, 1993a).

INFECTIOUS SKIN DISEASE

Bacterial skin disease

Bacterial skin disease is currently classified according to the depth of bacterial involvement in the skin. *Staphylococcus intermedius* is the most commonly isolated pathogen and treatment of this organism in the presence of other bacteria can cause dramatic improvement in clinical signs. Bacteria often become established secondary to other underlying problems including systemic disease, other skin disease, and local anatomical, environmental and immunological factors. Identification and correction of these factors are important in the management of these conditions.

Surface pyodermas
Acute moist dermatitis (pyotraumatic dermatitis)
This syndrome is seen commonly in thick-coated breeds in hot, humid weather, although the short-coated rottweiler also appears to be predisposed. Predisposing factors include allergic skin disease, flea infestation and otitis externa. Lesions are intensely pruritic and clinical signs are associated with self-trauma and secondary staphylococcal infection. Examination reveals a localized area of matted hair with erythema of the skin and a moist exudative surface (Fig. 47.6). Treatment involves clipping the hair, cleaning with mild antibacterial preparations and repeated application of topical glucocorticoids in a non-occlusive base. Mechanical restraint is a useful adjunct to therapy and parenteral glucocorticoids and antibiotics may be necessary in refractory cases. Extension to deep pyoderma (furunculosis) is a complicating factor in golden retrievers and Saint Bernards

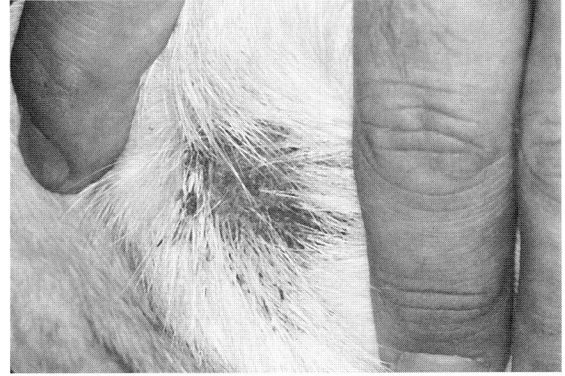

Figure 47.6 An area of acute moist dermatitis on the side of the face of a Labrador retriever with otitis externa. Photograph courtesy of Michael Herrtage. See colour plate.

(Reinke *et al.*, 1987). Systemic antibiotics without glucocorticoids are recommended in these cases.

Skin fold pyoderma
Increased moisture and friction in skin folds predisposes to secondary bacterial infection leading to erythema and self-trauma associated with moderate pruritus. Lesions may occur in tail folds (pugs, English bulldogs, Boston terriers), nasal folds of brachycephalic dogs, lip folds (spaniels, setters) and vulval folds of obese dogs with immature genitalia. Permanent cure requires surgical correction or in the case of vulval fold dermatitis, reduction in weight. Medical management as for pyotraumatic dermatitis is useful in alleviating the clinical signs.

Superficial pyodermas

Superficial pustular dermatitis
Non-pruritic skin disease with superficial pustules and papules primarily on the ventral abdomen, axilla and groin may occur in young dogs up to the age of sexual maturity (Fig. 47.7). Lesions should resolve in 10–14 days with topical antibacterial washes.

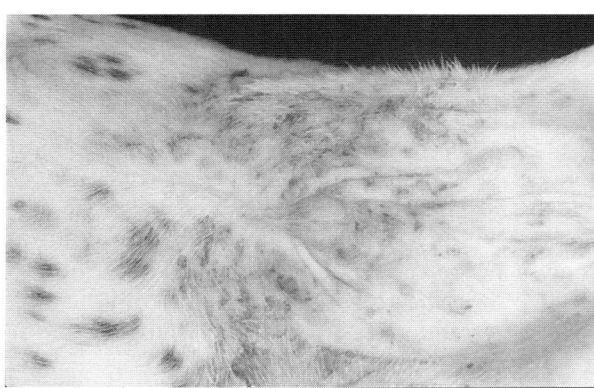

Figure 47.7 Superficial pustular dermatitis on the ventral abdomen of a 6-week-old pointer puppy. Photograph courtesy of Michael Herrtage. See colour plate.

Superficial bacterial dermatitis and folliculitis
Folliculitis is inflammation within the hair follicles resulting in papules, pustules and alopecia. The clinical presentation of this group of antibiotic-responsive diseases is variable as is the degree of pruritus. Animals may present with transient pustules, papules, epidermal collarettes, crusts and patchy alopecia or a combination of these changes, and a vigilant search for an underlying cause is required (Fig. 47.8). The lesions tend to recur. Diagnosis is often based on clinical signs, cytology

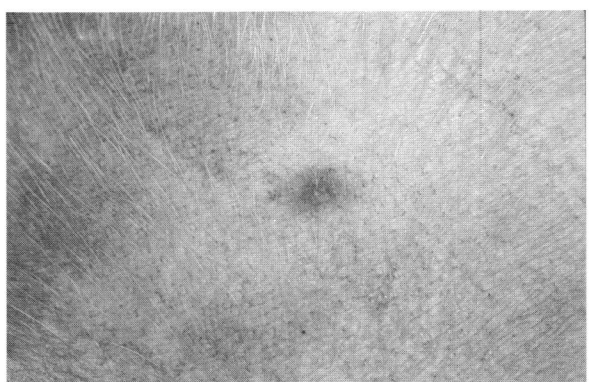
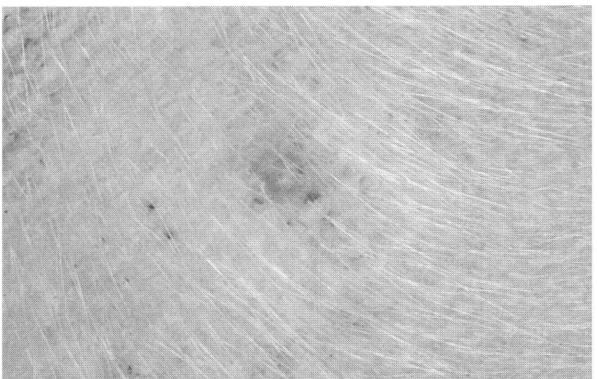
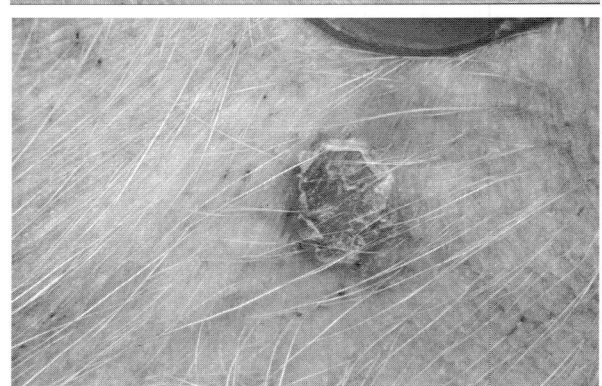
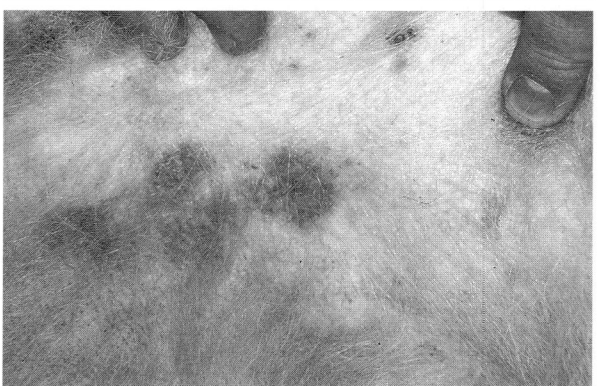

Figure 47.8 A papule (a), a pustule (b), an epidermal collarette (c) and pigmentation and crusting (d) in a dog with superficial bacterial folliculitis. Photographs courtesy of Michael Herrtage. See colour plate.

of pustule contents, and in recurrent cases, bacterial culture and sensitivity. Systemic antibiotics are generally indicated and may be selected empirically unless there is recurring disease. Narrow spectrum bacteriostatic or bactericidal antibiotics with activity against *Staph. intermedius* are desirable. Treatment should be given for a minimum of 21 days and for a further 5–7 days beyond clinical cure. Concurrent antibacterial washes applied twice weekly are recommended.

Deep pyodermas

Deep pyodermas commonly extend from areas of folliculitis. Furunculosis is the result of ruptured hair follicles releasing follicular contents (bacteria, keratin, sebum) into the dermis. A granulomatous foreign body reaction occurs resulting in pain, swelling, furuncles and draining sinuses.

Localized deep pyoderma

Areas of deep infection may be confined to the nose, pressure points, muzzle, chin, feet and perianal region. They present with pain, swelling, furuncles, crusts, draining sinuses and ulceration (Fig. 47.9). Both acral lick nodules and pyotraumatic dermatitis may have a component of furunculosis. *Staph. intermedius* is usually isolated from culture but Gram-negative invaders (*Escherichia coli*, *Proteus* spp.) may be present. Diagnosis is usually based on clinical signs but more complex cases should be biopsied and cultured. Localized deep pyoderma may complicate both demodicosis and dermatophytosis and these underlying causes should be ruled out with appropriate tests.

Generalized deep pyoderma

More generalized disease with draining sinuses and crusts may be seen in German shepherds,

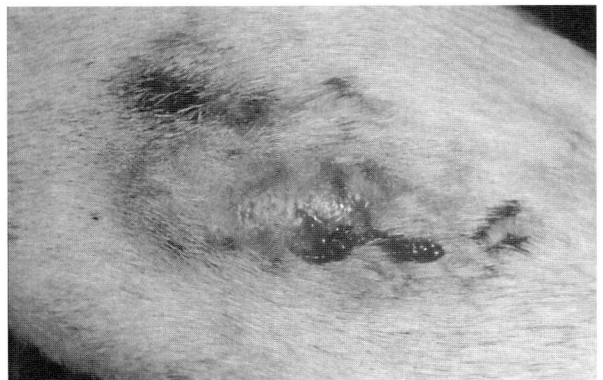

Figure 47.9 Localized area of deep pyoderma on the lateral aspect of the hindleg of a boxer. Photograph courtesy of Michael Herrtage. See colour plate.

English bull terriers and rottweilers among other large breed dogs. Lesions often occur on the lateral aspect of the limbs and feet (Fig. 47.10) and may be associated with fever, regional lymphadenopathy, anorexia and weight loss. Diagnosis is based on biopsy samples which

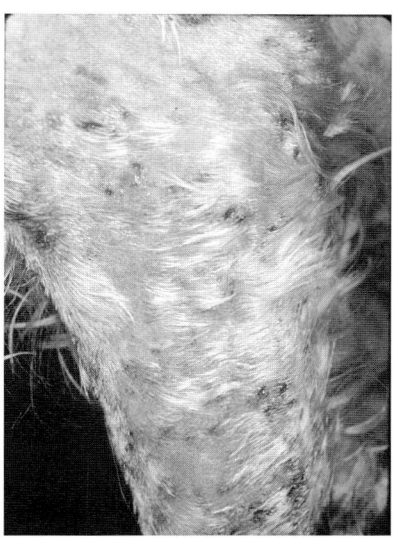

Figure 47.10 Generalized deep pyoderma in an Afghan hound. The hair on the forelimb has been clipped to show the discharging sinuses Photograph courtesy of Michael Herrtage. See colour plate.

should be submitted for histopathology and bacterial culture. A diligent search should be made to rule out the presence of underlying diseases such as hypothyroidism, hyperadrenocorticism (spontaneous or iatrogenic), neoplasia or other debilitating diseases. Demodex may also be involved. Aggressive systemic antibiotic treatment is required in generalized disease, pododermatitis or non-responsive local disease. Because of the depth of infection and the potential for local or systemic immunosuppression, bactericidal antibacterial agents should be selected based on the results of culture and sensitivity testing. The dose should be calculated for the dog's weight. Treatment should continue for 7–10 days beyond cure and may be necessary for 8–12 weeks.

Treatment of staphyloccal skin disease

Antibiotic therapy

Antibiotics used to treat bacterial skin disease are listed in Table 47.5. Concurrent glucocorticoid therapy is contraindicated.

Table 47.5 Antibiotics used for the treatment of bacterial skin disease

Drug	Spectrum	Activity	Dose	Comments
Erythromycin	Narrow	Bacteriostatic	10–15 mg kg^{-1} tid	May cause vomiting
Lincomycin	Narrow	Bacteriostatic	20 mg kg^{-1} bid	Cross resistance with erythromycin
Clindamycin	Narrow	Bacteriostatic	5.5–10 mg kg^{-1} bid	
Oxacillin	Narrow	Bactericidal	15–20 mg kg^{-1} tid	
Trimethoprim sulphonamides	Broad	Bactericidal	13–30 mg kg^{-1} bid	Potential for side effects
Clavulanic acid and amoxicillin	Broad	Bactericidal	11–22 mg kg^{-1} bid or tid	Higher dose rate required
Cephalexin	Broad	Bactericidal	20–30 mg kg^{-1} bid or tid	Drug of choice for deep pyoderma
Enrofloxacin	Broad	Bactericidal	2–5 mg kg^{-1} bid	Should be reserved for resistant cases

Topical antibacterial therapy

Washes

Topical therapy with antibacterial preparations is useful to remove scale, crust and exudate from the skin surface and reduce the number of bacteria. It may promote drainage of deeper lesions and reduce pain and pruritus. Prophylactic treatment may be useful for the treatment of recurrent superficial or deep pyoderma to reduce the severity and frequency of recurrence. Care must be taken to ensure that the product and frequency of treatment are not irritating or drying the skin. Products used for topical treatment of bacterial skin disease include chlorhexidine, benzoyl peroxide, ethyl lactate, povidone–iodine and hexitidine.

Two per cent chlorhexidine is non-irritant and non-drying with broad-spectrum antibacterial activity for 24–36 h after use. It may be used for both superficial and deep disease and can be used for long periods of time. Benzoyl peroxide (2.5–4%) has antimicrobial activity, is keratolytic, degreasing and has a follicular flushing effect. However, when used frequently, it can be irritant and drying. It is particularly useful in folliculitis and furunculosis cases. An emollient bath oil or humectant should be used concurrently. Povidone–iodine has antibacterial and antifungal activity lasting 6–8 h after application. However, it may cause irritation of the skin or contact allergy.

Topical treatment should be used 2–3 times weekly until clinical remission. Pododermatitis cases may require daily foot bathing.

Gels and creams

Localized pyodermas may be managed using non-occlusive topical preparations such as fucidin gel or mupirocin cream. Both penetrate well into granulomatous tissue and are bactericidal.

Mycobacterial skin disease

Atypical non-tuberculous *Mycobacterium* spp. have been isolated from cutaneous lesions in dogs. These fast-growing mycobacteria are opportunistic pathogens which contaminate wounds and whose pathogenicity is enhanced in adipose tissue. *Mycobacterium fortuitum*, *M. chelonei*, *M. phlei*, *M. smegmatis* and an as yet unidentified *Mycobacterium* species have been identified in canine lesions (Kunkle, 1990). Animals with a history of trauma present with nodules, swelling and discharging sinuses of the trunk, particularly the inguinal region. Diagnosis involves identification of organisms using acid fast stains in histopathological sections and culture of the mycobacteria from homogenized tissue samples. Treatment should be based on culture and sensitivity (Table 47.6). The disease has a tendency to recur although spontaneous regression may occur with *M. fortuitum* or *M. chelonei*.

A separate syndrome with multiple discrete nodules commonly affecting the ears has been recognized in Australia, New Zealand and South Africa. Intracellular acid fast organisms are identified on histopathology but culture of the organism has not been possible. These lesions resolve

Table 47.6 Drugs used in the management of atypical mycobacterial infections in dogs

Drug	Dose	Duration (weeks)
Gentamicin	2 mg kg^{-1} bid i.m.	2–4
Amikacin	5–7 mg kg^{-1} bid i.m.	2–4
Doxycycline	5–10 mg kg^{-1} sid to bid p.o.	4–6
Trimethoprim-sulphonamide	12–15 mg kg^{-1} bid p.o.	4–6
Enrofloxacin	5–15 mg kg^{-1} bid p.o.	3–4

After Kunkle (1990)

spontaneously (Kunkle, 1990).

Dermatophilosis

Dermatophilus congolensis may rarely colonize the skin of dogs secondary to trauma, immunosuppression or chronic maceration. Physical examination reveals adherent crusts in the haired portion of the skin and underlying erythema and ulceration when crusts are removed. Diagnosis is made by identification of the filamentous organisms on cytology and culture of crusts. Treatment requires clipping of the hair over the lesions and bathing in 2% lime sulphur, povidone–iodine or chlorhexidine for a minimum of two weeks. Amoxicillin or ampicillin (10–20 mg kg^{-1} bid) for 7–10 days may also be given.

Actinomycosis/nocardiosis

Actinomyces, an anaerobic commensal found in the mouth of many animal species and *Nocardia*, an aerobic environmental saprophyte, belong to a family of branching, filamentous bacteria (Actinomycetales). Cutaneous infection occurs secondary to trauma and is often associated with skin penetration by foreign bodies such as grass seeds. Animals present with fluctuant swellings which rupture and discharge serosanguineous to purulent exudate. Characteristic 'sulphur' granules may be evident in the discharge. Diagnosis is made by identification of organisms in sulphur granules or histopathological sections, and is confirmed by culture. Therapy of both diseases requires lavage, drainage and debridement of the lesions as well as long-term parenteral antibiotics. Penicillins (penicillin V 10 mg kg^{-1} qid per os) are the drugs of choice for actinomycosis and sulphonamides have been used to treat nocardiosis. There is, however, variation in the susceptibility of *Nocardia* spp. to antibiotics and poor correlation between *in vitro* and *in vivo* efficacy.

Fungal skin disease

Dermatophytosis

This superficial fungal disease is associated with invasion of keratinized structures (hair, claw, stratum corneum) by specially adapted fungi called dermatophytes. *Microsporum canis* and *Trichophyton mentagrophytes* are most commonly isolated from infected dogs although other dermatophytes cause sporadic disease. There is considerable geographical variation in the frequency of isolation of the different dermatophyte species (Lewis *et al.*, 1991; Sparkes *et al.*, 1993). Dermatophytosis is an important zoonosis. The pathogenesis is similar to that in the cat. Infection is by contact with infected animals or contaminated material in the environment. Disease is often self-limiting in healthy dogs and is more common in both young dogs and immunocompromised animals including those under treatment with glucocorticoids. Cutaneous changes are variable and depend on the degree of inflammation, although areas of alopecia and scale are commonly found. Diagnosis is made by Wood's lamp fluorescence, arthrospore identification within hair shafts and fungal culture.

Treatment of canine dermatophytosis should involve systemic, topical and environmental therapy. Griseofulvin is most often used but ketoconazole and itraconazole may be of value in some cases. Topical therapy with enilconazole, miconazole, chlorhexidine or povidone–iodine is useful in killing superficial organisms and reducing environmental contamination but is unlikely to affect fungal hyphae within hair shafts in the deeper portions of the follicle (DeBoer and

Moriello, 1995a). Hypochlorite bleach may be used for environmental decontamination.

Malassezia dermatitis

Malassezia pachydermatis is an opportunistic yeast pathogen that may cause significant skin disease. A number of breeds are predisposed including basset hounds, cocker spaniels, West Highland white terriers, dachsunds, poodles and Australian silky terriers, although regional differences are apparent (Dufait, 1983; Mason, 1992a; Plant *et al.*, 1992; Bond *et al.*, 1996). Other predisposing factors implicated include concurrent allergic diseases, keratinization disorders and poorly defined failures of skin immunity to the yeast (Mason, 1992a; Plant *et al.*, 1992; Bond *et al.*, 1996). Clinical signs may be generalized, often with a ventral distribution or localized to the feet, face, skin folds or perineum. Pruritus is common and is often severe. Examination of the skin reveals erythema, scale, hyperpigmentation and oily seborrhoea. Diagnostic criteria proposed for *Malassezia* dermatitis are the presence of abnormal numbers of the yeast in lesional skin and the clinical response accompanied by a reduction in yeast numbers following antifungal therapy (Bond and Lloyd, 1997).

Topical therapy twice weekly with selenium sulphide, enilconazole, miconazole and chlorhexidine is helpful. A shampoo containing 2% miconazole and 2% chlorhexidine has been shown to be very useful; this product has good activity against both the yeast and also staphylococci which frequently coexist with *Malassezia* in high numbers (Bond *et al.*, 1995b). Oral ketoconazole therapy (10 mg kg^{-1} bid) can be used in severe cases or if the owner is unable to bath the dog (Mason, 1992b). Any underlying diseases should be identified and corrected wherever possible. Recurrent cases which require long-term therapy are commonly seen.

Candidiasis

Candida albicans is a rare cause of chronic ulcerative lesions of the skin and oral mucosa in animals which are immunocompromised or have been treated with long-term broad-spectrum antibiotic therapy. Topical nystatin or miconazole and oral ketaconazole may be used for treatment.

Subcutaneous and systemic mycoses

These diseases are uncommon, difficult to treat and have a guarded prognosis. Diagnostic techniques involve identification of the organism either by cytology, histopathology with appropriate stains or fungal culture from a biopsy specimen.

Sporothrix schenkii may cause skin lesions in dogs secondary to penetrating wounds or trauma. Animals present with discrete ulcerated nodules or draining sinuses. Sporotrichosis is a human health risk but is treatable. Therapy includes the inorganic iodides, ketoconazole and itraconazole.

Pythiosis is a rare disease caused by a fungus of the genus *Pythium*. It is characterized by large granulomatous, ulcerative lesions with draining sinuses particularly of the limbs, tail base and perineum. Disease is reported in large breed dogs in subtropical zones of Australia and North America. Response to therapy is poor and surgical exision is often only palliative.

Eumycotic mycetoma is characterized by subcutaneous granuloma formation with multiple sinus tracts which discharge characteristic granules. Many fungi may produce this lesion including *Curvalaria* spp., *Madurella* spp., *Helminthosporium speciferum* and *Allescheria boydii*. Treatment is by surgical excision but response is poor. Prognosis may be improved by treatment with newer generation imidazole drugs.

Blastomycosis (*Blastomyces dermatitidis*) infection may be associated with draining sinuses and cutaneous granuloma formation of the face, nail bed or planum nasale. Skin lesions may occur as part of systemic spread from the respiratory tract. Disease is reported principally from North America. The prognosis is guarded but treatment with imidazoles (ketoconazole or itraconazole) has improved the prognosis.

Cryptococcus neoformans may rarely cause ulcerative, granulomatous skin lesions in dogs as part of systemic disease. Cutaneous manifestations are more common in the cat. Therapy of canine cryptococcosis is limited by the often severe neurological involvement and the inability of antifungal drugs to cross the blood–brain barrier. The newer imidazoles, fluconazole or itraconazole, are effective in human and feline cryptococcosis.

PROTOZOAL SKIN DISEASE

Leishmaniasis

Leishmania is a diphasic protozoan parasite with a blood sucking sandfly vector. Several species may cause disease in dogs although *Leishmania infantum* is the most commonly identified in Europe and Africa. Disease is epizootic in parts of the Mediterranean, East Africa, India, China, Central and South America. Infection of dogs in the UK and USA occurs after travel in these areas.

The organism is an obligatory intracellular parasite with an incubation period of one month to years after infection (Slappendel and Greene, 1990). Cutaneous signs are variable and occur in 90% of cases in combination with systemic signs. There are non-pruritic symmetrical areas of erythema, scale and ulceration of the feet, muzzle, pinna and periocular region. Abnormal growth of nails may be evident. Animals may also display weight loss, anorexia, uveitis, corneal oedema, proteinuria, lameness and epistaxis. Definitive diagnosis is made by demonstration of the organism in lymph node or bone marrow aspirates or skin biopsies.

In some countries, euthanasia is mandatory to decrease the reservoir for human infection. Treatment with pentavalent antimonial compounds (sodium stibogluconate, meglumine antimonate) combined with allopurinol may be indicated (Slappendel and Greene, 1990; Bravo *et al.*, 1993) but relapses occur and infected dogs may act as reservoirs for human infection (Ferrer, 1992).

PARASITIC SKIN DISEASE

Demodicosis

Small numbers of *Demodex canis* are thought to be part of the normal flora of canine hair follicles. Although the exact pathogenesis is not understood, it is generally accepted that there is a specific abnormality of T cell immunity which allows proliferation of the mites in young dogs. This defect is thought to have an hereditary component (Foley, 1991; Miller, 1992). Acquired immunoincompetence associated with systemic disease and glucocorticoid therapy may precipitate demodectic mange in adult or aged dogs.

Three forms of the disease are recognized.

Localized disease generally affects dogs less than one year of age with small non-pruritic areas of alopecia and scale which occur primarily on the face and forelegs. Lesions often resolve spontaneously in 6–12 weeks without treatment. Use of miticides is not recommended due to the potential for the development of resistance.

Generalized disease occurs most commonly in pure bred dogs with onset at less than 18 months of age, although adult onset demodicosis is recognized often with underlying systemic disease. There are multiple areas of patchy alopecia and scale (Fig. 47.11). Disease is generally considered non-pruritic although development of secondary bacterial infections with folliculitis and furunculosis can result in pruritus, regional lymphadenopathy, fever and anorexia (Fig. 47.12).

Pododermatitis occurs when demodicosis is confined to the feet especially in adult dogs. The condition is often painful and complicated by secondary bacterial infection (Fig. 47.13).

Diagnosis is by demonstration of increased numbers of adults or immature stages of *Demodex canis* on skin scrapings and hair pluckings. Generalized demodicosis and pododermatitis are treated with amitraz applied as a 0.05%

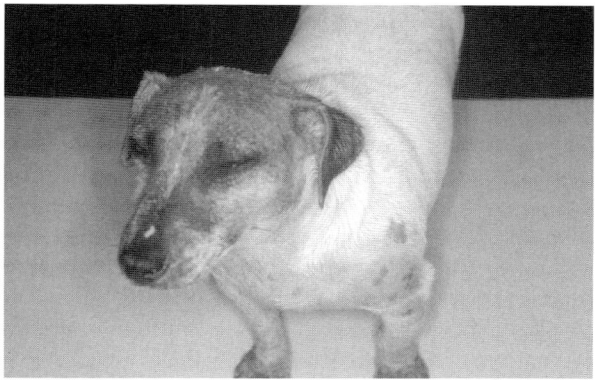

Figure 47.11 Generalized squamous demodicosis in a Jack Russell terrier. Photograph courtesy of Michael Herrtage. See colour plate.

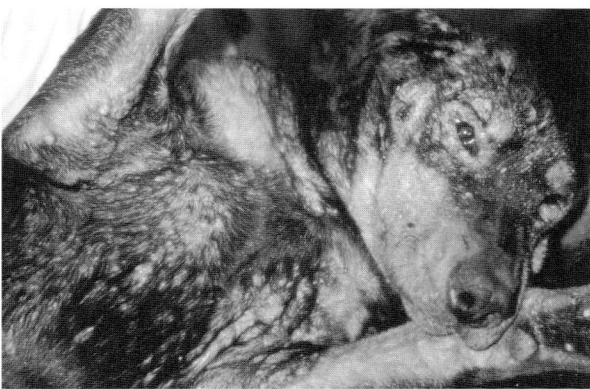

Figure 47.12 Generalized demodicosis with secondary bacterial furunculosis in a Doberman pinscher. Photograph courtesy of Michael Herrtage. See colour plate.

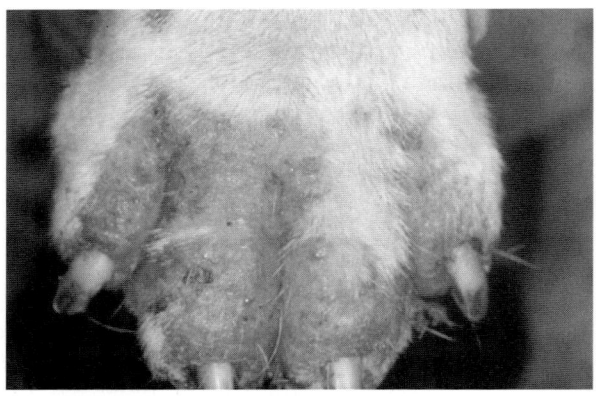

Figure 47.13 Demodicosis confined to the feet of an English bull terrier. Photograph courtesy of Michael Herrtage. See colour plate.

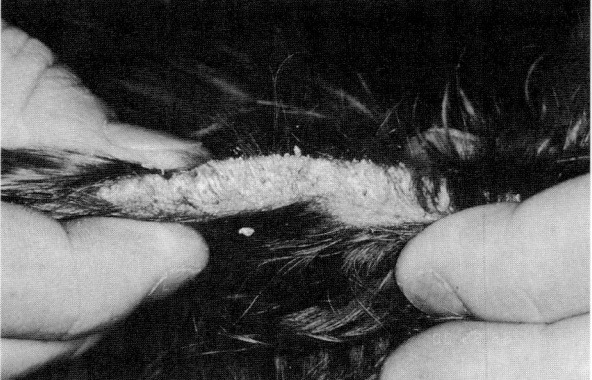

Figure 47.14 Alopecia and crusting of the edge of the pinna in an English springer spaniel with sarcoptic mange. Photograph courtesy of Michael Herrtage. See colour plate.

solution every 7 days. Treatment should continue until three negative skin scrapings are achieved at weekly intervals. The coat should be clipped to aid penetration of the amitraz. Benzoyl peroxide can be used for its descaling effect prior to miticidal treatment. Concurrent bactericidal antibiotics are recommended in cases with bacterial infections. Vitamin E has been reported to be effective in the treatment of generalized demodicosis with 147 of 149 cases resolving after use of oral vitamin E at 200 mg five times daily (Figueiredo et al., 1993). Results of further investigations have not been as encouraging (Griffin, 1987; Gilbert et al., 1992) although vitamin E may be of some benefit in reducing inflammation and appears to accelerate the response to topical amitraz therapy. Recent trials using daily milbemycin oxime (0.5–2 mg kg^{-1}) (Miller and Scott, 1991; Reedy and Garfield, 1991) or ivermectin (600 µg kg^{-1}) (Paradis and Ristic, 1993) have given encouraging results. Off-label use of these drugs has been suggested in chronic disease non-responsive to amitraz or where the dog and/or owner is unable to tolerate amitraz therapy.

Sarcoptic mange

Disease in dogs is associated with *Sarcoptes scabiei* var. *canis*. The parasite is host specific but can cause disease in aberrant hosts including humans. *Sarcoptes* is an obligate parasite with the entire 21-day life cycle occurring on the host. Infestation is associated with intense pruritus. Alopecia, papules and crusts with secondary self-trauma occur primarily on the pinna, elbows and hairless areas (Fig. 47.14). Diagnosis may be difficult to confirm even after multiple skin scrapings and a presumptive diagnosis is often made by response to therapeutic trial.

All dogs in the house should be treated with weekly acaricidal rinses. Organophosphates, amitraz and lime–sulphur may be used but resistance to organophosphates may be a problem (Moriello, 1992). Off-label use of ivermectin (200 µg kg^{-1} orally or by injection) is effective in the management of *Sarcoptes* (Paradis, 1989; Moriello, 1992) but it is contraindicated in rough collies, shelties and their crosses because of the risk of neurotoxicity. Neurotoxicity in other breeds has been reported sporadically.

Cheyletiellosis

Cheyletiella sp. live in the keratin layer of the epidermis and lay eggs which are attached to the hair by fine filaments. They are obligate parasites and spend the entire 35 days of their life cycle on the host, although adult females may survive ten days away from the host under appropriate conditions. Five species have been identified with *C. yasguri* considered to be the mite of dogs although transmission between host species does occur.

Disease occurs most commonly in young dogs with changes most evident on the dorsum. Pruritus is variable and may reflect development of hypersensitivity. Skin changes range from mild scale through to severe seborrhoea sicca and papules and crusting.

Diagnosis is made by microscopic identification of mites or eggs in coat brushings, superficial skin scrapings or acetate tape impressions.

Adult *Cheyletiella* mites are susceptible to a wide range of acaricides. All animals in a household should be treated weekly for six to eight treatments (Moriello, 1992). Off-label use of ivermectin is also effective (Foley, 1991; Moriello, 1992).

Trombiculidiasis

The six-legged larvae of *Trombicula autumnalis* (UK) and *Eutrombicula alfreddugesi* (USA) parasitize the feet, head, ears and ventrum of animals walked in fields or forests in endemic areas during summer/autumn. Infestation results in erythema, papules and crusting with the degree of pruritus depending on the development of hypersensitivity. Diagnosis is made by observation of the orange (0.2 mm) larvae. A single application of an acaricidal agent is usually sufficient for treatment. Other trombiculid species cause disease in different geographical locations.

Rhabditic dermatitis

Pelodera strongyloides is a free-living nematode found in damp soil or decaying organic material. Cutaneous migration of larvae through the feet and other contact areas results in erythema, papules and crusts and is associated with pruritus. Larvae may be found on deep skin scrapings or in biopsy specimens. Treatment involves removal of the animal from the source of infection. Ivermectin may be used with the provisos mentioned previously.

Hookworm dermatitis

Migration of hookworm larvae may result in erythema, alopecia, oedema and crusts in contact areas particularly the feet and footpads. Migrating larvae may not be found on skin scraping or histopathology although changes on histopathology are suggestive. Diagnosis is based on history of environmental contamination, gross appearance and demonstration of eggs or larvae on faecal flotation. Lesions of the feet are treated symptomatically using mild antibacterial soaks to remove crusts and systemic glucocorticoids to relieve pain and pruritus. The dog should be removed from the contaminated environment, faeces disposed of properly and dogs treated for adult hookworm to prevent recurrence.

Insect-mediated hypersensitivity

The stable fly (*Stomoxys calcitrans*) may bite the skin of dogs causing crusting and haemorrhagic skin lesions in animals which live outside. Lesions occur typically on the pinnal tip in prick-eared dogs or along the folded ear edge in other breeds, although lesions may occur elsewhere on the face and body where pre-existing skin disease exists. Treatment with topical antibiotics and steroids is recommended but prevention is difficult and is best achieved by housing the dog indoors. Numerous topical fly repellant preparations are available but need to be applied frequently to be beneficial. The number of flies may be reduced with environmental management and pyrethrin-based insecticides.

The importance of other fly species in producing hypersensitivity dermatitis in the dog is being evaluated (Griffin, 1993b). A syndrome affecting large breed, outdoor dogs and characterized histopathologically as eosinophilic furunculosis of the face has been reported (Gross, 1993; Curtis *et al.*, 1995). Affected dogs develop a papular eruption which progresses to swelling, nodules, ulceration and occasional fistulation. The disease is glucocorticoid responsive and an acute hypersensitivity reaction to arthropods is suspected.

NEOPLASTIC SKIN DISEASES

(See also Chapter 50)

The skin is the site for a wide range of primary tumours which are broadly classified as epithelial or mesenchymal or as tumours of melanin-producing cells depending on their tissue of origin (Tables 47.7 and 47.8). Secondary tumours which are metastases from non-cutaneous primary tumours are also described. The relative prevalence of cutaneous neoplasms is illustrated in Table 47.9.

Formulation of a therapeutic plan requires a definitive diagnosis using cytology, histopathology, investigation for metastases and determination of the extent of the primary tumour.

Mast cell tumours may occur in dogs of all ages and occur most commonly in brachycephalic breeds. Their gross appearance is extremely variable and they should be included in the differential diagnosis of all cutaneous masses. They also differ considerably in clinical behaviour. Well circumscribed, slow growing, solitary lesions are seen as are rapidly growing, poorly defined masses which metastasize early during the disease

Table 47.7 Canine epithelial tumours

Tumour origin	Tumour type
Epidermis	Basal cell carcinoma
	Squamous cell carcinoma
	Intracutaneous cornifying epithelioma
	Cutaneous papilloma
	Canine viral papilloma
Hair follicles	Pilomatrioma
	Trichoepithelioma
Sebaceous glands	Adenoma
	Adenocarcinoma
	Epithelioma
Sweat glands	Adenoma
	Adenocarcinoma
Perianal glands	Hepatoid adenoma
	Adenocarcinoma

Table 47.8 Canine mesenchymal tumours

Tumour origin	Tumour type	
Fibrous tissue	Fibroma	Fibrosarcoma
	Myxoma	Myxosarcoma
	Haemangiopericytoma	Undifferentiated sarcoma
Adipose tissue	Lipoma	Liposarcoma
Muscle	Leiomyoma	Leiomyosarcoma
Vascular/lymphatic tissue	Haemangioma	Haemangiosarcoma
	Lymphangioma	Lymphangiosarcoma
Peripheral nerves	Neurofibroma (Schwannoma)	
Lymphohistiocytic system	Histiocytoma	
	Cutaneous lymphoma	
	Transmissable venereal tumour	
Mast cells	Mast cell tumour	
Melanocytes	Benign and malignant melanoma	

course. Some tumours produce vasoactive amines which may cause local or systemic signs. (Treatment options are discussed in Chapter 50.)

Histiocytoma is a benign tumour occurring most commonly in dogs less than two years of age. It presents as a solitary, rapidly growing, well-circumscribed mass with alopecia and often ulceration. Lesions regress spontaneously.

Cutaneous lymphoma may occur in several forms. Epitheliotropic lymphoma is the result of T lymphocyte infiltration into the epidermis. The disease has a long clinical course and variable presentation but often appears as a pruritic skin disease with erythema, scale and ultimately raised plaques. Primary cutaneous lymphoma is the result of lymphoblast infiltration into the dermis. Clinical appearance is variable and the disease is rapidly progressive and responds poorly to treatment. Cutaneous lymphoma may also result from dissemination of lymphoma from another site.

Basal cell tumours arise from basal cells and are usually benign and solitary. They present as well circumscribed, raised masses which may become ulcerated often on the head and neck in older dogs. Prognosis following surgical removal is excellent.

Squamous cell carcinomas usually present as

Table 47.9 Relative prevalence (%) of common cutaneous neoplasms in dogs in Australia, USA and the UK

Neoplasm	Perth	Sydney[a]	Melbourne[b]	USA[c]	UK[d]
Mast cell tumour	16.1	16.1	17.6	21.3	19.2
Histiocytoma	15.6	13.8	12.2	2.5	6.0
Basal cell tumour	6.8	5.5	12.0	NS	4.1
Melanoma	5.5	5.5	6.8	5.0	6.3
Lipoma/liposarcoma	6.7	6.4	6.3	9.0	8.9
Squamous cell carcinoma	4.6	6.9	5.2	3.9	5.4
Fibroma/fibrosarcoma	8.0	7.3	6.3	9.1	9.7
Haemangioma/haemangiosarcoma	6.4	7.9	5.0	4.5	3.7
Haemangiopericytoma	2.8	7.3	4.1	3.2	4.2
Total case numbers	898	1000	1000	984	2616

After Burrows (1991). Data from [a]Rothwell *et al.* (1987), [b]Finnie and Bostock (1979), [c]Brodey (1970), [d]Bostock (1977).

solitary well-differentiated tumours with an ulcerated surface. They commonly occur on the digits and face and exposure to ultraviolet light may play a role in development of disease. Lesions also occur on the flanks and ventral abdomen of white dogs after chronic sun exposure. Metastasis usually occurs late in the disease although tumours on the digits are more aggressive with destruction of bone and metastases to local lymph nodes. Treatment options are dealt with in Chapter 50.

Intracutaneous cornifying epithelioma is a benign tumour arising from the epidermis in dogs less than five years of age. They present as solitary or multiple lesions of the trunk. Appearance is variable and they usually appear as firm subcutaneous masses with a central opening containing a keratinized plug or horn.

Canine viral papilloma is a contagious disease of young dogs caused by a papovavirus and resulting in multiple cauliflower masses or nodules especially of the oral cavity and head. Lesions usually resolve spontaneously as immunity develops.

ENDOCRINE DERMATOSES

(See also Chapter 39)

The dermatological lesions which characterize this group of diseases have a similar appearance clinically and histopathologically. There is usually non-pruritic skin disease with bilaterally symmetrical alopecia and hyperpigmentation with sparing of the head and limbs (Fig. 47.15). The coat is often dull, dry, easily epilated and fails to regrow after clipping. Information from the history and physical examination may provide a high index of suspicion for one disease in the group. Routine haematology, serum biochemistry and urinalysis are useful as screening tests.

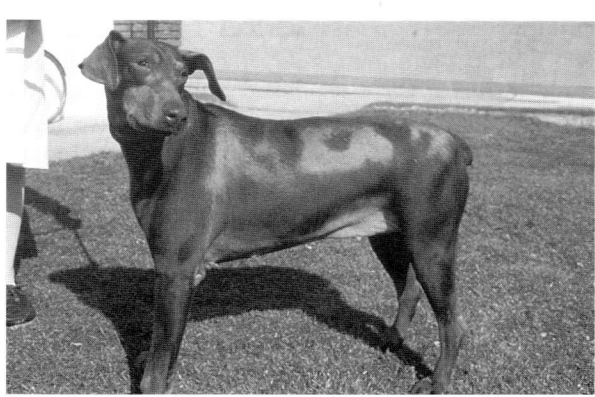

Figure 47.15 Bilaterally symmetrical, non-pruritic alopecia in a Doberman pinscher with hypothyroidism. The pattern of alopecia is typical for an endocrinopathy. Photograph courtesy of Michael Herrtage. See colour plate.

Hyperadrenocorticism

Clinical signs of spontaneous hyperadrenocorticism are associated with excessive production of cortisol by the adrenal cortex. This may be secondary to functional neoplasia of the adrenal cortex (adrenal dependent, ADH) but more commonly due to excess production of pituitary adrenocorticotrophic hormone (ACTH), (pituitary dependent, PDH). The latter syndrome may result from a functional pituitary neoplasm or failure of negative feedback of cortisol on ACTH production and release. Spontaneous disease affects middle-aged to older dogs with increased prevalence in poodles and dachshunds.

Cutaneous changes are similar to other endocrinopathies and comedones, thin comedones, thin skin and, less commonly, calcinosis cutis may be seen. Secondary bacterial and fungal infections and demodicosis may complicate hyperadrenocorticism. Systemic signs include polyuria, polydipsia, obesity, muscle weakness, a pendulous abdomen and testicular atrophy.

Haematology may reveal leucocytosis with neutrophilia, eosinopenia and lymphopenia. The urine specific gravity is usually less than 1.015 although the animal is often able to concentrate urine. Serum alkaline phosphatase is commonly elevated due to induction of a specific hepatic isoenzyme. Blood biochemistry may also reveal mild elevations in other hepatic enzymes (aspartate aminotransferase, alanine aminotransferase), hyperglycaemia and increased cholesterol.

Specific diagnostic procedures for diagnosis of hyperadrenocorticism include the low dose dexamethasone suppression test, ACTH stimulation test and measurement of urinary cortisol/creatinine ratio. Tests used to differentiate adrenal from pituitary disease include, where practical, measurement of ACTH levels, high-dose dexamethasone suppression test, abdominal radiography/ultrasonography and, where available, computed tomography or magnetic resonance scanning (Peterson, 1991; Nelson et al., 1991; Feldman and Mack, 1992).

Pituitary-dependent disease is most commonly managed by administration of o,p'-DDD (2,4' dichlorodiphenyldichloroethane) (mitotane) which causes necrosis of the zona fasciculata and reticularis of the adrenal gland (Feldman and Nelson, 1987a; Kintzer and Peterson, 1991). Other alternatives for treatment are oral ketaconazole 30 mg kg^{-1} in divided doses (Feldman and Nelson, 1992), tumour radiation (Mauldin, 1992) or surgery (hypophysectomy or bilateral adrenalectomy).

Adrenal neoplasia is most effectively managed by removal of the neoplastic adrenal gland. Ketaconazole or o,p'-DDD may alleviate the clinical signs (Feldman and Nelson, 1992).

Hypothyroidism

Canine hypothyroidism is associated most commonly with primary thyroid gland dysfunction. Disease occurs in middle-aged dogs with onset of signs from two to nine years. Dobermanns, boxers, Old English sheepdogs, Great Danes, Irish setters, miniature schnauzers, golden retrievers and dachshunds appear predisposed. Clinical signs are often vague and variable. Cutaneous signs suggestive of an endocrine disorder are present in approximately 50% of cases. Secondary pyoderma and seborrhoea may be evident. Dogs may display lethargy, exercise and temperature intolerance, weight gain, cardiac abnormalities, myxoedema especially of the face, and reproductive dysfunction.

Haematology may reveal normocytic, normochromic anaemia and cholesterol is often elevated on serum biochemical analysis. A reduction in plasma or serum total T4 in association with appropriate clinical signs is suggestive of hypothyroidism. A TSH stimulation test is still the most reliable method for diagnosis of hypothyroidism but diagnosis should not be based on this finding alone. Serum or plasma total T4 is measured before and six hours after administration of 0.1 u kg^{-1} of bovine TSH intravenously (Feldman and Nelson, 1987b). A TRH stimulation test may be performed if TSH is unavailable. More recently, assays of endogenous canine TSH have been developed; the predictive value of measuring TSH and thyroxine in a single blood sample is currently being investigated.

Administration of oral sodium thyroxine is the treatment of choice. An initial dose of 10 μg kg^{-1} twice daily is given for at least 12 weeks. Frequency and dose of thyroxine can be adjusted on the basis of serum total T4 levels measured four hours after medication (Nachreiner and Refsal, 1992).

Growth hormone responsive alopecia

Clinical signs of this condition are limited to the skin. The disease is seen most commonly in male dogs, particularly poodles, pomeranians, samoyeds, keeshonds and chow chows. Onset of signs is often between one and three years but animals may be older. No abnormality is evident on urinalysis, haematology or biochemistry and adrenal and thyroid function tests are within normal limits. Diagnosis is made by excluding other endocrinopathies or by performing a growth hormone stimulation test where this is available using xylazine or clonidine.

Treatment using human, bovine or porcine growth hormone supplementation is described but is limited by poor drug availability and potential for development of diabetes mellitus. As affected dogs are otherwise normal, treatment may not be indicated.

Sex hormone-related disease

Skin disease associated with aberrations in sex hormones is considered to be rare. This group includes several different clinical syndromes with variation in reproductive status, sex and disease presentation (Tables 47.10–47.12). Postulated mechanisms include absolute excess or deficiency of sex hormones and sex hormone imbalances. Many of these conditions are incompletely characterized.

Male dogs

Sertoli cell tumour of testes

Oestrogen may be produced by neoplastic Sertoli cells in testicles of male dogs resulting in enlargement of the prostate, signs of feminization (gynaecomastia, pendulous prepuce) and symmetrical alopecia initially of the perineum and ventrum. Boxers, weimeraners and Shetland sheepdogs appear to be predisposed and tumours occur most commonly in retained testicles. Treatment requires castration. Tumour metastases occur in about 10% of cases and bone marrow suppression resulting from increased oestrogen may occur.

Interstitial cell tumour of testes

Neoplastic interstitial cells may produce excess androgens. Tumours may be associated with seborrhoea oleosa, alopecia and hyperplasia of perianal and tail glands (Miller, 1989b; Schmeitzel, 1993).

Castration-responsive dermatoses

Symmetrical alopecia is described in the absence of feminization and in dogs with palpably nor-

Table 47.10 Sex hormone-related diseases affecting male dogs

(a) Diseases responsive to castration

Disease	Mechanism	Signs
Sertoli cell tumour of testes (especially retained testicles)	Increased oestrogens	• Boxers, Weimeraners, Shetland sheepdogs predisposed • Symmetrical alopecia ventrum/perineum • Feminization (gynaecomastia, pendulous prepuce) • Enlarged prostate • Metastases 10% • Bone marrow hypoplasia
Interstitial cell tumour of testes	Increased androgens	• Alopecia • Seborrhoea oleosa • Hyperplasia perianal/tail gland
Castration-responsive dermatoses		• Symmetrical alopecia • No feminization • Testes palpably normal • Malamutes/Siberian huskies • 'Woolly' coats, dark colours fade
Idiopathic male feminizing syndrome	Hypersensitivity to sex hormones? (Miller, 1989b)	• Signs as for Sertoli cell tumours • ± pruritus, seborrhoea, ceruminous otitis externa • Histopathology not compatible with endocrine disease

(b) Testosterone-responsive dermatoses

Signs	Treatment
• Symmetrical alopecia perineum/ventrum • Castrated or entire male dogs	Methyl testosterone 1 mg kg^{-1} (maximum 30 mg dog^{-1}) every other day. Response in 3 months

Table 47.11 Sex hormone-related disease affecting female dogs

Disease	Signs	Treatment
Telogen defluxion	• Alopecia 4–8 weeks post-partum • At parturition hormonal changes cause many hairs to enter telogen	Resolves spontaneously
Functional ovarian tumour/polycystic ovaries (?increased oestrogen)	• Alopecia/hyperpigmentation perineum/flanks • +/− seborrhoea, pyoderma, otitis externa • Enlarged vulva/nipples • May metastasize	Ovariohysterectomy
Oestrogen-responsive dermatoses	• Alopecia ventrum/perineum • Dogs spayed at a young age • ? especially Boxers and Dachshunds • Rare	Diethylstilboestrol 0.1–1 mg dog^{-1} p.o. sid for 3 weeks then off 1 week.

Table 47.12 Sex hormone-related diseases affecting both sexes

Disease	Signalment	Treatment
Adrenal syndrome	• Signs similar to growth hormone deficiency • May be associated with adrenocortical enzyme deficiency causing reduced cortisol and increased androgen/progestogen • Age onset 1–3 years • Especially chow chows, pomeranians, samoyeds • Diagnosis: cortisol/sex hormone levels after ACTH or hCG stimulation	? Desexing ? Growth hormone ? o,p'-DDD ? Ketaconazole
Seasonal flank alopecia	• Dobermanns, boxers, schnauzers and Airedale terriers • Occurs in neutered males and females • Seasonal alopecia/hyperpigmentation of the flanks followed by spontaneous regrowth of hair • Normal thyroid, adrenal, reproductive and growth hormone levels • May be related to photoperiod	Resolves spontaneously

mal testes. In Siberian huskies and malamutes, alopecia is preceded by the coat becoming 'woolly' and bleaching of coat colour (Miller, 1989b). Cutaneous signs resolve with castration.

Idiopathic feminizing syndrome
This is a rare disorder with clinical signs similar to those associated with Sertoli cell tumours although pruritus, seborrhoea and ceruminous otitis externa are often evident. The aetiology is unknown but may be related to hypersensitivity to sex hormones (Miller, 1989b). Histopathology is not compatible with endocrine disease. Treatment of choice is castration.

Testosterone-responsive dermatoses
Symmetrical alopecia initially involving the perineum and responsive to supplementation with testosterone is described in both castrated and entire male dogs.

Female dogs

Ovarian imbalance type 1
This term represents a rare disease of entire female dogs associated with functional ovarian tumours or polycystic ovaries and is presumed to be the result of excess oestrogen production. Alopecia and hyperpigmentation spread cranially from the perineum and flanks and are often associated with seborrhoea, pyoderma and otitis externa. Vulva and nipples are enlarged. Ovariohysterectomy resolves signs unless metastases have occurred.

Oestrogen-responsive alopecia
Alopecia of the ventral surface and perineum occurs rarely in female dogs spayed at a young age. Boxers and dachshunds appear to be at increased risk.

Diseases affecting both sexes

Adrenal syndrome

This disease is thought to be associated with an adrenocortical enzyme deficiency which results in reduced cortisol and elevated adrenal androgens and progestogens (Schmeitzel and Lothrop, 1990). Presentation is similar to growth hormone responsive disease and affects both male and female dogs with onset from one to three years. Chow chows, pomeranians and samoyeds may be predisposed and overlap may occur with growth hormone-responsive dermatoses (Schmeitzel, 1990). Measurement of cortisol and sex hormones after ACTH and human chorionic gonadotrophin administration may aid in diagnosis. Treatment is empirical; neutering, growth hormone, ketoconazole and o,p'-DDD have been recommended (Schmeitzel, 1993).

Seasonal flank alopecia

Seasonal flank alopecia is an uncommon syndrome characterized by seasonally recurrent bilateral non-pruritic alopecia and hyperpigmentation of the flanks which is followed by spontaneous hair re-growth. The condition occurs in both males and females whether neutered or entire. Predisposed breeds include dobermans, boxers, schnauzers and Airedale terriers. The aetiology is unknown but may be related to photoperiod. Affected dogs have been shown to have normal thyroid, adrenal, reproductive and growth hormone levels (Curtis et al., 1996).

Telogen defluxion

Generalized truncal alopecia may occur after a stressful episode such as generalized illness, fever or parturition. Hair loss is due to hair follicles simultaneously entering telogen and occurs 4–8 weeks after the initiating event. Signs resolve spontaneously.

IMMUNE-MEDIATED SKIN DISEASES

This group of skin diseases is considered to be rare representing less than 1% of all dermatological cases.

The pemphigus group

In this group of skin diseases, cutaneous signs are associated with formation of autoantibodies to desmosomal proteins. Breakdown of cohesion between cells results in pathological cleft formation. Accumulation of fluid within clefts leads to the formation of vesicles or bullae. These primary lesions are transient as canine epithelium is thin and the lesions are subject to trauma. Diagnosis is made by demonstration of intraepidermal clefting and the presence of acantholytic cells on histopathology of biopsy specimens. Immunostaining may support the diagnosis by demonstration of intercellular immunoglobulin and/or complement.

Pemphigus foliaceus is the most superficial of this group of diseases. Disease is reported in all breeds of dog but dobermanns, Newfoundlands, bearded collies and akitas appear to be affected most frequently. Onset of signs is usually from two to seven years and the disease is chronic in 75% of cases. Primary lesions of pustules are transient and animals usually present with crusting and erosions particularly on the face (especially over the bridge of the nose), ears and feet (Fig. 47.16). Footpads are often involved and generalized skin disease with scale, crusts and alopecia may occur with time.

Pemphigus erythematosus is similar to pemphigus foliaceus in appearance but lesions are generally confined to the planum nasale, bridge of the nose, periorbital region and ears. Antinuclear antibody (ANA) may be positive.

Pemphigus vulgaris primarily affects the oral cavity and mucocutaneous junctions although lesions may be generalized. Nail beds may be affected resulting in sloughing of nails. Secondary bacterial infection is common as are systemic signs of pyrexia, anorexia and weight loss.

Pemphigus vegetans is a rare disorder characterized by the formation of pustules which develop into papillomatous proliferations.

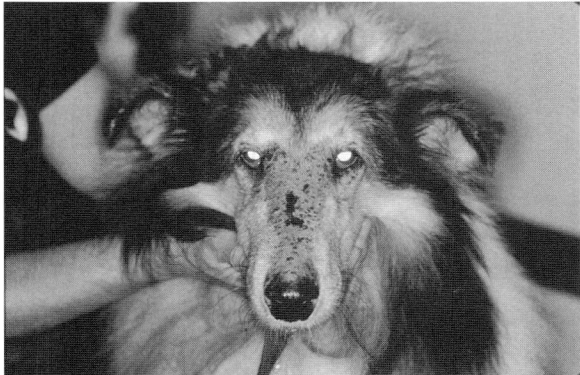

Figure 47.16 Alopecia, crusting and erosions on the bridge of the nose in a rough collie with pemphigus foliaceous. Photograph courtesy of Michael Herrtage. See colour plate.

Bullous pemphigoid

This is a rare disease associated with autoantibody directed against the basement membrane components. Disease may be more common in collies, Shetland sheepdogs and dobermanns. Clinical signs are similar to those of pemphigus vulgaris with ulceration of mucocutaneous junctions, the oral cavity, head, ears and inguinal skin (Fig. 47.17). Systemic signs may occur and chronic disease may be more generalized. Clefting occurs within the basement membrane and diagnosis is made on supportive histopathology and immunostaining. Other diseases which are characterized histologically by subepidermal vesicle formation and therefore resemble bullous pemphigoid, but which are associated with autoimmune responses directed against different structural proteins of the basement membrane have now been recognized (Olivry *et al.*, 1996).

Lupus group of diseases

The lupus group of diseases is associated with formation of immune complexes and deposition of these complexes around capillary beds and basement membranes leading to vasculitis. Diagnosis is based on compatible clinical signs and serology and the presence of a lichenoid infiltrate within the basement membrane zone.

Systemic lupus erythematosus is a multisystemic disease with a wide range of clinical presentations including cyclic fever, polyarthritis, glomerulonephritis, anaemia and dermatitis (see Chapter 44). Cutaneous changes are variable but commonly involve the face, ears and feet and present as erythema and crusting. Animals are usually antinuclear antibody (ANA) positive. The disease is multifactorial and the onset of signs occurs most commonly between two and four years of age.

Discoid lupus erythematosus presents as erythema and depigmentation of the planum nasale which may progress to crusts and ulceration. Disease may extend to the bridge of the nose, oral cavity and periorbital region and chronic cases have alopecia and scar formation. Dolicocephalic breeds appear predisposed and solar damage may play a role in disease. Animals are usually ANA negative.

Chronic depigmenting nasal dermatitis (Collie nose) clinically appears similar to discoid lupus with depigmentation of pigmented skin and crusting of the dorsum of the nose and planum nasale. Dolicocephalic breeds predominate and solar damage and immunological factors are implicated in the aetiology. An interface lichenoid infiltrate is seen on histopathology and ANA and immunofluorescence is negative. Oral prednisolone may give significant improvement in the condition but signs recur when the drug is withdrawn. Surgical reconstruction with rotation flaps to cover the abnormal area with viable haired skin provides an alternative to medical treatment (Stanley *et al.*, 1991).

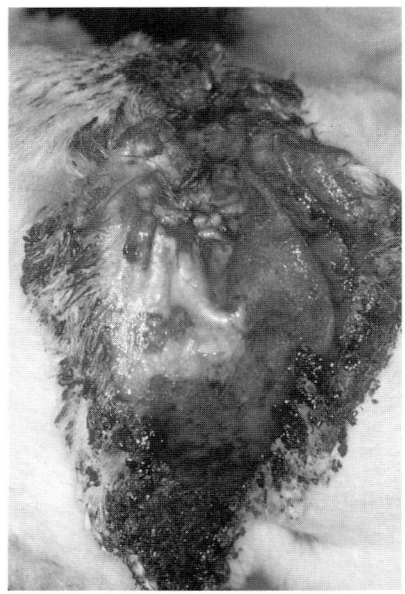

Figure 47.17 Ulceration of the oral cavity (a) and ear (b) of an Old English sheepdog with bullous pemphigoid. Photographs courtesy of Michael Herrtage. See colour plate.

Table 47.13 Sterile pustular dermatoses

Disease	Background	Pruritus	Immunostaining	Treatment
Subcorneal pustular dermatosis	More prevalent in miniature Schnauzers	Variable	Negative	Dapsone
Dermatitis herpetiformis	Associated with gluten enteropathy in humans	Severe	Positive	Dapsone
Superficial eosinophilic pustular dermatosis		Moderate/ severe	Negative	Anti-inflammatory glucocorticoids
Linear IgA dermatosis	Dachshunds	Variable	Positive	Anti-inflammatory glucocorticoids

Sterile pustular dermatoses

Several rare diseases with sterile pustular eruptions of the trunk have been described. The aetiology of these rare diseases has not been completely characterized although they are suspected to be immune-mediated. Primary lesions are transient and animals often present with epidermal collarettes, scale and crusts. The main clinical and diagnostic features of these diseases are listed in Table 47.13.

Uveodermatologic syndrome

This is a rare disease thought to result from a cell-mediated response against melanocytes. The disease is reported in young dogs of a number of breeds with a higher prevalence in akitas, chow chows, samoyeds and Siberian huskies (Morgan, 1989). Ocular signs secondary to uveitis usually precede skin changes which consist of depigmentation of hair (poliosis) and skin (vitiligo) particularly of eyelids, planum nasale, lips, scrotum and footpads. Rapidly depigmenting areas may become crusted and ulcerated.

Erythema multiforme and toxic epidermal necrolysis

Erythema multiforme usually occurs secondary to other diseases or drug administration and is characterized by acute onset of symmetrical skin lesions particularly of the ventrum and limbs. Cutaneous changes are variable but erythematous macules that spread peripherally and clear centrally are the hallmark of the disease. A more severe form characterized by vesicles, bullae and ulceration of the skin and mucous membranes is occasionally seen. Diagnosis is based on compatible histopathology and clinical history.

Toxic epidermal necrolysis is a rare, life-threatening disease which may be immune-mediated. It is often associated with underlying systemic disease or drug administration. Animals show pyrexia, anorexia and lethargy with vesiculobullous lesions of skin, oral cavity and mucocutaneous junctions that rapidly progress to severe ulceration.

Drug eruptions

Oral, parenteral or topical administration of drugs may occasionally result in cutaneous lesions as a result of immune-mediated reactions. The immune mechanism, type and distribution of lesions and histopathology is variable. History of drug administration may be helpful in diagnosis and lesions resolve upon withdrawal of the drug.

Uncommon immune-mediated skin diseases

Vasculitis

Deposition of immune complexes within blood vessel walls leads to inflammation, thrombosis, ischaemia and necrosis particularly of the extremities (digits, pinna and tail tip). The disease often occurs secondary to drug administration, infection or other chronic disease. Diagnosis is made on the basis of histopathological findings.

Cold agglutinin disease

Antibody (particularly IgM) with optimum binding below the animal's core temperature may be produced secondary to infection or neoplasia. The condition may also be idiopathic. Exposure to cold may lead to haemolysis and necrosis of the digits, tail tip and pinna secondary to vascular obstruction. A direct Coombs' test is positive at 4°C.

Juvenile cellulitis

This disease of unknown aetiology is presumed to have an immunological basis because of the response to immunosuppressive drugs and the histopathological appearance of the lesions. Disease affects dogs aged between 1 and 4 months and early signs of disease include submandibular lymphadenopathy and blepharitis. Cutaneous changes particularly of the muzzle and periorbital region include pustules, nodules, oedema, crusts and draining sinuses (Fig. 47.18). The feet, pre-

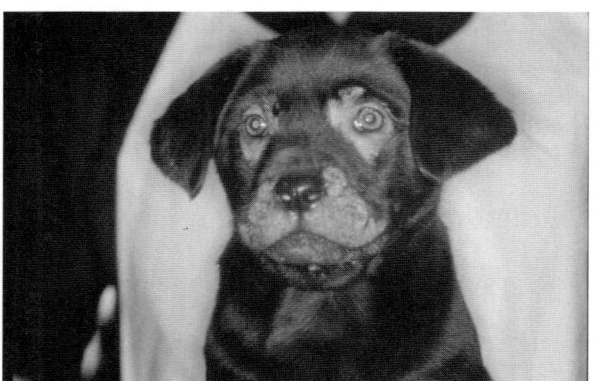

Figure 47.18 Juvenile cellulitis in a 10-week-old Labrador puppy. Photograph courtesy of Michael Herrtage. See colour plate.

puce and perianal region are occasionally affected. The disease responds rapidly to glucocorticoids and signs do not recur when the drug is withdrawn.

Canine familial dermatomyositis

Familial dermatomyositis is an inflammatory condition affecting skin, muscle and occasionally blood vessels that occurs almost exclusively in collies, Shetland sheepdogs and their related crosses. The disease is considered to be inherited although the exact aetiology is unknown and both immune-mediated disease (Schmeitzel, 1992) and infectious agents (Kunkle, 1992) have been implicated. The severity of the skin and muscle changes is variable as is the course of the disease. Signs may wax and wane spontaneously. Skin changes occur in dogs less than 6 months of age and include transient vesicles, erythema, ulceration and crusts of the face (muzzle and periocular region), ears, tail tip and over bony prominences of distal extremities. Myositis may be confined to temporal and masseter muscles resulting in atrophy and possibly difficulty in swallowing and mastication. Severe cases may show generalized muscle atrophy, retarded growth and mega-oesophagus.

■ Therapy of immune-mediated disease

Accurate diagnosis of immune-mediated disease is essential before commencement of immunosuppressive treatment due to the potential for drug side effects. Immune-mediated diseases associated with drug administration or underlying systemic disease may resolve without therapy if the underlying aetiology can be identified and corrected. Diseases, such as toxic epidermal necrolysis which involve large areas of skin or result in full thickness necrosis, may present with systemic signs and therefore require symptomatic and supportive therapy such as systemic antibiotics and intravenous fluid therapy.

Immunosuppressive therapy

Glucocorticoids

Immunosuppressive doses should be used initially: prednisolone, 1–2 mg kg^{-1} bid (20–40 mg m^{-2} bid); methylprednisolone, 0.8–1.5 mg kg^{-1} bid.

The glucocorticoid dose is reduced slowly over 8–10 weeks to achieve the lowest alternate day drug dose possible to prevent recurrence of clinical signs. The need for combination therapy should be considered if remission is not achieved within 14 days or if side effects of glucocorticoids become unacceptable.

Azathioprine

The immunosuppressive dose is 2.2 mg kg^{-1} sid or on alternate days in combination with glucocorticoids.

Azathioprine is useful in the management of the pemphigus group of diseases and lupus erythematosus (Rosenkrantz, 1993). Use of this drug may be associated with bone marrow suppression, pancreatitis and overgrowth with opportunist micro-organisms.

Chlorambucil

The immunosuppressive dose is 0.1–0.2 mg kg^{-1} sid or on alternate days.

Chlorambucil is used in combination with glucocorticoids or azathioprine/glucocorticoids. It may cause bone marrow suppression and gastrointestinal disturbances.

Cyclophosphamide

The immunosuppressive dose is 50 mg m^{-2} on alternate days.

This is a more potent alkylating agent which may be used alone or in combination with glucocorticoids. Use may be associated with leucopenia, haemorrhagic cystitis and gastrointestinal signs.

Chrysotherapy

Aurothioglucose should be used at 1 mg kg^{-1} week^{-1} intramuscularly.

Clinical response to administration of gold salts may take 6–8 weeks and combination with glucocorticoids is recommended. Use may be associated with a variety of side effects including drug eruptions, hepatic necrosis and thrombocytopenia.

Adjunctive therapies

Adjunctive therapies in the management of immune-mediated skin disease include supplementation with vitamin E and avoidance of exposure to ultraviolet light. Although vitamin E is of questionable efficacy it may reduce the need for more potent drugs. A combination of niacinamide and tetracyclines has been described as a treatment for discoid lupus erythematosus (White et al., 1992).

SKIN DISEASES ASSOCIATED WITH KERATINIZATION DISORDERS

Hepatocutaneous syndrome (necrolytic migratory erythema, superficial necrolytic dermatopathy)

Necrolytic migratory erythema is the term used to describe cutaneous signs most often associated with glucagon-secreting pancreatic tumours in humans. Although skin disease associated with functional pancreatic tumours has been reported in dogs (Gross et al., 1990; Miller et al., 1991; Bond et al., 1995a), the majority of canine cases are associated with severe vacuolar hepatopathy and diabetes mellitus hence the term hepatocutaneous syndrome. Disease tends to occur in older animals (mean 10.7 years). Cutaneous lesions most frequently involve footpads, mucocutaneous junctions (oral, ocular, genital and anal), pinna and pressure points and appear grossly as erosions and ulceration with erythema and crusting. Severe crusting and fissuring of the footpads results in lameness. Histopathological signs include a triad of parakeratosis, epidermal spongiosis and an infiltrate of inflammatory cells in the upper dermis. Cutaneous lesions and histopathology may resemble zinc-responsive dermatoses.

Diagnosis is based on histopathology of skin lesions and documentation of hepatic disease and/or diabetes mellitus. Alkaline phosphatase, alanine transaminase and fasting and postprandial bile acids may be increased. Hyperglycaemia and the presence of diabetes mellitus is variable and often develops after identification of cutaneous and hepatic pathology.

Humans with necrolytic migratory erythema show complete resolution of cutaneous signs following intravenous administration of amino acids. Amino acid levels were depressed in all cases where measured (Gross et al., 1993; Bond et al., 1995a). Egg yolks used as a dietary supplement in six dogs resulted in partial or complete resolution of cutaneous changes over a short time.

Glucocorticoids will improve the appearance of the skin but are contraindicated due to the frequent association of hepatocutaneous syndrome with hyperglycaemia and diabetes mellitus. Treatment must be considered palliative as it does not address the underlying aetiology. While the mechanism of the hepatic pathology is not understood, the prognosis for this condition is poor.

Zinc-responsive dermatoses

Animals with zinc-responsive disease present with erythema, exudation and thick crusts affecting the face (perioral and periocular regions, ears), pressure points, footpads and mucocutaneous junctions. Lymphadenopathy, lethargy and pyrexia may be evident. Two distinct clinical syndromes have been described. A genetic defect resulting in decreased intestinal zinc absorption is reported in Siberian huskies and Alaskan malamutes. Lesions often occur at puberty or during other periods of stress (Brown et al., 1978). Zinc-responsive disease may also occur in young growing dogs of large breeds fed high calcium or high fibre diets where the zinc is unavailable for absorption (Van den Broek and Thoday, 1986; Ohlen and Scott, 1986; Sousa et al., 1988).

Treatment involves supplementation with zinc sulphate 10 mg kg^{-1} day^{-1} or zinc gluconate as 1.5 mg elemental zinc kg^{-1} day^{-1}. Side effects of anorexia and vomiting are minimized if the zinc is given with food and by dividing the daily dose. A good quality commercial dog food should replace the existing diet if dietary inadequacies are identified.

Lethal acrodermatitis

This rare disease of English bull terriers is inherited as an autosomal recessive trait. Although the aetiology is unknown, zinc malassimilation is considered to be a contributing factor. Cutaneous signs are evident from six weeks of age and include scale, crusts and changes compatible with secondary bacterial folliculitis especially of the face, feet and pressure points. Retarded growth, gastrointestinal signs, ocular changes and increased susceptibility to infection are also evident. There is no response to zinc supplementation and death occurs by 15 months (Jezyk et al., 1986).

Fatty acid deficiency

Skin disease associated with fatty acid deficiency may result from long-term consumption of diets deficient in fat or stored inappropriately. Clinical signs may also be seen in animals with intestinal malabsorption, pancreatic exocrine insufficiency or bile salt deficiency. Dogs develop dry, dull coats and seborrhoea. Secondary bacterial infection may occur. Treatment involves correction of the diet if dietary inadequacies are found or supplementation with fatty acids.

Vitamin A-responsive dermatosis

Skin disease responsive to vitamin A supplementation but not associated with dietary vitamin A deficiency has been reported in cocker spaniels and sporadically in other breeds. Animals present with generalized scale, ceruminous otitis externa, hyperkeratosis of footpads and multifocal areas of crusts and frond-like keratinous plugs of the ventral thorax and abdomen. Diagnosis is by response to treatment with oral vitamin A (1000–2500 iu kg^{-1} day^{-1}). A response is seen in 3–8 weeks and treatment may be required for life. Synthetic retinoids (isotretinoin and etretinate) have been used to treat less common keratinization disorders such as sebaceous adenitis, schnauzer comedo syndrome and congenital lamellar ichthyosis. There may be some indications for isotretinoin as adjunctive therapy for epidermotropic lymphoma (Kwochka, 1989). Retinoids are difficult to obtain and expensive.

GENETIC/CONGENITAL DERMATOSES

Cutaneous asthenia (Ehlers–Danlos syndrome)

This hereditary group of diseases is the result of connective tissue abnormalities resulting in loose and abnormally fragile skin.

Canine ichthyosis

This is a rare hereditary disease resulting in marked scale and keratin projections of the skin and thickening of pads.

Colour dilution alopecia

This disease is the result of an hereditary ectodermal defect in animals with diluted coat colours. It has been described mainly in pure and cross-bred dogs with blue coat colour and occasionally in red and fawn-coloured dogs (dobermanns, dachshunds, Irish setters). Animals are born with normal coats and develop patchy alopecia, scale and dry hair between 8 weeks and 3 years of age. Changes are most obvious on the trunk and affect diluted colour hair only. Treatment is symptomatic and is directed towards secondary bacterial folliculitis.

Canine hereditary black hair follicle dysplasia

This condition is seen in black and black and white pure and cross-bred dogs and results in hypotrichosis, scale and dry, broken hairs in black coated areas only. No treatment is available.

Acral mutilation syndrome

This sensory neuropathy is an autosomal recessive disease of English pointers and German short-haired pointers. Affected pups excessively traumatize paws due to an absence of temperature and pain sensation. Lesions develop at between 3 and 5 months of age and no treatment is available.

SKIN DISEASES OF THE CAT

The spectrum of feline skin disease is expanding rapidly. Rather than a collection of syndromes, specific disease entities are now recognized and treated appropriately. Many of these skin diseases affect both the dog and cat. However, there are several reasons to consider feline skin disease separately.

- There are skin diseases unique to the feline species.
- Skin diseases affecting both the dog and cat may differ in prevalence. Recognition and investigation of these differences may give new insights into aetiology and pathogenesis. A common example is staphylococcal dermatitis which is common in the dog but rare in the cat.
- Treatment of skin disease in the cat is often limited by species idiosyncrasy. Grooming behaviour increases the chance of toxicity from topically applied drugs due to oral and gastrointestinal absorption. Toxicity of systemically administered drugs in the cat may occur secondary to prolonged biotransformation or increased sensitivity to certain drugs. Consequently, dermatological therapeutics may vary considerably compared to the dog.

ALLERGIC SKIN DISEASE

As in the dog, allergic skin disease in the cat produces pruritus. However, the clinical manifestation may differ considerably. A history of pruritus may be difficult to obtain. Owners recognize licking in the cat as normal behaviour and this may occur when the owner is absent. Consequently, symmetrical alopecia due to an instinctive pattern of grooming may be a major clinical sign of pruritic skin disease. The immunological basis of allergic skin disease in the cat remains to be elucidated. At present, IgE antibody has not been isolated but the presence of a reaginic antibody, possibly an IgG subclass, is suspected. Naturally occurring allergic contact dermatitis in the cat has not been documented.

In common with dogs, allergic dermatitis generally occurs in the 2–6-year age group (average 4 years) and has no gender predisposition. Several clinical syndromes have been described in the cat irrespective of the allergen or mechanism involved.

Papular dermatitis ('miliary' dermatitis)

The major lesion in this syndrome is the crusted papule which is easily palpated (Fig. 47.19). Histopathology reveals intraepidermal vesicle formation commonly infiltrated with eosinophils. The distribution of these lesions may provide information about the underlying cause. A lumbosacral distribution is more indicative of flea allergy dermatitis whereas involvement of the head and neck may indicate parasites with a tropism for this area (e.g. *Otodectes cynotis* or *Notoedres cati*) or food allergy/intolerance.

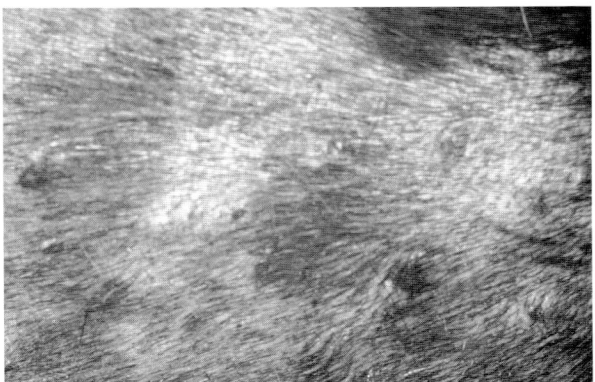

Figure 47.19 Papulocrustaceous reactions on the dorsum of a domestic short-haired cat with flea allergy dermatitis. The hair has been clipped to show the lesions. Photograph courtesy of Michael Herrtage. See colour plate.

Symmetrical alopecia

This is a frequently misunderstood syndrome in feline practice. Feline symmetrical alopecia, often without obvious signs of inflammation, may be an important sign of pruritus and self-trauma. The alopecia produced by overgrooming is often symmetrical and may affect the medial or caudal aspects of the thighs, the perineal area, the ventral abdomen, flanks and lumbosacral area (Fig. 47.20). Close observation reveals that the hair has been broken off and the shaft is not easily epilated. The alopecia is partial, never progresses to complete baldness, and in most cases, a velvety undercoat remains. This is contrary to the situation which occurs in endocrine skin disease.

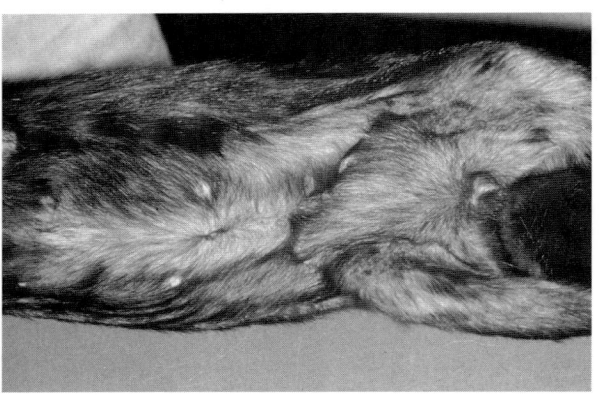

Figure 47.20 Diffuse symmetrical alopecia affecting the ventral abdomen and medial and caudal aspects of the hindlimbs in a domestic short-haired cat with flea allergy dermatitis. Photograph courtesy of Michael Herrtage. See colour plate.

Ulcerative dermatitis associated with self-trauma

This is less common than the two syndromes previously discussed. If pruritus is severe, scratching of accessible areas particularly the head and neck will result in marked ulceration and pyotraumatic dermatitis.

Eosinophilic granuloma complex

This is a poorly understood but important complex in which allergy plays a major part. This complex is discussed separately.

Allergy due to parasites

Flea allergy dermatitis

Flea allergy is the most common cause of 'miliary' dermatitis (Gross et al., 1986; Scott, 1987). The distribution often mimics that in the dog affecting rump, dorsum, tail head and thighs. However, miliary dermatitis of the neck and head regions has been reported in the cat (Muller et al., 1989b). Flea allergy dermatitis is also a major cause of symmetrical alopecia.

The pathogenesis of flea allergy is presumed to be similar to that in the dog. Diagnosis is based on a combination of clinical findings, demonstration of fleas or flea faeces in coat brushings, positive skin reactions to intradermal flea antigen and response to an appropriate insecticidal trial. Treatment involves removing the cause and control of self-trauma both of which are discussed at the end of this section.

Otodectic mange (Otodectes cynotis)

Ear mites are estimated to cause 50% of feline otitis externa. Much less frequently they parasitize other areas of the skin including the head, neck, dorsum and tail head regions. Hypersensitivity has been postulated as part of the pathogenesis (Powell et al., 1980). Miliary dermatitis is the common dermatological problem but pyotraumatic dermatitis may complicate the clinical picture. Diagnosis is based on identification of the mite/eggs in coat brushings and scrapings.

Mosquito/insect bite allergy

A specific seasonal papulocrustous dermatitis affecting the nose, muzzle and pinnae has been described secondary to mosquito bites (Mason and Evans, 1991). These lesions may progress to erosions and are associated with depigmentation. The footpads of affected cats may be ulcerated, swollen and hypopigmented. Peripheral eosinophilia and lymphadenopathy are observed. Histopathology suggests this syndrome may be a variant of the 'eosinophilic granuloma complex' with characteristics typical of insect bite hypersensitivity (Mason, 1993). Diagnosis is mainly aimed at evaluating the response to eliminating the cause. It is recommended that cats are kept in an insect-free environment. Cats protected by insect screening have shown resolution of signs within seven days (Mason, 1993).

Atopic dermatitis

Atopy in the cat has been difficult to characterize beyond a clinical description which mimics that in the dog. Although reaginic antibody is yet to be isolated, the clinical syndrome and its response to hyposensitization is well recognized by several authors (Scott, 1987; Kunkle, 1989; Prost, 1993). Atopy has been incriminated as the cause in 12.1% of miliary dermatitis cases and 12.5% of cats affected with eosinophilic plaque (Scott, 1987). Various degrees of peripheral eosinophilic infiltration may occur (Reedy, 1991). Symmetrical alopecia alone may be a clinical sign of atopy.

Diagnosis is dependent on intradermal skin testing and response to hyposensitization. The technique and choice of antigens are similar to those used for the dog. However, interpretation of skin testing results is more difficult as wheals are less erythematous and poorly circumscribed.

Food intolerance/allergy

The pathophysiology of this syndrome is not completely understood. Adverse reactions to food may involve hypersensitivity to food products, a non-specific physiological reaction to pharmacological or toxic agents in the diet or a combination of both. Reported prevalence rates of the syndrome vary but it is believed to be an uncommon cause of skin disease in the cat (Muller et al., 1989b; White and Sequoia, 1989; Rosser, 1993). Clinical signs include non-seasonal pruritus often affecting the head and neck (White and Sequoia, 1989; Rosser, 1993). Miliary dermatitis, symmetrical alopecia, eosinophilic plaque and ulcerative dermatitis secondary to severe self trauma may be seen (Baker, 1991). Diagnosis is made by feeding a restriction diet using a source of protein to which the cat has had minimal exposure. This may be home cooked or commercially prepared. There is controversy over the optimum time interval for which the diet should be fed. Although most authors recommend 3 weeks (White and Sequoia, 1989; Carlotti et al., 1990), a 9-week trial has been recommended by Rosser (1993b). A feline diet trial particularly if fed for longer periods, must provide adequate taurine. Confirmation of the diagnosis is made by improvement of clinical signs on the trial diet and provocation when the original diet is reinstituted. Intradermal and serological tests are of no value in the diagnosis of this syndrome.

Treatment of allergic skin disease

Treatment principles are similar to those used in the dog and consist of removing or decreasing the allergic burden (for example an insecticidal trial or restriction diet) and controlling self-trauma.

Insecticidal trial for fleas

Recommendations for controlling fleas on cats are as numerous as the products available. The aim should be to use the least toxic products to treat the affected cat, in contact animals and the environment. Care should be taken to use only those products licensed for use in the cat.

Anti-inflammatory therapy

Glucocorticoids

Cats appear to require higher therapeutic doses of glucocorticoids than dogs on a body weight basis. Oral prednisolone or methylprednisolone are recommended at double the canine dose rate, i.e. 2–4 mg kg^{-1}. Induction and alternate day dosing schedules are similar to those used in the dog.

Although cats are more tolerant of glucocorticoid side-effects than dogs, repeated use of depot glucocorticoids (for example methylprednisolone acetate) has produced iatrogenic hyperadrenocorticism (Scott et al., 1982). However, injectable depot glucocorticoids can be useful in cats which are difficult to dose orally as long as the potential for side effects is recognized. Dose rates may be decreased by using glucocorticoids in combination with antihistamines and essential fatty acids.

Antihistamines and essential fatty acids

Antihistamine therapy may be more useful in controlling self-trauma in the cat than in the dog. Chlorpheniramine (2 mg twice daily) has been reported to control up to 73% of pruritic cats (Miller and Scott, 1990) and to potentiate the effects of glucocorticoids. Clinical reports suggest that essential fatty acid supplements are efficacious in controlling pruritus in the cat (Harvey, 1991; Miller et al., 1993). Although there are no reports of synergism between antihistamines and essential fatty acids in the cat, combination antipruritic therapy would seem logical.

Megoestrol acetate

This progestogen has been used in feline inflammatory skin disease for two reasons: its anti-inflammatory effect and antianxiety properties. Although it is an effective antipruritic agent in the cat, it produces powerful adrenal suppression and chronic use has been associated with mammary gland hyperplasia/neoplasia, diabetes mellitus and iatrogenic hyperadrenocorticism. Its use has been superseded by combination antipruritic therapy.

Hyposensitization

Hyposensitization for atopy follows a similar protocol to that in the dog and has reported therapeutic benefit (Reedy, 1982; McDougal, 1986; Prost, 1993).

EOSINOPHILIC GRANULOMA COMPLEX

Traditionally, this complex encompasses three syndromes; the eosinophilic ulcer, plaque and collagenolytic granuloma. Although these entities have usually quite distinct histological patterns, the clinical and aetiological distinctions are less clear.

Indolent or eosinophilic ulcers

These lesions are well demarcated ulcers of the upper lip which may occur unilaterally or bilaterally (Fig. 47.21). The periphery is raised and surrounds a pinkish yellow ulcerated surface. There is a pleomorphic cell infiltrate seen on histopathology. Indolent ulcers are rarely accompanied by tissue or peripheral eosinophilia. Their cause is unknown but a response has been seen to antimicrobial therapy in some cases (Rosenkrantz, 1991). Cryosurgery, radiation therapy, surgical excision and immunosuppressive therapy using oral or intralesional glucocorticoid therapy have all been advocated.

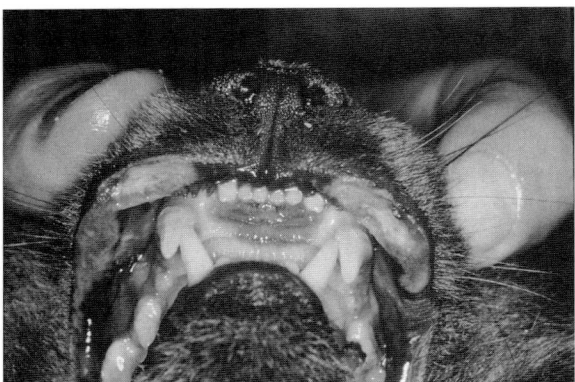

Figure 47.21 Eosinophilic ulcers affecting the upper lip of a domestic short-haired cat. Photograph courtesy of Michael Herrtage. See colour plate.

Eosinophilic plaque

This lesion consists of a raised demarcated lesion which may occur with any distribution (Fig. 47.22). It is associated with pruritus, tissue and circulating eosinophilia. Histopathologically there is spongiotic eosinophilic dermatitis

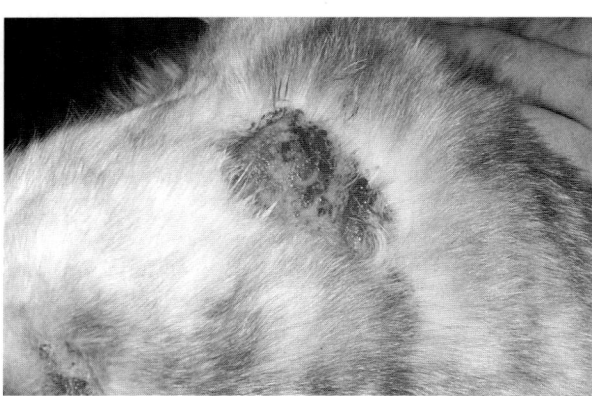

Figure 47.22 Eosinophilic plaque on the flank of a long-haired cat. Photograph courtesy of Michael Herrtage. See colour plate.

(Rosenkrantz, 1991). Hypersensitivity (e.g. to fleas, atopy, food) is most often incriminated in the pathogenesis of this lesion but non-specific trauma (mechanical or chemical) may induce similar signs (Kunkle, 1989). Management should be aimed at identifying an allergic cause, decreasing the allergic burden and controlling self-trauma with anti-inflammatory agents. Hyposensitization may be useful in those cats with positive intradermal skin test results (Kunkle, 1989; Prost, 1993).

Collagenolytic granuloma

This lesion is associated with degeneration of collagen and tissue eosinophilia, and is a deeper dermal reaction. Clinically, nodular granulomas may be seen within the oral cavity on the dorsum of the nose, pinnae and foot pads, or they may affect the skin in grooming areas producing a linear lesion along the medial aspect of forelegs or caudal aspect of thighs (Rosenkrantz, 1991; Mason and Evans, 1991). Occasionally, ulcerative lesions of the upper lip are more aggressive and have histopathological features in common with the collagenolytic granuloma group. Collagenolytic granulomas of the chin and lower lip ('button lip') may also occur (Kunkle, 1989). The postulated cause is hypersensitivity. Involvement of antigens which are introduced into the dermis by inoculation (insect bites), trauma or parasitic migration should be considered (Kunkle, 1989; Mason and Evans, 1991). Management is similar to that for eosinophilic plaque and includes a full investigation for allergic causes.

PSYCHOGENIC ALOPECIA (NEUROGENIC DERMATITIS)

Behavioural disturbances are well recognized as causes by which self-inflicted skin damage due to other aetiological agents is exacerbated. Anxiety may occur in susceptible cats when social patterns are disturbed. Separation anxiety, disruption of a stable family unit or territorial competition are examples. Certain breeds particularly the Siamese and Burmese appear to be predisposed (Fig. 47.23). The clinical expression is excessive hair licking and pulling with alopecia and occasional excoriation (Scott, 1990). Alopecia is often symmetrical. Pure psychogenic alopecia is uncommon and underlying causes of pruritus, especially allergy and ectoparasites, should be investigated and treated appropriately. Treatment using combinations of

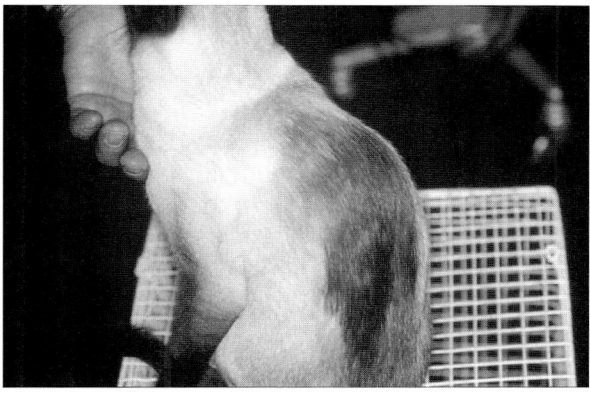

Figure 47.23 Psychogenic alopecia in a Siamese. There is diffuse alopecia along the back and the new hair has grown back with the point colour. Fleas etc. have been ruled out. Photograph courtesy of Michael Herrtage. See colour plate.

diazepam (1–2 mg kg^{-1} twice a day) and phenobarbitone (2–6 mg kg^{-1} twice a day) have been tried with variable success. The tricyclic antidepressant, clomipramine, may have a role in psychogenic dermatoses of the cat (Willemse, 1993).

INFECTIOUS SKIN DISEASE

Bacterial skin disease

Superficial bacterial dermatitis

Unlike the dog, superficial bacterial dermatitis and folliculitis in the cat is uncommon. The true prevalence is unknown as pustules and epidermal collarette formation are often not recognized clinically in this species. However, papular dermatitis and alopecia have been described in cases with histopathological evidence of neutrophilic folliculitis and in the absence of more common ectoparasitic and fungal causes (White, 1991). *Staphylococcus aureus* has been isolated on bacterial culture of biopsies from these cases. Histopathology may be required to make a diagnosis of folliculitis. Treatment consists of systemic antibacterial drugs, the choice of which should be based on culture and sensitivity results.

Deep bacterial dermatitis
Subcutaneous abscesses and cellutitis

The most common bacterial dermatitis in the cat occurs secondary to cat fight injuries. Pain and swelling of the affected area associated with pyrexia, lethargy and anorexia is characteristic. Rupture of the abscess leads to draining sinus tract formation. The onset is frequently seasonal and coincides with periods of increased cat activity in spring and autumn. The most common organisms isolated from bite abscesses are *Pasturella multocida*, *Streptococcus* sp., *Fusobacterium* and *Bacterioides* sp. (Scott, 1990). Rarely reported causes of feline abscesses include *Corynebacterium* spp., *Actinomyces* spp., *Nocardia* spp. and *Yersinia pestis* (DeBoer, 1991). Mycoplasma-like organisms (L forms) have been incriminated as a cause of recurring abscesses in a group of in-contact cats (Carro et al., 1989).

Cytological examination of samples obtained by fine needle aspiration is an important aid to diagnosis of any nodular lesion and will confirm the presence of an abscess. Bacterial culture and sensitivity from biopsy specimens is recommended if the abscess appears slow to heal. Routine culture techniques will not detect mycoplasma-like organisms. The therapeutic response to adequate gravitational drainage and treatment with penicillin V or synthetic penicillins for 7–10 days is usually brisk in the uncomplicated case. Infections with mycoplasma-like organisms (L forms) are rapidly responsive to oral tetracycline therapy (Carro et al., 1989).

Mycobacterial infections

Cutaneous tuberculosis (*Mycobacterium bovis*, *M. tuberculosis*) is an uncommon cause of dermal nodules and poorly healing abscesses in cats. Systemic signs referable to generalized lymphadenopathy, pulmonary and gastrointestinal involvement have been reported (Greene, 1990). Cats most commonly contract the infection from ingestion of *M. bovis*-infected milk. However, transmission from infected humans has been reported.

Another feline tuberculosis syndrome which presents primarily with dermatological signs has been reported in the UK (Gunn-Moore et al., 1996). The organism involved is believed to be *M. microti*, known to cause tuberculosis in voles. The postulated route of transmission to cats is by bite wounds from this sylvatic reservoir. Cutaneous nodules occasionally with involvement of underlying subcutaneous tissues, joint, muscle and/or bone are seen affecting the face, extremities, tail and perineum. Regional lymph node enlargement is common (Gunn-Moore and Shaw, 1997). Clinical and radiological signs referable to systemic involvement are less common but pulmonary lesions have been found in affected cats at post mortem. The zoonotic potential of this syndrome is unknown at present.

Diagnosis of feline tuberculosis may be made by

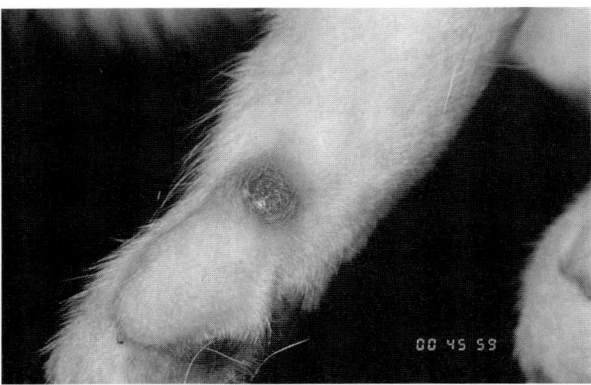

Figure 47.24 One of a number of nodules affecting a domestic short-haired cat with feline leprosy. Photograph courtesy of Michael Herrtage. See colour plate.

the demonstration of Ziehl-Nielsen-positive organisms in aspirates and/or biopsy specimens but confirmation requires culture. Appropriate handling of potentially tuberculosus material is necessary and identification of the organism by a specialist mycobacterial reference laboratory is recommended.

Once the organism has been identified, the zoonotic risk can be determined. Treatment of cats with classical tuberculosis due to *M. bovis* or *M. tuberculosis* is not recommended. Successful treatment of cats with the tuberculosis syndrome caused by *M. microti* has been reported using triple combination therapy of enrofloxacin, rifampicin and clarithromycin (Gunn-Moore and Shaw, 1997).

Feline leprosy is characterized by single or multiple non-painful nodules primarily affecting the face and extremities (Fig. 47.24). Draining sinus tracts, ulceration and regional lymphadenopathy may be present but systemic involvement is uncommon. The disease is more prevalent in cool, wet climates (New Zealand, Southern Australia, Great Britain) during the winter months. The aetiological agent is thought to be the rat leprosy bacillus (*M. lepraemurium*) but conclusive evidence is lacking (Wilkinson and Mason, 1991). Histopathology and cytology are useful diagnostic aids; multiple granulomas are present without caseation and multiple, acid-fast staining bacilli may be seen within the cytoplasm of macrophages. Bacterial culture and guinea-pig inoculation are negative differentiating this disease from cutaneous tuberculosis. Treatment regimes include surgical excision and chemotherapy with oral clofazimine (3–8 mg kg^{-1} once daily) for a 6-week induction course (White, 1991). Toxicity has been reported in cats treated with human leprosy drug regimes which include isoniazid and dapsone (Wilkinson and Mason, 1991).

Opportunistic mycobacterial infections in cats may be caused by the saprophytic, acid-fast growing organisms *Mycobacterium chelonei*, *M. fortuitum*, *M. phlei* and *M. smegmatis* (Kunkle, 1990). Transmission is through contamination of wounds particularly those associated with devitalized subcutaneous fat. Clinical signs include multiple granulomatous nodules with draining sinus tracts which are commonly distributed on the ventral abdomen, inguinal and lumbosacral areas. Infection with *M. smegmatis* or *M. smegmatis*-like organisms has a particular tropism for traumatized inguinal fat-pads. Multiple small punctate ulcers and draining sinus tracts are associated with pain, swelling, anorexia, lethargy and weight loss (Wilkinson and Mason, 1991). Diagnosis is based on the clinical presentation, cytology, histopathology and culture results. The number of acid-fast bacilli is variable and those associated with *M. smegmatis* infection may be more readily identified using Giemsa stain (Wilkinson and Mason, 1991). Organisms are associated with pyogranulomatous panniculitis and are often found surrounded by lipid vacuoles. Because of their lipophilic tendency, some bacilli may be removed by the routine histopathology fixation process, thus making them difficult to find. Culture is recommended from a biopsy specimen rather than exudate. The organism is relatively fast growing (3–5 days) (Kunkle, 1990).

Opportunistic mycobacteria are resistant to drugs used to treat tuberculosis and to many other antibiotics. *In vitro* efficacy may not reflect *in vivo* action due to the poor lipid solubility of many drugs (Wilkinson *et al.*, 1982). Treatment with doxycycline (25 mg orally per cat twice a day), fluquinolone antibiotics (enrofloxiacin 2.5 mg kg^{-1} orally three times a day) or clofazimine (3–8 mg kg^{-1} once daily) for prolonged periods of time (6–20 weeks) has been reported by various authors (Kunkle, 1990; DeBoer, 1991; Wilkinson and Mason, 1991) with varying degrees of success in individual cases. The combination of long-term systemic antibacterial therapy and aggressive surgical resection has been reported to be curative in five successive cases of *M. smegmatis* panniculitis in cats although considerable surgical expertise in reconstructive techniques may be required in advanced cases (Malik *et al.*, 1994).

Viral skin disease

Feline pox infection

Domestic cats are susceptible to infection with cowpox virus. The disease has been recognized

INFECTIOUS SKIN DISEASE

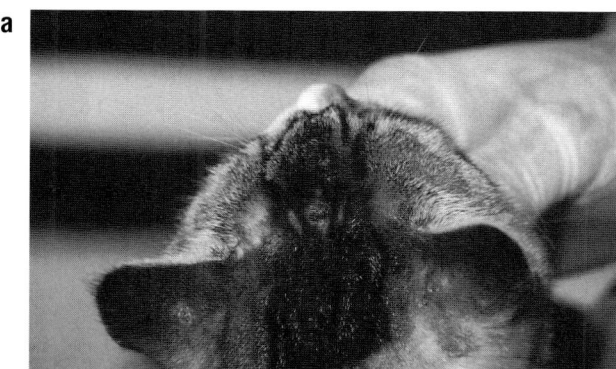

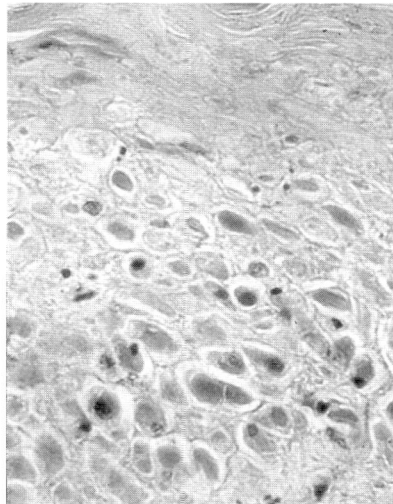

Figure 47.25 (a) Typical skin lesions of feline cowpox; (b) multiple intracytoplasmic eosinophilic inclusions in the epidermis of a cat with feline cowpox. Photograph courtesy of Michael Herrtage. See colour plate.

in most European countries and is most often seen in the autumn (Bennett, 1996). Small rodents are believed to be the reservoir hosts and bites the method of transmission. Clinical signs include ulcerated nodules affecting the distal extremities, face and tail base (Bennett *et al.*, 1986; Thomsett, 1989). Initially the lesions are pruritic but become painful following ulceration (Fig. 47.25). Systemic signs of pox infection are variable and may be rapidly progressive where glucocorticoids have been administered. Fever, lethargy, bronchopneumonia and pleuritis may be encountered in immunosuppressed cats. Diagnosis is based on skin biopsy and serology (Bennett *et al.*, 1985). Classic intracytoplasmic, eosinophilic inclusions are present in keratinocytes. Feline pox infection is usually self-limiting and recovery occurs within 4–6 weeks.

Treatment is tailored to controlling secondary bacterial infection. Glucocorticoids are contraindicated.

Other feline viral infections

Both *feline leukaemia virus* (FeLV) and *feline immunodeficiency virus* (FIV) infections have been associated with skin disease due to opportunistic organisms. Chronic poorly healing abscesses, pyoderma, atypical mycobacterial infections, cryptococcoses, and generalized parasitic infections such as demodicosis and notoedric mange have been reported in association with other systemic clinical signs. FeLV, the related sarcoma virus (FSV) and FIV, particularly in combination, are important in the pathogenesis of feline neoplasia; virally associated lymphoma and fibrosarcoma may affect the skin (Sparger, 1991). Diagnosis of FeLV infection is based on detection of viral antigen in blood, saliva or tears using ELISA and/or immunofluorescent antibody techniques. Feline immunodeficiency virus infection is diagnosed by detection of virally induced antibody using ELISA or CITE techniques. There is no specific antiviral therapy for either infection. However, appropriate treatment for opportunistic infections is recommended.

Occasionally, infection with *feline herpesvirus* or *calicivirus* may result in cutaneous manifestations. Ulcers may be present on the nasal philtrum and footpads (Flecknell *et al.*, 1979).

Fungal skin disease

Dermatophytosis

Dermatophytosis is a major cause of skin disease in the cat. The majority of infections are due to *Microsporum canis* (92–99%) with the higher prevalence occurring in catteries (Moriello, 1991; Sparkes *et al.*, 1993). Unlike other fungi, it is adapted to living on the hair and skin of cats and its presence often elicits minimal inflammatory reaction. The asymptomatic carrier state which may result presents a problem in both diagnosis and control. Factors predisposing to infection include age, self-trauma, ectoparasite infection, and the degree of environmental contamination. Cats less than one year of age are predisposed (Sparkes *et al.*, 1993). Commonly, diffuse alopecia with fractured, brittle hairs is present without clinical signs of inflammation (Fig. 47.26). Focal lesions are common on the head, neck and paws (Fig. 47.27). Pruritus may be a feature particularly

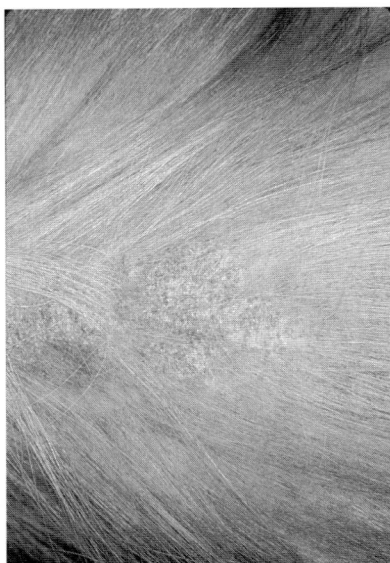

Figure 47.26 Diffuse alopecia along the dorsum in a Persian cat with *Microsporum canis* infection. Photograph courtesy of Michael Herrtage. See colour plate.

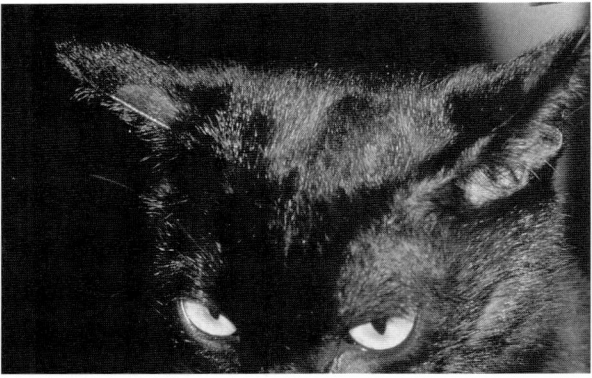

Figure 47.27 Focal lesions on the ears and face of a Burmese cat with *Trichophyton mentagrophytes* infection. The diffuse hair loss over the temporal region is normal in this breed. Photograph courtesy of Michael Herrtage. See colour plate.

if combined with ectoparasite infection. Occasionally a more severe inflammatory response may occur producing papular dermatitis, or rarely, dermal granuloma formation.

Sylvatic and geophilic dermatophytosis secondary to infection with *Trichophyton mentagrophytes*, *T. terrestre*, *T. ajelloi* and *Microsporum persicolor* is reported uncommonly in the cat (Wright, 1989). The clinical presentation is similar to that for *M. canis*.

M. canis is highly contagious and readily transmissible to humans. Definitive diagnosis is made by fungal culture from hair or biopsy specimens. In cats, Wood's lamp and direct microscopic examination of hairs for arthrospores are useful diagnostic aids if used correctly (Sparkes *et al.*, 1993).

Treatment of dermatophytosis is aimed at eliminating infection from affected animals, preventing spread and decontaminating the environment. Both topical and systemic medications are used. Griseofulvin is the systemic drug of choice. However, it is poorly absorbed and should be administered with a fatty meal. Griseofulvin is teratogenic and contraindicated in pregnant animals. Controversy exists regarding its dose and administration. Microsize formulations (10–25 mg kg^{-1} bid) for three to six weeks are most commonly recommended (Moriello, 1991). Griseofulvin toxicity has been increasingly recognized with leucopenia due to bone marrow suppression being the most serious. Recent reports indicate that side effects are not dose dependent although Helston *et al.* (1986) recommend not exceeding a total daily dose of 125 mg of microsize griseofulvin. Siamese, Abyssinian and Himalayan breeds appear predisposed. A possible interaction between griseofulvin and feline immunodeficiency virus in potentiating leucopenia is being investigated.

The imidazoles have been variously recommended for treatment of dermatophytosis. Ketoconazole is not recommended in cats due to toxicity and the presence of resistant strains (Moriello, 1991). Itraconazole is used in the treatment of human dermatophytosis. A recent comparative study of cats with experimentally induced *M. canis* infections showed itraconazole and griseofulvin to be equally effective (Moriello and DeBoer, 1995a).

Topical treatment with chlorhexidine (2%) and povidine–iodine solutions, enilconazole, natamycin and sodium bensuldazic acid appears to have minimal effect on the progression of disease (Wright, 1989; DeBoer and Moriello, 1995a). Lime sulphur dips although unpleasant to use have been recommended as an adjunct to systemic therapy (Moriello, 1991). If topical therapy is used, its efficacy particularly in long-haired cats may be increased by clipping.

Control measures consist of segregating affected animals until they have two negative brushings eight weeks apart (Wright, 1989). Disinfection of fomites including cages, baskets, runs and grooming equipment is essential. Steam sterilization or soaking in 10% formalin, 0.5% sodium hypochlorite, 0.5% chlorhexidine are alternatives (Wright, 1989; Moriello, 1991). Disposable contaminated items should be burnt. Environmental use of enilconazole in aqueous or fumigant vehicles has been reported. Samples taken from the environment of previously infected catteries were negative after enilconazole use (Palsson, 1991).

Fungal vaccines have been developed for use in the cat. Studies with experimental and commercial inactivated vaccines have given disappointing results (DeBoer and Moriello, 1995b; Moriello and DeBoer, 1995b) although this is an area of ongoing research and development.

Subcutaneous and systemic mycoses

Sporotrichosis

Sporothrix schenkii is a dimorphic fungus with a world-wide distribution. It is ubiquitous and infection occurs via wounds contaminated by soil or decaying vegetation. Sporotrichosis is recognized as a major pathogen of people and transmission of the disease by bite or scratch wounds from affected cats is reported (Dunstan et al., 1986). Early lesions in the cat may mimic cat fight abscesses and affect the extremities, head or base of tail. As the disease progresses, nodule formation with multiple draining sinuses occurs. Cavitating ulcers may develop which expose underlying muscle, tendons and bone. Infection remains localized or spreads along afferent lymphatic vessels to become disseminated. Other areas of skin may be affected following licking and grooming of lesions. Histologically, pyogranulomas are seen associated with large numbers of organisms. In cats, *Sporothrix* organisms are easily identified on impression smears of draining exudate.

Therapy with imidazoles particularly itraconazole is effective in many cases (Dunstan et al., 1986) but its zoonotic potential should be appreciated.

Other subcutaneous mycoses

Mycetoma syndromes are rare in the cat but actinomycotic and eumycotic mycetoma have been reported as in the dog (DeBoer, 1991).

Phaeohyphomycosis although uncommon has been reported more frequently in the cat than the dog. This syndrome is caused by pigmented fungi that do not form granules unlike the mycetoma group. Brown pigment is always found on culture growth and dark-walled septate hyphae may be seen on biopsy specimens. Fungal species incriminated in causing this syndrome include *Phialophora*, *Cladosporium* and *Alternaria*. Lesions usually consist of a solitary nodule on the extremities with draining sinus tracts or ulceration. Treatment is surgical excision.

Cryptococcosis

Cryptococcosis is caused by a saprophytic yeast-like fungus which develops a large capsule in affected tissue. *Cryptococcus neoformans* (var. *neoformans*, var. *gattei*) produces clinical signs primarily referable to the skin and respiratory tract in affected cats although involvement of the central nervous system and eye can occur. Multiple cutaneous ulcerative nodules commonly involve the head, bridge of nose and periocular regions. Upper respiratory tract signs referable to nasal granuloma formation are also common. Uveitis, optic neuritis, retinal detachment and neurological signs referable to the site of granuloma formation have been reported. Clinical signs are well reviewed by Ackerman (1988).

Diagnosis is made by cytological demonstration of the organism in the exudate or in periodic acid–Schiff-, Gomori- or Mayer-stained biopsy specimens. The organism may be cultured from both exudate and tissue samples. Serological detection of capsular antigen has been used in the diagnosis of feline cryptococcosis but lacks sensitivity (Barsanti, 1984). It may be useful in monitoring efficacy of treatment. Successful treatment using ketoconazole alone (10 mg kg^{-1} daily) and in combination with 5-flucytosine have been reported. The cryptococcal organism is highly sensitive to fluconazole and therapy (50 mg twice daily) produces dramatic resolution of the disease in cats (Malik et al., 1992).

Other systemic mycoses

Cutaneous lesions may accompany systemic signs of blastomycosis, histoplasmosis, coccidiodomycosis and trichosporonosis. All are rare diseases in the cat. Lesions are primarily related to granuloma formation with ulcerated nodules, draining sinus tracts and non-healing abscesses. Diagnosis is based on the presence of systemic signs typical of the mycosis suspected and demonstration of the causative agent on histopathology and culture of biopsy specimens. Imidazole therapy is the treatment of choice.

PARASITIC SKIN DISEASE

Parasites which are associated with allergic dermatitis have been discussed earlier.

Notoedric mange (*Notoedres cati*)

Notoedric mange is an uncommon contagious cause of pruritus in the cat and is responsible for isolated epizootic outbreaks in Europe. Miliary dermatitis of the pinnae, head and neck with associated pruritus may be initial signs but ulceration and crusting follow chronic infection. A more generalized distribution of lesions occurs in cats treated with immunosuppressive drugs or in cats which have intercurrent disease. Human infection has been reported (Scott and Horn, 1987). Diagnosis is by demonstration of mites and eggs in skin scrapings. Treatment with lime sulphur, organophosphates or carbamates in formulations appropriate for feline use for the duration of two mite life cycles (6 weeks) is curative. Ivermectin (200 µg kg^{-1} given subcutaneously) is highly effective although not registered for use in this species. All in-contact cats should be treated. The relative toxicity of ivermectin in cats is less than that for dogs and no breed idiosyncrasy has been reported (Hsu et al., 1989).

Cheyletiellosis

Cheyletiellosis is a common cause of scaling, partial alopecia and variable pruritus in the cat. *Cheyletiella blakei* is the usual species to infect cats but cross-infection with other species will occur. Cheyletiellosis is a zoonosis. Diagnosis is by demonstration of mites on clear adhesive tape preparations or skin scrapings. In some cases, mites may be difficult to find. Treatment using topical organophosphates, carbamates and lime sulphur are recommended. In multi-cat households or in cases where resolution is difficult, ivermectin is effective.

Demodicosis (*Demodex cati*, *Demodex* sp.)

Two types of demodex mite cause alopecia in the cat: *Demodex cati* and a short, rotund as yet unnamed species. The former inhabits hair follicles and may be found in otic cerumen. Feline demodectic mange is uncommon. Infection with *D. cati* is usually associated with systemic disease particularly FIV and FeLV infections. The non-follicular mite is found in the epidermis and is associated with more inflammation and pruritus. Hair loss may be focal or more generalized with a symmetrical distribution. It is associated with scaling erythema and comedone formation. Diagnosis of demodicosis is made by skin scrapings. Treatment and prognosis is dependent on investigation and exclusion of underlying disease. Off-label use of half strength amitraz (0.0125% solution administered weekly), lime sulphur, malathion or carbamate dips have been recommended (Medleau et al., 1988).

Other parasitic diseases

Trombiculidiasis, infection with *Lynxacarus radovsky* (cat fur mite) and *Dermanyssus gallinae* are reported causes of pruritus, regional alopecia (depending on the tropism of the parasite) and scaling. Diagnosis is by identification of mites or intermediate stages on skin scrapings, hair brushings and hair pluckings. Treatment with 2.5% lime sulphur, pyrethrin, pyrethroids or ivermectin (200–300 µg kg^{-1} subcutaneously or orally) and limiting exposure of cats to infected sources (fields, woodlands, poultry yards) is recommended.

ENDOCRINE DERMATOSES

Endocrinopathies causing skin disease in the cat are rare.

Feline endocrine alopecia

Endocrine abnormalities are an overdiagnosed cause of symmetrical alopecia in the cat. Feline endocrine alopecia (FEA) has been used to describe a symmetrical alopecia affecting the perineal, ventrum, inguinal regions and medial aspects of the hindlimbs. Male castrated cats are reportedly more affected. An endocrine cause in these cases has never been demonstrated and it is suggested this syndrome be renamed idiopathic symmetrical alopecia (Henfrey, 1993). Many cases are likely to be allergic with or without psychological involvement and all other causes should be ruled out before making a diagnosis of idiopathic symmetrical alopecia (ISA). Response of these cases to hormone preparations does not imply the cause is an endocrinopathy. Megoestrol acetate has powerful anti-inflammatory and anti-anxiety properties, and testosterone may produce psychogenic changes in anxious cats, which may be partially therapeutic in psychogenic alopecia. ISA is a diagnosis based on elimination of more common dermatopathies. Hair shafts should be examined for evidence of self-trauma. A skin biopsy to evaluate hair matrix activity may be indicated. An eosinophil count of greater than 1.5×10^9 l^{-1} excludes ISA in 92% of cases (Henfrey, 1993).

Other endocrinopathies

Thyroid disease

Confirmed naturally occurring, acquired hypothyroidism has only been reported in one case (Rand et al., 1993). This was associated with symmetrical alopecia, scaling and mucinosis. Kittens with congenital hypothyroidism may have an abnormal hair coat (retention of fluffy undercoat) but alopecia is not a feature (Jones et al., 1991). Iatrogenic hypothyroidism following bilateral thyroidectomy does not cause symmetrical alopecia although some hair loss may occur over the pinna.

Cutaneous signs associated with hyperthyroidism are uncommon although overgrooming and hair pulling may result in alopecia. An older cat with recent symmetrical hair loss, hyperactivity and weight loss should be evaluated for this disease.

Hyperadrenocorticism

This is an extremely uncommon disease in the cat. Bilaterally symmetrical alopecia with severe thinning and tearing of the skin in association with polyuria/polydipsia and pendulous abdomen may be seen. Concurrent diabetes mellitus is common and is often the major presenting sign (Nelson et al., 1988). Diagnosis is similar to that in the dog. Iatrogenic symmetrical alopecia has been seen in cats treated for long periods with megoestrol acetate (Kunkle, 1984).

NEOPLASTIC SKIN DISEASE

In the feline species, cutaneous neoplasia is second only to lymphoproliferative disorders in prevalence of cancer. The spectrum of tumour types is similar to that in the dog but there are several differences in prevalence, epidemiology and prognosis. Treatment modalities are extrapolated largely from canine protocols.

The prevalence of feline cutaneous neoplasms in different geographic locations is illustrated in Table 47.14.

Feline mast cell tumours

Mast cell tumours commonly occur as solitary nodules with an alopecic or ulcerated surface. They are most likely to be distributed on the head, neck and dorsal trunk. There is an age predilection for older male cats. The biological behaviour of this tumour varies. Although malignant mast cell tumours with a high degree of anaplasia, metastasis, paraneoplastic effects and recurrence after removal have been reported (Wilcock et al., 1986), the majority have a benign clinical course unlike their canine equivalent. Surgical excision is often curative and if recurrence occurs, it is not associated with dissemination (Buerger and Scott, 1987). Spontaneous remission has been reported with both solitary tumours and benign histiocytic mast cell tumours affecting young Siamese cats (Wilcock et al., 1986; Buerger and Scott, 1987). Therapy with systemic glucocorticoids is of debatable benefit. Where surgical excision is difficult, local treatment with cryotherapy or radiation is useful.

Fibroma/fibrosarcoma

These tumours are well represented in the cat. Multicentric feline sarcoma virus-induced

Table 47.14 Origin and relative prevalence (%) of feline cutaneous neoplasms

Tumour	Origin	New Zealand[a]	UK[b]	USA[c]
Squamous cell carcinoma	Epithelial	52	17.4	12.1
Basal cell carcinoma	Epithelial	18.5	14.8	N.S.
Fibroma	Mesenchymal	5.3	2.7	12.1
Mast cell tumour	Mesenchymal	3.3	7.7	7.3
Sebaceous adenoma	Epithelial	1.1	2.3	N.S.
Melanoma	Mesenchymal	0	2.7	6.3
Cutaneous lymphoma	Mesenchymal	0	2.7	N.S.
Lipoma	Mesenchymal	0	2.3	6.0
Haemangioma	Mesenchymal	0	0.3	2.3

[a]Lee (1987), [b]Bostock (1977), [c]Brodey (1970).

tumours may occur in kittens under four months of age. These are associated with concurrent feline leukaemia virus infection and the prognosis is grave.

More recently, an association between vaccination sites in the interscapular and thigh areas and development of soft tissue sarcomas has been recognized. The incidence of such vaccine site-associated sarcomas in the US has been estimated to be between 1:1000 and 1:10 000. Although certain types of killed vaccine have been incriminated, the current belief is that the adjuvant rather than the viral antigen is the trigger for neoplastic transformation of fibroblasts. The tumours enlarge rapidly, are locally invasive and tend to recur after removal (Lester *et al.*, 1996).

IMMUNE-MEDIATED DISEASES

Autoimmune diseases

The prevalence of immune-mediated dermatoses in the cat is similar to that in the dog (Scott *et al.*, 1987a). They account for only 1.4% of feline dermatoses.

Pemphigus foliaceus is the most common. In addition to crusting lesions of the face, ears, periocular regions and footpads, the nail beds and perimammary gland skin are commonly affected in cats. Both pemphigus vulgaris and pemphigus erythematosus have been reported in the cat but less commonly than pemphigus foliaceus (Scott *et al.*, 1987a). Diagnostic techniques are similar to those discussed for the dog.

Systemic lupus erythematosus is the second most common immune-mediated skin disease in cats. No age or gender predilections are reported although Siamese may be predisposed (Scott *et al.*, 1987a). The majority of cats present with systemic illness, fever and skin lesions affecting the ears, nailbeds and limbs in a symmetrical pattern. Both scaling and mucocutaneous ulcerative syndromes have been reported. Ulceration of lips and nasal philtrum is frequent. Antinuclear antibody is positive and histopathological findings of a hydropic and lichenoid interface dermatitis are supportive.

Toxic epidermal necrolysis and *erythema multiforme* are well recognized in the cat. Drug eruptions are believed to be the major causes in cats.

Cold agglutinin disease has been reported in the cat (Schrader and Hurvitz, 1983; Zulty and Kociba, 1990) and may be primary due to the inherent presence of cryoglobulin (IgM) autoantibody or secondary due to neoplastic or infectious disease such as haemobartonellosis or upper respiratory viral infection. Clinical signs include necrosis and sloughing of ear tips, paws, and distal tail. Diagnosis as in the dog is confirmed by a positive cold Coombs test. Bullous pemphigoid, discoid lupus erythematosus, pemphigus vegetans and vasculitis of immune-mediated origin have rarely been reported (Scott *et al.*, 1987b).

Treatment protocols are similar to that for the dog. Most feline cases of immune-mediated skin disease are responsive to glucocorticoids and control is more easily maintained due to the cats' greater resistance to side effects. Immunosuppressive doses of prednisolone for induction are twice those recommended for the dog (6.6 mg kg^{-1} daily). Alternate day prednisolone may give several years of remission. Aurothioglucose has also been used with success, alone or in combination with glucocorticoids.

Plasma cell pododermatitis

The aetiology and pathogenesis of this disease are unknown. An immune-mediated pathogenesis is suggested by basement membrane zone IgG deposition, positive ANA titres and the presence of intercurrent glomerulonephritis in some cases (Gruffydd-Jones *et al.*, 1980; Kunkle, 1984). An association with FIV infection has been reported (Guaguere and Prelaud, 1991).

Clinical presentation includes pain, lameness, fluctuant swelling of footpads followed by ulceration (Fig. 47.28). Systemic signs include pyrexia, anorexia and lymphadenopathy. Histopathology reveals marked infiltration of plasma cells and occasional leucocytoclastic vasculitis. Treatment

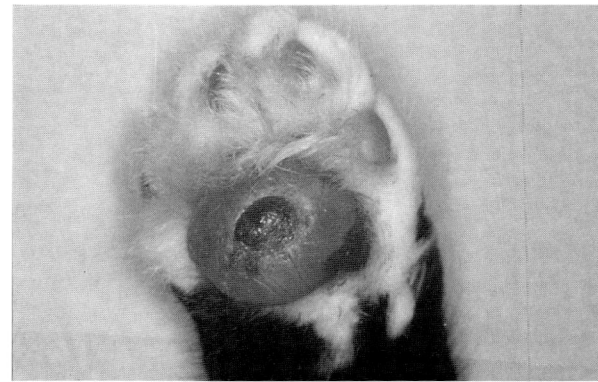

Figure 47.28 Plasma cell pododermatitis in a domestic short-haired cat. Photograph courtesy of Michael Herrtage. See colour plate.

with glucocorticoids and crysotherapy has been used but response should be interpreted in the light of spontaneous remission.

CONGENITAL AND GENETIC DERMATOSES

Skin diseases in this category can only be controlled by palliative therapy and are often associated with a poor prognosis. Where affected animals are part of a breeding programme, client consultation should include advice on neutering and investigation of pedigrees.

Cutaneous asthenia (*Ehlers–Danlos syndrome*) is an uncommon hereditary connective tissue disease characterized by hyperextensibility of the skin, laxity of joints, lack of cutaneous tensile strength, multiple full thickness lacerations associated with minimal trauma and subsequent scarring of lesions. Inherited recessive cutaneous asthenia is reported in the cat and biochemical analysis of defective collagen has confirmed a deficiency in procollagen peptidase in Himalayans (Counts and Byers, 1980).

Hereditary hypotrichosis has been reported as a cause of alopecia in the Siamese and Rex breeds. The Sphinx cat has been specifically bred for its lack of hair. Manipulation of the Rex mutation which prevents appropriate development of guard hairs produces alopecia in the Devon Rex. Histopathological examination of hair follicles reveals normal density of hair follicles, but hairs are in telogen and are unusually fragile. In Siamese and Sphinx with alopecia universalis, hair follicles are decreased in density. Cats with hypotrichosis are reluctant to groom. Consequently, scaling, greasy odour and excessive accumulation of sebaceous secretions are complications of the alopecia (Robinson, 1977).

Lentigo in ginger cats is a benign condition characterized by hyperpigmented macules of the eyelids, and perioral skin which become more pronounced with increasing age (Scott, 1987).

REFERENCES

Ackerman, L.J. (1988) Feline cryptococcosis. *Compendium on Continuing Education* **10**, 1049–1052.
Angarano, D.W. and MacDonald, J.M. (1992) Immunotherapy in canine atopy. In: *Current Veterinary Therapy* XI (Eds R.W. Kirk and J.D. Bonagura). W.B. Saunders, Philadelphia, pp. 505–508.
Baker, E. (1991) Food hypersensitivity. In: *Consultations in Feline Internal Medicine*. (Ed. J.R. August). W.B. Saunders, Philadelphia, pp. 97–100.
Baker, K.P. and Thomsett, L.R. (1990) Clinical examination and laboratory procedures. In: *Canine and Feline Dermatology* (Eds K.P. Baker and L.R. Thomsett). Blackwell Scientific Publications, Oxford, p. 56.
Barsanti, J.A. (1984) Cryptococcosis. In: *Clinical Microbiology of the Dog and Cat* (Ed. C.E. Greene). W.B. Saunders, Philadelphia, pp. 700–709.
Bennett, M (1996) Cowpox: an overview. *Veterinary International*, **2**, 12–21.
Bennett, M., Baxby, D., Gaskell, R.M., Gaskell, C.J. and Kelly, D.R. (1985) Laboratory diagnosis of orthopoxvirus infection in the domestic cat. *Journal of Small Animal Practice* **26**, 653–661.
Bennett, M., Gaskell, C.J., Gaskell, R.M., Baxby, D. and Gruffydd-Jones, T.J. (1986) Poxvirus infection in the domestic cat. Clinical and epidemiological observations. *Veterinary Record* **118**, 387–390.
Bibel, D.J., Aly R. and Shinefield, H.R. (1992) Antimicrobial activity of sphingosines. *Journal of Investigative Dermatology* **98**, 269–273.
Bond, R. (1997) *Malassezia pachydermatis* and canine skin disease. *Waltham Focus* **7**, 27–31.
Bond, R. and Lloyd, D.H. (1993) Combined treatment with concentrated essential fatty acids and prednisolone in the management of canine atopy. *Veterinary Record* **134**, 30–32.
Bond, R. and Lloyd, D.H. (1997) Skin and mucosal populations of *Malassezia pachydermatis* in healthy and seborrhoeic Basset Hounds. *Veterinary Dermatology* **8**, 101–106.
Bond, R., Thorogood, S. and Lloyd, D.H. (1994) Evaluation of two enzyme-linked immunosorbent assays as diagnostic aids for canine atopy. *Veterinary Record* **135**, 130–133.
Bond, R., McNeil, P.E., Evans, H. and Srebernik, N. (1995a) Metabolic epidermal necrosis in two dogs with different underlying diseases. *Veterinary Record* **136**, 466–471.
Bond, R., Rose, J.F., Ellis, J.W. and Lloyd, D.H. (1995b) Comparison of two shampoos for treatment of *Malassezia pachydermatis*-associated seborrhoeic dermatitis in Basset Hounds. *Journal of Small Animal Practice* **36**, 99–104.
Bond, R., Ferguson, E.A., Curtis, C.F., Craig, J.M. and Lloyd, D.H. (1996) Factors associated with elevated cutaneous *Malassezia pachydermatis* populations in dogs with pruritic skin disease. *Journal of Small Animal Practice* **37**: 103–107.
Bostock, D.E. (1977) Neoplasia of the skin and mammary glands in dogs and cats. In: *Current Veterinary Therapy* VI (Ed. R.W. Kirk). W.B. Saunders, Philadelphia, pp. 493–505.
Bravo, L., Frank, L.A. and Brenneman, K.A. (1993)

Canine leishmaniasis in the United States. *Compendium on Continuing Education* **15**, 699–708.

Breathnach, S.M. (1986) Do epidermotropic T cells exist in normal skin? A re-evaluation of the SALT hypothesis. *British Journal of Dermatology* **115**, 389–395.

Brodey, R.S. (1970) Canine and feline neoplasia. *Advances in Veterinary Science* **14**, 309–354.

Brown, R.G., Hoag, G.N., Smart, M.E. and Mitchell, L.H. (1978) Alaskan Malamute chondrodysplasia, V. Decreased gut zinc absorption. *Growth* **42**, 1–6.

Buerger, R.G. and Scott, D.W. (1987) Cutaneous mast cell neoplasia in cats: fourteen cases (1975–1985). *Journal of the American Veterinary Medical Association* **190**, 1440–1443.

Burrows, M. (1991) Skin tumours in the dog and cat – a West Australian perspective. In: *Proceedings of a Course in Small Animal Oncology*. Murdoch University Foundation for Continuing Veterinary Education, Perth, Western Australia, pp. 69–75.

Campbell, K.L. (1990) Effects of oral sunflower oil on serum and cutaneous fatty acids in seborrhoeic dogs. In: *Proceedings of Annual Meeting of the American Academy of Veterinary Dermatology and the American College of Veterinary Dermatology*, San Francisco, USA, p. 44.

Carlotti, D.N. and Costargent, F. (1994) Analysis of positive skin test in 449 dogs with allergic dermatitis. *European Journal of Companion Animal Practice* **4**, 42–59.

Carlotti, D.N., Remy, I. and Prost, C. (1990) Food allergy in dogs and cats. A review and report of 43 cases. *Veterinary Dermatology* **1**, 55–62.

Carro, T., Pederson, N.C., Beaman, B.L. and Munn, R. (1989) Subcutaneous abscesses and arthritis caused by a probable bacterial L-form in cats. *Journal of the American Animal Hospital Association* **194**, 1583–1585.

Counts, D.F. and Byers, B.F. (1980) Dermatosparaxis in a Himalayan cat. I Biochemical studies of dermal collagen. *Journal of Investigative Dermatology* **74**, 96–99.

Curtis, C.F., Bond, R., Blunden, A.S., Thompson, D.G., McNeil, P.E. & Whitbread, T.W. (1995) Canine eosinophilic folliculitis and furunculosis in three dogs. *Journal of Small Animal Practice* **36**, 119–123.

Curtis, C.F., Evans, H. and Lloyd, D.H. (1996) Investigation of the reproductive and growth hormone status of dogs affected by idiopathic recurrent flank alopecia. *Journal of Small Animal Practice* **37**, 417–422.

DeBoer, D.J. (1991) Non-healing cutaneous wounds. In: *Consultations in Feline Internal Medicine* (Ed. R. August). W.B. Saunders, Philadelphia, pp. 101–106.

DeBoer, D.J. and Moriello, K.A. (1995a) Inability of two topical treatments to influence the course of experimentally induced dermatophytosis in cats. *Journal of the American Veterinary Medical Association* **207**, 52–57.

DeBoer, D.J. and Moriello, K.A. (1995b) Investigations of a killed dermatophyte cell-wall vaccine against infection with *Microsporum canis* in cats. *Research in Veterinary Science* **59**, 110–113.

Dufait, R. (1983). *Pityrosporon canis* as the cause of canine chronic dermatitis. *Veterinary Medicine/Small Animal Clinician* **78**, 1055–1057.

Dunstan, R.W., Langham, R.F. and Reimann, K.A. (1986) Feline sporotrichosis: a report of five cases with transmission to humans. *Journal of the American Academy of Dermatology* **15**, 37–45.

Fakhri, A.B. and Lovell, J. (1979) In: *Miller's Anatomy of the Dog*, 2nd edn (Eds H. Evans and G. Christensen). W.B. Saunders, Philadelphia, p. 78.

Feldman, E.C. and Mack, R.E. (1992) Urine cortisol:creatinine ratio as a screening test for hyperadrenocorticism in dogs. *Journal of the American Veterinary Medical Association* **200**, 1637–1641.

Feldman, E.C. and Nelson, R.W. (1987a) Hyperadrenocorticism. In: *Canine and Feline Endocrinology and Reproduction* (Eds E.C. Feldman and R.W, Nelson). W.B. Saunders, Philadelphia, pp. 137–190.

Feldman, E.C. and Nelson, R.W. (1987b) Hypothyroidism. In: *Canine and Feline Endocrinology and Reproduction* (Eds E.C. Feldman and R.W. Nelson). W.B. Saunders, Philadelphia, pp. 55–87.

Feldman, E.C. and Nelson, R.W. (1992) Use of ketaconazole for control of canine hyperadrenocorticism. In: *Current Veterinary Therapy* XI (Eds R.W. Kirk and J.D. Bonagura). W.B. Saunders, Philadelphia, pp. 349–352.

Ferrer, L. (1992) Leishmaniasis. In: *Current Veterinary Therapy* XI (Eds R.W. Kirk and J.D. Bonagura). W.B. Saunders, Philadelphia, pp. 266–270.

Figueiredo, C., Viana, J.A. and Curi, P.R. (1993) Clinical evaluation of the effect of vitamin E in the treatment of generalised canine demodiocosis. In: *Advances in Veterinary Dermatology* II (Eds P.J. Ihrke, I.S. Mason and S.D. White). Pergamon Press, Oxford, pp. 247–261.

Finnie, J.W. and Bostock, D.E. (1979) Skin neoplasia in dogs. *Australian Veterinary Journal* **55**, 602–604.

Flecknell, P.A., Orr, G.M., Wright, A.I., Gaskell, R.M. and Kelly, D.F. (1975) Skin ulceration associated with herpesvirus infection in cats. *Veterinary Record* **104**, 313–315.

Foley, R.H. (1991) Parasitic mites of dogs and cats. *Compendium on Continuing Education (Small Animal)* **13**, 783–798.

Gilbert, P.A., Griffin, C.E. and Rosenkrantz, W.S. (1992) Serum vitamin E levels in dogs with pyoderma and generalised demodicosis. *Journal of the American Animal Hospital Association* **28**, 407–410.

Greene, C.G. (1990) Tuberculous mycobacterial infections. In: *Infectious Diseases of the Dog and Cat* (Ed. C.G. Greene). W.B. Saunders, Philadelphia, pp. 558–566.

Griffin, C.E. (1987) Treatment of demodicosis. In:

Proceedings of the 11th Kal Kan Symposium for the Treatment of Small Animal Diseases. Ohio State University College of Veterinary Medicine, p. 109.

Griffin, C.E. (1993a) Canine atopic disease. In: *Current Veterinary Dermatology. The Science and Art of Therapy* (Eds C.E. Griffin, K.W. Kwochka and J.M. McDonald). Mosby Year Book, Missouri, p. 99.

Griffin, C.E. (1993b) Detection of insect/arachnid specific IgE in dogs: comparison of two techniques utilising western blots as the standard. In: *Advances in Veterinary Dermatology* II (Eds P.J. Ihrke, I.S. Mason and S.D. White). Pergamon Press, Oxford, pp. 263–269.

Gross, T.L. (1993) Canine eosinophilic furunculosis of the face. In: *Advances in Veterinary Dermatology* II (Eds P.J. Ihrke, I.S. Mason and S.D. White). Pergamon Press, Oxford, pp. 239–246.

Gross, T.L., Kwochka, K.W. and Kunkle, G.A. (1986) Correlation of histologic and immunologic findings in cats with miliary dermatitis. *Journal of the American Veterinary Medical Association* **189**, 1322–1325.

Gross, T.L., O'Brien, T.D., Davies, A.P. and Long, R.E. (1990) Glucagon producing pancreatic endocrine tumours in two dogs with superficial necrolytic dermatitis. *Journal of the American Veterinary Medical Association* **197**, 1619–1622.

Gross, T.L., Song, M.D., Havel, P.J. and Ihrke, P.J. (1993) Superficial necrolytic dermatitis (necrolytic migratory erythema) in dogs. *Veterinary Pathology* **30**, 75–81.

Gruffydd-Jones, T.J., Orr, C.M. and Lucke, V.M. (1980) Footpad swelling and ulceration in cats: report on five cases. *Journal of Small Animal Practice* **21**, 381–389.

Guaguere, E. and Prelaud, P. (1991) Feline plasmocytic pododermatitis: clinical histopathological and immunological findings in 10 cases. In: *Proceedings of the 8th Annual meeting of European Society of Veterinary Dermatology*, Luxembourg, pp. 40–42.

Gunn-Moore, D.A., Jenkins, P.A. and Lucke, V.M. (1996) Feline tuberculosis: a literature discussion of 19 cases caused by an unusual mycobacterial variant. *Veterinary Record* **138**, 53–58.

Gunn-Moore, D.A. and Shaw S.E. (1997) Mycobacterial disease in the cat. *In Practice* 493–501.

Haines, D.M., Cooke, E.M. and Clarke, E.G. (1986) Avidin–biotin–peroxide complex immunohistochemistry to detect immunoglobulin in formalin-fixed skin biopsies in canine autoimmune skin disease. *Canadian Journal of Veterinary Research* **51**, 104–109.

Halliwell, R.E.W. (1987) Canine allergic skin disease. In: *Proceedings of the 11th Kal Kan Symposium for the Treatment of Small Animal Diseases*, Ohio State University College of Veterinary Medicine, p. 33.

Harvey, R.G. (1991) Management of feline miliary dermatitis by supplementing the diet with essential fatty acids. *Veterinary Record* **28**, 326–329.

Hay, R. J. (1992). Fungi and fungal infections of the skin. In: *The Skin Microflora and Microbial Skin Disease* (Ed. W.C. Noble). Cambridge, Cambridge University Press, pp. 232–263.

Helston, K.A., Nesbitt, G.H. and Caciolo, P. (1986) Griseofulvin toxicity in cats: literature review and report of seven cases. *Journal of the American Animal Hospital Association* **22**, 453–458.

Henfrey, J.I. (1993) Symmetrical alopecia in the cat. In: *BSAVA Manual of Small Animal Dermatology* (Eds P.H. Locke, R.G. Harvey and I.S. Mason). British Small Animal Veterinary Association, Cheltenham, pp. 114–120.

Hsu, W.H., Wellborn, S.G. and Schaffer, C.B. (1989) The safety of ivermectin. *Compendium on Continuing Education Small Animals* **11**, 584–588.

Jenkinson, D. M. (1989). Sweat and sebaceous glands and their function in domestic animals. *Advances in Veterinary Dermatology* **1**, 229–251.

Jezyk, P.F., Haskins, M.E., Mackay-Smith, W.E. and Patterson, D.F. (1986) Lethal acrodermatitis in Bull Terriers. *Journal of the American Veterinary Medical Association* **188**, 833–839.

Jones, B.R., Gruffydd-Jones, T.J. and Sparkes, A.H. (1991) Congenital hypothyroidism in the cat. *Bulletin of the Feline Advisory Bureau* **28**, 12–14.

Kintzer, P.P. and Peterson, M.E. (1991) Mitotane (o,p'-DDD) therapy of 200 dogs with pituitary dependent hyperadrenocorticism. *Journal of Veterinary Internal Medicine* **5**, 182–190.

Kunkle, G.A. (1984) Feline dermatology. *Veterinary Clinics of North America (Small Animal Practice)* **14**, 1065–1087.

Kunkle, G.A. (1989) Miliary dermatitis, eosinophilic granuloma complex, and symmetrical hypotrichosis as manifestions of allergy. *Current Veterinary Therapy* X (Ed. R.W. Kirk). W.B. Saunders, Philadelphia, pp. 583–586.

Kunkle, G.A. (1990) Atypical mycobacterial infections. In: *Infectious Diseases of the Dog and Cat* (Ed. C.E. Greene). W.B. Saunders, Philadelphia, pp. 569–572.

Kunkle, G.A. (1992) Canine dermatomyositis: a disease with an infectious origin. *Compendium on Continuing Education* **14**, 866–871.

Kwochka, K.W. (1989) Retinoids in dermatology. In: *Current Veterinary Therapy* X (Ed. R.W. Kirk). W.B. Saunders, Philadelphia, pp. 553–559.

Kwochka, K.W. (1990) Cell proliferation kinetics in the hair root matrix of dogs with healthy skin and dogs with idiopathic seborrhoea. *American Journal of Veterinary Research* **51**, 1570–1573.

Kwochka, K.W. and Rademakers, A.M. (1989) Cell proliferation of epidermis, hair follicles and sebaceous glands of Cocker Spaniels with idiopathic seborrhoea. *American Journal of Veterinary Research* **50**, 1918–1922.

Lee, E.A. (1987) Neoplastic skin disease. In: *Proceedings of Conference on Small Animal Dermatology*, New Zealand. Post Graduate

Foundation, Palmerston North, New Zealand, pp. 187–228.

Lester, S., Clemett, T. and Burt A. (1996) Vaccine site-associated sarcomas in cats: clinical experience and a laboratory review (1982–1993). *Journal of the American Animal Hospital Association* **32**, 91–95.

Lewis, D.T., Foil, C.S., Hosgood, G. (1991) Epidemiology and clinical features of dermatophytosis in dogs and cats at Louisiana State University: 1981–1990. *Veterinary Dermatology* **2**, 53–58.

Lloyd, D.H. and Garthwaite, G. (1982) Epidermal structure and surface topography of canine skin. *Research in Veterinary Science* **33**, 99–104.

Lloyd, D.H. and Mason, I.S. (1993) Fatty acid supplements and skin diseases (Workshop 14). In: *Advances in Veterinary Dermatology* II (Eds P.J. Ihrke, I.S. Mason and S.D. White). Pergamon Press, Oxford, pp. 455–458.

Malik, R.E., Wigney, D.I., Muir, D.B., Gregory, D.J. and Love, D.N. (1992) Cryptococcosis in cats: clinical and mycological assessment of 29 cases and evaluation of treatment using orally administered fluconazole. *Journal of Medical and Veterinary Mycology* **30**, 133–144.

Malik, R., Hunt, G.B., Goldsmid, S.E., Martin, P., Wigney, D.I., and Love, D.N. (1994) Diagnosis and treatment of pyogranulomatous panniculitis due to *Mycobacterium smegmatis* in cats. *Journal of Small Animal Practice* **35**, 524–530.

Mason, K.V. (1992a) Malassezia dermatitis and otitis. In: *Current Veterinary Therapy* XI (Eds R. Kirk and J. Bonagura). W.B. Saunders, Philadelphia, pp. 544–546.

Mason, K.V. (1992b). *Seborrhoeic dermatitis – the aetiology rediscovered*. Veterinary Dermatology Newsletter, British Veterinary Dermatology Study Group.

Mason, K.V. (1993) Clinical and pathophysiologic aspects of parasitic skin diseases. In: *Advances in Veterinary Dermatology* II (Eds P.J. Ihrke, I.S. Mason and S.D. White). Pergamon Press, Oxford, pp. 177–202.

Mason, K.V. and Evans, A.G. (1991) Mosquito bite-caused eosinophilic dermatitis in cats. *Journal of the American Veterinary Medical Association* **198**, 2086–2088.

Mauldin, G.N. (1992) Radiation therapy for endocrine neoplasia. In: *Current Veterinary Therapy* XI (Eds R.W. Kirk and J.D. Bonagura). W.B. Saunders, Philadelphia, pp. 319–321.

McDougal, B.J. (1986) Allergy testing and hyposensitisation for three common feline dermatoses. *Modern Veterinary Practice* **60**, 629–633.

Medleau, L., Brown, C.A. and Brown, S.A. (1988) Demodicosis in cats. *Journal of the American Animal Hospital Association* **24**, 85–91.

Miller, W.H. (1989a) Non-steroidal anti-inflammatory agents in the management of canine and feline pruritus. In: *Current Veterinary Therapy* X (Ed. R.W. Kirk). W.B. Saunders, Philadelphia, pp. 566–569.

Miller, W.H. (1989b) Sex hormone-related dermatoses in dogs. In: *Current Veterinary Therapy* X (Ed. R.W. Kirk). W.B. Saunders, Philadelphia, pp. 595–601.

Miller, W.H. (1992) Follicular disorders of the Doberman pinscher. In: *Current Veterinary Therapy* XI (Eds R.W. Kirk and J.D. Bonagura). W.B. Saunders, Philadelphia, p. 515.

Miller, W.H. and Scott, D.W. (1990) Efficacy of chlorpheniramine maleate for management of pruritus in cats. *Journal of the American Veterinary Medical Association* **197**, 67–70.

Miller, W.H. and Scott, D.W. (1991) Milbemycin in the treatment of generalised demodicosis in the dog. In: *Proceedings of the Annual Meeting of the American Academy of Veterinary Dermatology and the American College of Veterinary Dermatology*, Scottsdale, Arizona, p. 41.

Miller, W.H., Anderson, W.I. and McCann, J.P. (1991) Necrolytic migratory erythema in a dog with a glucagon-secreting endocrine tumour. *Veterinary Dermatology* **2**, 179–182.

Miller, W.H., Scott, D.W., Cayatte, S.M. and Scarlett, J.M. (1992) The influence of oral corticosteroids or declining allergen exposure on serological allergy test results. *Veterinary Dermatology* **3**, 237–244.

Miller, W.H., Scott, D.W. and Wellington, J.R. (1993) Efficacy of DVM Derm Caps liquid in management of allergic and inflammatory dermatoses of the cat. *Journal of the American Animal Hospital Association* **29**, 37–40.

Moore, F.M., White S.D., Carpenter, J.L. and Torchon, E. (1987) Localisation of immunoglobulin by the peroxidase method in autoimmune and non-autoimmune canine dermatopathies. *Veterinary Immunology and Immunopathology* **14**, 1–9.

Morgan, R.V. (1989) Vogt–Koyanagi–Harada syndrome in humans and dogs. *Compendium on Continuing Education* **11**, 1211–1218.

Moriello, K.A. (1991) Management of dermatophytosis in catteries. In: *Consultations in Feline Internal Medicine* (Ed. J.R. August). W.B. Saunders, Philadelphia, pp. 89–94.

Moriello, K.A. (1992) Treatment of sarcoptes and cheyletiella infestations. In: *Current Veterinary Therapy* XI (Eds R.W. Kirk and J.D. Bonagura). W.B. Saunders, Philadelphia, pp. 558–560.

Moriello, K.A. and DeBoer, D.J. (1995a) Efficacy of griseofulvin and itraconazole in the treatment of experimentally induced dermatophytosis in cats. *Journal of the American Veterinary Medical Association* **207**, 439–444.

Moriello, K.A. and DeBoer, D.J. (1995b) Feline dermatophytosis. *Veterinary Clinics of North America: Small Animal Practice* **25**, 901–921.

Muller, G.H., Kirk, R.W. and Scott, D.W. (1989a) Structure and function of the skin. In: *Small Animal Dermatology*, 4th edn. W.B. Saunders, Philadelphia, p.35.

Muller, G.H., Kirk, R.W. and Scott, D.W. (1989b) Immunologic disease. In: *Small Animal*

Dermatology, 4th edn. W.B. Saunders, Philadelphia, pp. 427–574.

Nachreiner, R.F. and Refsal, K.R. (1992) Radioimmunoassay monitoring of thyroid hormone concentrations in dogs on thyroid replacement therapy. *Journal of the American Veterinary Medical Association* **201**, 623–629.

Nelson, R.W., Feldman, E.C. and Smith, M.C. (1988) Hyperadrenocorticism in cats: seven cases (1978–1987). *Journal of the American Veterinary Medical Association* **193**, 245–250.

Nelson, R.W., Feldman, E.C. and Ford, S.L. (1991) Topics in the diagnosis and treatment of canine hyperadrenocorticism. *Compendium on Continuing Education* **13**, 1797–1805.

Nuttal, T.J. (1996) A retrospective study of hyposensitisation therapy at the Royal (Dick) School of Veterinary Studies. *Proceedings of the Third World Congress of Veterinary Dermatology*, Edinburgh, p. 50.

Ohlen, B. and Scott, D.W. (1986) Zinc-responsive dermatitis in puppies. *Canine Practice* **13**, 5–10.

Olivry, T., Fine, J.D., Dunston, S.L., Tenorio, A.P., Chasse, D., Monteiro-Riviere, N.A., Chen, M. and Woodley, D.T. (1996) Canine epidermolysis bullosa acquisita: circulating autoantibodies target collagen VII epitopes. *Proceedings of the Third World Congress of Veterinary Dermatology*, Edinburgh, p. 64.

Palsson, G. (1991) A treatment programme for ringworm in cats. *Svensk Veterinartidning* **43**, 709–712.

Paradis, M. (1989) Ivermectin in small animal dermatology. In: *Current Veterinary Therapy X* (Ed. R.W. Kirk). W.B. Saunders, Philadelphia, pp. 560–563.

Paradis, M. and Ristic, Z. (1993) Efficacy of daily ivermectin in dogs with generalised demodicosis. In: *Proceedings of the 10th European Society of Veterinary Dermatology Congress*, Aarlborg, Denmark, pp. 59–60.

Peterson, M.E. (1991) The use of endocrine testing in the diagnosis and treatment of endocrine disorders. Parts 1 and 2. In: *Proceedings of the Ninth Annual Veterinary Medical Forum of the American College of Veterinary Internal Medicine*, New Orleans, pp. 109–114.

Plant, J.D., Rosenkrantz, W.S., Griffin, C.E. (1992) Factors associated with a prevalence of high *Malassezia pachydermatis* numbers on dog skin. *Journal of the American Veterinary Medical Association* **201**, 879–885.

Powell, M.B., Weisbroth, S.H., Roth, L. and Wilhelmsen, C. (1980) Reaginic hypersensitivity in *Otodectes cynotis* infestation in cats and mode of mute feeding. *American Journal of Veterinary Research* **41**, 877.

Prost, C. (1993) Hypersensitivity to tobacco in six dogs and two cats. In: *Proceedings of the 10th European Society of Veterinary Dermatology Congress*, Aarlborg, Denmark, pp. 70–71.

Rand, J.S., Levine, J., Best, S.J. and Parker, W. (1993) Spontaneous adult onset hypothyroidism in a cat. *Journal of the American College of Veterinary Internal Medicine* **7**, 272–276.

Reedy, L.M. (1982) Results of allergy testing and hyposensitisation in selected feline skin diseases. *Journal of the American Animal Hospital Association* **18**, 618–623.

Reedy, L.M. (1991) Atopy. In: *Consultations in Feline Internal Medicine* (Ed. J.R. August). W.B. Saunders, Philadelphia, pp. 125–128.

Reedy, L.M. and Garfield, R.A. (1991) Results of a clinical study with an oral antiparasitic agent in generalised demodicosis. In: *Proceedings of the Annual Meeting of the American Academy of Veterinary Dermatology and the American College of Veterinary Dermatology*, Scottsdale, Arizona, p. 43.

Reinke, S.A., Stannard, A.A., Ihrke, P.J. and Reinke, J.D. (1987) Histopathological features of pyotraumatic dermatitis. *Journal of the American Veterinary Medical Association* **190**, 57–60.

Robinson, R. (1977) *Genetics for Cat Breeders*, 2nd edn. Pergamon Press, London, pp. 123–131.

Rosenkrantz, W.S. (1991) Eosinophilic granuloma confusion. In: *Consultations in Feline Internal Medicine* (Ed. J.R. August). W.B. Saunders, Philadelphia, pp. 121–124.

Rosenkrantz, W. (1993) Managment of immune mediated disorders. In: *BSAVA Manual of Small Animal Dermatology* (Eds P.H. Locke, R.G. Harvey and I.S. Mason). British Small Animal Veterinary Association, Cheltenham, pp. 270–275.

Rosser, E.J. (1993a) Food allergy in the dog: a prospective study of 51 dogs. In: *Proceedings American Academy of Veterinary Dermatology and American College of Veterinary Dermatology*, San Diego, p. 39.

Rosser, E.J. (1993b) Food allergy in the cat: a prospective study of 13 cats. In: *Advances in Veterinary Dermatology* II (Eds P.J. Ihrke, I.S. Mason and S.D. White). Pergamon Press, Oxford, pp. 33–39.

Rosser, E.J. (1993c). Diagnosis of food allergy in dogs. *Journal of the American Veterinary Medical Association* **203**, 259–262.

Rothwell, T.L.W., Howlett, C.R. Middleton, D.J., Griffiths, D.A. and Duff, B.C. (1987) Skin neoplasms of dogs in Sydney. *Australian Veterinary Journal* **64**, 161–163.

Scarff, D.H. and Lloyd, D.H. (1992) Placebo controlled cross over study of evening primrose oil in the treatment of canine atopy. *Veterinary Record*, **131**, 97–99.

Schmeitzel, L.P. (1990) Sex hormone related and growth hormone related alopecias. *Veterinary Clinics of North America (Small Animal Practice)* **20**, 1579–1601.

Schmeitzel, L.P. (1992) Canine dermatomyositis. An immune mediated disease with a link to canine lupus erythematosus. *Compendium on Continuing Education* **14**, 866–871.

Schmeitzel, L.P. (1993) Sex hormone related alopecias.

In: *Proceedings of Occasional Seminars in Dermatology*. Royal Veterinary College, North Mymms, UK, pp. 39–52.

Schmeitzel, L.P. and Lothrop, C.D. (1990) Hormonal abnormalities in Pomeranians with normal coat and those Pomeranians with growth responsive dermatosis. *Journal of the American Veterinary Medical Association* **197**, 1333–1341.

Schrader, L.A. and Hurvitz, A.I. (1983) Cold agglutinin disease in a cat. *Journal of the American Veterinary Medical Association* **183**, 121–122.

Scott, D.W. (1987) Feline dermatology 1983–1985. The secret sits. *Journal of the American Animal Hospital Association* **23**, 255–274.

Scott, D.W. (1990) Feline dermatology 1986–1988. Looking to the 1990s through the eyes of many counsellors. *Journal of the American Animal Hospital Association* **26**, 515–537.

Scott, D.W. and Buerger, R.G. (1988) Nonsteroidal anti-inflammatory agents in the management of canine pruritus. *Journal of the American Animal Hospital Association* **24**, 425–427.

Scott, D.W. and Horn, R.T. (1987) Zoonotic dermatoses of dogs and cats. *Veterinary Clinics of North America (Small Animal Practice)* **17**, 117–144.

Scott, D.W. and Miller, W.H. (1990) Nonsteroidal management of canine pruritus: chlorpheniramyne and a fatty acid supplement (DVM, Dermcaps) in combination and a fatty acid supplement at twice the manufacturer's recommended level. *Cornell Veterinarian* **80**, 381–384.

Scott, D.W., Manning, J.O. and Reimers, T.J. (1982) Iatrogenic Cushing's syndrome in the cat. *Feline Practitioner* **12**, 30–36.

Scott, D.W., Walton, D.K., Slater, M.R., Smith, C.A. and Lewis, R.M. (1987a) Immune-mediated dermatoses in domestic animals: ten years after. Part I. *Compendium Continuing Education* **9**, 424–434.

Scott, D.W., Walton, D.K., Slater, M.R., Smith, C.A. and Lewis, R.M. (1987b) Immune-mediated dermatoses in domestic animals: ten years after. Part II. *Compendium Contining Education* **9**, 539–549.

Scott, D.W., Miller, W. and Griffin, C. (1995) Immunologic skin diseases. In: *Small Animal Dermatology* (Eds D.W. Scott, W. Miller and C. Griffin). W.B. Saunders, Philadelphia, pp. 500–504.

Slappendel, R.J. and Greene, C.E. (1990) Leishmaniasis. In: *Infectious Disease of the Dog and Cat* (Ed. C.E. Greene). W.B. Saunders, Philadelphia, pp. 769–777.

Sousa, C.A., Stannard, A.A., Ihrke, P.J., Reinke, S.I. and Schmeitzel, L.P. (1988) Dermatosis associated with feeding generic dog food: 13 cases 1981–1982. *Journal of the American Veterinary Medical Association* **192**, 676–680.

Sparger, E.E. (1991) Feline immunodeficiency virus. In: *Consultations in Feline Internal Medicine* (Ed. J.R. August). W.B. Saunders, Philadelphia, pp. 543–550.

Sparkes, A.H., Gruffydd-Jones, T.J., Shaw, S.E., Wright A.I. and Stokes, C.R. (1993) Epidemiological and diagnostic features of canine and feline dermatophytosis in the United Kingdon from 1956 to 1991. *Veterinary Record* **133**, 57–61.

Stanley, B.J., Read, R.A., Eger, C.E. and Shaw, S.E. (1991) Bilateral rotation flaps for the treatment of chronic nasal dermatitis in four dogs. *Journal of the American Animal Hospital Association* **27**, 295–299.

Thomsett, L.R. (1989) Cowpox in cats. *Journal of Small Animal Practice* **30**, 236–241.

Van den Broek, A.H.M. and Thoday, K.L. (1986) Skin disease in dogs associated with zinc deficiency: a report on 5 cases. *Journal of Small Animal Practice* **27**, 313–323.

White, S.D. (1986) Cutaneous mycobacteriosis. In: *Current Veterinary Therapy* IX (Ed. R.W. Kirk). W.B. Saunders, Philadelphia, pp. 529–531.

White, S.D. (1991) Pyoderma in five cats. *Journal of the American Animal Hospital Association* **27**, 141–143.

White, S.D. (1992) Food hypersensitivity. In: *Current Veterinary Therapy* XI (Eds R.W. Kirk and J.D. Bonagura). W.B. Saunders, Philadelphia, pp. 513–515.

White, S.D. and Sequoia, D. (1989) Food hypersensitivity in cats: 14 cases (1982–1987). *Journal of the American Veterinary Medical Association* **194**, 692–695.

White, S.D., Rosychuk, R.A.W., Reinke, S.I. and Paradis, M. (1992) Use of tetracycline and niacinamide for treatment of autoimmune skin disease in 31 dogs. *Journal of the American Veterinary Medical Association*, **200**, 1497–1499.

Wilcock, B.P., Yager, J.A. and Zink, M.C. (1986) The morphology and behaviour of feline cutaneous mastocytomas. *Veterinary Pathology* **23**, 320–324.

Wilkinson, G.T. and Mason, K.V. (1991) Clinical aspects of mycobacterial infections of the skin. In: *Consultations in Feline Internal Medicine* (Ed. J.R. August). W.B. Saunders, Philadelphia, pp. 129–136.

Wilkinson, G.T., Kelly, W.R. and O'Boyle, D. (1982) Pyogranulomatous panniculitis in cats due to *Mycobacterium smegmatis*. *Australian Veterinary Journal* **58**, 77–78.

Willemse, A. (1993) Anti-obsessive therapy in companion animal dermatology. In: *Proceedings of the 10th European Society of Veterinary Dermatology Congress*, Aarlborg, Denmark, pp. 236–237.

Willemse, A., Van den Brom, W.E. and Rijnberk, A. (1984) Effect of hyposensitisation on atopic dermatitis in dogs. *Journal of the American Veterinary Medical Association*, **184**, 1277–1280.

Wright, A.I. (1989) Ringworm in dogs and cats. *Journal of Small Animal Practice* **30**, 242–249.

Yager, J.A. (1993) The skin as an immune organ. In: *Advances in Veterinary Dermatology* II (Eds P.J. Ihrke, I.S. Mason and S.D. White). Pergamon Press, Oxford, pp. 3–32.

Zulty, J.C. and Kociba, G.J. (1990) Cold agglutinins in cats with haemobartonellosis. *Journal of the American Veterinary Medical Association* **196**, 907–910.

48

Specific Infections of the Dog

I. A. P. McCandlish

The major canine infections	921	Infectious enteritis	939
Canine parvovirus infection	921	Contagious canine respiratory disease	941
Canine distemper	926	Neonatal infections and infectious infertility	944
Infectious canine hepatitis	930	Other viral infections	947
Leptospirosis	932	Other bacterial infections	948
Rabies	935	Protozoal infections	950
Adverse effects of vaccination	936	Rickettsial infections	953
Control of contagious diseases in veterinary premises	938		

Specific infections are still important causes of morbidity and mortality in dogs. This chapter concentrates on those infections which are commonly present in the British Isles or may be encountered in recently imported animals. Rather than being considered on an aetiological basis, the infections are considered according to the types of disease produced: the major, frequently fatal, usually contagious, systemic infections; infectious enteritis; contagious respiratory disease; neonatal infections; and infections due to other viral, bacterial, protozoal and rickettsial agents which present primarily as sporadic infections in individual animals.

THE MAJOR CANINE INFECTIONS

Standard immunization programmes have greatly reduced the prevalence of these diseases but unvaccinated dogs, especially in urban or semi-urban areas, maintain a continuing reservoir of infection. Disease control and elimination in kennels, especially those with a continuous throughput of pups, is often difficult, even with vaccination.

CANINE PARVOVIRUS INFECTION

Aetiology

Canine parvovirus type 2 (CPV-2), universally known simply as CPV, is a small, single-stranded DNA virus related to feline panleucopenia virus (Parrish and Carmichael, 1983) from which it possibly arose by mutation somewhere in the 1970s. The initial antigenic type was largely replaced by a more efficiently replicating type around 1980 and further minor antigenic shifts, as detected by monoclonal antibody panels, have also occurred (Parrish et al., 1985, 1988, 1991). These minor changes have not affected the main neutralizing epitopes so that vaccine efficacy has been unaffected. CPV-2 is unrelated to two other parvoviruses of dogs, the non-pathogenic canine adeno-associated virus, and canine minute virus (CPV-1) of uncertain but apparently limited pathogenicity.

CPV is extremely resistant, able to survive in faeces at room temperature for over a year and on contaminated ground for over 5 months (Gordon and Angrick, 1986). It is unaffected by detergents and most disinfectants.

Epizootiology

CPV is the commonest and most commonly fatal contagious canine disease. Evidence of CPV first appears in a few dog sera in Greece in 1974 (Koptopoulos et al., 1986). Its origin is unknown. Positive sera were recorded in Belgium in 1976 (Schwers et al., 1979) and by 1978, the virus had spread worldwide through a totally susceptible population (Carmichael and Binn, 1981). Initially, infection was commonest in kennels and two forms of disease, myocarditis (Robinson et al., 1979) and enteritis (Appel et al., 1979), were seen. By 1980, panzootics had occurred in most parts of the world and myocarditis, a consequence of neonatal infection, became increasingly rare as breeding bitches developed antibodies, either after natural infection or in response to vaccination. Since 1981, enteritis has been the main form of this now enzootic disease (McCandlish et al., 1981). Infection occurs by ingestion of virus in faeces or faecally contaminated material.

CPV enteritis is commonest in 6–12-week-old pups which have lost their maternally derived antibody (MDA) but have not yet developed active immunity. Although direct transmission does occur, the main source of infection is environmental contamination. Many cases occur in pups which are still in or have been recently purchased from kennels or pet shops. Other pups meet infection when allowed access to other dogs or areas where they have been and most unvaccinated animals have antibody by 6 months of age. Occasional cases occur in isolated adults brought into contaminated environments, e.g. boarding kennels or veterinary surgeries. An apparent seasonal incidence merely reflects seasonal variations in puppy populations.

Myocarditis is very rare, occurring only when pups of non-immune bitches or colostrum-deprived pups of bitches with low antibody titres encounter virus in the first few days of life. The few cases diagnosed at Glasgow University Veterinary School in the last few years have involved nosocomial infections in veterinary premises, e.g. pups of isolated bitches undergoing caesarean section. Such pups, with no maternal antibody, were born into a contaminated environment.

Pathogenesis

CPV pathogenesis is dominated by the small viral genome which limits replication to actively dividing cells (Macartney et al., 1984a,b; Meunier et al., 1985a,b). Oral infection is followed by uptake in the oropharyngeal lymphoid ring and Peyer's patches and initial replication takes place in dividing cells in thymus, spleen and lymph nodes at 1–3 days postinfection (DPI). Lymphocytolysis produces a plasma viraemia (primarily non-cell associated) from 3–4 DPI. Localization to mitotic intestinal crypt epithelium (4–5 DPI) results in cell destruction and shed of up to 10^9 virus particles per gram of faeces (5–6 DPI). As serum antibody titres rise, from 5 DPI, virus is eliminated first from lymphoid and other systemic sites and then from intestine. By the time maximal antibody titres are reached, 10–14 DPI, viral shedding has effectively stopped. Infection of pups with low residual MDA follows the same sequence but the timescale may be extended by up to 5 days (Macartney et al., 1988b).

The above sequence occurs in all infected dogs (Fig. 48.1). Whether enteritis (incubation period 5–10 days, usually up to 7 days) results depends on other factors, most importantly the degree of viraemia at 4 DPI and the intestinal crypt mitotic index at this time. If the index is low and only a few cells are destroyed, asymptomatic viral shed occurs. If the index is high and many cells are lysed, intestinal epithelial production is reduced and diarrhoea develops. At its most severe, there is crypt aplasia with mucosal collapse and denudation, secondary bacterial overgrowth and

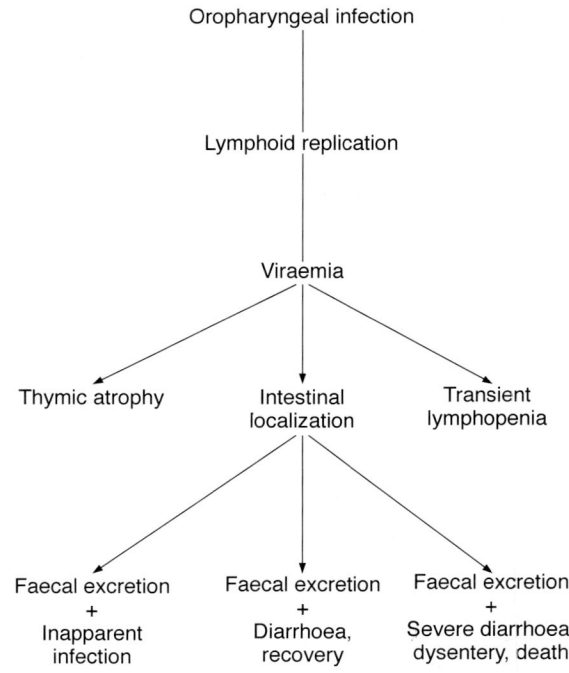

Figure 48.1 Pathogenesis of canine parvovirus enteritis.

invasion, and consequent dysentery, endotoxaemia and septicaemia. Vomiting is due to proximal small intestinal lesions, not gastritis.

Factors affecting viraemia include the weight of challenge and the activity and mass of lymphoid tissue. The large active thymus of pups may predispose to the severe disease seen in young animals. Of the many factors that affect intestinal mitotic rate, age, changes in intestinal flora and dietary regimes, and superficial intestinal infections are probably the most important.

Intestinal mitotic rate is very low in normal sucking pups, increases dramatically with weaning and the acquisition of a mature bowel flora and then settles to a stable, low to moderate rate. This can be increased by alterations in flora, dietary change, starving and refeeding, stress-induced corticosteroid release, and superficial mucosal infections which increase the rate of loss of surface epithelial cells. Severe disease is therefore most likely in recently weaned pups which have changed environments and/or have concomitant viral, bacterial or parasitic infections. Disease is more likely in adult animals if they are undergoing environmental or dietary change or are stressed in some other way, including undergoing surgery. Genetic factors may also contribute: Germanic breeds, especially rottweilers and Dobermanns, are particularly likely to develop severe disease (Glickmann *et al.*, 1985).

Although CPV lyses dividing haemopoietic cells, direct effects on blood parameters are few. Initial lymphocytolysis may cause a relative to absolute lymphopenia but this is usually over by the time intestinal signs are apparent. Marked neutropenia occurs with severe intestinal disease but is due partly to withdrawal of circulating and marrow stores of neutrophils to damaged intestinal mucosa, combined with the effects of secondary septicaemia and endotoxaemia.

Normal sucking pups infected in the first few days of life do not have a high enough crypt mitotic rate for enteritis to occur. However, cardiac myocytes are in their final phase of replication and support viral growth up to about 10 days of age. Although infection occurs early, evidence of myocarditis is seldom apparent before 3 weeks of age (Meunier *et al.*, 1984). The cardiac damage may have an immunological basis; it could represent a response to either persistent viral antigen or myocardial antigens exposed by viral-induced necrosis.

CPV might be expected to affect reproductive performance but no convincing evidence of this has been produced (Meunier *et al.*, 1981) and CPV has not been isolated from abortions or stillbirths. Only non-immune bitches infected during pregnancy would be at risk. Cerebellar hypoplasia is not associated with CPV and this may reflect a different viral trophism from feline parvovirus.

Clinical signs

Enteritis

The typical case of CPV enteritis is: slightly dull on day 1 of illness, anorexic and vomiting on day 2, diarrhoeic and dehydrated on day 3 (Fig. 48.2), and collapsed and dying with dysentery or getting better by day 4, but the severity and duration of disease varies enormously. Many dogs suffer only a few days depression, others do not vomit and many have a mild pasty or fluid diarrhoea with no evidence of blood. Fever is common only in severe cases. Enlarged mesenteric lymph nodes may be mistaken for foreign bodies or intussusceptions, especially in acutely ill vomiting pups which have not yet developed diarrhoea. Dehydration and weight loss can be very rapid. Pups seldom become susceptible before 4 weeks of age and most cases are in animals from 6 weeks to 6 months of age.

The disease course may be compressed especially in young pups (4–8 weeks) which can go from

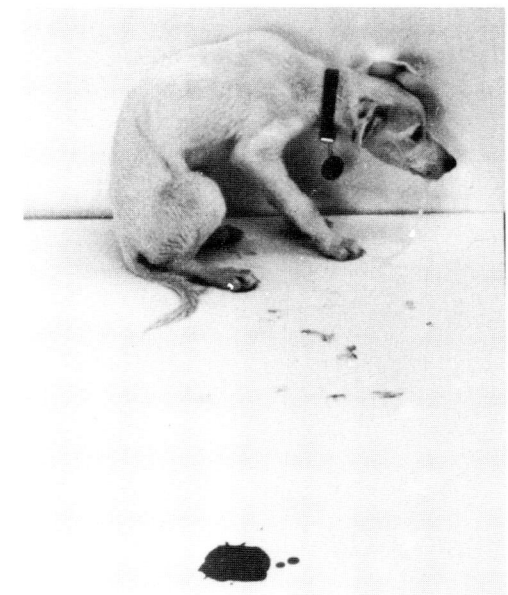

Figure 48.2 A 16-week-old pup with CPV enteritis. The pup is vomiting and has just produced a pool of dysenteric faeces. Reproduced with permission from McCandlish *et al.* (1981).

normality to death within 24 h. Toy breeds may become acutely dehydrated and die with few other clinical signs. Young pups and toy breeds may also become hypoglycaemic with terminal nervous signs. Recovery can be surprisingly rapid but may take 7–10 days or more in severely affected animals which have required intensive fluid therapy.

Most CPV infections are subclinical, even in pups. The average mortality rate in pups less than 12 weeks is about 10% although this can reach 100% in individual or groups of litters with predisposing factors such as build up of infection or concurrent superficial enteric infections. Mortality in adult dogs is less than 1%.

Since most infections in otherwise healthy, well-managed pups are subclinical, CPV can be introduced to a kennel and cycle silently. Disease may surface only if some change occurs, e.g. an undue build up of infection associated with increased puppy numbers or introduction of another minor enteric infection. A common source of contention is the pup which dies of CPV enteritis within 7–10 days of sale whereas pups still at the breeder's kennels remain well. Blood samples from the normal littermates often show high antibody levels indicating they have also been infected. However, they have not been subjected to the stress of sale, with change of environment and diet, and have, therefore, not developed clinical signs of disease. Such immune littermates make excellent replacements for the dead pup.

Myocarditis

The first indication of CPV myocarditis is often sudden death in fit, seemingly healthy pups 3–4 weeks of age. Playing or feeding pups collapse and die within minutes with pale mucosae and cold extremities. Some are found dead. Pups which reach veterinary attention are in acute cardiac failure with weakness, tachycardia, poor pulse, pallor or cyanosis and respiratory distress due to pulmonary oedema. Affected pups which reach 6–8 weeks may be stunted and in congestive cardiac failure with hepatomegaly and ascites (Fig. 48.3).

Some members of affected litters survive and lead apparently normal lives but others succumb to heart failure several months or years later. Unfortunately, it is impossible to predict which are likely to die and none can be sold as normal animals.

Diagnosis

The acute onset of severe diarrhoea or dysentery in dogs less than 1 year, and especially less than 6 months old, is suspicious. Older animals with similar signs are more likely to have canine haemorrhagic gastroenteritis or some other problem. Mild cases are indistinguishable from dietary upset and other infections. Viral identification is required for confirmation.

Reliable solid-phase enzyme-linked immunosorbent assay (ELISA) tests reveal antigen in faeces early in disease, but false negatives due to complexing of virus by antibody are increasingly common as illness progresses. High serum antibody levels are present in such cases and may be confirmatory in unvaccinated dogs or where high IgM levels can be demonstrated. Both faeces and blood samples may therefore be advisable for laboratory confirmation. The very rapid development of high serum titres often makes detection of a classic rising titre impossible. Vaccination can cause difficulties in interpretation of serological results.

Fatal cases are best confirmed by post mortem examination. The carcass is usually dehydrated, the thymus thin and lacy, and the mesenteric nodes swollen and oedematous. The intestines are thickened and inelastic with a granular serosal surface and variable congestion (Fig. 48.4); young pups often have blanched intestinal loops and the Peyer's patches may stand out as dark serosal spots. Histological examination of sections in 10% formalin from various small intestinal sites and lymphoid tissues will reveal diagnostic intestinal crypt (Fig. 48.5) and lymphoid lesions.

CPV myocarditis is suspected on a history of sudden deaths in 3–4-week-old pups. Post mortem at this age may reveal little other than pulmonary oedema but the diagnosis is readily

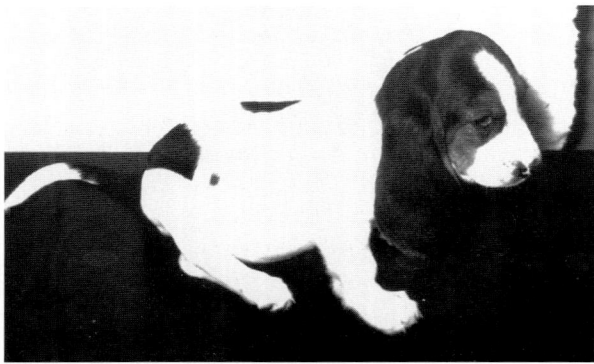

Figure 48.3 Two-month-old basset hound pup with CPV myocarditis. The pup was exercise tolerant. Marked abdominal enlargement due to ascites and hepatomegaly is apparent.

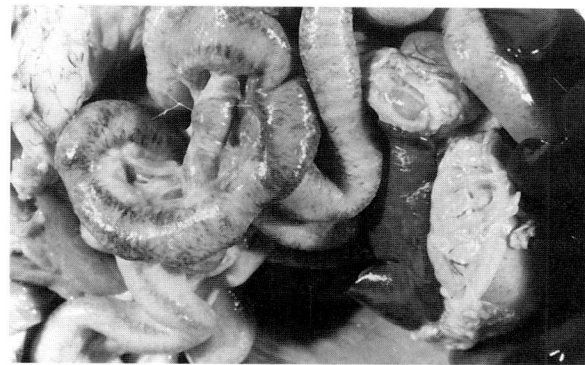

Figure 48.4 Abdominal contents in a fatal case of CPV enteritis. There is variable intestinal congestion, a very granular intestinal serosal surface and a few small fibrin strands extend between intestinal coils.

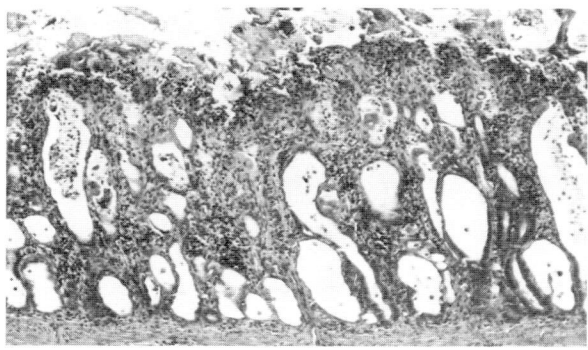

Figure 48.5 Histological appearance of CPV enteritis. The villi have been lost and the mucosal surface is composed of tissue debris and inflammatory cells. The surviving crypts are dilated and lined by flattened epithelial cells. (Haematoxylin and eosin × 100.)

confirmed by histological examination of heart muscle. Older pups may have enlarged hearts with pale foci or streaks in the myocardium; histology will reveal classic viral myocarditis with intranuclear inclusions. Cases in individual older pups with only myocardial scarring are difficult unless the litter history is known. Such pups usually have high serum titres but this is not diagnostic.

Treatment

Treatment of CPV enteritis is as for any gastrointestinal upset. Mild cases respond well to withholding solid food, with access to frequent small amounts of fluid, followed by a bland diet changed gradually to normal. More severe cases may require oral rehydration and antiemetics; antibiotics are not indicated unless there is pyrexia or other evidence of systemic disease. In severely dehydrated or dysenteric dogs, aggressive intensive therapy is required: intravenous fluids to replace both existing and continuing fluid losses; plasma volume expanders, whole blood or fresh frozen plasma, and glucocorticoids to reverse circulatory shock; broad-spectrum antibiotics to counter secondary bacterial invasion or endotoxaemia.

Antiemetics are essential in persistently vomiting dogs to prevent exhaustion as well as to control fluid loss but antidiarrhoeals are probably contraindicated, since slowing the rate of flow through the intestine may increase absorption of the bacterial endotoxins which contribute to clinical signs. CPV hyperimmune serum is not required but serum or plasma may contain anti-endotoxin which can be beneficial in dysenteric cases (Wessels and Gaffin, 1986). The rapid progression of disease in young pups and small breeds should always be considered before opting for out-patient therapy or postponing late night visits. Complete recovery can take up to 2 weeks.

Treatment of CPV myocarditis is non-specific, usually ineffective and not recommended.

Control

Both inactivated and modified live virus (MLV), homologous vaccines are available and effective (Carmichael et al., 1983; Wallace et al., 1985). MLV products based on feline parvovirus have been superseded due to poor performance (Thompson et al., 1988). Vaccination programmes can be started as early as 5–6 weeks of age but interference by MDA is very likely at this age and additional vaccine doses are required to ensure response (Pollock and Carmichael, 1982). Many breeding bitches have high antibody titres and low levels of MDA can be detected in up to 10–20% of 12-week-old pups (unpublished observations). Inactivated CPV vaccines and highly attenuated MLV products are readily blocked by even very low levels of MDA and repeated inoculation of these products at 2–3 week intervals up to 18 weeks of age may be necessary to ensure a protective response (Pollock and Coyne, 1993). More modern, less attenuated MLV vaccines (Churchill, 1988) may be better able to induce immunity in the face of low MDA, and, based on results obtained at Glasgow Veterinary School, administration of these products at 12 weeks of age gives adequate responses in 90–95% of pups.

Where the risk of infection is low, vaccination with a less attenuated vaccine strain at 8 weeks (or when first presented to a veterinarian), and again at 12 weeks will protect the majority of pups. Where 100% protection is regarded as essential, an additional vaccine at 16 weeks will induce immunity in the small proportion not responding at 12 weeks. Where there is a high risk of infection more frequent vaccine doses, e.g. 6, 9 and 12 weeks may be appropriate. Annual boosters are recommended but may not be necessary with modern products. MLV products should not be used in pregnant bitches.

In heavily contaminated kennels, high challenge by virulent virus will overcome MDA and induce disease several weeks before inactivated or highly attenuated MLV vaccines can induce immunity. Less attenuated vaccines are the products of choice in such kennels but, even with these products, their use must be combined with reduction of the burden of challenge to a point where vaccination has a reasonable hope of success. Thorough cleaning and disinfection are obvious measures although only formalin, bleach and glutaraldehyde-based products are likely to be effective. In Britain, several commercial preparations have been tested by the Ministry of Agriculture against CPV and these products carry specific recommendations for use. Breaking the infection cycle whereby each generation of pups picks up a little virus and passes out vast amounts in faeces is equally important. This can be achieved by a temporary break in breeding or by removing pups from the kennel at an early age before they become susceptible. Having a period when no susceptible pups are present also gives an opportunity for thorough cleaning of the puppy accommodation. If complete depopulation of puppy accommodation is impossible, then strict batching of litters with cleaning and disinfection of accommodation between batches will help reduce virus build-up. Care should be taken to prevent cross-infection between batches by human, animal or inanimate carriers.

Owners who have lost a pup with CPV and wish to replace it are better advised to buy an immune dog than to try to eliminate infection from their house and grounds. This can be achieved either by replacing the pup with a recovered/asymptomatic littermate, by buying an older fully vaccinated dog, or by finding a cooperative breeder who will hold a pup until a postvaccinal serological test shows protective levels of antibody (these vary depending on the test used and the laboratory should be asked for advice).

CPV myocarditis does not occur in the pups of bitches with high circulating antibody titres. Colostrum-deprived pups may be given hyperimmune sera, as may the neonate pups of bitches of uncertain antibody status which are likely to be exposed to infection, e.g. following caesarean.

CANINE DISTEMPER

Aetiology

Canine distemper virus (CDV) is a morbillivirus (family Paramyxoviridae) closely related to human measles, cattle rinderpest and the phocine (seal) distemper virus (Osterhaus and Vedder, 1988). CDV is a large enveloped single-stranded RNA virus. It is very susceptible to heat, light, detergents, acid (pH <4.4), and virtually any disinfectant. It does not persist for long outside infected dogs (Appel and Gillespie, 1972). The virus survives best at low temperatures with low humidity and is well preserved by freeze drying.

Epizootiology

Infection results mainly from inhalation of respiratory tract secretions either during dog-to-dog contact or by aerosol spread over a short distance (Krakowka et al., 1985). Ingested virus is also taken up by oropharyngeal macrophages but does not survive gastric acid. All infected dogs shed virus in all body secretions but excretion is short-lived in subclinical infections and even clinically affected dogs do not shed virus after recovery. Virus can persist for years in the nervous system but does not appear to be transmissible. Different laboratory strains vary in virulence but there is little work on varying pathogenicity of field strains.

Distemper is commonest in unvaccinated dogs in poorer urban areas. Most cases occur between 3 and 6 months of age as pups that have lost MDA start to be allowed out and encounter infection. The majority of 2-year-old unvaccinated urban dogs have antibody although few have ever shown signs of disease. Cases, at least in Glasgow, are more frequent in late winter and early spring.

Persistence of infection depends on the succession of susceptible pups that is readily available in poorer urban areas. In more affluent and less densely populated areas, distemper can disappear but, if vaccination programmes lapse, a large susceptible population may develop. Introduction of infection then results in local epizootics. Individual unvaccinated adults exposed to infection, e.g. in kennels, are clearly susceptible.

Disease also occurs in younger pups that have lost MDA and are exposed to virus. This is more likely in puppy farms or rescue kennels, which take in pups from a variety of sources, than in small or closed kennels. Transplacental and neonatal infections have been recorded (Krakowka et al., 1977) but are very uncommon as most breeding bitches have antibody either from vaccination or natural infection.

Pathogenesis

Inhaled virus is taken up by respiratory and oropharyngeal macrophages and has spread to tonsils, cervical and bronchial lymph nodes by 2 DPI (Appel, 1969). Further dissemination via mononuclear cells produces viral replication in spleen, thymus, and lymphoid tissue throughout the body by 4–7 DPI with an associated early pyrexia and absolute lymphopenia (Krawkowa et al., 1980).

Release of cell-associated and free virus from the lymphoid system allows spread of CDV to epithelial and nervous tissues at 8–10 DPI. The extent of spread and damage to these sites, and the ultimate outcome for the dog, depends on the interactions between the virus and the animal's immune system during the first week of infection (Fig. 48.6).

Extensive lymphocytolysis results in immunosuppression, poor cell-mediated immunity, and scant neutralizing antibody formation. Viral spread and multiplication is unchecked and extensive growth in epithelia results in classical 'catarrhal' distemper with respiratory, alimentary and oculonasal signs from 2 weeks postinfection (PI) onwards. Hyperkeratosis, although initiated at this stage, does not become obvious until at least 3 weeks PI. Dogs with severe catarrhal distemper are also likely to develop neurological disease from 4 weeks PI onwards. Immunosuppression also predisposes to secondary or concurrent infections which exacerbate or modify clinical signs, especially those involving the respiratory and alimentary tracts.

In contrast, dogs with minimal lymphoid lesions develop good cytotoxic cell-mediated responses and good neutralizing antibody (Appel et al., 1982). There is little spread to other sites, virus is rapidly eliminated from most tissues, and there are few or no clinical signs. A few of these dogs develop nervous disease months or even years later as a result of viral persistence in

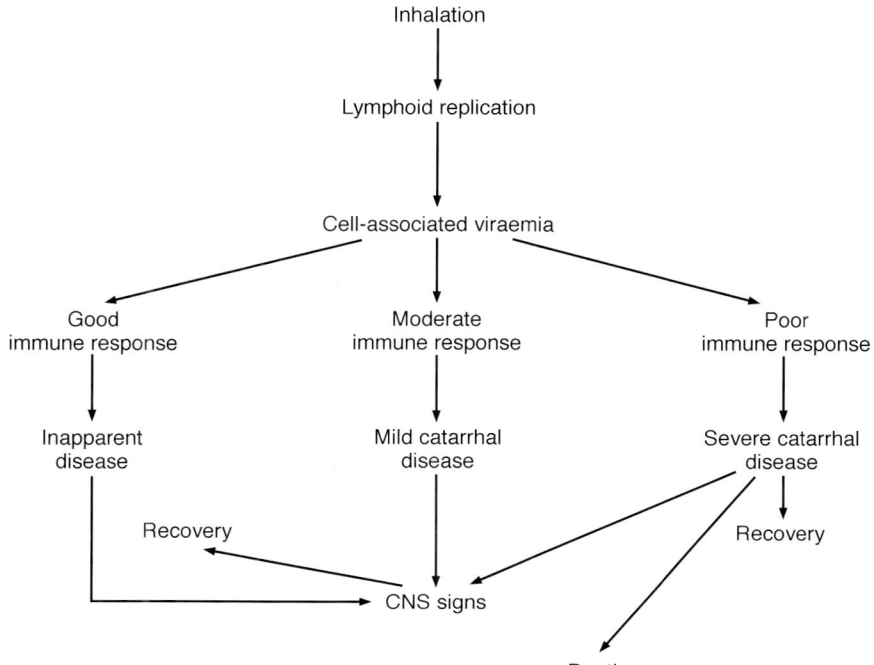

Figure 48.6 Pathogenesis of canine distemper.

the CNS and/or the development of immune responses to it (Vandevelde et al., 1986).

Clearly, many cases lie between these extremes. Such dogs may recover from catarrhal disease quite well, possibly as immunity develops more gradually and virus is eliminated. They may, nonetheless, develop hyperkeratosis or nervous signs.

In theory, since both CDV and CPV are lymphocytolytic and at least transiently immunosuppressive, exposure to either should predispose to severe disease if infected with the other. In practice, dual infections appear uncommon, possibly due to the different routes of infection.

Clinical signs

These are very variable, and may be influenced by factors such as age, condition, immune status and, possibly, viral strain. Probably 50–70% of infections are inapparent. Many others show only short-lived inappetance, fever, lymphadenopathy, and oculonasal discharge. A light cough, occasional vomiting or mild diarrhoea may occur. A definite clinical diagnosis is often impossible.

More severe cases start like the mild ones but signs persist and worsen. The oculonasal discharge becomes thick, mucoid or purulent with intensely congested conjunctivae and sclerae. The cough becomes harsh, moist and productive, and pneumonia with tachypnoea and harsh respiratory sounds develops. The tonsils and cervical nodes are usually enlarged and there is fluctuating fever. Persistent, pasty to slimy diarrhoea, sometimes containing flecks of blood, is very common and there is intermittent vomiting. A few cases become dehydrated or develop intussusceptions. These signs may come and go for several weeks. Hyperkeratosis and nervous signs appear from about 3 weeks after the onset of illness.

Definite hyperkeratosis (Fig. 48.7) occurs in up to 30% of severe cases. Initial mild thickening of the footpads, palpable as an 'edge' on dry pads, progresses to a thick 'wooden' layer which can be deeply fissured and painful. Similar changes occur on the rhinarium. The skin is often generally scurfy or flaky. Flat, circular pustules on glabrous abdominal skin are recorded, usually in younger pups, but these also occur independently of CDV. Dogs infected during development of their permanent dentition may show enamel hypoplasia (Fig. 48.8).

It is not possible to predict which dogs will develop neurological complications. Severely affected animals are more at risk but nervous signs do occur in otherwise asymptomatic cases. In a few dogs, nervous signs do not develop for months or even years after primary infection. Fits (seizures), chorea (myoclonus) and spinal cord deficits occur independently or in combination and severely affected dogs are often restless or distressed.

Seizures vary from short 'time-outs' or episodes of jaw-champing with excess frothy saliva to full-blown epileptiform convulsions with involuntary defecation and urination. Severely affected animals may develop general stupor or status epilepticus. Unilateral to symmetrical spinal cord deficits range from mild ataxia,

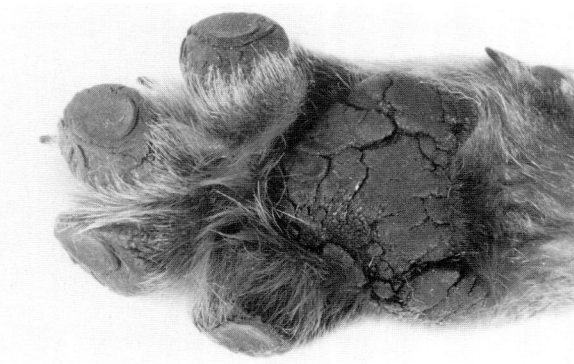

Figure 48.7 Hyperkeratosis of footpads in canine distemper. There are large distinct 'corns' on the digital pads and deep fissuring of the metacarpal pad. Reprinted with permission from Veterinary Notes for Dog Owners (Ed. T. Turner) (1990). Popular Dogs Publishing Co. Chapter 22 Viral and Bacterial Diseases, I.A.P. McCandlish.

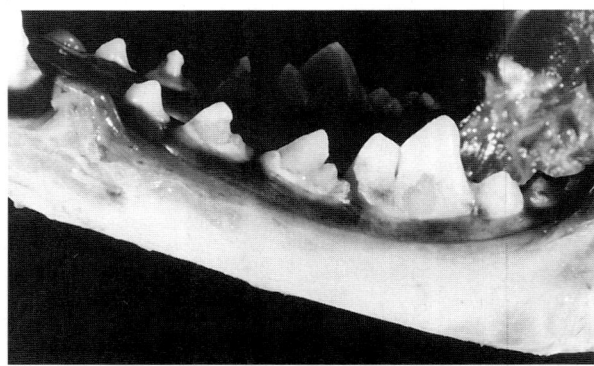

Figure 48.8 Enamel hypoplasia in canine distemper. There are well-defined defects in the enamel layer of premolars 2–4.

through hind limb paralysis with urinary and faecal incontinence to quadriplegia. Some spinal deficits improve with time. Chorea often affects a localized head or limb muscle group but may be more generalized. Chorea is usually, but not invariably, permanent and may be the only nervous sign to develop. CDV may also cause mild anterior uveitis, optic neuritis and focal retinal degeneration.

Neonatal infections cause acute fulminant encephalitis (Krakowka et al., 1985) and focal cardiomyopathy (Higgins et al., 1981) experimentally but are unusual in practice.

Diagnosis

Diagnosis on clinical grounds may be impossible in mild cases. In more severe cases, the combination of any four of the following should give rise to a presumptive diagnosis of CDV: conjunctival inflammation; respiratory signs; diarrhoea; illness of 3 weeks or longer; nervous signs. Hyperkeratosis with any two other features is also indicative of CDV (Lauder et al., 1954a).

Routine laboratory tests are unrewarding. Initial lymphopenia seldom persists and although viral inclusions can occur in both red and white blood cells their detection is exceptional. Neutrophilia may dominate in animals with secondary infections. Biochemical findings are non-specific.

Immunocytochemical detection of viral antigen in air-dried, acetone-fixed smears of conjunctival or tonsillar epithelium or urinary sediment is frequently advocated for diagnosis of acute cases but depends on access to a laboratory with appropriate antisera. Staining of similar smears using Giemsa type stains will sometimes reveal intracytoplasmic viral inclusion bodies but detection requires an experienced eye. False negatives are common with both techniques. Viral isolation is difficult and usually impractical: culture of nasal or oropharyngeal swabs, even in known cases, is almost always negative and the most reliable isolation method, direct culture of alveolar lavage fluid, is possible only if one has immediate laboratory access.

Unfortunately, serological tests, whether based on neutralization or ELISA assays, are also often difficult to interpret. Antibody titres in unvaccinated animals merely indicate exposure to the virus unless a fourfold rise in titre in paired samples or a predominantly IgM response can be demonstrated. Moreover, many clinical cases are immunosuppressed and have persistently low rather than the expected rising titres. Interpretation of results in vaccinated animals can be impossible. Detection of antibody (IgG) against CDV in cerebrospinal fluid (CSF) is virtually diagnostic in the absence of vascular damage or blood contamination, since it is produced locally and indicates viral replication within the brain (Johnson et al., 1988). Unfortunately, not all acutely infected animals develop brain lesions and CSF antibody. CSF samples should be submitted in plain tubes.

Thymic atrophy is the only consistent post mortem finding. Pneumonia, catarrhal enteritis and hyperkeratosis may be present but there are no gross nervous lesions (Lauder et al., 1954b). Tissues for histological confirmation (in 10% formalin) should include tonsil, lymph node, thymus or spleen, lung including a major bronchus, stomach, ileum, urinary bladder and brain, including the hind brain. Lesions are not always present in all tissues and inclusions may be hard to find. Snap-frozen fresh tissues for immunocytochemical detection of viral antigen are relevant only when a suitably equipped laboratory is available.

Treatment

Treatment is supportive and good nursing is essential. Dogs must be kept warm, dry, comfortable and clean; many prefer dim lighting. Broad spectrum antibiotics are indicated for dogs with severe upper respiratory signs or pneumonia. Hydration must be maintained, orally or systemically as appropriate, and antiemetics and antidiarrhoeals may be required. A light, high quality diet is indicated. Treatment of nervous signs should be directed at controlling convulsions if they develop; phenobarbitone is probably the drug of choice. There appears to be no advantage in using anticonvulsants prophylactically.

Up to half the cases with a definite clinical diagnosis die or are destroyed, usually because of uncontrolled seizures or paralysis. Chorea and occasional seizures are often well tolerated by both owners and dogs. The owners of dogs recovering from catarrhal disease should be warned of late onset nervous complications. Recovery may take two months or more.

Control

MLV vaccines are very effective in controlling CDV. Studies at Glasgow Veterinary School on

MDA in British pups have shown that 68% have lost MDA to distemper by 8 weeks, 86% by 9 weeks, 92% by 10 weeks, and virtually 100% by 12 weeks. Vaccination at 8 weeks of age or first presentation, and again at 12 weeks will, therefore, effectively protect the majority of pups when risk of infection is low. Where a higher risk exists, earlier and more frequent vaccination may be appropriate, e.g. 6, 9 and 12 weeks. Pups should be kept away from potential sources of infection for a week after their 12 week inoculation. A single inoculation should be effective over 12 weeks. Susceptible dogs known to have been exposed to CDV can be given rapid protection by intravenous administration of MLV vaccines within 3 days of exposure.

The scientific necessity for repeated annual booster vaccination is dubious. Certainly, the first booster vaccination should ensure protection for those dogs which may not have responded initially but there is evidence that immunity after such a booster can last at least 7 years (Appel and Gillespie, 1972). Revaccination may, however, be required to ensure acceptance by reputable boarding kennels.

Postvaccinal complications are rare. Encephalitis is the most serious and is associated with non-Ondestepoort vaccinal strains (Cornwell et al., 1988). MLV products should not be used in pregnant bitches and vaccination of bitches nursing neonate pups is probably best avoided (McCandlish et al., 1992). Failure of response is not as uncommon as was once believed and may be related to vaccine as well as to host factors.

Where distemper occurs in a kennel, the most important means of control is to stop the introduction of new susceptible dogs and subclinical cycling of infection. Ideally, the kennel should be depopulated, thoroughly cleaned and disinfected (quaternary ammonium compounds are effective) and left empty for 1 week. If dogs must be retained, all stock should be vaccinated, sick animals segregated, and no new dogs admitted until 1 month after the recovery of the last case; kennels should be cleaned and disinfected regularly. Owners who have lost a dog with CDV may acquire a new animal after 1–2 weeks provided their house is well cleaned and heated.

INFECTIOUS CANINE HEPATITIS

Aetiology

Infectious canine hepatitis (ICH) is caused by canine adenovirus type 1 (CAV-1), a medium-sized DNA virus resistant to solvents, detergents and quaternary ammonium compounds but inactivated by heat, phenols and ultraviolet light, i.e. more resistant than CDV but less than CPV (Appel, 1987). CAV-1 (Wright et al., 1971), and the closely related but serologically distinct CAV-2 (Swango et al., 1970), can also cause contagious canine respiratory disease. CAV-2 does not cause hepatitis (Swango et al., 1970).

Epizootiology

Clinical ICH is far rarer than either CPV enteritis or distemper, though serological evidence of infection in unvaccinated dogs is widespread. Most cases occur in individual dogs less than 6 months old. Some large kennels suffer regular losses from ICH in 6–12-week-old pups although usually only one or two pups in a litter become ill.

Infection spreads by direct or indirect contact with virus in urine, faeces or saliva. Faecal and salivary excretion is shortlived but urinary shedding lasts for up to 9 months. Inhalation of virus is also possible in cases with respiratory disease.

Pathogenesis

Most infections start with ingestion of virus and uptake in tonsils and Peyers patches (1 DPI). Spread to other lymphoid tissues, especially cervical and mesenteric nodes (3 DPI) results in early lymphadenitis, viraemia (3 DPI) and viral dissemination to endothelial cells and hepatocytes (Fig. 48.9), the major target sites (Appel, 1987).

Replication in endothelial cells gives a viraemic peak at 5–7 DPI. Virus also grows in reticulo-endothelial and mesothelial cells throughout the body. During this acute phase, ICH is characterized by fever and leucopenia. Widespread haemorrhages (Fig. 48.10) are also common and are due primarily to endothelial damage with a superimposed consumptive coagulopathy (disseminated intravascular coagulation, DIC). This bleeding tendency is exacerbated by failing liver function resulting in decreased production of clotting factors and accumulation of anticoagulant fibrin degradation products (Wigton et al., 1976).

Virus is present in hepatocytes (Fig. 48.11) from 5 DPI (Hamilton et al., 1966). Initial centrilobular necrosis becomes widespread causing acute hepatic failure and jaundice unless viral replication is limited by developing antibody. Virus also reaches other sites such as intestinal

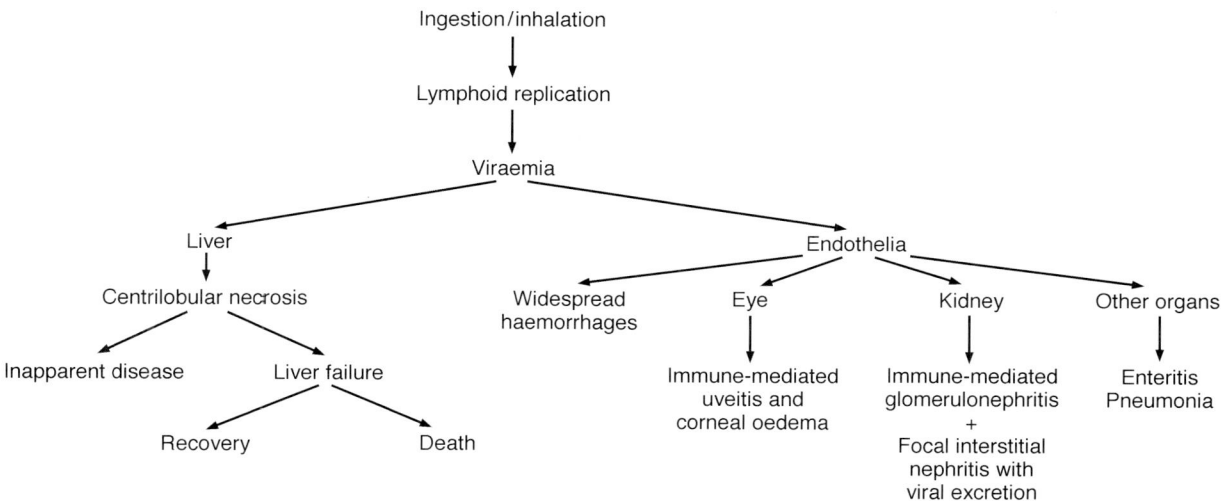

Figure 48.9 Pathogenesis of infectious canine hepatitis.

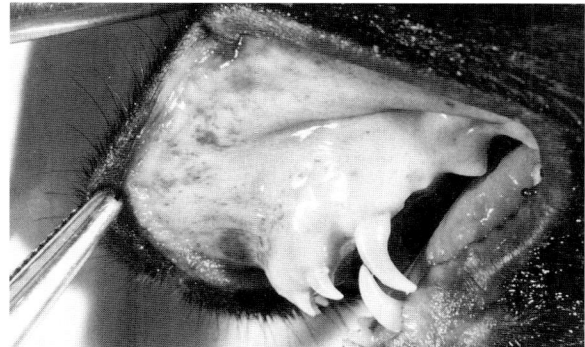

Figure 48.10 Many small punctate haemorrhages are present on the oral mucosa in this fatal case of ICH.

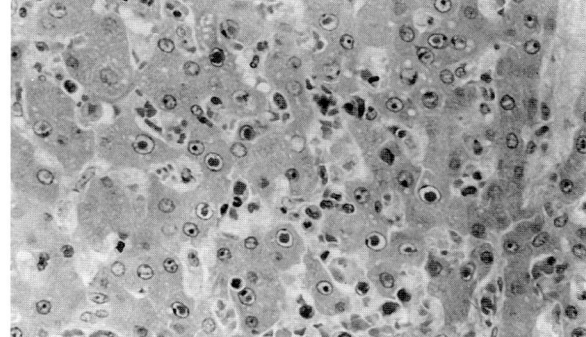

Figure 48.11 Liver in fatal ICH. Numerous large intranuclear inclusion bodies are present in hepatocytes. The nuclear membrane of affected nuclei is prominent. (Haematoxylin and eosin × 400.)

crypts, lung, salivary gland, eye and kidney from 5 DPI. Focal enteritis, bronchiolitis and pneumonia are common. Circulating antibody, detectable as early as 5 DPI, clears virus from vessels and most tissues by 10 DPI.

Up to 20% of cases develop corneal oedema (Fig. 48.12) 7–15 DPI. Early viral-induced lysis of uveal and corneal endothelial cells is followed by deposition of immune complexes and complement fixation (a type III hypersensitivity response) with exudation of fluid and inflammatory cells into the anterior chamber, damage to corneal endothelium and corneal oedema (Curtis and Barnett, 1983). One or both eyes may be affected. Most cases resolve within 2 weeks but a few dogs may have permanant corneal opacity.

In the kidney, immune complex deposition causes a transient glomerulonephritis at 7–15 DPI. More importantly, virus persists in renal tubular

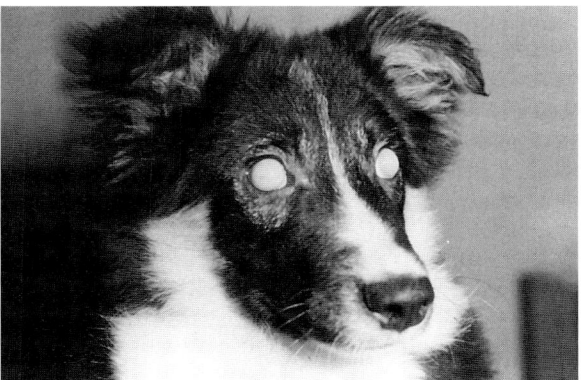

Figure 48.12 'Blue eye' – corneal opacity due to oedema in a 3-month-old Collie pup.

epithelium where it may induce focal interstitial nephritis (Wright, 1976) and be excreted for up to 6–9 months. It has been suggested that some cases of ICH progress to cirrhosis (Gocke *et al.*, 1970) but no convincing evidence has been produced.

Clinical signs

Dogs with ICH are dull, inappetant and acutely pyrexic (up to 41°C, 106°F) with lymphadenopathy and marked tonsillitis. Anterior abdominal pain and hepatomegaly are often accompanied by vomiting, a scanty, blood-tinged diarrhoea and tachypnoea. Severely affected dogs are collapsed, tachycardic and have pale mucous membranes; widespread petechiation or a more generalized haemorrhagic diathesis with epistaxis or haematuria may be evident. Terminal seizures or coma result from CNS haemorrhages and hepatic encephalopathy. Many acute cases die before showing evidence of jaundice but this can be intense in recovering dogs. Corneal oedema or 'blue-eye' can be regarded as a favourable prognostic sign since it indicates the development of a successful immune response.

The incubation period is about 4–6 days and dogs may be ill for a week or more. Peracute cases collapse and die so quickly that poisoning is often suspected. In contrast, a sudden 'blue-eye' may be the only indication of infection in some dogs. Most infections are inapparent.

Diagnosis

Laboratory tests may support a suspicion of ICH. Early leucopenia is followed by a reactive neutrophilia and lymphocytosis. Severe cases are often thrombocytopenic with prolonged clotting times. Indicators of hepatocellular damage, such as alanine and aspartate aminotransferase, and of cholestasis, such as alkaline phosphatase, increase dramatically in plasma with failing liver function and may remain elevated for 2–3 weeks after recovery. Moderate increases in bilirubin, bile acids or bromsulphthalein (BSP) retention may be noted even in non-jaundiced dogs. There is often mild proteinuria, bilirubinuria and/or haematuria.

Virus can be isolated from tonsillar swabs or clotted blood samples and paired serum samples will demonstrate a rising antibody titre. Infection with virulent virus induces higher antibody titres than does the homologous MLV vaccine.

Fatal cases are usually in good condition with moderately enlarged, intensely haemorrhagic lymph nodes, and a variably swollen, brightly congested or mottled liver with fibrin strands between the lobes. The gall bladder is often oedematous. There is usually fibrin rich or blood-stained fluid in serosal cavities and small haemorrhages are common on serosal and mucosal surfaces. Pneumonia is common in young pups. Histological examination of the liver and lymph nodes for viral inclusions is the easiest means of confirmation. Inclusions can also be found in Giemsa-stained impression smears of liver. Virus can readily be isolated from liver.

Treatment

Severe cases with compromised liver function and cardiovascular collapse require intravenous fluid replacement to replace fluid losses and for subsequent maintenance as well as correction of specific abnormalities such as hypoglycaemia or a high blood ammonia concentration. Dogs with coagulopathy may benefit from whole blood transfusions but anticoagulants may also be needed if there is evidence of disseminated intravascular coagulation. The prognosis in such cases is poor. Mild cases respond well to good supportive care over 7–10 days.

Control

MLV vaccines of both types CAV-1 and CAV-2 provide good protection against ICH and are normally given as combined products with CDV/CPV vaccines. As usual, regular boosters are recommended but may not be required. Some CAV-1 vaccine strains are shed in urine and cause occasional postvaccinal 'blue-eye'; neither problem occurs with CAV-2 strains. Inactivated CAV-1 vaccines are available but require two doses after 12 weeks of age and regular boosters to maintain immunity.

Infected kennels should be cleaned and disinfected. Known cases should be kept from contact with young pups until 1–2 weeks after the pups complete their vaccination course.

LEPTOSPIROSIS

Aetiology

Several serovars of *Leptospira interrogans* infect dogs (Van den Broek *et al.*, 1991) but the two most commonly associated with disease are *L. icterohaemorrhagiae* and *L. canicola*. These slender spiral bacteria are sensitive to light, drying and most disinfectants and survive best in moist conditions.

Epizootiology

Leptospirosis is now rare in developed temperate areas but is more common in semitropical regions. *L. icterohaemorrhagiae*, a rat pathogen, infects dogs by contamination of food or water with rat urine or by bites. *L. canicola*, a primary canine pathogen, spreads via infected dog urine; it appears to be more common in urban than rural areas and has a slight preponderance in males which are more likely to lick, than simply to sniff, urine. Both infections are zoonotic and cause serious human disease.

Pathogenesis

Infection is by ingestion of urine or urine-contaminated material with leptospiral penetration of intact mucosae or by invasion through cuts and abrasions, especially on the feet. Once in the blood, the bacteria multiply rapidly.

Multiplying *L. icterohaemorrhagiae* induce pyrexia, dullness, and degeneration of hepatocytes and endothelial cells. Hepatocellular damage and intrahepatic obstruction cause liver failure and jaundice whereas endothelial damage induces collapse, DIC and haemorrhage. The most severe cases die before jaundice and widespread haemorrhages become obvious at 6–8 DPI. Moderate nephritis and variable myositis, uveitis and meningitis are common. Antibody is detectable from about 7 DPI and eliminates infection from most sites by 10–12 DPI. Residual foci in renal tubules cause urine shedding for several months or longer.

With *L. canicola* infections, leptospiraemia induces pyrexia and dullness but damage to liver and endothelia is less marked. Antibody again eliminates the organisms from most sites by 10–12 DPI but many remain in renal tubules. Further bacterial damage to tubular epithelium in dogs with developing immunity induces infiltration of lymphocytes, macrophages and plasma cells around infected tubules (Morrison and Wright, 1976) and this infiltrate may be so massive as to induce acute renal failure (10–14 DPI). Less severe impairment of renal function is more common and most cases are asymptomatic. Leptospirae can be excreted for many months in untreated animals.

Some cross-over of clinical signs does occur, i.e. nephritis with *L. icterohaemorrhagiae* and hepatic dysfunction with *L. canicola*. *L. grippotyphosa* has been associated with chronic active hepatitis in one group of dogs (Bishop *et al.*, 1979). Infection of pregnant bitches with these or other serovars may result in infertility, abortions, stillbirths or weak pups (Ellis 1986).

Clinical signs

During early leptospiraemia, dullness, anorexia and pyrexia (up to 40°C, 104°F) may be accompanied by ill-defined muscle pain and weakness.

Dogs with peracute *L. icterohaemorrhagiae* infection may die from circulatory collapse with few specific signs. In slightly less severe cases, there is vomiting, which is often blood stained, scanty diarrhoea, which may be either blood stained or pale coloured, and widespread, mucosal and subcutaneous, petechial or ecchymotic haemorrhages. Swelling of the liver and possibly the kidneys causes severe abdominal pain and a few cases develop intussusceptions. Weight loss and dehydration can be marked. Initial pallor is replaced by increasingly severe jaundice. There may be terminal nervous signs due to hepatic encephalopathy. Mild cases show less severe evidence of liver and renal damage.

With *L. canicola* infections, the initial leptospiraemic phase is often mild but dogs may relapse or present with renal failure 7–10 days later. Dullness, anorexia, renal pain, thirst and vomiting are accompanied by oliguria or anuria in severe cases. Milder cases may be polyuric. As renal failure and the accompanying uraemia develop, vomiting becomes more marked, oral ulceration and an ammoniacal breath become apparent, and a scanty haemorrhagic diarrhoea develops. Terminally, there is severe dehydration, acidosis and collapse. Less severely affected animals may survive for some weeks before succumbing to terminal renal failure. Some dogs make an apparent full recovery only to present in chronic renal failure several months later.

Diagnosis

Routine biochemistry will confirm hepatic and/or renal failure. Haematology reveals an initial leucopenia progressing to reactive leucocytosis.

Severe *L. icterohaemorrhagiae* cases are thrombocytopenic and have variably increased clotting times (Navarro and Kociba, 1982). Confirmation of diagnosis requires detection of Leptospirae in blood or urine or demonstration of rising antibody titres in paired blood samples. Antibody levels following significant active infection are much higher than those achieved by vaccination so that single serum samples may be sufficient. Leptospiral culture is difficult and visualization of typical spiral organisms in fresh urine of untreated cases by dark ground or phase contrast microscopy is easier.

Post-mortem examination of fatal cases of *L. icterohaemorrhagiae* infection typically reveals a jaundiced carcass, widespread serosal and mucosal haemorrhages and a swollen bright bronze liver. Peracute cases are merely congested. Microscopy reveals diagnostic dissociation of hepatocytes (Fig. 48.13); focal nephritis and myositis, affecting both skeletal and cardiac muscle, are common. Dogs with acute nephritis due to *L. canicola* have swollen kidneys with white nodular interstital infiltrates, especially at the corticomedullary junction (Fig. 48.14), as well as changes due to uraemia such as erosive gastritis or intercostal pleuritis. Leptospirae can be demonstrated in tissues by special silver stains or immunocytochemical techniques as well as by culture.

■ Treatment

Cases with impaired hepatic and/or renal function need intensive supportive therapy with intravenous fluids. Whole blood and low-dose heparin may be needed in *L. icterohaemorrhagiae* cases with associated DIC. Penicillin rapidly abolishes leptospiraemia and aborts many infections before liver or renal damage becomes severe. Streptomycin and tetracycline are more effective in eliminating infection from renal tubules; they should be given for 10–14 days but must be used with caution in animals in renal failure.

■ Control

The use of inactivated vaccines in the standard vaccination programme appear effective in controlling leptospirosis although only low levels of antibody are produced and even these can be detected for comparatively short periods of time. At least two doses are needed but, since there is little risk of interference by MDA, inoculation at 8–9 weeks and again at 12 weeks is sufficient in low-risk areas. Annual revaccination is recommended. In semitropical areas with a high prevalence of disease, at least three initial doses are advised. Vaccination does not prevent asymptomatic shedding. Some countries, e.g. Australia and Sweden, require negative leptospiral titres before permitting import of dogs and such animals should not be vaccinated before testing.

Leptospiral vaccines are the most common cause of post-vaccinal anaphylaxis but this is usually induced by components of the culture media rather than the leptospirae. Experimental vaccines bases on purified outer envelope components have been produced (Bey and Johnson, 1982) and would be less likely to induce allergic reactions than conventional products.

All suspected cases of leptospirosis should be treated with great care to avoid human infection. Urine and blood from untreated cases are the

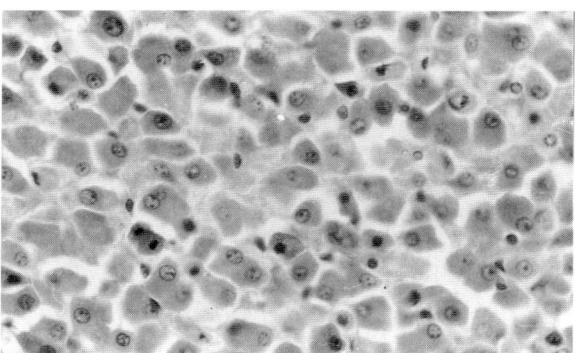

Figure 48.13 Liver in fatal *L. icterohaemorrhagiae* infection. There is widespread hepatocellular degeneration with dissociation or separation of hepatocytes from each other. (Haematoxylin and eosin × 450.)

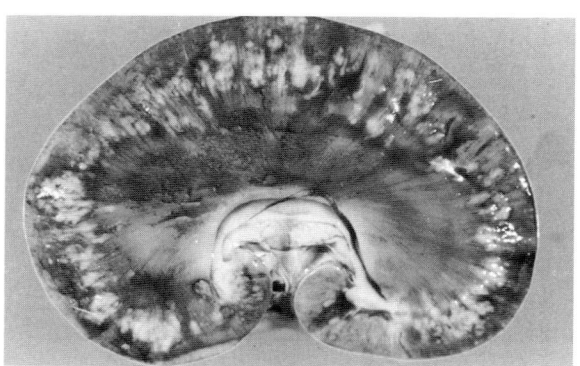

Figure 48.14 Kidney in fatal acute *L. canicola* infection. There are numerous white nodules concentrated in the deep renal cortex.

most likely sources of infection. Since leptospirae can penetrate intact mucosae and skin with minor scratches, splashes should be avoided and gloves worn. The presence of *L. icterohaemorrhagiae* in a kennel indicates that a higher level of rodent control is required.

RABIES

Aetiology

Rabies is caused by a large, bullet-shaped RNA lyssavirus (family Rhabdoviridae). Its outer envelope makes it sensitive to heat, light, detergents and disinfectants, and unable to survive for long outside its mammalian hosts. In addition to classical rabies virus, a number of rabies-related lyssaviruses have been identified, mainly in bats and small rodents in Africa and Northern Europe (WHO Expert Committee on Rabies, 1992), and these may also have the potential to cause neurological disease in man and larger mammals.

Epizootiology

Rabies is the oldest known canine disease and, being until recently almost invariably fatal in infected humans, it is also one which has been intensely investigated. A number of comprehensive reviews are available and provide detailed references (Baer and Wandeler, 1987; Clark and Prabhaker, 1985; WHO Expert Committe on Rabies, 1992).

Rabies occurs worldwide except in Australasia, Antartica and some islands and peninsular areas. Areas currently rabies free include the United Kingdom and Eire, Iceland, Japan, Taiwan, Norway and Sweden, and Spain and Portugal.

All mammals can be infected but susceptibility varies. Wild canidae are highly susceptible, domestic dogs moderately so. Rabies is perpetuated by wildlife reservoirs in all parts of the world, e.g. foxes in the northern hemisphere, skunks and raccoons in North America, bats in Central and South America. In Asia, Africa and Central and South America, feral and stray dogs are an additional reservoir.

Transmission is almost always via a bite wound. Respiratory infection occurs occasionally in bat caves where dark damp conditions allow the virus to survive in aerosols of infected saliva. Most human cases result from infected dog bites although in areas where canine vaccination is widespread, infected cats may be as much, if not more, of a problem than dogs. Even in areas with a wildlife reservoir, the domestic pet usually forms the link between man and wildlife.

Pathogenesis

Virus is inoculated into the tissues by a bite, replicates locally in muscle, then enters nerve axons at neuromuscular junctions or neurotendinal spindles and is transported along axons to the CNS. Once in the CNS, it spreads rapidly along neurones and induces behavioural abnormalities and progressive lower motor neurone deficits. Subsequent centrifugal spread along nerves from the brain results in localization in salivary glands and excretion in saliva.

The incubation period in dogs is usually 3–9 weeks but can be as short as 10 days or as long as 10 months. The incubation period is affected by the amount of implanted virus, the richness of local innervation and the distance from the wound to the CNS. Virus excretion can start before the onset of clinical signs but not all infected dogs excrete virus in saliva.

Clinical signs

The typical rabid dog shows an initial 2–3 day prodromal phase of altered temperament and behaviour: friendly dogs become shy and nervous, reserved animals suddenly affectionate. They are often pyrexic and may chew at the wound site. During the 1–7 day furious phase, the dog reacts excessively to most stimuli, may wander for long distances, and is spontaneously aggressive, attacking almost anything encountered. Early lower motor neurone signs are obvious as hind limb ataxia or paresis and partial paralysis of the lower jaw. Furious rabies is often absent or shortlived and, ultimately, dumb or paralytic rabies supervenes for the last 2–4 days. There is progressive paralysis: the lower jaw hangs open drooling saliva, swallowing is difficult, and the voice alters due to laryngeal paralysis; paraparesis progresses to paraplegia, quadriplegia, recumbency and terminal coma.

Death results from respiratory paralysis, usually within a week (occasionally 10–14 days) of initial signs. Atypical cases do occur, and recovery from experimental infection is recorded (Fekadu *et al.*, 1981), but naturally occurring rabies is generally regarded as invariably fatal.

Diagnosis

In endemic areas, rabies should be suspected in any dog with unexplained behavioural or nervous signs. The animal should be confined, observed and reported in accordance with local regulations. Dogs with typical signs are normally destroyed and their bodies or heads submitted for immuno-fluorescence testing of brain tissue. Apparently normal dogs which bite people should be observed for up to 3 weeks to see if rabid signs develop. Treatment is inappropriate. In rabies-free areas, a suspect case should be immediately isolated, confined and reported to local animal health authorities.

Control

In developed countries in which rabies is present, vaccination is often compulsory. Inactivated vaccines are given intramuscularly at 3–4 months, with a booster after 1 year, and thereafter annually or triennially as recommended. A few MLV products are available but postvaccinal encephalitis may occur, especially if these vaccines are administered to cats. The risk of postvaccinal encephalitis means that MLV products should never be used in exotic carnivores. Rabies occasionally occurs in vaccinated animals so vaccinated dogs bitten by rabid animals are usually revaccinated and confined for 3 months. Unvaccinated dogs in the same situation are often euthanased or confined for at least 6 months. Restrictions on dog movement may be enforced.

These measures have markedly reduced rabies in both humans and dogs in North America and Western Europe and recent successful oral immunization of European red foxes with recombinant vaccina-rabies vaccines may point the way to future wildlife control (Brochier et al., 1988). In less-developed countries, where rabies is endemic in dogs as well as wildlife and neither rabies vaccination nor dog control programmes operate effectively, rabies continues to take a heavy toll in humans as well as animals.

Some rabies-free countries now admit dogs and cats without quarantine provided they are certified as vaccinated. In other countries, such as Britain and Eire, quarantine of up to 6 months, even for vaccinated dogs, may still be enforced although the situation is under review. In Britain, quarantine is currently waived only for commercially traded breeding dogs of defined source which have never been in contact with wildlife, are clearly identified by microchip, and which have been shown serologically to have responded adequately to vaccination.

Since rabies virus is very labile, bites should be immediately and vigorously washed with soap or detergent. People bitten by known or suspected rabid animals should also receive prompt post-exposure prophylaxis with hyperimmune serum and human diploid vaccine, a regime which has proved highly effective in preventing the development of rabies.

ADVERSE EFFECTS OF VACCINATION

Adverse reactions to canine vaccines are unusual. Most are mild and transient but life-threatening problems can rarely arise. There are two main types of adverse reaction: those involving immunological mechanisms – the hypersensitivity reactions, and complications without an immunological basis which are probably more common. These are summarized in Table 48.1. Individual reactions are more common with some types of vaccines than others and particular dogs may be more at risk.

Non-immunological reactions

Probably the commonest adverse reaction is local irritation or tissue swelling at the site of inoculation. These arise most frequently with inactivated adjuvanted products. Postvaccinal abscesses usually indicate bad technique and hygiene rather than a vaccinal problem.

Mild pyrexia and dullness is sometimes recorded 1–2 days after administration of MLV products and is often ascribed to limited viral replication in lymphoid tissues. Such incidents are seldom reported and their true incidence is unknown. More severe disease may follow the use of MLV products in congenitally immunodeficient or immunosuppressed dogs, in neonate pups, or in exotic Canidae for which these products are incompletely attenuated. Shedding of MLV products with spread to in-contact animals has been recorded but reversion to virulence has not been demonstrated.

The most serious non-immunological adverse reaction is the development of postvaccinal encephalitis. This rare reaction is best recorded with MLV rabies and distemper vaccines. In America, it has been claimed that CDV-vaccinal encephalitis is predisposed to by combined

Table 48.1 Adverse effects of vaccination

Adverse reaction	Associated vaccines
Non-immunological	
• Local irritation	Inactivated, especially adjuvanted products
• Transient pyrexia	MLV products
• Clinical illness	Attenuated viral or bacterial products
• Postvaccinal encephalitis	MLV non-Onderstepoort vaccine strains, MLV rabies vaccines
• Shedding of vaccinal organism	MLV canine parvovirus and canine adenovirus vaccines. Intranasally administered vaccines
• Fetal malformation, abortion	MLV products if given during pregnancy
Immunological	
• Type I hypersensitivity (anaphylaxis)	Leptospiral vaccines
• Type II hypersensitivity (antibody dependent cytotoxicity)	MLV parvovirus vaccine – haemolytic anaemia MLV distemper vaccines – thrombocytopenia
• Type III hypersensitivity (immune complex or Arthus reaction)	MLV CAV-1 vaccines – blue eyes
• Type IV hypersensitivity (cell-mediated cytotoxicity)	Rabies vaccines of neural tissue origin

CDV–CPV vaccines or by concurrent infection with virulent CPV. However, in Britain, cases have arisen where neither of these factors have been present and these incidents have been associated with particular batches of vaccine; only non-Onderstepoort strains of distemper vaccine virus have been involved. Postvaccinal distemper encephalitis typically arises 7–10 days after inoculation as a sudden onset of nervous signs with ataxia, paresis and unusual aggressive or self-aggressive behaviour; signs referable to the alimentary and respiratory tract are unusual. A high prevalance of postvaccinal encephalitis was observed with a MLV canine coronavirus vaccine introduced in the USA in the 1980s and the product was quickly withdrawn from the market.

MLV products also have the potential to cross the placenta and, in theory, may cause problems from fetal malformation to abortion. They are not generally licensed for use in pregnant animals. No evidence has ever been produced that the use of live CPV vaccines in non-pregnant bitches or stud dogs has any subsequent effects on fertility.

Immunological reactions

Type I hypersensitivity reactions (acute/immediate hypersensitivity or anaphylaxis) are probably the best known immunological reaction and are certainly the most frightening. These occur most frequently with inactivated products, especially leptospiral vaccines, and may be induced by serum proteins or other substances in the inoculum rather than the vaccine components themselves. They may be more likely to occur in atopic animals. Type I reactions typically occur at second or subsequent inoculations. They may develop within minutes and are usually apparent within 1–2 h of administration. Local skin reactions occur but systemic anaphylaxis with vomiting, diarrhoea, dyspnoea, pallor and cardiac collapse is possible. The response to adrenaline, antihistamines and glucocorticoids is usually good. The suspected vaccine component should be removed from future vaccination courses and vaccines given only under close supervision. Antibody titres can be checked to see whether further booster vaccination is required.

Type III reactions are due to the deposition of antigen–antibody complexes in the wall of small vessels. This mechanism is responsible for the well-recognized phenomenon of anterior uveitis with corneal oedema which can follow the use of MLV CAV-1 vaccines. It is occasionally suggested that repeated booster vaccination of pet animals could lead to the development of more serious immune complex diseases such as glomerulonephritis but no association between the frequency of vaccination and the occurrence of such diseases has been shown.

Type II hypersensitivity reactions (antibody-dependent cytotoxicity) result from binding of inoculated antigen to host cells and subsequent destruction of cell and antigen by antibody. Cases of haemolytic anaemia and thrombocytopenia due to this mechanism have been reported following the use of MLV vaccines against parvovirus and distemper. Severe haemolysis or thrombocytopenia sufficient to induce a haemorrhagic diathesis would appear to be exceptionally rare but care should be taken in animals with pre-existing anaemia or haemorrhagic disorders. The suggestion that elective surgery should be delayed for a few weeks following vaccination is based on these reports.

Type IV delayed or cell-mediated hypersensitivity is rare but has been recorded following the use of rabies vaccines produced using nervous tissue.

In Britain, all suspect adverse reactions should be reported to the Veterinary Medicines Directorate of the Ministry of Agriculture, Fisheries and Food (MAFF), as well as to the manufacturer. A specific form is available from MAFF for this purpose. Conscientious reporting of adverse reactions by the profession allows early warning of problems associated with specific vaccines or vaccine batches, and is a compelling reason for keeping canine vaccination under veterinary control. Failure of response or vaccine 'breakdown' is regarded as an adverse reaction and should be reported in the same way.

CONTROL OF CONTAGIOUS DISEASES IN VETERINARY PREMISES

Acquisition of infection during a visit to or a stay in veterinary, or indeed medical, premises is a well-known hazard. Such nosocomial infections range from opportunistic infections of surgical wounds to potentially fatal contagious diseases. It may be impossible to prevent such infections completely but it is the responsibility of the veterinary surgeon to take reasonable precautions to prevent them and this is becoming more important as the tendency to resort to litigation increases.

Control of many opportunistic infections is readily achieved by good hygiene and disinfection (Greene, 1990), but control of contagious diseases can be more difficult. As mentioned above, almost the only cases of CPV myocarditis which we have seen in recent years have involved the pups of isolated, and usually unvaccinated, bitches which have been born by caesarean section where there is a strong probability that exposure to infection occurred in veterinary premises shortly after birth. Equally, we have encountered fatal cases of CPV enteritis in animals following surgery. Several colleagues have been faced with problems when it has been claimed that either CPV or CDV was introduced to previously unaffected kennels by animals which were exposed to infection during both short visits and longer stays in veterinary surgeries. In such circumstances, it may be important that a veterinary practice is able to demonstrate not necessarily that infection did not occur on its premises but that it took all reasonable and practicable precautions to control the spread of contagious disease.

First among such precautions is an awareness among both professional and lay staff of the risks of cross-infection. The problems that may arise from the extreme resistance of agents such as CPV which can result in indirect transmission of infection must be understood as must the potential for introduction of infection by subclinical cases or carrier animals.

Surgeries, kennels, waiting rooms and other areas where animals are held should be constructed so as to allow adequate cleaning and disinfection. Moreover, there should be a routine and regular procedure for cleaning and disinfection in all these areas, e.g. examination rooms should be cleaned and disinfected after every surgery and examination tables after every client. Having a written procedure means that all areas are considered, that there is no doubt as to policy for new members of staff, and that there is demonstrable practice concern for disease control. Appropriate disinfectants (particularly important for resistant organisms such as CPV) should be used at effective concentrations and for adequate periods of time. There should be an isolation area or facility for dealing with known or suspected cases of contagious diseases which must be managed as in-patients. Separate clothing, instruments and utensils should be used in such areas.

Equally important is warning clients of recognizable and preventable risks. This is particularly important in young pups presented for vaccination. These may, with advantage, be kept outside in the owner's car until they are due to be seen. If they do wait in a reception area, their owners should be advised not to allow them into contact with other animals which might be ill, or perhaps more importantly, with the owners (and children) of such animals. Unvaccinated animals should not be admitted except in emergency. This is particularly important for minor elective surgery but clearly there will be many times when the risk of contracting an infectious disease is far outweighed by the necessity to provide treatment.

Finally, if cases of nosocomial infections do occur, practice policy should be reviewed to determine if additional or stricter procedures should be implemented.

INFECTIOUS ENTERITIS

This general term is used for acute episodes of diarrhoea which are clearly transmissible. The most important cause, CPV-2, has already been discussed. However, infectious enteritis also occurs in kennels free from CPV-2 and in CPV-immune dogs. These other infections are considered here. Some cause significant disease on their own; others are generally mild. All may precipitate severe disease following CPV-2 infection.

Aetiology

Many viral, bacterial and parasitic agents have been isolated from dogs with acute enteritis (Table 48.2). Some are undoubtedly important, whereas others are uncommon, have little apparent pathogenicity, or are of unknown significance. Mixed infections are common. Zoonotic bacterial infections are particularly important. Helminth infections are unlikely causes of acute diarrhoea.

Epizootiology

Infectious enteritis is spread by direct contact and environmental contamination. It is commonest in kennels but also occurs in individual dogs. Infection may be acquired initially from contaminated food or water but subsequently spread by dog-to-dog transfer or environmental contamination. Infectious enteritis is more common, and generally more severe, in pups. Some specific information is available for particular agents.

Canine coronavirus (CCV) is closely related to feline coronavirus (and transmissible gastroenteritis virus of pigs). Canine strains may also infect cats. This enveloped RNA virus does not survive well outside the body and is difficult to isolate from other than very fresh material. Antibody to CCV is widespread (Binn *et al.*, 1981; Tennant *et al.*, 1991) but clinical disease is uncommon and severe disease even rarer (Carmichael and Binn, 1981). Immunity may be short lived and asymptomatic intermittent excretors may occur. Other viruses, such as rotavirus and astrovirus, are more resistant, may persist in the environment, and are probably significant mainly in young pups.

Table 48.2 Agents recovered from dogs with diarrhoea

A. Major systemic infections in which diarrhoea is a feature

Canine parvovirus type 2
Canine distemper virus
Canine adenovirus type 1

B. Agents confirmed as causing canine enteric pathology

Canine coronavirus	*Campylobacter* spp.	*Isospora* spp.
Canine rotavirus (pups)	*Salmonella* spp.	*Giardia* spp.
Canine parvovirus type 1 (neonates)		

C. Agents identified but of undetermined pathogenicity

Astrovirus	*E. coli*	*Cryptosporidium* spp.
Calicivirus	*Clostridium perfringens*	Other coccidial and
Herpesvirus	*Shigella* spp.	protozoan parasites
Parainfluenza virus	*Yersinia enterocolitica*	

Campylobacter species are Gram-negative curved bacilli which infect many mammals. *C. jejuni*, the most frequently isolated species in dogs, is uncommon in the faeces of healthy individuals but is more common in diarrhoeic single animals (Dillon *et al.*, 1987). The infection rate in groups, e.g. litters of pups or dogs in rescue shelters, can be much higher, whether animals are diarrhoeic or not (Bruce *et al.*, 1980). Many individual infections probably result from contaminated food but infection does spread through kennels. Most infections are mild or asymptomatic (Macartney *et al.*, 1988a) with severe clinical signs more likely in pups. Excretion persists for several weeks in untreated dogs. *C. jejuni* is one of the commonest causes of food poisoning in humans but infection can also be acquired from infected dogs.

Salmonella species are also Gram-negative bacilli with a wide host range. Isolates from dogs reflect the frequency of different *Salmonella* serotypes in the food animal population so that recently, for example, *Salmonella typhimurium* 204c has been a common canine isolate in our laboratories. Many infections are acquired from contaminated food or water but infection is also transmitted between dogs and zoonotic spread is possible. Although many infections are mild or asymptomatic, severe diarrhoea or dysentery with accompanying vomition can result, especially in pups. Young pups may become acutely septicaemic, with fever, collapse and death (Thompson and Wright, 1968), whereas infection in pregnant bitches may give rise to abortions, stillbirths and weak pups (Redwood and Bell, 1983). Recovered or asymptomatically infected animals may shed the organism for up to 6 weeks and true carriers with the potential to shed the organism many months later do occur. Late shedding is more likely if animals are stressed or suffer from other disease (Calvert, 1985).

Intestinal coccidia, most commonly *Isospora* spp. (usually *I. canis*, or *I. ohioensis*), are often considered non-pathogenic in dogs but heavy infections can cause illness especially in young pups and small breeds. Pups in crowded conditions of poor hygiene are most at risk (Lindsay and Blagburn, 1991). Coccidial oocysts are highly resistant and complete elimination is virtually impossible. The *Isospora* sp. most often involved do not affect humans. *Cryptosporidia* sp., a currently fashionable zoonotic coccidian parasite, is only occasionally detected in dogs. *Giardia* sp., another potentially zoonotic protozoan can also be detected in dogs (and cats), including normal animals (Kirkpatrick, 1988), but is perhaps more often associated with chronic than acute diarrhoea.

Pathogenesis

These superficial infections are acquired by ingestion and attach directly to intestinal mucosa. The viruses destroy absorptive villous epithelial cells causing variable villous stunting with diarrhoea if the reserve capacity of the intestine is exceeded (Keenan *et al.*, 1976; Johnson *et al.*, 1983). Bacteria may also cause villous stunting but bacterial toxins and inflammatory mediators may contribute to diarrhoea by causing fluid secretion into the gut lumen. Some bacteria, e.g. *Salmonella* spp. may cause severe mucosal destruction. In young pups, salmonellosis may cause septicaemia with focal necrosis and inflammation in many organs. Coccidia replicate in cells in the villous tips; light infections merely cause mild villous stunting but heavy synchronous infections can cause severe mucosal sloughing and dysentery.

Viral and bacterial incubation periods are short, usually 2–3 days. Coccidial replication takes longer, from 7 to 10 days. Unaffected crypt cells increase their mitotic rate to replace lost surface cells, and normal structure and function are usually restored within 4–7 days. The increased crypt mitotic rate makes these dogs especially susceptible to severe clinical disease if they should encounter CPV-2. CCV is usually excreted for up to 10–14 DPI whereas bacteria and coccidia may be excreted for several weeks. Further intermittent shedding of organisms can also occur. Immunity to superficial viral and bacterial infections is mediated mainly by local antibody production which may be of relatively short duration and is difficult to induce by systemically administered vaccines.

Clinical signs

Diarrhoea, the main and often only clinical sign, varies in severity from slightly soft faeces to profuse watery diarrhoea or even dysentery. The more severe cases may also be anorexic and fevered, may vomit, and can become dehydrated. In the most severe cases, total anorexia, depression, severe vomiting and profuse diarrhoea or dysentery may make clinical differentiation from parvovirus infection virtually impossible. No specific clinical signs are associated with individual agents although vomiting is perhaps more likely in animals with bacterial infections. Mortality is generally low provided good supportive therapy is given except in very young pups, toy breeds or animals with concurrent disease problems. Septicaemic salmonellosis can wipe out entire litters of young (4–8 week) pups with few clinical signs other than fever and collapse; anterior abdominal pain and even jaundice due to hepatic involvement may necessitate differentiation from ICH and leptospirosis.

Diagnosis

Most cases are mild and cannot be clinically differentiated in individual dogs from dietary upset. Severe cases are equally indistinguishable from CPV enteritis. Even when an infectious aetiology is apparent from the pattern of disease in a kennel, the agents responsible cannot be determined without laboratory investigation. This may be unwarranted in mildly affected individual dogs but should be undertaken in kennel outbreaks, when fatal cases occur, or if there is evidence of zoonotic spread.

Elimination of CPV-2 and identification of potential zoonoses are priorities. Rectal swabs or faecal samples should be submitted for bacterial culture. Faeces may be checked for CPV antigen by ELISA and similar tests for CCV may become available. Isolation of CCV requires very fresh faecal material but examination of paired sera, collected 2 weeks apart, should demonstrate a rising titre. Electron microscopy will reveal many viral agents in faeces but is seldom available for routine diagnosis. Coccidial and other oocysts can be identified in faeces by appropriate flotation techniques but trophozooites of protozoans such as *Giardia* are best visualized by direct microscopy of wet smears. In fatal cases, histopathology of fixed intestine will eliminate CPV, identify coccidia, and may indicate if superficial viral infections or bacteria are involved; intestinal contents may be checked for the presence of agents as described above.

Treatment

As with CPV enteritis, treatment is symptomatic, varying from 24 hours withdrawal of food to intensive care with intravenous fluid replacement. Antibiotics are only indicated if there is systemic illness or serious zoonotic risk and the choice of antibiotic should ideally be based on the results of faecal culture and known sensitivity patterns. However, many of our *Campylobacter* isolates have been resistant to the penicillins and sulphonamides but sensitive to the aminoglycosides, tetracyclines and erythromycin and treatment with such compounds has been effective in eliminating excretion of the organism in recovering animals. Antimicrobial treatment of salmonellosis has been controversial because of the supposed risk of prolonging excretion but is undoubtedly of value in animals with systemic signs of disease. Sulphonamides are probably the drugs of choice in coccidiosis but may be more effective as a prophylactic measure than for therapy of the disease.

Control

In kennels, measures for the control of CPV-2, i.e. thorough cleaning and disinfection, and batching of litters or groups of dogs will also control other agents which are generally less resistant. Complete elimination of coccidia may be impossible. *Salmonella* spp. and *Campylobacter* spp. may be introduced in food, and raw meat represents a potential source of infection. Inactivated vaccines against CCV have been developed but their efficacy remains to be proven. An MLV product introduced in America was withdrawn after fatal adverse reactions (Wilson *et al.*, 1986). Since CCV seldom causes severe disease or death, the case for general vaccination is debatable.

Few precautions are possible in individual dogs but raw meat should be fed with caution and spoilt or 'off' food should go in the bin, not the dog. Acute diarrhoea, especially in recently acquired pups, should be regarded as a potential human hazard. Affected animals should ideally be confined to an easily cleaned and disinfected area (preferably NOT the kitchen). Owners should be reminded to practise good personal hygiene and young children should not play with or handle sick animals.

CONTAGIOUS CANINE RESPIRATORY DISEASE

Contagious respiratory disease (CRD), generally known as kennel cough, is a syndrome of coughing due to tracheobronchitis which can be induced by several agents. Despite vaccination, it is still one of the commonest canine infections.

Table 48.3 Agents recovered from dogs with contagious respiratory disease

A. Systemic infections in which respiratory tract disease is a feature Canine distemper
B. Agents confirmed as causing significant respiratory tract disease *Bordetella bronchiseptica* Canine parainfluenza virus Canine adenoviruses
C. Agents of less important or undetermined significance *Mycoplasma* spp. Canine herpesvirus Canine reoviruses

Aetiology

Agents known to be associated with CRD are shown in Table 48.3 but it is probable that others remain to be identified.

Bordetella bronchiseptica is a frequent isolate and induces typical disease in non-immune dogs (Thompson *et al.*, 1976). Canine parainfluenza virus (CPIV), another common isolate (Binn *et al.*, 1970), also induces disease but this is generally mild and short lived. Both canine adenoviruses (CAV-1 and CAV-2) cause respiratory disease when given by aerosol (Swango *et al.*, 1970; Wright *et al.*, 1971), but are important mainly in unvaccinated pups. Other viruses are considered to be less important as they are isolated only occasionally and experimental infections are asymptomatic. Mycoplasmas appear to be normal upper respiratory tract commensals (Rosendal, 1982) which complicate lesions induced by other agents although a few strains may be rather more pathogenic (Rosendal, 1978). Other bacteria are usually considered to be secondary invaders. Mixed infections are common. This complex aetiology, together with the fact that immunity is short lived, means that individual dogs can suffer repeated attacks.

Epizootiology

CRD occurs when dogs from different sources are mixed. Disease is common in boarding kennels and rescue centres and release of infected dogs can lead to local outbreaks in neighbourhood pets. Disease often peaks in late summer towards the end of the holiday season. CRD also follows attendance at shows, training clubs, race meetings and even veterinary premises. The agents are spread mainly by direct contact or short distance aerosol transmission; most are sensitive to drying, light and disinfectants. Infection can also be spread by physical means, e.g. water or feeding bowls. *B. bronchiseptica* can infect many species, including humans and cats.

Small, relatively closed, breeding kennels may remain free for long periods. In contrast, large breeding kennels may suffer enzootic infection with few problems in adults but disease in successive litters of weaned pups.

Pathogenesis

Infection is by inhalation. *B. bronchiseptica* adheres to respiratory tract cilia causing rhinitis and tracheobronchitis (Thompson *et al.*, 1976). Pneumonia is unusual. Coughing becomes obvious 3–4 DPI and can last 7–10 days. The bacteria may stay in the airways for 12 weeks after infection (Bemis *et al.*, 1977). CPIV and other viruses multiply in nasopharyngeal and tracheobronchial epithelia causing mild, often asymptomatic disease (Appel and Percy, 1970). Clinical signs usually start at 4–7 DPI and last only a few days. Viral excretion has normally stopped by 14 DPI. *B. bronchiseptica* and CPIV infections appear synergistic: more severe and longer-lasting disease follows dual infection (Wagener *et al.*, 1984). Immunity to these surface infections is mediated mainly by local antibody and appears to be of relatively short duration, 12–18 months, even after natural infection.

CAV-1 and CAV-2 given via the respiratory tract in experimental infections induce necrotizing bronchiolitis. Pups with low levels of MDA which are immune to systemic ICH can still suffer from CAV respiratory disease. However, respiratory infection is aborted by high antibody levels, so that animals actively immune to ICH are normally also protected from CAV respiratory disease (Cornwell *et al.*, 1982, 1983).

Mixed infections, or infections complicated by mycoplasmas and secondary bacterial invaders can progress to pneumonia. Death is common only in neonates or immunosuppressed dogs. Occasional animals suffering repeated infections may develop chronic bronchial disease.

Clinical signs

The typical and often only sign of CRD is coughing which lasts from 2–3 days to 2–3 weeks. The cough is often harsh and irritating but sometimes moist and productive. Severely affected dogs suffer from paroxysms of coughing, often brought on by excitement or exercise, which end with retching. Owners may suggest the dog is trying to vomit (recently fed dogs may actually do so) or that there is some pharyngeal obstruction.

Sneezing, a serous or mucoid to mucopurulent nasal discharge, pharyngitis and enlargement of tonsils and local nodes can occur and may occasionally be the only findings. Most dogs remain bright. Pyrexia, anorexia and depression occur only if there is complicating pneumonia. This is more likely in the very young or very old, in animals with chronic problems such as cardiac failure, or in dogs with pre-existing respiratory disease such as tracheal collapse. Pups with CAV-induced disease are often tachypnoeic for a few days due to bronchiolitis but usually remain bright and active.

Most cases recover spontaneously and uneventfully within 2 weeks though some may take up to a month. A very few develop chronic bronchitis.

Diagnosis

The clinical signs are sufficiently characteristic to make a general diagnosis but early distemper must be considered in some cases.

Determination of the agents involved cannot usually be justified in individual cases and is difficult even in kennel outbreaks. Normal bacterial flora can interfere with isolation of *B. bronchiseptica* from nasal and pharyngeal swabs. Samples from the tracheal bifurcation are more reliable but are difficult to obtain without recourse to general anaesthesia. Virus isolation is likely to succeed only early in the course of infection. Serology can be undertaken but detection of rising titres is necessary since antibodies are widespread from both natural infection and vaccination and false negatives can occur.

Treatment

Owners may need reassurance more than their dogs need treatment. Most cases recover spontaneously. Antimicrobials are indicated if there is pyrexia, depression, other evidence of pneumonia, or a risk of transmission to more susceptible dogs. Ampicillin, oxytetracycline and trimethoprim–sulphonamide combinations are usually active against *B. bronchiseptica* and achieve reasonable levels in respiratory tract secretions. Systemic antibiotics should be given at maximal levels for at least 10 days (McCandlish and Thompson, 1976). Aerosolization of antibiotics such as kanamycin and gentamycin reduces the burden of *B. bronchiseptica* (Bemis and Appel, 1977) but is often impracticable.

Glucocorticoids and antitussives relieve harsh, irritating or paroxysmal coughing but are contraindicated in animals with pneumonia or moist productive coughs. Bronchodilators have also been used in dogs with paroxysmal cough but are of unproven efficacy. The value of mucolytics and expectorants in dogs with productive coughs is equally uncertain but they will cause no harm and can give an anxious owner something to do.

Avoiding excitement and exercise will help reduce a paroxysmal cough as will changing from a collar to a shoulder harness. Racing dogs should not resume full training until they have completely recovered.

Control

MLV-CAV vaccines against ICH provide good protection against CAV-associated respiratory disease and vaccines against both *B. bronchiseptica* and CPIV are also available. Since local immunity is more important than systemic responses with the latter two infections, intranasal vaccines should be more effective than parenteral preparations but even locally administered products are unlikely to induce 100% protection.

Live attenuated intranasal *B. bronchiseptica* vaccine is available in many countries either as a single component or a combined CPIV product (Shade and Goodnow, 1979; Chladek et al., 1981). Only a single inoculation is required initially but annual boosters are recommended. Since intranasal vaccines are not blocked by low levels of maternally derived antibody, and protection against *B. bronchiseptica* can be detected as early as 4 days after inoculation (Bey et al., 1981), these products may be of value both for early (from 6 weeks of age) vaccination of pups in kennels with enzootic disease and for providing rapid protection during disease outbreaks. Parenterally administered inactivated *B. bronchiseptica* and MLV CPIV products are also available in many countries. In general, two inoculations are recommended for the initial course with annual boosters but they are probably less effective than intranasal products in preventing shedding of infective agents (Emery et al., 1976; McCandlish et al., 1978).

Since immunity is short-lived, both primary and booster vaccinations against CRD in individual dogs should ideally be administered 1–2 weeks before anticipated challenge. It should be stressed to owners that although these products reduce the probability of CRD, they do not completely eliminate it.

Elimination of CRD, especially in boarding and rescue kennels, is impossible due to the multiple agents involved, the occurrence of asymptomatic infections or prolonged carriage, and the availablity of vaccines against only some agents. Good kennel design and management will help reduce the prevalence and severity of disease, whether or not vaccination is also undertaken. Small kennel blocks are preferable to larger ones and should be allocated on a rota basis so that new arrivals are not mixed with longer-term residents. Decreasing the population density and increasing the ventilation will prevent build up of infectious particles. If CRD does occur, care should be taken to prevent physical transfer of infection to other blocks. The affected block should be emptied, thoroughly cleaned and disinfected, then left for at least a week before admitting new animals.

NEONATAL INFECTIONS AND INFECTIOUS INFERTILITY

Up to 20% of pups die by 2 weeks of age, most in the first 7 days. Specific signs are unusual and since many pups gradually deteriorate, they are popularly known as 'fading pups'. Maternal and management factors such as starvation and hypothermia account for many deaths and congenital abnormalities for others. Probably no more than 20% are attributable primarily to infection. In many cases, no specific cause of death can be determined and factors such as fetal immaturity with low birth weights and poor pulmonary function due to inadequate surfactant may be involved (Blunden, 1986, 1988)

In theory, many agents associated with neonatal disease can be acquired transplacentally and can also cause embryonic death, abortion and stillbirth (Johnston and Raskil, 1987). These are shown in Table 48.4. *Brucella canis* infection, the main infectious cause of canine abortion, is dealt with separately. In practice, at least in Britain where *B. canis* does not occur, most neonatal infections appear to be acquired shortly after or during birth. Isolation of any agent from abortions and stillbirths is uncommon although this may mean only that any organisms involved are fastidious and unable to be detected by conventional isolation procedures: there is recent evidence that the notoriously fastidious CPV-1 (canine minute virus) can cause resorption and abortion (Carmichael *et al.*, 1991). Several organisms, such as streptococci and mycoplasmas, have historically been regarded as causes of endometritis and infertility but are also normal lower urogenital tract commensals and their role in reproductive disease requires re-evaluation. Unfortunately, investigation of canine abortion is undoubtedly hindered by the tendency of bitches to eat the evidence before it is noticed.

Neonatal infections

Aetiology

Organisms which may be found in dead neonates are also shown in Table 48.4.

Septicaemias or local bacterial infections, usually pneumonia or enteritis, are the commonest neonatal infections. Most are due to streptococci (in our experience often Lancefield Group G, occasionally B, L, or others), staphylococci (usually *Staph. intermedius*), *Pasteurella* spp., or *Escherichia coli* and other coliforms which are present in the environment or as commensals in healthy adults. Specific pathogens such as *Salmonella*, *Brucella* and *Leptospira* also occur but are uncommon whereas other organisms such as *Bacillus piliformis* (the cause of Tyzzer's disease) and *Yersinia enterocolitica* are rare.

Equally rare are infections with CPV-2, CDV and CAV, possibly because antibody is widespread in breeding bitches. Rotavirus has been found in pups with diarrhoea under 2 weeks of age but most infections appear mild. The only virus regularly associated with neonatal illness and death is canine herpesvirus (CHV) (Carmichael *et al.*, 1965; Cornwell *et al.*, 1966).

CHV is one of the less important causes of kennel cough in older pups and adults and has also been associated with local vaginal and penile lesions in adults (Poste and King, 1971). It grows best at 35–36°C and so is restricted to superficial mucosae in most dogs which have core temperatures >38°C. In neonates, however, the core temperature is only just over 37°C, and drops rapidly with chilling since pups cannot regulate their body temperature until 2–3 weeks of age. Infection of neonates can therefore result in systemic spread with extensive viral multiplication and tissue necrosis.

Table 48.4 Agents isolated from canine abortions and stillbirths or from pups dying in the neonatal period

A. **Viruses**	
(i) Shown to cause significant disease Canine herpesvirus Canine minute virus (CPV-1) Canine rotavirus	(ii) Uncommonly/rarely isolated CPV-2 CAV-1 CDV
B. **Bacteria**	
(i) Specific pathogens *Brucella* spp. *Campylobacter* spp. *Leptospira* spp. *Salmonella* spp. *Bacillus piliformis* *Yersinia enterocolitica*	(ii) Components of 'normal' flora *E. coli* *Mycoplasma* spp. *Staphylococcus* spp. *Streptococcus* spp. *Pasteurella* spp.
C. **Parasites** *Toxoplasma gondii* *Toxocara canis*	

Heavy prenatal infection with *Toxocara canis* exceptionally causes pneumonia and poor condition in pups less than 2 weeks old in association with visceral migration (Parsons, 1991). Transplacental transmission of *Toxoplasma gondii* (Capen and Cole, 1966) rarely results in disseminated neonatal disease with a variety of signs referable to involvement of the central nervous system, liver and lungs.

Epizootiology and pathogenesis

Most neonatal infections result from oronasal uptake either from the environment or from the bitch during or after whelping. Bacteria may also invade via the umbilicus or through skin abrasions or docking or declawing wounds. Dirty whelping accommodation increases the risk of infection.

Some bacteria are non-pathogenic for adults but may induce disease in neonates, e.g. enterotoxin-producing *E. coli* can probably cause profuse fluid diarrhoea in neonate pups just as they do in other species. Moreover, many organisms which are normal commensals or low-grade pathogens in adults grow rapidly in neonates, particularly if they are colostrum deprived, chilled or otherwise stressed. Pups derive only 5–10% of their dams' antibody titres by placental transfer and are susceptible to many infections until after adequate colostral absorption. Chilling allows systemic spread of CHV and also decreases non-specific defences against bacteria.

Localized infections such as enteritis or pneumonia do occur and may be associated with a wide range of organisms but there is often generalized spread and development of either septicaemia or endotoxaemia or multifocal inflammation and necrosis.

Clinical signs

Most pups with neonatal infections show broadly similar signs. The entire litter or only some of the pups may be affected. An initial failure to gain weight often goes unnoticed until the pup loses its normal sleek plump appearance, stops sucking and cries restlessly. Dehydration and laboured breathing may be noted. As the pup deteriorates, it becomes quiet and cold. Episodes of limb paddling, opisthotonus and periods of apnoea occur terminally. Close examination may reveal more specific signs such as diarrhoea, nasal discharge or a discharging navel. Many exudates are cleaned away by the bitch although she may also reject a sick pup. Small red or black sores under the chin or on the feet may indicate staphylococcal dermatitis and septicaemia.

Diagnosis

It is generally impossible to make an aetiological diagnosis of 'fading pups' on clinical grounds. Post-mortem examination is needed to rule out trauma and congenital defects; in some pups there may be evidence of mismothering such as persistence of meconium. Some pups are small with partially inflated lungs and may be immature. Others have empty, gas-filled stomachs and intestines and may not have been feeding successfully despite apparently sucking well.

CHV infection has a distinctive necropsy appearance. Most cases occur at 7–14 days of age. Small, grey, necrotic foci with haemorrhagic rims are seen in kidneys (Fig. 48.15), liver and lung. There are usually small haemorrhages on serosae, especially over the intestines, and the spleen and lymph nodes are often enlarged. The diagnosis can be confirmed by histological examination of major organs or virus isolation.

Acute staphyloccocal dermatitis occurs in pups as young as 3–4 days. Dark red or black, raised or swollen areas are found on the point of the chin (Fig. 48.16) and the backs of the feet, especially on the carpal pads; other areas, e.g. muzzle and ventral abdomen, are less commonly affected. Many of these pups develop staphylococcal septicaemia.

Other infections have few specific changes. There may be pneumonia, pleurisy, meningitis, enteritis or hepatic abscessation but congestion may be the only finding in septicaemia. Further histological and microbiological (usually bacteriological) investigations are required to determine the agent involved. Most septicaemias occur within the first 7 days of life.

In a substantial proportion of 'faded pups' no infectious or other cause can be found.

Treatment and control

Treatment of sick neonates is time-consuming, difficult and often unsuccessful. Puppy weights can be monitored from birth to detect problems early. Any pup failing to gain weight over 24 h should receive supplementary oral feeding with bitch milk substitute or 5–10% glucose. The pup must be kept dry and warm (environmental temperature 90°F). Urination and defecation must be induced by gentle perianal massage with warm wet cotton wool after feeding. Broad-spectrum antibiotics may be given. Pups with a poor sucking reflex can be fed by stomach tube (Hoskins, 1990) and dehydrated pups can be given fluids (50:50, Hartmann's solution:5% glucose subcutaneously at 1 ml 30 g^{-1}) but the prognosis for such pups is very poor.

CHV infection is sporadic and usually only single litters are affected. The whole litter may die and neurological deficits have been recorded in survivors (Percy et al., 1971). Bitches seldom produce more than one affected litter. Pups born shortly after an affected litter must be kept warm and may also be given immune serum prepared from the bitch which lost her pups. No vaccine is available.

Where there are repeated neonatal bacterial infections, prophylactic antibiotic treatment of pups at birth may help control losses. However, there is likely to be an underlying management problem and this must be carefully checked. Whelping accommodation must be clean, warm and draught-free. Heat lamps should be used with caution to avoid overheating the pups or causing discomfort to the bitch. Most importantly, pups should be encouraged to suck as soon as possible after birth to ensure maximal colostral uptake; hyperimmune serum can be given if the bitch has no or little milk. Puppy weight gain should be

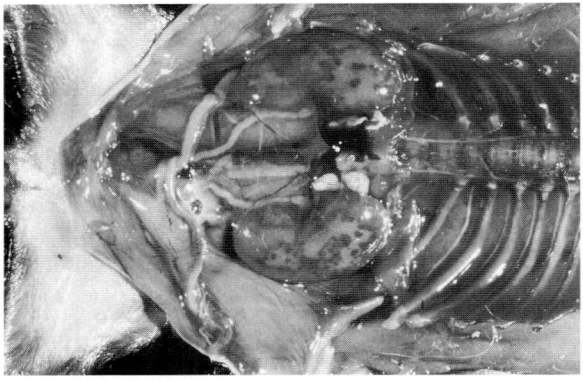

Figure 48.15 Canine herpesvirus infection. Multiple areas of necrosis give the kidneys a dramatic mottled appearance.

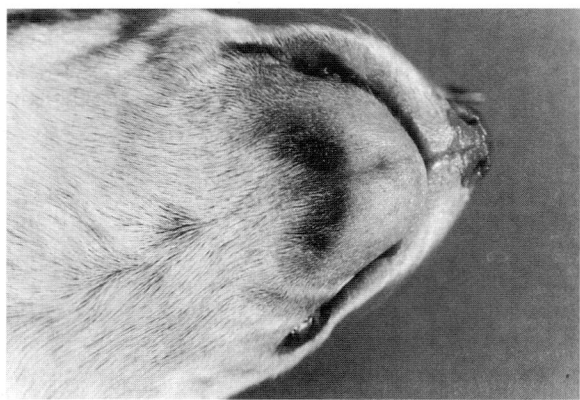

Figure 48.16 Staphylococcal dermatitis in a 7-day-old pup. Small raised dark nodules are present on the undersurface of the chin. The pup had died as a result of staphylococcal septicaemia.

monitored. Contact with other dogs should be kept to a minimum, particularly in mixed breeding and boarding kennels. This is particularly important when CRD occurs in a kennel since what is a minor respiratory infection in otherwise fit adults can prove fatal in neonates, either because of the introduction of CHV or because of severe bacterial pneumonia.

Canine brucellosis

Brucella canis occurs in the Americas and other parts of the world (Carmichael and Greene, 1990) but has not been identified in the UK. Infection causes infertility with abortion in bitches and testicular degeneration in dogs. Most cases arise by oronasal infection following exposure to heavily contaminated aborted material and vaginal secretions, but venereal transmission can occur and male urine may also be infective. Occasional cases of *B. abortus* infection follow access to contaminated cattle placentas or fetal tissues (Taylor *et al.*, 1975).

B. canis is taken up by phagocytes but is resistant to their normal killing mechanisms and actively multiplies in them. This results in a cell-associated bacteraemia which can last for 5 years. Systemic signs other than general lymphadenopathy and hyperglobulinaemia are uncommon. Discospondylitis, glomerulonephritis and uveitis occur occasionally but the main effects are in the reproductive tract. Abortion, usually about 2 weeks before term, is the commonest result of infection but early embryonic deaths, fetal resorption, stillbirths or weak pups also occur. Affected bitches have a greenish brown vaginal discharge for up to 6 weeks. In the male, epididymitis and orchitis cause spermatic abnormalities and infertility without loss of libido. The epididymis may be palpably enlarged and there is often secondary scrotal dermatitis.

Isolation from vaginal secretions or aborted material is straightforward on appropriate media. Isolation from low-grade bacteraemia is more difficult and several serological tests are used to detect infected dogs (Nicoletti and Chase, 1987). Identification and removal of infected animals is the main method of control in kennels. Treatment is difficult and, since *B. canis* is zoonotic, should only be undertaken after consultation with the owners. Infected pets should be neutered and treated with appropriate antimicrobials. Many antibiotics are ineffective *in vivo* and oral doxycycline combined with intramuscular gentamycin is probably the treatment of choice. Relapse is common and so dogs must be monitored for at least 6 months after the end of treatment.

OTHER VIRAL INFECTIONS

Aujesky's disease

Aujeszky's disease (pseudorabies) is a rare, almost invariably fatal canine infection caused by a porcine herpesvirus (Pensaert and Maes, 1987). Dogs are infected by eating raw pig meat or offal. Dog to dog transmission does not occur. The virus spreads along oral and other alimentary tract nerves to the brain causing inflammation of the myenteric plexuses and encephalitis, especially around cranial nerve nuclei, within 3–6 days. Clinical signs include altered behaviour, hypersalivation, dyspnoea and diarrhoea. Severe pruritus, usually of the head, occurs in many dogs. Constant rubbing and scratching (mad itch) causes skin swelling and excoriation. Paralysis, convulsions, and coma develop rapidly. Treatment is ineffective and death occurs within 24–48 h.

Canine papillomavirus

Viral papillomas or warts occur mainly in young dogs, most commonly in the mouth (Fig. 48.17) but also on skin and conjunctivae; different viral subtypes may affect different sites (Calvert, 1990). Viral papillomas are often multiple, develop rapidly for 1–2 months then regress spontaneously. Most vanish within a few months. Treatment is needed only if the warts become

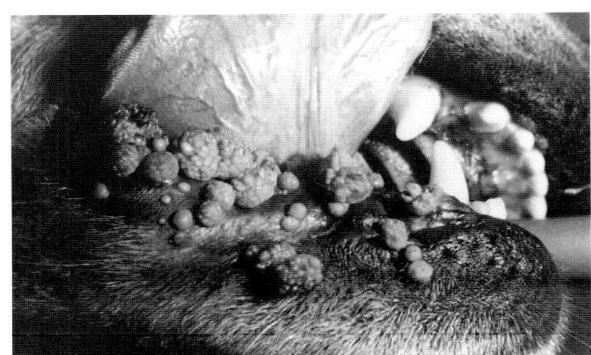

Figure 48.17 Oral papillomatosis in 9-month-old dog. There are numerous coalescing cauliflower-like warts on the lips.

traumatized or secondarily infected or are persistent. Surgical excision or cryosurgery are usually effective and removal of some may induce regression of the others. The efficacy of autogenous vaccines has never been convincingly demonstrated. Animals with heavy or persistent infections should be checked for underlying immunosuppression. Occasional transfer to other, usually young, dogs can occur but there is no risk to humans.

Other viruses

Dogs are susceptible incidental hosts for arthropod-borne viral infections in different parts of the world, e.g. louping-ill in the British Isles, equine encephalitis viruses in the Americas, but cases are very sporadic. Some human pathogens such as mumps and influenza viruses and even enteroviruses may also grow in dogs but canine infections appear to be incidental and asymptomatic.

Perhaps more significantly, several canine disease syndromes are suspected to be caused by as yet undefined viruses. These include a non-CAV, acute or persistent/chronic hepatitis, characterized by numerous acidophil cells (degenerate angular hepatocytes). This acidophil cell hepatitis can be transmitted by bacteriologically sterile cell-free liver filtrates but the suspected viral agent has not yet been isolated (Jarrett *et al.*, 1987). It is likely that future investigations of such syndromes will identify specific agents.

OTHER BACTERIAL INFECTIONS

Lyme borreliosis

Aetiology

Infection with *Borrelia burgdorferi*, a tick-borne spirochaete, was first recognized in people with inflammatory arthritis in Lyme, Connecticut in 1975. Canine cases were first recorded in 1984, and have been increasingly recognized in the USA, Britain and Europe. Infection in dogs is associated with acute to chronic non-erosive polyarthritis.

Epizootiology

Borreliosis is transmitted mainly by hard ticks, e.g. *Ixodes ricinus* in Europe. Infection of other arthropods, including fleas, and urinary excretion in infected mammals have been recorded but appear unimportant in transmission. In the UK, antibody titres are highest in dogs with known tick bites, and are generally higher in rural than urban animals (May *et al.*, 1991). Clinical disease appears rarer than the number of positive antibody titres might suggest and asymptomatic infection may be common.

Pathogenesis

The pathogenesis of borreliosis is poorly defined. In acute infections, tissue damage may be caused by interleukin-1 released from monocytes in response to bacterial lipopolysaccharide or by the early formation of immune complexes. Chronic disease appears to be due to persistent infection and the resultant immune-mediated disease. Synovial fluid from affected joints contains polymorphs and increased protein levels but bacteria are difficult to isolate. Nonetheless, appropriate antimicrobial treatment results in a fall in antibody titre and resolution of clinical signs.

Clinical signs

Clinical signs in dogs are largely limited to the locomotor system (Levy *et al.*, 1993). Acute cases are pyrexic and inappetant with lymphadenopathy and general stiffness. Lameness or pain is difficult to localize and may shift from leg to leg. The joints are seldom swollen. Chronic cases develop an intermittent or recurrent non-erosive inflammatory arthritis usually affecting two or more joints and often including the carpus. Focal tubular degeneration with urinary shedding and glomerulonephritis occurs in some animals and focal myocardial and endocardial inflammation has rarely been described. Neurological abnormalities are well recognized in humans but have only relatively recently been recorded in the dog (Mandel *et al.*, 1993).

Diagnosis

Lyme borreliosis should be considered in dogs with inflammatory arthropathy and fever, especially in tick-infested areas. Confirmation can be difficult since the signs are not pathognomonic, isolation of the organism is difficult, and antibody is widespread. A negative antibody result will help eliminate Lyme disease but a positive result is not diagnostic since antibody may mean simple exposure rather than true disease. High antibody levels may be more indicative but other causes of arthritis, such as rheumatoid disease, must be considered. Response to treatment may support a diagnosis of Lyme disease.

Treatment and control

Oral tetracycline (22 mg kg^{-1} tid) or ampicillin (20 mg kg^{-1} tid) for 10–14 days has been recommended, based on experience in humans, and may produce rapid relief from pain and lameness. Refractory chronic cases may respond to intravenous penicillin G (22 000 units kg^{-1} qid for 7 days). Non-steroidal anti-inflammatory agents can be used to manage pain but steroids are contraindicated since they may cause recrudescence of infection. Ticks should be removed as early as possible. An inactivated vaccine is now available in the United States for use in areas with high prevalance of infection (Levy et al., 1992).

Actinomycosis and nocardiosis

These are uncommon infections, more frequent in rural areas and usually affecting only one animal with occasional small clusters in working or hunting dogs. Two main syndromes occur (Hardie, 1990): first, subcutaneous pyogranulomatous cellulitis; second, severe pleurisy with empyema or less commonly peritonitis. Disseminated disease is rare. *Actinomyces* spp. are normal oral commensals whereas *Nocardia* spp. are soil saprophytes. Both are slender long Gram-positive organisms which form branching chains and both produce small yellow macrocolonies or 'sulphur granules'. *Nocardia* spp. are moderately acid fast whereas actinomycetes are not.

Subcutaneous lesions appear as irregular nodular masses with discharging necrotic tracts and are probably caused by implantation. There may be localized osteomyelitis. Treatment involves drainage, or possibly local excision and/or debridement, and appropriate antimicrobial therapy.

The route of infection in animals with pleurisy or peritonitis is seldom apparent; primary pneumonia or enteritis is rare. Dogs with serosal lesions are usually dull, fevered and anorexic. Pleurisy and empyema cause dyspnoea and exercise intolerance whereas peritonitis results in abdominal swelling and palpable masses. The serosae are covered by thick, reddish brown, velvety tissue (Fig. 48.18) and a copious dirty-brown to red, serosanguinous fluid is produced which may contain the classic 'sulphur' granules. Treatment requires surgical drainage and regular

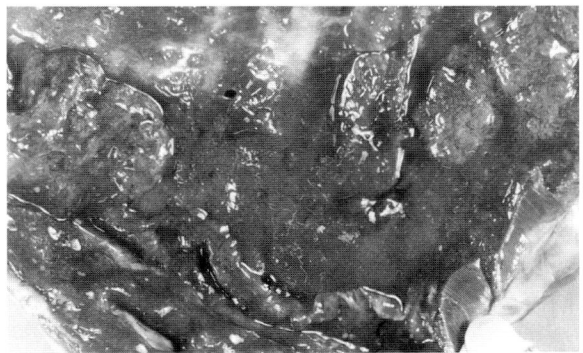

Figure 48.18 Parietal pleura from dog with actinomycosis. The pleura is covered by an irregularly thick layer of haemorrhagic granulation tissue.

lavage and antimicrobial therapy for up to 6–8 weeks. Choice of antibiotic should be based on culture and sensitivity tests but most cases of actinomycosis respond well to high doses of simple penicillins. Antibiotics such as clindamycin or erythromycin may be tried in refractory cases. Nocardosis is often more intractable; *in vitro* sensitivity may not reflect *in vivo* response but many cases respond to sulphonamides. Antimicrobials should be administered systemically but may also be included in lavage fluids provided care is taken to prevent overdosage. Early pleural infections respond much better than late-stage cases with extensive pleural thickening. Pleural stripping can be attempted in these cases.

Mycobacterial infections

Canine tuberculosis is rare. In developed countries, it is almost always the result of infection with *Mycobacterium tuberculosis* from human cases. As in humans, the canine disease is typified by chronic coughing, persistent pyrexia and weight loss (Liu et al., 1980). There are cavitating pulmonary masses with enlarged bronchial lymph nodes and serous pleural and pericardial effusions are common. Hypertrophic pulmonary osteopathy (Marie's disease) may develop. Intestinal lesions with enlarged mesenteric nodes or hepatic nodules are uncommon in dogs with human tuberculosis but granulomas are frequently found in the kidneys and organisms may be shed in urine. Diagnosis is primarily by demonstration of acid-fast organisms in aspirates and tissues. Treatment of dogs with tuberculosis is rarely undertaken but all cases must be followed up to trace the source – this is a zoonosis-in-reverse. *M. bovis* infections in dogs are very rare. They are caused by feeding infected milk or meat and result in chronic vomiting, diarrhoea, weight loss and enlarged mesenteric nodes.

Atypical mycobacterial infections are caused by free-living organisms of the *M. fortuitum-chelonei* or *M. avium-intracellulare* complexes. Infection usually follows implantation or wound contamination and results in localized, discharging subcutaneous granulomas (Gross and Connelly, 1983). Systemic spread is rare except in animals which are immunosuppressed or have intercurrent disease. Differentiation of the occasional systemic infection from classical tuberculosis depends on culture and identification of the organisms. Diagnosis of localized cutaneous lesions is most commonly made on biopsy as organisms are often sparse and aspirates may be negative. Culture on special mycobacterial media will allow typing of the organism and give guidance for antimicrobial therapy. Many atypical mycobacteria are resistant to standard antituberculosis drugs but may respond to quinolones. Surgical excision is probably the treatment of choice for localized skin lesions but recurrence is common unless wide excision is possible. If additional antimicrobial therapy is needed, laboratory guidance should be sought.

Tetanus

Tetanus is uncommon in dogs. It follows implantation of *Clostridium tetani* into deep wounds with anaerobic conditions suitable for multiplication and elaboration of the tetanospasmin toxin. This enters local or more distant motor nerves and spreads into and through the CNS, blocking inhibitory transmission to motor neurones and inducing spastic paralysis. Interference with autonomic nerves may result in vagal hyperactivity. Muscle stiffness can be localized around the original wound but generalized tetanus causes widespread muscle rigidity. The stiff limbs and contracture of facial muscles with 'lockjaw' and a 'sardonic grin' are diagnostic. Repeated muscle spasms and convulsions are followed by death from respiratory paralysis.

Early or localized cases usually respond to wound debridement and the administration of penicillin or metronidazole to prevent further toxin formation (Greene, 1990). Antitoxin can be given to neutralize circulating toxin but will not affect toxin which has already bound to nerves. Phenothiazines may be useful in controlling spasms as they depress excitatory impulses. Complete recovery may take over a month. Advanced cases which require phenothiazines and barbiturates to control spasms and convulsions and which also need intensive care to maintain vital functions, such as respiration and alimentation, carry a much poorer prognosis.

Botulism

Botulism in dogs arises from ingestion of preformed *Clostridium botulinum* toxin in contaminated foodstuffs, usually carrion or raw meat. Botulism is rare but is probably commonest in hound packs (Blakemore *et al.*, 1977). The toxin is absorbed from the stomach and intestines and binds to the presynaptic axon terminals of neuromuscular junctions, blocking acetylcholine release and inducing flaccid paralysis. There is progressive weakness and paralysis but pain sensation is not affected. Death is due to respiratory paralysis. As with tetanus, antitoxin neutralizes circulating but not bound toxin. Good nursing and supportive therapy to maintain fluid balance and nutrition will allow many mild cases to make a good recovery although this may take a few weeks. The toxin is heat sensitive and easily destroyed by thorough cooking.

PROTOZOAL INFECTIONS

Leishmaniasis

Aetiology and epizootiology

Leishmaniasis is a protozoal infection of many mammals, including humans. It occurs in warmer areas and is most prevalent in Central and South America, the Mediterranean basin and the Middle East. Two main forms, visceral and cutaneous, are recognized in humans but in the dog most cases have both skin and visceral abnormalities (Kontos and Koutinas, 1993). Organisms of the *Leishmania donovani* complex are most commonly isolated from dogs but other species do occur. Dogs, together with rodents, may act as a reservoir species for human infection in many areas. Infection is transmitted between animals, and between animals and humans, almost entirely by biting sandflies. However, direct zoonotic transmission is possible if infected canine body fluids or wound exudates are inoculated into man through abraded skin or puncture wounds, e.g. bites. Cases in Northern Europe and North America almost always involve imported animals (Longstaffe and Guy, 1986; Bravo et al., 1993). Infection can become established in new areas if suitable vectors exist.

Pathogenesis and pathology

Leishmania is an obligate intracellular parasite. In sandflies, it multiplies in gut cells as flagellated promastigotes which accumulate in the pharynx. These are inoculated into mammals when the fly bites, are taken up by macrophages and undergo repeated binary fission as non-flagellated amastigotes. They eventually kill the cell, and are released to parasitize yet more monocytes. Local multiplication is followed by spread to local lymph nodes and gradual dissemination through the body. The transmission cycle is completed when other sandflies are infected by ingestion of parasitized macrophages in blood or tissue fluid.

Overt disease may not develop for years, depending on the effectiveness of the host's cell-mediated (T-cell) immune response. General lymphadenopathy is one of the most consistent findings. Parasites are found in swollen mononuclear phagocytes in distended lymph node sinuses. T-cell areas are generally depleted but B-cell areas are expanded due to unregulated proliferation partly directed against *Leishmania* antigens but partly caused by non-specific polyclonal B-cell activation.

Spread to mononuclear phagocytes throughout the body causes splenic and hepatic enlargement, bone marrow dysfunction and anaemia, and alimentary, respiratory and ocular disease. Moreover, the marked B-cell reaction causes hyperglobulinaemia and immune complex disease. Glomerulonephritis with progressive renal failure is one of the commonest causes of death. Haemopoietic abnormalities also occur. Autoantibodies may induce haemolytic anaemia and thrombocytopenia whereas hyperglobulinaemia can interfere with fibrin polymerization and induce haemorrhagic diathesis with epistaxis, haematuria or melaena. Formation of cryoglobulins can cause precipitation and occlusion of small vessels in cold conditions with ischaemic necrosis of extremities.

Clinical signs

Canine leishmaniasis is a chronic multisystemic disease (Kontos and Koutinas, 1993). Skin lesions are usual. The face, especially round the eyes, nose and ears, and feet are often affected but lesions can be generalized. The hair is thin and brittle, the skin scaly, thickened and sometimes depigmented, and the nails are often long and brittle. Cutaneous or mucocutaneous plaques or nodules may develop and these may become eroded or more extensively ulcerated. Visceral disease commonly appears as generalized lymphadenopathy, weight loss and anorexia but clinical signs can be protean. Vomiting, diarrhoea, polyuria, polydipsia, epistaxis, and respiratory and ocular signs may all occur.

Diagnosis

Leishmaniasis should be suspected in dogs with skin disease, lymphadenopathy and other evidence of systemic disease. In non-endemic areas, the condition occurs in imported dogs, often after several years, and may be confused with lymphoid malignancy. Hyperglobulinaemia is characteristic but other biochemical changes are very variable. Anaemia, thrombocytopenia and lymphopenia are common. Lymph node and marrow aspirates will demonstrate the amastigotes in macrophages although a careful search is required in early cases. They are also visible on biopsy of skin nodules or lymph nodes (Fig. 48.19).

Treatment

Early cases with few visceral signs respond well to treatment but complete elimination of the organism is unlikely and relapses can be expected. The prognosis in cases with significant renal disease is

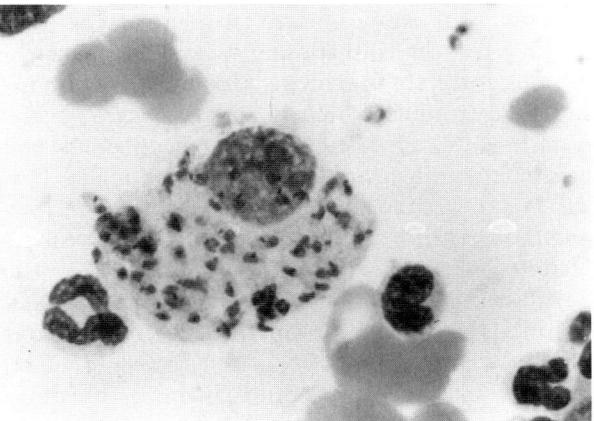

Figure 48.19 Leishmania amastigotes in cytoplasm of macrophage. Lymph node aspirate. (Giemsa × 1000.) Picture by courtesy of Dr P.E. McNeil.

poor. Sodium stibogluconate (30–50 mg kg^{-1}) or meglumine antimonate (100 mg kg^{-1}) can be given intravenously or subcutaneously daily for 3–4 weeks. Intramuscular administration of these drugs may induce muscle necrosis and should be avoided. Although the risk of direct human infection is low, it does exist, especially when dogs develop ulcerated and weeping lesions on the skin or, even more importantly, in the mouth. Great care must be taken in treating such dogs and owners must be warned of the risks.

Toxoplasmosis

Aetiology

Toxoplasma gondii is a protozoan parasite of worldwide distribution. Wild and domestic cats are the definitive hosts and produce oocysts in their faeces. Dogs, other mammals and birds are intermediate hosts in which only non-sexual parasitic forms are found, usually as encysted bradyzooites in body tissues.

Epizootiology and pathogenesis

Dogs are infected in two main ways: first, by eating oocysts from infected cats in faecally contaminated material and secondly, by eating tissue cysts from other intermediate hosts. Raw or undercooked meat, especially sheep meat, is the most likely source of tissue cysts but hunting dogs may acquire infection from prey animals. Ingestion of either oocysts or tissue cysts results in cyst breakdown, invasion through intestinal epithelium and dissemination of multiplying tachyzooites throughout the body. Actively dividing tachyzooites grow in and destroy many host cells but are eliminated from normal animals by host responses in about 3 weeks. Some tachyzooites form slow-growing tissue cysts containing bradyzooites which persist for many years. Tachyzooites can also cross the placenta and may cause fetal infection in pregnant animals. This appears to occur mainly during primary infection and subsequent pregnancies are usually unaffected.

Infection is more common than disease. Antibody is present in up to 30% of dogs and antibody prevalance increases with age (Dubey, 1987). Clinical disease is unusual and may require heavy infection or underlying immunosuppression (Dubey et al., 1989). Toxoplasmosis is often seen as a complication of distemper, especially in dogs with nervous signs. It has been suggested that immunosuppression allows breakdown of tissue cysts and recrudescence of infection. Disseminated toxoplasmosis occurs occasionally in young pups, between 6–12 weeks, and may reflect congenital transmission or infection of animals with poorly developed immune systems.

Disease is due to tissue necrosis caused by the rapid multiplication of tachyzooites. In young pups and immunosuppressed animals, focal necrosis is found in many organs, including liver, lungs, heart and kidneys. Serosal effusions are common. In older pups and adults, lesions are often resticted to muscles and nervous tissues.

Clinical signs

Generalized infection in pups or immunosuppressed dogs is rapidly progressive and affected animals may die within a week. Clinical signs are variable and include pyrexia, lymphadenopathy, vomiting and diarrhoea, coughing and respiratory distress, abdominal pain and jaundice, cardiac irregularities, uveitis and nervous signs such as head tilt, nystagmus, ataxia and fits.

In others, the disease is more chronic and neuromuscular problems predominate but can be variable. Ataxia, paresis and paralysis indicate spinal cord lesions whereas headtilt, nystagmus and seizures occur with cerebellar and cerebral lesions. Myositis may cause pain, wasting and paresis in the absence of CNS disease.

Diagnosis

Paired blood samples, taken 2 weeks apart, can be tested for toxoplasma antibodies. The classic Sabin–Feldman dye test, requires live organisms and can only be carried out in specialist laboratories. A fourfold rise with the second sample 1:64 or above is indicative of infection. More modern ELISA tests should allow detection of an IgM response consistent with recent active infection. The IgG response is usually high and may persist for several years; it indicates previous exposure rather than recent infection. In fatal cases, histopathology reveals tachyzooites and tissue cysts in affected organs. These must be distinguished from *Neosporum caninum*.

Treatment

Generalized toxoplasmosis in young pups is usually fatal. In older animals, treatment may be more successful. Clindamycin (3–13 mg kg^{-1} tid for 2 weeks) is probably the drug of choice and may be best given intramuscularly as high oral doses can cause gastrointestinal upset. Sulphonamides or synergistic combinations of sulphonamide (sulphadiazine 30 mg kg^{-1} bid) and pyrimethamine (0.5 mg kg^{-1} bid) by mouth for up to a fortnight can also be used.

Infected dogs pose no hazard to people provided infected dog tissues or fluids do not contaminate wounds. Owners of infected dogs should, however, be warned of the risks of cat faeces and uncooked meat for themselves as well as their dogs.

Neosporosis

Aetiology

Neospora caninum is a recently recognized protozoal parasite of dogs (Dubey, 1990). It forms tissue cysts similar to *T. gondii* and has probably been mistaken for toxoplasma in the past. A very similar, if not identical parasite is increasingly being recognized as a cause of abortion, and neonatal paresis and encephalomyelitis in cattle (Trees *et al.*, 1994). The life cycle of *N. caninum* is unknown but is assumed to be similar to *Toxoplasma*. Only tissue forms have been found in dogs and the definitive host in which oocysts develop has not been identified. Congenital transmission can occur in dogs. Antibody has been detected in up to 13% of UK dogs (Trees *et al.*, 1993).

Pathology

As in toxoplasmosis, multiplying tachyzooites cause cell necrosis and inflammation. Lesions occur mainly in skeletal muscles and nervous tissues, especially nerve roots, with some foci in heart, skin and subcutis, and other organs. Both tachyzooites and tissue cysts are found.

Clinical signs

The commonest finding is progressive ascending paralysis due to a polyradiculomyositis in both young (2–6 months) and older dogs. The hind limbs are often most severely affected. Muscle atrophy and stiffness progress to marked muscular rigidity with paralysis. Rigidity is caused partly by fibrosis of affected muscles and partly by nerve root lesions inducing lower motor neurone deficits. There may also be areas of dermatitis with subcutaneous nodules. Ascending lesions may cause cervical weakness, dysphagia and death.

Diagnosis

In an animal with suspicious clinical signs, a positive antibody test will help confirm the diagnosis. Clinical cases usually have titres ⩾ 800 by indirect fluorescent antibody tests. In other animals, the presence of antibody indicates exposure rather than disease with titres ⩽ 800. There is little cross-reaction with *T. gondii*. Muscle biopsies or CSF analysis may reveal thick-walled tissue cysts or individual tachyzooites lying free in cell cytoplasm. In comparison, toxoplasma cysts are thin-walled and tachyzooites are found in cytoplasmic vacuoles. Immunocytochemical stains will confirm which organism is involved. In fatal cases, histological examination of muscle, spinal cord and brain will confirm the diagnosis.

Treatment

Treatment as for toxoplasmosis has been suggested but is likely to be effective only if undertaken before muscle fibrosis and contraction have developed.

RICKETTSIAL INFECTIONS

Several forms of rickettsial infection may occur in the dog. These include: salmon poisoning disease of North Western America, in which the causative agent *Neorickettsia helminthoeca* is transmitted by a canine intestinal trematode which the dog acquires from eating raw or undercooked Pacific salmon; tick-transmitted Rocky Mountain spotted fever in Northern America and similar arthropod borne infections in Asia; and Q-fever which, although occurring in humans and a variety of domestic species worldwide, has only rarely been recognized in the dog. Neither salmon poisoning disease nor Rocky Mountain spotted fever has been recognized in British dogs, but one canine rickettsia, *Ehrlichia canis*, does occur in the Mediterranean basin and may be encountered in imported animals.

Ehrlichiosis

Aetiology

The obligate intracellular microorganism *Ehrlichia canis* is found in warm temperate and tropical areas worldwide and is transmitted between susceptible dogs by arthropod vectors, usually ticks (Woody and Hoskins, 1991). The organism is acquired by the tick when it feeds on an infected dog and it can then infect any other dog on which it subsequently feeds; fortunately, transovarial transmission to a new generation of ticks does not occur. Other *Ehrlichia* species are occasionally found.

Pathogenesis and clinical signs

Organisms inoculated by tick-bite are taken up by mononuclear cells in which they replicate by binary fission. The infection spreads via the mononuclear phagocyte system in a manner similar to that seen in leishmaniasis. Infected cells also cause damage to endothelia throughout the body causing vasculitis and a consumptive thrombocytopenia. A non-specific acute form of the disease with fever, anorexia and depression may be noted 1–3 weeks following initial infection but this is usually transient and most early infections are inapparent. Thrombocytopenia may be detected haematologically but overt bleeding problems are uncommon at this stage.

However, infection can persist intracellularly through a long subclinical phase before resurfacing as chronic problems many months or even years later. Persistent infection induces a marked but ineffective antibody response with generalized plasmacytosis and hyperglobulinaemia which, in combination with the continued vasculitis and thrombocytopenia, may result in bleeding problems. Mucosal and cutaneous petechiation, epistaxis and melaena may be noted as well as more common but non-specific findings of lethargy, anorexia and weight loss. Many animals are anaemic and, despite the bleeding problems, this is often non-regenerative as a result of erythroid hypoplasia. Megakaryocytic and myeloid hyperplasia may co-exist with erythroid hypoplasia during the acute and subclinical phases of the disease, but chronically or severely affected animals often show generalized marrow aplasia. Palpable lymphadenopathy and splenomegaly are unusual. A few animals develop obvious anterior uveitis or chorioretinitis, vague neurological signs or arthropathies.

Diagnosis

Intracytoplasmic inclusions or morulae, formed from closely packed masses of organisms can be found in circulating monocytes, or less commonly other white blood cells, especially during the earlier stages of infection but they are very difficult to detect in chronic cases. Serological testing is usually used to confirm the diagnosis in America where infection can be a problem. Histological findings in fatal cases are of marked plasmacytosis with perivascular cuffing by plasma cells in blood vessels throughout the body as well as focal haemorrhages. Unfortunately, the organisms are difficult to detect in formalin fixed tissues.

Treatment

Several agents have been successfully used to treat ehrlichiosis. Tetracycline (22 mg kg^{-1} tid for 2–3 weeks) is the usual drug of choice but doxycycline (5–10 mg kg^{-1} bid for 7–10 days) may be useful in animals which are refractory to tetracycline or suffer from relapses. Supportive therapy will also be required, including blood transfusions in severely anaemic animals and fresh blood or platelet-rich plasma in dogs with severe bleeding problems.

ACKNOWLEDGEMENTS

The author is indebted to her colleagues Dr Campbell Cornwell, Professor Andrew Nash, Dr David Taylor and, especially, Dr Hal Thompson of Glasgow University Veterinary School who have contributed greatly to this chapter through their advice in many discussions and friendly arguments.

REFERENCES

Appel, M. and Percy, D.H. (1970) SV-5 like parainfluenza virus in dogs. *Journal of the American Veterinary Medical Association* **156**, 1778–1781.

Appel, M.J.G. (1969) Pathogenesis of canine distemper. *American Journal of Veterinary Research* **30**, 248–292.

Appel, M.J.G. (1987) Canine adenovirus type 1 (infectious canine hepatitis virus). In: *Virus Infections of Vertebrates* Vol. 1: *Virus infections of carnivores* (Ed. M.J.G. Appel). Elsevier, Amsterdam, pp. 29–43.

Appel, M.J.G. and Gillespie, J.H. (1972) Canine distemper virus. In: *Virology Monographs* II (Eds S. Gard, C. Hallauer and K.F. Meyer). Springer-Verlag, New York, pp. 1–96.

Appel, M.J.G., Scott, F.W. and Carmichael, L.E. (1979) Isolation and immunisation studies of a canine parvo-like virus from dogs with haemorrhagic enteritis. *Veterinary Record* **105**, 156–159.

Appel, M.J.G., Shek, W.R. and Summers, B.A. (1982) Lymphocyte-mediated immune toxicity in dogs infected with virulent canine distemper virus. *Infection and Immunity* **37**, 592–600.

Baer, G.M. and Wandeler, A.I. (1987) Rabies virus. In: *Virus Infections of Vertebrates*, Vol. 1: *Virus infections of carnivores* (Ed. M.J.G. Appel). Elsevier, Amsterdam, pp. 167–182.

Bemis, D.A and Appel, M.J.G. (1977) Aerosol, parenteral and oral antibiotic treatment of *Bordetella bronchiseptica* infections in dogs. *Journal of the American Veterinary Medical Association* **170**, 1082–1086.

Bemis, D.A., Greisen, H.A. and Appel, M.J.G. (1977) Pathogenesis of canine bordetellosis. *Journal of Infectious Diseases* **135**, 753–762.

Bey, R.F. and Johnson, R.C. (1982) Leptospiral vaccines in dogs: immunogenicity of whole cell and outer envelope vaccines prepared in protein-free medium. *American Journal of Veterinary Research* **43**, 831–834.

Bey, R.F. Shade, F.J., Goodnow, R.A. and Johnson, R.C. (1981) Intranasal vaccination of dogs with live avirulent *Bordetella bronchiseptica*: correlation of serum agglutination titer and the formation of secretory IgA with protection against experimentally induced infectious tracheobronchitis. *American Journal of Veterinary Research* **42**, 1130–1132.

Binn L., Marchwicki, R.H., Eckermann, E.H. and Fritz, T.E. (1981) Viral antibody studies of laboratory dogs with diarrhoeal disease. *American Journal of Veterinary Research* **42**, 1665–1667.

Binn, L.N., Lazar, E.C., Helms, J. and Cross, R.E. (1970) Viral antibody patterns in laboratory dogs with respiratory disease. *American Journal of Veterinary Research* **31**, 697–701.

Bishop, L., Strandberg, J.D., Adams, J.R., Brownstein, D.G. and Patterson, R. (1979) Chronic active hepatitis in dogs associated with leptospires. *American Journal of Veterinary Research* **40**, 839–844.

Blakemore, W.F., Rees-Evans, E.T. and Wheeler, P.E.G. (1977) Botulism in foxhounds. *Veterinary Record* **100**, 57–58.

Blunden, A.S. (1986) A review of the fading puppy syndrome (also known as fading puppy complex). *Veterinary Annual* **26**, 264–269.

Blunden, A.S. (1988) Diagnosis and treatment of common disorders of newborn puppies. *In Practice* **10**, 175–184.

Bravo, L., Frank, L.A. and Brenneman, K.A. (1993) Canine Leishmaniasis in the United States. *Compendium on Continuing Education for the Practicing Veterinarian* **15**, 699–708.

Brochier, B., Thomas, I., Iokem, A., Gunter, A., Kalpers, J., Paquot, A., Costy, F. and Pastoret, P. P. (1988) A field trial in Belgium to control rabies by oral immunisation. *Veterinary Record* **123**, 618–621.

Bruce, D., Zochowski, W. and Fleming, G.A. (1980) *Campylobacter* infections in cats and dogs. *Veterinary Record* **107**, 200–201.

Calvert, C.A. (1985) Salmonella infection in hospitalised dogs: epizootiology, diagnosis and prognosis. *Journal of the American Animal Hospitals Association* **21**, 499–503.

Calvert C.A. (1990) Canine viral papillomatosis. In: *Infectious Diseases of the Dog and Cat* (Ed. C.E. Greene). W.B. Saunders, Philadelphia, pp. 288–290.

Capen, C.C. and Cole, C.R. (1966) Pulmonary lesions in dogs with experimental and naturally occurring toxoplasmosis. *Pathologia Veterinaria* **3**, 40–63.

Carmichael, L.E. and Binn, L.N. (1981) New enteric viruses in the dog. *Advances in Veterinary Science and Comparative Medicine* **25**, 1–37.

Carmichael, L.E. and Greene, C.E. (1990) Canine brucellosis. In: *Infectious Diseases of the Dog and Cat* (Ed. C.E Greene). W.B.Saunders, Philadelphia, pp. 573–584.

Carmichael, L.E., Strandberg, J.D. and Barnes, F.D. (1965) Identification of a cytopathic agent infectious for puppies as a canine herpesvirus. *Proceedings of the Society for Experimental Biology and Medicine* **120**, 644–650.

Carmichael, L.E., Joubert, J.C. and Pollock, R.V.H. (1983) A modified live canine parvovirus vaccine II: immune response. *Cornell Veterinarian* **73**, 13–29.

Carmichael, L.E., Schlaffer, D.H. and Hashimoto, A. (1991) Pathogenicity of minute virus of canines (MVC) for the canine fetus. *Cornell Veterinarian* **81**, 151–171.

Chladek, D.W., Williams, J.M., Gerber, D.L., Harris, L.l. and Murdock, F.M (1981) Canine parinfluenza–Bordetella bronchiseptica vaccine: immunogenicity. *American Journal of Veterinary Research* **42**, 266–270.

Churchill, A.E. (1988) Preliminary development of a live attenuated canine parvovirus vaccine from an isolate of British origin. *Veterinary Record* **122**, 334–339.

Clark, H.F. and Prabhaker, B.S. (1985) Rabies. In: *Comparative Pathobiology of Viral Diseases*, Vol. II (Eds R.G. Olsen, S. Krakowka and J.R. Blakeslee). CRC Press, Boca Raton, pp. 165–214.

Cornwell, H.J.C., Wright, N.G. Campbell, R.S.F. and Roberts, R.J. (1966) Neonatal disease in the dog associated with a herpes-like agent. *Veterinary Record* **79**, 661–662.

Cornwell, H.J.C., Koptopoulos, G., Thompson, H., McCandlish, I.A.P. and Wright, N.G. (1982) Immunity to canine adenovirus respiratory disease: a comparison of attenuated CAV-1 and CAV-2 vaccines. *Veterinary Record* **110**, 27–32.

Cornwell, H.C.J., Paterson, S.D., McCandlish, I.A.P., Thompson, H. and Wright, N.G. (1983) Immunity to canine adenovirus respiratory disease: effect of vaccination with an inactivated vaccine. *Veterinary Record* **113**, 509–512.

Cornwell, H.J.C., Thompson, H., McCandlish, I.A.P., Macartney, L. and Nash, A.S. (1988) Encephalitis in dogs associated with a batch of canine distemper (Rockborn) vaccine. *Veterinary Record* **112**, 54–59.

Curtis, R. and Barnett, K.C. (1983) The 'blue eye' phenomenon. *Veterinary Record* **112**, 347–353.

Dillon, A.R., Boosinger, T.R. and Blevins, W.T. (1987) Campylobacter enteritis in dogs and cats. *Compendium on Continuing Education for the Practicing Veterinarian* **9**, 1176–1183.

Dubey, J.P. (1987) Toxoplasmosis. *Veterinary Clinics of North America: Small Animal Practice* 17, 1389–1404.

Dubey, J.P. (1990) *Neosporum caninum*: a look at a new Toxoplasma-like parasite of dogs and other animals. *Compendium on Continuing Education for the Practicing Veterinarian* 12, 653–663.

Dubey, J.P., Carpenter, J.L., Topper, M.J. and Uggla, A. (1989) Fatal toxoplasmosis in dogs. *Journal of the American Animal Hospital Association* 25, 659–664.

Ellis, W.A. (1986) Leptospirosis. *Journal of Small Animal Practice* 27, 683–692.

Emery, J.B., House, J.A., Bittle, J.L. and Spotts, A.M. (1976) A canine parainfluenza viral vaccine: immunogenicity and safety. *American Journal of Veterinary Research* 37, 1323–1327.

Fekadu, M., Saddock, J.H and Baer, G.M. (1981) Intermittent excretion of rabies virus in the saliva of a dog two and six months after it had recovered from experimental rabies. *American Journal of Tropical Medicine and Hygiene* 30, 1113–1115.

Glickmann, L.J., Domanski, L.M., Patronek, G.J. and Visitainer, F. (1985) Breed related risk factors for canine parvovirus enteritis. *Journal of the American Veterinary Medical Association* 187, 589–594.

Gocke, D.J., Morris, T.Q. and Bradley, S.E. (1970) Chronic hepatitis in the dog: role of immune factors. *Journal of the American Veterinary Medical Association* 156, 1700–1705.

Gordon, J.C. and Angrick, E.J. (1986) Canine parvovirus: environmental effects on infectivity. *American Journal of Veterinary Research* 47, 1464–1467.

Greene, C.E. (1990) Tetanus. In: *Infectious Diseases of the Dog and Cat* (Ed. C.E. Greene). W.B. Saunders, Philadelphia, pp. 521–529.

Gross, T.L. and Connelly, M.R. (1983) Non-tuberculous mycobacterial skin infection in two dogs. *Veterinary Pathology* 20, 117–119.

Hamilton, J.M., Cornwell, H.J.C., McCusker, H.B., Campbell, R.S.F and Henderson, J.W.P. (1966) Studies on the pathogenesis of canine virus hepatitis. *British Veterinary Journal* 122, 225–238.

Hardie, E.M. (1990) Actinomycosis and nocardiosis. In: *Infectious Diseases of the Dog and Cat* (Ed. C.E. Greene). W.B. Saunders, Philadelphia, pp. 585–591.

Higgins, R.J., Krakowka, S., Metzler, A.E. and Koestner A. (1981) Canine distemper virus-associated cardiac necrosis in the dog. *Veterinary Pathology* 18, 472–486.

Hoskins, J.D. (1990) Nutrition and nutritional disorders. In: *Veterinary Pediatrics* (Ed. J.D. Hoskins). W.B. Saunders, Philadelphia, pp. 473–486.

Jarrett, W.F.H., O'Neil, B.W. and Lindholm, I (1987) Persistent hepatitis and chronic fibrosis induced by canine acidophil cell hepatitis virus. *Veterinary Record* 120, 234–235.

Johnson, C.A., Fulton, R.W., Henk, W.G and Cho, D. (1983) Gross and light microscopic lesions in gnotobiotic neonatal dogs inoculated with a canine rotavirus. *American Journal of Veterinary Research* 44, 1687–1693.

Johnson, G.C., Fenner, W.R. and Krakowka, S. (1988) Production of immunoglobulin G and increased antiviral antibody in cerebrospinal fluid of dogs with delayed onset canine distemper viral encephalitis. *Journal of Neuroimmunology* 17, 237–251.

Johnston, S.D. and Raskil, S. (1987) Fetal loss in the dog and cat. *Veterinary Clinics of North America: Small Animal Practice* 17, 535–554.

Keenan, K.P., Jervis, H.R., Marchwicki, R.H and Binn, L.N. (1976) Intestinal infection of neonatal dogs with canine coronavirus 1-71: studies by virologic, histologic, histochemical and immunofluorescent techniques. *American Journal of Veterinary Research* 37, 247–256.

Kirkpatrick, C.E. (1988) Epizootiology of endoparasitic infections in pet dogs and cats presented to a veterinary teaching hospital. *Veterinary Parasitology* 30, 113–124.

Kontos, V.J. and Koutinas, A.F. (1993) Old world canine leishmaniasis. *Compendium on Continuing Education for the Practicing Veterinarian* 15, 949–959.

Koptopoulos, G., Papadopoulos, O., Papanastasopoulou, M. and Cornwell, H.J.C.C. (1986) Presence of antibody cross reactive with canine parvovirus in the sera of dogs from Greece. *Veterinary Record* 118, 332–333.

Krakowka, S., Hoover, E.A., Koestner, A. and Ketring K (1977) Experimentally and naturally occurring transplacental transmission of canine distemper virus. *American Journal of Veterinary Research* 38, 919–922.

Krakowka, S., Higgins, R.J. and Koestner, A. (1980) Canine distemper virus: review of structural and functional modulations in lymphoid tissues. *American Journal of Veterinary Research* 41, 284–292.

Krakowka, S., Axthelm, M.K. and Johnson, G.C. (1985) Canine distemper virus. In: *Comparative Pathobiology of Viral Diseases*, Vol. II (Eds R.G. Olsen, S. Krakowka and J.R. Blakeslee). CRC Press, Boca Raton, pp. 137–164.

Lauder, I.M., Martin, W.B., Gordon, E.B., Lawson, D.D., Campbell, R.S.F and Watrach, A.M. (1954a) A survey of canine distemper. *Veterinary Record* 66, 607–611.

Lauder, I.M., Martin, W.B., Gordon, E.B., Lawson, D.D., Campbell, R.S.F and Watrach, A.M. (1954b) A survey of canine distemper. II: Pathology. *Veterinary Record* 66, 623–632.

Levy, S.A., Lissman, B.A. and Ficke, C. (1992) Field performance studies of *Borrelia burgdorferi* bacterin in three veterinary practices in borreliosis endemic areas. *Journal of the American Veterinary Medical Association* 202, 1834–1838.

Levy, S.A., Barthold, S.W., Dombach, D.M. and Wasmoen, T.L. (1993) Canine lyme borreliosis. *Compendium on Continuing Education for the Practicing Veterinarian* 15, 833–846.

Lindsay, D.S. and Blagburn, B.L. (1991) Coccidial parasites of dogs and cats. *Compendium on Continuing Education for the Practicing Veterinarian* **13**, 559–565.

Liu, S., Weitzman, I. and Johnson, G.C. (1980) Canine tuberculosis. *Journal of the American Veterinary Medical Association* **177**, 164–167.

Longstaffe, J.A. and Guy, M.W. (1986) Canine leishmaniasis – United Kingdom update. *Journal of Small Animal Practice* **27**, 663–671.

Macartney, L., McCandlish, I.A.P., Thompson, H. and Cornwell, H.J.C.C. (1984a) Canine parvovirus enteritis 1: clinical, haematological and pathological features of experimental infection. *Veterinary Record* **115**, 201–210.

Macartney, L., McCandlish, I.A.P., Thompson, H. and Cornwell, H.J.C.C. (1984b) Canine parvovirus enteritis 2: pathogenesis. *Veterinary Record* **115**, 453–460.

Macartney, L., Al-Mashat, R.R., Taylor, D.J and McCandlish, I.A.P. (1988a) Experimental infection of dogs with *Campylobacter jejuni*. *Veterinary Record* **122**, 245–249.

Macartney, L., Thompson, H., McCandlish, I.A.P. and Cornwell, H.J.C.C. (1988b) Canine parvovirus: interaction between passive immunity and virulent challenge. *Veterinary Record* **122**, 573–576.

Mandel, N.S., Senker, E.G., Schneider, E.M. and Bosler, E.M. (1993) Intrathecal production of *Borrelia burgdorferi*-specific antibodies in a dog with central nervous system Lyme borreliosis. *Compendium on Continuing Education for the Practicing Veterinarian* **15**, 581–586.

May, C., Carter, S.D., Barnes, A., Bell, S. and Bennett, D. (1991) Serodiagnosis of Lyme disease in UK dogs. *Journal of Small Animal Practice* **32**, 170–174.

McCandlish, I.A.P. and Thompson, H. (1976) Canine bordetellosis: chemotherapy using a sulphadiazine–trimethoprim combination. *Veterinary Record* **104**, 51–54.

McCandlish, I.A.P., Thompson, H. and Wright, N.G. (1978) Vaccination against canine bordetellosis: protection from contact challenge. *Veterinary Record* **192**, 479–483.

McCandlish, I.A.P., Thompson, H., Fisher, E.W., Cornwell, H.J.C.C., Macartney, L. and Walton, I.A. (1981) Canine parvovirus infection. *In Practice* **3**(3), 5–14.

McCandlish, I.A.P., Cornwell, H.J.C., Thompson, H., Nash, A.S. and Lowe, C.M. (1992) Distemper encephalitis in pups after vaccination of the dam. *Veterinary Record* **130**, 27–30.

Meunier, P.C., Glickmann, L.T., Appel, M.J.G. and Shin, S.J. (1981) Canine parvovirus in a commercial kennel: epidemiologic and pathological findings. *Cornell Veterinarian* **71**, 96–110.

Meunier, P.C., Cooper, B.J., Appel, M.J.G. and Slauson, D.O. (1984) Experimental viral myocarditis – parvovirus infection of neonatal pups. *Veterinary Pathology* **21**, 509–515.

Meunier, P.C., Cooper, B.J., Appel, M.J.G., Slauson, D.O. and Lanieu, M. (1985a) Pathogenesis of canine parvovirus enteritis: sequential virus distribution and passive immunisation studies. *Veterinary Pathology* **22**, 617–624.

Meunier, P.C., Cooper, B.J., Appel, M.J.G. and Slauson, D.O. (1985b) Pathogenesis of canine parvovirus enteritis: the importance of viraemia. *Veterinary Pathology* **22**, 60–71.

Morrison, I.A. and Wright, N.G. (1976) Canine leptospirosis: an immunopathological study of interstitial nephritis due to *Leptospira canicola*. *Journal of Pathology* **120**, 83–89.

Navarro, C.E.K. and Kociba, G.J (1982) Hemostatic changes in dogs with *Leptospira interrogans* serovar *icterohaemorrhagiae* infection. *American Journal of Veterinary Research* **43**, 904–906.

Nicoletti, P.L. and Chase, A. (1987) An evaluation of methods to diagnose *Brucella canis* in dogs. *Compendium on Continuing Education for the Practicing Veterinarian* **9**, 1071–1074.

Osterhaus, A.D. and Vedder, E.J. (1988) Identification of virus causing recent seal deaths. *Nature* **335**, 20.

Parrish, C.R. and Carmichael, L.E. (1983) Antigenic structure and variation of canine parvovirus type-2, feline panleucopenia virus and mink enteritis virus. *Virology* **129**, 401–414.

Parrish, C.R., O'Connell, P.H., Evermann, J.F. and Carmichael, L.E. (1985) Natural variation of canine parvovirus. *Science* **230**, 1046–1048.

Parrish, C.R., Have, P., Foreyt, W.J., Evermann, J.F., Senda, M. and Carmichael, L.E. (1988) The global spread and replacement of canine parvovirus strains. *Journal of General Virology* **69**, 1111–1116.

Parrish, C.R., Aquadro, C.F., Strassheim, M.L., Evermann, J.F. and Mohammed, H.O. (1991) Rapid antigenic type replacement and DNA sequence evolution of canine parvovirus. *Journal of Virology* **65**, 6544–6552.

Parsons J.C. (1991) Ascarid infections of cats and dogs. *Veterinary Clinics of North America: Small Animal Practice* **17**, 1307–1339.

Pensaert, M. and Maes, L. (1987) Pseudorabies virus (Aujezsky's disease). In: *Virus Infections of Vertebrates*, Vol. I: *Virus infections of carnivores* (Ed. M.J.G. Appel). Elsevier, Amsterdam, pp. 17–26.

Percy, D.H., Carmichael, L.E., Albert, D.M., King, J.M. and Jonas, A.M. (1971) Lesions in puppies surviving infection with canine herpesvirus. *Veterinary Pathology* **8**, 37–53.

Pollock, R.V.H. and Carmichael, L.E. (1982) Maternally-derived antibody to canine parvovirus: transfer, decline and interference with immunization. *Journal of the American Veterinary Medicine Association* **180**, 37–43.

Pollock, R.V.H. and Coyne, M.J. (1993) Canine parvovirus. *Veterinary Clinics of North America* **23**, 555–568

Poste, G. and King, N. (1971) Isolation of a herpesvirus from the canine genital tract: association with infertility, abortion and stillbirths. *Veterinary Record* **88**, 229–233.

Redwood, D.W. and Bell, D.A. (1983) *Salmonella panama*: isolation from aborted and newborn fetuses. *Veterinary Record* **112**, 362.

Robinson, W.F., Wilcox, G.E. and Flower, R.L.P. (1979) Evidence for a parvovirus as the aetiologic agent in myocarditis of puppies. *Australian Veterinary Journal* **55**, 294–295.

Rosendal, S. (1978) Canine mycoplasmas: pathogenicity of mycoplasmas associated with distemper pneumonia. *Journal of Infectious Diseases* **138**, 203–209.

Rosendal, S. (1982) Canine mycoplasma: their ecological niche and role in disease. *Journal of the American Veterinary Medical Association* **180**, 1212–1214.

Schwers, A., Pastoret, P.P., Burtonboy, G. and Thiry, E. (1979) Frequence en Belgique de l'infection a Parvovirus chez le chien avant et apres l'observation des primiers cas cliniques. *Annales Medicine Veterinaire* **123**, 561–565.

Shade, F.J. and Goodnow, R.A (1979) Intranasal immunisation of dogs against *Bordetella bronchiseptica*-induced tracheobronchitis (kennel cough) with modified live-*Bordetella bronchiseptica* vaccine. *American Journal of Veterinary Research* **40**, 1241–1243.

Swango, L.J., Wooding, W.L. and Binn, L.E. (1970) A comparison of the pathogenesis and antigenicity of infectious canine hepatitis virus and the A26/61 virus strain (Toronto). *Journal of the American Veterinary Medical Association* **156**, 1687–1699.

Taylor, D.J., Renton, J.P. and McGregor, A.B. (1975) *Brucella abortus* biotype I as a cause of abortion in a bitch. *Veterinary Record* **96**, 428–429.

Tennant, B.J., Gaskell, R.M., Jones, R.C. and Gaskell, C.J (1991) Prevalence of antibodies to four major viral diseases in dogs in a Liverpool hospital population. *Journal of Small Animal Practice* **32**, 175–179.

Thompson, H. and Wright, N.G. (1968) Canine salmonellosis. *Journal of Small Animal Practice* **10**, 579–582.

Thompson, H., McCandlish, I.A.P. and Wright, N.G. (1976) Experimental respiratory disease in dogs due to *Bordetella bronchiseptica*. *Research in Veterinary Science* **20**, 16–23.

Thompson, H., McCandlish, I.A.P., Cornwell, H.J.C.C., Macartney, L., Maxwell, N.S., Weipers, A.L., Wills, I.R.W., Black, J.A.C. and MacKenzie, A.C. (1988) Studies of parvovirus vaccination in the dog: the performance of live attenuated feline parvovirus vaccines. *Veterinary Record* **122**, 378–385.

Trees, A.J., Guy, F., Tennant, B.J., Balfour, A.H. and Dubey, J.P. (1993) Prevalence of antibodies to *Neosporum caninum* in a population of urban dogs in England. *Veterinary Record* **132**, 125–126.

Trees, A.J., Guy, F., Low, J.C., Roberts, L., Buxton, D. and Dubey, J.P. (1994) Serological evidence implicating Neospora species as a cause of abortion in British cattle. *Veterinary Record* **134**, 405–407.

Van den Broek, A.H.M., Thrushfield, M.V., Dobbie, G.R. and Ellis, W.A. (1991) A serological and bacteriological survey of leptospiral infection in dogs in Edinburgh and Glasgow. *Journal of Small Animal Practice* **32**, 118–124.

Vandevelde, M., Zurbriggen, A., Steck, A. and Bichsel, P. (1986) Studies on the intrathecal humoral immune response in canine distemper encephalitis. *Journal of Neuroimmunology* **11**, 41–51.

Wagener, J.S., Sobonya, R., Minnich, L and Taussig, L.M. (1984) Role of canine parainfluenza virus and *Bordetella bronchiseptica* in kennel cough. *American Journal of Veterinary Research* **45**, 1862–1866.

Wallace, B.L., Salsbury, D.L. and McMillen, J.K. (1985) In inactivated canine parvovirus vaccine: protection against virulent challenge. *Veterinary Medicine* **80**, 41–48.

Wessels, B.C. and Gaffin, S.L. (1986) Anti-endotoxin immunotherapy for canine parvovirus endotoxaemia. *Journal of Small Animal Practice* **27**, 609–615.

WHO Expert Committee on Rabies (1992) Eighth Report. WHO Technical Report Series, No 824, WHO, Geneva.

Wigton, D.H., Kociba, G.J. and Hoover, E.A. (1976) Infectious canine hepatitis: animal model for viral-induced disseminated intravascular coagulation. *Blood* **47**, 287–296.

Wilson, R.B., Holladay, J.A. and Cave, J.S. (1986) A neurologic syndrome associated with use of a canine coronavirus-parvovirus vaccine in dogs. *Compendium on Continuing Education for the Practicing Veterinarian* **8**, 117–124.

Woody, B.J. and Hoskins, J.D. (1991) Ehrlichial diseases of dogs. *Veterinary Clinics of North America: Small Animal Practice* **21**, 75–98.

Wright, N.G. (1976) Canine adenovirus: its role in renal and ocular lesions. *Journal of Small Animal Practice* **17**, 25–33.

Wright, N.G., Thompson, H. and Cornwell, H.J.C. (1971) Canine adenovirus pneumonia. *Research in Veterinary Science* **12**, 162–167.

FURTHER READING

Good reviews with comprehensive reference lists for virtually all canine infectious diseases are to be found in:

Greene, C.A. (Ed.) (1990) *Infectious Diseases of the Dog and Cat* (1990) W.B. Saunders, Philadelphia.

49

Infectious Diseases of the Cat

R. M. Gaskell and M. Bennett

Feline panleucopenia	959	Feline cowpox	974
Infectious upper respiratory disease complex	960	Other virus infections	976
Feline leukaemia virus	966	Cellulitis and abscess formation	977
Feline immunodeficiency virus	969	Other bacterial infections	978
Feline coronavirus infection	971	Miscellaneous infections	980
Enteric infections	973		

The aim of this chapter is to review the major infectious diseases of cats which are commonly encountered in the UK. Other, less common infections are also referred to which may occur in imported or quarantined animals or which are zoonotic.

FELINE PANLEUCOPENIA

Feline panleucopenia is a highly infectious disease found worldwide in domestic and big cats, and in some other species such as mink and racoon. However, in domestic cats in many parts of the world the disease has now largely been controlled by vaccination, and so clinical disease tends to occur only in animals from, for example, rescue catteries, where vaccination may not have been carried out.

Feline panleucopenia is caused by a parvovirus, a small, single-stranded DNA virus. Parvoviruses are very hardy and can readily survive outside their host. They are easily transmitted by personnel or on fomites and are resistant to many disinfectants. They may persist in infected premises for up to a year.

Pathogenesis

Infection is oronasal and the virus probably multiplies initially in oropharyngeal tissues (Greene and Scott, 1990; Gaskell, 1994). The virus then spreads to its main target tissues, the rapidly dividing cells of the bone marrow, lymphoid tissues, and intestinal epithelium, thus giving rise to the characteristic clinical signs of panleucopenia and enteritis. In fetal or newborn kittens, infection results in cerebellar hypoplasia and ataxia, whereas infection of the early embryo may result in resorption or abortion. The severity of disease is often made worse by secondary infections, for example in the gut, especially since the disease itself is immunosuppressive.

Clinical signs

Classic feline panleucopenia is primarily a disease of kittens, characterized by profound depression, pyrexia, anorexia, vomiting, dehydration, diarrhoea and often death (Carpenter, 1971; Greene and Scott, 1990). Diarrhoea may be a late sign and kittens may die before it becomes clinically apparent. Cats may be described as 'very depressed and sitting over a water bowl but not drinking'. Sometimes, however, the disease is much milder, with transient fever and leucopenia, and in many cases, infection is subclinical.

Feline ataxia, caused by infection of the fetal or neonatal cerebellum, is a non-progressive symmetrical ataxia often associated with an intention tremor. It is usually first recognized as kittens start to walk but in some cases may not be apparent until weaning. The severity varies according to the degree of cerebellar damage and not all the kittens in a litter are necessarily affected. The signs are non-progressive, and in many cases kittens learn to compensate and are able to live relatively normal lives. Such cats may be chronic virus excretors, however.

Overt abortion in cats is uncommon and embryonic death is usually apparent as reproductive failure. Feline panleucopenia virus infection and feline leukaemia virus infection are probably the two major infectious causes of feline reproductive failure. Care must be taken not to vaccinate pregnant cats with live feline panleucopenia vaccines.

Diagnosis

Diagnosis is often based on clinical signs, history and environment, and vaccination history. Demonstration of leucopenia is useful, but a definitive diagnosis is often only made at necropsy by histological examination of spleen, mesenteric lymph node, jejunum and ileum, or by virus detection. Virus is most readily isolated from faeces early in the disease or from spleen, mesenteric lymph node and intestinal mucosa collected at necropsy. The virus can be detected either by electron microscopy or by isolation in cell culture. However, the virus can be difficult to isolate and a negative result does not rule out the disease. Some, but not all, ELISA-based kits designed to detect canine parvovirus in faeces appear to work well for feline parvovirus. In cats which survive, demonstration of a rising antibody titre may also help to confirm the diagnosis.

Treatment

The treatment of enteric disease is largely supportive and includes the administration of fluids and use of antibiotics to control secondary bacterial infections; affected animals should be kept warm. Because of vomiting, impaired gut absorption and the immunosuppressive effects of the virus, a parenteral, bactericidal, broad spectrum antibiotic such as ampicillin or cephalosporin should be given. Antiemetics (e.g. acetylpromazine) may be useful in reducing fluid loss, but anticholinergic drugs (e.g. atropine) are not advisable because they can cause ileus. Nutritional supplements such as vitamins are sometimes given and hyperimmune antiserum may be useful. A blood transfusion may be considered in severely panleucopenic individuals. If the clinical signs are severe, however, the prognosis is poor.

During the later stages of the disease, if the cat appears to be recovering and gastroenteric signs have diminished, oral fluids and liquidized foods may be given. Oral or parenteral diazepam can also be used just before feeding to stimulate appetite.

Cats are often best nursed at home, but if hospitalized, scrupulous attention should be paid to hygiene and disinfection to avoid cross-infection.

Control

Both modified live and inactivated vaccines are available, and both have been very successful in controlling the disease (Povey, 1973; Gaskell, 1994). Modified live vaccines probably induce slightly better immunity and more rapid protection, but inactivated vaccines are entirely satisfactory and have the advantage that they can be used in pregnant queens. Immunity probably lasts for several years following the use of modified live vaccines, and for at least one year with inactivated vaccines. It is usually recommended that kittens are vaccinated initially at 12 weeks of age, when maternally derived antibody will have declined to non-interfering levels in most cats, with first boosters at one year of age and further doses at 1–2-year intervals depending on the type of vaccine used and the likelihood of exposure.

Management in the face of disease is based on vaccination and good hygiene. The virus is very resistant to many disinfectants and only hypochlorite (household bleach, diluted 1 in 32) or formaldehyde- or glutaraldehyde-based preparations are effective (Scott, 1980). Hypochlorite is best used with washing-up liquid to improve its cleaning properties. Thorough disinfection of the premises and all utensils is necessary. Despite this, persistence in the environment can still be a problem. Ideally the premises should be completely depopulated for several months. Failing this, cats should at least not be moved onto or from the premises and all breeding should stop. Live vaccines should be used to ensure rapid and strong immunity in the face of disease, except in pregnant queens, where inactivated vaccines should be given.

INFECTIOUS UPPER RESPIRATORY DISEASE COMPLEX

Despite the advent of vaccination in the mid-1970s, infectious respiratory disease in cats still occurs, although vaccination has probably reduced the overall severity of the condition seen.

Aetiology

The causes of infectious upper respiratory disease (URD) in cats are listed in Table 49.1, together with an estimate of their clinical significance. Feline herpesvirus 1 (FHV 1), also known as feline viral rhinotracheitis (FVR) virus, and feline calicivirus (FCV) are the two major causes of respiratory disease in cats (Gaskell and Dawson, 1994). Both are widespread in the cat population and have generally been considered to be of equal importance in causing the disease. In more recent years, however, we have observed a slightly higher isolation rate of FCV than expected compared to FHV 1 (Knowles et al., 1989). This may be explained in part by the antigenic diversity among FCV isolates compared to the one serotype of feline herpesvirus, and the consequent relative efficacy of the two vaccines.

The feline strain of *Chlamydia psittaci* can also cause mild respiratory signs but in general the major feature of *C. psittaci* infection is persistent or recurrent conjunctivitis (Wills and Gaskell, 1994). Feline reovirus has been shown to produce a mild, predominantly conjunctival disease experimentally but is probably not a very significant cause of naturally occurring URD.

Bacteria (e.g. staphylococci, streptococci, *Pasteurella* spp. and coliforms) and mycoplasmas are mainly important as secondary invaders, although a more primary role has been suspected for some *Mycoplasma* spp. The role of *Bordetella bronchiseptica* in feline URD is also currently being reassessed. It has been known for some time that this organism may be involved in respiratory disease in laboratory cat colonies, but more recently there have been a number of cases reported from cats in the field (Willoughby et al., 1991; Welsh, 1996) associated with *B. bronchiseptica* infection. It is not clear whether the organism is mainly important as a secondary pathogen or whether it plays a more primary role, as in dogs. Recently URD signs have been induced experimentally with *B. bronchiseptica* infection in specific-pathogen-free cats (Jacobs et al., 1993; Coutts et al., 1996) and studies have shown that infection with the organism in the general cat population is widespread (McArdle et al., 1994).

Finally, the pathogenicity of all agents, including secondary invaders, may be enhanced especially as a result of concurrent immunosuppressive illness, for example, infection with feline leukaemia virus (FeLV) or feline immunodeficiency virus (FIV).

Clinical signs

FHV infection is generally a severe disease characterized by pyrexia, sneezing, hypersalivation, conjunctivitis, and marked ocular and nasal discharges (Fig. 49.1; Gaskell and Dawson, 1994). More rarely, ulcerative keratitis, lingual or skin ulcers, lower respiratory tract involvement or generalized, multisystem infection may also occur.

Feline calicivirus infection is typically milder than FHV infection. General malaise is less

Table 49.1 The causes and significance of infectious respiratory disease in the cat

Agent	Clinical significance
Feline herpesvirus	One of two major causes. Clinical signs tend to be more severe
Feline calicivirus	One of two major causes. Usually mild clinical signs with oral ulcers
Feline *Chlamydia psittaci*	Approximately 30% cases of persistent conjunctivitis
Feline reovirus	Mild disease experimentally; probably of little clinical significance
Cowpox virus	Occasional respiratory/ocular signs but skin signs also usually present
Bordetella bronchiseptica	Some laboratory colonies; may also be important in the field
Other bacteria, e.g. staphylococci, streptococci, *Pasteurella* spp. and coliforms	Mainly secondary invaders
Mycoplasmas	Possibly primary, but usually secondary

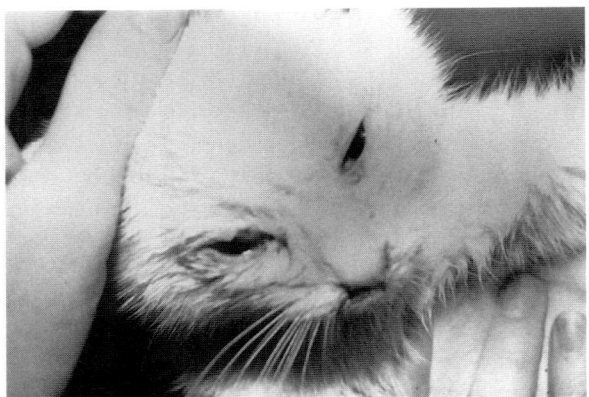

Figure 49.1 Oculonasal discharge in a cat infected with feline herpesvirus. See colour plate.

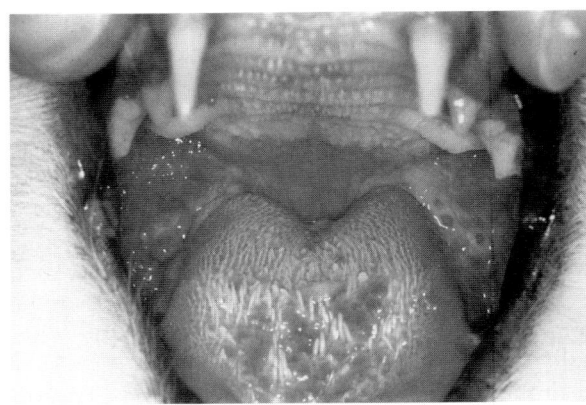

Figure 49.3 Chronic stomatitis and ulceration of the fauces associated with feline calicivirus infection. Photograph courtesy of Michael Herrtage.

common, discharges are usually much less copious, and ulceration of the tongue, hard palate or external nares is a characteristic feature (Fig. 49.2). Indeed such ulceration may occur unaccompanied by upper respiratory or ocular signs. Occasionally skin ulcers may occur. However, there are a large number of strains of FCV in comparison with the single strain of FHV and these may differ slightly in pathogenicity. Many strains of FCV induce a febrile lameness which may or may not be accompanied by respiratory and oral signs (Pedersen et al., 1983; Reubel et al., 1992; Dawson et al., 1993, 1994). Other strains have been described that induce a primary interstitial pneumonia, and with some isolates the infection is only subclinical. FCV may also be involved in the aetiology of chronic stomatitis (Fig. 49.3); in some studies a high proportion of cats with chronic stomatitis are FCV carriers (Thompson et al., 1984; Knowles et al., 1989) and it has now been shown that the virus may induce acute faucitis (Reubel et al., 1992). However, many cats with chronic oral disease are also infected with FIV and the role of each virus in inducing this syndrome is not clear.

C. psittaci is mainly a conjunctival pathogen (Wills and Gaskell, 1994). In the acute stages there is blepharospasm and marked ocular discharge, and the conjunctivae appear reddened and swollen. Initially only one eye may be affected, but usually both eyes are eventually involved. Mild URD may also occur, and although mild pulmonary lesions may be seen at necropsy, clinical signs of pneumonia are not usually seen. The conjunctivitis may persist for up to 6 weeks and, although most animals recover, recurrent or persistent signs may occur. Thus, although there may be considerable overlap between FHV, FCV and C. psittaci infection, some distinction may be drawn from the predominant clinical signs.

In studies where *Bordetella bronchiseptica* is the sole pathogen, clinical signs include pyrexia, sneezing, nasal discharge, submandibular lymphadenopathy, spontaneous or induced coughing and rahles at auscultation. Signs generally resolve within 10 days (Jacobs et al., 1993; Coutts et al., 1996). In many cases in the field, however, other factors such as stress, overcrowding and intercurrent disease may lead to more severe disease such as bronchopneumonia.

■ Diagnosis

Often an adequate diagnosis may be made on the basis of presenting clinical signs, but where a definitive diagnosis is required confirmatory lab-

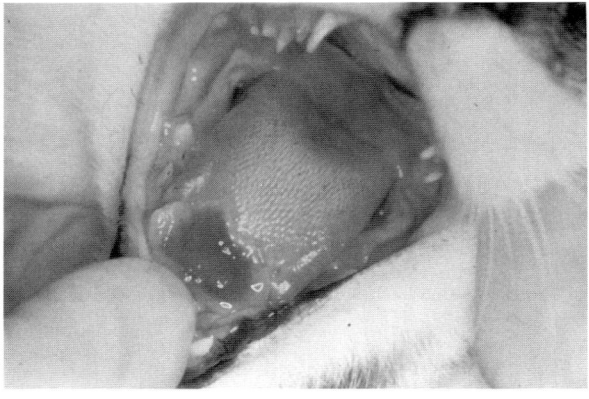

Figure 49.2 Tongue ulcers caused by feline calicivirus.

oratory tests are necessary. For the respiratory viruses, an oropharyngeal swab should be taken, placed in viral transport medium and sent by first class post to a laboratory for attempted virus isolation. Confirmatory tests for the presence of *C. psittaci* entail sending a conjunctival swab sent in special transport medium to an appropriate laboratory for attempted isolation of the organism or for testing by ELISA for the presence of antigen (Wills *et al.*, 1986). The conjunctival swab should be taken firmly to ensure the presence of epithelial cells in the sample. Conjunctival cytology to look for the presence of inclusion bodies is often difficult to interpret. More recently, PCR has been used in some laboratories for the diagnosis of both respiratory viruses and *C. psittaci* infection. *B. bronchiseptica* infection is best diagnosed from oral or nasal swabs sent in charcoal Amies transport medium to a laboratory for attempted isolation on selective medium such as charcoal–cephalexin agar.

Serology is generally not helpful in the diagnosis of respiratory virus infection because of widespread immunity from vaccination. However, serology can sometimes be helpful in establishing a possible diagnosis of *C. psittaci* infection in cats which have not been vaccinated against the disease.

Treatment

At present no antiviral drugs are in widespread use to control FHV 1 and FCV infections. However, 5-iododeoxyuridine (IUdR) has been used in cases of ulcerative keratitis associated with FHV 1 infection, and there are anti-herpesvirus drugs that have been developed for use in other species that may prove useful in FHV 1 infection, although at present none are licensed for use in animals. Trifluridine, for example, has good *in vitro* activity against FHV 1; acyclovir, however, does not inhibit FHV 1 replication.

Broad-spectrum antibiotics (such as ampicillin, potentiated sulphonamide and oxytetracycline) should be used to help control secondary bacterial infection and prevent chronic sequelae. Animals should be re-examined after 4–5 days and antibiotics continued if necessary. If there is no improvement after a week of treatment, bacterial culture and sensitivity testing should be performed. For *C. psittaci* or *B. bronchiseptica* infection oxytetracycline or doxycycline are the drugs of choice (see below).

Good nursing care is essential and is best given at home, since hospital intensive care requires an isolation unit and scrupulous hygiene to prevent cross-infection. Nebulizers and steam inhalation to clear airways are better tolerated by cats than nasal decongestants.

In severe cases, subcutaneous or intravenous fluids may be indicated for dehydration, and when anorexia is prolonged the use of a nasogastric tube may be indicated.

Epizootiology

Feline respiratory viruses

Both FHV 1 and FCV are highly successful pathogens of the cat, although infection is more common in colony animals than in individual household pets. Thus the disease occurs mainly in boarding catteries, breeding colonies, stray-cat homes or other situations where large numbers of cats have been brought together.

The feline respiratory viruses persist in the cat population in three main ways: firstly, by passing directly from acutely infected to susceptible animals. This depends on the presence of both sufficient susceptible animals in the population and sufficient opportunities for contact between them.

Secondly, they can persist in the environment. Although FHV and FCV can only survive outside a host for a relatively short time (FHV for up to 24 h, FCV for up to a week), it is nevertheless long enough for indirect transmission to occur, particularly within the close confines of a cattery where secretions may contaminate cages, feeding or cleaning utensils, or personnel. Aerosol transmission is thought to be relatively unimportant. Cats do not normally produce a fine particle infectious aerosol, although macrodroplets may be sneezed over a distance of 1–2 m.

Thirdly, the respiratory viruses may persist in the recovered cat by means of carriers. Despite vaccination, recent figures indicate that such carriers still seem to be widespread in the population and are of considerable importance as a source of virus. There are no known reservoir or alternative hosts for the viruses and vertical transmission does not seem to occur.

The carrier states are different for the two viruses (Gaskell and Dawson, 1994). In FHV infection at least 80% of cats become carriers. The virus is mostly latent, but periodically the cat undergoes episodes of virus shedding in oral and nasal secretions when it can infect other animals. These episodes of shedding may occur at any time, but are more likely to occur after a stress, such as a change of environment (for example, going to a cat show, to stud, or into a boarding cattery) or during lactation. Treatment with corticosteroids may also induce virus shedding. Virus shedding usually does not start until about a week after the stressful episode, and may then continue for up to two weeks. In some cases, shedding carriers may show mild clinical signs.

Unlike FHV carriers, FCV carriers shed virus more-or-less continuously in oral secretions. Such animals are therefore a constant source of infection to susceptible cats. After infection, most cats shed feline calicivirus for several weeks, but then, after a variable time, individual animals appear to eliminate the virus. However, some animals remain lifelong carriers. It has been found that FIV infection may increase both the amount and duration of shedding after FCV challenge (Dawson et al., 1991; Reubel et al., 1994).

FCV carriers may be classified into high, medium or low level carriers, depending on the amount of virus that they normally shed. Although all are infectious, virus is more easily spread from high level carriers. Low level carriers are not so infectious and may be more difficult to detect, requiring several oropharyngeal swabs to be taken over a period of 4–6 weeks. FCV carriers are very common in the general cat population; before vaccination was introduced, approximately 40% of colony cats, 25% of show cats and 8% of household pets were carrying the virus. Recent surveys have confirmed the virus is still widespread. Approximately 20% of general practice and hospital cases, examined for reasons other than respiratory disease, and 25% of apparently healthy show cats are positive for FCV (Knowles et al., 1989; Harbour et al., 1991; Coutts et al., 1994).

Feline C.psittaci *infection*

Although many species of animals and birds are susceptible to *C. psittaci* infection, there are a number of strains of the organism with different tropisms, pathogenicity and host specificity. Although some are zoonotic, the feline strain generally appears to be species specific. Like the feline respiratory viruses, chlamydial infection is probably transmitted mainly by direct or fomite contact with infectious discharges from acutely or chronically infected cats. Clinical signs may persist or recur for some time and shedding may persist for several months. The organism is found mainly in ocular secretions. Vaginal and rectal shedding has also been recorded in experimentally infected cats but the epidemiological significance of this is unknown.

Bordetella bronchiseptica *infection*

B. bronchiseptica is widespread in the cat population; surveys have shown that the majority of cats have antibody and the organism has been isolated from up to 11% of cats with or without respiratory disease (McArdle et al., 1994; Binns et al., 1995). Some of these cats appear to be clinically healthy carriers. Although infection is widespread, disease tends to occur in colony situations where other factors, such as stress and overcrowding and infection with other respiratory pathogens, may also play a role. Whether or not interspecies transmission (e.g. cats to dogs) occurs in the field has not yet been established.

Prevention and control

Viral respiratory disease

There are three types of vaccine available in the UK for the protection of cats against viral respiratory disease: modified live systemic, modified live intranasal and inactivated adjuvanted systemic (Gaskell, 1981, 1989; Gaskell and Dawson, 1994). Generally, such vaccines are reasonably effective in providing protection against clinical disease, though not necessarily against infection, and all may be used with reasonable confidence in routine vaccination programmes. However, they do have some limitations and control is best attempted through a combination of vaccination and management.

All household pets should be regularly vaccinated. Cats are most likely to be exposed to the respiratory viruses when entering a boarding cattery or a veterinary hospital. Ideally a friend or neighbour should feed the cat while the owner is on holiday to avoid stress and contact with other cats. If the cat does go to a boarding cattery, then it should be given a booster vaccination before entry unless it has been vaccinated within the previous 6 months.

All cats admitted to a boarding cattery should have an up-to-date vaccination record. Where vaccination has lapsed for longer than 18 months it is advisable to give a full course. In exceptional circumstances, when rapid protection is required, intranasal vaccine may be used. However, such vaccines may themselves induce mild clinical signs.

However, cattery owners should not rely solely on vaccination for disease control, since virus will inevitably be present in the cattery either from the occasional animal incubating the disease or, more likely, from carriers. Thus, precautions should still be taken to prevent any possible cross-infection and reduce the concentration of virus in the environment. A suitable disinfectant is a 1 in 32 dilution of hypochlorite (common bleach) in water with washing-up liquid. Cats should be housed individually unless they are from the same household and cages should have solid sides or be at least 1.5 m apart.

In disease-free breeding colonies cats should be vaccinated routinely. Inactivated vaccines are preferable, though if administered carefully, modified live vaccines should be satisfactory. Great care should be taken to avoid bringing virus into the colony; *any* cat with a history of respiratory disease or from a household with a history of respiratory disease may be a carrier. Cats can become infected subclinically under cover of maternal or vaccine-induced immunity. Cats entering the colony should be quarantined for 3 weeks with oropharyngeal swabs taken for virus isolation at least twice a week during this time. However this may still not detect a latent FHV-1 carrier or a very low-level FCV carrier. Since FIV infection seems to potentiate FCV infection, it is probably wise to test for FIV, and indeed FeLV, as well.

In breeding colonies where the disease is endemic, in some circumstances it may be feasible to restock the colony with virus-free cats and to employ a barrier system to keep the viruses out. However, in many situations, the only reasonable course is to attempt disease control. This may be done by:

1. Regular vaccination programmes including booster vaccination of queens either before mating or during pregnancy (if the latter, by using an appropriate inactivated vaccine only);
2. Avoiding the use of particular queens with a history of respiratory disease in their kittens;
3. Isolation of queens at least 3 weeks before kittening;
4. Early weaning of kittens into isolation away from their mother (ideally at 4–5 weeks) if it is likely she is a carrier;
5. Vaccinating all kittens as soon as maternally derived antibodies are at a non-interfering level (normally at nine or more weeks old);
6. In some cases, earlier vaccination, starting a week or so before past experience suggests that kittens generally become affected. Both intranasal and systemic vaccines have been suggested for this, but the intranasal vaccine is probably more useful in very young kittens as it may be better than some vaccines at overcoming maternally derived antibody. However, it is not licensed for use in kittens less than 12 weeks of age and thus should only be used after discussion with the owner, and if the colony is known to have some immunity to both respiratory viruses. Systemic vaccines should be given at 3-week intervals until 12 weeks of age, and the intranasal vaccine should be given, for example, at 4–5 weeks of age and then again at 12 weeks.

Vaccine reactions and breakdowns

Probably the most common reason for apparent vaccine reactions (i.e. when respiratory signs appear within a week or so of vaccination) is that the cat is already incubating the disease at the time of vaccination (Dawson and Gaskell, 1993). This is especially the case for young kittens which are generally vaccinated just as their maternally derived antibody wanes. There are also a number of other possible reasons for apparent vaccine reactions. For example, the cat might be a carrier, or a systemic vaccine may have inadvertently been given oronasally, in which case it may induce clinical signs. Experimentally it has been shown that some vaccine viruses given subcutaneously may spread to the oropharynx (Bennett *et al.*, 1989; Pedersen and Floyd-Hawkins, 1995).

Apparent vaccine breakdowns may also be explained in a number of ways. Even under ideal conditions, protection against disease is not necessarily complete in all animals. Vaccination does not eliminate infection from cats that are already carriers, and in general does not protect cats against the development of a carrier state. In addition, intercurrent disease (especially with FIV or FeLV), overwhelming infection or maternally-derived antibody may interfere with the vaccination programme.

It is also becoming increasingly apparent that present vaccines probably do not protect against all isolates of calicivirus and future vaccines may need to incorporate several complementary, cross-protective isolates. Finally it should be emphasized that apparent breakdowns may be due to infection with agents such as *C. psittaci* or *B. bronchiseptica* not included in the virus vaccines.

Feline Chlamydia psittaci *infection*

The prevention and control of chlamydial infection should be approached both by good management and the effective use of antibiotics. Since persistent or recurrent infection is common, all cats in a colony should be treated at the same time. Although several antibiotics may have some effect on the organism, the antibiotics of choice are oxytetracycline or doxycycline. Since the organism may generalize, systemic treatment should be given in addition to topical ophthalmic preparations. Treatment should also be continued for at least four weeks, or two weeks after clinical signs have disappeared, because the organism can be difficult to eradicate.

Both live and inactivated vaccines are available against *C. psittaci* infection. Although there has been discussion in the past as to the efficacy of such vaccines, more recent studies have indicated some protection against clinical disease, although not necessarily against infection or shedding of the organism.

Bordetella bronchiseptica *infection*

Although tetracycline and doxycycline are indicated in the acute phase of disease, treatment with doxycycline does not seem to eliminate infection from carriers (Coutts *et al.*, 1996). Prevention and control are probably best achieved therefore by good husbandry and hygiene measures which will reduce the level of infection in a household. An inactivated subunit vaccine against *B. bronchiseptica* infection in cats is available in some countries and, as in dogs, intranasal vaccines may also prove to be useful.

FELINE LEUKAEMIA VIRUS

Feline leukaemia virus (FeLV) is often cited as the most common infectious cause of death in young adult cats. It is a retrovirus in the mammalian type C retrovirus genus. Persistent infection eventually gives rise to one of several clinical syndromes including lymphosarcoma and other haemopoietic malignancies, immunodeficiency, anaemia and reproductive failure.

Pathogenesis

Virus is excreted from infected cats in saliva, urine, faeces and milk and the usual means of spread is by close contact and licking (Jarrett, 1994). Following infection, virus replicates in the oropharynx and may then spread to other lymphoid tissues, especially the bone marrow. Many cats mount an immune response which eliminates the virus at an early stage before it reaches the bone marrow.

In some cats, however, more extensive virus replication in the bone marrow can give rise to viraemia and widespread infection, especially in lymphoid tissues and the epithelial cells of the oropharynx, salivary glands and upper respiratory tract, with consequent virus excretion and transmission to other cats. At this stage cats may still mount an effective immune response and eliminate active infection (giving rise to a transient viraemia lasting between 2 days and 8 weeks), but some cats will develop persistent infection. It is these persistently infected cats which eventually go on to develop clinical disease.

The extent of virus spread varies according to the age of the cat and the dose of virus received. Fetuses and newborn kittens are the most susceptible to infection and congenital infection occurs in all kittens born to persistently infected queens. All such kittens will be persistently infected themselves. The susceptibility of kittens to infection decreases with age, such that it is unusual for persistent infection to develop in a cat over 16 weeks old. Cats with virus neutralizing (VN) antibodies are resistant to infection and VN antibody in colostrum can protect kittens, often for the first 4 weeks of life.

The dose of virus received depends largely on the kittens' environment. Among free range cats the amount of contact between excreting and susceptible cats is limited, the dose is therefore small and, although most cats become infected, very few develop persistent infection. In many multicat households, however, the degree of contact and therefore exposure to virus is high and in this situation up to 30% of kittens can become persistently infected.

Over half the cats which apparently recover from FeLV infection develop latent infection in bone marrow. Virus release from latent infections is generally too low to be detected or to infect epithelial cells and latently infected cats are therefore rarely sources of infection to other cats. However, virus excretion in milk has been recorded from a latently infected queen (Pacitti *et al.*, 1986). Latent infections are usually eliminated, although around 10% of cats can remain latently infected for at least three years (Pacitti 1987). For useful discussions of the mechanisms and pathogenesis of FeLV-related disease refer to Hoover and Mullins (1991) and Rojko and Kociba (1991).

Clinical signs

Persistent FeLV infection is associated with a high mortality rate. In one survey 85% of persistently viraemic cats died within 3.5 years of exposure compared with 15% of uninfected cats and in another survey 50% of cats developed FeLV-related disease and died within 6 months of diagnosis of persistent viraemia (McClelland et al., 1980). The clinical syndromes associated with FeLV infection are mainly associated with infection of the haemopoietic system although the exact pathogenic mechanisms are often not known. In addition, FeLV is often associated with reproductive failure.

Neoplasia

The most common haemopoietic malignancy in the cat is lymphosarcoma, which accounts for 90% of haemopoietic tumours and approximately one third of all feline tumours. Most cases of lymphosarcoma in the cat are associated with FeLV infection. Although some cats with lymphosarcoma, particularly alimentary lymphosarcoma, are not FeLV antigenaemic, epidemiological evidence suggests that some of these cases may be associated with past virus infection and it is worth checking the FeLV status of other cats in the household where such cases occur.

Feline lymphosarcoma can be divided into four main types: thymic lymphosarcoma, multicentric lymphosarcoma, alimentary lymphosarcoma and lymphoid leukaemia.

Thymic lymphosarcoma is mainly seen in cats under 3 years old and involves the thymus and sometimes local lymph nodes. Clinical signs include tachypnoea, dyspnoea, regurgitation and weight loss, due mainly to the space-occupying effects of the tumour. Pleural fluid containing neoplastic lymphoid cells is often present and may cause muffled heart sounds. It is often possible to palpate increased thoracic resistance. Diagnosis is based on radiography (Fig. 49.4), cytology of pleural fluid (Fig. 49.5) and testing for FeLV antigenaemia; 80% of cases are FeLV positive.

Multicentric lymphosarcoma is seen in cats with an average age of 4 years and is characterized by gross peripheral lymphadenopathy (Fig. 49.6) and an enlarged spleen. Affected cats are also often mildly anaemic. Diagnosis is by histopathological examination of lymph node biopsy. Approximately 60% of these cats are FeLV positive.

Alimentary lymphosarcoma is a disease of older

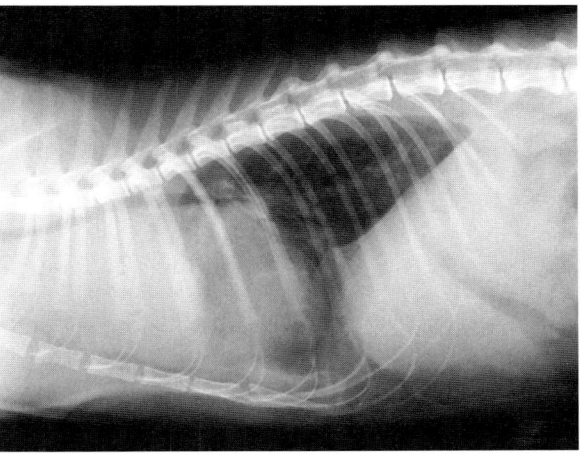

Figure 49.4 Lateral radiograph of a cat's thorax. The cranial mediastinal mass is a thymic lymphosarcoma. Photograph J.K. Dunn.

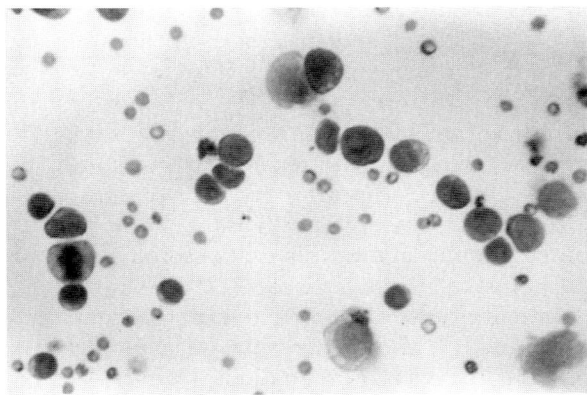

Figure 49.5 Pleural fluid from a cat with thymic lymphosarcoma containing a mixed population of medium-sized lymphocytes and larger lymphoblasts with prominent nucleoli. Note the variation in cell size and nuclear:cytoplasmic ratio. Photograph J.K. Dunn.

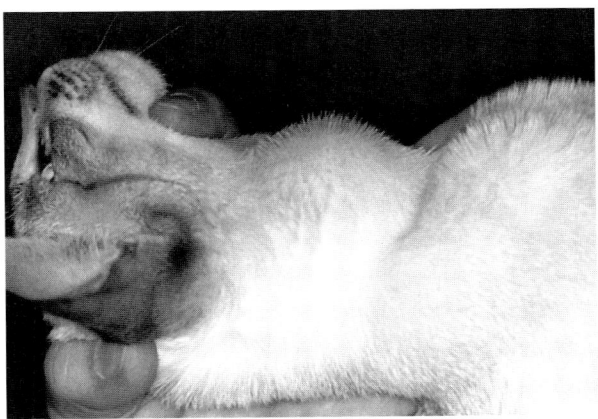

Figure 49.6 Marked enlargement of the submandibular and prescapular lymph nodes in a Siamese cat with multicentric lymphosarcoma. Photograph courtesy of Michael Herrtage.

cats (average age 8 years) characterized by the presence of abdominal masses, mainly between duodenum and colon, although sometimes the tumours are more diffuse. Mesenteric lymph nodes and occasionally the kidneys may also be involved. Clinical signs include anorexia, weight loss, vomiting (if there is high obstruction) or sometimes diarrhoea. Affected cats are often anaemic. Diagnosis is based on the clinical signs, abdominal palpation, radiography and laparotomy. Only 30% of cats with alimentary lymphosaroma are FeLV positive.

Lymphoid leukaemia primarily involves the bone marrow, and haematogenous spread of leukaemic cells often results in secondary infiltration of other organs such as the liver and spleen. The proliferation of neoplastic lymphocytes and lymphoblasts may also affect normal haemopoiesis. Thus, affected cats often have a raised white cell count and may be both anaemic and thrombocytopenic; the latter, if severe, may cause petechial haemorrhages on the skin and mucous membranes. Clinical signs include pyrexia, weakness, loss of appetite, often an enlarged spleen but rarely enlarged lymph nodes. Blood smears will often contain neoplastic cells. A bone marrow biopsy aspirate may also be useful. Approximately 60% affected cats are FeLV positive.

In addition to the above, lymphosarcoma may also involve the kidneys, nose, eyes, central nervous system (CNS) or skin.

Myeloid leukaemia is relatively uncommon and may involve granulocytes or erythroid cells or both. It arises in bone marrow but secondary neoplastic infiltrates may be found in the liver, spleen and lymph nodes. Clinical signs include progressive anaemia, intermittent pyrexia and weight loss. Thrombocytopenia may result in petechial haemorrhage, and leucopenia may cause immunosuppression and secondary infections. Diagnosis is based on bone marrow aspiration biopsy and haematology. The majority of affected cats are FeLV positive, the main exception being cats with eosinophilic leukaemia which are usually, but not always, FeLV negative (Swenson *et al.*, 1993).

Non-neoplastic FeLV related disease
Anaemia
Anaemia is relatively common in cats compared to other species and FeLV infection is probably the most important cause of anaemia in cats. It may be primary or the result of lymphoid or myeloid leukaemia interfering with normal haemopoiesis. Primary red cell aplasia causes a rapid onset, normocytic, normochromic, non-regenerative anaemia. The PCV often drops to less than 10% but the white cell count is normal. More rarely, anaemia may be associated with total marrow aplasia, with severe leucopenia and thrombocytopenia, weight loss, anorexia and pyrexia. FeLV-related haemolytic anaemia may also be common, but is usually mild and therefore often goes undiagnosed.

Immunosuppression
The pathogenic mechanism underlying FeLV-induced immunosuppression is complex and not at all well understood. It seems associated more with some strains of virus than others and the minor envelope protein p15E may play a role in its development. Immunosuppressed cats are susceptible to various secondary infections and the clinical signs may therefore be very similar to those described for FIV infection. Anaemia associated with *Haemobartonella felis* infection is more common in FeLV-infected cats than in uninfected cats and FeLV-infected cats are especially susceptible to respiratory and enteric infections. They may also be subject to non-healing skin wounds or persistent abscesses. An FeLV-associated 'panleukopenia-like' enteritis has also been reported.

Reproductive failure
FeLV is said to be the most common cause of reproductive failure in cats. Resorption of the fetus occurs at 3–5 weeks into pregnancy and may be accompanied by a slight vulval discharge. The precise mechanism of fetal damage is not known but may involve placentitis or endometritis. Infection of fetuses with FeLV can also be a cause of neonatal mortality (fading kittens).

∎ Treatment

Treatment of FeLV-related anaemias, immunosuppression and reproductive failure involves non-specific, supportive therapy only. Little success has been reported for treatment of either lymphoid or myeloid leukaemias. However, remission for 2 years for up to 60% of cats can be achieved by treatment of thymic and multicentric lymphosarcomas, although such cats still excrete virus. Several treatment protocols have been published, mainly involving long term treatment with cyclophosphamide, vincristine and prednisolone (Squires and Gorman, 1990). Cats should be carefully monitored for possible side effects of such therapy.

Testing and control

Several companies market ELISA, CITE or similar assays to test blood, serum, plasma or saliva for FeLV antigen and some laboratories use an immunofluorescence test to detect FeLV antigen in neutrophils. Some laboratories also offer a virus isolation service. Although agreement between ELISA-type assays, immunofluorescence tests and virus isolation on plasma or blood is good, some cats (approximately 10%) may be antigenaemic by ELISA but negative by virus isolation or immunofluorescence. The reasons for this are not entirely clear; some kits can give false positive results but some cats may have a focus of infection that releases antigen but not virus into the blood. ELISA-positive, virus isolation-negative cats are not thought to be a significant source of infection to other cats, although one such queen was shown to infect her kittens via the milk (Pacitti et al, 1986). Discordant cats should be isolated and re-tested in 12 weeks since some of them may have been undergoing a transient infection.

Control is best done by testing all the cats in a colony and separating those that are antigenaemic from those that are not. All the cats should then be tested 12 weeks later to distinguish persistently infected cats from those which are transiently infected. Any cats which test positive only on the second occasion need to be quarantined for a further 12 weeks before being retested. Cats which test positive on both occasions, i.e. persistently infected cats, should be removed from the colony. All the cats should be re-tested every 6–12 months. No cats should enter the colony during the test period, and thereafter all incoming cats should be tested and isolated for 12 weeks, and then re-tested before being allowed to mix with the other cats.

Several FeLV vaccines are available in the UK which require two initial immunizations three weeks apart and annual boosters. Cats can be first vaccinated at 8–9 weeks old. Under experimental conditions at least, available vaccines appear effective at preventing persistent infection in the majority of cats, but vaccination should not be used as a replacement for a test-and-remove policy for control in a colony.

FELINE IMMUNODEFICIENCY VIRUS

Feline immunodeficiency virus (FIV) is a lentivirus of cats related structurally, biochemically and genetically to human immunodeficiency virus (HIV), the cause of AIDS in humans. There is, however, no evidence of human infection with FIV.

Epidemiology

FIV is found world-wide. The virus has been isolated from domestic cats and closely related viruses have been found in other fields in zoos and the wild. The prevalence of infection in domestic cats varies with their disease status, life-style and age; generally about 20% of random 'sick cats' have antibody to FIV compared with less than 5% of healthy cats (Hopper et al., 1994). Many surveys have shown that the infection rate in males is at least twice that in females, that most infected cats are middle aged or old, and that infection is most common in free-roaming cats, feral cats, and multicat households (but not usually breeding or pedigree colony cats). In feral colonies and multicat households the prevalence of antibody ranges from 0 to 100%, with an average of 30% for feral cats and 50% for multicat households. Approximately 35% of cats in contact with an infected cat will have antibody.

The main route of virus transmission is thought to be through biting, although some instances of apparent vertical spread have been reported. Virus can be isolated not only from the lymphocytes of infected cats but also from the saliva, especially of clinically ill cats.

Clinical signs

FIV infection is associated with a variety of clinical signs or syndromes (Hosie et al., 1989; Pedersen et al., 1989), particularly chronic stomatitis and gingivitis, chronic respiratory disease, intermittent pyrexia, depression, lymphadenopathy, emaciation and, less frequently, chronic diarrhoea and chronic skin disease. Many cats also have ocular lesions or show signs of CNS infection. Haematological changes, especially anaemia, leucopenia and marked lymphopenia are common and many cats are hypergammaglobulinaemic.

Few studies have been done on the prevalence of FIV in specific disease syndromes, although several studies have suggested an association between FIV and feline calicivirus infection in cats with chronic stomatitis and gingivitis (Knowles et al., 1989; Tenorio et al.,1991; Waters et al., 1993). FIV should be strongly suspected in adult cats showing signs of chronic debilitating disease (especially chronic infection) and also in cats with neurological signs and/or behavioural changes.

Diagnosis

Diagnosis is based on antibody tests and virus isolation. ELISA and CITE tests are commercially available for the detection of antibody and some kits can be bought as combined FIV and feline leukaemia virus (FeLV) kits for practice laboratories. Some laboratories use in-house ELISAs or immunofluorescence assays, and some also use western blots or radioimmune precipitation assays (RIPA) to test for antibody. Antibody test results should be interpreted with care. Occasional 'false' negative results may be obtained as severely ill cats may have low or no detectable antibody – a similar phenomenon is seen in terminal AIDS in humans – and false positive results have also been reported with the ELISA and CITE kits. Because of the long period of asymptomatic infection before the development of clinical disease (see pathogenesis), many FIV-infected cats are perfectly healthy and it is important to remember that the detection of antibody does not necessarily mean that FIV is the cause of any current disease.

Virus isolation is very expensive. It involves the collection of 1–5 ml of heparinized blood into special media and culture of lymphocytes from the sample. It may take a month or more before the presence or absence of virus can be confirmed. Future developments, however, may include antigen capture ELISAs which work directly on saliva or blood, and more routine use of molecular techniques such as the polymerase chain reaction (PCR) for rapid virus detection.

Pathogenesis

A summary of some of the main features of the pathogenesis of FIV infection is shown in Fig. 49.7. Inoculation with FIV generally results in seroconversion by 3–4 weeks and the development of lymphadenopathy at around 6 weeks after infection. Some haematological changes may develop, especially lymphocytosis. This primary stage appears to be essentially self-limiting and lasts several months. Cats may have intermittent pyrexia and secondary infections, e.g. bacterial skin infections, and vaccination against other pathogens may not be effective at this stage of

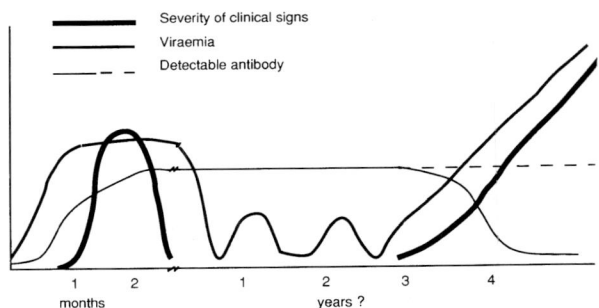

Figure 49.7 Possible pathogenesis of FIV infection.

infection. After a few months the lympadenopathy subsides and virus may become increasingly difficult to isolate with time.

End-stage disease usually does not develop for several years. The mechanism of the final immune suppression is not known. Like HIV, FIV infects T lymphocytes, especially CD4 T lymphocytes, macrophages and CNS cells, and a gradual decrease in CD4:CD8 T lymphocyte ratios and lymphoproliferation responses can be detected by about 10 months post-infection (Barlough *et al*, 1991).

Treatment and control

Treatment is based on nursing and treatment for secondary pathogens. Antibiotics can be used to help control secondary and opportunist bacterial infections. Corticosteroids or megoestrol acetate may also help moderate systemic signs but probably have little long-term beneficial effect. Some of the drugs being developed or used to treat HIV infection in humans also inhibit FIV in cell culture (Smyth *et al.*, 1994a) and some clinical effect has been claimed for 9-(2-phosphonomethoxyethyl) adenine (PMEA) and 3′-azido-3-deoxythymidine (AZT; zidovudine, Wellcome Foundation) in cats (Egberink *et al.*, 1991; Hartmann *et al.*, 1992). However, treatment of experimentally infected cats with AZT has generally given disappointing results (Hayes *et al.*, 1993; Meers *et al.*, 1993; Smyth *et al.*, 1994b) and we have had little success treating natural cases presented at Liverpool University Small Animal Hospital with AZT.

There is no FIV vaccine yet available for use in cats although several experimental vaccines are under development (Hosie, 1994). Attempts to control FIV infection therefore rely on prevention of cat-to-cat transmission. For pet cats kept singly or in small groups, prevention of roaming and fighting is probably the best, if not necessarily the easiest, way to reduce the risk of infection. Care should be taken when introducing new cats into a household if either the new cat or any existing cats are infected with FIV, as any fighting which follows will place all the cats at risk of infection. On the other hand, if a few cats in a stable multicat household in which fighting is rare are infected with FIV, then the risk of transmission may be small. Certainly, because of the long incubation period to disease, there is no humane reason why a cat should be killed simply because it is infected with FIV.

In a breeding colony with no evidence of FIV infection, it is best simply to avoid the introduction of seropositive cats. If the colony contains cats seropositive for FIV, it is probably best to separate or rehouse infected animals. Although queen-to-kitten transmission appears to be rare, it is inadvisable to breed from infected cats.

FELINE CORONAVIRUS INFECTION

Feline coronaviruses include both feline infectious peritonitis (FIP) virus and feline enteric coronavirus (FECV). All feline coronavirus (FCoV) isolates are very closely related both antigenically and genetically and all probably have the potential to induce either form of disease. Indeed, there is increasing evidence to suggest that FIP virus is a mutant of FCoV (Pedersen, 1995). FCoV is also very similar to canine coronavirus (CCV), which causes diarrhoea in dogs, and it is possible that CCV may be transmitted from dogs to cats (McArdle et al., 1992).

Clinical signs

Although infection with feline coronavirus (FCoV) can be associated with several clinical syndromes, most cats which become infected show no clinical signs at all and in some cases, only mild enteritis is seen. Feline enteric coronavirus infection is most common in kittens, particularly just after weaning, inducing a mild diarrhoea of a few days duration (Pedersen, 1995).

Some cases of FCoV infection, however, are much more severe and result in feline infectious peritonitis (Pedersen, 1995). Two forms of FIP occur – the 'wet' form, characterized by the accu-

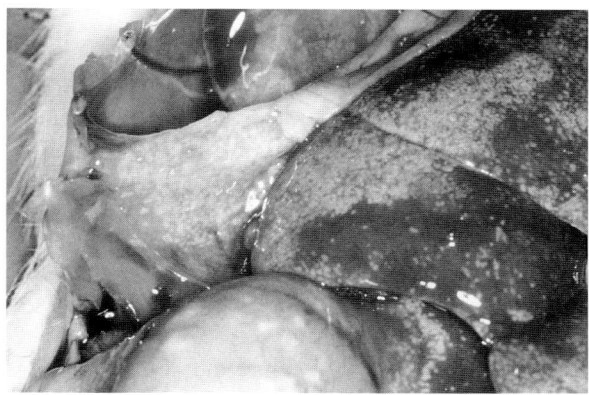

Figure 49.8 Multiple pyogranulomatous nodules on the surface of the liver, kidney and diaphragm in a cat with feline infectious peritonitis. Photograph courtesy of Michael Herrtage.

mulation of fluid in the body cavities, and the 'dry' form, characterized by granulomatous lesions in various body organs (Fig. 49.8). Both forms of the disease are invariably fatal.

The initial signs of both wet and dry FIP are similar, rather non-specific and often missed in field cases. They include mild pyrexia, anorexia and lethargy. In wet FIP these vague signs are followed by the development of ascites with weight loss, inappetence, depression, anaemia and death. As well as ascites, pleural and pericardial effusion occurs in about 20% of cases and in these cats tachypnoea and dyspnoea are prominent clinical signs. Jaundice is also sometimes seen, especially during the later stages of disease.

In dry FIP, granulomatous lesions develop in a variety of organs and clinical signs reflect the organs involved. Most frequently affected are organs in the abdominal cavity (particularly the liver and kidney), the CNS (dry FIP is the most common lesion of CNS in necropsy surveys) and eyes. The most common presenting signs are therefore chronic pyrexia, weight loss and depression. Involvement of the central nervous system may lead to a variety of neurological signs including ataxia, paresis, paralysis, disorientation, nystagmus and fits.

Although FIP is usually described as two discrete syndromes, wet and dry FIP are not mutually exclusive descriptions. Eye or CNS lesions may be clinically apparent in up to 10% of cases of wet FIP and many cats with wet FIP have some lesions of dry FIP at necropsy. There are also occasional reports of cats with wet FIP recovering but then developing dry FIP.

Pathogenesis

The main route of virus entry is oral with primary virus replication occurring in the tonsils and enterocytes. Transplacental transmission has occasionally been reported but does not appear to contribute significantly to the epidemiology of the disease.

The outcome of feline coronavirus infection depends both on the cat – its immune status and ability to mount an immune response to the virus – and the virus itself (Barlough and Stoddart, 1990; Pedersen, 1995). Some isolates of FoCV appear to be of lower virulence than others, but other factors such as the dose and route of infection may also play a role. Thus some cats will develop only subclinical infection, whereas others will develop mild enteritis or FIP. A complicating factor in the pathogenesis of FIP is that experimentally the disease has been shown to have an immune-mediated component. Thus cats with pre-existing antibody seem to develop enhanced disease following challenge with the virus. The role of this phenomenon in the pathogenesis of naturally occurring FIP is not known, but enhanced disease does not seem to occur in the field (Addie et al., 1995).

Rather than developing overt clinical disease or eliminating the virus, some cats seem to become virus carriers. The mechanism of this carrier state and the rates and times of virus excretion are not clear, though it has been shown by epidemiological studies that approximately one in three seropositive queens is likely to be a carrier and can transmit virus to her kittens (Addie and Jarrett, 1995). Such cats can obviously play an important role in the epidemiology of the disease in the field.

Diagnosis

The only way of making a definite diagnosis of FIP at present is by histopathology of tissues taken at necropsy or biopsy, for example of liver in wet FIP or of other affected organs in dry FIP (Barlough and Stoddart, 1990). In wet FIP, analysis of ascitic fluid is helpful in confirming a diagnosis. The fluid is characteristically yellow and tacky; it clots on standing and has a high globulin content.

Virus isolation, which should provide the ideal laboratory confirmation of diagnosis of FIP, is not usually possible from field cases. This is partly because many infected cats only shed low levels of virus (mainly before clinical signs appear) and partly because the virus is labile and many strains are difficult, if not impossible, to grow in cell culture. Alternative techniques, such as PCR, for detecting virus have been developed but need to be interpreted with care.

A great deal of reliance has been placed on serological techniques to diagnose FCoV infection but the results of such tests are difficult to interpret. Although high antibody titres have been said to indicate FIP virus infection and low titres to indicate enteric infection, this is not necessarily the case. Thus asymptomatic, recovered cats may develop high antibody levels whereas some cats with acute, wet FIP may have no detectable antibody.

Treatment

Nursing and symptomatic treatment, the use of corticosteroids or cyclophosphamide with antibiotics, and the removal of abdominal fluid from cats with wet FIP may provide temporary relief in some cats, but rarely produces a complete cure. A more permanent response to such treatments has been reported occasionally, but such cases are very rare and are very likely due to coincidental recovery rather than a result of treatment. Antiviral drugs which are effective against FCoV in cell culture (e.g. Weiss, 1995) seem not to work *in vivo*.

Epidemiology and control

The main source of infection within a colony of cats is probably carrier cats. From epidemiological studies it appears that one in three seropositive queens are carriers who can infect their offspring at around weaning (Addie and Jarrett, 1995). Other sources of infection are shedding kittens or other adult carriers within or introduced into the colony.

A temperature-sensitive intranasal vaccine is marketed in some parts of the world for use in cats 16 weeks of age and over (Christianson et al., 1989; Posterino-Reeves et al., 1992).

In colonies with endemic coronavirus infection, attempted eradication may only be worthwhile in the face of an outbreak of clinical disease or where subsequent infection can be kept out. Queens and kittens should be isolated for 12 weeks and then the kittens tested for antibody before they are allowed to join the rest of the colony (Addie and Jarrett, 1995). Where a queen is suspected of being a carrier, early weaning and removal of kittens from the queen into strict isolation will make it much more likely that the kittens remain free of infection. In coronavirus-free colonies, antibody testing and quarantine can be used to help prevent the introduction of carrier cats. However, FCoV is widespread and a coronavirus-free colony can be difficult to sustain.

Since FIP is, in general, a disease of low morbidity, an alternative approach is to accept FCoV infection is present and to reduce the risk factors which may precipitate disease by improving hygiene and minimizing stress (Pedersen, 1995).

It is wise to test colonies for FeLV infection since it has been shown experimentally that this can predispose FCoV-infected cats to the development of FIP.

ENTERIC INFECTIONS

Enteric virus infections

Feline panleucopenia

One of the main targets of panleucopenia virus are the villus crypt cells of the intestinal epithelium. Enteritis is therefore part of this disease syndrome, the clinical signs of which are described above.

Feline coronavirus

Again, feline coronavirus has a predilection for intestinal epithelium, in this case the tips of the villi. Generally only mild enteritis is seen. This virus can also induce feline infectious peritonitis and this is described above.

Feline rotavirus

Although infection is probably widespread, there are very few reports of rotavirus infection in cats and it is probably not a disease of major significance. The risk of infection in cats probably depends on the environment in which they live. Subclinical infection is probably most common, and when diarrhoea occurs it is usually only mild and transient. Young kittens in colonies are probably most at risk of developing clinical disease as they are more likely to meet infection earlier in life than most household pets. Nevertheless, it is always possible that more severe disease may occur if the situation is complicated by other pathogens or predisposing factors. Diagnosis is usually by detection of particles in faeces by electron microscopy but polyacrylamide gel electrophoresis may be more sensitive (Birch *et al*., 1985).

Feline astrovirus

Little has been published on the epidemiology or clinical significance of feline astrovirus infection, although one report suggests that less than 10% of cats in the UK have antibody (Harbour, 1990). Most isolations have been made from cats with persistent (4–14 days), green and watery diarrhoea, sometimes accompanied by vomiting, pyrexia and depression (Harbour, 1990). Diagnosis is usually by electron microscopy whereby characteristic five- or six-pointed star-shaped particles may be seen in faeces. Treatment is symptomatic.

Feline torovirus

The toroviruses are a group of viruses similar to the coronaviruses but with a characteristic rod- or doughnut-shaped core. Human and bovine toroviruses have been associated with diarrhoea but an equine virus appears to cause only asymptomatic infection. Recently, torovirus-like particles and antibody reacting with bovine toroviruses have been detected in cats. Although not reproduced experimentally, there is some evidence to link this virus in cats to a clinical syndrome involving diarrhoea and protrusion of the nictitating membrane (Muir *et al*., 1990). This syndrome is a common presentation of persistent diarrhoea in cats and is frustrating to treat, although eventually it is often self-limiting.

Enteric bacterial infections

Salmonellosis

Salmonellosis in cats is normally asymptomatic and clinical disease is usually associated with concurrent infections or immunosuppression. Surveys of the prevalence of *Salmonella* spp. in cat faeces vary between 1% and 18%; 7% of cats visiting University of Liverpool Small Animal Hospital were found to be excreting salmonellae. *S. typhimurium* is the serotype most frequently isolated. Clinical syndromes reported associated with salmonellosis include acute and chronic gastroenteritis, recurrent pyrexic episodes, vomiting, pneumonia, conjunctivitis, abortion, stillbirths and fading kittens. Severe infection and bacteraemia may cause endotoxaemia, depression, hypothermia and collapse. Transient bacteraemia may result in abscess formation in internal organs (such as the liver) with subsequent clinical signs appropriate to the organ involved. Treatment may include supportive fluid therapy in severe cases. Use of antibiotics should be avoided if possible as they may prolong shedding and select for resistance. If used, for example when animals are bacteraemic or endotoxaemic, antibiotics must be chosen based on the results of a sensitivity test as many salmonellae carry multiresistance plasmids (Wall *et al.*, 1995). Salmonellosis is one of the most common zoonotic infections and can cause severe illness or even death in humans, but it seems likely that cats are far less important as a source of human infection than are food animals and other humans, and the possibility of humans infecting cats should not be ignored.

Escherichia coli *infection*

Little is known about the role of *E. coli* in feline disease. *E. coli* forms part of the normal flora of the alimentary tract but it has been suggested that some cases of acute diarrhoea might be caused by *E. coli* strains capable of producing a verotoxin (Abaas *et al.*, 1989). *E. coli* can also be involved in pyelonephritis and acute cystitis and is also frequently isolated from abscesses and wounds. The antibiotics used to treat *E. coli* infections in cats should be chosen with regard to the site of the infection (for example, urinary tract, enteric or superficial infections) and the results of an antibiotic sensitivity test as antibiotic resistance is common.

Campylobacter *infection*

Cats can be infected with several species of *Campylobacter* although most reports concern the isolation of *C. jejuni*. Surveys suggest that approximately 5% of cats may be excreting *C. jejuni* in their faeces. There is no obvious correlation between infection and disease and it may be that most clinical campylobacteriosis is usually secondary to infection with other enteric pathogens such as coronaviruses or *E. coli*. Campylobacteriosis is a common cause of enteritis in humans, especially in young children, and cats and dogs are frequently blamed for human infection. Although owners should be warned of the zoonotic potential of campylobacteriosis if it is diagnosed in a cat, it is likely that cats, dogs and and their owners are more often infected from a common source.

Yersiniosis and pseudotuberculosis

Yersinia enterocolitica and *Y. pseudotuberculosis* can be isolated from the faeces of many animals, including cats and dogs. They generally cause no clinical signs in cats but both can cause severe disease in humans, especially in children. Often the source of human infection cannot be traced but there are reports of children becoming infected with *Y. pseudotuberculosis* through direct contact with cat faeces (Fukushima *et al.*, 1989). It may, therefore, be wise to treat cats shown to be shedding *Y. enterocolitica* or *Y. pseudotuberculosis* with tetracycline or potentiated sulphonamides.

Anaerobiospirillum

Anaerobiospirillum spp. are a normal part of the intestinal flora of cats and dogs, and in one survey were isolated from the faeces of 7/10 cats and 3/10 dogs. Their isolation in human faeces, however, is often associated with enteritis and diarrhoea in children. There are several reports providing good evidence of zoonotic spread from puppies to babies (Malnick *et al.*, 1989) and it is probable that cats can also be a source of human infection.

FELINE COWPOX

Aetiology

Cowpox virus is in the genus *Orthopoxvirus* in the family poxviridae (Baxby and Bennett, 1994). All orthopoxviruses are closely related and antigenically very similar. Cowpox virus should not be confused with pseudocowpox virus, a member of the genus *parapoxvirus* which also includes orf virus. Although both genera are members of the family poxviridae, the viruses in each genus have a different morphology and there is no clinically useful antigenic similarity between the two.

Epidemiology

Cowpox virus is only found in Europe and Eurasia. Despite its name, cowpox virus has never been very common in cattle and serosurveys reveal little evidence of bovine infection (unlike pseudocowpox virus which is endemic world-wide in cattle). The reservoir hosts of cowpox virus are wild rodents. The host rodent species vary geographically; voles and woodmice are probably the main host in Western Europe (Crouch *et al.*, 1995).

Cats are the most commonly recognized host of cowpox virus (Bennett et al., 1990a). They are thought to become infected when hunting. Most affected cats are adult and come from rural environments, and almost all are known by their owners to hunt small mammals. Most feline cases are seen in the autumn, presumably because small mammal populations are at their maximum size and are most active at that time of year. Cat-to-cat transmission can occur but generally causes only subclinical infection in the recipient cat. Cat-to-human transmission can also occur and approximately one half of human cases are due to contact with infected cats.

Cowpox virus has also been isolated from, and in some cases caused severe disease in, big cats, okapi, elephants, rhinoceroses and anteaters in European zoos.

Clinical signs

Most cats present with widespread skin lesions but many have a history of a recent, single skin lesion on the head, neck or a forelimb. The primary lesions vary in character from large abscesses or areas of cellulitis to small, scabbed papules or rodent ulcer-like lesions. Many owners describe the primary lesion as having developed from a small, bite-like wound.

The secondary skin lesions (see Fig. 47.25a) develop a few days to weeks after the primary lesion is first noticed. Secondary lesions first appear as small, randomly distributed dermal nodules, which over 3–5 days develop into ulcerated papules up to 1 cm diameter. These quickly develop scabs which dry and separate after a further 2–3 weeks. Lesions may be pruritic as they heal or if secondarily infected. New hair soon grows and most cats are completely recovered in 6–8 weeks.

Most cats exhibit no clinical signs other than skin lesions and a mild pyrexia but up to 20% may also develop a mild, serous nasal discharge, conjunctivitis or transient diarrhoea, and some cats may be depressed and anorexic. Transient systemic illness usually occurs only during the viraemic phase. More severe or longstanding systemic signs or delayed healing may result from secondary bacterial infection or immunodeficiency resulting from corticosteroid treatment, severe concurrent disease or infection with FeLV or FIV. Severe systemic signs, particularly pneumonia, suggest a poor prognosis and euthanasia might be considered.

Diagnosis

Clinical signs alone may enable diagnosis in some cases; differential diagnoses include cat bite abscesses, neoplasia, eosinophilic granuloma and miliary eczema. For laboratory confirmation, dry, unfixed scab material can be sent through the post without the need for special transport medium. Electron microscopy of scabs enables rapid diagnosis in most cases, whereas virus isolation produces a more sensitive and accurate result but make take up to two weeks. Tissue fixed in 5% formol–saline can be sent for histopathological examination (Fig. 47.25b). Serum can be tested for antibody in several ways; an immunofluorescent antibody test is now most frequently used in the UK.

Treatment and control

There is no specific treatment for cowpox. In most cats infection is self-limiting so treatment usually consists of broad-spectrum antibiotics to control secondary and concurrent bacterial infection. Corticosteroids should be avoided as they may exacerbate the condition. No vaccine is available and control of disease therefore relies largely on prompt diagnosis, isolation of affected individuals and reduction of contact with wild mammal reservoirs.

Public health aspects

About half of all cases of human cowpox can be traced to contact with infected cats (Baxby et al., 1994). Human disease usually consists of a single lesion on the hand or face. Human cowpox may also cause systemic illness with 'flu-like symptoms, and may require hospitalization especially if the patient is immunosuppressed. Smallpox vaccination may not provide complete protection against primary cowpox virus infection, although it might prevent more severe disease. Prior exposure to pseudocowpox or orf viruses does not, of course, provide protection.

Cat-to-human transmission is unlikely if basic hygienic precautions are taken. Veterinary surgeons and others handling infected cats should wear gloves and take care not to allow infected material into wounds or the eyes. Young children, the elderly and those with a pre-existing skin condition or debilitative or immunosuppressive disease should avoid contact with the cat while it remains infective (i.e. until the scabs have disappeared). If these elementary procedures are followed then the risk of human infection should be small, and it is rarely necessary to euthanize an affected cat on public health grounds.

OTHER VIRUS INFECTIONS

Rabies

Rabies occurs world-wide except in countries such as the UK where specific control measures have been taken. It is a disease which can affect virtually all mammals, though there are different reservoir hosts in different parts of the world. In Western Europe, the reservoir host is the fox, and domestic animals are infected through contact with this reservoir. Human exposure generally follows contact with infected domestic animals.

Rabies in cats generally has an incubation period of less than 2 months but occasionally may be up to six months or even longer. The clinical development of feline rabies typically involves prodromal, furious and then paralytic stages, each lasting a few days, but atypical disease is common. The prodromal phase is characterized by behavioural changes. Gradually the furious phase predominates, the cat becomes increasingly nervous, irritable and vicious and may show muscle tremors, flaccidity or incoordination. Difficulty in swallowing leads to drooling of saliva. During the final stage, generalized paralysis gradually develops ending in coma and death.

Vaccination is currently only allowed in the UK if the animal is to be exported or is to be put into quarantine. Permission to vaccinate is required from the local divisional veterinary officer (DVO). Rabies control measures in the UK are presently being reassessed.

If rabies is suspected in a cat, it must be reported to the DVO, local animal health inspector or the police. The suspect animal must never be moved from the premises until the Ministry of Agriculture, Fisheries and Food has completed its enquiries. The animal should be isolated in escape-proof accommodation and all personnel in contact with the animal should wash thoroughly in soap or detergent and water. All equipment and clothing which has been in contact with the animal should be sterilized. If anyone is bitten or scratched by a suspect case, the wound should be thoroughly washed with soap or detergent (not both) and water, and then cleaned with 70% ethanol, cetrimide or savlon. Immediate medical attention should be sought. The names and addresses of any contacts (e.g. animals in the waiting room) should be recorded and no further animals should enter the premises until permission has been obtained from the DVO.

Hantavirus

Hantavirus antibody in cats was first detected in laboratory-housed cats in Belgium, and recent surveys in Great Britain and Austria found serum antibody to *Hantavirus* in 5–10% of cats from a variety of disease and environmental backgrounds (Bennett *et al.*, 1990b; Nowotny, 1994). Hantaviruses are enzootic world-wide in wild and laboratory rodent populations and can also infect humans. The clinical significance of *Hantavirus* infection in cats is not known, although the British survey did suggest a possible association between *Hantavirus* antibody and non-specified chronic disease. In man, different strains of *Hantavirus* can cause a spectrum of clinical disease which includes mild or inapparent infection through to haemorrhagic fever and renal syndrome or acute pulmonary failure and death. However, there is currently little evidence to link cats directly with human infection.

Aujeszky's disease

Aujeszky's disease (pseudorabies, mad itch) is caused by a herpesvirus. The reservoir host is the pig, and cats can become infected by eating raw pork. Cats are not thought to transmit the disease themselves although they may shed virus in their oral and nasal secretions. Aujeszky's disease in cats is almost always fatal and often rapidly so. The first clinical signs seen include restlessness, anorexia and hypersalivation. Often no clinical signs will be seen in free roaming cats as they will run off to hide early in disease development (Maes and Penseart, 1987). Intense pruritus is often described as characteristic of Aujeszky's disease, but is often not seen in cats. Terminal signs, which develop usually within 48 h of the onset of clinical signs, include paralysis and coma. Some cats may die suddenly without showing any prior clinical signs.

Feline herpesvirus 2

A herpesvirus (FHV 2) which is serologically distinct from feline herpesvirus 1 has been isolated from cats in the USA. It has been implicated as a possible cause of feline urological syndrome (Fabricant, 1977) but these claims have not been substantiated. More recent antigenic and molecular studies on FHV 2 have shown it to be indistinguishable from the American type strain of bovid herpesvirus 4 (BHV-4) (Kruger et al., 1989). BHV-4 has been isolated from cattle with respiratory and reproductive disease in Europe but the European type strain of BHV-4 does not appear to infect cats (Thiry et al., 1991).

Feline syncytium-forming virus

Feline syncytium-forming virus (FeSFV) is a member of the foamy virus group (the spumavirinae) in the family Retroviridae. Spumaviruses have been isolated from many species, but they do not appear to be pathogenic; their main importance lies not in clinical medicine but as potential contaminants in research and vaccine production.

Other viruses

Influenza virus can infect cats following experimental inoculation and there is some serological evidence of natural feline infection. However, there is no evidence that cat-to-human transmission might occur, the reverse being more likely during human influenza pandemics. Several reports also exist of paramyxovirus infection of the CNS in cats; these infections have been associated with demyelinating encephalitis. Canine distemper virus (CDV) can induce subclinical infection in domestic cats both experimentally and in the field. In big cats, however, natural CDV infection has been associated with encephalitis. Borna disease virus has also been associated with non-suppurative meningoencephalomyelitis in cats.

CELLULITIS AND ABSCESS FORMATION

Abscesses and cellulitis are probably the most common infections encountered in cats. They are mostly due to bites and scratches received through fighting but wounds may also be caused by other means and the possibility of foreign bodies, including grass seed-heads and airgun pellets, should be investigated. Several bacterial species may be involved, including *Pasteurella multocida*, staphylococci, streptococci, *Bacteroides* spp., *Fusobacterium* spp. and sometimes *Actinomyces*, *Nocardia* or *Rhodococcus* spp. Enteric bacteria such as *E. coli* are also commonly found in wound infections.

The clinical signs vary according to the site and severity of the abscess. Bite or scratch wounds are generally found on the head, leg, back or base of tail and are usually painful and accompanied by pyrexia, depression, inappetence and enlarged local lymph nodes. Large, mature abscesses can be palpated but they may be not so obvious early in development and owners often notice only the systemic signs or behavioural changes. Diagnosis is based on the history and clinical and may be aided by haematology.

Treatment depends on the extent of infection and stage of development of the abscess. Antibiotics are generally unable to penetrate abscess walls, but may be useful for treating cellulitis and help prevent recurrence after drainage and other complications. The penicillins and their derivatives (ampicillin and amoxycillin) are effective against most abscess-forming bacteria. Cephalosporins, lincomycin, clindamycin and metronidazole are good second choices for their particular activity against anaerobes. In addition, a single injection of penicillin G given within 24 h of being bitten may prevent infection occurring. Surgical drainage should only be undertaken once the abscess has matured, a process which can be enhanced by the use of warm saline compresses.

If abscesses recur or persist, then a more thorough investigation is called for. An undetected foreign body may still be present or osteomyelitis may have developed and further surgery may be required. Alternatively, a persistent infection with Mycobacteria, *Nocardia* spp. or fungi may have developed, or the cat may be immunosuppressed by concurrent infection with feline immunodeficiency virus or feline leukaemia virus.

Actinomyces and *Nocardia* spp. are Gram positive, pleomorphic, facultative anaerobic bacteria. *Actinomyces* spp. are part of the normal flora of the oral cavity and respiratory tract, but *Nocardia* spp. are common soil saprophytes. Both can cause persistent pyogranulomatous lesions in cats and are most frequently isolated in association with abscesses, cellulitis and pyothorax. Actinomycosis and nocardiosis can be difficult to treat and whatever the site of the lesion, drainage and removal of pus is essential if subsequent antibiotic therapy is to be effective. *Actinomyces* spp. are usually susceptible to penicillins but, unlike many other anaerobes, are not sensitive to metronidazole. *Nocardia* spp. are often sensitive only to sulphonamides but, ideally, the choice of antibiotic would be based on an antibacterial sensitivity test.

OTHER BACTERIAL INFECTIONS

Streptococcal infections

Beta-haemolytic streptococci of Lancefield group G are part of the normal flora of the mucosae and skin of cats and kittens probably become infected at birth from their mother's genital tract through the umbilicus. In otherwise healthy kittens born of older queens, maternal antibody protects against clinical disease but in kittens born of younger or immunosuppressed queens, septicaemia and severe systemic disease, often culminating in death, may develop. In older kittens, up to about 6 months old, subclinical infection in the tonsils may develop into clinically apparent tonsillitis and cervical lymphadenopathy, but rarely more severe disease unless the cat is immunosuppressed. In addition, streptococci are frequently isolated from wounds and abscesses in adult cats and are common opportunist pathogens secondary to upper respiratory diseases.

Streptococci are susceptible to penicillins and early treatment with penicillin, together with cleansing of abscesses or wounds, is usually effective. In colonies with a history of neonatal disease, topical application of antiseptic to the navel and treatment at birth with a long-lasting penicillin or penicillin derivative may help prevent further disease.

In addition to group G streptococci, cats can also harbour asymptomatic infections of group A streptococci in their oropharynx. These infections are acquired from humans and can be transmitted back to humans. Hence a family pet may become a reservoir for human infection and the source of recurrent tonsillitis or pharyngitis in a family. Isolation of group A streptococci from a cat's oropharynx may be difficult. If a cat is suspected of being a source of human infection it may be advisable to treat the cat with penicillin or a cephalosporin even if isolation is not possible (Greene, 1988).

Tuberculosis, feline leprosy and other mycobacterial infections

Tuberculosis is a rare disease of cats. *Mycobacterium tuberculosis* and *M. bovis* infections are usually contracted through contact with infected humans, although cattle and certain wild mammals might be an alternative source of *M. bovis* infection in some areas. *M. avium* is a saprophyte found in soil and water and is only a very rare opportunist pathogen of cats.

Infection is usually subclinical and clinical signs, if they occur, generally reflect the location of granulomas. Chronic ulcerative infections of the oropharynx or respiratory tract may cause retching, a non-productive cough or dysphagia. Anorexia, wasting, vomiting or diarrhoea may accompany intestinal malabsorption owing to granuloma formation in the alimentary tract. Pleural or peritoneal effusions may also be present and intestinal infection often causes palpably enlarged mesenteric lymph nodes. Diagnosis is based on the history and demonstration of acid-fast organisms in biopsies of affected tissues or in smears of exudates. Isolation may be possible on special media but this can be a lengthy process. Radiography may reveal large granulomas in the respiratory tract or abdomen. Skin tests are usually ineffective in cats.

Although zoonotic spread from cats and dogs has not been reported, cats can excrete *M. tuberculosis* and *M. bovis* in exudates and faeces. Elderly or immunosuppressed owners might be particularly at risk and euthanasia should therefore be considered on public health grounds. Therapy is unlikely to be successful in cats.

Feline leprosy is caused by *M. lepraemurium* ('rat leprosy'). It is an uncommon condition thought to be contracted from rat bites. The lesions consist of nodular, sometimes ulcerated skin lesions on the head or extremities. Spread of the infection up a limb may be accompanied by swollen lymphatic vessels and draining lymph nodes. Diagnosis depends on finding acid-fast organisms in impression smears or biopsies. Treatment is by surgical removal, but dapsone at 50 mg twice a day for 2 weeks may be worth trying when complete surgical excision is not possible, although some toxic side effects have been reported with this drug in cats.

Various saprophytic *mycobacteria* have been isolated from superficial or, more rarely, deeper, persistent abscesses or granulomatous lesions of cats. Species isolated from these 'atypical' mycobacterial infections of cats include *M. fortuitum–M. chelonei* complex, *M. smegmatis* and *M. phlei*. The mycobacteria obtain entry through a wound into already damaged or infected tissue, and infection may be associated with immunosuppression. Diagnosis depends on the demonstration of acid-fast organisms in impression smears or biopsies. Treatment includes surgical removal of as much of the lesion as possible and antibiotic therapy for at least six weeks. Gentamicin, amikacin and potentiated sulphonamides have been used with apparent success, however the prognosis for such infections is guarded as recurrence is common.

Capnocytophaga (DF-2 and DF-2-like) infection

Capnocytophaga is a genus of fastidious, Gram-negative, pleomorphic bacilli originally known as dysgonic fermenter type 2 (DF-2) and DF-2-like organisms. They can be frequently isolated from the oropharynx and faeces of cats and dogs, in which they cause no disease. Human infection occurs through bites and scratches and is also usually asymptomatic. In immunocompromised individuals, however, they can cause septicaemia, severe systemic illness, meningitis, coma and death, and even in immunologically normal children may cause severe keratitis if inoculated into the eye by, for example, a cat scratch (August, 1988).

Tetanus

Feline tetanus is a very uncommon condition. Spastic paralysis, caused by the production of the toxin tetanospasmin by the organism growing anaerobically in a wound, first develops in muscles nearest the wound before the toxin's effects spread to involve more of the CNS. Cats can develop either generalized tetanus, characterized by stiffness of all limbs and contracture of facial muscles, or localized tetanus in which, for example, only one limb is affected. Treatment involves thorough debridement and cleansing of the wound and intravenous penicillin for at least five days together with good nursing and supportive therapy such as intravenous fluids. Antitoxin does not penetrate the CNS so its efficacy is debatable. Animals should be kept in a quiet and darkened room and disturbed as little as possible as they may be hyperaesthetic and particularly sensitive to sound.

Tyzzer's disease

This is a very rare disease of cats caused by *Clostridium piliformis*. Cats are thought to become infected through contact with rodents in which it is part of the normal intestinal flora. Clinical signs in cats include rapid onset of depression, abdominal pain, hepatomegaly and abdominal distension, jaundice and death within two days. A diagnosis is usually made post mortem.

Leptospirosis

Clinical feline leptospirosis is rare although antibody to leptospires can be detected in 5–20% of cats. Various serovars have been isolated from cats including *icterohaemorraghiae*, *pomona* and *bratislava*. Clinical signs, if present, include acute systemic illness or renal and hepatic disease. Cats have been shown to be capable of excreting the organism in urine for up to three months after experimental infection.

Mycoplasma infection

Mycoplasma felis can be isolated from many cases of upper respiratory tract disease in cats but is thought to be mainly a secondary pathogen. There is some evidence that it may also be a primary cause of conjunctivitis although it can often be isolated from the conjunctiva of healthy cats. *M. felis* has also been associated with reproductive disorders, pneumonia and pyothorax. The other *Mycoplasma* species most frequently isolated from cats is *M. gateae*. This organism appears to be part of the normal flora of the cat's oropharynx, respiratory and reproductive tracts. Other *Mycoplasma* species have also been isolated from cats, but their role in disease is not known.

Botulism

Experimental botulism has been described in cats, but the natural disease is very rare. The clinical signs included muscle weakness, paresis and flaccid paralysis. Treatment is primarily supportive; antibiotics, laxatives and enemas may help remove any ingested clostridia and toxins. The animal may have to be fed via a stomach tube or intravenously, and catheterization of the bladder may be necessary.

Plague

In some parts of North America, cats can become infected with the plague organism (*Yersinia pestis*) through contact with wild mammals or their fleas (Eidson *et al.*, 1991) and pass the infection on to humans, veterinary surgeons being particularly at risk. Plague has not been described in cats in Europe.

Cat scratch disease

Cat scratch disease (CSD) is a disease of humans characterized by usually benign, self-limiting lymphadenopathy. It is most commonly seen in children and is often associated with if not a cat scratch, then at least contact with a cat or dog. More severe disease or bacillary angiomatosis may be seen in AIDS patients. Two organisms have recently been identified as causes of CSD: *Bartonella henselae* and *B. quintana*. Both have been isolated from human CSD lesions. *B. henselae* can cause persistent bacteraemia in cats and may be transmitted by cat fleas (Koehler *et al.*, 1994), but the source of *B. quintana* is often not known. Long-term (30 days or more) treatment of infected cats with doxycycline or lincomycin may eliminate feline *B. henselae* infection.

MISCELLANEOUS INFECTIONS

Toxoplasmosis and other protozoal infections

The domestic cat is the definitive host for *Toxoplasma gondii* and one of the main sources for human infection in the UK. Clinical toxoplasmosis in the domestic cat is uncommon. Replication of the organism in the gut can be associated with mild diarrhoea in kittens, but most of the clinical signs of toxoplasmosis are caused by the development of cysts and granulomas in various tissues particularly the liver, lungs, lymph nodes, CNS and eyes. The clinical signs seen reflect the sites of lesions and the amount of tissue damage caused. The disease is most severe in neonatally infected kittens which often rapidly die of widespread systemic infection. More chronic disease is generally seen in older cats.

Definitive diagnosis is based on biopsy of affected tissues. Serology can be misleading since 40% of cats in the UK have antibody to *T. gondii* and acute disease can develop prior to detectable IgG antibody. Assays for IgM can therefore be useful for the early detection of acute infection and some cases of reactivation.

Transmission to humans from cats is by ingestion of sporulated oocysts excreted in cat faeces. The oocysts are hardy and can survive in contaminated material (e.g. cat litter or soil) for many months but are not infectious until sporulation which occurs at least 24 h after excretion. Human infection is usually asymptomatic, but in pregnant women infection can cause abortion or severe fetal abnormalities. To prevent infection from cats, pregnant woman should avoid contact with cat faeces or materials potentially contaminated by cat faeces. Thus they should not clean out cat litter, should wear gloves when gardening and carefully wash raw vegetables before eating them.

Cats can also be infected with *Isospora*, *Cryptosporidium* and *Giardia* spp. All have been associated with diarrhoea but can also be found in the faeces of apparently healthy cats. *Cryptosporidium* and *Giardia* spp. can also infect humans and cause diarrhoea but transmission from cats to people is rare.

Aspergillosis, cryptococcosis and other fungal infections

Aspergillosis is far less common in cats than in dogs. Although as in dogs it can cause chronic nasal disease, feline aspergillosis appears to be more often a systemic infection, and is usually associated with immunosuppression by FeLV, FIV or panleukopenia virus infections.

Cryptococcus neoformans is a fungus often found associated with bird, especially pigeon, guano. It can cause systemic infections in cats with the clinical signs reflecting the organ systems most severely affected. It is rarely reported in the UK.

Candida albicans is a common secondary pathogen particularly in chronic infections of the skin, ears and mucosal surfaces. As in humans, clinical candidiasis is often associated with immunosuppression.

Prototothecosis

Prototheca is a genus of algae, several species of which can be pathogenic to the cat (Tyler, 1990). It is found mainly in sewage from which it can contaminate drinking water, soil and food. Animal to animal spread does not occur. Infection is rare and usually associated with immunosuppression. Cats generally develop cutaneous nodules on the head or feet. Occasionally, however, systemic infection occurs causing intermittent, chronic, bloody diarrhoea, weight loss and signs of CNS and eye infection. Diagnosis depends on demonstration of the organism in biopsies or in smears of vitreous fluid, CSF or urine and by isolation on Sabaraud's media. Treatment is by surgical excision of skin lesions. There is no known effective treatment for systemic infection.

Q fever

Q fever is caused by *Coxiella burnetii*, a rickettsia which in Britain is maintained in wild and domestic animal populations by ingestion and inhalation of infective material such as placentas, urine and faeces. *C. burnetii* usually causes no disease in most of its hosts, the main exceptions being abortion in sheep and general malaise, pyrexia and pneumonia in humans. There have been several reports from North America of human Q fever contracted from parturient and aborting cats (Kosatsky, 1984).

Feline spongiform encephalopathy

This is a recently described condition of domestic and big cats involving slow, progressive degeneration of the CNS similar to that seen in scrapie in sheep and bovine spongiform encephalopathy (BSE) in cattle. Affected cats may show a range of behavioural and neurological signs including incoordination, loss of balance, hyperaesthesia, hypersalivation, intention tremor, muscle fasciculation and fitting (Gruffydd-Jones *et al.*, 1991; Peet and Curran, 1992; Willoughby *et al.*, 1992). The condition appears to be rare. The source of infection for cats is almost certainly bovine material: FSE has only been seen since the epidemic of BSE in cattle, and in mice behaves identically to BSE (Fraser *et al.*, 1994). In the UK, all naturally occurring spongiform encephalopathies, including FSE, are notifiable diseases.

REFERENCES

Abaas, S., Franklin, A., Kuhn, I., Orskov, F. and Orskov, I. (1989) Cytotoxin activity on Vero cells among *Escherichia coli* strains associated with diarrhea in cats. *American Journal of Veterinary Research* **50**, 1294–1296.

Addie, D.D. and Jarrett, O. (1995) Control of feline coronavirus infection in breeding catteries by serotesting, isolation and early weaning. *Feline Practice* **23**(3), 92–95.

Addie, D.D., Toth, S., Murray, G.D. and Jarrett, O. (1995) The risk of typical and antibody enhanced feline infectious peritonitis among cats from feline coronavirus endemic households. *Feline Practice* **23**(3), 24–32.

August, J.R. (1988) Dysgonic fermenter-2 infections. *Journal of the American Veterinary Medical Association* **193**, 1506–1508.

Barlough, J.E. and Scott, F.W. (1990) Effectiveness of three antiviral agents against FIP *in vitro*. *Veterinary Record* **126**, 556–558.

Barlough, J.E. and Stoddart, C.A. (1990) Feline coronaviral infections. In: *Infectious Diseases of the Dog and Cat* (Ed. C.E. Greene), W.B. Saunders, Philadelphia, pp. 300–312.

Barlough, J.E., Ackley, C.D., George, J.W., Levy, N., Acevedo, R., Moore, P.F., Rideout, B.A., Cooper, M.D. and Pedersen, N.C. (1991) Acquired immune dysfunction in cats with experimentally induced feline immunodeficiency virus infection: comparison of short term and long term infections. *Journal of Acquired Immune Deficiency Syndrome* **4**, 219–227.

Baxby, D. and Bennett, M. (1994) Cowpox virus. In: *Encyclopedia of Virology* (Eds R.G. Webster and A. Granoff), Academic Press, New York, pp. 261–267.

Baxby, D., Bennett, M. and Getty, B. (1994) Human cowpox; a review based on 54 cases 1969–93. *British Journal of Dermatology* **131**, 598–607.

Bennett, D., Gaskell, R.M., Mills, A., Knowle, J., Carter, S. and McArdle, F. (1989) Detection of feline calicivirus antigens in the joints of infected cats. *Veterinary Record* **124**, 329–332.

Bennett, M., Gaskell, C.J., Baxby, D., Gaskell, R.M., Kelly, D.F. and Naidoo, J. (1990a) Feline cowpox virus infection. *Journal of Small Animal Practice* **31**, 167–173.

Bennett, M., Lloyd, G., Jones, N., Brown, A., Trees, A.J., McCracken, C., Smyth, N.R., Gaskell, C.J. and Gaskell, R.M. (1990b) The prevalence of antibody to *Hantavirus* in some cat populations in Britain. *Veterinary Record* **127**, 548.

Binns, S.H., Dawson, S., Coutts, A.J., Bennett, M., Hart, C.A. and Gaskell, R.M. (1995) *Bordetella bronchiseptica* in cats: preliminary findings. *2nd European Congress of the Federation of European Companion Animal Veterinary Association*, p. 347.

Birch, C.J., Heath, R.L., Marshall, J.A., Liu, S. and Gust, I.D. (1985) Isolation of feline rotaviruses and their relationship to human and simian isolates by electropherotype and serotype. *Journal of General Virology* **66**, 2731–2735

Carpenter, J.L. (1971) Feline panleucopenia: clinical signs and differential diagnosis. *Journal of the American Veterinary Medical Association* **158**, 857–859.

Christianson, K.K., Ingersoll, J.D., Landon, R.M., Pfeiffer, N.E. and Gerber, J.D. (1989) Characterisation of a temperature sensitive feline infectious peritonitis coronavirus. *Archives of Virology* **109**, 185–196.

Coutts, A., Dawson, S., Willoughby, K. and Gaskell, R.M. (1994) Isolation of feline respiratory viruses from clinically healthy cats at UK cat shows. *Veterinary Record* **135**, 555–556.

Coutts, A.J., Dawson, S., Binns, S., Hart, C.A., Gaskell, C.J. and Gaskell, R.M. (1996) Studies on natural transmission of *Bordetella bronchiseptica* in cats. *Veterinary Microbiology* **48**, 19–27.

Crouch, A.C., Baxby, D., McClacken, C.M., Gaskell, R.M. and Bennett, M. (1995) Serological evidence for the reservoir hosts of cowpox virus in British wildlife. *Epidemiology and Infection* **115**, 185–191.

Dawson, S. and Gaskell, R.M. (1993) Problems with respiratory virus vaccination in cats. *Compendium on Continuing Education* **15**, 1347–1354.

Dawson, S., Smyth, N.R., Bennett, M., Gaskell, R.M., McCracken, C., Brown, A. and Gaskell, C.J. (1991) Effect of primary-stage feline immunodeficiency virus infection on subsequent feline calicivirus challenge in cats. *AIDS* **5**, 747–750.

Dawson, S., McArdle, F., Bennett, D., Carter, S.D., Bennett, M., Ryvar, R. and Gaskell, R.M. (1993) Investigation of vaccine reactions and breakdowns following feline calicivirus vaccination. *Veterinary Record* **132**, 346–350.

Dawson, S., Bennett, D., Carter, S.D., Bennett, M., Meanger, J., Turner, P.C., Carter, M.J., Milton, I. and Gaskell, R.M. (1994) Acute arthritis of cats associated with feline calicivirus infection. *Research in Veterinary Science* **56**, 133–143.

Egberink, H.F., Hartman, K. and Horzinek, M. (1991) Chemotherapy of feline immunodeficiency virus infection. *Journal of the American Veterinary Medical Association* **199**, 1485–1487.

Eidson, M., Thilsted, J.P. and Rollag, O.J. (1991) Clinical, clinicopathologic and pathologic features of plague in cats: 119 cases (1977–1988). *Journal of the American Veterinary Medical Association* **199**, 1191–1197.

Fabricant, C.G. (1977) Herpesvirus-induced urolithiasis in specific pathogen-free male cats. *Journal of the American Veterinary Medical Association* **38**, 1837–1842

Fraser, H., Pearson, G.R., McConnell, I., Bruce, M.E., Wyatt, J.M. and Gruffydd-Jones, T.J. (1994) Transmission of feline spongiform encephalopathy to mice. *Veterinary Record* **134**, 449.

Fukushima, H., Gomyoda, M., Ishikura, S., Nishio, T., Moriki, S., Endo, J., Kaneko, S. and Tsubokura, M. (1989) Cat contaminated environmental substances lead to *Yersinia pseudotuberculosis* infection in children. *Journal of Clinical Microbiology,* **27**, 2706–2709.

Gaskell, R.M. (1981) An assessment of the use of feline respiratory virus vaccines. In: *Veterinary Annual 21st Issue* (Eds C.S.G. Grunsell and F.W.G. Hill). Wright Scientechnica, Bristol, pp. 267–274.

Gaskell, R.M. (1989) Vaccination of the young kitten. *Journal of Small Animal Practice* **30**, 618–624.

Gaskell, R.M. (1994) Feline panleucopenia. In *Feline Medicine and Therapeutics* (Eds E.A. Chandler, C.J. Gaskell and R.M. Gaskell), Blackwell Scientific Publications, Oxford, pp. 445–452.

Gaskell, R.M. and Dawson, S. (1994) Viral-induced upper respiratory tract diseases. In: *Feline Medicine and Therapeutics* (Eds E.A. Chandler, C.J. Gaskell and R.M. Gaskell). Blackwell Scientific Publications, Oxford, pp. 453–472.

Greene, C.E. (1988) Zoonotic aspects of group A streptococcal infections in dogs and cats. *Journal of the American Animal Hospital Association* **24**, 218–222.

Greene, C.E. and Scott, F.W. (1990) Feline panleukopenia. In: *Infectious Diseases of the Dog and Cat* (Ed. C.E. Greene). W.B. Saunders, Philadelphia, pp. 291–299.

Gruffydd-Jones, T.J., Galloway, P.E. and Pearson, G.R. (1991) Feline spongiform encephalopathy. *Journal of Small Animal Practice* **33**, 471–476.

Harbour, D.A. (1990) Feline astroviral infections. In: *Infectious Diseases of the Dog and Cat* (Ed. C.E. Greene). W.B. Saunders, Philadelphia, pp. 313–314.

Harbour, D.A., Howard, P.E. and Gaskell, R.M. (1991) Isolation of feline calicivirus and feline herpesvirus from domestic cats 1980–1989. *Veterinary Record* **128**, 77–80.

Hartmann, K., Donath, A., Beer, B., Egberink, H.F., Horzinek, M.C., Hoffmann-Fezer, G., Thum, I. and Thefeld, S. (1992) Use of two virustatica (AZT, PMEA) in the treatment of FIV and FeLV seropositive cats with clinical symptoms. *Veterinary Immunology and Immunopathology* **35**, 167–175.

Hayes, K.A., Lafrado, L.J., Erickson, J.G., Marr, J.M. and Mathes, L.E. (1993) Prophylactic ZDV therapy prevents early viraemia and lymphocyte decline but not primary infection in feline immunodeficiency virus-inoculated cats. *Journal of Acquired Immune Deficiency Syndrome* **6**, 1270–134.

Hoover, E.A. and Mullins, J.I. (1991) Feline leukemia infection and diseases. *Journal of the American Veterinary Medical Association* **199**, 1287–1297.

Hopper, C.D., Sparkes, A.H. and Harbour, D.A. (1994) Feline immunodeficiency virus. In: *Feline Medicine and Therapeutics* (Eds E.A. Chandler, C.J. Gaskell and R.M. Gaskell). Blackwells Scientific Publications, Oxford, pp. 488–505.

Hosie, M. (1994) The development of a vaccine against feline immunodeficiency virus. *British Veterinary Journal* **150**, 25–39

Hosie, M., Sparkes, A. and Hopper, C. (1989) Feline immunodeficiency virus. *In Practice* **11**, 87–95.

Jacobs, A.A.C., Chalmers, W.S.K., Pasman, J., van Vugt, F. and Cuenen, L.H. (1993) Feline bordetellosis; challenge and vaccine studies. *Veterinary Record* **133**, 260–263.

Jarrett, O. (1994) Feline leukaemia virus. In: *Feline Medicine and Therapeutics* (Eds E.A. Chandler, C.J. Gaskell and R.M. Gaskell). Blackwell Scientific Publications, Oxford, pp. 473–487.

Knowles, J.O., Gaskell, R.M., Gaskell, C.J., Harvey, C.E. and Lutz, H. (1989) Prevalence of feline calicivirus, feline leukaemia virus and antibodies to FIV in cats with chronic stomatitis. *Veterinary Record* **124**, 336–338.

Koehler, J.E., Glaser, C.A. and Tappero, J.W. (1994) *Rochalimea henselae* infection; a new zoonosis with the domestic cat as reservoir. *Journal of the American Medical Association* **271**, 531–535.

Kosatsky, T. (1984) Household outbreak of Q-fever pneumonia related to a parturient cat. *Lancet* **ii**, 1447–1449.

Kruger, J.M., Osborne, C.A., Whetstone, C.A., Goyal, S.M. and Semlak, R.A. (1989) Genetic and serologic analysis of feline cell-associated herpesvirus-induced infection of the urinary tract in conventionally reared cats. *American Journal of Veterinary Research* **50**, 2023–2027.

Maes, L. and Pensaert, M. (1987) Pseudorabies virus (Aujeszky's disease). In: *Virus Infections of Carnivores* (Ed. M.J. Appel). Elsevier Science Publishers BV, Amsterdam, pp. 241–246.

Malnick, H., Jones, A. and Vickers, J.C. (1989) *Anaerobiospirillum*: cause of a new zoonosis? *Lancet* **ii**, 1145.

McArdle, F., Bennett, M., Gaskell, R.M., Tennant, B., Kelly, D.F., and Gaskell, C.J. (1992) Induction and enhancement of feline infectious peritonitis by canine coronavirus. *American Journal of Veterinary Research* **53**, 1500–1506.

McArdle, H.C., Dawson, S., Coutts, A., Bennett, M., Hart, C.A., Ryvar, R. and Gaskell, R.M. (1994) Seroprevalence and isolation rate of *Bordetella bronchiseptica* in cats in the UK. *Veterinary Record* **135**, 506–507.

McClelland, A.J., Hardy, W.D. Jr and Zuckerman, E.E. (1980) Prognosis of healthy feline leukemia virus infected cats. In: *Feline Leukemia Virus* (Eds W.D. Hardy, M. Essex and A.J. McClelland). Elsevier Science Publishers BV, Amsterdam, pp. 121–126.

Meers, J., Del Fierro, R.B., Cope, H.S., Greene, W.K. and Robinson, W.F. (1993) Feline immunodeficiency virus infection; plasma but not peripheral blood mononuclear cell virus titer is influenced by zidovudine and cyclosporin. *Archives of Virology* **132**, 67–81.

Muir, P., Harbour, D.A., Gruffydd-Jones, T.J., Howard, P.E., Hopper, C.D., Gruffydd-Jones, E.A.D., Broadhead, H.M., Clarke, E.M. and Jones, M.E. (1990) A clinical and microbiological study of cats with nictitating membrane protrusion and diarrhoea; isolation of a novel virus. *Veterinary Record* **127**, 324–330.

Nowotny, N. (1994) The domestic cat; a possible transmitter of viruses from rodents to man. *Lancet* **343**, 921.

Pacitti, A.M. (1987) Latent feline leukaemia virus infection: a review. *Journal of Small Animal Practice* **28**, 1153–1159.

Pacitti, A.M., Jarrett, O. and Hay, D. (1986) Transmission of feline leukaemia virus in the milk of a non-viraemic cat. *Veterinary Record* **118**, 381–384.

Pedersen, N.C. (1995) An overview of feline enteric coronavirus and infectious peritonitis virus infections. *Feline Practice* **23**(3), 7–20.

Pedersen, N.C. and Floyd-Hawkins, K. (1995) Mechanisms for persistence of acute and chronic feline calicivirus infections in the face of vaccination. *Veterinary Microbiology* **47**, 141–156.

Pedersen, N.C., Laliberte, L. and Ekman, S. (1983) A transient febrile limping syndrome of kittens caused by two different strains of feline calicivirus. *Feline Practice* **13**, 26–35.

Pedersen, N.C., Yamamoto, J., Ishida, T. and Hansen, H. (1989) Feline immunodeficiency virus infection. *Veterinary Immunology and Immunopathology* **21**, 111–129.

Peet, R.L. and Curran, J.M. (1992) Spongiform encephalopathy in an imported cheetah (*Acinonyx jubatus*). *Australian Veterinary Journal* **69**, 171.

Posterino-Reeves, N.C., Pollock, R.V.H. and Thurber, E.T. (1992) Long-term follow-up study of cats vaccinated with a temperature sensitive feline infectious peritonitis vaccine. *Cornell Veterinarian* **82**, 117–123.

Povey, R.C. (1973) Feline panleucopenia – which vaccine? *Journal of Small Animal Practice* **14**, 399–406.

Reubel, G.H., Hoffmann, D.E. and Pedersen, N.C. (1992) Acute and chronic faucitis of domestic cats. *Veterinary Clinics of North America* **22**, 1347–1360.

Reubel, G.H., George, J.W., Higgins, J. and Pedersen, N.C. (1994) Effect of chronic feline immunodeficiency virus infection on experimental feline calicivirus-induced disease. *Veterinary Microbiology* **39**, 335–351.

Rojko, J.L. and Kociba, G.J. (1991) Pathogenesis of infection by the feline leukemia virus. *Journal of the American Veterinary Medical Association* **199**, 1305–1310.

Scott, F.W. (1980) Virucidal disinfectants and feline viruses. *American Journal of Veterinary Research* **41**, 410–414.

Smyth, N.R., McCracken, C., Gaskell, R.M., Cameron, J.M., Coates, J.A.V., Gaskell, C.J., Hart, C.A. and Bennett, M. (1994a) Susceptibility in cell culture of feline immunodeficiency virus to 18 compounds. *Journal of Antimicrobial Chemotherapy* **34**, 589–594.

Smyth, N.R., Bennett, M., Gaskell, R.M., McCracken, C.M., Hart, C.A. and Howe, J.L. (1994b) 3'Azido-2',3'-deoxythymidine does not prevent feline immunodeficiency virus infection in domestic cats. *Research in Veterinary Science* **57**, 220–224.

Squires, R.A. and Gorman, N.T. (1990) Anti-neoplastic chemotherapy in cats. *In Practice* **12**, 101–111.

Swenson, C.L., Carothers, M.A., Wellman, M.L. and Kociba, G.J. (1993) Eosinophilic leukemia in a cat with naturally acquired feline leukemia virus infection. *Journal of the American Animal Hospital Association* **29**, 497–501.

Tenorio, A.E., Franti, C.E., Madewell, B.R. and Pedersen, N.C. (1991) Chronic oral infections of cats and their relationship to persistent oral carriage of feline calici-, immunodeficiency or leukemia viruses. *Veterinary Immunology and Immunopathology* **29**, 1–14.

Thiry, ME., Chappuis, G., Bublot, M., Van Bressem, M.F., Dubuisson, J. and Pastoret, P.-P. (1991) Failure to infect cats with bovine herpesvirus type-4 strain Movar 33/63. *Veterinary Record* **128**, 614–615.

Thompson, R.R., Wilcox, G.E., Clark, W.T. and Jansen, K.L. (1984) Association of calicivirus infection with chronic gingivitis and pharyngitis in cats. *Journal of Small Animal Practice* **25**, 207–210.

Tyler, D.E. (1990) Protothecosis. In: *Infectious Diseases of the Dog and Cat* (Ed. C.E. Greene). W.B. Saunders, Philadelphia. pp. 742–748.

Wall, P.G., Davis, S., Threlfall, E.J., Ward, L.R. and Ewbank, A.J. (1995) Chronic carriage of multidrug-resistant *Salmonella typhimurium* in the cat. *Journal of Small Animal Practice* **36**, 279–281.

Waters, L., Hopper, C.D., Gruffydd-Jones, T.J. and Harbour, D.A. (1993) Chronic gingivitis in a colony of cats infected with feline immunodeficiency virus and feline calicivirus. *Veterinary Record* **132**, 340–342.

Weiss, R.C. (1995) Treatment of feline infectious peritonitis with immunomodulating agents and antiviral drugs: a review. *Feline Practice* **23**(3), 103–106.

Weiss, R.C. and Tovio-Kinnucan, M. (1989) Inhibition of feline infectious peritonitis virus replication by recombinant human leukocyte (alpha) interferon and feline fibroblastic (beta) interferon. *American Journal of Veterinary Research* **49**, 1392–1335.

Welsh, R.D. (1996) *Bordetella bronchiseptica* infections in cats. *Journal of the American Animal Hospitals Association* **32**, 153–158.

Willoughby, K., Dawson, S., Jones, R.C., Symons, M., Daykin, J., Payne-Johnson, C., Gaskell, R.M., Bennett, M. and Gaskell, C.J. (1991) Isolation of *Bordetella bronchiseptica* from kittens with pneumonia in a U.K. breeding cattery. *Veterinary Record* **129**, 407–408.

Willoughby, K., Kelly, D.F., Lyon, D.G. and Wells, G.A.H. (1992) Spongiform encephalopathy in a captive puma (*Felis concolor*). *Veterinary Record* **131**, 431–434.

Wills, J. and Gaskell, R.M. (1994) Feline chlamydial infection. In: *Feline Medicine and Therapeutics* (Eds E.A. Chandler, C.J. Gaskell and R.M. Gaskell), Blackwell Scientific Publications, Oxford, pp. 544–551.

Wills, J., Millard, W.G. and Howard, P.E. (1986) Evaluation of a monoclonal antibody-based ELISA for detection of feline *Chlamydia psittaci*. *Veterinary Record* **19**, 418–420.

50

Principles of Cancer Therapy

J. M. Dobson

Introduction	985	Principles of radiation therapy	999
Tumour biology	985	Principles of anticancer chemotherapy	1005
The clinical approach to the cancer patient	988	Appendix I	1023
Cancer therapy	997	Appendix II	1023
Principles of oncological surgery	997		

INTRODUCTION

The diagnosis and management of cancer represents one of the major challenges facing the modern small animal veterinarian. There are many interrelated factors which have contributed to the increasing importance of cancer in companion animals over the past 10–20 years. Improved standards of welfare and health care have decreased death rates from infectious and other non-neoplastic diseases such that many animals now live to enjoy old age and suffer from a higher incidence of age-related disease, especially cancer. The perceived incidence of cancer in animals has also increased through advances in diagnostic techniques and the increasing use of cytology and histopathology. The actual incidence of tumours in companion animals is difficult to ascertain. In a major study on a defined population of animals the Tulsa Registry reported an incidence of 1126 cases of cancer per 100 000 dogs per annum and 470 cancers per 100 000 cats per annum (MacVean et al., 1978). Significant advances have been made in the treatment of cancer in animals, particularly in the development of techniques to improve the efficacy of surgical management of tumours, in the application of radiation therapy and in the use of cytotoxic drug therapy. Finally, the past 10–20 years have also seen a change in attitude of both the veterinary profession and the pet-owning public towards the problem of cancer in animals. Until recently a diagnosis of 'cancer' resulted in euthanasia of the patient. Today, many types of cancer can be managed successfully and, although a cure is not always possible, treatment can enable an animal to live a good quality of life for many months or years following the diagnosis of cancer.

The successful management of any disease depends on a basic understanding of the nature of that disease and this is especially important in the treatment of cancer. A great deal has been learnt about the biology, growth characteristics and causes of human and animal cancers during recent years, enabling more rational and effective treatments to be designed. Although the main purpose of this chapter is to discuss the principles of cancer therapy by surgery, radiation and chemotherapy, it is necessary to first consider the biology and behaviour of tumours.

TUMOUR BIOLOGY

It is generally accepted that the majority of naturally occurring cancers arise from the neoplastic transformation of a single precursor or stem cell. Although the events that lead to this neoplastic transformation are not fully understood, the basic change is related to disruption of the genetic mechanisms which normally control cell growth and differentiation. A number of regulatory cellular genes with oncogenic potential have been identified, these genes are termed oncogenes or tumour suppressor genes depending on their mode of action. External agencies, e.g. certain viruses, radiation, UV light, chemical carcinogens, may all act to cause cancer through interactions with these cellular genes, leading either to their up-grading (switching on) in the case of oncogenes or down-regulation (switching off) in the case of tumour suppressor genes. In the majority of cancers a sequence of several such genetic events or interactions, often occurring over a number of years, may be necessary before neoplastic transformation occurs (Wynford-Thomas, 1991).

Tumour cell populations

A tumour cannot be detected by palpation or radiography until it reaches approximately 1 cm in diameter or 0.5–1 g in weight, by which time it contains approximately 10^8–10^9 cells (Fig. 50.1). Cancer cells continually modify their properties during the process of growth, largely by small mutations occurring during cell division. Hence, although the cells in the tumour mass may share some features of the original precursor cell, they are heterogeneous in other properties such as the ability to metastasize. This heterogenicity is important in therapy because different cells within the tumour mass may be inherently more or less sensitive to cytotoxic drugs or to radiation.

Growth kinetics of a tumour

The dynamics of tumour growth are of considerable importance in tumour therapy. In the early stages of development most tumours grow rapidly, but, as with cells or bacteria in culture, the growth rate tends to slow down and reach a plateau as the tumour reaches larger proportions. For most tumours this plateau phase of growth is achieved at about the time that the tumour becomes clinically detectable (Fig. 50.1).

Growth fraction and doubling time (DT)

The growth characteristics of a tumour are usually described in terms of the 'tumour doubling time', i.e. the time it takes for a tumour to double in size. In early phases of growth the tumour doubling time is short, later, as the tumour becomes larger, doubling times lengthen. Tumour doubling time is a function of the number of actively dividing cells within the tumour, termed 'the growth fraction' (GF), and the time it takes for the dividing cells to complete the process of cell division, the 'cell cycle time'. During the early stages of tumour growth a high proportion of tumour cells are actively dividing, i.e. the growth fraction is high, but, by the time most solid tumours can be detected clinically, only a small proportion of the cells are dividing, i.e. the growth fraction is low. The growth fraction is important because most cytotoxic drugs act by interfering with the processes of cell division and are therefore only active against dividing cells.

The cell cycle

Cell division is a cyclical process with cells progressing through a series of well-defined stages of mitosis, growth, synthesis of DNA and further growth including preparation of the mitotic spindle (Fig. 50.2). Cells which are not actively dividing enter the 'G_0' or resting phase and may re-enter the cycle in response to a number of stimuli. Cells may be more or less sensitive to different drugs or to radiation at different stages of the cell cycle. For example, the vinca alkaloid drugs act by interfering with the formation of the mitotic spindle and are therefore 'cell cycle specific' agents acting on cells in the M (mitotic) phase of the cell cycle. The

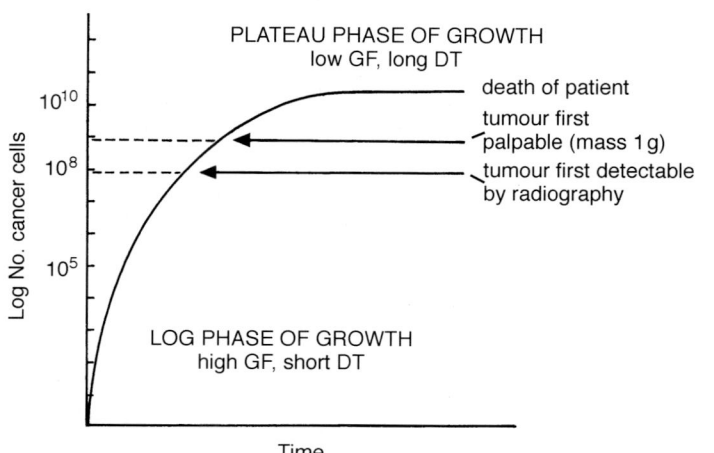

Figure 50.1 Growth kinetics of a tumour. Most tumours exhibit high rates of cell division in the early stages of growth. As the mass enlarges the growth rate and rate of cell division tend to be slowed by inhibitory factors until a plateau phase is reached. Tumours are not clinically detectable until relatively late in this sequence of events.

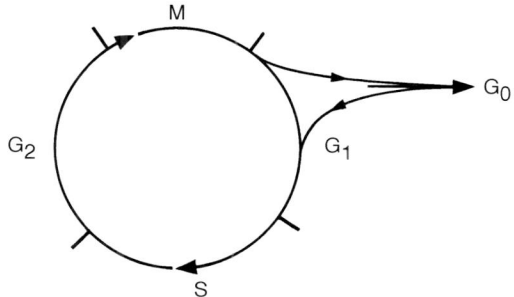

Figure 50.2 Cell growth and division follow an orderly sequence of events, described by the 'Cell Cycle'. The cell cycle is divided into five major stages: G_0, the resting phase; G_1, the intermitotic interval; S, the DNA synthesis phase; G_2, the premitotic interval and M, the mitotic phase.

alkylating agents, e.g. cyclophosphamide, are not cell cycle specific and act on all dividing cells. Cells also vary in their sensitivity to radiation according to the phase of the cell cycle. Cells in the M phase being most radiosensitive and those in the S (DNA synthesis) phase being most radioresistant. The resting (G_0) cells are also important in this context. Resting cells are relatively resistant to the actions of radiation and cytotoxic drugs and therefore form an important reservoir of cells from which the tumour may repopulate.

In summary, the popular concept of a tumour as a mass of homogeneous, rapidly dividing cells is incorrect. In reality the tumour cell population is quite heterogeneous and, by the time most tumours can be detected by palpation, the proportion of dividing cells is often less than that of normal body tissues such as skin, bone marrow or the gastrointestinal epithelium. The notable exception are tumours of the lymphoreticular system which maintain a high growth fraction despite a large tumour burden.

Tumour blood supply

One important factor influencing the growth pattern of a tumour is its blood supply. Most tumours derive their blood supply from vessels already present in adjacent host tissues by promoting growth of new vessels through the secretion of factors which promote angiogenesis. Although tumours may appear to be well vascularized and even haemorrhagic, in fact, tumour vasculature is generally inferior to that of normal tissues in terms of capillary density and ability to respond to physiological stimuli. For this reason many tumour cells exist in an environment of low oxygen tension and low pH, the latter resulting from build up of metabolic products. The nature of tumour vasculature has important implications in the delivery of drugs to a tumour and in radiation response.

Tumour behaviour

Neoplasms are traditionally classified according to their growth and behavioural characteristics as being benign or malignant (Table 50.1). Although

Table 50.1 Behavioural characteristics of benign and malignant neoplasms

	Benign	Malignant
Rate of growth	Relatively slow Growth may cease in some cases	Often rapid Rarely ceases growing
Manner of growth	Expansive Usually well-defined boundary between neoplastic and normal tissues. May become encapsulated.	Invasive Poorly defined borders, tumour cells extend into and may be scattered throughout adjacent normal tissues
Effects on adjacent tissues	Often minimal May cause pressure necrosis and anatomical deformity	Often serious Tumour growth and invasion results in destruction of adjacent normal tissues, manifest as ulceration of superficial tissues, lysis of bone
Metastasis	Does not occur	Metastasis by lymphatic, haematogenous routes and transcoelomic spread
Effect on host	Often minimal (can be life threatening if tumour develops in a vital organ, e.g. brain)	Often life-threatening by virtue of destructive nature of growth and metastatic dissemination to other, vital organs

Table 50.2 Cytological and histological features of malignancy

Cytological features	
Cell population	Pleomorphism
	Presence of mitoses, especially abnormal or bizarre forms
Cellular features	Large cell size/giant cells (anisocytosis)
	Poorly differentiated, anaplastic cells
	High nuclear to cytoplasmic ratio
Nuclear features	Large nuclear size, nuclear pleomorphism (anisokayrosis)
	Multiple nuclei (often of variable size)
	Hyperchromatic nuclei with clumping or stippling of chromatin
	Prominent and often multiple nucleoli of variable size and shape
Histological features	
Cellular features	As outlined for 'cytology'
Tumour architecture	Lack of structural organization of cells into recognizable form
Relationship with adjacent tissues	Invasion of cells into adjacent normal tissues
Evidence of metastatic behaviour	Tumour cells invading or present within lymphatics or venules

this division is useful for descriptive purposes, tumours display a spectrum of behaviour ranging from truly benign to highly malignant. Some tumours, e.g. oral acanthomatous epulis (basal cell carcinoma) and canine haemangiopericytoma, have local characteristics of malignancy but do not metastasize. Other tumours, e.g. mast cell tumours, can display a wide spectrum of behaviour ranging from benign to highly malignant. Histologically and cytologically a number of morphological features of a tumour can be used to predict its likely behaviour (Table 50.2) and the grade or histological appearance of the tumour in terms of mitotic rate, cellular and nuclear characteristics, is therefore important in prognosis.

The ability of malignant tumours to spread to and grow in distant organs is their most serious and life-threatening characteristic. The mechanisms involved in the process of metastasis are not fully understood. Current theories suggest that only certain clones of cells within a tumour develop the ability to metastasize but that these clones probably arise and disseminate in the early stages of that tumour's growth, often before the detection of the primary tumour (Hill, 1987).

Tumours may metastasize via the lymphatic route to local and regional lymph nodes or via the haematogenous route from where secondary tumours can subsequently develop in any body organ. In humans, different types of cancer show different target organ specificity for metastasis. For example, prostatic carcinoma tends to metastasize to bone; breast carcinoma to bone, brain, adrenal, lung and liver; and cutaneous melanoma to liver, brain and bowel. In small animals, the lungs are the most common site for the development of haematogenous secondary tumours but other sites including liver, spleen, kidneys, skin and bone should not be overlooked. Carcinomas and mast cell tumours usually metastasize by the lymphatic route and sarcomas and melanomas by the haematogenous route but tumours do not always follow expected patterns of behaviour and some tumours may spread by both lymphatic and haematogenous routes.

THE CLINICAL APPROACH TO THE CANCER PATIENT

The diagnostic evaluation of the patient is of great importance in the management of cancer. The initial approach to any patient with suspected cancer must be designed to achieve the following objectives:

1. To make a histological/cytological diagnosis of the nature and grade of the disease;
2. To determine the extent of the disease both in terms of local and distant spread;
3. To investigate and treat any tumour-related or concurrent complications which might affect the overall prognosis or the patient's ability to tolerate therapy.

A detailed history and careful physical examination of the animal is required from the outset of the case in order to meet these objectives. The temptation to concentrate only on the presenting mass must be avoided as this may lead to metastatic disease, tumour-related complications or concurrent disease being overlooked.

Investigative techniques

Although one can sometimes make an informed guess as to the likely nature of a tumour according to its site, gross appearance and history, *an accurate diagnosis can only be made upon microscopical examination of representative tissue or cells collected from the tumour.* Histological examination of needle, incisional or excisional biopsy samples is the most accurate method of cancer diagnosis. A biopsy provides the pathologist with the opportunity to examine the cellular components of the tumour, its architecture and its relationship to adjacent normal tissues. Careful thought must be given to the biopsy procedure. The technique used should provide a representative sample of tissue yet not predipose to local spread of the tumour nor complicate the subsequent treatment of the case (Table 50.3) (Else, 1989; White, 1991a). Cytology is increasing in popularity as a diagnostic technique and is useful in the investigation of neoplasia. Fine needle aspirates or impression smears from solid tumours and the cellular content of fluids collected from organs or body cavities can provide a great deal of information about the lesion and will often differentiate between inflammatory and neoplastic processes. The morphology of neoplastic cells will also often provide an indication of the likely histiogenesis of a tumour and its degree of malignancy. Fine needle aspiration is a quick and simple technique requiring a minimum of equipment which can easily be performed in practice (Figs 50.3a–d), however, cytological interpretation requires considerable skill and expertise. Many commercial clinical pathology laboratories will report on cytological samples and with practice most veterinarians should be able to use cytology to discriminate between reactive and neoplastic lesions and even to diagnose some particularly characteristic tumours, for example mast cell tumours.

In the cancer patient it is always preferable to achieve a diagnosis of tumour type and grade before embarking on therapy because only when the nature of the disease is known can the most effective therapy be prescribed.

Clinical staging

The stage or extent of a tumour is of equal importance to its histological type in determining prognosis and the feasibility of therapy. Successful treatment depends on eradication of all tumour stem cells, this can only be achieved if the extent of the disease is fully appreciated. It is, therefore, important to determine both the local extent of a tumour and to investigate the possibility of lymphatic or haematogenous metastasis as part of the initial evaluation of the cancer patient, prior to starting therapy. A number of clinical staging systems have been described and are widely used in human oncology. A TNM (T – tumour, N – nodes, M – metastases) system of clinical staging of animal tumours has been devised and is used at some centres (Fig. 50.4) (Owen, 1980). Whether or not such staging nomenclature is used, the underlying principles of assessing the extent of the primary tumour, the drainage lymph nodes and evaluating the patient for the presence of distant metastases are of paramount importance and a logical system for evaluation of the cancer patient must be followed (Table 50.4).

Table 50.3 Considerations for biopsy

• Procure a representative sample of the tumour	Avoid superficial ulcerations, areas of inflammation or necrosis Ensure adequate depth of biopsy, particularly for oral tumours Try to include tumour–normal tissue boundary in the biopsy sample
• Procedure should not predispose to local tumour recurrence or local spread	Minimize handling of tumour by adequate surgical exposure Ensure adequate haemostasis Minimize trauma to tumour and normal tissues Avoid contamination of normal tissue by surgical instruments
• Do not compromise subsequent therapy	Any biopsy procedure should be sited well within the margins of future excision

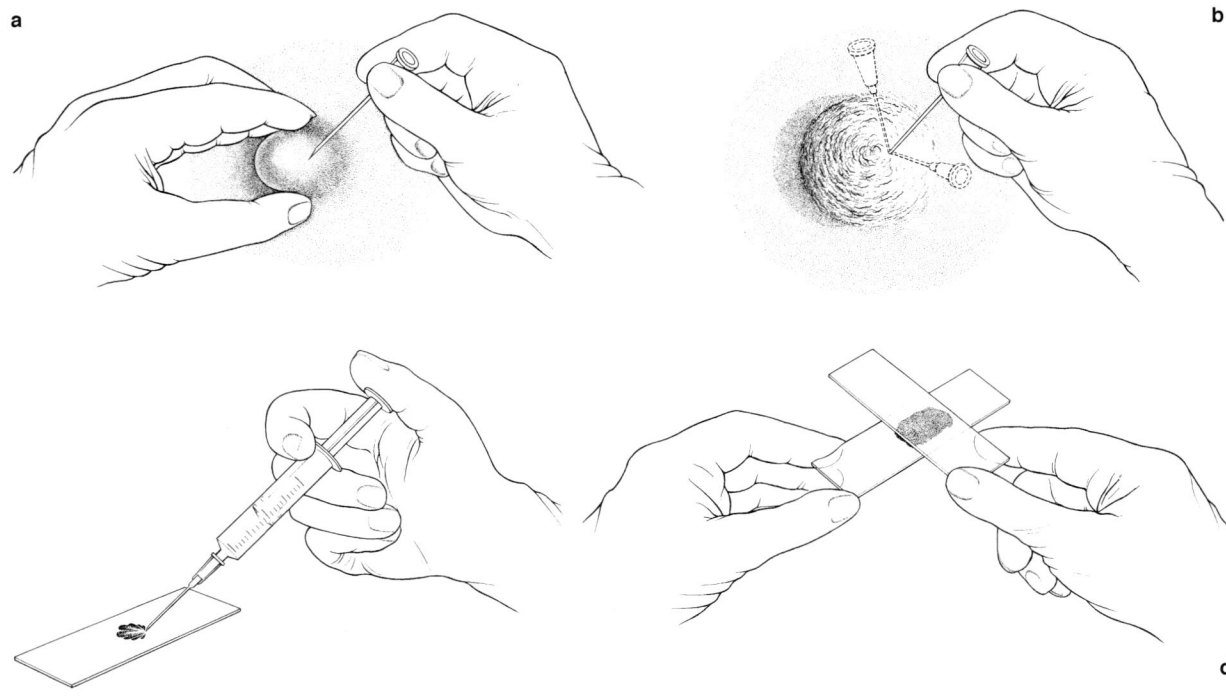

Figure 50.3 Diagrams depicting the sequence of events involved in collection of fine needle aspirate from an enlarged prescapular lymph node. (a) Following preparation of skin (as per venepuncture) the lymph node is located and immobilized in one hand. A 23G, 1 in hypodermic needle is introduced into the node. (b) A sample of cells is collected in the bore of the needle by stabbing the needle into the lesion several times, the needle being relocated in the lesion between 'stabs'. (c) The needle is withdrawn from the lesion and connected to an air filled syringe. The contents of the needle are blown onto a clean glass microscope slide. (d) A smear of the sample is made by gently drawing a second clean glass slide across the first.

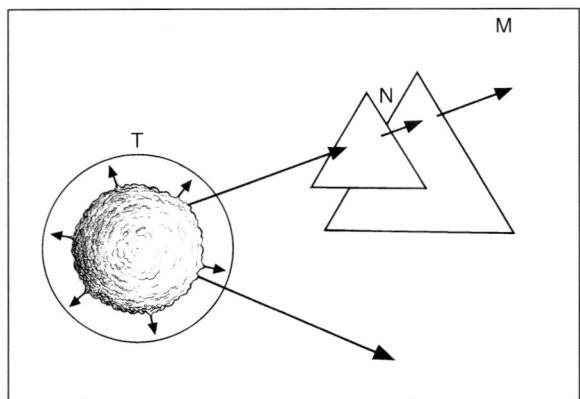

Figure 50.4 Schematic representation of the TNM system of tumour staging. 'T' represents the primary tumour mass, the size and degree of invasion of adjacent tissues must be assessed. 'N' represents the local and regional lymph nodes. 'M' represents potential sites of metastasis in distant organs. Redrawn from *BSAVA Manual of Oncology.*

Primary tumour

Malignant tumours tend to grow by invasion and many have microscopic extensions into adjacent normal tissues which cannot be appreciated by eye. Physical signs of local invasion are: diffuse, indistinct boundaries between normal tissue and tumour, fixation of the tumour mass in one or more planes and thickening of adjacent tissues. Some tumours, particularly soft tissue sarcomas, may, however, give the appearance of being well circumscribed and discrete due to the presence of a 'pseudocapsule' which is infiltrated by tumour cells. Hence, although the physical appearance of a tumour is important in determining its local extent, the information gained has to be taken in the context of the known growth behaviour of that type of tumour.

Other diagnostic techniques should be considered to aid in the evaluation of the primary tumour. Radiography can be useful in the assess-

Table 50.4 Methods for clinical staging of neoplasms

Technique	Primary tumour T	Local and regional lymph nodes N	Distant metastases M
Physical examination	To assess borders, mobility and depth	To assess size, texture, shape and mobility	Thorough physical examination of all systems – essential
Radiography	Important when tumour is adjacent to or involving bone, or for deeper tumours	Useful to assess internal lymph nodes, especially mediastinal and internal iliac (lymphangiography)	Right and left lateral thoracic films. Abdominal films may be useful to assess liver and spleen
Ultrasonography	Useful in assessment of deeper tumours, especially those in thoracic or abdominal cavities	Useful in assessment of deeper nodes	Ultrasonic assessment of liver, spleen and kidneys may detect nodular or diffuse neoplastic infiltrations
Endoscopy	Assessment of tumours involving hollow organs		
Aspirate/biopsy	Well-oriented biopsies may give information on depth of invasion of primary tumours	Cytology/histology may be required to distinguish between reactive and neoplastic lymph node enlargement	Cytology/histology of any suspicious lesion to confirm or exclude metastasis tumour
Haematological/biochemical investigations	Limited value in staging primary solid tumours, but essential for investigation of lymphoproliferative and myeloproliferative disease	Limited value	No specific tests or tumour markers to indicate metastases

ment of tumours adjacent to bone, particularly those in the oral cavity where the majority of malignant tumours invade the underlying bone. Contrast and plain radiography can also be useful in assessing less accessible tumours, e.g. those within nasal chambers or body cavities. Ultrasonography can be used to assess the extent of both superficial and deeper tumours and endoscopy can be useful in visual assessment of tumours involving hollow organs.

Lymph nodes

Local and regional lymph nodes must always be evaluated. Physical examination of the size and texture of superficial lymph nodes may indicate the presence of metastases (Fig. 50.5; Table 50.5) and radiography can assist in evaluating deeper nodes. Local lymph nodes may be enlarged as a result of reactive hyperplasia and cytological or histological evaluation of suspicious nodes may be required to distinguish between reactive hyperplasia and early nodal metastasis. It should be noted that focal metastatic deposits within a lymph node may be associated with secondary reactive changes in the rest of the node.

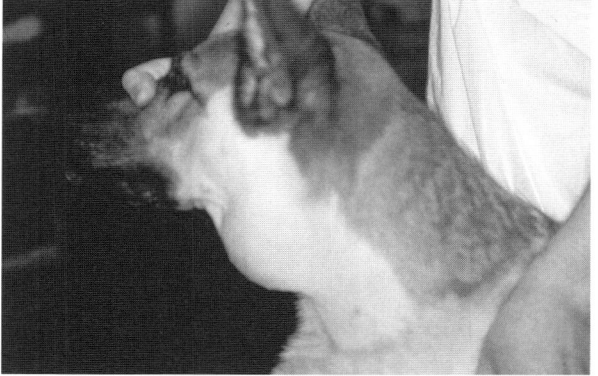

Figure 50.5 German shepherd bitch, presented with a grossly enlarged submandibular lymph node due to nodal metastasis of a mast cell tumour. The primary (poorly differentiated) mast cell tumour was located on the lower lip. See colour plate.

Metastases

Every attempt should be made to detect the presence of distant metastases during the initial evaluation of the cancer patient. The history, physical examination, thoracic radiographs and, where

Table 50.5 Features of reactive and neoplastic lymph node enlargement

Feature	Reactive hyperplasia	Tumour metastasis
Size	Slight to moderate enlargement	Slight to gross enlargement
Shape	Normal round–oval shape of node maintained	Node may become mis-shaped as tumour growth progresses
Texture	Soft to firm in texture	Firm to hard in texture
Mobility	Fully mobile with respect to adjacent tissues	Range from mobile in early stages to fixed in advanced disease
Cytology[a]	Mixed population of lymphocytes and lymphoblasts +/− neutrophils, plasma cells and macrophages	Neoplastic cells can usually be detected in cytological preparations

[a]Fine needle aspirates of suspicious lymph nodes are quick, cheap and simple to perform, and ultimately cytology or histology may be the only means of distinguishing between reactive hyperplasia and neoplastic enlargement of a lymph node.

available, ultrasonography are all useful screening procedures.

The lungs are the most common site for the development of secondary tumours in companion animals but discrete pulmonary tumours can only be detected on thoracic radiographs once they have reached the size of 0.5–10 cm in diameter. Right and left lateral thoracic radiographs should be included as a routine part of the initial work-up of any animal with a malignant tumour because the finding of pulmonary metastases leads to a poor prognosis (Fig. 50.6). The finding of a 'clear' thoracic film does not, however, exclude the possibility of micrometastases. Metastatic tumour in the liver, spleen or kidneys may be diffuse or nodular in distribution and may not significantly alter the shape or outline of those organs until the tumour reaches advanced stages. Ultrasonography is more useful than radiography in screening these organs (Fig. 50.7) but metastatic disease may also be below the threshold of ultrasonic detection.

Although it is important for the clinician to attempt to define the extent of a tumour as accurately as possible, it must be appreciated that because it is impossible to detect microscopic tumour extensions or deposits, there is a difference between the apparent clinical stage of a disease and its true pathological stage.

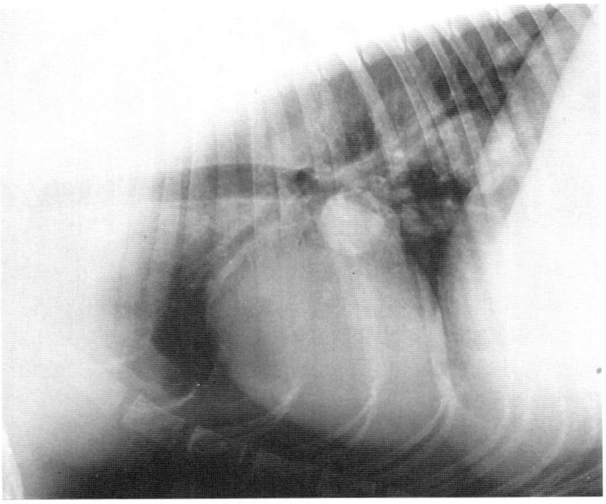

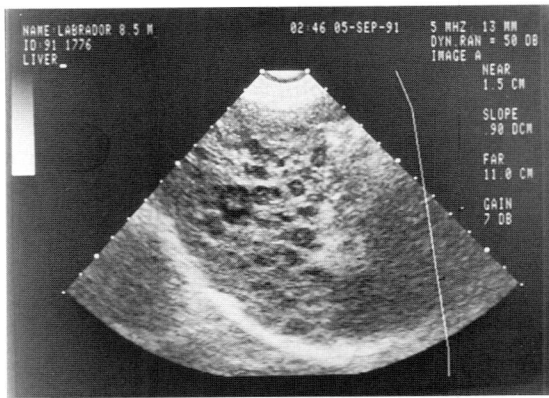

Figure 50.7 Ultrasonogram of liver showing multiple hypoechogenic areas correlating with metastatic tumours from a primary cutaneous mast cell tumour. Photograph courtesy of Michael Herrtage.

Tumour-related complications and concurrent disease

Tumours may be associated with a number of medical complications either resulting from the physical presence of the tumour or from products

Figure 50.6 Pulmonary metastasis. A right lateral thoracic radiograph from a dog with an osteosarcoma of the distal radius. A solitary pulmonary mass is seen overlying the base of the heart.

of the tumour which have effects on distant organs or body systems, these tumour-associated complications may be the presenting sign of the disease. Some of these conditions are life threatening and require emergency management; others, although not being immediately life-threatening, may affect the animal's ability to tolerate future treatment and influence the prognosis. It is therefore important that any such complication should be identified and treated.

Many animals presenting with cancer are elderly and may have concurrent cardiac, renal or hepatic dysfunction. The presence of these and/or other problems may also influence the prognosis and affect the patient's tolerance of treatment. All such problems should be fully addressed in the initial work-up.

Haematological complications

Neoplasms may cause a number of serious haematological complications through a variety of mechanisms which are summarized in Table 50.6. A routine haematological examination should therefore be included in the initial investigation of any cancer patient. The initial haematological assessment of the cancer patient is also very important to provide a basis from which to monitor the response to and toxicity of future treatment.

Anaemia is the most common haematological abnormality detected in cancer patients and this can vary from a mild to a very severe anaemia which may be regenerative or non-regenerative (Madewell and Feldman, 1980). A mild to moderate, normochromic, normocytic, non-regenerative anaemia is a common finding in animal cancer patients. This is usually an anaemia of chronic disease, postulated mechanisms of which include sequestration of iron (particularly in the bone marrow), shortened red blood cell lifespan, reduced erythropoietin activity or subnormal response to erythropoietin. The anaemia resulting from blood loss, haemolysis or lymphomyeloproliferative disease is often more severe and the resulting clinical signs (e.g. lethargy, depression) may be the reason for presentation of the animal.

Thrombocytopenia is a relatively common finding in myeloproliferative and lymphoproliferative disorders. Reduced platelet numbers may be found in up to 50% of dogs and cats with leukaemic conditions (Schlam et al., 1975; Morris et al., 1993). White blood cell counts may be normal, elevated or depressed in neoplastic conditions. A detailed consideration of diseases of the blood and blood-forming organs, covering neoplastic disease of these organs is to be found in Chapter 45.

Table 50.6 Haematological abnormalities associated with neoplasia

Primary	
Neoplastic invasion of the bone marrow/myelophthisis	Usually manifest as cytopenia: non-regenerative anaemia thrombocytopenia leucopenia
Secondary	
1. Tumour-mediated haematological abnormalities	Regenerative anaemia/thrombocytopenia may be associated with autoimmune haemolytic anaemia, or immune-mediated thrombocytopenia secondary to lymphoid neoplasia
	Microangiopathic anaemia, associated with fragmentation of red blood cells in haemangiosarcoma
	Sequestration of platelets in large abnormal tumour blood vessels, e.g. haemangiosarcoma
	Disseminated intravascular coagulopathy – triggered by many disseminated malignant tumours
2. Blood loss	Regenerative anaemia/thrombocytopenia haemorrhage from a tumour bleeding from gastroduodenal ulceration due to hypergastrinaemia or hyperhistaminaemia secondary to bleeding disorder

Metabolic and endocrine complications

Tumours can produce severe systemic or metabolic disturbances through the production of hormones or hormone-like substances which act on organs at sites distant from the primary tumour. The resulting clinical syndromes are termed 'paraneoplastic syndromes' and it is often this metabolic/endocrine disorder which alerts the owner to a problem, rather than detection of the underlying tumour (Giger and Gorman, 1984). Paraneoplastic syndromes can arise as a result of functional tumours of endocrine origin (Table 50.7) and a full discussion of the diagnosis and treatment of these syndromes can be found in Chapter 39. Various non-endocrine tumours can also produce and release hormones or hormone-like substances which have systemic effects (Table 50.8). Hypercalcaemia is the most common paraneoplastic syndrome recognized in the dog but is relatively rare in the cat.

Hypercalcaemia

Calcium is an important electrolyte involved in many physiological reactions in the body. It is especially important in maintaining the stability of excitable membranes, such that higher than normal concentrations of plasma calcium lead to decreased membrane excitability (Hille, 1982). The concentration of calcium in the extracellular fluid is normally maintained within a relatively narrow range by the combined actions of parathyroid hormone (PTH), calcitonin and vitamin D. The total serum calcium is equally distributed between that which is protein bound or complexed and that which is free or ionized. Only the ionized form of calcium is biologically active. The equilibrium between free and protein-bound calcium is dependent on the amount of plasma albumin and the acid–base balance (in acidic conditions the relative amount of ionized calcium is increased).

The most common cause of hypercalcaemia in the dog is neoplasia, although other, non-neoplastic causes do exist (e.g. hypoadrenocorticism) (Weller, 1984; Wotton and Pearson, 1988; Elliot et al., 1991). Cancer-associated hypercalcaemia results from the production of substances by haemopoietic and solid non-parathyroid neoplasms which stimulate bone resorption. Several hypercalcaemic factors produced by tumours have been identified including PTH, PTH-like substances, prostaglandins (PGE_2) and a lymphokine, osteoclast-activating factor (OAF) (Bockman, 1980; Mundy et al., 1985; Broadus et

Table 50.7 Syndromes associated with functional endocrine tumours

Syndrome	Tumour(s)	Clinical signs[a]
Hyperadrenocorticism (Cushing's syndrome)	Adrenal adenoma Adrenal adenocarcinoma Pituitary adenoma	Polydipsia/polyuria Polyphagia Coat changes: alopecia, calcinosis cutis Muscle weakness, Hepatomegaly Pendulous abdomen
Hyperthyroidism	Thyroid adenoma (cats) Thyroid adenocarcinoma (dogs and occasionally cats)	Polyphagia, polydipsia Weight loss, diarrhoea Tachycardia associated with hypertrophic cardiomyopathy Hyperexcitability
Primary hyperparathyroidism	Parathyroid adenoma	Due to hypercalcaemia – polydipsia/polyuria Anorexia, vomiting Muscle weakness Bradycardia/arrhythmias
Hypoglycaemia	Pancreatic islet (beta) cell tumour ('insulinoma')	Episodic weakness, collapse, disorientation and seizures
Hypergastrinaemia (Zollinger–Ellison syndrome)	Pancreatic gastrin producing neoplasm	Gastric and duodenal ulceration Vomiting (haematemesis)

[a]Only major clinical signs are included. The reader is referred to Chapter 39 for a more detailed discussion of these syndromes.

Table 50.8 Paraneoplastic syndromes resulting from non-endocrine tumours

Syndrome	Tumour(s)	Clinical signs
Hypercalcaemia	Lymphoid tumours, myeloid tumours Anal gland adenocarcinoma Solid tumours with skeletal metastases Other solid tumours	Polyuria/polydipsia Anorexia, vomiting Dehydration Muscular weakness, tremor Bradycardia
Hypoglycaemia	Hepatic tumours, especially hepatocelluar carcinoma Other tumours, especially large intra-abdominal tumours	Episodic weakness, collapse, disorientation and seizures
Hyperhistaminaemia	Mast cell tumours	Gastroduodenal ulceration Anorexia Vomiting, haematemesis, Melaena, anaemia
Syndrome of inappropriate ADH secretion	Associated with primary lung tumours in humans	Oedema/hyponatraemia

al., 1988). In many cases, however, the active substance is not known. In the dog, hypercalcaemia is most commonly associated with lymphoproliferative disorders (e.g. lymphoma), adenocarcinoma of the apocrine glands of the anal sac, other solid tumours with or without bone metastases and a functional adenoma of the parathyroid gland.

The clinical signs of hypercalcaemia are non-specific, reflecting the physiological importance of calcium in the function of many organ systems. The predominant clinical signs are polydipsia/polyuria, anorexia, vomiting, lethargy, depression and muscular weakness. These signs can be attributed to the effects of hypercalcaemia on the renal, gastrointestinal and neuromuscular systems, respectively. Hypercalcaemia can also affect the heart, resulting in bradycardia and arrhythmias. The renal effects of hypercalcaemia are of greatest importance. In the early stages hypercalcaemia affects the renal tubules causing an inability to concentrate urine which leads to hyposthenuria and polyuria with secondary polydipsia. The renal nephropathy is initially reversible but if the hypercalcaemia persists the renal damage becomes irreversible and eventually metastatic calcification of the renal tubular epithelium and basement membranes occurs (Osborne and Stevens, 1977). The renal effects of hypercalcaemia cause the animal to become dehydrated and hypovolaemic, further fluid loss may occur from vomiting. Renal failure caused by hypercalcaemia is therefore exacerbated by prerenal failure due to hypovolaemia and the animal becomes azotaemic.

Death due to renal or cardiac failure will follow unless the situation is corrected rapidly.

Treatment of hypercalcaemia

Immediate management of hypercalcaemia is aimed at rehydrating the patient. Sodium chloride (0.9%) is the fluid of choice. Restoration of circulating volume aids the lowering of the serum calcium by improving the glomerular filtration rate and assisting renal excretion of calcium. Once the animal is rehydrated, calcium excretion can be further promoted by saline diuresis (0.9% sodium chloride at 2–3 times maintenance rate) assisted by frusemide (Lasix™, Hoechst), intravenously, at a dose rate of 2 mg kg^{-1} bid or tid.

In hypercalcaemia associated with lymphoproliferative neoplasms, lowering of serum calcium can also be assisted by the use of glucocorticoids (prednisolone 2 mg kg^{-1} daily). These agents are cytotoxic to lymphoid cells and also reduce serum calcium by limiting bone resorption, reducing intestinal calcium absorption and enhancing renal excretion of calcium. The value of glucocorticoids in the treatment of hypercalcaemia associated with non-lymphoid neoplasms is debatable. Once the animal's condition is stabilized, treatment of the inciting cause of the hypercalcaemia is essential for long-term control.

There are a number of other agents which have been used in humans for the treatment of refractory hypercalcaemia, these include: mithramycin (25 μg kg^{-1}, single dose), calcitonin, i.v. infusion of phosphate solutions, phosphate enemas, sodium EDTA and peritoneal dialysis. More recently

Table 50.9 Treatment of hypercalcaemia

Objective	Action
1. Restore circulating volume	Intravenous fluid therapy 0.9% sodium chloride over 24 h
2. Reduce plasma calcium concentration	Saline diuresis: 0.9% NaCl at 2–3 × maintenance rate frusemide 2 mg kg^{-1} bid or tid Lymphoid tumours: glucocorticoids, e.g. prednisolone 2 mg kg^{-1} daily
3. Identify and treat inciting cause	Specific chemotherapy, surgery or radiation as appropriate

biphosphonates (disodium etidronate and disodium pamidronate) have been shown to be highly effective in the treatment of hypercalcaemia of malignancy. Rarely are any of these agents required in veterinary medicine as most cases of hypercalcaemia can be managed effectively by the strategy outlined in Table 50.9.

Hyperhistaminaemia and mast cell tumours

Mast cell tumours are very common in the dog and present a number of problems in diagnosis and treatment due to their very variable nature and clinical behaviour (O'Keefe, 1990). On occasion, and probably more commonly than is generally appreciated, these tumours are associated with systemic complications resulting from the release of histamine from tumour cells. The cytoplasmic granules of mast cells contain vasoactive amines and proteases including histamine and heparin. Degranulation and release of these mediators may occur spontaneously in some mast cell tumours or may be precipitated by manipulation of the tumour. The inflammatory mediators thus released may have both local and systemic effects. Local effects include oedematous swelling of the tumour and surrounding area, erythema and sometimes pruritus (Fig. 50.8). If significant amounts of heparin are present there may be a tendency for localized bleeding. The release of proteases may also cause delayed wound healing or wound breakdown following surgery.

A massive and sudden release of histamine could precipitate an anaphylactic reaction requiring emergency treatment with fluids, corticosteroids and antihistamines. Although this is extremely unusual, premedication of animals with antihistamine (e.g. diphenhydramine hydrochloride, 5–10 mg i.v.) prior to surgical manipulation of such tumours has been advocated by some

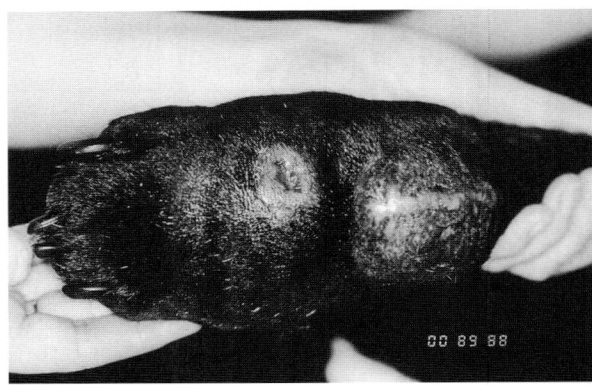

Figure 50.8 Mast cell tumour of foot associated with oedematous swelling and erythema. See colour plate.

authorities. A more common effect of hyperhistaminaemia occurs in the gastrointestinal tract. Up to 80% of dogs with mast cell tumours may develop gastroduodenal ulcers (Howard et al., 1969) as a result of hyperacidity secondary to hyperhistaminaemia (Fox et al., 1990). Histamine also causes hypermotility of the intestine, dilation of gastric blood vessels and increases endothelial permeability, the combination of which can lead to thrombosis and ischaemic necrosis of the gastric mucosa. Clinical signs vary according to the severity and duration of the problem and range from mild anorexia to vomiting, haematemesis, melaena and anaemia resulting from intraluminal bleeding. Ultimately the ulcers may perforate leading to peritonitis, collapse and death. Cimetidine (Tagamet™, Glaxo) 5–10 mg kg^{-1} tid (an H$_2$ antagonist) is strongly recommended in the management of such cases.

CANCER THERAPY

The demand for cancer therapy in small animals is undoubtedly increasing and, as a result of advances in therapeutic techniques, remarkable improvements in the survival rate of animals with malignant tumours can be achieved. The three main methods of cancer treatment in animals, as is the case in humans, are surgery, radiation and anticancer chemotherapy. Cancer therapy must always by tailored to suit the individual case, taking account of the biology, histology, grade and extent of that tumour. Clearly a cure, i.e. total eradication of all tumour stem cells, is the ultimate aim of cancer therapy but even the most effective methods of treatment currently available cannot be expected to achieve this aim in every case. The decision to treat an animal with cancer is one which must be made jointly by the veterinarian (bearing in mind the type of tumour, its extent, the facilities and experience available) and the owner. Owners must be counselled thoroughly in the nature of the disease, the prognosis, the options for treatment and the expectations of such treatment and should be given time to consider the options and reach a decision regarding their pets. The methods of cancer therapy which will be described in the remainder of this chapter are generally tolerated very well by animal patients provided that there are no pre-existing complications which make the patient more susceptible to toxicity.

PRINCIPLES OF ONCOLOGICAL SURGERY

Surgery is the most effective means of treatment for the majority of solid neoplasms in animals. The primary objective of surgical treatment of any tumour, be it benign or malignant, is to physically remove all the tumour cells. In most cases it will be necessary to include a margin of normal tissue in the surgical excision in order to achieve this aim. Failure of surgical treatment results either from the tumour being incompletely resected at the first attempt, in which case the tumour will regrow at or adjacent to the primary site, or from the tumour having metastasized to distant organs prior to surgical treatment, in which case the animal will subsequently develop further problems relating to metastatic tumour elsewhere. Surgery is rarely an effective or feasible means of managing disseminated disease and adjuvant chemotherapy is more appropriate in such cases. Local tumour recurrence is strongly influenced by the surgical approach and the main advances in surgical oncology have been in defining the margins of excision which are necessary to achieve eradication of different tumours and in developing techniques whereby such margins can be achieved. It is not the intent of this section to cover the surgical and reconstructive techniques used in oncology in detail, as these have been described elsewhere (White, 1991b). The following is a brief description of surgical techniques which have proved efficacious in the management of certain tumours.

Surgical approaches

Local excision

Truly benign tumours, e.g. fibroma, lipoma, mammary adenoma, can be cured by local surgical resection with a minimal margin of normal tissue (Fig. 50.9). Local surgical resection is a simple and straightforward procedure when lesions are small. A tumour which is left to enlarge will require a more major procedure at a later date.

Wide local excision

Locally invasive tumours, e.g. acanthomatous epulis, basal cell carcinoma, squamous cell carcinoma, are characterized by local extension of the tumour into adjacent normal tissues. In such cases

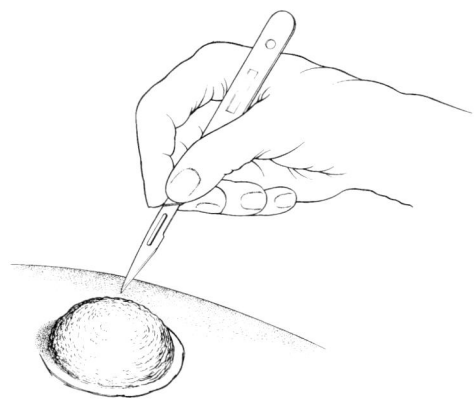

Figure 50.9 Local surgical excision (excisional biopsy). The tumour is excised through its immediate boundaries with a minimal border of surrounding tissue. Redrawn from *BSAVA Manual of Oncology* courtesy of Dr R.A.S. White.

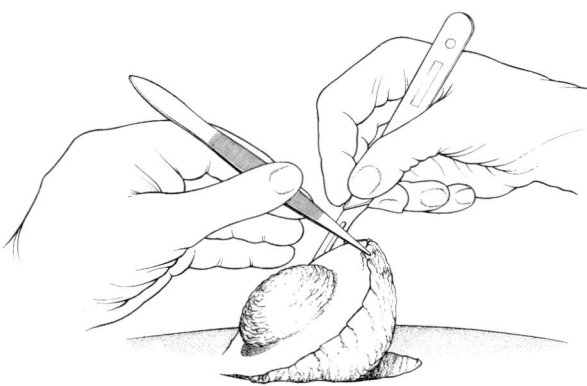

Figure 50.10 Wide local excision. The tumour is excised with a predetermined margin of surrounding tissue both lateral and deep to the tumour mass. Redrawn from *BSAVA Manual of Oncology* courtesy of Dr R.A.S. White.

local surgical excision is unlikely to remove all tumour cells and local recurrence will ensue unless a more aggressive surgical approach is adopted. Surgery is the treatment of choice for such tumours but wider margins of excision, including at least 1–2 cm of apparently normal tissues lateral and deep to the tumour are often required to achieve a successful outcome. Such a procedure is termed a 'wide local excision' (Fig. 50.10). For tumours sited on the chest or abdominal walls, achieving excisional margins of this magnitude is usually not difficult. Problems may arise, however, in the case of tumours sited on limbs or in the head region, particularly in the oral cavity. For tumours on limbs and the head, excisional margins can usually be achieved but, because of the lack of mobile skin and soft tissues, reconstructive techniques, e.g. skin grafting, may be necessary to close the resulting deficit. Tumours in the oral cavity present a particular problem because of their proximity to bone. Locally invasive tumours arising at this site frequently extend into the underlying bone such that successful surgery requires removal of portions of bone. Various techniques for mandibulectomy, premaxillectomy and maxillectomy have been well documented in the veterinary literature (Withrow and Holmberg, 1983; White *et al.*, 1985; Penwick and Nunamaker, 1987; Salisbury and Lantz, 1988). These procedures are very well tolerated in dogs and 1-year survival rates for animals with acanthomatous epulis are in the order of 90–100% (White and Gorman, 1989).

Compartmental excision

Finally, there are a group of solid tumours which are now recognized to infiltrate adjacent tissues so widely that even 1–2 cm excisional margins are not adequate to ensure complete removal of all tumour cells. This group includes moderately differentiated mast cell tumours and soft tissue sarcomas (e.g. fibrosarcoma, haemangiopericytoma). These tumours are not chemosensitive or radiosensitive and surgery remains the most effective treatment. Surgical removal of such tumours requires resection of every tissue compartment which the tumour involves, termed a 'compartmental' or 'en bloc' resection (Fig. 50.11). To achieve such a resection in tumours arising on the trunk invariably requires full thickness resection of either the abdominal or chest wall. The resulting deficits must be reconstructed using prostheses and skin flaps. In tumours arising in the proximal limb, it is sometimes possible to achieve an en bloc resection by removal of a muscle mass and overlying skin, leaving the animal with a functional limb. In other cases amputation may have to be considered.

All the surgical techniques described require careful planning especially when reconstructive techniques are involved. The treatment and the expected cosmetic and functional results should be fully discussed with the owner. It is therefore essential that the nature of the tumour is identified, preferably by biopsy (or cytology), before embarking on the definitive treatment. It is increasingly appreciated that the best chance of eradication of locally aggressive tumours is at the first surgical attempt. Subsequent surgical procedures are fraught with difficulties due to loss of normal anatomical relationships through scarring

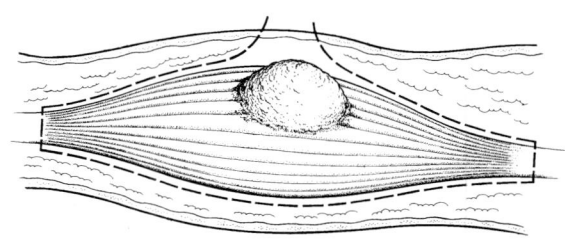

Figure 50.11 Compartmental resection. The tumour is resected together with the entire anatomic contents of the compartment in which it is contained. Fascial planes which are undisturbed by tumour invasion form the outer margins of the resection. Redrawn from *BSAVA Manual of Oncology* courtesy of Dr R.A.S. White.

PRINCIPLES OF RADIATION THERAPY

Ionizing radiation is widely used in the treatment of human cancer and is equally applicable to the treatment of the disease in small animals. Radiotherapy requires specialized equipment and facilities which are expensive to install and maintain. Consequently, the use of radiation therapy in animals is restricted to larger referral establishments. Although most veterinarians in practice will not have direct access to such facilities, it is important to review the principles and practice of radiation therapy, in order that suitable cases might be identified and referred at an appropriate stage.

The mode of action of radiation

Radiation is a form of energy which, when absorbed by living tissues, causes excitation and ionization of component atoms or molecules in the path of the beam. Subsequent chemical reactions result in breaking of molecular bonds and can result in cell death if molecules critical for cell viability are disrupted. The 'critical target' is generally regarded as being nuclear DNA but other molecules in other parts of the cell (e.g. proteins and lipids) may also be damaged and contribute to radiation-induced cellular injury (Hall, 1978).

Types of radiation used for therapy

A variety of ionizing radiations may be used for therapeutic purposes including X-rays, gamma rays and electrons (Table 50.10). There are essentially two techniques for the application of radiation to tumours. Radiation (X-rays, gamma rays and electrons) may be delivered in the form of an external beam of radiation directed into the tumour. Alternatively, radioactive substances which emit gamma or beta rays, may be applied to the surface of a tumour, implanted within the tumour or administered systemically to the patient. Each technique has advantages and disadvantages. Although external beam therapy is relatively safe for the operator, the equipment is expensive and multiple doses of radiation are required over a 4–6 week course of treatment (Fig. 50.12). Brachytherapy often offers better localiza-

Table 50.10 Techniques for radiotherapy

Technique	Source	Type of radiation	Characteristics and indications
External beam therapy 'teletherapy' administered as multiple fractions	Orthovoltage unit	X-rays 100–300 kV	Radiation of limited penetration with maximum dose on surface, preferential absorption by bone Superficial dermal/soft tissue tumours
	Linear accelerator	X-rays or electrons 4–20 MeV	Deeply penetrating radiation with skin sparing (max. dose below surface), uniform tissue absorption Deeper tumours, tumours adjacent to or involving bone
	Cobalt-60	Gamma-rays 1.25 MeV	Intermediate penetration with some skin sparing Deeper tumours as above
	Caesium-137	Gamma-rays 0.662 MeV	Intermediate penetration with some skin sparing Superficial treatments or implantation
	Strontium-90	Beta particles	Strontium applicator applied to surface, maximum depth of penetration 3–4 mm Very superficial tumours
Brachytherapy interstitial implantation or systemic administration continuous exposure	Gold-198	Gamma rays	Gold seeds applied via a surface mould or implanted within tumour
	Iridium-192	Gamma rays	Seeds or needles implanted into tumour
	Iodine-125	Gamma rays	Implanted permanently into tumour
	Iodine-131	Gamma and beta rays	Systemic administration – radioactive iodine preferentially taken up in thyroid, used in treatment of thyroid tumours
	Phosphorus-32	Beta rays	Systemic administration – preferential uptake in various tissues depending on chemical composition, e.g. phosphate salt – bone/bone marrow

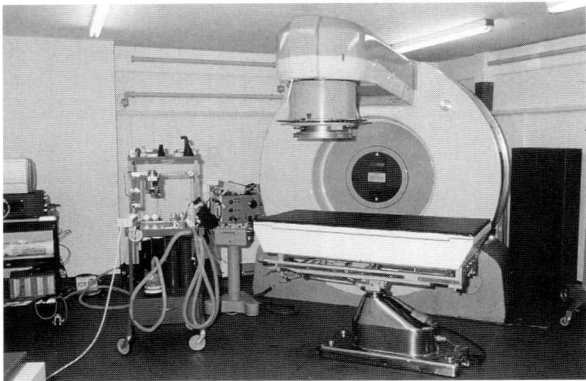

Figure 50.12 Linear accelerator.

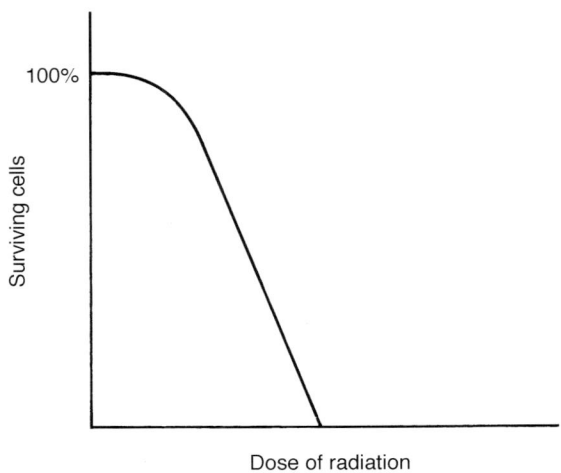

Figure 50.13 Mammalian cell survival curve postradiation (*in vitro*). Following a single exposure to radiation the number of surviving cells is proportional to the applied dose of radiation. (The shoulder at the start of the curve indicates that some radiation damage can be repaired.)

tion of the radiation and permits the delivery of high doses of radiation to the tumour with minimal normal tissue toxicity. However, the implant and the implanted patient present a radiation hazard for the operator and any staff caring for the patient. Radioactive isotopes can only be used on licensed premises and strict local rules for handling the isotope and patient must be applied. Both techniques require careful planning in consultation with medical physicists to ensure the required dose of radiation is delivered to the tumour (Thrall *et al.*, 1989).

The effects of radiation on living tissues

The response of living cells and tissues to radiation depends on the applied dose of radiation and the radiosensitivity of the cell population. Most normal and neoplastic cell populations show a typical cell survival curve with increasing cell death in response to increasing doses of radiation (Fig. 50.13). The shoulder at the start of the curve indicates that some radiation-induced cellular damage may be repaired. Radiosensitivity varies according to a number of factors, one of the most important being the growth fraction of the cell population. Dividing cells are generally more sensitive to radiation that non-dividing, differentiated cells. Thus tissues with a high proportion of dividing cells, e.g. bone marrow, gastrointestinal epithelium, are more radiosensitive than non-proliferating tissues, e.g. fibrous tissue and skeletal muscle. The same applies to tumours; those with a high growth fraction tend to be more sensitive to radiation than those with low growth fractions. Individual cells vary in their radiosensitivity as they pass through the phases of the cell cycle. Cells in the M (mitotic) phase of the cycle being most radiosensitive and those in the S (DNA synthesis) phase being most resistant. The resting (G_0) cells are also radioresistant. The oxygenation of cells is also thought to be significant in determining radiosensitivity. Tumour cells which exist at a low oxygen tension, i.e. hypoxic cells, may be 2.5–3 times less sensitive to radiation than normally oxygenated cells.

It is clear from the above that, although radiation is a potent means of causing cell death, it is not selective with respect to neoplastic cells. Radiation can be equally damaging to normal tissues, indeed, certain normal tissues may be more sensitive to radiation than many tumours. In order to be of therapeutic benefit, radiation must be used in such a way as to minimize normal tissue injury while achieving maximum tumour cell kill. One way in which this may be approached is by attempting to localize the radiation to the tumour. Radioactive implants and radiolabelled substances which are taken up by tumour cells (e.g. radioactive iodine for thyroid tumours) afford a degree of selectivity. With external beam radiation, the beam can be collimated to the area of the tumour and several treatment ports used in order to reduce the amount of entry and exit beam radiation affecting the surrounding normal tissues.

A further means of reducing normal tissue injury from external beam therapy is to 'fractionate' the treatment, that is to apply the radiation in multiple small doses over a long period of time rather than as one large dose. Following a single dose of radiation a number of changes will occur in the surviving cell population, these are referred to as the four 'Rs' of radiotherapy: repair, repopulation, redistribution and reoxygenation.

- *Repair* Both neoplastic and normal tissue cells have the ability to repair sublethal radiation damage and do so within hours of exposure.
- *Repopulation* Occurs through recruitment of surviving stem cells; again this applies to both normal and neoplastic tissues.
- *Redistribution* Because of their relative radioresistance, cells in the S phase of the cell cycle are more likely to survive a single dose of radiation than those in other phases. After a single dose of radiation most of the surviving cells will therefore be in or emerging from the 'S' phase. As these cells continue the process of cell division, they progress through the cell cycle and become more sensitive to a second dose of radiation.
- *Reoxygenation* Well-oxygenated tumour cells are more sensitive to radiation than hypoxic cells and less likely to survive a single dose of radiation. Death of oxygenated cells and increased blood flow following a dose of radiation may improve the oxygen status of previously hypoxic tumour cells thus rendering them more sensitive to a subsequent dose of radiation.

Hence, largely by virtue of the processes of reoxygenation and redistribution, tumour cell kill may be increased by delivering radiation in multiple small doses. Although normal tissue damage can be limited to some extent by allowing time for repair and repopulation between doses, repair and repopulation also occur in the tumour (Fig. 50.14). The optimum schedule for fractionation of radiation in clinical practice is not truly known but recent clinical trials in human patients have demonstrated considerable benefits in the delivery of two or three small fractions of radiation daily (Dische and Saunders, 1989). At the present time most radiation schedules for human patients use daily or alternate day treatments over a period of 4–6 weeks. In animals, where general anaesthesia is required for restraint of the patient during

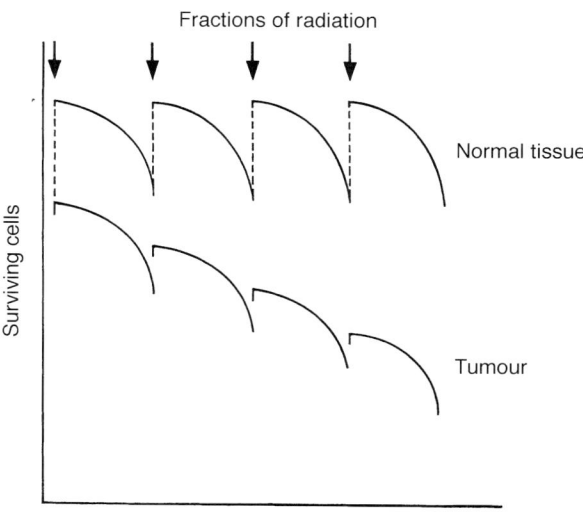

Figure 50.14 Tumour and normal cell survival following fractionated radiation. When multiple small doses (or fractions) of radiation are applied *in vivo* differences in the ability of tumours and normal tissues to repair radiation damage and repopulate, and the effects of re-oxygenation and redistribution (see text) allow a therapeutic effect.

treatment and where radiation facilities are not widely available, larger weekly or biweekly fractions tend to be used, although some centres are now treating animals on a daily basis.

Response to radiation

Although the chemical events leading to radiation-induced damage occur almost instantaneously, the biological expression of this injury may take days, weeks or even years to become apparent. Radiation therefore appears to have delayed actions in terms of both tumour response and normal tissue toxicity.

Tumour response

Tumours vary considerably in their response to radiation and different tumour types may be more or less sensitive to radiation (Table 50.11). It is debatable, however, whether this variation is solely due to differences in inherent cellular radiosensitivity or is more a feature of the growth characteristics and size of the tumour. Both factors probably play a role as tumours of the same histology may vary in their radiation response. In general, small, rapidly growing tumours tend to

Table 50.11 Relative radiosensitivity of common animal tumours

Relative radiosensitivity	Tumour
High	Lymphoproliferative disorders Myeloproliferative disorders Transmissible venereal tumour
Sensitive	Squamous cell carcinoma Basal cell carcinoma Adenocarcinoma (various)
Moderate	Mast cell tumours (variable) Malignant melanoma of the oral cavity
Low	Fibrosarcoma Osteosarcoma Chondrosarcoma Haemangiopericytoma

respond more favourably to radiation than large, slowly growing lesions where radiation treatment is unlikely to achieve more than a partial and temporary remission.

The desirable response to irradiation of a tumour is a complete disappearance of the tumour mass with no subsequent recurrence within a stated period of time, usually 2 years in small animals. Such a response would be deemed a 'cure', unfortunately this cannot be achieved in every case. Most tumours do, however, regress to some extent in response to radiation and, although the disease may not be cured, the palliation achieved will often allow a useful and pain-free extension of the animal's life. Because of the delay between treatment and response, tumour regression cannot usually be measured until several fractions of radiation have been delivered, i.e. 2–3 weeks after the start of therapy. In some cases the tumour may remain static or even increase slightly in size during the course of treatment. The regression of the tumour continues once the course of treatment is finished and the maximum or final response is not usually seen until 2–3 months after treatment. Persistence of a mass at the tumour site does not necessarily reflect a failure of treatment. The residual swelling may merely contain fibrous, stromal tissues which do not pose a threat to the patient. Tumours which have involved bone often promote a reactive proliferation of bone causing a swelling which will persist despite complete eradication of the tumour. In most cases where tumour regression is achieved the damaged and dead tumour cells are absorbed. In some tumours, however, areas of necrosis may become apparent after radiation and surgical debridement of such tissues may be required (Fig. 50.15).

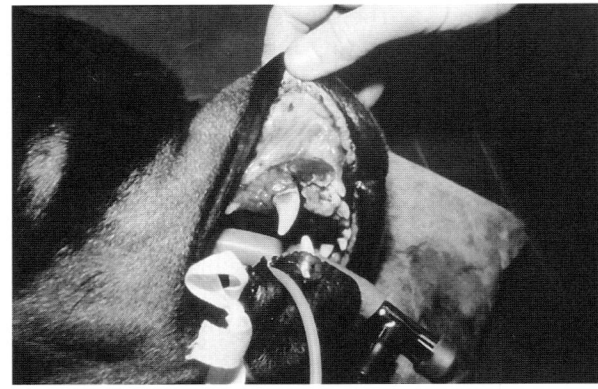

a

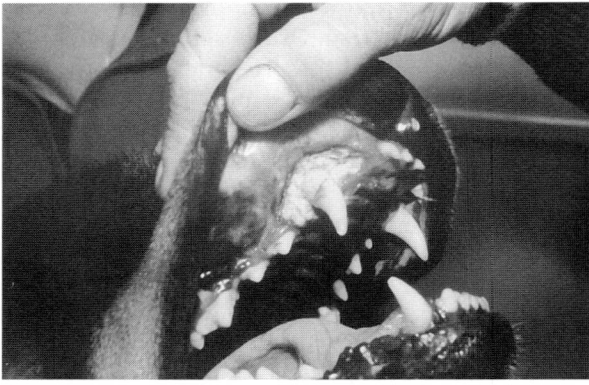

b

Figure 50.15 The typical response of an oral tumour to radiation therapy. Rottweiler with an osteosarcoma of the premaxilla, before treatment (a). The same dog at the end of a 4-week course of radiation therapy (b). The tumour has completely regressed but there remains necrotic bone at the tumour site which may require surgical debridement at a later date. See colour plate.

Normal tissue toxicity

In practice it is not usually possible to exclude all normal tissues from the field of radiation treatment, not least because generous margins are required to include any microscopic tumour extensions into adjacent tissues. In humans, radiation has a reputation for causing serious toxicity to the patient, however, radiation sickness and severe morbidity only arise when large areas of the body or vital organs are exposed to high doses.

In order to avoid such side effects, radiation is rarely used in this manner in the treatment of animals. Tumours most suitable for irradiation tend to be superficial or those sited on the extremities of the body. The skin, superficial connective tissues, mucous membranes (oral tumours) and bone are therefore the tissues most commonly included in the treatment field and some radiation-induced changes will occur in these tissues.

Radiation toxicity is usually divided into 'acute' reactions occurring during and shortly after the radiation treatment and 'late' reactions which are not observed for weeks or even months after treatment. This division is not absolute.

Acute radiation toxicity

Acute radiation reactions result from the death of actively dividing cell populations, e.g. epithelium of the skin and mucous membranes. Acute reactions range from a mild reddening or erythema of the skin/mucosa to vesiculation, desquamation and severe exfoliative dermatitis/necrosis. The latter is rarely seen with standard radiation schedules. In most cases erythema and a mild, superficial desquamation will occur and may cause the patient temporary discomfort (Fig. 50.16). These reactions usually resolve spontaneously as the normal cell population regenerates. Localized hair loss is a common result of irradiation of the skin in animals. This results from damage to the hair follicle epithelium at the time of treatment but the resulting alopecia does not usually occur until the existing hair is shed and not replaced (Fig. 50.17). Ultimately some hair usually regrows but this may be patchy and lacking pigmentation (Fig. 50.18).

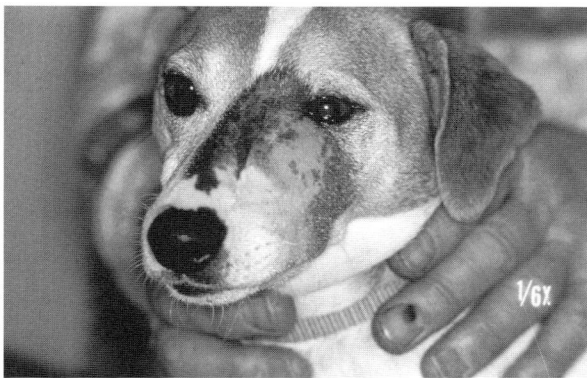

Figure 50.17 Post-radiation hair loss: alopecia is common in irradiated skin occurring weeks to months after radiation exposure. See colour plate.

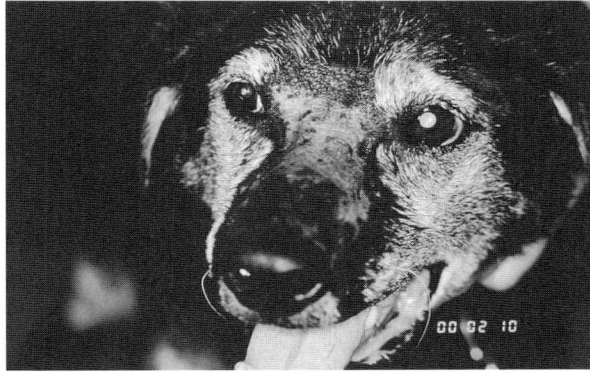

Figure 50.18 Patchy regrowth of hair: in many cases the hair will eventually regrow but this regrowth may be patchy and, as in the example shown, the hair may be grey/white. See colour plate.

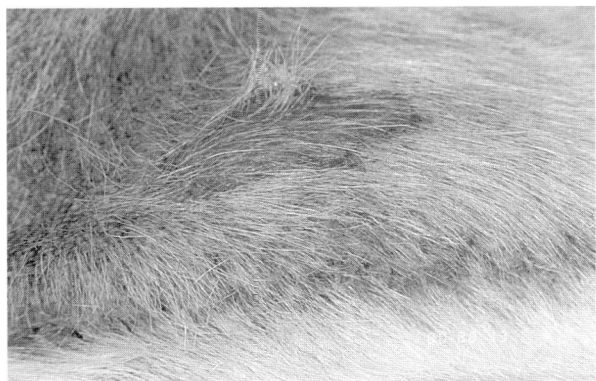

Figure 50.16 Acute radiation skin reaction: erythema and superficial desquamation of the skin may occur towards the end of a course of radiation treatment and in the immediate post-treatment period. These effects may cause temporary discomfort but usually resolve spontaneously as the normal tissues regenerate. See colour plate.

Late radiation toxicity

Late radiation reactions are less predictable and more serious. Late reactions tend to occur in slowly proliferating tissues, e.g. connective tissues and bone. In the skin, radiation induces fibrosis in the dermal connective tissues resulting in a thickened, rubbery texture and subsequently contraction of the skin and subcutis can occur. As a result of the fibrosis and vascular changes, irradiated skin and soft tissues can be very slow to heal and even the most minor surgical procedure can result in a non-healing, necrotic wound.

Osteonecrosis is a major concern in fields containing bone, particularly in cases where the bone is already compromised by tumour invasion. Late reactions in nervous tissues can also be a problem, irradiation of the spine should be avoided if at all possible as it can result in paralysis. Late radiation reactions can be very distressing as they are often irreversible and difficult to manage. For these reasons radiation protocols are usually designed to minimize the risk of serious late reactions, indeed, late radiation reactions are usually the dose-limiting factor in the radiation prescription.

Indications for radiation therapy in small animals

The main indication for radiation therapy in veterinary medicine is in the treatment of malignant tumours which, by virtue of their size or site, cannot be controlled by surgical means alone (Adams, 1991). Radiation is most effective and least toxic when used as a local treatment for superficial tumours or those on the extremities of the body. It is desirable that local and/or distant metastases are not present, although local lymph nodes can be included in the treatment fields. Because of the difficulties in localization and the risk of toxicity, tumours sited deep in the chest, abdomen or pelvis are not usually treated with radiation in animals. Benign tumours are often not very radiosensitive, and, because radiation is potentially carcinogenic, other means of treatment should always be sought to manage such tumours.

Tumours of the oral cavity, the nasal cavity and on the head, trunk and limbs are among those most commonly presented for radiation therapy (Fig. 50.19). The relative radiosensitivity of malignant tumours occurring at these sites is summarized in Table 50.11, but this should only be regarded as an approximate guide because the size and growth rate of the tumour will also influence response. Large, bulky tumours have a low growth fraction and are likely to contain significant numbers of hypoxic cells rendering them relatively radioresistant. The management of such tumours can be improved substantially by the combination of surgery and radiation (McLeod and Thrall, 1989). Radiation can be applied prior to, following or during surgery. At present, in veterinary medicine postoperative radiation is the most common method of combining these two modalities. Cytoreductive surgery reduces the tumour burden to microscopic levels leaving small numbers of well-oxygenated and rapidly proliferating cells which, in theory, should be sensitive to radiation. Radiation will, however, delay the healing of the surgical wound and must either be commenced immediately after surgery or once the wound has healed. The combination of radiation and surgery in this manner is potentially most beneficial in the management of problematic solid tumours, e.g. soft tissue sarcomas and intermediate grade mast cell tumours. It is preferable that radiation and surgery should be combined as a carefully planned therapeutic strategy. The use of radiation as an after-thought to salvage inadequate surgery is fraught with difficulties in planning and application and this practice is strongly discouraged.

Radiation may also be administered before surgery to decrease the tumour to more manageable proportions and 'sterilize' the tumour bed before surgical manipulation, thereby reducing the potential for local dissemination at the time of surgery. Preoperative radiation is increasingly

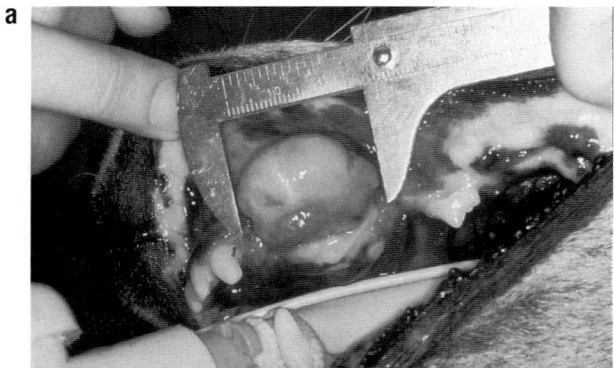
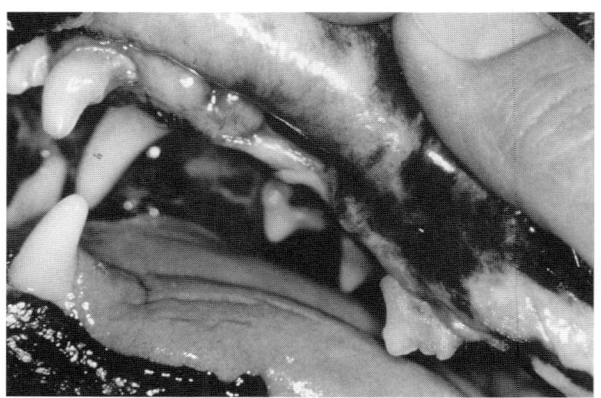

Figure 50.19 Radiation response. (a) Maxillary squamous cell carcinoma with extension into the nasal chamber preventing surgical management. (b) A complete regression of the tumour is achieved following 3600 cGy radiation delivered in 4 × weekly fractions. (This is the same dog as shown in Fig. 50.18). See colour plate.

used in the management of human cancers but veterinary experience of this technique is limited. The main problem with this combination is that irradiated soft tissues have poor tolerance of surgical manipulation and complications with wound healing may lead to dehiscence and necrosis.

Radiation may also be applied to unresectable tumours at the time of surgery. Surgical exposure of the tumour site and removal of sensitive tissues from the treatment field allows the application of high doses of radiation to tumours which are otherwise difficult to treat by radiation. Intraoperative radiation requires close proximity of surgical and radiation facilities and is not commonly practised in the veterinary field although the technique has been used in the treatment of a number of tumours including canine bladder carcinomas (Walker and Breider, 1987; Withrow et al., 1989).

PRINCIPLES OF ANTICANCER CHEMOTHERAPY

The use of cytotoxic or anticancer drugs in the treatment of cancer is a relatively new branch of veterinary medicine. In contrast to surgery and radiation which are only effective against local neoplastic disease, chemotherapy has the potential to act against systemic disease which is a major problem in oncology. Many cytotoxic drugs are now available for the treatment of human cancers and some of the major advances in human cancer therapy, for example in the treatment of childhood leukaemias and testicular cancers, have been achieved through the use of such drugs. In animals, chemotherapy has become established as the treatment of choice for lymphoproliferative and myeloproliferative diseases and significant increases in life expectancy can now be achieved in many of these conditions. The use of cytotoxic drugs in the treatment of other animal cancers is constantly being explored and as more drugs become available for veterinary use so the indications for chemotherapy in animals are likely to expand.

Cytotoxic drugs are highly potent agents and extreme care is required in all aspects of their use. Not only do they pose a danger to the patient but staff and owners should be aware of the potential hazards of exposure to these agents. Guidelines for safe handling of cytotoxic drugs are given later in this chapter. The therapeutic margin of most cytotoxic agents is extremely narrow and toxicity is the main dose-limiting factor. In humans, intensive medical care is often necessary to support the patient through periods of severe toxicity resulting from aggressive chemotherapy. Such intensive care is not routinely available or feasible in veterinary medicine and aggressive therapy which would result in serious toxicity to the patient also raises ethical questions. In veterinary practice treatment regimes and dosages are therefore a compromise between efficacy and toxicity. Careful consideration must always be given to the pharmacology and toxicity of the drug, the spectrum of its activity and the condition of the patient.

Mechanisms of action of cytotoxic drugs

Most cytotoxic drugs act on the processes of cell growth and division (Fig. 50.20); it therefore follows that the growth kinetics of a tumour are a major factor governing response to chemotherapy. Tumours with a high growth fraction are more likely to respond favourably to chemotherapy than those with a low growth fraction. The proportion of resting (G_0) cells is also important as these cells are resistant to the actions of cytotoxic drugs and therefore govern the ultimate response to therapy. Normal tissue toxicity follows a similar pattern: organs containing a high

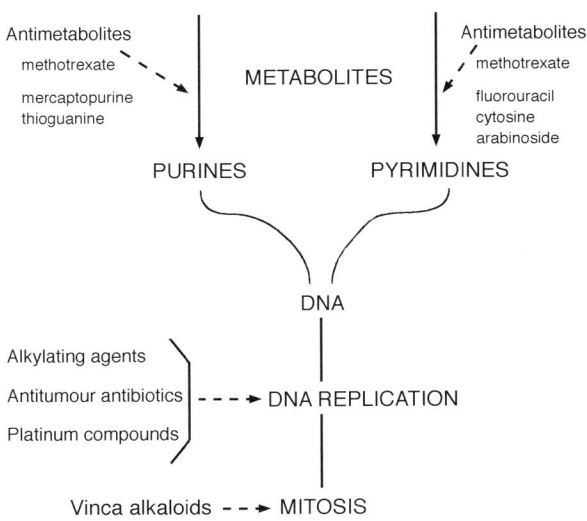

Figure 50.20 Summary of the mechanisms and sites of action of cytotoxic drugs.

proportion of dividing cells, e.g. bone marrow and the gastrointestinal epithelium, are most susceptible to drug-induced toxicity. The resting stem cell populations in these tissues are, however, relatively resistant to the actions of cytotoxic drugs and most cytotoxic drug toxicity is reversible.

Cytotoxic drugs are commonly divided into a number of classes each with characteristic sites or modes of action, antitumour activity and toxicity (see also Table 50.12 and Fig. 50.20).

Table 50.12 Anticancer drugs by group

Alkylating agents	
Nitrogen mustard derivatives	Cyclophosphamide
	Chlorambucil
	Melphalan
Ethenimine derivatives	Thiotepa
Alkyl sulphonates	Busulphan
Triazine derivatives	Dacarbazine
Nitrosureas	Carmustine
	Lomustine
Antimetabolites	
Antifolates	Methotrexate
Pyrimidine analogues	Cytosine arabinoside
	Fluorouracil
Purine analogues	Mercaptopurine
	Thioguanine
Antitumour antibiotics	
	Actinomycin D
	Bleomycin
	Daunorubicin
	Doxorubicin
	Epirubicin
	Mitoxantrone
	Mithramycin
	Mitomycin C
	Streptozotocin
Vinca alkaloids	
	Vincristine
	Vinblastine
Corticosteroids	
	Prednisolone
	Prednisone
Miscellaneous agents	
	L-Asparaginase/ cristantaspase
	Cisplatin
	Hydroxyurea

Alkylating agents

Alkylating agents are the most widely used cytotoxic agents in veterinary medicine. These drugs act by interfering with DNA replication and RNA transcription. They substitute alkyl radicals ($R\text{-}CH_2\text{-}CH_2$) for hydrogen atoms in the DNA molecule. Alkylation of nucleotide bases (e.g. the N^7 guanine of DNA) causes breaks, cross-linkages and abnormal base pairing in DNA. Alkylating agents also react with sulphydryl, phosphate and amino groups causing inhibition of enzymes involved in protein and nucleic acid synthesis. These actions of the alkylating agents are not cell cycle specific. Myelosuppression is the major side effect of these drugs, they may affect the gastrointestinal tract and can cause anorexia, vomiting and diarrhoea. Alkylating agents may also affect gametogenesis and cause alopecia in some breeds of dog.

Antimetabolites

Antimetabolites are a group of drugs which interfere with the normal metabolism of the cell. They are generally structural analogues of metabolites required for purine and pyrimidine synthesis and thus interfere with DNA and RNA synthesis by enzyme inhibition or by causing synthesis of non-functional molecules. Antimetabolites are cell cycle specific, acting during the S phase of the cell cycle. These agents all cause myelosuppression and may also affect the gastrointestinal tract causing anorexia, vomiting and diarrhoea. Renal and neurological toxicity are features of individual drugs (see individual agents).

Antitumour antibiotics

Antitumour antibiotics are derived from soil fungi, e.g. *Streptomyces*. These agents act by forming stable complexes with DNA thus inhibiting DNA synthesis and transcription. These actions are not cell cycle specific. Antitumour antibiotics have a particularly wide spectrum of antitumour activity. With the exception of bleomycin, antitumour antibiotics are myelosuppressive but they also cause a diverse range of selective toxicities (see individual agents).

Vinca alkaloids

The vinca alkaloids are plant alkaloids extracted from the periwinkle (*Vinca rosea* Linn). They bind to microtubular proteins (tubulin) and inhibit formation of the mitotic spindle, causing a metaphase arrest. These agents are thus cell cycle specific, acting during the M phase. Vinca alkaloids may have other cytotoxic effects on the cell which are less well documented, for example they may cause enzyme inhibition. Tubulin microtubules are also important in neurotransmission therefore neurological toxicity can occur.

Hormones

Hormonal manipulation has an important role in the management of breast, prostatic and endometrial carcinomas in humans. Although hormones clearly play a role in the development and growth of similar tumours in animals, the therapeutic value of hormonal manipulation has yet to be clearly demonstrated. Oestrogens and androgen antagonists may be of value in the management of certain hyperplastic or benign neoplastic conditions of the prostate and perianal hepatoid glands in the dog.

The corticosteroids prednisone and prednisolone are widely used in oncology. They have a cytotoxic action on haematological malignancies, particularly lymphomas. Their immunosuppressive activity is valuable in the management of certain tumour-related complications and finally, they have a role in the palliation of advanced disease.

Miscellaneous agents

There are a number of other agents with antitumour activity which do not fit into the previous groups. These include L-asparaginase (Cristantaspase) and platinum coordination compounds.

Doses of cytotoxic drugs are usually calculated as a function of body surface area (in M_2) rather than body weight because the blood supply to the organs responsible for detoxification and excretion (liver and kidneys) is more closely related to surface area than body weight. The calculation of body surface area from body weight and conversion tables for cats and dogs are provided in Appendix I. Details of all cytotoxic drugs included in the following text and tables are provided in an easy reference format in Appendix II. The dose rates, indications and side effects for these agents are only intended as an approximate guide to the use of these agents and more detailed information should be sought prior to their use. In the individual patient, the severity of the disease, haematological or metabolic complications and the presence of concurrent health problems must be fully addressed since all may influence the prognosis and the ability of the patient to tolerate cytotoxic drug therapy. Care must be taken in patients with compromised renal or hepatic function as impaired metabolism and excretion of the drug may result in increased toxicity.

The rationale of cytotoxic drug administration

The theoretical basis for cytotoxic drug regimes used in clinical practice has been established through years of laboratory and clinical research concerning the interaction of cytotoxic drugs and cancer cells *in vitro* and *in vivo*. Such work has led to the realization that the successful clinical application of cytotoxic drugs demands a different approach to that governing the administration of antibiotics and other pharmacological agents commonly used in practice.

The cell kill hypothesis

One of the most important and basic principles of anticancer chemotherapy is described by the 'Cell Kill Hypothesis' (Skipper et al., 1964). This states that cytotoxic drugs kill tumour cells by first-order kinetics: that is to say that a given dose of a cytotoxic drug kills a fixed percentage of the total tumour population as opposed to a set number of tumour cells. For example, if a given dose of a drug A kills 90% of tumour cells then it will reduce a tumour cell population of 100 million to 10 million, but if there are only 100 cells in a tumour the same dose of drug A will only reduce the number of tumour cells from 100 to 10. This theory therefore infers that, even a highly effective drug acting on a highly sensitive tumour cell population is unlikely to eradicate the tumour cell population in a single dose. In most clinical situations where tumours are known to be chemosensitive, a single treatment will achieve a log kill of 2 to 4.

The Cell Kill Hypothesis is essentially a theoretical model, it assumes a constant rate of growth for all tumour cells, that all tumour cells are equally chemosensitive and that the drug is equally distributed to all tumour cells. In the clinical setting these assumptions are not entirely accurate for reasons discussed earlier in this chapter. Furthermore, the toxicity of the drug to the patient is a major factor governing the dose of drug which can be administered. Nevertheless the Cell Kill Hypothesis does form the basis of two important principles of chemotherapy:

1. Maximum doses of anticancer drugs should always be used where possible.

2. Chemotherapy should be instituted when the tumour burden is at its lowest, i.e. when the tumour is first detected or, in the treatment of micrometastases, following surgical removal of the primary tumour.

Chemotherapy is unlikely to be effective if used as a last resort for the treatment of extensive and advanced disease.

In clinical practice a single dose of a single chemotherapeutic agent is clearly insufficient to eradicate a tumour. The most effective chemotherapeutic protocols employ a combination of cytotoxic agents delivered at timed intervals.

Single agent versus combination therapy

In most circumstances a combination of cytotoxic agents has proved to be more effective in the management of cancers than the use of a single agent. As a result of tumour cell heterogeneity many tumours contain cells which are inherently resistant to the actions of certain agents. By bombarding the tumour with a combination of agents which employ different mechanisms of action, the overall response can be enhanced. In addition, although all cytotoxic drugs have some damaging effects on normal tissues, different agents affect different normal tissues to varying degrees. Hence, if it is possible to combine drugs with different actions and toxicities, an additive tumoricidal effect can be achieved without an increase in toxicity. Most combination drug protocols have been designed according to these criteria, for example the COAP protocol, widely used in the treatment of multicentric lymphoma, employs:

Cyclophosphamide:	alkylating agent
Vincristine:	vinca alkaloid
Cytarabine:	antimetabolite
Prednisolone:	corticosteroid

Dosage and timing of treatments

The Cell Kill Hypothesis infers that it is desirable to administer the maximum possible dose of a drug to the patient. In practice, however, the dose of drug which can be administered is usually limited by normal tissue toxicity. In most circumstances the critical normal tissue is the bone marrow and, to a lesser extent the gastrointestinal epithelium. Fortunately, these normal tissues have a tremendous capacity for recovery from cytotoxic drug damage through processes of cellular repair and repopulation from recruitment of resting stem cells. In comparison, tumour cell populations have a reduced capacity for these reparative processes. Therefore, it is more beneficial to administer a cytotoxic drug at repeated intervals, allowing the normal tissues to recover between treatments than to use continuous therapy where the normal tissues are constantly exposed to the drug and unable to repair or repopulate (Fig. 50.21). The interval between treatments has to be carefully timed to allow for recovery of the normal tissues without expansion of the residual tumour population. If the time interval is too short, cumulative toxicity will occur resulting in leucopenia and thrombocytopenia, vomiting and diarrhoea. If the time interval is too long the tumour will repopulate and the benefit of the preceding treatment will have been lost.

The splitting of cytotoxic drug treatment into short intensive intervals is termed 'pulse' dosing and pulsed combination chemotherapy is now the most commonly used technique in the drug treatment of cancer. Certain chemosensitive tumours, for example lymphomas, often show a remarkable response following one or two courses of such therapy. Clinically this may be seen as a complete regression of the tumour and remission of any associated signs. It is important to appreciate that a clinical remission is not synonymous with cure. A complete clinical remission merely reflects a reduction in the tumour cell population from 10^{11} to 10^8 cells and unless treatment is continued there

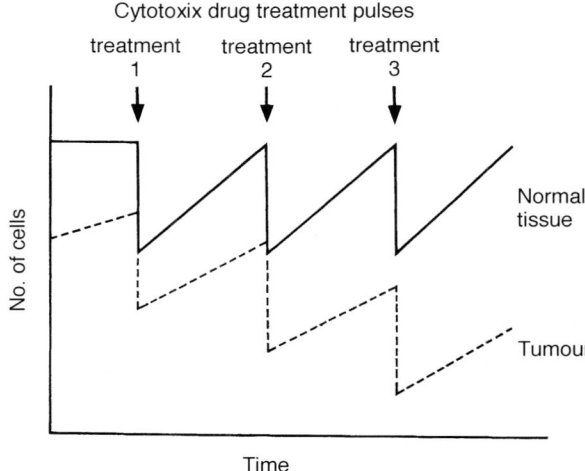

Figure 50.21 Theoretical basis for administration of cytotoxic drugs. If drug treatments can be sequenced to allow full recovery of normal tissues between treatments the reduced capacity for repair/recovery in the tumour results in increasing tumour cell kill.

will be a rapid expansion of the residual tumour mass resulting in a 'relapse' of the disease. Even the most chemosensitive of tumours usually require 6–12 months of aggressive chemotherapy to effect a cure.

Indications for chemotherapy in veterinary medicine

The main indication for chemotherapy in veterinary cancer medicine is in the treatment of systemic or disseminated malignant disease. In practice there are broadly two categories of disease where chemotherapy should be considered:

1. In the treatment of lymphoproliferative and myeloproliferative diseases which are generally systemic in nature;
2. As an adjunct to surgical and/or radiation treatment of the primary malignant tumours with a high risk of distant metastatic disease.

Lymphoproliferative and myeloproliferative disease

Definitions

The term 'lymphoproliferative disease' is used to describe all neoplastic conditions arising from lymphoid cells and includes all types of lymphoma (malignant lymphoma, lymphosarcoma), myeloma (multiple myeloma, plasma cell myeloma) and lymphoid leukaemias.

The term 'myeloproliferative disease' describes all non-lymphoid neoplastic conditions arising from the haemopoietic stem cell and includes all non-lymphoid leukaemias (e.g. acute myeloid leukaemia, chronic granulocytic or myelogenous leukaemia, polycythaemia vera) and primary myelofibrosis.

Chemotherapy is the treatment of choice for these conditions because of their systemic or widespread nature and because the tumours are usually sensitive to a wide range of cytotoxic drugs both as a result of a high growth fraction and inherent cell sensitivity.

Lymphoma (synonyms: malignant lymphoma, lymphosarcoma)

The disease

Lymphoma is the most common haemopoietic malignancy encountered in small animal practice, accounting for approximately 30% of all feline malignancies and 8–10% of all canine malignancies (Rosenthal, 1982; Priester and MacKay, 1980). The disease is characterized by a malignant proliferation of lymphoid cells and may arise in any organ containing lymphoid tissues and many non-lymphoid tissues, e.g. lymph nodes, thymus, alimentary system and skin. Thus different anatomic forms of the disease may be recognized (Table 50.13). Irrespective of the site of origin, the disease ultimately disseminates to involve other lymphoid and non-lymphoid tissues, particularly the spleen, liver, lungs and bone marrow. A clinical staging system can be used to describe the extent of the disease as shown in Table 50.14. Lymphoma may also be classified according to histological parameters, the cell type (e.g. lymphocytic or lymphoblastic) and cell distribution (e.g. nodular or diffuse) and according to the immunological type (e.g. T cell, B cell or null cell) (Moulton and Harvey, 1990).

Multicentric lymphoma is the most common form of the disease in the dog. Affected patients usually present with gross enlargement of one or more peripheral or superficial lymph nodes (Fig. 50.22). In our referral practice, most patients are presented with a generalized lymphadenopathy with or without hepatic and/or splenic involvement (i.e. Stage III or Stage IV disease). Approximately 30–50% of dogs presenting with

Table 50.13 Anatomic forms of lymphoma

Muliticentric
Thymic
Alimentary
Cutaneous
Solitary
(leukaemia)

Table 50.14 Clinical staging of canine multicentric lymphoma

Stage	Extent
I	Involvement limited to a single lymph node or lymphoid tissue in a single organ
II	Involvement of lymph nodes in a regional area +/− tonsils
III	Generalized lymph node involvement
IV	Hepatic and/or splenic involvement (+/− stage III)
V	Manifestations in the blood and/or involvement of bone marrow and/or other organ systems

From Owen (1980).

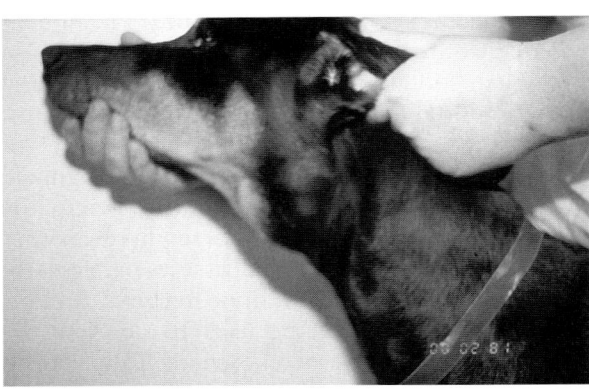

Figure 50.22 Canine multicentric lymphoma. This Dobermann was presented with generalized lymphadenopathy. The gross enlargement of submandibular lymph nodes is typical of that commonly seen in canine multicentric lymphoma. See colour plate.

multicentric lymphoma have metabolic or haematological complications, including dehydration, hypercalcaemia, anaemia, thrombocytopenia or white blood cell abnormalities. Approximately 10% of animals are presented in Stage V with bone marrow involvement (Dobson and Gorman, 1993).

Lymphoma is a common problem in the cat and the association with the feline retrovirus feline leukaemia virus (FeLV) is well documented (Hardy, 1981; Jarrett, 1994). Not all cats presenting with lymphoma are FeLV positive although serological and epidemiological evidence suggests that FeLV infection and retroviral transformation is an important causative agent in the vast majority of cases. The multicentric form of lymphoma is most common in middle-aged cats and approximately 50% of these cases will be FeLV positive. Thymic lymphoma is most common in young cats, aged 1–2 years, and 90% of such cases are FeLV positive. In elderly cats, the alimentary form of the disease is more common and a smaller

Table 50.15 Diagnostic investigation of multicentric lymphoma

Procedure	Comment
Lymph node aspirate or biopsy	Essential for diagnosis and classification of disease
Haematological evaluation	Essential full haematological evaluation includes: RBC, WBC and platelet counts RBC parameters differential WBC count
Biochemical 'screen'	Essential screen should include: urea, creatinine, alkaline phosphatase, alanine aminotransferase (ALT), aspartate aminotransferase (AST), & gamma glutamyl transferase (GGT), glucose and electrolytes (Na, K, Ca)
Radiography thorax and abdomen	Important if animal has respiratory signs or if there is evidence of organomegaly
Ultrasonography liver and spleen	Useful if animal has hepato/splenomegaly
Bone marrow aspirate or biopsy	Indicated in the case of haematological abnormalities
FeLV/FIV status	Essential in cats

proportion (approximately 35%) of these cases are FeLV positive (Jarrett, 1994). The FeLV status of an affected cat does not in itself affect treatment of that case although clearly there are ethical considerations if the cat is likely to come into contact with other, non-affected animals and the prognosis is worse for cats that are FeLV positive.

Diagnosis

The diagnosis of any form of lymphoma depends on the demonstration of malignant lymphoid cells by cytological or histological examination of affected tissues. Although the clinical presentation and history may be strongly suggestive of a diagnosis of lymphoma, particularly in the multicentric form of the disease, histological or cytological confirmation of the disease is essential. Further investigations are necessary to establish the extent of the disease and determine whether there are any tumour-related complications. The minimum requirements for the full investigation of a suspected case of lymphoma are summarized in Table 50.15. Although these investigations entail some time and expense, the future management of the case depends on the disease being correctly diagnosed and staged from the outset. Any tumour-related complications should be identified and treated appropriately at this time.

Therapy of lymphoma

Without treatment lymphoma is usually rapidly fatal and average survival times of 6–8 weeks are the norm. However, in both cats and dogs, lymphoma generally responds well to cytotoxic drug therapy (Rosenthal and MacEwan, 1990). A variety of chemotherapeutic protocols have been used in the treatment of canine lymphoma, many of which can also be used in the cat (Table 50.16; MacEwan et al., 1981; Madewell, 1985; Carter et al., 1987; Cotter and Goldstein, 1987; Postorino et al., 1989). In general, combination chemotherapy is more successful than single agent therapy but the results of treatment do not differ substantially with the different chemotherapeutic regimes

Table 50.16 Chemotherapeutic protocols used in the treatment of canine lymphoma

C.O.P. (high dose)
Cyclophosphamide: 250–300 mg m^{-2} p.o. every 21 days
Vincristine: 0.75 mg m^{-2} i.v. every 7 days for 4 weeks, then every 21 days
Prednisolone: 1 mg kg^{-1} daily p.o. for 4 weeks then on alternate days

C.O.P.A.
As above but with:
Doxorubicin: 30 mg m^{-2} i.v. in place of cyclophosphamide every 9th week

Cyclic combination therapy
Vincristine: 0.75 mg m^{-2} i.v. days 1 and 14
Asparaginase: 400 IU kg^{-1} i.m. day 1
Cyclophosphamide: 200–250 mg m^{-2} p.o. day 7
Methotrexate: 0.6–0.8 mg kg^{-1} i.v. day 21
Repeat cycle every 4 weeks except asparaginase (given for rescue only)
Chlorambucil may be used in place of cyclophosphamide for maintenance

C.O.A.P.
Cyclophosphamide: 50 mg m^{-2} p.o. every 48 h or on first 4 days of each week
Vincristine: 0.5 mg m^{-2} i.v. every 7 days
Prednisolone: 40 mg m^{-2} p.o. daily for 7 days then 20 mg m^{-2} every 48 h
Cytarabine: 100 mg m^{-2} i.v. daily on days 1–4
Maintenance: after minimum of 8 weeks, reduce above to alternate week treatment
Chlorambucil or melphalan may be used in place of cyclophosphamide
Doxorubicin or asparaginase may be used for rescue.

C.O.P. (low dose)
As for C.O.A.P. omitting cytarabine on days 1–4

Doxorubicin – single agent
Doxorubicin 30 mg m^{-2} i.v. every 3 weeks

Table 50.17 Clinical response to chemotherapeutic protocols used in the treatment of canine lymphoma

Protocol	Response rate (% CR)	Survival time	No. cases	Reference
C.O.P. (high dose)	75	6 months[a]	77	Cotter and Goldstein (1987)
C.O.P.A.	83	7 months[a]	46	Cotter and Goldstein (1987)
Cyclic combination therapy	89.9	219 days	59	MacEwan et al. (1981)
C.O.A.P	65	186 days	20	Madewell (1985)
C.O.P. (low dose)	56 (91[b])	245 days	43	Dobson and Gorman (1994)
Doxorubicin – single agent	76	270 days	21	Carter et al. (1987)
	59 (81[b])	230 days	37	Postorino et al. (1989)

[a]Remission time rather than overall survival time.
[b]Overall response rate, i.e. complete and partial response rate.

(Table 50.17). Whichever chemotherapy protocol is used approximately 70–80% of dogs with multicentric lymphoma will achieve a partial or complete clinical remission with average periods of remission in the order of 6–9 months. Overall survival times range from several weeks (in non-responding cases) to several years. Other forms of canine lymphoma may vary in their response to chemotherapy. Primary cutaneous lymphoma, for example, is a highly aggressive tumour and although the initial response to therapy may be favourable, this is usually short-lived.

In cats most forms of lymphoma respond to therapy; the multicentric and mediastinal forms are the most treatable with response rates in the order of 90% and remission times of 5–6 months (Cotter, 1983). In both cats and dogs, treatment of the alimentary form of lymphoma is often problematic. By the time the diagnosis is achieved the disease has often infiltrated large areas of bowel. Regression of the tumour in response to treatment does not necessarily result in restoration of normal bowel anatomy and function. Indeed, the rapid removal of lymphoma tissue from the intestines can lead to ulceration and perforation. The same problems may be encountered in the treatment of renal lymphoma in cats.

In practice the selection of a treatment protocol should be based upon the experience of the clinician, cost and the facilities available for monitoring and treating the patient. The C.O.P.(low dose) protocol is widely used because it causes minimal patient toxicity, the drugs are simple to administer and are relatively inexpensive. Great care must be taken in the administration of Doxorubicin to cats and for this reason the C.O.P. or C.O.A.P. protocols are favoured in this species.

Corticosteroids are included in many of the protocols for the treatment of lymphoma because of their cytotoxic effect on lymphoid cells. The sole use of corticosteroids will result in a significant regression of the disease in many instances but this response is usually short-lived. Corticosteroids are therefore a useful means of achieving short-term palliation of lymphoma and this approach may be indicated in cases where combined chemotherapy is not feasible or appropriate. Pretreatment with corticosteroids is *not* advisable, however, in cases where combined chemotherapy is to be used. The administration of corticosteroids before the initial work-up of the case can complicate the diagnosis and interpretation of laboratory results. Furthermore, it has been shown that cases which have received prior treatment with corticosteroids have significantly lower initial response rates and lower survival times than previously untreated cases (Dobson and Gorman, 1994).

The leukaemias

The term 'leukaemia' is applied to neoplastic conditions involving the bone marrow which arise from transformation of haemopoietic stem cells and result in leukaemia of the granulocytic, monocytic, erythroid and megakaryocytic as well as of the lymphoid cell series (Evans and Gorman, 1987; Sawyers et al., 1990). The terms 'acute' and 'chronic' are often used to describe the type or degree of cellular maturation of the leukaemia. 'Acute' refers to leukaemias of immature and poorly differentiated or 'blast' cells whereas 'chronic' reflects a leukaemia of well-differentiated, mature cells. The degree of maturity also reflects the course of the disease. Acute leukaemias are aggressive, life-threatening conditions which frequently follow a rapid course. Chronic leukaemias, although ultimately life-threatening, tend to follow a much more protracted course, and in some cases the initial diagnosis results from an incidental finding of a haematological abnormality. The most common forms of leukaemia diagnosed in the dog are acute lymphoblastic leukaemia (ALL), acute myelomonocytic leukaemia, acute myeloid leukaemia (AML), chronic granulocytic leukaemia (CGL) and chronic lymphocytic leukaemia (CLL). In the cat ALL, often associated with FeLV, is the most common (Gorman and Evans, 1987).

The clinical presentation and diagnosis of these conditions are described and discussed in Chapter 45.

Therapy of acute leukaemia

The treatment of animals with acute leukaemias is fraught with difficulties and is generally unsuccessful. In most cases the leukaemic destruction of the normal marrow elements results in severe haematological disturbances. Most patients presenting with either ALL or AML have varying degrees of anaemia, thrombocytopenia and leucopenia (neutropenia) either singly or in combination. In many cases there is also extensive infiltration of other organs, e.g. liver, resulting in metabolic disturbances. Although the neoplastic cells are often very chemosensitive, so too are any remaining normal myeloid cells and concurrent metabolic problems may further enhance the toxicity of chemotherapeutic agents. Unless the haematological and other problems can be managed effectively, the patient is likely to succumb to overwhelming infection, internal bleeding or organ failure.

Chemotherapeutic protocols which have been used in the treatment of ALL and AML are listed in Table 50.18. Vincristine is particularly useful because it causes minimal myelosuppression but is effective against a range of myeloid and lymphoid neoplasms. Antimetabolites and alkylating agents have also been used in various combinations but the doses of these myelosuppressive agents may require adjustment for individual patients. Intensive monitoring and medical

Table 50.18 Chemotherapeutic protocols used in the treatment of acute leukaemia

Acute lymphoblastic leukaemia
Basic protocol
Vincristine: 0.5–0.75 mg m^{-2} i.v. every 7 days
Prednisolone: 40–50 mg m^{-2} p.o., daily for 7 days then 20 mg m^{-2} every 48 h

Additional agents/combinations:
Cyclophosphamide: 50 mg m^{-2} p.o. every 48 h
or
Cytarabine: 100 mg m^{-2} i.v. daily for 2–4 days
or
Cyclophosphamide: 50 mg m^{-2} p.o. every 48 h
and
Cytarabine: 100 mg m^{-2} i.v. daily for 2–4 days
or
L-Asparaginase: 10 000–20 000 IU m^{-2} i.m. every 2–3 weeks

Acute myeloid leukaemia
Cytarabine: 100 mg m^{-2} i.v. in divided doses daily for 2–6 days
+/−
Prednisolone: 40–50 mg m^{-2} p.o., daily for 7 days then 20 mg m^{-2} every 48 h
+/−
Thioguanine: 50 mg m^{-2} p.o. daily or every 48 h
or
Mercaptopurine: 50 mg m^{-2} p.o. daily or every 48 h

Doxorubicin: 30 mg m^{-2} i.v. every 3 weeks
or 10 mg m^{-2} i.v. every 7 days

support are required for these patients. Blood transfusions can be used to manage severe anaemias and assist in the management of thrombocytopenia. Broad-spectrum antibiotic treatment, e.g. potentiated sulphonamides, should be administered to all neutropenic patients.

Most animals with acute leukaemias do not respond well to therapy and any remission or clinical improvement achieved is usually of short duration. The average survival time for both cats and dogs treated for acute leukaemias is in the order of 3–8 weeks. Matus *et al.* (1983) reported a series of 30 dogs with ALL treated with vincristine and prednisolone, the mean and median survival times were 68 and 19 days respectively.

Therapy of chronic leukaemia

Chronic leukaemias (CLL and CGL) carry a much more favourable prognosis than the acute forms of the disease. Indeed, chronic leukaemias are often detected as incidental findings following routine haematological examination for investigation of non-specific problems, e.g. lethargy, weight loss etc. In cases where the chronic leukaemia is not associated with any clinical signs, the question as to whether any treatment is indicated often arises and there may be justification for merely keeping the animal under observation with regular monitoring of haematological parameters. In many cases, however, the chronic leukaemia is associated with vague, non-specific signs of lethargy, mild anaemia or splenomegaly and in such cases or where the disease is associated with a monoclonal gammopathy, treatment is indicated. In animals the aim of treatment of chronic leukaemia is to restore the blood cell counts to the region of normality and to maintain this level by long-term maintenance therapy. The agents used and therapeutic approach are generally much less aggressive than in the management of other myeloproliferative or lymphoproliferative conditions. The alkylating agent chlorambucil is often cited as the drug of choice in the treatment of CLL and busulphan in CGL. Protocols used in the treatment of chronic leukaemias are listed in Table 50.19. Mean and

Table 50.19 Chemotherapeutic protocols used in the treatment of chronic leukaemia

---

Chronic lymphocytic leukaemia
Drug of choice:
Chlorambucil
   dose: 2–5 mg m^{-2}, p.o., daily for 7–14 days, then 2 mg m^{-2} every 48 h
   or: (20 mg m^{-2}, p.o., every 2 weeks)
+/
Prednisolone:
   40–50 mg m^{-2}, p.o., daily for 7 days then 20 mg m^{-2} every 48 h

Alternative induction protocol:
Cyclophosphamide: 200–300 mg m^{-2} once every two weeks (weeks 1 and 3)
Vincristine: 0.5–0.75 mg m^{-2} once every two weeks (weeks 2 and 4)
Prednisolone: 40–50 mg m^{-2}, p.o., daily for 7 days then 20 mg m^{-2} every 48 h
Maintenance: after 8 weeks, chlorambucil as above

Chronic granulocytic leukaemia
Hydroxyurea:
   dose: 40–50 mg kg^{-1} p.o. divided daily for 1–2 weeks then every 48 h
   (or: 80 mg kg^{-1} p.o. every 3 days to effect,[a] then reduce for maintenance)
   (or: 1 g m^{-2} daily p.o. to effect,[a] then reduce for maintenance)
+/
Prednisolone:
   40–50 mg m^{-2}, p.o., daily for 7 days then 20 mg m^{-2} every 48 h
Busulphan:
   dose: 2–6 mg m^{-2} p.o. daily to effect,[a] then reduce daily dosage for maintenance
+/
Prednisolone:
   40–50 mg m^{-2}, p.o., daily for 7 days then 20 mg m^{-2} every 48 h

---

[a] 'to effect' = until WBC count approaches the upper limit of normal. Maintenance therapy should aim to maintain the WBC count within 20–25 × 10^9 l^{-1}.

median survival times of 452 and 348 days, respectively, were reported from one series of 17 dogs with CLL treated with combinations of vincristine, prednisolone and chlorambucil (Leifer and Matus, 1986).

Myeloma (synonyms: multiple myeloma, plasma cell myeloma)

Myeloma results from a neoplastic proliferation of plasma cells (B lymphoctyes) predominantly in the bone marrow. The neoplastic cells often retain their secretory function and produce large quantities of immunoglobulins. On plasma protein electrophoresis this appears as a large, monoclonal 'spike' in the globulin fraction (Fig. 50.23) (MacEwan and Hurvitz, 1977). Animals with typical myelomas present with signs relating to hypergammaglobulinaemia and hyperviscosity in addition to haematological abnormalities resulting from the myelophthisis. In many cases myelomas also produce skeletal changes through localized resorption of bone resulting in multiple 'punched-out' or lytic lesions throughout the skeleton, most commonly affecting the pelvis, spine, ribs and proximal long bones (Fig. 50.24). Clinically this manifests as stiffness and skeletal pain. Hypercalcaemia may be associated with myeloma with or without skeletal changes. In humans, myeloma is also characterized by the presence of light chain proteins from immunoglobulin molecules in the urine. These are termed 'Bence–Jones' proteins and are strongly indicative of myeloma. In animals the presence of Bence–Jones proteinuria in myeloma cases seems to be very variable and myeloma should not be ruled out if Bence–Jones proteins are absent.

The diagnosis of myeloma in animals depends on demonstrating any of the previously mentioned features of the disease (i.e. monoclonal

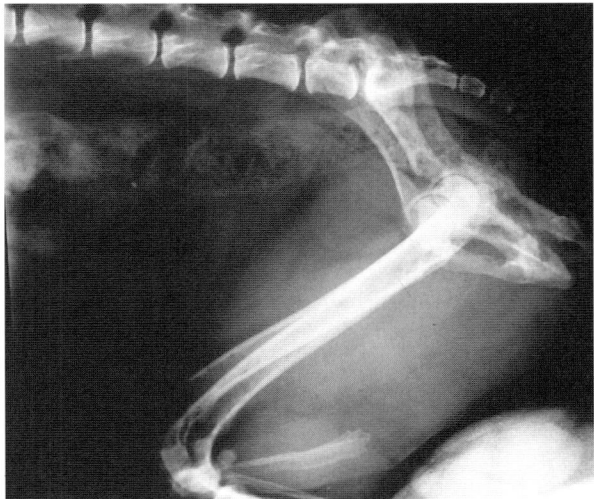

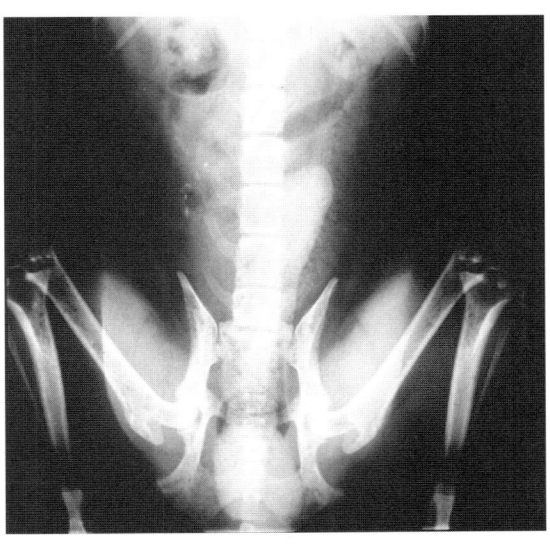

Figure 50.23 Serum electrophoretic trace on blood from a dog with a secretory myeloma; the monoclonal spike in the gamma-globulin region of the trace is strongly suggestive of myeloma.

Figure 50.24 (a and b) Radiographic changes associated with myeloma. These radiographs show diffuse osteolytic skeletal lesions in the pelvis, lumbar spine and femur of this dog.

Table 50.20 Chemotherapeutic protocols used in the treatment of myeloma

---
1. Induction
Melphalan: 1.5–2.0 mg m^{-2} p.o., daily for 3–6 weeks, then every 48 h
Prednisolone: 40 mg m^{-2} p.o. daily, reducing to 20 mg m^{-2} every 48 h depending on response
The aim of induction therapy is to lower plasma immunoglobulin concentration to within normal limits.

If response is not satisfactory, either:
  add: Vincristine: 0.5 mg m^{-2} i.v. every 7 days
  and/or replace melphalan with:
    Cyclophosphamide: 50 mg m^{-2} p.o. every 48 h
    Chlorambucil: 2–5 mg m^{-2} p.o. every 48 h

2. Maintenance
Using any of the combinations listed above, adjust dose rate and frequency to maintain plasma immunoglobulin concentration within normal limits.

---

gammopathy, skeletal lesions, hypercalcaemia) in addition to confirming the presence of neoplastic plasma cells in the bone marrow. Chemotherapy is the treatment of choice for myeloma and most protocols rely on a combination of an alkylating agent, either melphalan or cyclophosphamide, with prednisolone with or without vincristine (Table 50.20). In cases with hypergammaglobulinaemia, the plasma immunoglobulin concentration can be used as a guide to monitor the success of treatment and determine the frequency and dosage for maintenance therapy, the aim of treatment being to maintain the immunoglobulin concentration within normal limits. In cases of non-secretory myelomas, response and maintenance therapy are dictated by remission of other clinical signs and/or haematological toxicity. Although the prognosis for myeloma is guarded, most cases respond favourably to treatment and average survival times are in the order of 12 months or more (MacEwan and Hurvitz, 1977).

Adjuvant chemotherapy

The value of cytotoxic drugs in the sole treatment of other malignant tumours, e.g. carcinomas, sarcomas and melanomas, is limited because such tumours usually have a low growth fraction at the time of detection. Futhermore, the cell type may also be important in determining chemosensitivity and whereas most lymphoid and myeloid tumours are highly chemosensitive, most carcinomas respond poorly to chemotherapy and melanomas are notoriously refractory to cytotoxic agents. Cytotoxic drugs have an increasing role, however, in the management of some tumours as an adjunct to surgery and/or radiation therapy. The rationale of this approach is that surgery/radiation therapy are the most effective methods of removing the bulk of the tumour mass but can offer little to address the problem of distant metastases which, in the case of highly malignant tumours, develop early in the course of the disease. Systemic chemotherapy is indicated in association with surgical management of the primary tumour on the assumption that micrometastases are present and that cytotoxic drugs will be most effective against metastatic tumour colonies in their early stages of growth, i.e. before they become detectable. The same rationale applies to any residual tumour at the primary site.

Although adjuvant chemotherapy is used extensively in the management of human cancers, in animals it has mainly been used in the management of osteosarcomas and soft tissue sarcomas. The value of adjunctive chemotherapy in the management of the more malignant carcinomas in animals has been restricted by the toxicity of agents having activity against these types of tumour. Malignant melanomas are refractory to most cytotoxic drugs in all species.

Treatment of osteosarcoma

Osteosarcoma is a particularly aggressive and distressing tumour affecting the long bones of large to giant breed dogs. The primary tumour causes painful destruction of the long bone leading eventually to pathological fracture. Amputation of the limb only provides a temporary solution to the local pain. Osteosarcoma is a highly malignant tumour which metastasizes, primarily to the lungs, early in its course. For this reason, survival times are short with animals succumbing to metastatic pulmonary disease within 3–6 months of amputation (Brodey and Abt, 1976). Post-amputation survival times in these patients can be

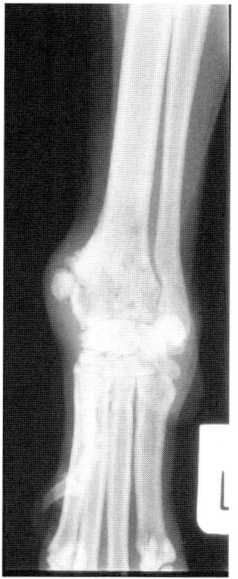 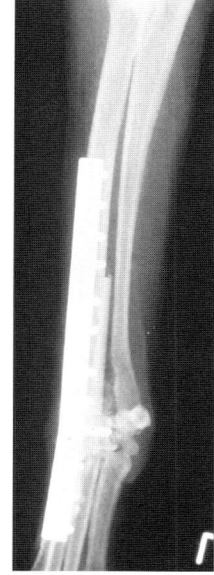

Figure 50.25 Limb salvage as a method of treatment for osteosarcoma of the distal radius in the dog. (a) Radiograph of a localized, early osteosarcoma of the distal radius. (b) The tumour and distal radius have been resected and replaced with a cortical bone graft, secured by a dynamic compression plate with carpal arthrodesis.

significantly increased by the use of doxorubicin and/or cisplatin (Shapiro et al., 1988; Maudlin et al., 1988). Amputation is very much a last resort, particularly in large breed dogs with limited life expectancy. More recently a number of surgical techniques have been developed to salvage the limb in these patients. This involves surgical resection of the affected bone and restoration of the limb by a variety of bone grafting techniques (Fig. 50.25) (LaRue et al., 1989). This approach may not be applicable in every case, but limb salvage has been relatively successful when combined with chemotherapy in selected cases.

Treatment of soft tissue sarcoma

Malignant tumours arising from mesenchymal connective tissues share a number of features in common irrespective of whether their origin is fibrous tissue, vascular tissues or adipose tissue. All are locally invasive and infiltrate widely into adjacent normal tissues. In this respect they require very wide margins of surgical excision. Malignancy varies throughout the group, some tumours, for example the canine haemangiopericytoma and well-differentiated fibrosarcoma, are slow growing and rarely if ever metastasize. Other members of the group are much more aggressive, they grow rapidly and have a high rate of distant metastasis, this is particularly true of haemangiosarcoma and poorly differentiated or anaplastic sarcomas. Although surgery and/or radiation is usually the treatment of choice for the primary tumour, adjunctive chemotherapy should be considered for the control of metastases in these aggressive tumours. Doxorubicin has proven activity against such tumours and may be used alone or in combination with vincristine and cyclophosphamide (the 'VAC' protocol, Table 50.21; Hammer et al., 1991) for this purpose. Indeed, doxorubicin or VAC may have some effect against the primary tumour in cases where surgery is not possible and, although a complete regression of the tumour may not be achieved, this combination can be very effective in the palliation of soft tissue sarcoma.

Treatment of mast cell tumours

Mast cell tumours present the clinician with great problems in both diagnosis and management because of their diverse and variable appearance and behaviour. Histological features, e.g. degree of cellular differentiation, mitotic rate, local invasion, can be used to grade mast cell tumours and this grading system does bear some relationship to the clinical behaviour of the tumour and prognosis. Well-differentiated tumours tend to be low grade and rarely metastasize whereas poorly differentiated tumours are usually locally aggressive tumours which disseminate widely. Intermediate grade tumours are usually only locally aggressive although metastasis can occur. Clearly there is an indication for systemic chemotherapy in the management of poorly differentiated mast cell tumours, however, the value of cytotoxic drugs for this purpose is the subject of continuing controversy. A favourable response may be seen after treatment with a combination of vincristine, cyclophosphamide and prednisolone but prednisolone alone may be equally effective in

Table 50.21 'VAC' protocol used in the treatment of soft tissue sarcoma

Day 1:	Doxorubicin:	30 mg m^{-2}, i.v.
	Cyclophosphamide:	100–150 mg m^{-2} i.v.
Days 8 and 15	Vincristine:	0.75 mg m^{-2}, i.v.
Repeat 3 weekly cycles		

Prophylactic antibiotic therapy with potentiated sulphonamides is advised.

achieving short-term palliation and control in these cases. No controlled clinical studies have been carried out to determine the true value of cytotoxic drugs in the management of poorly differentiated mast cell tumours.

Failure of chemotherapy – drug resistance

In clinical practice, anticancer drugs do not always achieve the desired effect in terms of tumour response and duration of response. In some cases the tumour may not respond to initial therapy; in others, the initial response appears to be good but the tumour eventually recurs despite continued treatment. Treatment failure may result from incorrect selection of drugs or dose rates. Even if a drug is administered at the correct dosage, the amount of drug reaching the tumour cells may not attain therapeutic concentrations if the blood supply to the tumour is compromised as often occurs in large, bulky tumours. Certain tumours are refractory to the actions of cytotoxic drugs from the outset. This may result from the growth kinetics of the tumour being inappropriate for the use of drugs, for example a slowly growing fibrosarcoma would not be expected to respond well to chemotherapy even with the use of aggressive therapeutic protocols. Some rapidly growing tumours may also fail to respond to therapy and in such cases it is surmised that the cell type of the tumour is inherently resistant to the actions of cytotoxic drugs. This is the case with many carcinomas and melanomas.

Acquired drug resistance

Tumour cells may acquire resistance to cytotoxic drugs in a number of ways (Curt et al., 1984). Cells may develop defective transport mechanisms which prevent entry of the drug into the cell, they may overcome the actions of cytotoxic drugs, e.g. alkylating agents by increased DNA repair, or use alternative metabolic pathways to overcome the actions of antimetabolites. Tumour cells may also develop mechanisms for inactivating cytotoxic agents. These mechanisms of drug resistance probably arise through mutations during the growth of the tumour and both the size of the tumour and its heterogeneity are important in this respect. The larger the tumour burden the greater the potential number of intrinsically resistant cells. Constant or repeated exposure of the tumour to a drug or combination of drugs selects for these existing resistant cells which eventually give rise to a tumour which is refractory to treatment. In some cases acquired drug resistance can be overcome by changing the treatment to a different cytotoxic agent with a different mechanism of action. For example, in the treatment of canine lymphoma, if the disease should relapse following a good initial response to C.O.P., doxorubicin may be successful as a 'rescue' treatment and further remissions can often be achieved in this way.

Multidrug resistance

The use of agents from different groups for rescue purposes does not always meet with success. A phenomenon of multidrug resistance (MDR) has been documented and is recognized as a major cause of treatment failure in human chemotherapy (Rothenburg and Ling, 1989). Multidrug resistance occurs when cells exposed to one type of cytotoxic agent not only develop resistance to the original agent but also become resistant to structurally unrelated agents with different mechanisms of action. For example, tumour cells which become resistant to doxorubicin are often also resistant to vincristine. Multidrug resistance appears to result from tumour cells developing the ability to actively export cytotoxic drugs out of the cell, hence preventing the accumulation of therapeutic levels of the agent within the cell. A cell surface P-glycoprotein (P-gp) associated with cell membrane transport systems which acts as an export pump for certain cytotoxic drugs, is expressed on MDR cell lines and the genes encoding for P-gp have been identified. MDR has been reduced in some MDR cell lines *in vitro* through the use of calcium channel blocking agents, e.g. verapamil (Merry et al., 1987). The clinical value of this finding has yet to be established. MDR is an important issue in cancer therapy and the subject of ongoing research.

Complications of chemotherapy

The potential toxicity of most cytotoxic drugs has already been discussed. Most of the drug schedules described in the previous section will be tolerated well by animals provided the patient does not have any complicating factors or underlying diseases. There are, however, a number of potential complications which can arise through the use of cytotoxic drugs many of which are life-threatening and may require emergency treatment. It is important that the clinician should be aware of such complications and that the animal is monitored regularly for any signs of toxicity. In this way potential problems can often be detected at an early stage and remedial action taken. Complications of chemotherapy can arise at any time during therapy. Some complications, e.g. hypersensitivity reactions, may occur immediately following administration of a drug, other complications, e.g. myelosuppression and gastrointestinal problems, usually occur early in the course of treatment within days to weeks of onset. In some cases delayed problems such as doxorubicin-induced cardiomyopathy may not occur for several months.

Tumour lysis syndrome

Tumour lysis syndrome (TLS) is fortunately relatively uncommon in veterinary cancer therapy. The syndrome describes a spectrum of severe metabolic disturbances resulting from lysis of tumour cells following cytotoxic drug treatment of patients with large burdens of extremely sensitive tumours, e.g. lymphoid and myeloid tumours (Couto, 1990). Induction therapy results in massive cell kill and release of cellular products into the circulation at a rate which exceeds the excretory capacity of the kidneys. This results in hyperkalaemia, hyperphosphataemia and hypocalcaemia, the combination of which may lead to acute renal failure, cardiac arrhythmias and death. Aggressive fluid therapy is necessary to promote excretion of the metabolic products and prevent renal failure. Although this syndrome is not very common, the clinician should be aware of tumour lysis syndrome as a possible complication in the treatment of animals with extensive lymphoproliferative or myeloproliferative disease, especially those patients with high WBC counts. These patients should be hospitalized and carefully monitored during the induction stage of therapy.

Anaphylaxis/hypersensitivity

Although hypersensitivity reactions to cytotoxic drugs are rare, a number of agents can produce such reactions when administered to animals. These include L-Asparaginase, doxorubicin, cisplatin and cytarabine. Most cytotoxic drug hypersensitivities are immune-mediated reactions but some drugs (e.g. doxorubicin) can degranulate mast cells directly and other agents may activate the alternative complement pathway.

The route of administration can affect the incidence of hypersensitivity reactions. L-Asparaginase may produce anaphylaxis in up to 30% of dogs when administered intravenously, for this reason it is recommended that the drug should always be given by the intramuscular route. Pretreatment with diphenhydramine can reduce the frequency of some drug reactions and this is usually recommended prior to doxorubicin infusion.

In the event of a hypersensitivity reaction administration of the drug should be stopped immediately, the animal should be treated with intravenous fluids, soluble corticosteriods, adrenaline and antihistamines. The animal should not be treated with the offending agent again.

Phlebitis and tissue necrosis

Many cytotoxic drugs for intravenous administration are intensely irritant and can cause severe local tissue necrosis following perivascular injection or extravasation from the intravenous injection site. Agents of concern in this respect are vincristine, vinblastine, doxorubicin and epirubicin. Doxorubicin and epirubicin are particularly irritant and extravasation of these agents can cause extensive necrosis and sloughing of skin, connective tissues, muscles and nerves. In order to minimize the risk of such an event, the animal must be adequately restrained and the drug administered via an intravenous catheter. The latter should be flushed with saline before and after administration of the agent.

In the event of perivascular leakage, the affected area should be aspirated immediately and flushed with physiological saline to try and remove as much of the agent as possible and to dilute any residual drug. Locally administered sodium bicarbonate (8.4% solution) will neutralize some agents and soluble corticosteroids (e.g. dexamethasone) may help stabilize cell membranes. Cold compresses may also help reduce the inflammatory response.

Myelosuppression and infection

Myelosuppression is the main dose-limiting factor in veterinary chemotherapy. Most cytotoxic drugs affect the replicating precursor cells of the bone marrow resulting in reduced production of blood cells. The duration and severity of the resulting cytopenia depends on the normal life-span of mature cells in the circulation. Hence granulocytopenia and thrombocytopenia present an earlier and more frequent complication than anaemia. Fortunately the resting stem cell populations are not affected by the actions of cytotoxic drugs and the marrow can, therefore, recover from cytotoxic damage once the agent is withdrawn. In practice, anaemia resulting from cytotoxic drug therapy is rare. A mild to moderate thrombocytopenia often occurs but is rarely severe enough to cause bleeding and neutropenia is the most common and the most serious complication of chemotherapy.

It is important that all animals receiving cytotoxic drugs have their blood cell counts monitored regularly. After a single infusion of a drug such as doxorubicin, the granulocyte count would be expected to fall to a nadir at 5–10 days and recover by 21 days. In this case a white blood cell count should be taken on day 21, to check that recovery has occurred prior to the next infusion of the drug. The duration of myelosuppression may be longer in drugs which do not have cell cycle specificity, for example, dacarbazine causes maximum myelosuppression at 2–4 weeks. If the patient is receiving a low-dose continuous treatment, the cell counts should be measured every 2 weeks where possible. Myelosuppression is considered to be severe when the total white blood cell count is less than $3.0 \times 10^9 \, l^{-1}$ and patients with neutrophil counts less than $1.0 \times 10^9 \, l^{-1}$ are at high risk for sepsis. In patients where the neutrophil count is less than $2.0 \times 10^9 \, l^{-1}$, cytotoxic treatment should be discontinued until the cell count recovers after which therapy may be re-instituted using 75% of the initial dose. In patients where the neutrophil count is of the order of $2-3 \times 10^9 \, l^{-1}$, the dose of cytotoxic drug should be reduced by 50% and the white blood cell count monitored carefully.

Neutropenia predisposes the cancer patient to infection which can have serious and life-threatening consequences. Infectious organisms may gain entry to the body through the respiratory, urogenital or gastrointestinal tracts, or through disruption of normal barriers (e.g. skin and mucosa) by the tumour. Absorption of enteric bacteria through damaged intestinal mucosa is the most common source of infection in animal cancer patients and *Escherichia coli* and *Klebsiella pneumoniae* are two of the most common pathogenic organisms.

Identification or detection of sepsis can be difficult in the neutropenic patient because the inflammatory response is altered by the neutropenia. Pyrexia is the most consistent sign of sepsis and although pyrexia may be due to tumour necrosis or other causes, in a neutropenic patient it should always be assumed that pyrexia is due to sepsis. Since defence mechanisms of the host are severely compromised, immediate treatment is required to prevent overwhelming infection and death. All cytotoxic drugs should be discontinued immediately, aggressive intravenous antibiotic therapy should be commenced with a combination of agents providing a broad spectrum of bacteriocidal activity, e.g. gentamycin and a cephalosporin or enrofloxacin. The patient should be maintained on intravenous fluids as necessary. Blood should be taken for aerobic and anaerobic culture and antibiotic therapy can subsequently be adjusted according to the results of culture and sensitivity.

Prophylactic antibiotic therapy is recommended in any neutropenic patient receiving chemotherapy or if there is an existing predisposition for infection, e.g. an exposed necrotic tumour. Care has to be taken in the selection of antibiotics for these patients. The normal intestinal flora affords a degree of protection against opportunist pathogens and disruption of this normal flora can predispose to bacterial overgrowth and systemic infection. Antimicrobial agents such as potentiated sulphonamides which have minimal effects on the gastrointestinal flora should be used in these circumstances.

Anorexia, vomiting and gastrointestinal toxicity

Many cytotoxic drugs can cause anorexia, vomiting and diarrhoea. This may occur as a direct result of the action of the drug on the oral, gastric and intestinal epithelium or as a result of non-specific myelosuppression. Death and desquamation of alimentary epithelium usually occurs 5–10 days after administration of the drug and leads to stomatitis, vomiting and mucoid or haemorrhagic diarrhoea. In the majority of cases such problems are self-limiting and the animal recovers spontaneously as the normal alimentary epithelium regenerates. Vomiting and diarrhoea can lead to dehydration and electrolyte imbalances and intravenous fluid therapy should be given in cases where the vomiting/diarrhoea is severe or prolonged. Mucosal injury can also predispose to systemic infection and parenteral antibiotics may be indicated, as discussed above.

Some drugs induce nausea and vomiting by stimulation of the chemoreceptor trigger zone, these include cisplatin and doxorubicin. Salivation and vomiting may occur during administration of these drugs but are more frequent within the first 24 hours of administration. Antiemetics, e.g. metaclopramide, are useful in the prevention or control of drug-induced vomiting and pretreatment with such agents is recommended before the administration of cisplatin.

Specific toxicity of individual agents

Several cytotoxic drugs which are regularly used in veterinary cancer medicine have specific toxic effects.

Cyclophosphamide-induced haemorrhagic cystitis

Haemorrhagic cystitis is a serious complication of cyclophosphamide therapy. Metabolites of cyclophosphamide (in particular acrolein) are excreted in the urine and have an irritant effect on the bladder mucosa. They cause an acute inflammation, often with profuse bleeding, and result in a sterile haemorrhagic cystitis. Haemorrhagic cystitis can occur at any time during cyclophosphamide therapy but is more common after administration of high doses of the drug or after long-term, continuous low-dose therapy. Haemorrhagic cystitis is also more common in patients with reduced urine output. The risk of haemorrhagic cystitis can be reduced by minimizing contact of the metabolites with the bladder epithelium through ensuring the patient is adequately hydrated, promoting fluid intake and encouraging the animal to empty the bladder frequently.

There is no specific therapy for cyclophosphamide-induced haemorrhagic cystitis. Cyclophosphamide therapy should be ceased immediately, supportive measures such as ensuring adequate hydration and the use of anti-inflammatory and antispasmodic agents may be helpful. Lavage of the bladder wall with cold saline may be beneficial and surgical debridement of mucosal deficits may be warranted in severe cases. A favourable response to intravesicular instillation of dimethyl sulphoxide (DMSO) has been reported in a small number of cases (Laing et al., 1988). The drug Mesna (Uromitexan™, Boehringer), reduces the production of acrolein and acts specifically with this metabolite in the urinary tract. Mesna may be administered simultaneously with cyclophosphamide to prevent haemorrhagic cystitis in human cancer patients. There is little experience of the value of this agent in animals.

Prolonged cyclophosphamide therapy may lead to an insidious and irreversible fibrosis of the bladder wall resulting in contraction of the bladder and urinary frequency or incontinence.

Doxorubicin-induced cardiomyopathy

Doxorubicin can cause both acute and chronic cardiac toxicity through effects on myocardial calcium metabolism.

Acute toxicity

Cardiac arrhythmias and ECG abnormalities often occur during and immediately following infusion of doxorubicin. In most cases these abnormalities are not associated with clinical signs, the heart reverts to normal rhythm shortly after the infusion and antiarrhythmic therapy is not required. On rare occasions ventricular arrythmias can occur and patients should always be carefully monitored throughout the infusion of the drug for this reason.

Chronic toxicity

Doxorubicin-induced cardiomyopathy is the result of a cumulative toxicity of doxorubicin on the myocardium which is irreversible. The development of cardiomyopathy is related to the total dose of doxorubicin administered. Although there is some interpatient variation serious toxicity usually occurs after a cumulative dose of 240 mg m^{-2} has been administered to a dog. Changes in myocardial contractility may be detected on ultrasonography at total doses as low as 180 mg m^{-2}. Electrocardiograph changes may also precede clinical (cardiac) signs of toxicity. Doxorubicin-induced cardiomyopathy results in a congestive heart failure which does not respond well to conventional treatment. For this reason the use of doxorubicin should be avoided in patients with existing cardiac disease and the total dose of 240 mg m^{-2} should not be exceeded in any patient.

Guidelines for the safe handling of cytotoxic drugs

The following notes are intended as guidelines to the precautions which should be taken to reduce the exposure of personnel to cytotoxic drugs when such agents are used in veterinary practice. Many cytotoxic drugs are carcinogens and mutagens, some are also teratogens. Many cytotoxic drugs are also extremely irritant and produce harmful local effects after direct contact with the skin or eyes. Detailed local rules and practices should be established for the safe handling of cytotoxic drugs at places where they are used. Cytotoxic drugs should not be handled by pregnant staff.

Cytotoxic drugs are commonly available in two forms: tablets or capsules for oral administration and powder or solutions for injection. There are three possible routes through which the agent may enter the body:

1. *Inhalation* may occur where an aerosol or airborne dust is generated due to poor technique or accident during manipulation.
2. *Ingestion* is unlikely to occur if good hygiene procedures are followed.
3. *Skin contact*: some drugs may be absorbed into the body through the skin if not removed by washing.

Tablets/capsules

In most cases these products are packed in sealed containers and many are now individually blister packed. Most tablets are further protected by an inert barrier coat. Such products do not therefore pose a hazard to staff or other personnel who may handle them unless they are mishandled or crushed.

General guidelines for the use of cytotoxic agents in tablet form

1. Tablets should not be broken or crushed and capsules should not be opened.
2. Disposable gloves should be worn when handling any tablet which does not have an inert barrier coat.
3. Where tablets are provided in individual wrappers, they should always be dispensed in this form.
4. In addition to the statutory requirements for the labelling of medicinal products, all containers used for dispensing cytotoxic drugs must be child-proof and carry a clear warning to keep out of the reach of children. Containers should also be clearly labelled with the name of the agent.
5. Staff and owners should receive clear instructions on the administration of tablets. Disposable plastic or rubber gloves should always be worn when administering these tablets because the protective barrier may break down on contact with saliva.
6. Always wash hands after handling any drug
7. Excess or unwanted drugs should be disposed of by incineration in a chemical incinerator.

Injectable solutions

The main risk for exposure to personnel arises during the preparation and administration of injectable cytotoxics, many of which are presented as freeze-dried material or powder, requiring to be mixed with a diluent. Potential dangers in the handling and manipulation of these products are the creation of aerosols during preparation/reconstitution of the solution and accidental spillage of solutions either onto work surfaces or body surfaces (skin, mucous membranes, eyes).

General guidelines for the safehandling of injectable cytotoxic drugs

1. The drug should only be reconstituted by trained personnel.
2. Reconstitution of the drug should only be performed in a designated area, well away from thoroughfares and food. Techniques should be used to prevent high pressure being generated within the vials and minimize the risk of creating aerosols. When excess air is expelled from a filled syringe it should be exhausted into a pad and not straight into the atmosphere.
3. Adequate protective clothing should be worn. This varies according to the agent. The minimum requirement should be suitable gloves and a gown with long sleeves to protect the skin, a protective visor or goggles to protect the eyes and a surgical mask to provide some protection against splashes to the face. It is preferable to reconstitute some cytotoxic drugs, e.g. doxorubicin, in a protective cabinet with external exhaust.
4. Administration: Luer lock fittings should be used in preference to push connections on syringes, tubing and giving sets. All animal patients must be adequately restrained for this procedure by trained staff. Fractious or lively animals may need to be sedated.
5. Waste disposal: Adequate care and preparation should be taken for the disposal of items (syringes, needles etc.) used to reconstitute and administer cytotoxic drugs. 'Sharps' should be placed in impenetrable containers specified for the purpose, solid waste (e.g. contaminated equipment, absorbent paper etc.) should be placed in double-sealed polythene bags. All such waste should be disposed of by high temperature incineration by a licensed authority.
6. In the event of spillage the following actions should be taken:
   (a) Personal protective equipment should be put on;
   (b) The spilt material should be mopped up with disposable absorbent towels (these should be damp if the spilt material is in powder form). The towels should be disposed of as above;
   (c) Contaminated surfaces should be washed with plenty of water.

Individual products vary with regard to irritancy

and potential carcinogenic, mutagenic and teratogenic hazard. Data sheets and health hazard sheets should be consulted before use of any such agent.

APPENDIX I: CONVERSION OF BODY WEIGHT TO SURFACE AREA

$$\text{Body surface area} = \frac{k \times \text{BWt(kg)}^{0.66}}{10^4}$$

Where $k = 10.1$ for dogs and $k = 10.0$ for cats.

Table 50.A1 Body weight:surface area conversion for dogs

kg	m²	kg	m²
0.5	0.06	26.0	0.88
1.0	0.10	27.0	0.90
2.0	0.15	28.0	0.92
3.0	0.20	29.0	0.94
4.0	0.25	30.0	0.96
5.0	0.29	31.0	0.99
6.0	0.33	32.0	1.01
7.0	0.36	33.0	1.03
8.0	0.40	34.0	1.05
9.0	0.43	35.0	1.07
10.0	0.46	36.0	1.09
11.0	0.49	37.0	1.11
12.0	0.52	38.0	1.13
13.0	0.55	39.0	1.15
14.0	0.58	40.0	1.17
15.0	0.60	41.0	1.19
16.0	0.63	42.0	1.21
17.0	0.66	43.0	1.23
18.0	0.69	44.0	1.25
19.0	0.71	45.0	1.26
20.0	0.74	46.0	1.28
21.0	0.76	47.0	1.30
22.0	0.78	48.0	1.32
23.0	0.81	49.0	1.34
24.0	0.83	50.0	1.36
25.0	0.85		

Table 50.A2 Body weight:surface area conversion for cats

kg	m²	kg	m²
2.0	0.159	3.6	0.235
2.2	0.169	3.8	0.244
2.4	0.179	4.0	0.252
2.6	0.189	4.2	0.260
2.8	0.199	4.4	0.269
3.0	0.208	4.6	0.277
3.2	0.217	4.8	0.285
3.4	0.226	5.0	0.292

APPENDIX II: FORMULARY OF CYTOTOXIC DRUGS IN TEXT AND TABLES

Alkylating agents

Cyclophosphamide

PoM **Cyclophosphamide** (Pharmacia and Upjohn)
PoM **Endoxana**™ (ASTA Medica)
US – **Cytoxan**™ (Mead-Johnson)

Available as: oral preparations: cyclophosphamide tablets, 50 mg (Cytoxan – 25 mg tablets)
parenteral preparations: cyclophosphamide powder (as hydrate) for reconstitution.
100 mg, 200 mg, other sizes available (reconstitute with sterile water and use within 2 h of preparation)

Indications: lymphoproliferative diseases and myeloproliferative diseases
multiple myeloma
(sarcomas and carcinomas)
(immunosuppression for immune mediated diseases)

Side effects: **myelosuppression**
gastrointestinal
urological (haemorrhagic cystitis)
alopecia

Dose: most commonly used:
50 mg m⁻² p.o. every other day or for the first 4 days of each week or:
100–300 mg m⁻² p.o. or i.v. every 3 weeks
(note maximum recommended dose for dogs, 250 mg m⁻²).
(Tables 50.16, 50.18–50.21)

Chlorambucil

PoM **Leukeran**™ (Glaxo Wellcome)

Available as: Chlorambucil tablets, 2 mg, 5 mg

Indications: chronic lymphocytic leukaemia
multiple myeloma
lymphoma (maintenance therapy)
(polycythaemia vera)
(immunosuppression for immune-mediated diseases)

Side effects: myelosuppression (reversible on stopping treatment)

Dose: 2–10 mg m⁻² p.o. every 24 or 48 h
(Tables 50.16, 50.19, 50.20)

Melphalan

PoM **Alkeran**™ (Glaxo Wellcome)

Available as:	melphalan tablets, 2 mg, 5 mg (injectable form is available)
Indications:	multiple myeloma lymphoproliferative disorders (mammary, ovarian and testicular carcinoma)
Side effects:	myelosuppression (may be delayed) gastrointestinal
Dose:	regimes vary according to condition treated, 1–5 mg m² p.o. daily or alternate day. (Tables 50.16, 50.20)

Busulphan

PoM **Myleran**™ (Glaxo Wellcome)

Available as:	Busulphan tablets, 500 μg, 2 mg
Indications:	chronic granulocytic leukaemia (polycythaemia vera)
Side effects:	myelosuppression, (pulmonary fibrosis – rare) (endocrinological – rare) (ocular – lens changes – rare)
Dose:	2–6 mg m^{-2} daily until WBC approaches upper limit of normal, then daily maintenance at reduced dosage to maintain WBC within $20–25 \times 10^9$ l^{-1}. (Table 50.19)

■ Antimetabolites

Methotrexate

PoM **Methotrexate** (Lederle)

Available as:	Oral preparations: methotrexate tablets, 2.5 mg, 10 mg Parenteral preps: methotrexate injection 2 mg ml^{-1}, 25 mg ml^{-1} and 50 mg and 500 mg powder for reconstitution
Indications:	lymphoproliferative and myeloproliferative diseases (transmissible venereal tumour) (Sertoli cell tumour) (soft tissue sarcoma and osteosarcoma)
Side effects:	myelosuppression gastrointestinal – can be severe renal tubular necrosis with high dose regimes
Dose:	see specific protocols low dose: 1–3 mg m^{-2} p.o. high dose with citivorum rescue – not recommended in animals due to toxicity (Table 50.16)

Cytarabine (cytosine arabinoside)

PoM **Cytarabine** (Non-proprietary) (other synonyms Ara-C)

Available as:	Injection: Cytarabine powder for reconstitution 100 mg, 500 mg, 1 g Alexan – cytarabine 20 mg ml^{-1}: 2 ml, 5 ml
Indications:	lymphoproliferative and myeloproliferative disease
Side effects:	myelosuppression gastrointestinal
Dose:	100 mg m^{-2} i.v. or s.c. daily for 2–4 days or 75 mg m^{-2} by i.v. infusion over 24 h (Tables 50.16, 50.18)

Mercaptopurine

PoM **Puri-Nethol**™ (Glaxo Wellcome)

Available as:	mercaptopurine tablets, 50 mg
Indications:	lymphoproliferative and myeloproliferative diseases
Side effects:	myelosuppression (gastrointestinal, nausea and vomiting – rare)
Dose:	50 mg m^{-2} by mouth every 24–48 h (Table 50.18)

Thioguanine

PoM **Lanvis**™ (Glaxo Wellcome)

Available as:	thioguanine tablets, 40 mg
Indications:	lymphoproliferative and myeloproliferative diseases
Side effects:	myelosuppression gastrointestinal, nausea and vomiting – rare
Dose:	50 mg m^{-2} by mouth every 24–48 h (Table 50.18)

■ Antitumour antibiotics

Doxorubicin hydrochloride (formerly Adriamycin™)

PoM **Doxorubicin Rapid Dissolution**™ (Pharmacia and Upjohn)
PoM **Doxorubicin Solution for Injection**™
US **Adriamycin** (Adria Labs)

Available as: Injection
Rapid dissolution – powder for reconstitution, 10 mg, 50 mg
Solution for injection – 2 mg ml^{-1}, 5 ml, 25 ml

Indications: lymphoproliferative and myeloproliferative diseases
soft tissue and osteogenic sarcomas (carcinomas)

Side effects: tissue irritant – severe perivascular reactions
myelosuppression
gastrointestinal
cardiac (acute and cumulative)
urologic – nephrotoxic in cats
alopecia
anaphylactic reactions

Dose: Dogs: 30–60 mg m^{-2} every 3 weeks to a maximum of 240–300 mg m^{-2} or
10 mg m^{-2} on days 1, 2 and 3 every 4 weeks
Cats: 20 mg m^{-2} every 3–6 weeks
(Tables 50.16, 50.18, 50.21)

Epirubicin – epi-doxorubicin

PoM **Pharmorubicin**™ (Pharmacia and Upjohn) (an analogue of doxorubicin)

Available as: powder for reconstitution, 10 mg, 20 mg, 50 mg

Indications: lymphoproliferative and myeloproliferative diseases
soft tissue and osteogenic sarcomas (carcinomas)

Side effects: tissue irritant – severe perivascular reactions
myelosuppression
gastrointestinal
cardiac (not as toxic as doxorubicin but caution is advised)
alopecia
anaphylactic reactions

Dose: Dogs: 30–60 mg m^{-2} every 3 weeks to a maximum of 240–300 mg m^{-2}
Cats: 20 mg m^{-2} every 3–6 weeks

Vinca alkaloids

Vinblastine

PoM **Vinblastine** (Non-proprietary)
PoM **Velbe**™ (Lilly)

Available as: injection, vinblastine sulphate powder for reconstitution, 10 mg

Indications: lymphoproliferative disorders (mammary and testicular carcinomas)

Side effects: myelosuppression
tissue irritant – perivascular reactions
neurological
gastrointestinal

Dose rate: 2.0–2.5 mg m^{-2} every 7 days.

Vincristine

PoM **Vincristine** (Non-proprietary)

Available as: injection, vincristine sulphate 1 mg m^{-1}; 1 ml, 2 ml injection, vincristine sulphate powder for reconstitution, 1 mg, 2 mg, 5 mg.

Indications: lymphoproliferative and myeloproliferative diseases
mast cell tumours
transmissible venereal tumour (thrombocytopenia)

Side effects: tissue irritant – perivascular reactions
peripheral and autonomic neuropathies
mild alopecia

Dose rate: 0.5–0.75 mg m^{-2} every 7 days.
(Tables 50.16, 50.18–50.21)

Hormones

Prednisolone

PoM **Prednsiolone** (non-proprietary)

Available as: tablets: 1 mg and 5 mg

Indications: lymphoproliferative and myeloproliferative disorders
mast cell tumours
brain tumours
management of complications of neoplasia
palliation of advanced neoplastic disease

Side effects: pancreatitis
diarrhoea
hyperadrenocorticism

Dose rate: 10–60 mg m^{-2} daily or every 48 h
(Tables 50.16, 50.18–50.20)

Miscellaneous agents

Platinum coordination compounds

Cisplatin

PoM **Cisplatin** (Non-proprietary).
US **Platinol**™ (Bristol-Myers)
(Diamminedichloroplatinum (II))

Available as: injection, cisplatin 1 mg m^{-1}, 10 ml, 50 ml, 100 ml

	injection, cisplatin, powder for reconstitution 10 mg, 50 mg (other sizes available)
Indications:	carcinomas soft tissue and osteogenic sarcoma
Side effects:	nephrotoxic, acute proximal tubular necrosis (cisplatin must be administered with intensive fluid diuresis) vomiting (myelosuppression)
Dose rate:	60–120 mg m^{-2} with prehydration and diuresis, every 3–4 weeks

L-Asparaginase

US, **Elspar**™ (M.S.D.)

Crisantaspase

PoM **Erwinase**™ (Speywood)

Available as:	injection, powder for reconstitution, 10 000 units
Indications:	lymphoproliferative disorders (melanoma and mast cell tumours)
Side effects:	hypersensitivity reactions (safest route of administration is intramuscular) haemorrhagic pancreatitis has been reported in dogs gastrointestinal
Dose rate:	10 000–40 000 IU m^{-2} every 7 days or as required (i.m). Premedicate with antihistamine if drug is to be administered i.v. or i.p. (Tables 50.16, 50.18)

Hydroxyurea

PoM **Hydrea**™ (Squibb)

Available as:	capsules, hydroxyurea 500 mg
Indications:	polycythaemia rubra vera chronic granulocytic leukaemia
Side effects:	myelosuppression
Dose rate:	50 mg kg^{-1} daily to effect or 80 mg kg^{-1} every 3 days, by mouth. (Table 50.19)

REFERENCES

Adams, W.M. (1991) Veterinary radiation therapy. *Compendium on Continuing Education* **13**, 262–273.

Bockman, R.S. (1980) Hypercalcaemia in malignancy. *Journal of Clinical Endocrinology and Metabolism* **9**, 317–333.

Broadus, A.E., Mangin, M., Ikeda, K., Insogna, K.L., Weir, E.C., Burtis, W.J. and Stewart, A.F. (1988) Humoral hypercalcaemia of cancer. *New England Journal of Medicine* **319**, 556–563.

Brodey, R.S. and Abt, D.A. (1976) Results of surgical treatment in 65 dogs with osteosarcoma. *Journal of the Veterinary Medical Association* **168**, 1032–1035.

Carter, R.F., Harris, C.K., Withrow, S.J., Valli, V.E.O. and Susaneck, S.J. (1987) Chemotherapy of canine lymphoma with histopathological correlation: doxorubicin alone compared to COP as first treatment regimen. *Journal of the American Animal Hospital Association* **23**, 587–596.

Cotter, S.M. (1983) Treatment of lymphoma and leukaemia with cyclophosphamide, vincristine and prednisolone: II treatment of cats. *Journal of the American Animal Hospital Association* **19**, 166–172.

Cotter, S.M. and Goldstein, M.A. (1987) Comparison of two protocols for maintenance of remission in dogs with lymphoma. *Journal of the American Animal Hospital Association* **23**, 495–499.

Couto, C.G. (1984) Haematologic abnormalities in small animal cancer patients. Part I Red blood cell abnormalities. *Compendium on Continuing Education* **6**, 1059–1065.

Couto, C.G. (1990) Management of complications of cancer therapy. Veterinary Clinics of North America. *Small Animal Practice* **20**, 1037–1051.

Cowell, R.L. and Tyler, R.D. (1989) *Diagnostic Cytology of the Dog and Cat*. American Veterinary Publications, California.

Curt, G.A., Clendeninn, N.J. and Chabner B.A. (1984) Drug resistance in cancer. *Cancer Treatment Reports* **68**, 87–99.

Dische, S. and Saunders, M.I. (1989) Continuous hyperfractionated accelerated radiotherapy (CHART). *British Journal of Cancer* **59**, 325–326.

Dobson, J.M. and Gorman, N.T. (1993) Canine multicentric lymphoma I: clinicopathological presentation of the disease. *Journal of Small Animal Practice* **34**, 594–598.

Dobson, J.M. and Gorman, N.T. (1994) Canine multicentric lymphoma II: comparison of response to two different treatment protocols. *Journal of Small Animal Practice* **35**, 9–15.

Elliot, J., Dobson, J.M., Dunn, J.K., Herrtage, M.E. and Jackson, K.F. (1991) Hypercalcaemia in the dog: a study of 40 cases. *Journal of Small Animal Practice* **32**, 564–571.

Else, R. (1989) Biopsy – special techniques and tissues. *In Practice* **11**, 27–34.

Evans, R.J. and Gorman, N.T. (1987) Myeloproliferative disease in the dog and cat. Definition, aetiology and classification. *Veterinary Record* **121**, 437–443.

Fox, L.E., Rosenthal, R.C., Twedt, D.C., Dubielzig, R.R., MacEwan, E.G. and Grauer, G.F. (1990) Plasma histamine and gastrin concentrations in 17 dogs with mast cell tumours. *Journal of Veterinary Internal Medicine* **4**, 242–246.

Giger, U. and Gorman, N.T. (1984) Oncologic emergencies in small animals Part II. Metabolic and endocrine emergencies. *Compendium on Continuing Education* **6**, 805–813.

Gorman, N.T. and Evans, R.J. (1987) Myeloproliferative disease in the dog and cat. Clinical presentations, diagnosis and treatment. *Veterinary Record* **121**, 490–496.

Hall, E.J. (1978) *Radiobiology for the Radiologist*. Harper & Row, New York.

Hammer, A.S., Couto, C.G., Filippi, J., Getzy, D. and Shank, K. (1991) Efficacy and toxicity of VAC chemotherapy (vincristine, doxorubicin, cyclophosphamide) in dogs with haemangiosarcoma. *Journal of Veterinary Internal Medicine* **5**, 160–166.

Hardy, W.D. (1981) The feline leukaemia virus. *Journal of the American Animal Hospital Association* **17**, 951–980.

Hefland, S.C. (1990) Principles and application of chemotherapy. *Veterinary Clinics of North America: Small Animal Practice* **20**, 987–1013.

Hill, R. (1987) Metastasis. In: *The Basic Science of Oncology* (Eds I.F. Tannock and R.P. Hill). Pergamon Press, New York, Oxford, 160–175.

Hille, B. (1982) Membrane excitability: action potential and ionic channels. In: *Physiology and Biophysics IV* 20th edn (Eds. T. Ruch and H. Patton). W.B. Saunders, Philadelphia.

Howard, E.B., Sawa, T.R. and Nielson, S.W. (1969) Mastocytomas and gastroduodenal ulceration. *Pathologia Veterinaria* **6**, 146–158.

Jarrett, O. (1994) Feline leukaemia virus. In: *Feline Medicine and Therapeutics*. 2nd edn (Eds E.A. Chandler, C.J. Gaskell and R.M. Gaskell). Blackwell Scientific Publications, Oxford.

Laing, E.J., Miller, C.W. and Cochrane, S.M. (1988) Treatment of cyclophosphamide-induced haemorrhagic cystitis in 5 dogs. *Journal of the American Veterinary Medical Association* **193**, 233–236.

LaRue, S.M., Withrow, S.J., Powers, B.E., Wrigley, R.H., Gillette, E.L., Schwars, P.D., Straw, R.C. and Richter, S.L. (1989) Limb sparing treatment for osteosarcoma in dogs. *Journal of the Veterinary Medical Association* **195**, 1734–1744.

Leifer, C.E. and Matus, R.E. (1986) Chronic lymphocytic leukaemia in the dog, 22 cases (1974–1984). *Journal of the American Veterinary Medical Association* **189**, 214–217.

MacEwan, E.G. and Hurvitz, A.I. (1977) Diagnosis and management of monoclonal gammopathies. *Veterinary Clinics of North America, Small Animal Practice* **7**, 119–132.

MacEwan, E.G., Brown, N.O., Patnaik, A.K., Hayes, A.A. and Passe, S. (1981) Cyclic combination chemotherapy of canine lymphosarcoma. *Journal of the American Veterinary Medical Association* **178**, 1178–1181.

MacVean, D.W., Monlux, A.W. and Anderson, P.S. (1978) Frequency of canine and feline tumors in a defined population. *Veterinary Pathology* **15**, 700–715.

Madewell, B.R. (1985) Canine lymphoma. *Veterinary Clinics of North America, Small Animal Practice*. **15**, 709–722.

Madewell, B. and Feldman, B. (1980) Characterization of anaemias associated with neoplasia in small animals. *Journal of the American Veterinary Medical Association* **176**, 419–425.

Matus, R.E., Leifer, C.E. and MacEwan, E.G. (1983) Acute lymphoblastic leukaemia in the dog: A review of 30 cases. *Journal of the American Veterinary Medical Association* **183**, 859–862.

Maudlin, G.N., Matus, R.E. and Withrow, S.J. (1988) Canine osteosarcoma: treatment by amputation versus amputation and adjuvant chemotherapy using doxorubicin and cisplatin. *Journal of Veterinary Internal Medicine* **2**, 177–180.

McLeod, D.A. and Thrall, D.E. (1989) The combination of surgery and radiation in the treatment of cancer. *Veterinary Surgery* **18**, 1–6.

Merry, S., Courtney, E.R., Fetherston, C.A., Kaye, S.B. and Freshney, R.I. (1987) Circumvention of drug resistance in human non-small cell lung cancer *in vitro* by verapamil. *British Journal of Cancer* **56**, 401–405.

Morris, J.S., Dunn, J.K. and Dobson, J.M. (1993) Canine lymphoid leukaemias and lymphomas with bone marrow involvement: a review of 24 cases. *Journal of Small Animal Practice* **34**, 72.

Moulton, J.E. and Harvey, J.W. (1990) Tumours of the lymphoid and haemopoietic tissues. In: *Tumours of Domestic Animals*, 3rd edn (Ed. J.E. Moulton). University of California Press, p. 231.

Mundy, G.R., Ibbotson, K.J. and D'Souza, S.M. (1985) Tumour products and the hypercalcaemia of malignancy. *Journal of Clinical Investigation* **76**, 391–394.

O'Keefe, D.A. (1990) Canine mast cell tumours. *Veterinary Clinics of North America: Small Animal Practice* **20**, 1105–1115.

Osborne, C.A. and Stevens, J.B. (1977) Hypercalcaemic nephropathy. In: *Current Veterinary Therapy* VI (Ed. R.W. Kirk). W.B. Saunders, Philadelphia, pp. 1080–1087.

Owen, L.N. (1980) *TNM Classification of Tumours in Domestic Animals*. World Health Organization, Geneva.

Penwick, R.C. and Nunamaker, D.M. (1987) Rostral mandibulectomy: a treatment for oral neoplasia in the dog and cat. *Journal of the American Animal Hospital Association* **23**, 19–25.

Postorino, N.C., Susaneck, S.J., Withrow, S.J., Macy, A.W. and Harris, C. (1989) Single agent therapy with adriamycin for canine lymphosarcoma. *Journal of the American Animal Hospital Association* **25**, 221–225.

Priester, W.A. and McKay, F.W. (1980) The occurrence of tumours in domestic animals. *National Cancer Institute Monograph* 54.

Rosenthal, R.C. (1982) Epidemiology of lymphosarcoma. *Compendium on Continuing Education* **4**, 855–860.

Rosenthal, R.C. and MacEwan, E.G. (1990) Treatment of lymphoma in dogs. *Journal of the American Veterinary Medical Association* **196**, 774–781.

Rothenberg, M. and Ling, V. (1989) Multi-drug resistance: molecular biology and clinical relevance. *Journal of the National Cancer Institute* **81**, 907–910.

Salisbury, S.K. and Lantz, G.C. (1988) Long-term results of partial mandibulectomy for treatment of oral tumours. *Journal of the American Animal Hospital Association* **24**, 285–294

Sawyers, C.L., Denny, C.T. and Witte, O.N. (1990) Leukaemia and the disruption of normal haematopoiesis. *Cell* **64**, 337–350.

Schlam, O.W., Jain, N.C. and Carroll, E.J. (1975) *Veterinary Haematology*, Lea & Febiger, Philadelphia, p. 554.

Shapiro, W., Fossum, T.W. and Kitchell, B.E. (1988) The use of cis-platin for treatment of appendicular osteosarcoma in dogs. *Journal of the Veterinary Medical Association.* **192**, 507–511.

Skipper, H.E., Schabel, F.M. and Wilcox, W.S. (1964) Experimental evaluation of potential anticancer agents XIII: on the criteria and kinetics associated with 'curability' of experimental leukaemia. *Cancer Chemotherapy Reports* **35**, 1.

Thrall, D.E., McLeod, D.A., Bentel, G.C. and Dewhirst, M.W. (1989) A review of treatment planning and dose calculation in veterinary radiation oncology. *Radiology* **30**, 194–221.

Walker, M. and Breider, M. (1987) Intra-operative radiotherapy of canine bladder cancer. *Veterinary Radiology* **28**, 200.

Weller, R.E. (1984) Cancer-associated hypercalcaemia in companion animals. *Compendium on Continuing Education* **6**, 639–646.

White, R.A.S. (1991a) Biopsy techniques. In: *BSAVA Manual of Small Animal Oncology* (Ed. R.A.S. White). BSAVA Publications, pp. 87–97.

White, R.A.S. (1991b) Oncological surgery. In: *BSAVA Manual of Small Animal Oncology* (Ed. R.A.S. White). BSAVA Publications, p. 113.

White, R.A.S. and Gorman, N.T. (1989). Wide local excision of acanthomatous epulides in the dog. *Veterinary Surgery* **18**, 12–14.

White, R.A.S., Gorman, N.T., Watkins, S.B. and Brearley, M.J. (1985) The surgical management of bone involved oral tumours in the dog. *Journal of Small Animal Practice* **26**, 693–708.

Withrow, S.J. and Holmberg, D.L. (1983) Mandibulectomy in the treatment of oral cancer. *Journal of the American Animal Hospital Association* **19**, 273–286.

Withrow, S.J., Gillette, E.L., Hoopes, P.J. and McChesney, S.L. (1989) Intra-operative irradiation of 16 spontaneously occurring neoplasms. *Veterinary Surgery* **18**, 7.

Wotton, P.R. and Pearson, G.R. (1988) Hypercalcaemia and malignancy in dogs. *Veterinary Annual* **28**, 233–238.

Wynford-Thomas, D. (1991) Oncogenes and anti-oncogenes: the molecular basis of tumour behaviour. *Journal of Pathology* **165**, 187–201.

FURTHER READING

Approved Code of Practice: Control of Substances Hazardous to Health and *Approved Code of Practice: Control of Carcinogenic Substances.* (1992). 3rd edn, COSHH Regulations 1988. HMSO, London.

Dobson, J.M. and Gorman, N.T. (1993) *Cancer Chemotherapy in Small Animal Practice.* Blackwell Scientific Publications, Oxford.

Gorman, N.T. (Ed) (1986) *Oncology.* Contemporary Issues in Small Animal Practice Series, Vol. 6. Churchill Livingstone, New York.

Guidance Notes MS21 from the Health and Safety Executive (1983) Precautions for the safe handling of cytotoxic drugs. HMSO, London.

Tannock, I.F. and Hill, R.P. (Eds) (1987) *The Basic Science of Oncology.* Pergamon Press, New York, Oxford.

White, R.A.S. (Ed) (1991) *BSAVA Manual of Small Animal Oncology.* BSAVA Publications.

51

Behaviour Problems

V. O'Farrell

Cognitive processes	1029	Problems of anxiety and stress	1039
Diagnosis and treatment of behaviour problems	1033	Prevention of problems	1041
Aggression	1037		

The incidence of behaviour problems in dogs is 40–50% and of serious problems 20–25% (Wilbur, 1976; Voith, 1985; O'Farrell, 1992). Although fewer cats than dogs present to veterinary surgeons with behaviour problems, Voith (1985) found owners reporting a comparable incidence (47% in cats versus 42% in dogs). Serious behaviour problems must be taken seriously. They can be life-threatening for the pet in the sense that they may lead to euthanasia. In addition, many behaviour problems which the owner chooses to tolerate may significantly impair the quality of life of the animal and/or owner. Many owners do not spontaneously consult their veterinary surgeon about behaviour problems, perhaps because they do not realize that they have anything to offer. It is therefore advisable to enquire routinely about behaviour, perhaps during general health checks.

In order to treat behaviour problems successfully, it is necessary to understand something of the processes underlying behaviour.

COGNITIVE PROCESSES

Thinking and learning

Dogs and cats tend to be regarded as family members and because they are such sensitive observers of human body language, there is a tendency for owners to ascribe to them human powers of thought. It is important, however, to recognize the limitations of their cognitive power. They cannot think in an abstract or symbolic way. They cannot understand language and they cannot reflect on the past or the future. There is, therefore, no point in warning them not to do something in the future (e.g. urinate in the owner's absence) or to remonstrate with them about something done in the past (e.g. having urinated when the owner was out). They are also incapable of learning or following a rule: for example, a dog may reliably walk to heel on the pavement because it has formed the habit of so doing, but it has not understood that it must not run in the road. Thus training a dog to behave in some desirable way must consist of getting it into the habit of performing in this way, rather than getting it to understand or showing it what to do. Therefore, the principle of human learning that much is learned from mistakes does not apply to learning in dogs and cats. In addition, neither dogs nor cats can be said to have a moral sense; they can have no concepts of right and wrong. It is, therefore, inappropriate and usually counterproductive for an owner to feel morally outraged by his dog's or cat's undesirable behaviour or to attribute to it complex moral motives such as revenge. Dogs and cats learn new behaviour in two ways: via classical conditioning or instrumental learning.

Classical conditioning takes place when a stimulus (technically known as the unconditioned stimulus) which naturally or instinctively provokes a reflex response (unconditioned response) is repeatedly paired with a previously neutral stimulus (conditioned response). Eventually the neutral stimulus on its own will provoke the reflex response (conditioned response). The best-known example of this phenomenon is its early demonstration by Pavlov, using dogs. The unconditioned stimulus used was food, the unconditioned response being salivation. At the same time as food was presented to the dogs, the bell was rung (conditioned stimulus). Eventually the dogs salivated when they heard the bell on its own. By and large, responses mediated by the autonomic nervous system are learned via classical conditioning, e.g. sexual responses, urination and defecation and emotional responses such as aggression or fear.

Instrumental learning applies to voluntary movements. Its basic principle is that if an action (response) performed in a certain situation (stimulus) is followed by a reward (reinforcement) when that situation occurs again the probability of the action being performed is increased. Dogs and cats are equally capable of instrumental learning, but because dogs tend to find more rewarding events which are under the owner's control (e.g. praise, tit-bits), the behaviour of dogs can be more easily altered by the owner. It is worth bearing in mind the following aspects of instrumental learning.

1. To be most effective, a reward must be delivered at the same time as the response to be learned or within one second afterwards.
2. Much problem behaviour in dogs is the result of instrumental learning and it is usually worth examining the situation in which the problem behaviour occurs for hidden rewards. This reward often turns out to be attention from the owner, even when this attention takes the form of anger.
3. Different schedules of reward are most effective at different stages of learning. When an animal is being taught a response, it will learn most quickly if the response is rewarded every time it occurs. Once a response is established, it is most resistant to extinction (unlearning) if it is rewarded at irregular intervals. This often applies to learned problem behaviour in dogs, such as begging for food at human mealtimes, where the owner is aware that the behaviour should not be rewarded, but occasionally does so.
4. Some events which are not intrinsically rewarding can act as rewards because of their learned association with intrinsically rewarding events. This phenomenon is known as secondary reinforcement. Thus, an owner can make a toy into a secondary reinforcer for his dog by arranging that the dog picking up the toy is a precondition of a pleasurable event such as being fed or getting attention from the owner. The toy can then be employed in the treatment of a range of behaviour problems (see below).

Punishment is the most over-used technique in the treatment of behaviour problems. It is often the method tried first by owners, whereas it should be a method of last resort. Although it occasionally is spectacularly successful, it has many possible pitfalls.

1. To stand any chance of being effective, punishment must be delivered within one second of the undesirable behaviour. There is, therefore, no point in taking a puppy to a puddle on the floor made half an hour previously and smacking it or shouting at a dog when the chewed remains of a slipper are discovered.
2. Even when delivered at the right time, there is a danger that the animal will associate the aversive stimulus with the wrong aspect of the situation. For example, an owner who shouts at a spraying cat may teach it to spray only when the owner is absent, rather than teaching it not to spray in the house.
3. The intensity of the punishment must be exactly right. If it is too strong it may provoke fear or aggression. If it is too weak it will be ineffective.
4. If punishment is repeated, the animal is likely to become habituated to it. This means that a stimulus which is effective in stopping undesirable behaviour the first time, may become ineffective on subsequent occasions.
5. Because of their past experience of punishment and because of their temperaments, individual animals vary in their reactions to the same punishing stimulus: what has no affect on one may frighten another severely.
6. The more motivated the animal is to perform an action, the greater the intensity of punishment required to stop it.
7. Punishment tends to increase anxiety. Therefore, if the behaviour is motivated by anxiety in the first place, punishment will make it worse.

From the foregoing, it can be seen that if punishment works, it works quickly: this explains the dramatic accounts of successful punishment (e.g. dogs permanently cured of food stealing by having a table cloth pulled from under them). Behaviour modification which relies on rewards, extinction, distraction and response substitution takes longer, but is more reliable. Where it is possible to use these methods they are, therefore, preferable to punishment. However, if there is no alternative to punishment, its effectiveness will be maximized if the following provisos are borne in mind.

1. The punishing stimulus is more appropriately viewed as a distracting stimulus: its aim is not to upset the animal, but to disrupt the undesirable behaviour and divert the animal's attention from it. Sometimes calling the animal's name is enough to achieve this aim. If not, a startling or novel stimulus is often effective, e.g. rape alarm, water pistol.
2. In most sequences of highly motivated behaviour, there is usually a moment at the beginning of the sequence (for example when a cat approaches a piece of furniture which it habitually scratches) where motivation is comparatively low and the animal can be distracted comparatively easily.
3. The most aversive feature of many punishing stimuli seems to be that they are unusual and unexpected. This is why 'all-purpose' startling stimuli soon become ineffective: their aversive power depends on their novelty. But it also means that thwarting the animal suddenly and unexpectedly in its purpose can be aversive in itself. Thus, if a door is unexpectedly shut in a dog's face as it runs out, or it is suddenly checked on an extending lead, it may be less eager to run out again. This seems to be the principle underlying the effectiveness of such devices as 'training disks' which make an unusual sound. Their successful use seems to depend on a pretraining schedule which pairs the sound with an unexpectedly frustrating experience.
4. After the undesirable behaviour has been successfully stopped by punishment or distraction, the animal should always be provided with another response which is intrinsically rewarding or which is rewarded by the owner.

Social behaviour

Many behaviour problems arise, particularly in dogs, because owners misunderstand their animals' instinctive social expectations or body language. Dogs and cats which, as puppies or kittens, have contact with human beings treat people throughout their lives as conspecifics who are assumed to share these expectations and body language.

Dogs are social animals which expect to live in packs. The behaviour of pack members towards one another is partly determined by the dominance hierarchy, a frequently misunderstood concept. In a pack of wolves or feral dogs, dominant animals tend to instigate activities and have prior claim over resources such as food. They tend to be older and heavier animals. However, the dominance hierarchy is not a rigid one (Lockwood, 1979); different members may be dominant in different circumstances. Also, individual wolves or dogs differ in the extent to which they are preoccupied with dominance. In dogs, certain breeds, such as the small Scottish terriers and guard dogs, tend to be more preoccupied with dominance, as do male dogs and spayed bitches. Dogs signal dominance and submission to their conspecifics by means of body language. Submission may be expressed by averting the gaze or the postures known as 'active submission' (Fig. 51.1) or 'passive submission' (Fig. 51.2). Dominance may be expressed by a typical body posture (Fig. 51.3); a dominant dog may also tend to take the social initiative with its owner and be unwilling to obey commands. Owners who need to reverse this relationship and assert their own dominant position should themselves seize this social initiative and reward only obedience to their commands (see dominance aggression below). Veterinary surgeons who try to enforce compliance in their canine patients by means of a dominant stance and tone of voice run the risk of an unproductive confrontation. A non-threatening manner is advisable.

Aggression is not an expression of dominance, but a sign that the dog feels that the normal conventions of behaviour have broken down. A dog which perceives itself as dominant in a relationship may attack if it feels its dominant body signals have not been appropriately responded to by a perceived subordinate; a subordinate dog may bite when frightened or cornered. Physical violence or threatening behaviour should therefore be avoided by both owners and veterinary surgeons.

It used to be thought that cats were solitary creatures which, once adult, sought the company

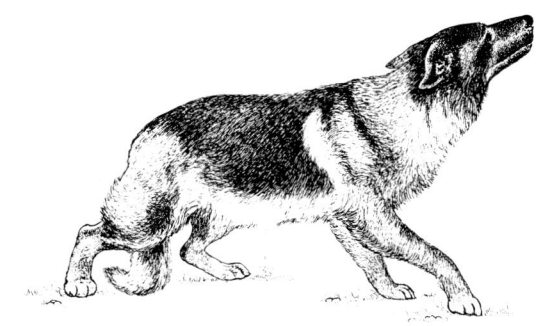

Figure 51.1 'Active submission' posture.

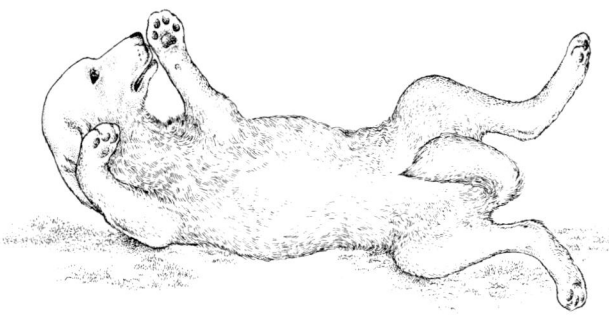

Figure 51.2 'Passive submission' posture.

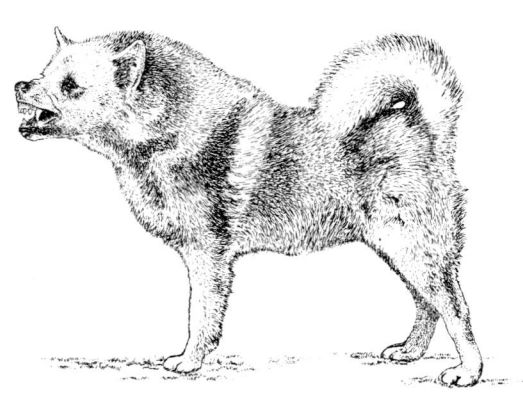

Figure 51.3 Typical dominant body posture.

of their own species only for the purposes of mating and breeding. However, it has now been demonstrated (e.g. Kerby and Macdonald, 1988) that when a food source is concentrated at one point feral cats may voluntarily form a colony. Similarly, owners of more than one cat report high levels of social interaction between the cats (Voith and Borchelt, 1986). There are individual differences in the sociability of pet cats, determined at least in part by genetic factors and early experience (Karsh, 1984). In feral cats, gender is also a determinant of sociability: colonies consist mainly of related females and their offspring, with mature males more loosely attached to several groups. It is likely, however, that in pet cats castration before maturity at least reduces this gender difference (Bradshaw, 1992).

Although groups of cats may include a 'despot' which claims preferential access to resources such as food, cats do not seem to display dominance and submission to each other so much as aggressive, threatening behaviour met with fear or defensive behaviour. As with the dog, aggression by the owner or veterinary surgeon is likely to be counterproductive. On the other hand, in contradistinction to dogs, taking the social initiative with cats is unlikely to improve the cat–owner relationship. Turner (1991) found that cats spend more time interacting with owners who initiate a lower proportion of these interactions.

Stress and anxiety

Like people, dogs and cats are subject to stress and anxiety. Some individuals are more susceptible than others. This is partly due to genetic factors (Murphree et al., 1967). Early environment is also important; kittens and puppies which are not handled by people or are reared in impoverished environments tend to be more fearful (Wilson et al., 1965; Agrawal et al., 1967). Anxiety may be manifested in the form of fear. Specific phobias may be learnt by classical conditioning. Thus a neutral stimulus, such as the veterinary surgeon, may come to arouse fear if paired with a painful or unpleasant medical procedure. Anxiety or stress may also result in over-excitement. This may be expressed in various ways: hyperactivity and barking (in dogs), urination and defecation or displacement activities. This latter is an ethological term used to describe parts of an instinctive behaviour pattern which are performed out of context and which seem to have a tension-relieving function for the animal. They are typically performed when the animal is in a state of conflict or frustration. When they become fixed and repetitive they are referred to as stereotypies. Common displacement activities include: tail chasing, digging, chewing, sexual mounting of inanimate objects (in dogs), self-mutilation and excessive grooming.

Developmental psychology

In the lives of both cats and dogs there is a sensitive period when experiences have a disproportionately large psychological effect; this period seems to last from approximately three to twelve weeks in the dog and two to seven weeks in the cat (Karsh and Turner, 1988). Animals not exposed to human beings during this period will rarely become properly tame and more subtle social handicaps appear in animals which have had restricted interactions.

Pet–owner relationships

As every veterinary surgeon in small animal practice is aware, there are wide variations in both the degree and kind of attachments between dogs or cats and their owners (Wilbur, 1976). The nature of the attachment can contribute both to the causation and maintenance of a problem and to the outcome of treatment. For example, only owners who are highly attached to their pets may be prepared to take the time and trouble required by many behavioural regimes. Voith (1985) has shown that cat owners are just as attached to their pets as are dog owners. Veterinary surgeons, however, tend to underestimate their clients' attachment to their pets (Catanzaro, 1988). This mistake seems more likely to occur with cat owners; O'Farrell (unpublished data) found that veterinary students consider dogs more rewarding pets than cats.

On the other hand, some highly attached owners may have unrealistic expectations of their pets. Owners who idealize their dogs report an unsatisfactory relationship with their own parent of the same sex (O'Farrell, 1994); this suggests that the dog is being used to compensate for an early deprivation in the owners' life. There is evidence that such inappropriate use of the dog can contribute to the development of behaviour problems. Dominance aggression is seen more often in dogs whose owners treat them as dependent children and displacement activities in dogs with anxious owners (O'Farrell, 1992).

DIAGNOSIS AND TREATMENT OF BEHAVIOUR PROBLEMS

Because of their training, veterinary surgeons are more apt to mistake a behavioural problem for a physical problem than vice versa. It may be useful to bear in mind that the diagnoses are not necessarily mutually exclusive. For example, a dog already showing dominance aggression may show aggression more readily because it is suffering from an ear infection. Also, the more chronic the physical disorder, the more likely it is to acquire behavioural components; a dog or cat which defecates in the house because of a gastrointestinal disorder may, out of habit, continue to do so after the physical condition has resolved. Dermatological disorders which are aggravated by licking or chewing may also benefit from a combined physical and behavioural approach.

The diagnosis and treatment of behavioural problems require a different approach from that required for physical problems. Although it may be possible to give the behaviour a descriptive label (e.g. dominance aggression), this label does not refer to a clinical entity, nor, on its own, does it imply a certain treatment procedure. To treat the problem effectively, it is necessary to assess all the factors operating, which will differ in each individual case. Similarly, the treatment programme itself must be tailored to individual needs. Most of the relevant information must be provided verbally by the owner, although observation of the dog or cat and its interaction with the owner is also necessary. For these reasons, it is usually advisable to set aside a longer time than would normally be spent on a veterinary consultation. In a diagnostic interview, it is usually advisable to cover the following areas.

Description of the problem

1. What exactly does the animal do? Do not be content with a general description of behaviour, such as 'nervous'. This may be ambiguous.
2. In what situations does the behaviour occur?
3. What happens following the behaviour? What the animal does is not usually as relevant as how the owners normally react, e.g. by inadvertently rewarding the behaviour in some way.

History of the problem

1. When and under what circumstances did it first occur?
2. What have the owners already done to treat the problem?

General information

1. What is the rest of the animal's behaviour like? Are there other problems?
2. What is the animal's daily routine? This can elicit information about owner attitudes. It can also provide clues about how the animal views its relationship with its owner: does the dog see itself as dominant? Is the cat very attached to its owner? The owner must be persuaded to be quite specific about his interactions with the animal. 'Then we go for a walk' is not enough, for example: it is necessary to know who initiates the walk.
3. What is the composition of the household and

the relationship of the animal with its other members?
4. What is the attitude of the owner and other family members towards the problem? This is probably the most important single prognostic factor. In most cases, if the owner is not prepared to spend time or to take the trouble, the treatment is unlikely to have a positive outcome. The prognosis is also guarded if there is disagreement over this question in the family.

Treatment should always be based on some kind of diagnosis, even a tentative one. The temptation to try out treatment methods on an empirical, ad hoc basis should be resisted: if an empirical treatment fails no knowledge has been gained. If a treatment based on a diagnosis fails, at least the diagnostic field is narrowed.

Treatment methods

Surgical

In cats, castration reduces or eliminates intermale aggression, urine marking and roaming in 80–90% of cases (Hart and Barrett, 1973). In dogs, roaming is reduced in 90% of cases, but intermale aggression, urine marking and mounting in only 50–60% of cases (Hopkins *et al.*, 1976). In dogs, the administration of an antiandrogen such as delmadione (Tardak, Syntex) may be useful in predicting the affect of castration on an individual. In bitches, there is no evidence that spaying is likely to have a beneficial effect on behaviour. On the contrary, it tends to increase dominance aggression in puppies already showing some aggression (O'Farrell and Peachey, 1990).

In cats other surgical treatments for spraying have been proposed, such as olfactory tractotomy (Hart, 1981) and bilateral ischiocavernosus myectomy (Komtebedde and Hauptman, 1990). These techniques must be regarded at present as experimental. As a treatment for territorial scratching, declawing is much less popular in Great Britain than in North America. Presumably this is partly due to the fact that a higher proportion of British cats go outdoors. There is evidence, however, (Landsberg, 1991), that most outdoor cats are not handicapped by declawing. On the other hand, territorial scratching is less likely than spraying to be an intolerable problem to most owners. All of these surgical interventions (olfactory tractotomy, ischiocavernosus myectomy and declawing) must significantly interfere with the cat's quality of life. Although in theory there might be cases where they are the only alternatives to euthanasia, other treatment methods or rehoming are almost always preferable and more appropriate.

The surgical treatment of a stereotypy by removal of one of the body parts involved (e.g. treatment of tail chasing by removing the tail) is absolutely contraindicated. Such an approach is hardly ever successful and the discomfort produced by the wound may well aggravate the problem.

Any attempt to alter behaviour by surgical means should always be immediately followed by behavioural treatment; there is otherwise a much higher risk of the undesirable behaviour continuing or reappearing.

Drug treatment

In general, it is best to reserve the use of medication for cases which are serious or at crisis point. Drugs should never be used without concurrent behavioural treatment. Compared with the wide range of drugs available for the psychiatric treatment of human beings, few are licensed for the treatment of behavioural disorders in small animals.

Until recently, the most widely prescribed was probably acepromazine maleate (Acetylpromazine, C-Vet). There is evidence that this reduces excitability more effectively than anxiety (Hart, 1985). In cases of anxiety two groups of drugs not licensed for animal use, the benzodiazepines, specially diazepam (Valium, Roche), and the tricyclic antidepressants, e.g. amitriptyline (Tryptizol, Morson), have been used successfully. For diazepam, a dose of 0.5–2.0 mg kg^{-1} has been recommended for dogs and 1–2 mg b.i.d. for cats; for amitriptyline, 2–4 mg kg^{-1} for dogs and 5–10 mg for cats (Marder, 1991). With diazepam, initial paradoxical effects such as hyperactivity have been reported. Animals should therefore be kept under supervision when these drugs are given for the first time. More recently, a combination of phenobarbitone (7.5 mg b.i.d. for cats and 2–3 mg kg^{-1} b.i.d. for dogs) and propranolol (5 mg b.i.d. for cats and 2–3 mg kg^{-1} b.i.d. for dogs) has also been found to be effective in reducing anxiety (Walker, personal communication).

In addition, long-acting opioid antagonists such as naltrexone (Nalorex, DuPont) have been found useful in the treatment of stereotypies.

In the last few years, the behavioural effects of megestrol acetate (Ovarid, Pitman-Moore) have become more widely known. In dogs, this is the drug of choice for the treatment of gender-related problems such as dominance aggression, mounting and urine-marking. Because of its effects on the limbic system, tending to make animals more tractable and equable in mood, the drug may be effective in a wider range of disorders where emotionality or over-arousal are contributing factors. In dogs, the recommended dose is 2 mg kg^{-1} daily for 2 weeks, followed by half that dose for a further 2 weeks; this dosage can safely be given to intact and castrated dogs and to spayed bitches.

In cats, megestrol can reduce urine spraying and intermale aggression (Hart and Hart, 1985). It can also be helpful in the treatment of stress-related disorders. In many cases, however, the risk of adverse metabolic and endocrinological effects (Henik et al., 1985) may outweigh the benefits; diazepam is a safer option and may reduce urine spraying (Cooper and Hart, 1992) and aggression as well as the more obvious symptoms of stress and anxiety. There is also evidence that buspirone is even more effective in reducing urine spraying (Hart et al., 1993).

Behavioural treatment

It should first be considered whether alterations are needed in the animal's general behavioural disposition? The alterations most commonly required are as follows.

1. In dogs, establishment of owner dominance. This is most obviously necessary when the dog is showing aggression. In addition, there are other behaviour problems, such as poor response to the owner's commands, which may also benefit from increasing owner dominance.
2. Reduction of stress: this should be attempted for animals showing symptoms of stress or anxiety. In addition to eliminating, where possible, specific sources of stress, all punishment should be stopped, the animal's routine made as stable as possible and the owner should try not to make the animal the focus of extremes of emotion.

To tackle the specific problem a number of strategies can be considered.

Remove or alter the stimulus

In most cases, it is worth starting by attempting to remove or alter the stimulus which elicits the problem behaviour, so that, if successful, the behaviour disappears. In some cases, particularly in cats, this may be all that is needed. In most cases, however, either the triggering stimulus cannot be removed because it is necessary to the animal's or the owner's life or it is not sufficient to remove it, because the problem behaviour will reappear in response to new stimuli. For example, excitement and barking in response to the telephone ringing may be temporarily eliminated by changing the sound of the ring, but it will usually reappear when the dog learns the meaning of the new sound. It is therefore necessary to break the connection between the triggering stimulus and the undesirable response. Broadly speaking, the methods of doing this (which are complementary rather than mutually exclusive) are as follows.

1. *Extinction*: the rewards for the undesirable behaviour are removed, e.g. a dog which pesters the family for tit-bits at meal times is ignored. This will not work on its own when the behaviour itself is enjoyable or self-rewarding, e.g. barking.
2. *Response substitution*: the animal is taught to respond to the triggering stimulus with an acceptable action rather than with the undesirable behaviour. For example, a dog might learn to sit in the hall when the bell rings rather than running to the door barking. This learning will take place more easily if:
  (a) The animal first learns the alternative response in circumstances where there are no competing responses (e.g. the dog is taught to sit in the hall when there is no door bell ringing);
  (b) The animal is highly motivated to perform the alternative response because:
     (i) the response obtains an attractive reward. The attractiveness of a reward can be enhanced by being made a secondary as well as a primary reinforcer (see section on Learning). Thus the dog might be rewarded for sitting in the hall with a toy which had previously been associated with enjoyable play sessions;
     (ii) the response is itself intrinsically enjoyable: responses which are motivated by the same instinct which prompts the instinctive behaviour have an advantage (e.g. pouncing on a toy mouse as an alternative to pouncing on human feet).

Systematic desensitization

This usually refers to a method of treating anxiety whereby the animal in a non-anxious state is presented with a version of the triggering stimulus which does not provoke anxiety. Starting with a very mild stimulus, the intensity of the stimulus can be gradually increased as treatment progresses. The method can also be applied to problems in which other states of high arousal are involved, e.g. excitement, aggression. In essence, the method consists of response substitution (see above), plus presentation of the triggering stimulus in gradually increasing degrees of intensity. Using the treatment of a phobia as an example, the animal is first put into a relaxed frame of mind. This might be achieved by petting it, feeding it tit-bits or by giving it a toy to play with, preferably preconditioned as a secondary reinforcer. The animal is then exposed to a version of the phobic stimulus which is so mild that it elicits either no anxiety at all or very mild anxiety which decreases quickly. This stimulus is presented to the animal several times. This procedure is repeated with stimuli of progressively greater intensities until a stimulus of normal intensity can be tolerated. Care should be taken to observe the following conditions.

1. Over the period of time when the treatment is being carried out, the animal should not be exposed to a normal version of the phobic stimulus. This may mean making special arrangements or postponing the treatment until an appropriate time (e.g. winter time for a thunder phobia).
2. Treatment should proceed very slowly and gradually. If the animal shows increasing, rather than decreasing anxiety in the presence of the stimulus, this is a sign that the treatment is proceeding too fast; that it should go back a few stages and proceed at a slower pace.

Thus the dog which barks at visitors is taught to sit in the hall first of all with no visitors approaching; the next step might be for it to sit while a visitor approaches the door and goes away without ringing the bell and so on.

Distraction

The dog is prevented from responding to the triggering stimulus by distracting it with a startling (and sometimes, unpleasant) stimulus. The effectiveness of this method is greatly increased if it is combined with response substitution. The effectiveness of the startling stimulus can be increased by preconditioning it: giving it a negative connotation by associating it with an unpleasant or frustrating experience (see section on punishment). Care should be taken not to upset or frighten the animal excessively as this may lead to behavioural side effects such as fear or aggression. In cases where the problem is caused by anxiety or stress, the distracting stimulus must be so mild as not to upset or frighten the animal at all.

Modifying owner attitudes

The successful treatment of a behavioural problem in a dog or cat usually involves a change in the owner's behaviour as well as that of the animal. Treatment plans which are theoretically correct from the point of view of the animal's behaviour frequently fail because the owner does not carry them out. It is therefore worth devoting attention to the factors which might facilitate or hinder a change of behaviour on the part of the owner. This does not mean that an owner is always responsible for his or her pet's behaviour problem: it is as important to recognize when an owner's attitude is not affecting the pet's behaviour as when it is affecting it. It is often tempting for a veterinary surgeon to dismiss a dog or cat's problem as being due to the 'neurosis' of the owner; this mental manoeuvre absolves him from the effort of puzzling further over the causes of the problem and of devising a treatment plan. Dog owners particularly are prone to encourage unwittingly a false solution of this kind, having taken to heart the often-quoted maxim that there are no bad dogs, only bad owners.

Correcting an owner's misinterpretations of his pet's behaviour is often an important prerequisite of change. For example, an owner may see his dog's destructiveness or his cat's spraying as a vengeful act, which may upset him unduly or lead to the inappropriate use of punishment. Sometimes it is clear that the owner's strong feelings about his pet are preventing him from accepting any re-interpretation of its behaviour or any alternative management regime.

However bizarre the veterinary surgeon may feel these attitudes to be, it is important that he tries to understand rather than to condemn them. Condemnation is likely to put the owner on the defensive. It is, therefore, advisable to refrain from general, judgemental comments (e.g. 'you spoil that dog' or 'you should be firmer with him') and concentrate on factual observations or recommendations about specific situations (e.g. 'it seems from what you tell me that you often reward the dog's barking by paying him attention' or 'try ignoring the dog when he pesters you').

Alternatives to treatment

Unfortunately, sometimes the veterinary surgeon hears about a behaviour problem for the first time when the owner requests euthanasia for it. There are occasions when it is clear that the veterinary surgeon should simply comply with this request, without suggesting treatment. These are usually situations in which (1) the animal is so dangerous that it would present an unacceptable hazard even if it engaged in the problem behaviour only rarely; and (2) there is no way of telling whether the problem behaviour has been eliminated other than waiting to see whether it recurs. An example of this situation might be a dog which has already severely bitten a young child in the household.

Another option is re-homing the pet. This is not usually advisable for dogs with serious problems, as they tend to recur in the new situation, perhaps after a few weeks. However, there are cases in which the dog's particular domestic situation or the personality of the owner seems to be making such a large contribution to the problem that this solution is worth trying. In cats, many serious problems are caused by the presence of another cat in the household. Re-homing these cats may be the best solution, but new homes for cats can be hard to find.

There are also less serious situations in which the veterinary surgeon may still feel inclined to comply immediately with the request for euthanasia, because given the uncertainty of the treatment outcome, this seems the kindest thing to do for a client who has already taken the painful decision. Certainly treatment is not worth attempting if the client is not motivated to undertake it. On the other hand, some owners are simply not aware that treatment is possible and, when the options are explained to them, such is the nature of their attachment to their pets, would prefer to attempt treatment; many feel that even if treatment fails they will at least have the satisfaction of knowing they have done everything possible.

AGGRESSION

Predatory aggression

This is usually directed against other species, although larger dogs sometimes treat smaller dogs as prey. Typically the attack is preceded by a chase, triggered by the victim running. In cats, the prey are usually birds or small mammals; owners are usually philosophical about this. Younger cats may chase or pounce on other cats or people as if they were prey, but in these cases the aggression is usually playful and not expressed in its full form. This is the most common form of aggression directed towards people (Borchelt and Voith, 1987). If they become a nuisance, these attacks are best treated by response substitution, by redirecting the aggression onto a toy. Owners should not attempt to hit the cat or push it away; the cat may interpret this behaviour as reciprocal play or, if alarmed, may exhibit defensive aggression. Nor should the cat be confined or isolated: playful cats need to be played with.

In dogs, predatory aggression is usually a problem when it is directed against mammals such as sheep or cats, inanimate moving objects such as cars or bicycles, or when it is directed against human beings. Dogs which are not familiar with babies may attack them, the attacks often being triggered by movements or sounds. As with predatory attacks on other species, a baby who is safe in one situation (say in a pram) may be at risk in another (for example, lying on the floor). Dogs, particularly those which are not used to babies, should therefore not be left alone with them.

Predatory aggression in dogs is difficult to treat, because it often involves victims whose own behaviour is difficult to alter; also it is an instinctive behaviour pattern which carries its own inbuilt reward. In addition, in many instances the effect of the behaviour is so disastrous that treatment has failed if it occurs again only once. However, a combination of the following methods may be tried.

1. Increasing the dominance and control of the owner over the dog (see section on the treatment of dominance aggression). This is appropriate if the chasing occurs when the owner is present.
2. Desensitization. The prey can be regarded as stimulus which causes arousal. The aim of the treatment then becomes to teach the dog to be calm in the presence of this previously arousing stimulus.
3. Punishment. This may be one of the situations in which punishing the behaviour can be an effective way of eliminating it, especially if the dog is of otherwise stable personality. Successful treatment of sheep-chasing has been reported using collars which deliver an electric shock, activated at a distance by radiotransmitter (e.g. Voith, 1984). Such treatment involves physical and psychological risk and should be carried out only under expert supervision.

Defensive aggression

This is aggression directed against a perceived threat. It can be categorized according to the kind of threat which elicits it.

Dominance aggression

Although it has been argued (e.g. Neville, 1991) that some cats show dominance in relation to their owners, from a practical point of view, this problem is confined to dogs. When directed against the owner, dominance aggression is usually provoked by an action by the victim which the dog perceives as threatening its dominant status. Examples of such actions are: trying to take something away from the dog, displacing it from its resting place, giving it a command or even merely patting, grooming or touching it. As well as reacting aggressively to such challenges, the dominant dog also displays a typical pattern of interaction with its owners: it takes the initiative in most of the interactions with the owner and is often slow to obey commands.

In order to treat dominance aggression, the owner must restructure his relationship with the dog. He should do this by ignoring its social approaches and requests. All the things the dog wants (for example, the owner's attention, being let out, being played with) should be used as rewards for obedience to the owner's commands. As far as possible, the owner should not let the dog decide how it will spend its time, but should keep the dog under his command, telling it to come with him, sit, stay etc.

Until the owner has gained some degree of dominance over the dog, he should as far as possible avoid the situations which provoke aggression. These should then be gradually re-introduced, as with systematic desensitization, taking care that at each stage no aggression is provoked.

When dogs in the same household fight, the cause is usually some ambiguity or change in the relative dominance status of the two dogs. To treat the problem, the owner should consistently reinforce the dominance status of one of the two dogs by always giving it preferential treatment.

Dominance aggression shown towards other dogs outside the household usually, but not always, involves male dogs. There may also be elements of territorial or protective aggression (see below). This behaviour can usually be distinguished from fear aggression by the enactment of a social exchange involving threats (although old enemies may not bother with this). Where a dog makes dominance attacks on other dogs, the owner should increase his own dominance over the dog. He should also systematically desensitize the dog to possible opponents using a head collar (e.g. Halti) and, if necessary, a muzzle. About 60% of cases of intermale aggression respond to castration (Hopkins et al., 1976).

Protective aggression

Both dogs and cats may protect their territory; dogs may also protect their owners. In the case of dogs, this may result in aggression towards visitors or strangers. Treatment should consist of systematic desensitization, using visitors who have been preinstructed to behave in progressively more provocative ways, and/or distraction and response substitution. Where appropriate, owner dominance should be increased.

Cats are often aggressive towards other cats which invade their territory. This can produce problems for cats living in the same household. Entire males showing this problem should be castrated; otherwise the problem is difficult to treat. A form of systematic desensitization, where the cats only meet under controlled conditions (e.g. with one of them caged), may be tried. Megestrol or diazepam may be helpful.

Fear-induced aggression

The hallmark of this type of aggression is that it is accompanied by fear: the animal may display a fearful body posture, with ears down. It typically occurs when the animal is physically restrained or cornered: for example during a veterinary consultation. In the case of dogs this may be exacerbated by practitioners who assume that the dog is mounting a dominance challenge and adopt the confrontational approach of shouting at or hitting the dog. The treatment of choice is systematic desensitization to the feared situation. In cats particularly, it may be a complicating factor in a problem which originates elsewhere: for example, a victim may respond to territorial aggression with fear-induced aggression.

Redirected aggression

Aggression may be displaced from the object which arouses it, onto neutral bystanders. Thus a dog or cat which is fighting with a member of its own species may attack an owner intervening in the fight. This tends to be a more serious problem in cats; their aggressive state of mind can persist for some time after the relevant incident.

Treatment should consist of removal, where appropriate, of the initial stimulus to aggression and systematic desensitization to the victim.

PROBLEMS OF ANXIETY AND STRESS

Phobias and nervousness

A monosymptomatic phobia in an otherwise normal animal usually responds well to systematic desensitization. More general nervousness (e.g. of going outside, of people), especially if caused by restricted exposure to the relevant stimuli when young, is not so easy to treat. If systematic desensitization and tranquillizing medication fail, it may be helpful to encourage the owner to work out a modus vivendi which is tolerable to all concerned, where the animal is not forced unnecessarily into the feared situations, but the owner does not become too preoccupied by the effect of his or her actions on the animal.

Overexcitement and displacement activities

Particularly in dogs, these may appear only in a specific situation, such as in a car or when visitors arrive. They may be treated by systematic desensitization to or removal of the triggering stimulus, ensuring that the excitable behaviour is not rewarded or distraction and response substitution. Thus excitement in the car might be treated by caging the dog so that it cannot see out of the window, not rewarding the excitement either with the owner's attention or with the progress of the journey (this may mean stopping the car whenever the excitement starts).

Destructiveness in the owner's absence in dogs is almost always caused by the stress of being parted from the owner; other manifestations of this stress are excessive barking or urination and defecation, which commonly occurs at night. Treatment should be aimed at decreasing the dog's dependence on the owner, who should pay less attention to the dog, especially immediately preceding and following a separation. He should also systematically desensitize the dog to separations, beginning with rewarding the dog for staying in another room. There should be no punishment of destructive behaviour.

Occasionally an animal may engage so constantly in displacement activities (e.g. tail chasing in dogs, excessive grooming in cats) that they cause damage to themselves or distress to their owners. In the author's experience, in dogs this is almost always linked with stress or disturbance in the owner or family. As well as treating the symptom behaviourly as outlined above, treatment should also be aimed at reducing the animal's overall level of stress; diazepam, amitriptyline or megestrol may be helpful here. Longer-acting opioid antagonists, such as naltrexone (Nalorex, Dupont) have also been found to reduce stereotypic behaviour (Dodman et al., 1988).

Inappropriate urination and defecation

Involuntary urination in dogs may occur as an expression of submission, along with a submissive body posture. It may also occur as a result of excitement, for example when the owner returns home. It can be treated by reducing the dominance threat or the excitement of the situation.

In dogs, normal urination (or, more rarely, defecation) indoors is often caused by faulty learning. Once having urinated in a particular spot, the stimuli there, including the scent mark left by the urine, tend to trigger the response of urinating again. Treatment consists of essentially the same procedure which should be employed in house-training a puppy; the habit of urinating in the correct place is built up by organizing the dog's life so that it urinates only in the desired place. It should be taken outside frequently, especially after meals, after sleep or when it sniffs the ground for scent marks.

In cats, normal urination indoors, or outside the litter tray, may occur because the cat has been deterred from going outside or from using its tray. Fear of a new cat in the neighbourhood, illness or infirmity may make it disinclined to go out. A cat may be unwilling to use a litter tray which is in too public a place or is too near its food dish, which is too dirty or which has a substrate of the wrong consistency. The problem may be improved by re-siting the trays, replacing them with covered 'igloos', cleaning them more often or changing the substrate; cats tend to prefer litter with fine granules. Punishment is counterproductive.

Both dogs and cats may engage in territorial urination. It is more common in males; small amounts of urine are involved, often deposited on vertical surfaces and cats usually, but not always, adopt a characteristic posture (Fig. 51.4). In dogs, although there may be no obvious stimulus, it may be triggered by the arrival of a strange dog or

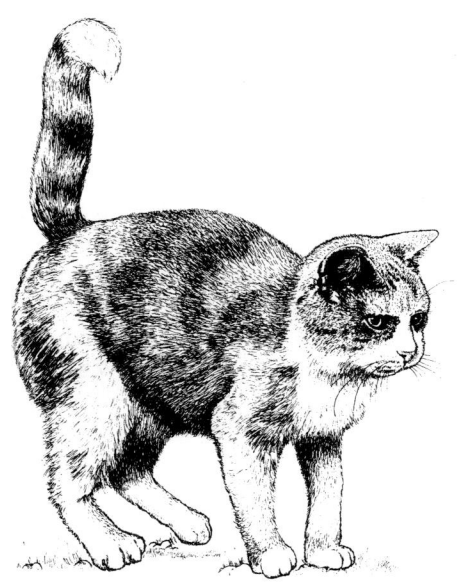

Figure 51.4 Cat showing characteristic territorial urination posture.

human visitor in the house. Once the triggering stimulus has been identified, the dog should be kept under supervision at the relevant times and provided with an alternative response.

Spraying is more common in multicat households; it may occur when new pets or people are added to the household, or when a cat flap is installed. It may also be the result of general stress or of frustration, for example when waiting in vain for the owner's attention. Treatment usually involves increasing the cat's sense of security. Cat flaps may have to be removed or the cat confined to a place where it feels secure: often a room where it does not spray. It is then gradually allowed access, under supervision, to the rooms where it used to spray.

In cats, castration is likely to reduce territorial urination; it may also be helpful in dogs. Otherwise, for cats, diazepam is the drug of first choice, followed by megoestrol acetate for cases which fail to respond. Megestrol may reduce territorial urination in dogs. For both species and for any kind of urination, the marks should be cleaned with a biological detergent, rather than disinfectant which is liable to leave its own scent mark.

Abnormal appetites

In dogs, coprophagia can be a problem. Although it is part of a dog's normal behavioural repertoire – bitches eat their puppies' faeces – many owners find it repugnant. The problem may be treated by supervising the dog at the relevant times and employing distraction and response substitution. If the faeces are the dog's own, the following modifications to the diet have been found to be helpful (McKeown et al., 1988):

1. an increase in fibre and protein and a decrease in carbohydrate content;
2. an iron supplement;
3. the addition of vegetable oil, increasing the dose over a week to 15 ml 4.5 mg body weight.

Cats, usually oriental breeds, sometimes eat wool and other fabrics. The causation of this behaviour is obscure, but it sometimes seems to form part of a prey catching/eating sequence, in that the cat brings the fabric to its food dish, or eats it immediately after its normal food. A dry diet or the addition of fibre to the diet may be helpful, as may meat with gristle attached to large bones.

Miscellaneous problems

Not coming back when called, on walks, is a common problem in dogs. Analysis of the interaction between dog and owner may reveal that the owner is punishing rather than rewarding the response of coming. Also these dogs have often learned to associate hearing the owner calling their names with the act of running away. To treat the problem the owner should frequently call the dog on walks, but only when the dog is likely to respond; he should not try to compete with rival attractions such as other dogs. The dog should always be rewarded when it comes. Increasing owner dominance may also be helpful. If the dog does run away, the owner should, where possible, resist the temptation to follow as this automatically puts the dog in the position of leader. He should walk away from the dog: it may also be necessary to do something intriguing such as talking to another dog or even lying down.

A common problem in cats is scratching vertical surfaces such as soft furnishings. This is essential self-maintenance behaviour for a cat but is also sometimes a form of territorial marking. It is best treated by providing the cat with a scratching post covered in material with a loose weave, placed close to the scratched furniture, which should be protected with, for example, a sheet of polythene. When the cat has transferred its sharpening to the post, this should be gradually moved away from the furniture.

PREVENTION OF PROBLEMS

As there is a genetic component in most behaviour problems, breeders of both dogs and cats bear a great deal of responsibility for prevention. They should resist the temptation to breed from animals with behavioural difficulties, however successful they are at shows. They should also arrange that, after the first two to three weeks of life, their litters are not kept in seclusion but are exposed to normal domestic sights and sounds and to a variety of people.

Similarly, owners, when they acquire a new puppy, should try to give it as much experience of the wider world as its vaccination programme will allow: it should, for example be taken for car rides. As soon as possible, it should mix with other dogs. Time spent with a new kitten or puppy is a good investment. Its life should be arranged so that undesirable behaviour is prevented. For puppies, training of positive responses, such as sitting on command, can begin early. Responses such as staying, which involve self-restraint, are more difficult for them and training of them should be delayed. Puppies should also be accustomed to gradually increasing lengths of separation from the owner. Allowing the puppy in the bedroom at night has, from a behavioural point of view, both advantages and disadvantages; the issue is often an emotive one and the veterinary surgeon should not allow his own prejudices to influence his advice.

REFERENCES

Agrawal, H.C., Fox, M.W. and Himwich, W.A. (1976) Neurochemical and behavioural effects of isolation rearing in the dog. *Life Science* **6**, 71–78.

Borchelt, P.L. and Voith, V.L. (1987). Aggressive behaviour in cats. *Compendium on Continuing Education for the Practicing Veterinarian* **9**, 49–57.

Bradshaw, J.W.S. (1992) *Behaviour of the Domestic Cat*. CAB International, Wallingford.

Catanzaro, T.G. (1988). A survey on the question of how well veterinarians are prepared to predict their client's human–animal bond. *Journal of the American Veterinary Medical Association* **192**, 1707–1711.

Cooper, L.C. and Hart, B.L. (1992). Comparison of diazepam with progestin for effectiveness in depression of spraying behaviour in cats. *Journal of the American Veterinary Medical Association* **200**, 797–801

Dodman, N.H., Schuster, L., White, S.D., Court, M.H., Parker, D. and Dixon, R. (1988) The use of narcotic agonists to modify stereotypic self-licking, self-chewing and scratching behaviour in dogs. *Journal of the American Veterinary Medical Association* **193**, 815–819.

Hart B.L. (1981) Olfactory tractotomy for control of objectionable urine spraying and urine marking in cats. *Journal of the American Veterinary Medical Association* **171**, 231.

Hart, B.L. (1985) Behavioural indications for phenothiazine and benzodiazepine tranquillizers in dogs. *Journal of the American Veterinary Medical Association* **186**, 1192–1194.

Hart, B.L. and Barrett, R.E. (1973) Effects of castration on fighting, roaming and urine spraying in adult male cats. *Journal of the American Veterinary Medical Association* **163**, 290.

Hart, B.L. and Hart, L.A. (1985). *Canine and Feline Behaviour Therapy*. Lee and Febiger, Philadelphia.

Hart, B.L., Eckstein, R.A., Powell, K.L. and Dodman, N.H. (1993) Effectiveness of buspirane on urine spraying and inappropriate urination in cats. *Journal of the American Veterinary Medical Association* **203**, 254–258.

Henik, R.A., Olson, P.N. and Roychuk, R.A.W. (1985). Progestogen therapy in cats. *Compendium on Continuing Education for the Practicing Veterinarian* **7**, 132–137.

Hopkins, S.G., Schubert, T.A. and Hart, B.L. (1976) Castration of adult male dogs: effects on roaming, aggression, urine marking and mounting. *Journal of the American Veterinary Medical Association* **168**, 1108.

Karsh, E.B. (1984) Factors influencing the socialisation of cats to people. In: *The Pet Connection* (Eds R. Anderson, B.L. Hart and L.A. Hart), University of Minnesota Press, Minnesota.

Karsh, E.B. and Turner, D.C. (1988) The human–cat relationship. In: *The Domestic Cat* (Eds D.C. Turner and P.B. Bateson). Cambridge University Press, Cambridge.

Kerby, G. and MacDonald, D.W. (1988) Cat society and the consequences of colony size. In: *The Domestic Cat: The Biology of Its Behaviour* (Eds D.C. Turner and P. Bateson), Cambridge University Press, Cambridge.

Komtebedde, J. and Hauptman, J. (1990) Bilateral ischiocavernosus myectomy for chronic urine spraying in castrated male cats. *Veterinary Surgery* **19**, 293–296.

Landsberg, G.M. (1991). Feline destruction and the effects of declawing. *Veterinary Clinics of North America* **21**, 265–279.

Lockwood, R. (1979) Dominance in wolves. In: *The Behaviour and Ecology of Wolves* (Ed. E. Klinghammer). Girland Press, New York.

Marder, A.R. (1991) Psychotropic drugs and behavioural therapy. *Veterinary Clinics of North America* **21**, 329–342.

McKeown, D., Luescher, A. and Machum, M. (1988) Coprophagia: food for thought. *Canadian Veterinarian* **28**, 849–850.

Murphree, O.D., Dykman, R.A. and Peters, J.E. (1967) Genetically determined abnormal behaviour in the dog; results of behavioural tests. *Conditioned Reflex* **2**, 199–205.

Neville, P.F. (1991) Treatment of behaviour problems in cats. *In Practice* **13**, 43–50.

O'Farrell, V. (1992) *Manual of Canine Behaviour*, 2nd edn. BSAVA Publications, Cheltenham.

O'Farrell, V. (1994) *Dog's Best Friend*. Methuen, London

O'Farrell, V. and Peachey, E. (1990) The behavioural effects of ovarohysterectomy on bitches. *Journal of Small Animal Practice* **31**, 595–598.

Turner, D.C. (1991) The ethology of the human–cat relationship. *Schweizer Archiv fur Tierheilkunde* **133**, 63–70.

Voith, V.L. (1984) Human/animal relationships. In: *Nutrition and Behaviour in Dogs and Cats* (Ed. R.L. Anderson). Pergamon Press, New York.

Voith V.L. (1984) Behavioural problems. In: *Canine Medicine and Therapeutics*, 2nd edn (Eds E.A. Chandler, J.B. Sutton and D.J. Thompson). Blackwell, Oxford.

Voith, V. (1985) Attachment of people to companion animals. *Veterinary Clinics of North America* **21**, 289–295.

Voith, V.L. and Borchelt, P.L. (1986) Social behaviour of domestic cats. *Compendium on Continuing Education for the Practicing Veterinarian* **8**, 637–644.

Wilbur, R.H. (1976) Pet ownership and animal control, social and psychological attitudes. Report to National Conference on Dog and Cat Control, Denver, Colorado.

Wilson, M., Warren, J.M. and Abbot, L. (1965) Infantile stimulation, activity and learning by cats. *Child Development* **36**, 833–853.

FURTHER READING

Borchelt, P.L. (1991) Cat elimination behaviour problems. *Veterinary Clinics of North America* **21**, 257–265.

Borchelt, P. and Voith, V. (1985) Punishment. *Continuing Education for the Practicing Veterinarian* **7**, 780–788.

Chapman, B.L. (1991) Feline aggression: classification, diagnosis and treatment. *Veterinary Clinics of North America* **21**, 315–328.

Luescher, U.A., McKeown, D.B. and Halip, J. (1991) Stereotypic or obsessive–compulsive disorders in dogs and cats. *Veterinary Clinics of North America* **21**, 401–415.

Marder, A.R. (1991) Psychotropic drugs and behavioural therapy. *Veterinary Clinics of North America* **21**, 329–342.

O'Farrell, V. (1992) Manual of Canine Behaviour, 2nd edn. British Small Animal Veterinary Association, Cheltenham.

O'Farrell, V. and Neville, P. (1994) *Manual of Feline Behaviour*. British Small Animal Veterinary Association, Cheltenham.

Turner, D.C. and Bateson, P.B. (1988) *The Domestic Cat*. Cambridge University Press, Cambridge.

Voith, V. and Borchelt, P. (1985) Separation anxiety in dogs. *Continuing Education for the Practicing Veterinarian* **7**, 42–52.

Voith, V. and Borchelt, P. (1985) Fears and phobias in companion animals. *Continuing Education for the Practicing Veterinarian* **7**, 209–218.

Voith, V. and Borchelt, P. (1985) Elimination behaviour and related problems in dogs. *Continuing Education for the Practicing Veterinarian* **7**, 537–544.

Index

Page numbers in **bold** refer to major discussions in the text, those in *italic* refer to figures and tables.

A

AB blood groups, 767, 811
Abdominal examination, 10
Abdominal pain, 67, **146–50**, *147*, 178, 505, 508
Abdominocentesis, *139*, **139–41**, 141, 150, 381–2, 456
Abducens nerve deficits, 234
Abortion, 586–7, 592–3, 944
Abscess, 152, **977–8**
Acaricidal therapy, 206
Acepromazine, 298, 460, 712, 1034
Acetylcholine receptor antibodies, 57, 223, 391
N-Acetylcysteine, 121, 788, 806
N-Acetylglucosaminidase, 619
Acetylpromazine, 49
Achalasia (cricopharyngeal dysphagia), 52, 388, 389
Achlorhydria, 424, 511
Achondroplasia, 728
Acral mutilation syndrome, 902
Acromegaly, 23, 78, 308, **530–1**, *531*, 581, 732
Actinomyces infection, 152, 300, 366, 887, 907, **949**, *949*, 977
Activated clotting time (ACT), 165
Activated partial thromboplastin time (APTT), 166, 183, 298, 782, 800, 801
Acute phase proteins, 29
Acyclovir, 860
Addisonian crisis, 107, 546, 548
Adenosine, 333
Adenosine diphosphate, 160
Adrenal cortical haemorrhage/infarction, 546
Adrenal cortical hormones, 544–5, *545*
Adrenal cortical neoplasia, 550, 894
Adrenal gland disorders, **545–61**
Adrenal glands, 544–5
Adrenal sex hormone imbalance, 192
Adrenal sex hormones, 544
Adrenal syndrome, 897
Adrenocortical insufficiency, idiopathic, 546
Adrenocorticotrophic hormone (ACTH), 527, 544, 545, 548, 549
Adrenocorticotrophic hormone (ACTH) stimulation test, 79, 223, 390, 548, 555–6, *556*

Adrenocorticotrophic hormone (ACTH)-secreting pituitary adenoma, 531
Adult respiratory distress syndrome (shock lung), 119, 120
Adynamic ileus, 431
Aelurostrongylus abstrusus, 359, *360*
Aeromonas aerogenes, 282
Afipia felis, 980
Afterload, 271–2
    heart failure, 274
Agalactia, 589
Aggression, 1034, 1035, **1037–9**
Alanine aminotransferase (ALT), 130, 133, 139, 259, 278, 461, **463**, 464, 480
Aldosterone, 72, 544, 545
    heart failure, 275
Aldosteronism, primary, 308
Alimentary lymphosarcoma, 967–8
Alimentary tract disease, **371–440**
    abdominocentesis, 381–2
    diagnostic imaging, 376–7
    endoscopy, 378–81, *379*
    exploratory coeliotomy, 382, *382*
    history-taking, 371–2
    laboratory investigations, 372–6
    physical examination, 372
Alimentary tract obstruction, 377, *378*
Alkaline phosphatase (ALP), 130–1, 133, 134, 139, 259, 278, 461, **463**, 464, 511
Alkylating agents, 1006, **1023**
Allergic skin disease
    cat, **903–6**
    dog, **880–3**
    treatment, 882–3, *882*, 905
Allergy testing, 879–80
Alopecia, **186–93**, *189*, 202, 203, *530*
    endocrinopathy, 186, *187*, 189, 192, 893, *893*, 894, 895, 896, 912
    focal, *191*
    growth hormone-responsive, 529–30, *530*, 894–5
    non-scarring disorders, 186, *187*
    post-radiation, 1003, *1003*
    pruritus, 188, 189, 190
    psychogenic (neurogenic dermatitis), 906–7, *907*
    scarring disorders, 186, 189
    symmetrical, *190*, 535, 552, 903, *904*
    therapy, 192–3
Alpha adrenergic blocking drugs, 309, 325

Ambulatory ECG (Holter monitoring), 223, 229, 260
Amikacin, 979
Amiloride, 323
Amino acid metabolism
    cat, 487
    hepatic encephalopathy, 458, *459*, 460
Aminosalicylates, 435
Amitraz, 206
Ammonia
    blood concentration, 132
    liver metabolism, 132, 457
        in cats, 487
        glutamate neurotransmission, 457–8, *458*
        metabolism in hepatic encephalopathy, 457, 458–60, 464
Ammonia tolerance test (ATT), 132, 460, 464–5, 472
Ammonium urate uroliths, 639, *639*, 641, 643, *643*, 645
Amoxycillin, 488, 733, 747, 887, 977
Amphotericin B, 639
Ampicillin, 135, 184, 284, 415, 484, 749, 887, 949, 963, 977
Amrinone, 324
Amylase, 139
    pancreatitis, 506, 507–8
Amyloidosis, 76
    kidney, 76, 178, 632, 634
    liver, 482–3
Anaemia, **107–17**, 118, 220, 222, 308, 461, **777–8**, **784–90**, 805–7
    chronic renal failure, 625, *625*, 777–8
    correction, 628
    classification, 112–13, *112*, *777*, *778*
    clinical manifestation, 107–8, 772
    haematological investigations, 109–12, *112*
    haemolytic, 113, *113*, 114, 785–7, 794, 805–6
        extrinsic, 114, *115*
    haemorrhagic, 113, *113*, 114, 373, 784–5, 805
    history-taking, 108, 771
    laboratory investigations, 109
    non-regenerative, **114–16**, *116*, 205, 373, 536, 777, 788–90, 791, 792, 794, 806–7
    pathophysiology, 107–8
    physical examination, 109

Anaemia (cont.)
  regenerative, *113*, **113–14**, 133, 373, 777, 784–8, 791, 792, 794, 805–6
  retinal vascular abnormalities, 852
  therapy, 116–17
Anaemia of chronic disease, 116, 789, 807, 993
Anaemia of inflammatory disease, 115, 777, 778
Anaerobiospirillum, 974
Anaesthesia, 24, 460
Anagen defluxion, 188
Anal sac abscess, 67
Anal sac disease, 439–40
Ancylostoma, 63, 421
Angiocardiography, 271
  congenital cardiac disease, 311, 314, *314*, 315–16, 317, 318, *319*
  dilated cardiomyopathy, 292–3
  hypertrophic cardiomyopathy, 295
Angiography, 106, 144–5
Angioneurotic oedema, 143
Angiostrongylosis, **306–7**, *359*
Angiostrongylus vasorum, 306, 359, *359*
  life cycle, 306–7, 359
Angiotensin converting enzyme (ACE), 72, 545
Angiotensin converting enzyme (ACE) inhibitors, 141, 288, 309, 323, 325, 629, 634
Angiotensin I, 545
Angiotensin II, 72, 275, 544, 545
Anisocoria, **855–7**, *856*
Anorchidism, 597
Anorectal disorders, **438–40**
Anorexia, **13–16**, *15*, 21, 52, 61, 75, 147, 256, 284, 401, 461, 505, 619, 771
  chronic renal failure, 624, 625
  complicating chemotherapy, 1020–1
Antacids, 50, 404
Antibiotic therapy, 424, 484, 488, 619
  bacterial endocarditis, 284
  bacterial infective (suppurative) arthritis, 747
  cancer treatment, 1006, **1024–5**
  cellulitis/abscesses, 977–8
  cholangitis-cholecystitis, 484
  diabetic ketoacidosis, 564
  discospondylitis, 748
  exocrine pancreatic insufficiency, 518
  gastric dilation and volvulus, 415
  jaundice, 135
  Lyme disease, 749
  osteomyelitis, 733
  prostatitis, 648
  pruritus, 199–200
  pyoderma, 885–6, *886*
  septic pleurisy, 366
  urinary tract infection, 185, 619, 637–9, *638*
  uveitis, 838
  vomiting, 50
Antibiotic-induced diarrhoea, 421
Anticoagulant rodenticide toxicity, 89, 108, 164, **800–1**, 809
Anticoagulants for blood samples, 773

Anticonvulsant drugs, 247
Antidiuretic hormone (ADH; vasopressin), 70, 71, 527, 532, 612
Antidiuretic hormone (ADH; vasopressin) response test, 79, 80–1, 533, 614, *615*
Antiemetics, 49–50, 404, 623, 628–9, 925
Antihistamines, 49, 882, *882*, 905, 996
Antihypertensives, 629, 634
Antimetabolites, 1006, **1024**
Antinuclear antibody (ANA), 36, 391, 727, 753, 783, 879
Antiphospholipid antibodies, 804
Antiplatelet antibodies, 36, 166, 782–3
Antipyretic drugs, *38*
Antithrombin III assay, 782
Antithrombin III deficiency, 804
Antithyroid drugs, 540
Anxiety, 1032, 1034, **1039–41**
Aonchotheca putorii, 407
Aortic regurgitation, 103
Aortic stenosis, 102, 103, 105, 219, 220, 259, 274, 277, **312–14**
  angiocardiography, 314, *314*
  echocardiography, 312–14, *313*
  electrocardiography, 312
  radiological examination, 312, *313*
Aortic thromboembolism, 690–1, 810
Aplastic anaemia, 788–9, 807
Appetite, 13, 16
APUDomas, 403, 408
Aqueous production and drainage, *839*
Arginine requirement in cats, 487
Arsenicals, 796
Arterial blood gases, 91, 97
Arterial hypoxaemia, 118–19
Arterial thromboembolism, **297–8**
Arteriovenous fistula, 144–5, 475
Arthrocentesis, 214, 726, *726*
Arthrogryposis, 704
Arthro-ophthalmopathy, 728
Arthroscopy, 214
Arthrotomy, 214
Ascending reticular activating system, 249
Ascites, 18, 105, **136–42**, *142*, 148, 256, 278, 300, 456, 457, 461, 474, 475, 486, 560
  abdominal fluid analysis, 139–41, *139*
  abdominocentesis, 139, 456
  differential diagnosis, *137*
  pathophysiological mechanisms, 136, **456**
Aseptic meningitis, 691
L-Asparaginase, 504, 1007, **1026**
Aspartate aminotransferase (AST), 130, 134, 139, 217, 221, *463*, 480
Aspergillosis, 36, 96, 289, 348, 684, 749, 980
  bone infection, 734
  brain, 678
  joint infection, 749
  nasal, 83, 84, 85, 347, 349–50, *349*
Aspiration pneumonia, 52, 54, 55, 89, 95, 119, **358–9**, 388, 390
Aspirin, 37, 38, 44, 161, 167, 293, 296, 298, 306, 633, 634, 712, 744, 800, 837

Assessment notes, 12
Asteroid hyalosis, 847
Astrocytomas, 676, 683
Ataxia, **232–5**, 236, 461
Atlantoaxial subluxation, 239, 685
Atopy, 194, 195, 196, 199, 200, 873, 874, 904
  skin disease, 880–1, *881*
Atrial fibrillation, 228, 229, 285, 288
  management, 332, 333, 334
Atrial natriuretic peptide, 72, 275, 276
Atrial septal defect, 274, **317**
Atrial standstill, persistent, 227, 228, 329, 330, 699
Atrioventricular (AV) block, 228, 329, *330*
Atrioventricular (AV) node, 255
Atrioventricular canal, common persistent, 317–18
Atrioventricular valve malformations, 102, 103, 104, **320**
Atrophic follicular disease, 186, *187*, *188*, 192
Atrophic gastritis, 406
Atropine, 49, 150, 329, 838
Atropine response test, 230
Atypical mycobacterial infections, 886, *887*, 908, **950**, 978–9
Aujesky's disease (pseudorabies), 678, 947, 976
Auscultation
  cardiac, 99, *99*, 257, *257*
  chest, 8, 9, 90, 95–6, 346–7, 361
Autoimmune haemolytic anaemia, 133, 152, **785–7**, *786*, 805
Axonopathy, progressive, 686
Azathioprine, 426, 428, 435, 504, 634, 752, 754, 787, 798, 837, 900

B

B lymphocytes, **151**, 768
Babesiosis, 109, 787–8
Bacillus piliformis, 421, 944, 979
Bacterial endocarditis, 30, 62, 103, 106, 119, **282–4**, 738, 747
Bacterial enteritis, 420–1
Bacterial infective (suppurative) arthritis, 746–7, *747*, 756–7
Bacterial skin disease, **883–7**, **907–8**
Bacterial (suppurative) myocarditis, 289, 298
Bacteroides, 425, 907, 977
Baermann flotation technique, 97
Ballotment for fluid thrill detection, 137
Barbiturates, 118, 246, 452, 458, 460, 678
  liver enzyme effects, 130, 131
Barium impregnated polyspheres (BIPS), 377–8, *378*, 424
Bartonella henselae, 980
Basal cell tumours, 892
Basal energy requirement (BER), 18
Basophilia, 780
Basophils, 767
Behaviour changes, **249–51**
Behaviour problems, **1029–41**
  diagnosis, 1033–4
  treatment, 1034–6

Behavioural therapy, 1035–6
Bence Jones proteinuria, 76, 617, 796
Benign idiopathic pericardial effusion, 299
Benign prostatic hyperplasia, 599, *599*, **646–7**
Bentiromide-para-aminobenzoic acid (BT-PABA) test, 64, 515, *515*
Benzimidazole, 407, 421
Benzocaine, 119
Benzodiazepines, 458, 460, 1034
Beta adrenergic agonists, 324, 328, 330
Beta adrenergic blocking drugs
 aortic stenosis, 314
 atrial fibrillation, 288
 heart failure, 327
 hypertension, 309, 629
 hypertrophic cardiomyopathy, 289, 296
 supraventricular tachyarrhythmias, 333
 ventricular arrhythmias, 335
Bethanechol, 391, 437
Biceps tendon luxation, 208
Bicipital tenosynovitis, 208
Bile, 58, 451–2, *452*
Bile duct carcinoma, 485
Bile duct cysts, 483
Bile reflux, 505
Bile salt (bile acid) metabolism, 451, *452*
Bile salt (bile acid) plasma levels, 131–2, 139, *463–4*, 473, 480
Biliary epithelium hyperplasia, 485
Biliary tract disease, 448, **483–6**
 history-taking, 461
 laboratory investigations, 462–6
 physical examination, 461–2
Biliary tract rupture, 485–6
Biliary tree anatomy, 448
Bilirubin, 126
 conjugation, 126, 454
 excretion, 126, *127*, 454, *454*, 455
 metabolism, 454–5, *454*, 487
 plasma assay, 128, 455
Bilirubinuria, 128–9, 133, 134, 454
Biliverdin, 126
Bismuth preparations, 50, 409, 419
Bite abscesses, cat, 907
Black hair follicle dysplasia, hereditary, 902
Bladder, 168, 169, 612–13, 651, *651*
Bladder neoplasms, 183, 644, 645, 1005
Bladder washes, 614
Blastomycosis, 678, 734, 738, 749, 888, 911
Bleeding disorders, **160–7**, *163*, 771
 cat, **809–10**
 dog, **800–4**
 haematuria, 183
 history-taking, 162, 771
 inherited, 108, 802–4, 810
 laboratory investigations, 164–7
  sample collection, 164
  screening tests, 164–7, *165*
 liver disease, 132, 460–1, 801
 physical examination, 164, 772
Bleeding time, 164, 165, 774
 buccal mucosal, *774*, 774
 cuticle, 774–5
Blepharitis, 827, *827*

Blink disorders, 857–8
Blood groups, 811
 cat, 767
 dog, 766–7, *767*
Blood pressure, 222, 307, *307*
Blood sampling, 772–3
Blood transfusion, 766, 767, **810–12**
Blood urea nitrogen, 616, *616*
Body weight conversion to surface area, 1023
Bone, 719–21
 growth, 721, *721*
 remodelling, 720
Bone biopsy, 215, 726–7
Bone cysts, 739
Bone disease, **719–40**
 cats, **739–40**
 classification, 727, *728*
 dogs, **727–39**
 history-taking, 723–4
 investigative techniques, 725–7
 physical examination, 724–5
Bone marrow aspiration, 34, 159, 166, 773–4, *774*
Bone marrow biopsy, 773–4, *774*
Bone marrow disorders, **765–812**
 complicating cytotoxic chemotherapy, 1019–20
Bone marrow examination (smears), 780
Bone marrow haematopoiesis, 765, *766*
 erythropoiesis, 766
 granulocytes, 767
 lymphocytes, 768
 monocytes, 767
 platelets, 768
Bone marrow hypoplasia/aplasia, 788–9, 807
Bone marrow neoplasia, **790–6**, **807–9**
Bone pain, 207, **214–16**, *215*
Bone scintigraphy, 725
Bone tumours, 683, **733–5**, *734*, 740, *740*
Bordetella bronchiseptica, 354, 942, 943, 961, 962, 963, **964**, 966
 tracheobronchitis, 93, 354, 355
Borrelia burgdorferi, 214, 289, 727, 748, 948
Botulism, 55, 688, **950**, 979
Bowel obstruction, 146
Boxer cardiomyopathy, 286–7
Brachial plexus avulsion, 690
Brachial plexus neuritis, 689
Brachial plexus tumour, 208
Brachytherapy, 999–1000
Bradycardia, *328*, **328–30**
Brain diseases, **674–81**
 anomalous, 674–5
 degenerative, 674
 idiopathic, 680
 inflammatory, 677–80
  infectious, 678–9
  non-infectious, 679–80
 metabolic, 675–6
 nutritional, 677
 toxic, 681
 vascular, 681
Brain lesions, 664–5, *664*

Brain trauma, 680
Brain tumours, 244, 245, 676–7, *677*
Brainstem lesions, 250, 664–5, *665*
Bromethalin toxicity, 681
Bromocriptine, 581
Bronchial collapse, 91, 353, **355–6**
Bronchial diagnostic procedures, 353–5
Bronchial disease, chronic, **356–7**, *357*, **358**
Bronchial sounds, 9
Bronchial-associated lymphoid tissue (BALT), 768
Bronchiectasis, 95, 357
Bronchitis, chronic, 94, 95, 96, 97, 120, 356–7
Bronchoalveolar lavage (BAL), 91, 97, 354
Broncho-oesophageal fistula, 54, 56, 89, 397
Bronchopneumonia, 9, 95, 96, 97, 119, **358**, 738
Bronchoscopy, 91, 97, 121, 353–4
Brucella canis, 584, 586, 597, 684, 944, 947
Brucellosis, 36, 480, 947
Brush border enzymes, 510–11, *511*
Bulbourethral glands, 594, 602
Bullous pemphigoid, 898, *898*
Buphthalmos, 823, *824*
Busulphan, 1014, **1024**

C
Cachexia, 18, 21
Calcareous (calcific) corneal degeneration, 835
Calcinosis cutis, 189, 552, 554
Calcitonin, 720, *720*, 721
Calcium blockers
 atrial fibrillation, 288
 chronic renal failure, 629
 heart failure, 327
 hypertension, 309
 hypertrophic cardiomyopathy, 296
 supraventricular tachyarrhythmias, 333
Calcium homeostasis, 541–2, 720, *720*
 chronic renal failure, 731
Calcium oxalate uroliths, 639, *639*, 641, 643, 645
Caloric testing, 235
Campylobacter sp., 62, 149, 374, 413, 434, 754
 enteritis, 420–1, 940, 941, 974
Cancer cachexia, 18
Cancer surgery, **997–9**
 compartmental excision, 998–9, *998*
 local excision, 997, *997*
 wide local excision, 997–8, *998*
Cancer therapy, **985–1026**
 biopsy, 989, *989*
 TNM staging, 989–92, *990*, *991*
 tumour-related complications, 992–6
  endocrine, 994, *994*
  haematological, 993, *993*
  metabolic, 994–6
Candidiasis, 888, 980
Canine adenovirus, 354, 355, 678, 930, 942, 944
 vaccination, 932, 943
  immunological reactions, 937

1046 INDEX

Canine distemper virus, 42, 89, 244, 245, 348, 373, **678**, 735, 789, *917*, **926–30**, *928*, 944, 977
   neurological disease, 239, 678, 928–9
   treatment, 929
   vaccinal encephalitis, 936, 937
   vaccination, 929–30
Canine herpesvirus, 480, 584, 944, 945, *946*
Canine papillomavirus, 947–8, *947*
Canine parainfluenza virus, 354, 355, 678, 942, 943
Canine parvovirus, 42, 43, 45, 63, 149, 371, 373, 418, 431, 678, 789, **921–6**, 944
   enteritis, 420, 922, 923–4, *923*, *925*, 938, 939, 940, 941
   myocarditis, 227, 289, 922, 924, *924*, *925*, 938
   treatment, 925
   vaccination, 925–6
Canine viral papilloma, 893
Capillary hydrostatic pressure, 142
Capnocytophaga infection, 979
Captopril, 288, 293, 296, 325, 629, 634
Carbergolamine, 581
Carbimazole, 540, 541
Carbohydrate malabsorption tests, 374
Carbohydrate metabolism, 58, 450, *451*, 561
Cardiac cachexia, 18, 105, 278
Cardiac catheterization, 271, 311, 314, *314*, 315, 316, 317, 318
Cardiac chambers, 262, 267, *267*, 268
   enlargement, *268*, *269*, 271, 276, 281, *281*
Cardiac conducting system, 255
Cardiac disease, acquired, **278–84**
Cardiac disease, congenital, 104, *105*, 227, *309*, **309–21**, 310
   control measures, 309–10
   cyanosis, 119, 120, 121
   right to left shunting, 119, 120, 124, 267, 310, 318, 320, 778
Cardiac dysrhythmias, 220, 222, **225–31**, *226*, 274, 560
   aortic stenosis, 312
   dilated cardiomyopathy, 285, 288
   echocardiography, 229–30
   electrocardiography, 228–9, 263–6
   extracardiac disease, 230
   hypertension, 308
   management, 230–1, *328*, **328–36**
   mechanisms, *225*
   thoracic radiography, 229
Cardiac examination, 8–9
Cardiac glycosides, 39, 287, 324–5
Cardiac innervation, 255–6
Cardiac murmurs, **99–106**, 120, 220, 221, 258–9, 310
   anaemia, 107–8, 772
   aortic stenosis, 312
   auscultation, 99, *99*
   bacterial endocarditis, 283
   causes, *100–1*
   classification, *102*, 103–4
   endocardiosis, 279

   patent ductus arteriosus, 310
   pathophysiology, 102–3
   physical examination, 8, 105
   pulmonary stenosis, 315
   tetralogy of Fallot, 318
   ventricular septal defect, 316
Cardiac neoplasms, 299–300
Cardiac size, 261–2
Cardiac tamponade, 136, 274, 277, 301
Cardiogenic shock, 107, 108, 119, 300
Cardiomyopathy of thyrotoxicosis, 298
Cardiotoxic drugs, 290, 299
Cardiovascular system, **255–336**
   cardiac catheterization/ angiocardiography, 271
   echocardiography, 270–1, *270*
   electrocardiography, 259–61
   history-taking, 256
   investigations, 259–71
   physical examination, 256–7
   radiological examination, 261–2
     cardiac chamber enlargement, 262, *267*, *268*, *269*
     cardiac size, 261–2
     caudal vena cava, 267
     great vessels, 267
     pulmonary patterns, 267
     pulmonary vasculature, 267
Carnitine requirement in cats, 487
Carpal joint disorders, 208, *210*, 725
Carprofen, 744–5
Castration, 23, 192, 646, 647, 648, 1034, 1040
Castration-responsive dermatoses, 895–6
Cat scratch disease, 980
Cataplexy, 680
Cataract, 844–6, *844*, *845*, *846*, 863
Catecholamines, 20, 458, 460
Cauda equina syndrome, 686
Cefuroxime, 415
Cellulitis, 907, **977–8**
Central blindness, 855, 865
Central core myopathy, 703
Central cyanosis, 118–19
Central diabetes insipidus, 74, 75, 78, **532**, **533–4**
   laboratory investigations, 80–1, 533, *533*, 615
Central venous pressure (CVP), 137–8, 144
Central visual pathway lesions, *856*
Central visual pathways, *855*
Cephalexin, 193, 284
Cephalosporins, 135, 733, 747, 785, 977
Cerebellar amyotrophies, 674
Cerebellar ataxia, 232–3, *232*
Cerebellar congenital malformations, 674
Cerebellar hypoplasia, 674–5
Cerebellar lesions, 665
Cerebral infarction, 308, 681
Cerebral thrombosis, 681
Cerebrospinal fluid (CSF) analysis, 235, 240, 246, 251, **668–70**, *670*, 678
Cerebrospinal fluid (CSF) collection, 668–9, *669*
Cervical spinal pain, 239

Cervicovaginal mucus arborization, 575
Cestodes (tapeworm) infection, 421
Charcot's joints (neuropathic arthritis), 756
Chediak–Higashi syndrome, 809
Chemodectoma, 290, 300, 302
Chemoreceptor trigger zone (CTZ), 39, 49
Cheyletiella (cheyletiellosis), 194, 195, 198, 203, 876, **890–1**, *912*
Chlamydia psittaci, 961
   conjunctivitis, 860
   feline infection, 961, 962, 963, **964**, **965–6**
Chlorambucil, 795, 901, 1014, **1023**
Chloramphenicol, 135, 484, 487, 488, 648, 678
Chlorinated hydrocarbons toxicity, 245, 246
Chlorpromazine, 49, 404, 452, 623, 785
Chlorthiazide, 533, 796
Cholangiohepatitis, 130, 488–9, *488*
Cholangiosarcoma, 689
Cholangitis, 486, **487**, **487–9**
Cholangitis-cholecystitis, 483–4
Cholecystokinin (CCK), 13, 400, 401, 452, 501, 561
Cholestasis, **452–5**
   cholangitis-cholecystitis, 484
   chronic cholangiohepatitis, 488
   diabetes mellitus, 481
   double gallbladder, 483
   extrahepatic, 453, *453*
   gallstones, 484
   intrahepatic, 453, *453*
   liver enzyme tests, 130–1
Cholestyramine, 431
Cholinesterase inhibitor insecticides, 505
Chondrodysplasia punctata, 728
Chondroma, 733
Chondrosarcoma, 683, 724
Chordae tendinae rupture, 274, 279, 281
Chorioretinitis, 851–2
Choroid plexus tumours, 677, *678*
Choroidal hypoplasia, 848
Chylothorax, **367**
Chylous effusions, 140, 365, 367
Ciliary conditions, 826–7
Ciliary dyskinesia, 357
Cimetidine, 50, 121, 394, 405, 411, 623, 629, 996
Cirrhosis, 76, 130, 204, 456, *468*, **468–70**, 478–1
Cisapride, 391, 394, 404, 409, 412, 431, 435, 437
Cisplatin, 725, 1007, 1017, **1025–6**
Classical conditioning, 1029–30, 1032
Clavulanic acid, 488, 733, 747
Cleft palate, 83, 385–6
Clindamycin, 422, 648, 688, 705, 952, 977
Cliteral hypertrophy, 585, *586*
Clomiphene citrate, 596
Clostridium botulinum, 688
Clostridium difficile, 421
Clostridium enterotoxin, 403, 421

Clostridium perfringens, 62, 63, 69, 374, 421
Clostridium spp., 425, 484
Clostridium tetani, 688, 950
Clot retraction, 166, 781
Clotrimazole, 350
Clotting (coagulation) assays, 781–2
  blood samples, 773
Clotting factor assays, 132, 134, 167, 782
Clotting factors, 460, 800, *801*
  coagulation cascade, *161*, **161–2**, **769–70**, *770*
Coagulation cascade, *161*, **161–2**, 461, **769–70**, *770*
Coat brushings, 197–8, 204, 876
Cobalamin serum level, 64, *373*, *374*, 425, 512
Coccidioidomycosis, 289, 421–2, 678, 734, 749, 911
Cognitive processes, 1029–33
Colchicine, 634
Cold agglutinin disease, 119, 900, 914
Colitis, 67, *433*, **433–5**
  idiopathic, 429, 434
Collagenolytic granuloma, 906
Collapse, **218–24**, *219*, 696
  definitions, 218
Collie eye anomaly, 848, *848*
Coloboma, 848, 854, 858
Colonic disease, **432–8**
Colonic microscopic anatomy, 433, *433*
Colonic motility, 432–3
Colonic neoplasia, 67, *438*, **438**
Colonic polyps, 438
Colonic water absorption, 432
Colonoscopy, 69, 381
Colony forming units (CFU), 765
Colour dilution alopecia, 189, 902
Coma, 249, 250
Comedones, 189, 203
Common bile duct infections, 483–4
Compartmental excision, 998–9, *998*
Complete heart block, 329, *330*
Computed tomography
  bone pain, 215
  brain lesions, 671
  consciousness level alteration, 251
  eye disease, 823
  head and neck disorders, 57
  joint pain, 212
  micturition abnormalities/urinary incontinence, 175
  nasal chamber disease, 85, 347
  seizures, 247
  spinal lesions, 241
Conception failure, 586, 592
Congestion, **123–5**
Conjunctival disease, **830–1**, **859–60**
Conjunctivitis, 830–1, *831*, 859
Consciousness level alteration, **249–51**, *250*
Constipation, 67, 147, 433, *436*, **436–7**, *437*, 438
Constrictive pericarditis *see* Pericardial fibrosis
Contact allergy, 200, 881–2

Contagious canine respiratory disease (kennel cough), **941–4**, *942*
Contractures, 709
  congenital, 704
Contrast radiography, 148
  abdominal pain, 148
  alimentary tract disease, 376
  defecatory tenesmus, 69
  diarrhoea, 64
  fever of unknown origin, 37
  intestinal obstruction, 424
  oesophageal disorders, 56
  regurgitation, 46, 56
  urinary tract disorders, 174, 183, 615
  vomiting, 46
Coombs' test *see* Direct antiglobulin test
Coonhound paralysis, 689
Copper storage hepatopathy, 75, **475–7**
Coprophagia, 1040
Cor pulmonale, 121, 277, **303–4**
Cor triatrium dexter, **321**
Corneal dermoids, 831–2, *832*, 860
Corneal disorders, **831–6**, **860–1**
Corneal dystrophy, **834–5**, *835*, 860
Corneal inclusion cysts, 835
Corneal lipid depositions, 835
Corneal neoplasia, 836
Corneal nigrum/necrosis (corneal sequestrum), 860–1, *861*
Corneal oedema, 834, *835*
Corneal opacity, congenital, 831
Corneal sequestrum (corneal nigrum/necrosis), 860–1, *861*
Corneal trauma, 834
Corneal ulceration, *833*, **833–4**
Corneal vascularization, *832*
Coronary reserve, 271
Corticotrophin releasing hormone, 544
Cortisol, 544
Corynebacterium sp., 282, 907
Costs, 11
Cough, chronic, *93*, **93–8**, *94*, 137, 256, 277, 345, 360
Cough reflex, 93–4
Coxiella burnetii, 981
Coxofemoral joint pain, 211, *211*
Crackles (rales), 9, 346, 347
Cramp in Norwich terriers, 704
Cranial drawer sign, 725
Cranial nerve deficits, 234, *387*
Cranial nerve tests, 663
Craniomandibular osteopathy, 736–7, *736*
Creatine kinase, 217, 221, 697, 699
Creatinine clearance, 614, 616–17
Creatinine serum levels, 616, *616*
Cricopharyngeal dysphagia (achalasia), 52, 388, 389
Cricopharyngeal stricture, congenital, 52
Cross-infection control, 938
Crusting disorders, **201–6**, *204*, *205*, *206*
Cryptococcosis, 84, 96, 244, 289, 348, 678, 749, 888, 911, 980
  bone infection, 734
  rhinitis, 349, *349*
Cryptorchidism, 597, 603, 874
Cryptosporidia, 63, 421, 422, 940, 980

Crystalline stromal dystrophy, 835, *835*
Crystalluria, 181–2, *182*, 618
Cushing's disease, 131, 707
  see also Hyperadrenocorticism
Cutaneous asthenia (Ehlers–Danlos syndrome), 902, 915
Cutaneous lymphoma, 892
Cutaneous tuberculosis, 907
Cuticle bleeding time, 165
Cyanosis, 90, **118–22**, 123, 220, 256
  central, 118–19
  congenital cardiac defects, 310, 315, 316, 318
  peripheral, 119
Cyclic haematopoiesis (neutropenia), 790
Cyclophosphamide, 108, 172, 189, 586, 634, 752, 754, 787, 794, 795, 798, 901, 1008, 1016, **1023**
  haemorrhagic cystitis, 1021
Cycloplegics, 837–8
Cyclosporin, 428, 634, 829
Cylinduria (urinary casts), 180–1, *181*, 618
Cyproheptadine, 298, 712
Cystic endometrial hyperplasia, 582–3, *583*, 591–2
Cystine uroliths, 639, *639*, 641, 643, 645
Cystitis, 76, 183
Cystography, 641
Cystoisospora diarrhoea, 421, 422
Cystometry, 175
Cystoscopy, 184, 615–16
Cytosine arabinoside, 794, 1008, **1024**
Cytotoxic chemotherapy, 39, 986, **1005–26**
  adjuvant treatment, 1016–18
  cell kill hypothesis, 1007–8
  classes of drugs, *1006*
  combination therapy, 1008
  complications, 779, 798, 1018–21
  dosage, 1007, 1008–9
  drug resistance, 1018
  haematological malignancy management, 1009–16
  mode of action, 1005–7, *1005*
  safety precautions, 1021–3
  treatment protocols, 1008–9, *1008*

D

Dacryocystitis, 829
Dancing Dobermann syndrome, 690
Dantrolene, 708
DAP format for progress notes, 12
Database (baseline information collection), **4–5**, *7*, **8–10**
DEA blood groups, 766–7, *767*, 811
Deafness, congenital, 680
Deep somatic pain, 146
Defecation, 66
  inappropriate, 1039–40
Defecatory tenesmus, **66–9**, *67*, *69*, 372, 433, 434, 438
Degenerative brain disease, 674
Degenerative joint disease, **741–6**, **755–6**
Degenerative muscle disorders, 686
Degenerative peripheral neuropathy, 686

Degenerative spinal cord disease, 239, 681–3, 685, 686
Dehydration, 42, 44
Delayed puberty, 577, 579, 589
Demodicosis, 152, 189, 194, 198, 203, 873, 876, *889*, **889–90**, *890*, 912, **912**
Dental disease, 83, 84, 383–4
Depigmenting nasal dermatitis, chronic (Collie nose), 898
Depression, 249, 250
Dermanyssus gallinae, 912
Dermatomyositis, familial, 703, 900
Dermatophilosis, 202, 887
Dermatophytosis, 188, 191, 193, 195, 198, 202, 203, 205, 873, **887–8**, **909–11**
Dermis, 873
Desferrioxamine mesylate, 415
Desmopressin (DDAVP), 533, 799
Detrusor instability, 175
Developmental psychology, 1032–3
Dexamethasone suppression test
  high dose, 557
  low dose, 79, 556, *556*
Diabetes insipidus, 74, **532–4**
  see also Central diabetes insipidus; Nephrogenic diabetes insipidus
Diabetes mellitus, 77, 78, 172, 221, 308, **561–7**, 708
  with acromegaly, 531
  complications, *564*, 687, 864
  dietary therapy, 564
  instability, 566–7, *567*
  insulin therapy, 564–5
  insulin resistance, 567, *567*
  ketoacidosis, 45, 562–4, *563*
  liver changes, 481–2
  monitoring therapy, 565–6
  obesity association, 24
  pancreatitis-associated, 508, 512
  polyuria/polydipsia, 75, 76
  primary/secondary causes, 561, *561*
  records, 566, *566*
  skin disorders, 203, 205
  transient luteal phase, 581
Diabetic neuropathy, 687
Diabetic retinopathy, 864
Diagnostic plan, 11
Diaphragmatic paralysis, 91
Diarrhoea, 17, 43, 45, **58–65**, 67, 137, 143, 147, 149, 372, **417–20**, 427, 433, 434, 461, 505
  acute, 59, 61
  antibiotic-induced, 421
  bacterial enteritis, 420–1
  causes, *418*
  chronic, 59, 418, *418*, 424, 425, 426
  chronic liver disease, 456
  complicating chemotherapy, 1020–1
  dietary, 419–20
  haemorrhagic, 422–3, *423*
  laboratory investigations, 62–5, 373, 374
  large bowel disease, *59*, *60*, *61*, 418
  parasitic infections, 421–2
  pathophysiology, 58–9, 417–18
  small bowel disease, *59*, *60*, *61*, 418
  sudden onset, 418, *418*
  treatment, 418–19, *419*
  viral enteritis, 420
Diazepam, 16, 24, 126, 175, 248, 435, 690, 1034, 1040
Dietary diarrhoea, 419–20
Dietary hypersensitivity, 419, **428–9**, 433–4
  see also Food allergy
Dietary trial, 57, 65
Diethylstilboestrol, 646
Diffuse bilateral cerebral disease, 249
Digestive processes, 58
Digoxin, 126, 296, 331, 332, 333, 334, 796
  dilated cardiomyopathy, 287–8, 293
  heart failure, 325
  toxicity, 287, 325, 329
Dilated cardiomyopathy, 102, 105, 106, 117, 136, 219, 227, 273, 274, 275, 277
  angiocardiography, 292–3
  atrial fibrillation, 285, 288
  cat, **291–3**
  dog, **284–8**, *286–7*
  echocardiography, 285–6, *286*, 292
  electrocardiography, 285, 291–2
  radiological findings, 285, *285*, *286*, 292, *292*
  treatment, 121, 287–8, 293
Diltiazem, 288, 296, 327, 333, 629
Dimethylsulphoxide, 634, 745
Diphallia, 601
Diphenhydramine, 49
Diphenoxylate, 419, 428, 435
Dipylidium caninum, 421
Dipyrone, 38, 785
Direct antiglobulin test (Coombs' test), 36, 133, 782, *783*, 787, 805
Dirofilaria immitis, 230, 304, 306, 359
Dirofilariasis, 89, 119, 267, 274, 277, **304–6**, *305*, 738, 780
  brain involvement, 679
  heart murmurs, 103
  lung disease, 94, 95, 359
  treatment, 306
Discharge summary, 12
Discoid lupus erythematosus, 898, 901
Discospondylitis, 239, *684*, **684**, *748*, 748
Disorientation (confusion), 249
Displacement activity, 1032, 1039
Disseminated intravascular coagulation (DIC), 167, 464, 788, **801–2**, 809–10
  antithrombin III deficiency, 804
  associated diseases, *802*
  gastric dilatation and volvulus, 414
  gastric mucosal damage, 403, 408
  haemorrhagic gastroenteritis, 423
  liver disease, 461
Distichiasis, 826, *826*, *827*
Distraction, 1036
Diuretics
  acute renal failure, 622
  glomerulonephropathy, 633
  heart failure, **321–3**
  potassium-losing, 322–3
  potassium-sparing, 323
  pulmonary oedema, 361
Doberman pinscher cardiomyopathy, 287
Dobutamine, 288, 293, 324, 332
Dog, physical examination, 5, *6–7*
Dog pox, 601
Dopamine, 288, 293, 330, 458, 499, 622
Doppler colour flow mapping, 271
Double contrast cystography, 174, 183
Double contrast gastrography, 47, *48*, 148, 377, 409
Double gallbladder, 483
Doxorubicin, 227, 755, 1012, 1017, 1018, 1019, **1024–5**
  cardiotoxicity, 290, 299, **1021**
Doxycycline, 954, 963, 966
Drug reactions
  bone marrow suppression, 798–9
  fever, 32
  keratoconjunctivitis sicca, 435
  pancreatitis, 504, 508
  platelet dysfunction, 800
  polyuria/polydipsia, 75
  skin eruption, 899
  vomiting, 44
Duodenal endoscopy, 380, 381
Duodenal juice analysis, 65, 381, 425
Dwarfing syndromes, 535, 729
Dysautonomia, 55, 68, 437, 690
Dyschezia, 67, 433, 434, 438
Dyschondrosteosis, 728
Dysmyelination of CNS, 675
Dysostoses, 729
Dysphagia, 51, **52–7**, 345, 372, 376, 384, **387–9**, 397, 696
  causes, *53*, 387, *387*
  diagnostic approach, *54*, 388
  physical examination, 55, 387–8
  treatment, 388–9
Dyspnoea, 9, **87–92**, 137, 221, 256, 285, 360, 363, 364, 365, 771, 772
  causes, 87
  immediate management, 90
  laboratory investigations, 90–2
  pathophysiology, 87–8
  physical examination, 90
  postural adaptations, 88, *89*
Dysuria, 168, 171, 177, 178, 185, 636, 643

E
Ears examination, 8
Ecchymotic haemorrhage, 109, 164, 772, 797, *797*
Echinococcus spp., 421
Echocardiography, 98, 270, **270–1**
  aortic stenosis, 312–14, *313*
  atrial septal defect, 317
  bacterial endocarditis, 283
  cardiac dysrhythmias, 229–30
  cardiac murmurs, 105–6
  collapse/episodic weakness, 222
  cyanotic congenital heart disease, 121
  dilated cardiomyopathy, 285–6, *286*, 292
  endocardiosis, 281
  fever of unknown origin, 34

hypertrophic cardiomyopathy, 289, 295, *296*
   patent ductus arteriosus, 311
   pericardial effusion, 301–2, *302*
   pulmonary stenosis, 315
   ventricular septal defect, 316
Eclampsia, postpartum, 244, 588, 593
Ectodermal congenital defects, 187
Ectoparasitic infestation, 194, 196, 198, 202, 203, 206, **889–91**, **911–12**
   alopecia, 186, 188, 191
   treatment, 192–3
Ectopic testes, 597
Ectopic ureter, 651, 653
Ectropion, 826, 858
Ehrlichiosis, 36, 152, 678, 789, 800, **953–4**
Eisenmenger's syndrome, 119, 316, **319–20**
Ejaculated fluid examination, 183, *183*, *184*
Elbow pain, 208, *209*
Electrocardiography, 98, **259–61**
   abnormal parameters, *262*
   ambulatory ECG (Holter monitoring), 223, 260
   aortic stenosis, 312
   ascites, 138
   atrial septal defect, 317
   atrioventricular heart block, *330*
   cardiac cycle relationship, *257*, 260–1
   cardiac dysrhythmias, 228–9, *263–6*, *332, 335*
   cardiac murmurs, 105
   collapse/episodic weakness, 222
   cor pulmonale, 303
   cyanotic congenital heart disease, 121
   dilated cardiomyopathy, 235, 291–2
   dirofilariasis (heartworm disease), 304
   endocardiosis, 281
   fever of unknown origin, 34
   hypertrophic cardiomyopathy, 288, 294
   hypoadrenocorticism, 548, *548*
   interpretation, 261
   mean electrical axis (MEA), 259, *260*
   normal parameters, *261*
   patent ductus arteriosus, 310–11
   pericardial effusion, 301
   pulmonary stenosis, 315
   restrictive cardiomyopathy, 297
   tetralogy of Fallot, 318
   ventricular septal defect, 316
   vomiting, 45
Electroencephalography, 247, 251
Electrolyte disturbances
   acute renal failure, 622–3
   diabetic ketoacidosis, 563–4
   diarrhoea, 63
   gastric dilatation and volvulus, 413
   myopathy, 687
   polyuria without polydipsia, 70
   regurgitation, 55
   vomiting, 42, 45, 49
Electromyography, 217, 224, 352, 674, **698**, 699
   micturition abnormalities/urinary incontinence, 175

spinal lesions, 238–9, 674
Electrophysiology, 230, 238–9, 671, 673
Electroretinography, 823
Elimination diets, 199
Emaciation, 18
Emphysema, pulmonary, 9
Enalapril, 288, 325, 629, 634
Encephalitis, 244, 246, 677–8
End-tidal capnography, 91, 97
Endocardiosis, 227, 277, **278–82**, *280*
   echocardiography, 281
   electrocardiography, 281
   heart failure, 277, 278
   radiological findings, 281, *281*
   therapy, *280*, 282
Endocrinopathy, **526–69**
   alopecia, 186, *187*, 189, 192, 893, *893*
   dermatoses, **893–7**, **912–13**
   obesity, 23–4
Endogenous pyrogen, 29, 31
Endoscopy
   abdominal pain, 149
   alimentary tract, 65, **378–81**, *379*
   larynx, 352
   nasal cavity, 348
   oesophageal disorders, 56–7
   vomiting, 47
Endotoxaemia, 37, 107, 149, 779
Energy requirement measures, 18
English cocker spaniel cardiomyopathy, 287
Enophthalmos, 824–5
Enrofloxacin, 415, 638, 648
Enteral feeding, 21
Enteritis, **417–23**
   haemorrhagic, 422–3
   infectious, 61, 62, 420–2, *939*, 939–41, **973–4**
Enterobacter, 34, 185
Enterococcus, 425
Enteropeptidases, 500, 505
Entropion, 825–6, *826*, 858, *859*
Enuresis, 168
Enzyme-linked immunosorbent (ELISA) test, 880
Eosinopenia, 780
Eosinophilia, 373, 780
Eosinophilic colitis, 434
Eosinophilic enteritis, 45, 373, 425–6, 429
Eosinophilic gastritis, 407
Eosinophilic granuloma complex, 385, 904, 905
Eosinophilic (indolent) ulcers, 905–6, *906*
Eosinophilic keratoconjunctivitis, 861
Eosinophilic meningoencephalitis, 246
Eosinophilic plaques, 196, 906, *906*
Eosinophilic pneumonia, 360, *360*
Eosinophils, 767
   response to disease, 780
Ependymomas, 683
Epidermal dysplasia, 202, 203
Epidermal self-renewal, 201, 872
Epidermis, 871–2, *872*
Epididymal disease, 599, 603
Epididymis, 597
Epididymitis, 599

Epilepsy, idiopathic, 219, 220, 242, 244, 245, 680
Epiphora, 829, 860
Epirubicin, 1019, **1025**
Episcleritis, 123, 836
Epistaxis, 84, 108, 164, 560, 771
Epoetin alfa, 628
Epulides, 385
Erysipelas, 746
Erysipelothrix rhusiopathiae, 282
Erythema multiforme, 899, 914
Erythrocytes *see* Red cells
Erythrocytosis, primary, 808
Erythromycin, 409, 412, 648, 757, 941
Erythropoiesis, 766
Erythropoiesis failure
   primary, 115, 788–9, 806–7
   secondary, 115–16, 789, 807
   therapy, 116–17
Erythropoietic prophyria, congenital, 806
Erythropoietin, 124, 613, 625, 766, 778
Erythropoietin assay, 124, 777
Escherichia coli, 62, 185, 282, 403, 425, 480, 484, 487, 584, 587, 592, 599, 647, 684, 944, 945, 974, 1020
   enteropathogenic, 374, 418, **421**
Essential amino acids, feline, 487
Essential fatty acid supplements, 882–3, 905
Ethylene glycol toxicity, 182, 245, 620, 622, 623, *623*
Eurytrema procyonis, 519
Eutrombicula alfreddugesi, 891
Excessive left ventricular moderator bands, 297
Exercise intolerance, 108, 312, 315, 318, 461, 551, 696, 697, 771
Exercise-induced weakness, 219
Exertional myopathy (cramp), 216, 708–9
Exfoliative vaginal cytology, 575, *576*
Exocrine pancreatic insufficiency, 59, 61, 425, **509–18**
   glucose intolerance, 512
   investigations, 63–4, 373, 374, 513–16
   nutritional status, 512–13
   pancreatic acinar atrophy, 509
   pancreatic regulatory peptides, 511–12
   small intestinal mucosa, 510–11, *511*
   treatment, 516–18
Exogenous pyrogens, 29
Exophthalmos, 823–4, *824, 825*
Exposure keratitis, 834
External beam radiation, 999
External genitalia disorders, 585–6, 592
Extinction, 1035
Extracellular fluid (ECF) osmolality, 71
Extradural tumours, 683, 687
Extramedullary haemopoiesis, 152
Extraocular muscles, *857*
Exudates
   ascites, 136, 139, *139, 140*
   pleural effusions, 365–6
Eye disease, 8, **820–66**
   cat, **858–66**
   diagnostic imaging, 823
   dog, **823–58**

Eye disease (cont.)
  history-taking, 820
  laboratory investigations, 822
  ophthalmological examination, 821–2
Eye position/movement disorders, 857, 865–6
Eyelid disease, 825–8, 858–9
Eyelid neoplasia, 827–8, 859

F

Facial nerve paralysis, 234
Factor VII deficiency, 804
Factor VIII assay, 167
Factor VIII deficiency (haemophilia A), 108, 162, 164, 167, **802–4**, *803*, **810**
Factor IX deficiency (haemophilia B; Christmas disease), **804**, **810**
Factor X deficiency, 804
Factor XI deficiency, 804
Factor XII (Hageman factor) deficiency, 810
Fading pups, 944, 945, 946
Faecal analysis, 45, 62, 63, 67, 149, 373–4
Faecal culture, 62, 68, 374
Faecal cytology, 63, 69
Faecal flotation for parasites, 97, 374, 422
Faecal impaction, 67
Faecal incontinence, 438–9
Faecal occult blood, 149, 374
Faecal proteolytic activity, 515–16, *516*
Famotidine, 394, 405
Fanconi syndrome, 76, 77, 636
Fasting energy metabolism, 20
Fat malabsorption, 374, 513
Fatty acid deficiency, 902
Feeding behaviour, 13
Feline allergic bronchitis, 118
Feline asthma, 91, 93, 94, 95
Feline astrovirus, 973
Feline calicivirus, 354, 961, **963–4**
  gingivitis-stomatitis-pharyngitis, 383, 962, *962*
  skin disease, 909
Feline cerebellar hypoplasia, 679–80
Feline coronavirus infection, **971–3**
Feline cowpox, 908–9, *909*, **974–6**
Feline enteric coronavirus infection, 971, 973
Feline herpes virus 1, 592, 961, *962*, **963–4**
Feline herpes virus 2, 977
Feline herpesvirus, 354, 384
  conjunctivitis, 859–60
  skin disease, 909
Feline hypersensitivity keratitis, 860
Feline immunodeficiency virus, 15, 56, 63, 84, 96, 109, 128, 373, 433, 771, 772, 784, 961, **969–71**
  colonic neoplasia, 438
  fever, 30
  gingivitis-stomatitis-pharyngitis, 383, 969
  skin disease, 909
  treatment, 970–1
Feline infectious anaemia, 805
Feline infectious peritonitis, 96, 132, 135, 244, 592, **678**

abdominal fluid, *141*, 971
control, 972–3
disseminated intravascular coagulation, 809
fever, 31, 36, 971
liver involvement, 489
neurological disease, 678, 971
pericardial effusion, 300, 971
pleural effusion, 366, 971
treatment, 972
see also Feline coronavirus infection
Feline ischaemic encephalopathy, 681
Feline leprosy, 907–8, 978–9
Feline leukaemia virus, 15, 56, 63, 84, 92, 96, 109, 116, 128, 152, 173, 373, 592, 771, 772, 784, 961, **966–9**
  colonic neoplasia, 438
  disseminated intravascular coagulation, 809
  enteritis, 420
  fever, 30
  gingivitis-stomatitis-pharyngitis, 383
  haemolytic anaemia, 805–6, 968
  haemopoietic neoplasms association, 807, 808, 809, *967*, **967–8**, **1010–11**, 1013
  immunosuppression, 968
  persistent latent infection, 966, 967
  pure red cell aplasia, 806, 968
  reproductive failure, 968
  skin disease, 909
  testing/vaccination, 969
  treatment, 968
Feline lower urinary tract disease, 24, 170, **643–6**, *644*
  obstructive *see* Urethral obstruction in cats
Feline lymphocytic cholangiohepatitis, 76
Feline panleucopenia, 42, 300, 592, **959–60**, 973
Feline parvovirus, 63, 420
Feline poxvirus, 195
Feline respiratory viruses, 348, **963–4**
  vaccines, 964–5
Feline spongiform encephalopathy, 981
Feline syncytium-forming virus, 977
Female reproductive disorders, **574–94**
  bitch, 577–89
  history-taking, 574
  investigative techniques, 575–6, *576*, *577*
  physical examination, 574–55
  queen, 589–94
Female reproductive endocrinology
  bitch, 577, *578*
  queen, 589, *590*
Feminizing syndrome, idiopathic, 896
Fenbendazole, 307, 359, 519
Ferritin, 111, 126, 784
Fetal resorption, 586–7, 592–3, 944
Fever, **28–38**, 90, 109, 123, 771
  adverse versus beneficial effects, 29
  intermittent (undulating), 29–30
  management, 37–8, *38*
  pathophysiology, 29
  remittant (septic), 30
  sustained (persistent), 30

see also Fever of unknown origin
Fever of unknown origin, **30–7**
  causes, 30–2, *32*
  criteria, 30
  diagnostic procedures, 34–7, *35*
  screening tests, 34
Fibrinogen assay, 167, 464, 782
Fibrinogen (fibrin) degradation products (FDPs), 167, 771, 782
Fibrinolysis, **162**, 770–1
Fibrocartilaginous embolism (ischaemic myelopathy), 685
Fibroma, 913–14
Fibrosarcoma, 385, 683, 724, 913–14
Filaroides ocleri, 359
Fine needle aspiration (FNA)
  haematuria investigation, 183, 184, *184*
  liver, 466
  lung lesions, 91, 354
  lymph node, 154, 775
  oesophageal disorders, 57
  prostatic disease, 174, 183, 184, *184*
  renal disease, 183, 184
  tumours, 989, *990*
Flea allergy, 190, 195, 196, 199, 874, 881, *882*, 904
Flea infestation, 194, 195, 198, 203, 905
Fluconazole, 350, 639, 888
Flucytosine, 639, 911
Fluid intake, 70
Fluid retention, 18
Fluid thrill, 137
Flunixin meglumine, 37, 44, 415, 745, 837
Fluoroscopy
  chronic cough, 96–7
  dyspnoea, 91
  hiatal hernia, 398
  oesophageal disorders, 56, 397
  swallowing evaluation, 56, 376–7
  tracheal/bronchial collapse, 353, 355
Flutamide, 647
Folate serum level, 64, 373, *374*, 425, 513
Follicle stimulating hormone (FSH), 527, 577
  male reproductive functions, 595, *596*, 602
Follicular dystrophy/dysplasia, 186, 187, 188, 189
Folliculitis, bacterial, 202
Food adverse reactions, 428–9
see also Dietary hypersensitivity
Food allergy, 199, 200, 381, 427, 874, 881, 905
Food idiosyncrasy, 429
Food intake regulation, 13
Food intolerance, 61, 65, 429, 881, 905
Food poisoning, 428
Forebrain lesions, 664, *665*
Forebrain tumours, 676
Foreign bodies
  gastric, 47, 410, *410*
  ingested, 44, 59, 61, 62, 64, 376
  inhaled, 30, 91, 96, 97, 356
  intestinal obstruction, 423, 424
  ocular, 830, 831, 834

oesophageal obstruction, 54, 55, 56, 57, **392–3**
oropharyngeal, 385
rectal, 67, 69
rhinitis, 348
salivary gland, 386
tracheal, 118
see also Linear foreign bodies
Forelimb oedema, 142
Fractional excretion, 618
Frank–Starling relationship, 271, 274, 275
Free T3 serum level, 536–7
Free T4 serum level, 536
Frontal sinuses, 83, 347
Frusemide, 75, 141, 287, 293, 295, 308, 361, 504, 622, 633
  heart failure management, 322–3
Functional (physiological) cardiac murmur, 102
Fundal disorders, 847–54, 864–5
Fundal neoplasms, 853
Fundoscopy, *821*
Fundus, 847–8, *847*, 863, *863*
Fundus inflammation, 851–2, *852*
Fungal culture, 877–8
Fungal infection, 980
  arthritis, 749, 757
  brain, 678
  lymph node granulomatous/pyogranulomatous response, 152, 155
  myocarditis, 289
  osteomyelitis, 734
  pneumonia, 96
  rhinitis, 349–50, *349*
  skin, 887–8, 909–11
  urinary tract infection, 639
Furunculosis, 873
Fusobacterium, 907, 977

G
GABA neurotransmission, 458
GABA/BZ receptor complex, 458, 460
Gait abnormalities, 697, 724
Galactostasis, 588–9, 594
Gallbladder duplication, 483
Gallbladder physiology, 452
Gallstones, 484–5
Gallop rhythms, 258
Gamma-glutamyltransferase (GGT), 131, 134, 139, **463**, 618–19
Gas exchange, 87–8, *89*
Gastric acid secretion, 401
Gastric allergy testing, 381
Gastric contents aspiration, 54
Gastric dilatation, isolated, 42, 146, 290, 413–14
Gastric dilatation and volvulus, 371, **413–16**
  electrolyte/acid–base disturbances, *413*
  management, 415–16
Gastric disease, **398–416**
Gastric emptying, 377, 400, 412, 414
Gastric foreign bodies, 47, 410, *410*
Gastric inhibitory peptide (GIP), 512, 561
Gastric lymphoma, 411

Gastric motility, 377, 399–400
  disorders, **411–12**, *412*
Gastric mucosal barrier, 399, *399*
  damage in ulcer pathogenesis, 407, 408
Gastric mucus production, 400–1
Gastric neoplasia, 405, 409, 410–11, *411*
Gastric outflow obstruction, 412–13, *413*
Gastric secretions, 400–1
Gastric ulcer biopsy, 409
Gastric ulceration, 147, **407–10**, *408*
Gastric volvulus, chronic, 416
Gastrin, 399, 400, 401
Gastrin releasing peptide (GRP), 499
Gastrinomas, 403, 408
Gastritis, acute, **401–3**, 625
  aetiology, 401, *402*
  secondary, 403
  treatment, 403–5
Gastritis, chronic, 405–7
  classification, *405*
  idiopathic, 406
  management, 409–10
  spiral organisms, 407
Gastritis, non-specific, 48–9
Gastroenteritis, 147
  haemorrhagic, 422–3, 429
  symptomatic therapy, 48–9
Gastrointestinal haemorrhage, 149, 373, 374
Gastro-oesophageal intussusception, 56, 397, *397*
Gastro-oesophageal reflux, 394
Gastroscopy, 47
Generalized seizures, 243
Generalized tremor syndrome (white shaker dog), 679, 691
Gentamycin, 757, 979
Giant axonal neuropathy, 686
Giardiasis, 63, 65, 374, **422**, 427, 940, 980
Gingivitis, 373, 383
Gingivitis-stomatitis-pharyngitis in cat, 383–4, 969
Glaucoma, 123, **839–42**, 863
  classification, *839*
  clinical signs, 839, *839*, 840
  medical treatment, 841, *841*
  primary, 839–41
    narrow (closed) angle, 839–41, *840*
    open angle, 841
  secondary, 841–2, *842*, *843*
  surgical treatment, 841, *842*
Glioma, 244, 676, *676*
Globoid cell leukodystrophy, 674, 686
Glomerulonephritis, 76, 178
Glomerulonephropathy, 78, 119, 139, 147, 149, 183, 303, 305, 617, **631–4**
  causes, *632*
Glossitis, 383
Glucagon, 13, 450, 561
  fasting energy metabolism/hypermetabolism, 20
Glucagonoma, 204
Glucocorticoid hormones, 450, 544
  stress leucocytosis, 779
Glucocorticoid therapy, 16, 24, 37, 38, 75, 504, 678, 682

allergic skin disease, 882, 905
autoimmune haemolytic anaemia, 787
colitis, 435
cytotoxic chemotherapy protocols, 1012
enema preparations, 435
gastric dilatation and volvulus, 415
gingivitis-stomatitis-pharyngitis in cat, 384
glomerulonephropathy, 634
hypoadrenocorticism, 549
  acute primary disease, 548
iatrogenic Cushing's disease, 189
immune-mediated skin disease, 900
liver enzyme effects, 130, 131
osteoarthritis, 743–4, 745–6, 756
pericardial effusion, 303
pruritus, 194, 195, 199, 200, 874–5, *874*
rheumatoid arthritis, 752
steroid hepatopathy, 481, *481*
uveitis, 836
withdrawal-associated hypoadrenocorticism, 549
Glucocorticoid-induced hepatopathy, 131
Glucose intolerance, 512
Glutamate dehydrogenase (GLDH), 130, 463
Glutamate neurotransmission, 457–8, *458*
Gluten-sensitive enteropathy, 429
Glyceryl trinitrate, 324
Glycogen storage diseases, 702–3
Glycosuria, 77, 179, **618**, 619
Gnathostoma spp., 407
Goitre, 534
Gold salts, 384, 752, 798, 901
Gonadotrophin releasing hormone (GnRH), 577
Gonioscopy, 822
Gracilis contractures, 709
Granulocytes, 767
Granulocytopathy syndrome, canine, 790
Granulomatous bowel disease, 32, 434
Granulomatous encephalitis, 246
Granulomatous gastritis, 407
Granulomatous meningoencephalitis, 244, 679
Great vessel assessment, 267
Griseofulvin, 193, 858, 887, 910
Growth deficiency, differential diagnosis, *529*
Growth hormone, 13, 527
  regulation of release, *528*
  reproductive disorders in bitch, 581
Growth hormone deficiency, 528, 729
Growth hormone therapy, 529, 530
Growth hormone-responsive alopecia, 529–30, *530*, 894–5
Growth regulation, 535
  see also Growth hormone
Guillain-Barré disease, 689
Gut peptides, 13
Gut-associated lymphoid tissue (GALT), 768

H
H_2 blockers, 394, 405, 415, 431, 629

Haemangiosarcoma, 290, 478, 683, 724
Haematemesis, 43, 108, 164, 373, 406, 407, 409, 771
Haematochezia, 67, 373, 433
Haematological disorders, **765–812**
   cat, 805–10
   dog, 784–804
   history-taking, 771
   investigative techniques, 772–5
   laboratory investigations, 775–80
   physical examination, 771–2
   tumour-related, 993, *993*
Haematological reference ranges, *775*
Haematopoiesis, **765–8**, *766*
Haematuria, 164, **176–85**, 614, 618, 619, 636, 639, 643, 644, 771
   causes, 176, *177*
   gross, 176
   history-taking, 177–8
   management, 184–5
   microscopic, 176
   urine analysis, 178–9
   urine culture, 182
   urine sediment examination, 179–82, *181*, *182*
Haemic cardiac murmur, 107, 772
Haemobartonella, 109
Haemobartonella canis, 787
Haemobartonella felis, 128, 805
Haemoglobin metabolism, 126, 454, 766
Haemoglobinaemia, 133
Haemoglobinopathies, congenital, 119
Haemoglobinuria, 108, 127, 133, 176, 618
Haemolytic anaemia, 107, 108, *113*, **113**, **114**, 127, 785, 805–6
   congenital in cat, 806
   extrinsic, 114, *115*
Haemolytic (prehepatic) jaundice, 132, 133, 134
Haemophilia A (factor VIII deficiency), 108, 162, 164, 167, **802–4**, *803*, 810
Haemophilia B (factor IX deficiency; Christmas disease), **804**, 810
Haemoptysis, 108, 771
Haemorrhage, 278
   abdominal pain, 149
   bleeding disorders, 164
   hypovolaemic shock, 108, 784
   physical examination, 109
Haemorrhagic anaemia, 107, 108, 113, *113*, 784–5, 805
   acute haemorrhage, 114, *114*
   chronic blood loss, 114, *114*
Haemorrhagic gastroenteritis, 422–3, 429
Haemostasis, **160–2**, 769–71, *769*
   coagulation cascade, 161–2, 769–70
   laboratory assessment, **780–4**
   primary, 160–1, *160*, 769
   secondary, 161, 769–70
   tertiary, 770
Haemostasis abnormalities *see* Bleeding disorders
Haemostasis function tests, **774–5**
Haemothorax, 364
Hair, 872
   macroscopic examination, 876

Hair growth cycle, 186, 535, 872, *873*
Hair plucks, 191, 197–8, 204
Hairballs (trichobezoars), 410
Hantavirus, 976
Harvest mite infestation, 195
Head examination, 5
Head and neck oedema, 143
Head tilt, 233
Head trauma, 245, 680
Heart failure, **271–8**
   cardiac function curve, *322*
   compensatory changes, 272, *273*, 274–5
      adaptive consequences, 276
      modifying mechanisms, 275–6
   congestive, 89, 91, 94, 95, 96, 98, 104, 106, 117, 119, 120, 123, 256, 267, 272, *273*, 277–8
      anaemia, 108
      ascites, 136, 137
      central venous pressure (CVP), 138
      congenital cardiac defects, 310, 316, 317
      dilated cardiomyopathy, 285
      endocardiosis, 277, 279, 281, 282
      hepatic congestion, 474
      left-sided, 277
      pericardial effusion, 300
      right-sided, 277–8
   functional classification, 278, *279*
   high output states, 274
   hypertrophic cardiomyopathy, 276, 277, 294
   left to right shunts, 277
   low output, 117, 272, *273*, 274, 278
   management, **321–8**
      diuretics, 321–3
      negative inotropic agents, 327–8
      positive inotropic agents, 326–7
      rest, 321
      vasodilator drugs, 324–5
   myocardial changes, 276
   pathophysiology, 272–7, *272*, *322*, *324–6*
      compliance failure, 274
      myocardial failure, 273
      pressure overload (afterload increase), 274, 275
      volume overload (increased preload), 273–4, 275
   pericardial disease, 277
   peripheral vasoconstriction, 276
   water/salt retention, 275, 276
Heart rate, maximum effective, 271
Heart sounds, 8, *257*, **257–8**
Heartworm *see* Dirofilariasis
Heat-stroke, 30, 38
Heinz bodies, 120, 121, 128, 766, 776, 788, 806
Helicobacter felis, 407
Helicobacter heilmanii, 407
Helicobacter pylori, 381, 403, 407
Helicobacter spp., 406, 407, 408
Hemiplegia/paresis, 236, 238
Hemivertebrae, 239
Heparin, 298, 798, 799
Hepatic arteriovenous fistula, 475

Hepatic congestion, **473–4**
Hepatic cysts, 483
Hepatic encephalopathy, 55, 75, 219, 221, **456–60**, 487, 675
   amino acid metabolism, 458, *459*, 460
   ammonia metabolism, 457, 458–60, 464
   congenital portosystemic shunts, 472, 473
   diagnosis, 459–60
   hypokalaemia, 459, *459*
   neurotransmitter dysfunction, 457–8
   potentiating drugs, 458, 460
   seizures, 243, 246
   treatment, 460
Hepatic fibrosis, 76, 130, 456
Hepatic lipidosis, 24, **489–91**, *490*
Hepatitis, 147, **467–70**
   acute, 467–8, *467*
   chronic, 456
   chronic active, 76, 135, **468–70**, *468*, *469*
   fulminant, 467
   infectious, **930–2**
   neonatal, 456, 471
   non-specific reactive, 480–1, *480*
Hepatocellular carcinoma, 477–8
Hepatocellular (intrahepatic) jaundice, 132, 133–4
Hepatocutaneous syndrome (necrolytic migratory erythema), 901
Hepatomegaly, 96, 105, 109, 278, 461, 462, 481
Hepatoportal fibrosis, congenital, 470–1
Hereditary ventricular arrhythmias, 227
Heterochromia irides, 836
Hexochlorophene toxicity, 681
Hiatal hernia, 52, 54, 56, *397*, **397–8**
Hickey–Hare test, 81
High altitude acclimatization, 124
Hindlimb lameness, 748
Hindlimb oedema, 143, 144
Hindlimb paralysis, 120, 297
Histiocytic colitis, 59, 434
Histiocytic gastritis, 407
Histiocytoma, 892
Histoplasmosis, 63, 69, 678, 734, 911
History taking, **4**, *6*
HLA-B27, 754
Holter monitoring (ambulatory ECG), 223, 229, 260
Hookworms, 421, 891
Hormone anticancer treatment, 1007
Horner's syndrome, 234, **856–7**, 865, *866*
   localization of lesions, *857*
Howell–Jolly bodies, 776, 805
Hunger, 13
Hyaloid artery, persistent, 847
Hydralazine, 309, 324
Hydrocephalus, 245, 250, 251, 674, *675*
Hydrochlorothiazide, 323, 533, 629
Hydrogen breath tests, 64, **374–5**, 425
Hydronephrosis, 178, 619
21-Hydroxylase deficiency, 192
Hydroxyurea, 426, 793, **1026**
Hymenal constrictions, 584
Hyperadrenocorticism, 23, 75, 76, 78, 92, 96, 172, 221, 303, 461, **549–60**, 732

adrenal-dependent, 550, 551, 557
   management, 560
alopecia, 188, 189, 192
clinical signs, 550–2
diagnostic imaging, 554–5, *554*
endocrine screening tests, 555–7, *555*
laboratory findings, 552–3, *553*
myopathy, 707
pathophysiology, 549–50, *550*
pituitary tumours, 531
pituitary-dependent, 549–50, *550*, 551, 557
   management, 557–60
screening tests, 79
skin disorders, 202, 205, **893–4**, 913
steroid hepatopathy, 481
stress leucogram, 779
Hyperaemia, **123–5**
Hyperammoniaemia, 221, 472–3, 487
   glutamate neurotransmission, 457–8, *458*
Hyperbilirubinaemia, **126–8**, *129*, 454, 455
Hypercalcaemia, 76, 221, *543*
   hyperparathyroidism, 543
   hypoadrenocorticism, 547
   pancreatitis, 505
   treatment, 544, 995–6
   tumour-related, 994–6, *996*
Hypercholesterolaemia, 506, 536, 633
Hypercoagulable states, 119, 633, 634
Hypereosinophilic syndrome, 425, *426*, 429
Hyperfibrinogenaemia, 633
Hypergammaglobulinaemia, 132
Hypergastrinaemia, 403, 408
Hyperglycaemia, 77, 221, 506, 508, 531, **675–6**
Hyperhistaminaemia, 996, *996*
Hyperkalaemia, 45, 244, 547
   acute renal failure, 619, 622, *622*
   myopathy, 707–8
   urethral obstruction in cats, 644, 645
Hyperlipidaemia, 23–4, 687
Hyperlipoproteinaemia, 244, 504
Hypermetabolism, 20–1
Hyperoestrogenism, 189, 308
Hyperparathyroidism, 308, **543–4**
   bone disease, 729–32, *730*, *731*
   chronic renal failure, 625, 628, 731
   primary, 78, 543
   secondary, 543
Hypersensitivity reactions, 194, 195, 196, 200, 203, 874
   cytotoxic drugs, 1019
   eosinophilia, 780
   insect-mediated, 891
   intradermal tests, 199
   serological tests, 199
   vaccination adverse reactions, 937–8
Hypertension, 24, 222, 274, **307–9**, 560
   chronic renal failure, 624, 626, 629
   glomerulonephropathy, 631, 632, 634
   treatment, 308–9, 629, 634
Hypertensive retinopathy, 852, 864, *864*
Hyperthermia, 30, 38, 244
   upper respiratory obstruction, 90, 96

Hyperthyroidism, 30, 75, 76, 78, 128, 259, 308, **538–41**, *539*, 732
   cardiac abnormalities, 298, 539, 540
   liver involvement, 489
   skin disorders, 203, 913
   treatment, 540–1
Hypertrophic cardiomyopathy, 105, 106, 274, 277, 278
   angiocardiography, 295
   cat, **293–6**, 297, 300, 539, 540
   dog, **288–9**
   echocardiography, 289, 295, *296*
   electrocardiography, 288, 294
   radiological examination, 288, 294–5, *295*
Hypertrophic gastritis, 406–7
Hypertrophic neuropathy, 686
Hypertrophic osteodystrophy *see* Metaphyseal osteopathy
Hypertrophic pulmonary osteopathy, 737–8, *738*
Hypervitaminosis A, 724, 731, 739–40, *739*
Hyphaema, 838–9, *838*, 863
Hypoadrenocorticism, 45, 46, 62, 63, 78, 108, 119, 274, **545–8**, 708
   electrocardiography, 548, *548*
   endocrine tests, 548, *555*, 557
   primary (Addison's disease), 221, **546–9**, *547*
   secondary, 549
Hypoalbuminaemia, 132, 138, 205, 456, 464, 480, 633
Hypocalcaemia, 221, 506, 542, *542*, 619
   postpartum/late pregnancy, 588, 593
   seizures, 244
   treatment, 541
Hypochondroplasia, 728
Hypofibrinogenaemia, 167, 804
Hypogastric nerve, 168
Hypoglycaemia, 219, 221, 243, 245, 548, 568, *569*, 587, **675**
Hypogonadism, 23, 595–6, 602
Hypokalaemia, 42, 563, 626
   chronic liver disease, 459, *459*
   diuretic-induced, 323
Hypokalaemic myopathy, 221, 687, 707–8, 710, *710*, 713
Hyponatraemia, 42, 547
Hypoparathyroidism, 244, **542–3**
Hypopituitarism, congenital, **528–9**, *529*, 535, 538, 729
Hyposensitization (immunotherapy), 883, 905
Hypospadias, 600, 603
Hyposthenuria, persistent, 79, 80–1
Hypotension, 222, 560
Hypothalamic-hypophyseal portal system, 526
Hypothalamus
   autonomic centres, 13, 14, 526
   pituitary function regulation, 526, *527*
   anterior lobe hormone release, 526
Hypothermia, 38
Hypothyroidism, 23, 56, 308, *535*, **535–8**
   alopecia, 188, 189, 192

congenital (cretinism), 188, 535, 536, 729
myopathy, 707
oestrus cycle abnormalities in bitch, 579
primary, 535
secondary, 535
skin disorders, 202, 205, **894**, 913
thyroid biopsy, 538
treatment, 538
Hypotrichosis, 186, 873, 915
Hypovolaemic shock, 107, 108, 117, 119, 272, 273, 274, 278, 784
   gastric dilatation and volvulus, 414
   hypoadrenocorticism, 547, 548
Hypoxia, 87, 88, *89*, 118, 222, 259
   liver damage, 482
   seizures, 244

I
Ibuprofen, 44, 744
Ichthyosis, 202, 873, 902
Icteric mucous membranes, 44
Icterus *see* Jaundice
IgA deficiency, 424
Iliac thrombosis, 297, 298
Immune-mediated dacryoadenitis, 829
Immune-mediated disorders, 30, 31, 152
Immune-mediated haemolytic anaemia, 36, 114, 127, 128, 135, 303
Immune-mediated joint disease, 31, 109, 152, **750–5**, **757–8**
   drug treatment, *752*, 758
Immune-mediated skin disease, **897–901**, **914–15**
   treatment, 900–1, 914
Immune-mediated thrombocytopenia, 36, 164, **796–8**, *797*
Immunodeficiency, 31, 36–7
Immunostaining, 878–9
Immunosuppressive therapy
   autoimmune haemolytic anaemia, 787
   colitis, 435
   eosinophilic enteritis, 426
   glomerulonephropathy, 634
   immune-mediated skin disease, 900–1, 914
   immune-mediated thrombocytopenia, 797–8
   inflammatory bowel disease, 428
   jaundice, 135
   joint disease, 752, 754
   uveitis, 837
Imperforate anus, 66, 440
Implantation failure, 586, 592
Incretin effect, 512
Infection
   chronic cough, 94, 95, 96
   complicating chemotherapy, 1020
   control in veterinary premises, 938–9
   fever of unknown origin, 30–1, 36
   lymphadenopathy, 152, 154, 155
   pancreatitis, 504
   reactive hepatitis, 480
   specific of cat, **959–81**
   specific of dog, **921–54**
   vomiting, 42, 44

Infectious arthropathies, 736–49
Infectious canine hepatitis, 467, **930–2**, *931*
  chronic active hepatitis following, 468
  corneal opacities, 931, *931*, 932
  vaccination, 932
Infectious enteritis, 59, 61, 62, *939*, **939–41**
Infectious myocarditis, **298**
Infectious skin disease, **883–91, 907–12**
Infectious upper respiratory disease complex, **960–3**, *961*, *962*
Inflammatory bowel disease, 32, 59, 61, 425, *427*, **427–8**, 429
Inflammatory myositis, **704–7**
Inflammatory response, 779, 780
Infraspinatus contractures, 709
Initial problem list, **10–11**
Insect-mediated hypersensitivity, 891, 904
Inspection, 5
Instrumental learning, 1030
Insulin, 13, 450, 452, 499, 561
  fasting energy metabolism/hypermetabolism, 20
  plasma levels, 223
Insulin resistance, 567, *567*
Insulin therapy, 562, **564–5**
Insulin-induced hyperglycaemia, 566
Insulinoma, 23, 245, 403, **568–9**, 687, 688
Interleukin-1 (IL-1), 29
Intermediate (intergrade) cardiomyopathy, 296
Intermittent (undulating) fever, 29–30
Intersexuality, *576*, 582, 583, 585, 591, 592
Interstitial cell tumours, 598, 895
Interstitial fluid colloid osmotic (oncotic) pressure, 142
Intervertebral disc disease, 148, 239, 408, 505
  spinal cord disease, 681–2, *681*
Intervertebral joint pain, 212, *213*
Intestinal function, 58
Intestinal lesion biopsy, 64, 65, 379
Intestinal obstruction, 61, 62, **423–4**
Intestinal pseudo-obstruction, 423
Intracutaneous cornifying epithelioma, 893
Intradermal skin testing, 879–80, *880*
Intradural-extramedullary tumours, 683
Intrahepatic cholestasis, 127, 128
Intrahepatic portal vein hypoplasia, congenital, 456
Intramedullary tumours, 683
Intraocular haemorrhages, 772, 797, *798*, 848
Intraocular pressure measurement, 822
Intrapericardial cysts, 300
Intrapericardial neoplasms, 299–300
Intravenous urography, 148, 174, 183, 615, 641
Intrinsic factor, 400
Intussusception, 69, 371, 376, *423*
Inulin clearance, 616
Investigative tests, 10, 11
Iris bombé, 841, 842, *842*
Iris coloboma, 836
Iris cysts, 838, *838*, 861
Iris hypoplasia, 836

Iris sympathetic nerve supply lesions, 856–7
Iron deficiency anaemia, 116, 117, 149, 373, 784, 789–90, 807
Iron metabolism tests, 111–12, *111*
Iron serum level, 111
Ischaemic myelopathy (fibrocartilaginous embolism), 685
Ischaemic myopathy, 712
Ischaemic pancreatitis, 505
Islet-acinar portal system, 499
Isoimmune haemolytic anaemia, 787, 806
Isoimmune thrombocytopenia, 799
Isospora, 940, 980
Itraconazole, 350, 888
Ivermectin, 306, 307, 350, 359, 912

J
Jaundice, 8, **126–35**, 454–5, 461–2
  biliary tract rupture, 486
  bilirubinuria, 128–9
  cholangitis-cholecystitis, 484, 487
  chronic cholangiohepatitis, 488
  classification, 132–3
  clinical/laboratory features, 133–4
  history-taking, 133
  intravascular haemolysis, 109, 127, 128
  laboratory investigations, 128–32
  liver damage tests, 129–31
    cholestasis, 130–1
    hepatocellular injury, 130
  liver function tests, 131–2
  management, 134–5
Joint disease, 719, **740–58**
  cats, **755–8**
  classification, *741*
  degenerative, 741–6, 755–6
  dogs, **741–55**
  history-taking, 723–4
  inflammatory, 746–55, 756–7
    immune-mediated, 750–5, 757–8
    infectious, 736–49
  investigative techniques, 725–7
  physical examination, 724–5
  traumatic, 741
Joint neoplasia, 755
Joint pain, 207, **208–14**
Joint scintigraphy, 212–13
Joints, **721–3**, *722*
Juvenile cellulitis, 900, *900*

K
Kaolin, 50
Kennel cough *see* Contagious canine respiratory disease
Keratinization defects, *201*, 202, 206, **901–2**
Keratinocytes, 871, 872
Keratitis, **832–4**
Keratoconjunctivitis, 123
Keratoconjunctivitis sicca, 435, 828–9, *828*, 860
Ketoconazole, 349, 350, 559–60, 647, 888, 889, 910, 911
Kidney, **612–13**, *613*
Klebsiella sp., 179, 403, 1020

L
Labrador retriever myopathy, 699–701, *700*
Lacrimal disorders, 828–9
Lactate dehydrogenase (LDH), 130, 217, 259, 463
Lactose intolerance, 61, 419
Lameness, 207, 208, 214, 724, 742, 755, 756
Langerhans cells, 767, 871, 872
Laplace's law, 272, 275
Laryngeal collapse, 353
Laryngeal disorders, **352–3**
Laryngeal function tests, 352
Laryngeal neoplasia, 54, 353
Laryngeal obstruction, 345, 352, 353
Laryngeal oedema, 118
Laryngeal paralysis, 54, 118, 221, 352–3, 690
Laryngeal stenosis, 353
Laryngitis, 352
Laryngoscopy, 56, 91
Larynx, 51, **351–2**
  diagnostic procedures, 352
  inspection, 346
Lead poisoning, 62, 116, 245, 246, 681
Learning, 1029–31
Legs examination, 8
Leishmania donovani, 889, 950
Leishmaniasis, 36, 152, 154, 203, 205, 749, 888–9, **950–2**, *951*, *951*
  treatment, 951–2
Lens, 842–3, *843*
Lens disorders, 842, **843–6**, 863
Lens luxation, 842, 843–4, *843*, 863
Leptospira canicola, 933, *934*
Leptospira grippotyphosa, 933
Leptospira icterohaemorrhagiae, 933, *934*, *934*, 935
Leptospira interrogans, 932
Leptospirosis, 678, 705, **932–5**, *934*, 944, 979
  treatment, 623, 934
  vaccination, 934
Lethal acrodermatitis, 202, 902
Leucocyte abnormalities, 790, 807
Leucocytes, 767, 768, 778–9
  reference ranges, *775*
Leucocytosis, 778–9
Leucopenia, 779
Leucotrichia, 189
Leukaemia, 791, 1009, **1012–13**
  acute lymphoblastic, 795, 809, 1013
  acute monocytic, 791
  acute myeloid (granulocytic), 791, 808, 968, 1013
  acute myelomonocytic, 791, 808, 1013
  aleukaemic (smouldering), 791
  basophilic, 794
  chronic granulocytic, 792, 808, 1013
  chronic lymphocytic, 795, 809
  cytotoxic chemotherapy, 1013–15, *1013*, *1014*
  feline leukaemia virus-associated, 968
  lymphocytic/lymphoid, 794–5, 809, 968
  megakaryoblastic, 791, 808

Leukaemoid reaction, 779
Leukodystrophy, 674
Leukoencephalomyelopathy, 674
Levamisole, 306, 307
Levothyroxine, 331, 538
Libido impairment, 596, 602
Lignocaine, 335–6
Lincomycin, 193, 977
Linear (string) foreign body, 8, 383, 424
Linguatula serrata rhinitis, 350
Lipase, 139, 506, 507
Lipid keratopathy, 835
Lipid metabolism, 20, 58, 450, *451*, 561
Lipoma, 683
Liposarcoma, 683, 724
Lips examination, 5
Lissencephaly, 245
Liver, **448–51**
   biliary tree anatomy, 448
   bilirubin metabolism, 126
   blood supply, 448–9
   detoxifying functions in cats, 487
   microanatomy, 449–50, *449*, *450*
   physiology, 450–1, *451*, 487
Liver biopsy
   hepatocellular (intrahepatic) jaundice, 134
   Menghini technique, 465–6
   portosystemic shunt localization, 473
   reactive hepatitis, 480
Liver damage assessment, 129–31
Liver disease, 32, 44, 46, 72, 78, **448–91**
   anaesthetic regimens, 460
   ascites, 456
   biopsy, 465–6
   blood coagulopathy, 460–1, 801
   cats, **486–91**
   cholestasis, 452–5
   dogs, **467–83**
   fine needle aspiration, 466
   gastritis/gastric ulceration, 403, 408
   history-taking, 461
   hypokalaemia, 459, *459*
   imaging techniques, 466
   laboratory investigations, 462–6
   laparoscopy, 466
   physical examination, 461–2
   portal hypertension, 455, 456
   systemic disease-associated, 479–83, 489–91
Liver enzymes, **462–3**
   anticonvulsant medication effects, 247
   ascites, 139
   cholestasis, 130–1
   hepatocellular injury, 130
   pancreatitis, 506
   peripheral oedema, 144
Liver function tests, 131–2
Liver tumours, 76, 456, **477–9**, *479*, 491
Local excision (excisional biopsy), 997, *997*
Loperamide, 419, 428, 431, 435
Lower motor neurone (LMN) lesions, 236, 238, 239, *239*, 664, 665–6, *666*, 667
Lower oesophageal sphincter, 51–2

Lower respiratory tract disease, **355–62**
   diagnostic procedures, **353–5**
   drug treatment, *362*
Lumbosacral stenosis/compression, 686
Lung contusion, 360
Lung neoplasia, 89, 94, 96
Lung sounds, 90, 95–6
Lungworms, 94, 95, 97, 354
Luteinizing hormone (LH), 527, 577, 589
   male reproductive functions, 595, *596*, 602
Lyme disease, 36, 214, 230, 678, 724, 757, **948–9**
   diagnosis, 749, 948–9
   joint involvement, 748–9, 948
   treatment, 749, 949
Lymph node biopsy, 159
Lymph node metastases, 152, 153, 158, *158*
   TNM staging, 991, *991*, *992*
Lymph nodes, 151, 768
Lymphadenopathy, 84, **151–9**, 772
   causes, 152–3, *153*
   fine needle lymph node aspiration (FNA), 154–5, *155*, 775
   investigations, 156–9
   management, 159
Lymphangiectasia, 61, 427, *430*, **430–1**
Lymphangiography, 145, 159
Lymphocytes, 37, 768
   response to disease, 779–80
Lymphocytic cholangitis, progressive, 130, 132, 135
Lymphocytic thyroditis, 535
Lymphocytosis, 779–80
Lymphoid hyperplasia, 155, *156*
   of glans, 601
Lymphoid system, 768
Lymphoma, 36, 44, 76, 109, 152, 153, 687, 1009
   anatomic forms, *1009*
   bone marrow aspiration, 159
   cytotoxic chemotherapy, 1011–12, *1011*, *1012*
   diagnostic investigations, 158–9, *1010*, 1011
   liver, 479, *479*, 491
   lymph node cytology, 155–6, *156*
      grading classification, 156, *157*, 158
   multicentric, 1009–10, *1010*
   reactive hepatitis, 480
   staging, *1009*
   see also Lymphosarcoma
Lymphopenia, 780
Lymphoproliferative disease, 108, 109, **794–6**, 799, 809, 1009
   cytotoxic chemotherapy, **1009–16**
Lymphosarcoma, 55, *366*, 395, 427, 683, 724, 755, 775
   colon, 438
   eye, 858, 863
   feline leukaemia virus-association, 967–8, *967*
   intestine, 373, 431, 432, *432*
   multicentric, **794**, 809, 967

   pericardial effusion, 300
   see also Lymphoma
Lymphoscintigraphy, 159
Lynxacarus radovsky, 912
Lysosomal storage disease, 674

M
α-Macroglobulins, 503, *503*, 771
Macropalpebral fissure, 825
Macrophages, 767–8
Magnetic resonance imaging
   brain lesions, 671
   consciousness level alteration, 251
   eye disease, 823
   head and neck disorders, 57
   micturition abnormalities/urinary incontinence, 175
   muscle pain, 216
   seizures, 247
   spinal lesions, 240–41
Maintenance energy requirement (MER), 18, 26–7
Malabsorption, 61, 62, 63, 425, 427, 431, 512
Malabsorption tests, 374
Malassezia dermatitis, 194, 196, 198, 199, 200, 202, **888**
Malassezia pachydermatis, 198, 202, 203, 205, 876
Male pseudohermaphrodites, 582, 591, 592
Male reproductive disorders, **594–604**
   dog, 595–602
   history-taking, 594
   investigative techniques, 595
   physical examination, 594
   tom, 602–4
Malignant histiocytosis, 755
Malignant hyperthermia, 30, 703, **708**, 714
Mammary gland disease, 588–9, 594
Mammary glands, 575
Mammary tumours, 589
Mandibular fracture, 14, 15, 208
Mannitol, 75, 622
Mast cell neoplasia, 873, 891–2, 913, 1004
   adjuvant chemotherapy, 1017–18
   gastritis/gastric ulceration, 403, 408
   hyperhistaminaemia, 996, *996*
Master problem list, 11
Masticatory muscle myositis, 208, 689–90, 706
Mastitis, 588, 594
Maxillary sinuses, 83, 347
Meal-induced thermogenesis, 27
Mean cell haemoglobin concentration (MCHC), 110
Mean cell volume (MCV), 110
Mean electrical axis (MEA), 259, *260*
Mediastinal disease, **362–7**
Mediastinal neoplasia, 363–4
Medulloblastoma, 677
Megacolon, 66, 67, 433, **436–8**, *437*
Megakaryoblasts, 162
Megakaryocytes, 162, 768
Megaloblastic anaemia, 116, 790, 807

Megaoesophagus, 52, 55, 56, 377, *389*, **389–91**, 689, 696, 699, 700, 707
  with pyloric dysfunction in cats, 413
  radiological examination, 390, *390*
Meglumine antimonate, 889, 952
Megoestrol acetate, 16, 24, 384, 549, 905, 1035, 1040
Melaena, 43–4, 108, 149, 164, 373, 406, 407, 410, 624, 625, 771
Melanocyte-stimulating hormone, 527
Melanocytes, 871
Melanoma, 385, 836
Melphalan, 796, 1016, **1024**
Ménétrière's disease, 406
Meningioma, 244, 676, *676*, 677, 683
Meningitis, 239, 246, 677–8, 685–6
  idiopathic, 679
Meningocele, 683
Meningomyelocele, 683
Mercaptopurine, **1024**
Mercury toxicity, 245
Mesodermal dysgenesis, 836
Metabolic bone disease, 727
  chronic renal failure, 625–6, *625*
  hyperparathyroidism, **729–32**, *730*, *731*
Metabolic brain disease, 249–50, 675–6
Metabolic epidermal necrosis, 203, 204, 205
Metabolic myopathies, **707–9**
Metacarpo(tarso)-phalangeal/interphalangeal joint pain, 208, *210*
Metaldehyde toxicity, 245, 246, 681
Metallosis of bone, 734
Metaphyseal osteopathy, 32, 362, 735–6, *736*
Methaemoglobinaemia, 119, 120
Methotrexate, 116, **1024**
Methylene blue, 121, 806
Methylprednisolone, 682, 900
Metoclopramide, 49–50, 380, 391, 394, 404, 409, 412, 431, 623
Metronidazole, 135, 422, 425, 428, 518, 681, 733, 977, 978
Microangiopathic (fragmentation) haemolytic anaemia, 114, 788, 806
Microphthalmos, 823, *823*
Microsporum canis, 876, 887, 909, 910, *910*
Microsporum persicolor, 203, 909–10
Micturition, 168
  inappropriate, 1039–40
Micturition abnormalities, **168–75**, 177, **649–53**
  causes, *169*, *650*
  diagnosis, 652–3
  drug treatment, *652*
  drug trial, 175
  history-taking, 171–2, 649–50
  laboratory investigations, 173–4
  management, 653
  pathophysiology, 168–70, 650–2
  physical examination, 172–3, 650
Miliary (papular) dermatitis, 196, 903
Milk allergy, 419
Mineralocorticoids, 544
Minute ventilation, 87
Mitochondrial myopathies, 701–2

Mitotane, 531, 557–9, 560
Mitotane-induced adrenocortical necrosis, 546
Mitral valve endocardiosis, 102, 104, 273, 279, 281, 282
Mitral valve incompetence, 102, 104, 277
Monocytes, 767–8
Monocytosis, 779, 780
Monoplegia/paresis, 236, 667–8
Monorchidism, 597, 603
Morphine, 118, 298
Motilin, 412
Motilin agonists, 404
Motility modifying anti-diarrhoeal drugs, 419, *419*, 428, 439
Motor neuronopathies, 687
Mucopolysaccharidoses, 674, 729, 739
Mucosal protectants, 404
Multidrug resistance, 1018
Multilobular osteoma, 733
Multiple cartilaginous bone disease, 729, 734
Multiple enchondromatosis, 728
Muscle atrophy, 724
Muscle biopsy, 217, 224, 239, 697–8
Muscle diseases, **695–714**
  acquired
    cat, 712–14
    dog, *704*, 704–10
  congenital
    cat, *710*, **710–11**
    dog, *698*, **698–704**
  degenerative, 686–7
  history-taking, 696
  investigative techniques, 697–8
  physical examination, 696–7
Muscle pain, 207, *216*, **216–17**
Muscle trauma, 216, 709
Muscle tumours, 709
Muscular dystrophy, 686, 698–9, 711
Myasthenia gravis, 54, 56, 118, 120, 223, **688–9**, *689*, 696
  acquired, 707, 712
  anti-acetylcholine receptor antibodies, 57, 689
  congenital, 702, 711
  Tensilon (Camsilon) test, 57, 689, 697, 702, 707
  treatment, 689
Mycetoma, 888, 911
Mycobacterial infections, **949–50**, **978–9**
  lymphadenopathy, 152, 154, 155
  skin, **886–7**, 907–8
  treatment, *887*, 908
Mycobacterium avium-intracellulare, 950
Mycobacterium bovis, 907, 950, 978
Mycobacterium chelonei, 886, 908, 950, 978
Mycobacterium fortuitum, 886, 908, 950, 978
Mycobacterium lepraemurium, 908, 978
Mycobacterium phlei, 886, 908, 978
Mycobacterium smegmatis, 886, 908, 978
Mycobacterium tuberculosis, 749, 907, 949, 978
Mycoplasma, 749, 944, 961, 979

  arthritis, 749, 757
  conjunctivitis, 860
  subcutaneous abscess, 907
Mycotic encephalitis, 246
Mycotic infections, 30, 36
Mydriatics, 837–8
Myelocele, 683
Myelodysplasia, 791, 793–4, 808
Myelofibrosis, 793, 1009
Myelography, 175, 239, 683
Myeloid metaplasia, 152
Myeloma, 36, 76, 683, 775, 795–6, 809, 852, 1009, *1015*, **1015–16**
  Bence–Jones proteinuria, 76, 617, 1015
  cytotoxic chemotherapy, 1016, *1016*
Myelophthisis, 789
Myeloproliferative disease, 108, 109, 775, 779, 799, 800
  acute, 791–2
  cat, 807–8
  chronic, 792
  classification, 791, *791*
  cytotoxic chemotherapy, 1009–6
  dog, 790–2
Myocardial disease, 117, 284
  primary
    cat, **291–8**
    dog, **284–9**
  secondary
    cat, **298–9**
    dog, **289–91**
Myocardial fibrosis, 274, 278
Myocarditis, **289–90**
  infectious, 298
Myoclonus, familial of Labrador retrievers, 690
Myoglobinuria, 176, 618, 708, 709
Myopathy, 54, 55, 56, 216, 667
  endocrine disease-associated, 707
  falling cavaliers, 703
  hereditary of Devon rex cats, 710–11
  hypothyroidism, 536
  metabolic, 707–9
  nutritional, 704, 712
  type II, 219
Myositis, 54, 55, 56, 148
  inflammatory, **704–7**
  masticatory muscles, 208, 689–90, 706
Myositis ossificans, 709, 713
Myotonia, 551–2, 686–7, 701, *701*, 711

N

Narcolepsy, 219, 680
Nares examination, 5, 346
Nasal anatomy, 82
Nasal aspergillosis, 83, 84, 85, 347, 349–50, *349*
Nasal cavity diagnostic procedures, 347–8
Nasal discharge, persistent, **82–6**, 351
  history-taking, 83
  investigations, 84–6, 348
  physical examination, 83–4, 347
Nasal flush, 85
Nasal mucociliary clearance, 82
Nasal neoplasia, 83, 84, 85, 347, 348, *350*, **350–1**, 1004

Nasal tissue biopsy, 85–6, 348
Nasolacrimal system disorders, 829
Nasopharyngeal disorders, 54
Nasopharyngeal polyps, 83, 85, 351, **385**
Nasopharynx, 51
    diagnostic procedures, 347–8
    examination, 382, 383
Natriuretic factors, 72
Neck examination, 8
Necrolytic migratory erythema (hepatocutaneous syndrome), 901
Nemaline myopathy, 711
Nematodes (roundworms), 421
Neomycin, 135
Neonatal infections, 944–7, *945*
Neoplastic transformation, 985–6
Neorickettsia helminthoeca, 953
Neosporosis, 230, 244, 289, 678, 688, **953**
    myositis, 705–6, *706*, 714, 953
Nephrogenic diabetes insipidus, 74, 532, 534, **634**
    laboratory investigations, 80–1, 533, *533*, *615*
Nerve conduction studies, 224, 239, 674
Nerve sheath tumours, 683, *683*, 687–8
Neuroaxonal dystrophy, 674
Neuroepithelioma, 683
Neurogenic dermatitis (psychogenic alopecia), 906–7, *907*
Neurological disease, **662–91**
    brain, **674–81**
    causes, *671*
    diagnostic investigations, 668–71, 673
    micturition abnormalities, 173
    multifocal, 691
    muscle/neuromuscular junction, **686–91**
    neurological examination, 662–4
    peripheral nervous system, **686–91**
    spinal cord, **681–6**
Neurological examination, 662–4, *662*, 696
    cranial nerve tests, *663*
Neurological syndromes, **664–8**
    head, 664–5
    spine, 665–7
Neuromuscular disorders, 67, 118
    dysphagia, 54, 55
Neuromuscular junction disorders, 667
Neuronal degeneration, 245
Neuro-ophthalmology, **855–8, 865–6**
Neuropathic arthritis (Charcot's joints), 756
Neuropeptide Y, 499
Neurotransmitters
    food intake regulation, 13
    hepatic encephalopathy pathogenesis, 457–8
    seizure activity, 242
Neurotrophic keratitis, 834
Neutropenia, 779
    complicating chemotherapy, 1019, 1020
Neutrophil function tests, 37
Neutrophils, 767, 779
Nitrates, 119
Nitric oxide, 400
Nitrites, 119
Nitroglycerine, 287, 293

Nocardiosis, 152, 155, 366, 734, 887, 907, **949**, 977
Nocturia, 74–5, 168
Non-steroidal anti-inflammatory drugs, 37–8, 44, 150, 164, 167, 207, 487, 756
    gastric dilation and volvulus, 415
    gastric effects, 401, **403**, **407–8**
    osteoarthritis, 743–4, 756
    platelet effects, 800
    uveitis, 837
Non-suppurative polioencephalomyelitis, 244
Non-ulcerative keratitis, 834
Noradrenaline, 28, 29, 458
Notoedres cati, 903, 911
Notoedric mange, 911–12
Nuclear sclerosis, 846
5'-Nucleotidase, 463
Nutritional bone disease, 729–31
Nutritional dermatoses, 203, 204
Nutritional myopathy, 704, 712
Nutritional retinal degeneration, 864, *865*
Nutritional support, 21
Nystagmus, 233, 235, **857**, *858*

O

Obesity, 16, 17, 18, **22–7**, 308, 504
    causes, 22–4, *22*, *23*
    complicated, *23*
    genetic factors, 22
    history-taking, 25
    management, 26–7, *26*
    physical examination, 25–6
Obstructive (posthepatic) jaundice, 132, 133, 134
Obstructive pulmonary disease, chronic, 9, 219, 274, 303
Obstructive uropathy, 178, 185
Ocular melanocytosis, 842
Oesophageal biopsy, 57
Oesophageal disease, **389–98**
Oesophageal diverticula, 56, 395–6, *396*
Oesophageal fistulae, 397
Oesophageal motility disorders, 396–7
Oesophageal neoplasia, 396
Oesophageal perforation, 392–3
Oesophageal stricture, 54, **394–5**, *395*
Oesophagitis, 14, 52, 54, *393*, **393–4**, *394*
    with pyloric dysfunction in cats, 413
Oesophagus
    anatomy, 51
    endoscopy, 379–80
    radiography, 46, 377
    swallowing physiology, 51–2
Oestrogen, 13, 164, 577, 580, 646, 789, 798
Oestrogen-responsive alopecia, 896
Oestrus cycle
    abnormalities in bitch, 579–80
    abnormalities in queen, 589–91
    endocrinology
        bitch, 577, *578*
        queen, 589, *590*
    hypothyroidism-associated abnormalities in bitch, 579
    investigative techniques, 575–6, *576*, *577*

    mammary changes, 575
    ovarian changes in bitch, 581
    vulval changes, 574
Oestrus induction, 579, 590
Oligospermia, 596
Ollulanus tricuspis, 407
Olsalazine, 435
Omeprazole, 405, 406, 623, 629
Oncogenes, 985
Ondansetron, 404
One stage prothrombin time (OSPT), 166, 183
Onion toxicity, 119
Ophthalmia neonatorum, 825
Ophthalmological examination, **821–2**
    haematological disorders, 772
Ophthalmoscopy, direct/indirect, 821, *821*
Optic atrophy, 854
Optic disc, 848
Optic disc disorders, 854
Optic nerve disorders, 854
Optic nerve hypoplasia, 854
Optic nerve neoplasms, 854
Optic neuritis, 854
Oral cavity
    physical examination, 8, 382, 383
    radiological examination, 376
Oral neoplasia, 384–5, 1004, *1004*
Oral protectants, 50
Oral squamous cell carcinoma, 385
Oral trauma, 384
Oral ulceration, 625
Orchitis, 597, 603
Organophosphate toxicity, 55, 245, 246, 681, 690
Oropharyngeal disease, 14, 15, 376, **382–7**
Oropharynx, 51
Orthopaedic examination, 724–5
Os penis disorders, 600, 601, 603
Osetochondrodysplasias, 730
Osteoarthritis, 24, 724, 747
    cat, **755–6**
    dog, **741–6**, *742*
    radiological features, 742, *742*
    treatment, 742–6, 756
        anti-inflammatory drugs, 743–6, *745*, 756
        surgery, 746
Osteochondrodysplasias, 728–9
Osteochondroma, 740
Osteochondrosis, 207, 724
Osteoclastoma (giant cell tumour), 724
Osteoma, 733
Osteomyelitis, 215, 216
    bacterial, 732–3, *732*
    mycotic, 734
Osteosarcoma, 683, 689, 724, 725, 740, 755
    adjuvant chemotherapy, 1016–17, *1017*
Otodectes cynotis, 194, 195, 876, 903, 904
Otodectic mange, 904
Ovarian agenesis, 581, 591
Ovarian cysts, 581–2, 591
Ovarian disease, 581–2, 591
Ovarian tumours, 582, 591
Ovaries, 581, 591
Overexcitement, 1039

Overfeeding, 16, 17
Overhydration, 70, 267
Overnutrition bone disease, 730–1
Ovulation, 577, 589
Ovulation failure, 580, 590
Ovulation induction, 580, 590
Oxygen transport, 88, 766
Oxygen-haemoglobin dissociation curve, 88
Oxytetracycline, 425, 518, 749, 963
Oxytocin, 527

P
P-glycoprotein, 1018
Pacemaker implantation, 329, 330
Packed cell volume (PCV), 109, 110, 775, 783
Palate disorders, 385–6
Pallor of mucous membranes, **107–17**, 220, 771
    anaemia *see* Anaemia
    cardiovascular causes, 117
Pancreas
    anatomy, *498*, **498–9**
        endocrine pancreas, 561
    biochemistry, 499–500
        zymogen activation, 500, *500*
    endocrine disorders, **561–9**
    exocrine disorders, **498–519**
    exocrine secretory physiology, 501
    exocrine secretory proteins, 58, 499, *499*
    neurohumeral regulation, 499
Pancreatic acinar atrophy, 509–10, 513
Pancreatic adenocarcinoma, 130, 518–19
Pancreatic duct, 498
Pancreatic duct obstruction, 504–5
Pancreatic flukes in cats, 519
Pancreatic ischaemia, 505
Pancreatic islets, **560**, **561**
    islet-acinar portal system, 499
Pancreatic polypeptide, 561
Pancreatic secretory trypsin inhibitor, 500, *500*
Pancreatitis, 24, 44, 46, **501–9**
    acute, 147, *148*, 149, 303, 408, 501
    aetiology, 504–5
    in cats, 502
    chronic, 501, 502, 510
    classification, *501*
    clinical signs, 505–6
    diagnosis, 505–8
    hereditary factors, 505
    history-taking, 505–6
    laboratory investigations, 506–8
    pancreatic enzyme levels, 506–7, *507*
    pathophysiology, 502–4, *502*, *503*
    radiographic signs, 506
    treatment, 508–9
Panosteitis, 32, 208, 215, 737, *737*
Papilloedema, 854
Papillomatosis, 947–8, *947*
Papular (miliary) dermatitis, 196, 903
Para-aminobenzoic acid (PABA) absorption test, 64
Paracetamol, 119, 120, 467

Paracetamol poisoning, 120, 121, 772, 788, 806
    treatment, 121–2
Paradoxical respiration, 88, 90, 95
Paradoxical vestibular syndrome, 234, 235
Paralysis, **236–41**
    clinical/neurological examination, 237–41
    definitions, 236
    diagnostic procedures, 239–41
    history-taking, 237
    localization of lesions, 236
    pathological lesions, 236–7
Paralytic ileus, 424
Paraneoplastic myopathy, 710
Paraneoplastic neuropathy, 688
Paraneoplastic syndromes, 362, 994, *994*, *995*
Paraoesophageal hiatal hernia, 397, 398
Paraphimosis, 601, 603
Paraplegia/paresis, 236, 238–9, *238*
Paraquat toxicity, 89, **361**
Parasitic disease
    brain involvement, 679
    chronic cough, 94, 95
    colitis, 433, 434
    diarrhoea, 59, 61, 63
    enteritis, 421–2
    eosinophilia, 780
    faecal flotation, 97
    gastritis, 407
    lower respiratory tract, 354, *359*, **359**
    rhinitis, 350
    skin disease, 889–91, 911–12
Parathyroid adenoma, 543, 731
Parathyroid carcinoma, 543
Parathyroid gland disorders, **542–4**
Parathyroid glands, 534, 541–2
Parathyroid hormone, 541, 542
    bone turnover, 720, *720*, 721
Paresis, 233–4, **236–41**
    clinical/neurological examination, 237–41
    definition, 236
    diagnostic procedures, 239–41
    history-taking, 237
    localization of lesions, 236
    pathological lesions, 236–7
Parosteal osteosarcoma, 740
Partial seizures, 243
Pasteurella, 907, 944, 977
Patellar luxation, 724, 725
Patent ductus arteriosus, 102, 103, 104, 105, 119, 220, 267, 274, 277, **310–12**
    echocardiography, 311
    electrocardiography, 310–11
    radiological examination, 311, *311*
Pectineus muscle hypotrophy, 704
Pectus excavatum, 89
Pelger–Hüet anomaly, 790
Peloderma strongyloides, 891
Pelvic fracture, 211
Pelvic nerve, 169
Pemphigus, 203, 897, *897*, 914
Penicillamine, 477

Penicillin, 623, 785, 887, 907, 934, 941, 949, 977, 978
Penicillium, 348, 349
Penile adhesions, 603
Penile disease, 600–2, 603–4
Penile frenulum, persistent, 600
Penile hypoplasia, 600, 603
Penile inflammation, 604
Penile lymphoid hyperplasia, 601
Penile neoplasms, 601, 604
Penis, 594, 597, 602
Pentosan polysulphate, 745
Pepsin, 400
Percussion, 9, 257
Perianal fistula, 440
Pericardial disease, 277, **299–303**
Pericardial effusion, 91, 117, 136, 274, 277, 278, **299–303**
    benign idiopathic, 299
    cat, 300
    causes, *300*
    clinical signs, 300–1
    dog, 299–300
    echocardiography, 301–2, *302*
    electrocardiography, 301
    examination of fluid, 302
    management, 302–3
    pericardiocentesis, 302
    pneumopericardiography, 301
    radiological findings, 301, *301*
Pericardial fibrosis (constrictive pericarditis), 300
Pericardial mesothelioma, primary, 300
Pericardiocentesis, 302
Pericarditis, 300
Perineal herniation, 66, 67, 68, 69
Periodontal disease, 152
Peri-oesophageal mass, 395
Periosteal proliferative polyarthritis, 757–8, *757*
Peripheral cyanosis, 119
Peripheral nerve biopsy, 239
Peripheral nerve disease, idiopathic, 690
Peripheral nerve disease, toxic, 690
Peripheral nerve trauma, 690
Peripheral nervous system disease, **686–91**
    degenerative, 686–7
    inflammatory, 688–90
    metabolic, 687
    neoplastic, 687–8
Peripheral neuromuscular system disorders, **667–8**
Peripheral oedema, **142–5**, *143*, 256, 632–3
    generalized, 142
    localized, 142–3
Peripheral vestibular disease, 680
Peritoneal dialysis, 508–9, 623
Peritoneal lavage, 381
Peritoneopericardial diaphragmatic hernia, congenital, 299, *299*
Pet-owner relationships, 1033
Petechial haemorrhage, 109, 164, 772, 797, *797*
Peyer's patches, 417, 428
Phaeochromocytoma, 30, 123, 308, 403, **560–1**

Phaeohyphomycosis, 911
Pharyngeal retching, 42, *43*
Pharyngitis, 383, 386
Pharynx
　anatomy, 51
　inspection, 346
Phenobarbitone, 16, 75, 116, 131, 247, 678, 680, 798, 929, 1034
Phenothiazines, 49, 247
Phenylbutazone, 44, 161, 167, 709, 744, 785, 789, 798, 800
Phenytoin, 16, 75, 116, 176, 247
Phimosis, 601, 603
Phobias, 1039
Phospholipase A_2, 506
Phthisi bulbi, 823, *824*
Physaloptera spp., 407
Physical examination, 4–5, 8–10, 24
　cat, 5, *6–7*
　check list, 5, *7*
　dog, 5, *6–7*
Physostigmine, 680
Pica, 16, 513, 771
Pigmentary keratitis, 834
Pilosebacious unit, 872–3, *873*
Pituitary disorders, **528–34**
Pituitary dwarfism *see* Hypopituitarism, congenital
Pituitary gland, 526–7
　anterior lobe, 526–7, *527*
　hormone release regulation, *526*, 527
　posterior lobe, 526, 527
Pituitary neoplasia, 531, 535, 550, 676
Placental retention, 587, 593
Placental site subinvolution, 588, 593
Plague, 979–80
Plasma cell myeloma, 724
Plasma cell pododermatitis, 914–15, *914*
Plasma colloid osmotic (oncotic) pressure, 142
Platelet abnormalities, **796–800**, 809
Platelet count, 166, *166*, 780–1
Platelet dysplasia, 800
Platelet factor 3, 160, 162, 768
Platelet factor 4, 160
Platelet function tests, 167, 781
Platelet-rich plasma transfusion, 798
Platelets, 768
　primary haemostasis, 160, 769
　production/release, 162, 768
　secondary haemostasis, 161
Pleural disease, **362–7**
　diagnostic procedures, 363
Pleural effusion, 91, 364–5, *365*
　dilated cardiomyopathy in cat, 292, 293
Pleural exudates, 365–6, *366*
Pleural fluid examination, 363
Pleural frictional sounds, 9
Pleural transudates, 365
Pleurisy, 148, 366, *366*
Pneumocystography, 174, 183
Pneumomediastinum, 363
Pneumonia, 92
Pneumonyssoides (Pneumonyssus) caninum rhinitis, 350
Pneumopericardiography, 301

Pneumothorax, 9, 91, 120, **364**
Pollakiuria, 168, 177, 613, 636, 643
Pollen allergy, 195
Polyarthritis, 148, 208, **211–12**, *213*, 724, 755, 757
　idiopathic canine, 36, **753–4**
Polycystic kidney disease, 178, 635–6
Polycythaemia, 119, 120, 123, **124–5**, 220, 244, 246, 308, **778**
　absolute, 124, 778
　relative, 124, 778
Polycythaemia vera (primary proliferative polycythaemia), 124, 778, **792–3**, *793*, 808
Polydipsia, **70–81**, 137, 143, 147, 461, 469, 472, 532, 551, 562, 619, 634
　causes, *73*
　differential diagnosis, *532*
　history-taking, 74–5
　laboratory investigations, 76–81, *79*
　physical examination, 75–6
Polymyopathy, 687, 712–13
Polymyositis, 216, 239, 704, 706–7, 714
Polyneuropathy, 667
　idiopathic, 689
Polyphagia, **16–17**, *17*, 61, 513, 551
Polyradiculoneuritis, 689
Polysulphated glycosaminoglycans, 745, 756
Polyuria, **70–81**, 137, 143, 532, 562, 613, 634
　acute renal failure, 621, 622, 623
　causes, *73*
　differential diagnosis, *532*
　history-taking, 74–5
　laboratory investigations, 76–81, *79*
　pathophysiology, 72, 74
　physical examination, 75–6
Porencephaly, 245
Portal hypertension, 278, 403, 455, 462
　arteriovenous fistula, 475
Portal vein hypoplasia, 470–1
Portal vein thrombosis, 456, **474–5**
Portography, 466, 473
Portosystemic shunts, 55, 76, 243, 245, 250, 456
　congenital, 471–3, *472*, 489
　shunt localization, 473, *473*, *474*
Positional strabismus, 233
Positive contrast urethrocystography, 174
Postpartum haemorrhage, 587, 593
Postpartum metritis, 587–8, 593
Postparturient disorders, 587–8, 593
Postural abnormalities, 724
Postvaccinal encephalitis, 936
Prazosin, 309, 325, 629
Prednisolone, 360, 409, 426, 428, 430, 469, 489, 518, 548, 549, 706, 744, 752, 754, 758, 787, 794, 795, 796, 797, 836, 900, 1008, 1016, **1025**
Pregnancy disorders, 586–7, 592–3
Pregnancy hypoglycaemia, 587
Preleukaemia, 791
Preload, 271–2
　heart failure, 273–4
Premature ovarian failure, 591
Prepubertal vaginitis, 584

Preputial adhesions, 603
Preputial discharge, 601–2
Preputial hair ring, 603–4
Preputial inflammation, 604
Priapism, 601, 603
Primidone, 16, 24, 75, 116, 131, 247, 798
Problem list, 10–11
Problem-oriented approach, 3, **4–12**
　assessment/progress notes, 12
　baseline information collection (database)
　　history, 4, *6*
　　physical examination, 4–5, *7*, 8–10
　discharge summary, 12
　initial problem list, 10–11
　plan formulation, 11
Problem-oriented veterinary medical records, 3
　baseline information collection (database), 4–5
Proctitis, 67, 439
Proctoscopy, 69
Progesterone, 577, 589
Progestogens, 16, 24, 485, 531, 580
Progress notes, **12**
Progressive retinal atrophy
　central (retinal pigment epithelial dystrophy), 850–1, *851*
　generalized, 850, *850*, *851*, 864, *865*
Prolactin, 527, 577, 589
　pseudopregnancy, 580, 581
Prolapsed globe, 825
Promegakaryocytes, 162
Propantheline bromide, 49, 175, 330
Propranolol, 288, 296, 333, 541, 629, 1034
Proprioception, 236
Proptosis, traumatic, 825
Prostate, 594, 597
　investigations, 174, 595
Prostate biopsy, 174
Prostate disease, 66, 69, 169, 171, 172, 174, 183, *183*, *184*, **599–600**, 603, **646–53**
Prostate gland infection, 183, 184
Prostate neoplasia, 174, 183, 600, *600*, 649
Prostatic abscess, 30, 648–9
Prostatic adenocarcinoma, **649**
Prostatic cysts, 600
Prostatic wash, 183, *183*, *184*, 614
Prostatitis, 76, 178, 599, **647–8**
α_1-Protease inhibitor, 503–4, *504*
Protein metabolism, 58, 561
　fasting energy metabolism/hypermetabolism, 20
Protein-losing enteropathy, 62, 143, 144, 145, 418, 427, **429–30**, *430*
Proteinuria, 149, 179, **617**
　acute renal failure, 619
　ascites, 139
　assessing significance, 77
　dirofilariasis, 305
　functional, 77
　glomerulonephropathy, 631, 633
　measurement, 617
　mechanisms, 76–7
　polyuria/polydipsia, 76
　tests, 76

Proteus, 179, 587, 641
Prothrombin time, 782, 800, 801
Protothecosis, 678, 980–1
Protozoal infection, **950–3**, 980
   brain disease, 678
   diarrhoea, 421–2
   myocarditis, 289
   myopathies, 705–6
   skin disease, 888–9
Protrusion of nictitating membrane-diarrhoea complex in cats, 420
Pruritus, 194–200, 202, 203, *874*, **874–5**
   alopecia, 188, 189, 190
   distribution patterns, *197*
   history-taking, 194–5
   laboratory investigations, 197–9
   management, 199–200
   physical examination, 195–6
   types of skin lesions, *196*, *197*
Pseudoanorexia, 14
Pseudocoprostasis, 436
Pseudomonas, 587
Pseudomonas aeruginosa, 282, 425, 602
Pseudopregnancy, 580–1, 588, 591, 594
Pseudorabies (Aujesky's disease), 678, 947, 976
Psychogenic alopecia (neurogenic dermatitis), 906–7, *907*
Psychogenic (primary) polydipsia, 74, 75
   laboratory investigations, 80, *615*
Psychogenic vomiting, 39
Ptyalism, 51, **52–7**, 384, 386
   clinical associations, *53*
   diagnostic approach, *54*
Pudendal nerve, 169
Puerperal tetany, 588, 593
Pug encephalitis, 679
Pulmonary contusion, 119, 120
Pulmonary diagnostic procedures, **353–5**
Pulmonary disease, 120
Pulmonary fibrosis, 9
Pulmonary function tests
   chronic cough, 97
   dyspnoea, 91
   lower respiratory tract disease, 355
Pulmonary haemorrhage, 360
Pulmonary hypertension, 119, 274
   congenital cardiac defects, 310, 316, 318, 320
Pulmonary neoplasia, **361–2**, *362*
Pulmonary oedema, 9, 105, 119, 256, 267, 277, **360–1**
   dilated cardiomyopathy, 285, 286
Pulmonary patterns, 267
Pulmonary scintigraphy, 355
Pulmonary stenosis, 103, 119, 259, 267, 274, 278, **314–16**, 317, 318
   angiocardiography, 315–16
   echocardiography, 315
   electrocardiography, 315
   radiological examination, 315, *315*
Pulmonary thromboembolism, 32, 92, 119, 267, 274, **362**
   cor pulmonale, 303
   glomerulonephropathy, 631, 632
   treatment, 304

Pulmonary vasculature assessment, 267
Pulse, 5
Pulse deficit, 8–9, 220
Pulse oximetry, 91, 97, 222
Pulsus paradoxus, 300
Punishment, 1030–1
Pupillary membrane, persistent, *823*, 836, 861
Pure red cell aplasia, 788, 806
Pyelonephritis, 30, 76, 78, 178, 183
Pyloric obstruction, 412–13
Pyloric stenosis, 42, 413
Pylorospasm, 413
Pylorus, 398
Pyoderma, 193, 195, 196, 200, 203
   deep, 885, *885*
   superficial
     dermatitis/folliculitis, 884, *884*
     pustular dermatitis, 884, *884*
   surface
     acute moist (pyotraumatic dermatitis), 883–4, *883*
     skin fold, 884
   treatment, 885–6, *886*
Pyogenic alopecia, 190
Pyometra, 75, 76, 78, 178, **582–3**, **591–2**, 779
Pyothorax, 30, 366, 779
Pyrantel, 421
Pyrethrin/pyrethroid toxicity, 55
Pyrexia *see* Fever
Pyridostigmine, 689, 702, 707, 712
Pyrimethamine, 705
Pyrogens, exogenous/endogenous, 29
Pythiosis, 888
Pyuria, 179–80

Q
Q fever, 981
Quadriceps contractures, 709
Quadriplegia/paresis, 236, 238, *238*
Quinidine, 325, 333, 785, 796

R
Rabies, 55, 244, **679**, **935–6**, 976
   neurological diseases, 678, 935
   vaccinal encephalitis, 936
   vaccination, 936, 976
Radioallergosorbent (RAST) test, 880
Radiography
   abdominal pain, 148
   alimentary tract disease, 376–7
   angiostrongylosis, 307
   aortic stenosis, 312, *313*
   ascites, 138
   atrial septal defect, 317
   bacterial endocarditis, 283
   bone pain, 214–15
   cardiac dysrhythmias, 229
   cardiac murmurs, 105
   cardiovascular disease, 261–2, 267–9
   chronic cough, 96
   collapse/episodic weakness, 222
   consciousness level alteration, 251
   cor pulmonale, 303
   cyanosis, 121

   defecatory tenesmus, 69
   dilated cardiomyopathy, 285, 292, *292*
   dirofilariasis (heartworm disease), 304–5, *305*
   discospondylitis, 748, *748*
   dyspnoea, 91
   endocardiosis, 281, *281*
   eye disease, 823
   female reproductive organs, 575
   haematological disorders, 775
   haematuria, 183
   hyperadrenocorticism, 554–5, *554*
   hypertrophic cardiomyopathy, 288, 294–5, *295*
   hypoadrenocorticism, 548
   intestinal obstruction, 424
   joint pain, 212–13
   larynx, 352
   lower respiratory tract, 353
   lymphadenopathy, 159
   mediastinal disease, 363
   megaoesophagus, 390, *390*
   micturition abnormalities/urinary incontinence, 173–4
   nasal cavity, 347
   nasopharynx, 347
   neurological disorders, 670–1
   oesophageal diverticuli, 396, *396*
   orthopaedic disorders, 725–6
   osteoarthritis, 742, *742*
   pancreatitis, 506
   patent ductus arteriosus, 311, *311*
   pericardial effusion, 301, *301*
   peripheral oedema, 144
   pleural disease, 363
   polycythaemia, 125
   polyuria/polydipsia, 78
   pulmonary oedema, 361
   pulmonary stenosis, 315, *315*
   restrictive cardiomyopathy, 297
   rheumatoid arthritis, 751, *751*
   seizures, 247
   spinal lesions, 237
   tetralogy of Fallot, 318, *319*
   upper airway assessment, 84–5
   urinary tract disease, 615
   urolithiasis, 182, 641
   ventricular septal defect, 316
   vomiting, 46–7
Radioisotope liver imaging, 466
Radiolabelled albumin excretion, 145
Radiosensitivity, 1000, 1001–2, *1002*
Radiotherapy, **999–1005**
   cell survival curve, 1000, *1000*
   fractionation, 1001, *1001*
   indications, 1004–5
   mode of action, 999
   techniques, 999–1000, *999*
   tissue effects, 1000–1
   toxicity to normal tissues, 1002–4
     acute reations, 1003, *1003*
     late reactions, 1003–4
   tumour response, 1001–2, *1002*
Rales (crackles), 9
Ranitidine, 50, 394, 405, 623, 629
Rapid gastric emptying, 412

Reactive arthritis, 754
Records, 3, 11, 12
Rectal agenesis, 440
Rectal cytology, 63
Rectal examination, 10
Rectal foreign body, 67, 69
Rectal neoplasia, 67
Rectal prolapse, 439
Rectal stricture, 439
Rectal temperature, 5
Rectal trauma, 67
Red cell antigens, 766–7
Red cell maturation defects, 789, 807
Red cell morphology, 775–6
  terminology, *776*
Red cell parameters, 775
Red cell parasites, 787–8
Red cell phosphofructokinase deficiency, 114, 788
Red cell pyruvate kinase deficiency, 114, 788
Red cells, 766
  response to disease, 777–8
Re-entry tachycardia, 330
Referred pain, 146, 147, 148, 208
Reflex dyssynergia, 175
Regenerative anaemias, *113*, **113–14**, 133, 373, 777, 784–8, 791, 792, 794, 805–6
Regurgitation, 39, 42, 51, **52–7**, 389, 390, 391, 396, 397
  causes, *43*
  clinical associations, *53*
  diagnostic approach, *54*
  oesophageal contrast radiography, 46
Reiter's syndrome, 754
Remittant (septic) fever, 30
Renal amyloidosis, 76, 178, 632, 634
Renal biopsy, 615, 621
Renal blood flow, 275
Renal concentrating mechanisms, 70, **71–2**
  impairment, *635*
Renal congenital defects, *635*, **635–6**
Renal cysts, 183
Renal dysplasia, 75, 635
Renal failure, acute, **619–23**
  causes, *620*
  management, 621–3
  urethral obstruction in cats, 644, 645
Renal failure, chronic, 44, 45, 62, 78, 108, 303, 619, **623–31**
  bone disease, 731, *731*
  causes, *624*
  clinical signs, *614*, 624
  diagnosis, 627
  drug dosage adjustment, 629, *630*, 631
  gastritis/gastric ulceration, 403, 408
  history-taking, 623–4
  hypertension, 274, 308
  hypoadrenocorticism, 547
  management, 627–31
    anaemia correction, 628
    antiemetics, 628–9
    antihypertensives, 629
    appetite enhancement, 628–9
    nutrition, 627–8, *627*
  transplantation, 631
  pancreatitis, 505
  pathophysiology, 624–6, *625*
  progression, 626, *626*
    monitoring, 629
  seizures (uraemic encephalopathy), 244
Renal function tests, 138, 618–19
Renal glycosuria, primary, 75
Renal hypoplasia, congenital, 76
Renal medullary washout, 72, 74
Renal neoplasia, 178, 183
Renal scintigraphy, 615, 617
Renal transplantation, 631
Renal tubular function, 72
Renin, 275, 544, 545, 613
Renin-angiotensin system, 72, 544–5
  acute renal failure, 620
  heart failure compensatory effects, 274–5
Renin-producing tumours, 308
Reperfusion injury
  acute renal failure, 621
  gastric dilation and volvulus, 415
Reproductive endocrinology
  dog, 595, *596*
  tom, 602
Reproductive system disorders, **574–604**
  female, **574–94**
  male, **594–604**
Respiratory centres, 87
Respiratory disease, **345–67**
  collapse/episodic weakness, 219, 220, 221, 222
  diagnostic approach, 347, *347*
  history-taking, 345
  physical examination, 345–7
  presenting signs, *346*
Respiratory distress, 87, *87*, 120, 220
Respiratory failure, 88, 345, 363
Respiratory rate, 5
Respiratory reserve capacity, 347
Respiratory sounds, 9, 104, 345, 346–7
Respiratory system examination, 9
Respiratory tract infection, 345
Response substitution, 1035
Restrictive cardiomyopathy, 296–7
Retained cartilaginous cores, 738, *738*
Reticulocyte counts, **110–11**, 776–7
Retinal degeneration, 864, *865*
Retinal detachment, 848, 853, *853*, *854*, 864
Retinal dysplasia, 848–50, *849*, 864
Retinal dystrophy/degeneration, inherited, 850–1
Retinal haemorrhages, 109, 164, 560, 772, 852, *864*, **864**
Retinal pigment epithelial dystrophy, 850–1, *851*
Retinal vascular abnormalities, 852
Retinal vasculature, 848
Retinopathy, hypertensive, 308
Retrograde urethrography, 183, 615, 641
Retropharyngeal abscess, 54, 55
Reverse sneezing, 82–3
Reverse T3 (rT3) serum level, 537
Rhabditic dermatitis, 891
Rhabdomyolysis, 76
Rhabdomyoma, 709
Rhabdomyosarcoma, 709
Rheumatoid arthritis, 36, **750–2**, *751*
Rheumatoid factor, 36, 727, 751
Rhinitis, **348–9**
  chronic, 351
  drug treatment, *351*
Rhinoscopy, 85
Rhinosporidium seeba rhinitis, 350
Rhinotomy, exploratory, 86
Rhodococcus sp., 977
Rickets, 730, *730*
Rickettsial disease, 678, **953–4**
Right aortic arch, persistent, **321**, 391, *392*
Rocky mountain spotted fever, 678, 679
Rotavirus, 420, 944, 973
Russell's viper venom time, 167

S
Salicylates, 126
Saliva production, 52
Salivary gland disease, 386–7
Salivary gland necrosis, 386
Salivary gland neoplasia, 386
Salivary mucocele, 386
Salmonella sp., 62, 149, 374, 418, 434, 754, 940, 944
  enteritis, 421, 940, 941, 973–4
Salmonella typhimurium, 940, 973
Salt retention, 275, 276
Sarcoptes scabiei, 194, 198, 876, 890
Sarcoptic mange, 890, *890*
Satiety, 13
Satiety centre, 13, 16, 24
Scabies, 194, 195, 198, 202, 203, 206
Scaling disorders, **201–6**
  histopathological features, *205*
  history-taking, 202–3
  laboratory investigations, 204–6
  management, 206, *206*
  pathophysiology, 201–2
  physical examination, 203–4
  symmetrical skin lesions, *204*
  trial therapy, 206
Scleral disorders, 836
Scleral neoplasia, 836
Scleritis, 836
Scorpion venom pancreatitis, 505
Scotty cramp, 690
Scrotal disease, 597–8
Seasonal dermatitis, 874
Seasonal flank alopecia, 189, 192, 897
Seasonal pruritus, 195
Sebaceous adenitis, 203
Sebaceous glands, 872–3
Seborrhoea, primary idiopathic, 202, 203
Secretin, 452, 501
Seizures, 220, **242–8**
  classification, 242–3
  definitions, 219
  extracranial causes, 243–4
  generalized, 243
  hepatic encephalopathy, 458
  history-taking, 245–6
  intracranial causes, 244–5

Seizures (cont.)
  partial, 243
  pathogenesis, 242
  physical examination, 246–7
  treatment, 247–8
Selective angiocardiography, 271
Semen analysis, 174, 595
Seminoma, 598
Semitendinosus fibrotic myopathy, 709
Sensory neuronopathies, 687
Septicaemia/bacteraemia, 152
  reactive hepatitis, 480
Serotonin, 13, 28, 29, 160, 399, 499
Sertoli cell tumour, 598, *598*, 895, 896
Sex hormone-related skin disease, 895–7, *895*
Shampoo treatments, *206*
Shigella sp., 754
Shock lung, 119, 120
Short bowel syndrome, 431
Shoulder joint pain, 208, *209*
Sialoadenitis, 386
Sialoliths, 386
Sick sinus syndrome, 219, 329, 330
Sinoatrial (SA) node, 255
Sinus arrhythmia, 256
Sinus bradycardia, 329
Sinus node dysfunction, 227, 228
Sinus tachycardia, 331
Sinusitis, chronic, 345, **351**
  Skeletal muscle, 695
  disorders *see* Muscle diseases
  fibre types, 695–6
  response to injury, 696
Skin, 201, 871–3
  examination, 189–90, 875
Skin biopsy, 191–2, 199, 205–6, 877, 878
Skin disease, **871–915**
  cat, **903–15**
  diagnostic procedures, 876–80
  dog, **880–902**
  genetic/congenital, 902, 915
  history-taking, 873–5, *874*
  hyperadrenocorticism, 552, *552*
  immune-mediated, 897–901, 914–15
  physical examination, 875
Skin impression/aspiration smears, 877
Skin infection, 186
  see also Pyoderma
Skin lesions, *196*, 875
Skin scrapings, 197–8, 204, 876
Skin tumours, **891–3**, *892*, *893*, *913*, **913–14**
Skin-associated lymphoid tissue (SALT), 872
Small intestinal absorptive/digestive processes, 416
Small intestinal bacterial overgrowth, 59, 61, 65, 373, 374, 381, **424–5**, 427
  exocrine pancreatic insufficiency, 511, 518
  microbiology, 425
  predisposing factors, 424–5
  short bowel syndrome, 431
  treatment, 425, 518

Small intestinal brush border enzymes, 381
Small intestinal disease, **416–32**
Small intestinal epithelium, 417, *417*
Small intestinal function tests, 64, 373, 374
Small intestinal motility, 417
Small intestinal motility disorders, 431
Small intestinal neoplasia, 431–2, *432*
Small intestinal permeability testing, 375–6, *375*, *376*
Small intestinal radiographic evaluation, 377
Small intestinal strangulation, 431
Smoke inhalation, 95
Sneezing, 82, 345
SOAP format for progress notes, 12
Social behaviour, 23, 1031–2, *1031*, *1032*
Sodium homeostasis, 70, 71, 72
Sodium nitroprusside, 324–5
Sodium restriction, 308
Sodium stibogluconate, 889, 952
Sodium sulphate, 121
Soft tissue sarcoma, 1017, *1017*
Somatostatin, 561
Sorbitol dehydrogenase, 463
Spermatic cord torsion, 598
Spermatocoele, 597–8
Spermatogenesis impairment, 596, 597, 602
Spina bifida, 683
Spinal cord disease, **681–6**
  anomalous, 683, 685
  cervical spine, 685–6
  degenerative, 681–3, 685, 686
  infectious, 684
  inflammatory, 684, 685–6
  lumbosacral spine, 686
  neoplasia, 683, *683*
  thoracolumbar spine, 686
  vascular, 685
  see also Spinal lesions
Spinal cord trauma, 684–5
Spinal cord tumours, 239, 683, *683*
Spinal dysraphism, 239, 683
Spinal lesions, 665–7
  localization, 665–6
  lower motor neurone (LMN) lesions, 664, 665–6, *666*
  severity assessment, 667
  upper motor neurone (UMN) lesions, 664, 665–6, *666*
  see also Spinal cord disease
Spinger spaniel rage syndrome, 680
Spirocera lupi, 396, 407, 738
Spironolactone, 141, 308, 323
Spleen, 768
Splenic torsion, 146
Splenomegaly, 109, 278, 462
Sporothrix schenkii, 888, 911
Sporotrichosis, 195, 911
Sprain injury, 741
Squamous cell carcinoma, skin, 893
Squamous prostatic metaplasia, 599
Staphylcoccus aureus, 282, 732, 907
Staphylococcal neonatal dermatitis, 946, *946*

Staphylococcus intermedius, 192–3, 198, 205, 641, 684, 875, 883, 885, 944
Staphylococcus sp., 34, 188, 484, 584, 592, 746, 748, 977
  enterotoxin, 403
  lymph node enlargement, 152
  urinary tract infection, 179
Status epilepticus, 242, 248
Stercobilin (urobilin), 126, 454
Stereotypies, 1034, 1035
Sterile pustular dermatoses, 899, *899*
Steroid hepatopathy, 481, *481*
Stifle joint pain, 211, *212*
Stillbirth, 944
Stomach
  contrast examination, 46, 377
  double contrast gastrogram, 47, *48*, 377
  endoscopy, 380, *380*, 381
  gastric mucosal barrier, 399
  gross anatomy, 398–9, *398*
  microscopic anatomy, 399, *399*
  motility, 399–400
Stomach decompression, 415
Stomatitis, 373, *383*, **383–4**
Storage diseases, 245, *672–3*, 674
Strabismus, **857**
Strain injury, 741
Stranguria, 168, 177, 178, 636, 643, 650
Streptococcus sp., 152, 358, 484, 584, 587, 592, 746, 907, 944, 977, **978**
  bacterial endocarditis, 282
Streptokinase, 298
Streptomycin, 135, 623, 934
Stress, 14, 1032, **1039–41**
  psychogenic (primary) polydipsia, 75
  urine glucose in cats, 77
Stress incontinence, 652
Stress leucogram, 779, 780
Stress testing, 222
Stridor, 90, 345
Stroke volume, 271
  heart failure, 272, 273
Struvite uroliths, 639, *639*, **641–2**
  feline lower urinary tract disease, 644, 645
Strychnine toxicity, 245
Stupor, 249, 250
Subcutaneous abscess, 907
Subcutaneous mycoses, 888, 911
Substance P, 499
Sucralfate, 404–5, 409
Sudden acquired retinal degeneration, 853
Sulphasalazine, 434–5
Sulphhaemoglobinaemia, 119
Sulphonamides, 119, 126, 135, 176, 193, 504, 785, 796, 798, 941, 953, 963, 979
Superficial bacterial dermatitis/folliculitis, 884–5, *884*, 907
Superficial keratitis, chronic (pannus), 834, *834*
Superficial lymph nodes examination, 8
Superficial pustular dermatitis, 884, *884*
Suppurative lymphadenitis, 152, 155

INDEX

Supraventricular tachyarrhythmias, **331–4**, *332*
   management, 332–4
Sustained (persistent) fever, 30
Swallowing, 51–2
   fluoroscopy, 56, 376–7
   phases, 51
   physiology, 51, 387
Sweat glands, 872–3
Swimmer puppies, 704
Symblepharon, 859
Sympathetic regulation
   cardiovascular system, 255–6
      heart failure, 274–5
   eye, 856
   fasting energy metabolism, 20
   pancreas, 499
   small intestine, 416
   stomach, 399, 400
   urinary continence, 168, 169
Synchisis scintillans, 847
Syncope, 108, 120, 220, 312, 315, 318, 336
   definition, 218
   prognosis, 223
Syneresis, 847
Synovial cell sarcoma, 755
Synovial fluid, 723
Synovial fluid analysis, 34, 283–4, *726*, **726**
Synovial joints, 721–3, *722*
Synovial membrane, 723
Synovial membrane biopsy, 214, 727
Systematic desensitization, 1036
Systemic lupus erythematosus, 31, 36, 109, **752–3**, 898, 914
Systemic mycoses, 888, 911
Systolic clicks, 258

T

T lymphocytes, **152**, 768
   epidermotropic, 872
   null cells, 152
   T helper (T_h) cells, 152
   T supressor (T_s) cells, 152
Tachycardia, **330–6**, 539, 772
   electrophysiological mechanisms, 330–1, *331*
Taenia spp., 421
Tamm–Horsfall mucoprotein, 617, 618
Tamoxifen, 596
Tapetal fundus, 847–8
Tarsal joint luxation/subluxation, 725
Tarsal joint pain, 211, *213*
Taurine deficiency
   dilated cardiomyopathy, 291, 292
   retinal degeneration, *864*, *865*
Taurine requirement in cats, 487
Tear overflow, 829, 860
^{99m}Technetium-labelled leucocyte scan, 37
Telogen defluxion (telogen effluvium), 188, 897
Temporomandibular joint pain, 14, 208, *208*
Tensilon (edrophonium chloride; Camsilon) test, 57, 223, 689, 697, 702, 707
Terbutaline, 331

Territorial scratching, 1034, 1041
Territorial urination, 1034, 1035, 1039–40
Testes, 596–7, 602
Testicular biopsy, 595
Testicular cysts, 597, *598*
Testicular degeneration, 603
Testicular disease, **597–8**, **603**
Testicular duct system aplasia, 599
Testicular function assessment, 595
Testicular tumours, 598, *598*, 603
   oestrogen-producing, 189, 192
Testosterone, 595, *596*, 602
Testosterone-responsive dermatoses, 896
Tetanus, 14, 688, **950**, 979
Tetracosatin test *see* Adrenocorticotrophic hormone (ACTH) stimulation test
Tetracycline, 135, 504, 907, 934, 941, 949, 954, 966
Tetralogy of Fallot, 105, 106, 119, 267, 278, 314, 316, **318–19**, 778
   electrocardiography, 318
   radiological examination, 318, *319*
Tetraparesis/plegia, 240, *240*
Therapeutic plan, 11
Thermoregulation, 28
Thiamine deficiency, 245, 246, 677
Thiazide diuretics, 504
Thioguanine, **1024**
Third eyelid (membrana nictitans) disorders, 829–30, *830*, 859, *859*
Third eyelid protrusion, 830, *831*, 859, *859*
Thirst, 71–2
Thirst centre, 71
Thoracic mass, 9
Thoracocentesis, 91, 363
Thoracotomy, exploratory, 363
Thorax examination, 8
Thrombin time (TT), 166–7, 782
Thrombocythaemia, essential, 794, 808
Thrombocytopenia, 109, 164, 166, 781, 796, 809, 993
   causes, *163*
   complicating chemotherapy, 1019
   immune-mediated, **796–8**, *797*
   pathogenesis, *797*
Thrombocytosis, 780–1
Thromboembolic disease, 120, 804, 810
Thrombolytic therapy, 298
Thrombopathia, inherited, 800
Thrombophlebitis, 119
Thromboxane A_2, 160, 631, 633, 768
Thymic tumours, 395, 689, 714, 967
Thymus, 768
Thyroid adenoma, 76, 298, 538
Thyroid atrophy, 535
Thyroid biopsy, 538
Thyroid carcinoma, 538
Thyroid function tests, 79, 106, 223, **536–8**, 540
Thyroid gland, 534–5, *534*
Thyroid gland disorders, **535–41**
Thyroid hormone-releasing hormone (TRH), 534
Thyroid hormone-releasing hormone (TRH) stimulation test, 537, *537*, 540

Thyroid hormones, 13, 534–5
   replacement therapy, 538
   role in metabolism, 535
Thyroid stimulating hormone (TSH), 527, 534
   canine hormone assay, 537–8
Thyroid stimulating hormone (TSH) stimulation test, 390, 537, *537*
Thyrotoxicosis *see* Hyperthyroidism
Thyroxine (T4), 13, 20, 126, 534, 535
Tick paralysis, 690
Tidal breathing flow-volume loop analysis, 352
Tissue plasminogen activator (t-PA), 298, 770
TNM staging, **989–92**, *990*, *991*
   lymph nodes, 991, *991*, *992*
   metastases, 991–2, *992*
   primary tumour, 990–1
Tonometry, 822
Tonsillar disease, 386
Tonsillar neoplasia, 95, 386
Tonsillitis, 386
Torovirus enteritis, 420, 973
Total hip replacement, 746
Total iron binding capacity (TIBC), 111
Total parenteral nutrition, 21
Total plasma protein (TPP) concentration, 109, 110, 783
   ascites, 138
   peripheral oedema, 144
Total red cell count, 109
   polycythaemia, 125
Total T3 serum level, 536–7
Total T4 serum level, 536, 540
Toxacara canis, 426, 945
Toxacara leonian, 421
Toxacara spp., 244, 421, 679
   reactive hepatitis, 480, 481
Toxic diarrhoea, 62
Toxic encephalopathy, 249–150
Toxic epidermal necrolysis, 899, 914
Toxic seizures, 245
Toxoplasmosis, 36, 56, 96, 97, 154, 230, 246, 289, 298, 300, 480, 587, 678, **679**, 688, 696, 945, 952, **952–3**, **980**
   diagnosis, 422, 952
   diarrhoea, 421–2
   myositis, 705, 714
   treatment, 705, 952–3
Tracheal collapse, 91, 94, 95, 96, 97, 118, 120, 353, **355–6**
Tracheal diagnostic procedures, 353–5
Tracheal foreign body, 118
Tracheobronchitis, infectious, **355**
Transcervical uterine canulation, 575
Transferrin, 111
Transferrin percentage saturation, 111, 784
Transitional cell carcinoma, 76
Transtracheal washes, 91, 97
Transudates
   ascites, 136, 139–40, *139*, *140*
   pleural effusions, 365, 366

Trauma
    alopecia, 186, 189, 193, 195, 198
        corneal injury, 834
        eyelid injury, 827
        globe injury, 835
        myocarditis, 289
        pancreatitis, 505
Trichiasis, 827
Trichinella, 705
Trichobezoars in cats, 410
Trichophyton mentagrophytes, 887, 909, *910*
Trichophyton spp., 909
Trichuris vulpis, 63, 68, 421, 433, 434
Tricuspid regurgitation, 317
Tricuspid valve dysplasia, 277–8, 320
Tricuspid valve endocardiosis, 279
Tricyclic antidepressants, 1034
Trigeminal nerve deficits, 54, 234
Trigeminal neuritis, 689
Triiodothyronine (T3), 20, 534, 535
Triiodothyronine (T3) suppression test, 540
Trimethoprim, 116, 638
Trimethoprim-sulfa, 422, 678
Trimethoprim-sulphadiazine, 184, 705, 785
Trimethoprim-sulphonamide, 508, 648
Trombicula autumnalis, 891
Trombiculidiasis, 891, 912
True hermaphrodites, 582, 585, 591
Trunk examination, 8
Trypanosoma, 230, 289
Trypsin, 500
Trypsin-like immunoreactivity (TLI), 63, 373, 506
        exocrine pancreatic insufficiency, 514–15, *514*
Trypsinogen, 500
Tryptophan, 13
Tuberculosis, 480, 738, 749, 949–50, 978–9
Tumour biology, 985–8
    benign/malignant behaviour, 987–8, *987*, *988*
    blood supply, 987
    cell heterogeneity, 986, 987
    growth kinetics, 986–7, *986*
Tumour biopsy, 989, *989*
Tumour lysis syndrome, 1019
Tumour necrosis factor (TNF), 29
Tumour suppressor genes, 985, 986
Tylosin, 425, 428, 430, 435, 518
Tyzzer's disease, 421, **979**

U
Ulcerative dermatitis with self-harm, 904
Ulcerative keratitis, 832–4, *832*, *833*
Ultrasonography
    abdominal pain, 149, *150*
    alimentary tract disease, 376
    ascites, 138
    defecatory tenesmus, 69
    diarrhoea, 64
    eye disease, 823
    female reproductive organs, 575
    haematuria, 183
    head and neck disorders, 56
    hepatocellular (intrahepatic) jaundice, 134
    hyperadrenocorticism, 555
    hyperparathyroidism, 543
    insulinoma, 569
    intestinal obstruction, *423*, 424
    intrathoracic masses, 56
    joint disorders, 213, 725
    liver disease, 466
    liver lymphoma, 479, *479*
    mediastinal disease, 363
    micturition abnormalities/urinary incontinence, 173–4
    pancreatitis, 506
    peripheral oedema, 144
    pleural disease, 363
    polyuria/polydipsia, 79
    portosystemic shunt localization, 473, *474*
    seizures, 247
    urinary tract disease, 615
    urolithiasis, 641
Uncinaria stenocephala, 421
Upper airway obstruction, 9, 120, 121, 221
Upper gastrointestinal tract endoscopy, 379–81
Upper motor neurone (UMN) lesions, 664, 665–6, *666*, *667*
Uraemic breath, 619, 624
Ureaplasma, 754
Urease activity test, 381
Ureteral calculi, 178
Ureteral ectopia, 171
Ureteral obstruction, 147
Ureteral rupture, 183
Ureters, 612
Urethral catheterization, 173
Urethral function, 168, 169
Urethral malignancy, 171, 172
Urethral obstruction in cats, 643–6, *644*
Urethral plug, 185, 644, 646
Urethral pressure profilometry, 175
Urethral prolapse, 601, *601*
Urethral rupture, 172, 183
Urethral sphincter incompetence, 171, 172, 650
Urethral stricture, 172
Urethral tumours, 183
Urge incontinence, 652
Urinalysis, **617**
    abdominal pain, 149
    acute renal failure, 619, 621
    alopecia with endocrinopathy, 192
    ascites, 139
    bacterial endocarditis, 283
    chronic renal failure, 627
    diarrhoea, 63
    feline lower urinary tract disease, 644–5
    haematological disorders, 784
    haematuria, 178–9
    lymphadenopathy, 158–9
    micturition abnormalities/urinary incontinence, 173
    peripheral oedema, 144
    polyuria/polydipsia, 76–8
    seizures, 246
    vomiting, 45
Urinary casts (cylinduria), 180–1, *181*, 618
Urinary continence, 168
Urinary corticoids/creatine ratio, 556
Urinary incontinence, **168–75**, 177
    causes, *170*, 651–2
    drug trial, 175
    history-taking, 171–2
    laboratory investigations, 173–4
    neurogenic/non-neurogenic, 170, 651
    overflow, 170
    paradoxical/obstructive, 170
    physical examination, 172–3
    polyuria/polydipsia, 74–5
Urinary tenesmus, 66
Urinary tract disease, **612–53**
    clinical signs, *613*
    history-taking, 613–14
    imaging, 615–16
    investigative techniques, 614–19
    laboratory investigations, 616–19
    physical examination, 614
    see also Feline lower urinary tract disease
Urinary tract infection, 77, 169, 172, 177, 618, **636–9**, 650, 748
    antibiotic therapy, 185, 619
    bacterial agents, 637, *637*
    feline lower urinary tract disease, 644, 645
    haematuria, 178, 179, 180, 182, 184
    management, 637–9, *638*, 645
Urinary tract neoplasia, 171
Urinary tract obstruction, 171, 172
Urinary tract tissue biopsy, 174–5
Urine collection, 614
Urine enzymes, 618–19
Urine formation, 612
Urine haemoprotein measurement, 618
Urine microbiology, 173, 182, 619
Urine osmolality, 77–8
Urine output, 70
Urine pH, **618**
    haematuria, 179
Urine protein:urine creatinine ratio (UP:UC ratio), 13, 77, 139, 179
Urine samples, 179
Urine sediment, **618**, 645
    bacteruria, 180
    crystalluria, 181–2, *182*
    cylinduria (urinary casts), 180–1, *181*
    epithelial cells, 180
    haematuria, 179–82
    pyuria, 179–80
Urine specific gravity, **617–18**, *618*
    polyuria/polydipsia, 77
Urine spraying/marking *see* Territorial urination
Urobilinogen, 126, 454
Urodynamic investigations, 175, 616
Uroflowmetry, 175
Urokinase, 298
Urolithiasis, 76, 146, 169, 171, 173, 174, 177, 180, 182, **639–43**, 650
    clinical signs, 639

composition of stones, 174, *639*, 640, *640*
diagnosis, 641
feline lower urinary tract disease, 644, 645, 646
haematuria, 184
history-taking, 639
imaging, 183
management, 641–3
pathophysiology, 640–1
radiological examination, 615
urinary tract obstruction management, 185
Ursodeoxycholic acid therapy, 485, 486
Uterine disease, 582–3, 591–2
Uterine horn aplasia, 582, 591
Uterine prolapse, 588, 593
Uterine stump pyometra, 30
Uterine tube aplasia, 582
Uterine tumours, 583, 592
Uterus, 581, 587, 591, 593
postpartum involution, 587, 593
Uveal disease, anterior, 836–9, 861–3
Uveal neoplasia, anterior, 838, 863
Uveitis, anterior, 123, 836–8, *836*, 861–3
causes, *837*, *862*, 862
clinical signs, *837*, 861, *861*, *862*
secondary glaucoma, 841, 842, *842*
sequelae, *837*
treatment, 836, 838, 862–3
Uveitis, posterior, 851–2, *852*, 864
Uveodermatological syndrome, 837, 899

V

Vaccination adverse reactions
cats, 965
dogs, 936–8, *937*
immunological reactions, 937–8
postvaccinal encephalitis, 936–7
Vagal manoeuvres, 230
Vagina, 581, 591
Vaginal aplasia, 584, 592
Vaginal cysts, 585
Vaginal disorders, 584–5, 592
Vaginal flora, 584
Vaginal hyperplasia, 584–5, *585*
Vaginal hypoplasia, 584
Vaginal neoplasia, 171, 585, 592
Vaginal prolapse, 585
Vaginitis, 584, 592
Vaginoscopy, 575
Valvular heart disease *see* Endocardiosis
Vascular brain diseases, 681
Vascular ring abnormalities, 52, **391–2**
Vascular spinal cord disease, 685
Vasculitis, 899
Vasculogenic shock, 107
Vasoactive intestinal peptide (VIP), 400, 499
Vasodilator drugs
arteriolar dilators, 324
balanced vasodilators, 324–5

chronic renal failure, 629
heart failure management, **324–5**
venodilators, 324
Vena cava assessment, 267
Vena caval obstruction, 142, 474
Venepuncture technique, 772–3
Venereal tumour, transmissible, 586, 602
Venous oxygen reserves, 271
Venous stasis, 119
Ventilation, 87
Ventilation/perfusion mismatch, 88, 119
Ventricular arrhythmias, 227, 228, 229, *334*, **334–6**, *335*
treatment, 335–6
Ventricular fibrillation, 334, 335
Ventricular septal defect, 102, 104, 119, 267, 274, 277, **316–17**, 318
angiocardiography, 316–17
echocardiography, 316
electrocardiography, 316
radiological examination, 316
Verapamil, 288, 309, 325
Vesicular sounds, 9
Vestibular ataxia, **233–5**
Vestibular constrictions, 584
Vestibular disease, **233–5**, *235*, 665, *665*
central, *234*
peripheral, *234*
Vinblastine, 1019, **1025**
Vinca alkaloids, 1006–7, **1025**
Vincristine, 586, 794, 798, 1008, 1013, 1016, 1018, 1019, **1025**
Viral arthralgia, 749
Viral arthritis, 757
Viral encephalitis, 246
Viral enteritis, 61, 62, 420
Viral myocarditis, 289
Viral skin disease, 908–9
Visceral pain, 146
Vitamin A deficiency, 731
Vitamin A-responsive dermatosis, 203, 206, 902
Vitamin D deficiency, 730, 731
Vitamin D metabolism, 542, 613
bone turnover, 720–1, *720*
chronic renal failure, 625–6, 731
Vitamin K antagonism, 800–1, 809
Vitamin K-dependent clotting factors, 134
Vitamin K^1 therapy, 801
Vitreal haemorrhage, 847
Vitreous disorders, 846–7
Vitreous, persistent hyperplastic primary, 846–7
Volume overload, 70
Volvulus, 42, 290, 431
Vomiting, **39–50**, 137, 143, 147, 372, 403, 405, 406, 407, 427, 434, 461, 505, 619
acute renal failure, 623
associated diarrhoea, 43, 45
associated nongastric conditions, *401*
causes, *40–1*

chronic renal failure, 624, 625, 628, 629
complicating chemotherapy, 1020–1
complications, 42
history-taking, 42–4, 52
laboratory investigations, 45–7
management, 47–50
pathophysiology, 39, 401, *402*
vestibular ataxia, 234
Vomiting centre, 39
direct stimulation, 39, 401
indirect stimulation, 39
Vomitus, 43, 45
von Willebrand's disease, 162, **799–800**, 809
von Willebrand's factor, 160, 768, 769
assay, 167, 781
Vulval aplasia, 592
Vulval congenital disorders, 585
Vulval hypoplasia, 586, *586*

W

Warfarin, 108, 164
Water balance, 70, 71
Water deprivation test, 79, 80, 533, 614, 615
Waterhammer pulse, 105, 310
Weakness, episodic, **218–24**
history-taking, 219–20
investigations, 221–4
physical examination, 220–1
Weight gain *see* Obesity
Weight loss, **18–21**, *19*, 67–8, 137, 148, 256, 461, 513, 539, 562, 771
Weight reduction programme, 26–7, *26*
Wheezes (rhonchi), 9, 346, 347
Whipple's triad, 568
Whipworms, 421
White shaker dog (generalized tremor syndrome), 679, 691
Whole blood clotting time (WBCT), 165, 781
Wide local excision, 997–8, *998*
Wobbler's syndrome, 685
Wood's lamp examination, 876–7

X

XX males, 582
Xylose absorption test, 64

Y

Yersinia enterocolitica, 421, 944, 974
Yersinia pestis, 907, 979
Yersinia pseudotuberculosis, 421, 974
Yersiniosis, 421, 754, 974

Z

Zidovudine (AZT), 970
Zinc-responsive dermatosis, 203, 206, 901–2
Zollinger-Ellison syndrome, 408
Zoonotic skin disease, 195, 203